Clinical
Cardiac Pacing
and Defibrillation

Clinical

Cardiac Pacing

and Defibrillation

2nd Edition

Kenneth A. Ellenbogen, M.D.
Director, Clinical Electrophysiology Section
Medical College of Virginia at Virginia Commonwealth University and
McGuire Veterans Affairs Medical Center
Richmond, Virginia

G. Neal Kay, M.D.
Director, Clinical Electrophysiology Section
Division of Cardiology
University of Alabama at Birmingham
Birmingham, Alabama

Bruce L. Wilkoff, M.D.
Director, Cardiac Pacing and Tachyarrhythmias Devices
Department of Cardiology
Director, Cardiovascular Computing Services
The Cleveland Clinic Foundation
Cleveland, Ohio

W.B. SAUNDERS COMPANY
A Harcourt Health Sciences Company
Philadelphia   London   Toronto   Sydney

W.B. SAUNDERS COMPANY
A Harcourt Health Sciences Company

The Curtis Center
Independence Square West
Philadelphia, Pennsylvania 19106

Library of Congress Cataloging-in-Publication Data

Clinical cardiac pacing and defibrillation / [edited by] Kenneth A. Ellenbogen,
G. Neal Kay, Bruce L. Wilkoff.—2nd ed.

p.   cm.

Rev. ed. of: Clinical cardiac pacing / [edited by] Kenneth A. Ellenbogen,
G. Neal Kay, Bruce L. Wilkoff. c1995.
Includes bibliographical references and index.

ISBN 0–7216–7683–9

1. Cardiac pacing. 2. Defibrillators. I. Ellenbogen, Kenneth A.
   II. Kay, G. Neal.   III. Wilkoff, Bruce L.   IV. Clinical cardiac pacing.
[DNLM: 1. Cardiac Pacing, Artificial. 2. Pacemaker, Artificial. 3. Defibrillators,
Implantable. WG 168 C6413 2000]

RC684.P3C54 2000   617.4′120645—dc21

DNLM/DLC   98–53093

Acquisitions Editor: Richard Zorab
Project Manager: Edna Dick
Production Manager: Denise LeMelledo
Illustration Specialist: Peg Shaw
Book Designer: Paul M. Fry

CLINICAL CARDIAC PACING AND DEFIBRILLATION   ISBN 0–7216–7683–9

Printed in the United States of America.

Last digit is the print number: 9   8   7   6   5   4   3   2   1

To my wife and family, Phyllis, Michael, Amy, and Bethany,
  for their patience, support and love.
To my parents, Roslyn and Leon,
  who instilled in me a thirst for learning.
To my students, teachers, and colleagues, who make each day an absolute delight.

KAE

To my teachers, colleagues, and students,
  who have taught me about cardiac pacing.
I am also indebted to the many members of the industry who have dedicated their
  professional careers to the design and improvement of pacing technology.
These individuals have greatly improved the therapy that clinicians can offer
  to their patients, undoubtedly resulting in an improvement in their lives.
Perhaps most important, this book is dedicated to my wife, Linda,
  for her patience and understanding during its preparation.

GNK

To my wife, Ellyn,
  and children Jacob, Benjamin, and Ephram
  for their godly and inspirational patience and support.
To my parents, Harvey and Glenna, for their unconditional love and insights.
To Yeshua, the Messiah, for his salvation,
  and His sustaining covenant love.

BLW

Contributors

Gregory M. Ayers, MD, PhD
InControl, Inc., Redmond, Washington
The Implantable Atrial Defibrillator: Basic Development to Clinical Implementation

Malcolm A. Barlow, MBBS
Fellow in Electrophysiology, University of British Columbia, Vancouver, British Columbia, Canada
Survival, Quality of Life, and Clinical Trials in Pacemaker Patients

S. Serge Barold, MB, BS, FRACP, FACC
Director of Research, North Broward Hospital District Electrophysiology Institute (EPI), Broward General Hospital, Fort Lauderdale, Florida
Timing Cycles and Operational Characteristics of Pacemakers

Peter H. Belott, MD
Clinical Instructor of Medicine, University of California at San Diego School of Medicine, San Diego; Medical Director, Pacemaker and Arrhythmia Center, El Cajon, California
Permanent Pacemaker and Implantable Cardioverter-Defibrillator Implantation

Alan D. Bernstein, MSc, EngScD
Adjunct Associate Professor, Department of Surgery, University of Medicine and Dentistry of New Jersey; Director of Technical Research, Department of Surgery, and Technical Director, New Jersey Pacemaker and Defibrillator Evaluation Center, Newark Beth Israel Medical Center, Newark, New Jersey
Pacemaker, Defibrillator, and Lead Codes

Wim Boute, BScEE
Director of Clinical Studies and Education, Vitatron, The Netherlands
Evoked QT Interval–Based and Intracardiac Impedance–Based Pacemakers

Charles L. Byrd, MD
Clinical Professor of Surgery, University of Miami School of Medicine, Miami; Attending Physician, Broward General Medical Center, Fort Lauderdale, Florida
Management of Implant Complications; Techniques and Devices for Extraction of Pacemaker and Implantable Cardioverter-Defibrillator Leads

David J. Callans, MD
Associate Professor of Medicine, University of Pennsylvania School of Medicine; Co-Director, Electrophysiology Laboratory, Hospital of the University of Pennsylvania, Philadelphia, Pennsylvania
Engineering and Clinical Aspects of Defibrillation Leads

A. John Camm, MD
Professor of Clinical Cardiology, St. George's Hospital Medical School; Consultant Cardiologist, St. George's Hospital, London, United Kingdom
An Overview of Sensors: Ideal Characteristics, Sensor Combination, and Automaticity

William J. Combs, MSEE
Medtronic Inc., Minneapolis, Minnesota
Activity Sensing and Accelerometer-Based Pacemakers

Stuart J. Connolly, MD
Professor, Faculty of Health Sciences, McMaster University, Hamilton, Ontario, Canada
Survival, Quality of Life, and Clinical Trials in Pacemaker Patients

Randolph A. S. Cooper, MD
Clinical Electrophysiologist, Wake Heart Associates, Wake Medical Center, Raleigh, North Carolina
The Implantable Atrial Defibrillator: Basic Development to Clinical Implementation

Ann M. Crespi, PhD
Technical Fellow, Medtronic, Inc., Minneapolis, Minnesota
Power Systems for Implantable Pacemakers, Cardioverters, and Defibrillators

George H. Crossley, III, MD
Associate Professor of Medicine, Cardiology Section, Department of Medicine, Wake Forest University, School of Medicine, Bowman Gray Medical Center, Winston-Salem, North Carolina
Follow-up of the Patient With a Defibrillator

Maria de Guzman, MD
Associate Professor of Medicine, Division of Cardiology, University of Southern California School of Medicine; Director of Electrocardiography, University of Southern California Medical Center, Los Angeles, California
Pacing for Acute and Chronic Atrioventricular Conduction System Disease

Parvin C. Dorostkar, MD
Assistant Clinical Professor of Pediatrics, Case Western Reserve Medical School; Director of Pediatric Electrophysiology, Rainbow Babies and Childrens Hospital, Cleveland, Ohio
Pediatric Pacing and Defibrillator Usage

Kenneth A. Ellenbogen, MD
Director, Clinical Electrophysiology Section, Medical College of Virginia at Virginia Commonwealth University and McGuire Veterans Affairs Medical Center; Professor of Medicine (Cardiology), Medical College of Virginia at Virginia Commonwealth University, Richmond, Virginia
Basic Physiology of Cardiac Pacing and Pacemaker Syndrome; Pacing for Acute and Chronic Atrioventricular Conduction System Disease; Pacing for Prevention of Tachyarrhythmias

Frederik Feith, MD, BScEE
Manager of Education, Vitatron, The Netherlands
Evoked QT Interval–Based and Intracardiac Impedance–Based Pacemakers

Michael S. Firstenberg, MD
Research Fellow, The Department of Cardiology, The Cleveland Clinic Foundation, Cleveland, Ohio
Cardiac Chronotropic Responsiveness

Seymour Furman, MD
Professor of Medicine and Surgery, Albert Einstein College of Medicine; Attending Physician, Department of Medicine and Department of Cardiothoracic Surgery, Division of Cardiology—Arrhythmia Service, Montefiore Medical Center, Bronx, New York
Introduction: History of Cardiac Pacing

Anne M. Gillis, MD
Professor of Medicine, University of Calgary; Medical Director of Pacing and Electrophysiology, Foothills Hospital, Calgary, Alberta, Canada
Sinus Node Disease

Michael R. Gold, MD, PhD
Associate Professor of Medicine, University of Maryland School of Medicine; Director, Cardiac Electrophysiology Service, University of Maryland Hospital, Baltimore, Maryland
Pacing in Patients With Heart Failure

H. Leon Greene, MD
Clinical Professor of Medicine, Division of Cardiology, Department of Medicine, University of Washington School of Medicine; Attending Physician, Harborview Medical Center, Seattle, Washington
Indications for Implantable Cardioverter Defibrillators: Clinical Trials

David L. Hayes, MD
Professor of Medicine, Mayo Medical School, Mayo Clinic and Mayo Foundation; Consultant, Division of Cardiovascular Diseases and Internal Medicine, Mayo Clinic, Rochester, Minnesota
Pacemaker and Implantable Cardioverter-Defibrillator Radiography; Electromagnetic Interference With Implantable Devices

Scott E. Hessen, MD
Clinical Assistant Professor of Medicine, Hahnemann University School of Medicine, Philadelphia; Medical Director, Electrophysiology Laboratory, Crozer Chester Medical Center, Upland, Pennsylvania
Engineering and Clinical Aspects of Defibrillation Leads

Fiona Hunter, PhD
Consultant, Cardiac Rhythm Management Laboratory, University of Alabama at Birmingham, Birmingham, Alabama
Principles of Defibrillation: Cellular Physiology to Fields and Waveforms

Raymond E. Ideker, MD, PhD
Professor of Medicine, Professor of Physiology, and Professor of Biomedical Engineering, University of Alabama at Birmingham, Birmingham, Alabama
Principles of Defibrillation: Cellular Physiology to Fields and Waveforms

Fredrick J. Jaeger, DO
Staff, Electrophysiology and Pacing Section; Director, Cardiac Arrhythmia Monitoring Laboratory, Cleveland Clinic Foundation, Cleveland, Ohio
Carotid Sinus Hypersensitivity and Neurally Mediated Syncope

Denise L. Janosik, MD, FACC
Associate Professor of Medicine, St. Louis University, St. Louis, Missouri
Basic Physiology of Cardiac Pacing and Pacemaker Syndrome

Bharat K. Kantharia, MD, MRCP
Assistant Professor, Division of Cardiology, Department of Medicine, Hahnemann University School of Medicine; Attending, Cardiac Electrophysiology, Hahnemann University Hospital, Philadelphia, Pennsylvania
Engineering and Clinical Aspects of Defibrillation Leads; Approach to Generator Change

David T. Kawanishi, MD
Associate Professor of Medicine, Division of Cardiology, University of Southern California School of Medicine; Director, Cardiac Catheterization Laboratory, University of Southern California Medical Center, Los Angeles, California
Pacing for Acute and Chronic Atrioventricular Conduction System Disease

G. Neal Kay, MD
Director, Clinical Electrophysiology Section, Division of Cardiology, University of Alabama at Birmingham, Birmingham, Alabama
Artificial Electrical Cardiac Stimulation; Rate-Adaptive Pacing Based on Impedance-Derived Minute Ventilation

Charles R. Kerr, MD
Head and Professor, Division of Cardiology, University of British Columbia, Vancouver, British Columbia, Canada
Survival, Quality of Life, and Clinical Trials in Pacemaker Patients

Mark W. Kroll, PhD
Senior Vice President, Technology and Design, St. Jude Medical Cardiac Rhythm Management Division, Sylmar, California
Testing of Implantable Defibrillator Functions at Implantation

Steven P. Kutalek, MD
Associate Professor of Medicine and Pharmacology, Hahnemann University School of Medicine; Director, Clinical Cardiac Electrophysiology, Hahnemann University Hospital, Philadelphia, Pennsylvania
Approach to Generator Change

Chu-Pak Lau, MD
Professor of Medicine, University of Hong Kong; Chief, Cardiology Division, Department of Medicine, Queen Mary Hospital, Hong Kong
An Overview of Sensors: Ideal Characteristics, Sensor Combination, and Automaticity; Evoked QT Interval–Based and Intracardiac Impedance–Based Pacemakers

Sarah S. LeRoy, RN, MSN
Pediatric Nurse Practitioner, University of Michigan Congenital Heart Center, University of Michigan Health System, Ann Arbor, Michigan
Pediatric Pacing and Defibrillator Usage

Sum-Kin Leung, MBBS (HK), FRCP (Edin)
Honorary Associate Professor (Medicine), Chinese University of Hong Kong; Consultant Cardiologist, Department of Medicine and Geriatrics, Kwong Wah Hospital, Hong Kong
An Overview of Sensors: Ideal Characteristics, Sensor Combination, and Automaticity; Evoked QT Interval–Based and Intracardiac Impedance–Based Pacemakers

Paul A. Levine, MD
Clinical Professor of Medicine, Loma Linda University School of Medicine, Loma Linda; Clinical Associate Professor of Medicine, University of California, Los Angeles; Vice President and Medical Director, St. Jude Medical Cardiac Rhythm Management Division, Sylmar, California
Pacemaker Diagnostics and Evaluation of Pacing System Malfunction

Margaret A. Lloyd, MD
Assistant Professor of Medicine, Mayo Medical School, Mayo Clinic and Mayo Foundation; Consultant, Cardiology, Mayo Clinic, Rochester, Minnesota
Pacemaker and Implantable Cardioverter-Defibrillator Radiography

Charles J. Love, MD
Associate Professor of Clinical Medicine, The Ohio State University School of Medicine; Deputy Director and Director of Clinical Affairs; Director, Arrhythmia Device Services, Ohio State University Division of Cardiology, Columbus, Ohio
Pacemaker Diagnostics and Evaluation of Pacing System Malfunction

J. March Maquilan, MD
Clinical Senior Instructor, Hahnemann University School of Medicine; Attending Cardiothoracic Surgeon, Hahnemann University Hospital, Philadelphia, Pennsylvania
Approach to Generator Change

Francis E. Marchlinski, MD
Professor of Medicine, Cardiovascular Division, Department of Medicine, University of Pennsylvania School of Medicine; Director, Cardiac Electrophysiology, University of Pennsylvania Health System, Philadelphia, Pennsylvania
Engineering and Clinical Aspects of Defibrillation Leads

Rahul Mehra, PhD
Senior Fellow, Atrial Fibrillation Research Division, Medtronic, Inc., Minneapolis, Minnesota
Pacing for Prevention of Tachyarrhythmias

Jay O. Millerhagen, MS
Guidant Corp., St. Paul, Minnesota
Activity Sensing and Accelerometer-Based Pacemakers

Harry G. Mond, MD, FRACP, FACC
Physician to the Pacemaker Clinic, Royal Melbourne Hospital, Melbourne, Victoria, Australia
Engineering and Clinical Aspects of Pacing Leads

Tibor Nappholz, BSc, BE
Telectronics Pacing Systems, Englewood, Colorado
Rate-Adaptive Pacing Based on Impedance-Derived Minute Ventilation

James P. Nelson, MSEE, MBA
Field Clinical Engineer, Guidant Corp., St. Paul, Minnesota
Pacemaker and ICD Pulse Generator Circuitry

Walter H. Olson, PhD
Director, Tachyarrhythmia Research, Bakken Fellow, Medtronic, Inc., Minneapolis, Minnesota
Sensing and Arrhythmia Detection by Implantable Devices

Victor Parsonnet, MD
Clinical Professor of Surgery, University of Medicine and Dentistry of New Jersey; Director, Division of Surgical Research, Department of Surgery, and Medical Director, New Jersey Pacemaker and Defibrillator Evaluation Center, Newark Beth Israel Medical Center, Newark, New Jersey
Pacemaker, Defibrillator, and Lead Codes

Robert W. Peters, MD
Professor of Medicine, University of Maryland School of Medicine; Chief of Cardiology, Department of Veterans Affairs Medical Center, Baltimore, Maryland
Pacing in Patients With Heart Failure

Shahbudin H. Rahimtoola, MD
Distinguished Professor of Medicine, Department of Medicine, University of Southern California Medical Center, Los Angeles, California
Pacing for Acute and Chronic Atrioventricular Conduction System Disease

David G. Reuter, MD, PhD
InControl, Inc., Redmond, Washington
The Implantable Atrial Defibrillator: Basic Development to Clinical Implementation

Dwight W. Reynolds, MD
Professor of Medicine and Director, Division of
  Cardiology, University of Oklahoma College of
  Medicine, Oklahoma City, Oklahoma
Permanent Pacemaker and Implantable Cardioverter-
  Defibrillator Implantation

Kenneth M. Riff, MD, MSEE
Vice President, Research and Monitoring Systems,
  Medtronic, Inc., Minneapolis, Minnesota
Monitoring Applications of Pacemaker Sensors

Sanjeev Saksena, MD, FACC, FCCC, FESC
Clinical Professor of Medicine, Robert Wood Johnson
  School of Medicine, New Brunswick; Director,
  Arrhythmia and Pacemaker Services, Eastern Heart
  Institute, General Hospital Center at Passaic, Atlantic
  Health System, Passaic, New Jersey
Pacing for Prevention of Tachyarrhythmias

Craig L. Schmidt, PhD
Manager, Battery Research, Medtronic, Inc., Minneapolis,
  Minnesota
Power Systems for Implantable Pacemakers, Cardioverters,
  and Defibrillators

Mark H. Schoenfeld, MD
Associate Clinical Professor of Medicine, Yale University
  School of Medicine; Director, Cardiac Electrophysiology
  and Pacemaker Laboratory, Hospital of Saint Raphael,
  New Haven, Connecticut
Follow-up of the Paced Patient

Gerald A. Serwer, MD
Professor of Pediatrics, University of Michigan Medical
  School; Director of Pacing, University of Michigan
  Congenital Heart Center, University of Michigan Health
  System, Ann Arbor, Michigan
Pediatric Pacing and Defibrillator Usage

Robert S. Sheldon, MD, PhD
Professor of Medicine, University of Calgary; Physician,
  Foothills Hospital, Calgary, Alberta, Canada
Carotid Sinus Hypersensitivity and Neurally Mediated
  Syncope

Richard B. Shepard, MD
Professor Emeritus of Surgery, Division of Cardiothoracic
  Surgery, University of Alabama at Birmingham,
  Birmingham, Alabama
Power Systems for Implantable Pacemakers, Cardioverters,
  and Defibrillators

Igor Singer, MBBS, FRACP, FACP, FACC, FACA
Professor of Medicine and Director of Electrophysiology
  and Pacing, University of Louisville, Louisville,
  Kentucky
Evaluation of Implantable Cardioverter-Defibrillator
  Malfunction, Diagnostics, and Programmers

Paul M. Skarstad, PhD
Medtronic, Inc., Minneapolis, Minnesota
Power Systems for Implantable Pacemakers, Cardioverters,
  and Defibrillators

Kenneth B. Stokes, BChem
Retired Director of Brady Leads Research, Medtronic, Inc.,
  Minneapolis, Minnesota
Artificial Electrical Cardiac Stimulation

Neil F. Strathmore, MBBS, FRACP
Clinical Instructor, University of Melbourne; Cardiologist,
  Royal Melbourne Hospital, Melbourne, Victoria,
  Australia
Electromagnetic Interference With Implantable Devices

Charles Swerdlow, MD
Clinical Associate Professor of Medicine, University of
  California, Los Angeles, School of Medicine; Research
  Scientist II, Cedars Sinai Medical Center, Los Angeles,
  California
Sensing and Arrhythmia Detection by Implantable Devices

Patrick J. Tchou, MD
Director, Cardiac Electrophysiology, The Cleveland Clinic
  Foundation, Cleveland, Ohio
Testing of Implantable Defibrillator Functions at
  Implantation

Darrel F. Untereker, PhD
Director of Technology and Senior Fellow, Medtronic, Inc.,
  Minneapolis, Minnesota
Power Systems for Implantable Pacemakers, Cardioverters,
  and Defibrillators

Gregory P. Walcott, MD
Assistant Professor of Medicine/Cardiology, University of
  Alabama at Birmingham, Birmingham, Alabama
Principles of Defibrillation: Cellular Physiology to Fields
  and Waveforms

Jay A. Warren, PhD
Vice President, Research and Development, Guidant/CPI,
  St. Paul, Minnesota
Pacemaker and ICD Pulse Generator Circuitry

Bruce L. Wilkoff, MD
Director of Cardiac Pacing and Tachyarrhythmias Devices,
  Department of Cardiology; Director, Cardiovascular
  Computing Services, The Cleveland Clinic Foundation;
  Associate Professor of Internal Medicine, Ohio State
  University School of Medicine, Cleveland, Ohio
Cardiac Chronotropic Responsiveness; Techniques and
  Devices for Extraction of Pacemaker and Implantable
  Cardioverter-Defibrillator Leads

Mark A. Wood, MD
Associate Professor of Medicine and Assistant Director,
  Cardiac Electrophysiology Laboratory, Medical College
  of Virginia, Richmond, Virginia
Sensing and Arrhythmia Detection by Implantable Devices

D. George Wyse, MD, PhD
Professor of Medicine (Cardiology), University of Calgary;
  Consultant Cardiac Electrophysiologist, Calgary Regional
  Health Authority, Calgary, Alberta, Canada
Indications for Implantable Cardioverter Defibrillators:
  Clinical Trials

Preface

Cardiac pacing and implantable defibrillators have had a great impact on the treatment of patients with cardiac arrhythmias. Since our first edition, the number of pacemakers and defibrillators being implanted in the United States and throughout the world has continued to increase. Since the first pacing system was implanted in 1958, this field has grown as its technology and indications expand and its sophistication increases. The sophistication of the cardiac devices now being implanted is exponentially greater than that of devices implanted more than three decades ago.

There are many consumers of pacemakers and defibrillator technology besides the patient. There are numerous physicians, including cardiologists, surgeons, internists, and emergency and family physicians, who care for these patients and need to evaluate the impact of this therapy on various medical conditions and treatments. In addition, nurses, engineers from pacemaker companies, and technical and sales representatives from these companies also interact with physicians and patients.

Our philosophy in putting together the second edition remains the same as that of our first effort. We have planned this book to emphasize the science of cardiac pacing and defibrillation and underline the importance of the fact that it is an interdisciplinary field. Physicians are part of a web of health professionals who need increasing amounts of information about implantable devices.

The evolution of cardiac pacing has inspired the publication of subspecialty journals, including *PACE, StimuCoeur, Journal of Cardiovascular Electrophysiology, Journal of Interventional Cardiac Electrophysiology, Cardiac Electrophysiology Review,* and *Europace,* as well as monographs and a number of new books on implantable devices. Several national and international conferences on pacing and defibrillation take place every year.

We have sought to meet the needs of many with this textbook. Clinicians, scientists, nurses, technicians, and engineers will find the information in these pages practical, authoritative, and helpful in better understanding this therapy. We are excited about the opportunity to present this material in a comprehensive scientific manner.

We gratefully acknowledge the invaluable assistance and encouragement of Richard Zorab of the W.B. Saunders Company for all his help in keeping the second edition on track. Jennifer Shreiner, his secretary, was a great facilitator of our communications. We owe a great debt of gratitude to our colleagues from the Medical College of Virginia and the McGuire Veterans Affairs Medical Center, the University of Alabama, and the Cleveland Clinic Foundation for their patience and support in shouldering the extra workload that allowed us to finish our chapters and editing on time.

Most importantly, we cannot thank enough our many contributors and their colleagues, who labored extensively, often taking time from family and other projects to finish their chapters. This large group of individuals deserves all the credit and thanks for making the second edition possible.

Our wonderful secretaries, Vera Wilkerson (Virginia Commonwealth University/Medical College of Virginia), Margaret Ho (Cleveland Clinic), and Dorothy Welch (University of Alabama) were invaluable for their contributions to help get this project completed.

We only hope that this textbook will stand as a valuable tool and reference, helping clinicians, scientists, and engineers make the decisions that improve patients' lives. We hope this book serves as a resource to all these people for many years to come.

KENNETH A. ELLENBOGEN
G. NEAL KAY
BRUCE L. WILKOFF

Contents

Introduction: History of Cardiac Pacing

Seymour Furman

The history of heart block and what has been called Stokes-Adams disease (syndrome) runs through the past 300 years of medical history. Initially, the syncopal episodes, which are part of the syndrome, were considered to be a category of epilepsy. "Epilepsy" associated with a slow pulse was first described at the beginning of the 18th century. Before Stokes described 7 cases, 11 other case descriptions had been made, 1 by Adams.[1]

The earliest recorded description of what can now be regarded as bradycardia with syncope was by the Slovene Marko Gerbec (1658 to 1718) (in Latin, *Marcus Gerbezius*) who wrote, "I noticed something even more unusual about the pulse of two patients, one of whom, a melancholic, a hypochondriac, otherwise basically healthy, had such a slow pulse that the pulse of healthy person would beat three times before his pulse would beat for a second time: . . . Otherwise the man had been robust, precise in his movements, but very sluggish, frequently dizzy, and from time to time subject to mild epileptic seizure."[2]

Further descriptions of slow pulse with syncope, all categorized as epilepsy variants, were provided by Morgagni in 1769: "He was in his sixty-eighth year, of a habit moderately fat, and of a florid complexion, when he was first seized with the epilepsy, which left behind it the greatest slowness of pulse, and in like manner a coldness of the body."[3] Other descriptions were made by Spens in 1793,[4] by Burnett in 1824,[5] and the following by Adams in 1826,[6] "An officer in the revenue, aged 68 years, . . . was just then recovering from the effects of an apoplectic attack. . . . What most attracted my attention was, the irregularity of his breathing, and remarkable slowness of pulse, which generally ranged at the rate of 30 in a minute. . . . November 4, 1819, he was suddenly seized with an apoplectic attack, which in two hours carried him off. . . ." In 1846, William Stokes[7] described seven cases, including case I—repeated pseudoapoplectic attacks, not followed by paralysis: slow pulse, with

valvular murmur. Stokes' further case descriptions associated syncope with slow cardiac rate and cardiac standstill as the cause of syncope. His reports were remarkably modern in perceptions and associations, which, because they had not been made by earlier workers, makes the first position of his name appropriate. In 1890, Huchard proposed the name Stokes-Adams disease, believing that Stokes' description was so far superior to Adams' or that of anyone else as to properly be the first.[8] At that time, the term *heart block* had not yet been coined.

Electrical stimulation by electric eels and the electric organ of the torpedo have been used therapeutically.[9, 10] Widespread electrical stimulation therapy during the 19th century was encouraged by individual cases of successful resuscitation and Volta's[11] invention of the battery to produce electricity, Galvani's[12] electrical stimulation of vertebrate muscle, Aldini,[13] his nephew, of mammalian muscular stimulation, and Bichat's[14] stimulation of the severed heads of guillotine victims. During the second half of the 19th century, research laboratory investigation of cardiac electrophysiology led to experimental mammalian[15] and human[16] cardiac stimulation and recommendations concerning routine therapeutic use of electrical stimulation.[17]

Gaskell[18] demonstrated in 1883 that atrioventricular conduction in the tortoise was not a function of the nervous system but that the cardiac depolarization began in the atrium and spread across atrial tissue to the atrioventricular groove and then to the ventricle. By 1899, Wilhelm His Jr. published an extensive analysis of a single patient with Stokes-Adams syndrome to demonstrate the independent contraction of atrium and ventricle, the ventricular bradycardia and asystole during the attack itself.[19] In its title, the names of Adams-Stokes disease and the condition of heart block were linked. His had earlier identified the conduction bundle that bears his name and in 1895 had demonstrated that cutting it with a cataract knife produced atrioventricular

(AV) block.[20] By 1906, Erlanger had demonstrated with electrocardiography (ECG)[21] and in the laboratory that Stokes-Adams disease was closely associated with heart block.[22] He had devised a technique for controlled and reproducible production of AV block, with which his studies were accomplished.[23] By 1908, Lewis[24] was able to synthesize the information which had accumulated over the previous decade and provide an analysis in which block of the AV conduction system and episodic asystole were the causes of Stokes-Adams disease. Until this time, only asystole had been considered to be the cause of syncope, but in 1922, Kerr and Bender[25] demonstrated that ventricular fibrillation also is a cause. An ECG review by Parkinson and colleagues[26] in 1941 assembled the ECGs of patients with heart block, asystole, and syncope in a fashion that can be readily recognized today.

From the end of the 19th century to the middle of the 20th century, many publications described the cardiac rhythms associated with heart block and Stokes-Adams syndrome. Autopsies of patients dying from or with heart block,[27] the clinical events associated with chronic heart block,[28] and the effect of medications on the associated bradycardia[29] and during episodes of syncope[30] were described. The clinical events associated with heart block and Stokes-Adams syndrome included ECG demonstration of AV dissociation,[31] syncope as a result of asystole,[32] and ventricular fibrillation.[33] Autopsy of patients who died from Stokes-Adams disease and diseases such as diphtheria[34] and Chagas' disease,[35] as causes of heart block, as well as patients included in the later descriptions of Lev[36] and Lenegre[37] of the sclerosis of the AV conduction system, were progressively added. With the introduction of ECG at the beginning of the 20th century,[38] ECG descriptions of AV block demonstrated continued atrial activity but with cessation of ventricular activity[39] or ventricular tachycardia[40] after ventricular bradycardia or arrest. The high morbidity associated with Stokes-Adams disease became recognized, as did the mortality rate, which was about 50% in the year following its diagnosis.[41] By midcentury, the variety of rhythmic diagnoses was well established, as was therapy with agents such as barium chloride,[42] epinephrine,[43] atropine,[44] isoproterenol,[45] and corticosteroids.[46] None of the electrical therapy used earlier and beginning to be developed by midcentury was directed toward treating Stokes-Adams syndrome or heart block; rather, it was directed toward treating undifferentiated cardiac arrest.

In 1927, Marmorstein of Odessa (Soviet Union) described catheter stimulation of the right ventricle through a dog's jugular vein and of the left ventricle through the carotid artery,[47] after which he disappeared. Nothing further was made of these findings. Mark C. Lidwill, an Australian anesthesiologist, had recorded ECGs at the time of patient death and found idioventricular rhythm and the failure of the normal cardiac pacemakers. Lidwell appeared to be aware that cardiac muscle could be made to contract with intracardiac epinephrine and electrical stimulation and worked with Edwin H. Booth, a physicist, to design a portable device powered by being plugged into "a lighting point." One stimulating pole was a skin pad soaked with a strong salt solution and the other a needle insulated except at its tip to be plunged into the heart. A switch allowed change of polarity, the rate was variable between 80 and 120 bpm, and

the output ranged from 1.5 to 120 V. In 1929, Lidwill reported to the Australasian Medical Congress in Sydney, Australia: "The method was tried in two or three cases and was completely successful in the case of a stillborn infant. . . . At the end of ten minutes the current was stopped and it was found that the heart would beat of its own accord. The child recovered completely and is now living and quite healthy."[48] No other records, photographs, or devices exist.

Between 1929 and 1932, Hyman[49, 50] in New York attempted emergency stimulation with a cardiac pacemaker designed to be carried on the back of an associate. He referred anecdotally to Lidwill's earlier work but had no reference and was in error about the inventor's name (whom he referred to as Gould). A hand-cranked magneto, such as that used to produce electricity to start an automobile, powered the Hyman device. Cardiac stimulation was achieved by means of a needle electrode plunged through the chest wall into the heart. Success was reported, and the technique received significant local press coverage. Hyman, however, could not convince a manufacturer to commercialize the device until the local New York branch of the Siemens Company accepted the project at the end of the 1930s. A battery-powered device was completed in about 1942 but could not be delivered to the United States from Germany because the two countries were then belligerents. Hyman had unsuccessfully attempted to convince the United States Navy, in which he served, of his pacemaker's value for resuscitation of the injured and wounded. The Navy declined the opportunity, and the United States Air Force eventually destroyed the Siemens plant in Nürnberg at which the Hyman device was stored. The device was lost, and only a photograph of a "black box" remains.

In 1931, Werner Forssmann,[51] a trainee in urology, introduced a urologic catheter into his heart through the basilic vein, observing its passage through his body with a fluoroscope and a mirror. The technique was developed as a diagnostic tool by André Cournand and Dickinson W. Richards[52] during the 1940s, who aspirated blood for oxygen saturation, measuring intracardiac pressures and recording intracardiac electrograms. The three shared the 1956 Nobel Prize for medicine for the invention of cardiac catheterization.

The Second World War was crucial to the development of many technologies, including cardiac pacing. Previously, the heart was deemed inviolate and cardiac surgery impossible. Prewar cardiac surgery[53, 54] for congenital cardiac disease actually involved surgery on the adjacent great vessels. During the war, Harken[55, 56] developed techniques for surgical removal of intracardiac foreign bodies and demonstrated that the heart could be routinely and successfully operated on without cardiopulmonary bypass, which then did not exist, and helped change the intellectual climate concerning cardiac surgery.

■ BASIC TECHNOLOGIC INNOVATIONS

The following basic technologic innovations led to the development of the modern cardiac pacemaker-defibrillators:

1. The dry electrolytic capacitor (widely used in electric circuits), which stores continuous flows of smaller amounts of electricity for episodic discharge as a stimulus by a

cardiac pacemaker and much larger amounts for cardiac defibrillators, was patented by Samuel Ruben in 1926.[57]

2. The mercury-zinc cell, with a flat and sustained output voltage and large electrical capacity for its weight and size, was particularly useful for powering electronic circuits and was also invented by Ruben during the Second World War, largely for military use. It was patented in 1947.[58]

3. The transistor and diode were invented at Bell Laboratories in 1947 and 1949, respectively. Both allowed construction of an electronic circuit sufficiently small to be implanted.[59, 60]

4. The lithium-iodine cell was invented in 1968 and patented in 1972.[61] It was designed to overcome the brief longevity in electronic applications (including pacemaker) of the mercury-zinc cell, which also evolved hydrogen during production of electricity, so that an implantable pacemaker could not be hermetically sealed, by then recognized as a serious shortcoming[62] (Table 1).

■ PACEMAKER POWER SOURCES

From the beginning of pacemaker development, a wide variety of power sources were evaluated, but few met the required standards. Three essential requirements exist for a pacemaker power source:

1. The output must be renewable, that is, a secondary (rechargeable) cell or, if primary, of sufficiently great longevity, so that when completely implanted, it permits an acceptable interval between device replacements.

2. The output must present a flat voltage, relative to body temperature, so that the circuit can be designed to the voltage developed by the cell or battery.

3. Consumption of the power source should be readily detectable so that sudden and unpredictable power source failure does not occur.

The Hyman device, intended for ambulatory resuscitation, derived its power from a magneto, then widely available to develop the electricity to start an automobile engine by hand cranking. The Hyman pacemaker was hand cranked to be operated.

Two later devices (described later), designed for sinoatrial pacing by Hopps and transcutaneous pacing by Zoll, were powered by 110- to 120-V line current. In 1958, Reynolds, in Colombia, developed a vacuum tube circuit pacemaker powered by a 6-V lead acid battery, with electrodes implanted by thoracotomy.

Implantable Power Sources

Mercury-zinc. This cell was used in all primary cell pulse generators developed from 1960 until about 1972 or 1973.

Nickel-cadmium. Rechargeability was a feature of the 1958 implantable pulse generator and was used in other devices experimentally until 1973.[63] Aside from the derivatives of the 1958 unit, the next successful model was developed by Fischel and associates,[64] made available commercially by Pacesetter Systems Inc., and first implanted in a human on February 10, 1973. Eventually, 10,022 pacemakers were implanted, with the last on October 19, 1984. During the fall of 1999, approximately 800 units were still functioning in patients, many for more than 20 years.

Lithium–cupric sulfide. This cell was invented in 1973, adapted for pacemaker use by the Cordis Corporation, and first implanted in patients in 1977. It was a major pulse generator power source until 1989. Some devices were still in service as of early 1998.

Lithium-iodine. Invented in 1968, a 3-ampere/h cell (702E) was incorporated into a hermetically sealed pacemaker in 1972. The earliest implantable units were manufactured by L'Ectromedici Medicale (LEM) in Italy[66] and soon thereafter by Cardiac Pacemakers Inc. (CPI) in the United

Table 1. Ancillary Technology

Device	Inventor (Organization)	Date	Significance
Dry electrolytic capacitor	Ruben (Ruben Labs)	1926*	Output circuit requirement for all PM, ICD
Mercury-zinc cell	Ruben (Ruben Labs)	1947†	First working pacer power source
Transistor (bipolar point contact)	Bardeen and Brattain (Bell Labs)	1947‡	Essential for circuit miniaturization
Junction diode and junction transistor	Schockley (Bell Labs)	1949§	Essential for circuit miniaturization
Lithium-iodine cell	Moser and Schneider (Catalyst Research Div. MSA)	1968#	The present standard pacemaker power source
Lithium-silver vanadium oxide cell	Liang, Bolster, and Murphy (WGL)	1981¶	The present standard ICD power source

PM, pacemaker; ICD, implantable cardioverter-defibrillator.

*Linford HB: Samuel Ruben—Acheson Medalist. J Electrochem Soc 11C, Jan 1971; Owens BB, Salkind AJ: Key events in the evolution of implantable pacemaker batteries. *In* Owens B (ed): Batteries for implantable biomedical devices. New York, Plenum Press, 1968.

†Ruben S: US Pat. 2,422,045, 1947.

‡Bardeen J, Brattain WH: The transistor, a semi-conductor triode. Physiol Rev 74:230, 1948.

§Schockley W: Theory of P–N junctions in semiconductors and P–N junction transistors. Bell Syst Tech J 28:435, 1949.

#Moser JR: Solid state lithium iodine primary battery. US Pat. 3,660,193, 1972. Schneider AA, Moser JR: US Pat. 3,674,562, 1972.

¶Liang CC, Bolster ME, Murphy RM: US Pat. 4,310,609, 1982.

Courtesy of A.J. Salkind, DSc.

States.[67] The cell is capable of fabrication into a variety of sizes and has allowed the present marked reduction in pulse generator size. It does not evolve hydrogen during the production of electricity and therefore allows hermetic sealing of the pulse generator, itself a major contribution to pulse generator stability and reliability.[62]

Plutonium (Pu 238). Urged on by Parsonnet because of the brief longevity of mercury-zinc–powered pacemakers, the first plutonium (half-life, 86 years)-powered nuclear pacemakers were implanted during 1972.[68] Some 3000 were eventually implanted worldwide, and many are still functioning after 20 to 25 years. Nuclear pacemakers were manufactured in France, the United States, the United Kingdom, the Federal Republic of Germany (Promethium), the Soviet Union, and possibly elsewhere. The prolonged longevity of lithium anode cells and the regulatory burden placed on nuclear isotopes have caused cessation of nuclear pacemaker manufacture.

Promethium (Pm 147). This isotope, with a half-life of 2.6 years, was capable of powering a pacemaker for less than 10 years.[69] Once lithium-iodine–powered pulse generators were introduced, it fell into disuse (Fig. 1).

Competing Power Sources

Confronted with the brief longevity of cardiac pacemakers available in the early years after the first implantations, a variety of power sources were investigated as alternatives to the mercury-zinc cell, including the following:

Biogalvanic. These included a battery of dissimilar metals in the subcutaneous tissue to develop an electromotive force[70] and piezoelectric crystals surrounding the aorta, which, in a self-perpetuating way, would produce electricity to power a pulse generator by the force of contraction of the previous heart beat,[71] the energy of glucose oxidation,[72] and skeletal muscle contraction.

Other chemical batteries. These included rechargeable nickel-cadmium cells fabricated into a useful commercial product,[73] rechargeable mercury-zinc cells,[74] and most recently, cells with a lithium anode, which have come to dominate pacemaker construction.[75]

■ CLINICAL CARDIAC PACING

The impetus for modern cardiac pacing was the development of cardiac surgery, not with the intention of pacing heart block or the Stokes-Adams syndrome, but rather with the intention to treat sudden cardiac arrest and, later, AV block resulting from repair of congenital defects. In 1948, newly returned from Canadian military service during World War II, Wilfred G. Bigelow of Toronto General Hospital undertook the development of techniques to repair congenital cardiac lesions with controlled hypothermia, during which, he believed, metabolism would be so diminished that circulatory arrest could be tolerated.[76] Bigelow was joined by John Callaghan, a young surgical trainee who had recently completed a year as a medical officer in the Canadian North and was knowledgeable about the effects of whole body hypothermia and its management for patient survival. During a series of experiments, they determined that, in the process of rewarming, control of the cardiac rate was important, so that the profound bradycardia that occurred during hypothermia could be controllably accelerated as metabolic needs increased.

John R. Hopps of the National Research Council of Canada, who had been recruited to develop cooling and rewarming equipment for the hypothermia, was assigned to develop a cardiac-stimulating capability.[77] A stimulator[78] and catheter electrode[79] were developed, designed to stimulate the sino-

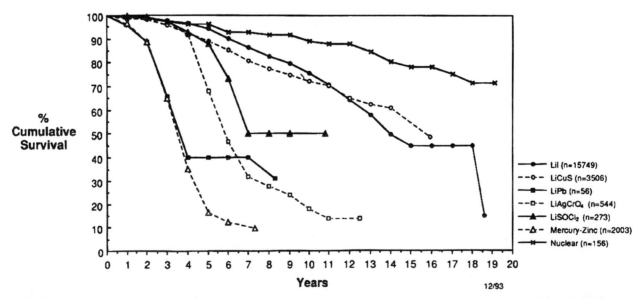

Figure 1. Cumulative survival over a 20-year period with lithium, mercury-zinc, and nuclear power sources of pacemakers. Fifty percent of the pulse generators had failed either by power source depletion or circuit failure, as follows: mercury-zinc, 3.5 years; lithium-lead, 3.5 years; lithium silver chromate, 5.5 years; lithium thionyl chloride, 7.0 years; lithium iodine, 12.5 years; lithium cupric sulfide, 13.0 years; nuclear, 50% survival not reached during follow-up period. (Modified from Song S: The Bilitch report: Performance of implantable cardiac rhythm management devices. PACE 17:692–708, 1994.)

atrial node and to be introduced through the external jugular vein of a dog. The atrial pacing technique was used in animals[80] and clinically during cardiac repair. Sinoatrial node pacing was attempted in several (probably five) patients who had suddenly collapsed, possibly as a result of acute myocardial infarction, perhaps with AV block. Because only the sinoatrial region of the right atrium—never the right ventricle—was paced, that effort failed, was abandoned, and was not reported. The atrial pacing technique, and a brief film, were presented at an American College of Surgery meeting in Boston in 1950, at which time Paul M. Zoll became aware of the technique and subsequently corresponded with Bigelow during the time he was developing his own pacing system.

Zoll had considered that stimulating the ventricle would cause it to contract and that such stimulation could be effective through the intact chest wall. He reported the technique in 1952[81] and demonstrated using ECG that the heart would beat in response to an adequate amplitude stimulus delivered across the intact chest. An output of about 70 to 150 V was required, and stimulation was variable in rate between 30 and 120 stimuli per minute. Two disk electrodes, about 1 inch in diameter, were placed anteriorally and left laterally near the cardiac apex and were held in place by a rubber strap that encircled the chest.

Conductive electrolyte solution between the electrode and the skin reduced the resistance to electrical flow. Still, skin burns below and adjacent to the electrode were common. Stimulation caused painful contractions of the skeletal muscles of the chest and upper abdomen. Such stimulation was difficult to tolerate, frequently required sedation, and could be used only briefly. The longest reported duration was 7 days of episodic stimulation,[82] which did not allow patient activity, except when the pacemaker was in place but not actually stimulating. Operation was entirely manual, activating the device and deactivating it, and setting output and stimulation rate. Power was derived from line current, to which patient and device were tethered, although later during the 1950s a portable battery-operated device was introduced.

Zoll continued to promulgate the external transcutaneous pacemaker throughout his career,[83] introducing an improved version with a longer pulse duration and larger and more efficient electrodes many years later.[84] He also entered into the competition to develop an implantable pulse generator during the early 1960s (see later).

In 1955 Arne Larsson, a Swedish electrical engineer, developed severe myocarditis attributed to eating infected oysters. Intermittent heart block followed with rates between about 40 and 70 bpm and with recurrent syncope on a daily basis. Digitalis was administered, which increased the frequency and severity of the syncope. Work became difficult and then impossible. The patient's disorder was diagnosed as AV block with Stokes-Adams episodes, and his wife increasingly despaired of his survival. She read in the newspaper of pacing techniques being evaluated and importuned her husband's cardiologist to apply them.[85] Those techniques involved myocardial wires and an external pulse generator. Dr. Ake Senning, the cardiac surgeon at the Karolinska Hospital in Stockholm, was approached but decided that such an approach would be unsatisfactory because of the risk of recurrent infection. He and Rune Elmqvist, who was himself a physician and engineer who designed medical equipment, had been considering an implantable pulse generator. Urged on by the impetus of Larsson's grave illness and Mrs. Larsson's ceaseless pressure, Elmqvist designed and built two identical models of an implantable nickel-cadmium–powered pulse generator. Two stainless steel myocardial sutures were used as the bipolar electrode. On October 8, 1958, Senning implanted the pacemaker by thoracotomy. It failed after about 6 hours. The second, identical unit was then implanted and functioned for about 8 days, when it too failed.[86] Larsson, whose condition had by this time stabilized to fixed complete heart block and thereafter involved fewer syncopal episodes, was left without a pacemaker until a mercury-zinc powered unit was implanted by thoracotomy on November 4, 1961. Wife and husband remain alive as of November 1999 (Table 2).

Three additional Elmqvist-designed rechargeable unipolar units, with a flat disk electrode, were implanted. On February 3, 1960 in Montevideo, Uruguay, Drs. Roberto Rubio and Orestes Fiandra implanted one in a 40-year-old woman, who survived with a functioning device for 9 months until she died of sepsis from infection of the thoracotomy wound.[87] At least two models were implanted in London by Harold Siddons, one on March 31, 1960,[88] which functioned for about 10 months[89] and a second on an uncertain date, which

Table 2. The First Implanted Pacemakers

Inventors	Power Source	Electrode	Date of Implantation	Date of Implant Failure
Senning, Elmqvist	NiCd—rechargeable	Bare wires	10/8/58	10/8/58
Glenn, Mauro, Eisenberg	Radiofrequency	Bare wires	1/29/59	2/19/59
Abrams, Light, Wood	Radiofrequency	Bare wires	2/13(?)/60	?
Fiandra, Rubio, Elmqvist	NiCd—rechargeable	1-cm disk	2/3/60	10/20/60
Siddons, Elmqvist	NiCd—rechargeable	1-cm disk	3/31/60	10 mo
Chardack, Greatbatch	HgZnO	Hunter-Roth	6/6/60	18 mo
Zoll, Belgard	HgZnO	Bare wires	11/7/60	?
Kantrowitz	HgZnO	Bare wires	5/5/61	Patient died 5/9/61
Nathan, Keller*	HgZnO	Ventricle—Chardack Atrium—flat spiral	6/22/62	?
Lagergren	HgZnO	Endocardial	6/5/62	?
Parsonnet	HgZnO	Endocardial	10/6/62	12/15/62

HgZnO, mercury-zinc; NiCd, nickel-cadmium.
*Atrial synchronous.

functioned for only 22 hours. Because the electrodes of the first two and later three implants were different, the early failure of the first two pulse generators may have been related to lead and not to the pulse generator.

By the late 1950s, the concept of an implantable pacemaker was being seriously considered. A conference held on September 10, 1958 at Rockefeller University in New York, convened by Vladimir Zworykin, PhD, of the Radio Corporation of America (RCA), a co-inventor of television, and chaired by Carl Berkely of the Rockefeller Institute, explored the state of the existing art and science of cardiac pacing. Suggestions from some of the presenters that an implantable device was a conceivable approach to the long-term management of Stokes-Adams disease were opposed to the concept of episodic transcutaneous stimulation, as needed, which was espoused by Zoll. (Most of the then recognized workers in the field from the United States participated, including Zoll, Wegria, Bakken, Hellerstein, Kossman, Morse, Stephenson, Weirich, and others.) Cardiac arrest, for example, during a surgical procedure, or other cardiac standstill was not clearly distinguished from asystole associated with complete heart block and Stokes-Adams syndrome.

The symposium reviewed the appropriate pacing rate, whether atrial synchrony was desirable for maximum cardiac efficiency, and other issues of cardiac output. Zoll emphasized his external pacing technique, a radiofrequency stimulator he was in the process of developing, and the problem of continually rising myocardial stimulation thresholds, with only several weeks of continuous pacing, in dogs. Hellerstein strongly supported atrial synchrony, whereas Zoll, clearly the most prominent pacemaker-involved investigator present, believed it to be of little value. Although the development of an implantable pulse generator was discussed and supported by Berkely, Weirich, and Hellerstein, support for a portable, external transcutaneous stimulator for episodic emergency use was strong. The design of a potential implantable device was stated possibly to be "electrical, mechanical or chemical."

Events were moving so quickly, however, that most of those present (Zoll, Weirich, and Bakken excepted) contributed little of permanence to the field. Transvenous pacing, already accomplished in New York, was not mentioned, and neither Glenn of New Haven nor Chardack or Greatbatch of Buffalo (all geographically proximate) or other overseas workers such as Cammilli or Leatham and Davies were involved.[90]

Soon at least three teams were in the process of developing a wholly implantable device, which each designed to be powered by mercury-zinc cells. The groups were headed by Kantrowitz of Brooklyn,[91] Zoll of Boston,[92] and Chardack, Gage, and Greatbatch of Buffalo, New York.[93] Wilson Greatbatch, an electrical engineer, had worked in the research laboratory at Cornell University in Ithaca and later participated in a joint engineering-medical group in Buffalo. He and Drs. William Chardack and Andrew Gage eventually began a project for the development of an implantable pacemaker built in a shed on Greatbatch's property. The first 45 patients had pulse generators powered by 10 mercury-zinc cells (13.5 V) and a single transistor circuit.[94] They accomplished the first complete implantation of leads and pulse generator, as the second stage of a two-stage procedure,

on June 6, 1960.[93] The Zoll group completed their first implantation on November 7, 1960,[92] and the Kantrowitz group on May 5, 1961.[91] With the Chardack-Greatbatch implant, and their subsequent agreement with Medtronic for manufacture, the era of implantable cardiac pacing began.

Early in 1958 Jorge Reynolds, an engineer from Bogota, Colombia, attended the Miami meeting of the American Association for Thoracic Surgery. C. Walton Lillehei introduced Reynolds to William Chardack (who with Wilson Greatbatch, was engaged in developing an implantable pacemaker) and to Paul Zoll, who had already clinically demonstrated transcutaneous pacing. Reynolds returned home and began to design a pacemaker system. An implantable device was not feasible; thus, he designed a stimulator in which the timing mechanism was a 78-rpm phonograph with a brush on the rotating disk that made 78 contacts per minute and allowed current flow from a 100-A, 12-V automobile battery.

Although this initial device was successful in animal experimentation, later devices used more conventional electron tubes, transformers, and a multivibrator to set the timing. Electrodes were made of helical coils of pure platinum insulated with silicone rubber and sutured onto the heart by means of thoracotomy. The first patient had implantation by thoracotomy with the two electrodes placed as close as possible to the epicardial surface of the right ventricular apex. The electronics and automobile battery were external and weighed about 45 kg (about 100 lb); the unit was moved on a handcart used to transport oxygen tanks. Four patients were eventually paced in this way, and by the end of 1959, local manufacture began of external transistorized pacemakers powered first by carbon-zinc cells and later by 9-V cells. A 9-V battery could power such external pacemakers with transcutaneous epicardial electrodes for about 15 days before battery replacement was required. Infection at the skin entrance was said to be readily controlled. Radiofrequency pacemakers were also developed and used locally. Eventually, some 2800 external pacemakers were used throughout Colombia and other South American countries before imported mercury-zinc–powered pacemakers replaced local manufacture.[95]

Because of economic difficulties, pacemakers were also manufactured at the Dante Pazzanese Institute in Sao Paulo, Brazil in the Department of Cardio-Thoracic Surgery under the supervision of Decio Kormann. Between 1965 and 1976, some 3000 mercury-zinc–powered implantable pacemakers were manufactured, until local commercial production and importation began. Manufacture in Montevideo by Fiandra, in Bogota by Reynolds, and in Brazil by Kormann represented the beginning of cardiac pacing in South America. Each persisted in development, manufacture, and distribution of devices when pacemakers were otherwise commercially unavailable.[96]

■ RADIOFREQUENCY

Radiofrequency systems were developed around the world, and at least five were implanted in humans. The systems were based on the demonstration by Verzeano[97] that adequate electrical energy could be transmitted by radiofrequency emission to stimulate a biologic system, and later by Mauro[98] that an implanted radiofrequency system could be used for neurologic stimulation. The first human cardiac radiofrequency stimulator developed by Glenn in 1958[99] was a direct adaptation of the Mauro and Eisenberg stimulator.[100] Energy was transmitted from the passive implanted receiver by wire electrodes[101] and later also by transvenous leads.[102] Such stimulating systems were also developed and implanted by Cammilli[103] in Florence, Italy, by Abrams in Birmingham, UK[104] (manufactured by Lucas), by Siddons and Davies in London,[105] by Reynolds in Colombia, by Suma in Japan,[106] by Barr in Israel,[107] and by others. The evaluation of radiofrequency transmission of energy was a popular (though not widely employed) concept before the achievement of a totally implanted power source. During radiofrequency pacing, electrical energy is transmitted across the intact skin by an antenna held in place by adhesive. The external pulse generator comprised the power source and electronic circuit. All systems were asynchronous in operation. Several had external rate and amplitude controls. In each instance, decoupling, that is, movement of the antenna relative to the implanted receiving module, frequently caused cessation of pacing.

In 1956 Lillehei at the University of Minnesota, Minneapolis began the use of cross-circulation and then cardiopulmonary bypass with a bubble oxygenator to repair congenital cardiac lesions and atrial and ventricular septal defects in children.[108] Some 10% of those who underwent ventricular septal defect repair developed complete heart block, which usually manifested instantly when the offending suture had been placed. This had a high mortality rate, which Lillehei attempted to treat with intravenous isoproterenol and external pacing, using the Zoll transcutaneous technique.[109] Closed chest stimulation was painful, required continuous immobilization and prolonged periods of sedation, and was ultimately unsatisfactory. Intravenous isoproterenol increased the ventricular rate but required constant careful monitoring to avoid inadequate administration and bradycardia or excessive administration and tachycardia. The surgical team experimented with the placement of Teflon-insulated stainless steel surgical sutures[110] into the myocardium, which were then connected to the lowest possible output of the Zoll pacemaker.

If a suture electrode was required postoperatively, a large-bore needle was placed through the chest wall into the left ventricular myocardium, and a steel suture electrode was placed, then connected to the line-operated pacemaker. Some patients with heart block reverted to satisfactory AV conduction after several weeks. In other patients, AV block persisted permanently, and these cases usually ended as fatalities. A 1957 winter storm produced a power failure in Minneapolis, threatening the lives of children maintained on line-operated pacemakers. Because the hospital did not then have a backup power supply, Lillehei asked Earl Bakken, then working for the surgical research laboratory, as a representative of his recently founded firm Medtronic, to design a battery-powered external pacemaker. This was accomplished by modifying the design of a battery-powered metronome circuit, a description of which had recently been published in the magazine *Popular Electronics*. The pacemaker-dependent children were then maintained with the wire suture electrodes and an external, battery-powered pacemaker. Both devices were associated with progressive fibrosis at the myocardial level and the development of a high stimulation threshold, referred to as *exit block*.[111]

Transvenous Pacing

When open heart surgery was to begin at Montefiore Hospital (Bronx, NY), it was recognized that a means was required for pacing the heart should heart block result. Experiments on producing heart block and pacing the heart with myocardial wires and a pulse generator, designed at the hospital, were begun. Furman, a surgical resident assigned to assist in developing the open heart surgical program and a cardiac pacing technique, had also been performing cardiac catheterization. He added a wire to the lumen of a Cournand catheter and passed it into the right ventricle through the external jugular vein of a dog on March 12, 1958, with successful pacing of the heart from the right ventricular endocardial surface.[112] When pacing was successfully and reproducibly demonstrated in animals, the technique was shown to the chief of cardiology, John B. Schwedel, who recognized its possibilities and determined to foster it.

A patient with acquired complete heart block and an idioventricular rate of about 30 bpm required resection of a carcinoma of the colon. On July 16, 1958, a Cournand electrode catheter was passed into the patient's right ventricle through the right basilic vein with fluoroscopic control, and pacing was achieved for 2 hours during the operation. He was weaned from stimulation at the conclusion of the procedure, and the catheter electrode was removed. The patient returned to complete heart block with idioventricular rhythm. He subsequently successfully underwent prostatectomy without a pacemaker and died suddenly on the following day, July 31, 1958.

On August 18, 1958 a second patient, bedridden and ill with chronic rheumatic heart disease, atrial fibrillation with slow ventricular response, severe electrolyte imbalance, and syncope, underwent electrode placement through the left basilic vein. He had been paced across the intact chest wall, had sustained severe mental deterioration, and had lost bladder and bowel control and the ability to recognize anyone or to speak. Right ventricular pacing was continued until November 21, 1958, by which time the patient had been continually paced for 13 weeks and 5 days. Electrolyte imbalance had been reversed, and he had recovered from his mental and neurologic deficits and was ambulatory. He was discharged from the hospital with atrial fibrillation and a sustainable unpaced ventricular rate.[113] He had several recurrences, requiring briefer periods of pacing and survived until February 18, 1962.

By January 15, 1961, the technique, which had been supported in the cardiac catheterization laboratory under the direction of Doris J.W. Escher, was established. The ability to successfully pace the heart transvenously, with prolonged survival, was proved with 25 patients paced for various durations. Complications were technical, including lead displacement and fracture, infection of a lead that exited through the skin, electronic and pacemaker battery failure, but not thrombosis, thromboembolism, or rising stimulation thresholds. Patients were paced for prolonged periods with a battery-powered external pulse generator designed for postoperative use.[114] Of the first 25 patients, 7 sustained transvenous pacing with an external pulse generator for 23 to 86 months. Thirteen of the 25 survived more than 6 months, including one each for 106 months, 232 months, 240 months, and 315 months. Those patients whose lives had extended into the implant era received implants at their own request.[115]

Lagergren coupled an endocardial lead with an implantable pulse generator and achieved a wholly implanted transvenous system on June 5, 1962[116] in Stockholm, Sweden. Parsonnet accomplished full transvenous implantation in the United States on October 6, 1962.[117] A wholly implantable transvenous system was commercially introduced by Chardack and Medtronic during 1965.[118] From that time, the progressive worldwide change from thoracotomy to transvenous implantation occurred.

The race to develop an implantable device was under way in 1959 in both the United States and Europe. Three power sources dominated the first units implanted in humans: rechargeable cells, radiofrequency energy transmission, and mercury-zinc batteries. The rechargeable and radiofrequency models had a component external to the body as part of the system. Only the mercury-zinc primary cell was entirely independent of an external component (i.e., fully implanted), but it required surgical replacement of the pulse generator when it was exhausted. Estimates at the time of design of the mercury-zinc units were that they would last about 5 years before battery depletion occurred.[93] The best mean longevity for any mercury-zinc cell pulse generator ever implanted (except for one infrequently used model) was about 30 months. The first mercury-zinc models failed before 1 year.

Pacing Modes

Cardiac stimulation by most of the earliest workers was continuous, with pacing manually switched either on or off. The operator determined whether continued pacing was required or, by observing an ECG, whether the patient's heart had resumed a spontaneous rhythm. Even at the earliest time, different pacing modes were being used. While Zoll intended to pace the ventricles across the intact chest wall, Bigelow, Callaghan, and Hopps paced the sinoatrial node area, that is, the atrium. This was done because they did not consider heart block during their cardiac stimulation; rather, they planned to accelerate the bradycardia induced by whole body hypothermia.

Leatham and Davies, regarding their external transcutaneous pacemaker reported in 1956, decided that automatic onset and termination of stimulation was an important function. Accordingly, they designed a second stimulator with those characteristics: "The warning device sounds an alarm (inserted as an additional contact on relay B) or sets the automatic stimulator into action if for a pre-determined time no QRS has been received." And later, "A spontaneous beat from the patient, however, will be received by the warning device and will cut off the stimulator."[119] For a time, external pacemakers manufactured in the United States required wholly manual operation, but by 1958 Electrodyne-Zoll external transcutaneous pacemakers had an automatic "on" capability, but were without automatic pacing cessation.

The earliest battery-operated external pacemakers, intended for stimulating the heart through epicardial wires or transvenous leads, were also wholly asynchronous in operation. This was also true for all of the radiofrequency or induction pacemakers and the earliest of the wholly implantable devices, either rechargeable or with mercury-zinc cells. Nevertheless, the concept of atrial synchrony and its lure as a potentially physiologic mode was recognized early.

At least three atrial synchronous systems were reported in animal experiments in 1957,[120] 1959,[121] and 1960[122] before the first human system by Nathan and associates,[123] in 1963, was manufactured commercially by the Cordis Corporation and named Atricor. That system was unipolar and wholly implanted by thoracotomy, had a single atrial lead and two ventricular leads (one redundant as a spare), and was powered by five mercury-zinc cells. It was the first implantable (or widely available) pacemaker sensitive to cardiac function and as such was revolutionary in concept and application. The atrial lead did not stimulate but transmitted the P wave to the pulse generator, which, after an AV delay, triggered a ventricular stimulus. Lower and upper rate limits, AV delay, and atrial refractoriness were set at manufacture in this entirely nonprogrammable model. In the absence of sensed atrial events, the unit was set to a lower rate of 50 or 60 bpm, depending on the model. This mode (VAT) was available well into the lithium era and was eventually programmable in rate and output.

The Atricor sensed only a single (atrial) channel. Because it was introduced before the era of transvenous implantation in the United States and required an atrial lead applied to the epicardial surface of the atrium, implantation was by thoracotomy, usually left anterolateral. It was soon recognized that the atrial synchronous mode could often substitute for a ventricular noncompetitive pacemaker, which was then otherwise unavailable. Because the patient with intermittent heart block commonly has a PR interval longer than the pacemaker AV delay when in a period of 1:1 conduction, the atrial synchronous mode was occasionally used for that purpose. This model was competitive with spontaneous, usually ectopic, ventricular activity because it was not sensitive to the ventricle. The earliest pacemaker-induced and pacemaker-mediated arrhythmias were documented with the Atricor pacemaker model.

Another atrial synchronous system was later developed in Sweden and implanted by a mixed transvenous route. Transvenous pacemaker implantation had been introduced in Sweden by Lagergren in 1962[124] and rapidly became the standard route. In 1965, Carlens,[125] an otolaryngologist, had conceived of mediastinoscopy for biopsy of the lymph nodes at the tracheal bifurcation, which could be approached from an incision in the suprasternal notch. The space lies between the bifurcation of the trachea posteriorly and the left atrium anteriorly. An electrode similar to the ventricular-stimulating electrode can detect the P wave at that point. An atrial synchronous mercury-zinc–powered pacemaker was constructed and implanted partially transvenously and partially by mediastinoscopy.[126] Ventricular rate variation based on maintenance of atrial synchrony and linked to the atrial rate was initially intuitively based. Hemodynamic studies by Samet,[127] Benchimol,[128] and especially Karlof[129] established the relationship of atrial synchrony and rate variation to cardiac output. The series of Karlof[130] publications (1966 to 1974) demonstrated that, with exercise, an increase in cardiac rate unassociated with atrial synchrony produced, in the presence of complete heart block, an equivalent increase in cardiac output. This finding was the concept central to the eventual development of rate modulation sensors.

In 1967, Bilitch and colleagues[131] published a single, well-documented case, which had a major impact on the development of cardiac pacing. It demonstrated ventricular fibrillation resulting from an asynchronous pacemaker stimulus falling on the vulnerable portion of the T wave of an elderly patient with an acute myocardial infarction. The logic of this event was that a pacemaker should sense the existence of a QRS complex and avoid competitive stimulation. Soon thereafter, Berkovits[132] introduced a pacemaker sensitive to electrical events of ventricular (the chamber being stimulated) origin that he labeled on "demand." As with previous devices, a minimum stimulation rate was set, but when a QRS was detected, the pacemaker withheld its stimulus and resumed its timing cycle. The atrial synchronous pacemaker had encouraged the concept that a stimulus might be competitive and yet harmless if it fell into the absolute refractory portion of ventricular depolarization. The manufacturers of atrial synchronous pacemakers designed systems that sensed the ventricle rather than the atrium and stimulated the ventricle, in response to the sensed ventricular event, without any delay. This resulted in an established pacing rate and a response in which the stimulus was triggered to fall harmlessly into a QRS at the instant it was sensed.[133] By 1966, two noncompetitive single-chamber systems were available. One inhibited pacemaker output in the presence of a spontaneous event; the other triggered a stimulus. Both were commercially successful for several years.

By 1970, the advantages of atrial synchrony and of noncompetitive pacing had become apparent. Because only a single sensing channel was possible, Berkovits modified his demand pacemaker to stimulate the atrium without sensing it and then to stimulate the ventricle after an AV delay, in the demand mode.[134] In the presence of a sinus rhythm at a rate less than the pacemaker stimulation rate, atrial synchrony was restored. He named this device Bifocal Demand.[135] By the end of 1970, implantable pacemakers were available in six different pacing modes: VOO, AOO, VAT, VVI, VVT, and DVI.

In 1973, Parsonnet, Furman, and Symth, in an Intersociety Commission for Heart Disease Resources (ICHD) report on Cardiac Pacing,[136] introduced the concept of the three-position code of pacemaker function. The need to sense the chamber being paced, the ventricle, became progressively more apparent and intellectually dominant, as did the value of atrial synchrony and rate variation. Medtronic Model 2409, the ASVIP (Atrial Sensing Ventricular Inhibited Pacing) pacemaker, which sensed two channels (atrium and ventricle), provided atrial synchrony and noncompetitive ventricular pacing and was introduced in 1979 but received only limited interest.[137, 138] It was the first unit to provide atrial synchrony and ventricular inhibition, a new mode (VDD). It was also the unit that demonstrated a new, pacemaker-mediated arrhythmia, the endless-loop tachycardia (e.g., pacemaker-mediated re-entry tachycardia, pacemaker re-entry tachycardia).[139]

This and subsequent VDD systems used two leads: atrial and ventricular. A simultaneous development was that of the single lead that could sense, but not pace, atrial activity. A single lead for atrium and ventricle had long been considered a potentially important innovation. The "crown of thorns" lead of multiple atrial fronds[140] and that of an atrial lead component that bent away from the ventricle[141] were eventually unused. Antonioli[142] introduced a ventricular lead in 1979 with an integral atrial electrode in a fixed position within the atrium and achieved atrial synchrony. He continued its development to sense individual P waves and provide full atrial synchrony.[143] Later a device was introduced into clinical evaluation, the RS4, with a single lead designed by Goldreyer[144] that he named Orthogonal. This VDD mode sensed the atrium and stimulated the ventricle at the atrial rate but not on a 1:1 basis, a technique called *rate responsive* by the manufacturer.[145] The technique was an attempt to overcome the presumed difficulties of intermittent atrial undersensing and loss of 1:1 atrial synchrony by responding to overall, not individual, atrial activity and by matching the atrial rate and stimulated ventricular rate by means of a prolonged time constant, so that a rate increase or decrease, especially in the event of an unsensed P wave, would be moderated. The unsensed P wave would not cause the next interval to be at the lower rate limit. The device never achieved commercial release, and the Orthogonal lead was later modified to become a successful component of clinical and commercially successful VDD systems that did provide 1:1 atrial synchrony.

Rogel[146] in 1965 and Irnich[147] in 1975 proposed a pacemaker mode that combined the capability of the DVI mode of atrial pacing and ventricular pacing and sensing and the VAT mode of atrial sensing and ventricular pacing into a kind of "universal" pacemaker that would pace and sense both the atrium and the ventricle. In 1977 model SP0069BV, an experimental pacemaker that met the DDD designation as having "universal" function, was initially implanted. It has been invented by Funke[148] and had the ability to sense and pace both the atrium and the ventricle. The first commercial models were Medtronic model 7000 and Cordis model 233D.

The hemodynamics of cardiac function had long been of interest to the pacemaker community. The ability to control the atrial rate, the ventricular rate, the association between the two, whether 1:1 synchronization or some other ratio was achieved, the delay between atrial contraction and ventricular contraction, the timing relationships between right and left atrium and right and left ventricle, the effect of rest and exercise, erectness or recumbency, and the pressure relationships within the atrium and ventricle all led productively to the extensive and repetitive evaluation of the cardiac hemodynamics with and without cardiac pacing. Atrial function and its contribution to overall cardiac function had been debated by physiologists since Harvey's description of the circulation. Gesell[149] provided experimental data, as did Erlanger, Lewis, and Wenckebach, but it was the advent of the cardiac pacemaker that provided much of the information now available. One conclusion derived from Karlof's[129] and other authors' later investigations was that, with exercise and a nonfailing myocardium, cardiac output is directly related to cardiac rate.

In 1975, Funke[150] described, without clinical use, a pacemaker for which the stimulation rate was linked to the respiratory rate. This was determined by an intrapleural piezoelectric microphone to detect changes in intrapleural pressure. In 1976, Cammilli[151] clinically implanted a pacemaker that sensed changes in blood pH and demonstrated increases in stimulation rate associated with activity. He did not continue this effort. Rickards and Norman,[152] who recognized the changes in the QT interval with activity, developed the first clinically and commercially available rate-modulated ventricular pacemaker. Although Bazett had described variation in duration of the QT interval many years earlier,[153] Rickards recognized the relation to activity and demonstrated that the QT interval duration was modulated with catecholamine level and could be measured and converted into a sensor for use in a pacemaker. Thus, Cammilli, and somewhat later Rickards, introduced the concept of the rate-modulated single-chamber (VVIR) ventricular pacemaker. Because the QT interval has ventricular function only, this pacemaker could not be used for atrial rate-modulated pacing. The algorithm for QT sensor operation required several modifications, so that other sensors continued to be sought. Rossi[154] introduced another respiratory rate-modulated pacemaker in which a lead from the pulse generator directed subcutaneously across the chest measured the respiratory rate by measuring impedance changes. This model was commercially available for about a decade after its introduction. A central venous temperature-measuring sensor achieved commercial availability but is no longer available.[155] Other sensors have subsequently been developed, but in 1998, three sensors were in clinical use: the piezoelectric sensor in several configurations, a minute ventilation impedance–mediated sensor, and the stimulus-T or QT sensor.

Anderson[156] of Medtronic developed the concept of the piezoelectric activity sensor, which could be placed within the case of the pulse generator. This was placed within an existing VDD pacemaker then in clinical use. The electrical signals developed by the sensor mimicked those of the atrial lead, derived directly from the atrium. With atrial sensing no longer needed because electrical signals related to activity were derived from within the pulse generator itself, the device was used as a single-lead ventricular (or atrial) stimulator. The piezoelectric sensor in a variety of configurations has become, by far, the most popular sensor now in use. Placement of a sensor in a DDD pacemaker in 1989 completed the sequence of pacemaker modes with the DDDR unit, now the most advanced and sophisticated of the pacemaker units available.

■ FUTURE IMPLICATIONS

In the new millenium, following development of sensors, lithium power sources, and dual chamber pacing, new directions for cardiac stimulation are being evaluated. The immediate future is the stimulation of both ventricles and evaluation of the effect of biventricular pacing for the control of congestive heart failure. Biatrial pacing and biventricular pacing will also be evaluated for greater efficacy in control of heart failure and perhaps in arrhythmia management to add to more conventional antitachycardia pacing and defibrillation. Parts of the myocardium will be stimulated differentially and the normal cardiac depolarization pattern will be extensively modified to change the pattern, timing, and strength of contraction. The implanted device, now sensitive to cardiac electrograms and exercise and activity sensors to yield a change in stimulation rate, will become sensitive to other physiologic and artificial functions so that it will transmit physiologic and other data, yet to be defined, about the patient in whom it is implanted. Transmission of right ventricular and pulmonary artery pressures is obvious, but the development of left ventricular stimulation and sensing,

transmission of left sided hemodynamics, and assessment of left ventricular contractility will follow soon.

Pacemaker telemetry is substantially of the operation of the device itself and adds only recording, memory, and transmission of the electrical signals associated with cardiac function (ECG and EGM). Newer telemetry will detect and transmit even smaller electrical signals and convert chemical and hemodynamic events and conditions into electrical signals to change the character of stimulation and allow transmission of a much broader base of information. There is no doubt that computer and electronic technology, upon which modern cardiac stimulation is based, is evolving very rapidly. The multilead, multichamber, technologically complex cardiac stimulator of a quarter century hence will be unrecognizably different from today's device and establish itself as a major contributor to management of cardiac patients with and without conduction disturbances. These devices will evaluate the cardiac effect of the change in stimulation and modify electronic function accordingly. Self-regulatory stimulation will finally become a reality.

REFERENCES

1. Lewis JK: Stokes-Adams disease: An account of important historical discoveries. Arch Intern Med 101:130–142, 1958.
2. Music D, Rakovec P, Jagodic A, Cibic B: The first description of syncopal attacks in heart block. PACE 7:301–303, 1984.
3. Morgagni G: Letter the ninth, which treats epilepsy. *In* De Sedibus et Causis Morborium, 1761. (The Seats and Causes of Diseases, translated by Benj Alexander). London, Millar & Cadell, 1762, p 92.
4. Spens T: History of a case in which there took place a remarkable slowness of the pulse. Medical Commentaries (Edinburg) 7:463, 1793.
5. Burnett, W: Case of epilepsy, attended with remarkable slowness of the pulse. Med Chir Trans 13:202, 1827.
6. Adams R: Cases of diseases of the heart accompanied with pathological observations. Dublin Hosp Rep 4:396, 1827.
7. Stokes R: Observations on some cases of permanently low pulse. Dublin Q J Med Sci 2:73, 1846.
8. Huchard H: Le maladie de Stokes-Adams. Bull Med (Paris) 4:937–940, 1890.
9. Wilson G: On the employment of the electric eel, *Gymnotus electricus,* as a medical shock machine by the natives of Surinam. Rep Br Assoc Adv Sci. 1859–1860, p 158.
10. Walsh J: On the electrical property of the torpedo. Philos Trans; 63:461, 1773.
11. Volta A: On electricity excited by the mere contact of conducting substances of different kinds. In a letter to Sir Joseph Banks, March 20, 1800.
12. Galvani L: De viribus electricitatis in motu musculari, commentarius. Bologna Institute Scientia 1791.
13. Aldini G: General Views on the Application of Galvanism of Medical Purposes. London, J Callow, 1819, p 96.
14. Bichat MFX: Recherches Physiologiques sur la Vie et la Mort. Paris, Brosson, Gabon & Cie, 1800.
15. Du Bois-Reymond E: Untersuchungen Uber Thierische Electricitat Berlin, Reimer, 1848–1884.
16. McWilliam JA: Electrical stimulation of the heart in man. Br Med J 1:348–350, 1889.
17. Von Ziemssen H: Studien uber die Bewegungsvorgange am menschlichen Herzen, sowie uber die mechanische und elektrische Erregbarkeit des Herzens und des Nervusphrenicus. Deutsches Arch fur Klin Med 30:270–286, 1881–1882.
18. Gaskell WH: On the innervation of the heart, with especial reference to the heart of the tortoise. J Physiol 4:43–127, 1883.
19. His W Jr: Ein Fall von Adams-Stokes' scher Krankheit mit ungleichzeitigem Schlagen der Vorhof und Herzkammern (Herzblock). Deutsches Arch fur Klin Med 64:316–331, 1899.
20. His W: Zur geschichte des atrioventricul-bundels nebst bemerkungen uber die embryonale Herztetigkeit. Klin Wochenschr 12:569–574, 1933.
21. Erlanger J: On the physiology of heart-block in mammals, with espe-

cial reference to causation of Stokes-Adams disease. Part II. On the physiology of heart block in the dog. J Exp Med 8L8–32, 1906.

22. Erlanger J: On the physiology of heart-block in mammals, with especial reference to causation of Stokes-Adams disease. Part I. Observations on an instance of heart block in man. J Exp Med 7:676–724, 1905.

23. Erlanger J, Blackman JRL: Further studies on the physiology of heart-block in mammals: Chronic auriculo-ventricular heart-block in the dog. Heart 1:177, 1910.

24. Lewis T: A lecture on the occurrence of heart block in man and its causation. Br Med J 2:1798–1802, 1908.

25. Kerr WJ, Bender WL: Paroxysmal ventricular fibrillation with cardiac recovery in a case of auricular fibrillation and complete heart-block while under quinidine sulphate therapy. Heart 10:269–281, 1922.

26. Parkinson J, Papp C, Evans W: The electrocardiogram of the Stokes-Adams attack. Br Heart J 3:171–199, 1941.

27. Cohn AE, Holmes GM, Lewis T: Report of a case of transient attacks of heart-block, including a post mortem examination. Heart 2:241–248, 1911.

28. Levine SA, Matton M: Observations on a case of Stokes-Adams syndrome, showing ventricular fibrillation and asystole lasting five minutes, with recovery following the intracardiac injection of adrenaline. Heart 12:271–279, 1926.

29. Laslett EE: Two cases of paroxysmal bradycardia (total). Q J Med 5:377–387, 1912.

30. Rowe JC, White PD: Complete heart block: A follow-up study. Ann Intern Med 49:260–270, 1958.

31. Froment R, Gonin A: Les syncopes du bloc auriculo-ventriculaire: Considerations sur leur semeiologie et leur pathogenie. Paris Med 1:375–380, 1938.

32. Levine SA, Matton M: Observations on a case of Stokes-Adams syndrome, showing ventricular fibrillation and asystole lasting five minutes, with recovery following the intracardiac injection of adrenaline. Heart 12:271–279, 1926.

33. Roe BB, Katz HJ: Complete heart block with intractable asystole and recurrent ventricular fibrillation with survival. Am J Cardiol 15:401–403, 1965.

34. Fleming GB, Kennedy AM: A case of complete heart-block in diphtheria with an account of post-mortem finding. Heart 2:77–83, 1910.

35. Rosenbaum MB, Alvarez AJ: The electrocardiogram in chronic chagasic myocarditis. Am Heart J 50:492–527, 1955.

36. Lev M: Anatomic basis for atrioventricular block. Am J Med 37:742, 1964.

37. Lenegre J: Les blocs auriculo-ventriculaires completes chroniques: Etudes des causes et des lesions a propos de 37 cas. (Chronic complete atrioventricular blocks: Study of causes and lesions apropos of 37 cases). Mal Cardiovasc 3:311–343, 1962.

38. Einthoven W: Ueber die Form des menschlichen Electrocardiogramms. Pflugers Arch 60:101–123, 1895.

39. Schwartz SP, Schwartz LS: The Adams-Stokes syndrome during normal sinus rhythm and transient heart block I. The effects of isuprel on patients with the Adams-Stokes syndrome during normal sinus rhythm and transient heart block. Am Heart J 106:849–861, 1959.

40. Eraklis AJ, Green WT, Watson CG: Recurrent paroxysms of ventricular tachycardia following mitral valvuloplasty. Ann Surg 161:63–66, 1965.

41. Johansson BW: Longevity in complete heart block. Ann N Y Acad Sci 167:1031–1037, 1969.

42. Cohn AE, Levine SA: The beneficial effects of barium chloride on Adams-Stokes disease. Arch Intern Med 36:1–12, 1925.

43. Linenthal AJ, Zoll PM: Prevention of ventricular tachycardia and fibrillation by intravenous isoproterenol and epinephrine. Circulation 1963; 27:5–11.

44. Lister JW, Stein E, Kosowsky BD, et al: Atrioventricular conduction in man: Effect of rate, exercise, isoproterenol and atropine on the PR interval. Am J Cardiol 16:516–523, 1965.

45. Chandler D, Clapper MI: Complete atrioventricular block treated with isoproterenol hydrochloride. Am J Cardiol 3:336–342, 1959.

46. Friedberg CK, Kahn M, Scheuer J, Bleiter S: Adams-Stokes syndrome associated with chronic heart block: Treatment with corticosteroids. JAMA 172:1146–1152, 1960.

47. Marmorstein M: Contribution a l'etude des excitation electriques localises sur le coeur en rapport avec la topographie de l'innervation due coeur chez le chien. J Physiol Pathol 25:617–625, 1927.

48. Mond HG, Sloman JG, Edwards RH: The first pacemaker. PACE 5:278–282, 1982.

49. Hyman AS: Resuscitation of the stopped heart by intracardiac therapy. Arch Intern Med 46:553–568, 1930.

50. Hyman AS: Resuscitation of the stopped heart by intracardiac therapy. IV. Further use of the artificial pacemaker. U S Navy Med Bull 33:205–214, 1935.

51. Forssmann W: Die sondierung des rechten herzens. Klin Wochenschr 8:2085–2087, 1929.

52. Cournand A: Catheterization of the right auricle in man. Proc Soc Exp Biol Med 46:462–466, 1941.

53. Blalock A, Taussig HB: The surgical treatment of malformation of the heart in which there is pulmonary stenosis or pulmonary atresia. JAMA 128:189–202, 1945.

54. Carfoord C, Nylin G: Congenital coarctation of the aorta and its surgical treatment. J Thorac Surg 14:347–361, 1945.

55. Harken DE: A review of the activities of the thoracic center for the III and IV hospital groups, 160th general hospital European theater of operations, June 10, 1944, to Jan. 1, 1945. J Thorac Surg 15:31–43, 1946.

56. Harken DE, Williams AC: Foreign bodies in and in relation to the thoracic blood vessels and heart: Migratory foreign bodies within the blood vascular system. Am J Surg 72:80–90, 1946.

57. Ruben S: US Patent 2,422,045 (1947).

58. Linford HB: Samuel Ruben-Acheson Medalist. J Electrochem Soc 11C, Jan 1971.

59. Bardeen J, Brattain WH: The transistor, a semiconductor triode. Physiol Rev 74:230, 1948.

60. Schokley W: The theory of p-n junctions in semiconductors and p-n junction transistors. Bell Sys Tech J 28:435, 1949.

61. Schneider A, Moser J, Webb THE, Desmond JE: A new high energy density cell with a lithium anode. Proc US Army Signal Corps Power Sources Conf, Atlantic City, NJ, 1970.

62. Tyers GFO, Brownlee RR: The non-hermetically sealed pacemaker myth, or Navy-Ribicoff 22,000—FDA-Weinberger 0. J Thorac Cardiovasc Surg 71:253–254, 1976.

63. Furman S, Raddi WJ, Escher DJW, et al: Rechargeable pacemaker for direct myocardial implantation. Arch Surg 91:796–800, 1965.

64. Fischell RE, Lewis KB, Schulman JH, Love JW: A long-lived, reliable, rechargeable cardiac pacemaker. In Schaldach M and Furman J (eds): Advances in pacemaker technology, New York/Heidelberg, Springer-Verlag, 1975, pp 357–382.

65. Levine P: Personal communication, May 17, 1999.

66. Antonioli GE: Lithium pacemaker: The first clinical experience. PACE 13:363–370, 1990.

67. Lillehei RC, Romero LH, Beckman CB, et al: A new solid state, long life, lithium powered pulse generator. Ann Thorac Surg 18:479–489, 1974.

68. Parsonnet V, Myers GH, Gilbert L, et al: Clinical experience with nuclear pacemakers. Surgery 78:776–785, 1975.

69. Schmidt TH, Kowalewski H, Matheson WE, et al: Promethium and plutonium as fuel isotopes in radionuclide batteries. Digest of the Tenth International Conference on Medical and Biologic Engineering. Dresden, GDR, 1973, p 341.

70. Roy OZ, Wehnert RW: Biogalvanic energy sources. In Thalen HJT (ed): Cardiac pacing. Proceedings of the 4th International Symposium: Van Gorcum & Comp, BV Assen, 1973, pp 209–215.

71. Parsonnet V, Myers G, Zucker IR, Lotman H: The potentiality of the use of biologic energy as a power source for implantable pacemakers. Ann N Y Acad Sci 111:915–921, 1964.

72. Warner H, Robinson BW: A glucose fuel cell. Digest of the Seventh International Conference on Medical and Biologic Engineering, Stockholm, 1967, p 520.

73. Love JW, Lewis KB, Fischell RE, Schulman J: Experimental testing of a permanent rechargeable cardiac pacemaker. Ann Thorac Surg 17:152–156, 1974.

74. Tyers GFO, Foresman RA Jr, Part CD, et al: Preclinical testing of a redundant, rechargeable cardiac pacemaker. J Thorac Cardiovasc Surg 62:763–768, 1971.

75. Greatbatch W, Lee JH, Mathias W, et al: The solid-state lithium battery: A new improved chemical power source for implantable cardiac pacemakers. IEEE Trans Bio-Med Eng 18:317–324, 1971.

76. Bigelow WG: Cold hearts: The Story of Hypothermia and the Pacemaker in Heart Surgery. Toronto, Ontario, McClelland and Stewart Limited, 1984.

77. Hopps JA: Passing pulses. The Pacemaker and Medical Engineering: A Canadian Story. Ottawa, Ontario, Publishing Plus Limited, 1995.

78. Hopps JA, Bigelow WG: Electrical treatment of cardiac arrest: A cardiac stimulator-defibrillator. Surgery 36:833–849, 1954.

79. Hopps JA: The development of the pacemaker. PACE 4:106–108, 1981.

80. Bigelow WG, Callaghan JC, Hopps JA: General hypothermia for experimental intracardiac surgery: The use of electrophrenic respirations, an artificial pacemaker for cardiac standstill, and radio-frequency rewarming in general hypothermia. Ann Surg 132:531–539, 1950.

81. Zoll PM: Resuscitation of the heart in ventricular standstill by external electric stimulation. N Engl J Med 247:768–771, 1952.

82. Douglas AH, Wagner WP: Ventricular control by artificial pacemaker for 7 days with recovery. JAMA 157:444–446, 1955.

83. Falk RH, Zoll PM, Zoll RH: Safety and efficacy of noninvasive cardiac pacing: A preliminary report. N Engl J Med 309:1166–1168, 1983.

84. Zoll PM, Zoll RH, Falk RH, et al: External noninvasive temporary cardiac pacing: Clinical trials. Circulation 71:937–944, 1985.

85. Larsson A, Larsson AM: Personal interview. September 14, 1997.

86. Elmqvist R, Senning A: An implantable pacemaker for the heart. *In* Smyth CN (ed): Proceedings of the Second International Conference on Medical Electronics. Paris, June 24–27, 1959, pp 253–254. London, Iliffe & Sons, 1960.

87. Fiandra O: The first pacemaker implant in America. PACE 11:1234–1238, 1988.

88. Siddons AHM, Humphries O'N: Complete heart block with Stokes-Adams attacks treated by indwelling pacemaker. Proc Roy Soc Med 54:237–238, 1961.

89. Siddons AHM: Long-term artificial cardiac pacing: Experience in adults with heart block. Ann Roy Coll Surg Eng 32:22–41, 1963.

90. Jeffrey K: Conference on artificial pacemakers and cardiac prosthesis. Sponsored by the Medical Electronics Center of the Rockefeller Institute, 1958. PACE 16:1445–1482, 1993.

91. Kantrowitz A, Cohen R, Raillard H, et al: The treatment of complete heart block with an implanted controllable pacemaker. Surg Gynecol Obstet 115:415–420, 1962.

92. Zoll PM, Frank HA, Zarsky LR, et al: Long-term electrical stimulation of the heart for Stokes-Adams disease. Ann Surg 154:330–346, 1961.

93. Chardack WM, Gage AA, Greatbatch W: A transistorized, self-contained implantable pacemaker for the long-term correction of complete heart block. Surgery 48:643–654, 1960.

94. Chardack WM, Gage AA, Federico AJ, et al: Clinical experience with an implantable pacemaker. Ann N Y Acad Sci 111:1075–1092, 1964.

95. Reynolds J: The early history of cardiac pacing in Colombia. PACE 11:355–361, 1988.

96. Kormann D: Personal interview. October 23, 1995.

97. Verzeano M, Webb RG Jr, Kelly M: Radio control of ventricular contraction in experimental heart block. Science 128:1003, 1958.

98. Mauro A: Technique for *in situ* stimulation. Yale Biophys Bull 1:2, 1948.

99. Glenn WWL, Mauro A, Longo E, et al: Remote stimulation of the heart by radio-frequency transmission. N Engl J Med 261:948–951, 1959.

100. Eisenberg L, Mauro A, Glenn WWL, Hageman JH: Radio frequency stimulation: A research and clinical tool. Science 147:578–582, 1965.

101. Widmann WD, Glenn WWL, Eisenberg L, Mauro A: Radio-frequency cardiac pacemaker. Ann N Y Acad Sci 111:992–1006, 1964.

102. Glenn WWL, Furman S, Gordon AG, et al: Radio-frequency controlled catheter pacemaker. N Engl J Med 275:137–140, 1966.

103. Cammilli L, Pozzi R, Drago G, et al: Remote heart stimulation by radio-frequency for permanent rhythm control in the Morgagni-Adams-Stokes syndrome. Surgery 52:765, 1962.

104. Abrams LD, Hudson WA, Lightwood R: A surgical approach to the management of heart-block using an inductive coupled artificial cardiac pacemaker. Lancet 1:1372–1374, 1960.

105. Siddons AHM: Long-term artificial cardiac pacing: Experience in adults with heart block. Ann Roy Coll Surg Engl 32:22–41, 1963.

106. Suma M, Fujimori Y, Mitsui T, et al: Direct induction pacemaker. Digest of the Sixth International Conference on Medical Electronic and Biological Engineering. Tokyo, 1965, p 96.

107. Barr IM, Yerushalmi S, Blieden L, Neufeld HN: Endocardial radio-frequency pacemaking. Israel J Med Sci 1:1018–1021, 1965.

108. Allen P, Lillehei CW: Use of induced cardiac arrest in open heart surgery. Minn Med 40:672–676, 1957.

109. Barnard CN, DeWall RA, Varco RL, Lillehei CW: Pre and postoperative care for patients undergoing open cardiac surgery. Dis Chest 35:194–212, 1959.

110. Weirich WL, Paneth M, Gott VL, Lillehei CW: Control of complete heart block by use of an artificial pacemaker and a myocardial electrode. Circ Res 6:410–415, 1958.

111. Lillehei CW, Gott VL, Hodges PC, et al: Transistor pacemaker for treatment of complete atrioventricular dissociation. JAMA 172:2006–2010, 1960.

112. Furman S, Robinson G: The use of an intracardiac pacemaker in the correction of total heart block. Surg Forum 8:245–248, 1958.

113. Furman S, Schwedel JB: An intracardiac pacemaker for Stokes-Adams seizures. N Engl J Med 261:943–948, 1959.

114. Furman S, Escher DJW, Schwedel JB, Solomon N: Transvenous pacing: A seven year review. Am Heart J 71:408–416, 1966.

115. Furman S: Recollections of the beginning of transvenous cardiac pacing. PACE 17:1697–1705, 1994.

116. Lagergren H, Johansson L, Landegren J, Edhag O: One hundred cases of treatment for Adams-Stokes syndrome with permanent intravenous pacemaker. J Thorac Cardiovasc Surg 50:710–714, 1965.

117. Zucker IR, Parsonnet V, Gilbert L, Asa MM: Dipolar electrode in heart block. JAMA 184:549, 1963.

118. Furman S, Escher DJW, Solomon N, Schwedel JB: Implanted transvenous pacemakers. Ann Surg 164:465–474, 1966.

119. Leatham A, Cook P, Davies JG: External electric stimulator for treatment of ventricular standstill. Lancet 2:1185–1189, 1956.

120. Folkman MJ, Watkins E: An artificial conduction system for the management of experimental complete heart block. Surg Forum 8:331–335, 1957.

121. Stephenson SE, Edwards WH, Jolly PC, Scott HW: Physiologic P-wave cardiac stimulator. J Thorac Cardiovasc Surg 38:604–609, 1959.

122. Kahn M, Senderoff E, Shapiro J, et al: Bridging of interrupted A-V conduction in experimental chronic complete heart block by electronic means. Am Heart J 59:548–559, 1960.

123. Nathan DA, Center S, Wu C-Y, Keller JW: An implantable synchronous pacemaker for the long term correction of complete heart block. Circulation 27:682–685, 1963.

124. Lagergren H: How it happened: My recollection of early pacing. PACE 1:140–143, 1978.

125. Carlens E, Johansson L, Karlof I, Lagergren H: New method for atrial-triggered pacemaker treatment without thoracotomy. J Thorac Cardiovasc Surg 50:229–232, 1965.

126. Carlens E: Mediastinoscopy: A method for inspection and tissue biopsy in the superior mediastinum. Dis Chest 36:343–352, 1959.

127. Samet P, Bernstein WH, Nathan DA, Lopez A: Atrial contribution to cardiac output in complete heart block. Am J Cardiol 16:1–10, 1965.

128. Benchimol A, Duenas A, Liggett MS, Dimond EG: Contribution of atrial systole to the cardiac function at a fixed and at a variable ventricular rate. Am J Cardiol 16:11–21, 1965.

129. Karlof I: Haemodynamic effect of atrial triggered versus fixed rate pacing at rest and during exercise in complete heart block. Acta Med Scand 197:195–206, 1975.

130. Karlof I: Haemodynamic studies at rest and during exercise in patients treated with artificial pacemaker. Acta Med Scand 565:1–24, 1974.

131. Bilitch M, Cosby RS, Cafferky EA: Ventricular fibrillation and competitive pacing. N Engl J Med 276:598–604, 1967.

132. Lemberg L, Castellanos A, Berkovits BV: Pacemaking on demand in AV block. JAMA 191:12–14, 1965.

133. Neville J, Millar K, Keller W, Abidskov JA: An implantable demand pacemaker [Abstract]. Clin Res 14:256, 1966.

134. Castillo CA, Berkovits BV, Castellanos A Jr, et al: Bifocal demand pacing. Chest 59:360, 1971.

135. Furman S, Reicher-Reiss H, Escher DJW: Atrioventricular sequential pacing and pacemakers. Chest 63:783–789, 1973.

136. Parsonnet V, Furman S, Smyth NPD: Implantable cardiac pacemakers: Status report and resource guideline. A report of the Intersociety Commission for Heart Disease Resources. Am J Cardiol 34:487–502, 1974.

137. Den Dulk K, Lindemans FW, Bar FW, Wellens HJJ: Pacemaker related tachycardias. PACE 5:476–485, 1982.

138. Bathen J, Gunderson T, Forfang K: Tachycardias related to atrial synchronous ventricular pacing. PACE 5:471–475, 1982.

139. Furman S, Fisher JD: Endless loop tachycardia in an AV universal (DDD) pacemaker. PACE 5:486–489, 1982.

140. Wainwright R, Crick J, Sowton E: Clinical evaluation of a single-pass implantable electrode for all modes of pacing. The "crown of thorns" lead. PACE 6:210–220, 1983.

141. Lajos T: Transvenous physiologic pacing: A new atrioventricular electrode. PACE 5:264–267, 1982.
142. Antonioli GE, Grassi G, Baggioni GF, et al: A simple P-sensing ventricle stimulating lead driving a VAT generator. *In* Meere C (ed): Cardiac pacing. Montreal, PaceSymp, 1979, Chap. 34.9.
143. Antonioli GE: Single lead atrial synchronous ventricular pacing: A dream come true. PACE 17:1531–1547, 1994.
144. Goldreyer BN, Olive AL, Leslie J, et al: A new orthogonal lead for P-synchronous pacing. PACE 4:638–644, 1981.
145. Shapland JE, MacCarter D, Tockman B, Knudson M: Physiologic benefits of rate responsiveness. PACE 6:329–332, 1983.
146. Rogel S, Mahler Y: The universal pacer: A synchronized-demand pacemaker. J Thorac Cardiovasc Surg 61:466–471, 1971.
147. Irnich W: The ideal pacemaker. *In* Harthorne JWH, Thalen HJTh (ed): Boston Colloquium on Cardiac Pacing. The Hague, Netherlands, Martinus Nijhoff Medical Division, 1977, pp 111–122.
148. Funke HD: Die optimierte sequentielle Stimulation von Vorhof und Kammerein neuartiges Therapiekonzept zur Behandlung bradykarder Dysrhythmien. Herz Kreislauf 10:479–483, 1978.
149. Gesell RA: Auricular systole and its relation to ventricular output. Am J Physiol 29:32–63, 1911.
150. Funke HD: A cardiac pacemaker with activity-dependent frequency regulation. Biomed Tech 20:225–228, 1975.
151. Cammilli L, Alcidi L, Papeschi G: Un nuovo pacemaker sensibile alle necessita metaboliche. Osp Lt Chir 28:85, 1975.
152. Rickards AF, Norman J: Relation between QT interval and heart rate: New design of physiologically adaptive cardiac pacer. Br Heart J 45:56–61, 1981.
153. Bazett HC: An analysis of the time-relations of electrocardiograms. Heart 7:353–367, 1920.
154. Rossi P, Plicchi G, Canducci G, et al: Respiratory rate as a determinant of optimal pacing rate. PACE 6:502–507, 1983.
155. Jolgren D, Fearnot N, Geddes L: A rate responsive pacemaker controlled by right ventricular blood temperature. PACE 7:794–801, 1984.
156. Anderson K: Personal interview. May 10, 1997.

Basic Concepts of

Cardiac Pacing and

Defibrillation

Chapter 1

Artificial Electrical Cardiac Stimulation

Kenneth B. Stokes and G. Neal Kay

The fundamental basis for cardiac pacing is myocardial stimultion, a complex biophysical process. An understanding of the factors that influence myocardial stimulation is important for all clinicians involved in the care of patients with implantable pacemakers. Thus, although this chapter focuses on artificial electrical stimulation, it also includes contributions from such diverse disciplines as cellular biology, cardiovascular physiology, electrode physics and chemistry, electrical and mechanical engineering, pharmacology, and pathology. Electrostimulation is first reviewed on the cellular level. Next, the design and function of pacing electrodes is discussed, including the principles of strength–duration relationships, strength–interval relationships, constant-current versus constant-voltage pacing, anodal versus cathodal stimulation, unipolar versus bipolar stimulation, pacing impedance, pharmacologic and metabolic effects on stimulation threshold, and the practical aspects of pacemaker programming. The fundamental principles of newly emerging multisite pacing for tachyarrhythmia prevention and improvement in hemodynamics are reviewed. Finally, the clinical relevance of each of these fundamental factors is discussed in the context of managing patients with implanted pacemakers.

■ CELLULAR ASPECTS OF MYOCARDIAL STIMULATION

The Phospholipid Bimembrane

Biologic tissues, such as nerve and muscle, respond to an electrical stimulus with a self-regenerating wave of electrical depolarization that is out of proportion to the strength of the stimulus. This property is known as excitability.[1] Excitable tissues are characterized by a separation of charge across the cell membrane. Thus, it is the cell membrane that determines the fundamental property of excitability. The cell membrane

of the cardiac myocyte is composed principally of phospholipids, cholesterol, and proteins.[2] The membrane phospholipids have a charged polar headgroup and two long hydrocarbon chains arranged as shown in Figure 1–1. The cell membrane is arranged as two layers of phospholipids with their hydrophobic aliphatic chains oriented toward the aqueous phase (periphery) and their polar headgroup regions toward the periphery. Because the membrane is composed of two layers of phospholipids, the polar regions interface with the aqueous environments inside and outside the cell. The lipid-soluble hydrocarbon chains are forced away from the aqueous phase to form a nonpolar interior. The close packing of the phospholipid molecules functions as a barrier, preventing the passive diffusion of charged ions and molecules through the membrane. The high density of charged polar headgroups determines the dielectric properties of the membrane. This allows a large voltage gradient to exist across the membrane, which is essential for maintenance of the myocyte resting potential and the property of excitability.

Determinants of the Resting Transmembrane Potential

There are relatively large gradients of individual ion concentrations across the cardiac cell membrane.[3] The extracellular/intracellular gradient mmol/L:mmol/L for Na^+ is approximately 145 mmol/L:10 mmol/L, whereas that for K^+ is about 4.5 mmol/L:140 mmol/L. In the absence of a cell membrane, each cation would rapidly move in a direction determined by the concentration gradient. The diffusion force tending to move K^+ out of and Na^+ into the cell is proportional to the concentration gradients of those ions, respectively. The potential energy attributable to the diffusion force (PE_d) tending to move K^+ out of the cell is given by the following equation:

(1) $PE_d = RT \, ln[K^+]_i/[K^+]_o,$

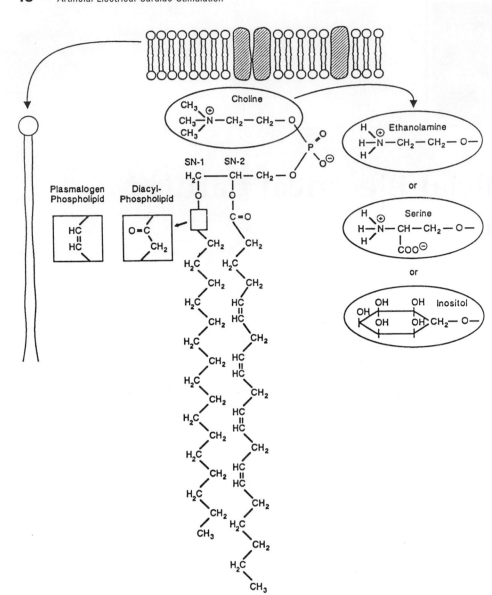

Figure 1-1. Sarcolemma structure and phospholipid composition. The lipid bilayer containing two membrane proteins is shown at the top of the figure. The detailed structure of the phospholipids is shown below. All of the aliphatic hydrocarbon groups on the sn-2 position are fatty acids that are covalently bound in the form of esters. The aliphatic hydrocarbon groups at the sn-1 position include either O-acyl esters or vinyl ethers. (From Creer MH, Dabmeyer DJ, Corr PB: Amphipathic lipid metabolites and arrhythmias during myocardial ischemia. *In* Zipes DP, Jalife J [eds]: Cardiac Electrophysiology: From Cell to Bedside. Philadelphia, WB Saunders, 1990, pp 417–432.)

where R is the gas constant, T is the absolute temperature, *ln* is the natural logarithm, $[K^+]_i$ is the concentration of potassium ion inside the cell, and $[K^+]_o$ is the concentration of potassium ion outside the cell. Thus, if the ratio of K^+ inside the cell to K^+ outside the cell is large, the potential energy across the membrane is large. The separation of charged ions from the inside to the outside of the cell results in an electric potential across the membrane. In resting cardiac cells, the intracellular cytoplasm has a measured potential of about -90 mV, compared with that of the extracellular fluid. This electric force tends to move positively charged ions such as K^+ and Na^+ to the inside of the cell and negatively charged ions such as chloride (Cl^-) to the outside of the cell in proportion to the potential gradient. The potential energy attributable to the electric force (PE_e) tending to move K^+ into the cell is expressed as follows:

$$(2) \quad PE_e = zFV_m,$$

where z is the valence (the number of positive or negative electronic charges) of the ion, F is the Faraday constant (96,500 coulombs/equivalent) and V_m is the transmembrane potential difference (measured in millivolts). During equilibrium, the total of the potential energies due to diffusion and electric forces is zero, and no net ionic movement occurs. Thus, the sum of equations 1 and 2 set to zero yields the Nernst equation, which describes the potential that must exist for K^+ to be in equilibrium across the membrane of a resting cardiac cell:

$$(3) \quad V_m(K^+) = -26.7 \; ln[K^+]_i/[K^+]_o,$$

or in more familiar $\log_{10}$ terms, $V_m(K^+) = -61.5 \log[K^+]_i/[K^+]_o$. Using known values for intracellular and extracellular K^+, $V_m(K^+) = -90$ mV. When equation 3 is solved using Na^+ concentrations, a $V_m(Na^+)$ of $+50$ mV is obtained. Thus, it is the equilibrium potential for potassium ion (not sodium ion) that is the major factor responsible for the resting transmembrane potential. This suggests that the resting membrane is more permeable to K^+ than to Na^+. The Goldman constant field equation (modified by Hodgkin and Katz) describes how these and other ions contribute to V_m[4]:

(4) $\quad V_m = \dfrac{-RT}{F} \ln \dfrac{P_K{}^+[K^+]_i + P_{Na}{}^+[Na^+]_i + P_{Cl}{}^-[Cl^-]_o + ...}{P_K{}^+[K^+]_o + P_{Na}{}^+[Na^+]_o + P_{Cl}{}^-[Cl^-]_i + ...}$

where, $P_K{}^+$, $P_{Na}{}^+$ and $P_{Cl}{}^-$ are the cell membrane permeabilities for the respective ions. Using physiologic concentrations, this equation yields a transmembrane potential of -90 mV (the equilibrium potential for K^+). Equation 4 describes how resting potentials vary as sodium and potassium ion concentrations are changed. Because there is a passive leak of charged ions through pores in the membrane, the resting potential is maintained by two active transport mechanisms that exchange Na^+ ions for K^+ and Ca^{2+} ions. These membrane pores are discussed in more detail later.

■ PROPAGATION OF AN ELECTRICAL STIMULUS

Artificial lipid membranes in their pure form are electric insulators. It is the presence of specialized protein molecules in the membrane that allows it to be conductive.[5, 6] These proteins determine the metabolic characteristics of the membrane and provide both active and passive transport of ions and molecules, which results in ionic currents. When an electric current is applied to a cardiac cell membrane, the current propagates away from the site of the stimulus. This propagation from the stimulus occurs both passively (analogous to conduction of current along a low-resistance wire) and actively (with a self-regenerating wave of action potentials that is triggered within the myocardium). Both passive and active propagation are important electrical properties of the myocardium.

Cable Theory of Passive Stimulus Propagation

A cardiac myocyte can be thought of as a one-dimensional cable (Fig. 1–2).[7] The membrane can be conceptualized as a

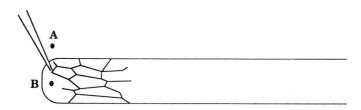

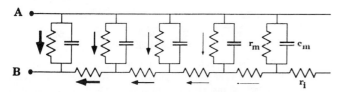

Figure 1–2. Equivalent circuit for a single fiber composed of electrically coupled single cells placed in an electrically conductive medium. A constant current is made to flow from A to B through the surface membrane and along the fiber core. Small voltage changes are produced to ensure constant values of the resistors. (From Weidmann S: Passive properties of cardiac fibers. *In* Rosen MR, Jause MJ, Wit AL [eds]: Cardiac Electrophysiology: A Textbook. Mt. Kisco, NY, Futura, 1990, pp 29–35.)

simplified circuit composed of a capacitor (with the ability to store charge) and a resistor (opposing the flow of current) in parallel. When a constant-current stimulus is applied at a site along the membrane, most of the charge initially flows into the capacitor. Eventually, the charge on the capacitor reaches a steady level. As current continues to be applied, it flows through the resistors across the membrane (R_m) and through the inside of the cell (R_i). In a simple resistance-capacitance circuit, two constants determine passive conduction, the *time constant* and the *length constant*. In this model of passive electrotonic membrane conductance, the capacitor is charged along an exponential time course, with 64% of the final charge being reached after time constant (T), assuming that there is no current flowing in the opposite direction. The change in voltage (V) across the membrane as a function of distance (X) will be as follows:

(5) $\quad V_x = V_{x=0}\,(e^{-x/a})$,

where a is the length constant of the fiber, the distance over which voltage drops by a factor of e, or about 37% of its original value at the site of stimulation. If r_m is the membrane resistance times unit length (Ω-cm) and r_i is the longitudinal resistance per unit length (Ω/cm), the length constant (a) becomes defined by the following equation:

(6) $\quad a = \sqrt{\dfrac{r_m}{r_i}}$

In a cable, total membrane charge still changes exponentially, but the region near the site of the applied stimulus (X=0) changes more quickly, and the region beyond this site (X=a), more slowly. The specific membrane capacity (C_m) is as follows:

(7) $\quad C_m(F/cm^2) = T\,(sec)/R_m\,(\Omega\text{-}cm^2)$,

where R_m is the specific membrane resistance. A single Purkinje fiber typically has an internal resistance that is two to three times greater than that of blood. The specific membrane resistance of a Purkinje fiber is on the order of 10^4 Ω-cm². The time constant of the surface membrane is on the order of 10 msec and the membrane capacity is about 1 μF/cm².[8]

When a current is made to flow through a row of several different cells, specialized regions of the membrane, called *gap junctions* or *intercalated disks*, provide low-resistance communication between cells. A junctional area of 1 cm² has a resistance of about 0.1 Ω.[9, 10] Thus, in *normal* myocardium, these cell-to-cell contacts offer negligible resistance, the major part of the resistance being in the cellular cytoplasm. Under pathologic conditions such as hypoxia or ischemia, however, the gap junctions become a major hindrance to axial current flow, preventing leakage of current to injured cells.[11, 12] Conduction velocity in the longitudinal axis of fiber orientation is much more rapid (three to five times) than in the transverse axis. Expression of gap junction proteins, such as connexon 43, may change with several factors, including the presence of cardiac arrhythmias. For example, the distribution of connexon 43 becomes disorganized within atrial myocardium with the occurrence of atrial fibrillation, thereby changing the characteristics of cell-to-cell propagation.

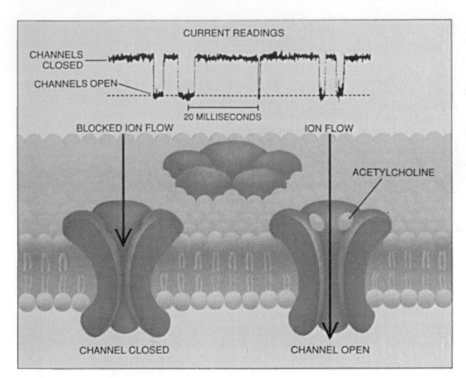

Figure 1–3. Receptor channels found at the neuromuscular end plate open in response to the transmitter acetylcholine. When no acetylcholine is present, effectively no current passes through a channel. When acetycholine binds to the receptor, an elementary current of a few picoamperes flows. The measured durations of the current and the intervals between them vary because the interaction of acetylcholine molecules with the receptors is governed by probability. (Illustrations by Dana Burns-Pizer from The patch clamp technique by E Neher and B Sakmann, March 1992. Copyright © 1992 by Scientific American, Inc. All rights reserved.)

■ ACTIVE ELECTRICAL PROPAGATION IN THE HEART

Ion Channels

The membrane proteins have numerous functions, including those of ion channels and signal transducers. The concept of ion channels was proposed in the 1950s by Hodgkin and Huxley.[1] It was not until the introduction of the patch clamp technique by Neher and Sakmann in 1976, however, that the properties of these channels could be studied directly.[13, 14] Currently it is known that there are two basic types of ion channels, distinguished by the factors that control opening and closing of the channel. For example, ion channels at muscle fiber endplates are *chemically* gated by specific transmitters (Fig. 1–3). The opening of these channels is triggered by the binding of acetylcholine, whereas their closing is induced by its unbinding. In neuronal axons, conduction is mediated by faster, *voltage*-gated channels. These channels respond to differences in electrical potential across the membrane (between the inside and outside of the cell). Voltage-gated channels for sodium, potassium, and calcium appear to operate in similar ways, sharing many of the same structural features. In addition, each type of channel can be subdivided into several subtypes with different conductance or gating properties.

Voltage-gated channels open in response to an applied potential. The source of this voltage can be an action potential propagated from an adjacent cell, or the electric field of an artificial pacemaker. If depolarization of the membrane exceeds a threshold voltage, an action potential is triggered, resulting in a complex cascade of ionic currents flowing across the membrane into and out of the cell. As a result of this flow of charge across the membrane, the potential gradient across the membrane (Fig. 1–4) changes in a characteristic pattern of events that produce the cardiac action potential.

Selective membrane-bound proteins (ion channels) determine the passive transmembrane flux of an individual ion species. The transmembrane currents determine or influence cellular polarization at rest, action potential depolarization and repolarization, conduction, excitation–contraction cou-

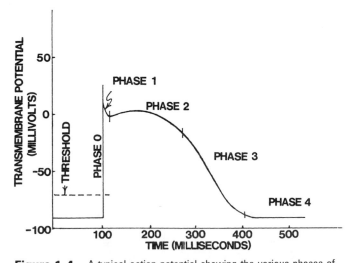

Figure 1–4. A typical action potential showing the various phases of depolarization and repolarization. In phase 0 (depolarization), Na^+ rapidly enters the cell through fast channels. In phase 1, the initial repolarization is primarily the result of activation of a transient outward K^+ current and inactivation of the fast Na^+ current. In phase 2 (plateau), the net current is very small, although the individual currents are about an order of magnitude larger. Phase 3 (final repolarization) completes the cycle with the Na^+-K^+ pump bringing the membrane potential to a stable point at which inward and outward currents are again in balance. (From Stokes K, Bornzin G: The electrode–biointerface [stimulation]. *In* Barold S [ed]: Modern Cardiac Pacing. Mt. Kisco, NY, Futura, 1985, pp 33–78.)

pling, and myofibril contraction. The channels that regulate transmembrane conductance of Na$^+$ and Ca^{2+} are voltage gated. The sodium channel is a large protein molecule composed of approximately 1830 amino acids.[15] It contains four internally homologous repeating domains. These are thought to be arranged around a central water-filled pore that is lined with hydrophilic amino acids. It is estimated that there are 5 to 10 Na$^+$ channels per square micron of cell membrane. When a change in the membrane potential to about -70 to -60 mV occurs (the threshold potential), four to six positively charged amino acids move across the membrane in response to a change in the electric field. This causes a change in the channel protein's conformation, resulting in opening of the channel. After a single Na$^+$ channel changes to the open conformation, about 10^4 Na$^+$ ions enter the cell. Upon depolarization of the membrane, the Na$^+$ channels remain open for less than 1 msec. After rapid depolarization of the membrane, the Na$^+$ channel again changes to the closed conformation. In addition to the Na$^+$ channel, specialized proteins are suspended in the cell membrane that have differential selectivity for K$^+$, Ca^{2+}, and Cl$^-$ ions with markedly different time constants for activation and inactivation.

In contrast to Purkinje fibers, sinus and atrioventricular (AV) node cells are characterized by action potentials with slower rates of depolarization. In these structures, depolarization is primarily mediated by inward Ca^{2+} conductance through specialized Ca^{2+} channels. There are two types of Ca^{2+} channel in the mammalian heart: the L and T types. The L-type channels are the major voltage-gated pathway for entry of Ca^{2+} into the myocyte, and they are heavily modulated by catecholamines.[16] The T-type channels contribute to spontaneous depolarization of the cell associated with automaticity (pacemaker currents). The pore of the Ca^{2+} channel has a functional diameter of about 0.6 nm, larger than sodium channels (0.3 to 0.5 nm).[17] The selectivity for Ca^{2+} is high, up to 10,000-fold greater than that for Na$^+$ or K$^+$. The key elements are high-affinity binding sites for Ca^{2+}, positioned along a single file pore. "Elution" of a Ca^{2+} ion occurs when another Ca^{2+} ion enters and is selectively bound.

The resting membrane potential and cellular polarization are maintained by pumping Na$^+$ ions out of the cell and K$^+$ ions into the cell. The Na$^+$-K$^+$ ATPase pump moves three Na$^+$ ions out of the cell in exchange for two K$^+$ ions moved into the cell.[18-20] The basic unit of the Na$^+$-K$^+$ ATPase protein (pump) consists of one α- and one β-subunit. The α-subunit is large, with 1016 amino acids, spanning the entire membrane, whereas the β-subunit is a smaller glycoprotein. There appear to be about 1000 pump sites per square micron of cardiac cell membrane. The fully activated pump cycles about 50 to 70 times per second (an interval of 15 to 20 msec/cycle). Similarly, the Na$^+$-Ca^{2+} pump moves three Na$^+$ ions out of the cell in exchange for one Ca^{2+} ion.[21, 22] Thus, both transport mechanisms result in the *net* movement of one positive charge out of the cell, polarizing the membrane with the maintenance of a negatively charged interior. The function of both exchange mechanisms is dependent on the expenditure of energy in the form of high-energy phosphates and is susceptible to interruptions in aerobic cellular metabolism (such as during ischemia).

The Cardiac Action Potential

When the voltage gradient across the membrane of a myocyte decreases such that the inside of the cell becomes less negatively charged with respect to the outside of the cell, a critical voltage is reached (termed the *threshold voltage*). At threshold the cell membrane suddenly undergoes a further depolarization that is out of proportion to the intensity of the applied stimulus. This abrupt change in the potential across the membrane is the start of a cascade of inward and outward currents that together are known as an *action potential*.[23] The cardiac action potential is an enormously complex event and consists of five phases[24]: phase 0, the upstroke phase of rapid depolarization; phase 1, the overshoot phase of initial rapid repolarization; phase 2, the plateau phase; phase 3, the rapid repolarization phase (see Fig. 1–4); phase 4, in which cells with spontaneous pacemaker activity are characterized by a slow, spontaneous depolarization of the membrane until the threshold potential is again reached and a new action potential is generated.

Phase 0—Rapid Depolarization

The upstroke of the action potential is triggered by a decrease in the potential gradient across the membrane to the threshold potential of -70 to -60 mV. Upon depolarization of the membrane to the less negative threshold voltage, the Na$^+$ channels open, resulting in an influx of positively charged ions (the inward Na$^+$ current) and rapid reversal of membrane polarity. The rate of depolarization in phase 0 ranges from 800 V/sec in Purkinje cells to 200 to 500 V/sec in atrial and ventricular myocytes. In these cells, the inward Na$^+$ current is primarily responsible for phase 0 of the action potential. In sinoatrial and atrioventricular nodal cells, where the inward Ca^{2+} current predominates, the upstroke velocity of phase 0 is much lower (20 to 50 V/sec).

Phase 1—Inital Repolarization

After voltage-dependent activation of the Na$^+$ current in phase 0, the membrane potential rapidly changes from negative to positive. The increased conductance of Na$^+$ is rapidly followed by voltage-dependent inactivation. Phase 1 is characterized by the transient outward K$^+$ current. The outward movement of K$^+$ is a major contributor to the various repolarization phases. It is complex and has a number of discrete pathways.[25, 26] Most K$^+$ currents demonstrate *rectification*, that is, decreased K$^+$ conductance with depolarization. The K$^+$ currents include the instantaneous inward rectifier K$^+$ current, the outward (delayed) rectifier K$^+$ current, the transient outward currents, and ATP-, Na$^+$-, and acetylcholine-regulated K$^+$ currents. The initial repolarization, however, is mainly the result of activation of a transient outward K$^+$ current and inactivation of the fast inward Na$^+$ current. The transient outward K$^+$ current has two components: one component is voltage gated and the other is activated by a local rise in Ca^{2+}.[27]

Phase 2—Plateau

The net current during the plateau phase is apparently small, although the individual currents are about an order of magnitude larger.[28] Among the inward currents are the slowly activating Na$^+$ current, a Ca^{2+} current, and an Na$^+$-Ca^{2+}

exchange current. Outward currents include a slowly activating K^+ current, a Cl^- current, a more rapidly activating K^+ current, and the Na^+-K^+ electrogenic pump. During phase 2 of the action potential, the cardiac cell cannot be excited by an electrical stimulus, regardless of its intensity (the *absolute refractory period*).

Phase 3—Final Repolarization

Deactivation of inward Na^+ and Ca^{2+} currents occurs earlier than the K^+ currents, favoring net repolarization of the membrane. When the membrane is sufficiently repolarized, an inward K^+ rectifier current is progressively activated, resulting in a regenerative increase in outward currents and an increasing rate of repolarization. Repolarization is also accomplished by the function of the Na^+-K^+ ATPase pump. The membrane potential eventually becomes stable, so that inward and outward currents are again in balance and the resting potential re-established. Between the end of the plateau phase and full repolarization, the cell is partially refractory to electrical stimulation. During this period (the *relative refractory period*), a greater stimulus intensity is required to generate an action potential than is required after full recovery of the resting membrane potential. For clinical measurement of myocardial refractoriness (the *effective refractory period*), stimulation of the heart is usually performed at twice the threshold current as determined during late diastole.

Phase 4—Automaticity and the Conduction System

Automaticity is the property of certain cells to initiate an action potential spontaneously. It has been known for centu-

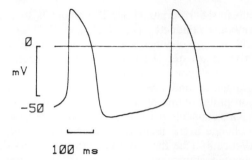

Figure 1–6. Spontaneous activity recorded in a single sinoatrial myocyte. The slow diastolic "pacemaker" depolarization extends from the maximum diastolic potential of −71 mV to the threshold for action potential onset, about −54 mV. (From DiFrancesco D: The hyperpolarization-activated current, I_f, and cardiac pacemaking. *In* Rosen MR, Jause ML, Wit AL [eds]: Cardiac Electrophysiology: A Textbook. Mt. Kisco, NY, Futura, 1990, pp 117–132.)

ries that the heart can exhibit spontaneous contraction even when completely denervated. Leonardo da Vinci observed that the heart could "move by itself."[29] William Harvey reported that pieces of the heart could "contract and relax" separately.[30] Many cells within the specialized conduction system have the potential for automaticity. Not all parts of the heart, however, possess this property. In fact, cells in different areas of the heart have different transmembrane potentials, thresholds, and action potentials. Fast responses are characteristic of ordinary working ventricular muscle cells and His-Purkinje fibers (resting membrane potential −70 to −90 mV with rapid conduction). Normal sinus and AV nodal cells have slow responses, with resting potentials of −40 to −70 mV and slow conduction velocities. Those cells, or group of cells, with the fastest rate of spontaneous membrane depolarization during phase 4 are the first to reach threshold potential and initiate a propagated impulse. Thus, cells with the steepest slope of phase 4 become the heart's natural pacemaker. Ordinary working myocardial cells are usually not automatic. Normally, depolarization is initiated at the sinoatrial node (Fig. 1–5).[31, 32] Action potentials from an isolated sinoatrial node cell are shown in Figure 1–6.[33] Rather than maintaining a stable resting membrane potential, the repolarization of the action potential is followed by a slow depolarization from about −71 to −54 mV, the threshold to initiate another action potential. This slow, spontaneous depolarization drives cardiac automaticity. In the case of atrioventricular nodal cells, the fast upstroke is carried predominantly by an inward Ca^{2+} current. Repolarization is caused by delayed activation of the K^+ current. The balance of inward and outward currents determines the net "pacemaker" current and is finely regulated by both adrenergic and cholinergic neurotransmitters. In the presence of AV block or abnormal sinoatrial nodal function, AV junctional cells in the region of the proximal penetrating bundle usually assume the role of pacemaker at rates slower than that of the sinus node. In the absence of disease in the AV junction, the escape rhythm occurs with a frequency that is about 67% of the sinus rate.[34]

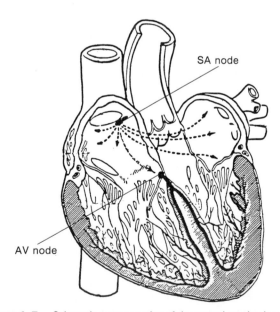

Figure 1–5. Schematic representation of the normal conduction system of the heart. The cycle begins at the sinoatrial (SA) node, propagating a wave of depolarization across the atrium. As the stimulus enters the atrioventricular node, its conduction slows. This allows complete contraction of the atria before the impulse reaches the ventricles. As the impulse enters the His bundle, conduction velocity increases. The impulse is then transmitted through the left and right bundle branches and the Purkinje fibers throughout the right and left ventricular endocardial shells.

■ ARTIFICIAL INDUCTION OF SELF-PROPAGATING MYOCARDIAL CURRENTS

Theories of Artificial Cardiac Stimulation

For an electrical stimulus to trigger a self-propagation wave of depolarization within the myocardium, an electric field of sufficient intensity must be applied between the two stimulating electrodes. There are two major theories about how an electrical stimulus induces a self-propagating wavefront of depolarization within myocardium. The *current density* theory maintains that the critical factor required to induce a regenerative wavefront of depolarization is the magnitude of current flowing through a given mass of myocardium between the stimulating electrodes. Thus, in this theory, the stimulation threshold is a function of current density (A/cm^3) in the excitable myocardium underlying the electrode.[35-38] The competing *electrical field* theory holds that the critical factor affecting myocardial depolarization is the magnitude of the electric field (V/cm^3 in viable tissue) that is induced in the myocardium beneath the stimulating electrode.[39, 40] Ideally, these theories are related by Ohm's law:

$$(8) \quad V = IR,$$

where V is the stimulus voltage, I is the current, and R is the total resistance to current flow. Thus, the greater the potential difference between two electrodes, the greater the current flow at the electrode–tissue interface. The total energy of a pacing stimulus is determined by the voltage and the current as well as the duration of the stimulus:

$$(9) \quad E = VIt,$$

where E is the stimulus energy and t is the pulse duration. For a constant voltage pulse generator, equation 9 can be expressed as follows:

$$(10) \quad E = \frac{V^2t}{R}$$

The stimulation threshold of isolated cardiac myocytes has been shown to depend on their orientation within an electric field. The threshold is lowest when the myocytes are oriented parallel to the field and highest when the axis of the myocytes is perpendicular to the field.[41] It is clear that myocardial stimulation may be induced with anodal or cathodal stimulation, or both, although with somewhat different characteristics. Perhaps because of the absence of a generally accepted theory of electrical stimulation, there is widespread confusion in the scientific literature regarding the measurement of stimulation threshold. Various investigators have used many different parameters to express stimulation threshold, including current (mA), potential (V), energy (μJ), charge (μC), pulse width (msec), and voltage quantity (V-sec).[42-48] For the purposes of this chapter, we define stimulation threshold as *the minimum stimulus amplitude at any given pulse width required to consistently achieve myocardial depolarization outside the heart's refractory period.*[36] Thus, stimulation thresholds measured with a constant-voltage (CV) generator are presented in volts and those of a constant-current generator (CI) are presented in milliamperes.

■ STRENGTH–DURATION RELATIONSHIPS

Chronaxie, Rheobase, Energy, and Pulse Duration Thresholds

The intensity of an electrical stimulus (measured in volts or milliamperes) that is required to capture the atrial or ventricular myocardium is dependent on the time that the stimulus is applied, the pulse duration.[49, 50] This interaction of stimulus amplitude and pulse duration defines the strength–duration curve (Fig. 1–7). The voltage or current amplitude required for endocardial stimulation has an exponential relation to the pulse duration, with a relatively flat curve at pulse durations of greater than 1 msec and a rapidly rising curve at pulse durations of less than 0.25 msec. Because of this fundamental property, a stimulus of short pulse duration must be of much greater intensity to capture the myocardium than a longer-duration pulse. Conversely, increasing the pulse width beyond 1 msec (along the flat portion of the curve) has little influence on the intensity of the stimulus that is required for capture. Thus, it is not acceptable to express the stimulation threshold in terms of pulse amplitude without also defining the pulse duration that was used. The shape of the strength–duration curve is influenced by several factors, including the site of electrical stimulation (transesophageal or endocardial), the type of stimulus that is used (constant-current or constant-voltage), and the stimulation frequency.

Hoorweg, in 1892, used a voltage source, galvanometer, and low-leakage capacitors to conduct quantitative stimulation studies.[51] He found that the voltage at which a capacitor must be charged to cause a depolarization of nerves and muscles was an inverse function of capacitance, as follows:

$$(11) \quad V(C) = aR + b/C,$$

where V(C) is the voltage (V) as a function of capacitance (C), R is resistance, and a and b are coefficients that vary with the specimen (tissue) tested. Hoorweg determined that there was only one specific capacitor for which energy at stimulation threshold was a minimum. He also determined that the threshold charge was a linear function, "intersecting the y-axis above zero." It should be pointed out that Hoorweg apparently did not have the capability to measure thresholds at very short pulse durations because in reality the threshold charge increases toward infinity as the pulse duration approaches zero. In 1901, Weiss reported a linear relationship between threshold charge and the duration of current flow.[52] He called this relationship the "formule fondamentale," expressed as follows:

$$(12) \quad Q(t) = \int^t I_t dt = at + b,$$

where Q(t) is the charge (Q) as a function of pulse duration (t), I$_t$ is the current during pulse duration t, and a and b are coefficients depending on the specimen (type of tissue). Weiss also noted that the threshold energy varies as a function of the shape of the stimulus pulse, whereas the quantity of electricity (charge) at threshold remains constant. In 1909, Lapique pointed out that at infinitely long pulse widths, there is a "fundamental threshold."[53] He called this the *rheobase*. Thus, rheobase is defined as *the lowest stimulus current or voltage that results in capture of the heart at an infinitely long pulse duration.* Lapique also noted that the ratio a/b in the Weiss equation is a time constant that characterizes the tissue (i.e., the time constant of the cell membrane). He called this time constant *chronaxie*. He then redefined the Weiss equation as follows:

$$(13) \quad I_t = a + \frac{b}{t} = I_{rheobase}\left(1 + \frac{t_{chronaxie}}{t}\right),$$

where I_t is the current (I) during the pulse duration (t), $I_{rheobase}$ is the rheobase current (the lowest possible current threshold with t equal to infinity), and $t_{chronaxie}$ is the chronaxie time. Chronaxie is defined as *the threshold pulse duration at twice rheobase amplitude*, as shown in Figure 1–7. Lapique also determined that stimulation at the chronaxie pulse width approaches the minimum threshold energy.[54] Although Nernst proposed the concept that the energy for stimulation is a constant, this is not correct[55] as shown in Figure 1–7.

Lapique's modification of the Weiss equation can be further modified in terms of charge (Q), as follows[56]:

$$(14) \quad Q = I_{rheobase}t + (I_{rheobase} \times t_{chronaxie}).$$

At very short pulse widths, equation 14 approaches the limit of chronaxie multiplied by rheobase. The lower this product, the lower the charge necessary to stimulate the heart. Thus, the two most important reference points on a current or voltage strength–duration curve are rheobase and chronaxie. Although true rheobase typically requires pulse widths of 10 msec or greater, an *apparent* rheobase is usually measured at pulse widths of 1.5 to 2 msec. This means that the chronaxie obtained by finding the pulse width at twice the *apparent* rheobase is slightly low, representing an *apparent* chronaxie value. Nonetheless, these apparent values are clinically useful because most constant voltage instrumenta-

tion does not allow measurements at pulse widths of more than 1.5 to 2 msec. From Figure 1–7, it is evident that the lowest possible pulse width is desirable to minimize charge drain (because the pulse generator's battery has a finite number of charges). Too low a pulse duration, however, puts thresholds close to the steeply ascending limb of the voltage or current curve, where slight fluctuations could risk loss of capture. Irnich recommended that chronaxie, or the pulse duration slightly to the left of chronaxie, is the most efficient for both pacing and defibrillation.[57, 58] In most cases, chronaxie appears to represent the best overall compromise between adequate safety and generator longevity. Irnich found that chronaxie varies as a function of stimulation mode, generator impedance, electrode size, shape, and material, and time since implantation.

To insist that thresholds can be measured in microjoules or milliseconds is to deny the fact that rheobase is a critical part of the strength–duration relationship. Regardless of the pulse duration or energy used, one cannot stimulate the heart unless the stimulus *amplitude* (either voltage or current) exceeds rheobase.[59] For example, if rheobase is achieved with a pulse amplitude of 0.5 V and 10 msec, the pulse at this point on the strength–duration curve will have 5 μJ of energy with a 500-Ω lead. A 0.4-V, 20-msec pulse on a 500-Ω lead has 6.4 μJ energy (28% greater than the "threshold" energy at 10 msec), but cardiac capture will not be achieved. A 100-msec pulse at 0.4 V has 32 μJ energy (540% greater than "threshold" energy at 10 msec) but still will not capture the heart for the same reason. No matter how far the pulse duration is extended (with increased energy), the myocardium will not be captured unless the stimulus amplitude is at least the rheobase value. Thus, there is probably no such thing as an energy threshold, per se, although one can calculate the energy of the pulse at threshold.[48]

Practical Application of the Strength–Duration Relationship to Threshold Measurement

The strength–duration relationship requires the clinician to measure the stimulation threshold at a specific amplitude and pulse duration. Clinically, the threshold can be measured by either (1) decreasing the amplitude of the constant-voltage stimulus at a constant-pulse duration until loss of capture (voltage threshold), or (2) decreasing the pulse width at a constant-voltage (pulse width threshold). The stimulation threshold is defined clinically as the lowest amplitude (voltage or current) or pulse duration that results in consistent capture of the myocardium, depending on whether the voltage or pulse width is decremented. It is important to keep in mind that the pulse width threshold is actually the pulse duration on the strength–duration curve where the programmed stimulus amplitude is at threshold. If, however, the pulse voltage or current is less than rheobase, myocardial capture will not occur, regardless of the pulse width. Thus, the term *pulse duration threshold* is a misnomer for voltage or current threshold at a particular pulse duration.

Examination of the strength–duration curve suggests that one must be careful to consider its shape when programming an implantable pacemaker. For example, if the pulse duration threshold is 0.5 msec at an amplitude of 2 V, programming the pacemaker to a pulse duration of 1 or even 1.5 msec

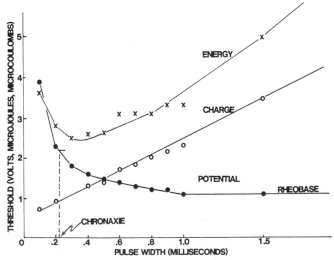

Figure 1–7. Relationships between chronic ventricular canine constant voltage strength–duration curves expressed in terms of potential (V), charge (μC), and energy (μJ) for a tined unipolar lead with an 8-mm² polished ring-tip electrode. Thresholds are measured at gain of capture. Rheobase is the current or voltage threshold to the right that is independent of pulse width. Chronaxie is the pulse width at twice the rheobase. (From Stokes K, Bornzin G: The electrode–biointerface [stimulation]. *In* Barold S [ed]: Modern Cardiac Pacing. Mt. Kisco, NY, Futura, 1985, pp 33–78.)

provides a very small margin of safety (Fig. 1–8). Instead, doubling the stimulus amplitude to 4 V at a pulse duration of 0.5 msec would provide an adequate margin of safety. In contrast to this example, consider the same patient in whom the pulse duration threshold was 0.15 msec at a pulse amplitude of 3.5 V. In this patient, increasing the pulse width to 0.45 msec would also provide an adequate safety margin. The reason that a three-fold increase in pulse width is not adequate in the first example but is acceptable in the second relates to its location on the strength–duration curve. As a general rule, programming the pulse generator to twice the voltage threshold near the chronaxie pulse duration usually provides an efficient output pulse with an adequate safety margin.

Capture Hysteresis (Wedensky Effect)

The threshold stimulus amplitude that is measured by decreasing the voltage or current until loss of capture occurs has been noted by several authors to be less than that determined by increasing the stimulus intensity from a subthreshold amplitude until capture is achieved. This apparent hysteresis in threshold determined by incrementing and decrementing the stimulus amplitude has been termed the *Wedensky effect*.[60] Although the mechanism for this observation

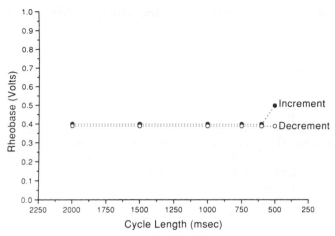

Figure 1–9. Pacing thresholds determined by gradually incrementing and decrementing the pulse amplitude until gain and loss of capture, respectively, are demonstrated in a patient with complete atrioventricular block. The pacing threshold was determined at cycle lengths of 2000, 1500, 1000, 750, and 500 msec and a constant-pulse duration of 2.0 msec. To prevent variation in the cycle length during incrementing and decrementing pulse amplitudes, a backup pulse was delivered at 25 msec. Note that the threshold values determined in this manner are similar with increments and decrements of the stimulus amplitude. Thus, the Wedensky effect may be marginal when the pacing cycle length is maintained at a constant value.

was not clear until recently, this concept has enjoyed widespread acceptance. Langberg and colleagues used programmed stimulation with precisely timed stimuli to examine this phenomenon and noted no demonstrable capture hysteresis at pacing cycle lengths of greater than 400 msec.[61] These authors concluded that the Wedensky effect was related to asynchronous pacing in the relative refractory period when incrementing the stimulus intensity, as compared with synchronous late diastolic stimulation during decrementation of the stimulus amplitude until loss of capture. We have confirmed these observations using constant-voltage pacing in which asynchronous pacing was prevented while increasing the stimulus intensity until capture was achieved (Fig. 1–9).

Effect of Pacing Rate on Stimulation Threshold

Hook and coworkers reported a significant increase in ventricular pacing threshold in 10 of 16 patients at 400 msec and in 15 of 16 at 300 msec (relative to a pacing cycle length of 600 msec).[62] The phenomenon was not observed at every trial (e.g., 12 of 72 trials at 400 msec). The patients were all candidates for implantable defibrillators, and many (9 of 12) were receiving antiarrhythmic drugs. The leads were bipolar (a pair of epicardial corkscrews in 11 patients, an endocardial screw-in lead in 5 patients).

The atrial stimulation threshold has also been shown to vary as a function of pacing rate.[63, 64] Katsumoto and associates reported that 29 of 36 patients exhibited atrial constant-current (CI) current and energy threshold variations as a function of pacing rate in the 60- to 120-bpm range using activated vitreous carbon electrodes.[65] Kay and colleagues

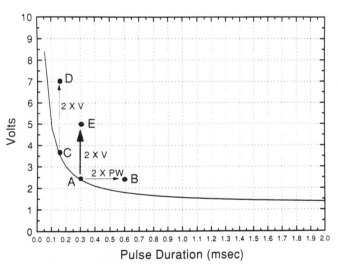

Figure 1–8. Programming of the pulse amplitude and pulse duration based on analysis of the strength–duration curve in a patient evaluated at the time of pulse generator replacement (6 years after lead implantation). The rheobase voltage was 1.4 V with a chronaxie pulse duration of 0.30 msec. Note that the stimulation threshold, determined by decreasing the stimulus amplitude at a constant pulse duration of 0.5 msec, was about 2 V (point A). Doubling of the pulse duration on the relatively flat portion of the strength–duration curve (point B) provides little safety margin of ventricular capture. In contrast, consider a threshold value on the steeply ascending portion of the strength–duration curve (point C). Doubling the pulse amplitude doubles the safety margin on this portion of the curve, but it lies very close to the curve (point D). An appropriate setting for the chronic pacing pulse might be achieved by doubling the pulse amplitude from point A to point E. Also note that a similar programmed setting would have been obtained had the pulse duration been tripled from point C. Thus, the shape of the strength–duration curve has an important influence on the choice of the amplitude and duration of the pacing pulse.

also found significant human atrial threshold changes as a function of pacing rate (between 125 and 300 bpm) using constant voltage stimulation.[66] They found a significant increase in rheobase voltage, chronaxie, and minimum threshold energy at pacing rates of more than 225 bpm using platinized (low polarizing) unipolar electrodes. They also determined strength–interval curves and found no correlation between atrial effective refractory period and rheobase voltage, chronaxie, or rate-dependent changes in either of these values. They concluded that the phenomenon is probably related to the "opposing effects of decreasing cycle length on the action potential duration and the slope of the strength–interval curve. Thus, if the pacing interval shortens to a greater extent than the refractory period and pacing stimuli are delivered during the ascending limb of the strength–interval curve (the relative refractory period), the diastolic threshold will increase."

The increase in stimulation threshold with increasing stimulation rate probably has minimal implications for bradycardia pacing. It is important for antitachycardia pacing, however, because threshold must be measured at rates required to interrupt the arrhythmia. In addition, the safety factors used with antitachycardia pacemakers must be based on thresholds measured at the clinically appropriate rates rather than during pacing at resting rates.

Stability of Strength–Duration Curves and the Distorting Effect of Polarization

None of the relationships published in the last 100 years has exactly duplicated the capacitively coupled, constant-voltage strength–duration curves that have been measured empirically with various types of electrodes. This may, in part, be due to the confounding effect of polarization, which varies significantly with electrode size, shape, surface finish, material, and so forth. Another problem, however, is that the voltage and current strength–duration relationships, typically plotted on linear coordinates, are really logarithmic (Fig. 1–10).[67] When plotted in this manner, the strength–duration curve for CI stimuli is now seen as a straight line up to rheobase (because polarization is not "seen" with CI pacing). The CV strength–duration curve for a highly polarizing polished platinum electrode is a straight line at pulse widths less than 0.5 msec (Fig. 1–11). At these pulse durations, the curve is not significantly distorted by polarization. The CV strength–duration curve for a modern low polarizing electrode approaches a straight line within the pulse durations of clinical significance ($\leq$1 msec). These data and Figures 1–7 and 1–12 help to demonstrate the distorting effects of polarization on strength–duration curves (and both rheobase and chronaxie). Within the linear portion, all these logarithmic curves have about the same slope (m):

$$(15) \quad I(CI) = Bt^m,$$

or

$$(16) \quad V(CV) = At^m,$$

where B is a (CI) constant and A is a (CV) constant that determines the location of the curve (on the y-axis). If we include the effects of electrode polarization, it is apparent that the strength–duration curve for CV pacing at pulse durations less than rheobase must be as follows:

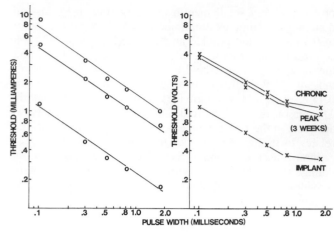

Figure 1–10. Logarithmic plots of canine ventricular constant current *(left)* and constant voltage *(right)* strength–duration curves for a passively fixed, atraumatic, unipolar lead with an 8-mm² polished platinum ring-tip at various implant times. (From Stokes K, Bornzin G: The electrode–biointerface (stimulation). *In* Barold S [ed]: Modern Cardiac Pacing. Mt. Kisco, NY, Futura 1985, pp 33–78.)

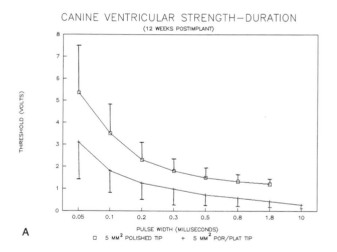

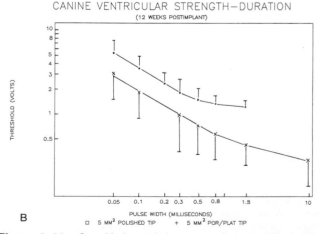

Figure 1–11. Capacitively coupled constant-voltage strength–duration curves on linear *(A)* and logarithmic *(B)* coordinates for 5-mm² polished *(top line)* and porous platinized *(lower line)* platinum electrodes.

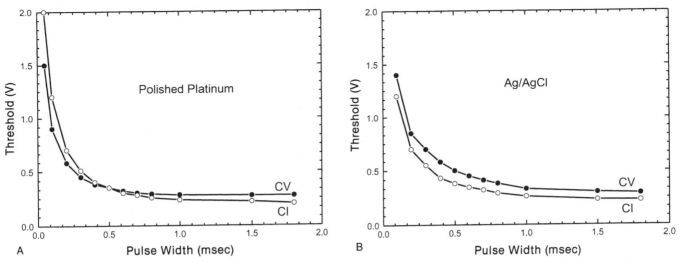

Figure 1–12. Constant-current compared with constant-voltage canine ventricular strength–duration curves for passively fixed, atraumatic electrodes. *A,* Polarizing, 8-mm² polished ring-tip electrode. *B,* Non-polarizing, Ag/Ag⁺,Cl⁻ 8-mm² electrode.

(17) $V = At^m + V_{pol}(t)$,

where $V_{pol}(t)$ is the voltage due to polarization (V_{pol}) as a function of pulse width (t).

The slope of the strength–duration curves for passively fixed, atraumatic leads does not change with time after implantation (see Fig. 1–10). The acute, peak, and chronic mean thresholds of five ventricular and three atrial passively fixed, atraumatic leads in 77 canines had a (log_{10}) slope of about -0.60 ± 0.07 V/msec.[67] The correlation coefficient for these relationships is typically more than 0.99 at pulse durations of less than 0.5 msec for polished electrodes and of less than 1.0 msec for low polarizing designs. Traumatic electrodes (such as those with active fixation) in our canine experience typically have a lower slope immediately after implantation, but this shifts to about the same -0.60 V/msec value within days as the acute trauma to the electrode–tissue interface heals.

Because strength–duration curves are typically plotted on linear rather than logarithmic coordinates, changes in voltage and current threshold after implantation are usually seen as a shift upward and to the right. In most cases, chronaxie, being related to the slope of the curve (the tissue's time constant), does not change significantly with time. Cornacchia and colleagues, however, have shown that administration of propafenone shifts the strength–duration curve *and* chronaxie to the right.[68] Thus, measurement of the strength–duration relationship may be required after the administration of antiarrhythmic drugs.

Some older pulse generator designs have attempted to compensate for the gradual decline in stimulus voltage that occurs as a consequence of battery depletion by automatic "stretching" of the pulse duration to maintain the stimulus energy at a nearly constant value. Although this feature is designed to prevent loss of capture, increasing the pulse duration from a programmed value of 0.5 msec adds relatively little to the pacing safety margin because this approaches an essentially flat portion of the strength–duration curve. In fact, this automatic increase in pulse duration actually accelerates battery depletion. As a result, many newer pulse generators have abandoned this approach to battery depletion in favor of automatic regulation of stimulus voltage to ensure constant stimulus amplitude despite declining battery voltage.

■ STRENGTH–INTERVAL RELATIONSHIPS

In addition to the strength–duration relationship previously discussed, voltage and current stimulation thresholds also vary as a function of the coupling interval of the stimulus to prior beats and to the stimulation frequency used for the basic drive train. A typical constant-current ventricular strength–interval curve is shown in Figure 1–13. At relatively long extrastimulus coupling intervals (>270 msec), the intensity of the extrastimulus that is required for ventricular capture is relatively constant, approaching the rheobase value. At shorter extrastimulus coupling intervals (<250 msec), however, the intensity of the extrastimulus must be increased for it to elicit myocardial capture.

The exponential rise in amplitude required for capture at short coupling intervals is the result of encroachment into the refractory period of the myocardium. During the *relative* refractory period (corresponding to the repolarization phase of the action potential), the myocardium can be induced to generate a new action potential if the stimulus has sufficient intensity. During the *absolute* refractory period (corresponding to the plateau phase of the action potential), no depolarization can be effected, regardless of the stimulus intensity. The strength–interval curve of atrial and ventricular myocardium is shifted to the left at shorter basic drive cycle lengths. Therefore, the *effective* refractory period, which is generally measured at a pulse duration of 2 msec and an amplitude that is twice late diastolic threshold, decreases as a function of the pacing cycle length. At relatively slow pacing rates (less than 200 bpm), there is relatively little interaction of the strength–duration and strength–interval curves. As discussed previously, however, at rapid pacing rates (>225 bpm), pacing stimuli during the basic drive may encounter the relative refractory period. If the stimulus amplitude becomes subthreshold, 2:1 capture of the myocardium results.

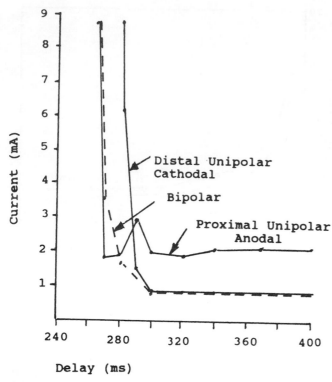

Figure 1–13. Strength–interval curves. Unipolar distal cathodal, unipolar proximal anodal, and bipolar strength–interval curves during an acute study in a patient with a temporary bipolar lead (equal-sized cathode and anode). The bipolar and unipolar anodal refractory periods are equal and shorter than unipolar cathodal. (From Mehra R, Furman S: Comparison of cathodal, anodal, and bipolar strength–interval curves with temporary and permanent pacing electrodes. Br Heart J 41:468, 1979.)

■ CONSTANT-CURRENT VERSUS CONSTANT-VOLTAGE STIMULATION

A CI generator delivers a (current) pulse that is usually a square wave. That is, the leading edge of the pulse (I_{le}) equals the trailing edge (I_{te}). The current delivered by a CI pulse generator is independent of pacing impedance to the limits of the power source (Fig. 1–14). If impedance decreases, the resultant voltage automatically decreases to keep current constant. In the presence of a high-resistance circuit, such as with a partial lead fracture, the limits of the power source are reached, and the battery is said to be saturated. In this instance, the battery cannot generate enough voltage to maintain a preset level of current, resulting in delivery of a lower current than is programmed. Although under normal operating conditions the current waveform is rectangular, the resultant voltage waveform is not. It starts out with an initial leading edge voltage (V_{le}) but increases as a function of pulse duration to a larger trailing edge voltage (V_{te}; Fig. 1–15). At the end of the pulse, an immediate drop in voltage equal to V_{le} is observed, followed by an exponential decay back to baseline. The voltage rise during the pulse (called the *overvoltage*) is caused by an increase in pacing impedance due to electrode polarization, and the afterpotential is caused by the gradual dissipation of that polarization.

Today, all implantable pulse generators are capacitively coupled, approximately CV devices. At the beginning of the

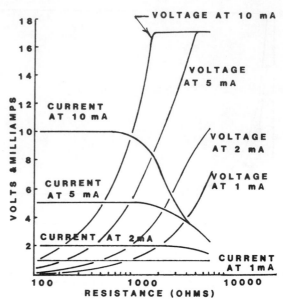

Figure 1–14. The effects of pacing impedance on constant-current leading edge waveform amplitudes using a Medtronic model 5880A external pulse generator. Current is independent of impedance until the battery is "saturated." This occurs when the voltage cannot increase any more to keep current constant. (From Barold SS, Winner JA: Techniques and significance of threshold measurement for cardiac pacing. Chest 70:760, 1976.)

pulse, the fully charged capacitor delivers a leading edge voltage that is constant regardless of impedance, as long as the impedance is high enough (Fig. 1–16). The voltage drops during the pulse to the trailing edge value. This change in voltage over the pulse duration ("droop") is directly proportional to the total charge delivered (Q^*, measured in coulombs) and is inversely proportional to the capacitance of the pulse generator (C_{pg}, measured in farads), or approximately as follows:

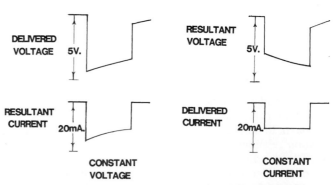

Figure 1–15. Voltage and current waveforms from a capacitively coupled constant-voltage implantable pulse generator (Medtronic model 7000A, *left*) and the constant-current mode output of an external research stimulator (Medtronic model 1356, *right*). A unipolar lead with a polished platinum, 8-mm² ring-tip is used in conjunction with a 900-mm² titanium anode in 0.18% NaCl solution. The voltage across the lead is measured against a 100-mm² Ag/AgCl electrode to eliminate the anode's polarization from the waveform. (From Stokes K, Bornzin G: The electrode–biointerface (stimulation). In Barold S [ed]: Modern Cardiac Pacing. Mt. Kisco, NY, Futura 1985, pp 33–78.)

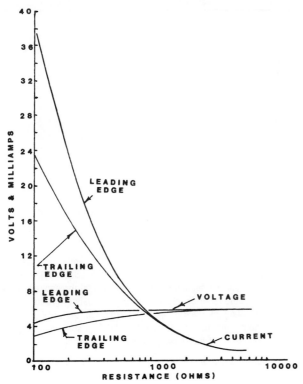

Figure 1–16. The effect of pacing impedance on capacitively coupled constant-voltage leading and trailing edge waveform amplitudes using a Medtronic model 5950 pulse generator. The leading edge voltage remains constant as a function of pacing impedance$\geq$200 Ω. The trailing edge of the voltage waveform, however, changes slightly with impedance up to about 1000 Ω. Current falls significantly with increasing impedance. Any constant-voltage source may no longer be constant at very low pacing impedances because the battery becomes unable to supply enough current to maintain a steady voltage. These very low impedance values are not likely to be encountered clinically on a properly functioning pacing system. (From Barold SS, Winner JA: Techniques and significance of threshold measurements for cardiac pacing. Chest 70:760, 1976.)

(18) $V_{le} - V_{te} = Q^*/C_{pg}$.

Charge is also a function of impedance or resistance, as follows:

(19) $Q = It = \dfrac{Vt}{R}$

(in a simple resistive circuit), or Vt/Z_p (in a complex nonlinear circuit, such as a pacemaker, where Z_p is the total pacing impedance). Therefore, the CV droop is also a function of pacing impedance (Z_p) as follows:

(20) $V_{le} - V_{te} = \dfrac{V^*t}{Z_pC_{pg}}$,

where V^* is the total voltage applied (the area under the waveform bounded by (V_{le} and V_{te}). With a very high impedance lead, therefore, the voltage pulse is almost rectangular ($V_{le} = V_{te}$). With low pacing impedance, the droop is steeper because more current is drained from the output capacitor. Thus, the current begins with a high initial value in a CV generator but decreases to the trailing edge, as a function of the pulse duration. With very low impedance values

($<$200 Ω), the battery may not be able to supply enough current to maintain a constant voltage. Leads for CV generators, therefore, are designed to have as high an impedance as is efficiently practical to minimize current drain.

Constant current (CI) thresholds are related to constant voltage (CV) thresholds by impedance. However, impedance is not linear with pulse duration but increases with polarization. Therefore, CI strength–duration curves can have slightly different shapes than CV curves. Irnich, for example, pointed out that (with polished electrodes) typical CI chronaxie values are almost twice those found with CV stimulation (see Fig. 1–8).[47] Most modern endocardial leads have relatively low polarizing electrodes (such as those with iridium oxide, fractal, platinized platinum, or "activated" carbon surfaces). These tend to have lower-voltage rheobase and somewhat higher chronaxie than highly polarizing electrodes (see Figs. 1–10 and 1–12).[69] In fact, a nonpolarizing electrode made from Ag/Ag$^+$,Cl$^-$ has the same shape strength–duration curve for CV and CI stimulation (see Fig. 1–12). Therefore, polarization affects the value of CV chronaxie. This accounts for most of the differences between the shapes of CV and CI strength–duration curves.

■ MONOPHASIC AND BIPHASIC WAVEFORMS

If we omit the postpulse recharge, most pacing stimuli are monophasic. Abrupt reversal of polarity during the stimulus (biphasic waveform), however, has been demonstrated to decrease the voltage threshold required for atrial and ventricular defibrillation.[70] Knisely and colleagues studied the effect of biphasic and triphasic stimuli on excitation threshold in rabbit and frog ventricles (Fig. 1–17).[71] At very long pulse

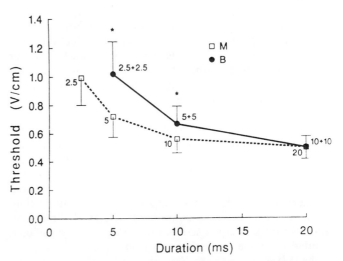

Figure 1–17. Monophasic (M) and biphasic (B) strength–duration curves obtained in strips of frog ventricular myocardium superfused with a solution containing 3 mmol/L of potassium. At a pulse duration of 20 msec, there is no significant difference in the rheobase threshold. Note that the monophasic waveform produces a lower threshold than the biphasic waveform at pulse durations of 5 msec and less. Thus, although the monophasic and biphasic waveforms have a similar rheobase, chronaxie is less with monophasic than with biphasic stimuli. ms, millisecond. (From Knisely SB, Smith WM, Ideker RE: Effect of intrastimulus polarity reversal on electric field stimulation thresholds in frog and rabbit myocardium. J Cardiovasc Electrophysiol 3:239, 1992.)

durations (20 msec), there was no difference in the stimulation threshold for monophasic and biphasic stimulus waveforms. Thus, reversal of waveform polarity during the stimulus did not affect rheobase voltage. At shorter pulse durations (2.5 msec), however, the threshold voltage was significantly greater for biphasic than for monophasic waveforms. Thus, the chronaxie pulse duration was significantly increased by an intrastimulus polarity reversal. Although biphasic stimuli decrease the voltage required for defibrillation, the excitability threshold for bradycardia pacing at clinically relevant pulse durations appears to be increased using biphasic pulses. Thus, bradycardia pacing stimuli are monophasic. This must not be confused with prestimulus or poststimulus "conditioning" or "fast-recharge" pulses, which are designed not to interfere with the pacing stimulus per se.

Another method that has been proposed to lower the stimulation threshold involves the use of overlapping biphasic waveforms.[72] This configuration uses unipolar anodal and cathodal pulses delivered to two closely spaced electrodes such that the pulses of opposite polarity overlap with a high-voltage gradient between the electrodes. This method has been suggested as a means to reduce the stimulation threshold of noncontact electrodes within the right atrium. However, threshold is said to be achieved at only 1 pulse. That is, if capture occurs with 2V positive and 2V negative pulses, threshold is said to be 2V, not 4V. Current drain is also high because of the use of 2 stimuli.

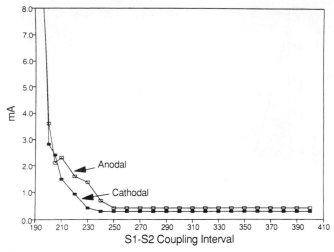

Figure 1–18. Anodal and cathodal ventricular strength–interval curves are demonstrated in a patient with atrioventricular block with unipolar constant-current stimuli. Note that the anodal threshold is slightly higher than the cathodal threshold at coupling intervals of greater than 250 msec. At coupling intervals of less than 210 msec, the anodal threshold is about equal to the cathodal threshold. In some patients, the anodal threshold may not decrease ("dip") to a value that is less than the cathodal threshold.

■ ANODAL AND CATHODAL STIMULATION

Generally speaking, anodal stimulation is associated with properties that are less desirable than cathodal stimulation. If the stimulating electrode is a unipolar cathode, the strength–interval curve has a shape that is similar to a strength–duration curve. The shape of the typical anodal strength–interval curve is somewhat different from that of a cathodal curve (Fig. 1–18). Given equal-sized electrodes, the anodal stimulation threshold is generally somewhat greater than that for cathodal stimulation at long coupling intervals. With progressively more premature coupling intervals, there is a dip in the anodal curve to threshold values less than those of the cathodal curve. At still more premature coupling intervals, the anodal curve rises steeply (as observed with cathodal stimulation).[73] The "dip" phenomenon is not always seen.[74] If the electrodes of a bipolar lead are of equal size, or if the anode is smaller than the cathode, it is possible to stimulate earlier in the cardiac cycle (in the relative refractory period) than with unipolar cathodal stimulation. This may occur because the threshold for anodal stimulation with electrodes of equal size is lower than that for cathodal stimulation in the strength–interval curve at shorter pulse widths.[73, 74]

That anodal stimulation can generate tachyarrhythmias in ischemic or electrolyte unbalanced hearts is well documented.[75–78] This is one of several reasons that implantable bipolar leads are designed with considerably larger anodes than cathodes. In fact, it is commonly thought that the bipolar anode needs to be large enough so that anodal stimulation is prevented. It is unlikely that this actually prevents anodal stimulation, however, because most pulse generators are set at outputs much higher than threshold such as 5 V and 0.5 msec with a 0.5 V, 0.5 msec cathodal stimulation threshold. Even a 50 mm² anode probably reaches threshold at a stimulus intensity well below 5 V and 0.5 msec. It is likely that delivery of the stimulation pulse with many bipolar leads actually results in capture of the myocardium at both the cathode and the anode. Thus, there is probably more to the size relationship between cathode and anode than is known. Many newer bipolar leads have smaller anodes because the cathodes are smaller. The anode:cathode ratio should be maintained and, of course, the designs should be supported with strength–interval tests. Bipolar pacing with equal-sized electrodes is common in temporary pacing and implanted epicardial systems (in which two unipolar leads are often used for bipolar pacing). The clinician must keep in mind the arrhythmogenic possibilities of such combinations.

Another reason that anodes should be relatively large is to preclude unacceptable corrosion rates. Platinum, for example, does not corrode under the cathodic current densities used in pacing, but anodic potentials can cause corrosion. The proximal electrode (anode) of a bipolar pacing lead, therefore, is made large enough to ensure that current density is too low to affect significant corrosion. Careful examination of explanted platinum polished distal tips (cathodes) often reveals rough surfaces that are the result of corrosion. Although this seems contradictory, it is easily explained. The distal tip is a cathode during its *stimulation* pulse. Some generators also have a fast recharge pulse after the stimulus to neutralize the afterpotential. Because the polarity of the fast recharge is reversed, this portion of the pulse is actually anodal. Thus, as the "cathode" size decreases, corrosion increases eventually to unacceptable levels. Nonetheless, excellent canine performance has been reported with electrodes as small as 0.6 mm² in geometric surface area.[79] When the electrode is porous, the surface area of the electrolyte interface is actually large despite the small volume encompassed by the geometric surface. This reduces the current density at the electrolyte–metal interface to a level below that required for corrosion by the fast-recharge pulse.

■ UNIPOLAR AND BIPOLAR STIMULATION

All pacing systems require a negatively charged cathode and a positively charged anode to complete the electrical circuit. Thus, in reality, all pacemakers are bipolar. The unipolar pacemaker has one electrode in the heart and one relatively large electrode remote from the heart, usually on the pulse generator can. Bipolar pacemakers have both the cathode and the anode in (or on) the chamber of the heart to be paced and sensed. There has been a great deal of debate regarding the relative merits of unipolar versus bipolar pacing, most of which relates to issues other than stimulation. The effects of unipolar and bipolar configurations on sensing are profound and are covered in Chapter 2. The engineering aspects are equally important and are discussed in Chapter 3. At one time, it was generally accepted that bipolar leads had higher stimulation thresholds than unipolar leads. This statement, based on old technology, is approximately true only if both electrodes are of equal size. In this case, the output voltage delivered by the pulse generator is divided equally between the two electrodes, causing the measured threshold to be higher. This can be corrected by making the cathode relatively small and the anode relatively large. This produces the largest potential difference across tissue adjacent to the cathode, reducing the stimulation threshold. It also makes the anode a relatively poor stimulating electrode, reducing the arrhythmogenic potential compared with a bipolar lead with equal-sized electrodes.

In practical terms, the anode must be at least three times larger than the cathode to produce bipolar thresholds that are statistically equivalent to unipolar.[80] It has become standard practice in the design of pacing leads to ensure that the anode is at least 4.5 times larger than the geometric surface area of the cathode. The bipolar electrode spacing can also be important, especially for sensing (see Chap. 2). It is generally accepted, for example, that as the electrodes are moved closer together, the signal-to-noise ratio, resistance to crosstalk, and median frequency of the sensed signal increase, whereas signal amplitude may decrease. If the spacing is too close, transvenous electrode pairs can have high stimulation thresholds as current can be shunted between the two electrodes, effectively producing a short circuit. In his classic thesis, De Caprio determined that the optimum bipolar spacing (for sensing) was about 8 mm.[81]

■ MULTISITE PACING

Although transvenous pacing has been traditionally performed from the right atrium and right ventricular apex, several studies have suggested that stimulation of the left-sided chambers may be a useful therapy for selected clinical disorders. For example, simultaneous pacing of both the right and left atrium through the coronary sinus may decrease the frequency of paroxysmal atrial fibrillation or atypical atrial flutter.[82] Although coronary sinus leads have been used since 1970 for atrial pacing, right atrial pacing with J-shaped leads has long been the standard method because of

improved pacing thresholds and easier implantation.[83] Bi-atrial pacing from the atrial septum or Bachman's bundle has also been reported.[84] Implantation of permanent pacing leads in the cardiac veins via the coronary sinus has also been reported as a method for chronic left ventricular stimulation.[85] Although epicardial left ventricular pacing using standard myocardial leads has been studied as a method for biventricular pacing for the treatment of congestive heart failure, it requires a more extensive operation than a transvenous approach. Transvenous stimulation of the left ventricle requires placement of the lead into a branch of the cardiac venous circulation, usually the anterior interventricular or posterolateral veins. The electrical properties of chronic stimulation of both the right and left ventricles are complex. The complexity of dual veniricular stimulation has been reported in canine studies.[86]

In canine studies bipolar leads were placed transvenously into a distal epicardial ventricular branch of the great cardiac vein. The distal electrode was a 5.8-mm^2 porous, platinized hemisphere with a steroid coating. A transvenous lead was also placed at the right ventricular apex. Two varieties of right ventricular apex electrodes were used, one with a 4-mm^2 platinized target tip and the other with a 1.2-mm^2 steroid-eluting tip. Several modes of stimulation were compared (Tables 1–1, 1–2, and 1–3). One configuration (ventricular split bipole) used two unipolar leads and an adapter such that the electrode in one chamber was the cathode, whereas the electrode in the other chamber served as the anode. The second configuration (dual-cathode) joined the left and right ventricular electrodes in parallel as a common cathode. The anode was the pulse generator can. The thresholds as a function of time after implantation are shown in Figure 1–19. The single chamber chronic coronary venous left ventricular thresholds were two to three times higher than the right ventricular single chamber values. The threshold for simultaneous capture of both the right and left ventricles was similar to the unipolar left ventricular threshold. Similar findings were observed regardless of whether the anode was the pulse generator can or a ring electrode in the right ventricle. In contrast, with the ventricular split bipole configuration, the threshold for combined capture of both ventricles was much higher, leading to exit block (>5 V) in many cases.

Table 1–1. Canine Thresholds (V) at 0.5 msec, 12 Weeks Postimplant (n = 13)

Chambers Paced	Unipolar LV	Unipolar RV	Unipolar DCO
1	1.8 ± 1.2	0.9 ± 0.2	0.9 ± 0.2
2			2.0 ± 1.4
1	2.6 ± 1.9	0.9 ± 0.5	1.1 ± 0.6
2			3.3 ± 2.0
	Bipolar RV −, LV +	**Bipolar LV −, RV +**	**Bipolar DCO −, RV Ring +**
1	1.4 ± 0.5	2.0 ± 0.9	1.0 ± 0.4
2	7.2 ± 3.5	3.5 ± 1.0	1.7 ± 0.9
1	1.4 ± 1.0	3.0 ± 1.6	NA
2	8.5 ± 3.0	4.6 ± 2.3	NA

LV = Left ventricular coronary vein; RV = right ventricular apex; DCO = dual cathodal output.

Unipolar Canine RVA & LVCV Thresholds Vs Time

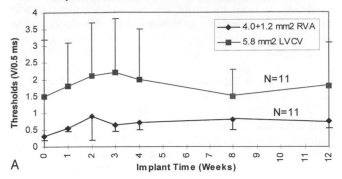

A

**Unipolar Canine RV & LV Thresholds for 5.8 mm²
CapSure SP Electrodes**

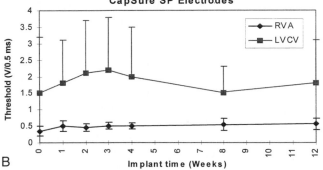

B

Figure 1–19. Unipolar canine right ventricular apex and left cardiac vein ventricular thresholds as a function of implant time. In the upper panel, the leads are paired in each canine with a 5.8 mm² left ventricular lead, and pooled data in the right ventricle from 1.2 and 4.0 mm² electrodes. Pooling was allowed because there was no statistically significant difference between the two electrode's thresholds ($p \ll 0.5$). In the lower panel, the left ventricular lead is compared with one of the same design in different animals. In both cases, the left ventricular thresholds are about twice those of the right-sided leads.

The pacing impedance with the dual-cathode configuration was 43% lower than the average of the two single-chamber values. When a small electrode with high imped-ance (1.2 mm²) was paired with a larger electrode (4 mm²), the dual-cathode impedance was 51% lower than the average of the two unipolar impedances values. Pacing impedance in the ventricular split bipole configuration was markedly higher than that for either electrode alone.

Thus, it appears that thresholds for dual ventricular stimu-

Table 1–2. Canine Pacing Impedance at 2.5V/0.5 msec, 12 Weeks Postimplant

Unipolar LV	Unipolar RV	Unipolar DCO
790 ± 118	734 ± 190	433 ± 68
829 ± 642	1193 ± 297	488 ± 157
Bipolar RV−, LV+	**Bipolar LV−, RV+**	**Bipolar DCO−, RV Ring+**
1193 ± 186	1014 ± 157	410 ± 64
1863 ± 745	1216 ± 806	NA

LV = left ventricular coronary vein; RV = right ventricular apex; DCO = dual cathodal output.

Table 1–3. Canine R-Wave Amplitudes (MV) 12 Weeks Postimplant

Unipolar LV	Unipolar RV	Unipolar DCO
13 ± 4	26 ± 4	14 ± 2
13 ± 4	26 ± 4	14 ± 7
Bipolar RV−, LV+	**Bipolar LV−, RV+**	**Bipolar DCO−, RV Ring+**
29 ± 4	35 ± 7	NA
29 ± 4	29 ± 4	NA

LV = Left ventricular coronary vein; RV = right ventricular apex; DCO = dual cathodal output.

lation may be lowest when two approximately equal-sized electrodes are used as a dual-cathode configuration and the anode is a ring electrode in the right ventricle. Certainly, the ventricular split bipole configuration is not optimal. In con-trast to stimulation, sensing favored the ventricular split bipole configuration because the left ventricular R waves measured in the cardiac veins were about half the amplitude of right ventricular apex electrograms. With a dual-cathode configuration, the R wave was comparable to the smaller unipolar left ventricular electrogram. With the ventricular split bipole configuration, the R wave was slightly larger than the right ventricular electrogram. Therefore, the optimal configuration for sensing was not the same as that for simu-lation.

■ DESIGN FEATURES OF PACING ELECTRODES THAT AFFECT PERFORMANCE

The performance of pacing electrodes is the major determi-nant of the stimulus threshold. Therefore, the stimulation characteristics of the electrode determine the margin of safety between the stimulus intensity that is delivered by the pulse generator and that required for myocardial stimulation. The electrodes also determine the pacing impedance, another factor that strongly influences pulse generator longevity. In addition to providing myocardial stimulation, the electrodes determine the sensing characteristics of the pacing system.[87] In this section, the size, surface structure, and biologic re-sponse to electrodes that are critical factors for the design of pacing electrodes are discussed. Some secondary effects,

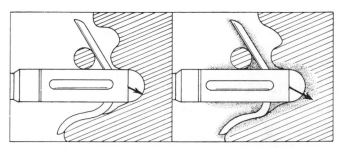

Figure 1–20. Schematic representation of a simple collagenous capsule around the electrode, which separates it from excitable tissue. In effect, the fibrous tissue now becomes a "virtual electrode" with radius r + d, where r is the (spherical) electrode's radius and d is the thickness of fibrous tissue. (From Stokes K, Bornzin G: The electrode–biointerface (stimulation). *In* Barold S [ed]: Modern Cardiac Pacing. Mt. Kisco, NY, Futura, 1985, pp 33–78.)

including shape, spacing, fixations, and material, are also reviewed.

Size of the Stimulating Electrode (Geometric Surface Area)

It has been observed that stimulation threshold varies as an inverse function of the size or geometric surface area of the stimulating electrode.[39, 40, 88, 89] Irnich argued that, in theory, the chronic stimulation threshold of a spherical electrode should decrease as its radius (geometric surface area) decreases to a minimum value. As the radius of the electrode decreases below that minimum value, chronic threshold should begin to increase. Thus, the electric field strength (E) necessary for stimulation is a function of the potential (V) applied to a spherical electrode of radius, r. For a given applied potential, the smaller the radius of the electrode, the more intense is the electric field generated in the underlying myocardium. In this analysis, the strength of the electric field that is required to stimulate myocardium was assumed to be a universal constant (expressed in V/cm). If the minimum field intensity required to initiate depolarization is greater than that generated by the delivered stimulus, the applied voltage must be increased to achieve threshold. Conversely, if electrode radius is increased, the field strength may not be sufficient to capture the heart without increasing the applied voltage.

It has long been recognized that stimulation threshold increases during the first several weeks after lead implantation. This increase in threshold is related to the development of a conductive but nonexcitable fibrotic capsule with approximate mean thickness (d) that forms around the electrode, separating it from normal, excitable myocardium (Fig. 1–20).[39, 40, 90, 91] The fibrous capsule is a biologic response to the presence of the foreign body, in this case an electrode. It is not a response to the electrical stimulus.[92] In reality, therefore, (r + d) describes the dimensions of the effective or "virtual electrode," as defined by Furman and associates.[36] If the stimulus voltage is held constant, the field strength varies as a function of the thickness of the inexcitable capsule. Thus, higher voltages must be applied to maintain the intensity of the field at the interface of the virtual electrode and the excitable myocardium, so that chronic thresholds (for steroid-free electrodes) must be higher than

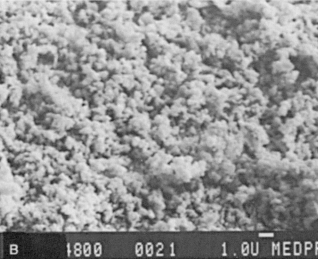
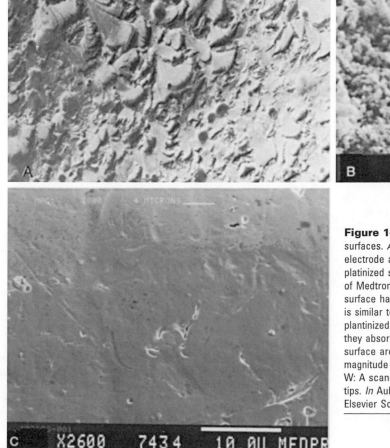

Figure 1–21. Electron micrographs of microporous electrode surfaces. *A*, Activated carbon surface of Siemans model 412S/60 electrode at about 8000 magnifications. *B*, Medtronic model 4011 platinized surface at 6900 magnifications. *C*, Polished platinum surface of Medtronic model 6971 at 7000 magnifications. The polished platinum surface has little microstructure. Its actual microscopic surface area is similar to its apparent or geometric surface area (8 mm²). The plantinized platinum surface is composed of particles so small that they absorb visible light and the surface appears black. The true surface area of the interface, therefore, must be many orders of magnitude greater than the geometric surface area. (*A* from Seeger W: A scanning electron microscopic study on explanted electrode tips. *In* Aubert AE, Ector H [eds]: Pacemaker Leads. Amsterdam, Elsevier Science Publishers, 1985, pp 417–432.)

the implant values. This theory was modeled by Irinch,[39, 40] as follows:

$$(21) \quad E = \frac{V}{r}\left[\frac{r}{(r + d)}\right]^2$$

Equation 21 is lacking a crucial parameter required by the strength–duration relationship time. According to Irnich, the equation is based on measurements taken at a pulse duration of 1 msec.[93] Holding everything else constant, the capsule thickness is the same for a large electrode radius as for a small one. If, for example, two electrodes of different radii (r = 0.5 mm and 5 mm) develop a 1-mm thick capsule (d), the electrode with smaller actual radius will be associated with a greater percentage increase in the radius of the virtual electrode (r + d) than will the larger electrode (300% versus 20%, respectively). This helps to explain the observation that smaller electrodes have lower acute thresholds but develop a greater rise in threshold over time.[91, 94] There is a point (r = d), at which chronic threshold reaches a minimum. According to equation 21, when d is greater than r, thresholds increase. Therefore, there is a theoretical minimum spherical electrode radius at which thresholds must reach their minimum value. Irnich found this to be r = 0.72 mm with polished electrodes. In reality, because most electrodes are not spherical, the relationship between stimulation threshold and electrode radius is more complex. Therefore, electrode size is usually discussed in terms of geometric surface area.

Relationship of Electrode Size and Sensing Performance

As discussed in Chapter 2, the amplitude of the electrogram that is sensed by the amplifier of the pulse generator is less than the amplitude of the available signal in the myocardium. The attenuation of the signal is related to the ratio of the source impedance (of the electrode–myocardial interface) and the input impedance of the sensing amplifier. The higher the source impedance, the more the signal amplitude is attenuated for a given input impedance. Signal attenuation, however, can be greatly minimized by increasing the input impedance of the sense amplifier so that the ratio of the source impedance to the input impedance is very large.

In the early 1970's, a 5-mm² Elgiloy Microtip electrode was marketed. This electrode was later removed from the market because of poor sensing.[95] Although acceptable electrogram amplitudes were measured on an oscilloscope (with very high input impedance), there was a relatively high rate of failure to sense when this lead was implanted in combination with certain pulse generators. Although this electrode had good stimulation thresholds and about 1000 Ω pacing impedance, it also had about 5000 Ω sensing (source) impedance. Because the pulse generators of one manufacturer had a very low sensing amplifier input impedance (10,000 Ω), about one third of the actual electrogram amplitude was attenuated in the amplifier (see Chap. 2). Thus, the idea that "small electrodes do not sense well" was born, when in reality the problem was in the amplifier design.[94, 96] The significance of such impedance mismatch was not generally recognized at the time, however. It is now recognized that small porous and microporous electrodes provide both excel-

lent stimulation thresholds and sensing performance when combined with modern pulse generators that have much higher input impedance than earlier models.

Electrode Surface Structure (Interfacial Surface Area)

Based on animal studies, it has been claimed that electrodes with pores that allow tissue ingrowth have thinner fibrous capsules and somewhat lower chronic thresholds than solid or polished surfaces.[97–100] These claims have been somewhat controversial when applied to humans.[101–104] Pore structures of certain dimensions are known to promote rapid tissue ingrowth (Fig. 1–21).[105] It has been argued that this provides rapid stability of the electrode at its interface with the myocardium and prevents electrode motion that otherwise may result in tissue irritation and high chronic stimulation thresholds. On the other hand, properly designed tines and myocardial screws provide immediate stability and good chronic threshold performance. Activated carbon electrodes are reported to have porosity on the order of 10 nm (Fig. 1–22).[106]

The endocardial Target Tip electrode, introduced in 1983, had several grooves in a hemispherical, 8-mm² electrode that provided regions of high electric field strength and promoted endocardial stability.[107] The surface was platinized to produce micron-sized surface microporosity (see Fig. 1–21). Although fibrotic tissue cannot grow into such small structures, these microporous electrodes had significantly lower chronic thresholds than their otherwise equivalent porous and polished counterparts.[105, 106, 108–111] It appears that the chronic thresholds of porous and microporous electrodes are

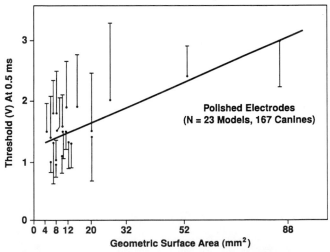

Figure 1–22. Chronic (12-week) canine ventricular (gain of capture) thresholds (V) at 0.5 msec as a function of polished platinum electrode geometric surface area (N = 23 models, 167 animals). The correlation is fair at about 0.82. The slope is about 0.02 V/mm². There are no significant differences in thresholds for geometric electrode surface areas between 26 mm² and 4.5 mm² (the smallest tested). the thresholds of 53 and 85 mm² polished (endocardial) electrodes were significantly higher than those of the rest of the group. There were no significant differences between endocardial and myocardial electrodes or as a function of electrode shape. (From Stokes K: The effects of ventricular electrode surface area on pacemaker lead performance. *In* Adornato E, Galarsi A [eds]: The '92 Scenario on Cardiac Pacing. Rome, L Pozzi, 1992, pp 505–514.)

superior to those of polished surfaces. The argument that ingrowth of tissue into the electrode prevents motion to result in a less irritating interface with the myocardium remains unproved, however.

Multivariant Effects of Electrode Size, Shape, Material, and Surface Structure

If we add the effects of electrode shape, surface structure, size, location, and chemical composition to electrode size, the number of permutations becomes excessive for a typical scientific analysis of each factor. The combined effects of a wide range of platinum electrode geometric surface areas, shapes, and surface structures on chronic (12-week) unipolar canine ventricular thresholds has been studied, which allows us to evaluate their individual effects.[112–113] As shown in Figure 1–23, the correlation between threshold and geometric surface area for polished electrodes of 85, 53, and 26 mm² is fair (r = 0.83), with decreasing threshold as a function of decreasing size. The slope of the curve was about 0.02 V/mm². Between about 4.5 mm² (the smallest tested) and 26 mm², however, the size–threshold correlation for polished electrodes is negligible, and no statistically significant differences can be demonstrated, regardless of electrode shape. The correlation coefficient between chronic thresholds and electrode size for *porous* electrodes ranging in geometric surface area from 10 mm² (the largest tested) to about 1.5 mm² is only 0.083 (no correlation; Fig. 1–24). We were unable to discriminate to a statistically significant level between porous and microporous surfaces in this analysis. Surface areas below 1.5 mm² produced dramatically increas-

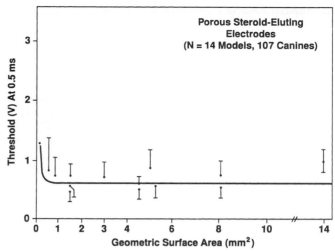

Figure 1–24. Chronic (12-weeek) canine (gain of capture) ventricular thresholds (V) at 0.5 msec as a function of porous steroid-eluting electrode geometric surface area. The curve includes 14 designs (107 animals). No significant relationship (correlation = 0.041) between electrode surface area and chronic threshold between 14 mm² (the largest tested) and about 0.6 mm² was found. The slope of the curve at more than 0.6 mm² was only 0.017 V/mm². Thresholds rose as a function of geometric surface area of less than 0.6 mm². (From Stokes K: The effects of ventricular electrode surface area on pacemaker lead performance. *In* Adornato E, Galarsi A [eds]: The '92 Scenario on Cardiac Pacing. Rome, L Pozzi, 1992, pp 505–514.)

ing thresholds. The *porous, steroid-eluting* population of electrodes (Fig. 1–25) also showed no significant relationship between geometric electrode surface area and chronic threshold between 14 mm² (the largest tested) and about 0.6 mm². The correlation coefficient between surface area

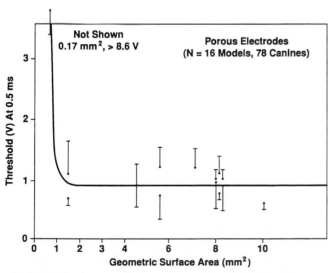

Figure 1–23. Chronic (12-week) canine ventricular (gain of capture) thresholds (V) at 0.5 msec as a function of porous electrode geometric surface area. This series includes 16 designs (N = 78 animals). The term *porous* refers to totally porous, porous surface, microporous, and DCD electrodes. The correlation coefficient in the geometric surface area range of 10 mm² (the largest tested) and about 1.5 mm² is only 0.083 (no correlation). The slope of the curve at 1.5 mm² or greater is 0.006 V/mm². Surface areas of less than 1.5 mm² produced dramatically increasing thresholds. (From Stokes K: The effects of ventricular electrode surface area on pacemaker lead performance. *In* Adornato E, Galarsi A [eds]: The '92 Scenario on Cardiac Pacing. Rome, L Pozzi, 1992, pp 505–514.)

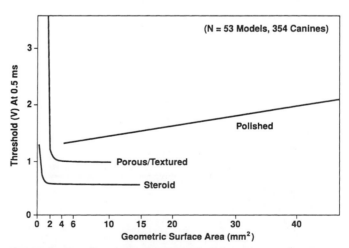

Figure 1–25. Chronic (12-week) canine ventricular thresholds (V) at 0.5 msec as a function of geometric surface area from Figures 1–22 to 1–24, shown without data points or error bars for clarity (53 unipolar ventricular lead models; N = 352 canines). These three populations are significantly different from each other. (From Stokes K: The effects of ventricular electrode surface area on pacemaker lead performance. *In* Adornato E, Galarsi A [eds]: The '92 Scenario on Cardiac Pacing Rome, L Pozzi, 1992, pp 505–514.)

and threshold for this group of electrodes was only 0.041 (no correlation). Stimulation thresholds rose dramatically as a function of geometric surface area for electrodes smaller than 0.6 mm².

All three curves relating stimulation threshold to geometric electrode surface area are shown in Figure 1–26 on the same scale (without error bars) for comparison. Within the limits defined previously, these three populations of electrodes are significantly different from one another. Thus, it is clear that the major determinant of chronic stimulation threshold within clinically useful ranges is not so much the electrode size, geometric surface area, or shape as its surface structure (interfacial surface area) and the property of steroid elution. This analysis strongly suggests that the reason these factors have a significant influence on chronic stimulation threshold is related to their effects on inflammation at the myocardial interface (the foreign body response).

■ THRESHOLD CHANGES AS A FUNCTION OF TIME FOLLOWING LEAD IMPLANTATION

It is well known that stimulation thresholds change as a function of time after implantation, typically rising to a peak value after several weeks.[114–117] With older polished electrodes, some patients had thresholds that evolved over longer periods (as long as 6 months).[118] Luceri and colleagues observed that after the acute rise in stimulation threshold, 43% of 120 patients had stable chronic thresholds for up to 8 years.[119] Seventeen percent of patients had decreasing chronic thresholds at a rate of 5% decrease per year, and 19% had rising thresholds at a rate of 14% per year. Twenty percent of the patients had thresholds that

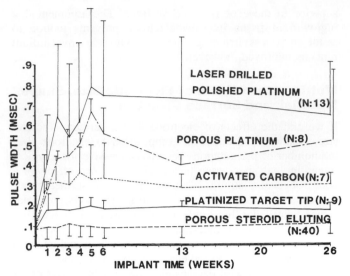

Figure 1–27. Loss of capture pulse duration human ventricular thresholds as a function of implant time for a series of unipolar leads with 8 mm² geometric surface area electrodes.[106] These threshold values appear to be typical of that type of electrode, not unique to the particular manufacturer. The top curve is a polished electrode with holes drilled in it by a laser. Its performance appears to be similar to that of polished electrodes in general. The second curve is porous surface platinum, next is microporous carbon, then microporous plantinized platinum (with grooves), and, at the bottom, platinized, porous platinum with steroid.

varied widely around a stable mean. Some typical acute to chronic changes as a function of time in the canine are shown in Figure 1–27 for passively fixed 8-mm² ventricular and 11-mm² atrial polished platinum electrodes. Atrial thresholds typically rise to a peak within 1 week, then decrease substantially. The chronic atrial threshold is often substantially lower than the chronic ventricular value. The ventricular thresholds have a lower peak value, and in many cases, this peak may not be apparent for 3 or 4 weeks. It is clear that there is a wide range of variability in chronic stimulation thresholds between patients with this type of electrode. Therefore, one cannot assume that the threshold course will be typical for any given patient.

Polished electrodes are still used in some transvenous screw-in and epicardial or myocardial leads. In addition, there are still many patients in whom the older polished electrodes are implanted. Thus, the preceding discussion is still useful today. For modern leads, however, polished electrodes are obsolete. Modern fixation electrodes have a porous or microporous surface structure. Most also elute a glucocorticosteroid. As shown in Figure 1–28, the technologic progression from polished to porous to microporous to steroid-eluting electrodes has significantly reduced the evolution of stimulation threshold as a function of time after implantation.[107] In fact, as can be determined from the follow-up data available, the thresholds of porous and microporous steroid-eluting leads do not change significantly with increasing time after implantation.[106, 120–122] The reasons for threshold changes as a function of time and electrode design are to be found in the foreign body response to the electrodes.

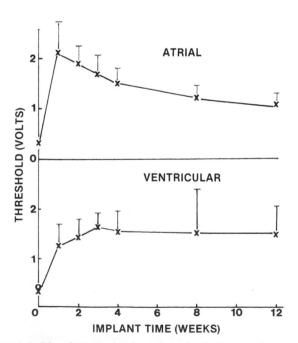

Figure 1–26. Acute to chronic canine gain of voltage capture threshold changes at 0.5 msec as a function of time after implantation for unipolar leads with passively fixed, atraumatic, polished platinum, 11-mm² atrial *(upper)* and 8-mm² ventricular *(lower)* electrodes.

▪ THE ELECTRODE–TISSUE INTERFACE AND THE FOREIGN BODY RESPONSE

Passively Fixed Leads With Steroid-Free Polished Electrodes

The body's response to an implanted device is relatively well characterized.[123, 124] Figure 1–29 shows schematically what ordinarily happens at an implantation site as a function of time. If one analyzes the tissues adjacent to canine ventricular endocardial atraumatic electrodes as a function of time after implantation, the evolution depicted in Figure 1–29 is typically observed (with one exception). In the first 1 to 3 days, there is no evidence of cellular inflammation, and thresholds do not change significantly. This lack of a cellular response in the first few days is an exception to the classic view of surgical wound inflammation. In a surgical wound, polymorphonuclear leukocytes normally are present during this period to scavenge necrotic debris, bacteria, and so on. The lack of polymorphonuclear leukocytes adjacent to atraumatic endocardial electrodes is explained only by the fact that the electrode is placed quite far from the surgical wound.

The classic view of inflammation holds that the initial event is dilation of blood vessels and alteration in the vascular endothelium resulting in increased permeability. This increased perfusion and permeability of the blood vessel walls allows plasma to leak into the surrounding tissue, producing edema. Because plasma and serum are more conductive than myocardium, pacing impedance decreases almost immediately after lead implantation. After about 2 to 3 days, a mixed cellular inflammation begins to appear in the tissues surrounding the electrode, and the stimulation threshold begins to rise. Tissue inflammation reaches its peak in about a week, with clearly evident interstitial edema

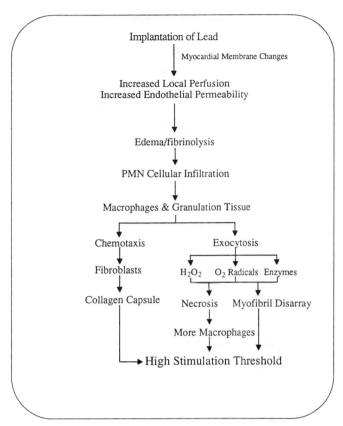

Figure 1–29. Schematic representation of the inflammatory process and foreign body response to lead implantation. This has been correlated approximately with time after implantation of a cardiac pacemaker lead, based on our histologic studies of canine electrode-tissue sites.

and cellular necrosis. Pacing impedance typically reaches its minimum value at the inflammatory peak (about 1 week), after which it increases as the edema resolves. The stimulation threshold may or may not reach its peak at the same time as the nadir of pacing impedance.

After the early, mixed cellular reaction, the inflammatory response is characterized by a gradual accumulation of macrophages that reach the electrode surface, adhere, and become activated. The major function of the macrophage is to phagocytose dead or foreign cells and particles by the process of endocytosis (Fig. 1–30).[125] In the case of a large foreign object, such as a pacing electrode, the process of endocytosis is impossible. In this case, the macrophage tries to destroy the large foreign body by the process of exocytosis, the extracellular release of enzymes and oxidants. Macrophages spread over the electrode surface, often differentiating into foreign body giant cells. Their lysosomes migrate to the membrane surface, releasing hydrolytic enzymes and oxidants into the surrounding tissue and onto the electrode surface. Additional macrophages settle on the foreign body giant cells and are activated. Myocytes adjacent to the electrode–tissue interface are bathed in a "soup" of inflammatory mediators resulting from exocytosis. These mediators of the inflammatory response dissolve the subcellular collagen beams, struts, and nets that hold the myocytes in the normal orderly array of myocardium.[126]

After 3 to 4 weeks (for a stable, biocompatible device),

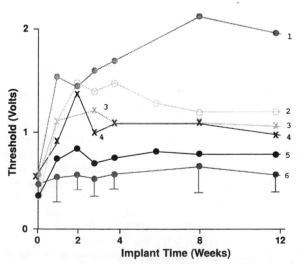

Figure 1–28. Canine ventricular voltage thresholds at 0.5 msec of 8-mm² unipolar, transvenous, tined leads as a function of implant time. 1. Polished platinum ring-tip (manufacturer A). 2. Polished platinum ring-tip (manufacturer B). 3. Porous surface platinum hemisphere (manufacturer C). 4. Porous surface titanium hemisphere (manufacturer B). 5. Platinized Target Tip (manufacturer B). 6. Steroid-eluting titanium porous surface electrode (manufacturer B).

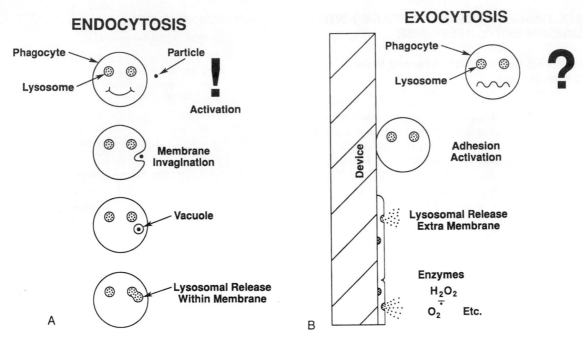

Figure 1–30. *A*, Schematic representation of phagocytosis by endocytosis. A small particle is attached to the macrophage's membrane. The membrane invaginates, encapsulating the particle in a membrane-lined vesicle. The vesicle and lysosome migrate toward each other, and their membranes fuse. The particle is then destroyed by lysosomal enzymes and oxidants. *B*, Schematic representation of the process of "frustrated phagocytosis" by exocytosis, or the acute foreign body response on the device surface resulting in lysosomal release of inflammatory mediators on the device surface and into the adjacent tissue.

the more global inflammatory response has essentially resolved with the development of a collagenous capsule surrounding the electrode. If the electrode is biocompatible and stable relative to the myocardium, there are few further significant visible histologic changes in the adjacent tissues after this period. The stimulation threshold of a polished electrode may still be at or just past the peak phase in the ventricle, however. Thresholds may subsequently decrease, remain stable, or increase, depending on the intensity of the chronic foreign body response at the electrode-tissue interface.

Chronic atraumatic polished electrodes (Fig. 1–31*A*) typically have a layer of foreign body giant cells on their surface. These are covered by a layer (or layers) of macrophages that can be surprisingly thick. This cellular component of the capsule is not an acute, transient phenomenon but has been observed on electrodes up to 13 years after implantation in our canine studies. These cells are covered by a layer of collagen that is oriented along the surface of the electrode. The myocytes adjacent to the collagen layers are disarrayed and interspersed with collagen fibers that are radially oriented with respect to the surface of the electrode. There may also be circular "holes" in this layer of disoriented myocytes, which appear to be infiltrated with fatty material. We have observed groups of macrophages with fused membranes (foreign body giant cells) enveloping bundles of myocardial fibers adjacent to the electrode 1 to 4 weeks after implantation. Based on our unpublished work, the presence of this fatty infiltration and its location and severity depend on the stability, myocardial location, and shape of the electrode relative to the vector of myocardial contraction. Outside the disarrayed myofiber zone, one finds normally ori-

ented myocardium. Thus, it is clear that the concept of a simple fibrous capsule (Irnich's "d") separating the electrode surface from viable myocardium does not completely describe this complex biologic response and its effect on pacing.

Passively Fixed Leads With Porous and Microporous Electrodes

Electrodes with pores on the order of 10 to 100 μm in size allow the ingrowth of collagen as a result of chronic inflammation. Thus, in a sense, macroporous electrodes promote inflammation. In addition, the chronic capsule surrounding porous electrodes can be associated with significant myofibrillar disarray (see Fig. 1–31*B*). Despite these factors, porous electrodes are associated with a relatively thin collagenous capsule. Histologic study of the chronic tissue reaction surrounding porous electrodes has shown that inflammatory cells are usually not found on the surface of the electrode. Rather, the active cellular component of the fibrous capsule is located *within* the pores and is removed with the device during the tissue-trimming operation. Similarly, microporous electrodes tend to have few cells on their surfaces with well-healed interfaces (see Fig. 1–31*C*). We have found that the chronic tissue interface with the Target Tip design has an active cellular component deep in the grooves of the electrode (see Fig. 1–31*D*). The smooth outer surface, however, interfaces directly with collagen.

Passively Fixed Leads With Steroid-Eluting Electrodes

It has long been recognized that systemically administered glucocorticosteroids decrease both acute and chronic stimulation thresholds. Indeed, the administration of oral or parenteral glucocorticosteroids to patients with exit block may allow the stimulation threshold to decrease to a level that maintains effective pacing. Initially, it was believed that the threshold-lowering effect of systemic glucocorticoid therapy was due to effects on the myocyte membrane and sodium and potassium "retention."[127] Steroid-eluting leads, in which dexamethasone sodium phosphate or acetate is gradually released from a reservoir within or around the electrode, are standard for permanent pacing. It has been conclusively demonstrated that steroid elution decreases chronic thresholds. Despite the clear clinical benefits of steroid elution on the evolution of stimulation thresholds, the mechanism of this effect is less well understood.[128] Athough steroid-eluting, porous electrodes tend to have thinner capsules than polished platinum electrodes, the capsule surrounding a steroid-eluting lead can be difficult to differentiate from steroid-free electrodes in blind analyses. The capsule surrounding a steroid-eluting lead is characterized by minimal cellularity between the collagen and electrode surface and minimal myofibrillar disarray.

Effect of Glucocorticoids on the Evolution of Pacing Thresholds

Glucocorticosteroids are known to stabilize the membranes of phagocytes, such as the macrophage, through interaction with surface receptors, inhibiting release of lysosomal contents.[129] It has been shown, however, that dexamethasone and its derivatives have no significant electrical effects on myocyte membranes.[130, 131] It is probable that the salutary effect of systemic glucocorticoids on stimulation threshold is the result of inhibition of the release of inflammatory mediators from the cellular components of the fibrous capsule. When steroid therapy is discontinued, the release of inflammatory mediators resumes and stimulation thresholds once again increase. The same phenomenon minimizes inflammation (foreign body response) on and adjacent to the surface of a steroid-eluting electrode. Acute stabilization of macrophage membranes on the electrode surface reduces or minimizes lysosomal release, thereby minimizing myofibrillar disarray and myocyte membrane damage. Chronic steroid elution suppresses the slow, insidious leakage of inflamma-

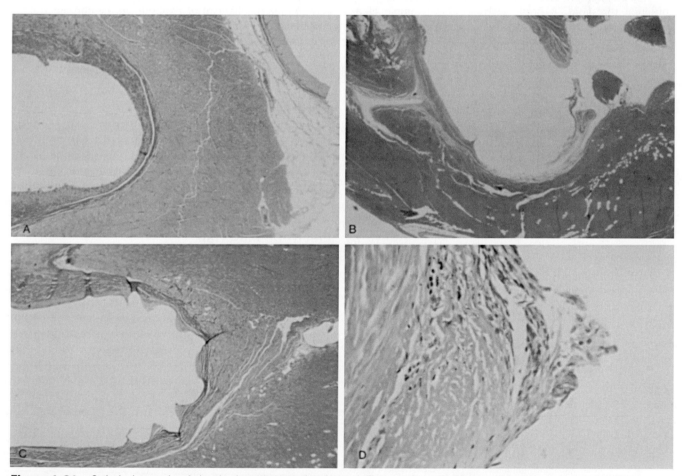

Figure 1–31. Optical micrographs of chronic electrode–tissue interfaces. *A,* The capsule surrounding a polished electrode *(upper left)* has a relatively thick layer of activated phagocytic cells, including foreign body giant cells on the surface, with macrophages further out. Collagenous material encapsulates these cells, with fibrous stringers extending outward into the myocardium. *B,* Myofibrillar disarray is seen between the collagenous capsule and normal myocardium. The capsule surrounding a porous electrode *(upper right)* appears to be thinner. The active cellular component of the capsule and some of the collagen, however, have been removed with the electrode to facilitate trimming of the tissues. *C,* A microporous (Target Tip) electrode–tissue interface is shown in the lower left section of the micrograph. Note the thin fibrous capsule over the external surfaces and at the ridges. *D,* Some macrophages are seen deep in the Target Tip electrode's grooves at higher magnification.

tory mediators, thereby preventing threshold increase, without the risk of systemic side effects.

Pathologic Changes Due to Mechanical Instability at the Myocardial–electrode Interface

Mechanically unstable electrodes can provoke a significant pathologic response in the myocardium. Consider, for example, a transvenous corkscrew electrode that "rocks" at the interface with the endocardium because the lead behind it is too stiff. In some cases, large pockets of activated macrophages may develop on either side of the helix, resulting in the formation of a "preabscess." In other cases, thick collagenous capsules form, then differentiate into cartilage and, if the instability is severe enough, bone. Because active-fixation myocardial electrodes interfere with the contractile motion of the adjacent myofibers, myocardial degeneration with fatty infiltration may result in patterns that are clearly related to this mechanical interference. For example, the center of a myocardial helix may fill in with fatty "cells." A myocardial pin may provoke myocardial degeneration and fatty infiltration as well. Thus, mechanical instability at the electrode–myocardial interface may produce marked histologic and physiologic effects that result in deterioration of stimulation threshold. A particularly notable example of a lead with a high potential for exit block was the Telectronics model 330-801 active-fixation lead. This lead used an electrically inactive helix and a platinum-iridium electrode. The presence of a stiff metal J-shaped retention wire increased the stiffness effect of this lead, with a high incidence of exit block (about 10%).

■ SOME SECOND-ORDER EFFECTS OF ELECTRODE DESIGN

Spatial and Size Relationships Between Electrode Pairs

It was established previously that, within clinically relevant limits, porous and microporous electrode size and shape per se have no significant effect on the chronic stimulation thresholds (at least with steroid-free electrodes). Nonetheless, the size and shape of the electrode can still be important factors under certain circumstances. For example, a small

displacement can affect the performance of a smaller electrode because its high-density field influences relatively few cells.[39, 40] A larger electrode is not as threshold efficient, but perforation is less likely, and small displacements have less effect on lead performance. That ring-tip electrode design is essentially a small electrode made into a large shape.[132] This allows high electric field strength coverage of a larger number of myocardial cells, while affording a lower probability of perforation than a lead with a smaller tip. Although myocardial screws, barbs, hooks, and so forth are traumatic to the underlying myocardium, these electrodes all have points that serve as sources of high field strength. Thus, myocardial electrodes can have good chronic performance, assuming that the lead is not so stiff as to apply undue force on the electrode–myocardial interface.

Electrode Fixation

The most efficient electrode design has poor long-term performance if it is mechanically unstable, resulting in both high stimulation thresholds and histopathologic evidence of excessive trauma. For chronically stable, steroid-free electrodes in canines, however, we have found no correlation between the mechanism of fixation and the chronic stimulation threshold (Table 1–4). Given similar geometric surface areas, we found comparable chronic canine ventricular thresholds with tined, flanged, screw-in, and hook-in polished electrodes, whether endocardial or myocardial. These results have been confirmed by human studies in both the atrium and ventricle.[133–135] Thus, the hypothesis that fixation remote from the electrode stimulation site is necessary for low chronic thresholds does not appear to be valid.[136, 137] It has not been established whether this is also true for steroid-eluting electrodes. A variety of leads are available, however, that combine active fixation and steroid elution. The low-term pacing thresholds of these leads are much lower than those for similar models without steroid elution.

Electrode Materials

To minimize inflammation and its subsequent effects on stimulation threshold, electrodes for permanent pacing should be biocompatible and resistant to chemical degrada-

Table 1–4. Chronic (12-week) Unipolar Canine (Constant-Voltage) Thresholds (V_{thr}) of Polished Platinum Electrodes at 0.5 msec versus Fixation Mechanism

Model No.	Insertion Fixation	Electrode Location Shape	Surface Area (mm²)	Stimulation Threshold (V_{thr})	n	p vs 6971[a]
6901	Endocardial flange	Endocardial cylinder	11	1.9 ± .77	11	.2
6950	Endocardial long tines	Endocardial cylinder	11	1.6 ± .48	4	>.5
6961	Endocardial short tines	Endocardial ring	8	1.8 ± .69	9	.35
6971	Endocardial medium tines	Endocardial ring	8	1.5 ± .57	8	—
4016	Endocardial helix	Myocardial helix	10	1.1 ± .30	6	.1
6959	Endocardial helix	Endocardial ring	13	1.3 ± .42	8	.4
6955	Endocardial helix	Myocardial helix	10	1.6 ± .51	10	>.5
4951	Epicardial hook	Myocardial hook	10	1.5 ± .44	10	>.5
6917	Epicardial helix	Myocardial helix	12	1.4 ± .53	17	>.5

[a]$p < .05$ considered statistically significant.
From Stokes K, Bornzin G: The electrode-biointerface (stimulation). *In* Barold S (ed): Modern Cardiac Pacing. Mt. Kisco, NY, Futura, 1985, pp 33–78.

tion. Many materials, such as platinum, titanium, titanium oxide, titanium nitride, carbon, tantalum pentoxide, iridium, and iridium oxide have been shown to be acceptable for use as pacing electrodes.[138–140] Even silver, which is toxic in neurologic tissue, and certainly not corrosion resistant, has been used successfully in the heart as an electrode.[133] Titanium and tantalum have been known to acquire a surface coating of oxides, which, it has been argued, may impede charge transfer at the electrode interface. To prevent this, titanium has been coated with platinized platinum or vitreous carbon. Others accept the concept that the oxide layer acts as the dielectric of a capacitor, such that no charge is transferred across the dielectric during stimulation. In any case, titanium oxide electrodes are highly corrosion resistant, and these combinations have been found to have excellent long-term performance as pacing electrodes.[141–145]

Some theories have held that the foreign body reaction is a response to the electrode material per se.[99, 146] Therefore, many attempts have been made to improve thresholds through the use of more biocompatible materials. For example, it has been claimed that pyrolytic carbons are more biocompatible and produce lower chronic thresholds than platinum.[99, 102, 103, 136] Besides having a different composition, these electrodes are also microporous. When similar electrodes are polished, we have found that the chronic canine thresholds are not significantly different from polished platinum. There can be no doubt that proper electrode material selection is necessary to prevent unacceptable toxic responses or corrosion. At this point, however, there does not appear to be a biocompatible electrode composition that significantly improves thresholds.

Of course, not all conductive materials are suitable for use as electrodes. Certain materials, such as zinc, copper, mercury, nickel, and lead, are associated with toxic reactions in the myocardium and are unsuitable for use in permanent pacing leads.[133] Stainless steel materials are highly variable in composition and microstructure, with great variability between production lots. Electrodes made from one lot may be acceptable, whereas those made from another lot may corrode unacceptably. Because some of the corrosion products may be inflammatory or toxic, high thresholds may occasionally occur with these materials. Thus, stainless steel materials are no longer used for implantable electrodes. The polarity of the electrode may also have an important influence on its chemical stability. For example, Elgiloy, a non-noble and highly polarizing metal alloy, has been acceptable as a cathode. When used as an anode, however, this alloy is susceptible to a significant degree of corrosion. As a result, Elgiloy does not appear to be used as an electrode material today.

The materials presently used for permanent pacing electrodes include platinum-iridium, titanium (oxide), platinum- or carbon-coated titanium, platinized platinum, vitreous carbon, and iridium oxide. The platinized platinum, "activated" carbon, and iridium-oxide electrodes are associated with a reduced degree of polarization. A negligible degree of corrosion occurs with these materials. The vitreous carbon electrodes have been improved by roughening the surface, a process known as activation that increases the surface area of the interface, thereby reducing polarization. Fractal coating of the distal electrode has been introduced as a method for reducing electrode polarization. This technique involves coating the distal electrode with a microscopic granular structure that produces a complex surface.

Electrode Location (Epicardial, Endocardial, Myocardial)

As shown previously in canine ventricles for electrodes without steroid elution, the site of fixation has no effect on stimulation thresholds. Similarly, epicardially applied corkscrews, transvenous corkscrews, and passively fixed endocardial electrodes all tend to have about the same chronic thresholds in canines (see Table 1–4). Most epicardial or myocardial leads are used in pediatric pacing patients, in whom threshold complications are relatively frequent.[147, 148] It is generally perceived that epicardial or myocardial electrodes without steroid elution have a less desirable threshold performance than endocardial leads. One reason that epicardial and myocardial leads have lagged behind endocardial passively fixed lead performance is because of the mechanical limitations involved. Transvenous active-fixation and epicardial leads are significantly more complex and more difficult to design with all the attributes needed to produce low chronic stimulation thresholds. Nonetheless, there is no inherent reason that transvenous activate-fixation or myocardial electrodes should not perform as well as or better than endocardial systems.

The first transvenous steroid-eluting active-fixation lead (Medtronic model 5078) was bipolar, with an electrically inactive fixed helix surrounding a 5.8-mm² porous, platinized cathode. This lead had excellent electrical performance in both the atrium and ventricle.[149–152] There were some difficulties with helix distortion and entrapment in some cases, however, resulting in the abandonment of the design. Next, an extendible-retractable design was developed that is currently in widespread use for active-fixation permanent pacing. Medtronic models 4068 polyurethane insulated) and 5068 (silicone insulated) have been shown to have significantly lower pacing thresholds than comparable models without steroid elution.[153–156] Similar findings have been reported with the St. Jude model 1388T lead with an extendable-retractable helix and steroid-elution.[157] Although active-fixation steroid-eluting leads provide significantly reduced pacing thresholds than standard active-fixation leads, the thresholds tend to be slightly higher than for passive-fixation steroid-eluting leads.[158] Steroid elution has also been applied to epicardial leads, with a significant reduction in long-term pacing threshold as compared with steroid-free leads.[159]

■ PACING IMPEDANCE

Impedance (Z) is a complex phenomenon, which is poorly understood in the pacing community and often confused with resistance (R). Indeed, resistance is usually a good first approximation of impedance. Nonetheless, a reasonable understanding of the fundamental concepts in pacing requires a basic understanding of impedance. Impedance is defined as the *sum of all forces opposing the flow of current in an electric circuit*. In most circuits, impedance is defined as follows:

$$(22) \quad Z = \sqrt{R^2 + (A_i - A_c)^2},$$

where R is the sum of the resistances that follow Ohm's law $(R = V/I)$ and A_i is the inductive reactance,

(23) $\quad A_i = 2\pi f L,$

and A_c is the capacitive reactance,

(24) $\quad A_c = \dfrac{1}{2\pi f C}.$

The frequency of the signal (f) is measured in hertz, the inductance (L) in henrys, and the capacitance (C) in farads. In pacing, however, the inductance is usually considered to be too small to be of significance, so the induction reactance (A_2) is ignored. Some argue that there can be no such entity as impedance in a DC circuit because frequency is (by definition) zero. Pacing stimuli, however, are not DC signals. They do have significant frequency components when analyzed by fast Fourier transform, as shown in Figure 1–32. Thus, the term *impedance* is correctly applicable to the pacing stimulus. Pacing impedance (Z_p), therefore, is typically represented as follows:

(25) $\quad Z_p = \sqrt{R^2 + \left(\dfrac{1}{2\pi f C}\right)^2}.$

Although impedance can be very complicated, we will try to simplify it by examining the components separately. This will be facilitated by referring to a simplified equivalent circuit for pacing impedance shown in Figure 1–33.

Pacing Resistance

There are a number of resistances in the total pacemaker circuit, including the resistances of the conductor wires, the tissue between the electrodes, and the electrode–tissue interfaces (remember, there are always two electrodes). The resistance of the conductor wire leading to the stimulating

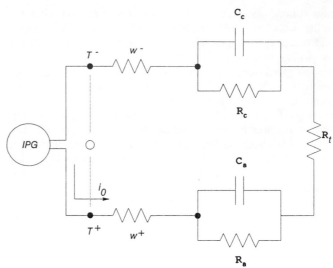

Figure 1–33. A simplified equivalent circuit for a cardiac pacemaker. T^- and T^+ are the negative (cathode) and positive (anode) terminals of the pulse generator (in a unipolar device, T^+ is inside the can). R_w^- is the resistance of the conductor wire leading to the distal tip of the lead (cathode), whereas R_{w+} is that leading to the bipolar lead's proximal ring electrode or the unipolar pulse generator's can. R_t is the resistance of the tissue between the bipolar lead's two electrodes, or the lead tip to the pulse generator can in a unipolar system. R_c is the ohmic polarization of the cathode, whereas R_a is that of the bipolar anode or unipolar generator can. C_c is the capacitance of the cathode, whereas C_a is that of the anode (can). The equivalent circuit is the same for unipolar and bipolar systems, but the values for some of the components differ.

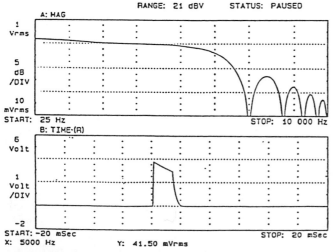

Figure 1–32. Frequency analysis of a stimulating pulse. *Bottom,* A capacitively coupled constant-voltage pacing pulse (about 1.8 V, leading edge) in the time domain. *Top,* A fast Fourier transformation of the same pulse in the frequency domain. (From Schaldach M [ed]: The stimulating electrode. *In* Electrotherapy of the Heart. Berlin, Springer-Verlag, 1992, p 153.)

electrode (R_w), is usually a significant value, typically in the range of 50 to 150 Ω. The resistance of the conductor wire leading to the anode (R_w) may be significant, as for a bipolar lead (typically, 50 to 150 ω), or may be insignificant, as for a unipolar pacing system, approaching zero. The resistance of the tissue (R_t) can vary, depending on the electrode spacing. It will be relatively low for a bipolar lead (about 50 Ω) but significantly higher for a unipolar system (about 150 Ω). The resistance of the electrode–tissue interface depends on the geometric surface area of the electrodes. Because efficient cathodes are relatively small, the resistance at the cathode–tissue interface (R_c) can be relatively high (e.g., roughly 250 Ω for an 8-mm² hemispheric electrode), whereas that of the anode (R_a) should be much less (e.g., 100 Ω for a bipolar lead and <5 Ω for a unipolar pacemaker).

When the pacing pulse is turned on, several events occur almost immediately. Unless the electrode is a perfect capacitor, electrochemical reactions must occur at the electrode surface–electrolyte interface for charge to be transferred from an electronic to an ionic medium. As the stimulus is initiated, the majority of carriers, such as Na^+ and Cl^-, rapidly conduct charge away from the interface. This is observed as the initial fast rise or leading edge (l_e) of the pulse wavefom, where $R = V_{le}/I_{le}$, as shown in Figure 1–34. The leading edge resistance at the cathode is R_c in Figure 1–34, and that at the anode is R_a. Sometimes, this leading edge resistance is referred to as *ohmic polarization.*

Electrode Capacitance

When a metal is placed in an electrolyte solution, a potential is developed at the electrolyte–metal interface. This can be observed by placing a pacing lead in a saline-filled beaker. If the electrode is tapped against the glass, surprisingly large voltage spikes can be seen on an oscilloscope connected to the lead terminal and a reference electrode in the beaker. In 1879, Helmholtz suggested that a layer of ions exists on the surface of an electrode that is surrounded by a layer of oppositely charged ions in the solution.[160] This theory is theromodynamically inadequate, however, so the diffuse double layer was proposed by Stern in 1924.[159, 161] A more recent model of the double layer was described by Devanathan and colleagues.[161] In this model, a layer of water molecules adsorbs to the surface of the electrode. A second layer is formed of hydrated ions and more water (Fig. 1–35). In physiologic electrolytes, these ions include Na^+ and Cl^- in major concentrations *(majority carriers)*. Other ions present in lower concentrations *(minority carriers)* include hydronium (H_3O^+), hydroxyl (OH^-), and phosphate ($HPO_4^=$). These layers have relatively high dielectric constants and form an interface that behaves electrically like a capacitor (C_c and C_a in Fig. 1–33). Thus, the commonly used and simplified model of pacing impedance (Z_p) includes a capacitor and resistor in parallel, both in series with resistances.

Electrode Polarization

When the pulse is turned on, majority carriers are rapidly depleted near the electrode surface. Minority carriers must then carry charge across the capacitive double layer. Because the minority carriers are also rapidly depleted, more ions

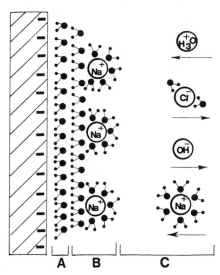

Figure 1–35. Hypothesized structure of the double layer at an uncharged *(left)* and charged *(right)* cathodic electrode interface. Region A contains a layer of surface hydration. Region B contains a second, more loosely held hydration layer with hydrated ions. Based on electrostatic considerations, layer B has a high dielectric constant, approaching that of pure water. It has a thickness of less than 10Å. Region C is bulk solution. (From Stokes K, Bornzin G: The electrode–biointerface (stimulation). *In* Barold S [ed]: Modern Cardiac Pacing. Mt. Kisco, NY, Futura, pp 33–78.)

must diffuse into the region from relatively remote areas.[162] As pulse duration increases, the voltage required to push current past the capacitive barrier also increases. This phenomenon is presented in schematic form in Figure 1–35 and in graphic form in Figure 1–36. Because the voltage rise is dependent on the concentration of majority and minority carriers, this phenomenon is known as *concentration polarization* (CP). Mindt and Schaldach reported that the magnitude of CP may be as large as 5 to 20 F/cm² for polished electrodes.[163]

As a result of concentration polarization, there are local accumulations and depletions of ionic species, such as H_3O^+, OH^-, Cl^-, Na^+ and so on, which are slightly separated from their counter-ions. A large force (voltage) is required to separate ions slightly without precipitation. Thus, a significant increase in potential (termed *overvoltage*) can occur that is a function of pulse duration during a CI pulse. When the pulse is turned off, the ohmic polarization instantaneously disappears, as shown by a trailing edge drop equal in magnitude to the leading edge of the pulse. A slow decay of potential occurs, as shown in Figures 1–34 and 1–36. This slow decay is the result of the diffusion of the polarized ions back to electroneutrality.

Optimizing Impedance

The effects of impedance on the pacing system are significant. On the positive side, high impedance reduces current drain from the battery, increasing its longevity. From this standpoint, the higher the pacing impedance, the better. On the negative side, electrode polarization during the pulse contributes nothing to stimulation. More potential must be

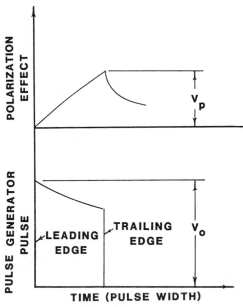

Figure 1–34. The effect of polarization *(upper diagram)* has been seperated from the capacitively coupled constant-voltage pacing pulse *(lower diagram)* to help clarify the electrical manifestation of electrode polarization. At the leading edge of the pulse, polarization is essentially zero. With time (pulse duration) the voltage due to polarization (sometimes called *polarization overvoltage*, V_p) increases. When the pacing pulse is shut off, polarization overvoltage decays exponentially as a result of diffusion. (From Stokes K, Bornzin G: The electrode–biointerface [stimulation]. *In* Barold S [ed]: Modern Cardiac Pacing. Mt. Kisco, NY, Futura, pp 33–78.)

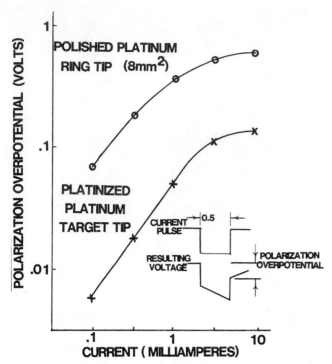

Figure 1–36. Polarization as a function of applied current was studied using an 8-mm² platinized Target Tip electrode and an 8-mm² polished platinum ring-tip in 0.18% saline solution. Polarization overvoltage was defined as shown in the lower right inset. (From Stokes K, Bornzin G: The electrode–biointerface (stimulation). *In* Barold S [ed]: Modern Cardiac Pacing. Mt. Kisco, NY, Futura, pp 33–78.)

applied to overcome the effects of polarization, raising the measured stimulation threshold. In addition, the afterpotential resulting from electrode polarization can interfere with sensing. Therefore, the ideal pulse would have no polarization and would be all resistance. The way the resistance is distributed in the system, however, can also have markedly different effects, making the stimulating pulse either efficient or inefficient with an unnecessarily higher threshold and a lower safety factor. To clarify these issues, we need to examine the electrode–tissue interface impedance and conduction losses.

Optimum Impedance at the Electrode–Tissue Interface

The resistance (ohmic polarization) of the stimulating electrode is inversely and exponentially proportional to the size of the electrode and the temperature and conductivity of the tissue.[164, 165] For all practical purposes, we can assume that in vivo temperature and conductivity are essentially constant. Therefore, maximizing the resistance may be accomplished simply by decreasing the geometric surface area of the electrode, as illustrated in Figure 1–37. A simple size reduction alone, however, has the negative effect of increasing polarization impedance. Thus, the way in which electrode size is reduced is critically important.

Electrode polarization is represented mathematically as the capacitive reactance (equation 24). At any given fre-

quency, therefore, the ideal electrode has very high capacitance, so that the reactance (polarization) approaches zero. For a given electrode material (as a first approximation), capacitive (C) is essentially a function of the interfacial surface area (A_i):

$$(26) \quad C = \frac{eA_i}{d},$$

where e is the dielectric constant of the double layer and d is its thickness. Because e and d are essentially constants in vivo, the capacitance of the electrode varies as a function of the surface area of its interface (A_i). How does one change a very large surface area into a small geometric volume? Initially, this was accomplished by making the electrodes porous.[90–93] Microporous electrodes, such as activated carbon or platinized platinum, have even higher real surface area.[67, 99, 116] This is equivalent to taking a large sheet of paper and crumpling it into a small ball. Thus, we find that the polarization overvoltage of polished electrodes is greater than that of porous, which is greater than that of microporous electrodes because the capacitance of microporous surfaces is greater than that of porous surfaces and still greater than that of polished surfaces.

Another approach to the problem of decreasing polarization is to use a material that supplies its own majority charge carriers. An example is the silver–silver chloride electrode in chloride solution. The majority carrier, in this case chloride, cannot be depleted. Chloride evolves at the cathode and is formed at the anode. Thus, voltage across the electrode interface has a waveshape essentially identical to that of the applied constant current, and the electrode is said to be nonpolarizing. Unfortunately, there does not appear to be a suitable nonpolarizing (charge carrier–supplying) electrode material available for permanent implantation. Silver–silver chloride electrodes, for example, are not used for permanent pacing because the anode erodes and the AgCl eventually dissolves from the cathode.[153, 167] Thus, the ideal, practical

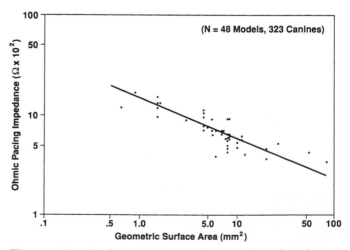

Figure 1–37. Leading edge ohmic polarization or electrode resistance of chronic (12 weeks' postimplantation) canine ventricular leads measured with a Medtronic model 5311 PSA as a function of the unipolar cathode's geometric surface area. Each data point is a population of canines testing one lead design. The study includes 323 animals and 48 lead models.

stimulating electrode is made of a corrosion-resistant, biocompatible material, with small geometric size and very high interfacial surface area, thereby affording very high capacitance.

Conductor Resistance and Conduction Losses

A simple and commonly used method of increasing the system impedance without adding electrode polarization is to use higher-resistance lead conductors. On the positive side, this reduces current drain from the battery. However, increasing resistance in the wire also increases the stimulation threshold and reduces the safety factor. Based on Kirchoff's law, the current in a circuit (assuming 100% efficiency) must be the same at every point at any given instant. Therefore, based on Ohm's law, the voltage must be divided at points in the circuit, proportional to the resistance. When we use the word *voltage*, we really mean a potential *difference* between the cathode relative to the anode. A pulse generator programmed to deliver a 5 V output pulse really develops a 5 V potential at the cathode, relative to the anode. That being the case, the voltage available at the stimulating cathode must be less than the generator is actually programmed to deliver by an amount that is proportional to the resistance of the conductor wire (R_{cw}). The voltage divider principle as applied to the cathode of a pacemaker system can be reduced to the following:

$$(27) \quad V_c = V_o \left(1 - \frac{R_w}{Z_p} \right),$$

where V_c is the voltage at the cathode, V_o is the voltage output of the pulse generator, R_w is the resistance of the conductor wire, and Z_p is the total pacing impedance.[168] If the total pacing impedance in a hypothetical unipolar pacemaker circuit is 500 Ω and the resistance of the conductor to the cathode (R_w) is zero, then the potential between the cathode surface and unipolar anode (the pulse generator can) is the same as the output voltage of the pulse generator. If the conductor resistance is 150 Ω and all else in the circuit is held constant, the total impedance increases to 650 Ω. This reduces current drain, prolonging longevity of the pulse generator battery, compared with the 500 Ω system. It also reduces the voltage available at the cathode surface by 150/650, or 23%. Thus, if the clinician sets the pulse generator output pulse at 5 V, in reality only 3.8 V is produced between the electrodes in contact with the heart. In this case, the safety factor may be less than the clinician believes.

Voltage division also affects stimulation threshold. Again, consider the hypothetical unipolar pacemaker in which the resistance of the conductor wire joining the pulse generator to the stimulating electrode is zero, the total impedance is 500 Ω, and the stimulation threshold is 1 V. If the conductor resistance is increased to 150 Ω, thereby increasing the total pacing impedance to 650 Ω, the measured threshold would increase by 30% (1.3 V). At first, this may not seem significant. In some situations, however, it could cause the clinician to program to higher outputs, resulting in unnecessarily higher current drains and reduced battery longevity. If one accepts the current density theory of pacing or uses a CI generator, the effect of the conductor wire resistance cannot be dismissed. The resistance in a conductor causes some of the current to be wasted as heat. This is expressed as the power (P) loss, which is expressed by the following:

$$(28) \quad P = I^2 R.$$

The energy (E) wasted as heat due to conductor resistance is as follows:

$$(29) \quad E = Pt,$$

where t is the time that the pulse is applied (the pulse duration). In fact, these equations give exactly the same percentage losses as voltage divison.[155] Therefore, regardless of how one views the basic mechanism of myocardial stimulation, increased resistance in the lead conductor represents a waste of energy. Thus, it is clear that although high pacing impedance may be desirable, impedence should be maximized at the electrode–tissue interface, not as resistance in the lead conductors. The ideal lead has as low as practical resistance in its conductors. It does not matter whether the system is unipolar or bipolar, the principles are the same.

■ PHARMACOLOGIC EFFECTS ON CARDIAC STIMULATION

Antiarrhythmic Drugs

Several types of antiarrhythmic drugs have been demonstrated to increase stimulation thresholds in both humans and animals. Type 1 drugs decrease Na^+ conductance and decrease the rate of rise of the action potential. Thus, it should be no surprise that these agents may increase the threshold for pacing. Type 1A drugs, such as quinidine[169] and procainamide,[170] may result in increased thresholds, especially when administered in high doses.[171] Type 1C drugs, such as encainide, flecainide, and propafenone, have been associated with increased pacing thresholds.[172–176] The increase in stimulation threshold with these drugs has been demonstrated to correlate with the change in QRS duration. In addition to the type 1 agents, propranolol has been demonstrated to result in an increase in pacing threshold when administered intravenously.[177] Amiodarone, lidocaine, tocainide, and verapamil have been reported to have minimal effects on pacing threshold, although we have seen one patient with congenital heart disease in whom amiodarone reproducibly increased the pacing threshold to the point of exit block.[165]

■ METABOLIC EFFECTS ON CARDIAC STIMULATION

Stimulation thresholds may rise during sleeping or eating, factors associated with withdrawal of sympathetic tone and increased vagal tone.[170, 178] In contrast, factors associated with increased sympathetic tone, such as exercise or assumption of the upright posture, are associated with a decrease in threshold. The myocardial stimulation threshold is increased by several metabolic abnormalities, including hypoxemia, hypercarbia, metabolic alkalosis, and metabolic acidosis. Hughes and colleagues noted an increase in pacing threshold of more than 70% by either metabolic acidosis or alkalosis.[179] In the presence of respiratory or cardiac arrest, the pacing threshold may increase by well more than 100%, resulting in loss of capture despite the use of a conventional safety margin. Because of this observation, antitachycardia pacing devices, such as pacemakers and implantable cardioverter-defibrillators, are often designed to deliver high-intensity stimuli during antitachycardia pacing or after a high-energy shock. In patients undergoing implantation of a cardioverter-defibrillator, Khastgir and colleagues were unable to demonstrate an increase in pacing threshold 10 and 60 seconds after defibrillation.[180] Ventricular fibrillation was electrically induced, however, and defibrillation was promptly performed under controlled circumstances in this study.

In the presence of a primary respiratory arrest, pacing stimuli may not capture the myocardium until adequate ventilation and pH balance are restored. Thus, careful attention to respiration and pH must be maintained during anesthesia in patients with implanted pacemakers to ensure continued myocardial capture. Ischemia produces variable effects on stimulation threshold, depending on the location of pacing electrode relative to the ischemic myocardium. In the presence of acute myocardial ischemia, the resting membrane potential decreases (cells become partially depolarized), the action potential upstroke velocity decreases, and the action potential duration dramatically shortens. In the presence of metabolic blockade with 2,4-dinitrophenol, Delmar noted an upward shift in the strength–duration curve, indicating an increase in the current required for capture at all pulse durations.[181] Thus, if the stimulating electrode is located in an ischemic region, the stimulation threshold would be expected to increase. With further ischemia and infarction, the myocardial threshold may rise dramatically. This may be seen clinically in patients who develop an acute inferior myocardial infarction with right ventricular infarction in whom a previously implanted pacemaker may suddenly lose capture. If the stimulating electrode is located in a nonischemic region (such as the right ventricle), however, activation of the the sympathetic nervous system may reduce the pacing threshold.

Hyperkalemia has been shown to increase the stimulation threshold when the serum K^+ concentration exceeds 7 mEq/L.[182, 183] In contrast, in the presence of hypokalemia, intravenous K^+ may decrease the pacing threshold and restore capture of a subthreshold pulse.[184] In addition, the reduced excitability during hyperkalemia can be corrected by the intravenous administration of calcium.[185] Hyperglycemia in the range of 600 mg/dL may increase stimulation thresholds by as much as 60%.[186] Thus, patients with diabetes or renal failure, conditions associated with the potential for altered glucose metabolism and electrolyte abnormalities, may need a larger safety margin than other patients. Hypothyroidism has also been demonstrated to increase pacing thresholds, an effect that is reversible with thyroxine replacement.[187, 188] As stated previously, glucocorticosteroids have been shown to decrease stimulation thresholds and have been used to treat exit block acutely and chronically.[189] Endogenous and synthetic catecholamines are effective in lowering pacing thresholds.[190, 191] The effect of intravenous epinephrine and isoproterenol is to decrease stimulation threshold initially, followed by an increase. Intravenous and sublingual isoproterenol have been demonstrated to reverse high pacing thresholds related to antiarrhythmic drug toxicity.[192]

■ CALCULATING BATTERY LONGEVITY AND PROGRAMMING GENERATORS FOR OPTIMUM PERFORMANCE

A pacemaker battery is a source of electric charge (measured in coulombs). Current (measured in amperes) is the rate at which charge flows in a circuit, as follows:

$$(30) \quad 1 \text{ } Ampere = 1 \frac{Coulomb}{Second}$$

Pacemaker batteries are rated in terms of their quantity of charge (currrent × time) or in units of ampere-hours. The longevity (L) of the battery is the *deliverable* charge capacity (Q_c) divided by the rate at which charge is consumed, as follows:

$$(31) \quad \text{Longevity (yr)} = \frac{Q_c \times 10^6}{8760 \text{ (hr/yr)} \times (I_c + I_l)},$$

where I_c is the current drained by the pulse generator circuitry and I_l is the current drained through the lead to the patient.[155] Note that I_C and I_l are "continuous" measures of current, not the current per each pacing pulse. The current drained by the circuit is a function of the circuit design and is not programmable by the clinician. The deliverable battery capacity is also a fixed parameter and not clinically adjustable. Thus, the clinician has only one parameter that can be adjusted to affect battery longevity: the current being transmitted through the lead (I_l). The lead current is given as follows:

$$(32) \quad I_l = \frac{V^2_o T}{Z_p V_b CL \times 10^{-6}},$$

where V_o is the generator output voltage, t is the pulse duration, Z_p is the pacing impedance, V_b is the battery voltage, and CL is the cycle length (msec).[155] The pacing impedance and the battery voltage are also not clinically adjustable. Thus, the only parameters of the output pulse that the clinician may adjust to optimize battery longevity are V_o (amplitude in volts) and t (pulse duration in milliseconds). In addition, significant improvement in battery longevity can be made by decreasing the frequency that pacing pulses are delivered, such as by programming the upper and lower pacing rates, the AV delay, hysteresis, and pacing mode.

Adequate Margin of Safety

A pacemaker must be operated within a reasonable safety factor that ensures capture of the myocardium by the delivered pulse. Because the output pulse is a fixed value, the safety margin must change with spontaneous variation in stimulation threshold. We need to know, therefore, how much thresholds actually change in the acute to chronic period as well as chronically on an hour-to-hour and day-to-day basis. The safety factor (SF) for pacing has been defined as a function of the output voltage of the pulse generator (V_o) divided by the stimulation threshold voltage (V_{thr}), as follows:

$$(33) \quad SF = V_o / V_{thr}$$

Alternatively, we can think of safety factors as a percentage:

$$(34) \qquad SF = 100 \left(\frac{V_o - V_{thr}}{V_{thr}} \right).$$

Thus, if V_o is 2.5 V and V_{thr} is 1 V, the SF = 2.5:1 or 150%. Both of these indices are valid, although the simple ratio (equation 33) is easier to use. Many pulse generators are implanted at the factory preset for pulse amplitude and duration. Clinicians may set the pulse generator output pulse values higher at implantation, then measure the stimulation threshold about 6 weeks later. The chronic output pulse is then programmed based on these chronic results. Settings as low as 2.5 V and 0.5 msec at implantation appear to ensure capture for most adult patients with modern microporous, steroid-eluting leads, but higher values should be used with older technology leads. This is not necessarily the situation with children, who experience a higher rate of exit block because of their active inflammatory responses. Because of the unique inflammation-suppressing properties of steroid-eluting electrodes, these are indicated for pediatric pacing whenever possible.[116, 193, 194] The safety factors provided during the peak threshold phase are highest for steroid-eluting porous electrodes and lower for (in descending order) microporous electrodes, porous electrodes, and polished-tip electrodes, based on data represented in Figures 1–27 and 1–28. There may also be situations in which the patient's pacemaker must be set at the maximum output at implantation (e.g., if the patient will not be available for follow-up). In these cases, an acceptable balance of safety margin and battery longevity will be obtained with a setting of 2.5 V and 0.5 msec a steroid-eluting electrode, or a setting of up to 5 V and 0.5 msec with other leads.

Modern perception of the range of chronic circadian threshold variation is based mainly on the work of Sowton and associates[195] (published in the mid-1960s), Preston and coworkers[196] (the late 1960s), and Westerholm (1971).[197] The first two studies used CI generators and reported thresholds in terms of energy. Because the computed energy "thresholds" could have been a reflection of changes in impedance, the actual variation in voltage threshold cannot be determined from these studies. Westerholm, who reported both voltage and energy data, noted substantial circadian variation in both parameters. In all of these studies, the leads were primarily epi/myocardial with polished electrodes. These human data, however, may be of marginal relevance to modern CV generators and porous, steroid-eluting electrodes.

We have found no significant threshold changes in adult canines using modern chronic atrial or ventricular leads as a function of eating, sleeping, or exercise.[198] This finding is supported by Kadish and coauthors, who found no changes in chronic human pacing thresholds during a 24-hour period in four of five patients studied.[199] Although in one patient, threshold at 0.6 msec changed from 1 to 1.5 V between 3:00 and 6:00 PM, these investigators concluded that "ventricular pacing thresholds do not show substantial diurnal variability." Grendahl and Schaanning also found minimal variation in pacing threshold during the day, after meals, or during sleeping or physical activity.[200] Shepherd and colleagues reported a large, transient increase in stimulation threshold in a child during two successive summers that were presumed to be related to a summer cold.[201] The effects of

various drugs on thresholds have been reported, but neither the test protocols nor the results have been consistent.[202] Thus, there appears to be little in the literature to support the statistical validity of any particular safety factor.

On the basis of the earlier report of Preston and colleagues, Barold and associates suggested that V_o/V_{thr} must be at least 1.75 to ensure an adequate safety margin, assuming a 50% increase in energy at threshold throughout the day.[203] Ohm and colleagues studied threshold evolution as a function of implant duration for an 8-mm² polished platinum ring electrode and found that this lead had a peak threshold of 2.2 ± 0.75 V at 0.5 msec pulse duration 2 weeks after implantation.[204, 205] Assuming an output setting of 5 V and 0.5 msec pulse duration, the average patient had a V_o/V_{thr} of 2.3 during threshold peak. The 98th percentile patient (mean ± 2 standard deviations) had $5V/(2.2 + 2 \times 0.75 \text{ V})$ or about a 1.35 safety margin at peak threshold. To the best of our knowledge, exit block with that lead at an output setting to 5 V and 0.5 msec and 2 weeks after implantation was extremely rare. Therefore, it seems reasonable that even safety margins as low as 1.35 may be acceptable for many patients. Nonetheless, unusual and unpredictable situations may occur that justify higher values.[188] The presently accepted chronic safety factor is at least 2:1. This appears to be adequate for most patients. In patients who are highly dependent on a pacemaker, an even higher safety margin may be appropriate. In other patients, such as those who are not pacemaker dependent, values as low as 1.35:1 may be acceptable.

Programming Voltage Versus Pulse Width for Maximum Pulse Generator Longevity

A common clinical concern for programming of the pulse generator to optimize battery longevity relates to whether it is more useful to program the amplitude or the duration of the output pulse. Based on equation 32 and on examination of the strength–duration relationship, it is more efficient to reduce the voltage output of the pulse (V_o), because the current drain varies as the square of voltage. Figure 1–38

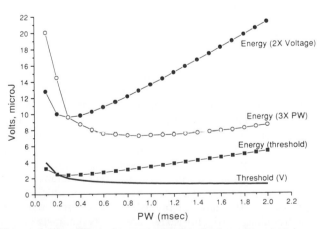

Figure 1–38. Effect of programming the stimulus voltage to twice threshold (at a constant pulse duration) or programming the pulse width to three times the threshold value (at the threshold voltage) on current drain and safety margin. See text for discussion.

illustrates the effect of doubling the threshold voltage (at a constant pulse width) or tripling the threshold pulse width (without changing voltage) on current drain. In this example, the rheobase voltage was determined to be 1 V and the chronaxie duration was 0.3 msec. The stimulation threshold was 4 V at a pulse duration of 0.1 msec or 2 V at 0.3 msec. Tripling the pulse duration at 4 V to 0.3 msec provides an adequate (2:1) safety margin with a current of 8 mA/pulse (4.8 μA continuous current) and a stimulus energy of 9.6 μJ. Similarly, doubling the threshold voltage at a pulse duration of 0.3 msec from 2 to 4 V gives an identical current drain (8 mA/pulse, or 4.8 μA) and safety factor. If the patient has a higher threshold, for example 2 V at 1 msec, doubling the voltage or tripling the pulse width would still give the same current drain (12 μA). The safety factor, however, would be significantly different. Tripling the pulse width would provide a marginal (at best) safety margin because theshold is approaching rheobase on the flat portion of the strength–duration curve. It is necessary to double the voltage in this case to ensure a 2:1 safety margin. The foremost consideration for programming voltage and pulse duration is patient safety.

Summary

Perhaps the most important concept for programming an implantable pacing system is a thorough understanding of the strength–duration relationship. Modern pulse generators allow the clinician to program both the pulse amplitude (in volts) and the pulse duration (in milliseconds). The stimulation threshold is a function of both these parameters. The exponential shape of the strength–duration curve must always be considered when programming the output pulse to ensure an adequate margin of safety between the delivered stimulus and the capture threshold. For example, pulse durations of 1 msec and greater are located on the flat portion of the strength–duration curve, whereas pulse durations of less than 0.15 msec are on the steeply rising portion of the curve. The practical importance of this can be appreciated by considering two points on the strength–duration curve shown in Figure 1–8. If the clinician determines the threshold to occur at point A (2 V and 0.5 msec) by decrementing the stimulus voltage at a constant-pulse duration, programming the pulse duration to 1 msec (point B) provides very little margin of safety. Similarly, if the threshold is measured to be at point C (3.5 V and 0.15 msec) by decrementing the pulse duration at a constant voltage, doubling the stimulation voltage to 7 V (point D) also provides a poor safety margin. When one considers the shape of the strength–duration curve, a more appropriate programmed setting would be provided by doubling the threshold voltage at a pulse duration of 0.5 msec (point E, 4 V and 0.5 msec). As a genral rule, if the threshold is determined by decrementing the stimulus voltage, an adequate margin of safety can be assumed by doubling the voltage if the pulse duration used was greater than 0.3 msec.

The two most important points on the strength–duration curve (rheobase and chronaxie) are easily estimated with modern pulse generators (see Fig. 1–8). Rheobase can be estimated by decrementing the output voltage at a pulse duration of 1.5 to 2 msec. Chronaxie can then be estimated by determining the threshold pulse duration at twice the rheobase voltage. If the threshold is determined by decrementing the pulse duration, an adequate safety margin can be assumed by tripling the pulse duration only if the threshold is 0.15 msec or less. If the rheobase and chronaxie are measured, doubling the threshold voltage at the chronaxie pulse duration provides an excellent method for programming a pacing system. Although programming the output of a pulse generator must first ensure patient safety, conservation of battery life is an important consideration. As a general rule, in the choice between decreasing pulse width or voltage, it is more energy efficient to reduce the voltage output of the pulse because the current drain varies as the square of voltage. As stated previously, doubling the pulse amplitude quadruples the current drain, whereas doubling the pulse width only doubles the current drain.

The clinician must also consider the acute to chronic evolution of the stimulation threshold when programming the pulse generator at the time of the implantation. Because there is typically an acute rise in threshold during the first several weeks after lead implantation, the voltage and pulse duration may need to be programmed to higher values than would be needed for chronic pacing. The physician is wise to re-evaluate the stimulation threshold after the acute rise (and subsequent fall) that may occur after implantation. For most patients, the pacing system can be programmed to chronic output settings at a follow-up evaluation about 6 weeks after lead implantation. Although these recommendations may not be applicable to patients receiving a steroid-eluting lead, a degree of caution is probably warranted. The importance of drug and electrolyte effects on the strength–duration curve should also be appreciated. For patients requiring antiarrhythmic drug therapy, the stimulation threshold should be measured after drug initiation to ensure an adequate margin of safety for pacing. Similarly, patients who are more likely to experience alterations in electrolyte concentration (such as patients with renal failure) may require that their pacemaker be programmed with a greater margin of safety. Perhaps most important, the degree that the heart is dependent on pacing to sustain life or prevent severe symptoms must be factored into the choice of a programmed margin of safety. For pacemaker-dependent patients, a pacing pulse that is at least 2.5 times the chronic capture threshold is generally recommended. In contrast, patients who are unlikely to experience severe symptoms should failure to capture occur may have their pacemaker programmed to a lower margin of safety (about two times threshold). The effect of pacing rate on the stimulation threshold should also be considered for patients requiring antitachycardia pacing. For patients requiring pacing rates in excess of 250 pbm, the pacing threshold should be measured at all rates likely to be used for antitachycardia pacing to ensure capture.

Modern implantable pulse generators use a CV output circuit. Because the current resulting from a CV pulse is inversely related to the pacing impedance, a high (conductor) resistance lead decreases the current drain on the pulse generator battery but also reduces the margin of safety. Thus, in the presence of very high resistance (such as a conductor fracture), the current and voltage between the electrodes decrease, often resulting in failure of the pulse to capture the myocardium. In contrast, in the presence of a lead insulation failure, the impedance of the pacing circuit decreases, resulting in an increase in the current and little change in the stimulation threshold (depending on the size of the breach versus the electrode size). Pacing impedance is determined by four factors: (1) resistance in the conductor wire, (2) polarization at the electrode–tissue interface, (3) resistance (or ohmic polarization) at the electrode–tissue interface, and (4) resistance of the tissues between the electrodes. The first two of these factors are energy inefficient, decreasing current available for stimulation, whereas the third factor decreases current drain without decreasing the efficiency of stimulation. Thus, the ideal electrode would have high resistance at the electrode–tissue interface but low resistance in the conductor wire and low polarization.

REFERENCES

1. Hodgkin AL, Huxley AF: A quantitative description of membrane current and its application to conduction and excitation in nerve. J Physiol (Lon) 117:500–544, 1952.
2. Corr PB: Contribution of lipid metabolites to arrhythmogenesis during early myocardial ischemia. In Rosen MR, Janse MJ, Wit AL (eds): Cardiac Electrophysiology: A Textbook. Mt. Kisco, NY, Futura 1990, pp 720–722.
3. Kleber AG: Sodium-potassium pumping. In Rosen MR, Janse MJ, Wit AL (eds): Cardiac Electrophysiology: A Textbook. Mt. Kisco, NY, Futura, 1990, pp 37–54.
4. Hodgkin AL, Katz B: The effect of sodium ions on the electrical activity of the giant axon of the squid. J Physiol (Lond) 108:37, 1949.
5. Bean RC: Protein-mediated mechanisms of variable ion conductance in thin lipid membranes. Membranes 2:409–477, 1973.
6. Haydon DA, Hladky SB: Ion transport across thin lipid membranes: A critical discussion of mechanisms in selected systems. Q Rev Biophys 5(2): 187–282, 1972.
7. Weidmann S: Passive properties of cardiac fibers. In Rosen MR, Janse MJ, Wit AL (eds): Cardiac Electrophysiology: A Textbook. Mt. Kisco, NY, Futura, 1990, 29–35.
8. Mobley BA, Page E: The surface of sheep cardiac Purkinje fibres. J Physiol (Lond) 220:547–563, 1972.
9. Metzger P, Weingart R: Electric current flow in cell pairs isolated from adult rat hearts. J Physiol (Lond) 366:1177–195, 1985.
10. Stewart JM, Page E: Improved steriological techniques for studying myocardial cell growth: Application to external sarcolemma, T system, and intercalated disks of rabbit and rat hearts. J Ultrastr Res 65:119–134, 1978.
11. Hofmann H: Interaction between a normoxic and a hypoxic region of guinea pig and ferret papillary muscles. Circ Res 56:876–883, 1985.
12. Kleber AG, Riegger CB, Janse MJ: Electrical uncoupling and increase of extracellular resistance after induction of ischemia in isolated, arterially perfused rabbit papillary muscle. Circ Res 61:271–279, 1987.
13. Neher E, Sakmann B, Steinbach JH: The extracellular patch clamp: Method for resolving currents through individual open channels in biological membranes. Plugers Arch Eur J Physiol 375:219, 1978.
14. Neher E, Sakmann B: The patch clamp technique. Sci Am 266(3): 44–51, 1992.
15. Ebihara L: The sodium current. In Rosen MR, Janse MJ, Wit AL (eds): Cardiac Electrophysiology: A Textbook. Mt. Kisco, NY, Futura, 1990, pp 63–74.
16. Hartcl HC, Duchatelle-Gourdon I: Structure and neural modulation of cardiac calcium channels. J Cardiovasc Electrophysiol 3:567–578, 1992.
17. Tsien RW: Calcium channels in the cardiovascular system. In Rosen MR, Janse MJ, Wit AL (eds): Cardiac Electrophysiology: A Textbook. Mt. Kisco, NY, Futura, 1990, pp 75–89.
18. Thomas RC: Electrogenic sodium pump in nerve and muscle cells. Physiol Rev 52:563–594, 1972.
19. Glitsch HG: Electrogenic Na pumping in the heart. Annu Rev Physiol 44:389–400, 1982.
20. Gadsky DC: The Na/K pump of cardiac cells. Annu Rev Biophys Bioeng 13:373–398, 1984.
21. Mullins IJ: The generation of electric currents in cardiac fibers by Na/Ca exchange. Am J Physiol 236:C103–110, 1979.
22. Hilgemann DW: Numerical approximations of sodium-calcium exchange. Prog Biophys Mol Biol 51:1–45, 1988.
23. Carmeliet E: The cardiac action potential. In Rosen MR, Janse MJ, Wit AL (eds): Cardiac Electrophysiology: A Textbook. Mt. Kisco, NY, Futura, 1990, pp 55–62.
24. Hoffman BF, Cranefield PF: Electrophysiology of the Heart. New York, McGraw-Hill, 1960.
25. Binah O: The transient outward current in the mammalian heart. In Rosen MR, Janse MJ, Wit AL (eds): Cardiac Electrophysiology: A Textbook. Mt. Kisco, NY, Futura, 1990, pp 93–106.
26. Joho RH: Toward a molecular understanding of voltage-gated potassium channels. J Cardiovasc Electrophysiol 3:589–601, 1992.
27. Coraboeuf E, Carmeliet E: Existence of two transient outward currents in sheep cardiac Purkinje fibers. Pflugers Arch 392:352–359, 1982.
28. Cohen IS, Datyner N: Repolarizing membrane currents. In Rosen MR, Janse MJ, Wit AL (eds): Cardiac Electrophysiology: A Textbook. Mount Kisco, NY, Futura, 1990, pp 107–116.
29. Bottazzi F: Leonardo as physiologist. In Leonardo da Vinci. London, Leisure Arts, 1964, pp 373–387.
30. Harvey W: De Motu Cordis. Translated by D. Whitteridge. The Movement of the Heart and Blood, Oxford, Blackwell, 1628.
31. Keith A, Flack M: The form and nature of the muscular connections between the primary divisions of the vertebrate heart. J Anat Physiol 41:172–189, 1907.
32. Irisawa H: Comparative physiology of the cardiac pacemaker mechanism. Physiol Rev 58:461–498, 1978.
33. DiFrancesco D: The hyperpolarization-activated current, I_f, and cardiac pacemaking. In Rosen, MR, Janse ML, Wit AL (eds): Cardiac Electrophysiology: A Textbook. Mount Kisco, NY, Futura, 1990, pp 117–132.
34. Urthaler F, Isobe JH, James TN: Comparative effects of glucagon on automaticity of the sinus node and atrioventricular junction. Am J Physiol 227:1415–1421, 1974.
35. Furman S, Parker B, Escher DJW: Decreasing electrode size and increasing efficiency of cardiac stimulation. J Surg Res 11:105, 1971.
36. Furman S, Hurzler P, Parker B: Clinical thresholds of endocardial cardiac stimulation: A long-term study. J Surg Res 19:149, 1975.
37. Angello DA, McAnulty JH, Dobbs J: Characterization of chronically implanted ventricular endocardial pacing leads. Am Heart J 107(6): 1142–1145, 1984.
38. Geddes LA, Bourland JD: The strength-duration curve. IEEE Trans Biomed Eng BME-32(6):458–459, 1985.
39. Irnich W: Considerations in electrode design for permanent pacing. In Thalen HJT (ed): Cardiac Pacing. Proceedings of the IVth International Symposium On Cardiac Pacing. Assen, The Netherlands, Van Gorcum, 1973, p 268.
40. Irnich W: Engineering concepts of pacemaker electrodes. In Schaldach M, Furman S (eds): Advances in Pacemaker Technology. New York, Springer-Verlag, 1975, p 241.
41. Bardou AL, Chenais J-M, Birkui PJ, et al: Directional variability of stimulation threshold measurements in isolated guinea pig cardiomyocytes: Relationship with orthogonal sequential defibrillating pulses. PACE 13:1590–1595, 1990.
42. Preston TA, Fletcher RD, Lucchesi BR, Judge RD: Changes in myocardial thresholds: Physiologic and pharmacologic factors in patients with implanted pacemakers. Am Heart J 74:235–242, 1967.
43. Katsumoto K, Niibori I, Takamatsu T, Kaibara M: Development of glassy carbon electrode (dead sea scroll) for low energy cardiac pacing. PACE 9 (6 P II):1220–1224, 1986.
44. Mond H, Stokes K, Helland J, et al: The porous titanium steroid eluting electrode: A double blind study assessing the stimulation threshold effects of steroid. PACE 11(2):214–219, 1988.
45. Hill WE, Murray A, Bourks JP, et al: Minimum energy for cardiac pacing. Clin Phys Physiol Meas 9(1):41–46, 1988.
46. Breivik K, Ohm O-J, Engedal H: Acute and chronic pulse-width thresholds in solid versus porous tip electrodes. PACE 5:650–657, 1982.
47. Irnich W: The chronaxie time and its practical importance. PACE 3:292–301, 1980.
48. Barold SS, Stokes KB, Byrd CL, McVenes R: Energy Parameters in cardiac pacing should be abandoned. PACE 20:112–121, 1996.
49. Dressler L, Gruse G, von Knorre GH, et al: The optimization of the pulse delivered by the pacemaker. PACE 2:282, 1979.
50. Chaptal AP, Ribot A: Statistical survey of strength-duration threshold curves with endocardial electrodes and long-term behavior of these

electrodes. IN Meere C (ed): Proceedings, VI World Symposium on Cardiac Pacing. Montreal, PACESYMP, 1979, p 21–2.

51. Hoorweg JL: Condensatorentladung und auseinandersetzung mit du Bois-Reymond. Pflugers Arch 52:87–108, 1892.

52. Weiss G: Sur la Possibilité de render comparable entre les appareils cervant à l'excitation électrique. Arch Ital Biol 35:413, 1901.

53. Lapique L: Definition experimentale de l'excitabilité. C R Soc Bil 67:280, 1909.

54. Lapique L: La Chronaxie et ses Applications Physiologiques. Paris, Hermann et Cie, 1938.

55. Nernst W: Zur theorie des elektrischen reizes. Pflugers Arch 122:275–314, 1908.

56. Ripart A, Mugica J: Electrode-heart interface: Definition of the ideal electrode. PACE 6(P II):410–421, 1983.

57. Irnich W: Elektrotherapie des Herzens. Berlin, Fachverlag Schiele & Schon, 1976.

58. Irnich W: The chronaxie time and its practical importance. PACE 3:292, 1980.

59. Bernstein AD, Parsonnet V: Implications of constant energy pacing. PACE 6(6):1229–1233, 1983.

60. Wedensky NE: Uber die Beziehungzwischen Reizung und erregung im Tetanus. St. Petersburg, Ber Akad Wiss, 54:96, 1887.

61. Langberg JJ, Sousa J, El-Atassi R, et al: The mechanism of pacing capture hysteresis in humans [Abstract]. PACE 15:577, 1992.

62. Hook BC, Perlman RL, Callans JD, et al: Acute and chronic cycle length dependent increase in ventricular pacing threshold. PACE 15:1437–1444, 1992.

63. Plumb VJ, Karp RB, James TN, Waldo AL: Atrial excitability and conduction during rapid atrial pacing. Circulation 63:1140–1149, 1981.

64. Buxton AE, Marchlinski FE, Miller JM, et al: The human atrial strength-interval relation: Influence of cycle length and procainamide. Circulation 79:271–280, 1989.

65. Katsumoto K, Niibori T, Watanabe Y: Rate dependent threshold changes during atrial pacing: Clinical and experimental studies. PACE 13:1009–1019, 1990.

66. Kay GN, Mulholland DH, Epstein AE, Plumb VJ: Effect of pacing rate on human atrial strength-duration curves. J Am Coll Cardiol 15(7): 1618–1623, 1990.

67. Stokes K, Bornzin G: The electrode–biointerface (stimulation). In Barold S (ed): Modern Cardiac Pacing. Mount Kisco, NY, Futura, 1985, pp 33–78.

68. Cornacchia O, Maresta A, Nigro P, et al: Effect of propafenone on chronic ventricular pacing threshold in patients with steroid-eluting (capture) and conventional leads. Eur J Cardiac Pacing Electrophysiol 2:A88, 1992.

69. Garberoglio B, Inguaggiato B, Chinaglia B, Cerise O: Initial results with an activated pyrolytic carbon tip electrode. PACE 6:440, 1982.

70. Jones JL, Jones RE, Balasky G: Improved cardiac cell excitation with symmetrical biphasic defibrillation waveforms. Am J Physiol 253:H1418–H1424, 1987.

71. Knisley SB, Smith WM, Ideker RE: Effect of intrastimulus polarity reversal on electric field stimulation thresholds in frog and rabbit myocardium. J Cardiovasc Electrophysiol 3:239–254, 1992.

72. Tse HF, Lau CP, Leung SK, et al: Single lead DDD system: A comparative evaluation of unipolar, bipolar and overlapping biphasic stimulation and the effects of right atrial floating electrode location on atrial pacing and sensing thresholds: PACE 19:1758–1763, 1996.

73. Mehra R, Furman S: Comparison of cathodal, anodal, and bipolar strength-interval curves with temporary and permanent pacing electrodes. Br Heart J 41:468–476, 1979.

74. Kay GN: Basic aspects of cardiac pacing. In Ellenbogen KA (ed): Cardiac Pacing. Cambridge, MA, Blackwell Scientific, 1992.

75. Preston TA: Anodal stimulation as a cause of pacemaker-induced ventricular fibrillation. Am Heart J 86:366–372, 1973.

76. Wiggers CJ, Wegria R, Pinera B: Effects of myocardial ischemia on fibrillation threshold: Mechanism of spontaneous ventricular fibrillation following coronary occlusion. Am J Physiol 131:309–316, 1940.

77. Mehra R, Furman S, Crump JF: Vulnerability of the mildly ischemic ventricle to cathodal, anodal and bipolar stimulation. Circ Res 41:159–166, 1977.

78. Bilitch M, Cosby RS, Cafferry EA: Ventricular fibrillation and competitive pacing. N Engl J Med 276:598–604, 1967.

79. Stokes K, Bird T, Taepke R: A new low threshold, high impedance microelectrode. In Antonioli GE, Reufeut AE, Ector H (eds): Pacemaker Leads. Amsterdam, Elsevier, 1991, pp 543–548.

80. Bird T, Stokes K: Ventricular electrode spacing and anode size [Abstract 205]. Revue Europeene De Technologie Biomedicale 3(12):63, 1990.

81. De Caprio V: Endocardial electrograms from transvenous pacemaker electrodes. Ph.D. Thesis (biomedical engineering), Polytechnic Institute of New York, 1977.

82. Saksena S, Prakash A, Hill M, et al: Prevention of atrial fibrillation with chronic dual-site right atrial pacing. J Am Coll Cardiol 28:687–694, 1996.

83. Moss AJ, Rivers RJ: Atrial pacing from the coronary vein: Ten-yer experience in 50 patietns with pervenous pacemakers. Circulation 57:103–106, 1978.

84. Bailin S, Adler S, Guidice H, et al: Bachmann's bundle pacing for the prevention of atrial fibrillation: Initial trends in a multi-center randomized prospective study. PACE 22(4, part II):727, 1999.

85. Daubert C, Ritter P, Cazeau S, et al: Permanent biventricular pacing in dilated cardiomyopathy: Is a totally endocardial approach technically feasible? PACE 19:699, 1996.

86. McVenes R, Stokes K: Alternative pacing sites: How the modern technology deals with this new challenge. In Antonioli GE (ed): Pacemaker Leads 1997. Bologna, Monduzi Editore, 1997, pp 223–228.

87. Ripart A, Fletcher R: Sensing. In Ellenbogen KA, Kay GN, Wilkoff B (eds): Clinical Cardiac Pacing. Philadelphia, WB Saunders, 1992.

88. Barold SS, Ong LS, Heinle RA: Stimulation and sensing thresholds for cardiac pacing: Electrophysiologic and technical aspects. Prog Cardiovasc Dis 24:1, 1981.

89. Smyth NPD, Tarjan PP, Chernoff E, et al: The significance of electrode surface area and stimulating thresholds in permanent cardiac pacing. J Thorac Cardiovasc Surg 71:559, 1976.

90. Parsonnet V, Zucker IR, Kannerstein ML: The fate of permanent intracardiac electrodes. J Surg Res 6:285, 1966.

91. Thalen HJTh, Van den Berg JW: Threshold measurements and electrodes of the cardiac pacemaker. Acta Pharmacol Nederl 14:227, 1966.

92. Akyurekli Y, Taichman GC, White DL, et al: Myocardial responses to sutureless epicardial lead pacing. In Meere C, (ed): Proceedings, VI World Symposium on Cardiac Pacing. Montreal, PACESYMP, 1979.

93. Irnich W: Personal communication.

94. Adamec R, Lasserre B, Simonet F, et al: Behaviour of epimyocardial stimulation threshold after heart pacemaker implantation using sutureless electrodes. In Meere C (ed): Proceedings, VI World Symposium on Cardiac Pacing, Montreal, PACESYMP, 1979.

95. Hughes H, Brownlee R, Tyres G: Failures of demand pacing with small surface area electrodes. Circulation 54:128, 1976.

96. Antonioli EG, Baggioni FG, Grassi G: Intracardiac electrogram parameters, electrode surface area and pacer input impedance: Their correlations. J Ital Cardiol 10(5):536–553, 1980.

97. Wilson GJ, MacGregor DC, Bobyn JD, et al: Tissue response to porous-surface electrodes: basis for a new atrial lead design. In Moore C (ed): Proceedings, VI World Symposium on Cardiac Pacing, PACESYMP, 1979.

98. Amundson D, McArthur W, MacCarter D, et al: Porous electrode-tissue interface. In Moore C (ed): Proceedings, VI World Symposium on Cardiac Pacing, PACESYMP, 1979.

99. Amundson DC, McArthur W, Moshaffafa M: The porous endocardial electrode. PACE 2:40, 1979.

100. MacGregor DC, Wilson GJ, Lixfeld W, et al: The porous surface electrode: A new concept in pacemaker lead design. J Thorac Cardiovasc Surg 78:281, 1979.

101. Breivik K, Ohm O-J, Engedahl H: Acute and chronic pulse-width thresholds in solid versus porous tip electrodes. PACE 5:650, 1982.

102. Berman ND, Dickson SE, Lipton IM: Acute and chronic clinical performance comparison of porous and solid electrode design. PACE 5:67, 1982.

103. Freud GE, Chinaglia B: Sintered platinum for cardiac pacing. Int J Artif Organs 4:238, 1981.

104. MacCarter DM, Lundberg KM, Corstjens JP: Porous electrodes: Concept, technology and results. PACE 6:427, 1983.

105. MacGregor DC, Pilliar RM, Wilson GJ, et al: Porous metal surfaces: A radical new concept in prosthetic heart valve design. Trans Am Soc Artif Intern Organs 22:646, 1976.

106. Elmqvist H, Schuller H, Richter G: The carbon tip electrode. PACE 6:436, 1983.

107. Bornzin GA, Stokes KB, Wiebusch WA: A low-threshold, low-polarization plantinized endocardial electrode [Abstract]. PACE 6:A-70, 1983.

108. Heineman F, et al: Clinical comparison of available "low threshold leads" [Abstract]. Proceedings, Xth Congress of European Soc Cardiol. Vienna, August 1988.

109. Beck-Jansen P, Schuller H, Winther-Rasmussen S: Vitreous carbon electrodes in endocardial pacing. *In* Meere C (ed): Proceedings, VI World Symposium on Cardiac Pacing. Montreal, PACESYMP, 1979, p 29–9.

110. Richter GJ, Weidlich E, Sturm FV, et al: Non-polarizable vitreous carbon pacing electrodes in animal experiments. *In* Meere C (ed): Proceedings, VI World Symposium on Cardiac Pacing. Montreal, PACESYMP, 1979.

111. Midel MG, Jones BR, Brinker JA: A comparison of platinized grooved electrode performance with ring-tip electrodes. PACE 12:752–756, 1989.

112. Stokes K: The effects of ventricular electrode surface area on pacemaker lead performance. *In* Adornato E, Galassi A: The '92 Scenario on Cardiac Pacing. Rome, Edizioni Luigi Pozzi, 1992, pp 505–514.

113. Stokes KB, Bird T, Gunderson B: The mythology of threshold variations as a function of electrode surface area. PACE 14(11):1748–1751, 1991.

114. Pearce JA, Bourland JD, Neilsen W, et al: Myocardial stimulation with ultrashort duration current pulses. PACE 5:52–58, 1982.

115. Meyers GH, Parsonnet V: Engineering in the Heart and Blood Vessels. New York, Wiley-Interscience, 1989.

116. Hurzeler P, Furman S, Escher DJW: Cardiac pacemaker current thresholds versus pulse duration. *In* Silverman HT, Miller IF, Salkind AJ (eds): Electrochemical Bioscience and Bioengineering. Princeton, NJ, Electrochemical Society, 1973, p 124.

117. Barold SS, Winner JA: Techniques and significance of threshold measurement for cardiac pacing. Chest 70:760, 1976.

118. Brownlee WC, Hirst R: Six years experience with atrial leads. PACE 9(6 P II):1239–1242, 1989.

119. Luceri RM, Furman S, Hurzeler P, et al: Threshold behavior of electrodes in long-term ventricular pacing. Am J Cardiol 40:184, 1977.

120. Mond H, Stokes K: The electrode–tissue interface: The revolutionary role of steroid elution. PACE 15(1): 95–107, 1992.

121. Ohm O-J, Breivik K: Pacing leads. *In* Gomez FP, et al (eds): Cardiac Pacing. Electrophysiology. Tachyarrhythmias. Madrid, Editorial Grouz, 1985, pp 971–985.

122. Hoff PI, Breivik K, Tronstad A, et al: A new steroid-eluting electrode for low-threshold pacing. *In* Gomez FP, et al (eds): Cardiac Pacing. Electrophysiology. Tachyarrhythmias. Mount Kisco, NY, Futura, 1985, pp 1014–1019.

123. Anderson JM: Inflammation, wound healing and foreign body response. *In* Biomaterial Science, An Introductory Text, Society for Biomaterials, San Diego, 1990.

124. Anderson JM: Inflammatory response to implants. ASAIO 11(2):101–107, 1988.

125. Henson PM: Mechanisms of exocytosis in phagocytic inflammatory cells. Am J Pathol 101:494–514, 1980.

126. Robinson TF, Cohen-Gould L, Factor SM: Skeletal framewok of mammalian heart muscle: Arrangement of inter- and pericellular connective tissue structures. Lab Invest 29(4), 482–498, 1983.

127. Preston TA, Judge RD: Alteration of pacemaker threshold by drug and physiologic factors. Ann N Y Acad Sci 167:686–692, 1969.

128. Stokes K, Anderson J: Low threshold leads: The effect of steroid elution. *In* Antonioli GE (ed): Pacemaker Leads. Amsterdam, Elsevier, 1991, pp 537–542.

129. Sibille Y, Reynolds HY: Macrophages and polymorphonuclear neutrophils in lung defense and injury. Am Rev Respir Dis 141:471–502, 1990.

130. Benditt DG, Kriett JS, Ryberg C, et al: Cellular electrophysiologic effects of dexamethasone sodium phosphate: Implications for cardiac stimulation with steroid-eluting electrodes. Int J Cardiol 22(1):67–73, 1989.

131. Stokes KB, Kriett JM, Gornick CA, et al: Low-threshold cardiac pacing electrodes. *In* Frontiers of Engineering in Health Care—1983. Proceedings, Fifth Annual Conference IEEE Engineering in Medicine and Biology Society, 1983.

132. Mond H, Sloman JG, Cowling R, et al: The small tined pacemaker lead: Absence of displacement. *In* Meere C (ed): Proceedings, VI World Symposium on Cardiac Pacing. Montreal, PACESYMP, 1979, p 29–5.

133. Baker JH, Shepard RB, Plimb VJ, Kay GN: Effects of fixation mechanism and electrode material on atrial stimulation threshold: Long-term evaluation in 338 patients [Abstract]. PACE 15:54, 1992.

134. Cornacchia D, Jacopi F, Fabbri M, et al: Comparison between active screw in and passive leads for permanent transvenous ventricular pacing [Abstract]. PACE 6:A56, 1983.

135. El Gamal M, Van Gelder L, Bonnier J, et al: Comparison of transvenous atrial electrodes employing active (helicoidal) and passive (tined J-lead) fixation in 116 patients [Abstract]. PACE 6:205, 1983.

136. Kay GN, Anderson K, Epstein AE, Plumb VJ: Active fixation atrial leads: Randomized comparison of two lead designs. PACE 12:1355–1361, 1989.

137. Rasor NS, Spickler JW, Clabaugh JW: Comparison of power sources for advanced pacemaker applications. *In* Proceedings, 7th Intersociety Energy Conversion Engineering Conference, Washington, DC. Amer Chem Cos 1972, 752.

138. Hirshorn MS, Holley LK, Hales JR, et al: Screening of solid and porous materials for pacemaker electrodes. PACE 4:380, 1981.

139. Schaldah M: New pacemaker electrodes. Trans Am Soc Artif Intern Organs 17:29, 1971.

140. Helland J, Stokes K: Nonfibrosing cardiac pacing electrode. US Patent 4033357, February 17, 1976.

141. Elmqvist H, Schuller H, Richter G: The carbon tip electrode. PACE 6:436, 1983.

142. Thuesen L, Jensen PJ, Vejby-Christensen H, et al: Lower chronic stimulation threshold in the carbon-tip than in the platinum-tip endocardial electrode: A randomized study. PACE 12:1592–1599, 1989.

143. Bornzin GA, Stokes KB, Wiebush WA: A low threshold, low polarization, platonized endocardial electrode. PACE 6:A-70, 1983.

144. Mugica J, Duconge B, Henry L, et al: Clinical experience with new leads. PACE 11:1745–1752, 1988.

145. Djordjevic M, Stojanov P, Velimirovic D, et al: Target lead-low threshold electrode. PACE 9:1206–1210, 1986.

146. Timmis GC, Helland J, Westveer DC, et al: The evolution of low threshold leads. Clin Prog Pacing Electrophysiol 1:313, 1983.

147. Stokes KB: Preliminary studies on a new steroid eluting epicardial electrode. PACE 11:1797–1803, 1988.

148. Hamilton R, Gow R, Bahoric B, et al: Steroid-eluting epicardial leads in pediatrics: Improve epicardial thresholds in the first year. PACE 14:2066, 1991.

149. Stokes K, Frohling G, Bird T, et al: A new bipolar low threshold steroid eluting screw-in lead. Eur J Cardiac Pacing Electrophysiol 2:A89, 1992.

150. Schwaab B, Frohling G, Schwerdt H, et al: Longterm follow-up of a bipolar steroid eluting pacing lead with active and passive fixation. *In* Antoniolo GE (ed): Pacemaker Leads 1997. Bologna, Monduzzi Editore, 1997, pp 361–364.

151. Schwaab B, Frohling G, Schwerdt H, et al: Long-term follow-up of three microporous active fixation leads in atrial position. *In* Antoniolo GE (ed): Pacemaker Leads 1997. Bologna, Monduzzi Editore, 1997, pp 365–368.

152. Schwaab B, Frohling G, Schwerdt H, et al: Atrial and ventricular pacing characteristics of a steroid eluting screw-in lead. *In* Antoniolo GE (ed): Pacemaker Leads 1997. Bologna, Monduzzi Editore, 1997, pp 383–388.

153. Stokes K, Frohlig G, Bird T, Hess D, Ruta R: A new bipolar low threshold steroid eluting screw-in lead [Abstract]. Eur JCPE 2(2):A89, 1992.

154. Brinker J, Crossley G, Hurd H, et al: Multicenter randomized controlled study of a new bipolar steroid eluting active fixation lead. PACE 16:946, 1993.

155. Crossley GH, Kay GN, Ferguson B, et al: Treatment of patients with prior exit block using a novel steroid eluting active fixation lead. PACE 17:870, 1994.

156. Brinker J, Crossley G, Reynolds D, et al: Chronic performance of a bipolar steroid eluting active fixation lead: A multicenter randomized trial. PACE 17:853, 1994.

157. Love C, Rumin H, Lundeen T, et al: Experience with a new endocardial screw-in lead in atrial and ventricular application (Pacesetter Model 1388T). PACE 20:1149, 1997.

158. Menozzi C: Comparison between latest generation steroid-eluting screw-in and tined leads: Long term follow-up. *In* Antoniolo GE (ed): Pacemaker Leads 1997. Bologna, Monduzzi Editore, 1997, pp 389–394.

159. Nurnberg JH, Schopper H, Busscher U, et al: Retrospective comparison of epicardial steroid-eluting and conventional leads for pacing after corrective surgery in congenital heart disease. PACE 20:1193, 1997.

160. Moor WJ: Physical Chemistry. Englewood Cliffs, NJ, Prentice-Hall, 1972, p 510.
161. Conway BE: Theory and Principles of Electrode Processes. New York, Ronald Press, 1965, p 33.
162. Kahn A, Greatbatch W: Physiologic electrodes. *In* Ray C (ed): Medical Engineering. Chicago, Year Book Medical, 1974, p 1073.
163. Mindt W, Schaldach M: Electrochemical aspects of pacing electrodes. *In* Schaldach M, Furman S (eds): Advances in Pacemaker Technology. New York, Springer-Verlag, 1975, p 297.
164. Lindemans FW, Denier van der Gon JJ: Current thresholds and luminal size in excitation of heart muscle. Cardiovasc Res 12:477, 1977.
165. Irnich W, Gebhardt U: The pacemaker-electrode combination and its relationship to service life. *In* Thalen HJTh (ed): To Pace or Not to Pace, Controversial Subjects in Cardiac Pacing. The Hague, Martin Nijhoff, 1978, p 209.
166. Piersma BJ, Calhoon SW Jr, Greatbatch W: Some comparisons of Pt and Ti physiological electrodes. *In* Silverman HT, Miller IF, Salkind AJ (eds): Electrochemical Bioscience and Bioengineering. Princeton, NJ, Electrochemical Society, 1973, p 133.
167. Greatbatch W: Metal electrodes in bioengineering. CRC Crit Rev Bioeng 5:1, 1981.
168. Stokes K, Bird T, Taepke R: High pacing impedance. Efficient or wasteful [Abstract 452]. PACE 14:730, 1991.
169. Wallace AG, Cline RE, Sealy WC, et al: Electrophysiologic effects of quinidine. Circ Res 19:960–969, 1966.
170. Gay RJ, Brown DF: Pacemaker failure due to procainamide toxicity. Am J Cardiol 34:728–731, 1974.
171. Moss AJ, Goldstein S: Clinical and pharmacological factors associated with pacemaker latency and incomplete pacemaker capture. Br Heart J 31:112, 1969.
172. Hellestrand KJ, Burnett PJ, Milne JR, et al: Effect of the antiarrhythmic agent flecainide acetate on acute and chronic pacing thresholds. PACE 6:892, 1983.
173. Salel AF, Seagren SC, Pool PE: Effects on encainide on the function of implanted pacemakers. PACE 12:1439, 1989.
174. Montefoschi N, Boccadamo R: Propafenone induced acute variation of chronic atrial pacing threshold. A case report. PACE 13:480–483, 1990.
175. Huang SK, Hedberg PS, Marcus FI: Effects of antiarrhythmic drugs on the chronic pacing threshold and the endocardial R wave amplitude in the conscious dog. PACE 9:660, 1986.
176. Bianconi L, Boccadamo R, Toscano S, et al: Effects of oral propafenone therapy on chronic myocardial pacing threshold. PACE 15:148–154, 1992.
177. Kubler W, Sowton E: Influence of beta-blockade on myocardial threshold in patients with pacemakers. Lancet 2:67, 1970.
178. Preston TA, Fletcher RD, Lucchesi BR, Judge RD: Changes in myocardial threshold: Physiologic and pharmacologic factors in patients with implanted pacemakers. Am Heart J 74:235, 1967.
179. Hughes HC, Tyers GFO, Torman HA: Effects of acid-base imbalance on myocardial pacing thresholds. J Thorac Cardiovasc Surg 69:743–752, 1975.
180. Khastgir T, Lattuca J, Aarons D, et al: Ventricular pacing threshold and time to capture postdefibrillation in patients undergoing implantable cardioverter-defibrillator implantation. PACE 14:768–772, 1991.
181. Delmar M: Role of potassium currents on cell excitability in cardiac ventricular myocytes. J Cardiovasc Electrophysiol 3:474–486, 1992.
182. Gettes LS, Shabetai R, Downs TA, et al: Effect of changes in potassium and calcium concentrations on diastolic threshold and strength-interval relationships of the human heart. Ann N Y Acad Sci 167:693–705, 1969.
183. Lee D, Greenspan K, Edmands RE, et al: The effect of electrolyte alteration on stimulus requirement of cardiac pacemakers. Circulation 38:124, 1968.
184. Walker WJ, Elkins JT, Wood LW, et al: Effect of potassium in restoring myocardial response to a subthreshold cardiac pacemaker. N Engl J Med 271:597, 1964.
185. Surawicz B, Chelbus H, Reeves JT, et al: Increase of ventricular excitability threshold by hyperpotassemia. JAMA 191:71–76, 1965.
186. Westerholm CJ: Threshold studies in transvenous cardiac pacemaker treatment. Scand J Thorac Cardiovasc Surg 8(Suppl):1, 1971.
187. Schlesinger Z, Rosenberg T, Stryjer D, et al: Exit block in myxedema, treated effectively by thyroid hormone replacement. PACE 3:737–739, 1980.
188. Basu D, Chatterjee K: Unusually high pacemaker threshold in severe myedema: Decrease with thyroid hormone therapy. Chest 70:677–679, 1976.
189. Nagatomo Y, Ogawa T, Kumagae H, et al: Pacing Failure due to markedly increased stimulation threshold 2 years after implantation: Successful management with oral prednisolone. A case report. PACE 12:1034–1037, 1989.
190. Haywood J, Wyman MG: Effects of isoproterenol, ephedrine, and potassium on artificial pacemaker failure. Circulation 32(Suppl II):110, 1965.
191. Katz A, Knilans TK, Evans JJ, Prystowsky EN: The effects of isoproterenol on excitability, supranormal excitability and conduction in the human ventricle (Abstract). PACE 14:710, 1991.
192. Levick CE, Mizgala HF, Kerr CR: Failure to pace following high dose anti-arrhythmic therapy: Reversal with isoproterenol. PACE 7:252–256, 1984.
193. Stokes KB, Church T: The elimination of exit block as a pacing complication using a transvenous steroid-eluting lead. Proceedings, VIII World Symposium on Cardiac Pacing and Electrophysiology. Jerusalem, 1987; and PACE. 10(3) Pt II: 748, (Abst. 475), 1987.
194. Till JA, Jones S, Rowland E, et al: Clinical experience with a steroid eluting lead in children [Abstract]. Circulation 80:389, 1989.
195. Sowton E, Norman J: Variations in cardiac stimulation thresholds in patients with pacing electrodes. Digest of the 7th International Conference on Medical and Biological Engineering. Stockholm, 1967.
196. Preston TA, Fletcher RD, Luchesi BR, et al: Changes in myocardial threshold: Physiologic and pharmacologic factors in patients with implanted pacemakers. Am Heart J 74:235–242, 1967.
197. Westerholm C-J: Threshold studies in transvenous cardiac pacemaker treatment. Scand J Thorac Surg Suppl 8 (Supl): 1–35, 1971.
198. McVenes R, Lahtinen S, Hansen N, Stokes K: Physiologic and drug induced changes in cardiac pacing and sensing parameters [Abstract 324]. Eur JCPE 2(2): A86, 1992.
199. Kadish A, Kong T, Goldberger J: Diurnal variability in ventricular stimulation threshold and electrogram amplitude [Abstract]. Eur JCPE 2(2):A86, 1992.
200. Grendahl H, Schaanning CG: Variations in pacing threshold. Acta Med Scand 187:75–78, 1970.
201. Shepherd R, Kim J, Colvin E, et al: Pacing threshold spikes months and years after implant [Abstract 308]. PACE 14:694, 1991.
202. Barold S: Effect of drugs on pacing thresholds. *In* Antonioli GE, et al (eds): Pacemaker Leads 1991. New York, Elsevier, 1991, pp 73–86.
203. Barold SS, Ong LS, Heinle RA: Stimulation and sensing thresholds for cardiac pacing: Electrophysiologic and technical aspects. Prog Cardiovasc Dis. 24:1, 1981.
204. Ohm O-J, Breivik K: Pacing leads. *In* Gomez FP, et al (eds): Cardiac Pacing. Electrophysiology Tachyarrhythmias. Madrid, Editorial Grouz, 1985, pp 971–985.
205. Hoff PI, Breivik K, Tronstad A, et al: A new steroid-eluting electrode for low-threshold pacing. *In* Gomez FP, et al (eds): Cardiac Pacing Electrophysiology. Tachyarrhythmias. Mount Kisco, NY, Futura, 1985, pp 1014–1019.
206. Creer MH, Dobmeyer DJ, Corr PB: Amphipathic lipid metabolites and arrhythmias during myocardial ischemia. *In* Zipes DP, Jalife J (eds): Cardiac Electrophysiology: From Cell to Bedside. Philadelphia, WB Saunders, 1990, pp 417–432.
207. Seeger W: A scanning electron microscopic study on explanted electrode tips. *In* Aubert AE, Ector H (eds): Pacemaker Leads. Amsterdam, Elsevier, 1985, pp 405–410.
208. Schaldach M: The stimulating electrode. *In* Schaldach M (ed): Electrotherapy of the Heart. Berlin, Springer-Verlag, 1992, p 153.
209. Stokes K, Anderson J: Low threshold leads: The effect of steroid elution. *In* Antonioli GE, Reufeut AE, Ector H (eds): Pacemaker Leads. Amsterdam, Elsevier, 1991, pp 537–542.

Principles of Defibrillation: Cellular Physiology to Fields and Waveforms

Gregory P. Walcott, Fiona Hunter, and Raymond E. Ideker

Electrical defibrillation is the only practical means for halting ventricular fibrillation. Although it has been known for more than a century that application of an electric shock directly to the myocardium causes ventricular fibrillation and that the heart can be returned to normal rhythm by subsequent application of a shock of greater magnitude,[1–3] our knowledge of the mechanisms underlying the process of defibrillation was slow in developing. It was only with the relatively recent introduction of novel techniques for the analysis of action potentials and activation sequences[4–8] that greater insight into the physiology of both fibrillation and defibrillation has been achieved. It is hoped that this insight will result in a higher success rate for external defibrillation and improved design of implantable cardioverter-defibrillators.

A large part of current research is dedicated to determining the underlying reason for the success or failure of a defibrillating shock. Ventricular fibrillation is maintained by multiple activation fronts that are constantly moving in a pattern of re-entry. Characteristics of the activation pattern and action potential are thought to be important determinants of whether a shock will successfully defibrillate the heart. A successful defibrillating shock is thought to extinguish most of these activation fronts, permitting the resumption of coordinated responsiveness.[9–13] For the defibrillating shock to be completely successful, this must be accomplished without creating an environment that promotes susceptibility to reinitiation of fibrillation.[12, 13] It has been established that the *distribution* of the potential gradient created by the defibrillation shock is of great importance and that a minimum potential gradient throughout the ventricular myocardium is required for successful defibrillation.[14–16]

Fundamentally, defibrillation is thought to be realized through an electrical pulse causing an alteration in the transmembrane potential of the myocyte. It most likely requires a rapid induction of changes in the transmembrane potential of the myocytes in a critical mass of myocardium (75% to 90% of the myocardium in dogs).[11, 14, 16] Because this represents a large mass of tissue, depolarization must be achieved at a considerable distance from the stimulating electrode. To gain an understanding of this complex far-field process, various mathematical models have been generated, and the predictions of computer simulations have been compared with physiologic findings. Both discontinuities in the anisotropic properties of the extracellular and intracellular domains, as described by the bidomain model,[17, 18] and highly resistive discontinuities in the intracellular space (e.g., collagenous septae), as described in the secondary source model,[19–21] may contribute to the far-field changes in the potential gradient that halt the activation fronts of fibrillation.

The mechanisms underlying degeneration into fibrillation in failed shocks remain incompletely understood. Residual wandering wavelets,[22] nonuniform refractoriness,[23] and areas of low potential gradient in which critical points form[15] may be the sources of propagating wavefronts that can incur fibrillation through re-entry. Centrifugal propagation from ectopic foci induced by the defibrillation shock may also play a role, especially in the atrium.[13]

In this chapter, we expand on the subjects mentioned previously. We discuss some of the characteristics of ventricular fibrillation that are thought to be important to understanding defibrillation and some of the characteristics of shocks that lead to successful defibrillation, such as waveform shape and electrode configuration. We then trace a shock from its origin at the defibrillation electrodes to how it is distributed through the heart, to how it affects the transmembrane potential, and finally to how it leads to the successful cessation of fibrillation.

■ FIBRILLATION

To understand defibrillation, it is necessary to have an understanding of fibrillation. Knowing the basic characteristics of ventricular fibrillation and whether it is maintained by re-entrant or focal activity, as well as knowing the characteristics of the action potential and the excitability of the fibrillating tissue, helps to define the therapy that will be successful in stopping the arrhythmia.

Ventricular fibrillation has been characterized as progressing through four stages based on high-speed cinematography of electrically induced fibrillation in dog hearts[24] (Fig. 2–1). A brief *undulatory,* or tachysystolic, stage of only 1 to 2 seconds' duration occurs first. It is characterized by three to six undulatory contractions that resemble a series of closely occurring systoles and involve the sequential contraction of large areas of the myocardium. This is followed by a second stage of *convulsive incoordination,* in which more frequent waves of contraction sweep over smaller regions of the myocardium. Because the contractions in each region are not in phase, the ventricles are pulled around in a convulsive manner. It is during this stage of fibrillation that the implantable cardioverter-defibrillator shocks are given—10 to 20 seconds after the onset of fibrillation. In the third stage of *tremulous incoordination,* the independently contracting areas of the ventricular surface become even smaller, giving the heart a tremulous appearance. Tremulous incoordination lasts for 2 to 4 minutes before the fourth and final stage of *atonic fibrillation* occurs. Atonic fibrillation develops within 2 to 5 minutes after the onset of fibrillation and is characterized by the slow passage of feeble contraction wavelets over short distances. With time, the number of quiescent areas increases. Ischemia plays a role in the development of the third and fourth stages because the fibrillating heart remains in the second stage if the coronary arteries are perfused with oxygenated blood.[25, 26] Ventricular fibrillation resolves spontaneously if less than a critical mass of the myocardium is involved (about 25% of the myocardium in dogs).[27]

Driving the mechanical activity of the heart during fibrillation is the electrical activity of the myocardium. The electrical activity of the heart during fibrillation has been studied using both extracellular and optical recordings. Several groups have suggested that fibrillation is maintained by re-entry. In most cases, re-entry appears to be caused by "wandering wavelets" of activation, in which activation fronts follow continually changing pathways from cycle to cycle. In some studies, the activation sequence appears moderately repeatable from cycle to cycle, following approximately the same pathway.[28, 29] Occasionally, a spiraling pattern of functional re-entry emanates from the same region for several cycles. Sometimes, the central core of these spiral waves can meander across the heart.[8] At other times, new re-entrant activation fronts are generated when one front interacts with another during its vulnerable period.

Knowing that the arrhythmia is maintained by re-entry suggests that the way to halt the arrhythmia is by causing wavefronts to collide and extinguish each other, either by exciting tissue in front of wavefronts to cause collisions and wavefront block or by exciting tissue at the core of the spiral wave to extinguish these waves.

Several classification schemes for atrial fibrillation have been developed. On the basis of the characteristics of the complexes in bipolar atrial electrocardiograms from patients in atrial fibrillation, Wells and associates[30] divided atrial fibrillation into four types (Fig. 2–2). Type I atrial fibrillation is characterized by atrial electrograms that show discrete complexes of variable morphologies separated by an isoelectric baseline free of perturbation (see Fig. 2–2). Type II atrial fibrillation is characterized by discrete beat-to-beat atrial electrogram complexes of variable morphology but without an isoelectric baseline. Type III atrial fibrillation is characterized by atrial electrograms that demonstrate neither discrete complexes nor isoelectric intervals. Type IV atrial fibrillation is characterized by atrial electrograms consistent with type III atrial fibrillation, alternating with periods of atrial electrograms consistent with type I atrial fibrillation and occasionally type II atrial fibrillation. In contrast to the stages of ventricular fibrillation described previously, these types of atrial fibrillation do not represent stages in the progression of fibrillation in that one type does not necessarily progress to the next type. Any one of the types of patterns can be observed initially, and the pattern of atrial fibrillation can change from a more organized type to a less organized type, or vice versa. Using high-resolution mapping, Konings and colleagues[31] determined that there was a wide spectrum of complexity of the activation patterns observed during atrial fibrillation in humans. Classification according to criteria of complexity indicated three types of atrial fibrillation, each of which was associated with a different average fibrillation PP interval (174, 150, 136 msec, respectively).[32] Activation characterized by broad wavefronts that propagate rapidly and without significant conduction delay was classified as type 1 atrial fibrillation. Delayed conduction and intra-atrial conduction blocks resulting in a more complex pattern was classified as type II atrial fibrillation. A highly complex pattern of activation involving three or more wavelets and frequent re-entry was classified as type III atrial fibrillation.

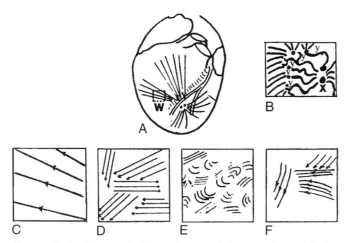

Figure 2–1. Diagrams indicating the spread of waves observed in the analysis of motion pictures during the four stages of fibrillation described by Wiggers. *A,* Spread of wavefront during initial, undulatory stage. *B,* Theoretical passage of impulses from point *x* to form a wave front at *y.* *C* through *F,* Appearance of contraction waves in small rectangular area W, magnified. *C,* Undulatory stage. *D,* Convulsive stage. *E,* Tremulous stage. *F,* Atonic stage. (From Wiggers CJ: Studies of ventricular fibrillation caused by electric shock: Cinematographic and electrocardiographic observations of the natural process in the dog's heart: Its inhibition by potassium and the revival of coordinated beats by calcium. Am Heart J 5:351–365, 1930.)

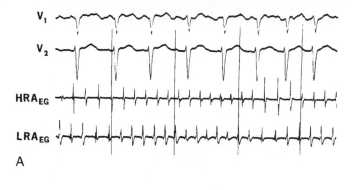

A

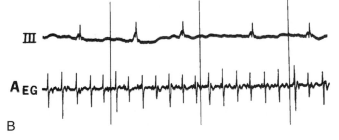

B

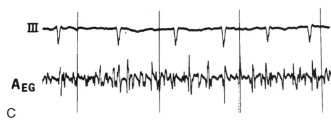

C

Figure 2–2. The four types of atrial fibrillation described by Wells and colleagues. *A,* ECG leads V1 and V2 recorded simultaneously with a filtered (12–500 Hz) bipolar atrial electrogram from the high right atrium (HRA$_{EG}$) and from the low right atrium (LRA$_{EG}$) during type I atrial fibrillation. Lead V1 shows a coarse atrial fibrillation pattern. The relative timing of the two atrial electrograms is sequential and not simultaneous. *B* to *D,* ECG lead III recorded simultaneously with a bipolar atrial electrogram (A$_{EG}$). *B,* Type II atrial fibrillation. *C,* Type III atrial fibrillation. *D,* Type IV atrial fibrillation. Note the change in pattern from an initial type III to a type I. (From Wells JL Jr, Karp RB, Kouchoukos NT, et al: Characterization of atrial fibrillation in man: Studies following open heart surgery. PACE 1:426–438, 1978.)

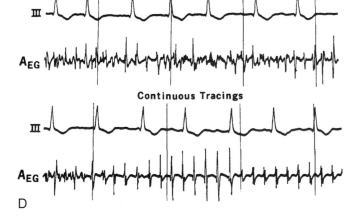

Continuous Tracings

D

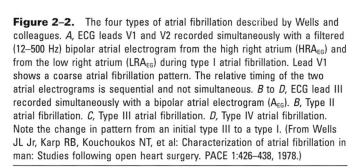

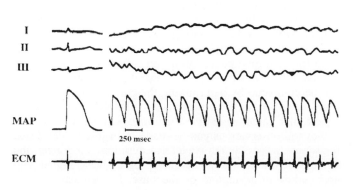

Figure 2–3. Recording taken during ventricular fibrillation in a human. Leads I, II, and III are body surface electrocardiograms. Note that there is no period of diastole between action potentials. MAP, right ventricular monophasic action potentials; ECM, local bipolar electrogram. (From Swartz JF, Jones JL, Fletcher RD: Characterization of ventricular fibrillation based on monophasic action potential morphology in the human heart. Circulation 87:1907–1914, 1993.)

The Cellular Action Potential and the Excitable Gap During Fibrillation

In the past few years, our knowledge of the characteristics of the action potentials during fibrillation has increased greatly. This is a direct result of the introduction of techniques for recording of action potentials in whole hearts either in vivo or in perfused isolated hearts.[4–6, 8, 33] During fibrillation, the action potentials are altered; the action potential duration is decreased, the action potential upstroke is slowed and of decreased magnitude (decreased dV/dt), the plateau phase is abbreviated, and diastolic intervals are abbreviated or absent (Fig. 2–3). During the first few seconds of ventricular fibrillation and atrial fibrillation, the activation rate is quite rapid; the mean cycle length of ventricular fibrillation in patients undergoing defibrillator implantation was measured to be 213 ± 27 msec.[6] Diastolic intervals are rarely seen during early fibrillation, and the upstroke of most action potentials occurs before the transmembrane potential has returned to baseline from the previous action potential. The demonstration of an *excitable gap* in fibrillating atrial tissue[34] and evidence of an excitable gap in fibrillating ventricular tissue[35] suggest that there are periods late in the action potential in the fibrillating myocardium during which an electrical stimulus can capture a portion of the fibrillating myocardium. Knowing that there is an excitable gap suggests that there is an opportunity to stimulate the tissue just in front of a fibrillation wavefront to cause wavefront block.

As described in Chapter 1, the electrical activity of the heart is controlled ultimately by ion channels located in the cell membrane of the myocyte. It has been established that both the voltage-gated fast channels (Na^+) and slow channels (Na^+ and Ca^+) are active during the first few seconds of ventricular fibrillation.[5] The fast channel activity is indicated by the rapidity of the upstroke of the action potential (phase 0) during early fibrillation and its sensitivity to administration of the Na^+ channel blocker, tetrodotoxin. As fibrillation proceeds, the upstrokes of the action potentials become increasingly slower, with a decreased dV/dt_{max}, but the action potentials remain sensitive to tetrodotoxin until 1 to 5 minutes after initiation of fibrillation. A transition then occurs in which the action potential upstrokes become insensitive to tetrodotoxin. This suggests that the propagation of the action potential is no longer mediated primarily by the fast voltage–gated sodium channels and may be mediated by slow voltage–gated calcium channel activity in the later stages of fibrillation.[4] The activation complexes recorded from the ventricular myocardium remain active only as long as the coronary arteries are perfused with oxygenated blood, suggesting that ischemia may be responsible for the loss of the fast channel activation during prolonged ventricular fibrillation.[25]

■ DEFIBRILLATION

Successful defibrillation can reflect either the immediate cessation of all activation fronts or the cessation of activation fronts after two to three cycles,[10, 36] followed by the coordinated beating of the heart. Unsuccessful defibrillation can reflect a failure to inhibit the fibrillating activation fronts or the resumption of fibrillating activation fronts after their initial inhibition. As previously mentioned, applying a powerful electrical shock to the heart is the only reliable means of stopping fibrillation.

Waveforms, Current Strength, and Distribution During Defibrillation

The two most common waveform shapes used clinically are the *monophasic* and *biphasic* waveforms. In monophasic waveforms, the polarity of the shock is constant at each electrode for the entire duration of the electrical shock. In biphasic waveforms, the polarity of the shock changes at each electrode part way through the defibrillation waveform. Many studies, in both animals and humans, have shown that biphasic waveforms can defibrillate with less current and energy than monophasic waveforms in both internal and transthoracic defibrillation configurations.[37–40] Within each type, waveforms can be described as truncated exponential or damped sinusoidal shapes. Most implantable cardioverter-defibrillators (ICDs) use truncated exponential biphasic waveforms. In contrast, most external defibrillators to date use damped sinusoidal waveforms. Because of the inductor necessary to shape the damped sinusoidal monophasic waveform, these defibrillators tend to be large and heavy. More recently, smaller, lighter external defibrillators have been developed that use truncated exponential biphasic waveforms similar to those used in ICDs. Damped sinusoidal biphasic waveforms are used in external defibrillators in Russia and, similar to truncated exponential biphasic waveforms, have been shown to have an improved efficacy over monophasic waveforms.[41, 42]

Not all biphasic waveforms are superior to monophasic waveforms, however. For example, if the second phase of the biphasic waveform becomes much longer than the first phase, then the energy required for defibrillation increases and can eventually rise to a level above the energy required to defibrillate with a monophasic waveform with duration equal to the first phase of the biphasic waveform.[40, 43, 44] The optimum duration of the two phases of the biphasic waveform depend on the electrode impedance and the defibrillator capacitance.[45–48]

Several groups have shown that for square waveforms, defibrillation efficacy follows a strength–duration relationship similar to cardiac stimulation[49, 50]; as the waveform gets longer, the average current at the 50% success point becomes progressively less, approaching an asymptote called the *rheobase*.[51] On the basis of this observation, several groups have suggested that cardiac defibrillation can be mathematically modeled using a parallel resistor–capacitor (RC) network to represent the heart[46, 52–54] (Fig. 2–4). Empirically, it has been determined that the time constant for the parallel RC network is in the range of 2.5 to 5 msec.[46, 47, 53] In one version of the model,[53] a current waveform is applied to the RC network. The voltage across the network is then calculated for each time point during the defibrillation pulse. The relative efficacy of different waveform shapes and durations can be compared by determining the current strength that is necessary to make the voltage across the RC network reach a particular value, called the *defibrillation threshold*.

Several observations can be made from this model. First, for square waves, as the waveform duration gets longer, the voltage across the network gets progressively higher and approaches an asymptote or rheobase. For truncated expo-

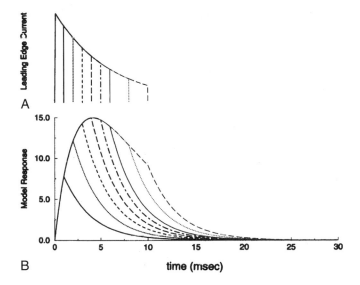

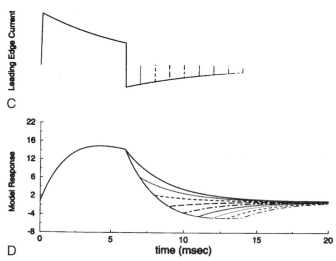

Figure 2–4. The response of a parallel resistor-capacitor network representation of the heart to monophasic and biphasic truncated exponential waveforms with a time constant of 7 msec. The parallel resistor-capacitor network has a time constant of 2.8 msec. *A,* The input monophasic waveforms. Leading edge current of the input waveform was 10 A. The waveforms were truncated at 1, 2, 3, 4, 5, 6, 8, and 10 msec. *B,* The model response, V(t). Initially, as the waveform gets longer, V(t) increases until it reaches a maximum at about 4 msec, after which V(t) begins to decrease. *C,* The input biphasic waveforms. Leading edge current was 10 A. Phase 1 was truncated at 6 msec. Phase 2 was truncated after 1, 2, 3, 4, 5, 6, 7, and 8 msec. *D,* the model response does not change polarity until phase 2 duration is longer than 2 msec.

nential waveforms, however, the model voltage rises, reaches a peak and then, if the waveform is long enough, begins to decrease (see Fig. 2–4). Therefore, the model would predict that monophasic exponential waveforms should be truncated at a time when the peak voltage across the RC network is reached. Current or energy delivered after that point is wasted. In supporting this prediction, strength–duration relationships measured in both animals[53] and humans[55] do not approach an asymptote but rather reach a minimum and

remain constant as the waveform gets longer. This minimum occurs over a range of waveform durations and does not extend indefinitely. Schuder and colleagues[56] showed that if the duration of a waveform gets too long, then defibrillation efficacy decreases.

Second, the model predicts that the heart acts as a low-pass filter.[54] Therefore waveforms that rise gradually should have an improved efficacy over waveforms that turn on immediately. This prediction has been shown to hold true for external defibrillation,[57] internal atrial defibrillation,[58] and internal ventricular defibrillation.[59] Ascending ramps defibrillate with a greater efficacy than do descending ramps.[59, 60]

Several groups have suggested that the optimal first phase of a biphasic waveform is the optimal monophasic waveform.[45, 48] If this is true, then what does the model predict as the "best" second phase of a biphasic waveform? Empirically, it appears that the role of the second phase is to return the model voltage response back to zero as quickly as possible to maximize the increased efficacy of the biphasic waveform over that of the monophasic waveform with the same duration as phase one of the biphasic waveform. If the network voltage does not reach zero or if it overshoots zero, efficacy is lost.[45, 53] Swerdlow and colleagues[47] have shown in humans that the "best" second phase of a biphasic waveform is one that returns the model response close to zero.

Together, these ideas allow the clinician to choose optimal capacitor sizes and phase durations for truncated exponential biphasic waveforms, the most commonly used waveforms in ICDs. The capacitor has to be large enough to be able to raise the network voltage to its threshold value and still hold enough charge to drive the network voltage back to zero. For a 40-Ω interelectrode impedance and a network time constant of 2.8 msec, the minimum capacitor size that can accomplish this is 75 μF.

The location of the defibrillation electrodes affects the magnitude of the shock necessary to defibrillate the heart. Typically, 200 to 360 J of energy is necessary for successful defibrillation when the defibrillation electrodes are located on the body surface, as occurs in transthoracic defibrillation with a damped sinusoidal monophasic waveform. Less energy is required for a truncated exponential biphasic waveform.[61] However, only about 4% to 20% of the current that is delivered to transthoracic defibrillation electrodes ever reaches the heart. Indeed, when the defibrillation electrodes are placed in the heart, usually only 20 to 34 J of energy is required, and this may be as low as only a few joules when very large, contoured epicardial electrodes are used.[40, 62] The strength of the shock also varies for different locations on or in the heart; epicardial patches defibrillate with a lower shock energy than do transvenous electrode configurations.[63]

Although defibrillation efficacy is usually described by some measure of defibrillation shock strength—either energy, voltage, or current—little insight into the mechanisms of defibrillation can be made from these measures. Knowing how the current (or voltage) of a defibrillation shock is distributed over the heart allows a much deeper understanding of how defibrillation occurs. Several studies have been performed that measure the potential gradient distribution throughout the heart during a defibrillation shock.[14, 64, 65] The potential gradient is a measure of the difference in voltage produced by a shock at any point in the heart as compared with a nearby point. The potential gradient is therefore measured in volts per centimeters of tissue. At a region with a high potential gradient, the difference in voltage at any point from an area 1 cm away from this point is high. Regions of low potential gradient have a measured voltage that is similar to that of nearby points.

These studies show, for most electrode configurations, an uneven distribution, with areas of high potential gradient near the defibrillation electrodes and areas of low potential gradient in regions distant from the defibrillating electrodes. It has been hypothesized that a minimum potential gradient must be attained for successful defibrillation to occur and that this requirement is independent of the current applied or the electrode configuration.[15, 16] The minimum potential gradient required for defibrillation is lower for biphasic (4 V/cm) than for monophasic waveforms (6 V/cm).[16] Thus, a minimum potential gradient of 6 V/cm was required for successful defibrillation using a 10-msec truncated exponential monophasic waveform in the open-chest dog model.[16] Similar findings were observed using a 14-msec truncated exponential monophasic waveform and multiple electrode configurations.[15]

Following a shock that fails to defibrillate ventricular fibrillation, the site of earliest activation immediately after the shock can be mapped and related to the electric field that was produced by a shock. The sites of earliest activation after a failed shock occur in the areas of lowest potential gradient.[15, 16] In contrast, a minimum potential gradient of 4 V/cm was required for successful defibrillation using a truncated exponential biphasic waveform. Because a higher shock strength is required to induce a higher potential gradient, biphasic shocks successfully defibrillate with lower energy than monophasic shocks because a lower-voltage gradient is required.

The requirement for a minimum potential gradient may reflect the need for a shock to prevent the generation of new activation fronts that can result in reinitiation of fibrillation.[66] Comparison of the potential gradients and the sites of activation for various shock strengths indicate that postshock activation occurs at numerous sites throughout the ventricle when the shock strength is much lower than that needed for defibrillation (Fig. 2–5).[67] As the shock strength and consequently the potential gradient are increased, activation occurs only in the region in which the potential gradient is lowest. At shock strengths just lower than those required for defibrillation, postshock activation arises in a limited number of myocardial regions. The activation fronts arising from these regions of low potential gradient then propagate to activate the other regions of the myocardium for a few cycles before re-entry occurs, activation becomes disorganized, and fibrillation is reinitiated. Although postshock activation sites can still arise in regions of lowest potential gradient after a shock slightly greater than that required for defibrillation, the cycles of activation that originate from these sites are slower. These activations terminate after a few cycles without reinitiating fibrillation.[66, 67]

So far, we have discussed how defibrillation can fail because a shock is of insufficient strength. What happens if a defibrillation shock gets very large? At high shock strengths, the probability of defibrillation success begins to decrease again. It is thought that at large strengths, defibrillation shocks can have detrimental effects on the heart.

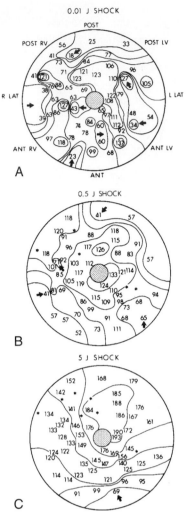

Figure 2–5. Epicardial isochronal maps of first activation after unsuccessful shock episodes. A polar projection of the ventricles is shown, with the stippled region in the center representing an apical defibrillation electrode and with the atrioventricular groove at the periphery. Numbers represent locations of electrodes with satisfactory recordings and give time of activation for those locations expressed in milliseconds from the time of onset of the shock. Asterisks indicate electrode sites where adequate recordings were not obtained. Isochronal lines are 20 msec. apart. Arrows indicate early sites of activation. Panels *A, B,* and *C* show maps following a 0.01-J shock, a 0.5-J shock, and a 5-J shock, respectively. With increasing shock energy, the number of early sites decreases, first at the apex and then at the base, whereas the time interval between the shock and activation times at early sites increases. Ant, anterior; L, left; Lat, lateral; Post, posterior; R, right; V, ventricle. (From Shibata N, Chen P-S, Dixon EG, et al: Epicardial activation following unsuccessful defibrillation shocks in dogs. Am J Physiol 255:H902–H909, 1988.)

Increasing the shock strength to very high levels (>1000 V with transvenous electrodes) can result in activation fronts arising from regions of high potential gradient that reinduce ventricular fibrillation.[68] Cates and coworkers[69] showed that, for both monophasic and biphasic shocks, increasing shock strength does not always improve the probability of successful defibrillation and may in fact increase the incidence of postshock arrhythmias. Chapman and associates[70] showed in dogs that the time until the heart recovered hemodynamically after a defibrillation episode was shorter for biphasic than for monophasic shocks. Further, they showed that hemodynamic recovery took longer after high energy shocks than after low energy shocks. Reddy and colleagues[71] showed that transthoracic defibrillation with biphasic shocks resulted in less postshock electrocardiographic evidence of myocardial dysfunction (injury or ischemia) than standard monophasic damped sinusoidal waveforms, without compromise of defibrillation efficacy.

One mechanism that has been implicated in the means by which shocks cause damage to the myocardium is *electroporation,* the formation of holes or pores in the cell membrane. Electroporation may occur in regions in which the shock potential gradient is high (>50 to 70 V/cm) and may even occur in regions where the potential gradient is much less than 50 V/cm.[72] The very high voltage can result in disruption of the phospholipid membrane bilayer and the formation of pores that permit the free influx and efflux of ions and macromolecules. Electroporation can cause the transmembrane potential to change temporarily to a value almost equal to that of the plateau of the action potential, which is characteristic of massive ion exchange. During the plateau phase, the cell is paralyzed electrically, being both unresponsive and unable to conduct an action potential. Exposure of the myocardium to yet higher potential gradients, probably >150 V/cm, results in arrhythmic beating, and at very high potential gradients, necrosis may occur.[73]

The shape of the waveform alters the strength of the shock at which these detrimental effects occur. Use of a 10-msec truncated exponential monophasic waveform for ventricular fibrillation in dogs resulted in conduction block in regions where the potential gradient was more than 64 ± 4 V/cm.[74] Shocks that created even higher potential gradients in the myocardium of 71 ± 6 V/cm were required for conduction block when a 5-msec/5-msec truncated exponential biphasic shock was used. Addition of a second phase to a monophasic waveform, thereby making it a biphasic waveform, reduced the damage sustained by cultured chick myocytes compared with that induced by the monophasic waveform alone.[75] Thus, biphasic waveforms are less apt to cause damage or dysfunction in high-gradient regions than are monophasic waveforms.

Models Proposed to Explain the Induction of Changes in the Transmembrane Potential Throughout the Heart During a Defibrillation Shock

A shock in the form of a square wave given across the defibrillation electrodes appears almost immediately as a square wave in the extracellular space of the heart. The defibrillation shock appears in the extracellular space of the heart almost immediately and without significant distortion because the extracellular space throughout the body is primarily resistive, with little reactive component. Phase delays and alterations of the appearance of the shock wave occur in the transmembrane potential, however, owing to the capacitance and ion channels of the membrane of the myocyte.[76] Consequently, a square wave shock can elicit an exponential change in the transmembrane potential (Fig. 2–6).

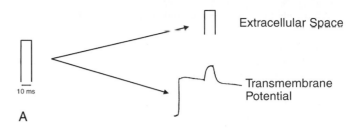

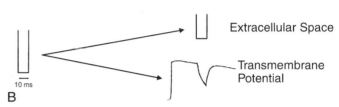

Figure 2–6. The effect of a square wave shock on the extracellular potential and the transmembrane potential. The square wave shock appears immediately as a relatively undistorted square wave in the extracellular space. It appears as an exponentially increasing change in the transmembrane potential. When given during the action potential plateau, as shown in the figure, the depolarization obtained when a shock of one shock polarity is delivered has a different magnitude and time course compared with the hyperpolarization obtained when a shock of the opposite polarity is delivered. (From Walcott GP, Knisley SB, Zhou X, et al: On the mechanism of ventricular defibrillation. PACE 20:422–431, 1997.)

The nonlinear behavior of the membrane caused by the ion channels also affects the outcome of reversing the polarity of the defibrillation shock. Reversing the polarity of the defibrillation shock may reverse the sign of the change in the transmembrane potential in some regions of the myocardium, and the nonlinear behavior of the membrane can alter the magnitude and the time course of this change. As discussed previously, reversing the polarity of the shock may not reverse the sign of the change in the transmembrane potential in all regions of the heart; some areas may be hyperpolarized upon both shock polarities.[77] This behavior may reflect the nonlinear behavior of the membrane ion channels.

Several models have been formulated in an attempt to explain the mechanisms by which the defibrillation shock is distributed throughout the myocardium such that it effectively restores coordinated, effective action potentials. As yet, none of the models adequately describes all of the experimental findings regarding the changes in the action potential that occur during defibrillation. It is well established experimentally that changes in the transmembrane potential can occur at a distance of many centimeters from the defibrillating shock electrodes. These changes in transmembrane potential can result in new action potentials or prolongation of the action potential as described previously.[23, 78] Direct excitation can be observed,[23] even at great distances from the electrode (>30 mm)[79] or across the entire heart.[80] A critical mass of the heart must be captured for effective defibrillation.[11, 81]

Although the one-dimensional cable model described in Chapter 1 adequately describes the generation of self-propagating action potentials close to an electrode as required for pacemaking, it fails to account for the far-field changes observed during defibrillation. During stimulation or defibrillation, this model predicts that the tissue near the anode should be hyperpolarized, whereas the tissue near the cathode should be depolarized.[82] The magnitude of the hyperpolarization and depolarization, however, decreases exponentially with the distance from the electrodes according to the membrane space constant (the distance at which the hyperpolarization or depolarization has decreased by 63%). For cardiac tissue, the space constant is only 0.5 to 1 mm.[82, 83] Therefore, the one-dimensional cable equations predict that tissue more than 10 space constants, about 1 cm, away from the defibrillation electrodes should not directly undergo changes in transmembrane potential because of the shock field. That is, new action potentials should not arise by direct excitation at distances greater than 1 cm from the electrodes. Thus, this model fails to describe the experimentally observed global distribution of action potentials during defibrillation.

Therefore, several additional mathematical formulations have been proposed, including the sawtooth model,[20, 84–86] the bidomain model,[87] and the formation of secondary sources at barriers in the myocardium,[19, 88] to explain how a defibrillation shock affects the transmembrane potential a long distance away from the shocking electrodes. In the simplest formulations of these models, the extracellular and intracellular spaces are considered to be low-resistance media and the membrane to be a high-resistance medium in parallel with capacitance. The simple case models incorporate only passive myocardial properties. Recently, the models have been rendered more realistic by the addition of active components to represent the ion channels in the membrane, gap junctions, and membrane discontinuities.[89, 90] By convention, the current is defined as the flow of positive ions from the anode to the cathode.

The Sawtooth Model

The one-dimensional cable model has two low-resistance continuous spaces that conduct current from the shock, the intracellular and the extracellular, separated by a high-resistance cell membrane. In the sawtooth model, the intracellular space is divided by a series of high-resistance barriers, the gap junctions. Because of these high-resistance barriers, current moving in the intracellular space is forced to exit into the extracellular space and re-enter the cell on the other side of the barrier. Exit and re-entry of the current from the intracellular domain results in hyperpolarization near the end of the cell closest to the anode and depolarization near the end of the cell closest to the cathode. A tracing of the changes in transmembrane potential along a fiber during the shock should, therefore, resemble the teeth of a saw, with each tooth corresponding to an individual cell[20, 84–86] (Fig. 2–7). Increases in the junctional resistances are predicted to increase the magnitude of the potential changes at the ends of the cells.[20] Although gap junctions are of low resistivity, they can present significant junctional resistance under certain conditions, such as hypoxia[91, 92] and calcium depletion.[93] As the resistance of the gap junctions increases, it is pre-

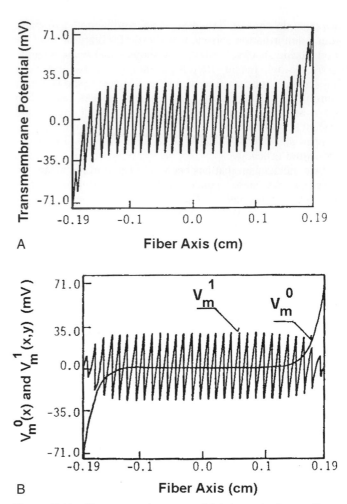

Figure 2–7. The transmembrane potential during a shock according to the sawtooth model. *A,* The transmembrane potential shown is a summation of the membrane potential profile of the cable model and the periodicity arising from the periodic changes in intracellular resistances. The anode is to the left and the cathode is to the right in this one-dimensional model. The fiber is divided into 31 cells of equal length separated by junctions of high resistance. In the figure, the junctional resistance is much higher than is thought to occur in cardiac fibers to allow the sawtooth pattern to be seen. *B,* The two parts of the summation shown in panel *A* are shown. V_m^0, the transmembrane potential profile of the cable model; V_m^i, the periodicity arising from the periodic changes in the intracellular resistance. (Adapted from Krassowska W, Pilkington TC, Ideker RE: Periodic conductivity as a mechanism for cardiac stimulation and defibrillation. IEEE Trans Biomed Eng 34:555–560, 1987.)

dicted that the current passes preferentially through the cell membrane.

The sawtooth model adequately describes the requirement for a minimum potential gradient because the magnitude of the hyperpolarization and polarization at the ends of the cells is directly proportional to the strength of the stimulus. It also adequately describes the generation of action potentials at a distance from the electrodes and the differences in threshold stimuli between cathodal and anodal stimulation.

Sawtooth changes in transmembrane potential have been observed in preparations of isolated cardiomyocytes[94, 95]; however, such a pattern in isolated cells would be consistent with the cable model. This pattern has not been observed in a syncytium of cardiac cells.[19, 96, 97]

Although the resistivity of the gap junctions at the boundaries between the cells may not adequately explain the physiologic effects of defibrillation, the resistivity of other intracellular discontinuities and interruptions may well play a role. Most theories concerning the generation of action potentials and their propagation across the ventricle, such as the bidomain theory described later, consider the myocardium a uniform electrical continuum. This assumption does not take into account the discontinuities of the intracellular domain, where the myocardium is interrupted by barriers such as connective tissue septae, blood vessels, and scar tissue. As described previously for the sawtooth model, on encountering such a barrier, the intracellular current must leave the intracellular space, cross the barrier, and re-enter the intracellular domain on the other side. Depolarization should occur on one side of the barrier and hyperpolarization on the other side. Therefore, the barrier acts as if it is a set of electrodes during the shock, becoming a secondary source of action potentials (Fig. 2–8). These secondary sources are important causes of depolarization and hyperpolarization throughout the myocardial tissue during a shock.[19] The resistive barriers act in a manner similar to that described for the sawtooth model. In this case, however, the resistive barriers represent larger discontinuities, which tend to increase with age and cardiac hypertrophy.[98]

Computer simulations have shown that cathodal stimulation delivered to the myocardium near an oval scar results in three distinct activation fronts: the primary activation front and secondary fronts at the distal and proximal edges generated by the exit and re-entry of current from the intracellular and extracellular spaces (see Fig. 2–8).[99] Optical recording techniques have been used to directly record changes in transmembrane potentials throughout a monolayer of ventricular myocytes.[19] Localized regions of depolarization and hyperpolarization were observed that coincided with discontinuities in the monolayer that resulted in slow conductance. The significance of secondary sources has also been demonstrated in whole hearts by mapping of potentials and determination of shock thresholds before and after the generation of a transmural lesion in the myocardial wall of dogs.[88] Generation of the lesion resulted in the development of a region of direct activation in the area of the lesion in addition to the region of direct activation resulting from the stimulating electrode observed before the lesion. Furthermore, the strength of the shock required to cause direct activation in the area of the lesion was less than half of that required before generation of the lesion (Fig. 2–9).

The effects of secondary sources obviously have major implications for the probability of successful defibrillation at different shock strengths in individual patients, particularly elderly patients, and the potential for re-entry. Furthermore, the size and placement of operative lesions may play a significant role in the success of subsequent defibrillation.

The Bidomain Model

The bidomain model is an extension of the one-dimensional cable model into two or three dimensions. That is, the extracellular and intracellular spaces are represented as single, continuous domains extending in two or three dimensions that are separated by the highly resistive cell membrane[87] (Fig. 2–10). If the conductivities of the intracellular and extracellular spaces are constant in all directions, then the model collapses to the one-dimensional cable model. *Anisotropy* refers to how conductivities change with the direction of myocardial fiber orientation. Clerc[100] has shown that conductivity is higher in the direction parallel to the long axis of myocardial fibers (longitudinal) than in the direction perpendicular to the fibers (transverse) for both the intracellular and extracellular spaces. If conductivities change with direction, but change the same for the intracellu-

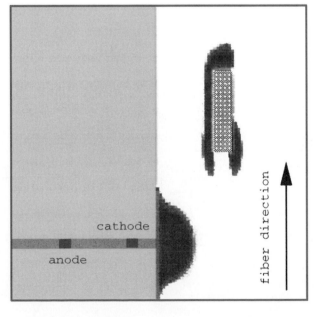

Figure 2–8. Secondary sources adjacent to a scar elicited by a single large pacing pulse as seen in a computer model. The right region is the myocardium with a rectangular scar *(stippled region)*. The left region is the blood pool with a pacing catheter in it. Notice that a pacing pulse depolarizes not only the tissue near the cathode but also that near the scar. (From Street AM: Effect of connective tissue embedded in viable cardiac tissue on propagation and pacing: Implications for arrhythmias. Durham NC: Duke University, Dept. of Biomedical Engineering, 1996, p 134.)

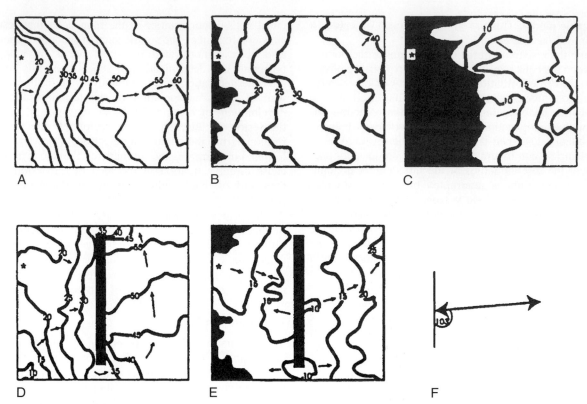

Figure 2–9. Isochronal activation maps following cathodal stimulation before and after creating a transmural incision that caused secondary sources adjacent to the lesion. Isochrones are drawn at 5-msec intervals timed from the onset of S1 or S2 stimulus. Arrows represent direction of activation. Darkened regions represent areas directly activated by the stimulus. Black vertical bars represent the approximate location of the transmural incision. *A,* S1 stimulus delivered before incision. *B,* 75-mA S2 stimulus delivered before incision. *C,* 250-mA S2 stimulus delivered before the incision. *D,* S1 stimulus delivered after incision. *E,* 75-mA S2 stimulus delivered after incision. *F,* Orientation of long axis of myocardial fibers. (From White JB, Walcott GP, Pollard AE, et al: Myocardial discontinuities: A substrate for producing virtual electrodes to increase directly excited areas of the myocardium by shocks. Circulation 97:1738–1745, 1998.)

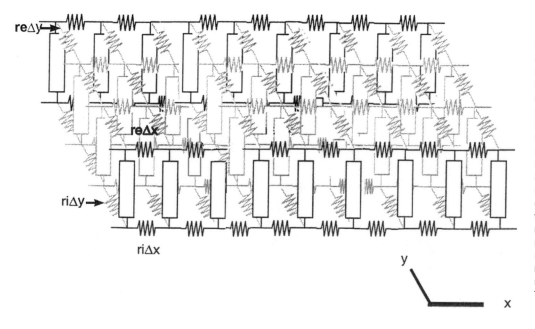

Figure 2–10. A circuit diagram of a two-dimensional bidomain model. The top of the resistor network represents the extracellular space; the bottom of the network represents the intracellular space. ReΔx represents the extracellular resistivity in the x direction. ReΔy represents the extracellular resistivity in the y direction. RiΔx and riΔy represent the intracellular resistivities in the x and y directions. The rectangles represent the cell membrane. For a passive model, the rectangle would be replaced by a parallel resistor-capacitor network. For an active model, the rectangle would be replaced by a membrane ion model.

lar and extracellular spaces, the bidomain model collapses to the one-dimensional cable model.

Studies have shown that the anisotropy ratio is about 3:1 in the extracellular space and 10:1 in the intracellular space. When these anisotropy ratios are used, the bidomain model begins to give new insights into how shocks change the transmembrane potential. Similar to the one-dimensional cable model, the bidomain model predicts that hyperpolarization occurs in tissues under the extracellular anodal electrode. Likewise, depolarization occurs in tissue under the extracellular cathodal electrode. Unlike the one-dimensional cable model, the bidomain also predicts that depolarization occurs along the long axis of the myocardial fibers at distances just a few millimeters from the anode. A similar effect is predicted to occur at the cathode, with hyperpolarization at distances of a few millimeters.[101, 102] Therefore, the effect on the transmembrane potential near the shocking electrode is predicted to be much more complicated by the bidomain model than by the one-dimensional cable model.

The power of the bidomain model, however, is that it hypothesizes that there should be changes in the transmembrane potential, either hyperpolarization or depolarization, across the entire heart. In this model, the change in transmembrane potential elicited by the shock depends on the distribution of intracellular and extracellular current that is affected by the change in potential gradient with distance, the distance from the electrode, and the orientation of the myocardial fibers. Experimental studies have shown that there is a complex pattern of transmembrane potential changes during the delivery of a defibrillation shock similar to those predicted by the bidomain model.[77, 103, 104]

The secondary source and bidomain models may not be mutually exclusive; rather, both may contribute to the changes in transmembrane potential. The exact mechanism by which an electrical pulse results in defibrillation remains incompletely understood at the level of the cell membrane and the ion channels. As the transmembrane potential attains values closer to the typical resting transmembrane potential than the usual minimum of -65 mV observed in fibrillating myocytes, this may allow the voltage-gated Na^+ channels to recover sufficiently and the myocytes to regain full excitability.

The Effect of the Defibrillating Shock Field on the Cellular Action Potential

The final common pathway of changes in the transmembrane potential caused by a defibrillation shock is to affect the shape and duration of the cellular action potential. The shock can have one of three effects on the myocardium, depending on the local strength of the shock and its timing with respect to the local action potential. If the shock is delivered during the plateau, then there will be little or no change in the action potential. If the shock is strong enough and delivered relatively late during the action potential, then it will initiate a new action potential. A shock that is strong enough but delivered during early phase 3 of the action potential will modify and prolong an ongoing action potential without initiating an entirely new action potential (Fig. 2–11).

A defibrillation shock has to do two things to defibrillate the heart successfully. First, it must stop most or all activation wavefronts on the heart. Second, it must not reinitiate fibrillation. The extension of refractoriness hypothesis helps

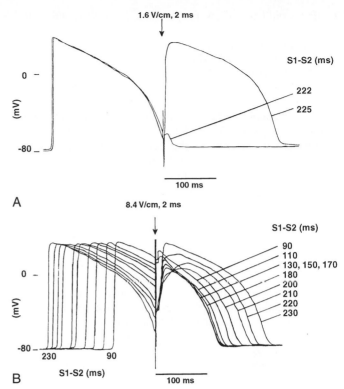

Figure 2–11. Transmembrane recordings from a guinea pig papillary muscle showing an all-or-none response to a weak field stimulus and action potential prolongation in response to a larger stimulus. *A,* Recordings that illustrate the response to an S2 stimulus of 1.6 V/cm oriented along the fibers. The S1–S2 stimulus intervals for each of the responses are indicated to the right of the recordings. The responses are markedly different even though the change in S2 timing was only 3 msec. An S1–S2 interval of 222 msec caused almost no response, whereas an interval of 225 msec produced a new action potential. *B,* A range of action potential extensions produced by an S2 stimulus generating a potential gradient of 8.4 V/cm oriented along the long axis of the myofibers. The recordings were obtained from the same cell as in panel *A.* The action potential recordings, obtained from one cellular impairment, are aligned with the S2 time. An S1 stimulus was applied 3 msec before phase zero of each recording. The longest and shortest S1–S2 intervals tested, 230 and 90 msec, respectively, are indicated beneath their respective phase-zero depolarizations. The S1–S2 intervals for each response after S2 are indicated to the right. (From Knisley SB, Smith WM, Ideker RE: Effect of field stimulation on cellular repolarization in rabbit myocardium: Implications for reentry induction. Circ Res 70:707–715, 1992.)

to explain how a shock can stop fibrillation. A shock can prolong the refractory period of an action potential without triggering a new action potential if it is of a sufficient strength and is delivered at an appropriate interval with respect to the upstroke.[23, 105] If the first activation front that forms after a defibrillation shock encounters tissue with an extended refractory period, the front will be stopped because it cannot propagate into the region of refractory tissue. This is called the *extension of refractoriness hypothesis for defibrillation.*

Also, a defibrillation shock must not restart fibrillation. If only part of the front encounters tissue with an extended refractory period, only part of the front will be halted. The rest of the activation front will propagate forward and will eventually move into the area that could not be stimulated or that would not allow propagation (unidirectional block). This process of stimulating some tissue and creating unidirectional block in adjacent regions creates a re-entrant circuit that eventually breaks down into fibrillation. The *critical point* is that point at which critical shock strength intersects a critical level of refractoriness, leading to the formation of a re-entrant circuit.[106–108]

To understand better how re-entrant circuits and critical points are formed after a defibrillation shock, studies have examined the behavior of the heart after the delivery of a shock during a paced ventricular rhythm.[107] Shocks were used to initiate ventricular fibrillation during the vulnerable period of the paced rhythm. A large premature S2 stimulus was delivered through a long narrow electrode oriented perpendicular to an activation front arising from an S1 stimulus (Fig. 2–12). S2 shocks were given to scan the vulnerable period after the last S1 stimulus. At an appropriate S1 to S2 coupling interval, a re-entrant circuit formed and continued for several cycles before breaking down into fibrillation. The initial postshock activation front circled a point at which a shock potential gradient field of 5 to 6 V/cm for a 10-msec monophasic shock intersected tissue that was just passing out of its refractory period to a 2-mA local stimulus. This intersection formed a critical point.

The intersection of a particular potential gradient level with a particular refractory state divides the tissue into four regions centered around the critical point (see Fig. 2–12C). The region to the left of the critical point was still in its refractory period and was not directly excited by the shock. The region to the right of the critical point had recovered enough to be directly excited by the S2 stimulus. Above the critical point, the shock had no effect on the refractory period of the tissue, whereas below the critical point, the shock prolonged the refractory period of the tissue. Therefore, an excitation wavefront propagated from the upper right quadrant of the mapped region across the top half of the plaque. Because of the prolongation of refractoriness in the tissue below the critical point, and excitation wavefront was unable to propagate across the bottom half of the plaque directly. As this tissue recovered, the excitation wavefront from the top half of the plaque entered the area at the bottom half and re-excited the tissue, creating a re-entrant circuit around the critical point.

Recent studies provide some insight into why the activation pattern observed in Figure 2–12 occurs. When the myocardium is field stimulated with a shock field whose potential gradient is less than the critical value for that waveform, an all-or-none response is observed (see Fig. 2–11). If the stimulus is applied with a coupling interval greater than the refractory period, a new action potential is generated. If the coupling interval is shorter than the refractory period, almost no response is seen. When the shock field strength is greater than a critical value, a whole gradation of responses is observed, depending on the coupling interval. As the coupling interval is made shorter, a smaller response occurs. However, even these smaller responses prolong refractoriness. It is this prolongation of refractoriness adjacent to directly stimulated myocardium that leads to unidirectional block and ultimately to the formation of critical points and of functional re-entrant circuits. If fibrillation is initiated

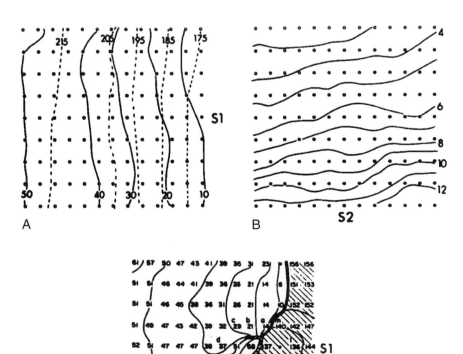

Figure 2–12. Initiation of reentry and ventricular fibrillation after orthogonal interaction of myocardial refractoriness and the potential gradient field created by a large stimulus. *A,* Distribution of activation times during the last S1 beat *(solid lines)* and recovery times to a local 2-mA stimulus *(dashed lines)* in milliseconds after this activation. *B,* S2 stimulus field (V/cm). *C,* Initial activation pattern just after the S2 stimulus. The hatched region is thought to be directly excited by the S2 stimulus field. (From Frazier DW, Wolf PD, Wharton JM, et al: Stimulus-induced critical point: Mechanism for electrical initiation of reentry in normal canine myocardium. J Clin Invest 83:1039–1052.)

by the re-entrant pathway formed whenever a critical point is created within the myocardium, then the shock strength of a successful defibrillation shock should be above that at which no critical points are formed.

Ideker and associates[109] examined the potential gradient and degree of refractoriness at the critical point for a series of monophasic and biphasic waveforms and compared these values with the defibrillation threshold. Monophasic waveforms lasting 1, 2, 3, 8 and 16 msec were delivered, as were biphasic waveforms in which both phases were of equal duration, and the total duration of both phases together was 2, 4, 8, and 16 msec. The defibrillation threshold decreased as the potential gradient at the critical point decreased and as the degree of refractoriness at the critical point decreased. Therefore, the waveform that induced a critical point located where both the potential gradient and the degree of refractoriness were lowest, that is, the 4/4-msec biphasic waveform, had the lowest defibrillation threshold. This observation may explain why some waveforms defibrillate at lower voltages than others.

The mechanism for the formation of critical points described here may be too simplistic in light of the complex ways that a shock can affect the transmembrane potential. Furthermore, the requirement that a critical point not be formed for a shock to succeed may be too stringent. Several studies have shown that a shock can still succeed in defibrillating, even if it creates rapid postshock activation for one or two cycles, suggesting that for successful defibrillation, it may not be necessary to prevent the creation of critical points and re-entry. Rather, it is only necessary that the re-entrant circuits die out in one or two cycles before secondary re-entry occurs. Further research is necessary to understand these phenomena more completely.

REFERENCES

1. Prevost JL, Battelli F: Sur quelques effets des décharges électriques sur le coeur des Mammifères. Comptes Rendus des Seances, Academi des Sciences 129:1267–1268, 1899.
2. Beck CS, Pritchard WH, Feil HS: Ventricular fibrillation of long duration abolished by electric shock. JAMA 135:985–986, 1947.
3. Zoll PM, Linenthal AJ, Gibson W, et al: Termination of ventricular fibrillation in man by externally applied electric countershock. N Engl J Med 254:727–732, 1956.
4. Akiyama T: Intracellular recording of in situ ventricular cells during ventricular fibrillation. Am J Physiol 240:H465–H471, 1981.
5. Zhou X, Guse P, Wolf PD, et al: Existence of both fast and slow channel activity during the early stage of ventricular fibrillation. Circ Res 70:773–786, 1992.
6. Swartz JF, Jones JL, Fletcher RD: Characterization of ventricular fibrillation based on monophasic action potential morphology in the human heart. Circulation 87:1907–1914, 1993.
7. Witkowski FX, Penkoske PS, Kavanagh KM: Activation patterns during ventricular fibrillation. In Zipes DP, Jalife J, (eds): Cardiac Electrophysiology: From Cell to Bedside. Philadelphia, WB Saunders, 1995, pp 539–544.
8. Gray RA, Jalife J, Panfilov AV, et al: Mechanisms of cardiac fibrillation: Drifting rotors as a mechanism of cardiac fibrillation. Science 270:1222–1225, 1995.
9. Wiggers CJ: The physiologic basis for cardiac resuscitation from ventricular fibrillation: Method for serial defibrillation. Am Heart J 20:413–422, 1940.
10. Mower MM, Mirowski M, Spear JF, et al: Patterns of ventricular activity during catheter defibrillation. Circulation 49:858–861, 1974.
11. Zipes DP, Fischer J, King RM, et al: Termination of ventricular fibrillation in dogs by depolarizing a critical amount of myocardium. Am J Cardiol 36:37–44, 1975.
12. Chen P-S, Shibata N, Wolf PD, et al: Epicardial activation during

successful and unsuccessful ventricular defibrillation in open chest dogs. Cardiovasc Rev Rep 7:625–648, 1986.
13. Gray RA, Ayers G, Jalife J: Video imaging of atrial defibrillation in the sheep heart. Circulation 95:1038–1047, 1997.
14. Chen P-S, Wolf PD, Claydon FJ, III, et al: The potential gradient field created by epicardial defibrillation electrodes in dogs. Circulation 74:626–636, 1986.
15. Wharton JM, Wolf PD, Smith WM, et al: Cardiac potential and potential gradient fields generated by single, combined, and sequential shocks during ventricular defibrillation. Circulation 85:1510–1523, 1992.
16. Zhou X, Daubert JP, Wolf PD, et al: Epicardial mapping of ventricular defibrillation with monophasic and biphasic shocks in dogs. Circ Res 72:145–160, 1993.
17. Henriquez CS: Simulating the electrical behavior of cardiac muscle using the bidomain model. Crit Rev Biomed Eng 21:1–77, 1993.
18. Fishler MG, Sobie EA, Thakor NV, et al: Mechanisms of cardiac cell excitation with premature monophasic and biphasic field stimuli: A model study. Biophys J 70:1347–1362, 1996.
19. Gillis AM, Fast VG, Rohr S, et al: Spatial changes in transmembrane potential during extracellular electrical shocks in cultured monolayers of neonatal rat ventricular myocytes. Circ Res 79:676–690, 1996.
20. Plonsey R, Barr RC: Inclusion of junction elements in a linear cardiac model through secondary sources: Application to defibrillation. Med Biol Eng Comput 24:137–144, 1986.
21. Fast VG, Rohr S, Gillis AM, et al: Activation of cardiac tissue by extracellular electrical shocks: Formation of 'secondary sources' at intercellular clefts in monolayers of cultured myocytes. Circ Res 82:375–385, 1998.
22. Moe GK, Abildskov JA, Han J: Factors responsible for the initiation and maintenance of ventricular fibrillation. In Surawicz B, Pellegrino ED (eds): Sudden Cardiac Death. New York, Grune & Stratton, 1964.
23. Dillon SM, Mehra R: Prolongation of ventricular refractoriness by defibrillation shocks may be due to additional depolarization of the action potential. J Cardiovasc Electrophysiol 3:442–456, 1992.
24. Wiggers CJ: Studies of ventricular fibrillation caused by electric shock: Cinematographic and electrocardiographic observations of the natural process in the dog's heart: Its inhibition by potassium and the revival of coordinated beats by calcium. Am Heart J 5:351–365, 1930.
25. Worley SJ, Swain JL, Colavita PG, et al: Development of an endocardial-epicardial gradient of activation rate during electrically induced, sustained ventricular fibrillation in the dog. Am J Cardiol 55:813–820, 1985.
26. Opthof T, Ramdat Misier AR, Coronel R, et al: Dispersion of refractoriness in canine ventricular myocardium: Effects of sympathetic stimulation. Circ Res 68:1204–1215, 1991.
27. Garrey WE: The nature of fibrillatory contractions of the heart: Its relation to tissue mass and form. Am J Physiol 33:397–414, 1914.
28. Ideker RE, Klein GJ, Harrison L, et al: Epicardial mapping of the initiation of ventricular fibrillation induced by reperfusion following acute ischemia [Abstract]. Circulation 58:II–64, 1978.
29. Rogers J, Usui M, KenKnight B, et al: Recurrent wavefront morphologies: A method for quantifying the complexity of epicardial activation patterns. Ann Biomed Eng 25:761–768, 1997.
30. Wells JL Jr, Karp RB, Kouchoukos NT, et al: Characterization of atrial fibrillation in man: Studies following open heart surgery. PACE 1:426–438, 1978.
31. Konings KTS, Kirchof CJHJ, Smeets JRLM, et al: High-density mapping of electrically induced atrial fibrillation in humans. Circulation 89:1665–1680, 1994.
32. Allessie MA: Reentrant mechanisms underlying atrial fibrillation. In Zipes DP, Jalife J (eds): Cardiac Electrophysiology: From Cell to Bedside. Philadelphia, WB Saunders, 1995, pp 562–566.
33. Gray RA, Jalife J: Self-organized drifting spiral waves as a mechanism for atrial fibrillation [Abstract]. Circulation 94:I–94, 1996.
34. Allessie M, Kirchhof C, Scheffer GJ, et al: Regional control of atrial fibrillation by rapid pacing in concious dogs. Circulation 84:1689–1697, 1991.
35. KenKnight BH, Bayly PV, Gerstle RJ, et al: Regional capture of fibrillating ventricular myocardium: Evidence of an excitable gap. Circ Res 77:849–855, 1995.
36. Witkowski FX, Penkoske PA, Plonsey R: Mechanism of cardiac defibrillation in open-chest dogs with unipolar DC-coupled simultaneous activation and shock potential recordings. Circulation 82:244–260, 1990.

37. Bardy GH, Ivey TD, Allen MD, et al: A prospective randomized evaluation of biphasic versus monophasic waveform pulses on defibrillation efficacy in humans. J Am Coll Cardiol 14:728–733, 1989.

38. Block M, Hammel D, Böcker D, et al: A prospective randomized cross-over comparison on mono- and biphasic defibrillation using nonthoracotomy lead configurations in humans. J Cardiovasc Electrophysiol 5:581–590, 1994.

39. Chapman PD, Vetter JW, Souza JJ, et al: Comparison of monophasic with single and dual capacitor biphasic waveforms for nonthoracotomy canine internal defibrillation. J Am Coll Cardiol 14:242–245, 1989.

40. Dixon EG, Tang ASL, Wolf PD, et al: Improved defibrillation thresholds with large contoured epicardial electrodes and biphasic waveforms. Circulation 76:1176–1184, 1987.

41. Gurvich NL, Markarychev VA: Defibrillation of the heart with biphasic electrical impulses. Kardiologiia 7:109–112, 1967.

42. Walcott GP, Melnick SB, Chapman FW, et al: Comparison of monophasic and biphasic waveforms for external defibrillation in an animal model of cardiac arrest and resuscitation [Abstract]. J Am Coll Cardiol 405A, 1995.

43. Tang ASL, Yabe S, Wharton JM, et al: Ventricular defibrillation using biphasic waveforms: The importance of phasic duration. J Am Coll Cardiol 13:207–214, 1989.

44. Feeser SA, Tang ASL, Kavanagh KM, et al: Strength-duration and probability of success curves for defibrillation with biphasic waveforms. Circulation 82:2128–2141, 1990.

45. Kroll MW: A minimal model of the single capacitor biphasic defibrillation waveform. PACE 17:1782–1792, 1994.

46. Kroll MW: A minimal model of the monophasic defibrillation pulse. PACE 16:769–777, 1993.

47. Swerdlow CD, Fan W, Brewer JE: Charge-burping theory correctly predicts optimal ratios of phase duration for biphasic defibrillation waveforms. Circulation 94:2278–2284, 1996.

48. Walcott GP, Walker RG, Krassowska W, et al: Choosing the optimum monophasic and biphasic waveforms for defibrillation [Abstract]. PACE 17:789, 1994.

49. Blair HA: On the intensity-time relations for stimulation by electric currents. II. J Gen Physiol 15:731–755, 1932.

50. Lapicque L: In L'Excitabilité en Fonction du Temps. Paris, Libraire J. Gilbert, 1926, p 371.

51. Mouchawar GA, Geddes LA, Bourland JD, et al: Ability of the Lapicque and Blair strength-duration curves to fit experimentally obtained data from the dog heart. IEEE Trans Biomed Eng 36:971–974, 1989.

52. Irnich W: The fundamental law of electrostimulation and its application to defibrillation. PACE 13:1433–1447, 1990.

53. Walcott GP, Walker RG, Cates AW, et al: Choosing the optimal monophasic and biphasic waveforms for ventricular defibrillation. J Cardiovasc Electrophysiol 6:737–750, 1995.

54. Sweeney RJ, Gill RM, Jones JL, et al: Defibrillation using a high-frequency series of monophasic rectangular pulses: Observations and model predictions. J Cardiovasc Electrophysiol 7:134–143, 1996.

55. Gold MR, Shorofsky SR: Strength-duration relationship for human transvenous defibrillation. Circulation 96:3517–3520, 1997.

56. Schuder JC, Stoeckle H, West JA, et al: Transthoracic ventricular defibrillation in the dog with truncated and untruncated exponential stimuli. IEEE Trans Biomed Eng 18:410–415, 1971.

57. Walcott GP, Melnick SB, Chapman FW, et al: Comparison of damped sinusoidal and truncated exponential waveforms for external defibrillation [Abstract]. J Am Coll Cardiol 27:237A, 1996.

58. Harbinson MT, Allen JD, Imam Z, et al: Rounded biphasic waveform reduces energy requirements for transvenous catheter cardioversion of atrial fibrillation and flutter. PACE 20:226–229, 1997.

59. Hillsley RE, Walker RG, Swanson DK, et al: Is the second phase of a biphasic defibrillation waveform the defibrillating phase? PACE 16:1401–1411, 1993.

60. Schuder JC, Rahmoeller GA, Stoeckle H: Transthoracic ventricular defibrillation with triangular and trapezoidal waveforms. Circ Res 19:689–694, 1966.

61. Bardy GH, Marchlinski FE, Sharma AD, et al: Multicenter comparison of truncated biphasic shocks and standard damped sine wave monophasic shocks for transthoracic defibrillation. Transthoracic Investigators. Circulation 94:2507–2514, 1996.

62. Karlon WJ, Eisenberg SR, Lehr JL: Effects of paddle placement and size on defibrillation current distribution: A three-dimensional finite element model. IEEE Trans Biomed Eng 40:246–255, 1993.

63. Block M, Hammel D, Isburch F, et al: Results and realistic expectations with transvenous lead systems. PACE 15:665–670, 1992.

64. Tang ASL, Wolf PD, Claydon FJ, III, et al: Measurement of defibrillation shock potential distributions and activation sequences of the heart in three-dimensions. Proc IEEE 76:1176–1186, 1988.

65. Tang ASL, Wolf PD, Afework Y, et al: Three-dimensional potential gradient fields generated by intracardiac catheter and cutaneous patch electrodes. Circulation 85:1857–1864, 1992.

66. Chen P-S, Wolf PD, Melnick SD, et al: Comparison of activation during ventricular fibrillation and following unsuccessful defibrillation shocks in open chest dogs. Circ Res 66:1544–1560, 1990.

67. Shibata N, Chen P-S, Dixon EG, et al: Epicardial activation following unsuccessful defibrillation shocks in dogs. Am J Physiol 255:H902–H909, 1988.

68. Walker RG, Walcott GP, Smith WM, et al: Sites of earliest activation following transvenous defibrillation [Abstract]. Circulation 90:I–447, 1994.

69. Cates AW, Wolf PD, Hillsley RE, et al: The probability of defibrillation success and the incidence of postshock arrhythmia as a function of shock strength. PACE 17:1208–1217, 1994.

70. Chapman FW, El-Abbady TZ, Walcott GP, et al: Dysfunction following transthoracic defibrillation shocks in dogs [Abstract]. PACE 20:1128, 1997.

71. Reddy RK, Gleva MJ, Gliner BE, et al: Biphasic transthoracic defibrillation causes fewer ECG ST-segment changes after shock. Ann Emerg Med 30:127–134, 1997.

72. DeBruin KA, Krassowska W: Electroporation and shock-induced transmembrane potential in a cardiac fiber during defibrillation strength shocks. Ann Biomed Eng 26:584–596, 1998.

73. Schuder JC, Gold JH, Stoeckle H, et al: Transthoracic ventricular defibrillation in the 100 kg calf with symmetrical one-cycle bidirectional rectangular wave stimuli. IEEE Trans Biomed Eng 30:415–422, 1983.

74. Yabe S, Smith WM, Daubert JP, et al: Conduction disturbances caused by high current density electric fields. Circ Res 66:1190–1203, 1990.

75. Jones JL, Jones RE: Decreased defibrillator-induced dysfunction with biphasic rectangular waveforms. Am J Physiol 247:H792–H796, 1984.

76. Walcott GP, Knisley SB, Zhou X, et al: On the mechanism of ventricular defibrillation. PACE 20:422–431, 1997.

77. Clark DM, Rogers JM, Ideker RE, et al: Intracardiac defibrillation-strength shocks produce large regions of hyperpolarization and depolarization [Abstract]. J Am Coll Cardiol 27:147A, 1996.

78. Zhou X, Wolf PD, Rollins DL, et al: Effects of monophasic and biphasic shocks on action potentials during ventricular fibrillation in dogs. Circ Res 73:325–334, 1993.

79. Daubert JP, Frazier DW, Wolf PD, et al: Response of relatively refractory canine myocardium to monophasic and biphasic shocks. Circulation 84:2522–2538, 1991.

80. Colavita PG, Wolf PD, Smith WM, et al: Determination of effects of internal countershock by direct cardiac recordings during normal rhythm. Am J Physiol 250:H736–H740, 1986.

81. Zhou X, Daubert JP, Wolf PD, et al: Size of the critical mass for defibrillation [Abstract]. Circulation 80:II–531, 1989.

82. Weidmann S: Electrical constants of trabecular muscle from mammalian heart. J Physiol 210:1041–1054, 1970.

83. Kléber AG, Riegger CB: Electrical constants of arterially perfused rabbit papillary muscle. J Physiol 385:307–324, 1987.

84. Plonsey R, Barr RC: Effect of microscopic and macroscopic discontinuities on the response of cardiac tissue to defibrillation (stimulating) currents. Med Biol Eng Comput 24:130–136, 1986.

85. Krassowska W, Frazier DW, Pilkington TC, et al: Potential distribution in three-dimensional periodic myocardium. II. Application to extracellular stimulation. IEEE Trans Biomed Eng 37:267–284, 1990.

86. Krassowska W, Pilkington TC, Ideker RE: Potential distribution in three-dimensional periodic myocardium. I. Solution with two-scale asymptotic analysis. IEEE Trans Biomed Eng 37:252–266, 1990.

87. Tung L: A Bidomain Model for Describing Ischemic Myocardial DC Potentials. Cambridge, MA; MIT Press, 1978.

88. White JB, Walcott GP, Pollard AE, et al: Myocardial discontinuities: A substrate for producing virtual electrodes to increase directly excited areas of the myocardium by shocks. Circulation 97:1738–1745, 1998.

89. Trayanova N: Discrete versus syncytial tissue behavior in a model of cardiac stimulation. I: Mathematical formulation. IEEE Trans Biomed Eng 43:1129–1140, 1996.

90. Trayanova N: Discrete versus syncytial tissue behavior in a model of

cardiac stimulation. II. Results of stimulation. IEEE Trans Biomed Eng 43:1141–1150, 1996.

91. Kieval RS, Spear JF, Moore EN: Gap junctional conductance in ventricular myocyte pairs isolated from postischemic rabbit myocardium. Circ Res 71:127–136, 1992.

92. Shaw RM, Rudy Y: Electrophysiologic effects of acute myocardial ischemia: A mechanistic investigation of action potential conduction and conduction failure. Circ Res 80:124–138, 1997.

93. Shaw RM, Rudy Y: Ionic mechanisms of propagation in cardiac tissue: Roles of the sodium and L-type calcium currents during reduced excitability and decreased gap junction coupling. Circ Res 81:727–741, 1997.

94. Knisley SB, Blitchington TF, Hill BC, et al: Optical measurements of transmembrane potential changes during electric field stimulation of ventricular cells. Circ Res 72:255–270, 1993.

95. Windisch H, Ahammer H, Schaffer P, et al: Optical multisite monitoring of cell excitation phenomenon in isolated cardiomyocytes. Pflungers Arch 430:508–518, 1995.

96. Zhou X, Ideker RE, Blitchington TF, et al: Optical transmembrane potential measurements during defibrillation-strength shocks in perfused rabbit hearts. Circ Res 77:593–602, 1995.

97. Wikswo JP Jr, Lin S-F, Abbas RA: Virtual electrodes in cardiac tissue: A common mechanism for anodal and cathodal stimulation. Biophys J 69:2195–2210, 1995.

98. Sommer JR, Scherer B: Geometry of cell and bundle appositions in cardiac muscle: Light microscopy. Am J Physiol 248:H792–H803, 1985.

99. Street AM, Plonsey R: Activation fronts elicited remote to the pacing site due to the presence of scar tissue. Proceedings of the 18th Annual International Conference of the IEEE Engineering in Medicine and Biology Society, Amsterdam: Institute of Electrical and Electronics Engineers, Inc.; Piscataway, NJ, 1996, p 358 (CD ROM).

100. Clerc L: Directional differences of impulse spread in trabecular muscle from mammalian heart. J Physiol 255:335–346, 1976.

101. Wikswo JP Jr: Tissue anisotropy, the cardiac bidomain, and the virtual cathode effect. *In* Zipes DP, Jalife J (eds): Cardiac Electrophysiology: From Cell to Bedside. Philadelphia, WB Saunders, 1995, pp 348–362.

102. Knisley SB: Transmembrane voltage changes during unipolar stimulation of rabbit ventricle. Circ Res 77:1229–1239, 1995.

103. Efimov IR, Cheng Y, Van Wagoner DR, et al: Virtual electrode-induced phase singularity: A basic mechanism of defibrillation failure. Circ Res 82:918–925, 1998.

104. Efimov IR, Cheng YN, Biermann M, et al: Transmembrane voltage changes produced by real and virtual electrodes during monophasic defibrillation shock delivered by an implantable electrode. J Cardiovasc Electrophysiol 8:1031–1045, 1997.

105. Knisley SB, Smith WM, Ideker RE: Effect of field stimulation on cellular repolarization in rabbit myocardium: Implications for reentry induction. Circ Res 70:707–715, 1992.

106. Winfree AT: When Time Breaks Down: The Three-Dimensional Dynamics of Electrochemical Waves and Cardiac Arrhythmias. Princeton, NJ, Princeton University Press, 1987.

107. Frazier DW, Wolf PD, Wharton JM, et al: Stimulus-induced critical point: Mechanism for electrical initiation of reentry in normal canine myocardium. J Clin Invest 83:1039–1052, 1989.

108. Chen P-S, Wolf PD, Dixon EG, et al: Mechanism of ventricular vulnerability to single premature stimuli in open-chest dogs. Circ Res 62:1191–1209, 1988.

109. Ideker RE, Alferness C, Hagler J, et al: Rotor site correlates with defibrillation waveform efficacy [Abstract]. Circulation 84:II–499, 1991.

110. Krassowska W, Pilkington TC, Ideker RE: Periodic conductivity as a mechanism for cardiac stimulation and defibrillation. IEEE Trans Biomed Eng 34:555–560, 1987.

111. Street AM: Effect of connective tissue embedded in viable cardiac tissue on propagation and pacing: Implications for arrhythmias. Durham NC, Duke University, Dept. of Biomedical Engineering, 1996; p 134.

Chapter 3

Sensing and Arrhythmia Detection by Implantable Devices

Mark A. Wood, Charles Swerdlow, and Walter H. Olson

The ability of a pulse generator to appropriately sense electric signals that originate in the myocardium is dependent on the electrophysiologic properties of the underlying myocardium, the characteristics of the electrodes in contact with the heart, the conductors within the lead, and the sensing amplifier in the pulse generator. Each of these components has an important influence on the sensing performance of the pacing system. In addition to these components that must detect electric events in the myocardium, the timing circuits in the pulse generator must reject unwanted electric signals, such as far-field cardiac events, skeletal myopotentials, and interference that originates in the environment. This chapter focuses on the fundamental factors of myocardial sensing and their clinical application to cardiac pacemakers and implantable cardioverter-defibrillators (ICDs).

■ THE INTRACARDIAC ELECTROGRAM

Origin of the Intracardiac Electrogram

A fundamental property of excitable tissues such as myocardium is the ability to maintain a resting electric potential across the cell membrane. In the case of a normal ventricular myocyte, the interior of the cell is electrically negative with respect to the outside and has a resting potential gradient of approximately −90 mV across the membrane. In the absence of electric currents within the myocardium, two electrodes placed on the outside of a cardiac myocyte in its resting state would record the same electric potential (+90 mV) with respect to the inside of the cell. *Relative to each other*, there would be no net potential difference between the electrodes (Fig. 3–1). Thus, in the resting state, this pair of electrodes would record no electric signal.

In addition to the property of separation of charge across the cell membrane, the normal myocardium is characterized

by the ability to generate self-propagating action potentials that result from a complex cascade of electric currents that flow across the membrane through specialized ion channels and between cells through intercalated disks. Consider the sequence of electric events recorded by a pair of electrodes placed at separate endocardial sites as a depolarizing wave of action potentials sweeps through the underlying myocardium

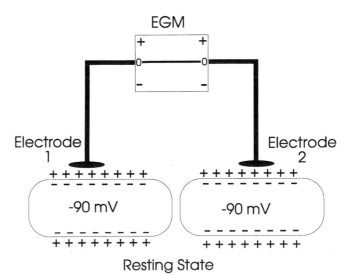

Figure 3–1. Schematic representation of two electrodes recording from two myocytes in the resting polarized state. Both cells have a gradient of 90 mV across the membrane, and the interior of the cell is electrically negative with respect to the outside of the cell. Although both electrode 1 and electrode 2 record from the electrically positive outside of the cell, with respect to one another, they record the same charge. Thus, because both electrodes record the same charge, the electrogram (EGM) recorded between these electrodes shows no deflection from neutral.

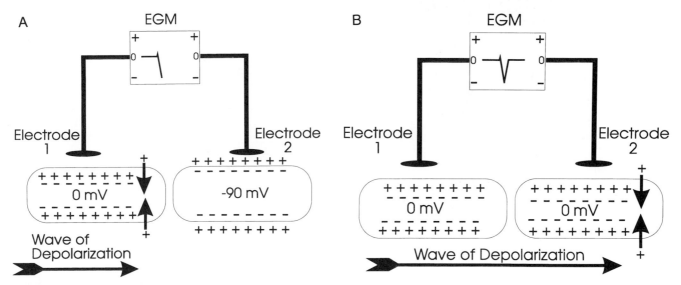

Figure 3–2. *A,* The effect of a wave of action potentials is demonstrated as it travels from left to right in this figure. Note that as the wave of depolarization progresses, positively charged Na$^+$ ions move from the outside to the inside of the cell, causing the inside of the cell to become charged to about 0 mV with respect to the outside. Although the cell under electrode 1 is depolarized and shows no separation of charge across the membrane, it is electrically negative relative to the cell under electrode 2. Because the two electrodes record different charges, there is a potential difference between them, and a negative (downward) deflection is recorded in the electrogram (EGM). *B,* The wave of depolarization advances over the cell on the right, causing the same transmembrane potential (0 mV) in the cells under both electrode 1 and electrode 2. The electrogram records no difference in potential between electrodes 1 and 2, and the deflection returns to baseline.

(Fig. 3–2). As the wave of depolarization moves from left to right in this figure, electrode 1 suddenly shifts from recording the positively charged outside of the underlying cell to recording a potential that is about 0 mV relative to the inside of the cell (see Fig. 3–2A). Although the inside and outside of the myocardial cells underlying this electrode are approximately electrically neutral, electrode 1 has suddenly become electrically negative relative to electrode 2. The electrogram recorded between these electrodes at this precise moment inscribes a brisk downward (negative) deflection. As the depolarizing wave continues to advance, so that the myocardium under electrode 2 also becomes depolarized (see Fig. 3–2B), the two electrodes record similar absolute voltage, and the electrogram returns briskly to the baseline. Thus, as this diagram illustrates, it is the *difference in electric potential between two electrodes* produced by electric currents within the myocardium that generates the intracardiac electrogram.

Figure 3–3 illustrates how the orientation of two electrodes relative to a wavefront of depolarization can have a dramatic influence on the intracardiac electrogram. In Figure 3–3A, if the interelectrode axis is oriented parallel to the wavefront of depolarization, a brisk electrogram is inscribed. In contrast, if the two electrodes are oriented exactly perpendicular to the wavefront (see Fig. 3–3B), both electrodes record from the electrically positive outside of the resting myocytes. As the wavefront of depolarization passes directly under both electrodes, the electric potential of the myocardium suddenly shifts to about 0 mV. *Relative to each other,* however, there is *no difference in electric potential* between the electrodes. Thus, if two electrodes record precisely the same electric charge at all times, no intracardiac electrogram is generated.

Unipolar Versus Bipolar Electrograms

Thus far we have considered only the electric signals recorded from a pair of electrodes in contact with the myocardium, that is, the bipolar sensing configuration. Unipolar pacing systems use one electrode in contact with the myocardium (usually the cathode) and another electrode in contact with the pulse generator case (usually the anode). Although there are clinically important differences between bipolar and unipolar sensing, the same basic principles of sensing apply to both configurations.[1–5] The differences in these configurations result from the fact that a unipolar system records the difference in potential between a more widely spaced pair of electrodes and that one electrode is not in contact with the heart. As the depolarizing wave advances toward the electrode in contact with the myocardium, this electrode becomes slightly positive relative to the electrode on the pulse generator case (Fig. 3–4A). As the depolarizing wave passes directly under the electrode in contact with the myocardium, this electrode suddenly becomes negatively charged relative to an electrode that is remote from the heart, and a brisk negative deflection is inscribed in the electrogram (see Fig. 3–4B). As the wavefront passes away from the intracardiac electrode, the electrogram returns to baseline.

Because electrograms represent the difference in potential between two electrodes over time, the unipolar sensing configuration is also influenced by other electric signals that are nearer to the electrode that is not in contact with the heart. For example, unipolar atrial electrograms are more likely to record large far-field cardiac signals, such as R waves, than are bipolar electrograms. Events nearer the extracardiac electrode, such as skeletal myopotentials, affect this electrode more than the intracardiac electrode and also inscribe their electric signals in the unipolar electrogram. Thus, unipolar

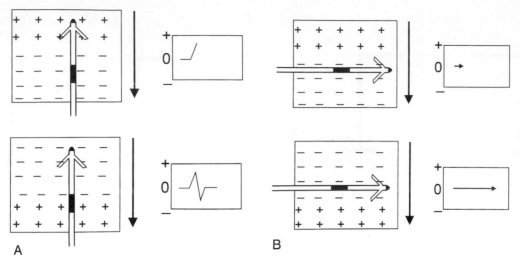

Figure 3–3. The effect of interelectrode axis on a bipolar electrogram. *A,* A wavefront of activation spreads parallel to the interelectrode axis of a bipolar lead. Note that as the wave of positive charges advances toward the tip electrode *(top)*, a brisk positive deflection is inscribed in the electrogram. As the wave of activation spreads past the ring electrode, the electrogram shifts abruptly from positive to negative before returning to baseline. *B,* The interelectrode axis is perpendicular to the spread of activation. Note that the wave of activation reaches the tip and ring electrodes simultaneously, with no net difference between the electrodes at any point *(top* and *bottom)*. Therefore, the electrogram does not show a deflection from baseline. This diagram illustrates the importance of interelectrode axis on the morphology of the intracardiac electrogram.

sensing has the potential disadvantages of greater susceptibility to unwanted far-field intracardiac signals and skeletal myopotentials.

A bipolar electrogram can be considered as the instantaneous difference in potential between two unipolar electrograms recorded from two intracardiac electrodes and a common remote indifferent electrode. In mathematical terms, the bipolar electrogram is equal to the unipolar electrogram from electrode 1 minus the unipolar electrogram from electrode 2: $BiEGM = UniEGM_1 - UniEGM_2$. This relationship explains the diminished susceptibility of bipolar recordings to extracardiac signals because the two electrodes in close proximity are likely to record simultaneously similar extraneous potentials, which are then canceled. Because of this

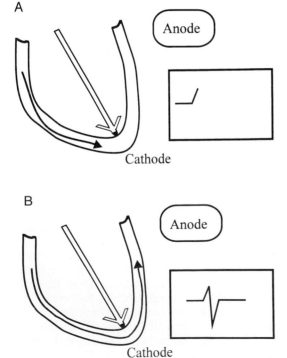

Figure 3–4. *A,* Demonstration of the concept of unipolar sensing. Note that there are actually two electrodes, one located within the heart (cathode) and one located outside the heart in contact with the pulse generator case (anode). As a wavefront of activation advances toward the intracardiac electrode *(arrow)*, the electrogram records a positive deflection. At the moment the wavefront passes the cathode *(B)*, the electrogram suddenly shifts from positive to negative before returning to baseline as the wave spreads away.

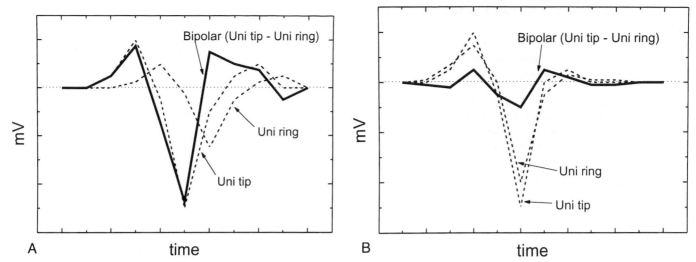

Figure 3–5. The relationship between unipolar and bipolar electrograms recorded between the tip and ring electrodes of a bipolar pacing lead. *A*, The unipolar ring electrogram is equal to exactly half the amplitude of the unipolar tip electrogram. Note that there is a phase shift in the timing of activation, the tip electrogram being activated earlier than the ring electrode. The bipolar electrogram is equal to the unipolar tip electrogram minus the unipolar ring electrogram at all times. Because there is a difference in the amplitude and timing of the unipolar tip and ring electrograms, the bipolar electrogram has acceptable amplitude. *B*, The unipolar ring electrogram has an amplitude that is only slightly less than that of the unipolar tip electrogram. In addition, there is essentially no phase shift. Although both unipolar electrograms demonstrate acceptable amplitude for sensing, the bipolar electrogram shows both diminished amplitude and diminished slew rate.

fact, unipolar electrograms may also be less susceptible to the orientation of the interelectrode axis in some cases than are bipolar electrograms. For example, Figure 3–5*A* illustrates unipolar electrograms recorded from the tip and ring electrodes of a bipolar pacing lead. The unipolar tip electrogram has an amplitude that is equal to twice the unipolar ring electrogram. There is a phase shift in the moment of activation (the intrinsic deflection), however, as the wave of depolarization travels beneath the tip electrode earlier than the ring electrode. The bipolar electrogram is equal to the difference in potential at each point in time between the tip and ring electrodes. If the unipolar tip and ring electrograms have similar amplitude and timing, however, the difference in potential between the electrodes is small, and the bipolar electrogram may be of much lower amplitude than either unipolar electrogram alone (see Fig. 3–5*B*).

Electrogram Waveforms, Amplitude, and Slew Rate

The *intrinsic deflection* of an electrogram is the rapid downstroke of the electrogram that occurs as the myocardium directly underlying the electrode suddenly becomes electrically negative during depolarization. Furman and colleagues[2] noted that 58% of unipolar endocardial electrograms at lead implantation were biphasic, with an initial upstroke followed by a downstroke, such that the R and S waves were roughly equal. In 30% of cases, the electrogram was predominantly monophasic negative, and in 12%, it was monophasic positive. The acute ventricular electrogram may demonstrate a current of injury with an elevated ST segment that later disappears.[2] The intracardiac electrogram is characterized in clinical practice in terms of its amplitude (measured in millivolts) and its slew rate (measured in volts per second).

Both factors are important determinants of whether an electric event will be sensed by the pacemaker.

Figure 3–6 illustrates the minimum amplitude and slew rate that should be accepted at lead implantation to ensure appropriate sensing. The amplitude of an electrogram depends on several factors, including the mass of myocardium underlying the electrode, the contact of the electrode with the myocardium, the orientation of the electrode with respect

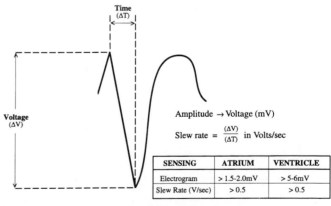

SENSING	ATRIUM	VENTRICLE
Electrogram	> 1.5-2.0mV	> 5-6mV
Slew Rate (V/sec)	> 0.5	> 0.5

Figure 3–6. The major clinical descriptors of an intracardiac electrogram are illustrated. The amplitude of the electrogram is the difference in voltage recorded between two electrodes and is measured in millivolts. The slew rate is equal to the first derivative of the electrogram (dV/dt) and is a measure of the sharpness of the electrogram. Slew rate is measured in volts per second. In general, the amplitude of the electrogram should be greater than 1.5 to 2.0 mV in the atrium and at least 5 to 6 mV in the ventricle at the time of lead implantation to ensure adequate sensing. The slew rate should be at least 0.5 V/sec in both the atrium and the ventricle.

to the axis of depolarization, and the presence of any inexcitable tissue between the myocytes and the electrode. Because the right ventricle typically has a much greater mass of myocytes than the right atrium, the ventricular electrogram usually has a much greater amplitude than the atrial electrogram. Electrodes that are in contact with infarcted myocardium or that become encapsulated with a thick layer of fibrotic tissue typically demonstrate a lower amplitude than electrodes directly in contact with healthy myocytes.

The slew rate represents the maximal rate of change of the electric potential between the sensing electrodes. Mathematically, the slew rate is the first derivative of the electrogram (dV/dt) and is a measure of the change in electrogram voltage over time. The slew rate is thus directly linked to the electrogram amplitude and duration. In general, an electrogram with an acceptable amplitude usually has an acceptable slew rate. Nevertheless, there are exceptions to this rule, so that both parameters should be measured with a pacing system analyzer at the time of lead implantation. Figure 3–7 demonstrates the interaction of electrogram amplitude, slew rate, and sensitivity threshold with respect to whether an electrogram is sensed by the sensing amplifier of a pacemaker or ICD. Note that electrograms of very low amplitude are not sensed, regardless of the slew rate. Because of filtering by the sensing circuitry, electrograms with an amplitude that exceeds the sensitivity threshold are not sensed if the slew rate is inadequate. There is a further interaction between the programmed sensitivity threshold and the adequacy of the slew rate, with greater slew rates required for appropriate sensing when the sensitivity threshold is programmed to a higher value.

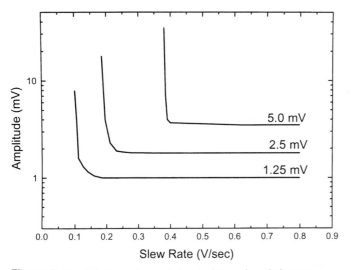

Figure 3–7. This figure demonstrates the interaction of electrogram amplitude (mV) and slew rate (V/sec) at three sensitivity settings for the Medtronic Spectrax sensing amplifiers. Note that with a programmed sensing threshold of 1.25 mV, electrograms with an amplitude of more than 1 mV will be sensed provided that the slew rate is at least 0.15 V/sec. If the slew rate is less than 0.1 V/sec, the amplitude must be greater to allow the electrogram to be sensed. At higher sensitivity threshold settings, greater amplitudes and slew rates are required for sensing by an electrogram.

Evolution of Electrograms Over Time

Like stimulation thresholds, intracardiac electrograms typically evolve during the first several weeks after lead implantation. The amplitude of the intracardiac electrogram usually declines to a nadir during the first several days to weeks after lead implantation before increasing to a chronic value that is slightly lower than that noted at implantation.[3–5] This decrease in electrogram amplitude is related to the development of a layer of inexcitable tissue surrounding the electrode in contact with the myocardium. This fibrotic capsule effectively increases the distance between the surface of the electrode and the excitable myocardium in which the electric signals arise.

Platia and Brinker[5] reported that the mean atrial unipolar electrogram amplitude decreased from 3.5 mV at implantation to 2.2 mV 1 month after implantation before returning to a chronic value of 3.2 mV at 13 months. For ventricular unipolar electrograms, there was a slight decrease in the amplitude from 13.5 mV at implantation to 10.1 mV at 1 month, before a chronic value of 13.0 mV was recorded at 13 months. DeCaprio and colleagues[1] reported that unipolar ventricular electrograms showed a reduction in amplitude from a mean of 12.4 ± 5.2 mV at implantation to 12.1 ± 5.3 mV during chronic follow-up. The change in slew rate was more significant, with a reduction from 3.5 V/sec at implantation to 2.3 V/sec at chronic follow-up. Bipolar electrograms demonstrated similar evolutionary changes, with a decrease in amplitude from 13.4 to 10.5 mV and a decrease in slew rate from 3.6 to 2.2 V/sec.

The evolution of electrogram amplitude is often more dramatic with active-fixation leads, in which atrial undersensing may occur during the first several days after lead implantation despite adequate electrogram amplitudes at implantation. To account for these changes in electrogram amplitude over time, the filtered electrogram recorded at lead implantation should be at least twice the sensitivity threshold that will be programmed in the pulse generator. This is especially true for electrodes with relatively traumatic active-fixation mechanisms. The addition of corticosteroid elution to pacing leads tends to attenuate the evolution of electrograms over time.[6] Because of this, it may be possible to accept a somewhat lower margin between the sensitivity setting in the pulse generator and the filtered electrogram amplitude at lead implantation if passive-fixation, corticosteroid-eluting leads are used.

Frequency Spectra of Intracardiac Electrograms

The electrogram that is recorded between two electrodes may register changes in voltage from sources other than the underlying myocardium, such as skeletal muscles and environmental interference.[7] In addition, some electrical events in the heart, such as the T wave, may exhibit large intracardiac electrogram amplitudes that are undesirable to sense. Fortunately, the frequency spectrum of these unwanted sources differs from that of myocardial depolarizations. This allows selective filtering to exclude unwanted signals (Fig. 3–8).

The spectrum of frequencies of an intracardiac electro-

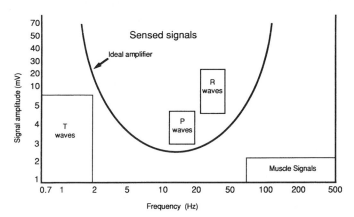

Figure 3–8. Schematic representation of the frequencies that are most typical of T waves, P waves, R waves, and myopotentials. An ideal sensing amplifier would have maximum sensitivity to signals with frequencies ranging from 10 to 40 Hz (typical of P waves and R waves) and decreased sensitivity to signals with very low (T waves) or very high (myopotentials) frequencies. In reality, there is often an overlap between the frequencies of myopotentials and the desired P waves and R waves.

gram can be studied by fast Fourier transformation, a technique that transforms the waveform into a series of sine waves and plots the energy content of the signal as a function of frequency. Myers and associates[4] studied the bandwidth of intracardiac ventricular electrograms in 30 patients using a physiologic recorder and electrodes of varying size. They defined the bandwidth of the signal as the point at which the amplitude spectrum has decreased to one fourth of its peak value. The bandwidth of the ventricular electrogram ranged from as narrow as 5 Hz to as wide as 116 Hz, depending on the size of the electrode and the loading conditions of the sense amplifier (see Sensing Impedance). In general, small electrodes demonstrated a wider electrogram bandwidth than large electrodes at a low-input impedance of the sensing amplifier but little difference at high-input impedance.

Kleinert and colleagues[8] reported that ventricular unipolar electrograms contained maximal energy in the frequencies ranging from about 10 to 50 Hz. The peak energy of the intracardiac R wave was centered at about 25 to 30 Hz. The T wave in the intracardiac ventricular electrogram has a much lower range of frequencies, the peak energies being located below 3 Hz. Atrial electrograms are characterized by a frequency spectrum that is similar to that of the ventricular electrogram, with typical energies in the range of 10 to 50 Hz. The peak energies are centered at about 20 to 30 Hz. The far-field R wave in the unipolar atrial electrogram is typically composed of lower frequencies, ranging from 5 to 20 Hz. It is therefore possible for pacemaker sensing circuits to attenuate the low frequencies that are characteristic of the T wave or far-field R wave by filtering without interfering with P-wave or R-wave sensing. Myopotentials typically have a higher frequency spectrum than P waves or R waves, with maximal energies in the range of 50 Hz. Although myopotentials contain more high-frequency components, there is considerable frequency overlap between R waves and P waves and signals generated by the pectoralis muscle. In general, myopotentials have a lower amplitude than ventricular electrograms; however, this is not true for P waves.

Therefore, although some components of myopotentials can be effectively filtered, unipolar pacing systems remain susceptible to myopotential inhibition.

Processing the Intracardiac Electrogram

Filtering of Intracardiac Signals

To improve the signal-to-noise ratio of intracardiac signals, sensing amplifiers incorporate filters that are intended to reject unwanted signals while allowing appropriate sensing of P waves and R waves.[9, 10] Ideally, the filter would allow the intrinsic deflection in the atrium and ventricle to pass while removing T waves, far-field cardiac events (such as R waves in the atrial electrogram), skeletal myopotentials, or afterpotentials. Figures 3–9 and 3–10 illustrate the effect of different filtering frequencies on the waveform of right atrial and right ventricular electrograms. Note that as the high-pass filter (designed to attenuate frequencies lower than this setting while allowing higher frequencies to "pass") is increased, there is a decrease in the amplitude of the electrogram.

Klitzner and Stevenson[9] studied the effect of high-pass filters on the ventricular electrogram in patients with right

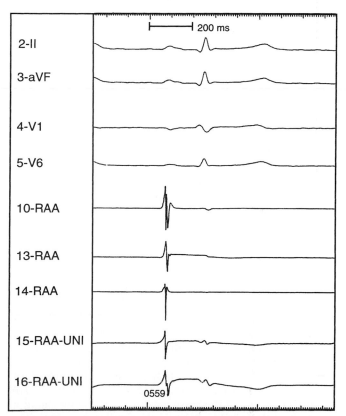

Figure 3–9. The effect of filtering on the electrogram recorded from the right atrial appendage (RAA). From top to bottom, surface electrocardiograph leads II, aVF, V₁, and V₆ are recorded simultaneously with bipolar electrograms filtered at 30 to 500 Hz (10-RAA), 0.05 to 100 Hz (13-RAA), and 100 to 2000 Hz (14-RAA). A notch filter designed to remove 60-Hz alternating current (AC) signals is used for the uppermost RAA electrogram. The two bottom tracings illustrate unipolar recordings with filter settings of 0.05 to 100 Hz and 0.05 to 1000 Hz (15-RAA-UNI and 16-RAA-UNI, respectively).

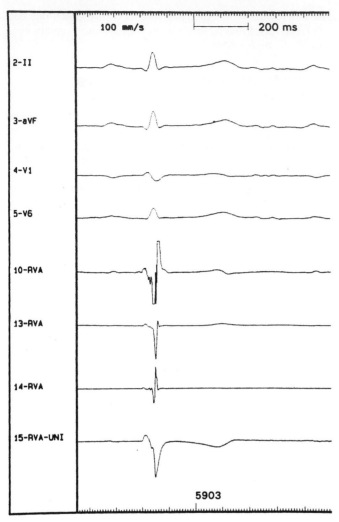

Figure 3–10. Effect of filtering on the right ventricular apex (RVA) electrogram. From top to bottom, four surface electrocardiographic leads (leads II, aVF, V₁ and V₆) are displayed, with intracardiac electrograms recorded at the RVA. Filter settings for the RVA electrograms (*top* to *bottom*) are as follows: bipolar, 30 to 500 Hz with notch filtering (10-RVA); bipolar, 0.05 to 100 Hz without notch filtering (13-RVA); bipolar, 100 to 2000 Hz without notch filtering (14-RVA); and unipolar, 0.05 to 1000 Hz (15-RVA-UNI).

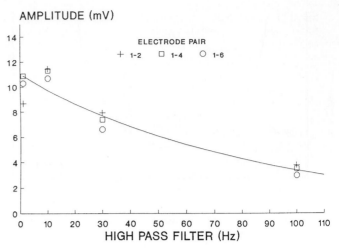

Figure 3–11. The effect of high-pass filtering on the amplitude of right ventricular intracardiac electrograms in humans. Note that as the high-pass filter is increased in frequency from 0.05 to 100 Hz, the amplitude of the electrogram is progressively reduced. (From Klitzner TS, Stevenson WG: Effects of filtering on right ventricular electrograms recorded from endocardial catheters in humans. PACE 13:69, 1990.)

ventricular catheters and noted that an increase in the high-pass filter from 1 to 10 Hz had little effect on the electrogram amplitude (from 9.0 to 11.2 mV) or duration (from 35 to 39 msec). However, a high-pass filter of 30 Hz decreased the ventricular electrogram amplitude to 8.2 mV and the duration to 34 msec. An increase in the high-pass filter to 100 Hz further decreased the amplitude to 4 mV and the duration to 24 msec (Fig. 3–11). Decreasing the low-pass filter (designed to attenuate signals with high frequencies, allowing lower frequencies to "pass") from 2500 Hz to 100 Hz had no effect on electrogram amplitude or duration.

Permanent pacemakers use analog filters that have a *center frequency* at which the signal is least attenuated (Fig. 3–12). At frequencies above and below the center frequency, the signal amplitude is decreased. In other words, for any programmed sensitivity threshold setting, signals above or below the center frequency must have a greater amplitude to be sensed than signals in the center frequency range.

The center frequency of the sensing amplifier that is measured is markedly dependent on the waveform used for testing. The sine-squared test waveform has been most commonly used for evaluating sensing circuits, although manufacturers have not agreed on a consistent approach. Using different test waveforms to determine the amplitude

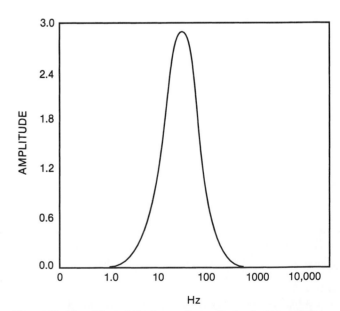

Figure 3–12. Effect of filtering on the amplitude of an intracardiac electrogram that will be sensed for a modern permanent pulse generator. The size of the signal actually sensed by the sensing amplifier is shown on the ordinate as a function of signal frequency on the abscissa. Note that the signal frequency for which the amplifier is most sensitive *(center)* is about 30 to 40 Hz.

of a signal that will be sensed by the pulse generator results in a variance of up to 100% in the sensing threshold for an electrogram between manufacturers. Because of this, the same ventricular electrogram may be measured very differently by the pulse generator of different manufacturers. In addition, the ability of a pulse generator to reject unwanted signals is influenced by the test waveform that is used.[7] Thus, skeletal myopotentials that are effectively rejected by one pulse generator may be readily sensed by another (Fig. 3–13).

This discussion of filtering has important clinical implications at the time of pacemaker implantation. One cannot assume that an electrogram that is recorded on a physiologic recorder with a wide bandpass filter and high-input impedance will accurately reflect the filtered electrogram that is actually sensed by the pulse generator.

Afterpotentials

After delivery of a stimulation pulse, the myocardium in contact with the stimulating electrode becomes electrically charged as current is transferred from the electrode to the myocardium. For a cathodal pulse, the negatively charged electrode in contact with the endocardium becomes surrounded by positively charged ions (such as Na^+ and H_3O^+), whereas negatively charged ions (such as Cl^-, HPO_4^{2-}, and OH^-) are electronically repelled from the electrode. This *polarization* at the electrode–tissue interface begins at the start of the pacing pulse and increases to the end of the stimulus. After the pacing stimulus, the degree of polarization gradually dissipates as ions re-establish electric neutrality. Polarization thus represents a voltage source in the tissues that may be sensed as an electric signal of opposite polarity to the stimulation waveform (Fig. 3–14).

Polarization is related to several factors, including the amplitude and duration of the stimulation pulse and the radius, surface area, geometry, surface structure, and chemical composition of the electrode. The magnitude of afterpo-

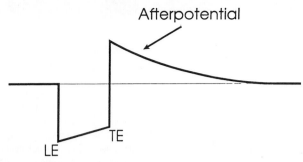

Figure 3–14. Diagram of a constant-voltage pacing pulse (downward deflection) with leading edge (LE) and trailing edge (TE) voltage and a resultant afterpotential of opposite polarity. Afterpotentials may interfere with sensing, especially if the stimulus is of high amplitude and duration.

tentials depends on the polarization properties of the electrode and decreases with increasing microscopic surface area. The chemical content of the electrode also has a major effect on polarization, with afterpotentials being reduced by materials that have low polarization properties. The materials presently used for permanent pacing electrodes include platinum-iridium, titanium (oxide), platinum- or carbon-coated titanium, platinized platinum, vitreous carbon, and iridium oxide. The platinized-platinum, "activated" carbon, and iridium oxide electrodes greatly reduce the degree of polarization. The vitreous carbon electrodes can be manufactured by a process known as *activation*, which increases the electrode surface area by roughening the surface, thereby reducing polarization. To reduce afterpotentials and prevent loss of stimulation efficiency related to polarization at rapid pacing rates, manufacturers have introduced "rapid recharge" circuits following pacing stimuli. For example, Medtronic, Inc. (Minneapolis) has used a recharge period after delivery of the pacing stimulus in which the output capacitor is allowed to recharge from the accumulated polarization in the myocardium over a period of 8 msec.[11] This allows the polarization to dissipate at the electrode–tissue interface and reduces afterpotentials (Fig. 3–15).[12]

Unless suitable blanking of the sense amplifiers is em-

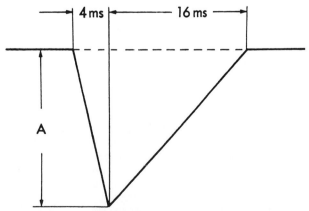

Figure 3–13. Proposed test signal waveform for testing sensing amplifiers. A 20-msec test signal with a 4-msec initial downward deflection and a 16-msec upward deflection was found by Irnich to best reflect the characteristics of intracardiac electrograms. The 4/16 msec test signal proposed to Irnich was changed by ISO, CENELEC to 2/13 msec. (From Irnich W: Intracardiac electrograms and sensing test signals: Electrophysiological, physical, and technical considerations. PACE 8:870, 1985.)

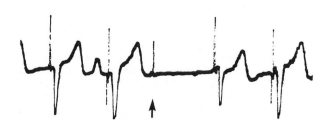

Figure 3–15. Surface electrocardiographic tracing made from a patient with a Medtronic Spectrax pulse generator that incorporates a rapid recharge pulse after sensed ventricular events. The first two complexes represent VVI pacing stimuli. The third complex demonstrates an attenuated stimulus artifact *(arrow)* that is the result of a rapid recharge pulse delivered synchronously with a sensed ventricular event. This artifact could easily be mistaken for noncapture of a pacing stimulus. (From Barold SS, Kulkarni H, Thawani AJ, et al: Electrocardiographic manifestations of the rapid recharge function of pulse generators after sensing. PACE 11:1215, 1988.)

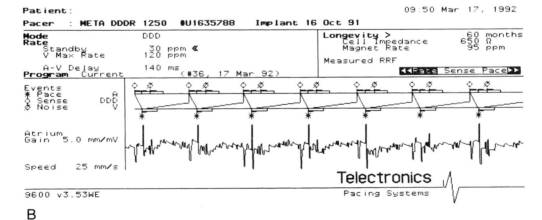

Figure 3–16. Crosstalk in a patient with a DDD pacemaker. In this patient, the ventricular blanking period had been shortened with an atrial stimulus amplitude of 7.5 V and a pulse duration of 2.0 msec because of a high stimulation threshold. The first six complexes show atrial pacing followed by ventricular pacing. The seventh complex from the left shows an atrial pacing stimulus and inhibition of the ventricular pacing stimulus due to sensing of afterpotentials from the atrial lead by the ventricular sensing channel. Crosstalk is most likely to occur in the presence of an atrial stimulus of high amplitude and duration combined with a sensitive ventricular sensing setting.

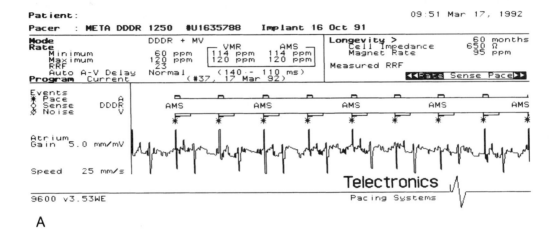

Figure 3–17. Inappropriate automatic mode switching (AMS) demonstrated by sensing of the far-field ventricular electrogram with the Meta DDDR model 1250 pulse generator. There is bipolar atrial and ventricular sensing. *A,* DDDR pacing with programmer printouts showing simultaneous tracings of the events recorded by the pacemaker and the intracardiac atrial electrogram. AMS occurred during the events recorded in panel *A.* The atrial electrogram shows prominent voltage corresponding to the ventricular stimulus artifact. Following this are the smaller voltages of the far-field paced ventricular electrogram. Soon after this appear the larger voltages of the retrograde atrial electrogram, another potential cause of AMS. *B,* When the pacemaker is reprogrammed to the DDD mode, AMS does not occur because the sensed far-field paced ventricular electrogram is beyond the AMS window and is interpreted as noise. Sensing in the postventricular atrial refractory period (PVARP) with resetting of the atrial refractory period now occurs, but there is no retrograde atrial deflection in the atrial electrogram. This fact confirms that the far-field paced ventricular electrogram was responsible for the AMS and not the retrograde P wave (VMR, ventricular maximum rate or upper tracking rate; RRF, rate-response factor). (From Mond H, Barold SS: Dual-chamber, rate-adaptive pacing in patients with paroxysmal supraventricular tachyarrhythmias: Protective measures for rate control. PACE 16:2168, 1993.)

ployed, afterpotentials can be sensed by the pulse generator and can inappropriately inhibit pacing output. If a high stimulation amplitude is used, afterpotentials may also be sensed by the amplifier in the opposite chamber. For example, afterpotentials resulting from atrial stimulation may be sensed by the ventricular sense amplifier of a dual-chamber pacemaker and may inappropriately inhibit ventricular output, a phenomenon known as *crosstalk* (Fig. 3–16). Crosstalk is more likely to occur with a wide interelectrode distance and therefore is much more common with unipolar than with bipolar sensing configurations. Thus, the combination of an atrial stimulus with high amplitude and a ventricular sense amplifier programmed to high sensitivity is especially likely to generate crosstalk.

To avoid crosstalk, the ventricular sense amplifier is temporarily disabled (blanked) immediately after delivery of the atrial pacing stimulus. The duration of the ventricular blanking period may be a programmable parameter, and values of 25 to 50 msec are most commonly used. The phenomenon of *reverse crosstalk,* in which the atrial sense amplifier detects far-field electric events in the ventricle, may also occur.[13] Reverse crosstalk may become clinically manifest with dual-chamber pacemakers that offer automatic mode reversion algorithms designed to switch from the DDD or DDDR mode to the VVI or VVIR mode in response to atrial tachyarrhythmias (Fig. 3–17). In the presence of high atrial sensitivity, the far-field R wave in the atrial electrogram can result in inappropriate mode switching.

Blanking and Refractory Periods

As the preceding discussion demonstrates, it is not possible to distinguish the desired components of an electrogram from unwanted signals by filtering alone. Therefore, pulse generators use the expected timing of atrial and ventricular activation as a means of improving signal discrimination. To ignore the depolarizations and afterpotentials induced by pacing stimuli, the atrial and ventricular sensing amplifiers are disabled for a brief period after the pacing stimulus. This interval is called the *blanking period* and for the ventricle is generally 20 to 50 msec in duration. This temporary inactivation prevents sense amplifier saturation by the high-input voltage of the pacing stimulus. Saturation of the amplifier

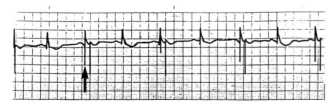

Figure 3–18. Loss of atrial sensing with apparent ventricular undersensing and ventricular pacing. Note that in the second complex, an atrial pacing stimulus follows the P wave because of undersensing in the atrium. The atrial pacing stimulus occurs at the start of the ventricular QRS complex. The ventricular electrogram is not sensed because of blanking in the ventricular sensing amplifier immediately following an atrial pacing stimulus. This sequence is repeated in the fourth, sixth, and eighth complexes. Atrial undersensing may lead to apparent ventricular undersensing because the ventricular blanking period does not permit sensing of electric signals for a period of 10 to 40 msec after an atrial output pulse.

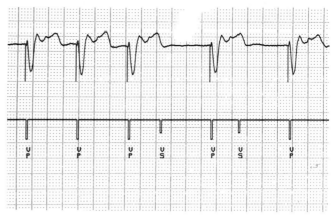

Figure 3–19. Marker channel from a VVI pacemaker. A surface electrocardiogram lead is shown as the top tracing with the marker channel from the pacemaker programmer on the bottom. The first three complexes show ventricular pacing (VP) with capture. The pauses following the third and fourth complexes result from T-wave oversensing (VS) demonstrated by the marker channel.

would necessitate a period of recovery before the amplifier can again become functional. The blanking of the amplifier allows it to be re-enabled immediately without the delay of recovery. Thus, if an electric event occurs within this blanking period, it will not be sensed. In dual-chamber pacing systems, both the atrial and ventricular sense amplifiers are blanked immediately after a pacing stimulus in either chamber (Fig. 3–18).

To avoid sensing of T waves and far-field events by the ventricular sense amplifier, a programmable *refractory period* is employed (Fig. 3–19). During the refractory period, the sense amplifier remains enabled because amplifier saturation is not expected to occur. The pulse generator, however, will not respond to electric signals that exceed the programmed sensitivity threshold value during the refractory period. Events during the refractory period may be sensed for tachyarrhythmia detection algorithms but generally do not alter the timing cycles. Combined with filtering, blanking and refractory periods have greatly reduced the incidence of T-wave and far-field sensing. Nevertheless, programming of the refractory period to an inappropriately short duration may allow T-wave sensing, especially if a very sensitive sensing threshold value is programmed.

The programmed refractory period is especially important for proper function of AAI pacemakers in which far-field R waves or even T waves may be sensed. Thus, the atrial refractory period must be longer than the paced PR interval as measured by the intracardiac atrial electrogram. This interval must include the entire intracardiac R wave to avoid far-field sensing. The atrial refractory period of an AAIR pacemaker is usually in the range of 325 to 450 msec. For unipolar AAIR pacemakers, an even longer refractory period may be necessary to avoid oversensing of far-field T waves. This situation can be even more complex with AAIR pacing systems because the PR interval may prolong with excessively rapid atrial pacing rates, especially if the rate-adaptive sensor is programmed overly aggressively. Rate-adaptive pacemakers have the additional complication of increasing the lower pacing rate in response to output of the sensor.

Thus, if the refractory period is longer than the pacing interval at the upper programmed pacing rate, asynchronous pacing may occur at high sensor-indicated rates.

Refractory and blanking periods are required in both the atrial and ventricular sensing amplifiers of dual-chamber pacemakers. After the atrial pacing stimulus, the atrial and ventricular sensing amplifiers are blanked for a period to avoid sensing afterpotentials. After the postatrial blanking period in the ventricular channel, the ventricular sense amplifier is alert for the occurrence of an intrinsically conducted QRS complex. Delivery of a ventricular pacing stimulus or the occurrence of an intrinsic ventricular beat activates a blanking period followed by a refractory period in the ventricular sensing amplifier to avoid afterpotentials and T-wave oversensing. After a ventricular paced or sensed event, the atrial sense amplifier also enters a postventricular atrial blanking period of 100 to 160 msec followed by a *postventricular atrial refractory period* (PVARP). The atrial blanking period is designed to avoid oversensing of ventricular pacing stimuli and far-field R waves, whereas the PVARP is designed to avoid sensing retrogradely conducted atrial activation that may follow ventricular activation or ventricular premature depolarizations. The net result is a period of refractoriness in the atrial sense amplifier known as the *total atrial refractory period* (TARP), which is equal to the atrioventricular (AV) delay plus the PVARP: TARP = AV delay + PVARP.

The duration of the TARP has profound implications for atrial sensing and tracking of the atrium at high sinus rates (Fig. 3–20). To allow appropriate recognition of very rapid atrial signals associated with pathologic arrhythmias, such as atrial fibrillation, many newer dual-chamber pacemakers with mode-switching algorithms allow electric signals that occur after the atrial blanking period but within the PVARP to be logged into atrial rate counters without being tracked.[14] Such sensing within the PVARP may also avoid the occurrence of asynchronous atrial pacing at high sensor-indicated pacing rates.

Because the AV delay of most current dual-chamber pacemakers shortens in response to increasing atrial rates or sensor input, the TARP also shortens. Several manufacturers now offer dual-chamber pacemakers that also shorten the PVARP with increasing atrial or sensor-indicated rates, fur-ther reducing the TARP during exercise. The result of these newer algorithms is that the programmed upper tracking rate can be more safely increased while providing protection from retrogradely conducted atrial beats and the initiation of pacemaker-mediated tachycardia at lower heart rates. Appropriate recognition of pathologic atrial arrhythmias is also enhanced, improving the sensitivity of mode-switching algorithms.

Sensing Impedance

As discussed previously, the intracardiac electrogram originates from electric currents in the myocardium underlying the pacemaker lead. The electric signal, however, may become distorted as it is transmitted by the pacing lead to the sensing amplifier. The theoretical model for understanding pacemaker sensing has been described as a voltage source (the myocardium) in series with a resistor and a capacitor that are in parallel (Fig. 3–21). The three components of sensing impedance include tissue resistance (R_t), Faraday resistance (R_F), and Helmholtz capacitance (C_H). The total sensing impedance (Z_S) is approximated by the following equation:

(1) $Z_S = R_t + [R_F/(1 + C_H R_F)]$

The tissue resistance (R_t) can be measured in the standard manner as the ratio of current to voltage: $R_t = \dfrac{V}{I}$. Tissue resistance is related to the ohmic resistance of the lead conductor and the resistance of the myocardium; it typically ranges from 300 to 1000 ohms (Ω) for a permanent pacing lead. The Faraday resistance represents the impediment to current flow across the tissue–electrode interface and is indirectly related to the surface area of the electrode. Ohm[15] measured the Faraday resistance at the tissue–electrode interface and found it to range from as low as 7.7 kΩ for the large surface area ring electrode of a bipolar lead (48 mm^2) to as high as 87 kΩ for a tip electrode measuring 11 mm^2. The Helmholtz capacitance (C_H) is the polarization capacitance at the tissue–electrode surface and is related to the frequency content of the signal. Capacitance (C) is the ratio of charge (Q) to voltage (V) (C = Q/V). Therefore, for a high-capacitance electrode, a large amount of charge can be stored on the electrode without generating a significant voltage. Capacitance is directly related to the surface area of the

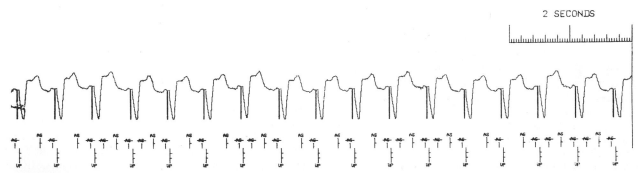

Figure 3–20. An example of the usefulness of intracardiac marker channels in a patient with a DDD pacemaker. The surface electrocardiogram demonstrates ventricular pacing at the upper rate limit during atrial flutter. The atrial marker channel demonstrates atrial events that were sensed within PVARP (-AS-) and atrial events sensed outside PVARP (AS). Note that following a ventricular pacing stimulus (VP), some atrial electrograms are not sensed, resulting in apparent electrogram dropout because the atrium is blanked for a period following delivery of a ventricular pacing stimulus. Only atrial signals recorded outside PVARP (AS) are tracked.

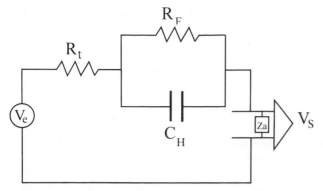

Figure 3–21. Schematic representation of sensing impedance. The electric signal in the myocardium is a voltage source (V$_e$). The tissue resistance (R$_t$) represents the impediment to flow of current through the myocardium, the electrode, and the lead conductors. The Faraday resistance (R$_F$) is related to the transfer of charge from the myocardium to the electrode. The tissue–electrode interface is also capable of storing charge, represented by a Helmholtz capacitor (C$_H$). Thus, sensing impedance is represented by a resistor (R$_t$) in series with a resistor (R$_F$) and a capacitor (C$_H$) that are in parallel. The current then flows through the input impedance of the sensing amplifier (Z$_a$). The amplitude of the signal that is actually sensed by the sense amplifier (V$_S$) is somewhat less than the amplitude of the electrogram at its source in the myocardium (V$_e$). The greater the input impedance of the sense amplifier in relation to the sensing impedance, the less the electrogram is attenuated.

electrode and generally ranges from 1 to 10 mF. The greater the polarization capacitance of the electrode, the lower the sensing impedance (Z$_S$). Polarization capacitance is dependent on the surface area of the electrode, the surface structure, and the electrode materials. Electrodes with low polarization properties have a high Helmholtz capacitance.

The higher the frequency of the signal, the lower the capacitance (and the higher the sensing impedance). A resistance-capacitance circuit may also introduce electrogram distortion, such that the electrogram is effectively filtered. The lower frequency limit (f) of such a filtering effect of an electrode is determined by the following formula:

$$(2) \quad f = \frac{1}{2} \pi R_F C_H,$$

where R$_F$ is the Faraday impedance and C$_H$ is the Helmholtz capacitance. Ideally, the low-frequency filtering effect of an RC circuit should be less than the range of frequencies expected for P waves and R waves (10 to 40 Hz). For low-capacitance electrodes, f is increased compared with high-capacitance electrodes and may result in effectively filtering frequencies within the desired range of R waves and P waves. For example, Fischler[16] found that the lower-frequency cutoff of low-capacitance electrodes (leads made from elgiloy) may be as high as 15 Hz in the presence of a low-input impedance of the sensing amplifier (20 kΩ). Therefore, to avoid distortion of the electrogram, the electrode should have a high capacitance.

Sensing impedance is important to understand because it relates to the amplitude of the electrogram that is actually sensed by the pulse generator. The voltage of the signal that is sensed by the pulse generator (V$_S$) is directly related to the input impedance of the sense amplifier (Z$_A$) and inversely related to the total sensing impedance (Z$_S$) by the following formula:

$$(3) \quad V_S = \frac{Z_A}{Z_A + Z_S} \times V_E,$$

where V$_E$ is the voltage of the electrogram at its source in the myocardium. Thus, if Z$_A$ is equal to Z$_S$, then V$_S$ would be equal to ½ V$_E$. In other words, if the sensing impedance is equal to the input impedance of the amplifier, the electrogram sensed by the pulse generator would be only half the amplitude of the electrogram in the myocardium. Such an attenuation of the electrogram amplitude by an input impedance that is too low or a sensing impedance that is too high is referred to as *impedance mismatch*. To minimize the attenuation of the electrogram by impedance mismatch, the input impedance of the sensing amplifier must be increased to a value that is far greater than the sensing impedance. If the input impedance is infinite, no attenuation of the electrogram would occur. Physiologic recorders usually have an input impedance of 500 to 1000 kΩ and produce little attenuation of the electrogram. The input impedance of modern pacemaker sense amplifiers is typically 25 to 40 kΩ, thus minimizing impedance mismatch and electrogram distortion.

Effects of Leads on Sensing
Electrode Size and Configuration

The radius of an electrode has important effects on stimulation threshold but lesser influence on the amplitude of the sensed electrogram. The higher Faraday resistance, lower Helmholtz capacitance, and higher sensing impedance of smaller electrodes should theoretically degrade sensing. In practice, small electrodes provide electrograms that are equivalent in amplitude and slew rate to larger electrodes, provided that the input impedance of the sensing amplifier is sufficiently high.[15, 16] Clinical evaluation demonstrated equivalent sensing characteristics among leads with 8- to 1.5-mm tip electrodes.[17, 18] Similarly, the interelectrode distance of a bipolar pacing lead has little effect on the amplitude and slew rate of the intracardiac electrogram but does have a major effect on the duration of the electrogram.[1] The greater the separation of electrodes, the longer the duration of the electrogram. This results from greater far-field sensing with wider electrode separation. Conversely, very small electrodes with close interelectrode spacing produce electrograms with a short duration and attenuated far-field signals.

To further minimize far-field signals and improve signal-to-noise discrimination, Goldreyer and colleagues[19, 20] developed an orthogonal pacemaker lead that incorporated a pair of platinum-iridium electrodes placed perpendicular to the long axis of the catheter (Fig. 3–22). The orthogonal electrodes "float" within the atrial cavity without necessarily contacting the endocardial surface. The mean P-wave amplitude recorded from such electrodes was 2.4 ± 1.7 mV with a far-field R wave of only 0.07 mV. The surface area of the orthogonal electrodes had an important effect on the amplitude of the atrial electrogram, with a mean P wave of 2.0 ± 0.77 mV for electrodes with a 0.8-mm^2 surface area and 1.32 ± 0.27 mV for 10-mm^2 surface area electrodes. The duration of the bipolar orthogonal electrogram was only 15 to 20 msec. Thus, the advantage of orthogonal electrodes is the excellent signal-to-noise discrimination provided by the rejection of far-field events.

When incorporated onto a ventricular lead, orthogonal atrial electrodes or floating atrial ring electrodes allow for

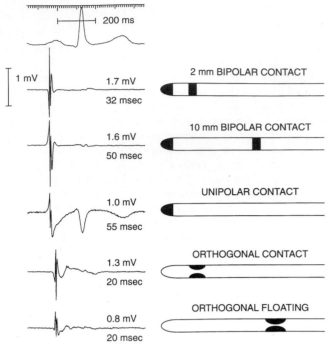

Figure 3–22. Effects of electrode configurations on the atrial endocardial electrogram. The electrograms are obtained from a single patient with two catheters placed simultaneously in the right atrial appendage. One catheter has 2-mm ring electrodes *(top three tracings)* and the other catheter has 1-mm orthogonal electrodes. The surface electrocardiogram tracing is shown at the top of the figure. Time and voltage amplitude scales are shown. For each electrode configuration *(right),* the corresponding electrogram is shown *(left),* with the peak-to-peak amplitude (in mV) and electrogram duration (in msec) labeled. Contact refers to electrodes in contact with the atrial tissue. Floating refers to noncontact electrodes in the atrial chamber. Note that greater ring electrode spacing from 2 to 10 mm prolongs the electrogram duration without altering the amplitude. The unipolar electrogram shows a wider and diminished atrial electrogram and a prominent far-field ventricular electrogram as well. The orthogonal electrode configurations provide electrograms of lesser amplitude and shorter duration than the ring electrodes.

VDD or DDD pacing using a single lead.[21–24] In large studies of floating atrial electrodes, the P-wave amplitude decreases by about 40% to 50% immediately after implantation, but thereafter chronic sensing thresholds are stable over time.[25, 26] In the same patients, P-wave amplitude from floating electrodes (2.5 ± 0.8 mV) are smaller than from passive-fixation leads (4.2 ± 0.35 mV) in the atrial appendage.[26] The disadvantages of orthogonal single-pass lead designs are the complexity of a multiconductor lead with its attendant reliability concerns, high pacing thresholds, lower P-wave amplitude, and greater postural P-wave variation compared with endocardial contact electrodes.[27]

Lead Positions

For electrodes in contact with the endocardium, the amplitude of the sensed electrogram appears to be little influenced by the intracardiac lead position, assuming lead stability. Sensing characteristics are similar at implantation and chronically between leads positioned in the right ventricular outflow tract and the right ventricular apex.[28] Similarly, atrial

leads positioned in the right atrial appendage, right atrial septum, and low posterior right atrium all provide comparable atrial electrogram amplitudes.[29, 30] The right atrial appendage, however, has been reported to yield the greatest atrial electrogram amplitude and slew rate compared with other atrial sites.[31] For floating atrial electrodes, optimal sensing is usually obtained from the high or middle right atrium.[26]

The chronic sensing and pacing characteristics of epicardial leads are inferior to those of endocardial leads owing to exuberant fibrous capsule formation that results in exit block in up to 26% of implanted leads.[32] The introduction of steroid-eluting epicardial lead designs has greatly improved chronic pacing thresholds, with no pacing failure in early reports.[33, 34] Although the chronic sensing function of these leads is not well described, sensing failure is not mentioned. Data from the clinical trial of the Medtronic Model 4965 steroid-eluting unipolar epicardial electrode show atrial and ventricular electrogram amplitudes of 2.4 ± 1.6 and 5.9 ± 2.8 mV, respectively, at implantation in 275 patients (256 children).[35] The sensing thresholds did not change in either chamber over 12 months of follow-up. Steroid-eluting bipolar epicardial electrodes have shown excellent short-term sensing characteristics in immature dogs.[36]

Left atrial and left ventricular sensing can be achieved chronically with leads positioned in the coronary sinus and cardiac veins.[37, 38] Left atrial sensing appears to be optimal in the proximal to middle coronary sinus.[38] Left ventricular sensing is best in the distal coronary sinus or distal cardiac veins (Fig. 3–23).[37] Standard or specially designed leads have been used for coronary sinus positions.[37] A canted lead tip design orients the electrode toward the left atrium or ventricle and improves lead stability (Fig. 3–24). Small-diameter tineless ventricular leads facilitate access to the distal coronary venous branches. Using specialized lead designs, left ventricular pacing is achieved in 82% of patients, compared with 53% using standard leads.[37] Coronary sinus atrial electrogram amplitudes of 2 to 2.5 mV may be achieved chronically with ventricular electrograms of 9 to 13 mV recorded from the cardiac veins.[37, 39–41] Coronary venous lead stability is problematic, especially for atrial sensing.[40]

Cardiac electrical activity can also be monitored through implanted, leadless, extracardiac devices. The Insertable Loop Recorder (Medtronic, Minneapolis, MN) incorporates two electrodes in the elongated can (6 × 1.6 cm) of a passive monitor-only device that is placed subcutaneously in the pectoral region.[42] Because of the extracardiac electrode positions, an electrocardiographic (ECG) lead rather than an intracardiac electrogram is recorded. This device functions as an event monitor being activated manually by the patient to freeze up to 40 minutes of ECG data in loop memory.

Unipolar Versus Bipolar Sensing Performance

Theoretically, the sensing characteristics of unipolar and bipolar pacing systems should differ substantially.[43] In clinical practice, however, the amplitude and slew rates are similar for unipolar and bipolar systems.[44, 45] Furman and colleagues[2] reported that unipolar and bipolar ventricular electrograms were similar in amplitude (12.19 versus 11.75 mV) and slew rate (2.82 versus 2.82 V/sec), although the unipolar electrogram is characterized by a greater current of

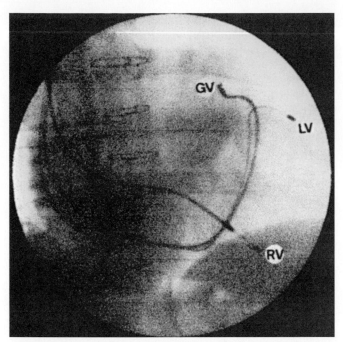

Figure 3–23. Anteroposterior fluoroscopic view of permanent pacemaker lead positions for pacing and sensing the left ventricle. Three leads are shown. One lead is in a standard position in the right ventricular apex (RV), and two leads are positioned through the coronary sinus. A bipolar lead is positioned in the proximal great cardiac vein (GV) to pace the anterobasilar left ventricle. A smaller-diameter unipolar lead rests in an anterolateral cardiac vein (LV) to pace the left free wall. (From Daubert C, Ritter P, Le Breton H, et al: Permanent left ventricular pacing with transvenous leads inserted into the coronary veins. PACE 21:239–245, 1988.)

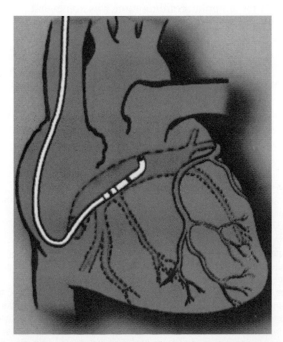

Figure 3–24. A specially designed Medtronic model 2188 coronary sinus lead for left atrial pacing and sensing. The canted lead tip is rotated to orient the electrode toward the atrium for optimal sensing and pacing. The distal angulation also serves to stabilize the lead within the coronary sinus.

injury (2.62 versus 1.64 mV) and T-wave amplitude (2.41 versus 1.60 mV) than the bipolar configuration. These authors found that atrial unipolar endocardial electrograms had a mean amplitude of 4.83 ± 2.21 mV, with an average slew rate of 1.18 V/sec. The far-field R wave of the unipolar atrial electrogram measured 2.21 mV in amplitude, with a slew rate of only 0.13 V/sec.

In a study by Nielsen and associates[44] using 74 patients with polarity programmable pacemakers, bipolar R waves were 7.78 ± 2.4 mV, and unipolar R waves were 7.67 ± 2.1 mV at implantation. During chronic followup, no significant differences between unipolar or bipolar sensing were found. Similar results have been described for atrial sensing, although bipolar sensing thresholds have been described as superior in some studies. Kay and colleagues[46, 47] found mean atrial electrogram amplitudes to be 4.6 mV for bipolar and 3.1 mV for unipolar leads at implantation in 28 patients. Atrial slew rates were similar for the two lead types.

Within individual patients, however, there may be significant differences between unipolar and bipolar sensing. De Caprio and coworkers[1] reported similar mean ventricular electrogram amplitude in 49 patients. The bipolar electrogram, however, was larger in 49% of patients, and the unipolar electrogram was larger in 43% of patients.

Despite similar sensing thresholds, there are important differences between unipolar and bipolar sensing in clinical practice. These differences include the longer electrogram duration and greater vulnerability of the unipolar configuration to sensing far-field events, myopotentials, and electromagnetic interference. Far-field oversensing is particularly problematic for unipolar atrial sensing.[45]

Brouwer and colleagues[48] measured matched unipolar and bipolar electrograms in 22 patients with bipolar atrial leads. P-wave amplitudes were similar (3.25 ± 1.23 mV unipolar versus 3.28 ± 1.09 mV bipolar), but the amplitude of far-field R waves was much lower for bipolar sensing (0.35 ± 0.32 mV bipolar versus 1.38 ± 0.65 mV unipolar). Atrial leads positioned lateral in the high right atrium had similar atrial electrograms to those recorded in the right atrial appendage. Leads placed inferior in the lower right atrium had much larger far-field R waves.

These shortcomings of unipolar sensing limit the highest programmable unipolar sensitivity in pacemakers and preclude the use of unipolar leads in most tachyarrhythmia detection algorithms.

Active Versus Passive Fixation
The method of lead stabilization, active or passive, has no significant effects on sensing characteristics in most studies. Using a variety of both active- and passive-fixation ventricular leads in 302 patients, Cornacchia and colleagues[49] found no significant difference in acute or chronic sensing thresholds between the different designs. Similarly, no difference in acute atrial sensing thresholds was found in 116 patients receiving either acute- or passive-fixation leads.[49] These findings were recently reiterated for modern steroid-eluting screw-in and tined leads in both the atrium and ventricle. In 57 patients, no significant differences in sensing were found in either chamber between the two lead designs at 1 year of follow-up.[50]

Steroid-Eluting Leads
Despite reducing chronic pacing thresholds, steroid elution appears to have no clinically significant effects on the sens-

ing characteristics of endocardial leads. In a study of 451 patients, Santini and Seta[51] found no difference in chronic atrial sensing thresholds between steroid-eluting and non–steroid-eluting unipolar leads; however, ventricular sensing thresholds were improved with steroid-eluting leads. No effect on chronic ventricular sensing thresholds by steroid-eluting leads has been described by others.[52] In a comparison of two active-fixation leads of similar design except for steroid-elution capabilities, Crossley and colleagues[53] found that atrial stimulation thresholds were significantly decreased with the steroid-eluting lead but that sensing characteristics remained similar. Similar results have been reported for steroid-eluting versus non–steroid-eluting tined atrial leads.[54] As described previously, however, the sensing characteristics of epicardial leads may be greatly enhanced by steroid-eluting electrodes.

Drug and Metabolic Effects on Sensing

The effects of various metabolic abnormalities and pharmacologic agents on pacing thresholds are well described. Much less information is available concerning the effects of these conditions on the sensing functions of permanent pacing systems, however. In general, factors that reduce intracardiac electrogram amplitude, slow conduction velocity, or diminish slew rate have the potential to produce sensing abnormalities. Either oversensing or undersensing can result from changes in the intracardiac electrogram. Undersensing may result from reduction in electrogram amplitudes or slew rate after myocardial infarction at the electrode–tissue interface or from drug and electrolyte effects.[55] These same influences can produce oversensing as well. By prolonging the intracardiac electrogram duration beyond blanking periods, ischemia or antiarrhythmic drugs can produce double counting of the QRS complex (Fig. 3–25).[56] Similarly, drugs that prolong the PR or QT intervals beyond the refractory periods may result in oversensing. Reduction in electrogram amplitude may dramatically increase the sensitivity of automatic gain or threshold control devices. This higher sensitivity may then allow sensing of far-field events.

Electrogram Changes During Exercise, Respiration, and Posture

The effect of exercise on the atrial electrogram has been studied by Frohlig and colleagues[57] in 33 patients with dual-chamber pacemakers. In this study involving bicycle exercise with telemetered atrial electrograms, 29 of the pacemakers were unipolar and 4 were bipolar, and all leads were of the active-fixation, screw-in variety. Six of 33 patients developed atrial undersensing during exercise at sensitivity values that were adequate at rest. There was a decline in the mean atrial electrogram amplitude from 6.4 ± 1.9 mV at rest to 5.6 ± 1.9 mV during exercise, whereas the slew rate decreased from 1.35 ± 0.45 V/sec to 1.18 ± 0.45 V/sec ($P < .001$). The decrease in atrial electrogram amplitude ranged up to 41%, and the slew rate decreased by as much as 51%. In general, the frequency content of the atrial electrogram was characterized by an increase in low-frequency and a decrease in high-frequency signals. Thus, a complete evaluation for suspected inappropriate sensing may require the use of exercise or ambulatory electrocardiographic monitoring.

Similar decreases averaged 33.8%, and up to 56% of these were reported in 11 children.[58] Other studies by Shandling[59] and Schuchert[60] did not find significant changes between rest and exercise. Decreases in atrial electrogram amplitude are not caused by atrial rate alone or by β-blockade.[61] Studies by Varriale[62] and Chan[63] of VDD/R leads with "floating" atrial electrodes showed significant decreases with exercise, 19.5% and 11.6%, respectively, and maximum decreases of up to 60% to 75%. The P-wave amplitudes did increase significantly during full inspiration, during full expiration, and for erect posture.[59]

Substantial respiratory variations in the amplitude of the ventricular intrinsic deflection and slew rate are illustrated in Figure 3–26.[63] Respiratory variation in ventricular electrogram amplitude was a mean of 9.7% for unipolar atrial electrograms and 11.5% for bipolar atrial electrograms.[2] The effect of respiration on ventricular electrograms was less, although the unipolar configuration was somewhat less susceptible to respiratory changes than the bipolar configuration (about 5.3% unipolar and about 9.4% bipolar). A consistent reduction of the atrial electrogram amplitude by 16.6% for DDDR and 12.8% for VDD/R pacing occurred during the relaxation phase of the Valsalva maneuver.[46, 63] The very large decreases in atrial electrogram amplitude for some patients in these studies may put into question the standard practice of using sensitivities that are twice the sensing limit.

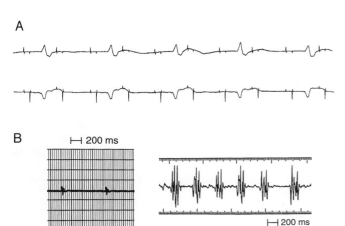

A

B ⊢ 200 ms

⊢ 200 ms

Figure 3–25. Myocardial ischemia causing undersensing and oversensing. *A,* Two-lead telemetry tracing from a patient with a permanent DDD pacemaker hours after a massive anterior and inferior myocardial infarction. There is complete loss of ventricular sensing and capture, probably owing to infarction at the lead–myocardial interface. *B,* Ventricular electrograms from a Ventritex V100C defibrillator before *(left)* and during *(right)* acute anterior myocardial infarction. The electrograms were recorded at different gains from two different programmers. The electrogram amplitudes of the two recordings are comparable. Before the infarction, the electrogram duration was 80 msec, and during the infarction, the duration increased to 180 msec. The patient presented with chest pain and repeated inappropriate cardioverter-defibrillator shocks during sinus rhythm due to double counting of each prolonged ventricular electrogram, which extended beyond the ventricular refractory period. (From Ellenbogen KA, Wood MA, Gilligan DM: Evaluation of "inappropriate" ICD shocks in an asymptomatic patient following myocardial infarction. PACE 19:254–255, 1996.)

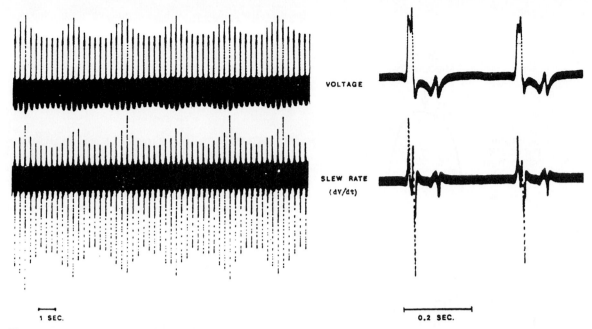

VOLTAGE

SLEW RATE
(dV/dt)

1 SEC.

0.2 SEC.

Figure 3–26. Respiratory variations of intracardiac electrogram amplitude and slew rate (dV/dt) are typically about 10% for the atrium and ventricle. These variations result from beat-to-beat changes in stroke volume caused by respiration or movement at the electrode tissue interface. (From Furman S, Hurzeler P, DeCaprio V: Cardiac pacing and pacemakers. III. Sensing the cardiac electrogram. Am Heart J 93:794–801, 1977.)

■ CLINICAL ASPECTS OF PACEMAKER SENSING

Assessment of Sensing at Pacemaker Implantation

For clinicians involved in the care of patients with permanent pacemakers, evaluation of sensing begins at the time of pacemaker implantation. Measurement of a sensing threshold is typically performed using a pacemaker system analyzer (PSA). Ideally, the PSA used to obtain these measurements should have filter settings identical to those found on the pulse generator being implanted. PSAs from various manufacturers use different filtering and waveform calibrations and may report either peak-to-peak or base-to-peak electrogram amplitude to best emulate the function of their respective implanted devices.

Although the correlations between electrogram amplitudes are high among different manufacturers' PSAs, the absolute amplitudes reported from the same patients can vary dramatically,[64] especially for atrial electrograms. The reported atrial electrogram amplitude may vary by 50% between different manufacturers' PSAs. In addition, the coefficient of variation between repeated measures with the same PSA may be as great as 31%.[64] For these reasons, the sensing characteristics of the PSA and the implanted device should match as closely as possible; even so, the PSA measures are a rough estimate of in vivo pacemaker function.

To avoid future problems with oversensing or undersensing in the pacing system, it is necessary to obtain the best possible intracardiac signal at the time of implantation. The peak-to-peak ventricular electrogram at implantation should be larger than 6 mV and should have a slew rate greater than 0.75 V/sec. The atrial electrogram should ideally be greater than 1.5 mV and should have a slew rate of at least 0.5 V/sec. An electrogram of borderline amplitude may be adequate for sensing if the slew rate is satisfactory. However, an electrogram with inadequate amplitude will not be sensed regardless of slew rate.

It is important to remember that the amplitude and frequency spectrum of the electrogram can change with time. A 15% to 20% decrease in R-wave amplitude and a 25% to 50% decrease in R-wave slew rate may be seen with maturation of the electrode–tissue interface (Fig. 3–27).[1, 2] At implantation, there is a significant increase in both P-wave and R-wave amplitude with screw-in (active) fixation leads that peaks about 20 to 30 minutes after implantation[65] (Fig. 3–28). There is typically no significant change in P-wave or R-wave amplitude with the passive-fixation leads during the first 30 minutes after lead implantation. Each lead position should be evaluated with multiple determination of P- or R-wave amplitude to document lead stability and to exclude spurious values.

Evaluation for oversensing can be performed using the PSA sensing indicator with the unit set to maximum sensitivity. Most PSAs do not allow for the extremely high sensitivities (down to 0.15 mV) available in contemporary permanent pacemakers, however. The use of atrial or ventricular triggered modes at high unipolar output can precisely identify the sensed events on the ECG monitor at the time of implantation (Fig. 3–29). This technique provides a particularly graphic display of the sensing functions for the implanting physician. For further evaluation of sensing at implantation, some PSAs are capable of printing the filtered intracardiac electrogram for direct measurement (Fig. 3–30). Alternatively, the intracardiac electrogram can be measured directly on a physiologic recorder using sterile connectors to inter-

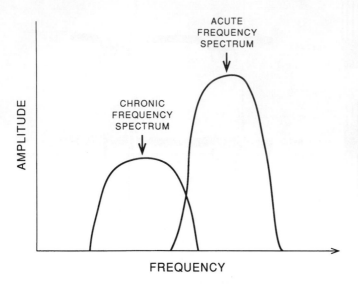

Figure 3–27. The effect of lead evolution on the amplitude and frequency spectrum of intracardiac electrograms. The amplitude of the electrogram can be expected to decrease between implantation and chronic follow-up, and a shift will occur in the frequency spectrum to lower frequencies. These changes in the electrogram may lead to undersensing in some patients despite adequate electrogram characteristics at the time of lead implantation.

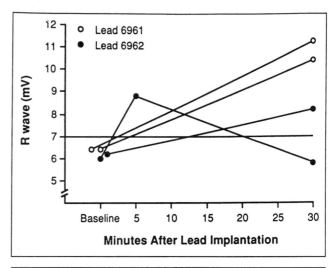

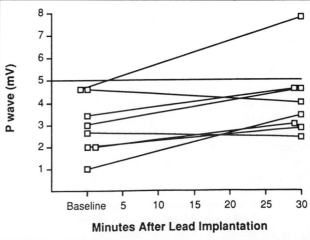

Figure 3–28. Effect of time on amplitudes of R waves *(top)* and P waves *(bottom)* immediately after implantation of active-fixation pacing leads. Note that R-wave amplitudes in four patients that were less than 7 mV immediately after lead implantation showed increases by 30 minutes after implantation. Also note that the atrial electrogram amplitude in most patients increased from baseline to a higher level 30 minutes after implantation of the lead. (From de Buitleir M, Kou WH, Schmaltz S, et al: Acute changes in pacing threshold and R- or P-wave amplitude during permanent pacemaker implantation. Am J Cardiol 65:999, 1990.)

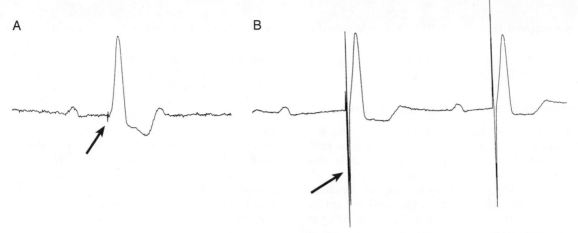

Figure 3–29. The use of triggered mode to assess sensing function at DDD pacemaker implantation. The patient undergoing implantation has a temporary ventricular pacer because of complete heart block *(A)*. A small pacing artifact is seen *(arrow)*. At atrial lead implantation the "P wave" measured 3.6 mV by the pacemaker system analyzer. The possibility of oversensing the temporary pacemaker output prompted the use of AAT mode *(B)*. In AAT mode, atrial pacing was simultaneous with the temporary ventricular pacing output *(arrow)*, indicating that the atrial sensed event is actually the far-field pacing stimulus and not the P wave.

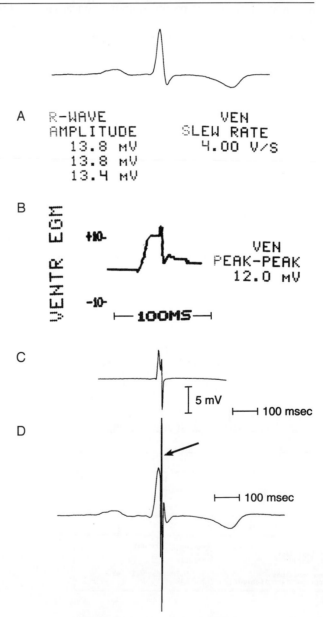

Figure 3–30. Evaluation of ventricular sensing at implantation. All measures were made from the same patient. The surface electrocardiogram is shown at the top of the figure. *A,* Measured R-wave amplitude from the pacemaker system analyzer (PSA). Note the variation in the measured R wave from 13.4 to 13.8 mV. The slew rate is excellent at 4.0 V/sec. *B,* The telemetered ventricular electrogram from the same PSA with an estimated peak-to-peak amplitude of 12 mV. *C,* The ventricular electrogram as recorded by a physiologic recorder with filters from 30 to 500 Hz. The amplitude (11 mV) is determined by the gain calibration from the recorder. *D,* Use of triggered mode (VVT) from the PSA to assess ventricular sensing. The PSA is set to a lower rate below the intrinsic rate, and sensitivity is set to 8 mV. The large pacing artifact *(arrow)* during the QRS indicates sensing at this point. The R-wave amplitude detected by the PSA is therefore ≥8 mV.

face with the recorder (see Fig. 3–30). This technique does not provide the same electrogram filtering as the permanent pacemaker, however, and the measured value is typically less than that reported by the PSA.[64]

Assessment of Sensing After Implantation

Sensing can be evaluated using a number of different techniques after implantation of a modern pacing system. In the absence of a reliable escape rhythm, sensing of intrinsic cardiac signals may be difficult or impossible, especially for devices lacking temporary programming or automated analysis functions. In patients with a stable intrinsic atrial or ventricular rhythm, sensing can be tested by monitoring the surface ECG for the presence of atrial or ventricular demand pacing stimuli during the patient's spontaneous rhythm. To assess the amplitude of the intrinsic intracardiac electrogram measured by the sensing amplifier, the lower pacing rate is programmed below the patient's intrinsic rate. The sensitivity value is then increased (to a less sensitive setting) until inhibition of pacing is lost, and pacing output artifacts are observed (Fig. 3–31A).

Bipolar pacing stimuli may be difficult to detect on the surface ECG. Reprogramming to unipolar pacing or high bipolar output may help visualize the pacing stimulus. In some pulse generators, sensitivity threshold testing is automated, with the programmer displaying the surface ECG and marker channels while decreasing the sensitivity of the sensing amplifier after a fixed number of beats (see Fig. 3–31B). In patients with AV block who have DDD pacemakers, the atrial sensing threshold may be tested by programming the lower rate and AV delay to values that ensure atrial tracking and ventricular pacing. The atrial sensitivity threshold is then programmed to less sensitive values (either manually or by automated testing) until atrial tracking is lost, indicating that the intrinsic atrial electrogram is less than the programmed atrial sensing threshold (see Fig. 3–31C).

Sensing can also be effectively evaluated by programming the pulse generator to the triggered mode (i.e., VVT or AAT) and observing the ECG for the timing of pacing stimuli relative to intrinsic electrical events, such as P waves, R waves, or T waves. In Figure 3–32, AAT pacing shows atrial pacing atrifacts coincident with P waves at a programmed sensitivity of 1 mV. As the sensitivity threshold is increased (to a less sensitive value), the atrial pacing stimuli

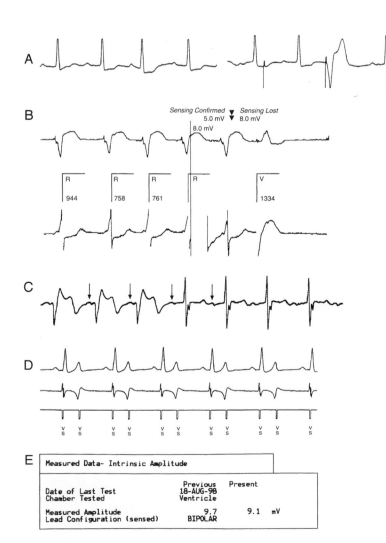

Figure 3–31. Evaluation of sensing after device implantation. *A, left,* Surface electrocardiogram (ECG) lead recording from a patient with a VVI pacemaker with lower rate set to 50 bpm and sensitivity at 1.4 mV. No pacemaker output is seen. *Right,* After reprogramming to 5.6 mV, ventricular pacing at the lower rate limit is noted, indicating loss of sensing at this programmed value. *B,* Automated ventricular pacemaker programmer sensing test. The surface ECG *(top),* marker channel *(middle),* and ventricular electrograms *(bottom)* are displayed by the programmer. The programmer automatically reduces the pacemaker sensitivity throughout the test until the operator confirms loss of sensing. There is reprogramming from 5 to 8 mV sensitivity at the marker after the fourth QRS. Undersensing of the fifth complex occurs as indicated by the absence of response on the marker channel. The last QRS complex is a paced event at the lower rate limit (indicated by V or the marker channel and a different ECG complex). *C,* Determination of atrial sensing threshold by loss of ventricular tracking in DDD mode. The tracing is obtained from a single-channel telemetry monitor. The first three complexes show ventricular tracking of P waves *(arrow)* at a pacemaker sensitivity of 2.8 mV. With reprogramming to atrial sensitivity of 4 mV, there is loss of atrial sensing manifest as discontinuation of ventricular pacing (fourth QRS complex) because atrial tracking can no longer take place. There is no atrial or ventricular pacing because the pacemaker lower rate limit is less than the R-R interval in sinus rhythm. *D,* Pacemaker programmer printout showing surface ECG *(top),* telemetered intraventricular electrograms *(middle),* and marker channel *(bottom).* A ventricular electrogram amplitude of 12 mV can be estimated by the calibration of 2 mV/mm given by the programmer at this gain. Note that the marker channel demonstrates T-wave oversensing. *E,* Numeric values of the ventricular electrogram amplitude (9.1 mV) provided by the pacemaker programmer after pacemaker interrogation. The device stores the last previously determined value in memory for easy comparison.

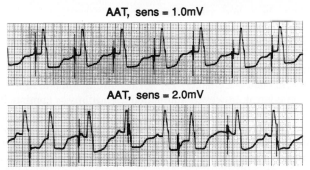

AAT, sens = 1.0mV

AAT, sens = 2.0mV

Figure 3–32. Usefulness of the AAT pacing mode to determine atrial sensing. In the upper panel, an atrial sensitivity setting of 1 mV is programmed. Note that atrial pacing stimuli are delivered simultaneously with sensed P wave. Note also that the P wave begins slightly before the pacing stimulus, indicating that the stimuli are triggered by sensed atrial events occurring after onset of the surface electrocardiographic P wave. In the lower panel, the atrial sensitivity has been reprogrammed to 2 mV. Atrial pacing stimuli are now delivered asynchronously, indicating that the intrinsic P-wave amplitude must be less than the programmed value of 2 mV.

occur asynchronously at the lower rate limit, indicating failure to sense the intrinsic P wave at the programmed value. In the presence of oversensing, the triggered mode allows for recognition of T-wave sensing (manifested by VVT pacing stimuli synchronous with the T wave), make-and-break potentials (manifested by pacing stimuli that are randomly distributed throughout the cardiac cycle), or far-field sensing. The AAT mode is especially helpful for evaluating suspected

far-field R-wave sensing, which can be identified by atrial pacing stimuli delivered synchronously with both the P waves and the R waves.

The clinical evaluation of pacemaker sensing has been greatly simplified by the incorporation of telemetered intracardiac electrograms and marker channels into the display of pacemaker programmers (see Fig. 3–31B and D). The capability to display the surface ECG, intracardiac electrograms, and marker channels simultaneously allows the clinician to visualize both the signals the pacing system is sensing and the pulse generator's interpretation of these electric events. The telemetered electrogram can be calibrated and measured, and the sensitivity threshold value can be approximated from the measured amplitude of the signal. It should be stressed, however, that the amplitude of the electrogram telemetered by the programmer and the amplitude of the signal that is sensed by the sensing amplifier may be different. The filtered, processed, and displayed waveforms do not exactly correspond to the processing by the pulse generator's sensing amplifiers. Numeric values of the sensed atrial or ventricular electrogram amplitude are reported by some programmers (see Fig. 3–31E). This format is necessary in devices using automatic gain or threshold control and that therefore do not function at a fixed sensitivity setting.

Special Sensing Functions

Amplification: Fixed Gain and Automatic Adjustment

The primary functional operations within the sensing system of a pacemaker or ICD are shown in Figure 3–33. The raw signal coming from the leads, connector, and hermetic feedthroughs encounters protection circuitry, such as zener

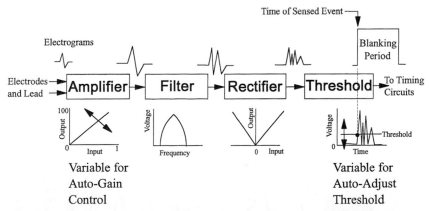

Figure 3–33. A functional block diagram for a pacemaker or implantable cardioverter-defibrillator (ICD) sense amplifier. The electrogram signal from two implanted electrodes is amplified for subsequent processing; bandpass filtered to reduce T waves, myopotential, and interference; rectified to make signal polarity unimportant; and compared with the sensing threshold voltage. At the instant the processed signal exceeds the sensing threshold voltage, a sensed event is declared to the timing circuits and is indicated by a marker pulse on the electrocardiogram recording. The sense amplifier is turned off or blanked for 20 to 100 msec so that each depolarization is sensed only once. For pacemakers, the programmed sensitivity controls the constant sensing threshold voltage *(vertical arrows)*. For ICDs, the amplifier gain (slope of input versus output) or the sensing threshold voltage is automatically adjusted according to the amplitudes of the depolarizations. This is necessary to avoid T-wave oversensing because ventricular sense amplifiers in ICD are about 10 times more sensitive than pacemaker sense amplifiers. In actual circuits, some functions, such as amplification and filtering, may be integrated.

diodes, before reaching the amplifier. Sense amplifiers for bradycardia pacemakers use programmable fixed gain and threshold. ICDs need to use much more sensitive amplifiers to sense VF reliably, and this often causes T-wave oversensing for fixed gain and threshold devices.[66–68]

To solve this problem, ICDs use either *automatic gain control* or *autoadjusting threshold* to adjust the sensitivity dynamically for reliable sensing of ventricular fibrillation (VF) without oversensing T waves in sinus rhythm or other inappropriate signals.[69] Automatic gain control is a feedback system that attempts to keep the amplifier output signal amplitude constant for any input signal and then uses a fixed threshold to sense the R waves. In contrast, autoadjusting threshold uses constant amplification. The peak amplitude of the R waves provides the feedback for adjusting the starting amplitude of a time-decaying threshold. Both systems have an "attack" time that determines how rapidly the gain or threshold can increase as well as a "decay" time for gain or threshold decreases.

For the automatic gain control method, the amplifier gain, which is the slope of the line relating the amplifier input and output, varies according to the signal amplitude, whereas the threshold voltage is fixed. For autoadjusting threshold, the amplifier gain is fixed, and the horizontal line representing the threshold voltage, shown on the right of Figure 3–34, varies according to peak signal amplitude and the time since an R wave was last sensed.

The principal difference between automatic gain control and autoadjusting threshold is that automatic gain control amplifies all signal and noise equally, whereas autoadjusting threshold adjusts the threshold for a filtered and rectified signal. Although this difference suggests a theoretical benefit for the autoadjusting threshold approach, the clinical significance of this difference, if any, has not been studied.

Practical amplifiers have a limited dynamic range; therefore, the electrogram is saturated or clipped when it exceeds a maximum value. Amplifiers must recover quickly after pacing pulses and defibrillation shocks, reject large DC offsets due to electrode polarization, and reject common mode noise applied to both inputs. They also must have high signal-to-noise ratios but use only a few microamperes of battery current.

Permanent pacemakers do not require automatic amplification control; however, automated algorithms to continually monitor and adjust sensing thresholds may optimize sensing in response to limited spontaneous changes in electrogram amplitude. One such algorithm employs two simultaneous sensing levels: the programmed sensitivity (inner target) and a value twice the programmed value (outer target) (Fig. 3–35).[70] Sensed electrograms exceeding both target values result in a decreased sensitivity. Signals exceeding only the inner target increase sensitivity. In this manner, a 2:1 sensing margin is maintained.

Sensing the Evoked Response

The ability to sense local myocardial depolarization (the evoked response) after a pacing stimulus allows for confirmation of myocardial capture. Sensing of the evoked response, however, is obscured by the decaying polarization afterpotential, which follows the pacing stimulus.[71] This polarization artifact can be attenuated by use of high capacitance, low polarization leads or by use of multiphasic pacing impulses to neutralize the postpacing polarization capacitance. The ventricular depolarization evoked response reaches maximal amplitude about 45 msec after the pacing stimulus. The evoked repolarization artifact is measurable within 350 msec of the pacing stimulus.[71]

Several systems are now in use to detect the depolarization evoked response. The Pacesetter Autocapture (St. Jude Medical, Sunnyvale, CA) algorithm employs bipolar sensing after unipolar pacing to verify ventricular capture.[72] After the pacing impulse, sensing is blanked for 15 msec to prevent amplifier saturation (Fig. 3–36). From 15 to 62 msec

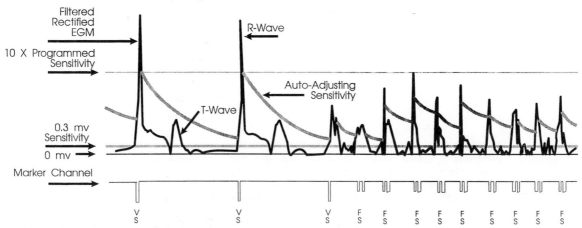

Figure 3–34. The autoadjusting threshold concept used to avoid oversensing T waves in sinus rhythm while still sensing very-low-amplitude ventricular fibrillation electrograms. The filtered and rectified electrogram for two sinus beats followed by spontaneous ventricular fibrillation has superimposed on it the autoadjusting sensitivity. For large R waves, the threshold jumps up to 10 times the programmed sensitivity (0.3 mV) and decays with a time constant of about 500 msec. Note that for the sinus beats, this threshold is larger than the T waves, so that oversensing is avoided. When ventricular fibrillation begins, the smaller R waves keep the threshold at a lower value, which allows sensing or R waves that are even smaller than the T waves in sinus rhythm. Marker channel symbols indicate the cycle lengths as ordinary ventricular senses (VS) or fibrillation senses (FS).

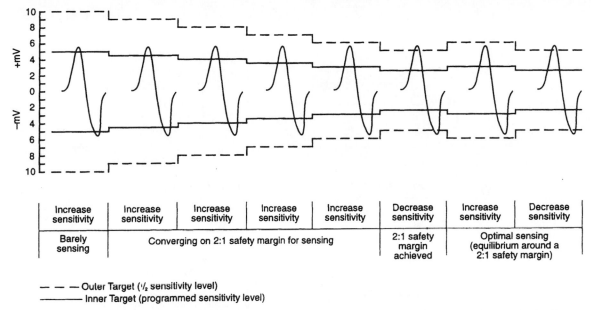

Increase sensitivity	Increase sensitivity	Increase sensitivity	Increase sensitivity	Increase sensitivity	Decrease sensitivity	Increase sensitivity	Decrease sensitivity
Barely sensing	Converging on 2:1 safety margin for sensing				2:1 safety margin achieved	Optimal sensing (equilibrium around a 2:1 safety margin)	

— — — Outer Target (½ sensitivity level)

———— Inner Target (programmed sensitivity level)

Figure 3–35. Autosensing algorithm for permanent pacemaker to maintain 2:1 sensing safety margin. See text for details. (From Castro A, Liebold A, Vincent J, et al: Evaluation of autosensing as an automatic means of maintaining a 2:1 sensing safety margin in an implanted pacemaker. PACE 19:1708–1713, 1996.)

after the pacing stimulus, the evoked response sensing window is open. Sensing during this interval confirms capture, whereas failure to sense results in a high-amplitude backup pulse delivered 62 msec after the initial output. In clinical trials, the chronic ventricular evoked response amplitude averaged 10 mV, with an average R wave of 18 mV.[73] This particular algorithm requires use of a low polarization pacing lead and is currently in use for ventricular pacing only. This algorithm allows for beat-to-beat tracking of ventricular capture.

Alternatively, the repolarization artifact can be neutralized by applying a triphasic pacing stimulus.[74, 75] An initial positive voltage (precharge) is followed by a negative output (stimulus) that depolarizes the myocardium. A positive voltage (postcharge) completes the triphasic waveform. If properly balanced, the positive and negative voltages neutralize the charge accumulation at the electrode–tissue interface, thereby minimizing the polarization artifact. The complex nonlinear behavior of the electrode–tissue interface necessitates extensive feedback processing and electrogram template matching to maintain charge balancing, however. Atrial-evoked responses of 3.1 ± 1.4 mV, with P waves of 5.6 ± 3.0 mV, are measurable with this system.[76]

A novel approach to detection of the evoked response does not attempt to attenuate the polarization artifact. This algorithm uses the standard sense amplifier circuitry to discriminate the evoked response from lead polarization. The circuitry is sensitive to reversal of the sign of the slew rate and to an increase in the magnitude of the slew rate, neither of which should result from the methodical exponential decay of the polarization artifact alone (Fig. 3–36).[77] This algorithm offers the potential benefit of working with any pacing lead regardless of polarization characteristics, and it does not require extensive signal processing.

■ SENSING AND DETECTING ATRIAL DYSRHYTHMIAS

The Atrial Electrogram During Atrial Dysrhythmias

Compared with sinus rhythm, ectopic atrial activation and atrial dysrhythmias can alter the amplitude, frequency content, slew rate, and morphology of the atrial electrogram. Retrograde atrial activation during ventricular pacing reduces atrial electrogram amplitude and slew rate by up to 50% compared with sinus rhythm in most patients.[78] These electrogram changes are more pronounced for high right atrial lead positions than for sites in the atrial appendage or low right atrium.[79]

The atrial electrogram frequency content is not significantly altered by retrograde atrial activation.[80] Analysis of electrogram turning-point morphology or first differential coefficient of slew rate has been used to discriminate sinus electrograms from those recorded during retrograde and ectopic atrial activation in small groups of patients.[81] Less sophisticated visual morphologic analysis does not effectively discriminate sinus from ectopic atrial electrical activity.[82]

Atrial electrical activity during atrial fibrillation is characterized by extreme temporal and spatial variability. Electrical activity tends to be most organized when recorded from the trabeculated right atrial appendage and is more disorganized in the smooth right atrium or coronary sinus.[83] The amplitude, width, and morphology of atrial electrograms during fibrillation varies markedly at and between anatomic locations.[84, 85] Compared with sinus rhythm, the electrograms recorded from a single atrial site during atrial fibrillation show a broader frequency content and a reduction in mean electrogram amplitude. Karagueuzian and colleagues[86] dem-

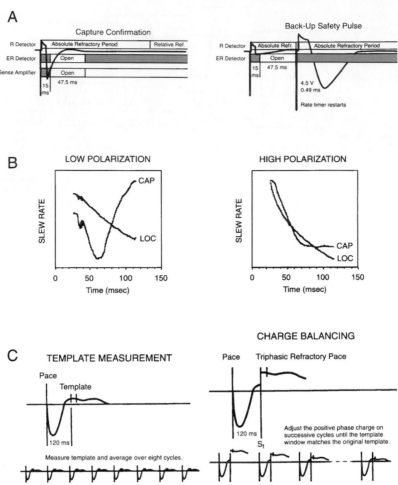

Figure 3–36. Three methods for detecting the ventricular evoked response to document ventricular capture after a pacing stimulus. *A,* Pacesetter Autocapture algorithm. *Left,* Fifteen milliseconds after the ventricular pacing stimulus *(venticle line),* the sense amplifier and evoked response (ER) detection circuit are opened for 47.5 msec. An electrogram sensed in this window *(dark line)* represents the ventricular evoked response, confirming capture. *Right,* After the first pacing stimulus, no electrogram is detected during the ER detection window, indicating failure to capture. A high-output stimulus is then delivered 62.5 msec after the first. ER detection is not attempted for this stimulus. The afterpotential is minimized by use of a low polarization lead. (Courtesy of Pacesetter, St. Jude Medical, Sunnyvale, CA.) *B,* Medtronic, Inc. algorithm using the magnitude and reversal of the slew rate to detect ventricular capture. With loss of capture (LOC), the slew rate of the potential recorded after pacing represents only the afterpotential that always follows a consistent exponential decay. Deviations from this decay represent the ER of capture (CAP). *Left,* Reversal of the sign and increasing magnitude of the slew rate with a low polarization lead are evident with capture. *Right,* With a high polarization lead, the change in the sign and plateau in slew rate magnitude deviate from LOC. (Courtesy of Medtronic, Inc., Minneapolis, MN.) *C,* Charge balancing system showing template measurement and feedback adjustment. *Left,* During pacing-induced depolarization, a template of the ER is generated from eight depolarizations. A hardware feedback circuit operates continuously to eliminate charge accumulation on the output capacitor. *Right,* After the 120-msec template window, a second triphasic stimulus (St) is delivered during myocardial refractoriness. The precharge phase is adjusted until the template window matches the original template and the afterpotential is minimized. (From Feld GK, Love CJ, Camerlo J, et al: A new pacemaker algorithm for continuous capture verification and automatic threshold determination. Elimination of pacemaker afterpotential utilizing a triphasic charge balancing system. PACE 15:171–178, 1992.)

onstrated that during sinus rhythm in dogs, the atrial electrograms contained discrete frequency bands within the spectrum from 0 to 25 Hz. During atrial fibrillation, the frequency spectrum broadened to 0 to 50 Hz and became more continuous. In humans, the spectral components of electrograms from two separate atrial (or ventricular) sites show greatly reduced spectral coherence during fibrillating as opposed to nonfibrillating rhythms.[87]

A comparison of atrial electrogram amplitudes in sinus rhythm, atrial fibrillation, and flutter was reported by Wood and coworkers[85] in 69 patients. In this study using temporary pacing catheters in the high right atrium or appendage, the mean electrogram amplitude fell from 1.59 ± 1.36 mV in sinus rhythm to 0.77 ± 0.58 mV in atrial fibrillation ($P < .0001$). The mean electrogram amplitudes in both atrial fibrillation and atrial flutter were highly correlated to the amplitudes in sinus rhythm. In atrial flutter the mean amplitude was 1.58 ± 1.81, compared with 1.81 ± 2.09 mV during sinus rhythm ($P < .0001$). The coefficient of variance of electrogram amplitude was similar for sinus rhythm and atrial flutter ($18.8 \pm 12.7\%$ versus $22.3 \pm 10.0\%$, respectively) but markedly increased for atrial fibrillation ($41.6 \pm 9.2\%$, $P < .0001$ versus sinus) (Fig. 3–37). The likelihood of any patient demonstrating very-low-amplitude atrial elec-

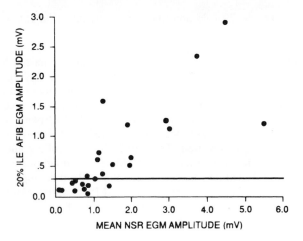

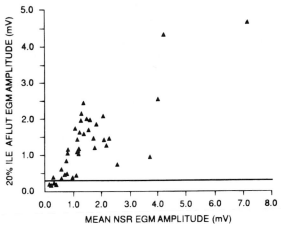

Figure 3–38. Twentieth percentile (20% ILE) electrogram (EGM) amplitudes versus mean normal sinus rhythm (NSR) atrial electrogram amplitudes for patients with atrial fibrillation (AFIB) and atrial flutter (AFLUT). *Top,* For 25 patients with atrial fibrillation, the 20th percentile electrogram amplitude is ≤0.3 mV (reference line) only when the mean sinus amplitude is ≤1.5 mV. *Bottom,* For 44 patients with atrial flutter, the 20th percentile electrogram amplitude is ≤0.3 mV only when the sinus amplitude is ≤0.5 mV. These very-low-amplitude electrograms may be undersensed at conventional pacemaker sensitivity settings. (From Wood MA, Moskovljevic P, Stambler BS, Ellenbogen KA: Comparison of bipolar atrial electrogram amplitude in sinus rhythm, atrial fibrillation, and flutter. PACE 19:150–156, 1996.)

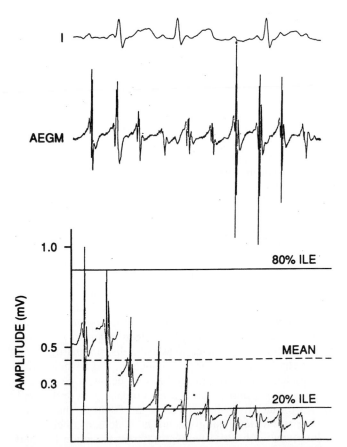

Figure 3–37. Extreme atrial electrogram amplitude variability during atrial fibrillation. *Top,* Ten consecutive atrial electrograms (AEGM) were recorded from a patient using a temporary catheter. *Bottom,* The mean, 80th percentile (80% ILE), and 20th percentile (20% ILE) electrogram amplitudes are shown. The 20th percentile electrogram amplitudes are 0.18 mV, representing very-low-amplitude signals.

trograms (<0.3 mV) during atrial fibrillation or flutter was associated with the mean sinus electrogram amplitudes (Fig. 3–38). The 20th percentile of the measured electrogram amplitudes in atrial fibrillation was 0.3 mV or less in 65% of patients with a mean sinus electrogram amplitude of 1.5 mV or less. No patient with sinus P waves of more than 1.5 mV had 20th percentile atrial electrograms of less than 0.3 mV. The 20th percentile electrogram amplitude in atrial flutter was 0.3 mV or less in 33% of patients who had a mean sinus electrogram amplitude of < 0.5 mV and in none who had a sinus amplitude of more than 0.5 mV.

The electrode spacing and position of atrial leads have dramatic effects on the characteristics of the recorded atrial fibrillation electrograms.[86, 88] Baerman and associates[88] demonstrated that the atrial fibrillation electrogram amplitude was increased 20-fold and that the calculated atrial rate was slower with electrodes in contact with the atrial endocardium compared with floating atrial electrodes. Wider spacing of contact electrodes increased the measured atrial rate but had little effect on electrogram amplitude. Significantly higher probability density function (PDF) values were obtained for narrowly spaced electrodes in endocardial contact, compared with free-floating or wider spaced contact electrodes. The median frequency value was not changed by differing electrode spacing or position. These differing electrode configurations can result in inconsistent abilities to diagnose atrial fibrillation based on rate and PDF criteria. By reducing atrial rate, median frequency, amplitude, and PDF, antiarrhythmic drugs may also interfere with the detection of atrial fibrillation based on these parameters.[89]

Detecting Atrial Fibrillation by Implanted Devices

The accurate detection of atrial tachyarrhythmias is essential to the function of mode-switching pacemakers, dual-chamber pacing ventricular defibrillators, and atrial defibrillators. This ability represents a considerable challenge for these devices, however. Any atrial tachycardia detection algorithm must contend with wide variations in atrial rate, electrogram amplitude, electrogram morphology, and frequency content, especially during atrial fibrillation. In addition, these devices must exclude far-field signals at high sensitivities and employ banking periods that do not mask the atrial arrhythmias.

Requirements for Atrial Tachycardia and Atrial Fibrillation Detection

Antiarrhythmic devices detect atrial tachycardia flutter and fibrillation (AT and AF, respectively) to perform different functions:

- Dual-chamber pacemakers mode switch to prevent inappropriate tracking of AT/AF[90-93]
- Dual-chamber ventricular ICDs may detect instances of AT/AF that otherwise satisfy ventricular rate criteria to withhold inappropriate ventricular therapy[94, 95]
- Atrial ICDs detect atrial fibrillation for atrial defibrillation[96-100]

These functions make different demands on atrial tachyarrhythmia detection algorithms. Dual-chamber pacemakers must detect AT/AF rapidly and with high sensitivity to prevent symptomatic, inappropriate tracking at the upper rate limit. Dual-chamber ICDs must discriminate rapidly between ventricular tachyarrhythmias and instances of AT/AF that satisfy ventricular rate criteria to ensure patient safety. Some inappropriate detection of AT/AF is considered an acceptable price to maintain high sensitivity for detecting ventricular tachyarrhythmias. In contrast, atrial ICDs must detect atrial fibrillation with high specificity to minimize painful and potentially proarrhythmic therapy. Rapid detection is less important because atrial fibrillation is usually clinically stable and may terminate spontaneously after hours to days. Ideally, an atrial ICD should permit therapy for long-duration AT/AF while withholding therapy from self-terminating AT/AF. To achieve this goal, it must detect atrial fibrillation continuously for extended periods of time. The difficulties imposed by the last requirement may be appreciated by

comparison with detection requirements for ventricular ICDs. Although ventricular ICDs detect ventricular fibrillation continuously only for periods of less than 10 seconds, undersensing of ventricular fibrillation due to varying or low-amplitude electrograms remains an occasional but serious problem.[101-103] Electrograms in atrial fibrillation also have varying and even lower amplitudes than those in ventricular fibrillation.[85, 104]

Dual-chamber and atrial ICDs may discriminate between AT and AF to deliver antitachycardia pacing for AT. Therefore, these devices must determine the atrial rate and rhythm accurately. This requirement mandates that postventricular blanking of the atrial sense amplifiers be minimized to a value insufficient to blank far-field R waves. Thus, either the atrial electrode must not record far-field R waves or the detection algorithm must prevent sensing of far-field R waves from causing inappropriate detection of AT/AF.

Mode Switching

Current mode switching pacemakers and ICDs use two basic detection algorithms to sense atrial tachyarrhythmias. One such algorithm counts the number of atrial sensed events occurring below a preprogrammed interval. When a preprogrammed number of short intervals is reached, mode switching occurs. Reversion of atrial tracking occurs when a programmed number of intervals exceeding the detection interval occur. This type of algorithm responds quickly to atrial arrhythmias but may produce more intermittent ventricular tracking in atrial fibrillation. The second type of algorithm follows a calculated atrial rate. This rate is determined by incrementing or decrementing a calculated running interval by fixed amounts in response to each sensed PP interval. For example, the Medtronic Thera DR 7960 decrements the calculated mean atrial interval by 24 msec for each PP interval shorter than the programmed tachycardia detection interval and increments the calculated interval by 8 msec for each interval longer than the tachycardia detection interval. This unequal increment and decrement of the mean atrial interval serves to maintain mode switching during periods of signal dropout. When the calculated rate is above the detection rate, mode switching is operational. This type of algorithm is slower to activate and inactivate mode switching but may provide less variation in ventricular pacing rate during atrial fibrillation.

Enhancements of these mode switching algorithms using activity sensors to define "nonphysiologic" atrial rates or abrupt changes in the atrial rate are incorporated in some devices. The timing of the atrial electrogram in relation to the RR interval can be used to assist in discriminating among atrial arrhythmias, retrograde conduction, and far-field events in dual-chamber pacing defibrillators (see later). Some dual-chamber pacing defibrillators use automatic gain or threshold control for atrial sensing. Whether the feature reduces oversensing and undersensing has not been demonstrated.

Problems with atrial tachyarrhythmia detection by mode switching devices and defibrillators may include both undersensing and oversensing. Undersensing of the arrhythmias may result from intermittent failure to sense (drop out) of very low amplitude atrial electrograms in atrial fibrillation (Fig. 3–39). Although some authorities suggest programming a 3 to 3.5-fold safety margin based on the sinus sensing

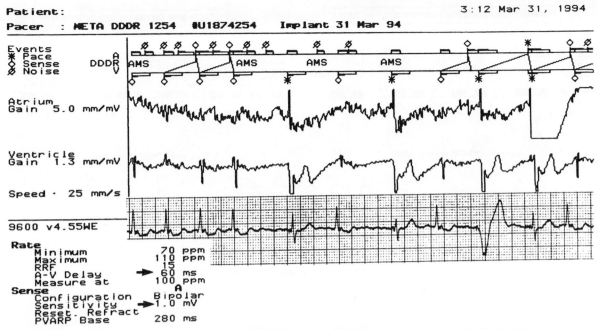

Figure 3–39. Failure of automatic mode switching (AMS) as a result of atrial undersensing in atrial fibrillation. This programmer printout from a Telectronics Meta 1254 shows a ladder diagram for atrial (A—*top*) and ventricular (V—*bottom*) events. Beneath this are atrial electrograms, then ventricular electrograms and the corresponding surface electrocardiogram tracing. With atrial sensitivity at 1 mV, there is undersensing of ongoing atrial fibrillation in the middle of the tracing, denoted by the absence of sensed and noise events on the atrial marker channel. As a result, reversion to atrial tracking occurs at the end of the tracing. (From Ellenbogen KA, Mond H, Wood MA, Barold SS: Failure of automatic mode switching: Recognition and management. PACE 20:268–275, 1997.)

threshold, atrial sensitivity must be programmed to less than 1 mV to maintain mode switching in most patients regardless of atrial electrogram amplitude in sinus rhythm.[105–107] The very high atrial sensitivity (to 0.15 mV) available in many devices can largely overcome signal dropout but may facilitate far-field sensing of the T or R wave, double counting of atrial paced events, and noise sensing, thus leading to false detection of atrial arrhythmias.[108–110]

The difficulty in balancing between oversensing and undersensing based on sensitivity programming has been demonstrated by Leung and coworkers.[110] In this study, high sensitivities to minimize intermittent tracking of AF produced oversensing in 57% of patients. At low sensitivities to reduce oversensing, 50% of patients experienced intermittent tracking of AF, and 9% had failure to mode switch. In addition, oversensing may occur in 50% of patients with unipolar atrial leads at sensitivities to allow detection of atrial fibrillation.[111, 112] These leads should therefore be avoided in devices designed to detect atrial arrhythmias.

More problematic than signal dropout, however, is undersensing of organized atrial arrhythmias, especially atrial flutter, by the intermittent or continuous occurrence of atrial electrograms during the blanking periods.[113, 114] This may lead to complete failure to mode switch or to oscillation in and out of mode switching as the mode switch criteria are intermittently fulfilled. The durations of the postatrial and postventricular atrial blanking periods impose mathematical limits on the rates of regular atrial tachycardias that can be consistently detected (Fig. 3–40). For devices with atrial blanking throughout the AV delay and contiguous with the onset of the postventricular atrial blanking period (PVABP),

the device will be unable to sense on a 1:1 basis regular atrial tachyarrhythmias with cycle lengths shorter than the sum of the AV delay and PVABP. Mode-switching failure may occur when the interval between sensed atrial events exceeds the tachycardia detection interval. Some devices allow sensing during part of the AV delay but do not prevent the problem. Devices that use calculated atrial rates may be less prone but are not immune to this behavior.

The detection of atrial arrhythmias by implantable devices may be optimized by device programming and other factors (Table 3–1). At implantation, the use of closely spaced, bipolar endocardial leads carefully placed in the high right atrium or appendage provides the largest electrogram amplitude for sensing while minimizing far-field signals. Regardless of the sinus sensing threshold, programmed sensitivities of 0.15 to 1.0 mV are typically needed to detect atrial fibrillation consistently. If programmable, atrial blanking periods should be made as short as possible while still preventing oversensing. If blanking occurs throughout the AV delay, this parameter should be programmed as short as possible to minimize the total atrial blanking period, which can limit the detection of atrial flutter. If blanking occurs during part of the AV delay, lengthening the AV delay is also possible to force a flutter wave to fall into the sensing period between the postatrial and postventricular atrial blanking periods. The detection criteria for arrhythmia detection (e.g., detection rate, number of rapid cycles, reversion criteria) should be highly programmable to individualize detection for each patient. Algorithms that are quick to mode switch are preferred by most patients.[115] For mode switching devices with counter-type algorithms, mode switching after

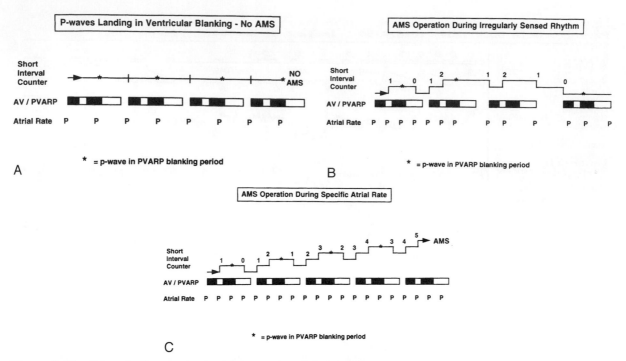

Figure 3–40. Schematic diagrams showing failure to mode switch during regular and irregular atrial rhythms. In each panel, the short interval counter is shown at the top, and the atrial blanking periods during the atrioventricular delay (AV) and PVARP *(dark segments)* are shown in the middle. The actual occurrence of atrial electrograms (P) is shown at the bottom. *A,* For a regular atrial tachycardia such as atrial flutter, every other atrial electrogram may fall within an atrial blanking period. The short interval counter is not incremented in this case, and mode switching fails to occur. *B,* For irregular atrial rhythms such as atrial fibrillation, some atrial electrograms fall within the blanking periods, whereas others are sensed to advance the counter. Pauses in the rhythm or signal dropout may cause long intervals, causing the counter to decrement to zero, so that mode switching does not occur. *C,* With rapid atrial tachyarrhythmias or shortened blanking periods, enough atrial electrograms fall outside the blanking periods to activate mode switching eventually as the short interval counter reaches 5. Mode switching is delayed, however, owing to the occurrence of electrograms within blanking periods that decrement the counter. (From Ellenbogen KA, Mond H, Wood MA, Barold SS: Failure of automatic mode switching: Recognition and management. PACE 20:268–275, 1997.)

five or fewer rapid atrial beats appears to be optimal. Finally, data logging and electrogram storage are useful to document device function.[114]

Atrial Fibrillation Detection in an Atrial Defibrillator

The Metrix atrial ICD (InControl, Guidant Corp., St. Paul, MN) performs intermittent off-line analysis of a two-channel, 8-second segment recorded from a right ventricular bipole and a right atrial–coronary sinus bipole.[116] Nominally, this analysis is performed every 20 minutes. The analysis is performed in two steps (Fig. 3–41). In the first step, the algorithm determines the presence or absence of sinus rhythm by determining the percentage of time that a right atrial–coronary sinus bipolar signal is isoelectric. R waves detected on the ventricular channel are blanked in the analysis of the right atrial–coronary sinus channel to prevent detection of far-field R waves. If the total of these "quiet intervals" is more than a programmable percentage (nominally, 25%), the rhythm is classified as sinus rhythm. If it is less than this percentage, a second "baseline crossing" analysis is performed. The algorithm determines the number of baseline crossings of the right atrial–coronary sinus bipolar signal during a part of the ST segment, from 60 to 200 msec after the R wave on the right ventricular bipole. The baseline crossing count is the average number of baseline crossings per R wave. Atrial fibrillation is detected if the average

baseline crossing count exceeds the programmed value (nominally, 2). Because this system does not pace the atrium, blanking periods do not interfere with detection of atrial fibrillation.

The performance of this algorithm has been reported. Sra and coworkers[96] reported 92% sensitivity for detection of atrial fibrillation and 100% specificity for detection of sinus rhythm in 11 patients studied in the electrophysiology laboratory. Tse and colleagues[117] reported inappropriate detection of sinus tachycardia in 3 of 51 patients (6%) during follow-up. Wellens and colleagues[100] reported that sensitivity for detection of atrial fibrillation was 92% in 2240 tests of the detection algorithm.

The Metrix system has several important limitations. First, atrial pacing is not provided. Second, if automatic therapy is programmed, it delivers a shock as soon as atrial fibrillation is detected and R-wave synchronization occurs. For this reason, it usually is programmed to deliver only patient-activated therapy and is thus of limited value in patients with asymptomatic atrial fibrillation. Atrial electrograms are evaluated only during the ECG ST segment, so that the precise rate and regularity of the atrial rhythm cannot be determined. Because detection is performed intermittently, continuous atrial fibrillation cannot be distinguished from sequential, self-terminating episodes. Furthermore, atrial tachyarrhythmia is not detected, atrial fibrillation is not

Table 3–1. Factors Affecting Mode Switching

Atrial Electrogram

Amplitude
Cycle length
Amplitude variation
Frequency content

Atrial Lead

Bipolar versus unipolar
Electrode spacing
Lead position

Pacemaker Features

Programmed sensitivity
Mode-switching algorithm
  Counter based
  Calculated atrial rate based
Blanking periods
Atrial tachycardia detection rate

Other

Antiarrhythmic drugs
Far-field sensing
Rate-response settings, upper tracking rate (some devices)

detected during ventricular-paced rhythm, and a coronary sinus electrode is required.

Atrial Tachyarrhythmia Detection in a Combined Atrial and Ventricular Defibrillator

The dual-chamber Jewel AF (Medtronic) algorithm diagnoses specific arrhythmias by the PR Logic algorithm described later in this chapter. In this algorithm, one sequence of couple codes is specific for atrial tachyarrhythmia with 2:1 atrioventricular conduction. The algorithm's second P:R pattern analysis method is an AT/AF Evidence Counter based on the number of sensed atrial electrograms in consecutive RR intervals. This counter is used in combination with the median atrial cycle length to provide high specificity for detecting atrial tachyarrhythmias with N:1 atrioventricular conduction and those that do not have repeating couple codes, such as AF/AT with variable atrioventricular conduction. The AT/AF Evidence Counter increments or decrements for each RR interval. It increments if there are two or more paced or sensed atrial events per RR interval and if an RR interval with one atrial event follows an RR interval with two or more atrial events. Otherwise, it decrements (Fig. 3–42). Similar, more rapidly responding atrial evidence counters are used in conjunction with other information to withhold ventricular therapy for rapidly conducted atrial tachyarrhythmia or atrial fibrillation and mode switch from DDD to DDI pacing.

The AT/AF Evidence Counter operates in two different modes for preliminary and sustained detection. Preliminary detection occurs when the count reaches 32, initiating an AT/AF episode. The episode timer begins to increment, and the Evidence Counter switches to the sustained-detection mode in which AT/AF remains detected if the count is 27 or greater and the atrial rate criterion remains fulfilled. The maximum value of the counter is 47.

Termination of Device-Defined Atrial Arrhythmia Episodes: A device-defined atrial arrhythmia episode ends

with detection of *sinus rhythm,* which is defined as five consecutive RR intervals that fulfill the sinus rhythm PR pattern, or 3 minutes of unclassified atrial rhythm with a median rate less than the programmed AT detection rate. The sustained-detection mode, combined with tolerance for periods of unclassified atrial rhythm, is intended to prevent inappropriate episode termination despite some atrial undersensing during AT/AF.

Far-Field R-Wave Discrimination: To ensure accurate detection of atrial rate and rhythm, the ICD has minimal postventricular atrial blanking (none after sensed ventricular events; 30 msec after paced ventricular events). This constraint, combined with autoadjusting atrial sensitivity, may result in inappropriate atrial sensing of far-field R waves. The detection algorithm uses the fact that the pattern of far-field R waves in sinus rhythm produces a measured 2:1 atrioventricular ratio with a characteristic alternation of measured PP intervals to discriminate it from 2:1 AV conduction of regular AT. It detects far-field R waves by a combination of three factors: exactly two atrial events in each RR interval, stable and short interval between the R wave on the ventricu-

Step 1: Quiet (Isoelectric) Interval

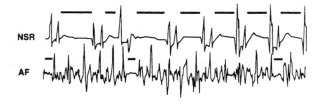

Step 2: Baseline Crossing

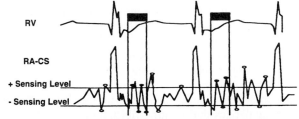

Figure 3–41. Atrial fibrillation detection algorithm for the InControl Metrix defibrillator. In the first step, the algorithm determines the presence or absence of sinus rhythm by determining the percentage of time that a right atrial–coronary sinus bipolar signal is isoelectric. This stage is intended to be highly sensitive to the presence of nonsinus rhythms. If the total of these "quiet intervals" is more than a programmable percentage, the rhythm is classified as sinus rhythm. If it is less than this percentage, a second "baseline crossing" analysis is performed. This analysis is intended to be highly specific for atrial fibrillation (AF). The algorithm determines the number of baseline crossings of the right atrial–coronary sinus bipolar signal during a part of the ST segment. The baseline crossing count is the average number of baseline crossings per R wave. AF is detected if the average baseline crossing count exceeds the programmed value (nominally, 2.0). Because this system does not pace the atrium, blanking periods do not interfere with detection of AF.

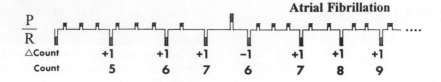

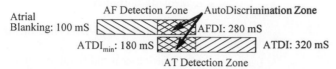

Figure 3–42. Atrial fibrillation detection for the Medtronic Jewel AF defibrillator. *Upper panel,* The atrial tachycardia/atrial fibrillation (AT/AF) evidence counter, which is an up–down counter that increases when there are two or more Ps in the RR interval and decreases after the second RR interval that has only zero or one P. This counter is able to tolerate some undersensing of AF and is specific for greater than 1:1 tachycardias. AT is initially detected if the median atrial cycle length is in the AT zone (180–450 msec nominal) and the AT/AF evidence counter for the P:R pattern reaches 32. *Lower panel,* The atrial fibrillation and atrial tachycardia detection zones that may overlap. If the median atrial cycle length occurs in the overlap between the atrial fibrillation and atrial tachycardia zones, an autodiscrimination algorithm decides whether it is one or the other based on the irregularity of recent PP intervals. At a ventricular event, the difference between the shortest and longest of the last 12 atrial cycle lengths is compared with 25% (nominal) of the median atrial cycle length. If this difference is greater than the percentage of the median atrial cycle length for six of the last eight ventricular events, then the rhythm is called AF; otherwise, it is labeled as atrial tachycardia by the device.

lar channel and the far-field R wave on the atrial channel, and stable alternation in the interval between P wave and far-field R wave. If all three criteria are met, the atrial electrogram following the short PP interval is classified as a far-field R wave and excluded from the AT/AF Evidence Count (Fig. 3–43).[118]

AT/AF Autodiscrimination: AT/AF detection zones may overlap. The AT/AF overlap zone is the range of cycle lengths greater than or equal to the minimum cycle length in the atrial tachyarrhythmia zone and less than the atrial fibrillation detection interval. If the median atrial cycle length is in this overlap zone, the atrial rhythm is classified as atrial tachyarrhythmia if it is regular or atrial fibrillation if it is not (Fig. 3–44). The purpose of this autodiscrimination feature is to permit antitachycardia pacing for fast, regular atrial arrhythmias, including periods when the atrial rhythm regularizes during atrial fibrillation.

Several features of this dual-chamber ICD system combine to permit continuous detection of atrial fibrillation for extended periods: (1) a closely spaced, atrial sensing bipole[118a]; (2) autoadjusting sensitivity with a short time constant; (3) minimal blanking of the atrial sense amplifier to prevent atrial undersensing; and (4) a detection algorithm that continues to detect AF despite undersensing. In a recent study of this ICD,[119] stored data appropriately recorded 91 AT/AF episodes longer than 1 hour for a total 2942 hours of continuous detection of AT/AF. Holter recordings validated continuous detection for 112 hours (Fig. 3–45).

Detection and Discrimination of Atrial Tachyarrhythmias: In a recent study of 80 patients, the true-positive rate was 98% for detection of spontaneous AF (n = 132)

and 87% for detection of spontaneous AT (n = 165). All inappropriate detections were caused by limitations of the algorithm for rejection of far-field R waves and lasted less than 5 minutes. Discrimination of AT versus AF permitted delivery of painless antitachycardia pacing, which successfully treated 45% of all AT episodes and 42% of regular atrial tachyarrhythmias in the AF zone.

Clinical Guidelines.

1. PR Logic performs best when the atrial electrode is positioned to minimize far-field R waves. This requires an implant-support device that displays the atrial bipolar signal continuously.

2. Optimal programming of AT/AF detection intervals differs from optimal programming of the mode-switching interval in DDD pacemakers. If atrial blanking is minimal, the atrial tachyarrhythmia detection interval should be set slightly greater than the anticipated interval rather than slightly less than the minimum sinus cycle length. This will reduce inappropriate detection due to far-field R waves without compromising detection of atrial tachyarrhythmia. Programming too low a value for the AT detection interval, however, may result in underdetection of AT despite adequate atrial sensing.

3. Inappropriate detection of sinus tachycardia with far-field R waves as AT/AF is a transient phenomenon that need not result in inappropriate therapy. Restricting therapy to AT/AF episodes of longer than 10 minutes should prevent inappropriate therapy. In contrast, ventricular ICDs usually deliver inappropriate therapy if inappropriate detection occurs.

4. In patients without a history of ventricular tachyarrhythmias, the VF Detection Interval and the Supraventricu-

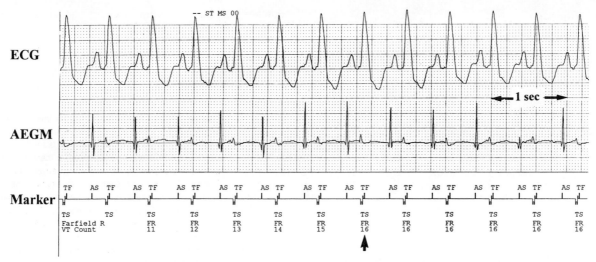

Figure 3–43. Oversensing of far-field R waves as P waves on the atrial channel is more likely for dual-chamber defibrillators than for dual-chamber pacemakers because the atrial blanking period after a ventricular event is reduced or eliminated to enhance sensing of atrial tachyarrhythmias. The atrial bipolar electrogram (AEGM) shows far-field R waves that are being sensed. The Gem DR and Jewel AF have an algorithm for ignoring far-field R waves during sinus tachycardia that uses consistent alternation of PP intervals (>30 msec), low RP interval variability (<50 msec), and consistent R-P intervals (<20 msec from the average RP). For every RR interval, there must be exactly two atrial events. The consistent alternation of PP intervals is needed to avoid rejecting 2:1 atrial flutter rhythms. One of the P waves must be close to the R waves (P-R < 60 msec or R-P < 160 msec). These criteria must be met for 10 of the last 12 RR intervals to reject P events as far-field R waves. If far-field R waves had not been rejected by this algorithm, then inappropriate detection would have occurred when the ventricular tachycardia counter reached 16 *(arrow)*.

lar Tachycardia Minimum Cycle Length (SVT Limit) should nominally be programmed to a low value (e.g., <280 msec). These patients are not generally at risk for ventricular tachycardia, and PR Logic discriminates poorly between ventricular and atrial tachyarrhythmias in the ventricular fibrillation zone.

Shock Synchronization

Synchronization of shocks to bipolar electrograms is important to prevent initiation or reinitiation of ventricular tachycardia or fibrillation by shocks delivered in the vulnerable period of the cardiac cycle. Design principles for shock synchronization algorithms are different for atrial and ventricular ICDs. *Ventricular ICDs* attempt to synchronize VT/VF therapy to a sensed R wave but will deliver ventricular fibrillation shocks even if synchronization cannot be confirmed because of the possibility that low-amplitude ventricular fibrillation electrograms are undersensed. In contrast, synchronization algorithms for atrial ICDs must err on the side of specificity. They deliver shocks with ventricular

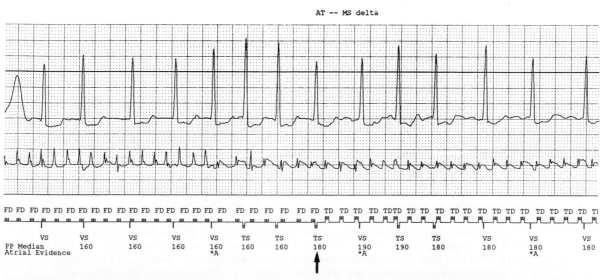

Figure 3–44. Discriminating atrial fibrillation from atrial tachycardia can be based solely on the median atrial cycle length. See text for details.

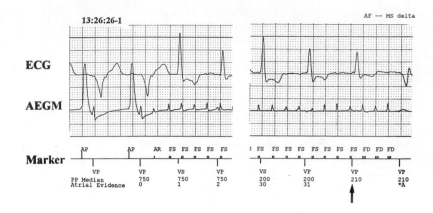

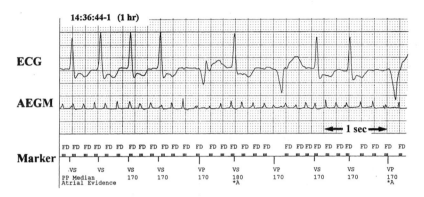

Figure 3–45. Holter monitor recording illustrating continuous detection of atrial fibrillation (AF). Surface electrocardiogram (ECG), telemetered bipolar atrial electrogram (AEGM), and telemetered marker channel are shown. Upward marks correspond to atrial events, and downward marks correspond to ventricular events. The two lines below the marker channel indicate the median PP interval for the last 12 atrial events and the value of the (AT/AF) Evidence Counter. *A,* shows the onset of atrial fibrillation at 13:26:26 and initial detection of atrial fibrillation after 32 ventricular events *(arrow).* Double atrial markers (FS) change to triple atrial markers (FD). *B,* A sample of the rhythms after 1 hour of continuous recording. One low-amplitude P wave is undersensed. During continuous detection of AF, triple atrial markers are displayed regardless of the PP interval.

proarrhythmic potential (Fig. 3–46) to patients who do not have spontaneous ventricular arrhythmias. Further, standalone atrial ICDs such as the Guidant Metrix are incapable of detecting or treating device-induced VT/VF. Because the vulnerable period may extend to the next R wave during sinus tachycardia[120] or rapidly conducting atrial fibrillation,[121] synchronized shocks to R waves that end short RR intervals may be proarrhythmic (Fig. 3–47).

Atrial ICDs are designed to deliver shocks only after a minimum synchronization interval of about 500 msec

Figure 3–46. Proarrhythmia caused by inappropriate shock during rate-only detection. *A,* The top left tracing shows electrograms recorded from high-voltage leads (HVA-HVB) of a Medtronic Model 7223 ICD during sinus rhythm. The top right tracing shows the initial stored electrogram from the treated tachycardia. The electrograms in these two panels are essentially identical, indicating that the treated arrhythmia is supraventricular. Note that the electrogram during tachycardia is clipped at the maximum amplitude of 8 mV. The lower panels are "Flashback Interval" plots of the RR-interval cycle lengths before rate-only detection of ventricular fibrillation (VF), which occurs at the right side of each panel. The interval number before detection is plotted on the abscissa, and the corresponding interval is plotted on the ordinate. The lower left panel shows 2000 RR intervals before detection. A tachycardia is present throughout. Shortly after the 400th interval, the rhythm accelerates gradually in a manner typical of sinus tachycardia and decreases below the programmed VF detection interval of 340 msec. The lower right panel shows this gradual acceleration on an expanded scale during the last 100 intervals before detection. Cycle-length measurements are truncated to the nearest 10 msec. *B,* Stored electrogram during therapy of the tachycardia detected in panel A. The first VF shock (VF Rx 1) results in widening of the electrogram without change in the cycle length of 330 msec. This is probably due to shock-induced right bundle-branch block, which was documented in this patient at electrophysiologic testing. The tracing is discontinuous at the end of the first line and continuous thereafter. Shocks 2, 3, and 4 resulted in no change in rate or electrogram morphology. On the second line, the fifth VF shock (VF Rx 5) induced VT with a cycle length of 280 msec, despite appropriate synchronization to the nadir of the R wave. The sixth VF shock (VF Rx 6) accelerated the VT to a cycle length of 210 msec. This rhythm terminated spontaneously 21 seconds later, and sinus tachycardia with a wide electrogram resumed *(asterisk).* No additional shocks were delivered during these 21 seconds because the maximum number of therapies per zone is six in this implantable cardioverter-defibrillator. The patient reported that during exertion, he experienced multiple shocks followed by syncope. The programmed shock strength was 24 J for the first shock and 34 J for subsequent shocks.

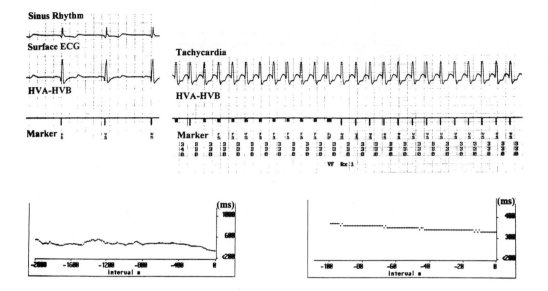

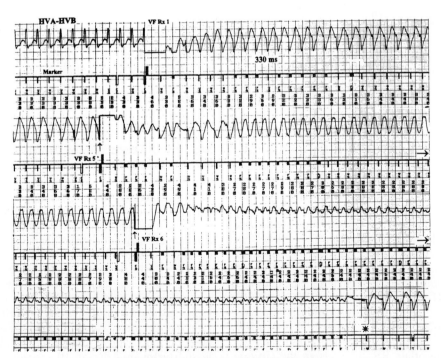

Figure 3–46. *See legend on opposite page*

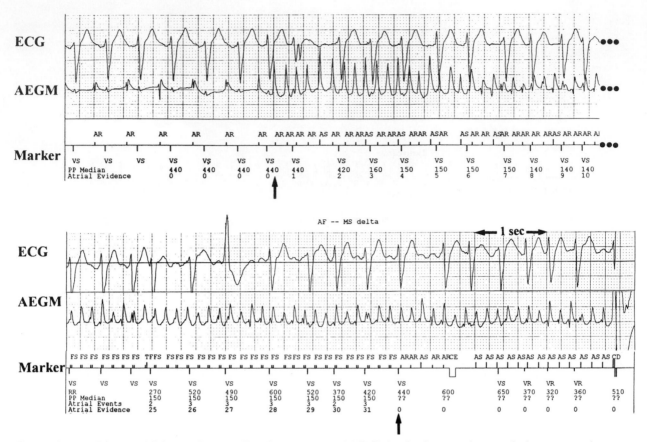

Figure 3–47. Telemetered Holter monitor recording of spontaneous atrial fibrillation that began at the arrow in the upper panel as shown by the atrial electrogram (AEGM) that is reliably sensed except for one P wave with inadequate slew rate. The atrial evidence counter begins incrementing after the arrow and continues on the lower panel (not continuous) until 32 ventricular beats accumulate, resulting in atrial fibrillation detection at the arrow. The delay to therapy was programmed to zero minutes and hours, so that charging was immediate and completed after only 600 msec (broad marker pulse). The synchronization algorithm waited until a long interval occurred (550 msec) to deliver the shock to the atrial pathway, indicated by the shock marker symbol, which initially goes upward for an atrial shock (Jewel AF).

(see Fig. 3–47). In addition, the Metrix ICD uses two additional checks to prevent proarrhythmic shocks. First, shocks are synchronized to R waves only if they are detected both on the right ventricular bipolar electrogram and the right ventricular tip–to–coronary sinus electrogram. Second, a qualifying R wave must not end a long–short sequence, which increases the risk of proarrhythmia. To achieve this goal, the Minimum Synchronization Interval is defined as the interval between the later of the S-wave components of the preceding QRS complex sensed on both channels and the earlier of the two Q-wave components of the next QRS complex. If the SQ interval for synchronization is less than 800 msec, the synchronized SQ interval must be within 140 msec of the preceding QQ interval. This algorithm has been highly specific for appropriate RR intervals in the electrophysiology laboratory[122] and in clinical trials in patients with structurally normal hearts.[100] It has not been tested in patients with left bundle-branch block, which causes consistently short SQ intervals compared with QQ intervals and might prevent synchronization. It has also not been evaluated critically in challenging circumstances, such as electromagnetic interference and lead failures.

Sensing and Detection of Ventricular Tachycardia and Fibrillation Electrograms in Ventricular Tachycardia and Fibrillation

Ectopic beats may have lower-amplitude R waves than sinus rhythm R waves, as shown in Figure 3–48, but the reverse may also be true. For monomorphic ventricular tachycardia, Ellenbogen and colleagues[67] found a 14% decrease in the mean amplitude for epicardial electrograms but only a 5% decrease for endocardial electrograms.

The ventricular fibrillation amplitudes decreased by 25% for epicardial signals but by 41% for endocardial electrograms, as shown in Figure 3–49. During ventricular fibrillation, the mean electrogram amplitude did not change, but in 60% of individual episodes the amplitude changed by at least a factor of 2 during 10 seconds. Analysis of their data tables shows that ventricular fibrillation amplitude was less than or equal to 1 mV in 11 of 69 episodes (16%) in 6 of 21 patients (29%). These very-low-amplitude ventricular fibrillation electrograms are of particular concern for design of ICD sensing systems. Figure 3–50 shows examples of the highly variable electrograms, all from separate patients, that have very different intrinsic deflections, amplitudes, slew

CHART SPEED 25.0 mm/s

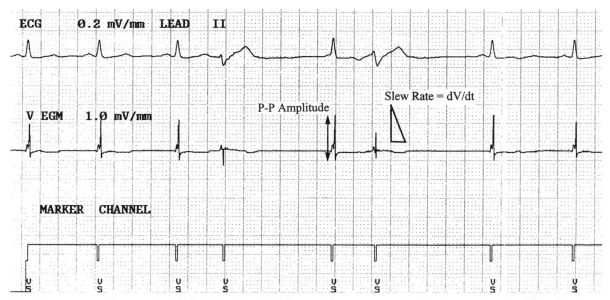

Figure 3–48. An electrocardiogram (ECG) lead II, a bipolar right ventricular electrogram (EGM) and a marker channel with pulses that show when sensing occurs. The QRS on the ECG is about 1 mV, which is typical. There are also two paraventricular contractions (PVCs) (the fourth and sixth complexes) with similar shapes but different amplitudes. On the V-EGM, the peak-to-peak amplitude of the sinus R waves are 10 to 12 mV. The slew rate is the maximum slope (dV/dt) on the intrinsic deflection when the depolarization wavefront passes the electrode tip. The slew rate is difficult to measure at standard paper speed but is typically 0.5 to 3.0 V/sec. Slew rate is a simple way to estimate the frequency content of a signal. The sinus beat in the center between the two PVCs has the main intrinsic deflection during the last part of the ECG QRS complex. Note that the sinus R waves on the V-EGM have an early deflection and a notch that are within the surface ECG. A small early deflection is also seen on the V-EGM for the PVCs. The amplitude of the main intrinsic deflection of the PVC is less than that of the sinus rhythm R wave. The electrograms have distinctly different morphologies. The leading edge of the sense marker pulses indicates the instant that sensing occurs. Each R wave on the V-EGM is appropriately sensed at the initial deflection for 0.3 mV sensitivity. If the programmed sensitivity were raised to 2 or 3 mV, sensing would probably be delayed until the main intrinsic deflection of the R wave. This delay is of little practical consequence except to electrocardiographers, who expect it to happen at the initial deflection on the QRS. Each R wave is sensed only once because sensing is blanked for 120 msec after each ventricular sense. P-P, peak to peak

Figure 3–49. Mean peak-to-peak amplitude of ventricular electrograms during induced ventricular fibrillation (VF) and normal sinus rhythm (NSR). Mean electrogram amplitudes were calculated during VF at 1, 5, and 10 seconds of VF. Avg, average; Epi, epicardial; ICEGM, intracardiac electrogram; sec, second; Trans, transvenous. (From Ellenbogen KA, Wood MA, Stambler BS, et al: Measurement of ventricular electrogram amplitude during intraoperative induction of ventricular tachyarrhythmias. Am J Cardiol 70:1017–1022, 1992.)

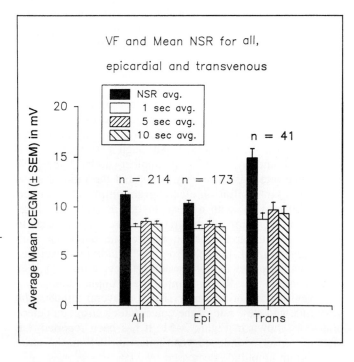

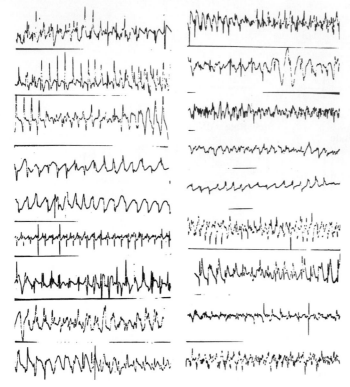

Figure 3–50. Unfiltered human bipolar electrograms showing induced ventricular fibrillation during cardioverter-defibrillator implantation in 20 patients. Note the wide variation in amplitudes and slew rates among these different patients. The morphology of each bipolar depolarization often changes several times on most of these strips. This may cause some oversensing of ventricular fibrillation, which is acceptable because it will result in more prompt detection.

■ SENSING OF VENTRICULAR FIBRILLATION BY IMPLANTABLE CARDIOVERTER-DEFIBRILLATORS

The primary challenge for sensing of ventricular fibrillation is to prevent undersensing during the episode while avoiding oversensing of cardiac or extracardiac signals during regular rhythm.

Figure 3–52 shows a histogram of manually measured ventricular fibrillation cycle lengths (*unhatched bars*) and sensed (0.3 mV) cycle lengths (*hatched bars*) for the same episodes. These two superimposed histograms match well. Sense amplifier blanking was 120 msec. The histograms both have peaks at about 200 msec and a range from 130 to 300 msec for patients who are not taking antiarrhythmic drugs. Occasional ventricular fibrillation oversensing and variability of the cycle lengths due to sensing different parts of the electrogram waveshapes is common. Cycle lengths of greater than 300 msec usually represent occasional brief undersensing during the episode. If the amplitude of the sinus-rhythm R wave at implant is more than 5 mV, nominal sensitivity settings do not result in underdetection of ventricular fibrillation.[126] Patients with low-amplitude R waves may require higher sensitivity settings to ensure reliable sensing of ventricular fibrillation. This may result in T-wave oversensing.

Although detection counting algorithms are designed to permit some undersensing of ventricular fibrillation, rare cases of undersensing have resulted in serious delays in detection or detection failure. It is well recognized that ventricular fibrillation electrograms with extremely low amplitude and slew rate may cause sufficient undersensing to result in clinical underdetection. This has been reported following an apical infarction at the site of the endocardial sensing electrodes that required repositioning of the lead.[127]

rates, and morphologies. As described later, rapidly varying electrogram amplitudes in ventricular fibrillation may cause clinically significant undersensing despite automatic gain control[123] or autoadjusting threshold. Inspection of these electrograms during implant should focus on possible large beat-to-beat amplitude variability that may cause ventricular fibrillation undersensing. If this is found, such areas with fractionated conduction may warrant lead tip repositioning.

The correlation between sinus rhythm electrogram amplitudes and ventricular fibrillation electrogram amplitudes was poor (r = 0.19) in one study.[67] Although a stronger correlation was found (r = 0.70) in another study,[124] the 95% confidence intervals were very large, and the ratio of sinus to ventricular fibrillation electrogram amplitudes ranged from 0.29 to 1.05, with a mean of 0.5 ± 0.20. The large interpatient variation of this ratio makes it impractical to estimate ventricular fibrillation electrogram amplitude with any precision from sinus electrograms in individual patients. The practical effect of this variability is to require at least 5-mV peak-to-peak R-wave amplitude at implantation.

If ventricular fibrillation persists for several minutes, the amplitude and slew rate of the epicardial electrogram deteriorates, as shown in Figure 3–51. It has been reported that after the onset of induced ventricular fibrillation, the atrial electrogram amplitude decreased by 31%.[125]

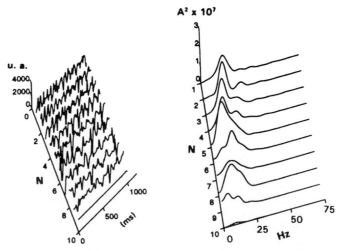

Figure 3–51. *Left,* ventricular fibrillation recordings made at 30-second intervals for the first 5 minutes of ischemia from an epicardial electrode. *Right,* The amplitude power spectra as a function of frequency for these same signals. The signal amplitude is zero on the last sequence of the graph because the ventricular fibrillation spontaneously terminated. (From Chorro FJ, Guerrero J, Cánoves J, et al: Quantification of the modifications in the dominant frequency of VF under conditions of ischemia and reperfusion. PACE 21:1716–1723, 1998.)

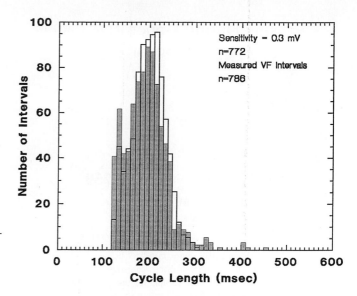

Figure 3–52. Sensed cycle lengths of human ventricular fibrillation electrograms by an implantable cardioverter-defibrillator (ICD) sensing system are compared with manual cycle length measurements of the same signals from many patients. Two histograms are superimposed. The unshaded vertical bars show the manually measured cycle lengths during ventricular fibrillation (786 intervals); the shaded bars show the intervals sensed by the ICD (772 intervals). Intervals of less than 120 msec, the blanking period, were not permitted. Note that there was some oversensing for intervals of less than 180 msec, a slight amount of undersensing for intervals between 180 and 280 msec, and a small number of long intervals greater than 280 msec that represent undersensing during ventricular fibrillation. The peak in the histograms occurs at about 220 msec.

It is less well appreciated that electrograms with rapidly varying amplitude may also cause sufficient undersensing to result in underdetection, despite the presence of many electrograms with sufficient amplitude to be sensed. This occurs because abrupt changes in electrogram amplitude variability may not be tracked by the automatic gain control[123] or autoadjusting threshold, as shown on the right side of Figure 3–53. In this situation, underdetection may be resolved by repositioning the sensing lead to obtain a more uniform, although lower-amplitude, ventricular fibrillation electrogram.

In dual-chamber ICDs, sensing may be restricted to short periods of the cardiac cycle because of the combined effects of postpacing blanking periods during high-rate pacing and

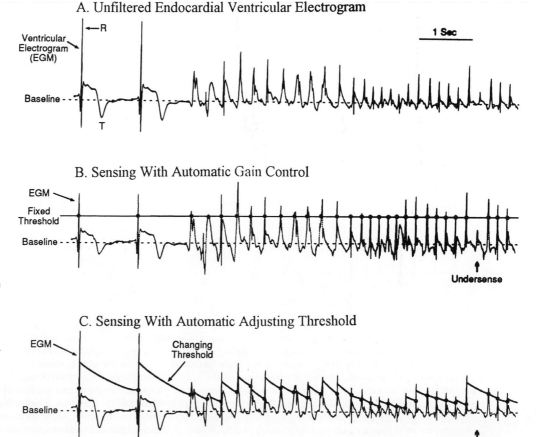

Figure 3–53. Sinus rhythm and ventricular fibrillation signals are shown for the raw electrogram in panel *A,* for automatic gain control in panel *B,* and for automatic adjusting threshold in panel *C.* In panel *B,* the small electrograms are amplified compared with those in panel *A,* and the sensing is shown by the dots where the signal crosses the fixed threshold. In panel *C,* the electrograms are the same as in panel *A,* the threshold varies according to the amplitude of the electrogram, and sensing is again shown by the dots where the signal crosses the variable threshold.

VT Sensing During Upper Rate Pacing
Worst Case Scenario

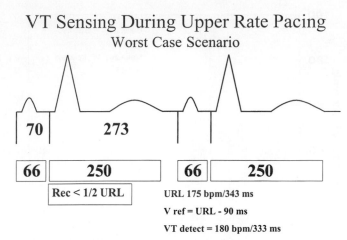

Rec < 1/2 URL

URL 175 bpm/343 ms

V ref = URL - 90 ms

VT detect = 180 bpm/333 ms

Figure 3–54. Modified DDDR upper rate limit behavior with automatic gain control envelopes. Dual-chamber rate-responsive pacing at the maximum sensor upper rate limit of 175 bpm for the Ventak AV II shows that postatrial pace blanking of 66 msec and postventricular pace blanking of 250 msec allow only a small window to initiate sensing of a spontaneous ventricular tachyarrhythmia. Such a tachyarrhythmia could hide in these paced blanking periods for many paced cycles until the first ventricular sense occurs to inhibit the dual-chamber pacing. (From personal communication with Dr. Marshall Stanton, 1992.)

ventricular blanking after atrial paced events needed to avoid crosstalk in some dual chamber systems (Fig. 3–54). If a sufficient fraction of the cardiac cycle were blanked, ventricular fibrillation depolarizations could be systematically undersensed. Such undersensing may be decreased by shortening of the postpacing ventricular blanking period, but this may result in T-wave oversensing, as shown in Figure 3–55. To date, there have been no clinical reports of ventricular fibrillation undersensing due to high-rate pacing in dual-

chamber ICDs or rate-responsive single-chamber ICDs. Kulkamp and colleagues[128] showed that the time to detection of induced ventricular fibrillation was not significantly different for the dual-chamber VENTAK AV (Guidant, St. Paul, MN) when pacing DDD at 150 bpm and the single-chamber Mini ICD when pacing VVI at 100 bpm.

Undersensing and Oversensing During Regular Rhythm

The requirement for reliable sensing of variable and low-amplitude electrograms during ventricular fibrillation creates inherent conflicts that may result in undersensing or oversensing during regular rhythm.

Undersensing

Automatic gain control and autoadjusting threshold may cause sensing errors during sinus rhythm.[129–131] Spontaneous increases in the amplitude of R waves in sinus rhythm or during nonsustained ventricular tachyarrhythmia may reset automatic gain control, resulting in undersensing of subsequent sinus rhythm and inappropriate bradycardia pacing. In some devices such inappropriate bradycardia pacing has been proarrhythmic, resulting in initiation of sustained ventricular tachyarrhythmia.[130] This occurred because the automatic gain control abruptly increased (150%) or decreased (67%) the gain after a fixed number of different beats or passage of a fixed time. Sinus rhythm amplitude decreases of 39% after premature beats[129] also caused undersensing of sinus R waves and inappropriate bradycardia pacing that induced VT[131] without change in automatic gain.

T-Wave Oversensing

ICDs have been observed to oversense T waves.[132, 133] T-wave oversensing after paced beats reduces the effective bradycardia pacing rate and may inhibit antitachycardia pac-

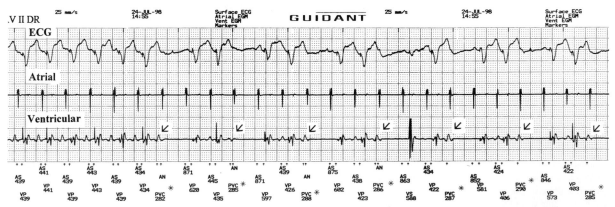

Figure 3–55. Real-time recordings during treadmill exercise testing are shown from surface electrocardiogram lead II, atrial bipole, ventricular integrated bipole, and marker channel in a pacemaker-dependent patient with high-grade atrioventricular block and normal sinus node function. The patient has a dual-chamber pacing defibrillator. This test was performed because the patient complained of exercise-induced near syncope. The programmed ventricular sensitivity was set to the least sensitive value of 0.44 mV. At heart rates of more than 140 bpm, T-wave oversensing *(arrows)* occurred and resulted in inhibition of ventricular output. Oversensed T-waves are classified as paraventricular contractions on the marker channel (PVC*). This oversensing occurs because of a combination of two factors: First, the postventricular blanking period is shortened at high rates to maintain a window to sense the onset of ventricular tachycardia or fibrillation; this feature is not programmable. Second, automatic gain control is set to the maximum value after paced ventricular events. At the nominal sensitivity setting of 0.18 mV, exercise testing demonstrated high-grade AV block at sinus rates of more than 130 bpm.

ing or cause antitachycardia pacing to be delivered at the wrong rate, resulting in shocks for ventricular tachyarrhythmia that could be terminated by pacing.[103, 131] T-wave oversensing during sinus tachycardia may result in inappropriate detection of ventricular tachyarrhythmias and fibrillation. T-wave oversensing can also cause inappropriate confirmation or synchronization of shocks. The latter may result in a shock delivered during the vulnerable period and induce ventricular tachyarrhythmia. T-wave oversensing may be reduced by lengthening the ventricular refractory period.

Oversensing of Noncardiac Signals

Electromagnetic interference from an electronic antitheft device has resulted in inappropriate sensing, detection, and shocks.[134] Inappropriate sensing, detection, and shocks also have been reported following telemetry[135] and magnet tests.[136] Bradycardia-dependent sensing of diaphragmatic myopotentials has resulted in inappropriate inhibition of bradycardia pacing and delivery of spurious shocks. This type of oversensing has been reported only for integrated bipolar electrodes.

Oversensing Due to Lead Insulation Failure

Myopotential oversensing leading to inappropriate detection and shocks is a common presentation of sensing-lead insulation failure.

Oversensing of Far-Field R Waves

In dual-chamber ventricular ICDs, low-amplitude P waves may require programming to high atrial sensitivities. This may result in sensing of far-field R waves on the atrial channel. Oversensing of far-field R waves presents unique problems for dual-chamber atrial ICDs, as described later.

Postshock Sensing

Postshock sensing is crucial to redetection after unsuccessful tachyarrhythmia therapy and to accurate detection of tachyarrhythmia termination. The first implantable defibrillator used a single electrode pair for sensing and shocking. Winkle and coworkers[137] first described considerable postshock signal distortion on spring-patch shocking electrodes but only minimal postshock distortion on separate standard bipolar electrodes used only for sensing. *Electroporation,* the process by which shocks create microscopic holes in the cardiac cell membranes near the shocking electrode, has been proposed as the mechanism for postshock distortion of electrograms recorded from high-voltage electrodes.[138] For two large surface area (125 mm²) endocardial catheter shocking electrodes separated by 5 mm, substantial postshock decreases in R wave amplitudes and increases in pacing thresholds persist for up to 10 minutes.[139, 140] Recordings from separate sensing electrodes during transthoracic shocks showed that these effects were localized to electrodes used for both shocking and sensing. Another study also found no significant postshock changes in R-wave amplitudes on standard bipolar epicardial sensing electrodes.[141]

Several studies have shown that postshock sensing is better for true bipolar sensing electrodes than for integrated bipolar sensing electrodes in which one sensing electrode is a high-voltage coil. Integrated bipolar electrodes have longer ventricular fibrillation redetection times and significantly

more unsensed beats during ventricular fibrillation than dedicated bipolar sensing.[142] Studies with Endotak 60 (Guidant, St. Paul, MN) series leads reported failure to sense ventricular fibrillation after shocks associated with decreases in sinus rhythm electrograms from 10.5 mV preshock to 1.9 mV postshock.[143] The electrograms did not fully recover for up to 2 minutes after the shock. This lead uses integrated bipolar sensing between the pacing tip electrode and the right ventricular shocking coil, which are separated by 6 mm. A subsequent report showed smaller decreases in electrogram amplitude for Endotak 70 series leads with 12-mm spacing between the electrodes.[144]

■ DETECTION ALGORITHMS FOR SINGLE-CHAMBER VENTRICULAR IMPLANTABLE CARDIOVERTER-DEFIBRILLATORS

Tiered-therapy ICDs have up to three programmable rate-detection zones that permit programming of zone-specific therapies and detection enhancements. ICDs use digital circuits and microprocessors to classify each ventricular cycle length into one of these zones. Detection algorithms then analyze a series of recent cycle lengths with concurrent and serial calculations, logic, and counting. ICD detection algorithms for ventricular fibrillation are designed to have high sensitivity despite reduced specificity, because the consequences of underdetecting ventricular fibrillation are so grave. This basic philosophy pervades all aspects of detection processes from initial detection through episode termination.

In contrast, detection algorithms for ventricular tachycardia must balance the risks of underdetection with the painful and potentially proarrhythmic consequences of inappropriate therapy. A high-specificity detection algorithm is appropriate for hemodynamically stable, slower ventricular tachycardia because the risks of underdetection are low and the probability of rate-zone overlap with SVT is high. For these reasons, tiered-therapy ICDs include detection-enhancement algorithms to discriminate ventricular tachycardia from SVT. In contrast to detection algorithms for hemodynamically stable ventricular tachycardia, a high-sensitivity algorithm is appropriate for faster tachycardia (e.g., cycle length <300 msec) because the risks for underdetection are high and the probability of rate-zone overlap with SVT is low.

Ventricular Rate Detection Algorithms

Because some undersensing of ventricular fibrillation electrograms cannot be eliminated with either autogain or autothreshold methods, ventricular fibrillation detection counting algorithms must tolerate some degree of undersensing. Initial detection in the fastest (ventricular tachycardia) zone occurs when a certain percentage (typically, 70% to 80%) of intervals in a sliding window (usually 10 to 24 intervals) fulfill the programmed rate criterion. The type of counter used in the ventricular fibrillation zone can only increase or decrease by 1 for each event.

Guidant ICDs also use this X of Y counting in the slower (ventricular tachycardia) zones. Medtronic ICDs use a counter that is reset to zero by a single normal sensed event in the ventricular tachycardia zone. This type of counter requires that each one of a consecutive series of intervals has a cycle length less than the programmed detection interval for ventricular tachycardia. This consecutive-interval counting method diminishes inappropriate detection of atrial fibrillation without compromising sensitivity for detection of monomorphic ventricular tachycardia.[145] Ventricular tachycardia with highly variable cycle lengths, however, may be underdetected. St. Jude ICDs use a method for classifying intervals that depends not only on the latest interval but also on the average of the current interval with the previous three intervals. A potential advantage of this method is that averaging minimizes the effects of intermittent undersensing (Fig. 3–56).

These three counting algorithms were compared by applying them to large numbers of simulated rhythms with a wide range of two-rhythm parameters, mean cycle lengths, and standard deviation of cycle lengths.[102] The Medtronic algorithm was superior at rejecting simulated atrial fibrillation, highly variable rhythms near the zone between slow ventricular tachycardia and no detection. Each algorithm was tested for consistency of rhythm classification by applying it to 10 rhythms with different random number generator seeds but equal rhythm parameters for each combination of cycle lengths and standard deviation of cycle lengths tested. Consistency values were 83% for the Guidant algorithm, 82% for the Medtronic algorithm, and 71% for the St. Jude algorithm. Counters may be independent in each zone, or sensed events in one zone may increment counters for all slower zones. This latter approach minimizes the risk for prolonged detection times if successive ventricular tachycardia intervals are classified in different zones. Alternative methods for classifying rhythms that straddle zone boundaries use a combined-count or summation criterion.[102]

In addition to these algorithms for initial detection of ventricular tachycardia or fibrillation, ICDs use confirmation algorithms to confirm the persistence of either condition after capacitor charging, synchronization algorithms to synchronize shocks to R waves, redetection algorithms to detect arrhythmias after delivered therapy, and episode-termination algorithms to redetect normal rhythm. Redetection refers to detection after delivery of therapy to determine whether the arrhythmia has terminated, accelerated, or continued unchanged. A redetected arrhythmia may accelerate or decelerate from one tachyarrhythmia zone to another or accelerate or decelerate but remain within the same zone. In general, confirmation and redetection algorithms are less restrictive than initial detection algorithms. Redetection may be delayed briefly after delivery of therapy to allow for transient delays in arrhythmia termination after antitachycardia pacing or postshock nonsustained ventricular tachycardia.

Extended High-Rate, Antitachycardia Pacing Time-Out, and Sustained Rate Duration Features

Some manufacturers apply safety-net methods to treat tachyarrhythmias that persist longer than a programmed "sustained" or "extended" duration. St. Jude ICDs have an Extended High Rate (EHR) detection algorithm that limits the duration of redetections and low-energy therapies to a programmable time period. The EHR timer starts when the average cycle length is less than a separate programmable EHR detection interval that is nominally equal to the Tach A interval. If the programmable timer (10 seconds to 5 minutes) expires and the tachycardia persists, the low-energy tachycardia therapies are abandoned, and ventricular fibrillation therapy is initiated. This feature ensures that VF therapy is delivered if a tachyarrhythmia persists longer than the programmed EHR time. A programmable feature (SVT Discriminator Inhibition of EHR), however, restricts EHR only to rhythms classified as ventricular tachycardia by SVT-VT discrimination features described later.

Guidant ICDs have a somewhat similar Antitachycardia Pacing Time-Out feature that instructs the ICD to omit any remaining antitachycardia pacing therapy in a zone and to initiate programmed shock therapy for that zone. Guidant ICDs also have a Sustained Rate Duration (SRD) override that allows programmed therapy to be delivered in the lowest zone of a multizone device when an episode of tachycardia is sustained for a programmable period beyond Duration, but detection enhancements inhibit therapy. The principal utility of this feature is to prevent ventricular tachycardia underdetection by detection enhancements designed to discriminate ventricular tachycardia from SVT. The fundamental premise is that ventricular tachycardia will continue to satisfy the rate criterion for the programmed duration, whereas the ventricular rate during sinus tachycardia or atrial fibrillation may decrease below the rate boundary during this period. The limitation of the sustained-duration override is delivery of inappropriate therapy when SVT exceeds the programmed duration. This is particularly problematic for patients with atrial flutter.

Programming Zones and Durations for Detection

Programming Detection Zone Boundaries

The physician should program the minimum required number of detection zones. Single-zone programming is appropriate for patients whose only clinical arrhythmia is ventricular fibrillation or poorly tolerated, rapid ventricular tachycardia. The safety margin for detection is estimated by the difference between the programmed ventricular fibrilla-

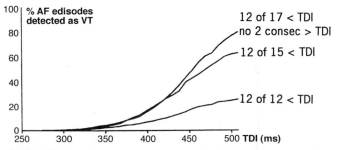

Figure 3–56. Four ventricular rate-only algorithms were compared using 482 episodes of atrial fibrillation and 260 episodes of ventricular tachycardia. The algorithm with the best specificity for the ventricular tachycardia zone used consecutive counting requiring all RR intervals to be less than the ventricular tachycardia detection interval, even after lengthening this programmable detection interval to maintain sensitivity. (From Anderson MH, Murgatroyd F, Hnatkova K, et al: Performance of basic ventricular tachycardia detection algorithms in implantable cardioverter defibrillators: Implications for device programming. 20 (Pt I):2975–2983, 1997.)

tion detection interval and the appropriate percentile (typically, 70% to 80%) of intervals for the specific "X of Y" counting used. In the absence of antiarrhythmic drugs, the 75th percentile is less than 200 msec in more than 99.5% of ventricular fibrillation episodes when true bipolar sensing is used.[102] A programmed detection interval of 320 msec will ensure detection of ventricular fibrillation despite moderate undersensing and prevent detection of most cases of sinus tachycardia in adults, but it may permit detection of atrial fibrillation with a rapid ventricular rate.

For the patient with ventricular tachycardia, two-zone programming is required. When consecutive-interval counting is used, the detection interval should be at least 40 msec greater than the expected cycle length. Adequate width of the ventricular tachycardia zone is also required to prevent underdetection of irregular ventricular tachycardia if consecutive-interval counting is used, even in the presence of a combined count criterion. If the ventricular tachycardia detection zone is too narrow, occasional intervals longer than the detection interval reset the ventricular tachycardia counter and may prevent the combined count from being fulfilled.

The complexity of three-zone programming should be reserved for patients who have two distinct rates of ventricular tachycardia that require different methods of antitachycardia pacing or patients with dual-chamber Medtronic ICDs who have rapidly conducted atrial fibrillation, as described later. Some experts advocate programming the lowest zone as a "monitor-only zone," with detection on and therapies off. Physicians who choose this approach should be aware that interactions between the counter in the monitor-only zone and the next highest zone may decrease the number of intervals required for detection in the higher zone and that detection enhancements may be restricted in the higher zone.

For three-zone Medtronic ICDs, fast ventricular tachycardia (FVT) via ventricular fibrillation type of detection is recommended when a patient has a fast, pace-terminable ventricular tachycardia with cycle lengths that may overlap with some of the cycle lengths during ventricular fibrillation (range, 240–310 msec). This FVT via ventricular tachycardia type of detection is recommended when a patient has both a slow, hemodynamically stable ventricular tachycardia and another faster ventricular tachycardia that requires a more aggressive set of therapies but does not substantially overlap the range ventricular fibrillation cycle lengths (>310 msec) (Fig. 3–57).

Programming Duration or Number of Intervals for Detection and Redetection

In patients who have frequent, long episodes of nonsustained ventricular tachycardia, nominal values for these parameters should be increased to prevent unnecessary capacitor charging and resultant premature battery depletion. Patients with long QT syndrome may benefit from such programming. Post-therapy redetection should be delayed sufficiently to prevent unnecessary and potentially proarrhythmic therapy for self-terminating arrhythmias. Redetection of ventricular tachycardia should be delayed beyond nominal values for patients in whom ventricular tachycardia is well tolerated, but antitachycardia pacing is not.

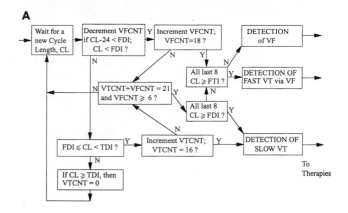

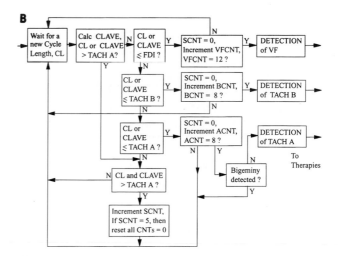

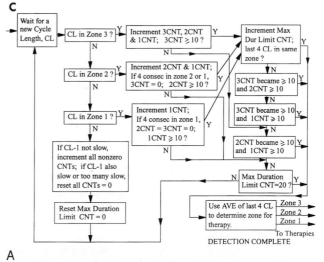

Figure 3–57A. Panel *A*, Simplified detection algorithm flowcharts. Panel *A*, Medtronic, Inc. Jewel 7219.

Illustration and legend continued on following page

Stability and Onset Algorithms for SVT-VT Discrimination in Single-Chamber Devices

When tiered-therapy ICDs detect VT only by rate criteria, inappropriate therapy for SVT occurs in 45% of those who receive therapy (Fig. 3–58).[146] The problem of inappropriate therapy is greater for tiered-therapy ICDs than it was for

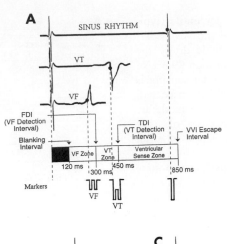

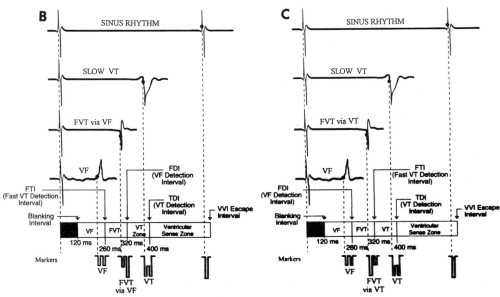

B

Figure 3–57A *Continued.* Panel *B*, Ventritex, Inc. Cadence V100. Panel *C*, Cardiac Pacemakers, Inc. Ventak PRx 1700. Each flowchart takes in new cycle lengths (CL) on the left and may detect a tachyarrhythmia in one of three zones labeled as VF, fast VT, or VT for the Jewel 7219; VF, Tach B, or Tach A for the Cadence; and Zone 3, Zone 2, or Zone 1 for the PRx. Integer event counters with various prefixes are labeled *CNT. Programmable integers for the duration of sustained tachyarrhythmias are shown as integer constants with nominal values. *Increment* means to increase an integer counter by 1, and *decrement* means to decrease a counter by 1. CLAVE is the average of the last four CLs. CL-24 means the 24th previous CL, and CL-1 means the previous CL. For each new CL, each algorithm is processed, and if a tachyarrhythmia is not detected on that CL, the algorithm returns to get another CL, and the process repeats. Nominal values were assumed when possible, and various optional algorithms, such as Stability, Onset, Extended High Rate, and so forth, were not included for the sake of simplicity.

Figure 3–57B The classification of each sensed cycle length by the Medtronic implantable cardioverter-defibrillator (ICD) is shown for VF and VT zones in panel *A*. Sensed events between 120 msec and the fibrillation detection interval (FDI) are classified as VF and marked by a short double marker, as shown in panel *A*. Longer sensed intervals between the FDI and the tachycardia detection interval (TDI) are classified as VT cycle lengths marked by tall double markers. Still longer cycle lengths greater than the TDI are classified as normal sensed events, such as sinus rhythm. In panel *B*, the VF zone is divided into a VF zone and a fast VT zone by the fast tachycardia interval (FTI) denoted by a short–long marker in panel *B*. In panel *C*, the VT zone is divided into a fast VT zone and a slow VT zone by the FTI, and a fast VT cycle length is denoted by a long–short marker in panel *C*.

early ICDs because the probability of rate overlap between the target ventricular tachycardia and SVT is greater; pacing therapies delivered during SVT may induce ventricular tachycardia,[147] and cardioversion may induce atrial fibrillation, which may in turn be sensed as ventricular tachycardia and treated with pacing, reinitiating ventricular

tachycardia.[103, 147–149] For these reasons, tiered-therapy ICDs include detection-enhancement algorithms to discriminate ventricular tachycardia from SVT.

The first generation of tiered-therapy ICDs included two such algorithms. Interval-stability (stability) algorithms attempt to discriminate ventricular tachycardia from atrial

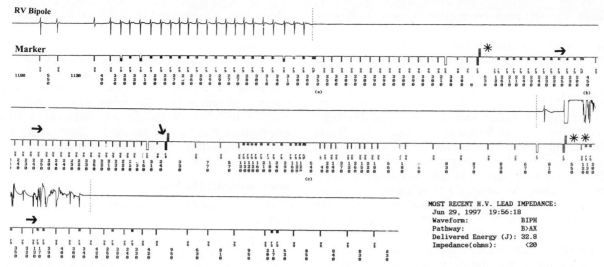

Figure 3–58. Complex causes of inappropriate detection and therapy. This patient, who had an abdominally implanted cardioverter-defibrillator (Medtronic Jewel 7218), complained that he received multiple shocks for arrhythmias that previously had been terminated by one or two shocks. Stored electrograms from right ventricular bipole and marker channel are shown. The left side of the top panel shows the onset of an irregular tachycardia with a mean cycle length of 290 msec. Electrogram morphology during the tachycardia varies slightly on a beat-to-beat basis and is similar to two (probably supraventricular) electrograms, the first electrogram on the tracing and the first electrogram at the right side of the second panel. The rhythm irregularity and electrogram morphology suggest that the rhythm is a rapidly conducted atrial arrhythmia. The marker channel shows that the first delivered 15-J shock (down–up CD marker) toward the right of the top panel accelerates the rhythm to a regular rhythm with a mean cycle length of 230 msec. This rhythm is probably ventricular tachycardia, although 1:1 conduction of an atrial arrhythmia due to postshock sympathetic enhancement of atrioventricular conduction cannot be excluded. Electrograms are not telemetered during charging and are telemetered intermittently during redetection. A 24-J shock terminates this rhythm, but two beats later, rapid signals are detected. Many intervals are just longer than the ventricular blanking period of 120 msec suggesting the presence of electronic noise. This results in redetection of ventricular fibrillation (VF). Because shocks after the first shock in this episode are committed, the third 34-J shock is delivered in sinus rhythm near the right side of the second panel. Postshock intervals show a transient period of short intervals, including some near the ventricular blanking period of 120 msec. Postshock electrograms show high-frequency electronic signals characteristic of electronic noise. These terminate before redetection of VF can occur. Telemetry showed that the lead impedance for the high-voltage pathway (coronary sinus to right-ventricle plus subcutaneous patch) was 20, indicating an insulation failure. At surgery, the coronary sinus coil electrode had an insulation failure in the pocket adjacent to the pulse generator, which was not an active can device. Postshock oversensing of noise was caused by shorting of some of the high-voltage discharge into the sensing circuits of the device. This example illustrates multiple problems: inappropriate detection of rapidly conducted atrial fibrillation in the VF zone, ventricular proarrhythmia caused by an inappropriate shock, shock-induced sensing of electronic noise caused by insulation failure of a high-voltage lead, and delivery of a noncommitted shock in sinus rhythm.

fibrillation by rejecting irregular arrhythmias that fulfill rate criteria. Sudden-onset (onset) algorithms attempt to discriminate sinus tachycardia from ventricular tachycardia by rejecting tachycardias in which the rate increases gradually.[150–154] Optimal programming of onset and stability can reduce inappropriate therapy of SVT by more than 80% with less than 1% underdetection of hemodynamically stable ventricular tachycardia.[147, 149, 155]

Stability Algorithms

The Medtronic stability algorithm operates when the ventricular tachycardia count reaches 4 by comparing the latest interval with each of the three previous intervals. If the absolute value of any of these interval differences is greater than the programmed stability interval in milliseconds, the VT counter is reset to zero. This resetting of the ventricular tachycardia counter must occur often enough to avoid inappropriate detection.

The Guidant stability algorithm calculates RR interval differences throughout the duration of the tachycardia. From the time of initial detection until the end of duration, it computes on a beat-to-beat basis a weighted-average variance of RR interval differences in which more recent intervals are weighed more heavily than earlier intervals. If, at the end of initial duration, the cycle length variance is greater than the programmed value, the rhythm is declared unstable and therapy is inhibited. The ICD continues to analyze stability as long as the rate criterion remains satisfied. Therapy is delivered as soon as the cycle length variance is less than the programmed value.[156]

This stability algorithm may also be used to discriminate regular ventricular tachycardia from the irregular type to determine if antitachycardia pacing or shock therapy should be delivered. The St. Jude stability algorithm measures the stability delta as the difference between the second longest and second shortest intervals in a group of recent intervals defined by the interval-stability window size. This window size (nominally, 12) must be less than the selected number of intervals for any tachycardia detection. VT therapy is withheld if the measured stability is more than the programmed value (nominally, 50 msec). The St. Jude stability algorithm may be used together with a Sinus Interval History

(SIH) count. The SIH count (nominally, 2; range, 1–9) is the maximum number of sinus intervals that can occur during a tachyarrhythmia classified as ventricular tachycardia. An SIH count of zero would correspond to consecutive-interval counting.

Onset Algorithms

The Guidant onset algorithm finds the maximum difference between adjacent intervals for the five intervals on each side of the lowest rate boundary. When this maximum difference exceeds the programmable onset parameter of 9% to 34%, the algorithm selects the shorter of these two intervals as the pivot interval. Then, the difference between the average of the four intervals before the pivot interval and three of the four intervals starting with the pivot interval must also be greater than the programmable 9% to 34% to satisfy the onset criterion. St. Jude ICDs compare the average interval to previous averages, and the difference must exceed the programmable sudden onset delta of 50 to 500 msec (nominally, 100 msec). Older Medtronic ICDs compared the average of the latest four events to the average of the previous four events and used a percentage change threshold.[157]

Clinical Studies

Onset and stability enhancements have been studied in detail.[147, 149, 155, 158] Studies of interval-stability during ventricular tachycardia have reported mean cycle length differences of 7%,[159] decreasing variability over time,[160] more variability for slower ventricular tachycardias, and at the onset of ventricular tachycardia.[161] In the absence of antiarrhythmic drugs, stability algorithms are highly specific for rejecting atrial fibrillation with ventricular rates of less than 170 min^{-1} while producing minimal delays in detection of monomorphic ventricular tachycardia.[147] Antiarrhythmic drugs may decrease the interval stability of monomorphic ventricular tachycardia.[162, 163] Appropriately programmed stability algorithms delay, but almost never prevent, detection of monomorphic ventricular tachycardia because rhythm stability is evaluated continuously.

In contrast, onset algorithms prevent detection of ventricular tachycardia if the rhythm is not classified correctly by the initial evaluation.[155, 162] This occurs under the following conditions: (1) ventricular tachycardia occurs during sinus tachycardia without abrupt onset, (2) it occurs with abrupt onset but during sinus tachycardia with cycle length in the VT zone; (3) the initial ventricular tachycardia cycle length exceeds the ventricular tachycardia detection interval followed by gradual acceleration across this detection boundary; or (4) undersensing occurs at the onset of ventricular tachycardia. For this reason, some investigators recommend that onset algorithms be programmed in conjunction with a sustained-duration override to prevent ventricular tachycardia underdetection.

Ventricular Electrogram Morphology Analysis

Morphology algorithms, which discriminate ventricular tachycardia from SVT based on electrogram morphology, provide an alternative method for discriminating SVT from ventricular tachycardia that does not depend on a correct classification of one or a few intervals. Morphology algorithms were not applied in early ICDs because the required

calculations exceeded the capability of the microprocessors in these devices. However, morphology of QRS complexes in the surface ECG has been used for several decades in Holter monitor scanners and intensive care monitoring units. The surface ECG integrates the electrophysiology of both ventricles, but bipolar intracardiac electrograms record primarily local activation and therefore do not contain the same types of morphologic information. Intracardiac far-field R electrograms may be more useful for discriminating ventricular tachycardia from SVT than local bipolar electrograms.[164, 165]

Investigational Methods

A review of methods of morphology analysis may prove instructive:

- The computationally demanding correlation waveform analysis (CWA) method[166, 167] has been widely used to distinguish SVT from ventricular tachycardia. CWA is often used as a basis for evaluating other methods because it is amplitude and baseline invariant. Down sampling of 250 samples/sec digitized data by 5:1 with preservation of extrema before CWA had negligible effects on the results.[168]

- Several computationally simpler methods (bin area method, normalized area of difference, and the derivative area method) have been shown to be comparable to CWA.[169]

- Further reductions in computation were achieved with signature analysis that finds the fraction of samples that are outside template window boundaries.[170, 171]

- Another method, called gradient pattern detection (GPD), approximates the wave shape with a series of signed straight lines with quantified lengths.[172, 173]

- A similar method, temporal electrogram analysis (TEA), uses the sequence and duration of signal excursions above or below positive or negative thresholds.[174]

- A time-sequenced adaptive algorithm uses linear prediction of electrogram morphology for the entire cycle to find a relative increase in an error function at the onset of ventricular tachycardia followed by a decrease in the error function by the 20th beat of ventricular tachycardia.[175]

- A step function model for the pulse shape near the peak of the R wave in the electrogram has been proposed to classify electrogram morphologies.[176] An area of difference method superimposes an unknown waveform over a stored template waveform and sums the area between the two curves.[177] With a limited number of acute bipolar electrograms, this method gave patient-specific separation of SVT and ventricular tachycardia.

- The integrated electrogram evoked response, called the paced depolarization integral (PDI), showed promise for discriminating between SVT and VT.[178]

- An artificial neural network with a multilayer feed-forward architecture used waveform morphology and heart rate to classify electrogram morphology without patient-specific decision thresholds and templates.[179]

Many practical issues may limit the utility of these wave shape measurements when used to supplement rate detection algorithms; however, additional electrodes are not required. Clearly, bundle-branch block or any type of aberrant conduction may confound these measurements. Electrogram amplitudes and morphologies undergo considerable change during the first few months after implantation owing to growth of a fibrotic capsule over the electrodes and lead. Appropriate filtering of electrograms before any waveform analysis is clearly important. Sympathetic tone, exercise, heart rate, lead maturation, and other sources of variability are known to alter the amplitude and shape of intracardiac electrograms.[180–184]

Clinical Methods

The first ICD morphology algorithm for SVT–ventricular tachycardia discrimination compared electrogram width during tachycardia with the width during sinus rhythm as defined by a programmable slew rate.[185] This electrogram-width algorithm has limited specificity in the presence of fixed bundle-branch block, rate-related bundle-branch block, and varying electrogram slew rates. It has limited sensitivity in patients with narrow-complex ventricular tachycardia.

More sophisticated morphology algorithms have been evaluated recently. The St. Jude template-matching algorithm compares each bipolar sensing electrogram in the morphology window (nominally, 8 electrograms) to a stored template based on the number of peaks, sequence of peaks, peak polarity, amplitude, and width. Before this comparison, each complex is aligned with the template based on its dominant peak polarity. If the dominant peak polarity of the test complex does not match that of the template, the test complex is shifted, and an attempt to align the electrograms is repeated. Complexes are judged by % Template Match, which indicates the degree of similarity that must exist between a complex and a template for them to be considered a match (nominally, 70%). No. Template Match indicates the number of complexes in the window that must match the template for the morphology discriminator to indicate SVT (nominally, 5).

This algorithm was compared with rate-only detection using a library of stored electrograms.[186] This algorithm reduced inappropriate detection of SVT by 94% while retaining a 98% sensitivity for ventricular tachycardia. It has been implemented in an ICD (Angstrom MD Model V-1900, Ventritex, St. Jude Medical, Sunnyvale, CA). Clinical data have not yet been reported.

A two-step algorithm incorporating electrogram width in the first step and a sequence of four locally maximum positive and negative values was tested in the electrophysiology laboratory.[187] While retaining 100% sensitivity for ventricular tachycardia, this algorithm rejected 94% of sinus tachycardia and 92% of atrial fibrillation. Early ICDs used different morphology algorithms to discriminate monomorphic VT from polymorphic ventricular tachycardia and ventricular fibrillation. The PDF and its digital counterpart, the Turning Point Morphology (TPM) algorithm, use the concept that ventricular fibrillation has less isoelectric line than other rhythms.[188, 189] The Guidant morphology algorithm (TPM) provides more aggressive therapy if the electrogram has less isoelectric time than a threshold percentage designed to avoid noise. Clinical experience with the PDF concept has shown that it may reduce sensitivity and delay detection of fast monomorphic ventricular tachycardias (cycle length <250 msec) that have isoelectric segments but need to be shocked.[137, 189–193] The PDF uses the entire cardiac cycle, so

that it increases even when only cardiac rate increases. It is also susceptible to large T waves and ST segments.

Another published technique uses threshold crossings to create a binary sequence and a probability distribution to perform sequential hypothesis testing that trades off detection accuracy for time-to-detection.[194, 195]

Zones for Detection Enhancements

Guidant detection enhancements are programmable only in the lowest zone of a multizone device. Medtronic enhancements are programmable in zones that use consecutive-interval counting (ventricular tachycardia and FVT via VT). St. Jude enhancements are available in a zone of cycle lengths bounded by the Sinus-Tach A boundary on the slow end and an independently programmable SVT Upper Limit on the fast end. The minimum SVT Upper Limit is 5 msec plus the Fib cutoff.

Programming Detection Enhancements

Single-chamber detection enhancements should be programmed only in rate zones that correspond to hemodynamically stable ventricular tachycardia. Stability algorithms should be programmed in patients with hemodynamically stable monomorphic ventricular tachycardia who are at risk for atrial fibrillation with a ventricular rate in the ventricular tachycardia zone. Recommended programmed values are 40 msec for Medtronic ICDs[147] and 24 to 40 msec for the Guidant ICDs[149, 155, 158] when nominal intervals or durations for detection are used. Less strict values are required for patients taking type I or III antiarrhythmic drugs.[162, 163]

Onset algorithms may be programmed in patients with hemodynamically stable monomorphic ventricular tachycardia who are at risk for sinus tachycardia with a rate in the ventricular tachycardia zone despite maximally tolerated β-blocker therapy. Recommended values for programming onset algorithms are 84% to 88% for older Medtronic ICDs[147] and 9% for Guidant ICDs. The reported incidence of underdetection of ventricular tachycardia using these settings is 0.5% for Medtronic ICDs and 5% to 10% for Guidant ICDs.[155, 158] Onset algorithms should be programmed only in conjunction with a sustained-duration algorithm or if the patient-specific risk of failure to detect ventricular tachycardia in the ventricular tachycardia zone is judged acceptable. Brugada and colleagues,[155] reported results of optimal programming of Guidant onset and stability algorithms in conjunction with the sustained-duration override in patients with hemodynamically stable ventricular tachycardia. The sustained-duration override increased sensitivity for detection of ventricular tachycardia from 90% to 100% but also increased inappropriate therapy of SVT from 4% to 18%. No patient had syncope during the delay in ventricular tachycardia therapy until the end of the sustained-duration period that occurred in 10% of ventricular tachycardia episodes.

The recommended programmed values for the Medtronic electrogram width algorithm are the maximum slew rate that measures all sinus rhythm electrograms within a 12-msec range and a width threshold of 4 msec greater than the maximum measured width in sinus rhythm. Reprogramming is required in most patients.[185] Morphology algorithms may be programmed in patients with hemodynamically stable monomorphic ventricular tachycardia who are at risk for any SVT in the ventricular tachycardia zone. They may be particularly valuable for discrimination of ventricular tachycardia from atrial flutter and as an alternative to onset algorithms for discrimination of sinus tachycardia from ventricular tachycardia.

Data regarding interactions among various detection enhancements (onset, stability, and morphology) are limited. Combinations of these enhancements should be programmed with caution in the absence of a sustained-duration feature.

■ DUAL-CHAMBER DETECTION OF VENTRICULAR TACHYARRHYTHMIAS

Dual-Chamber Algorithms: Background

Dual-chamber detection algorithms use atrial and ventricular timing data to discriminate SVT from ventricular tachycardia. Ideally, analysis of PP, PR, RR, and RP intervals should permit improved discrimination of SVT from ventricular tachycardia. During tachycardia, the finding of atrioventricular dissociation with a ventricular rate greater than the atrial rate is diagnostic for ventricular tachycardia. During ventricular tachycardia, if retrograde conduction to the atrium is present, it may be 1:1, 2:1, or retrograde Wenckebach.

Early studies in patients undergoing electrophysiologic testing showed that up to one third of those with slow, hemodynamically stable ventricular tachycardia had 1:1 retrograde conduction. In supine, sedated ICD patients, however, the incidence of 1:1 retrograde conduction during induced ventricular tachycardia has varied from 0% to 4.4%.[23, 24] The occurrence of 1:1 SVT with long atrioventricular times may lead to misclassification of SVT as ventricular tachycardia.[196] Pre-existing atrial tachyarrhythmias or atrial tachyarrhythmias that begin after the onset of ventricular tachycardia, however, may complicate accurate determination of the relationship between atrial and ventricular electrograms.

The first algorithm for comparing atrial and ventricular events to discriminate ventricular tachycardia and SVT for most tachyarrhythmias was published in 1979.[197, 198] For tachycardias with a 1:1 atrioventricular relationship, chamber of sudden onset was used for paroxysmal 1:1 tachycardias. If onset was not sudden, then sinus tachycardia was diagnosed. A weakness of this method is that ventricular tachycardia initiated by SVT will be classified as SVT.

Another algorithm used the effect of a single atrial extrastimulus delivered with a prematurity of 80 to 120 msec to classify tachycardia with the 1:1 AV relationship.[199] These atrial extrastimuli failed to alter the subsequent RR intervals by more than 10 msec in 22 VTs but shortened the subsequent RR interval for conducted SVTs.[200, 201] This extrastimulus method, however, may classify SVT as ventricular tachycardia if the extrastimulus blocks at the AV node. It may classify ventricular tachycardia as SVT if ventricular capture occurs. Further, atrial extrastimuli may be proarrhythmic in either the atrium or the ventricle.

Morphologic data may also be used to discriminate tachyarrhythmias with 1:1 AV relationships. Correlation waveform analysis successfully discriminated antegrade from retrograde atrial depolarization wave shapes for 1:1 tachycardias but required 19 patient-specific thresholds.[202]

As noted previously, orthogonal electrodes may be useful for discriminating antegrade from retrograde atrial conduction.

Other investigators have evaluated algorithms based on a neural network morphology classifier with a decision tree for timing analysis[203] and a multiway sequential hypothesis testing algorithm that calculates a likelihood function from PR intervals as they are received.[204] ICD manufacturers have developed dual-chamber detection algorithms with markedly different design philosophies. One manufacturer uses atrial data only to prevent onset and stability algorithms from withholding appropriate therapy but not to improve specificity of ventricular tachycardia therapy. Two manufacturers have developed algorithms that use dual-chamber data to discriminate ventricular tachycardia from SVT. Details of these algorithms and preliminary results have been reported.[94, 95, 119, 205] Next is a review of the key features of the algorithms of two major U.S. ICD manufacturers (Guidant and Medtronic).

P-R Logic Pattern and Rate Analysis—Gem DR

The dual-chamber detection algorithm in Medtronic dual-chamber ICDs (Model 7271 Gem DR and Model 7250 Jewel AF) is based on several basic design principles. The high sensitivity of single-chamber, rate-only detection is retained as the underlying basic detection algorithm. The dual-chamber algorithm withholds detection of VT/VF only if it can positively identify a specific SVT. The algorithm uses information recorded during at least several RR intervals to diagnose rhythms. This minimizes the effects of undersensing or oversensing in either the atrium or the ventricle and avoids the uncertainty of the onset rhythm to permit accurate detection of ventricular tachycardia induced by or occurring simultaneously with SVT. The physician-programmable parameters are minimal and clinically relevant. The range of cycle lengths over which dual-chamber detection applies is programmable independently of the ventricular tachycardia and ventricular fibrillation detection zones.

The algorithm has four key elements: (1) the pattern of atrial and ventricular events, (2) atrial and ventricular rates, (3) regularity of ventricular intervals, and (4) presence or absence of atrioventricular dissociation. It uses two methods of dual-chamber pattern analysis. The first P:R pattern analysis method discriminates SVT from VT by use of syntactic P:R pattern recognition and contextual-timing analysis.[94, 205, 206] The fundamental units of this method are couple codes that represent the number and timing of P waves in two consecutive RR intervals. Sequences of couple codes identify specific rhythms (Fig. 3–59). The second P:R pattern analysis method is an AT/AF Evidence Counter. The algorithm has been reviewed recently.[207]

The elements of P and R event pattern analysis and timing analysis are combined to detect and treat VT/VF as shown in (Fig. 3–60). If RR rate detection occurs and the median RR interval is more than the programmable SVT minimum RR interval, the possibility of double (simultaneous atrial and ventricular) tachyarrhythmias is first assessed by evidence of atrioventricular dissociation and, in the ventricular tachycardia zone, regularity of the ventricular rate. If a double tachycardia is identified, ventricular tachycardia or ventricular fibrillation therapy is delivered. If not, specific criteria for AF/AT, sinus tachycardia, and other 1:1 SVT criteria are evaluated sequentially. If none of these SVTs are

COUPLE CODE SYNTAX ANALYSIS

Figure 3–59. Pattern analysis for PR Logic dual-chamber ventricular tachyarrhythmia detection algorithm. For the last two RR intervals, the number and timing of P waves are used to classify the current R wave as one of 19 couple codes represented by the letters of the alphabet shown. P waves may be in the junctional zone from 80 msec before the R wave to 50 msec after the R wave, the antegrade zone from 50% of R-R interval to 80 msec before the R wave, or the retrograde zone from 50 msec after the R wave to 50% of R-R. Pure sinus tachycardia is AAAAA--. Sinus tachycardia is permitted to deviate from pure sinus tachycardia by the syntactic strings of letters, such as ABCEA, which is one representation for a paraventricular contraction as shown on the marker channel rhythm at the bottom.

- Couple codes for overlapping pairs of RR intervals

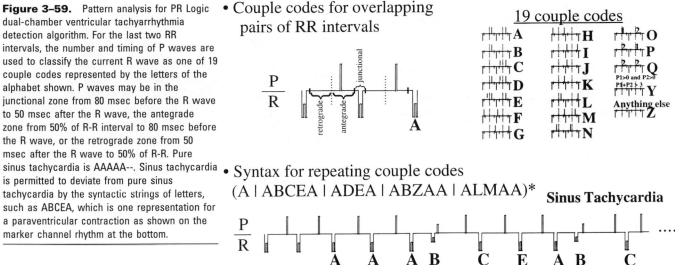

- Syntax for repeating couple codes
  (A | ABCEA | ADEA | ABZAA | ALMAA)* **Sinus Tachycardia**

Medtronic GEM DR

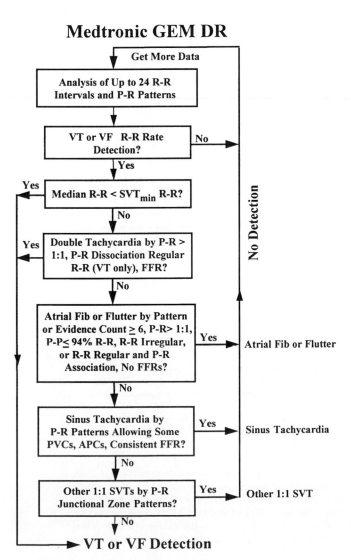

Figure 3–60. Block diagram for detection of ventricular tachycardia (VT) or ventricular fibrillation (VF) by the Gem DR dual-chamber implantable cardioverter-defibrillator. After each new R wave is sensed, at the top, analysis of the R:R, P:P, and P:R patterns and timing occurs, single-chamber RR rate detection is tested, and rhythms with median RR intervals of less than the programmable supraventricular tachycardia (SVT) minimum cycle length are detected without considering the dual-chamber algorithm. If double tachycardia (VF/VT/FVT plus SVT) is not detected, the three dual-chamber criteria for atrial fibrillation/atrial flutter, sinus tachycardia, and other 1:1 SVTs are tested. If any one of these three SVT rhythms is recognized, inappropriate detection is avoided. If none of these SVTs can be positively identified, however, detection occurs to maintain high sensitivity for VT and VF detection.

positively identified, ventricular tachycardia or ventricular fibrillation must be detected.

Clinical results of this algorithm have been reported for 1092 arrhythmias recorded in 300 patients.[196] Of these, 214 (20%) had median cycle length less than the programmed minimum SVT cycle length and were detected by the single-chamber algorithm. Of the remaining 878 arrhythmias classified by the dual-chamber algorithm, all 585 sustained episodes of ventricular tachycardia and ventricular fibrillation were classified correctly, one nonsustained episode of double tachycardia was misclassified as SVT for two beats, and 73% of 292 SVT episodes were classified correctly. The principal causes of misclassification of SVT were intermittent atrial detection of far-field R waves (42%), sinus tachycardia with first-degree atrioventricular block misclassified as ventricular tachycardia with 1:1 ventriculoatrial dissociation because of timing of the P wave in the zone of retrograde conduction (30%), and incorrect detection of rapidly conducted atrial fibrillation in the ventricular fibrillation zone as double tachycardia (11%). Thirty of 32 episodes of AF/AT (94%) conducted in the ventricular tachycardia zone were diagnosed correctly. However, the Other 1:1 SVT rule rejected only one of seven atrial or atrioventricular node reentrant tachycardias. Figure 3–61 illustrates the performance algorithm.

Atrial View Enhanced Onset and Stability—VENTAK AV

The VENTAK AV dual-chamber detection algorithm detects the presence of SVT and withholds therapy in the lowest zone of a multizone device only on the basis of single-chamber onset and stability algorithms. As in Guidant single-chamber ICDs, therapy is always delivered in this zone when the Sustained Rate Duration timer expires. The two dual-chamber detection enhancements, AFib Rate Threshold and V Rate > A Rate, provide an additional level of certainty regarding inhibition of therapy for rapidly conducted atrial arrhythmias. The sole function of these enhancements is to prevent the onset and stability algorithms from withholding appropriate therapy during the Sustained Rate Duration period. Thus, compared with Guidant single-chamber ICDs, these algorithms accelerate delivery of therapy that would otherwise have been delayed until the Sustained Rate Duration timer expired.

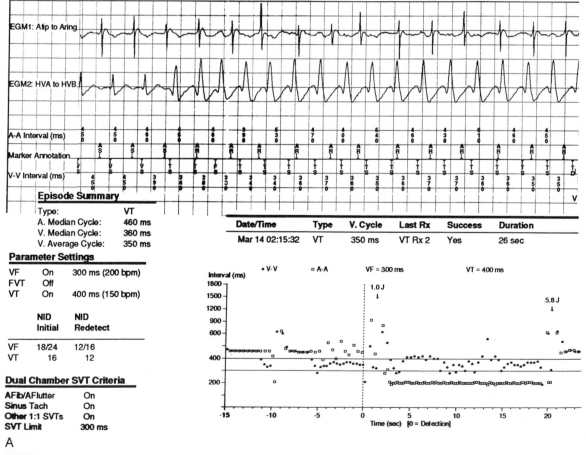

Figure 3–61. *A,* Detection of spontaneous ventricular tachycardia (VT) with clear PR dissociation, a distinct morphology change on the coil-to-can stored far-field electrogram, a not very sudden onset owing to pre-existing sinus tachycardia and somewhat unstable ventricular cycle lengths. Note that during PR dissociation, all of the P waves are accurately sensed even though they occur immediately after a ventricular sense. The interval plot shows that a four beat run of VT occurred before about six sinus beats that preceded the sustained VT. The atrial cycle lengths during VT were somewhat altered by the VT. The first therapy was a 1-J cardioversion that induced atrial flutter, which was terminated by a 5.8-J shock (Gem DR ICD).

The AFib Rate Threshold enhancement (nominally, 200 bpm) is used in conjunction with the stability algorithm. It is intended to permit therapy for irregular ventricular tachycardia in the absence of evidence of atrial fibrillation. The V Rate > A Rate enhancement is an inhibitor override that uses the relationship between average atrial and ventricular rates to overrule either or both the onset and stability inhibitors. It supersedes these inhibitors if the average ventricular rate exceeds the average atrial rate by more than 10 bpm.[208] It is intended to permit therapy for gradual-onset ventricular tachycardia without 1:1 ventriculoatrial conduction. Ventricular tachycardia that occurs without abrupt onset will remain untreated until the end of the Sustained Rate Duration timer if it either has sustained 1:1 ventriculoatrial conduction or occurs in the presence of a simultaneous atrial tachyarrhythmia. The diagram in Figure 3–62 shows the logic used in the VENTAK AV for the two new dual-chamber enhancements.

Figure 3–63 shows examples of this algorithm. To date, its clinical performance has not been evaluated critically.

Programming Dual-Chamber Detection Enhancements

In the Medtronic Gem DR, all three three SVT rejection criteria (Sinus Tachycardia, AF/AT, Other 1:1 SVT) are programmable independently as "on" or "off." The "SVT Limit" is the minimum cycle length at which the dual-chamber detection algorithm is applied. In the Guidant VENTAK AV series, the AFib Rate and V Rate > A Rate enhancements are also programmable "on" or "off." These features apply only in the lowest zone of a multizone programming because they are linked intrinsically to the single-chamber enhancements onset and stability.

Results of the Gem DR[119, 196] clinical trials have resulted in several insights regarding optimal programming of PR Logic:

- The Other 1:1 SVT rule should be programmed off until atrial lead stability is ensured because application of this rule with an atrial lead dislodgment to the ventricle could inhibit therapy for ventricular tachycardia. The Sinus

Text continued on page 121

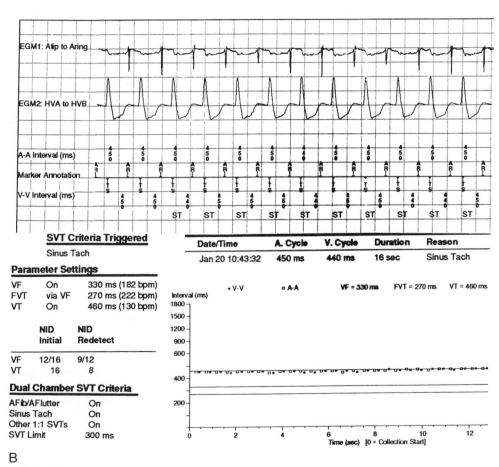

Figure 3–61 *Continued. B,* Appropriate rejection of 1:1 sinus tachycardia with no therapy. The coil-to-can stored ventricular electrogram has a wide R wave indicative of bundle-branch block. The ST annotations begin on the third ventricular beat, indicating that a ventricular rate algorithm would have detected ventricular tachycardia on this beat and given inappropriate therapy. The ST annotations continue as long as the sinus tachycardia algorithm is the reason for withholding therapy. The interval plot shows a 1:1 tachycardia that is just below the tachycardia detection interval that was programmed to 460 msec. The duration of this sinus tachycardia was 16 seconds (Gem DR ICD).

Illustration continued on following page

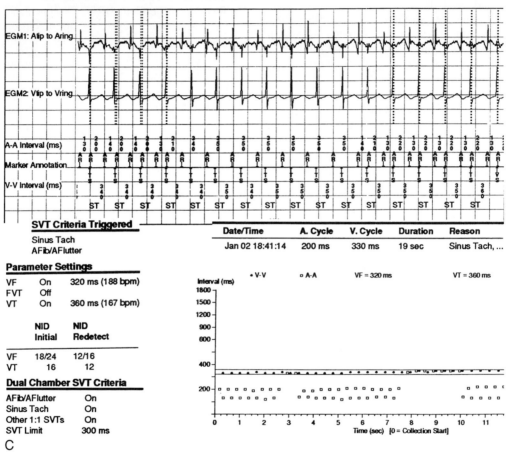

Figure 3–61 *Continued.* *C,* Appropriate rejection of sinus tachycardia indicated by the ST annotations in the presence of substantial far-field R-wave oversensing on the atrial channel. The far-field R waves are clearly visible on the stored atrial electrogram, and they are consistently sensed at the beginning and end of the strip. In the middle of the strip, however, the oversensing of far-field R waves stopped for seven beats. The interval plot shows the alternation of short atrial cycle lengths that is characteristic of far-field R-wave oversensing (Gem DR ICD).

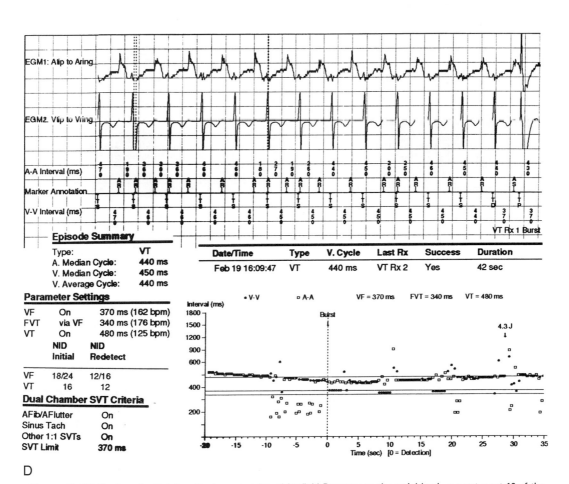

D

Figure 3–61 *Continued.* *D,* Intermittent oversensing of far-field R waves on the atrial lead may not meet 10 of the 12 criteria for far-field R waves as shown in this figure, resulting in inappropriate detection of ventricular tachycardia (VT). The gaps in the alternating pattern are sufficiently inconsistent to make the rhythm indeterminant, which forces the classification of ventricular tachycardia for safety. Contrast this strip with panel *B,* in which the far-field oversensing was intermittent, was not recognized, and resulted in inappropriate detection and therapy (Gem DR ICD).

Illustration continued on following page

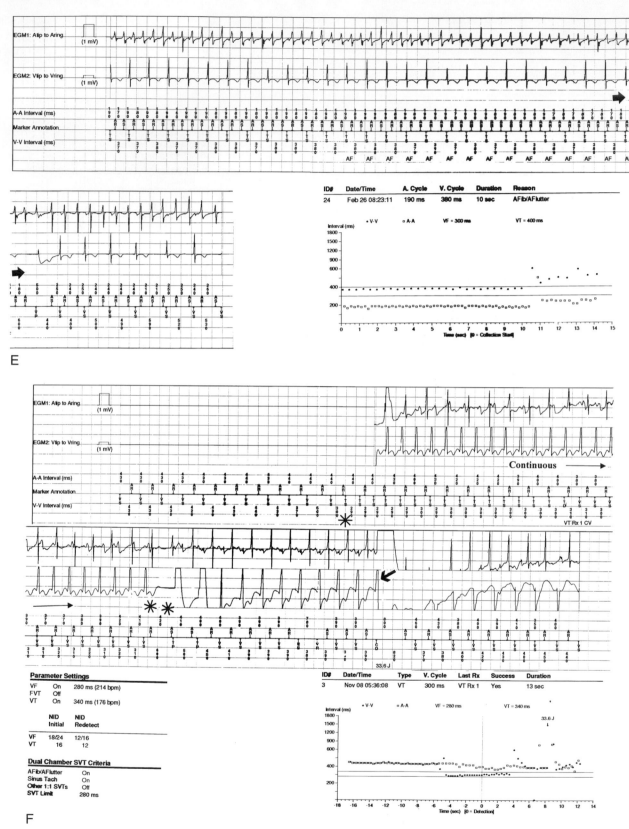

Figure 3–61 Continued. *See legend on opposite page*

Guidant VENTAK AV III DR

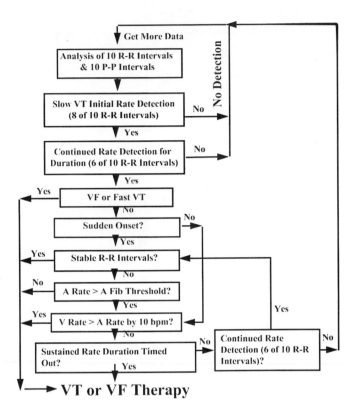

Figure 3–62. The VENTAK AV dual-chamber detection algorithm modifies R-R interval. Stability and Onset algorithms using atrial rate information. If all detection enhancements are programmed "on," then for each ventricular event, the 10 most recent PP and RR intervals may be analyzed if ventricular rate detection initially finds 8 of 10 RR intervals in the slow ventricular tachycardia (VT) zone and then at least 6 of 10 R-R intervals remain in the slow VT zone. If the dual-chamber analysis in the slow VT zone finds that the ventricular rate is greater than the atrial rate by at least 10 bpm, detection occurs. Otherwise, if the atrial rate is greater than the atrial fibrillation rate threshold and the RR intervals are not stable, detection is withheld. If the atrial rate is not greater than the atrial fibrillation rate threshold, detection still can be withheld if the R-R intervals are stable and there was sudden onset of the short R-R intervals.

Figure 3–61 *Continued.* E, Atrial flutter with 2:1 atrioventricular conduction was appropriately rejected based on the consistent PR association and stable rates in both the atrium and the ventricle. In the middle of the strip, the atrial fibrillation (AF) annotations begin because there are 16 ventricular beats in the ventricular tachycardia (VT) zone. Near the end of this continuous strip, the atrial rhythm slows as shown on the interval plot, and there is one ventricular paced beat followed by 2:1 and 3:1 conduction at ventricular rates that are less than the VT zone (Gem DR). F, Atrial bipole, right ventricular bipole, and marker channel are shown. Onset of ventricular tachycardia (VT) *(asterisk)* during sinus tachycardia activates electrogram recordings. VT with atrioventricular (AV) dissociation is detected toward right side of top panel (TD) when 16 consecutive intervals are less than the programmed detection interval of 340 msec and the dual-chamber pattern grammar does not make a specific diagnosis of supraventricular tachycardia. Detection of VT initiates capacitor charging. Spontaneous termination of VT occurs in the middle panel *(two asterisks)*, and sinus tachycardia resumes at a cycle length of 390 msec. The confirmation algorithm of this implantable cardioverter-defibrillator (ICD) requires only that one of the first four consecutive intervals after capacitor charging ends (CE) is less than the programmed detection interval, plus 60 msec. Because the post-VT sinus tachycardia cycle length is only 50 msec greater than the detection interval of 340 msec, the ICD incorrectly confirms the presence of VT. Dual-chamber evidence of sinus tachycardia is not considered in this confirmation algorithm. The bottom panel shows ICD programming *(left)* and interval plot *(right)*. A-A and V-V markers show onset of VT with AV dissociation, sinus acceleration during VT, and spontaneous termination of VT (Gem DR ICD).

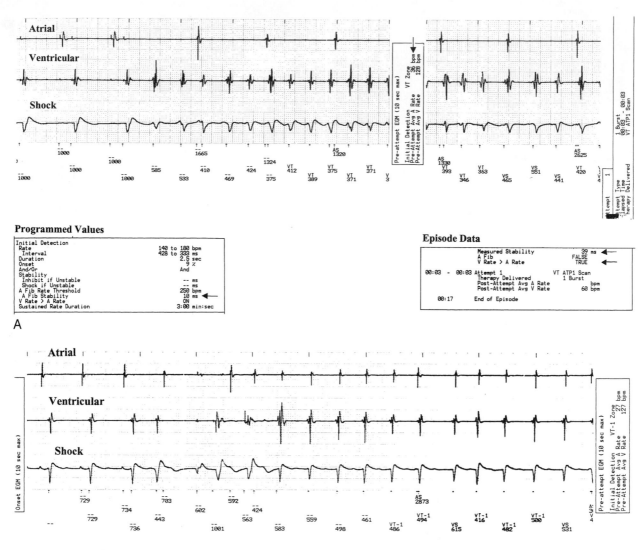

Figure 3–63 *A,* Stored electrograms from atrial bipole, ventricular integrated bipole, and high-voltage channel (right ventricular coil to superior vena cava coil plus can) are shown together with relevant programmed values *(bottom left)* and stored episode data *(bottom right).* The programmed value of stability is 10 msec *(arrow at lower left).* Irregular ventricular tachycardia (VT) with measured stability of 39 msec *(top arrow at lower right)* is detected without delay for Sustained Rate Duration because "V Rate > A Rate" is evaluated correctly as true *(bottom arrow at lower right).* Note that atrial rate is measured inaccurately at 36 bpm *(vertical arrow)* because one of the atrial electrograms *(asterisk)* falls in the 87-msec postventricular atrial blanking period. A proposed strategy for improving rejection of atrial fibrillation over that achieved by single-chamber devices is to program stability to a strict value that will reject all atrial fibrillation (such as 10 msec in this example) and rely only on "V Rate > A Rate" to discriminate VT from atrial fibrillation. This method cannot be used in patients who have VT with 1:1 ventriculoatrial conduction. Undersensing caused by postventricular atrial blanking during rapidly conducted atrial fibrillation might also cause inappropriate therapy. The sensitivity and specificity of this strategy are under evaluation. (Courtesy of Dr. Paul Dorian, Toronto, Canada.) *B,* Stored electrograms from atrial bipole, ventricular integrated bipole, and high-voltage (right ventricular coil to superior vena cava coil plus can) are shown. Two paraventricular contractions initiate atrioventricular nodal re-entrant supraventricular tachycardia (SVT) *(arrows).* Only one of the atrial electrograms in SVT is sensed *(asterisk).* The remainder time in the 87-msec postventricular atrial blanking period. At the time of inappropriate detection, the average ventricular rate was measured at 127 bpm, and the average atrial rate was measured at 27 bpm. "V Rate > A Rate" was evaluated incorrectly as true because of the postventricular atrial blanking period (VENTAK AV II).

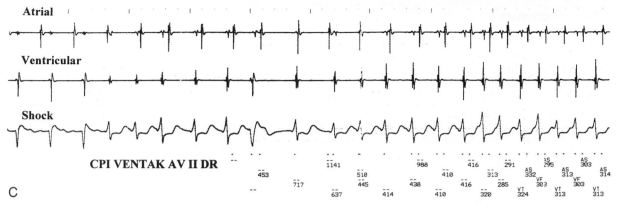

Figure 3–63 *Continued. C,* Stored electrograms from atrial bipole, ventricular integrated bipole, and high-voltage (right ventricular coil to superior vena cava coil plus can) are shown. The first three sinus beats are followed by a six-beat run of nonsustained ventricular tachycardia (VT). Two beats later, VT with 1:1 ventriculoatrial conduction resumes. This episode terminated after 13 seconds. It was not detected as VT because "V Rate > A Rate" was evaluated correctly as false (VENTAK AV II).

Tachycardia and AF/AT rules can be programmed safely at implantation.

- The Sinus Tachycardia rule provides reliable rejection of sinus tachycardia in both the ventricular tachycardia and ventricular fibrillation zones, provided that first-degree atrial ventricular block is not present and far-field R waves are not sensed intermittently. To ensure reliable discrimination of sinus tachycardia from ventricular tachycardia, the atrial sensing threshold must be programmed to a value high enough to prevent sensing of far-field R waves.
- The AF/AT rule provides reliable rejection of atrial fibrillation and atrial tachycardia in the VT zone but not in the ventricular fibrillation zone. Thus, in patients at risk for rapidly conducting AF/AT, the Fibrillation Detection Interval should be programmed to as low a value as is safe. An FVT via VT zone should be programmed for hemodynamically unstable ventricular tachycardia to retain high specificity for rejection of rapidly conducting AF/AT.
- The SVT Limit should be programmed to less than the shortest cycle length at which SVT is likely to conduct. The cycle lengths of ventricular tachycardia and ventricular fibrillation are not relevant to programming of this feature.

Clinical Comparison of Single-Chamber and Dual-Chamber Detection

To date, dual-chamber and single-chamber detection enhancements have not been compared prospectively. Initial reports indicate that nominal programming of first-generation dual-chamber detection algorithms perform comparably to optimal programming of single-chamber detection enhancements (see Table 3–1).[95, 119, 196]

Dual-chamber detection has several specific advantages:

1. Nominal programming of dual-chamber algorithms is simpler than optimal patient-specific programming of single-chamber algorithms. Single-chamber detection enhancements have been applied infrequently in clinical practice because optimal programming is complex and device specific.

2. Physicians may be more concerned about actively causing underdetection of ventricular tachycardia by specific programming than they are about inherent ICD limitations of painful and potentially proarrhythmic, inappropriate shocks. Guidant dual-chamber algorithms prevent delays in therapy until the end of sustained duration that may occur as a result of underdetection by onset or stability algorithms. Physicians may be more willing to program these enhancements in dual-chamber ICDs because they are less likely to result in substantial delays in detection or failed detection.

3. In contrast to single-chamber detection enhancements, which are limited to one or more ventricular tachycardia zones, Medtronic dual-chamber algorithms may be applied in both ventricular tachycardia and ventricular fibrillation zones.

4. Dual-chamber algorithms that analyze PP, RR, P, and PR pattern and rate improve discrimination of AT from ventricular tachycardia and correctly classify irregular ventricular tachycardia without 1:1 ventriculoatrial conduction.

5. It is likely that they will improve discrimination of sinus tachycardia from ventricular tachycardia.

Dual-chamber electrograms may increase physician confidence in the analysis of stored electrograms.

At present, limitations of dual-chamber algorithms include atrial sensing problems (e.g., far-field R waves) leading to rhythm misclassification; tradeoffs between problems of crosstalk versus undersensing caused by cross-chamber blanking periods; discrimination of ventricular tachycardia with 1:1 ventriculoatrial conduction from sinus tachycardia or other 1:1 SVTs; and discrimination of simultaneous ventricular tachycardia and SVT (double tachycardia) from rapid, regular conduction of atrial tachyarrhythmias.

It is not yet known in which patients the additional complexity, expense, and battery drain of a dual-chamber ICD is justified solely to improve discrimination of ventricular tachycardia from SVT. Patients will not benefit, however, if sinus tachycardia or atrial arrhythmias are not conducted at a cycle length of less than the longest programmed detection interval.

Future Developments

Future developments for dual-chamber ICD detection algorithms may include the addition of ventricular or atrial depolarization morphology analysis to complement the P and R wave timing analysis. Premature atrial test stimuli[201] may be used to aid the diagnosis of the 1:1 tachyarrhythmias. Finally, advances in signal processing,[209] computational capabilities, and adaptive systems made possible by advances in microelectronics are likely to allow more comprehensive systems to be developed.

REFERENCES

1. De Caprio V, Hurzeler P, Furman S: A comparison of unipolar and bipolar electrograms for cardiac pacemaker. Circulation 56:750, 1977.
2. Furman S, Hurzeler P, De Caprio V: Cardiac pacing and pacemakers. III. Sensing the cardiac electrogram. Am Heart J 93:794, 1977.
3. Parsonnet V, Myers GH, Kresh YM: Characteristics of intracardiac electrograms. II. Atrial endocardial electrograms. PACE 3:406, 1980.
4. Myers GH, Kresh YM, Parsonnet V: Characteristics of intracardiac electrograms. PACE 1:90, 1978.
5. Platia EV, Brinker JA: Time course of transvenous pacemaker stimulation impedance, capture thresholds, and intracardiac electrogram amplitude. PACE 9:620, 1986.
6. Mond HG, Stokes KB: The electrode-tissue interface: The revolutionary role of steroid elution. PACE 15:95, 1992.
7. Irnich W: Intracardiac electrograms and sensing test signals: Electrophysiological, physical, and technical considerations. PACE 8:870, 1985.
8. Kleinert M, Elmqvist H, Strandberg H: Spectral properties of atrial and ventricular endocardial signals. PACE 2:11, 1979.
9. Klitzner TS, Stevenson WG: Effects of filtering on right ventricular electrograms recorded from endocardial catheters in humans. PACE 13:69, 1990.
10. Steinhaus DM, Foley L, Knoll K, Markowtiz T: Atrial sensing revisited: Do bandpass filters matter? PACE 16:946, 1993.
11. Medtronic, Inc.: Spectrax SX 5984, 5984 LP, 5985 Technical Manual. Minneapolis, Medtronic, Inc., 1984.
12. Barold SS, Kulkarni H, Thawani AJ, et al: Electrocardiographic manifestations of the rapid recharge function of pulse generators after sensing. PACE 11:1215, 1988.
13. Mond HG, Barold SS: Dual chamber, rate adaptive pacing in patients with paroxysmal supraventricular tachyarrhythmias: Protective measures for rate control. PACE 16:2168, 1993.
14. Lau CP, Tai YT, Fong PC, et al: Atrial arrhythmia management with sensor controlled atrial refractory period and automatic mode switching in patients with minute ventilation sensing dual chamber rate adaptive pacemakers. PACE 15:1504, 1992.
15. Ohm O-J: The interdependence between electrogram, total electrode impedance, and pacemaker input impedance necessary to obtain adequate functioning of demand pacemakers. PACE 2:465, 1979.
16. Fischler H: Polarization properties of small-surface-area pacemaker electrodes: Implications on reliability of sensing and pacing. PACE 2:403, 1979.
17. Wiegard UKH, Bode F, Potratz J, et al: Effects of surface area reduction in steroid eluting leads: A comparison of four modern bipolar electrodes. PACE 20:1444, 1996.
18. Ellenbogen KA, Wood MA, Gilligan DM, et al: Steroid-eluting high impedance pacing leads decrease short- and long-term current drain: Results from a multicenter clinical trial. PACE 22:39–48, 1999.
19. Goldreyer BN, Olive AL, Leslie J, et al: A new orthogonal lead for P synchronous pacing. PACE 4:638, 1981.
20. Goldreyer BN, Knudson M, Cannom DS, Wyman MG: Orthogonal electrogram sensing. PACE 6:464, 1983.
21. Papouchado M, Crick JCP. Evaluation of atrial signals from a single lead VDD pacemaker. PACE 19:1772–1776, 1996.
22. Ovsyshcher IE, Katz A, Rosenbeck S, et al: Single lead VDD pacing: Multicenter studies. PACE 19:1768–1771, 1996.
23. Ray JL, Ghelbazouri FE, Tribouilloy C: Dual chamber pacing with a single lead system: Initial clinical results. PACE 19:1777–1779, 1996.
24. Curzio G, and the Multicenter Study Group: A multicenter evaluation of a single pass lead VDD pacing system. PACE 14:434, 1991.
25. Rosenheck S, Sharon Z, Liebowitz D, Gotman M: Two-year follow up in pediatric and adult patients with single pass lead VDD pacing systems. Am J Cardiol 81:1054–1055, 1988.
26. Manolis AG, Dragios D, Katsivas A, et al: Acute P wave amplitude detection by a bipolar floating electrode with passive fixation comparative study. PACE 20:1452, 1997.
27. Toivonen L, Lommi J: Dependence of atrial sensing function on posture in a single-lead atrial triggered ventricular (VDD) pacemaker. PACE 19:309–313, 1996.
28. Le Hellos, Lelong B, Hacot J, et al: Medium term follow up with right ventricular outflow tract pacing in patients with dilated cardiomyopathy. PACE 20:1538, 1997.
29. Bailin SJ, Johnson WB, Solinger B: Permanent atrial septal pacing and stability: Long term results. PACE 20:1053, 1997.
30. Saksena S, Prakash A, Hill M, et al: Prevention of recurrent atrial fibrillation with chronic dual site atrial pacing. J Am Coll Cardiol 28:687–694, 1996.
31. Timmis GC, Westneer DC, Gadowski G, et al: The effect of electrode position on atrial sensing for physiologically responsive cardiac pacemakers. Am Heart J 108:909–916, 1984.
32. Villafare J, Austin E: Cardiac pacing problems in infants and children: Results of a 4-year prospective study. South Med J 86:784–788, 1993.
33. Karpawich PR, Stokes KB, Procter K, et al: Improved epimyocardial pacing: Initial experience with a new bipolar, steroid eluting, high impedance lead design. PACE 20:2032–2037, 1994.
34. Karpawich PR, Hakimi M, Arciniegas E, Cavitt DL: Improved chronic epicardial pacing in children: Steroid contribution to porous platinized electrodes. PACE 15:1151–1157, 1992.
35. Medtronic 4965 database. Minneapolis, Medtronic Inc., 1996.
36. Karpawich PR, Stokes KB, Helland JR, et al: A new low threshold platinized epicardial pacing electrode: Comparative evaluation in immature canines. PACE 11:1139–1148, 1988.
37. Daubert C, Ritter P, Le Breton H, et al: Permanent left ventricular pacing with transvenous leads inserted into the coronary veins. PACE 21:239–245, 1998.
38. Kutarski A, Oleszczak K, Poleszak K, et al: Coronary sinus: The second standard lead position for permanent atrial pacing. PACE 20:1530, 1997.
39. Daubert C, Ritter P, Cazeau S, et al: Permanent biventricular pacing in dilated cardiomyopathy: Is a totally endocardial approach technically feasible? PACE 19:699, 1996.
40. Gras D, Mabo P, Daubert C, et al: Left atrial pacing: Technical and clinical considerations. In Barold SS, Mugica J (eds): Recent Advances in Cardiac Pacing: Goals for the 21st Century. Armonk, NY, Futura, 1997, p 4.
41. Daubert C, Cazeau S, Ritter P, et al: Transvenous lead insertion for permanent biventricular pacing. PACE 20:1518, 1997.
42. Krahn AD, Klein G, Yee R, Norris C: Maturation of the sensed electrogram amplitude over time in a new subcutaneous implantable loop recorder. PACE 20:1686–1690, 1991.
43. Mond H: Unipolar versus bipolar pacing: Poles apart. PACE 14:1411–1424, 1991.
44. Nielsen AP, Cashion R, Spencer W, et al: Long-term assessment of unipolar and bipolar stimulation and sensing thresholds using a lead configuration programmable pacemaker. J Am Coll Cardiol 5:1198–1204, 1985.
45. Schuchert A, Cappato R, Kuck K-H, Meinertz T: Programmable polarity: Effects on pacing and sensing of bipolar steroid-eluting leads. PACE 19:2099–2102, 1999.
46. Griffin JC: Sensing characteristics of the right atrial appendage electrode. PACE 6:22–25, 1983.
47. Kay GN, Epstein AE, Plumb VJ: Comparison of unipolar and bipolar active fixation atrial pacing leads. PACE 11:544–549, 1998.
48. Brouwer J, Nagelkerke D, Den Heijer P, et al: Analysis of atrial sensed far-field ventricular signals: A reassessment. PACE 20:916–922, 1997.
49. Cornacchia D, Fabbri M, Finzi C: Comparison between active screw in and passive leads for permanent transvenous ventricular pacing. PACE 6:A-56, 1983.
50. Spampinato A, Nobile A, Cornacchia D, et al: Clinical trial of last generation bipolar steroid eluting catheters: Comparison between screw in vs tined lead. PACE 20:1444, 1997.
51. Santini M, Seta F: Do steroid-eluting electrodes really have better performance than other state-of-the-art designs? The Italian Multicenter Study Group on low output stimulation. PACE 16:722–728, 1993.
52. Schuchert A, Kuck K-H: Benefits of smaller electrode surface area (4 mm²) on steroid-eluting leads. PACE 14:2098–2104, 1991.

53. Crossley G, Brinker JA, Renolds D, et al: Steroid elution improves the stimulation threshold in an active fixation atrial permanent pacing lead: A randomized, controlled study. Model 4068 Investigators. Circulation 92:2935–2939, 1995.

54. Wish M, Swartz J, Cohen A, et al: Steroid-tipped leads versus porous platinum permanent pacemaker leads: A controlled study. PACE 13:1887–1890, 1990.

55. Gay RJ, Brown DF: Pacemaker failure due to procainamide toxicity. Am J Cardiol 43:728–732, 1974.

56. Ellenbogen KA, Wood MA, Gilligan DM: Evaluation of "inappropriate" ICD shocks in an asymptomatic patient following myocardial infarction. PACE 19:254–255, 1996.

57. Frohlig G, Schwendt H, Schieffer H, Bette L: Atrial signal variations and pacemaker malsensing during exercise: A study in the time and frequency domain. J Am Coll Cardiol 11:806, 1988.

58. Ross B, Zeigler V, Zinner A, et al: The effect of exercise on the atrial electrogram voltage in young patients. PACE 14:2092–2097, 1991.

59. Shandling A, Florio J, Castellanet M, et al: Physical determinants of the endocardial P wave. PACE 13:1585–1589, 1990.

60. Schuchert A, Kuck K-H, Bleifeld W: Stability of pacing threshold, impedance, and R wave amplitude at rest and during exercise. PACE 13:1602–1608, 1990.

61. Rosenheck S, Schmaltz S, Kadish A, Morady F: Effect of rate augmentation and isoproterenol on the amplitude of atrial and ventricular electrograms. Am J Cardiol 66:101–102, 1990.

62. Varriale P, Chryssos B: Atrial sensing performance of the single-lead VDD pacemaker during exercise. J Am Coll Cardiol 22:1854–1857, 1993.

63. Chan C-C, Lau C-P, Leung S-K, et al: Comparative evaluation of bipolar atrial electrogram amplitude during everyday activities: Atrial active fixation versus two types of single pass VDD/R leads. PACE 17:1873–1877, 1994.

64. Wilson JH, Siegmund JB, Johnson R, et al: Pacing system analysers: Different systems—different results. PACE 17:170–20, 1994.

65. de Buitleir M, Kou WH, Schmaltz S, et al: Acute changes in pacing threshold and R- or P-wave amplitude during permanent pacemaker implantation. Am J Cardiol 65:999, 1990.

66. Singer I, Adams L, Austin E: Potential hazards of fixed gain sensing and arrhythmia reconfirmation for implantable cardioverter defibrillators. PACE 16:1070–1079, 1993.

67. Ellenbogen KA, Wood MA, Stambler BS, et al: Measurement of ventricular electrogram amplitude during intraoperative induction of ventricular tachyarrhythmias. Am J Cardiol 70:1017–1022, 1992.

68. Callans DJ, Hook BG, Marchlinski FE: Effect of rate and coupling interval on endocardial R wave amplitude variability in permanent ventricular lead systems. J Am Coll Cardiol 22:746–750, 1993.

69. Brumwell DA, Kroll K, Lehmann MH: The amplifier: Sensing and depolarization. *In* Kroll MW, Lehman MH (eds): Implantable Cardioverter Defibrillator Therapy: The Engineering–Clinical Interface. Norwell, MA, Kluwer Publishing, 1996, pp 275–302.

70. Castro A, Liebold A, Vincente J, et al: Evaluation of autosensing as an automatic means of maintaining a 2:1 sensing safety margin in an implanted pacemaker. PACE 19:1708–1713, 1996.

71. Bolz A, Hubman M, Hardt R, et al: Low polarization pacing lead for detecting the ventricular-evoked response. Medical Progress Through Technology 19:129–137, 1993.

72. Clarke M, Liu B, Schuller H, et al: Automatic adjustment of pacemaker stimulation output correlated with continuously monitored capture thresholds: A multicenter study. PACE 21:1567–1575, 1998.

73. Zrenner B, Schmitt C, Mussig D, et al: Chronic recording of monophasic action potentials by an implanted dual chamber pacemaker. PACE 20:1536, 1997.

74. Feld GK, Love CJ, Camerlo J, Marsella R: A new pacemaker algorithm for continuous capture verification and automatic threshold determination: Elimination of pacemaker afterpotential utilizing a triphasic charge balancing system. PACE 15:171–178, 1992.

75. Vonk BF, Van Oort G: New method of atrial and ventricular capture detection. PACE 21:217–222, 1998.

76. Curtis AB, Maas SM, Domijan A, et al: A method for analysis of the local atrial evoked response for determination of atrial capture in permanent pacing systems. PACE 14:1576–1581, 1991.

77. Unpublished data. Minneapolis, Medtronic, Inc., 1998.

78. McAlister HF, Klementowicz PT, Calderon EM, et al: Atrial electrogram analysis: Antegrade versus retrograde. PACE 11:1703–1707, 1988.

79. Wainwright R, Davies W, Tooley M: Ideal atrial lead positioning to detect retrograde atrial depolarization by digitization and slope analysis of the atrial electrogram. PACE 7:1152–1158, 1984.

80. Timmis GC, Westveer DC, Bakalyar DM, et al: Discrimination of antegrade from retrograde atrial electrograms for physiologic pacing. PACE 11:130–140, 1988.

81. Davies DW, Wainwright RJ, Tooley MA, et al: Detection of pathological tachycardia by analysis of electrogram morphology. PACE 6:200–208, 1986.

82. McAlister HF: Atrial electrogram analysis: Antegrade versus retrograde. PACE 11:1703–1707, 1988.

83. Roithinger FX, Sippensgroenewegen A, Karch MR, et al: Organized activation during atrial fibrillation in man: Endocardial and electrocardiographic manifestations. J Cardiovasc Electrophysiol 9:451–461, 1998.

84. Konings KTS, Smeets LRM, Penn OC, et al: Configuration of unipolar atrial electrograms during electrically induced atrial fibrillation in humans. Circulation 95:1231–1241, 1997.

85. Wood MA, Moskovljevic P, Stambler BS, Ellenbogen KA: Comparison of bipolar atrial electrogram amplitude in sinus rhthym, atrial fibrillation and atrial flutter. PACE 19:150–156, 1996.

86. Karagueuzian HS, Khan SS, Peters W, et al: Nonhomogeneous local atrial activity during acute atrial fibrillation: Spectral and dynamic analysis. PACE 13:1937–1942, 1990.

87. Ropella KM, Sahakian AV, Baerman JM, Swiryn S: The coherence spectrum: A quantitive discriminator of fibrillatory and nonfibrillatory cardiac rhythms. Circulation 80:112–119, 1989.

88. Baerman JM, Ropella KM, Sahakian AV, et al: Effect of bipole configuration on atrial electrograms during atrial fibrillation. PACE 13:78–87, 1990.

89. Ropella KM, Sahakian AV, Baerman JM, Swiryn S: Effects of procainamide on intra-arterial electrograms during atrial fibrillation: Implications for detection algorithms. Circulation 77:1047–1054, 1988.

90. Levine P, Bornzin G, Barlow J, et al: A new automode switch algorithm for supraventricular tachycardias. PACE 17:1895–1899, 1994.

91. Bonnet J, Brusseau E, Limousin M, Cazeau S: Mode switch despite undersensing of atrial fibrillation in DDD pacing. PACE 19:1724–1728, 1996.

92. Ricci R, Puglisi A, Azzolini P, et al: Reliability of a new algorithm for automatic mode switching from DDDR to DDIR pacing mode in sinus node disease patients with chronotropic incompetence and recurrent paroxysmal atrial fibrillation. PACE 19:1719–1723, 1996.

93. Kamalvand K, Tan K, Kotsakis A, et al: Is mode switching beneficial? A randomized study in patients with paroxysmal atrial tachyarrhythmias. J Am Coll Cardiol 30:496–504, 1997.

94. Gillberg J, Brown M, Stanton M, et al: Clinical testing of a dual chamber atrial tachyarrhythmia detection algorithm. Computers in Cardiology 57–60, 1996.

95. Nair M, Saoudi N, Kroiss D, Letac B: Automatic arrhythmia identification using analysis of the atrioventricular association. Circulation 95:967–973, 1997.

96. Sra J, Maglio C, Chen V, et al: Atrial fibrillation detection in humans using the METRIX atrial defibrillation system. J Am Coll Cardiol 27:375A, 1996.

97. Lau CP, Tse HF, Lok NS, et al: Initial clinical experience with an implantable human atrial defibrillator. PACE 20:220–225, 1997.

98. Maglio C, Akhtar M, Blanck Z, et al: Atrial fibrillation detection and synchronization during atrial fibrillation in patients with implanted atrial defibrillator. Circulation 96:522, 1997.

99. Seidl K, Jung W, Werling C, et al: Performance of the AF detection and R-wave synchronization for the Metrix automatic implantable atrial defibrillator. Eur Heart J 18 (Suppl):322, 1997.

100. Wellens HJ, Lau CP, Luderitz B, et al: Atrioverter: An implantable device for the treatment of atrial fibrillation. Circulation 98:1651–1656, 1998.

101. Jung M, Manz M, Moosdorf R, Luderitz B: Failure of an implantable cardioverter-defibrillator to redetect ventricular fibrillation in patients with a nonthoracotomy lead system. Circulation 86:1217–1222, 1992.

102. Olson W: Safety margins for sensing and detection: Programming tradeoffs. *In* Kroll M, Lehmann M (eds): Implantable Cardioverter Defibrillator Therapy: The Engineering-Clinical Interface. Norwell, MA, Kluwer Academic Publishers, 1996, pp 389–420.

103. Reiter MJ, Mann DE: Sensing and tachyarrhythmia detection problems in implantable cardioverter defibrillators. J Cardiovasc Electrophysiol 7:542–558, 1996.

104. Kerr C, Mason M: Amplitude of atrial electrical activity during sinus rhythm and during atrial flutter-fibrillation. PACE 8:348–355, 1985.

105. Gross JN, Uri M, Ben-Zur MD, et al: Effectiveness of automatic mode change is dependent on atrial sensitivity settings. PACE 18:884, 1995.

106. Ricci R, Puglisi A, Azzolini P, et al: How should atrial sensitivity be programmed in automatic mode switching pacemakers? PACE 20:1063, 1997.

107. Palma EC, Kedarnath V, Vankawalla V, et al: Effect of varying atrial sensitivity, AV interval, and detection algorithm on automatic mode switching. PACE 19:1734–1739, 1996.

108. Seidl K, Meisel E, VanAgt E, et al: Is the atrial rate episode diagnostic feature reliable in detecting paroxysmal episodes of atrial tachyarrhythmias? PACE 21:694–700, 1998.

109. Frolig G, Kinderman M, Heisel, et al: Mode switching without atrial tachyarrhythmias. PACE 19:592, 1996.

110. Leung SK, Lau CP, Lam C, et al: How should atrial sensitivity be programmed for optimal automatic mode switching? J Am Coll Cardiol 29:149A, 1997.

111. Weigand UKH, Schier H, Bode F, et al: Should unipolar leads be implanted in the atrium? A Holter electrocardiographic comparison of threshold adapted unipolar and high sensitive bipolar sensing. PACE 21:1601–1608, 1998.

112. LeWalter T, Schimpf R, Jung W, et al: Prospective evaluation of mode switch behaviour in patients with dual chamber pacing and unipolar atrial leads: Relevance of atrial fibrillation/flutter potentials and myopotential triggering. PACE 19:642, 1996.

113. Ellenbogen KA, Mond H, Wood MA, Barold SS: Failure of automatic mode switching: Recognition and management. PACE 20:268–275, 1997.

114. Ellenbogen KA, Wood MA, Mond H, Barold SS: Clinical applications of mode-switching for dual chamber pacemakers. *In* Singer I, Barold SS, Camm AJ (eds): Non-Pharmacologic Therapies for the 21st Century: The State of the Art. Armonk, NY, Futura, 1998, 819–844.

115. Kamalvand K, Tan K, Kotsakis A, et al: Is mode switching beneficial? A randomized study in patients with paroxysmal atrial tachyarrhythmias. J Am Coll Cardiol 30:496–504, 1997.

116. Kim J, Boeck J, White H, et al: An atrial fibrillation detection algorithm for an implantable atrial defibrillator. Computers in Cardiology 169–172, 1995.

117. Tse HF, Lau CP: Efficacy of AF detection and safety of R-wave synchronized shocks for the Metrix automatic implantable atrial defibrillator. J Am Coll Cardiol 31:38A, 1998.

118. Wolpert C, Jung W, Scholl C, et al: Electrical proarrhythmia: Induction of inappropriate atrial therapies due to far-field R wave oversensing in a new dual chamber defibrillator. J Cardiovasc Electrophysiol 9:859–863, 1998.

118a. Brouwer JG, Nagelkerke D, Den Heijer P, et al: Analysis of atrial sensed far-field ventricular signals: A reassessment. PACE 20:916–922, 1997.

119. Swerdlow C, Sheth N, Olson W: Clinical performance of a pattern-based, dual-chamber algorithm for discrimination of ventricular from supraventricular arrhythmias. PACE 21:892, 1998.

120. Cohen TJ, Liem BL: A hemodynamically responsive antitachycardia system. Circulation 82:394–406, 1990.

121. Ayers GM, Alferness CA, Ilina M, et al: Ventricular proarrhythmic effects of ventricular cycle length and shock strength in a sheep model of transvenous atrial defibrillation. Circulation 89:413–422, 1994.

122. Sra J, Maglio C, Dhala A, et al: Feasibility of atrial fibrillation detection and use of a preceding synchronization interval as a criterion for shock delivery in humans with atrial fibrillation. J Am Coll Cardiol 28:1532–1538, 1996.

123. Bardy GH, Ivey TD, Stewart R, et al: Failure of the automatic implantable defibrillator to detect ventricular fibrillation. Am J Cardiol 58:1107–1106, 1986.

124. Leitch J, Yee R, Klein G, et al: Correlation between the ventricular electrogram amplitude in sinus rhythm and in ventricular fibrillation. PACE 13:1105–1109, 1990.

125. Kopp DE, Gilkerson J, Kall JG, Wilber DJ: Effect of ventricular fibrillation on atrial electrograms. Circulation 90:I–177, 1994.

126. Michelson BI, Igel DA, Wilkoff BL: Adequacy of implantable cardioverter-defibrillator lead placement for tachyarrhythmia detection by sinus rhythm electrogram amplitude. Am J Cardiol 76:1162–1166, 1995.

127. Personal Communication with Dr. Marshall Stanton, 1992.

128. Kuhlkamp V, Mortensen PT, Dornberger V, et al: A randomized controlled clinical trial comparing VF detection time between the VENTAK AV acute study device and the VENTAK MINI. PACE 20:1094, 1997.

129. Callans DJ, Hook BG, Marchlinski FE: Effect of rate and coupling interval on endocardial R wave amplitude variability in permanent ventricular sensing lead systems. J Am Coll Cardiol 22:746–750, 1993.

130. Callans DJ, Hook BG, Marchlinski FE: Paced beats following single nonsensed complexes in a "codependent" cardioverter defibrillator and bradycardia pacing system: Potential for ventricular tachycardia induction. PACE 14:1281–1287, 1991.

131. Callans DJ, Hook BG, Kleiman RB, et al: Unique sensing errors in third-generation implantable cardioverter-defibrillators. J Am Coll Cardiol 22:1135–1140, 1993.

132. Singer I, DeBorde R, Veltri EP, et al: The automatic implantable cardioverter defibrillator: T wave sensing in the newest generation. PACE 11:1584–1591, 1988.

133. Vlay SC, Moser SA, Seifert F: Sensing aberration by the automatic implantable cardioverter defibrillator during intraoperative testing. PACE 11:331–335, 1988.

134. Santucci PA, Haw J, Trohman RG, Pinski S: Interference with an implantable defibrillator by an electronic anti-theft surveillance device. N Engl J Med 339:1371–1374, 1998.

135. Gottlieb C, Miller JM, Rosenthal ME, et al: Automatic implantable defibrillator discharge resulting from routine pacemaker programming. PACE 11:336–338, 1988.

136. Kim SG, Furman S, Matos JA, et al: Automatic implantable cardioverter/defibrillator: Inadvertent discharge during permanent pacemaker magnet tests. PACE 10:579–582, 1987.

137. Winkle RA, Bach SM, Echt DS, et al: The automatic implantable defibrillator: Local ventricular bipolar sensing to detect ventricular tachycardia and fibrillation. Am J Cardiol 52:265–270, 1983.

138. Bardy GH: Ensuring automatic detection of ventricular fibrillation. Circulation 86:1634–1635, 1992.

139. Yee R, Jones DL, Jarvis E, et al: Changes in pacing threshold and R wave amplitude after transvenous catheter countershock. J Am Coll Cardiol 4:543–549, 1984.

140. Yee R, Jones DL, Klein GJ: Pacing threshold changes after transvenous catheter countershock. Am J Cardiol 53:503–507, 1984.

141. Bardy GH, Olson WH, Ivey TD, et al: Does unsuccessful defibrillation adversely affect subsequent AICD sensing of ventricular fibrillation? PACE 11:485, 1988.

142. Goldberger JJ, Horvath G, Donovan D, et al: Detection of ventricular fibrillation by transvenous defibrillating leads: Integrated versus dedicated bipolar sensing. J Cardiovasc Electrophysiol 9:677–688, 1998.

143. Jung W, Manz M, Moosdorf R, et al: Failure of an implantable cardioverter-defibrillator to redetect ventricular fibrillation in patients with a nonthoracotomy lead system. Circulation 86:1217–1222, 1992.

144. Jung W, Manz M, Pfeiffer D, et al: Change in amplitude of endocardial electrograms following defibrillator discharge: Comparison of two lead systems. J Am Coll Cardiol 21:128A, 1993.

145. Anderson M, Murgatroyd F, Hnatkova K, et al: Performance of basic ventricular tachycardia detection algorithms in implantable cardioverter defibrillators: Implications for device programming. PACE 20:2975–2983, 1997.

146. Nunain S, Roelke M, Trouton T, et al: Limitations and late complications of third-generation automatic cardioverter-defibrillators. Circulation 91:2204–2213, 1995.

147. Swerdlow CD, Chen PS, Kass RM, et al: Discrimination of ventricular tachycardia from sinus tachycardia and atrial fibrillation in a tiered-therapy cardioverter-defibrillator. J Am Coll Cardiol 23:1342–1355, 1994.

148. Pinski SL, Fahy GJ: The proarrhythmic potential of implantable cardioverter-defibrillators. Circulation 92:1651–1664, 1995.

149. Schaumann A, von zur Muhlen F, Gonska BD, Kreuzer H: Enhanced detection criteria in implantable cardioverter-defibrillators to avoid inappropriate therapy. Am J Cardiol 78:42–50, 1996.

150. Olson WH, Bardy GH, Mehra R, et al: Comparison of different onset and stability algorithms for detection of spontaneous ventricular arrhythmias. PACE 10:439, 1987.

151. Swerdlow CD, Chen PS, Kass RM, et al: Discrimination of ventricular tachycardia from sinus tachycardia and atrial fibrillation in a tiered-therapy cardioverter-defibrillator. J Am Coll Cardiol 23:1342–1355, 1994.

152. Fisher JD, Goldstein M, Ostrow E, et al: Maximal rate of tachycardia development: Sinus tachycardia with sudden exercise vs. spontaneous ventricular tachycardia. PACE 6:221, 1983.

153. Mercando AD, Gableman G, Montefiore JD, et al: Comparison of the rate of tachycardia development in patients: Pathologic vs sinus tachycardia. PACE 11:516, 1988.

154. Brown JP, Gillette PC, Goh TH, et al: Discrimination of tachycardia by rate of onset. Computer Interpretation of the ECG XI, Engineering Foundation 98–101, 1986.

155. Brugada J, Mont M, Figueiredo M, et al: Enhanced detection criteria in implantable defibrillators. J Cardiovasc Electrophysiol 9:261–268, 1998.

156. Ventak PRx Model 1700 Physician's Manual. St. Paul, MN, Cardiac Pacemakers, 1992.

157. PCD Jewel Model 7219 Technical Manual. Minneapolis, Medtronic, Inc., 1993.

158. Neuzner J, Pitschner HF, Schlepper M: Programmable VT detection enhancements in implantable cardioverter defibrillator therapy. PACE 18:539–547, 1995.

159. Geibel A, Zehender M, Brugada P, et al: Changes in cycle length at the onset of sustained tachycardias: Importance for antitachycardiac pacing. Am Heart J 115:588–592, 1988.

160. Volosin KJ, Beauregard LM, Baviszewski R, et al: Spontaneous changes in ventricular tachycardia cycle length. J Am Coll Cardiol 17:409–414, 1991.

161. Olson WH, Bardy GH: Cycle length and morphology patterns at the onset of spontaneous ventricular tachycardia and fibrillation. PACE 9:284, 1986.

162. Swerdlow CD, Ahern T, Chen PS, et al: Underdetection of ventricular tachycardia by algorithms to enhance specificity in a tiered-therapy cardioverter-defibrillator. J Am Coll Cardiol 24(2):416–424, 1994.

163. Le Franc P, Kus T, Vinet A, et al: Underdetection of ventricular tachycardia using a 40 ms stability criterion: Effect of antiarrythmic therapy. PACE 20(12):2882–2892, 1997.

164. Callans DJ, Hook BG, Marchlinski FE, et al: Use of bipolar recordings from patch-patch and rate sensing leads to distinguish ventricular tachycardia from supraventricular rhythms in patients with implantable cardioverter defibrillators. PACE 1991; 14:1917–1922, 1991.

165. Block M, Neuzner J, Bocker D, et al: Initial clinical experience with a new multiprogrammable implantable cardioverter-defibrillator. PACE 16:1913, 1993.

166. Collins SM, Arzbaecher RC: An efficient algorithm for waveform analysis using the correlation coefficient. Computers and Biomedical Research 14:381–389, 1981.

167. DiCarlo LA, Jenkins JM, Kreigler C: Discrimination of ventricular tachycardia from ventricular fibrillation by morphologic analysis of electrograms. Computers in Cardiology, IEEE Computer Society 201–204, 1991.

168. Steinhaus BM, Wells RT, Greenhut SE, et al: Detection of ventricular tachycardia using scanning correlation analysis. PACE 13:1930–1936, 1990.

169. Throne RD, Jenkins JM, DiCarlo LA: A comparison of four new time domain techniques for discriminating monomorphic ventricular tachycardia from sinus rhythm using ventricular waveform morphology. IEEE Trans Biomed Eng 38:561–570, 1991.

170. Greenhut SE, Steinhaus BM, Murphy AJ: Comparison of a new template matching algorithm, correlation, and area of difference methods for detection of ventricular tachycardia. Computers in Cardiology 1991, IEEE Computer Society 371–374, 1991.

171. Greenhut SE, Deering TF, Steinhaus BM, et al: Separation of ventricular tachycardia from sinus rhythm using a practical, real-time template matching computer system. PACE 15:2146–2153, 1992.

172. Davies DW, Wainwright RJ, Tooley MA, et al: Detection of pathological tachycardia by analysis of electrogram morphology. PACE 9:200–208, 1986.

173. Tooley MA, Davies DW, Nathan AW, et al: Recognition of multiple tachyarrhythmias by rate-independent means using a small microcomputer. PACE 14:337–340, 1991.

174. Paul VE, O'Onunain S, Malik M, et al: Temporal electrogram analysis: Algorithm development. PACE 13:1943–1947, 1990.

175. Finelli CJ, Li PC, Jenkins JM, et al: The time-sequenced adaptive algorithm: Application to morphological adaptation and arrhythmia onset detection. Computers in Cardiology 1991, IEEE Computer Society 205–208, 1991.

176. Turner TR, Thomson PJ, Cameron MA: Statistical discriminant analysis of arrhythmias using intracardial electrograms. IEEE Trans Biomed Eng 40(9):985–989, 40(11):1189, 1993.

177. Langberg JJ, Gibb WJ, Auslander DM, et al: Identification of ventricular tachycardia with use of the morphology of the endocardial electrogram. Circulation 77:1363–1369, 1988.

178. Belz MK, Ellenbogen KA, Camm AJ, et al: Differentiation between monomorphic ventricular tachycardia and sinus tachycardia based on the right ventricular evoked potential. PACE 15:1661–1666, 1992.

179. Farrugia S, Yee H, Nickolls P: Implantable cardioverter defibrillator electrogram recognition with a multilayer perceptron. PACE 16:228–234, 1993.

180. Jenkins JM, DiCarlo LA, Chiang CJ, et al: Impact of filtering upon ventricular tachycardia identification by correlation waveform analysis. PACE 14:1809–1814, 1991.

181. Finelli CJ, DiCarlo LA, Jenkins JM, et al: Effects of increased heart rate and sympathetic tone on intraventricular electrogram morphology. Am J Cardiol 68:1321–1328, 1991.

182. Ross BA, Zinner A, Ziegler V, et al: The effect of exercise on the atrial electrograms in humans. J Am Coll Cardiol 9:32A, 1987.

183. Paul VE, Bashir Y, Murphy T, et al: Variability of the intracardiac electrogram: Effect on specificity of tachycardia detection. PACE 13.1925–1929, 1990.

184. Rosenheck S, Schmaltz S, Kadish AH, et al: Effect of rate augmentation and isoproterenol on the amplitude of atrial and ventricular electrograms. Am J Cardiol 66:101–102, 1990.

185. Klingenheben T, Sticherling C, Skupin M, Hohnloser SH: Intracardiac QRS electrogram width—an arrhythmia detection feature for implantable cardioverter defibrillators: Exercise induced variation as a base for device programming. PACE 21:1609–1617, 1998.

186. Shieh M, Clem L, Malden L, et al: Improved supraventricular and ventricular tachycardia discrimination using electrogram morphology in an implantable cardioverter defibrillator. Ital J Cardiol 1998; 28(Suppl 1):245–251, 1998.

187. Gold M, Hsu W, Marcovecchio A: A new tachyarrhythmia discrimination algorithm for implantable defibrillators. Circulation 98:I–192, 1998.

188. Langer A, Heilman MS, Mower MM, et al: Considerations in the development of the automatic implantable defibrillator. Med Instrum 10:163–167, 1976.

189. Routh AG, Larnard DJ, et al: The probability density function as an arrhythmia discriminator in cardiac electrogram analysis. Miami Technicon International Conference IEEE TH0206:19–22, 1987.

190. Gamache CL, Redd RM, Janosik DI, et al: Analysis of probability density function by programmed electrical stimulation. J Am Coll Cardiol 15:200A, 1990.

191. Tomaselli GF, DeBorde R, Griffith LSC, et al: The role of AICD probability density function in tachycardia discrimination: An in vivo study. Cardiostimulation 12:125, 1990.

192. Hemmer WL, Weismuller P, Lass M, et al: Morphology sensing for tachycardia detection: Reliability of PDF in the Ventak P AICD. Herz Schrittmacher 10:187–195, 1990.

193. Toivonen L, Viitasalo M, Jarvinen A, et al: The performance of the probability density function in differentiating supraventricular from ventricular rhythms. PACE 15:726–730, 1992.

194. Thakor NV, Zhu YS, Pan KY, et al: Ventricular tachycardia and fibrillation detection by a sequential hypothesis testing algorithm. IEEE Trans Biomed Eng 37:837–843, 1990.

195. Thakor NV, Natarajan A, Tomaselli GF: Multiway tachyarrhythmia detection algorithm. Computers in Cardiology, IEEE Computer Society 227–230, 1992.

196. Wilkoff B, Gillberg J, Hillman S, Larsen J: Clinical Experience with detection of spontaneous ventricular arrhythmias by a new dual chamber defibrillator in a multicenter study. Circulation 98:1507, 1998.

197. Jenkins JM, Wu D, Arzbaecher RC: Computer diagnosis of supraventricular and ventricular arrhythmias. Circulation 60(5):977–987, 1979.

198. Arzbaecher R, Bump T, Jenkins J, et al: Automatic tachycardia recognition. PACE 7 (3 Pt II):541–547, 1984.

199. Munkenbeck FC, Bump TE, Arzbaecher RC: Differentiation of sinus tachycardia from paroxysmal 1:1 tachycardias using single late diastolic atrial extrastimuli. PACE 9 (1 Pt I):53–64, 1986.

200. Jenkins J, Noh KH, Bump T, et al: A single atrial extrastimulus can distinguish sinus tachycardia from 1:1 paroxysmal tachycardia. PACE 9 (6 Pt II):1063–1068, 1986.

201. Arzbaecher R, Polikaitis A: Dual chamber tachycardia identification. PACE 16 (Pt II):1110, 1993.

202. Throne RD, Jenkins JM, Winston SA, et al: Discrimination of retrograde from anterograde atrial activation using intracardiac electrogram waveform analysis. PACE 12 (10):1622, 1989.

203. Leong PHW, Jabri MA: Matic: An intracardiac tachycardia classification system. PACE 15 (9):1317–1331, 1992.

204. Thakor NV, Natarajan A, Tomaselli GF: Multiway sequential hypothesis testing for tachyarrhythmia discrimination. IEEE Trans Biomed Eng 41 (5):480–487, 1994.

205. Brown M, Gillberg J, Stanton M, et al: Acute human testing of a dual chamber ventricular tachyarrhythmia detection algorithm at Mayo Clinic. Computers in Cardiology 61–64, 1996.

206. Kaemmerer W, Olson W: Dual chamber tachyarrhythmia detection using syntactic pattern recognition and contextual timing rules for rhythm classification. PACE 18:872, 1995.

207. Olson W: Dual chamber sensing and detection for implantable cardioverter-defibrillators. *In* Singer S, Barold SS, Camm A (eds): Nonpharmacologic Therapy of Arrhythmias for the 21st Century: The State of the Art. I. Armonk, NY, Futura, 1998, pp 385–421.

208. Technical Manuals: Models 1810, 1815, Ventak AV Dual Chamber ICD. St. Paul, MN, Guidant, Inc., 1998.

209. Shkurovich S, Sahakian AV, Swiryn S: Detection of atrial activity from high-voltage leads of implantable ventricular defibrillators using a cancellation technique. IEEE Trans Biomed Eng 45 (2):229–234, 1998.

Engineering and Clinical Aspects of Pacing Leads

Harry G. Mond

The implantable cardiac pacemaker is an integrated and highly sophisticated system composed of one or more leads and a pulse generator. Pacemaker leads, which interface the sophisticated electronics in the pulse generator with the heart, play a crucial role in delivering the output pulse from the pulse generator to the myocardium, and the intracardiac electrogram from the myocardium to the sensing circuit of the pulse generator. With rate-adaptive cardiac pacing, the lead may also be an integral part of the artificial sensor. In comparison with the marked advances in pulse generator and sensor technology, advances in pacing leads have occurred relatively slowly. Perhaps the most significant developments in pacing leads have been in the design of electrodes. Problems still exist, however, with lead conductors, insulators, and fixation mechanisms, which need to be solved to achieve the reliability and ease of use that will be required for fully automatic pacing systems of the future. This chapter addresses the engineering of cardiac pacing leads and the clinical application of this technology.

■ LEAD POLARITY

Controversy has continued unabated for more than 30 years with respect to which cardiac pacing system, unipolar or bipolar, is superior.[1] Compared with their unipolar counterparts, early bipolar leads were large, cumbersome, and difficult to implant. Today, with major technologic and engineering advances, bipolar leads approximate unipolar designs in size and ease of insertion. By strict definition, all electrical circuits, including those of a pacemaker, are bipolar. To complete the circuit, electrons flow from the cathode to the anode. When applied to transvenous leads, the terms *unipolar* and *bipolar* simply indicate *the number of electrodes in contact with the heart* (Fig. 4–1). A unipolar lead has only one electrode (the cathode), located at the tip. Current flows from the negatively charged cathode to the

heart and returns to the anode (the pulse generator) to complete the circuit. In contrast, a bipolar lead has both electrodes within the heart, separated by a short distance from each other at the distal end. The tip electrode is the cathode, and a proximal ring electrode serves as the anode. If the voltage gradient (or current density) in the myocardium in contact with the cathode is of sufficient intensity, myocardial stimulation and cardiac contraction result (see Chapter 1).

In reality, the differences between unipolar and bipolar pacing are relatively minor. Both configurations are reliable for long-term pacing in both the atrium and the ventricle. Unipolar and bipolar leads have seen waves of popularity that have reflected the state of the art at the time, the local availability of leads and pulse generators, and individual physician preferences. Today, however, there is a growing worldwide trend toward the increased use of bipolar leads,

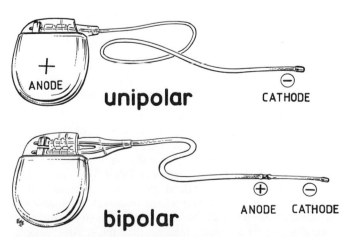

Figure 4–1. Diagram demonstrating differences between unipolar and bipolar lead systems. See text for details.

although unipolar pacing leads remain popular in Europe. The principal differences between these two electrode configurations are discussed in the following sections.

Size

Historically, bipolar transvenous leads were thicker and stiffer than unipolar leads. This made them harder to insert at the venous entry site and more cumbersome to manipulate through the cardiac chambers. There was also fear that these thicker, stiffer leads would obstruct venous channels, compromise tricuspid valve function, or perforate the heart. The original bipolar designs had two parallel conductors individually encased in a large double-lumen insulated tube. At the proximal end of the lead was a bulky bifurcated bipolar connector. Today, bipolar pacing leads have become almost as thin as their unipolar counterparts. These engineering advances are discussed later in this chapter.

Repair

In general, there is little difficulty repairing a standard unipolar lead, particularly one insulated with silicone rubber. The extravascular section of the lead can be cut short and a new connector attached by the use of a connector replacement kit. The repair of a bipolar lead is extremely difficult. With a bifurcated connector, one pole can be capped if the other is suitable for unipolar pacing. The repair, however, becomes more complicated or impossible with modern coaxial bipolar leads, especially with polyurethane insulation.

Stimulation Threshold

In general, the larger the anode, the lower the total pacing impedance. Because the anode is larger with a unipolar pacing system (the pulse generator casing) than with a bipolar system (the proximal electrode), the total impedance is less. Theoretically, unipolar leads with only one conductor should also have lower ohmic resistance than a bipolar lead. Thus, with unipolar pacing and a constant-voltage generator, there should be a lower voltage threshold than with bipolar pacing. In reality, modern pacing leads—whether they are unipolar or bipolar—have very small, low polarization cathodes, which play a much more important role in determining overall pacing impedance than the larger anode. Because of this, bipolar leads offer only marginally higher impedance than unipolar leads, and the stimulation thresholds are very low with both configurations.[2]

Sensing of Intracardiac Electrograms

For many years, it was widely believed that unipolar pacing systems were superior to bipolar systems with respect to sensing of intracardiac signals. This was suggested by early studies with temporary leads, usually in the setting of an acute myocardial infarction or after open heart surgery.[3, 4] With its larger interelectrode distance, the unipolar system "sees" more of the heart in which to detect a spontaneous intracardiac electrical event. In contrast, the small interelectrode distance of a bipolar lead restricts the sensing zone to a limited area of myocardium. Modern implantable pacing systems are different with respect to sensing of spontaneous

intracardiac signals than earlier designs. Comparative studies of unipolar and bipolar sensing configurations have shown comparable ventricular electrogram amplitudes and slew rates.[5–8] These reported studies have also shown that, irrespective of the sensing polarity, ventricular electrogram amplitudes and slew rates usually exceed the standard limits of the sensing circuit by a comfortable margin. In contrast, atrial potentials may have very low amplitudes, particularly in elderly patients, who are the main recipients of cardiac pacemakers. Despite this, in comparative studies, bipolar atrial sensing has not been inferior to unipolar sensing,[9, 10] and on occasion it may actually be superior.[11]

Far-Field Sensing

The atrial sense amplifier of a dual-chamber or atrial (AAI) pacemaker may demonstrate apparent inappropriate sensing that is related to far-field signals arising in the ventricles. Although such far-field R waves usually have small amplitude in the atrial electrogram, in the presence of high atrial sensitivity settings, such signals may be inappropriately interpreted as atrial depolarizations. Generally, this is more likely to occur if the tip of the atrial lead is positioned near the tricuspid valve. Because all leads sense the dipole between anode and cathode, a bipolar lead with closely spaced electrodes is less likely to record far-field electrical signals than is a unipolar lead, wherein the electrodes are widely spaced. Bipolar leads positioned within the right atrial appendage have been shown to have significantly smaller far-field ventricular signals than do unipolar leads in the same position,[12] despite a similar size of the atrial component of the unipolar and bipolar electrograms. Sensed, far-field electrical signals may also result in inappropriate mode switching in pacemakers with these algorithms.[13] Thus, bipolar leads have a clear advantage with respect to decreasing the size of far-field cardiac signals.

Crosstalk

Crosstalk is an alteration in pacemaker timing induced by the sensing in one chamber of a signal originating in the opposite cardiac chamber.[14] The most commonly described model of crosstalk is the inappropriate sensing of the atrial-pacing stimulus by the ventricular channel in dual-chamber pacing. The resultant inhibition of ventricular output may be either intermittent or persistent and can be life-threatening in the pacemaker-dependent patient with complete heart block. Because of the larger amplitude of the pacing stimulus, crosstalk is far more common with unipolar than with bipolar dual-chamber pacing systems.[14–23] Crosstalk with bipolar dual-chamber systems is rare and, when present, is probably related to residual polarization (afterpotentials) and noise in the sensing circuit.[17–20]

Skeletal Muscle Myopotential Oversensing

Unipolar pacing systems are far more susceptible to skeletal myopotential sensing and consequent inhibition than are bipolar systems. Such inhibition represents the most common source of unipolar oversensing, although its clinical importance in terms of patient symptoms and well-being remains controversial.[24–33] Skeletal myopotential inhibition is common with unipolar atrial lead systems, because of the necessity to use high sensitivity settings. With unipolar dual-chamber systems, inappropriate sensing of skeletal myopotentials may result in inhibition of atrial and ventricular outputs,[34–36] or inappropriate triggering of the ventricle may result in loss of atrioventricular synchrony and pacemaker-mediated tachycardia.

Extracorporeal Oversensing

Electromagnetic interference (EMI) from a source outside the body may enter a pacemaker sensing circuit either directly into the pulse generator or through the lead. Because the pulse generator is shielded by a metal case, direct penetration by EMI is uncommon. The antenna effect of the lead remains a potential problem, although significant cases of oversensing of EMI are rare and are limited to a small number of environmental situations. In theory, unipolar pacing leads should be more sensitive than bipolar leads to EMI, because of the larger interelectrode distance that amplifies the antenna effect.[37, 38] This may be of significance with the higher sensitivity settings that are often required for atrial sensing. With DDD pacing, EMI may result in pacemaker-mediated tachycardia, which, although annoying, is usually transient and benign.

Right Ventricular Perforation

Because of their stiffness, certain models of bipolar leads were more prone to right ventricular perforation.[39] The problem became evident when implanting physicians who were comfortable leaving a generous curve of a unipolar lead in the ventricle used the same technique with a bipolar lead. The stiff distal end of the lead may damage the endomyocardium and in some cases can result in ventricular penetration and perforation. Factors influencing the forces transmitted to the cardiac wall include the interelectrode distance, the cathode size and shape, the lead conductor, and the insulation materials. As discussed later, certain leads with polyurethane insulation are very stiff and more prone to right ventricular penetration and perforation. This problem can be overcome with careful implantation techniques and the use of newer silicone rubber–insulated and polyurethane-insulated leads with more flexible tips.[39]

Skeletal Muscle Stimulation

The proximity of adjacent skeletal muscle to the anode of a unipolar pulse generator may result in undesirable stimulation of this skeletal muscle. The resultant muscle twitching is usually prevented at the time of implantation by positioning the anode toward the subcutaneous tissues, away from the pectoralis muscle. Minor, but nevertheless annoying, skeletal muscle stimulation may still occur with unipolar pacing, especially if high stimulation voltages are used. Skeletal muscle stimulation is not a problem with bipolar pacing systems, unless there is a break in the insulation that allows current to stimulate nearby muscle tissue.

Depth of the Pulse Generator Pocket

Because of the potential for local skeletal muscle stimulation from the anode, unipolar pulse generators cannot be buried deep to skeletal muscle unless very low voltages are programmed. This problem is most evident in elderly patients with very little subcutaneous tissue or in the young patient in whom a cosmetic result is particularly important. Bipolar pacemakers are not prone to such problems. For children or very thin adults in whom a submuscular pocket is desirable, bipolar leads are a virtual requirement to prevent muscle stimulation.

Stimulus Artifact Size

The unipolar stimulus artifact recorded on the surface electrocardiogram (ECG) is significantly larger than a bipolar stimulus of equal voltage (Fig. 4–2). Because of this difference, bipolar pacemakers can be difficult to test by electronic means that depend on surface ECG electrodes to measure the pacing rate and pulse width from the stimulus. On occasion, it may be difficult to determine from the ECG whether a rhythm is bipolar pacing or is a spontaneous rhythm propagated with a wide QRS complex. This problem in interpretation may arise during routine testing, during ECG monitoring, or during analysis of a Holter monitor. In these situations, temporary programming to the unipolar configuration can be helpful.

Polarity Programming Flexibility

A bipolar lead connected to a pulse generator with programmable lead polarity permits noninvasive switching between

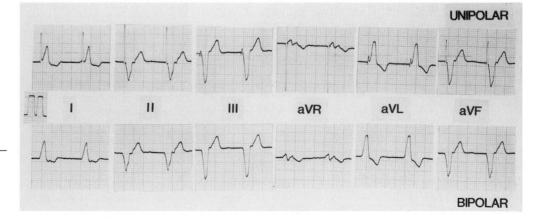

Figure 4–2. Six-lead electrocardiograms demonstrating differences between unipolar and bipolar pacing. Note the large stimulus artifact with unipolar pacing.

either polarity for pacing and sensing. Most modern pacemakers offer separately selectable polarities for pacing and sensing in both the atrium and ventricle.[1] Programming to unipolar pacing is particularly important in bipolar lead systems with failure of the inner insulation or fracture of the outer (anodal) conductor. This permits, at least on a temporary basis, intact unipolar pacing and sensing. The ability to separately program the polarity configuration for pacing and sensing also allows the advantages of either configuration to be exploited while minimizing its disadvantages.

Vulnerability to Ventricular Arrhythmias

There is the theoretical risk of ventricular fibrillation whenever a pacemaker stimulus is delivered into the vulnerable period of the ventricle. Experimentally, the ventricular fibrillation threshold is lower with anodal or bipolar stimulation than with conventional unipolar cathodal stimulation.[40] Despite these laboratory observations, no clinical differences between permanent unipolar and bipolar systems have been reported with respect to the risk of inducing ventricular arrhythmias.

Special Pacing Systems and Implantable Cardioverter-Defibrillator Interactions

Because of the specific sensing requirements of automatic antitachycardia pacemakers and implantable cardioverter-defibrillators (ICD) with pacing capability, these systems must be bipolar to minimize inappropriate sensing of far-field and extracardiac signals. The implantation of a separate dual-chamber pacemaker and an ICD is best accomplished with a bipolar pacemaker to (1) minimize the chances of oversensing of pacing stimuli by the ICD, which may result in the delivery of inappropriate shocks; or (2) inhibit appropriate ICD shocks during ventricular fibrillation because of pacing stimuli. Unipolar pacemakers can inhibit detection of ventricular fibrillation if the pacing stimuli decrease the automatic sensitivity of the ICD. The delivery of an appropriate shock from an ICD may, with some pulse generators, result in polarity switching of the pulse generator from bipolar to unipolar pacing. Indeed, some authors are so concerned about the use of unipolar pacing in patients with ICDs as to recommend the banning of unipolar leads.[41] To a large extent, these problems have been overcome with ICDs that have dual-chamber pacing capabilities.

A number of sensor-driven pacing systems, such as those that use impedance measurements (minute ventilation), require a bipolar lead. In others, such as the evoked QT interval sensor, unipolar pacing is preferred but can be incorporated into a polarity programmable bipolar pacing system.[42]

Reliability

Perhaps the most important reason for choosing a unipolar pacing lead concerns the issue of long-term reliability. Theoretically, the more complex a lead design and the more components that are required for its manufacture, the greater the chances for its failure. Unipolar leads, which may have only six to eight components, are easier to fabricate than are bipolar leads, which have more than twice as many components. Lead designs that incorporate a rate-adaptive sensor and transvenous defibrillation leads that also provide

pacing and sensing capabilities may have more than 40 components. Not surprisingly, unipolar leads have a record of fewer mechanical failures than comparable bipolar leads.

During the past decade, there has been an increasing incidence of insulation failure, particularly in certain types of polyurethane-insulated bipolar leads.[43] Despite this, excellent long-term survival has been documented with other types of bipolar leads insulated with other types of polyurethane[44, 45] or silicone rubber.[43] Reliability of pacing leads is also influenced by implantation techniques. For example, use of the subclavian vein puncture for lead insertion exposes it to the risk of crush injury as the lead passes between the clavicle and first rib, particularly with bipolar leads.[46, 47] Using the cephalic vein as the lead entry site avoids the clavicle–first rib failure mechanism but does not completely protect the lead from failure related to suturing the anchoring sleeve or to intrinsic degradation of polyurethane.[48]

As new lead designs are developed, a clear objective must be to improve reliability, particularly with the more complex bipolar or multipolar varieties. Ideally, all leads should perform reliably for the lifetime of the patient. A summary of the differences between bipolar and unipolar pacing systems is shown in Table 4–1. If reliability were comparable, bipolar leads would be preferable in almost all respects.

■ THE PACING ELECTRODE

Electrode Size

The earliest transvenous pacing leads had large stimulating electrodes with surface areas approximating 100 mm^2.[49] Such electrodes presented a large surface area to the endocardium that resulted in a very low pacing impedance, generally in the order of 250 ohms (Ω). Because current flow is inversely related to impedance, the current drain with these leads was excessive. In addition, because the current was dispersed

Table 4–1. Polarity Preference: Unipolar Versus Bipolar

Pacemaker Characteristic	Bipolar	Unipolar
Lead size		+
Lead repair		+ +
Stimulation threshold	0	
Cardiac myopotential sensing	0	
Far-field sensing	+ +	
Crosstalk	+ + +	
Skeletal myopotential oversensing	+ + +	
Extracorporeal (electromagnetic interference) oversensing	+ +	
Right ventricular perforation		+ +
Local skeletal muscle stimulation	+ + +	
Depth of pulse generator pocket	+ + +	
Stimulus artifact size		+ +
Programming flexibility	+ + +	
Vulnerability to ventricular arrhythmias		+
Special pacing systems and implantable cardioverter-defibrillator interactions	+ + +	
Reliability		+ +

0, no significant difference; +, not significant but preferable; + +, significant but not an important preference; + + +, significant and important preference.

over a large surface area, the resulting stimulation threshold was often high. By reducing the cathodal surface area, high current densities and lower stimulation threshold levels were obtained, together with improved longevity of the power source because of a higher impedance at the electrode–tissue interface.[50–54] By the late 1970s most pacing lead designs had cathodes with surface areas in the range of 8 to 12 mm² and impedance measurements of 400 to 800 Ω. At that time, further reduction in cathode size was regarded as undesirable because of the theoretical concerns of microdislodgment due to the small electrode surface area. Nevertheless, leads with 4- to 6-mm² electrodes and later with less than 2-mm² electrodes and with more than 1000 Ω of impedance and extremely low stimulation thresholds were introduced and found to be safe for long-term pacing and sensing.[55–57]

There are limits to the reduction of the electrode surface area. For example, small geometric surface area polished electrodes demonstrate significant polarization potentials, which decrease pacing efficiency. In theory, extremely small surface area electrodes may also compromise sensing of cardiac myopotentials. This, however, depends on low input impedance of the sense amplifier, which does not occur today. Extremely small electrodes may also be more likely to penetrate or perforate the myocardial wall. This problem can be exacerbated when the distal portion of the lead is relatively stiff.[39]

Polarization and Electrode Porosity

The ideal pacemaker lead should have high electrode–tissue impedance, low ohmic resistance of the conductor, and low polarization. The term *polarization* refers to the electrochemical impedance generated at the electrode–tissue interface (see Chapter 1). Electrical current within metal conductors is ohmic, or due to the flow of electrons. In body tissues, however, current flow is due to the movement of charged molecules or ions. At the electrode–tissue interface, there is a transfer of ohmic energy to ionic energy, and an intense chemical reaction occurs. This polarization is due to the alignment of oppositely charged particles and is a capacitance effect. It explains the change in impedance that occurs during delivery of the pacing stimulus. At the leading edge of the constant-voltage stimulus, polarization is not present,

and the capacitance is zero. During the stimulus, the capacitance increases to reach its maximum at the trailing edge of the stimulus. The capacitance gradually decreases after the stimulus, as a result of the dissipation of ions back to electrical neutrality.

The accumulation of ions in the myocardium gives rise to the afterpotential that is typically recorded after a pacing stimulus. This electrochemical polarization effect increases as the geometric electrode surface area is reduced. Polarization impedance is also dependent on the time that has elapsed since lead implantation, the electrode materials, the electrode surface structure, the current delivered (increases with low current), the pulse width (increases with extended pulse width), the electrode chemistry, and the stimulation polarity.[54, 58] Whereas the polarization effect can represent 30% to 40% of the total pacing impedance, this contribution may be as high as 70% for some smooth surface, small area electrodes.[54]

An early attempt to produce a low polarization electrode was the differential current density (DCD) design. This used a small insulating or dielectric, saline-filled container that was composed of silicone rubber or Teflon. A hole or holes were drilled at the distal end, permitting contact of an enveloped large surface area electrode with the endocardium.[59–61] The current density at the hole was high, but there was no direct electrode–tissue interface and thus virtually no polarization effect. Because of design problems, these electrodes did not gain clinical acceptance. The trade-off between low stimulation thresholds resulting from electrodes with a small radius and the effects of polarization was addressed by designing electrodes with a complex surface structure. During the late 1970s it was recognized that a porous electrode was, in a sense, an extension of the differential current density electrode concept and had low polarization properties.[62] With porous electrodes, the geometric electrode radius can be made small, yet the electrode surface area is in reality large because it includes the internal spaces within the electrode pores.

The original porous electrode consisted of sintered platinum-iridium fibers, giving the appearance of a fine wire mesh. Because the whole electrode was composed of these fibers, this was referred to as a *totally porous* electrode (Fig. 4–3).[63] The other form of porous electrode involved surface

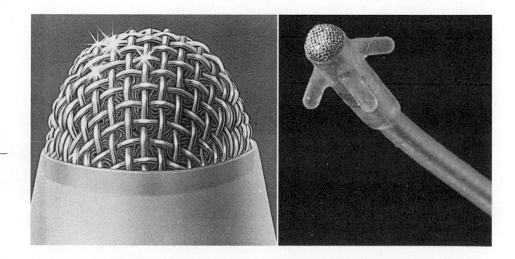

Figure 4–3. Totally porous electrode. (Courtesy of Cardiac Pacemakers Inc., St. Paul, MN.)

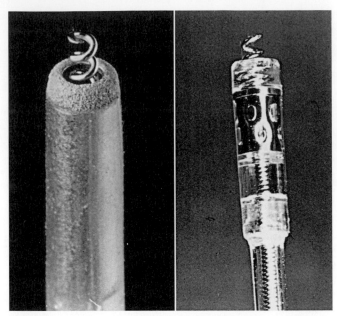

Figure 4–4. Active-fixation leads. *Left,* Electrically inert screw emerging from a porous electrode. *Right,* Electrically active screw. (*Left* courtesy of Telectronics, a division of St. Jude Medical, Sylmar, CA; *right* courtesy of Medtronic, Minneapolis, MN.)

treatment of a solid electrode and was referred to as a *porous surface* electrode. The pores can be created in a number of ways, such as sintering a metal powder or microspheres onto a solid metal substrate. The result is an interconnecting network of pores uniformly distributed throughout the coating.[64] Depending on the surface porosity, such electrodes may be *macroporous* (constructed with small spheres), or *microporous* (using a fine metal powder). Platinum electroplating using platinum powder is a way of producing a microporous surface on an electrode. The electrode appears black because the surface particles are smaller than the wavelength of visible light, which is therefore absorbed. Large microsurface areas can also be created by coating the electrode with platinum-iridium[65] or titanium nitride[66] or by thermal bonding of iridium oxide onto a titanium substrate.[67]

Studies comparing porous electrodes with solid-tip electrodes generally have shown that the porous designs have superior stimulation thresholds and sensing characteristics.[68-73] A porous surface cathode can also be incorporated into an active-fixation lead (Fig. 4–4). The screw, which passes through the center of the porous electrode, is used for lead fixation, but not for stimulation or sensing.[74, 75] It is also possible to create a microporous surface on an endocardial[76] or epimyocardial screw electrode.[77]

Low polarization leads can also be created, by etching or texturizing the electrode surface.[78, 79] A variation uses pores drilled with a laser into a mushroom- or dish-shaped electrode. These pores create both areas of low polarization and zones of high current density. Clinical studies of laser-drilled pores have shown lower chronic stimulation thresholds,[80] although higher than with other porous designs.[81] A development in porous electrode technology has been fractal coating.[82] The titanium electrode is totally covered with iridium hemispheres. On top of these hemispheres, smaller hemi-

spheres are applied again and again, enlarging the active surface area 1000-fold. These fractal coated leads have very low polarization properties.

Electrode Composition

The composition of the electrode can be crucial to its long-term function. Electrode corrosion or degradation may occur over time. Some metals, such as stainless steel[83] and zinc,[84] are clearly unacceptable because their excessive corrosion releases metal ions into the electrode–tissue interface, causing an excessive foreign body reaction and a thick perielectrode fibrous capsule. Platinum is relatively nonreactive but acts as a catalyst for the breakdown or reformation of water, depending on whether electrons are consumed (anode) or given up (cathode). Alloying platinum with 10% iridium increases its mechanical strength without altering its electrical performance.[80] For many years, polished platinum and platinum-iridium were the most common materials used in the cathode position (Fig. 4–5). With the success of porous electrodes, platinum powder was used to create a low polarization porous electrode by being sintered onto platinum. Another cathode material widely used in the past was Elgiloy (Elgin National Watch Company, Elgin, IL), an alloy of cobalt, iron, chromium, molybdenum, nickel, and manganese.[83] Elgiloy, however, cannot be used as the anode in bipolar leads because of its potential for excessive corrosion. Both platinum-iridium and Elgiloy cathodes show minor corrosion over time, although no adverse clinical effects have been documented.[85]

In Europe and in the United States, carbon has been extensively used as a material for cathodes because of its acceptable stimulation thresholds and relatively low polarization properties. Normal carbon or graphite is mechanically weak, is brittle, and has poor wear resistance.[86] In contrast, vitreous carbon, a highly purified pyrolytic form of carbon, has excellent mechanical strength, biocompatibility, and complete inertness to body tissues.[87, 88] A disadvantage of vitreous carbon is excessive polarization loss,[89] which can be overcome by treating the surface with an oxidation process called *surface activation*.[86-90] Animal studies have shown only minor tissue reactions with vitreous carbon,

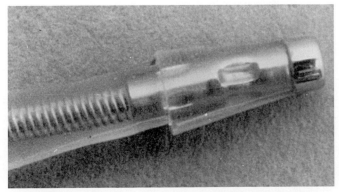

Figure 4–5. Lead with a wedge or flange passive-fixation device and a polished platinum iridium electrode. (Courtesy of Medtronic, Minneapolis, MN.)

compared with the reaction surrounding platinum-iridium electrodes.[61, 86, 89–91]

Numerous short-term and long-term studies have testified to the excellent stimulation thresholds achieved with activated carbon electrodes, particularly when compared with polished platinum-iridium electrodes.[85, 89, 92–94] The *glassy carbon electrode* is also microporous but differs from other commercially available carbon electrodes by having a smooth, glassy luster.[95] Titanium, titanium oxide, titanium alloys, iridium-oxide–coated titanium, and especially titanium nitride, in a variety of shapes and sizes, have become popular for use as cathode materials because of their reported low stimulation thresholds and acceptable polarization losses.[59, 63, 96–102] This includes a platinum-coated titanium, steroid-eluting electrode. The low chronic stimulation thresholds obtained with this electrode, however, appear to result from the properties of steroid elution rather than the electrode's configuration or materials.[103]

Electrode–Tissue Interface

The rise in stimulation threshold that normally follows lead implantation results from inflammation at the electrode–tissue interface.[104] The magnitude of this rise in stimulation threshold is unpredictable and in some cases excessive. In these situations, it is necessary to use relatively high voltage outputs, at least for the first 3 months after implantation. As the inflammatory process subsides and a fibrous capsule is formed, the stimulation threshold usually falls to a chronic plateau level that is often considerably higher than at implantation. Inflammation is the crucial factor that must be controlled to achieve a consistently low stimulation threshold after implantation.[103]

In the design of pacing electrodes, a number of basic bioengineering principles that influence the stimulation threshold are important. As discussed, the cathode should be small enough to produce a high current density and electric field strength. The electric field strength decreases, however, as a function of the square of the distance between the electrode surface and the tissue to be stimulated. Consequently, the electrode radius should optimally be equal to or less than the thickness of the fibrous capsule that inevitably envelops it. If the electrode is smaller than the fibrous capsule, the stimulation thresholds actually increase.[99] To ensure good clinical performance, the lead must also provide adequate fixation for the electrode. The development of fixation mechanisms, such as tines, has greatly reduced the risk of electrode dislodgment.[105] In addition, tissue ingrowth into porous and grooved electrodes may also enhance mechanical stability and ensure intimate electrode contact with the endocardium at the electrode–tissue interface.

The mechanical design of the lead is also important for the control of the inflammation. The electrode should be stable and lie gently against the endocardium, causing as little physical irritation as possible. A lead design that allows excessive pressure to be imparted to the distal electrode can traumatize the endomyocardium and provoke an accelerated inflammatory response. In some cases, lead stiffness can result in myocardial ischemia and ventricular perforation.[39] Because of the effect of lead stiffness on chronic stimulation thresholds, the mass of the distal portion of the lead should be as small as possible, but not so small as to act as a penetrating needle point. To prevent further trauma at the electrode–tissue interface, softer forms of silicone or polyurethane may be used for the distal portion of endocardial leads.

Physical methods aimed at preventing irritation at the electrode–tissue interface should also be considered. Ripart and Mugica[106] have suggested interposing an inert biocompatible conductor material, such as a hydrogel, between the electrode and endocardium both to reduce mechanical irritation and to present to the endocardium a contaminant-free electrode. It has long been known that a perfectly clean electrode gives a lower stimulation threshold than one contaminated with dust, fiber material, glove powder, or other contaminants collected during manufacture, particularly in the pores of the electrode. A variation of the clean electrode concept is the ion-exchange membrane, which permits free flow of current, but the membrane protects the endocardium from the irritating effects of the electrode and contaminants.[107] Such membranes can be impregnated with anti-inflammatory drugs such as glucocorticosteroids. Another way of coating the electrode is to use blood-soluble materials such as mannitol or polyethylene glycol. Once in the circulation the material dissolves, leaving a contaminant-free electrode.

The use of local pharmacologic agents is a novel and highly effective way to counter the inflammatory reaction at the electrode–tissue interface. For research purposes, drug delivery systems that dispense controlled doses of pharmacologic agents directly at the electrode–tissue interface have been developed and used in animal studies.[108, 109] The agents that have been studied include anti-inflammatory drugs, anticoagulants, and drugs that prevent the formation of an extracellular matrix. Apart from glucocorticosteroids, no consistent improvement in stimulation threshold has been found, and in some cases significant deterioration in stimulation threshold has occurred. For example, heparin inhibits fibrin formation and prevents the development of a protective fibrous barrier during acute inflammation, thus allowing more physical damage to occur.[108] Other agents that prevent extracellular matrix formation without altering the inflammatory response, namely tunicamycin and *cis*-hydroxyproline, also cause an elevation in stimulation threshold,[109] indicating that prevention of inflammation was the most important consideration in reducing the chronic stimulation threshold. From these studies, it is not surprising that glucocorticosteroid-eluting electrodes, because of their potent anti-inflammatory action, result in a significant reduction in peak and chronic stimulation threshold levels after implantation.[108, 109]

For implantable pacing leads, dexamethasone sodium phosphate was found to be much more effective than prednisolone.[104] Prednisolone has a high affinity for protein, rendering the protein-bound drug pharmacologically inactive. The early edema at the electrode–tissue interface is protein-rich; therefore, minute amounts of prednisolone released by a drug-eluting device may be immediately inactivated.[104] Dexamethasone sodium phosphate, which does not have a high affinity for protein, has been used clinically in a number of pacing leads with steroid-eluting electrodes. The original design was composed of a platinum-coated titanium electrode.[110] Immediately behind the porous electrode lies an internal chamber containing a plug of silicone rubber compounded with 1 mg or less of dexamethasone sodium phosphate. This plug is referred to as a steroid and silicone rubber *monolithic controlled release device* (MCRD). The internal chamber communicates with the outer surface of the electrode and the adjacent electrode–tissue interface through a porous channel (Fig. 4–6).

Extensive experience with the steroid-eluting electrode, both in the experimental animals and in humans, has demonstrated very low acute and chronic stimulation thresholds in both the atrium and ventricle, with virtual elimination of the early postoperative peak.[103, 111–119] In particular, excellent results have been obtained in children (a group known to have a high incidence of elevated stimulation thresholds)[120] and in patients with a previous history of high threshold exit block.[121, 122]

The precise role of dexamethasone sodium phosphate in this first-generation electrode was initially uncertain. It was considered that the unique design and materials of the electrode were responsible for the favorable results. It has now been demonstrated conclusively, however, that it is the steroid that prevents the stimulation threshold rise.[103, 123, 124] The effect of glucocorticosteroids in lowering the stimulation threshold has been shown to persist for at least a 10-year clinical follow-up period.[123]

The action of glucocorticosteroid at the electrode–tissue interface is not completely understood, but the drug is believed to have a stabilizing effect on the membranes of macrophages lying within the pores of the electrode, on the channel connecting the MRCD plug to the electrode–tissue interface, and on the electrode surface.[125] The resident macrophages within the fibrous capsule are believed to be long-lived with little turnover. The glucocorticosteroid prevents or at least retards lysosomal release, mitigating the release of oxidants, oxygen free radicals, hydrolytic enzymes, and other inflammatory mediators that can damage myocardium. It is this damage to myocytes that is probably responsible for most of the increase in stimulation threshold.

Considering the amount of steroid present in the MRCD plug, it is hard to understand how such a small quantity of steroid could have such a profound and lasting effect on the stimulation threshold. To understand this, the dynamics of steroid elution in vivo must be considered. This includes the drug's solubility, its concentration gradient, and the path length through which it must diffuse. Immediately after implantation, the steroid concentration gradient is high, and

a significant portion of the available drug can dissolve and diffuse to the electrode–tissue interface. Because of its relatively low concentration, the presence of steroid does not entirely prevent the foreign body response. Unlike the in vitro situation, steroid loss is impeded by thrombosis in the elution channel and acutely in the electrode pores. Chronically, there is incorporation of a fibrous tissue layer, which fills the elution channel and pores with collagen. The resultant volume that the steroid can dissolve into is extremely small, and the collagen-filled elution channel presents a long diffusion path. The steroid solution within the pores rapidly becomes saturated. Most of the drug, therefore, remains in its solid state within the MCRD, thus preserving its stability.[123] Once in the collagen-packed space, the steroid attaches to specific receptors on the macrophages, and there appears to be little if any washout or steroid loss. Consequently, the chronic elution rate from the MCRD is miniscule, and from the steroid analysis data, 14% of the steroid theoretically still remains within the MCRD at 20 years.[123] In light of this, it seems more than likely that the adequate steroid elution will last the lifetime of most patients who receive such pacing leads.

Steroid-eluting electrodes also demonstrate excellent implantation and long-term R-wave amplitudes and telemetered electrograms.[113, 115, 119, 120, 126–128] Superior R-wave sensing has been demonstrated with steroid-eluting electrodes when compared with standard electrodes.[129, 130] Steroid-eluting electrodes have also shown superior P-wave sensing compared with platinized porous-platinum electrodes.[117]

The first-generation steroid-eluting electrode was composed of platinum-coated titanium. Without steroid elution, this electrode is associated with relatively high, unpredictable stimulation thresholds, appreciably higher than a platinized porous-platinum electrode.[131] With steroid elution, these leads were associated with low chronic stimulation thresholds that had been unprecedented with any other lead design. Thus, the utility of steroid elution has been universally accepted.

Controversy remains regarding whether a steroid-eluting electrode is really necessary because almost comparable chronic data can be presented with electrodes composed of microporous carbon, platinized porous-platinum, and iridium-oxide–coated titanium. All steroid-free electrodes still tend to develop an unpredictable acute peak stimulation threshold, which makes it necessary to program pulse gener-

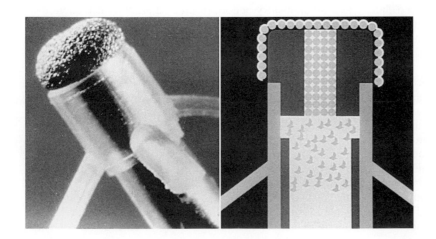

Figure 4–6. *Left,* First-generation porous, platinum-covered titanium, steroid-eluting electrode. *Right,* Cross-sectional diagram of the same electrode, demonstrating the silicone rubber plug impregnated with dexamethasone sodium phosphate lying immediately behind the electrode and connected to it by a channel. (Courtesy of Medtronic, Minneapolis, MN.)

Stimulation Threshold (Volts)

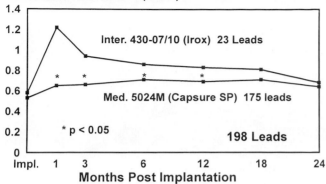

Figure 4–7. Mean bipolar stimulation thresholds for 198 ventricular leads to compare a porous steroid-eluting, 5.8-mm² platinized platinum electrode (Medtronic 5024M Capsure SP, 175 leads) with a conventional porous 8-mm² iridium oxide–coated titanium electrode (Intermedics 430-07, 430-10 Irox, 23 leads). During the first 3 months after implantation, the Irox lead showed a typical rise in stimulation threshold, falling to a plateau a little higher than the Capsure SP lead. At 18 months, there was no statistical difference between the two lead types, and at 24 months, the stimulation thresholds were almost identical. Med, Medtronic; Inter, Intermedics, Angleton TX; Impl, implantation.

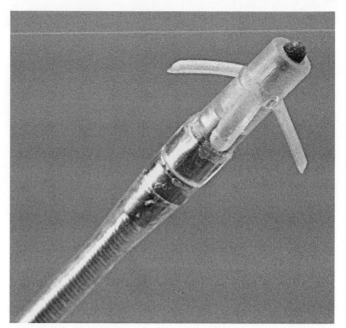

Figure 4–8. A 1.2-mm² platinized porous-platinum steroid-eluting electrode. Note the protective ring of silicone rubber immediately behind the electrode to prevent perforation. (Courtesy of Medtronic, Minneapolis, MN.)

ators at implantation at 5-V output and at 0.5-msec pulse width to ensure an adequate margin of safety (Fig. 4–7). Despite the low mean chronic stimulation thresholds with these non–steroid-eluting electrodes, unpredictable rises in chronic stimulation threshold still occur.[132] With steroid-eluting electrodes, significant chronic stimulation threshold rises have not been reported, provided mechanical causes, such as myocardial penetration, perforation, or lead dislodgment, have been excluded. Patients in whom a steroid-eluting electrode is implanted that is coupled with a good lead design and implantation technique can be safely paced from the day of implantation at 2.5 V. When stimulation threshold measurements are measured regularly, most patients with steroid-eluting electrodes can be safely paced at 1.6 V.[133] The ability to use these low-current drains safely has important ramifications for pulse generator longevity and size, especially with dual-chamber and rate-responsive systems. As discussed earlier, steroid-eluting electrodes are clearly superior to other electrodes for patients with previously documented exit block, and they should be used whenever such patients are encountered.

With the technical and clinical information that is available regarding stimulation threshold and polarization, a number of new leads have been designed with more advanced electrodes. Steroid-eluting, platinized microporous-platinum electrodes with 5.8-mm² and 1.2-mm² surface areas have demonstrated lower stimulation thresholds than those of the original platinum-coated titanium design (Figs. 4–8 and 4–9).[57, 134–138] They also provide higher lead impedance than their predecessors. The design of extremely small electrodes is crucial. Because the electrode surface area is so small, the distal end may resemble a sharp arrowhead, which may either perforate the thin right ventricular wall or fail to make contact with the endomyocardium. To prevent perforation, a silicone rubber protection collar to blunt the distal end can be placed around the electrode (see Fig. 4–8). However, an

occasional high threshold exit block is to be expected,[139] although this should be weighed against a superior performance from this electrode compared with its predecessors.

Because of the early need for atrial screw-in leads, it was always assumed that stimulation thresholds in the atrium

Stimulation Threshold (Volts)

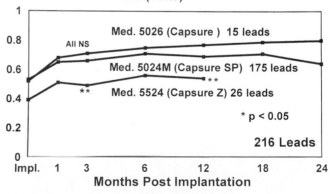

Figure 4–9. Mean bipolar stimulation thresholds for 216 ventricular leads to compare three generations of Medtronic porous steroid-eluting electrodes. The first generation (Capsure model 5026, 15 leads) has an 8-mm² platinum-coated titanium electrode; the second generation has a 5.8-mm² platinized porous-platinum electrode (Capsure SP model 5024M, 175 leads); and the third generation has a 1.2-mm² platinized porous-platinum electrode (Capsure Z model 5524, 26 leads). All electrodes have only a minimal rise in stimulation threshold after implantation. As the electrode surface area becomes smaller, the measured mean stimulation threshold falls. Med, Medtronic; Impl, implantation; NS, not significant between Capsure and Capsure SP; **refers to statistical significance between Capsure Z and both Capsure and Capsure SP.

Stimulation Thresholds (Volts)

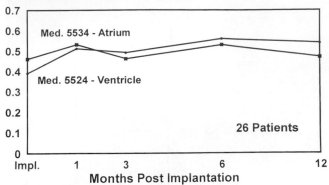

Figure 4–10. Mean bipolar stimulation thresholds for 52 leads (26 atrial and 26 ventricular) in 26 patients, to compare the mean stimulation thresholds between atrium and ventricle using the same 1.2-mm² platinized porous-platinum, steroid-eluting electrode (Capsure Z models 5534 and 5524). The atrial stimulation thresholds at implantation were slightly higher, but by 3 months after implantation, the reverse is seen. See text for explanation. Med, Medtronic; Impl, implantation.

were higher than in the ventricle and that this was an electromechanical feature of the thin-walled right atrium. More recently, long-term follow-up studies of tined, passive-fixation, atrial appendage leads have shown that atrial J-shaped steroid-eluting leads can be easily and reliably placed in the right atrial appendage and that very low stimulation thresholds can be achieved.[111, 116] When compared with identical electrodes placed in the ventricle in the same patients, atrial stimulation thresholds are slightly higher at implanta-

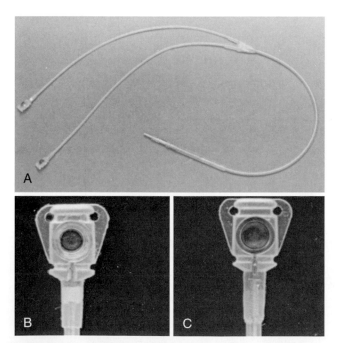

Figure 4–11. *A,* Bipolar, platinized porous-platinum steroid-eluting epicardial electrodes. *B* and *C,* Detailed views of the electrodes with cathode on the left and anode on the right. (Courtesy of Medtronic, Minneapolis, MN.)

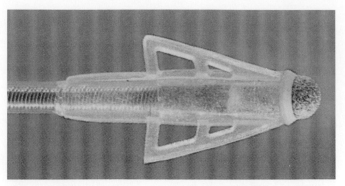

Figure 4–12. Porous-platinum iridium, steroid-eluting fined lead. Immediately behind the electrode is a silicone rubber collar impregnated with steroid. (Courtesy of Telectronics, a division of St. Jude Medical, Sylmar, CA.)

tion, but within 3 months, they become marginally lower than in the ventricle (Fig. 4–10).[140] This can be explained in the way the leads lie in the heart. Ventricular electrodes are placed against the apical wall and may physically irritate the endocardium. Atrial appendage leads, however, hang in the appendage, and provided that the electrode makes contact with the wall, endocardial irritation is kept to a minimum.

A steroid-eluting epicardial lead has also been described.[141, 142] Unlike other permanent pacing leads implanted using a transthoracic approach, the electrode is not a helical screw; therefore, this lead is not myocardial. The electrode is a platinized porous-platinum button-shaped configuration, which can be duplicated into a bipolar configuration (Fig. 4–11). As with the original transvenous steroid-eluting electrode, there is a silicone rubber plug impregnated with dexamethasone sodium phosphate behind the electrode. Both animal and clinical pediatric data have shown encouraging results,[143–146] although long-term performance may depend on other characteristics of epicardial leads, such as the conductors.

A silicone rubber plug within the electrode is not the only method by which steroid can be delivered to the electrode–tissue interface. Another electrode design uses a porous ceramic or silicone rubber collar impregnated with dexamethasone sodium phosphate. This drug-eluting collar is positioned immediately proximal to the tip electrode (Fig. 4–12). Data in humans have shown a significant reduction in stimulation thresholds in both the atrium and ventricle for both unipolar[147–152] and bipolar[153–155] leads. An advantage of such a design would be a steroid-eluting active-fixation screw-in lead (discussed later).

As stated earlier, steroid can be impregnated into an ion-exchange membrane. Clinical studies using carbon and titanium nitride electrodes have shown very low stimulation thresholds at implantation, with almost no elevation in stimulation thresholds; however, there were no differences in these studies between electrodes with and without steroid after the first 3 postimplantation months.[156–158]

■ LEAD FIXATION

Transvenous leads are attached to the endocardium either actively or passively. Active-fixation leads incorporate devices that invade the endomyocardium, whereas passive-fixation leads promote fixation by indirect means. When correctly implanted, both fixation mechanisms result in an extremely low incidence of lead dislodgment.

Passive Fixation

The first attempt to attach a fixation device to a lead was with the use of a wedge or flange at the tip (see Fig. 4-5). Although this probably reduced the incidence of lead dislodgment, carefully controlled studies were never performed.[159] Other early passive-fixation electrodes included a helifix electrode[160] and a balloon-tip lead,[161] both of which were not commercially successful because of difficulties with implantation and a high incidence of perioperative and postoperative complications.[162] During the late 1970s, small tines positioned immediately behind the electrode were shown to have a low incidence of lead dislodgment, and these remain the most popular passive-fixation design (see Fig. 4-3, 4-6, and 4-8).[163] Variations of this concept include wings, cones, and fins (see Fig. 4-12). Such passive-fixation devices are extensions of the insulation material, which become entrapped within cardiac trabeculae, particularly in the right atrial appendage and right ventricle.

Active Fixation

Transvenous, active-fixation leads are composed of a screw at the distal end of the lead, which may or may not be electrically active. They can be classified as fixed exposed screws, protected screws, and retractable and extendable screws.[164] The original designs had a fixed, unprotected screw, which could damage venous and intracardiac structures during lead insertion. To overcome this, a protective bullet-shaped covering, such as mannitol, can be used.[164] After insertion into the venous channels and heart, the mannitol dissolves within a few minutes, allowing the bare screw to be secured in the appropriate chamber. Such leads have also been designed with steroid elution using dexamethasone acetate.[165]

The major active fixation design available, however, is the retractable and extendable screw-in lead, which has become popular for atrial use (see Fig. 4-4).[166] This design uses a variety of mechanisms to extend and retract the screw, including an implement to turn the connector pin, which in turn is mechanically and electrically connected to the electrically active screw helix by means of the conductor. An attempt to isolate the screw electrically from the conductor was unsuccessful.[167] A screwdriver stylet has also been used to extend and retract the screw.[155]

Not all active-fixation leads can be retracted once inserted. In one design, the screw must be retracted manually outside the body and then extended from within its protective covering at the distal end of the lead using a standard stylet.[168] This is performed immediately before fixation.

Unlike tined leads, all active-fixation leads traumatize the endomyocardium. This may result in significant elevations of stimulation thresholds after implantation.[169] In an unsuccessful attempt to achieve better long-term stimulation thresholds, the screw was electrically insulated and protruded centrally from a porous ring-shaped cathode (see Fig. 4-4). Although the electrode itself was passive, continual rubbing

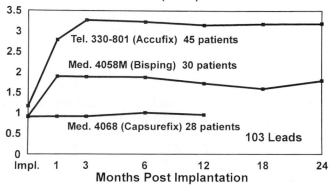

Stimulation Thresholds (Volts)

Figure 4-13. Mean bipolar stimulation thresholds for 103 atrial leads to compare three designs of active-fixation screw-in electrodes. The electrically inert screw with the porous electrode (Accufix model 330-801, 45 patients) has the highest mean chronic stimulation thresholds, all above 3 V. The electrically active screw (Bisping model 4050M, 30 patients) also performs poorly, with a mean chronic stimulation threshold close to 2 V. The screw-in lead with the steroid-eluting collar (Capsurefix model 4068, 28 patients) performs like all other atrial steroid-eluting leads. There is no rise in mean stimulation threshold, which remains at about 1 V. Tel, Telectronics; Med, Medtronic; Impl, implantation.

against the endocardium resulted in even higher stimulation thresholds than the electrically active screw design (Fig. 4-13). It is also possible to have an electrically active screw protruding through a porous electrode, allowing both components to act as the cathode. A steroid-eluting collar surrounding the base of the screw (Fig. 4-14)[170–173] and a monolithic controlled-release device immediately behind the screw[76] have each demonstrated significantly improved stimulation thresholds in active-fixation leads (see Fig. 4-13). A novel design using a standard porous steroid-eluting electrode lying centrally and surrounded by a fixed nonretractable screw has shown results comparable to those of the tined steroid-eluting electrode. This is not surprising, however, because the electrode is totally unrelated to the fixation mechanism.[174]

Epimyocardial leads are all active-fixation leads. Although most have a helical screw, stab-on fishhook designs have been available for pediatric use for a long time. All designs have a high incidence of complications—in particular, high threshold exit block.[175]

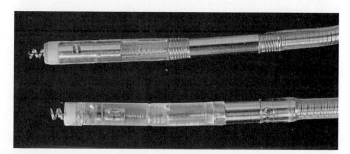

Figure 4-14. Transvenous, screw-in active-fixation leads with steroid-eluting collars immediately behind the screw. (*Top,* courtesy of Telectronics; *bottom,* courtesy of Medtronic, Minneapolis, MN.)

■ LEAD CONDUCTORS

The conductor of a pacing lead is composed of wire that conducts the electrical current from the pulse generator to the stimulating electrode. Unipolar leads require one conducting coil, whereas bipolar leads require two. Conductors are also responsible for transfer of the sensed cardiac signals (intrinsic or evoked) from the electrodes to the sensing amplifier of the pulse generator. An early and reliable conductor used in the 1960s was composed of four tinsel ribbons of stainless steel wrapped around a central Terylene core. This multistrand lead provided redundant current pathways and had immense flexibility and a low incidence of conductor fracture. Transvenous implantation of this lead was difficult because there was no method for stiffening the lead to guide the tip to the apex of the right ventricle. Consequently, a major advance in pacemaker implantation was the introduction of helically coiled conductors. These were composed of a single strand of a tightly coiled wire wound around an empty core, which allowed the passage of a stainless steel stylet to the tip electrode. The introduction of stylets for stiffening the lead greatly improved the ease of implantation. Such leads were prone to fracture at stress points such as sites where anchoring ligatures were applied, where the conductor entered a lead connector, and where the lead was encased in an endocardial bridge within the heart. In these situations, the point of fracture was a fulcrum, with one side of the conductor moving separately from the other. Thus, one side of the conducting wire was in tension while the other was in compression. To make the conductor more flexible and to create redundancy, two or more wires were constructed in a multifilar coil arrangement (Fig. 4–15).

The original conductor materials were stainless steel or platinum. These materials were later replaced with more corrosion-resistant alloys that have better fatigue resistance, such as MP35N, an alloy of nickel, chromium, cobalt, and molybdenum. To reduce the resistance to current flow further, specialized conductors were designed, including DBS (drawn brazed strand)[176] and DFT (drawn filled tube) designs. These wires were composed of a central core of highly conductive material, such as silver, surrounded by a more durable corrosion-resistant material, such as MP35N (see

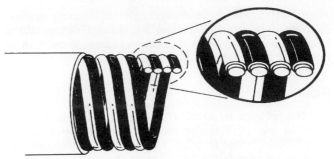

Figure 4–16. Schematic representation of single-coil multiconductor technology. Each conductor strand is individually coated with a thin layer of insulator. The multiconductor single helical coil is then insulated again with a thicker conventional insulator. (Courtesy of Telectronics, a division of St. Jude Medical, Sylmar, CA.)

Fig. 4–15). The resistance of such conductors may be only several ohms and less than 10% of MP35N alone. Modern conductors undergo intense fatigue and fracture testing by continual bending of the lead to a specific angle or over a specified radius. In recent years, conductor fractures have become less common, and they now represent only a small proportion of chronic pacing lead complications. The most common cause of conductor fracture in clinical practice today is related to subclavian crush injury.

Bipolar transvenous leads obviously require two conductors. The original configuration used a parallel arrangement in double-lumen insulation tubing with a single insulator surrounding both conductors. A major improvement was the coaxial design. This permits the creation of a much smaller circumference lead body with a single inner lumen for stylet control and an even distribution of insulating material around the outer conductor. The inner coil connects to the cathodal tip and is separated from the outer coil by an inner insulating tube. Such leads are only slightly thicker than unipolar designs. Because of the complexity of these designs, the long-term reliability of coaxial bipolar leads appears to be less than for unipolar leads.

The recent development of *coated wire technology* has permitted the manufacture of thin bipolar leads that have outside diameters as small as those of unipolar leads. The technique involves coating single strands of conductor wire with a thin layer of polymer insulation. Two or more conductors can be grouped together into a multifilar, single coil, which is then placed within another insulative tube to form a lead body with virtually the same flexibility and handling characteristics as a unipolar lead (Fig. 4–16). For example, with a quadrifilar coil, two of the insulated wires can be connected to the cathodal electrode, and the other two are connected to the anodal electrode of a bipolar lead. The thinness of the design should eliminate the complications seen with traditional bipolar leads, including the occurrence of subclavian crush injury and the problems associated with stiffness discussed earlier. At implantation, the leads handle like unipolar leads. For surgeons accustomed to the thicker, stiffer lead body, positioning of an atrial lead in the atrial appendage can be more difficult. Clinically, the leads in both the atrium and ventricle perform satisfactorily.[177–179] Another thin bipolar design is composed of two parallel conductors in a double-lumen silicone tubing. The cathode conductor is

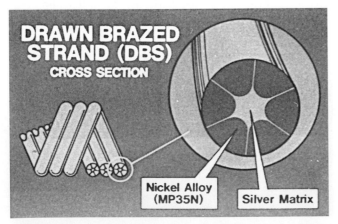

Figure 4–15. Cross-section of a drawn brazed strand lead conductor, showing the silver matrix surrounded by MP35N. (Courtesy of Medtronic, Minneapolis, MN.)

a typical multifilar nickel alloy coil, which permits passage of a stylet. The parallel anode connector is a small-diameter cabled nickel alloy wire, which has very little impact on the overall lead diameter. Early clinical experience has been encouraging.[180]

Nonmetals, such as plastics or carbon, can also be used as the conductors in pacing leads.[181] Because of the problems of conductor fracture, a *fail-safe lead* has been suggested by Green,[182] in which a standard primary conductor is surrounded by a secondary conductor medium, such as a liquid gel or paste. Because such materials are not readily available, and the leads could be difficult to manufacture and sterilize, lead manufacturers have opted to stay with and improve the reliability of the proven coil conductors.

Unlike endocardial leads, epimyocardial leads do not require a stylet for implantation. Thus, there is considerably more flexibility in the design of epicardial conductors. Most epimyocardial leads use a tinsel wire conductor. Despite this, lead conductor fractures remain a significant problem with epimyocardial leads because of the greater stresses imposed by the movement of the heart, diaphragm, and abdominal muscles. Epicardial lead fracture has been a particular problem in children.

■ LEAD INSULATION

The lead insulation extends from the lead connector to the cathode tip and, in a bipolar lead, is interrupted by the anode ring. The lead collar, used to secure the lead at the venous entry site, is usually manufactured with lead insulation material. One of the earliest insulating materials for permanent pacemaker leads was polyethylene. This material had excellent biocompatibility and reasonable biostability. As an insulator for pacing leads, however, polyethylene was stiff, thick, and difficult to bond; abraded with nonpolished metals; and had poor long-term performance.[183]

Silicone Rubber

During the 1960s, silicone rubber (MDX4-4515-50A) became popular as an insulating material for pacing leads. Although the material is highly biocompatible and biostable, it has relatively low tear strength and could be easily damaged during surgery using sharp instruments or tight ligatures. To compensate for the relatively low tear strength of silicone rubber, a thick layer of insulation was required, making the lead diameter considerably larger than that of leads designed with polyethylene. Another disadvantage of silicone rubber is its high coefficient of friction, making it difficult to pass one lead over another during implantation of two leads for dual-chamber pacing. This potential disadvantage of silicone rubber has been overcome by the technique of surface polishing or coating the lead with a highly lubricous material called *fast-pass coating*. During the late 1970s, a stronger and tougher high-performance silicone rubber insulator (ETR Q747-50A) was introduced that allowed the manufacture of thinner silicone rubber leads. Lead manipulation, however, could be difficult because of the tendency for the insulator to stretch or elongate if the lead was pulled back after entrapment in the trabeculae or chordae. The stiffening stylet was then unable to reach the tip of the lead if further manipulation was required.

Polyurethanes

Polyurethane, a generic name for a large family of synthetic polymers, was introduced as an insulating material for transvenous pacing leads in 1978.[184] As a group, the polyurethanes exhibit high tensile and tear strengths, flexibility, and a low coefficient of friction when wetted with blood.[185] Polyurethanes, when compared with silicone rubber, have more than an 18-fold lower friction coefficient, making them much easier to insert and pass along venous channels.[186] Their other advantages include biocompatibility, noncarcinogenicity, and low thrombogenicity, much like silicone rubber.[187] Unfortunately, many polyurethanes rapidly degrade in the body as a result of enzymatic activity. Others cannot be extruded and injection molded into insulation tubing that is suitable for pacing leads. One group, Pellethane 2363 (Upjohn Co., CPR Division, Torrance, CA) was found to be biostable and suitable for pacing lead insulation.

The properties of polyurethanes vary according to the *soft* and *hard* segments of the polymer molecular chain. The soft segments are composed of polyether or polyester chains and the hard segments of urea or urethanes. Structurally, segmented polyurethanes are composed of a core of hard segments surrounded by soft skin made up of soft segments. The hard and soft segments are thermodynamically immiscible, thus tending to separate. It is this structural feature that determines the mechanical and surface properties of polyurethane.[188]

Because it was possible to manufacture thin polyurethane insulating tubing suitable for pacing leads, polyurethane leads became extremely popular. By 1981, however, a number of disturbing reports appeared, questioning the long-term integrity and reliability of this insulating material. These reports described in vivo degradation of implanted polyurethane, with surface cracking and subsequent insulation failure.[189–194]

Polyurethane Failure Mechanisms

Continuing research revealed that some polyurethane insulation failures were at least in part related to specific manufacturing processes in certain leads using the polyurethane insulating material Pellethane 80A. The tendency of the hard and soft segments to separate creates inherent stresses in segmented polyurethanes.[188] These in turn can be intensified during manufacture and in particular during the cooling process after extrusion. Here, the molten polymer is forced through a die or into a mold, after which it is rapidly cooled. Polyurethane tubing manufactured by the extrusion technique causes the surface molecules to cool quickly and thus contract, resulting in considerable surface tension. At the same time, the core molecules remain hot and therefore in compression. The result is the creation of a zero stress boundary or neutral axis between the surface and the core, the depth of which depends on the manufacturing process.[191] The final result of this process is surface cracking or crazing of the polyurethane. The cracking and crazing can be further exacerbated by continuing lead manufacturing such as expansion and shrinking of the insulator during the conductor coil insertion,[195] stretching and bonding, as well as surface trauma during and after implantation. In the biologically corrosive environment of the human body, lipid and protein may deposit onto the damaged polyurethane, causing swelling that disrupts the surface organization.[191] This continuing insulation degradation process, referred to as *environmental stress cracking* (ESC), may lead to insulation failure when the cracking propagates through the full thickness of the insulator to the conductor.

Explanted leads using Pellethane 80A insulation have demonstrated varying degrees of ESC. The most minor and common change is referred to as *surface frosting* and appears as a whitish haze. This does not result in functional clinical insulation failure. The crack depth is typically 2.5 to 30 μm and is worst in areas subjected to applied strains either during manufacture or implantation.[191] With time, in the presence of environmental stresses, this may progress to insulation failure. A more significant ESC change seen in explanted leads occurs in areas where excessive strains are applied during manufacture or at implantation, such as close to the lead connector (Fig. 4–17) or where ligatures are placed around the lead.[48] This change may also occur where the lead insulation sits between the clavicle and first rib when the lead is introduced by subclavian puncture.[46, 47] Although the subclavian venous access route is frequently blamed for the failure of polyurethane leads, there is nevertheless a high failure rate when the cephalic vein is used and when care is taken with ligatures around the suture collar.[196] Severe frosting may also be seen in intracardiac portions of the lead extracted for other reasons. Such patches may occur where the lead turns to enter the right ventricle from the right atrium. In these areas, endocardial tunnels may form around the lead, where contact is made with the inner wall of the heart, resulting in excessive stresses on the insulation. It is likely, therefore, that those intracardiac sites may also be responsible for insulation failures.

Metal-induced oxidation (MIO) is another reported mechanism of insulation failure. MIO is a process of oxidative degradation of the polyurethane insulation and involves a reaction of the polymer with oxygen that is believed to be released by hydrogen peroxide, which comes from inflammatory cells on the outer surface of the lead.[197] For the reaction to occur, a catalyst is required. These catalysts are

probably metallic corrosion products from the conductor, which accumulate after ingress of body fluids onto the lead.[195] Although this fluid may come from breakdown of the insulation, fluid ingress has also been reported with breakdown of the bonding at the electrode-insulation junction and with stylet perforation during implantation.[198] Clinically, there may be failure of the insulation of unipolar leads or both the inner and outer insulation of bipolar leads. To minimize MIO, conductors can be barrier coated.[43] The objective is to cover the conductor coil with a submicroscopic layer of platinum, which is inert and minimizes the potential for metal ion release and hence interaction with the insulation materials.[199]

As a result of the information gathered on the causes and mechanisms of ESC and MIO, manufacturing changes were instituted to overcome the problems found with the polyurethane Pellethane 80A.[200] Despite this, questionable long-term implant performance continues to plague some of the more recent generations of bipolar leads that use the same Pellethane 80A polyurethane.[43, 196, 201–205] Unipolar leads have not shown an increased incidence of insulation problems, apart from those caused by trauma at surgery or at ligature sites.[206–208] Unipolar leads insulated with Pellethane 80A probably suffer the same degradation of the insulating material. The difference between unipolar and bipolar leads insulated with this material is that there are generally no clinical consequences to insulation failure with unipolar leads; bipolar leads, in contrast, may develop a complete short, resulting in loss of pacing and sensing.

Most available polyurethane-insulated leads use Pellethane 55D. This polyurethane is stiffer and harder than Pellethane 80A because it has significantly fewer polyether segments.[209] Pacing leads using Pellethane 55D insulation are consequently much stiffer than those of a similar size using Pellethane 80A and can therefore be more prone to perforation of the right ventricle.[39] Long-term clinical results of Pellethane 55D have shown its improved biostability performance over Pellethane 80A.[44, 210, 211]

Questions remain about whether a polyurethane controversy still exists. Early-model Pellethane 80A–insulated leads demonstrated unacceptable clinical failure rates as a result of well-recognized problems with the insulation. Only time will tell whether these problems with Pellethane 80A can be corrected. Pellethane 55D–insulated leads, however, are free of the degradation problems of Pellethane 80A–insulated leads, but the stiffness of the Pellethane 55D leads makes them more prone to right ventricular perforation. They may be suitable, however, for use in the atrium. Ongoing reports of Pellethane 80A lead failures are still appearing in the literature and are not specific to manufacturer.[212] Table 4–2 provides a comparison of the physical parameters of the types of silicone rubber and polyurethane used as insulators in pacing leads.

New varieties of polyurethane are continually being investigated, and combinations of silicone rubber and polyurethane may be clinically acceptable. The major body of the lead may be composed of polyurethane, but at the distal end, where the lead lies inside the ventricle, the insulation may be a softer silicone rubber. Another alternative is to place a barrier of silicone rubber or other materials between the polyurethane and the conductor. The silicone rubber and polyurethane combinations may also be composed of a thin,

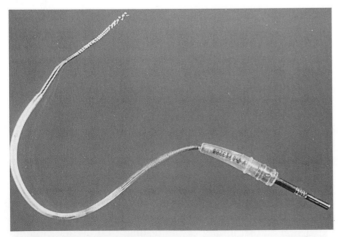

Figure 4–17. Proximal end of a transvenous, polyurethane-insulated lead demonstrating marked crazing, shown as dense white patches on the insulator surface. This bipolar lead also has a unique in-line connector, which is not low profile.

Table 4–2. **Lead Insulator Comparisons**

Physical Parameters	Common Insulation Types			
	Polyurethane Pellethane 2362-80A	Polyurethane Pellethane 2362-55D	Silicone Rubber MDX4-4515-50A	Silicone Rubber ERT Q747-50A
Durometer hardness	82A	55D	52A	50A
Ultimate tensile strength (psi)	4500	6900	1350	1300
Ultimate elongation (%)	550	390	450	900
Tear strength (psi)	470	650	80	230

tough protective outer coating of polyurethane over thin high-performance silicone rubber in a coaxial arrangement.[200]

J-Shaped Retention Wire Fracture

The most publicized lead controversy in recent years has surrounded the Accufix/Encor leads. This type of controversy is unique in lead technology and is indirectly related to lead insulation. In 1988, the Cordis Corporation of Miami developed and marketed a J-shaped atrial-appendage active-fixation lead (the 329-701). During this period, the company was purchased by Telectronics of Sydney, Australia, and to conform to the IS-1 BI standard (see later discussion), the lead connector was modified, renamed the Accufix 330-801, and approved by the United States Food and Drug Administration. Between 1988 and 1994, an estimated 40,860 of these leads were implanted worldwide. During late 1994, a small number of the active-fixation, steroid-eluting collar-design leads, the Accufix DEC 033-812, were also implanted.

During November 1994, Telectronics issued a worldwide voluntary recall and safety alert on all these lead models because of reports of fracture of a memory retention wire used to maintain the J shape. The electrically inert, 8.75-cm J-shaped retention wire lies deep to the outer insulation, is welded at its distal end to the anodal band, and is free at its proximal end (Fig. 4–18). Retention wire fracture does not appear to interrupt normal lead function. Once fractured, the ends of the retention wire can perforate and protrude through the lead insulation and migrate outside the lead, damaging surrounding intracardiac and extracardiac tissues (Fig. 4–19). Deaths from cardiac and vascular tears have been reported. In addition, the J-shaped retention wire can embolize to the pulmonary circulation.

Immediately after the voluntary safety alert, Telectronics established a Physician Advisory Committee to formulate patient management protocols. To achieve this, an international multicenter study was initiated to determine the incidence and severity of the fracture problem using chest radiographs and later cardiac fluoroscopy. These ongoing studies, comprising 1865 patients in the multicenter study and elsewhere, have been the most extensive, thorough, and expensive pacemaker investigations ever undertaken.[213] With the sale of Telectronics to St. Jude Medical (St. Paul, MN) in 1997, the Accufix Research Institute was established to continue monitoring the problem.

One of the first reports from the Physician Advisory Committee classified the fluoroscopy appearances into four groups and recommended management according to these appearances and other risk factors (Table 4–3). The other risk factors included the following:

Patient age and gender: Unless there are overriding comorbidities, patients younger than 40 years of age should have the lead extracted. The older the patient, the greater the risk associated with lead extraction. Elderly frail women are at greatest risk.

Implantation date: The longer the implantation time, the higher the risk of retention wire fracture.

Fluoroscopic appearance: Leads with a more open J shape are at a higher risk of retention wire fracture.

There are potential risks associated with monitoring patients by fluoroscopic examination. Young patients facing a lifetime of fluoroscopic examinations may develop cumulative effects from the irradiation. There is also a risk

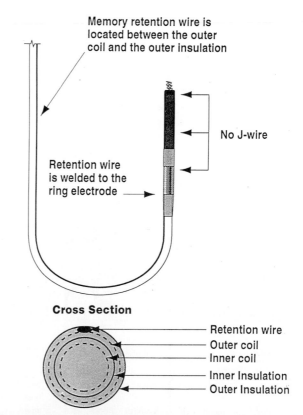

Figure 4–18. Schematic diagram of a bipolar Telectronics Accufix lead to show the J-shaped memory retention wire, welded to the anode ring and lying between the outer coil and the outer insulation. (Courtesy of Accufix Research Institute, Sydney, Australia.)

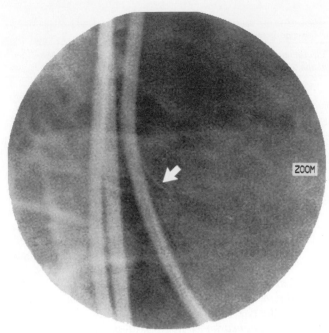

Figure 4–19. Cardiac fluoroscopic image of an implanted Telectronics Accufix lead, to demonstrate a fracture in the J-shaped memory retention wire, with one of the fractured ends having perforated the insulation and migrated out into the right atrial cavity (group IV). (Courtesy of Accufix Research Institute, Sydney, Australia.)

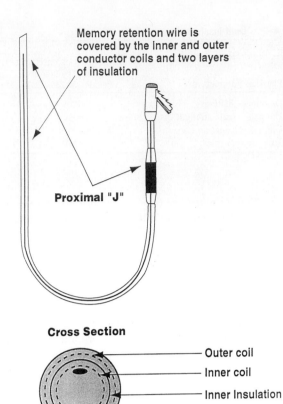

Figure 4–20. Schematic diagram of a bipolar Telectronics Encor lead to show the J-shaped memory retention wire, which extends to the distal electrode and lies deep to inner coil.

(<1% per month) of progressing from "no fracture" to any other fracture group between screenings. Progression from no fracture to cardiac tamponade in 2 weeks has been reported. On the basis of the results of fluoroscopic screenings in the multicenter study, the rate of progression from group I to a higher group is 2% per 6-month interval, after the initial screening. The rate of progression from group II to a higher group is 5.5% per 6-month interval, and it appears that the incidence is *not* decreasing.[213–216]

As of September 1998, a total of 39 retention wire injuries had been reported. Six cases were fatal. The median time from implantation to injury was 27 months. The main clinical presentation has been pericardial effusion and cardiac tamponade. Other trauma have included intracardiac thrombosis and pulmonary embolism,[217] tricuspid valve laceration, aortic erosion, and migration of fractured retention wire, particularly to the lungs.[213, 218]

Of particular concern is the incidence of lead extraction complications. By May 1998, a total of 113 major intravascular extraction complications had been reported. In 15 cases, the complications were fatal. Serious injuries have included tearing of the atrium, subclavian vein, and superior vena cava.[213]

The J-shaped retention wire is not unique to the Accufix family of active-fixation leads. The unipolar and bipolar J-shaped passive-fixation tined Encor leads also have J-shaped retention wires. Unlike the Accufix leads, in which the retention wire was located immediately deep to the outer insulation, the retention wire in the Encor models lies within the cathode conductor (Fig. 4–20). The design of the Encor

Table 4–3. Classification of Fluoroscopic Appearance of Telectronics Accufix Lead Models with J-Shaped Retention Wires

Life Expectancy	Fracture Classification			
	Group I	*Group II*	*Group III*	*Group IV*
	No fracture suspected	Fracture suspected; wire does not protrude through the outer insulation	Fracture suspected; wire protrudes through the outer insulation	Fracture suspected; a fragment of wire has migrated from the lead.
Longer* (younger or those with no comorbidities)	Monitor or consider extraction	Strongly consider extraction	Strongly consider extraction	Evaluate on a case-by-case basis
Shorter (elderly or those with comorbidities)	Monitor	Monitor or consider extraction	Evaluate on a case-by-case basis	Evaluate on a case-by-case basis

*For patients <40 yr of age, strongly consider extraction unless comorbidities provide a contraindication.

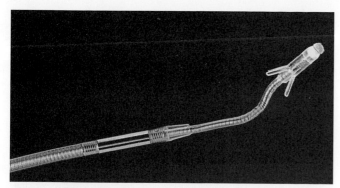

Figure 4–21. Telectronics Encor DEC lead, removed at the time of initial implantation, because of a deformity seen under fluoroscopy at the distal end of the lead. The implantation was difficult, and the lead deformity probably occurred while passing the lead through an introducer. It was this type of lead trauma at implantation that resulted in the memory retention wire deformity and ultimately fracture.

retention wire varies among specific models but is longer than that in the Accufix leads (about 11.6 cm) and extends from its attachment to the cathode proximally. The reason for the differences among the lead designs relates to the action of the Accufix screwdriver stylet, which would be ineffective if the retention wire were located deep to the cathodal conductor. Fracture and protrusion associated with the bipolar Encor retention wire appear to be related to the way the lead is implanted (Fig. 4–21). Between 1984 and 1995, about 23,540 bipolar Encor leads were distributed worldwide. Fluoroscopy is recommended on at least one occasion to visualize the J shape and the distal end of the lead. Five classes (A to E) are recognized to determine the status of the retention wire, and the terms *straight, curved, kinked,* and *severed* are used to define the contour of the interclectrode region of the lead.

By August 1997, 37 protrusions had been identified, and there had been one fatal injury and eight nonfatal complications. Six major extraction complications had been reported, but no reports of retention wire protrusion had been made with the unipolar Encor lead models.[213]

Unlike all other mechanical pacing lead failures, the Accufix and Encor problem necessitates possible lead extraction rather than abandonment. After the initial medical and media outcry, the Accufix and Encor saga settled into a well-organized routine of follow-up and extraction. However, this was not before a run of unnecessary lead extractions in elderly group I patients, who experienced a high incidence of complications, including death.[219]

■ SINGLE-PASS LEADS

With the popularity of dual-chamber pacing, it was not surprising that a single lead pacing system would be developed to overcome the need for two separate leads. By definition, a single-pass lead incorporates both the atrial and ventricular leads within a single lead body.[220] The main limiting factor of a single-pass lead is the necessity for the atrial electrode to make contact with the atrial wall to permit atrial pacing. Attempts over the years to pace both the atrium and the ventricle with a single lead produced a variety of exotic,

cumbersome, and frightening designs, none of which were accepted commercially.[221–223] Because of this, most single-pass leads are suitable only for atrial sensing with the atrial-synchronous, ventricular pacing mode (VDD). The development of the modern bipolar, single-pass lead has had a long and extensive evolution, the technical aspects of which have been comprehensively documented by Antonioli.[224] There are now a number of well-established requirements for successful VDD pacing.[224] These include the following:

Patient selection: High-degree atrioventricular block with normal sinoatrial function. Sinus bradycardia below the low rate of the pacemaker may result in the pacemaker syndrome because the VDD pacing mode is actually VVI pacing at the lower rate limit. A normal right atrial size and no supraventricular tachyarrhythmias are desirable.

Implantation procedures: The atrial dipole should lie close to the middle to high atrial wall to permit acceptable bipolar atrial sensing. Considerable work has gone into the development of the ideal bipolar atrial dipole for these leads, which is between 5 and 10 mm.

Programming: VDD pulse generators suitable for single-pass leads require a wide range of atrial sensitivity settings, postventricular atrial refractory periods, and atrioventricular delays. The low rate must be lower than the sinus rate to prevent pacemaker syndrome. It is this concern that limits the use of single-pass VDD pacing.[225]

With the widespread use of single-pass leads, favorable reports on long-term[226] and pediatric[227] use have been published. Another advance involves the use of a steroid-eluting ventricular electrode.[228]

Despite the initial lack of success, the search for a single-pass lead with atrial pacing capabilities (DDD) continues. A single-pass tined, single-stylet lead with an atrial J-shaped component activated by stylet withdrawal, after the distal ventricular component is positioned, is undergoing preclinical evaluation.[229] Another intriguing design has a distal active-fixation atrial electrode, and the body of the lead is looped through the tricuspid valve. The proximal ring electrode lies against the ventricular endocardium.[230]

Questions remain about whether an intra-atrial floating bipolar electrode can be used to pace the atrium consistently at a reasonable stimulation threshold, to overcome the limitations of VDD pacing, and to widen the indications for available single-pass leads. In a study using single-pass leads and standard atrial pacing techniques, just over half of the patients had effective atrial stimulation in the upright position, but the stimulation thresholds were high, and there was a significant incidence of side effects.[231] A new stimulation technique involves a novel form of overlapping biphasic pulses on a bipolar two-ring atrial electrode.[232, 233] The first unipolar square wave pulse is applied to the distal electrode and is positive. The second pulse, which is negative, is applied to the proximal electrode, and the delay between the two pulses, which is programmable, is from 0 to 1 msec. Care must be taken in choosing the lead with the most appropriate distance between the atrial and unipolar ventricular electrodes. Early results indicate chronic stimulation thresholds in excess of those desirable for chronic long-term atrial pacing. Possible troublesome complications include loss of atrial pacing during inspiration and stimulation of the diaphragm.[225] Such complications may be of less concern with temporary pacing.[234]

■ LEAD CONNECTORS

The lead connector connects the lead to the pulse generator. The original pacing leads had no specialized connector. A small area of conductor at the proximal end was exposed and attached directly to the pulse generator using a small set-screw.[235] On occasion, the set-screw had a sharp cutting end, and exposure of the conductor was not necessary. This was tedious, time-consuming, and unreliable. Consequently, a proliferation of unique connectors was developed. Eventually two similar and reliable unipolar connector designs emerged, one 5 mm in diameter and the other 6 mm. Both required an appropriate pulse generator connector port, although the smaller size could be adapted to fit the larger. For bipolar pacing, two unipolar connectors were necessary.

A major improvement in lead connectors was the low-profile, in-line bipolar design. An in-line connector places both electrical terminals on a single lead pin, with an insulating barrier separating the anode from the cathode. Because it was crucial to prevent short circuiting between the terminals, a number of unique designs was introduced during the early 1980s. These designs were not always low in profile and were in some cases cumbersome (see Fig. 4–17). With unique in-line designs, it was difficult or impossible to modify the connector to suit pulse generators for which it is not designed. The connector and pulse generator compatibility problem became a major clinical concern, particularly during pulse generator replacement. In some cases, large and unreliable adaptors were used, but on other occasions a new lead was required. Not surprisingly, a plea for standardization was made.[236-238]

With the initial impetus coming from the German Pacing Group, pacemaker manufacturers were urged to develop a low-profile, in-line connector standard that would be suitable for both unipolar and bipolar leads.[239] Early progress was slow, because of the concern that a connector standard would be enforced without regard to future evolutionary developments. This would restrict future innovation in lead and pulse generator design, rather than enhance it.[240]

By late 1985, a low-profile 3.2-mm unipolar and bipolar pacemaker lead connector designated Voluntary Standard #1, or VS•1, was ratified.[241] Pacemaker intercompany rivalry, however, resulted in three variations of lead connector and pulse generator connector cavity variations: the VS•1, VS•1A, and VS•1B. Not surprisingly, these variations were not totally interchangeable. The differences were mainly related to bipolar leads and concerned the length of the lead connector pin and the presence or absence of sealing rings on the lead (Fig. 4–22). A VS•1 standard specifies sealing rings on the lead; VS•1A is similar, but the lead pin is longer, as is the receiving port in the pulse generator. The receiving port of the VS•1B pulse generator has both sealing rings and a long receiving port. Although a long connector pin (VS•1A or VS•1B) fits into the short receiving port of the VS•1 pulse generator, the proximal anodal ring contact of the connector may not mate correctly with the anodal terminal of the pulse generator. As a consequence, bipolar pacing and sensing may not be possible. To many pacemaker implantation surgeons, these subtle differences were not ob-

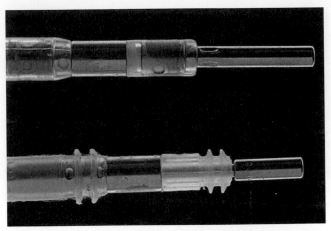

Figure 4–22. *Top,* 3.2-mm VS•1B lead connector with long connector pin and no sealing rings. Sealing rings are required in the pulse generator. *Bottom,* IS-1 lead connector. Note the short lead pin and sealing rings. (Courtesy of Medtronic, Minneapolis, MN.)

vious until confronted with lead and pulse generator incompatibility either perioperatively or postoperatively during pacemaker testing. Such errors are expensive and potentially hazardous to the patient.

Sealing rings are an integral part of the insulating mechanism of low-profile in-line connectors. They do not need to be on the lead connector; they can also reside within the receiving port of the pulse generator. Engineering principles usually demand that sealing rings, which could be damaged, should reside on the component to be replaced, in most cases the pulse generator. A pulse generator connector block with sealing rings, however, is significantly larger than one without them.

With these controversies in mind, a joint IEC and International Standards Organization (ISO) International Pacemaker Standards Working Group (ISO TC150/SC2/WG2 and IEC 62D/WG6) set about to define a formal international connector standard. The VS•1 lead connector design was adapted by the group to yield a standard that called for a low-profile connector with sealing rings on the lead, with the option of having additional sealing rings inside the pulse generator connector cavity. This final standard, designated IS-1 UNI for unipolar leads and IS-1 BI for bipolar leads, is now the official international lead connector standard (see Fig. 4–22).

To help with the problem of VS•1 and IS-1 incompatibility, there is flexibility for the manufacturers of pulse generators in respect to the length of the bore for the lead pin within the connector cavity and the presence or absence of sealing rings in the connector cavity. Therefore, before pulse generator replacement, the implantation surgeon must check the compatibility of the implanted lead and the proposed pulse generator.

In addition, the IS-1 standard calls for unipolar and bipolar lead connectors to be interchangeable. To prevent a unipolar lead from being inadvertently attached to a bipolar nonpolarity programmable pulse generator, the labeling for both lead and pulse generator must be carefully inspected. To prevent damage to a unipolar IS-1 lead connector from the anode set-screw of a bipolar connector, a protective ring may be present over the unipolar lead connector at the

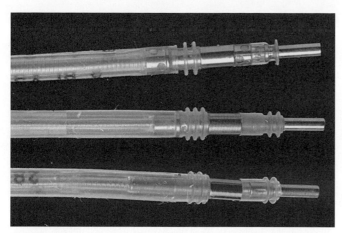

Figure 4–23. Three lead connectors to demonstrate the similarity between unipolar and bipolar IS-1 connectors. With unipolar connectors, there is an anodized protective ring to prevent the anodal set-screw of a bipolar pulse generator from damaging the connector. *Top,* bipolar. *Middle,* unipolar. *Bottom,* unipolar. (*Top* and *bottom,* courtesy of Telectronics, a division of St. Jude Medical, Sylmar, CA; *middle,* courtesy of Medtronic, Minneapolis, MN.)

appropriate position (Fig. 4–23). This ring, however, may be mistaken for a true anode terminal and the lead regarded as bipolar. Although the manufacturer's intentions are good, the results at surgery may be potentially disastrous. In terms of backward compatibility of the IS-1 leads to older pulse generators, unipolar and bipolar low-profile connectors can be easily converted to the standard 5-mm unipolar design by the use of a sleeve.

■ CORONARY SINUS PACING

Atrial pacing from the coronary sinus using specialized pacing leads was reported as early as the 1960s.[242, 243] With the development of specialized automatic tachycardia reversion pacing systems in the early 1980s, the placement of leads in the atria became critical. To interrupt a re-entry circuit in the left atrium, the lead was required to be positioned near the mouth of the coronary sinus, and thus an interest developed once again in this form of pacing. For a permanent pacing lead to be positioned in the coronary sinus, the cathode should lie about 4 cm behind the tip of the lead and have a 60-degree angle behind that. The lead between the tip and the cathode is stiffened, usually with conductor coil (Fig. 4–24). In this way, the lead lies within the body of the coronary sinus, with the tip at the entrance of the great cardiac vein and the cathode close to the coronary sinus orifice.[243] Although most of these early leads were unipolar, bipolar versions were available with variable interelectrode spacing.[244]

Despite the minor resurgence in coronary sinus pacing in the 1980s, this form of pacing never became established once right atrial appendage and active-fixation leads became popular. A number of significant problems was also reported. Pacing thresholds were frequently elevated both at implantation and over the long term because the electrode did not make contact with the sinus wall. Frequently, both the atrial and ventricular electrograms were sensed, leading to inap-

propriately slow atrial pacing. Because there was no fixation device, the lead and cathode could move during the cardiac and respiratory cycles, leading to alternate pacing in the atrium and ventricle.[244] Coronary sinus perforation and pericardial tamponade were also reported.[245]

With the more recent interest in biatrial pacing, there has been a resurrection of coronary sinus pacing in a number of centers in Europe and the United States. One recent design uses a distal cathode with two 45-degree angles, one behind the anode and the other immediately behind the tip of the cathode.[246] The purpose of these angles is to enable close contact of the cathode and the sinus wall. There has been experience in placement of this lead in the distal, middle, and proximal coronary sinus; however, because of dislodgment, only middle or distal placement is recommended.[246]

The coronary sinus has also been used for biventricular pacing. Using a standard lead, distal cathodal pacing with the lead pushed as far as possible into the coronary sinus results in left ventricular pacing through the great cardiac vein.[247] This principle has been used to establish biventricular pacing with the other lead in the right ventricle. Great cardiac vein placement is technically difficult and time-consuming, and both specially designed and standard leads have been used.[248–250]

Because current dual-chamber pulse generators cannot accept more than two pacing leads, the use of complicated dual-chamber pacing systems with three or four transvenous leads introduces a number of unresolved problems with pacing hardware. Pacing either the atria or ventricles from two sites (biatrial and biventricular if both, or bifocal if in the same chamber) can be achieved using a DDD pulse generator and a very short atrioventricular delay. These systems, however, become complicated when dual-chamber atrioventricular pacing is required. One system uses one lead as the cathode, and the other has the anode connected to the pulse generator by a Y-shaped connector. This does not necessarily produce reliable pacing of both chambers because of anodal high-threshold exit block. Although much work is being done in this regard, appropriate Y-shaped adapters have not been designed.[249] The resurgence of interest in coronary sinus lead placement is an exciting new development in physiologic pacing. Its success, however, awaits the design of new, complicated pulse generator connector blocks that are able to accept three or four pacing leads.

■ CONCLUSIONS

Remarkable advances have been made in the design of pacing leads. The most important change has been the devel-

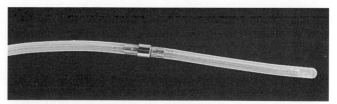

Figure 4–24. Unipolar coronary sinus lead. The cathode lies about 4 cm from the tip of the lead. Note that the conductor and hence the stylet pass through the cathode to the tip of the lead. This allows the tip of the lead to be rigid during placement and semirigid after placement. (Courtesy of Cordis, Miami, a division of Telectronics, St. Jude Medical, Sylmar, CA.)

opment of small, porous, steroid-eluting electrodes that provide extremely low chronic stimulation thresholds and that have low polarization characteristics. It is important to remember the less heralded advances in conductor and insulator technology. These advances have resulted in safer, more reliable leads. In addition, the remarkable international and intercompany cooperation in the development of the IS-1 lead connector standard has been a major improvement in the clinical practice of cardiac pacing. Future developments in pacing leads are likely to occur in the placement of leads in branches of the coronary venous circulation for pacing nontraditional pacing sites, further refinements in high-impedance electrodes, and greater attention to lead extractibility.

REFERENCES

1. Mond HG: Unipolar versus bipolar pacing: Poles apart. PACE 14:1411, 1991.
2. Mond H, Strathmore N, Hunt P, et al: Bipolar and unipolar permanent pacing leads: Which is superior? PACE 12:678, 1989.
3. Barold SS, Gaidula JJ: Failure of demand pacemaker from low-voltage bipolar ventricular electrograms. JAMA 215:923, 1971.
4. Yates JD, Preston TA: Failure of demand function in temporary epicardial bipolar pacemaker systems. Ann Thorac Surg 15:135, 1973.
5. Breivik K, Ohm O-J, Engedal H: Long-term comparison of unipolar and bipolar pacing and sensing, using a new multiprogrammable pacemaker system. PACE 6:592, 1983.
6. Czermin J, Kaliman J, Laczovics A, et al: Unipolar versus bipolar pacing: A prospective, intra-patient, long-term study. PACE 10:663, 1987.
7. Binner L, Richter P, Wieshammer S, et al: Bipolar versus unipolar mode in dual chamber pacing: Comparison of myopotential interference, acute and long-term pacing and sensing thresholds. PACE 10:646, 1987.
8. DeCaprio V, Hurzeler P, Furman S: A comparison of unipolar and bipolar electrograms for cardiac pacemaker sensing. Circulation 56:750, 1977.
9. Klementowicz P, Andrews C, Furman S: Superior bipolar sensing: A prospective study. J Am Coll Cardiol 9:31A, 1987.
10. Masterson M, Yuzcu EM, Maloney JD, et al: Atrial pacing and sensing: Unipolar versus bipolar. Seven different leads compared. PACE 10:435, 1987.
11. De Boer H, Kofflard M, Scholtes T, et al: Differential bipolar sensing of a dual chamber pacemaker. PACE 11:158, 1988.
12. Griffin JC: Sensing characteristics of the right atrial appendage electrode. PACE 6:22, 1983.
13. Mond H, Barold SS: Dual chamber, rate-adaptive pacing in patients with paroxymal supraventricular tachyarrhythmias: Protective measures for rate control. PACE 16:2168, 1993.
14. Levine PA, Venditti FJ, Podrid PJ, et al: Therapeutic and diagnostic benefits of intentional crosstalk mediated ventricular output inhibition. PACE 11:1194, 1988.
15. Young TE, Byrd CL, Winn CM, et al: Crosstalk update in state-of-the-art pacemakers. PACE 8:791, 1985.
16. Irwin M, Cameron D, Louis C, et al: Crosstalk-stimulation of the ventricle in the implanted dual unipolar system. PACE 11:508, 1988.
17. Reynolds D, Combs W, Bennett T: "Crosstalk" in bipolar DDD pacemakers. PACE 10:734, 1987.
18. Midei MG, Levine JH, Walford GD, et al: Incidence of myopotential interference and crosstalk inhibition in unipolar and bipolar dual chamber pacemakers. PACE 10:1010, 1987.
19. Sweesy MW, Batey RL, Forney RC: Crosstalk during bipolar pacing. PACE 11:1512, 1988.
20. Combs WJ, Reynolds DW, Sharma AD, et al: Cross-talk in bipolar pacemakers. PACE 12:1613, 1989.
21. Byrd CL, Schwartz SJ, Gonzales M, et al: Rate responsive pacemakers and crosstalk. PACE 11:798, 1988.
22. Barold SS, Falkoff MD, Ong LS, et al: Arrhythmias caused by dual-chambered pacing. In Steinbach K, Glogar D, Laszkovics A, et al (eds): Cardiac Pacing. Proceedings of the Seventh World Symposium on Cardiac Pacing. Vienna, Darmstadt, Steinkopff Verlag, 1983, p 505.
23. Barold SS, Falkoff MD, Ong LS, et al: Timing cycles of DDD
pacemakers. In Barold SS, Mugica J, (eds): New Perspectives in Cardiac Pacing. Mount Kisco, NY, Futura, 1988, p 69.
24. Mymin D, Cuddy TE, Sinha SN, et al: Inhibition of demand pacemakers by skeletal muscle potentials. JAMA 223:527, 1973.
25. Ohm O-J, Bruland H, Pederson OM, et al: Interference effect of myopotentials on function of unipolar demand pacemakers. Br Heart J 36:77, 1974.
26. Redd R, McAnulty J, Phillips S, et al: Demand pacemaker inhibition by isometric skeletal muscle contraction. Circulation 49(Suppl 3):241, 1974.
27. Gribbin B, Abson CP, Clarke LM: Inhibition of external demand pacemakers during muscular activity. Br Heart J 36:1210, 1974.
28. Anderson ST, Pitt A, Whitford JA: Interference with function of unipolar pacemaker due to muscle potentials. J Thorac Cardiovasc Surg 71:698, 1976.
29. Jacobs LJ, Kerzner JS, Diamond MA, et al: Myopotential inhibition of demand pacemakers: Detection by ambulatory electrocardiography. Am Heart J 101:346, 1981.
30. Jacobs LJ, Kerzner JS, Diamond MA: Pacemaker inhibition by myopotentials detected by Holter monitoring. PACE 5:30, 1982.
31. Furman S: Electromagnetic interference. PACE 5:1, 1982.
32. Hauser RG: Bipolar leads for cardiac pacing in the 1980s: A reappraisal provoked by skeletal muscle interference. PACE 5:34, 1982.
33. Secemsky SI, Hauser RG, Denes P, et al: Unipolar sensing abnormalities: Incidence and clinical significance of skeletal muscle interference and undersensing in 228 patients. PACE 5:10, 1982.
34. Echeverria HJ, Luceri RM, Thurber RJ, et al: Myopotential inhibition of unipolar AV sequential (DVI) pacemaker. PACE 5:20, 1982.
35. Fetter J, Hall D, Hoff GL, et al: The effects of myopotential interference on unipolar and bipolar dual chamber pacemakers in the DDD mode. Clin Prog Electrophysiol Pacing 3:368, 1985.
36. Zimmern SH, Clark MF, Austin WK, et al: Characteristics and clinical effects of myopotential signals in a unipolar DDD pacemaker population. PACE 9:1019, 1986.
37. Exworthy KW: Electromagnetic compatibility of pacemaker systems. In Meere C (ed): Proceedings of the Sixth World Symposium on Cardiac Pacing. Montreal, 1979, Chap. 35-7.
38. Reis R: Potential interference with medical electronic devices. Bull N Y Acad Med 55:1216, 1979.
39. Cameron J, Ciddor G, Mond H, et al: Stiffness of the distal tip of bipolar pacemaker leads. PACE 13:1915, 1990.
40. Merx W, Han J, Yoon M: Effects of unipolar cathodal and bipolar stimulation of vulnerability of ischemic ventricles to fibrillation. Am J Cardiol 35:37, 1975.
41. Weiss DN, Zilo P, Luceri RM, et al: Should unipolar pacemaker leads be banned? Lessons from pacemaker/implantable cardioverter defibrillator interactions. PACE 20:237, 1997.
42. Molajo AO, Burgess L: Comparison of paced evoked response sensing of transvenous porous platinum ventricular leads during unipolar and bipolar pacing. PACE 12:678, 1989.
43. Medtronic, Inc: Product performance report. September 1997.
44. Furman S, Benedek ZM, and the Implantable Lead Registry: Survival of implantable pacemaker leads. PACE 13:1910, 1990.
45. Hayes DL: Pacemaker polarity configuration: What is best for the patient? PACE 15:1099, 1992.
46. Jacobs DM, Fink AS, Miller RP, et al: Anatomical and morphological evaluation of pacemaker lead compression. PACE 16:434, 1993.
47. Magney JE, Flynn DM, Parsons JA, et al: Anatomical mechanisms explaining damage to pacemaker leads, defibrillator leads, and failure of central venous catheters adjacent to the sternoclavicular joint. PACE 16:445, 1993.
48. Sweesy MW, Forney CC, Hayes DL, et al: Evaluation of an in-line bipolar poyurethane ventricular pacing lead. PACE 15:1982, 1992.
49. Mond H: The Cardiac Pacemaker: Function and Malfunction. New York, Grune & Stratton, 1973, p 60.
50. Furman S, Parker B, Escher DJW: Decreasing electrode size and increasing efficiency of cardiac stimulation. J Surg Res 11:105, 1971.
51. Smyth NPD, Tarjan PP, Chernoff E, et al: The significance of electrode surface area and stimulating thresholds in permanent cardiac pacing. J Thorac Cardiovasc Surg 71:559, 1976.
52. Lindesmans FW, Zimmerman ANE: Cardiac current, voltage, charge and energy thresholds as functions of electrode size and impulse duration. In Meere C (ed): Proceedings of the Sixth International Symposium on Cardiac Pacing. Montreal, 1979, Chap. 3.2.
53. Furman S, Garvey J, Hurzeler P: Pulse duration variation and electrode

size as factors in pacemaker longevity. J Thorac Cardiovasc Surg 69:382, 1975.

54. Barold SS, Ong LS, Heinle RA: Stimulation and sensing thresholds for cardiac pacing: Electrophysiologic and technical aspects. Prog Cardiovasc Dis 24:1, 1981.

55. Mond H, Holley L, Hirshorn M: The high impedance dish electrode: Clinical experience with a new tined lead. PACE 5:529, 1982.

56. Schuchert A, Kuck KH: Benefits of smaller electrode surface area (4 mm^2) on steroid-eluting leads. PACE 14:2098, 1991.

57. Ellenbogen KA, Wood MA, Gilligan DM, et al: Steroid-eluding high-impedance pacing leads decrease short- and long-term current drain: Results from a multicenter clinical trial. PACE 22:39, 1999.

58. Tyers GFO, Torman HA, Hughs HC Jr: Comparative studies of "state of the art" and presently used clinical cardiac pacemaker electrodes. J Thorac Cardiovas Surg 67:849, 1974.

59. Parsonnet V, Gilbert L, Lewin G, et al: A nonpolarizing electrode for endocardial stimulation of the heart. J Thorac Cardiovasc Surg 56:710, 1974.

60. Hein F, Blaser R, Thull R, et al: Electrochemical aspects of pacing electrodes (discussion). *In* Watanabe Y (ed): Cardiac Pacing. Proceedings of the Fifth International Symposium. Tokyo, Exerpta Medica, 1977, p 510.

61. Timmis GC, Helland J, Westveer DC, et al: The evolution of low threshold leads. Clin Prog Pacing Electrophysiol 1:313, 1983.

62. Amundson DC, McArthur W, Mosharrafa M: The porous endocardial electrode. PACE 2:40, 1979.

63. MacCarter DJ, Lundberg KM, Corstjens JPM: Porous electrodes: Concept, technology and results. PACE 6:427, 1983.

64. MacGregor DC, Wilson GJ, Lixfeld W, et al: The porous-surfaced electrode: A new concept in pacemaker lead design. J Thorac Cardiovasc Surg 78:281, 1979.

65. Skalsky M, McMichael A, Maddison D, et al: Evaluation of a new low polarisation, high impedance Pt/Ir coated porous 6 mm^2 dish electrode. PACE 8:788, 1985.

66. Kreyenhagen P, Helland J: Evaluation of a titanium nitride coated tip electrode. *In* Antonioli GE, Aubert AE, et al (eds): Pacemaker Leads 1991. Proceedings of the Second European Conference on Pacemaker Leads. Ferrara, Italy, Elsevier, 1991, p 451.

67. Adler S, Spehr P, Allen J, et al: Chronic animal testing of new cardiac pacing electrodes. PACE 13:1896, 1990.

68. Breivik K, Ohm O-J, Dregelid E, et al: Electrophysiological characteristics of porous electrodes versus solid ones. PACE 4:A-5, 1981.

69. Tayler D, Oakley D, Rowbotham D, et al: Comparison of a porous electrode tipped with a conventional endocardial pacing lead. PACE 4:A-76, 1981.

70. Bobyn JD, Wilson GJ, Mycyk TR, et al: Improved electrophysiological performance using a new porous-surfaced ventricular endocardial pacing electrode. PACE 4:A-82, 1981.

71. Powell L, McEachern M, Elrod P, et al: Atrial endocardial porous and non-porous electrodes: A comparative study. Clin Prog Electrophysiol Pacing 4(Suppl):41, 1986.

72. Heinemann F, Davis M, Helland J: Clinical performance of a pacing lead with a platinized target-tip electrode. PACE 7:471, 1984.

73. Djordjevic M, Stojanov P, Velimirovic D: Target lead: Low threshold electrode. PACE 9:1206, 1986.

74. Mond H, Hua W, Wang CC: Atrial pacing leads: The clinical contribution of steroid elution. PACE 18:1601, 1995.

75. Ormerod D, Walgren S, Berglund J, et al: Design and evaluation of a low threshold, porous tip lead with a mannitol coated screw-in tip ("sweet tip"). PACE 11:496, 1988.

76. Love C, Frumin H, Lundeen T, et al: Experience with a new endocardial steroid screw-in lead in atrial and ventricular applications (Pacesetter Model 1388T) [Abstract]. PACE 20:1149, 1997.

77. Karpawich PP, Stokes KB, Helland JR, et al: A new low threshold platinized epimyocardial pacing electrode: Comparative evaluation in immature canines. PACE 11:1139, 1988.

78. Hirshorn MS, Holley LK, Skalsky M, et al: Characteristics of advanced porous and textured surface pacemaker electrodes. PACE 6:525, 1983.

79. Window B, Thompson A, Sharples F, et al: Sputter technology: A technique for producing low polarisation surfaces. PACE 10:743, 1987.

80. McMichael A, Wilson A, Mond H, et al: A two year evaluation of two laser-porous electrodes. PACE 10:743, 1987.

81. Heinemann F, Coppess M, Stokes K, et al: Clinical comparison of "high tech" pacemaker leads. Clin Prog Electrophysiol Pacing 4(Suppl):43, 1986.

82. Schaldach M, Bolz A, Breme J, et al: Acute and long term sensing and pacing performance of pacemaker leads having TiN electrode tips. *In* Antonioli GE (ed): Pacemaker Leads. Amsterdam, Elsevier, 1991, p 441.

83. Thalen HJTh, van den Berg JW, van der Heide JN, Nieven J: The Artificial Cardiac Pacemaker. London, William Heinemann Medical Books Ltd, 1969, p 161.

84. Hirshorn MS, Holley LK, Hales JRS, et al: Screening of solid and porous materials for pacemaker electrodes. PACE 4:380, 1981.

85. Parsonnet V, Villanueva A, Driller J, et al: Corrosion of pacemaker electrodes. PACE 4:289, 1981.

86. Richter GJ, Weidlich E, Sturm FV, et al: Non-polarizable vitreous carbon pacing electrodes in animal experiments. *In* Meere C (ed): Proceedings of the Sixth World Symposium on Cardiac Pacing. Montreal, Pacesymp, 1979, Chap 29.13.

87. Elmqvist H, Schueller H, Richter G: The carbon tip electrode. PACE 6:436, 1983.

88. BeckJansen P, Schuller H, Winther-Rasmussen S: Vitreous carbon electrodes in endocardial pacing. *In* Meere C (ed): Proceedings of the Sixth World Symposium on Cardiac Pacing. Montreal, Pacesymp, 1979, Chap 29.9.

89. Gargeroglio B, Inguaggiato B, Chinaglia B, et al: Initial results with an activated carbon tip electrode. PACE 6:440, 1983.

90. Ripart A, Mugica J: Electrode-heart interface: Definition of the ideal electrode. PACE 6:410, 1983.

91. Mugica J, Henry L, Attuel P, et al: Clinical experience with 910 carbon tip leads: Comparison with polished platinum leads. PACE 9:1230, 1986.

92. Pioger G, Ripart A: Clinical results of low energy unipolar or bipolar activated carbon tip leads. PACE 9:1243, 1986.

93. Pioger G, Mugica J: Five years experience with 1527 carbon tip leads: Comparison with polished platinum leads. PACE 9:283, 1986.

94. Thuesen L, Jensen PJ, Vejby-Christensen, et al: Lower chronic stimulation threshold in the carbon-tip than in the platinum-tip endocardial electrode: A randomized study. PACE 12:1592, 1989.

95. Katsumoto K, Niibori T, Takamatsu T, et al: Development of glassy carbon electrode (Dead Sea Scroll) for low energy cardiac pacing. PACE 9:1220, 1986.

96. Moracchini PV, Cappelletti F, Melandri PF, et al: Titanium oxide tip electrode: A solution to minimize polarization and threshold increase. PACE 8:A-85, 1985.

97. Greatbatch W: Implantable Active Devices. 3. Electrodes and Leads. Clarence, NY, Greatbatch Enterprises, 1983, pp 1–37.

98. Schaldach M, Hubman M, Weikl A, et al: Sputter-deposited TiN electrode coatings for superior sensing and pacing performance. PACE 13:1891, 1990.

99. Irnich W: Engineering concepts of pacemaker electrodes. *In* Schaldach M, Furman S (eds): Advances In Pacemaker Technology. New York, Springer-Verlag, 1975, p 241.

100. Kreyenhagen P, Helland J, Forino R: Assessment of a tip electrode coated with titanium nitride [Abstract]. PACE 14:629, 1991.

101. Tang C, Yeung-Lai-Wah JA, Qi A, et al: Initial experience with a co-radial bipolar pacing lead. PACE 20:1800, 1997.

102. DelBufalo AGA, Schlaepfer J, Fromer M, et al: Acute and long-term ventricular stimulation thresholds with a new, iridium oxide-coated electrode. PACE 16:1240, 1993.

103. Mond H, Stokes K, Helland J, et al: The porous titanium steroid eluting electrode: A double blind study assessing the stimulation threshold effects of steroid. PACE 11:214, 1988.

104. Mond H, Stokes KB: The electrode-tissue interface: The revolutionary role of steroid elution. PACE 15:95, 1992.

105. Mond H, Sloman G: The small tined pacemaker lead: Absence of dislodgement. PACE 3:171, 1980.

106. Ripart A, Mugica J: Electrode-heart interface: Definition of the ideal electrode. PACE 6:410, 1983.

107. Guerola M, Lindegren U: Clinical evaluation of membrane-coated 3.5 mm^2 porous titanium nitride electrodes. *In* Aubert AE, Ector H, Stroobandt R (eds): Euro-pace '93 Monduzzi Editore, 1993, p 447.

108. Stokes K, Bornzin G: The electrode-biointerface: Stimulation. *In* Barold SS (ed): Modern Cardiac Pacing. New York, Futura, 1985, p 33.

109. Brewer G, McAuslan BR, Skalsky M, et al: Initial screening of bioactive agents with potential to reduce stimulation threshold. PACE 11:509, 1988.

110. Stokes KB, Bornzin GA, Wiebusch WA: A steroid-eluting, low-threshold, low-polarising electrode. *In* Steinbach K, Glogar D, Laszkovics A, et al (eds): Cardiac Pacing. Proceedings of the Seventh World Symposium on Cardiac Pacing. Vienna, Darmstadt, Steinkopff Verlag, 1983, p 369.

111. Kruse I, Terpstra B: Clinical experience with a steroid-eluting electrode for atrial and ventricular pacing. *In* Aubert AE, Ector H (eds): Pacemaker Leads. Amsterdam, Elsevier Science Publishers BV, 1985, p 255.

112. Hoff PI, Breivik K, Tronstad A, et al: A new steroid-eluting lead for low-threshold pacing. PACE 8:A-4, 1985.

113. Kruse IM: Long-term performance of endocardial leads with steroid-eluting electrodes. PACE 9:1217, 1986.

114. Church T, Martinson M, Rueter J, et al: A multi-center clinical trial of unipolar steroid-eluting electrodes. PACE 10:659, 1987.

115. Cuddy TE, Rabson JLR, Bucher DR, et al: A comparison of threshold performance in bipolar and unipolar steroid-eluting electrodes. PACE 10:434, 1987.

116. Aonuma K, Iesaka Y, Nogami A, et al: Long term improvement of atrial pacing threshold and sensitivity with steroid tip leads: A comparative study between steroid and target tip lead. PACE 11:510, 1988.

117. Pirzada FA, Moschitto LJ: Steroid-eluting electrodes: Four year experience. PACE 14:695, 1991.

118. Pirzada FA, Moschitto LJ, DiOrio D: Long term follow up of steroid eluting electrodes. Cardiostim 90. RBM 12:105, 1990.

119. Helloco A, Lelong B, Leborgne O, et al: Clinical experience with steroid endocardial lead in permanent atrial pacing. Cardiostim 90. RBM. Seventh International Congress, Nice, 12:105, 1990.

120. Till JA, Jones S, Rowland E, et al: Clinical experience with a steroid eluting lead in children. Circulation 80:389, 1989.

121. Stokes K, Church T: The elimination of exit block as a pacing complication using a transvenous steroid eluting lead. PACE 10:748, 1987.

122. Petitot JC, Metivet F, Lascault G, et al: What improvement with the Medtronic steroid eluting lead 4003? Cardiostim 90. RBM 12:108, 1990.

123. Mond H, Stokes KB: The steroid-eluting electrode: A 10-year experience. PACE 19:1016, 1997.

124. Tronstad A, Hoff PI, Ohm O-J: Myocardial excitability thresholds of a new steroid lead compared to two non-steroid leads: A double blind study. PACE 10:754, 1987.

125. Sibille Y, Reynolds H: Macrophages and polymorphonuclear neutrophils in lung defence and injury. Am Rev Respir Dis 141:471, 1990.

126. Greve H, Heuer H, Peters W: Intra- and postoperative data of the Medtronic electrodes target tip 4011-58 and steroid 4003. Clin Prog Electrophysiol Pacing 4(Suppl):42, 1986.

127. Vardas PE, Kenny RA, Ingram A: Acute and chronic performance of new technology versus conventional endocardial pacing leads. Clin Prog Electrophysiol Pacing 4(Suppl):38, 1986.

128. Schuchert A, Hopf M, Kuck KH, et al: Chronic ventricular electrograms: Do steroid eluting leads differ from conventional leads? PACE 13:1879, 1990.

129. Bucking J, Schwartau M: The effect of localized steroid elution from a pacemaker electrode on the pacing threshold and intracardiac R wave amplitude (translated). Herzschrittmacher 5:27, 1985.

130. Timmis GC: "Meet the Experts" presentation at the North American Society of Pacing and Electrophysiology meeting, May 1986. Reproduced in Medtronic Inc. literature "Think System," MC 871503, September 1987, and "Capsure Leads: The Drug, Technology, and Benefits Abstracted," MC 870675, 1987.

131. Mond HG: Development of low stimulation-threshold, low-polarization electrodes. *In* Barold SS, Mugica J (eds): New Perspectives in Cardiac Pacing, vol 2. Mount Kisco, NY, Futura, 1991, p 133.

132. Jones BR, Midei MG, Brinker JA: Does the long term performance of the target tip electrode justify reducing a pacemaker's nominal output? PACE 9:299, 1986.

133. Hiller K, Rothschild JM, Fudge W, et al: A randomized comparison of a bipolar steroid-eluting lead and a bipolar porous platinum coated titanium lead. PACE 14:695, 1991.

134. Mond H, Hunt P, Hunt D: A second generation steroid eluting electrode. Cardiostim 90. RBM. Seventh International Congress, Nice, 12:62, 1990.

135. Pioger G: Low surface area electrodes: Comparison between Synox 60 BP (1.3 mm^2), Capsure Z 5034 (1.2 mm^2) and Stela BT26 (2 mm^2):158 cases [Abstract]. PACE 20:1443, 1997.

136. Danilovic D, Breivik K, Hoff PI, et al: Clinical performance of steroid-eluting pacing leads with 1.2-mm^2 electrodes. PACE 20:2799, 1997.

137. Uwe KH, Bode F, Potratz J: Effects of surface reduction in steroid-eluting leads: A comparison of four modern bipolar electrodes [Abstract]. PACE 20:1444, 1997.

138. Pioger G, Botte M, Defaye P, et al: Clinical study of 419 mini-tip permanent pacing leads (1.2 mm^2): One year results of a French multicentric study [Abstract]. PACE 20:1211, 1997.

139. Johnson B, Voegtin L, Greene C, et al: Clinical performance of the 5034 ventricular lead: A balance of consequences of a new high impedance lead? [Abstract]. PACE 20:1150, 1997.

140. Hua W, Mond HG, Strathmore N: Chronic steroid eluting lead performance: A comparison of atrial and ventricular pacing. PACE 20:17, 1997.

141. Stokes KB: Preliminary studies on a new steroid eluting epicardial electrode. PACE 11:1797, 1988.

142. Karpawich PP, Hakimi M, Arciniegas E: Improved chronic epicardial pacing in children: Steroid contribution to porous platinised electrodes. PACE 15:1151, 1992.

143. Kugler JD, Fetter J, Fleming W: A new steroid-eluting epicardial lead: Experience with atrial and ventricular implantation in the immature swine. PACE 13:976, 1990.

144. Johns JA, Fish FA, Burger JD, et al: Steroid-eluting epicardial pacing leads in pediatric patients: Encouraging early results. J Am Coll Cardiol 20:395, 1992.

145. Hamilton R, Bahoric B, Griffiths J, et al: Steroid eluting epicardial leads in pediatrics: Improved epicardial thresholds in the first year. PACE 14:633, 1991.

146. Johns JA, Fish FA, Burger JD, et al: Steroid-eluting epicardial pacing leads in pediatric patients: Encouraging early results. PACE 14:633, 1991.

147. Wilson A, Cowling R, Mathivanar R, et al: Drug eluting collar: A new approach to reducing threshold. Cardiostim 90 Nice. RBM. Seventh International Congress, Nice, 12:61, 1990.

148. Brewer G, Mathivanar R, Skalsky M, et al: Composite electrode tips containing externally placed drug releasing collars. PACE 11:1760, 1988.

149. Mathivanar R, Anderson N, Harman D, et al: In vivo elution of drug eluting ceramic leads with a reduced dose of dexamethasone sodium phosphate. PACE 13:1883, 1990.

150. Crossley GH, Bubien R, Dailey SM, et al: Chronic stimulation threshold with a drug eluting collar electrode: Long term follow up. PACE 14:628, 1991.

151. Wilson A, Kay N, Padeletti L, et al: A multicentre study of steroid eluting collar leads. PACE 14:629, 1991.

152. Schuchert A, Kuck KH: Benefits of smaller electrode surface area (4 mm^2) on steroid eluting leads. PACE 14:2098, 1991.

153. Skalsky M, Mathivanar R, Anderson N, et al: Threshold performance of bipolar leads with a drug eluting collar (DEC). Cardiostim 90. RBM. Seventh International Congress, Nice, 12:108, 1990.

154. Mond HG, Hua W, Wang CC: Atrial pacing leads: The clinical contribution of steroid-elution. PACE 18:1601, 1995.

155. Hua W, Mond H, Sparks P: The clinical performance of three designs of atrial pacing leads from a single manufacturer: The value of steroid elution. Eur J Cardiac Pacing Electrophysiol 6:99, 1996.

156. Wiegand UKH, Potratz J, Luninghake F, et al: Electrophysiological characteristics of bipolar membrane carbon leads with and without steroid elution compared with a conventional carbon and a steroid-eluting platinum lead. PACE 19:1155, 1996.

157. Guerola M, Lindegren U: Long term clinical evaluation of 3.5 mm^2 porous titanium-nitride electrodes with a layer of ion-exchange membrane, with and without steroids [Abstract]. PACE 17:773, 1994.

158. Svensson O, Karlsson J-E, Binner L, et al: Comparison of threshold values between steroid and nonsteroid unipolar membrane leads. PACE 17:2008, 1994.

159. Mond H: The Cardiac Pacemaker. New York, Grune & Stratton 1983, p 75.

160. Bergdahl L: Helifix, an electrode suitable for transvenous and ventricular implantation. J Thorac Cardiovasc Surg 80:794, 1980.

161. Sloman JG, Mond HG, Bailey B, et al: The use of balloon-tipped electrodes for permanent cardiac pacing. PACE 2:579, 1979.

162. Bennett D, Bray C, Ward C, et al: Comparison of 2 types of active fixation electrodes. PACE 4:A-32, 1981.

163. Mond H, Sloman G: The small tined pacemaker lead: Absence of dislodgement. PACE 3:171, 1980.

164. Stokes KD: Recent advances in lead technology. *In* Barold SS, Mugica J (eds): New Perspectives in Cardiac Pacing. Mount Kisco, NY, Futura, 1988, pp 217.

165. Greco OT, Ardito RV, Martinelli M, et al: Sweet Tip Rx: A new type of atrial active fixation lead [Abstract]. PACE 20:1462, 1997.

166. Bisping HJ, Kreuzer J, Birkenheier H: Three year clinical experience with a new endocardial screw-in lead with introduction protection for use in the atrium and ventricle. PACE 3:424, 1980.

167. MacGregor DC, Wilson GJ, Dutcher RG, et al: A new positive fixation endocardial pacemaker lead using an extendable retractable helix. *In* Meere C (ed): Proceedings of the Sixth World Symposium on Cardiac Pacing. Montreal, 1979, Chap. 29.14.

168. YP fractally coated screw-in lead. Biotronik Gmbh & Co. Berlin, Germany.

169. Mond H, Ong TW, Strathmore N, et al: Atrial Pacing Leads: Active or Passive Fixation. Cardiac Society of Australia and New Zealand, Christchurch, New Zealand, August 1993.

170. Crossley GH, Brinkler JA, Reynolds D, et al: Steroid elution improves the stimulation threshold in an active-fixation atrial permanent pacing lead. Circulation 92:2935, 1995.

171. Spampinato A, Nobile A, Cornacchia D, et al: Clinical trial of last generation bipolar, steroid-eluting catheters: Comparison between screw-in vs tined lead [Abstract]. 20:1444, 1997.

172. Heil RW: Preclinical evaluation of a positive fixation lead with steroid eluting collar containing mixed form of steroid [Abstract]. PACE 18:1818, 1995.

173. Freedman RA, Marks M, Ruffy R, et al: Chronic electrical performance of two manufacturers' active fixation leads: Long-term improvement in atrial and ventricular capture thresholds associated with steroid elution [Abstract]. PACE 19:719, 1996.

174. Frohlig G, Schwaab B, Schwerdt H: A new steroid-eluting screw-in electrode. PACE 17:1134, 1994.

175. Hamilton RM, Chiu C, Gow RM, et al: A comparison of two stab-on unipolar epicardial pacing leads in children. PACE 20:631, 1997.

176. Upton JE: New pacing lead conductors. *In* Meere C (ed): Proceedings of the Sixth World Symposium on Cardiac Pacing. Montreal, 1979, Chap. 29.6.

177. Adler SC, Forster AJ, Sanders RS, et al: Thin bipolar leads: A solution to problems with coaxial bipolar designs. PACE 15:1986, 1992.

178. Breivik K, Danilovic D, Ohm O-J, et al: Clinical evaluation of a thin bipolar pacing lead. PACE 20:637, 1997.

179. Tang C, Yeung-Lai-Wah JA, Qi A, et al: Initial experience with a co-radial bipolar pacing lead. PACE 20:1800, 1997.

180. Grammage MD, Swoyer J, Moes R, et al: Initial experience with a new design parallel conductor, high impedance, steroid-eluting bipolar pacing lead [Abstract]. PACE 20:1229, 1997.

181. Chisholm AW, Cameron JR, Froggart GM, et al: A new long life electrode. PACE 4:A-85, 1981.

182. Green GD: Pacemaker leads. Impulse: A publication of Cardiac Pacemakers Inc., June 1976.

183. Dolezel B, Adamirova L, et al: In vivo degradation of polymers. Biomaterials 10:96, 1989.

184. Stokes K, Cobian K, Lathrop T: Polyurethane insulators, a design approach to small pacing leads. *In* Meere C (ed): Proceedings of the Sixth World Symposium on Cardiac Pacing. Montreal, 1979, Chap. 28-2.

185. Guerin P: Use of synthetic polymers for biomedical application. PACE 6:449, 1983.

186. Scheuer-Lesser M, Irnich W, Kreuzer J: Polyurethane leads: Facts and controversy. PACE 6:454, 1983.

187. Stokes K: The biostability of polyurethane leads. *In* Barold SS (ed): Modern Cardiac Pacing. Mount Kisco, NY, Futura, 1985, p 173.

188. Pande GS: Thermoplastic polyurethanes as insulating materials for long-life cardiac pacing leads. PACE 6:858, 1983.

189. Parins DJ, Black KM, McCoy KD, Horvath NJ: In vivo degradation of a polyurethane. Cardiac Pacemakers Incorporated, publication, 1981.

190. Stokes K: The long term biostability of polyurethane leads. Stimucoeur Medical 10:205, 1982.

191. Byrd CL, McArthur W, Stokes K, et al: Implant experience with unipolar pacing leads. PACE 6:868, 1983.

192. Scheuer-Leeser M, Irnich W, Kreuzer J: Polyurethane leads: Facts and controversy. PACE 6:454, 1983.

193. Timmis GC, Westveer DC, Martin R, et al: The significance of surface changes on explanted polyurethane pacemaker leads. PACE 6:845, 1983.

194. Round Table Discussion. The polyurethane controversy. PACE 6:459, 1983.

195. Phillips R, Frey M, Martin RO: Long-term performance of polyurethane pacing leads: Mechanisms of design-related failures. PACE 9:1166, 1986.

196. Irwin M, Graham KJ, Hayes D, et al: Does the venous route used for lead placement effect the incidence of lead failure? PACE 15:571, 1992.

197. Stokes K, Urbanski P, Upton J: The in vivo auto-oxidation of polyether polyurethanes by metal ions. J Biomater Sci Polym Ed 1:207, 1990.

198. Davis M, Stokes K: Polyurethane cardiac pacing: Six years experience. Cardiostim '84.

199. Medtronic Report: Ensuring and evaluating pacing lead performance. Medtronic News 20:21, 1992.

200. Stokes KB, Church T: Ten-year experience with implanted polyurethane lead insulation. PACE 9:1160, 1986.

201. Woscoboinik JR, Maloney JD, Helguera ME, et al: Pacing lead survival: Performance of different models. PACE 15:1991, 1992.

202. Fletcher R, McManus C, Keung E, et al: The Veterans Affairs Lead Registry: 10 year follow-up. PACE 15:512, 1992.

203. Hayes DL, Graham KJ, Irwin M, et al: A multicenter experience with a bipolar tined polyurethane ventricular lead. PACE 15:1033, 1992.

204. Sweesy MW, Forney CC, Hayes DL, et al: Evaluation of an in-line bipolar polyurethane ventricular pacing lead. PACE 15:1982, 1992.

205. Zweibel S, Gross J, Furman S: Long-term clinical experience of patients implanted with two types of bipolar polyurethane ventricular leads [Abstract]. PACE 20:1153, 1997.

206. Pirzada FA, Seltzer JP, Blair-Saletin D, et al: Five-year performance of the Medtronic 6971 polyurethane endocardial electrode. PACE 9:1173, 1986.

207. Hayes DL, Stokes KB, Helland J: Clinical survivorship and failure mechanisms of polyurethane pacing leads. PACE 8:779, 1985.

208. Beyersdorf F, Kreuzer J, Schmidts L, et al: Examination of explanted polyurethane pacemaker leads using the scanning electron microscope. PACE 8:562, 1985.

209. Stokes KR, Frazer AW, Carter EA: The biostability of various polyether polyurethanes under stress. ANTEC'84. 1073, 1984.

210. Telectronics Lead Performance Report. Denver, Telectronics Pacing Systems Inc., 1991.

211. Byrd CL, Schwartz SJ, Wettenstein E: Chronic analysis of polyurethane leads. PACE 8:A-83, 1985.

212. Zweibel, Gross J, Furman S: Long-term clinical experience of patients implanted with two types of bipolar polyurethane ventricular leads [Abstract]. PACE 20:1153, 1997.

213. Important information about Telectronics Accufix and Encor Atrial "J" leads. A publication of the Accufix Research Institute. May 1998.

214. Lloyd MA, Hayes D, Holmes DR Jr: Atrial "J" pacing lead retention wire fracture: Radiographic assessment, incidence of fracture and clinical management. PACE 18:958, 1995.

215. Lau C, MacPherson M, Nishimura SC, et al: Natural history of the Accufix 330-801 recall: A conservative approach [Abstract]. PACE 20:1190, 1997.

216. Kennergren C, Flinck A, Walfridsson H, et al: Telectronics Accufix, J-shaped atrial leads 033-812 and 330-801: Is the problem of J-wire fractures decreasing? [Abstract]. PACE 20:1189, 1997.

217. Lau C, Nishimura SC, Oxorn D, et al: Is this the natural history of the retention wire? A case report. PACE 20:1373, 1997.

218. Kao H-L, Wang S-S, Chen W-J, et al: Migration of a fractured retention wire in the pulmonary artery from an active fixation atrial lead. PACE 18:1966, 1995.

219. Parsonnet V: The retention wire fix. PACE 18:955, 1995.

220. Mond H: The Cardiac Pacemaker: Function and Malfunction. New York, Grune & Stratton, 1983, p 87.

221. Babotai I, Turina M: A new atrio-ventricular electrode [Abstract]. PACE 2:A-84, 1979.

222. Lajos TZ, Wanka J: Transvenous atrial pacing with a new electrode. J Thorac Cardiovasc Surg 69:575, 1975.

223. Sowton E, Crick J: The crown of thorns: A single pass electrode for physiologic pacing [Abstract]. PACE 4:A-95, 1981.

224. Antonioli G: Single lead atrial synchronous ventricular pacing: A dream come true. PACE 17:1531, 1994.

225. Roelke M, Harari D, Meyerowitz EJ, et al: VDD pacing mode: An acceptable alternative to DDD [Abstract]. PACE 19:568, 1996.

226. Folino AF, Buja G, Ruzza L, et al: Long-term follow-up of patients with single lead VDD stimulation. PACE 17:1854, 1994.

227. Rosenheck S, Elami A, Amikam S, et al: Single pass lead VDD pacing in children and adolescents. PACE 20:1961, 1997.
228. Schuchert A, Van Langen H, Michels K, et al: Comparison of electrical characteristics between a steroid-eluting single pass VDD lead and a standard steroid-eluting ventricular lead. PACE 20:1787, 1997.
229. Morgan K, Bornzin GA, Florio J, et al: A new single pass DDD lead [Abstract]. PACE 20:1211, 1997.
230. Hirschberg J, Ekwall C, Bowald S: DDD pacemaker system with single lead (SLDDD) reduces intravascular hardware: Long-term experimental study [Abstract]. PACE 19:601, 1996.
231. DiGregorio F, Morra A, Bongiorni M, et al: A multicenter experience in DDD pacing with single-pass lead [Abstract]. PACE 20:1210, 1997.
232. Hartung WM, Strobel JP, Taskiran M, et al: "Overlapping bipolar impulse": Stimulation using a single lead implantable pacemaker system first results [Abstract]. PACE 19:601, 1996.
233. Lucchese F, Halperin C, Strobel J, et al: Single lead DDD pacing with overlapping biphasic atrial stimulation: First clinical results [Abstract]. PACE 19:601, 1996.
234. Newby KH, Barold H, Tomassoni G, et al: Dual chamber pacing with a single pass multipolar temporary electrode lead: Electrogram amplitude and pacing in the atria from free floating proximal electrodes [Abstract]. PACE 19:719, 1996.
235. Mond H: The Cardiac Pacemaker: Function and Malfunction. New York, Grune & Stratton, 1983, pp 71–75.
236. Furman S: Lead connectors [Editorial]. PACE 12:1, 1989.
237. Irnich W: Pacemaker standards [Editorial]. PACE 12:269, 1989.
238. Furman S: Connectors [Editorial]. PACE 13:567, 1990.
239. Executive Committee of the German Working Group on Cardiac Pacing, Communication to Professor K Steinbach, European Working Group on Cardiac Pacing. June 1985.
240. Doring J, Flink R: The impact of pending technologies on a universal connector standard. PACE 9:1186, 1986.
241. Calfee RV, Saulson SH: A voluntary standard for 3.2 mm unipolar and bipolar pacemaker leads and connectors. PACE 9:1181, 1986.
242. Moss AJ, Rivers RJ, Kramer DH: Permanent pervenous atrial pacing from the coronary vein: Long term follow up. Circulation 49:222, 1974.
243. Ellenstad MH, Messenger J, Greenberg P, et al: The use of coronary sinus pacing. In Thalen HJT, Harthorne JW (eds): To Pace or Not to Pace, The Hague, Martinus Nijhoff, 1978, p 156.
244. Mond H: The Cardiac Pacemaker: Function and Malfunction. New York, Grune & Stratton, 1983, p 86.
245. Kitamura K, Jorgensen CR, From AHL: Transvenous atrial and ventricular pacing from the coronary sinus complicated by perforation and cardiac tamponade. Chest 60:95, 1971.
246. Daubert C, Leclercq C, Le Breton H, et al: Permanent left atrial pacing with a specifically designed coronary sinus lead. PACE 20:2755, 1997.
247. Bai Y, Strathmore N, Mond H, et al: Permanent ventricular pacing via the great cardiac vein. PACE 17:678, 1994.
248. Daubert C, Ritter P, Gras D: Use of specifically designed coronary sinus leads for permanent left ventricular pacing: Preliminary experience [Abstract]. PACE 20:1054, 1997.
249. Barold SS, Cazeau S, Mugica J, et al: Permanent multisite cardiac pacing. PACE 20:2725, 1997.
250. Daubert JC, Cazeau S, Ritter P, et al: Transvenous lead insertion for permanent biventricular pacing [Abstract]. PACE 20:1518, 1997.

Chapter 5

Engineering and Clinical Aspects of Defibrillation Leads

Bharat K. Kantharia, David J. Callans, Scott E. Hessen, and Francis E. Marchlinski

An implantable cardioverter-defibrillator (ICD) was first implanted surgically in a human subject on February 4, 1980 by Mirowski and colleagues.[1] Since then the role of ICDs in the management of patients with malignant ventricular tachyarrhythmia has become well established.[2-5] ICD lead technology and implantation methods have changed substantially during the past two decades. This chapter outlines important design and engineering characteristics of ICD leads, with a focus on how ICD lead system technology and implantation methods have evolved.

■ HISTORICAL PERSPECTIVE

Hopps and Bigelow[6] laid the scientific foundation for internal transvenous defibrillation in 1954. In their initial prototypes, the detection of ventricular fibrillation (VF) was accomplished by a change in the phasic nature of the pressure curve monitored using a transducer mounted on the tip of a transvenous catheter in the right ventricle. Successful detection and treatment of VF was accomplished using this system in dogs and baboons.[6]

Clinical studies performed during open heart surgery proved the feasibility of defibrillation with endocardial leads in humans.[7] The initial ICD was manufactured by Medrad Inc. (Pittsburgh, PA) and was designed to recognize ventricular fibrillation using a single transcardiac electrogram morphology signal called *probability density function* (PDF). The signals were obtained from the shocking leads, which were a titanium epicardial left ventricle (LV) cup or patch electrode and a large-caliber titanium spring coil lead in the superior vena cava (SVC).[1] The implantation procedure thus mandated a thoracotomy. To improve detection of ventricular tachycardia, a separate rate-sensing lead for rate counting was added to the PDF morphology sensing, still obtained from the shocking electrodes.[8] Important limitations of this system included frequent high-energy requirements for defi-

brillation, migration of the spring coil lead, and SVC thrombosis.[2, 9] Because of the need for a thoracotomy for placement of the patch lead and the frequent need for additional epicardial patch leads to achieve an acceptably low defibrillation threshold (DFT), a fully epicardial defibrillation lead system evolved.[3, 10, 11] This lead system typically consisted of two large patch leads for defibrillation, with epicardial screw-in leads used for sensing of the ventricular rate. Successful implantation with adequate DFTs using a monophasic shock waveform could be achieved in more than 95% of patients with this system. Because of the need for thoracotomy in patients who were often hemodynamically compromised, significant morbidity and mortality were associated with implantation of the epicardial ICD lead system.

The first nonthoracotomy lead system was implanted in late 1986. This system consisted of a transvenous defibrillating lead (Endotak) manufactured by Cardiac Pacemakers Inc. (CPI, St. Paul, MN), and a subcutaneous patch. The role of the subcutaneous patch was, in part, to control the direction of the shock pulses given through the lead system. The early endocardial leads consisted of platinum-tip electrodes and two coiled titanium-shocking electrodes. These first-generation endocardial defibrillation leads had a higher failure rate because of lead fractures.[12] As a result of the high fracture rate, the widespread clinical use of nonthoracotomy lead ICD systems was delayed for several years.

In the early 1990s, investigational nonthoracotomy lead systems were again being evaluated. Medtronic, Inc. (Minneapolis, MN) evaluated a multilead nonthoracotomy system (Transvene) consisting of endocardial leads in the right ventricle (RV), SVC, or coronary sinus. CPI redesigned the Endotak lead and launched further clinical trials of transvenous ICD implantation. This single nonthoracotomy lead had two defibrillating coil electrodes positioned at the RV apex and SVC. Finally, Telectronics, Inc. (Sydney, Australia) began evaluating a nonthoracotomy ICD lead system (Enguard PFX). This system consisted of a RV lead for combined sensing, pacing, and defibrillation, coupled with a separate tined atrial pacing and defibrillation lead.

DFTs were frequently high using these different endocardial leads when coupled with a monophasic shocking waveform.[13–21] Auxiliary subcutaneous patch leads were frequently required to achieve an acceptable DFT. Furthermore, it could be anticipated that a thoracotomy with epicardial patch lead placement would be required for successful ICD implantation in up to 15% of patients. With the development of more effective biphasic shock waveforms and the incorporation of the "active can" as part of the shock delivery system, a single transvenous endocardial shocking lead is typically all that is required for successful ICD system implantation.[22–25] Uncommonly, additional subcutaneous patch or array leads are still required to achieve an adequate DFT in patients with a high DFT.[26, 27] Even more rarely, a thoracotomy with epicardial patch lead placement is necessary.

■ IMPLANTABLE CARDIOVERTER-DEFIBRILLATOR LEAD SYSTEMS

Technical Aspects

Unlike pacemaker leads, ICD leads have the function of delivering a high-voltage shock for defibrillation in addition to pacing and sensing functions. Therefore, despite some technologic similarities, ICD leads must be designed differently from pacemaker leads. Nonetheless, the application of the vast technologic experience gathered from pacemaker leads has helped in design of the present state-of-the-art ICD leads. Like pacemaker leads, ICD leads are composed of electrodes, conductors, insulating coating, connectors, and a fixation mechanism. The distal tip of almost all ICD leads incorporates an electrode that remains in electrical contact with the heart for sensing of the cardiac activity. The conductors are the coils of wires that conduct the electrical currents between the electrodes and the ICD pulse generator. The lead insulation is provided by biocompatible and biostable compounds, usually silicone or polyurethane. The connectors are the portions of leads that connect the lead to the ICD pulse generator. The fixation mechanisms designed to stabilize the lead within the heart are classified as active (as with a retractable screw-in helix mechanism that engages the myocardium) or passive (as with flexible tines that wedge the lead within trabeculae in the right ventricle). ICD leads with steroid-eluting tip electrodes are also available. These technologic aspects of the ICD leads and their components are discussed further in their appropriate sections in this chapter.

Lead Sensing

The ICD system's sensing ability depends on (1) characteristics of the lead–tissue interface; (2) the input amplifier characteristics, such as filtering and gain; and (3) the detection and classification algorithm. Both normal electrical impulses, such as during sinus rhythm, and abnormal signals, such as during VF, need to be sensed reliably. As indicated previously, the first sensing system that was used clinically was

based on the analysis of the PDF. In this system, the proportion of time during the cardiac cycle that the sensed electrogram was electrically quiet (near the isoelectric line) was continuously analyzed. This concept is based on the observation that organized cardiac rhythms, such as sinus rhythm, are characterized by a sharp divergence of the electrogram above or below the isoelectric line during the QRS complex, with a greater portion of the cycle nearly isoelectric during the diastolic interval. The proportion of the cardiac cycle spent by the input electrogram between two amplitude limits located near zero potential is then measured. In contrast to sinus rhythm, a disorganized arrhythmia, such as VF, is characterized by a lower proportion of the cardiac cycle near the isoelectric line, with absence of a repeatable peak amplitude. Thus, PDF recognized this absence of a time peak at the zero potential segments as an indication of VF. Ventricular tachycardia (VT) is characterized by a wide QRS complex with a lower proportion of the cardiac cycle near the isoelectric line than during a narrow QRS.

Despite these observations, there is some overlap between VT and sinus rhythm when the sensed vector indicates a relatively narrow QRS complex during VT and when there is a relatively wide QRS during bundle branch block or intraventricular conduction delay. Thus, PDF is sensitive for VF but may fail to detect VT reliably.[28] Furthermore, problems with oversensing have been observed because of the lack of specificity of the PDF paradigm when sensing is accomplished from the high-voltage shocking electrodes in patients with a wide QRS complex.

Device modifications were implemented early after the initial implantation of ICDs with PDF to allow sensing of VT and VF by monitoring of the heart rate as well as the PDF. A rate-sensing bipolar electrode was added to the system. Separate epicardial or endocardial bipolar rate-sensing leads were used to improve sensitivity and specificity of arrhythmia detection.[8, 9, 13] Subsequently, the probability density function was eliminated as a requirement for arrhythmia detection, although this feature has been retained as an option to differentiate VT from supraventricular tachycardia (SVT) when there is overlap in the ventricular rate of these arrhythmias.

With the epicardial ICD lead system, two unipolar screw-in leads placed no farther than 1 cm apart are used for bipolar sensing. To maximize electrogram amplitude, an attempt should be made to position the leads in a parallel axis to the propagation wavefront based on the basis of fiber orientation. The epicardial rate-sensing leads are commonly placed on the LV because the greater mass increases the amplitude of the bipolar electrogram. Rate-sensing leads, however, may be screwed into the RV if the LV myocardium is infarcted or otherwise grossly scarred. In the absence of studies directly comparing the epicardial and endocardial sensing of ventricular tachyarrhythmias, endocardial sensing is assumed to be superior based on the experience with epicardial sensing and pacing in patients with pacemakers.[13]

The endocardial transvenous rate-sensing lead can be a dedicated bipolar sensing lead or an integrated lead incorporating shocking and sensing elements (Fig. 5–1). In the *dedicated bipolar* sensing lead, sensing is accomplished between the electrode at the tip of the lead and a ring electrode placed 1 to 2 cm proximal from the tip. In the *integrated* sensing lead, rate sensing occurs between the tip electrode

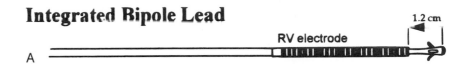

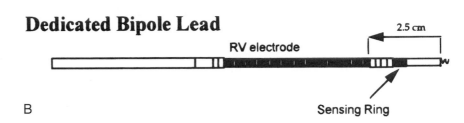

Figure 5-1. Comparison of typical electrode positioning and tip electrode to right ventricular (RV) electrode distance (pullback distance) for integrated (panel *A*) versus dedicated (panel *B*) bipolar sensing.

and the RV defibrillation electrode. The difference between dedicated bipolar and integrated sensing designs is largely a function of interelectrode distance and size of the proximal anodal electrode. To minimize far-field sensing, the distance between the tip electrode and the most distal portion of the RV coil electrode is minimized for integrated sensing leads (a factor known as *pullback distance*). The pullback distance is the distance between the lower active edge of the RV defibrillation electrode and the RV apex. The pullback distance is characteristically smaller in integrated bipolar leads and larger in dedicated bipolar leads. Minimization of pullback distance resulting from an integrated lead affects both sensing and defibrillation efficacy. A short pullback distance is considered to provide a lower DFT because the shocking lead can more closely approximate the RV apex.[29] Notably, however, an integrated lead system can result in inferior sensing characteristics as a result of greater susceptibility to far-field signals, such as P waves or smaller intracardiac ventricular electrograms owing to the shortened interelectrode distance.

A number of reports have documented problems with VF redetection after failed shocks when the distance between the tip and the shocking electrode was 0.6 cm.[30–32] Natale and coworkers[32] noted that delays in redetection of VF with an integrated bipolar system may still be present, albeit rarely, even when the tip to shocking electrode distance is 1.2 cm, which is the current industry standard. A recent study by Goldberger and colleagues[33] suggested that only minor differences of uncertain clinical significance in primary detection and redetection of VF existed when comparing dedicated and integrated bipolar sensing systems with tip to coil spacing of 18.3 mm. These investigators identified wide interindividual differences that were observed regardless of the recording configuration. Of note, the minor differences in detection and redetection times noted were observed only with a maximum sensitivity of 1.2 mV, a sensitivity threshold that is typically greater than that programmed for most ICD systems.

It appears that there is not a significant inherent sensing advantage of one recording system over the other for most patients given current standards regarding interelectrode spacing, filtering, and sensitivity settings in commercially available ICD lead systems. Two exceptions are worth noting, however. For patients with a small RV in which the RV coil electrode may straddle the tricuspid valve, an integrated

sensing lead may detect atrial electrograms as ventricular signals. This may result in inhibition of ventricular pacing when the ventricular sensitivity is high (such as automatically occurs during ventricular pacing). Second, some patients with a previously implanted ICD require concomitant pacing. If a separate pacemaker is implanted in a patient with a pre-existing integrated sensing ICD, it may be more difficult to obtain a pacing lead position that minimizes crosstalk between the pacemaker and the ICD than when a dedicated bipolar sensing ICD lead is used. In this situation, device–device interactions can be avoided by upgrading the ICD to a newer generation of device with the appropriate pacing functions.

Lead Pacing Function

The pacing function of the current generation of ICDs is frequently as important as defibrillation for an increasing number of patients with significant bradyarrhythmia or pace-terminable VT. The epicardial screw-in leads are generally suboptimal in their pacing performance with high pacing thresholds and the all-too-common development of exit block.[13] Leads with a steroid-eluting tip, which minimizes the increase in pacing threshold as a result of fibrotic encapsulation, are now available for both endocardial and epicardial rate sensing and pacing. With reduction of fibrotic reaction around the tip, improvement in sensing function is also expected.

Defibrillation Leads

Effective defibrillation requires that high-energy shocks depolarize or hyperpolarize a critical mass of the heart.[34–37] The number, location, size, polarity, and type of ICD lead, as well as the specific type of defibrillating waveforms, may all affect defibrillation.[22–25, 38–45] As noted earlier in this chapter (Fig. 5–2), epicardial patches were the primary shocking system used throughout the 1980s. Epicardial patch leads are still occasionally used, especially when effective defibrillation with nonthoracotomy lead systems cannot be achieved. Typically, two patches are placed inside or outside the pericardium, with one over the posterolateral wall or the apex of the LV and the other onto the RV or the right atrium (RA), so that the maximum ventricular mass between the two electrodes is included. The placement of the patch leads

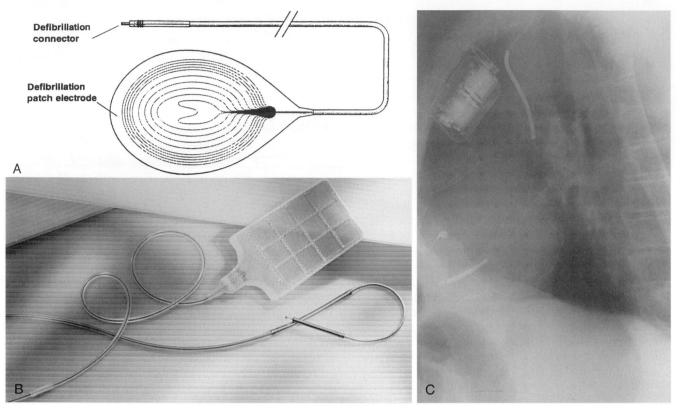

Figure 5–2. ICD patch leads for subcutaneous and epicardial application (see text). *A,* Schematic illustration of oval shaped patch electrode manufactured by St. Jude's/Ventritex Inc. *B,* Photograph of rectangular shaped patch manufactured by Guidant/CPI Inc. *C,* Radiographic image of lateral view of the chest with one of two epicardial patches outlined.

thus mandates an operative procedure to enter the thoracic cavity.

Surgical approaches for patch lead placement typically involve a lateral thoracotomy or median sternotomy. Subcostal and subxiphoid approaches have also been used. Early and late perioperative pulmonary complications, such as atelectasis, infection, atrial fibrillation, and pleural effusions, are common. Additional complications associated with intrathoracic patch lead placement, such as hemorrhage, pericarditis, pericardial constriction, patch erosion, patch dislodgment, and lead fractures, have been documented.[3, 4, 46–52]

Epicardial patches characteristically consist of a titanium or aluminum alloy mesh with a conductor of drawn brazed strand (DBS) stainless steel and silver composite. The back of the electrode and the conductor are insulated with silicone or polyurethane. Epicardial patches are available in different sizes and shapes, depending on the manufacturer. Selection of the optimal size and location for patch lead placement frequently occurs in the operating room setting on the basis of surgical access to the heart and the size of the heart. Animal testing, coupled with clinical experience, suggests that large patches (>25 cm²) provide a higher-voltage gradient in the shock field over a greater mass of the ventricles, resulting in a lower DFT.[53] Large electrodes also reduce impedance, resulting in greater flow of current between the electrodes.

High current density, on the other hand, can result in complex electrochemical reactions at the lead–tissue interface.[54] This phenomenon of edge effect, in which very high current density is concentrated at the edges of the shocking electrodes, can potentially cause tissue damage and failure of electrical propagation into the high current regions. However, the clinical significance of this phenomenon has not been documented for epicardial patch leads. Although concern was expressed that large patches might potentially interfere with the LV wall motion and function, documented abnormalities have been uncommon. The large patches may also insulate the heart from an external defibrillation shock and have been reported to increase energy requirements for defibrillation using nonthoracotomy lead systems.[37, 55, 56] Occasionally, because of a suboptimal DFT, more than two patches may be necessary. Implantation of multiple-patch electrodes is made possible with the use of Y connector, which couples two of the patches, making them electrically common. This parallel connection as a common cathode or anode to deliver shocks may occasionally lower the DFT further.[57]

Endocardial defibrillation leads are almost exclusively used with newly implanted ICD systems (Fig. 5–3, Tables 5–1 to 5–4). The availability of biphasic shocking waveforms delivered with the pulse generator can acting as one active electrode and an endocardial shocking coil as the other electrode virtually guarantees an acceptable DFT and a successful implant.[22–25] Endovascular leads coupled with monophasic shocks during initial implantation using nonthoracotomy lead systems did not produce this same track record of success. As a result, complex combinations of lead systems exist in the patient population who received an ICD

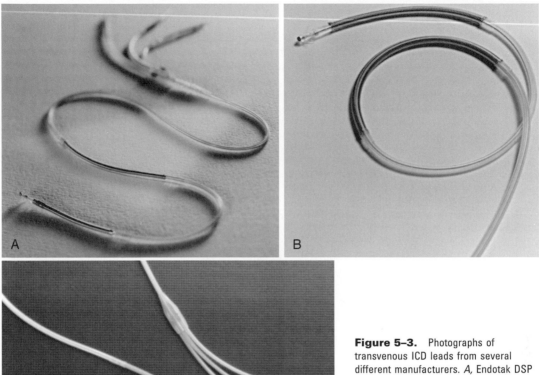

Figure 5–3. Photographs of transvenous ICD leads from several different manufacturers. *A*, Endotak DSP lead (Courtesy of Guidant/CPI Inc.). *B*, Sprint 6942 lead (Courtesy of Medtronic Inc.). *C*, SPL lead (Courtesy of St Jude's/Ventritex Inc.).

Table 5–1. Specification of Endotak Lead*

Feature	Lead Model	
	Endotak C 70/110	*Endotak DSP 70/120*
Position	RV/SVC	RV/SVC
Fixation	Tines	Tines
Lengths	100 cm (0070, 0072, 0074)	100 cm (0093, 0095)
	70 cm (0113, 0115)	110 cm (0097), 70 cm (0123, 0125)
Connectors	4.75-mm ring seal, bifurcated	IS-1 bipolar, pace/sense
	6.1-mm ring seal high voltage	DF-1 high voltage
Insulation	Silicone	Silicone
Tube design	Multilumen	Multilumen
Tip electrode	Porous	Porous
Electrode surface area	9 mm $\times$ mm tip	8 mm $\times$ mm tip
	379 mm $\times$ mm distal coil	450 mm $\times$ mm distal coil
	617 mm $\times$ mm proximal coil	660 mm $\times$ mm proximal coil
	10,000 mm $\times$ mm MINI HC shell	10,000 mm $\times$ mm Mini HC shell
Interelectrode spacing	11.7 cm (0070), 14.7 cm (0072)	15 cm (0093, 0123)
	17.7 cm (0074)	18 cm (0095, 0097, 0125)
Coil length	RV = 4.5 cm, SVC = 7.0 cm	RV = 4.5 cm, SCV = 7 cm
	RV coil = 0.90 Ω for 65-cm lead	RV coil = 1.12 Ω for 65-cm lead
Conductor resistance	SVC coil = 0.49 Ω for 65 cm	SVC coil = 0.85 Ω for 65-cm lead

*Manufacturer: Guidant/CPI Corp., St. Paul, MN.
RV, right ventricle; SVC, superior vena cava.

Table 5-2. Specification of Transvene and Sprint Leads

	Lead Model		
Feature	**Transvene 6934S**	**Transvene 6936**	**Sprint 6932**
Position	RV	RV	RV
Fixation	4 tines (2.5-mm lenght)	Screw-in (2-mm helix)	4 tines (2.5-mm length)
Lengths	65 cm and 110 cm	65, 75, 110 cm	65, 75, 100 cm
Connectors	IS-1 bipolar, pace/sense	IS-1 bipolar, pace/sense	IS-1 bipolar, pace/sense
	DF-1 high voltage	DF-1 high voltage	DF-1 high voltage
Insulation	Silacure (silicone)	Inner layer 55D polyurathane middle/outer layer 80A polyurathane	Silacure (silicone)
Tip electrode	Steroid eluting	Nonsteroid eluting	Steroid eluting
Electrode surface area	8 mm × mm tip	10 mm × mm helix	5.8 mm × mm tip
	27 mm × mm ring	37 mm × mm ring	37 mm × mm ring
	208 mm × mm coil	426 mm × mm coil	350 mm × mm coil
	10,800 mm × mm Jewel/Jewel Plus shell	8600 mm × mm MicroJewel II shell	8600 mm × mm MicroJewel II shell
	9200 mm × mm MicroJewel shell	9200 mm × mm MicroJewel II shell	9200 MicroJewel shell
	8600 mm × mm MicroJewel II shell		
Interelectrode spacing	Tip-ring 9 mm	Tip-ring 12 mm	Tip-ring 9 mm, ring coil 6.2 mm
	Ring-coil 6.3 mm	Ring-coil 6.3 mm	Tip-coil 19 mm
Sensing type	True bipolar	True bipolar	True bipolar
Defibrillation coil	RV	RV	RV
Coil length	5 cm	5 cm	5 cm
Diameter	12F body (3.9 mm)	10F body (3.3 mm)	7.8F body (2.6 mm)
	2.5-mm tip	3.5-mm head, 1.6-mm helix	3.05-mm coil, 2.7-mm tip
Conductor barrier	No specific coating	Encase coil coating	
Conductor resistance	108 Ω at 65 cm (bipolar pacing)	113 Ω at 65 cm (bipolar pacing)	49 Ω at 65 cm (bipolar pacing)
	2.1 Ω at 65-cm (defibrillation)	2.8 Ω at 65 cm (defibrillation)	0.83 Ω at 65 cm (defibrillation)

*Manufacturer: Medtronic, Minneapolis, MN.
RV, right ventricle.

Table 5-3. Specification of TVL Leads*

	Lead Model		
Features	**TVL (RV01, RV-1101, RV02)**	**TVL SVC (SV-1101, SV01, SV02, SV03)**	**TVL (SP01, SP02, SP03, SP04)**
Position	RV	SVC	RV
Fixation	Tines	Tines	Tines
Lengths	100 cm (RV01, RV-1101)	100 cms (SV01)	70 cm SP01, SP02
	67 cm (RV02)	110 cms (SV-1101)	100 cm SP03, SP04
		45 cms (SV02)	
		55 cms (SV03)	
Connectors	IS-1 (3.2 mm) pace/sense		IS-1 (3.2 mm) pace/sense
	DF-1 (3.2 mm), defibrilation		DF-1 (3.2 mm) defibrilation
Insulation	Stainless stell	Silicone	Silicone
Connector	Pacing tip 1.8 mm	Stainless steel	MP35N
Electrode diameter	Defibrillation 3 mm	2.4 mm	Pacing tip 1.8 mm
			Defibrillation 3 mm
Electrode surface area	Pacing tip 6 mm × mm tip		Distal defibrillation 480 mm × mm
	Defibrillation 470 mm × mm	550 mm × mm	Prox defibrillation 671 mm × mm
Interelectrode spacing	11 mm		
Electrical resistance			
Pace	63 Ω RV01, RV-1101, 37 Ω RV02		58 Ω SP01, SP02;
			83 Ω SP03, SP04
Sense	11 Ω RV01, RV-1101, 9.4 Ω RV02		18Ω SP01, SP02
			20 Ω SP03, SP04
Defibrillation	3.5 Ω RV01, RV-1101, 2.1 Ω RV02	SV-1101, 4 Ω	3.1 Ω SP01, SP02 (prox defib)
		SV01, 3.4 Ω	2.1 Ω SP01 (prox defib)
		SV02, 2 Ω	1.9 Ω SP02 (prox defib)
		SV03, 2.2 Ω	3.7 Ω SP03 (prox defib)
			3.5 Ω SP04 (prox defib)

*Manufacturer: Ventritex, St. Jude Medical, Sunnyvale, CA.
RV, right ventricle; SVC, superior vena cava.

Table 5–4. Specification of Intervene Leads*

Feature	Lead Model	
	Intervene, 497-19/497-20	Intervene, 497-22
Position	RV	
Fixation	497-19, tines; 497-20: screw-in	SV
Pacing electrode		—
Pacing electrode		
Shape	Slotted/ring	—
Surface area	8 mm × mm	—
Material	IROX	—
Defibrillation electrode		
Length	5 cm	5 cm
Shape	Trifilar coil	Trifilar coil
Surface area	4.4 cm × cm	4.4 cm × cm
Material	IROX	IROX
Lead body		
Inner coil (pacing)		
Coil construction	Trifilar coil	Trifilar coil
Material	Nickel-cobalt alloy	Niclel-cobalt alloy
Insulation	Silicone	Silicone
Diameter	3.0 mm × mm	3 mm × mm
Connectors		
Pacing connector		—
Material	Silicone	—
Diameter	3.2 mm × m (IS-1)	—
Pin diameter	1.6 mm	—
Defibrillator connector		
Material	Silicone	Silicone
Diameter	3.2 mm × mm (DF-1)	3.2 mm × mm (DF-1)
Pin diameter	1.25 mm	1.25 mm

*Manufacturer: Sulzer/Intermedics, Angelton, TX.

RV, right ventricle; SVC, superior vena cava; IROX, iridium-oxide–coated titanium.

folding of the lead after implantation. The lead body consists of a wire mesh between the clamp-and-crimp tube and is welded to the electrode mesh connecting the electrode to a conductor cable. A molded, silicone rubber strain relief, which houses the clamp-and-crimp tube, is bonded to both the patch sheets and the silicone rubber tubing of the lead body. The conductor runs through the tubing's single lumen and is crimped to a terminal pin at the connector end. The embedded electrode is radiopaque, which allows the patch position to be seen with a chest radiograph or fluoroscopy (Fig. 5–2).

The subcutaneous patch electrode can be positioned at the apex or prepectoral region subcutaneously or placed behind the lattissimus dorsi muscle on the left. The prepectoral and left posterior locations enhance the efficacy of the monophasic shock waveform.[67, 68] Care must be instituted in placing the patch lead. If the insulated backing side of the subcutaneous patch electrode is positioned facing the heart with the coil side away from the heart, then there may be insufficient energy available for reliable defibrillation. Current ICD system technology has eliminated the need for subcutaneous patch electrodes for most patients by making the ICD generator can electrically active.[25]

The subcutaneous array (Fig. 5–4) consists of three electrically common multifilar coil elements that combine to form one electrode with a large surface area. The three-pronged array elements are joined by insulated cable at a molded silicone yoke. The cable runs through a single lumen that is crimped to a terminal pin at the connector end. The array is tunneled subcutaneously in a posterior direction just inferior to the lateral rib margins (Fig. 5–4). The array provides a large surface area for defibrillation that can be directed posteriorly to provide a more favorable redistribution of defibrillation current to the LV apex and free wall. Studies using the array show a consistent decrease in monophasic DFT by 5 to 20J.[26, 27]

As previously noted, the high DFTs observed in the studies of nonthoracotomy defibrillation lead systems were related to monophasic waveforms. Amiodarone therapy and larger LV mass were found to be the predictors of high monophasic DFTs.[52] The success and simplicity of implantation of nonthoracotomy defibrillation lead systems has been markedly improved by using biphasic shock waveforms.[22–24] With current generator devices using biphasic shock waveforms, most of the energy is delivered with an initial pulse. The polarity reverses with the second pulse, which delivers the balance of the available energy. When waveform characteristics are optimized for efficiency, it takes (on average) 44% less energy to defibrillate tachyarrhythmias with the biphasic waveform than with a monophasic waveform.[22]

A detailed description of the commercially available endovascular leads that are currently implanted is provided in Tables 5–1 to 5–4. For most endocardial leads, titanium or platinum-iridium alloy is used because of high biocompatibility and conductivity. However, there are some potential drawbacks to these metals. Formation of metallic oxides during high-voltage shocks in the case of titanium and increased metal fatigue in the case of platinum-iridum alloys are potential disadvantages of these materials. Carbon in a highly purified pyrolytic form is biocompatible and nearly inert to the body tissue. This form of carbon fiber can be produced with a diameter of 10 to 50 millimicrons with a

system in the first half of the 1990s. Of the three transvenous systems (RV–SVC electrodes,[58–62] RA–chest wall electrodes,[59–62] and RV–chest wall patch electrodes[63]), only the RV–SVC approach has been used in humans, coupled with monophasic shocking systems. However, adequate defibrillation thresholds with this dual endovascular shocking system were obtained by only 20% to 60% of implants. Even when a separate shocking lead and electrode were placed in the coronary sinus, adequate DFTs using a monophasic shocking waveform were not uniformly achieved. Attention was drawn to certain factors, such as position and configuration of the leads and the polarity during the shock, to overcome the problem of high monophasic DFTs. In some patients, it was possible to improve the DFT by positioning the coil electrode well above the high RA,[64] by delivery of sequential defibrillation pulses,[65, 66] or by reversing polarity such that the RV coil functioned as the anode.[38]

Monophasic DFTs were often lowered by the addition of a subcutaneous or submuscular patch or a subcutaneous electrode array. These extrathoracic electrodes typically serve as the anode for defibrillation. The subcutaneous patch electrode, similar to the epicardial patch, consists of a conductive mesh laminated and sewn between two silicone rubber sheets, one of which contains windows that expose the mesh. The reinforced silicone rubber backing inhibits

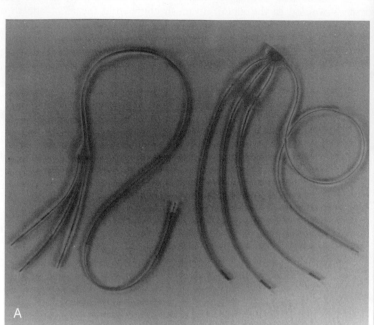
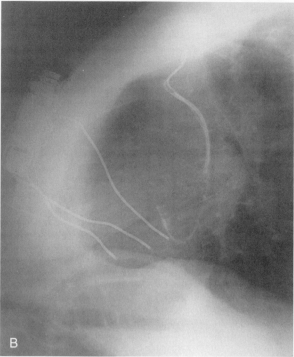

Figure 5–4. Photograph of subcutaneous array is shown on the left. (Courtesy of Guidant/CPI Inc.). Radiographic image of the lateral view of the chest showing characteristic position of array leads that increase surface area for defibrillation.

conductivity of up to 100,000 siemens/cm. A fiber strand 0.5 mm in diameter comprises a multitude of these tiny individual fibers. The fiber strand can be woven together to form a mesh. Because of a highly complex surface structure (maximizing surface area) and low polarization characteristics, the carbon fibers exhibit lower impedance for defibrillation.

Investigations with carbon fiber leads have suggested superiority of the new braided carbon electrodes over conventional metallic electrodes.[69–71] Reductions in pacing thresholds and electrode polarization have been demonstrated in pacing leads that are coated with iridium oxide (IROX), a low polarizing material.[72] The microporousness of IROX coating enhances the effective surface area of the electrode–myocardial interface. By virtue of the low polarization property of IROX, reduction in shock-induced polarization is expected. The IROX coating, therefore, markedly improves current flow through the heart for shocks of similar voltage. Significant reduction in DFTs has been demonstrated using IROX-coated leads in the experimental swine model.[73]

Engineering and Design Aspects for Endocardial Leads That May Influence Defibrillation Efficacy

Lead designs and technologic engineering aspects of conductors, insulators, fixation mechanisms, and connectors play key roles in determining the efficacy of the ICD leads.[74–76] Such features as conductor materials, wire thickness, number of wire filars, and lead diameter are selected to provide optimal lead functioning in terms of stiffness, handling char-

acteristics, lead resistance, fatigue life, and delivery of therapy. As a result, certain design decisions are made that enhance or diminish the lead efficacy.[29] In addition to the potential value of new coating and lead materials discussed previously, the following principles may enhance the defibrillation efficacy of an endovascular lead.

Minimize electrode pullback (see Fig. 5–1). As discussed, the electrode pullback (i.e., the shortest distance between the active surface of the RV defibrillation electrode and the apex of the heart) depends on the physical design of the lead and is referred to as *design pullback*. Leads using an integrated bipole between the tip and RV defibrillator electrode for rate sensing and pacing typically have shorter design pullback distances. With a longer pullback, a rise in defibrillation energy to up to 40% has been demonstrated for monophasic shock waveforms.[77] Shortening the pullback distance with integrated bipolar sensing systems to values less than 1 cm appears to lead to problems with VF redetection and should be avoided.[30–33]

Deliver current to the apex. Current distribution from the RV defibrillation electrode depends on two design factors: (1) the termination method in which the internal lead conductor is connected to the RV electrode, and (2) the resistance of the RV electrode. The transvenous endocardial defibrillation electrodes are constructed with a proximal termination technique, which connects the high-voltage conductor inside the lead body to the proximal end of the RV defibrillation electrode. An additional low-resistance (0.1 Ω) internal shunting wire connecting the proximal and distal ends of the RV electrode results in a balanced current delivery along the RV electrode, with

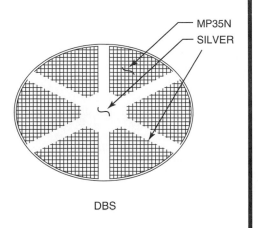 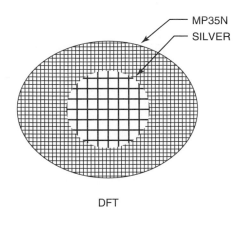

Figure 5–5. Composite wire defibrillator conductors. *Left,* A cross-section of a drawn brazed strand (DBS) conductor. The low-resistance silver is typically drawn between and around high-strength MP35N, an alloy of nickel, cobalt, chromium, and molybdenum. *Right,* A drawn filled tube (DFT) conductor. The high-resistance shell (MP35N or titanium) is filled with low-resistence metals, such as silver.

the greatest current leaving the end of the electrode at its conductor termination.

Minimize energy loss in the lead. Some of the energy delivered by the ICD pulse generator is lost in the lead conductors. This is directly proportional to the total lead body resistance and the square of the electric current passing through the system. Therefore, the lead designed to impart low resistance will yield high defibrillation energy (see Conductors).

Use large, efficient electrodes. Efficient defibrillation depends on the surface area of the defibrillation electrodes. If the surface areas of the defibrillation electrodes are too small, they limit the current delivery. Because there are limitations to increasing the length of conventional RV defibrillation electrodes, an effective larger defibrillation area can be accomplished by lengthening the SVC electrode and by increasing the diameter of the SVC electrode in a two-electrode lead system.[37] A larger overall defibrillation electrode surface area is also produced by making the pulse generator can an active shocking electrode, adding a subcutaneous or submuscular patch electrode, or adding a subcutaneous array.[25]

Conductors

When a voltage difference is applied to a wire, current flows in inverse proportion to the resistance of the conducting material. Since the resistance to current flow in a lead conductor is not zero, an amount of energy proportional to the resistance is wasted in the form of heat. The defibrillator conductors, by virtue of the requirement to deliver a high voltage, require a low resistance to minimize voltage losses in the wires. Because resistance is reduced with a conductor of greater cross-sectional surface area, measures to reduced resistance usually improve the characteristics of metal fatigue and corrosion resistance.

Most pacing leads use multifiler MP35N as the material for conductors, an alloy of nickel, cobalt, chromium, and molybdenum. This material has excellent fatigue and corrosion resistance but has too high resistance for defibrillation. Two so-called composite wires, drawn brazed strand (DBS) and drawn filled tube wire are routinely used for ICD leads

(Fig. 5–5). These composite wires incorporate the low resistivity of metals such as silver with the strength of stainless steel, titanium, or MP35N. DBS is used in the Endotak lead, and the drawn filled tube is in the Transvene and EnGuard leads.

To improve flexibility and fatigue resistance, the wires are further formed into coils, as in the drawn filled tube conductor, or twisted into small-diameter cables, as in DBS conductor. Although coiling enhances the fatigue life and flexibility, it also increases the length of the wire and thus its resistance. For drawn filled tube conductors, the resistance is a function of the wire diameter, amount of silver, diameter of the coil and number of filers in the conductor. In drawn filled tubes, the core consists of silver, which is usually not welded. Therefore, crimping of the wire to the terminal pin and defibrillation electrode is used. This crimp joint must be strong enough to withstand insertion and withdrawal forces at the defibrillator header.

For integrated function of pacing, sensing, and transvenous defibrillation, the lead coils can be arranged either in concentric or parallel paths (Fig. 5–6). Coils also provide a

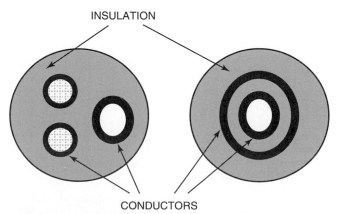

Figure 5–6. Potential lead construction configurations. *Left,* Parallel construction with central lumen for stylet insertion in drawn filled tube coil (open conductor). *Right,* Typical concentric lead construction.

lumen for the passage of a stylet for use during implantation and extraction of the endocardial transvenous lead. For an epicardial patch, a multiwire DBS cable is used as the conductor. This provides a low-resistance conductor with fatigue resistance. In some cases, the DBS cable is insulated with polytetrafluoroethylene (PTFE, or Teflon) to provide additional electrical insulation between the conductors.

Insulators

The insulator tubing must provide a high resistance (minimum of 50,000 Ω) to prevent any leakage of current between conductors in the lead. Polyurethane is one insulating material used for pacemaker and ICD leads. It has excellent biocompatibility. It also provides a high tensile strength, good flexibility, and low coefficient of friction. Each of these factors contributes favorably to the handling characteristics of polyurethane. Unfortunately, some forms of polyurethane (especially Pellethane 80A) degrade in the body by mechanisms such as environmental stress cracking and metal ion oxidation. The performance of improved polyurethane products is expected to be better but remains unproved.

Silicone rubber has also been extensively used as insulator in pacing and ICD leads. Silicone is also used as the backing material for epicardial and subcutaneous patches. Silicone is highly biocompatible and biostable but has relatively low tear strength and could be easily damaged by a tight ligature or a sharp instrument. In general, silicone-insulated leads must be of greater diameter than polyurethane leads. Silicone may also abrade if the lead remains in constant contact with an edge of the pulse generator, resulting in insulation breach. Additionally, because of its high coefficient of friction, it is difficult to pass one silicone lead over another. This potential disadvantage of silicone has been overcome by surface polishing or coating the lead with a highly lubricious material. Despite these limitations, silicone remains a material with a proven record of reliability for pacing and ICD leads.

Connectors

The connectors secure the lead to the pulse generator both mechanically and electrically. In early ICD leads, there was no standard for the connectors. Superficially, they looked like 5-mm unipolar pacemaker leads with a larger 6-mm-diameter sealing surface. Most manufacturers' leads were only 100% compatible only with their own generators. There is a trend toward standardization to enable interchangeability of the leads and pulse generators from different manufacturing companies. Presently, the defibrillator lead connector standard ISO-11318 is commonly referred to as DF-1 and the sense and pace lead connector as IS-1, the same as for permanent pacing leads.

Fixation Mechanism

The method for ensuring mechanical stability of the lead within the heart may be either passive or active (Fig. 5–7). Passive-fixation leads use flexible tines of silicone or polyurethane that are designed to engage trabeculae within the RV as a means of securing the lead within the heart. Active-

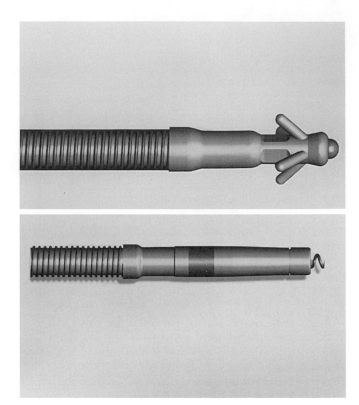

Figure 5–7. Fixation mechanisms for transvenous ICD leads. (Courtesy of Medtronic, Minneapolis, MN.)

fixation leads use an extendable-retractable metallic helix at the distal tip, which is advanced into the endomyocardium.

Both types of fixation mechanism have advantages and disadvantages. With active screw-in fixation, the lead can be positioned and secured in areas other than the RV apex. This is an important consideration in patients with a separate permanent pacemaker in which the ventricular pacing lead is positioned at the RV apex. Active-fixation leads may be positioned at a wide variety of sites within the RV to minimize the amplitude of a pacing stimulus in the sensed ventricular electrogram, reducing the chances of a device–device interaction. For patients with congenital heart disease in whom the defibrillation lead must be positioned in an anatomic LV, active-fixation leads are preferred because of the absence of trabeculae.

The tined, passive-fixation mechanism permits fibrotic ingrowth and thus develops maximum holding power. The main disadvantage of the tined leads is the inability to place the lead in locations other than the ventricular apex. Also, lead removal of a chronic tined lead may be difficult because the distal end of the lead is of far greater diameter than more proximal portions.

Fixation of the lead is also accomplished at the venous puncture site using a suture sleeve and within the device pocket. By virtue of their length, the ICD leads can easily be kinked within the defibrillator pocket. Excessive kinking can result in connector failure as well as insulation failure. Hence, extreme care should be taken to minimize kinking of the lead within the pocket or the tunnel region. Epicardial and subcutaneous patch leads often have suture sites with holes, dimples, or mesh reinforcement designs. If patches are not sutured in place, crinkling or folding of the electrode may occur, resulting in lead failure.

Adapters

Adapters are necessary in cases when multiple defibrillation electrodes or different lead systems and generators are used. These adapters and extenders must be designed with the same diligence required for the leads and generators. Attention should be paid to the sealing rings because leakage may occur across the seals. Older adapters have used an uncured medical adhesive to seal the setscrews, leading to an unacceptable risk of failure. In most cases, adapter failure is manifested clinically by the occurrence of inappropriate shocks from the ICD owing to detection of "make-break" potentials in the sensed electrogram. Modern adapters use a setscrew seal similar to that used in the pulse generator.

Implantation Techniques and Special Considerations

In most centers, electrophysiologists who have had extensive supervised training in pacemaker and defibrillator implantation perform ICD implantation.[78, 79] The implantation technique is essentially similar to the implantation of permanent pacemakers. To avoid potential risks of pneumothorax, hemothorax, and tendency for crush fracture of the lead at the costochondral junction, the technique of cephalic vein cutdown is preferred. This technique, however, involves more surgical dissection. Furthermore, a small vein may not accommodate a large-diameter ICD lead. In these cases, puncture of the subclavian or axillary veins is accomplished with Seldinger's technique, and the lead is introduced into the heart with the use of a peel-away introducer.

After the lead has been introduced, it is placed in the RV using similar techniques for the pacemaker lead implantation. At this point, pacing and sensing parameters are assessed. An R-wave amplitude of at least 5 mV with a slew rate of greater than 0.75 V/sec is recommended. Although the correlation between the ventricular electrogram amplitudes during sinus rhythm and VF is not well defined,[80, 81] it is generally believed that electrogram amplitudes during VF are larger if greater electrogram amplitudes are recorded during sinus rhythm. Furthermore, a sensed signal amplitude of more than 5 mV recorded during sinus rhythm makes it more likely that the sensing electrode is in reasonable proximity to viable myocardium. A pacing threshold of less than 1.5 V measured at a pulse width of 0.5 msec is also desired. We also routinely check for evidence of diaphragmatic stimulation with higher pacing stimulus amplitude. The pace and sense lead impedance measured at 5 V should be between 400 and 1200 Ω. A breach in the insulator or coil fracture should be suspected with lower and higher impedance, respectively.

We also routinely perform and recommend a synchronized low-energy (1 J) test shock to assess the integrity of shocking leads. A shocking lead impedance in the range of 35 to 70 Ω is usually acceptable. Notably, lead impedance measurements are manufacturer specific, and an awareness of appropriate values for each system is required. For patients with an inadequate DFT, a reversal in lead polarity is initially attempted after documenting that the RV lead is located as apically as possible. A persistent elevation in DFT may necessitate an additional endocardial lead. Endocardial leads are usually added only if a single-coil RV shocking lead has been used. A subcutaneous array or patch lead may also be necessary.

Insertion of a subcutaneous array requires a small incision at the level of the left nipple or the fifth left intercostal space. A pathway for each limb of the array is then created using a blunt-tipped malleable dilator. The introducer sheath is then placed over the dilator. The dilator is then removed, and the limb of the array is inserted into the sheath. The sheath is then peeled away. The procedure is repeated to insert the other limbs of the array along the course of the fourth, fifth, and sixth intercostal spaces. The arrays are then sutured to the chest wall fascia. To place a subcutaneous patch, a more lateral incision toward the axilla is made, and a subcutaneous pocket is created. The center of the patch is then placed at the level of the fifth intercostal space in such a way that the exposed coils face the heart without the edges of the patch curling up. It is especially important to suture the edges of the subcutaneous patch to the underlying muscular fascia to avoid distortion of the lead during healing.

Lead Complications

Advances in ICD generator and lead technology have contributed to a marked decline in the complication rate from the ICD therapy; however, lead-related complications remain common. From a total of nine studies, an overall 12.7% cumulative incidence of ICD lead-related complications has been reported.[76] Both early and late complications for both epicardial and endocardial lead systems have been described.[3, 4, 46–51, 82–87] The early postoperative complications related to epicardial lead implantation include a perioperative mortality rate of 1.5% to 5.6%, bleeding, acute pericarditis, atrial arrhythmias, patch displacement, patch hematoma, and pneumothorax or hemothorax during subclavian vein puncture for SVC lead insertion. The long-term complications of the epicardial patch leads include patch erosion, patch dislodgment, patch crumpling, fracture, infection, and constrictive pericarditis.

The overall incidence of lead-related complications with transvenous leads in a review of published series has been 6.8%, ranging from 2% to 28%.[85] Wide variation in the incidence of the lead-related complications might be related to multiple factors, including short or incomplete follow-up, differences in technique of implantation, manufacturing-specific component problems, and the lack of diagnostic capabilities of some ICD models. These complications include lead dislodgment, insulation break, crush or compression fractures, sensing malfunction, ventricular perforation, formation of intracardiac thrombi, and pulmonary emboli and infection.

Lead dislodgment or migration remains a significant complication and has been reported in up to 10% of ICD implants.[13, 85, 86] Dislodgment occurs most commonly shortly after implantation and may occur with both passive- and active-fixation leads. In fact, the lowest dislodgment rate noted has been with the Endotak C lead.[86, 87] Presumably the large size and weight are responsible for the low dislodgment rate for the Endotak leads. Dislodgment of the transvenous lead may also occur in patients with twiddler's syndrome.[88]

Lead dislodgment may manifest clinically as failure to sense, failure to pace, or failure to defibrillate, with potentially catastrophic results.

Lead insulation break or fractures have been reported in up to 3.1% of implants and may be anticipated in more than 5% of implants during long-term follow-up.[76] Typically, insulation defects manifest as inappropriate shocks due to oversensing of noise (Fig. 5–8). A breach in insulation from insulation erosion or fracture results in shunting of the current and thus reduces the efficacy of the shock. To avoid lead fracture from the subclavian crush syndrome, implantation through the cephalic vein or a more lateral percutaneous approach to subclavian or axillary venipuncture is recommended.[86] Manifestations of a complete fracture include increased pacing thresholds or failed defibrillation and high impedance.

Undersensing of ventricular tachyarrhythmias still occurs with endocardial lead systems. A problem involving sensing and redetecting ventricular tachyarrhythmias immediately after defibrillation can occur, particularly with older integrated sensing leads (Endotak 60 series). This is thought to be due to the high-voltage field resulting in local myocardial stunning, conduction delays in the myocardial tissue receiving high energy shocks, and significant changes in electrogram amplitudes and slew rates in the tissue near the shocking electrodes.[76, 89, 90] The time course and voltage-dependent effects of high- and low-shock energies on electrogram amplitudes were studied by Gottlieb and colleagues.[91] In their study, a consistent and predictable voltage and time-dependent reduction in postshock endocardial R-wave amplitude recorded by means of integrated and true bipolar nonthoracotomy lead systems was observed. No significant postshock reduction in the R-wave amplitude was seen in the true bipolar sensing or the integrated bipolar sensing leads after low-energy (5 J) shocks. With higher-energy shocks (30 J), however, there was a significant reduction in the endocardial R-wave amplitude recorded from the integrated system during the first 20 seconds after the discharge as compared with the true bipolar sensing system.[91]

Unique sensing errors, such as inappropriate inhibition of bradycardia pacing due to T-wave oversensing when the lead system is used for pacing, have also been described.[92] Pacemaker–ICD interactions leading to ICD double counting of the pacing stimulus and the local intracardiac electrogram may cause inappropriate shocks. Undersensing of VT by the ICD as a result of the ICD sensing of the pacemaker stimuli during VF has also been observed. With appropriate precautions, these complications can be virtually eliminated.[93, 94]

There has been a decline in infection rate since a nonthoracotomy prepectoral implantation approach has been introduced. Less damage to tissue, smaller and fewer leads, shorter procedure times, and increasing experience of the implanting physicians are some of the reasons for the reduction in infection rate. In addition to appropriate antibiotic therapy, ICD lead infection usually necessitates ICD system explanation. Extraction of endocardial defibrillation leads can be performed reliably using locking stylets and telescopic sheaths manufactured by Cook Pacemaker Corp. (Leechburg, PA).[95] Excimer laser energy has been used to remove scar tissue around the pacemaker leads. The technique uses laser sheaths (Spectranetics Corp., Colorado Springs, CO), which dissolves the scar tissue around the lead using laser energy directed by means of fiber optics. The feasibility of this technique to extract chronic transvenous defibrillator leads has been demonstrated.[96, 97]

Lead Follow-Up

Routine follow-up of patients with an ICD is necessary to identify both early and late lead complications. Chest radiographs provide useful surveillance information on lead integrity and are suggested yearly. We recommend a regular outpatient follow-up at 3- to 6-month intervals for patients with ICD devices to facilitate appropriate identification, di-

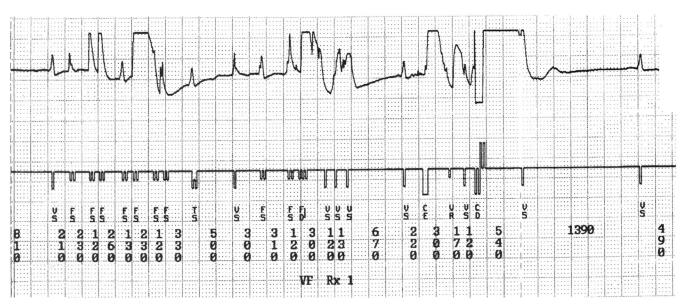

Figure 5–8. Intracardiac electrograms showing evidence of electrical noise consistent with evidence of a lead integrity problem before implantable cardioverter-defibrillator shock.

agnosis, and troubleshooting of ICD lead malfunction.[98] The frequency of follow-up visits should, however, be individualized.

The integrity of the pace and sense lead may be tested through noninvasive threshold and impedance measurements and compared with industry standards and the prior results of follow-up for each patient. Pacing thresholds, sensed R-wave amplitude, and qualitative assessment of the intracardiac electrogram and impedance values should always be compared with previously recorded values to identify evidence suggesting early problems with lead integrity or displacement of the lead. A marked deviation in the pacing and sensing parameters suggest a problem with lead integrity or dislodgment. Documenting appropriate high-voltage defibrillation impedance after a spontaneous or induced arrhythmia event leading to an ICD discharge is crucial for assessing the integrity of the defibrillation lead. High-voltage impedance values of greater than 100 Ω suggests lead conductor fracture, whereas low-impedance values of less than 25 Ω suggest insulation failure. A large disparity in the programmed and delivered energy after shock delivery should suggest lead conductor failure.

Sensing is assessed during spontaneous rhythm and during any event leading to ICD therapy. Unexpected or frequent shocks or shocks that fail to terminate ventricular arrhythmias should alert the physician to the possibility of lead dysfunction, which can be documented from the stored diagnostic information from the ICD device (see Fig. 5–8). Shocks occurring during specific movements or postures suggest oversensing or noise detection due to lead fracture. If adequate or inappropriate sensing is suspected but not documented because of limited diagnostic capabilities of the ICD device, electrophysiologic testing with assessment of sensing during VF and VT may be required. Presently, there is neither consensus nor guidelines for performing noninvasive programmed stimulation at regular intervals to test for integrity of the shocking leads in the absence of spontaneous arrhythmic events or systems that can automatically provide such diagnostic information. We consider such testing appropriate at least every 2 years.

Future Systems

Future improvements in ICD generator design and ICD lead technology are expected. New lead designs should be aimed at reducing the fibrotic reactions within the heart, which may result in new arrhythmogenic foci and a deterioration of the intracardiac electrogram.[99] A decrease in the fibrotic reaction would also make the lead extraction easier in the setting of lead disruption and infection. Small flexible steroid-eluting leads using low polarization electrodes may minimize increases in the pacing threshold. The effects of steroid elution on myocardial fibrosis surrounding the shocking coils is unproved. Lead technologies that incorporate the potential for rapid extraction should be considered.

New lead designs, such as braided carbon electrodes and IROX-coated leads, may prevent potential problems caused by localized trauma by high current density near the defibrillating electrodes and may help improve efficacy. Hemodynamic sensors, which could be integrated with the ICD leads, are being evaluated. Leads that have the ability to index hemodynamic variables to arrhythmic events should permit

more aggressive therapies with a high-energy shock for VTs with hemodynamic instability and antitachycardia pacing for more stable VT.

Finally, devices with dual-chamber atrial and ventricular pacing, sensing, and shocking capabilities are now routinely implanted in appropriately selected patients.[100–102] In addition, the diagnostic value of the atrial recordings has been confirmed. In future systems atrial leads will undoubtedly be developed that can also produce effective low-energy atrial defibrillation.

REFERENCES

1. Mirowski M, Reid PR, Mower MM, et al: Termination of malignant ventricular arrhythmias with an implanted automatic defibrillator in human beings: N Engl J Med 303:322–324, 1980.
2. Marchlinski FE, Flores BT, Buxton AE, et al: The automatic implantable cardioverter defibrillator: Efficacy, complications and device failure. Ann Intern Med 104:481–488, 1986.
3. Kelly PA, Cannon DS, Garan H, et al: The automatic implantable cardioverter defibrillator: Survival in patients with malignant ventricular arrhythmias. J Am Coll Cardiol 11:1278–1286, 1988.
4. Winkle RA, Mead RH, Ruder MA, et al: Long term outcome with the automatic implantable cardioveter defibrillator. J Am Coll Cardiol 13:1353–1361, 1989.
5. Moss AJ, Hall WJ, Cannon DS, et al. For the Multicenter Automatic Defibrillator Implantation Trial: Improved survival with an implanted defibrillator in patients with coronary disease at high risk for ventricular arrhythmia. N Engl J Med 335:1993–1940, 1996.
6. Hopps JA, Bigelow WG: Electrical treatment of cardiac arrest: A cardiac stimulator/defibrillator. Surgery 36:833–849, 1954.
7. Mirowski M, Mower MM, Gott VL, et al: Feasibility and effectiveness of low energy catheter defibrillation in man. Circulation 47:79–85, 1973.
8. Winkle RA, Bach SM, Echt DS, et al: The automatic implantable defibrillator: Local ventricular bipolar sensing to detect ventricular tachycardia and fibrillation. Am J Cardiol 52:265–270, 1983.
9. Reid PR, Mirowski M, Mower MM, et al: Clinical evaluation of the internal automatic cardioverter defibrillator in survivors of sudden cardiac death. Am J Cardiol 51:1608, 1983.
10. Echt DS, Armstrong D, Schmidt P, et al: Clinical experience, complications and survival in 70 patients with automatic implantable cardioverter/defibrillator. Circulation 71:289–296, 1985.
11. Manolis AS, Rastegar H, Estes NAM: Automatic implantable cardioverter defibrillator: Current status. JAMA 262:1362–1368, 1989.
12. Tullo NG, Saksena S, Krol RB, et al: Management of complications associated with a first-generation endocardial lead system for implantable cardioverter-defibrillators. Am J Cardiol 66:411–415, 1990.
13. Gold MR, Shorofsky SR: Transvenous defibrillation lead systems: J Cardiovasc Electrophysiol 7:570–580, 1996.
14. Schwartzman D, Concato J, Ren JF, et al: Factors associated with successful implantation of nonthoracotomy defibrillation lead systems. Am Heart J 131:1127–1136, 1996.
15. Sra J, Natale A, Axtrell K, et al: Experience with two different nonthoracotomy system for implantable defibrillator in 170 patients. PACE 17:1741–1750, 1994.
16. Kopp DE, Blakeman BP, Kall JG, et al: Predictors of defibrillation energy requirements with nonepicardial lead system. PACE 18:253–260, 1995.
17. Bardy GH, Allen MD, Mehra R, et al: Transvenous defibrillation in humans via the coronary sinus. Circulation 81:1252–1259, 1990.
18. Yee R, Klein GJ, Leitch JW, et al: A permanent transvenous lead system for an implantable pacemaker cardioverter-defibrillator: Nonthoracotomy approach to implantation. Circulation 85:196–204, 1992.
19. Zipes DP, Roberts D: Results of the international study of implantable pacemaker cardioverter-defibrillator: A comparison of epicardial and endocardial lead systems. Circulation 92:59–65, 1995.
20. Saksena S, and the PCD Investigators and Participating Institutions: PACE 16:202–207, 1993.
21. Brooks R, Garan H, Torchiana D, et al: Determinants of successful nonthoracotomy cardioverter-defibrillator implantation: Experience in 101 patients using two different lead systems. J Am Coll Cardiol 22:1835–1842, 1993.

22. Neuzner J, et al: Effect of biphasic waveform pulse on endocardial defibrillation efficacy in humans. PACE 17:207–212, 1994.

23. Block M, Hammel D, Bocker D, et al: A prospective randomized cross-over comparison of mono- and biphasic defibrillation using nonthoracotomy lead configuration in humans. J Cardiovasc Electrophysiol 5:581–590, 1994.

24. Natale S, Sra J, Axtell K, et al: Preliminary experience with a hybrid nonthoracotomy defibrillating system that includes a biphasic device: Comparison with standard monophasic device using the same lead system. J Am Coll Cardiol 24:406–412, 1994.

25. Bardy GH, Johnson G, Poole JE, et al: A simplified, single-lead unipolar transvenous cardioversion-defibrillation system. Circulation 88(2):1–5, 1993.

26. Jordaens L, Vertogen P, Belleghem YV: A subcutaneous lead array for implantable cardioverter defibrillators. PACE 16:1429–1433, 1993.

27. Higgins SL, Alexander DC, Kuyper CJ, et al: The subcutaneous array: A new lead adjunct for the transvenous implantable cardioverter defibrillator to lower defibrillation thresholds. PACE 18:1540–1548, 1995.

28. Mirowski M, Mower MM, Langer A, et al: The automatic implantable defibrillator: A new avenue. In Bricks W, Loogen F, Schulte HD, Seipel L (eds): Medical and surgical management of tachyarrhythmias. Berlin, Springer-Verlag, 1980, p 71.

29. Lang DJ, Heil JE, Hahn SJ, et al: Implantable cardioverter defibrillator lead technology: Improved performance and lower defibrillation thresholds. PACE 18(Pt II):548–559, 1995.

30. Reiter M, Mann D: Sensing and tachyarrhythmia detection problems in implantable cardioverter defibrillators. J Cardiovasc Electrophysiol 7:542–558, 1996.

31. Callans D, Swarna U, Schwartzman D, et al: Postshock sensing performance in transvenous defibrillation lead systems: Analysis of detection and redetection of ventricular fibrillation. J Cardiovasc Electrophysiol 6:604–612, 1995.

32. Natale A, Sra J, Axtell K, et al: Undetected ventricular fibrillation intravenous implantable cardioverter-defibrillators: Prospective comparison of different lead system—device combinations. Circulation 93:91–98, 1996.

33. Goldberger JJ, Horvath G, Donovan D, et al: Detection of ventricular fibrillation by transvenous defibrillating leads: Integrated versus dedicated bipolar sensing. J Cardiovasc Electrophysiol 9:677–688, 1998.

34. Mower MM, Mirowski M, Spear JF, et al: Patterns of ventricular activity during catheter defibrillation. Circulation 49:858–861, 1974.

35. Dillon SM: Optical recordings in the rabbit heart show that defibrillation strength shocks prolong the duration of depolarization and the refractory period. Circ Res 69:842–856, 1991.

36. Witkowski FS, Penkoske PA, Plonsey R: Mechanism of cardiac defibrillation in open-chest dogs using unipolar DC-coupled simultaneous activation and shock potential recordings. Circulation 82:244, 1990.

37. Wharton JM, Wolf PD, Chen PS, et al: Is an absolute minimum potential gradient required for ventricular defibrillation? Circulation 74(Suppl II):342, 1990.

38. Ideker RE, Wolf PD, Alferness C, et al: Current concepts for selecting the location, size and shape of defibrillation electrodes. PACE 14(I):227–240, 1991.

39. Strickberger SA, Hummel JD, Horwood LE, et al: Effect of shock polarity on ventricular fibrillation threshold using a transvenous lead system. J Am Coll Cardiol 24:1069–1072, 1994.

40. Saksena S, Mehra AH, et al: Prospective comparison of biphasic and monophasic shocks for implantable cardioverter-defibrillators using endocardial leads. Am J Cardiol 70:304–310, 1992.

41. Wyse DG, Kavanagh KM, Gillis AM, et al: Comparison of biphasic and monophasic shocks for defibrillation using a nonthoracotomy system. Am J Cardiol 71:197–202, 1993.

42. Saksena S, Luceri R, Krol RB, et al: Endocardial pacing, cardioversion and defibrillation using a braided endocardial lead system. Am J Cardiol 71:834–841, 1993.

43. Swartz JF, Fletcher RD, Karasik PE: Optimization of biphasic waveforms for human nonthoracotomy defibrillation. Circulation 88:2646–2654, 1993.

44. Werner J, Manz M, Moosdorf R, et al: Clinical efficacy of shock waveforms and lead configuration for defibrillation. Am Heart J 127:985–993, 1994.

45. Trappe HJ, Fieguth HG, Pfitzner P, et al: Epicardial and nonthoracotomy defibrillation lead systems combined with a cardioverter defibrillator. PACE 18(Pt II):127–132, 1995.

46. Almassi GH, Chapman PD, Troup PJ, et al. Constrictive pericarditis associated with patch electrodes of the automatic implantable cardioverter defibrillator. Chest 92:369–371, 1987.

47. Manolis AS, Rastegar H, Estes NAM: Automatic implantable cardioverter defibrillator: Current status. JAMA 262:1362–1368, 1989.

48. Bardy GH, Gregg MG, Johnson G, et al: Intraoperative identification of lead fracture during automatic implantable cardioverter defibrillator replacement. J Electrophysiol 3:75–80, 1989.

49. Mittleman RS, Mack K, Rastegar H, et al: Inappropriate shocks and elevation of defibrillation thresholds in a patient with automatic defibrillator patchsilastic erosion and titanium mesh fraying. PACE 1452–1455, 1991.

50. Brady PA, Friedman PA, Trusty JM, et al: High failure rate for an epicardial implantable cardioverter-defibrillator lead: Implications for long-term follow-up of patients with an implantable cardioverter-defibrillator. J Am Coll Cardiol 31:616–622, 1998.

51. Bakker PFA, Hauer RNW, Wever EFD: Infections involving implanted cardioverter defibrillator devices. PACE 15(III):654–658, 1992.

52. Almassi GH, Olinger GN, Wetherbee JN, et al: Long-term complications of implantable cardioverter defibrillator lead system. Ann Thorac Surg 55:888–892, 1993.

53. Mehra R, DeGroot PJ, Norenberg MS: Energy waveforms and lead systems for implantable defibrillators. In Luderitz B, Saksena S (eds): Interventional Electrophysiology. Mount Kisco, NY, Futura, 1991, pp 377–394.

54. Yabe S, Smith WM, Daubert JM, et al: Conduction disturbances caused by high current density electric fields. Circ Res 66(5):1190–1203, 1990.

55. Walls JT, Schuder JC, Curtis JJ, et al: Adverse effects of permanent cardiac internal defibrillator patches on external defibrillation. Am J Cardiol 64:1144–1147, 1989.

56. Lerman BB, Deale OC: Effect of epicardial patch electrodes on transthoracic defibrillation. Circulation 81(4):1409–1414, 1990.

57. Fromer M, Brachman J, Block M, et al: Efficacy of automatic multimodal device therapy for ventricular tachyarrhythmias as delivered by a new pacing cardioverter defibrillator. Circulation 86:363–374, 1992.

58. Yee R, Zipes DP, Gulamhusein S, et al: Low energy countershock using an intravascular catheter in an acute cardiac care setting. Am J Cardiol 50:1124–1129, 1982.

59. Schuder JC, Stoeckle H, West JA: Relationship between electrode geometry and effectiveness of ventricular defibrillation in the dog with catheter having one electrode in right ventricle and other electrode in superior vena cava, or external jugular vein or both. Cardiovasc Res 7:629–637, 1973.

60. Jackmann WM, Zipes DP: Low energy synchronous cardioversion of ventricular tachycardia using a catheter electrode in a canine model of subacute myocardial infarction. Circulation 66:187–195, 1982.

61. Kallok MJ, Wibel FH, Bourland JD, et al: Catheter electrode defibrillation in dogs: Threshold dependence on implant time and catheter stability. Am Heart J 109:821–826, 1985.

62. Schuder JC, Stoeckle H, Gold JH, et al: Ventricular defibrillation in the dog using implanted and partially implanted electrode system. Am J Cardiol 33:243–247, 1974.

63. Mirowski M, Mower MM, Staeven WS, et al: Standby automatic defibrillator: An approach to prevention of sudden coronary death. Arch Intern Med 126:158–161, 1970.

64. Saksena S, Tullo NG, Krol RB, et al: Initial clinical experience with endocardial defibrillation using an implantable cardioverter/defibrillator with a triple-electrode system. Arch Intern Med 149:2333–2339, 1989.

65. Yee R, Jones DL, Klein GJ, et al: Sequential pulse countershock between two transvenous catheters: Feasibility, safety and efficacy. PACE 12:1869–1877, 1989.

66. Hsia HH, Kleiman RB, Flores BT, et al: Comparison of simultaneous versus sequential defibrillation pulsing technique using a nonthoracotomy system. PACE 17:1222–1230, 1994.

67. Saksena S, DeGroot P, Krol RB, et al: Low energy endocardial defibrillation using an axillary or pectoral thoracic electrode location. Circulation 88:2655–2660, 1993.

68. Schwartzman D, Jadonath RL, Preminger MW, et al: The importance of subcutaneous patch position on the defibrillation threshold for nonthoracotomy defibrillation lead systems. Circulation 88:I–216, 1993.

69. Alt E, Theres H, Heinz M, et al: A new approach towards defibrillation

electrodes: Highly conductive isotropic carbon fibers. PACE 14(II):1923–1928, 1991.

70. Fotuhi P, Alt E, Callihan R, et al: Endocardial carbon braid electrodes: New approach to lowering defibrillation thresholds. PACE 16:1919, 1993.

71. Elmqvist H, Schueller H, Richter G: The carbon tip electrode. PACE 6:436, 1983.

72. Del Bufulo AGA, Schlaepfer J, Fromer M, et al: Acute and long-term ventricular stimulation thresholds with a new iridium oxide-coated electrode. PACE 16:1240–1244, 1993.

73. Nicbauer MJ, Wilkoff B, Yamanouchi Y, et al: Iridium oxide-coated defibrillation electrode reduced shock polarization and improved defibrillation efficacy. Circulation 96:3732–3736, 1997.

74. Timmis GC. The electrobiology and engineering of pacemaker leads. *In* Saksena S, Goldschlager N (eds): Electrical Therapy for Cardiac Arrhythmias: Pacing Antitachycardia Devices, Catheter Ablation. Philadelphia, WB Saunders, 1990, pp 3–90.

75. Accorti PR: Leads technology. *In* Singer I (ed): Implantable Cardioverter Defibrillator. Armink, NY, Futura, 1994, pp 179–206.

76. Nelson RS, Gilman BL, Shapland JE, et al: Leads for the ICD. *In* Kroll MW, Lehmann MH (eds): Implantable Cardioverter Defibrillator Therapy: The Engineering and Clinical Interface. Kluwer Academic Publishers, 1906, pp 173–204.

77. Heil JE, KenKnight BH, Derfus DL, et al: Sensing strategies dramatically affect defibrillation efficacy of endocardial based lead systems in swine [Abstract]. PACE 17:785, 1994.

78. Hammel D, Block M, Konertz W, et al: Surgical experience with defibrillator implantation using nonthoracotomy leads. Ann Thorac Surg 55:685–693, 1993.

79. Strickberger SA, Hummel JD, Daoud E, et al: Implantation by electrophysiologists of 100 consecutive cardioverter defibrillators with nonthoracotomy lead systems. Circulation 90:868–872, 1994.

80. Ellenbogan KA, Wood MA, Stambler BS, et al: Measurement of ventricular electrogram amplitude during intraoperative induction of ventricular tachyarrhythmias. Am J Cardiol 70:1017–1022, 1992.

81. Leitch JW, Yee R, Klein GJ, et al: Correlation between the ventricular electrogram amplitude in sinus rhythm and in ventricular fibrillation. PACE 13:1105–1109, 1990.

82. Saksena S, Mehta D, Krol RB, et al: Experience with a third generation implantable cardioverter defibrillator. Am J Cardiol 67:1375–1384, 1991.

83. Manolis AS: Implantable cardioverter-defibrillator lead systems. *In* Estes NAM, Manolis AS, Wang PJ (eds): Implantable Cardioverter-Defibrillators. New York, Marcel Dekker, Inc., 1994, pp 607–633.

84. Elefteriades JA, Biblo LA, Batsford WP, et al: Evolving patterns in the surgical treatment of malignant ventricular tachyarrhythmias. Ann Thorc Surg 49:94–100, 1990.

85. Lawton JS, Wood MA, Gilligan DM, et al: Implantable transvenous cardioverter defibrillator leads: The dark side. PACE 19:1273–1277, 1996.

86. Schwartzmann D, Nallamothu N, Callans DF, et al: Postoperative lead-related complications in patients with nonthoracotomy defibrillation lead system. J Am Coll Cardiol 26:776–786, 1995.

87. Hauser RG, Kurschinski DT, McVeigh K, et al: Clinical results with nonthoracotomy ICD systems. PACE 16:141–148, 1993.

88. Mehta D, Lipsius M, Suri RS, et al: Twiddler's syndrome with the implantable cardioverter-defibrillator. Am Heart J 123:1079–1082, 1992.

89. Jung W, Manz M, Moosdorf R, et al: Failure of an implantable cardioverter defibrillator to redetect ventricular fibrillation in patients with a nonthoracotomy lead system. Circulation 86:1217–1222, 1992.

90. Berul CI, Callans DJ, Schwartzman DS, et al: Comparison of initial detection and redetection of ventricular fibrillation in a transvenous defibrillator system with automatic gain control. J Am Coll Cardiol 25:431–436, 1995.

91. Gottlieb CD, Schwartzman DS, Callan DJ, et al: Effects of high and low shock energies on sinus electrograms recorded via integrated and true bipolar nonthoracotomy lead systems. J Cardiovasc Electrophysiol 7:189–196, 1996.

92. Callans DJ, Hook BG, Kleiman RB, et al: Unique sensing errors in third-generation implantable cardioverter-defibrillators. J Am Coll Cardiol 22:1135–1140, 1993.

93. Blanck Z, Niazi I, Axtell K, et al: Feasibility of concomitant implantation of permanent transvenous pacemaker and defibrillator systems. Am J Cardiol 74:1249–1253, 1994.

94. Brooks R, Garan H, McGovern BA, et al: Implantation of transvenous nonthoracotomy cardioverter-defibrillator system in patients with permanent endocardial pacemakers. Am Heart J 129:45–53, 1995.

95. Kantharia B, Pennington J, Kleinman D, et al: Feasibility of extraction of endocardial implantable cardioverter defibrillator leads. PACE 21:4(Pt II):970, 1998.

96. Krishan SC, Vassolas G, Epstein LM: Initial experience with a laser sheath to extract chronic transvenous defibrillator leads. J Am Coll Cardiol 31(2 Suppl A):120A, 1998.

97. Niebauer MJ, Al-Khandra A, Chung MK, et al: The Spectranetics laser sheath reduces extraction time for nonthoracotomy defibrillator leads. J Am Coll Cardiol 31(2 Suppl A):120A, 1998.

98. Rosenthal ME, Alderfer JT, Marchlinski FE: Troubleshooting suspected ICD malfunction. *In* Kroll M, Lehmann MH (eds): Implantable Cardioverter-Defibrillator Therapy: The Engineering Clinical Interface. Dordrecht, The Netherlands, Kluwer Academic Publishers, 1996, pp 435–476.

99. Epstein A, Anderson P, Kay GN, et al: Gross and microscopic changes associated with a nonthoracotomy implantable cardioverter defibrillator. PACE 15:382, 1992.

100. Geelen P, Lorga F, Chauvin M, et al: The value of DDD pacing in patients with an implantable cardioverter defibrillator. PACE 20(Pt II):177–181, 1997.

101. Lavenge T, Daubert J-C, Chauvin M, et al: Preliminary clinical experience with the first dual chamber pacemaker defibrillator. PACE 20(Pt II):182–188, 1997.

102. Mattke S, Fiek M, Markewitz A, et al: Comparison of a unipolar defibrillation system with a dual lead system using an enlarged defibrillation anode. PACE 19:2083–2088, 1996.

Chapter 6

Power Systems for Implantable Pacemakers, Cardioverters, and Defibrillators

Darrel F. Untereker, Richard B. Shepard, Craig L. Schmidt, Ann M. Crespi, and Paul M. Skarstad

This chapter provides the clinician with information about power systems (batteries and capacitors) used in implantable pacemakers and defibrillators. Batteries and capacitors are the sources of the energy used to operate these devices. Batteries are active devices that convert chemical energy into electric energy, whereas capacitors are passive devices that temporarily store energy, often to increase the available power (rate of energy delivery) in an electric circuit. The purpose of this chapter is to communicate background and clinically useful information pertaining to these power-related components. We hope this will help physicians in managing their patients who have implanted pacemakers and defibrillators. The chapter describes the basic principles and terminology of batteries and capacitors. It also discusses some important factors to be considered in the design of these components and how they relate to the clinical characteristics of implantable device performance.

The battery is conceptually different from the other components of an implantable pacing or defibrillator system. In principle, the other components of pacing systems are designed to last indefinitely. The available chemical energy of the battery, however, is consumed during its normal use. Thus, the battery has a finite service life because it contains a fixed amount of the active chemicals that furnish its energy. As the pacemaker or defibrillator is used, the battery's remaining energy supply is reduced. Eventually, the output voltage falls to a level that is insufficient to operate the device. When this happens, the battery is no longer useful and must be replaced. At present, the only practical way to produce a reliable device is to make the power source an integral part of the pulse generator. Thus, the entire pulse generator must be replaced to renew the battery.

Whereas batteries transform chemical energy into electric energy, capacitors are energy-storage devices. Capacitors are used in electronic devices for two major purposes. One is to control the timing of events. The second is to intermittently boost the power capability of electronic circuits. It is the second reason that is of principal interest here. Thus, the capacitors in an implantable cardioverter-defibrillator (ICD) allow the device to deliver a therapeutic, high-voltage, high-energy shock to the heart in a few milliseconds, a feat that the battery could not do by itself.

We believe that clinicians need to understand the major properties and limitations of implantable device batteries and capacitors as well as how these affect the treatment of patients. This understanding is one facet of the knowledge needed for optimal patient management.

■ DEFINITIONS

Some basic definitions relating to batteries and capacitors are listed here. They are listed to provide a common ground for reading this chapter. The reader may wish to refer to these definitions when needed.

Oxidation: Any process by which a chemical entity, such as an atom, ion, radical, or compound, loses electrons.

Reduction: Any process by which a chemical entity, such as an atom, ion, radical, or compound, gains electrons.

Anion: A negatively charged ion. It is attracted to positively charged ions and repelled by negatively charged ions.

Cation: A positively charged ion. It is attracted to negatively charged ions and repelled by positively charged ions.

Conduction: The movement of charge under the influence of an electric field. There are two fundamental forms of conduction. One is electronic, in which electrons are the charge carriers, and the second is ionic, in which charged chemical species (ions) are the charge carriers. Usually, metals and semiconductors are electronic conductors, whereas solutions and some nonmetallic substances are ionic conductors.

Anode: (a) The electrode at which oxidation occurs in an electrochemical cell; (b) The material that undergoes oxidation in an electrochemical cell; (c) The electrode that furnishes electrons to the external circuit, thus the negative terminal of a spontaneously discharging galvanic cell. In a capacitor, the plate that loses electrons and has a net positive charge.

Cathode: (a) The electrode at which reduction occurs in an electrochemical cell; (b) The material that undergoes reduction in an electrochemical cell; (c) In a spontaneously discharging galvanic cell, the positive terminal that attracts electrons from the external circuit. In a capacitor, the plate that has gained electrons and has a net negative charge.

Galvanic cell: A device that is capable of spontaneously transforming chemical energy into electric energy. Examples are flashlight batteries and fuel cells.

Battery: A galvanic cell; or a group of galvanic cells connected in series, in parallel, or in a series–parallel combination for the purpose of increasing their voltage or current capability.

Capacitor: A passive energy-storage device that stores energy in a dielectric medium.

Dielectric: A nonconductive (insulating) material or vacuum.

Half-cell potential: A numerical value expressed as a voltage (vs. an arbitrary reference electrode) that characterizes a substance's tendency to either oxidize or reduce.

Stoichiometry: The numerical relationship between atoms or molecules that exactly react with one another.

Rate capability: The ability to deliver a sustained current of a certain magnitude (this should not be confused with pacing rate).

Energy density: The energy content of a battery or capacitor based on volume or mass.

Power: The rate at which energy is made available or consumed; here, from a battery or capacitor.

Deformation: A nonideal behavior in a capacitor whereby the amount of charge required to bring the capacitor voltage to a specified value is greater than would normally be necessary because the capacitor has not been used for an extended period.

Dielectric strength: The ability of a dielectric material to maintain a voltage difference across a given thickness of the material. Dielectric strength is also the minimum voltage that will cause a dielectric insulator in a capacitor to break down (fail).

■ BATTERIES

Basic Function and Electrochemistry of Batteries

Energy Storage in Batteries

A battery converts chemical energy into electric energy. The source of this energy is the electrochemical reactions that occur within the battery. The amount and type of the materials participating in these reactions are the primary factors that determine the deliverable energy content of a battery.

Chemical Reactions

During a chemical reaction, substances interact to form reaction products. For example, in burning, the fuel combines with oxygen from the air to form combustion products. These usually include water, carbon dioxide, and perhaps

other species. The fuel is oxidized during this process. Oxygen from the air is reduced. The exact amounts of each are determined by the stoichiometry of the reaction. Equations 1 to 4 are examples of different types of reactions in which oxidation and reduction occur. They are called *redox reactions* and show the exact relationships between the reactants.

(1) $\quad 2H_2 + O_2 \rightarrow 2H_2O$ (formation of water)

(2) $\quad 2C_6H_6 + 15O_2 \rightarrow 12CO_2 + 6H_2O$
$\qquad\qquad\qquad\qquad$ (burning of benzene)

(3) $\quad 4Fe + 3O_2 \rightarrow 2Fe_2O_3$ (rusting of iron)

(4) $\quad 2Li + I_2 \rightarrow 2LiI$
$\qquad$ (discharge of a lithium-iodine pacemaker battery)

Chemical reactions like these occur spontaneously because the products are in a lower energy state than the reactants. The difference in energy appears as heat in the case of combustion or rusting. A battery or galvanic cell is designed to convert much of this energy difference between the reactants and the products into electric energy rather than heat.

Electron Transfer

A battery operates because the electrons transferred during a redox reaction are channeled from one terminal of the battery through the circuit and back to the battery through its other terminal. The maximum work these electrons can do outside the battery is related to the difference in "free energy" of the reactions, a thermodynamic quantity. Chemical reactions, such as those in equations 1 to 4, show reactants on the left side of the equation and products on the right side. In concept, these reactions can be thought of as the sum of two partial, or "half," reactions, which are written so that two half reactions add together to describe the complete chemical event. For example, equation 4 shows the chemical reaction that describes the discharge of the most common battery system used to power bradycardia pacemakers. Equations 5 and 6 show the two half reactions that, when added together, describe the principal part of the electrochemical reaction that occurs during discharge of a lithium-iodine battery. In this case, the total reaction also includes the two ions that combine to form a solid material, LiI.

(5) $\quad Li \rightarrow Li^+ + e^-$ (oxidation of lithium)

(6) $\quad I_2 + 2e^- \rightarrow 2I^-$ (reduction of iodine)

Half-Cell Potentials

Half-cell equations, like equations 5 and 6, indicate what reactions can occur. Half-reaction equations, however, give no information about the likelihood that any reaction will actually occur. The thermodynamic tendency for a reaction to occur is measured by its half-cell potential (see previous section, Definitions).

Table 6–1 shows the potentials associated with some half-cell reactions used in battery systems. The most positive values are for substances that give up electrons easily and become more positively charged (oxidized). These materials are typically metals. Substances with more negative half-cell potentials have a tendency to accept electrons. These materials gain electrons and reduce their charge.

Table 6–1. Standard Oxidation Potentials of Some Common Substances

Redox Reaction		Half-Cell Potential
Li	$\rightarrow$ Li$^+$ + e$^-$	3.05
Na	$\rightarrow$ Na$^+$ + e$^-$	2.71
Mg	$\rightarrow$ Mg^{2+} + 2e$^-$	2.37
Al	$\rightarrow$ Al^{3+} + 3e$^-$	1.66
Zn	$\rightarrow$ Zn^{2+} + 2e$^-$	0.76
Co	$\rightarrow$ Co^{2+} + 2e$^-$	0.28
H	$\rightarrow$ 2 H$^+$ + 2e	0.00
Ag	$\rightarrow$ Ag^{2+} + e$^-$	-0.79
I	$\rightarrow$ ½I$_2$ + e	-0.54
2 Br$^-$	$\rightarrow$ Br$_2$ + 2e$^-$	-1.07
2 H$_2$O	$\rightarrow$ O$_2$ + 2H$^+$ + 4e$^-$	-1.23
2F$^-$	$\rightarrow$ Fi$_2$ + 2e$^-$	-2.65

Major Chemical and Electrical Components of Batteries

Figure 6–1 schematically shows a simple battery. The major parts of a battery are the anode, the cathode, and the electrolyte. The anode and cathode must be physically separated, and both must be in contact with the electrolyte, which is often a solution.

Anode and Cathode

The two major battery components involved in the electrochemical reaction during discharge of a galvanic cell are the anode and the cathode. The anode, which is often a metallic substance, furnishes electrons to the external circuit, whereas the cathode, which is usually not a metal, receives them.

It can be confusing to think of an anode in a battery as being negative, and the cathode positive, because the pacing stimulus occurs at the cathode tip of the lead and is a negative pulse. However, the terminology is not inconsistent.

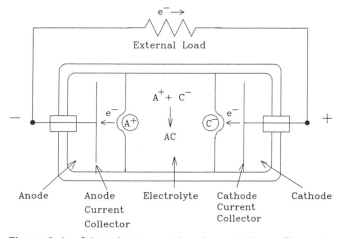

Figure 6–1. Schematic representation of a sealed battery. The anode material is on the left, the cathode material on the right, and the electrolyte in the middle of the cell. The discharge reaction is A + C → AC. In this example, both A$^+$ and C$^-$ are mobile ions, and the discharge product, AC, is insoluble and precipitates in the electrolyte solution. In this figure, connections to the interior of the cell are made through feedthroughs.

Oxidation always occurs at an anode and reduction at a cathode. In a spontaneously discharging electrochemical cell (a battery), oxidation at the anode delivers electrons to the external circuit, and the battery anode is thus negative. These electrons cause electrochemical reduction to occur in the solution surrounding the pacing lead tip (the cathode).

Electrolyte

The anode and the cathode are separated by the electrolyte, which is a crucial component of the battery. As the battery discharges, it furnishes electrons at one terminal, pushes them through an external circuit, and receives them at a second terminal. If this were all that happened, the discharge process would not occur for long because a large positive charge would quickly develop near the anode–electrode interface, and an equally large negative charge would develop on the cathode side. The build-up of these charges would suppress further reaction. It is the electrolyte that prevents this from happening by allowing the accumulating opposite charges at the two electrodes to migrate and neutralize each other. The requirement for an electrolyte is that it conduct ions but not electrons. If the electrolyte conducted electrons as well as ions, the battery would be internally shorted, just as it would if a wire were directly connected to the positive and negative terminals. Many battery electrolytes are solutions, but some are solids. This is discussed further later.

Discharge Product

The discharge product of any cell reaction must accumulate somewhere within the battery. Just where it collects depends on the relative mobility of the migrating ions and the solubility of the discharge product in the electrolyte. In many common batteries, the discharge product collects within a porous cathode structure, but in the important lithium-iodine implantable battery system, the discharge product accumulates near the anode surface. This is discussed later.

Stoichiometry and Cell Balance

Physical separation of the anode and cathode is required for a battery to be functional. The left side of Figure 6–1 shows the anode, which will lose electrons to form A$^+$ ions; the right side shows the cathode, which will gain electrons to form C$^-$ ions as the battery discharges. These processes occur in concert. The electrons generated on the anode side of the battery are consumed on the cathode side. Thus, there is a specific ratio of the anode and cathode materials that react to form the discharge product. A cell that contains exactly the required ratio of anode and cathode materials is said to be a *balanced cell*. Most medical batteries are not designed with the stoichiometric ratio of the active cathode and anode materials. This is done for two reasons. One is to increase operational safety, and the second is to provide controllable and gradual end-of-service characteristics.

The maximum energy content of a battery is fixed by the amount of anode and cathode materials in the cell. This energy may appear as heat or electricity, depending on the specific battery chemistry, the design of the battery, and the manner in which it is discharged; however, the total amount of energy delivered is invariant. Thus, the more energy that appears as heat, the less is available to power an electrical device. The efficiency of converting chemical energy to electric energy is high for devices like pacemakers, which require very small amounts of current, but, as shown later, this efficiency decreases dramatically for devices like defibrillators, which demand very high currents.

Cell Thermodynamics and Kinetics

The operation of any battery is dependent on both thermodynamic and kinetic processes. *Thermodynamics*, in this context, refers to whether a chemical reaction can or is likely to occur. *Chemical kinetics*, on the other hand, refers to how fast the reaction actually proceeds. In general, thermodynamic properties relate to the theoretical limits of battery operation, whereas kinetics often determine how much of the energy can be delivered and at what voltage and current.

Cell Voltage and Current

The voltage of a single cell can be calculated from fundamental thermodynamic quantities. The theoretical voltage is calculated from the half-cell potentials for the anode and cathode reactions. This is the voltage that is measured when there are no kinetic limitations, a condition that occurs only when an insignificant amount of current is being drawn from the battery. This is called the *open-circuit voltage*. In practice, the open-circuit voltage can be measured using a high-impedance voltmeter that draws almost no current from the battery during the measurement process.

Chemical Kinetic Limitations

As soon as current is drawn from the battery, some chemical kinetic limitations start to be observed. With the onset of current flow, for example, the voltage at the battery terminals is diminished compared with the open-circuit value. At the extreme, only the cell kinetics and internal resistance of the battery limit the current that flows from the battery into a complete short circuit. Both the chemistry and the design of the battery determine the relationship between load-circuit voltage and current drawn from the battery. A typical relationship is shown in Figure 6–2.

Open-Circuit and Short-Circuit Voltages and Currents

In Figure 6–2, the load voltage approaches the open-circuit voltage as the current approaches zero. At the other extreme, the maximum (short-circuit) current is observed when the load voltage approaches zero. How rapidly the curve in Figure 6–2 changes with current depends on the particular battery chemistry and how the battery is designed. For example, a lead-acid battery for automotive use is constructed of very conductive materials and is designed with large, high surface area electrodes (anode and cathode) so that extremely high currents can be drawn from it to run an engine's starter. On the other hand, a transistor radio battery is designed with small electrodes to manage the relatively low currents that are typical of small portable electronic devices.

For any specific battery, the output voltage and the current are closely related. However, there is no fundamental relationship between voltage and current that holds for all batteries. Even for the same chemical components, the shape of a battery's current–voltage curve, like the one shown in Figure 6–2, is strongly dependent on the design of the battery.

Temperature Effect on Battery Function

The characteristics of a battery also change with temperature. For many applications, battery specifications must be devel-

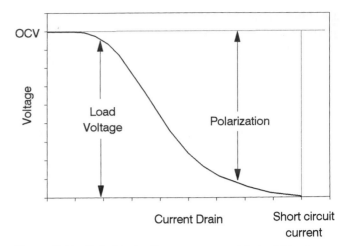

Figure 6–2. Typical load voltage versus current drain plot for a battery. The load voltage is always less than the open-circuit voltage. Current drain increases toward the right. The maximum cell voltage is obtained at zero current, and the maximum current drain occurs at zero load voltage. The exact shape of the plot depends on the chemistry and design of the battery.

oped to cope with the entire range of temperatures over which the battery is expected to operate. In general, battery performance is at an optimum between 10° and 50°C, and it deteriorates at either higher or lower temperatures. A battery's voltage becomes lower at colder temperatures, and cell kinetics are generally much slower under colder conditions; thus, the ability of a normal battery to supply current is typically greatly diminished at low temperatures. At higher temperatures, reaction rates increase beyond what is desirable. These reactions can harm a battery and lead to premature failure. Fortunately, implantable devices operate at the relatively constant body temperature of about 37°C, so they are not normally subject to either high or low temperatures. Even for implantable medical devices, however, there are situations during manufacturing, shipping, delivery, and sterilization in which the power source may be exposed to temperatures that are different from body temperature. Engineers must take these conditions into account when designing and choosing power sources.

Battery Terminology

Capacity

The fundamental unit of battery capacity is the coulomb (1.6×10^{19} electrons), which is the amount of charge delivered by 1 ampere (A) of current in 1 second. In the context of implantable devices, a more practical unit of capacity is the ampere-hour (Ah), which represents the charge carried by a current of 1 ampere flowing for 1 hour. A battery for an implantable medical device usually has a capacity rating of between 0.5 and 2.0 Ah. Many papers have been written about the proper way of determining and specifying the capacity of a medical battery.[1–3] No single method is uniquely correct. What is important to the physician who is interested in comparing the capacities of different pacemaker and defibrillator batteries is to pay careful attention to the assumptions and methods that were used to estimate the capacity. Various methods produce numbers ranging from theoretical values that can never be achieved in the field to very realistic values that are based on detailed models or accelerated testing. In general, more optimistic numbers are obtained from theoretical calculations based only on the amount of active materials in the battery. More sophisticated methods account for known limitations or limited availability of the components within the battery. For example, most batteries are not able to use all of their active components before they cease to function. A prediction that does not take this into account is too optimistic. In addition, other limitations come into play. For example, the load-circuit voltage always decreases as the battery is used. Because the electronic circuits of a pulse generator can operate only above a specified minimum voltage, the cell capacity that is generated below this voltage is not usable and should not be counted in a projection of battery life. Self-discharge and other parasitic chemical reactions further reduce the amount of energy a battery will deliver.

Estimating the deliverable capacity of implantable medical batteries is made especially difficult by their long service life. The time frame for the operation of most implantable medical devices is so long (5 to 10 years) that real-time measurements of capacity are not practical. Therefore, accelerated tests and models are typically used to estimate the amount of deliverable capacity in these batteries before they are put into clinical use. Fortunately, technology in this area has improved a great deal, and it is now possible to make quite accurate projections of battery capacity.[4–6]

Energy Density

The fundamental unit of energy is the joule (J). This is the energy given to 1 coulomb of charge that is accelerated by a difference in potential of 1 V. One joule is also the energy transferred by 1 watt (W) of power in 1 second. Just as battery capacity is often measured in ampere-hours, battery energy is often expressed in watt-hours (Wh) instead of joules.

An additional battery parameter of interest to clinicians and implantable device designers is energy density, a parameter that can be expressed on the basis of either mass or volume. For medical applications, volume is usually more important than mass, so ratings based on volumetric energy density are most commonly used. The time integral of the product of voltage and current divided by the total volume of the battery is its energy density. The energy density of a battery can be approximated by the product of average voltage and nominal capacity divided by volume (or mass if desired). Modern batteries for pacemakers have energy densities as high as 1 Wh/cm^3, including the case.

The deliverable energy density of a battery obviously depends on its chemistry, but it also depends to a large extent on its construction. A battery's energy density is maximized when all extraneous materials in the battery are minimized and the amounts of active anode and cathode materials are in the stoichiometric ratio for the discharge reaction. However, a battery designed for maximum energy density would, in most instances, not meet other important requirements, including safety, optimal reliability, and longevity. A medical battery designer attempts to make energy density as large as possible while still meeting all these other requirements.

Battery Structure and Related Functional Characteristics

Current Collector

The current collector makes the connection between the positive or negative terminal of the battery and its respective active electrode inside the cell. A current collector is usually a wire connected to a screen, or a grid that is embedded in the anode or cathode material of the battery. The current collector often also serves as a structural member of the battery to provide physical integrity and strength to that electrode. The size of the current collector is sometimes used as a design parameter to limit the maximum current that can be drawn from a cell. This minimizes the risks from an inadvertent short of the electrodes during battery manufacture or assembly into a pulse generator. Some medical batteries use the case of the cell as the current collector for the cathode.

Separator

The separator is often confused with the electrolyte. The electrolyte is the medium that conducts ions within the battery, whereas the separator is a physical, structural member of the cell that keeps the anode and cathode materials apart, thus preventing shorting of the cell. All batteries need an electrolyte, but not all batteries require a separator. A separator is usually needed in batteries that contain liquid electrolytes. Without a separator in these batteries, there would be little to stop the anode from shorting to the cathode if the cell were squeezed or if there were any internal movement of the electrodes during use (which can result from volume changes during discharge). The separator is made of a material that has a porous structure so that the electrolyte solution can fill the pores and ions can move between the anode and cathode sides of the battery. Flashlight batteries use paper separators. Medical batteries with liquid electrolytes use porous polymer films that do not react with other components of the battery system. A medical battery with a separator is the lithium-silver vanadium oxide battery used to power implantable defibrillators.

Internal Impedance

Electrical impedance and resistance are important battery properties that play a crucial role in the clinical performance of many implantable devices. The terms *impedance* and *resistance* are often used interchangeably, although impedance is calculated using a time-varying current, whereas resistance is calculated using a constant current. The difference between resistance and impedance can be important to electrical circuit designers.

Hermetic Seal

Most batteries need to be sealed, but few batteries other than those used for implantable medical devices and aerospace applications need to be so well sealed that they are truly hermetic (i.e., gas tight). Hermeticity implies the use of welded construction and glass or similar feed-throughs to make electrical connections between the inside and the outside of the battery. This is necessary to prevent slow interchanges of materials between the battery and its surroundings. For example, batteries using lithium electrodes must be sealed to prevent water from entering the case. In addition, some of the components used inside medical lithium batteries are volatile and could be corrosive or damaging if they leaked out. Medical batteries are typically considered hermetically sealed if the leak rate for a test gas (usually helium) out of the battery is less than 1×10^{-7} cm³/sec at 1 atmosphere helium pressure difference between the inside and the outside of the cell.

Nonideal Battery Behavior

The previous discussion has focused on the principles and nomenclature of battery operation. It is also important to understand some of the things that limit the ability of a battery to power an implantable device. Several important nonideal processes are discussed in the following paragraphs.

Polarization

Polarization is any process that causes the voltage at the terminals of a battery to drop below its open-circuit value when it is providing current. Internal resistance is one important cause in some types of batteries. This is well illustrated in Figure 6–3 for the lithium-iodine battery.

This figure shows the discharge voltage versus capacity curve at four rates of constant-current discharge. The differences between these curves are mainly due to the voltage drop associated with internal resistance of the battery.

Another cause of polarization is the development of a concentration gradient within the battery. As a battery discharges, the ions in the electrolyte must move to maintain electrical neutrality. If they cannot move quickly enough, concentration gradients develop within the battery. A concentration gradient lowers the cell's load voltage because the half-cell potentials at the anode and cathode are logarithmically related to the ratio of the reactant and product concentrations.

Similarly, the electron transfer rate from the redox reaction may not be able to occur as rapidly as the external demand requires. In such cases, the maximum rate of discharge of the battery becomes governed by the rates at which the redox reactions can occur. When current is drawn from a battery, all of these processes occur to some extent. The net effect of these kinetic limitations is always observed as a decrease in the voltage at the terminals of the battery.

Self-Discharge

Self-discharge is the spontaneous discharge of a cell or battery by an internal chemical reaction rather than through useful electrochemical discharge. We have all seen the effects of self-discharge at one time or other. The flashlight that does not work when needed after a prolonged storage time is a good example. One mechanism by which self-discharge can occur involves a slow direct reaction between the anode and the cathode. Other self-discharge processes may involve reactions between either the anode or the cathode and another substance in the battery, such as the solvent in the electrolyte. A typical example would be a reaction between the anode and the electrolyte solvent to form a passive film or a gas. The zinc–mercuric oxide batteries used to power the first implantable pulse generators produced hydrogen gas by such a process. The need to let this gas leak out of the pacemaker slowly was one reason why the electronic circuitry in the early pulse generators was encapsulated in epoxy. These parasitic reactions are usually very slow, but because medical batteries are expected to operate for many years, their accumulated effects can be appreciable. Although it is difficult to measure the very slow rate of self-discharge reactions, techniques such as microcalorimetry, which can detect the small amounts of heat that are involved, have been used for this purpose.[7, 8] The rate of heat generation can be used to calculate the rate of self-discharge by applying thermodynamic principles and equations.

Classification of Batteries

Batteries may be classified in many ways. For example, batteries may be categorized by application, functional characteristics, chemistry, or the physical state of some component. One fundamental distinction is between primary and secondary batteries.

Primary Batteries

Primary batteries can be used only once. They are not designed to be recharged. Familiar examples of primary batteries are zinc-carbon dry cells, alkaline zinc–manganese dioxide flashlight batteries, zinc–mercuric oxide batteries used in early pacemakers, lithium-iodine batteries used to power most modern cardiac pacemakers, and lithium-silver vanadium oxide batteries used to power defibrillators.

Secondary Batteries

Secondary batteries can be repetitively discharged and charged. The distinction between primary and secondary batteries is important, particularly because attempts to charge a primary battery can be dangerous. Familiar examples of secondary batteries include the lead acid batteries used in automobiles and the cadmium–nickel oxide ("Ni-Cad") and metal hydride–nickel oxide batteries widely used in portable electronics devices (e.g., cellular telephones, power tools, and lap-top computers). Rechargeable cadmium–nickel oxide batteries were used to power some cardiac pacemakers built

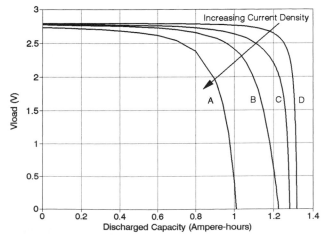

Figure 6–3. Load voltage versus capacity plot for lithium-iodine battery discharged at four magnitudes of constant current. Curve A = 40 µA/cm², curve B = 20 µA/cm², curve C = 10 µA/cm², and curve D = 2 µA/cm². The deliverable capacity decreases with increasing current in this current range because of increasing effects of polarization.

in the 1970s. Today, cadmium–nickel oxide battery technology is being phased out of many applications because of its potential for environmental contamination with toxic cadmium-containing materials when the battery is thrown away. Cadmium–nickel oxide also suffers from poor reversibility under different charging and discharging conditions ("memory effect"). This battery chemistry is being replaced by the metal hydride–nickel oxide battery, which has voltage and current characteristics similar to those of the cadmium–nickel oxide system, plus a significantly greater energy density and a greatly reduced environmental hazard.

A newer rechargeable battery system is also being developed based on lithium-ion technology. This technology, which is approximately 10 years old, incorporates a lithium intercalated carbon anode (intercalation is an association, not a true chemical bond) and a lithium intercalated metal oxide cathode (such as CoO_2). The lithium ion is "passed" from the anode to the cathode during discharge and from the cathode to the anode during charge. The cell discharge occurs at an average voltage as high as 3.7 V. These batteries have already proven to be able to be cycled (one cycle is one charge and one discharge) up to 1000 times, while still retaining 80% of their initial discharge capacity. The lithium-ion chemistry is currenty being considered for use in several types of implantable medical devices. As of this writing the energy density of the lithium-ion system is about half that of a typical lithium primary battery, and its long-term low-rate reliability is still being assessed. The indications so far are that this is a very safe battery system. The most attractive feature of this technology arises from its cycle life. While the energy density of a lithium-ion battery may only be half that of a typical lithium primary battery, the *total* energy delivered (e.g., over a conservative 200 cycles) is 100 times that of its primary counterpart. It is expected that this secondary battery system will thus be attractive for medical uses when the capacity required is so great that ordinary lithium batteries would need to be too large to be implanted. Some applications under current study are implantable pain control and cardiac assist devices.

Further discussion of secondary battery technology in this chapter is limited because such cells are not being used in medical devices that are currently implanted. The interested reader can find a good presentation of secondary battery technology in references 9 to 11.

Aqueous and Nonaqueous Batteries

Another broad distinction between types of batteries is based on the choice of the electrolyte solvent. Batteries with aqueous electrolytes include many systems using zinc, lead, cadmium, aluminum, or magnesium anodes. Examples include zinc–mercuric oxide batteries, cadmium–nickel oxide rechargeable batteries, zinc-air batteries, and alkaline zinc–manganese dioxide flashlight batteries. Clinicians are probably familiar with the zinc-air battery, which is commonly used to power hearing aids.[12] This is an unusual battery system because it uses oxygen from the air as the active cathode chemical. The oxygen is reduced at a carbon electrode that is exposed to the air outside the battery via a small hole in the case. The use of oxygen from the air makes this battery system attractive because the battery can be small.

Water is an excellent solvent for salts and forms electro-lyte solutions with excellent ionic conductivity. However, water cannot be used as a component of long-lived batteries employing lithium or sodium anodes because these very active metals undergo rapid reaction with water to form hydrogen gas and an alkali hydroxide. Because of such reactions, alkaline metal anode batteries use nonaqueous solvents that react minimally with these metals. Most lithium-based batteries employ a mixture of organic ethers and esters as solvents for the electrolyte. For example, lithium–manganese dioxide batteries, which are widely used to power automatic cameras, use mixtures containing dimethoxyethane, in which lithium trifluoromethane sulfonate or lithium perchlorate is dissolved, to make the electrolyte. A few lithium batteries, however, are designed with solid ceramic or polymeric electrolytes. These electrolytes are solid ion-conducting materials and do not require any solvent.

Implantable Battery Design Requirements

Implantable medical devices must be thought of as a system. Longevity, end-of-service indications, and even basic reliability depend on optimal integration of the battery with the other components of the pulse generator. The type of battery selected for a particular application is determined by several crucial requirements. Without question, the main requirement in battery selection for implantable devices is high reliability. Other significant requirements include the longevity of the device (directly related to energy density and circuit design) and an appropriate indication of impending battery depletion (end-of-service warning). These are discussed in detail later.

The basic considerations when designing a battery for an implantable medical device include the electronic technology of the device that it will power and the voltage and current variations that will be required by the circuit, the therapy, and the individual patient. The desired longevity of the device must also be established. Once these application requirements are formulated, the current, voltage, and capacity requirements of the battery can be determined. An important limitation is the physical space—both volume and shape—within the pulse generator that can be allotted to the battery. Once this is determined, the required energy density can be calculated, and various battery systems and designs can be considered and evaluated.

Battery Chemistry

Different chemical systems have different battery characteristics. Voltage, energy density, and inherent current capability are all primarily functions of the battery chemistry. The chemistry of the battery must be chosen to match the needs of the application. For cxample, the rate of energy consumption differs markedly between pacemakers and defibrillators, and sometimes even between atrial and ventricular defibrillators. Pacemakers use very small amounts of energy when they stimulate the heart, on the order of 15 μJ. Defibrillators, on the other hand, deliver a much larger amount of energy when they discharge, as much as 40 J. Although the sizes of the batteries used in defibrillators and pacemakers are not greatly different, a pacemaker battery could never come close to supplying energy at the rate required to power a defibrillator. Likewise, the defibrillator battery would be a poor choice to power a pacemaker, although it could easily supply the current needed. The high-power design of a defibrillator battery has a significantly lower energy density than that of a pacemaker battery, perhaps by a factor of three. Thus, if a defibrillator battery were used for pacing and everything else were equal, it would need to be three times as big as a pacemaker battery to obtain the same longevity. Additionally, a high-current cell poses more inherent safety risks (such as gross overheating from an internal short) than does a low-current cell, so there are still other reasons for matching the battery to the application as closely as possible.

Cell Balance

An ideal battery would contain the exact stoichiometric ratio of the active anode and cathode substances plus a small amount of electrolyte. In practice, however, batteries are built with one electrode in excess of the other. For medical batteries in use today, the anode is the electrode in surplus by 5% to 25%. Having an unbalanced cell with excess anode leads to both a more gradual and a more predictable decline of the cell voltage as the cell approaches depletion than if the cell was stoichiometrically balanced.

The amount of electrolyte is also crucial to the long-term performance of batteries with liquid electrolyte. Minor parasitic or self-discharge reactions can consume significant amounts of some components of the electrolyte over time. Thus, a battery must contain a sufficient amount of electrolyte so that it can operate reliably over its entire intended service life.

Power Requirements

Another important consideration in designing an appropriate battery for a device is the peak power requirement. The battery must be capable of supplying the required power without a large drop in load voltage. The lithium-iodine battery, for example, has a relatively high internal resistance, which increases even more as the battery is discharged. Its primary use is as a power source for implantable cardiac pacemakers, which typically have peak power demands on the order of 100 to 200 μW. Under these conditions, the lithium-iodine battery can maintain an adequate voltage even when its internal resistance reaches several thousand ohms. On the other hand, an implantable cardiac defibrillator may have peak power requirements about 10,000 times greater than those of a pacemaker, and a lithium-iodine battery would be incapable of meeting these requirements. This difference in peak power capability may be made more obvious by realizing that if all of the lithium-iodine batteries ever produced were connected in an optimal series-parallel combination, they would operate fewer than 10 100-W light bulbs. In contrast, it would take only about 100 defibrillator batteries in an appropriate series-parallel combination to light the same 10 100-W bulbs. It appears that the power and current demands for bradycardia pacemakers will be increasing in the near future because of more use of telemetry and proposed features such as multisite pacing. This is causing pacemaker designers to consider chemistries other than lithium-iodine as power sources for new products.

Average Versus Instantaneous Current Drain

A pacing circuit uses a small capacitor to buffer the current drain on the battery. The pacing pulse is delivered to the heart by discharge of this capacitor through the pacing lead for a relatively short interval (i.e., the pacing pulse width). The battery then charges this capacitor at a relatively low rate between pacing pulses. The use of a capacitor as a buffer allows the battery to supply short bursts of power that may be more than two orders of magnitude higher than it could deliver directly. Thus, electronic buffering reduces the instantaneous power demands placed on the battery. It also allows the use of battery designs with reduced anode and cathode surface areas and improved volumetric efficiency. The same principle applies to the use of batteries to charge the large capacitors used to deliver a defibrillation shock to the heart from an ICD, even though the magnitudes of the current and voltage are much greater.

Shape, Size, and Mass Constraints

Finally, all of these requirements (longevity, end-of-service indication, peak power, and so on) must be balanced against dimensional and mass constraints. The mass, dimensions, and shape of an implantable pulse generator are extremely important for safe implantation in children and for aesthetic reasons in many adults. In the case of ICDs, recent improvements in packaging and circuit technology have made it possible to produce ICDs that are small enough to be implanted routinely in the pectoral region of the chest.

The ratio of volume to surface area in the battery is an important factor. The performance of a battery of fixed volume can vary substantially depending on its electrode surface area-to-volume ratios. The operating current and longevity demanded of the battery determine both the minimum areas and the amounts of the anode and the cathode needed. On the other hand, the area-to-volume ratio must not be made too large or the battery will be costly to make and will have a diminished energy density. Thus, these parameters can be changed only within certain ranges without jeopardizing either the long-term performance or the reliability of the battery. The battery design selected for a particular device not only must meet electrical performance requirements but also must ensure an acceptable longevity for the pulse generator, be small enough for implant use, and have a good aesthetic appearance.

Relationship Between Current Drain and Battery Size

The relationship between average current and required battery size is not one of direct proportionality. For example, decreasing the average current by 50% does not permit a 50% reduction in battery size without compromising longevity. As battery size is decreased, packaging efficiency also decreases because an increasing fraction of the battery weight and volume is composed of inactive materials (case, electrode separator material, current collectors, and so on). Also, the cell is not balanced; there is an excess of lithium anode. In essence, this excess lithium is also an inactive material that reduces the packaging efficiency. This effect is most severe if the size reduction is accomplished by thinning the battery, which has been the trend in recent years. If battery size reduction is accomplished only by decreasing thickness, only a minimal decrease in the inactive material content inside the cell occurs because the mass and volume of the case, any separator material, and current collectors are largely unchanged. Thus, if a cell is made thinner, its capacity and energy density suffer far more than might be expected by the change in volume alone. A careful consideration of factors like these is always needed. The situation is even more complicated for applications like ICDs, in which there are both low power demands for pacing and device operation and high power demands for the defibrillation therapy.

Relationship Between Energy Density and Current Drain

Usable energy density is also a function of the current demand on the cell. This is particularly true for a battery such as the lithium-iodine battery, which has inherently high internal impedance. As the current drawn from the cell is increased, the resulting voltage drops significantly (see Fig. 6–3) and reduces the length of time during which the cell can provide current at or above the minimum voltage necessary to operate the electronic circuits. Thus, useable energy density, which is directly proportional to the area under the discharge (voltage vs. capacity) curve, is also reduced. For batteries like those used to power ICDs, this is not as important an issue because the internal resistance of these batteries is very low.

Effect of Clinical Needs and Patient Preferences on Battery Design

Marketing trends, which are intertwined with clinical needs, also impose important limitations on the size and shape of batteries. For example, a thin, small pulse generator is a major clinical requirement for infants. For adults, a somewhat larger pulse generator with a greater battery capacity may be desirable for increased device longevity. The recent improvements in the delivery of defibrillation therapy by transvenous leads was one factor that prompted a greater push to minimize the size of ICDs so that they could be implanted in the upper chest wall like a bradycardia pacemaker. A major aspect of deciding the size, shape, and weight of an implantable device is being sure that the battery is not optimized without consideration of medical and patient factors. For example, the battery should not be optimized for device longevity without weighing the consequences of making the device larger or thicker. This is because device size can be related to erosion, comfort, or even patient acceptance because of aesthetic appearance.

Medical Battery Design Issues and the Management of the Patient

The Battery and Longevity of the Pulse Generator

Longevity is typically defined as the interval between implantation of the device and detection of the end-of-service indicator. Battery longevity can vary dramatically among patients because of the programmed parameters and frequency of therapy. Thus, the longevity requirement in battery design is typically linked to a specified set of nominal conditions. The minimum battery capacity required to achieve the specified longevity can be calculated from the average current needed for this nominal set of conditions. The following equation relates the longevity of the pulse generator, L, to the deliverable capacity of the battery, Q, and the average pacing current, I.

$$(7) \quad L = \frac{Q}{8766 \cdot I}$$

The unit of L is years, Q is in milliampere-hours (mAh), and I is in milliamperes (mA). The conversion factor 8766 (365.25 days per year × 24 hours per day) is needed because longevity is expressed in years, not hours.

Parasitic Battery Capacity Losses

Other than delivering therapy to the patient, there are numerous additional drains on battery capacity. First, self-discharge and possibly other parasitic losses of the anode or cathode begin from the date of battery manufacture and continue throughout use. Although small, these losses may not be insignificant over the service life of the device. For example, the lithium-iodine battery may lose 10% of its capacity over the life of an implant because of the direct reaction of lithium and iodine. The solvent in liquid electrolyte batteries may slowly react with the lithium anode until there is not enough solvent left in the cell for it to function. Second, some current is required to power the circuit before implantation of the device. Hence, some allowance must be made for capacity consumed during the expected period of shelf life between manufacture and implantation. Finally, substantial battery capacity must also be kept in reserve to continue to power the device after the end-of-service indicator has been detected. For example, a device that requires a 72-month longevity and a 6-month end-of-service interval would need additional battery capacity of at least 8% (i.e., $6/72 \times 100$) more than the value calculated from equation 7 just to accommodate the end-of-service period.

Longevity of Pulse Generators

Two primary factors determine the longevity of an implanted pulse generator. The first factor is related to the size, design, and chemistry of the battery. The second factor is related to the rate at which the battery is discharged (i.e., the average current). The general relationships among battery size, average current, and longevity are obvious: larger batteries and lower current drains increase longevity. Because of better pacing electrodes and better electronic circuits, the average current drain for bradycardia devices has decreased substantially during the past decade. The trend throughout the evolution of cardiac pacemakers has been that reduced current demands lead to smaller batteries and pulse generators while maintaining relatively constant longevity. There is some expectation that this trend will continue, but the path to lower current often has a sawtooth-like profile as new features and therapeutic modalities temporarily increase the required current. A good example is the increase in current demand that occurred when technology moved from single- to dual-chamber pacemakers. The same sort of trend can be expected for defibrillators as their electronic circuits are improved and the average threshold for defibrillation becomes lower. The entire situation for ICDs is complicated, however, because of the unpredictable mixture of bradycardia and tachyarrhythmia therapies and the constant need to have a very high power capability in any device that may be required to deliver a defibrillation shock.

Overhead Current

The battery must also supply the static (or overhead) current that is needed to power the electronic components even when no stimulating therapy is being delivered. The overhead current for bradycardia devices has actually increased as these devices have become more complicated; at the same time, advances in electronic technology have substantially reduced the static current drain for tachycardia devices. The static current for all devices is now about 10 μA. As a first approximation, static or overhead current can be considered to be independent of the programmed settings of the pulse generator when calculating longevity or considering its effect on battery behavior.

Effect of Pulse Width on Pacing Current

Increasing the pacing rate, pulse width, or pulse amplitude increases the average pacing current. Some of these relationships, however, are highly nonlinear. For example, as shown later, doubling the pacing stimulus voltage quadruples the current drain on the battery. The average pacing current (not including overhead current) is directly proportional to the pacing rate. However, the effect of pulse width on the average pacing current is not linear. Recall that the pacing pulse results from the discharge of a capacitor through a nominally resistive load (i.e., the electrode–heart interface). This capacitor produces a pulse in which the current decays exponentially with time, as shown for two different pulse widths in Figure 6–4A and B.

Thus, the time-dependent behavior of the current during the pacing pulse is given by the following equation:

$$(8) \quad I = \frac{V_A}{R_H} e^{\frac{1}{R_H C}}$$

where V_A is the amplitude at the beginning of the pacing pulse, R_H is the resistance of the heart, C is the value of the capacitor that delivers the pacing pulse, and t is the time since the beginning of the pacing pulse. In Figure 6–4A and B, the pulse widths are t_w and $t_{w/2}$, respectively. The area under each current–time curve gives the total charge delivered during the pulse. Although the width of the pulse in Figure 6–4B is half that of the pulse in Figure 6–4A, the charge delivered by this pulse is considerably more than half that of the longer pulse. The exact ratio of the charge delivered in the two cases depends on the values of the resistance and capacitance. Nevertheless, reducing the pulse width by a given fraction always reduces the average pacing

current by a substantially smaller fraction because of the exponentially decaying shape of the pacing stimulus current curve.

Effect of Pulse Amplitude on Pacing Current

The definition of pacing pulse amplitude may vary somewhat among manufacturers of implantable pulse generators. For our purposes, *pulse amplitude* is defined as the voltage delivered to the heart at the beginning of the pacing pulse (leading-edge voltage). As stated earlier, the area under the current–time curve gives the charge delivered per pulse. Thus, doubling the amplitude doubles the current and the total charge delivered to the heart. It also might appear that because the charge per pulse is doubled, the average pacing current drawn from the battery would also be doubled. However, the impact on the pacing current is much larger than that, as seen from the following argument. The energy per pacing pulse is defined by the following equation:

$$(9) \quad E = V_A \cdot I_A \cdot t_w$$

In this equation, V_A is the average pacing stimulus output voltage of the pulse generator, I_A is the average pacing current delivered to the heart, and t_w is the pulse width. If we consider the lead–electrode–heart interface to be mainly resistive, Ohm's law, $I = V/R$, can be substituted in equation 9. When this is done, it becomes the following:

$$(10) \quad E = (V_A^2/R_H) t_w$$

Here, R_H is the effective ohmic load of the heart and lead. From this equation, it is readily apparent that energy consumption increases with the square of the output voltage. Because the battery supplies all of the energy delivered to the heart at a relatively constant voltage, any increase in energy is accompanied by a proportional increase in current drawn from the battery. Thus, the average pacing current is proportional to the square of the pacing stimulus voltage. In fact, this is the best situation; additional energy losses occur when the stimulus voltage is programmed to a higher level because the electronic processes for increasing the stimulus voltage are not 100% efficient.

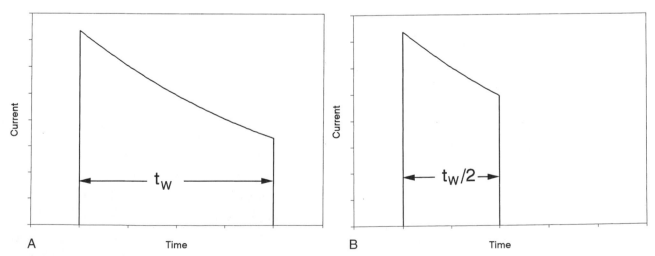

Figure 6–4. Comparison of charge delivered to the heart as the pacing pulse width is shortened. The two cases in *A* and *B* assume a discharge into the same patient. The pulse width, t_w, is typically between 0.2 and 1.5 msec, and the maximum current is between 2 and 15 mA, depending on the pulse generator output voltage and the lead–heart interface resistance.

Effect of Ohmic Load on Pacing Current

Finally, it is important to consider the effect of the lead resistance, R_H, on the average pacing current. In a sense, the term *lead resistance* is really a misnomer. The resistance of the lead itself is relatively small (50 to 100 Ω), and most of the resistance actually arises at the electrode–tissue interface (500 to 1000 Ω or more). The factors affecting the impedance of this interface are discussed in Chapter 1. In general, the average pacing current is approximately inversely proportional to the sum of the actual lead and tissue interface resistance. Thus, there is a substantial interest in lead technologies that can increase the impedance of the electrode–tissue interface, thereby decreasing the pacing current, while at the same time maintaining a constant, or even a reduced, pacing threshold voltage.

Summary of Programming Effects on Longevity of Bradycardia Pulse Generators

In summary, the wide range of pacing parameters that can be programmed can have a dramatic effect on the current drain from the battery in an implanted pulse generator. For example, in the same patient, a pacemaker with a 6-year longevity under nominal pacing parameters may reach its replacement time in 2 years at one extreme of programmed amplitude and pulse width or after more than 10 years at the other extreme. This is why the relationships between the programmed pacing parameters and the pacing threshold need to be considered quantitatively when the clinician is judging alternative programmable pulse generator settings or discussing predictions of future pulse generator replacement with the patient.

Considerations for Longevity of Implantable Cardioverter-Defibrillators

Most of the arguments concerning bradycardia pacemakers also apply to ICDs. However, ICDs are much more complicated than typical pacemakers, and it is not nearly as easy to generalize about the effect of different factors on their longevity. In general, the two most important factors to consider are the defibrillation threshold, which determines the amount of energy consumed during the delivery of each high-voltage therapy, and the frequency of tachyarrhythmia events compared with time spent pacing the heart. It is possible for the longevity to vary by a factor of two to three as a result of these issues alone. This is discussed further later.

Battery End-of-Service Indication

End-of-service requirements result from the need to indicate impending battery depletion in both pacemakers and defibrillators in a manner that allows the patient and physician adequate time to replace the device. In general, this requires a battery to have some measurable characteristic, such as voltage or impedance, that is related to its state of discharge. The pulse generator end-of-service indication must occur well before the battery loses so much voltage that it cannot sustain cardiac pacing or perform defibrillation. Again, this requirement is typically linked to a specific set of nominal pacing or defibrillation parameters. A detailed knowledge of the variations in battery performance, changes in load current with pulse generator settings, and accuracy of the end-of-

service measurement circuitry is necessary to ensure that these requirements will be met.

Elective Replacement Indicator

All modern implantable pulse generators have an *elective replacement indicator* (ERI) that alerts the clinician to impending battery depletion and allows adequate time for replacement of the device. This point is also referred to as the *recommended replacement time* or the *end-of-service point*. As a general rule, the indicator is designed to occur at least 3 months before the battery voltage drops to a level at which erratic pacing or the loss of capture results.

Methods for Monitoring State of Battery Discharge

Several means are used to monitor a battery's state of discharge.

Battery Voltage

The most common method measures battery voltage. Historically, this was accomplished by comparing the battery voltage to a diode reference voltage generated by the pacemaker circuitry. The ERI was triggered when the battery voltage dropped below the reference level. Most modern devices incorporate a voltage measurement circuit in the form of an analog-to-digital converter. The digitized battery voltage can be compared with a value stored in a nonvolatile memory to trigger the ERI, or it can be telemetered to the programmer where the comparison is made.

For lithium-iodine batteries, the battery voltage remains relatively constant throughout most of its discharge under low load conditions. This is shown in the voltage versus capacity curve in Figure 6–5. This figure also shows the resistance of this battery as it discharges. Notice that the resistance changes from a modest value at the beginning of service to a large value when it is nearly depleted.

Because the battery voltage is relatively constant for much of the pulse generator's useful life, the telemetered voltage may not be particularly useful for estimating its

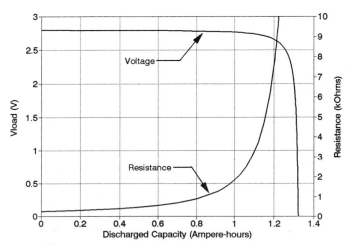

Figure 6–5. Relationships among voltage, resistance, and delivered capacity for a lithium-iodine battery. The voltage remains reasonably constant throughout the service life of the battery, whereas the resistance builds up steadily with discharge. Note the rapid fall-off in voltage as the resistance rapidly increases near the end of service life.

remaining service life until the end-of-service time draws near. On the other hand, the measured voltage may be useful for determining the battery's ability to remain above the ERI voltage after reprogramming to a higher current.

Voltage characteristics differ for different battery chemistries. Therefore, the clinician should not assume a familiarity with one model of implantable device or that one type of battery can be applied to another device or battery chemistry. For example, the lithium-iodine battery has a fairly flat discharge curve throughout most of its life at pacing currents. Its ERI is chosen somewhere on the knee of the discharge curve. The exact voltage chosen depends on the expected average drain current for that particular device at the end of the implant's service life. Other battery chemistries, however, have voltage characteristics much different from those of lithium-iodine. The lithium-silver vanadium oxide battery presently used in ICDs has two distinct voltage regions before the typical ERI voltage. The region after the second plateau is sloped. The switch from the second plateau to the sloped discharge region is used as the ERI trigger in some devices using this battery chemistry. This voltage is much less sensitive to current variances than is the voltage chosen for a lithium-iodine battery because the internal resistance of this battery is much lower than the lithium-iodine battery.

Battery Impedance

Battery impedance is another parameter used to signal the elective replacement point. Battery impedance is generally much less dependent on current than is battery voltage and may convey more information about the battery's state of discharge. For example, although the voltage of a lithium-iodine battery remains relatively constant through most of its discharge, its impedance increases continuously and especially rapidly as the battery approaches depletion (see Fig. 6–5). At depletion, battery impedance is useful not only for signaling the elective replacement point but also for providing an estimate of remaining service life. This feature has been incorporated into some pacemaker designs. Battery impedance is determined by measuring the voltage drop across a known resistor within the pulse generator, and then applying Ohm's law.

Consumed Charge as Indicator of Remaining Battery Use Time

A final method used to indicate remaining battery life has been to measure the cumulative sum of the charge removed from the battery. This is accomplished by monitoring the current drawn from the battery or the current and voltage (i.e., energy) delivered to the heart. This method requires an accurate knowledge of the original deliverable capacity of the battery because the technique actually measures the capacity already used, and the amount left must be calculated by subtracting this number from the initial capacity.

Elective Replacement Indicator Triggering

The relatively high resistance of power sources such as the lithium-iodine battery results in a battery voltage that is highly dependent on current. Thus, any large changes in average battery current in pulse generators that use battery voltage to indicate the elective replacement point (even if temporary) may drop the battery voltage below the ERI trigger value. Such changes in current can occur as a result of rate-responsive pacing, magnet-rate pacing, telemetry, and so on. This could also occur during electrophysiologic studies with noninvasively programmed stimulation (NIPS), in which the pacemaker is used to interrupt an episode of tachycardia by delivering short bursts of very high rate pacing. Because the ERI is usually latched (stored) when it is triggered, these temporary increases in current can cause a premature appearance of the ERI. The amount of service life lost to these premature triggers is typically relatively small (see the extreme example given later in this chapter). In most cases, devices are designed to make it possible to reset an ERI that has been prematurely triggered. In some devices, the ERI is inhibited during temporary high-current events to circumvent some of the issues described previously. In ICDs, the ERI is usually based on the battery voltage or the time required to charge the capacitor. Typically, the battery voltage is measured during normal sensing and pacing operation and not during a defibrillation therapy, when the battery voltage is much lower. Because of the low internal resistance of ICD batteries, there is little effect of pacing parameters on the triggering of ERI in these devices. Alternatively, some ICDs base their ERI determination on the time required to charge the output capacitor. This approach is possible because the lithium-silver vanadium oxide batteries used presently have a reduced power capability as they approach depletion.

Clinical Indicators of the Battery Replacement Time

The clinical indicators of battery depletion vary widely among manufacturers of pulse generators. In fact, there are often significant variations among various models provided by a single manufacturer. Some of the more common indicators are listed below.

1. Stepwise change in pacing rate. Elective replacement time is indicated by a change in the pacing rate to a predetermined fixed rate (such as 65 beats per minute [bpm]) or a fractional change in rate (such as a 10% decrease from the programmed rate).

2. Stepwise change in magnet rate. The magnet-pacing rate decreases in a stepwise fashion related to remaining battery life.

3. Pacing mode change. DDD and DDDR pulse generators may automatically revert to another mode, such as VVI or VOO, to reduce current drain and extend battery life.

4. Pulse width stretching. Some pulse generators increase the width of the pacing pulse to compensate for decreasing pulse amplitude associated with declining battery voltage. Pulse width stretching has also been used as an indicator of imminent ERI.

5. Telemetered battery voltage or impedance. In modern pacemakers, the battery voltage or the battery impedance can be telemetered out to the programming device. This information can be useful in estimating remaining battery life or in indicating an imminent ERI by algorithms performed outside the pulse generator.

All manufacturers provide technical manuals containing tables or graphs that indicate the relationship between battery voltage or impedance and the estimated remaining service life of the device. This time period differs for different loads on the battery as influenced by pacing rates and stimulus currents, as discussed previously.

The Elective Replacement Indicator in Practice

The ERI is both extremely useful and, if used uncritically, potentially misleading in some patients. The object of having an ERI is to allow the use of the pulse generator as long as is safely possible. Some pertinent questions must be addressed by the clinician when considering elective pulse generator replacement based on the ERI:

1. How does the ERI for this particular pulse generator manifest itself?

2. Because the goal is to replace the pulse generator not too long before its continued use becomes unsafe, what is the definition of safe in terms of pacing loss for the patient in question?

3. What factors other than the need for pacing must be considered in making a decision about the timing of pulse generator replacement in this patient (such as the temporary presence of infection or other intercurrent illness)?

Concerns for the Patient if Pacing Ceases

Having a probable expectation of the clinical consequences of loss of pacing in a particular patient is critically important. Patients who are most pacemaker dependent must be considered for early replacement of the pulse generator, usually as soon as ERI is detected. If the pacing threshold is very high, the output voltage of the pulse generator may decrease below the level necessary for capture before the ERI appears or reaches its nominal value. For example, the output voltage of some pulse generators starts to decrease when the magnet rate begins to decrease. If the normal magnet rate is 100 bpm and the ERI magnet rate is 85 bpm, pacing capture in patients with very high thresholds may be lost when the magnet rate reaches 92 bpm rather than 85 bpm. Whether the potential loss of capture occurs or not depends on (1) the relationship between the magnet rate and the actual output voltage of the pulse generator at the programmed output voltage setting, and (2) the actual pacing threshold for the patient in question. It is worth noting that reprogramming the pulse generator to a higher output voltage near its expected end-of-service life has an especially great effect on reducing the remaining service life of the pulse generator if it is powered by a lithium-iodine battery. The result of increasing the output is both an increase in current drain due to the higher output and a large increase in polarization voltage because of the high internal resistance. These two effects combine to shorten the remaining service life more than might be expected.

In some rate-responsive pulse generators, the magnet rate may indicate that the ERI time has been reached immediately after implantation. This occurs during pacing at high voltage (7.5 V) into leads with normal impedance. Reprogramming of the pulse generator to 5 V restores the magnet rate to its beginning-of-life value. Proof that the battery is not depleted can be obtained by telemetry of the battery impedance.

Pulse Width Stretching Effects on Safety of Pacing

Certain pulse generators increase the pulse width as the battery output voltage decreases to maintain a nearly constant energy of the pacing pulse. This feature is intended as both a marker of battery status and a safety factor. The battery and stimulus output voltages decrease over time with cell depletion. Having the pulse generator automatically increase the stimulus duration helps to maintain the safety margin of the output pulse compared with the pacing threshold. The pacing stimulus strength–duration curve, however, is curvilinear. Increases in pulse duration provide little margin of safety if the pulse amplitude is near rheobase (see Chapter 1). Therefore, when the threshold voltage has decreased enough to reach or nearly reach the rheobase, further pulse width stretching provides little additional safety margin even though the pulse energy continues to increase, and thus depletes the remaining battery capacity even faster.

Common Sense Clinical Guidelines

The points discussed previously translate into two clinical guidelines that bear on the relationships between the status of the patient and the status of the pulse generator battery at ERI: (1) The physician should replace the pulse generator sooner than he or she otherwise would if the clinical history or present situation suggests that something serious may happen to the patient in question if pacing capture is lost; and (2) in such a situation, the pulse generator (or the pulse generator and lead) should be changed even sooner if the pacing threshold is high. The time to change the pulse generator for life-preserving purposes cannot be decided on the basis of pulse generator and battery specifications alone.

Battery Failure Modes and Methods of Assessing Reliability

A detailed understanding of all of the processes that occur in a battery, along with careful, meticulous manufacturing and extensive testing for verification, is needed to ensure battery reliability. Tables 6–2 and 6–3 list the impact of some major failure mechanisms on important battery characteristics and the principal methods that are used to eliminate them.

Battery Chemistries Used in Implantable Devices

Table 6–4 qualitatively compares various power sources that have been used in past or current pacemakers and defibrillators. In this table, 0 is the poorest rating, and 5 is the best.

Table 6–2. Battery Failure Mechanisms and Methods of Control

Failure Mechanism	Methods of Control
High internal resistance	Choice of electrolyte
	Consistent manufacturing
Electrolyte loss and gas formation	Choice of electrolyte
	Dry electrolyte
	Enough electrolyte in cell
Internal short	Good manufacturing processes
	Good battery design
	Fusible separator
	Controlled contact area
External short	Fuse
	Care in handling
Manufacturing variations	Robust cell design
	Consistent manufacturing

Table 6-3. Effect of Failure Mechanisms on Medical Battery Properties

Failure Mechanism	Capacity Loss	Voltage Drop	Hermeticity Loss	Case Swelling	Unpredictable End of Service
Water in cell	X	X			
Films on electrodes		X			X
Electrolyte loss				X	X
Feedthrough corrosion	X	X			
Gas formation				X	X
Internal short	X			X	
External short	X		X		X
Manufacturing variances		X			

When implantable pacemakers were first developed in the late 1960s, lithium and other high-energy density batteries did not exist. The first implantable pacemaker used a nickel–cadmium oxide battery, which was used as a primary battery. That implant lasted only a few hours. However, the concept of the battery-powered pacemaker was proved. The most advanced power source for portable electronic devices at that time was the zinc–mercuric oxide battery that had been developed for military applications during World War II. It became the battery of choice by default and remained so until the mid-1970s.

Mercury Cells

The zinc–mercuric oxide (or mercury) battery has good energy density and high current capability but a low voltage (just more than 1 V). Early pacemakers were designed to use up to five or six mercury cells in series. The circuits and the pacing leads then in use put relatively high current and voltage demands on the individual cells within the pulse generator. In addition, this multiple-cell configuration allowed the pacemaker to continue to operate if one of the cells in the series configuration failed. Unfortunately, this happened unpredictably and frequently. The longevity of pacemakers using mercury cells was typically between 1 and 3 years. These cells self-discharged and generated hydrogen gas. The pulse generators of that day were encapsulated in epoxy rather than being hermetically sealed, in part so that the small amounts of hydrogen gas produced could diffuse out of the pulse generator. Even more troublesome was the propensity of this chemistry to develop a metallic mercury

short through the separator. Such an event soon left that cell completely discharged and behaving much like a piece of solid wire. This is why the strategy of the extra cell in series was needed. In a short time, the lithium cells completely displaced the zinc–mercuric oxide batteries from implantable applications.

Lithium Cells

The advent of lithium batteries in the early 1970s resulted in a dramatic revolution in cardiac pacing. Lithium was chosen as the anode material for several reasons. First, it has a high-capacity density, 2.06 Ah/cm^3. Lithium also forms many electrochemical couples that have appropriate stability, adequately fast discharge kinetics, and high energy density. The lithium chemistries used in permanent pacemakers included three chemistries with liquid organic electrolytes: lithium-silver chromate, lithium-cupric sulfide, and lithium-manganese dioxide; one chemistry with a liquid cathode component, lithium-thionyl chloride; and one chemistry that behaved almost like a solid-state battery, lithium-iodine. The chemistries of these battery systems are discussed in detail in reference 13.

Types of Lithium Cells

Although none of the several varieties of lithium batteries developed for implantable medical use proved to be inherently unreliable, only the lithium–iodine system remains in widespread use for cardiac pacing today. The lithium–cupric sulfide and lithium–silver chromate batteries had some attractive features, although they are no longer used today.

Table 6-4. Comparison of Characteristics of Implantable Medical Battery Systems

System	High Voltage	High Current	High Power	Low Self-Discharge	High Energy Density	Degree of Rechargeability	Highly Predictable Discharge	Highly Inherent Reliability
Zn/HgO	1	4	4	2	2	0	2	2
Li/I$_2$	3	1	1	4	4	0	4	4
Li/MnO$_2$	3	3	4	3	3	0	4	3
Li/SOCl$_2$	4	3	4	2	4	0	3	3
Li/CuS	2	3	3	3	3	0	4	3
Li/SVO	3	4	4	3	3	0	3	2
Ni/CdO	1	4	4	2	2	5	3	2
Ni/H$_2$	1	4	4	2	2	5	3	2
Nuclear	0	1	1	5	5	0	5	5
Li/V$_2$O$_5$	3	4	3	2	3	0	2	3

For all parameters, 0 = poor and 5 = best.

The type of lithium–manganese dioxide cells used in the late 1970s is also no longer made; however, newer versions of this system are beginning to be used again to power some implantable cardiac pacemakers with higher power requirements, such as optical sensors that measure mixed venous oxygen saturation. These sensors require battery currents in the range 0.1 to 1 mA at 2 V to power light-emitting diodes. Lithium-iodine batteries cannot provide this level of power without a significant loss of energy density. Thus, the longevity of a pulse generator needing high-current pulses is significantly less if it uses a low-current battery than if it uses a higher current battery, such as lithium-manganese dioxide. For similar reasons, lithium–thionyl chloride batteries are still used in some implantable pulse generators for neurologic and drug-delivery applications.

Nuclear Batteries

The evolutionary path to the lithium battery was not without it side branches. One of the most interesting of these was the development of nuclear batteries to power cardiac pacemakers. About 3000 nuclear-powered pacemakers were implanted between 1970 and 1982.[14] Two types of nuclear batteries have been used in pacemakers. The first type works by the β-voltaic effect. A β-emitter, such as promethium-147, gives off electrons that impinge on a semiconductor, producing an electric current. In the second type, the heat evolved during nuclear decay is converted to electric energy via a thermopile. Plutonium-238 was commonly used in this type of power source. Both power sources are described in reference 13. The great advantage of nuclear power sources is their longevity and extreme reliability. The half-life of plutonium-238 is 88 years. In practical terms, a pulse generator powered by a nuclear source should last the life of the patient. Like many other power sources, however, nuclear batteries are no longer being used in implantable devices. Safety and regulatory requirements were the principal reasons for their demise. The rigorous and time-consuming follow-up requirements were a major inconvenience for manufacturers, physicians, and patients alike, all of whom were held responsible for tracking the regulated power source and then returning it to the manufacturer when it was no longer being used. In addition, the extreme longevity of nuclear power sources is in itself a problem. A patient with a functioning 20-year-old pacemaker cannot benefit from continuing advances made in pacemaker technology, which typically changes substantially every 5 years. Also, nuclear batteries are relatively large and expensive. Their size was competitive with the zinc–mercuric oxide batteries of the 1960s, but they cannot compete with modern 1-Wh/cm³ primary lithium batteries.

Rechargeable Cells

The goals of small volume, light weight, and long service life appeared to be matched to rechargeable batteries, and one device of this type was manufactured commercially. About 5000 rechargeable nickel oxide–cadmium battery-powered pacemakers were implanted in the 1970s.[10] These pacemakers functioned much more reliably than the mercury-zinc units in use at that time. Most of these rechargeable pulse generators were eventually replaced over a 15-year period because of the need for more versatile pulse generators powered by primary lithium batteries.[15]

Rechargeable batteries did not have continuing commercial success in pacemakers for two main reasons. First, advances in electronics reduced the current drain of pulse generator circuits enough that designers could make an acceptably small pacemaker with a primary battery. The lower energy density of rechargeable batteries (0.2 Wh/cm³, compared with 1 Wh/cm³ for lithium-iodine batteries), combined with a high rate of self-discharge, made rechargeable batteries less attractive. They no longer provided a volume savings when the high-energy density lithium batteries became available. Another disadvantage was their need to be recharged about once a week. Thus, candidates for rechargeable pacemakers needed to meet the requirements for being mentally, physically, and emotionally able to recharge their pacemaker reliably. For elderly patients, remembering to recharge the battery was a potential problem with rechargeable batteries. It appears unlikely that a new rechargeable battery chemistry will replace lithium primary batteries in bradycardia pulse generators in the near future. The higher power requirements for some new devices, however, are raising an interest in the use of rechargeable lithium batteries.

The Lithium-Iodine Battery

The lithium-iodine battery has been used in most cardiac pacemakers manufactured during the past two decades.[16] The first implant of a pacemaker powered by a lithium-iodine battery occurred in 1972.[17] About 5 million lithium-iodine–powered pacemakers have been implanted. There are many factors favoring the use of this battery system. When the current demand is low, lithium-iodine batteries have a high energy density and a low self-discharge, resulting in good longevity and small size. The inherent high impedance of the lithium-iodine battery has not been a major disadvantage because the current required by modern pacemaker circuits is so low, typically about 10 μA. (Note that the much greater stimulus current is drawn from a capacitor, which can charge for a long time between pacing pulses, compared with its discharge time.) The voltage and impedance characteristics of this lithium cell also allow the clinician to monitor the approaching end-of-service indication. This battery system is simple and elegant in concept and is inherently resistant to many common modes of failure, as discussed later. As a result, lithium-iodine batteries have attained a record of reliability unsurpassed among electrochemical power sources.[16]

Lithium-Iodine Cell Structure

Most lithium-iodine batteries consist of an anode of lithium coated with a thin film of poly-2-vinylpyridine (P2VP) and a cathode composed of a thermally reacted mixture of iodine and P2VP. Although lithium-iodine batteries are sensitive to moisture during manufacture, they can be safely and reliably manufactured in rooms maintained at low relative humidity (1%).

Figure 6–6 shows a cut-away view of a typical lithium-iodine battery. In general, batteries for powering bradycardia pacemakers all have a single, central anode that is surrounded by cathode material. Such a battery has a fairly small electrode area and thus a rather modest current-delivering capability, but small currents are all that have been needed for bradycardia pacemakers in the past. Visible in

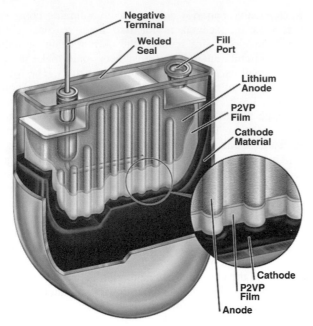

Figure 6–6. Cut-away view of a typical lithium-iodine battery showing its internal construction. Easily identifiable interior parts include the anode feedthrough, the anode current collector (wire), the cathode, the P2VP film on the anode, and the port where the cathode material is poured into the cell. The connection to the cathode is through the battery case.

this figure are the central anode with an embedded current collector wire and the iodine cathode that fills much of the volume inside the battery. This figure also shows several other important structures. One of these is the electric feedthrough that connects the anode to the outside of the cell. The case serves as the site of the electrical connection to the cathode, which is in direct contact with the inside of the container. Another visible feature is the fillport. The fillport is the means by which the cathode mixture is introduced into the cell. The fillport is welded shut after the cathode is put in the cell.

Electrochemical Properties of Lithium-Iodine Cells

When lithium-iodine batteries are manufactured, the iodine initially reaching the surface of the lithium reacts directly with the lithium, yielding lithium iodide. This reaction needs to proceed only to a small extent before the surface of the lithium is covered by lithium iodide, and the reaction rate slows greatly. The voltage of the cell rises quickly, as this layer forms, to 2.8 V, which is characteristic of the lithium-iodine couple. Lithium iodide is an electronic insulator with a high enough lithium-ion conductivity to act as a solid electrolyte in the cell. The cell potential, 2.8 V, is not simply the difference in the two half-cell potentials for the lithium and iodine couples given in Table 6–1. The values in Table 6–1 were calculated for the case in which Li^+ and I^- are dissolved ions. In the lithium-iodine battery, which contains no solvent, the two ions combine to form solid lithium iodide salt. Because lithium iodide is a lower-energy material than the dissolved ions, the cell has a larger voltage than if the ions were dissolved in a solution. The lithium iodide produced as the cell discharges is also the electrolyte in this

system. It accumulates near the surface of the anode because it is not soluble in the cathode mixture. Because the product of the direct reaction of the anode and cathode is also the electrolyte, a breach of the electrolyte layer in a cell simply results in the creation of more electrolyte. Thus, the electrolyte is said to be *self-healing*. This characteristic contributes to the high reliability of this battery.

The iodine in the cathode is made conductive by reaction with poly-2-vinylpyridine (P2VP). The reaction products form a viscous, conductive, two-phase liquid polyiodide plus excess crystalline iodine material.[18] Practical batteries are made with cathode compositions in the range of 20 to 50 parts of iodine per part of P2VP by weight. As the cell discharges, the crystalline iodine is consumed first, followed by iodine from the conductive liquid phase.

The resistivity of lithium iodide to lithium ion transport is significant; in practice, the measured resistance of the cell is less than what would be expected from the build-up of a planar lithium iodide layer. This can be attributed to the polyvinyl pyridine coating originally on the anode surface. The polyvinyl pyridine reacts with lithium and iodine to produce a small amount of a liquid that enhances the conduction of the discharge product and also causes the lithium iodide to grow in a slightly irregular form.[19] The resistance of the electrolyte in a lithium-iodine cell increases during the course of discharge from a few hundred ohms to several thousand ohms.[20] Early in life, the removal of the solid iodine from the cathode, as the cell discharges, actually increases the conductivity of the cell. As iodine is removed from the conductive liquid phase, however, the resistivity of the remaining material increases by several orders of magnitude before the cell is completely discharged. This effect is primarily responsible for the battery's high resistance in the later part of its service life. This is a fundamental characteristic of this battery system and limits its application to uses that do not require very high or very frequent bursts of current, especially toward the end of its service life.

Discharge Curve for the Lithium-Iodine Battery

Figure 6–7A and B shows the characteristic shapes of the voltage and resistance curves as a function of discharge for a typical lithium-iodine battery. The most salient characteristic of these curves is the initial slow change of each parameter followed by a rapid change near the end of discharge. The point where the resistance curve becomes noticeably steeper corresponds to the point in the discharge where the crystalline iodine becomes depleted from the two-phase cathode mixture. Before this point, the resistance change is dominated by the growing electrolyte. Beyond it, the cathode rapidly dominates the resistance of the cell as the cathode becomes lower in iodine content. The region of discharge dominated by cathode resistance is used to signal the approaching end of service for most pacemakers.

Effects of Current Drain on Deliverable Capacity From Lithium-Iodine Cells

The high energy density of the lithium-iodine battery may be negated if the application requires frequent periods of high current drain. This is because there is an optimal average current for the operation of this (or any) battery. Figure 6–8 shows a plot of the deliverable capacity versus the log of average current drain for a typical lithium-iodine battery.

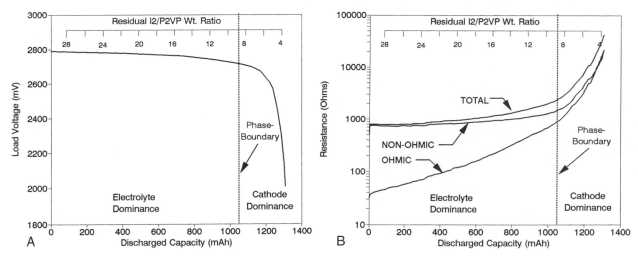

Figure 6–7. *A,* Voltage capacity plot for lithium-iodine battery during discharge. The superimposed scale shows residual I_2/P2VP weight ratio (starting at 50:1). The dashed vertical line defines the boundary between the two-phase and the single-phase cathode regions where the electrolyte and cathode, respectively, dominate the internal resistance. *B,* Resistance capacity plot analogous to part *A*. The ohmic and nonohmic contributions to the internal resistance are shown along with their sums.

The maximum in this curve is the optimal operating point for this battery for maximum deliverable capacity. Comparison of these curves for different battery systems and even sizes and designs of a single type of battery can help a device designer choose the best power source. Consider the following example: in the typical conditions encountered in an implanted cardiac pacemaker, a lithium–manganese dioxide battery has a volumetric efficiency of about 80% of that of a lithium-iodine battery. If the application requires frequent, intermittent current pulses at a 10-fold increase in magnitude, however, the overall deliverable energy density of the lithium–manganese dioxide battery may become greater than that of the lithium-iodine battery. The following are examples of implantable devices that might require a large intermittent current drain from the battery. One is a pulse generator that uses a sensor (like a physiologic oxygen saturation sensor) for pacemaker rate-response control, or a pacemaker designed for simultaneous multisite pacing (to increase cardiac output in congestive heart failure patients), or possibly even one designed to transmit information frequently about a patient's condition to an external device.

Comparison of Pacemaker and Defibrillator Batteries

Implantable defibrillators deliver up to 40 J to the heart in a few milliseconds. By contrast, the energy required to stimulate the heart in bradycardia pacing is on the order of 1 to 10 µJ over a 1-msec or less time frame. The time needed to charge the capacitor before the shock is delivered depends on the ability of the battery to sustain a very high current (up to 4 A) during this period. Thus, the implantable defibrillator requires a high peak-power battery. The energy delivered by the battery is the product of the battery voltage and the charge on the capacitor, or power multiplied by time. Working in reverse, the power required to charge the defibrillator for a 30-J shock in 10 seconds is 3 W. This assumes that all the energy in the capacitor is delivered to the heart, which is nearly the case for many modern implantable defibrillators.

The design of defibrillator batteries is different from that of a bradycardia battery. Figure 6–6, which was discussed previously, shows a cut-away view of a typical battery used to power a pacemaker. This battery has small and rather thick electrodes. Contrast this figure with Figure 6–9, which shows an analogous cut-away for a defibrillator battery.

The battery in this figure has very different construction. To begin with, it does not have a single central anode. Instead, it has wound layers of anode and cathode material separated by a thin layer of porous material. Both the anode and cathode layers are also very thin, in contrast to the much thicker anode and cathode layers in the low-rate bradycardia battery. The design of the defibrillator battery with large, thin electrodes gives this battery the capability to deliver the large amount of current needed to charge the high-voltage capacitors in the defibrillator quickly.

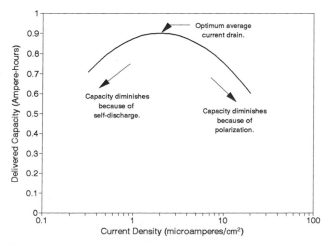

Figure 6–8. Capacity versus log current–drain curve for typical lithium-iodine medical battery showing that deliverable battery capacity has a maximum value because of the competing effects of self-discharge and polarization.

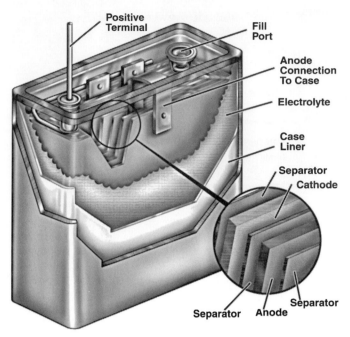

Figure 6–9. Cut-away view of a typical high-rate defibrillator battery showing a wound construction in which a "sandwich" containing anode, separator, and cathode is rolled, flattened, and fitted inside the battery case. This type of battery uses a liquid electrolyte to ensure high internal conductivity. In the battery shown here, the anode is connected to the case, and the cathode is connected to the feedthrough. Notice the multiple connections to the cathode to ensure low internal resistance.

Defibrillator Battery Impedance

A further requirement is that the battery must deliver the high power level while maintaining a high voltage. In other words, the battery cannot polarize (decrease in voltage) to a great extent. To accomplish this, the battery must have low internal impedance. Two design features are the keys to attaining low impedance. First, these batteries must contain a very conductive liquid electrolyte, in contrast to the solid electrolyte found in lithium-iodine batteries. Because the liquid electrolyte has no mechanical integrity, a porous separator sheet is used to keep the anode and cathode apart. Second, the anode and the cathode need to have large surface areas that lower the current density and hence also the impedance due to the electrochemical reactions occurring. Because of the high currents required to charge the ICD capacitor, a substantial metallic current collector must be embedded in each active electrode of the battery to minimize voltage loss within the electrodes themselves. These features give the battery low impedance, but at the expense of increased volume. The deliverable capacity density of a defibrillator battery is typically 0.2 Ah/cm³, compared with 0.5 Ah/cm³ in lithium-iodine pacemaker batteries. This difference in energy density is a function of the different cell designs required by the vastly different power requirements for the two applications. Battery designers are working to increase the capacity density of high-rate cells through more efficient packaging, minimization of inert materials, and optimization of the battery electrodes. It is unlikely, however, that any design optimization can overcome all the limitations inherent to a high-rate battery design.

Energy Losses in Defibrillators

The charge and discharge processes in a cardiac defibrillator have numerous inefficiencies that result in a substantial disparity between the chemical energy consumed in the battery and the electric energy delivered to the heart. The charging circuit, for example, has a finite level of resistance and other voltage losses inherent to the operation of certain components (e.g., diodes). These translate into energy lost to heat as the capacitor is charged and later discharged. Similarly, there is a small amount of energy lost in the leads because of their finite resistance as the discharge occurs. The large defibrillation capacitors themselves contribute to some energy losses in the device, as described later. Finally, the most significant loss of energy is associated with the battery itself. Batteries in ICDs are designed to be as small as possible, which means that they tend to be operated near their maximum power capability. An ideal power source operates at maximum power when the load placed on the power source matches the internal resistance of the power source. This well-known concept is often referred to as *impedance matching*. In terms of energy efficiency, it means that when a power source is operating at maximum power, only half of the total energy consumed is delivered to the external load. The remainder of the energy is dissipated as heat in the power supply. As a rule of thumb, it is useful to approximate the energy loss in an ICD battery as a result of the defibrillation therapy as about 50%. Considering all of these contributions, the overall efficiency of the battery/charging-circuit/capacitor/lead system is, at best, only about 35%. That is, only about a third of the chemical energy consumed in the battery is actually delivered to the heart. In many instances, the overall efficiency is less than 25%. The energy content of a typical ICD battery is on the order of 20,000 J. If the ICD delivered a 35-J shock, a system operating at 25% efficiency would consume 140 J (about 0.7% of the total battery energy).

One-Cell and Two-Cell Defibrillator Designs

The first ICDs were all powered by a 6-V battery consisting of two 3-V cells in series. In general, this was done because charging circuits operate with increased efficiency (less energy loss) when powered by a higher voltage source. The main disadvantage of a two-cell battery is a loss of volumetric efficiency resulting from the additional packaging and interconnects of the two individual cells. Recent improvements in charging-circuit efficiency have made it possible to power an ICD with one cell. The single-cell battery, however, must contain about the same total energy and deliver about the same power as its two-cell predecessor. In effect, it is similar to placing the two cells in parallel within the same battery case rather than having them in series. Thus, most of the gain in volumetric efficiency is associated with the advantage of a single container, which may require less inert materials that lower the battery's energy density.

An ICD powered by a single cell, however, may or may not be the most volumetrically efficient device design. The volume savings afforded by a single battery package may be negated by additional battery capacity required to compensate for decreased efficiency of the charging circuit or the need for a higher power capability. Other design goals, such as a desired shape for the ICD, are often the overriding factors in the choice between a single or two cells in series to power the device.

Defibrillator Volume and Clinical Performance

Dramatic reductions in ICD volumes have occurred in the past few years. Most of these reductions have been a result of improved charging circuit performance, reduction of bradycardia pacing current because of more efficient circuits, improved volumetric efficiency of batteries and capacitors, and improved packaging efficiency of all the components in the ICD. It is also possible, however, to achieve significant volume reductions by trading off longevity, charge time, or maximum shock energy. These choices can translate into lower battery or capacitor volume, and thus a smaller device.

Defibrillator Battery Chemistry and Characteristics

The first implantable defibrillators were powered by batteries that had a lithium anode and a vanadium oxide cathode.[21, 22] These batteries had some limitations, however, in terms of reproducible discharge characteristics and a higher than desirable rate of self-discharge. Currently, lithium batteries that have a silver vanadium oxide (SVO) cathode power all ICDs.[23–25] The SVO cathode provides a reasonable balance between good energy density, good rate capability, and a gradual loss of voltage as the cathode is depleted. Although alternative cathode materials are likely to be developed and implemented in future devices, it is worthwhile to consider a number of discharge characteristics of the Li-SVO battery.

Typical discharge behavior for the Li-SVO battery is shown in Figure 6–10*A* and *B*. On both figure parts, the uppermost curve represents the battery voltage during normal sensing and bradycardia pacing operations. This is sometimes referred to as the *background voltage*. It is this background voltage that is typically monitored by the ICD and reported by means of telemetry. Its fall below a specified value may also be used as an ERI, as is sometimes done in a bradycardia pacemaker. Because of the high power capability (i.e., low internal resistance) of these batteries, there is

relatively little dependence of the background voltage on pulse generator settings. This is in sharp contrast to the behavior described for the lithium-iodine batteries used to power bradycardia pacemakers.

The background voltage for the Li-SVO battery is relatively independent of ICD model and manufacturer. The voltage slopes gently from about 3.25 V at the beginning of the battery's life to about 3.15 V at about 30% depth of discharge. This is followed by a region of more rapidly declining voltage, which levels off at a value of about 2.6 V at about 50% depth of discharge. This 2.6-V region is very flat, sloping less than 0.1 V until about 85% depth of discharge. After this, the background voltage resumes a more rapid decline throughout the remainder of useful battery life. For devices that employ a two-cell battery (i.e., two cells connected in series), the telemetered battery voltage doubles the values described previously.

The battery voltage during the period when the output capacitor is being charged is much lower than the background voltage. This is shown in Figure 6–11, which depicts the typical voltage of a two-cell Li-SVO battery before, during, and after the charging of a defibrillator capacitor. This is often referred to as the *pulse voltage* or *load voltage* of the battery. The lower curve on Figure 6–10*A* depicts the load voltage as a function of discharge capacity. The actual value of the load voltage is highly dependent on the ICD design and programmed parameters. The general trend of a gradually decreasing load voltage throughout the life of the battery, however, is typical of all Li-SVO batteries (and most other battery chemistries). As the battery approaches the end of its useful life, the loss of load voltage becomes much more rapid.

The declining load voltage is associated with both the declining background voltage and slightly increasing internal resistance of the battery. The decline in load voltage is indicative of reduced battery power and is accompanied by a corresponding increase in the time required to charge the output capacitor. Typical charge time behavior is shown in the lower curve of Figure 6–10*B*. Again, the specific charge time values vary significantly from one ICD model and

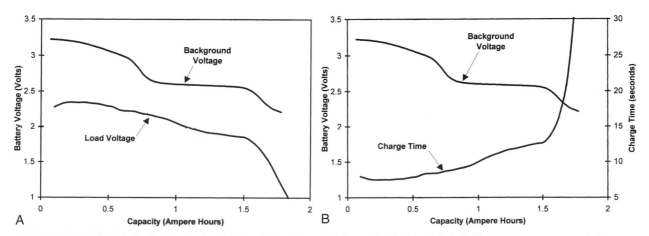

Figure 6–10. *A*, Typical voltage capacity plot for a lithium-silver vanadium oxide single-cell battery. The upper curve represents the battery voltage during monitoring and pacing activities. The lower curve represents the battery voltage whenever capacitor charging is occurring. *B*, Similar plot to part *A* except that the lower curve represents the time required to charge the capacitor at various states of battery discharge.

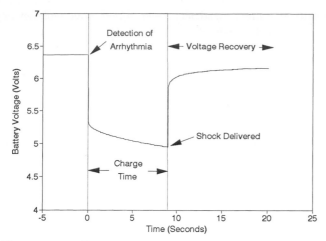

Figure 6–11. Typical voltage–time curve showing a two-cell defibrillator battery voltage during the course of delivering a defibrillator shock. The left-hand side shows the voltage before and during detection, the middle section during charging of the high-voltage capacitor, and the right-hand section the voltage recovery after delivery of the defibrillation shock.

manufacturer to another. However, the general trend of a gradually increasing charge time throughout device life is typical. Most significant is the rapid increase in charge time as the battery reaches the end of its useful life. The clinical importance of this lies in the fact that longer charge times may occur over the life of the ICD, resulting in a greater chance of syncope during ventricular arrhythmias and possibly a higher defibrillation threshold (DFT).

Elective replacement of the ICD is typically indicated either by the background voltage or charge time. In the case of an ERI based on background voltage, it is important for the clinician to be aware of the long voltage plateau in the region of 2.6 V (5.2 V in a two-cell battery). The elective replacement voltage is normally set just below this value, in the region of 2.55 to 2.45 V. There has been some tendency for ICDs to be explanted prematurely because of the clinician's concern about the remaining longevity when the telemetered battery voltage is close to the ERI voltage. Inspection of Figure 6–10A and B shows, however, that the device continues to perform well throughout this entire region of discharge. Thus, the telemetered voltage being "close" to the ERI value should not normally cause undue concern because ICDs are carefully designed to provide an adequate period of safe operation after elective replacement has been indicated. The period of safe operation, however, would be appreciably shortened if the patient were prone to frequent periods of multiple shocks.

Clinical Implications of Battery Design on Defibrillation Therapy

A number of factors make it difficult to compare the performance characteristics of one ICD directly to another. Some of these issues arise because of the different ways manufacturers define their specifications or the size of the defibrillation capacitors they choose to put in their devices. Probably the most significant item to remember is that the time required for charging the device to deliver a defibrillation

shock should not be used to compare one ICD to another without assessing other parameters. This results from the charging time being a sensitive function of both the charging circuit and battery designs, as well as from how well these components are engineered to work together. The clinician should also be aware that charge times are generally quoted for formed capacitors (see later section, Capacitors). Charge times for capacitors that have not been recently formed can be up to 40% longer for the first pulse.

Finally, there can be a significant increase in charge time as the device approaches ERI and also in the post-ERI region. These increases are associated with the reduced power capability of the battery as it approaches depletion and, in some cases, may also be associated with a gradual increase in battery resistance over time. These battery characteristics are dependent on battery design and manufacturer. As discussed earlier, the energy removed from the battery during each charge of the output capacitor represents a significant fraction of its total energy (on the order of 0.5% to 1.0%). Hence, the longevity of a defibrillator has a strong dependence on the frequency of the shock therapy. This is further complicated in modern ICDs that routinely perform other functions, such as bradycardia pacing, in addition to providing defibrillation shocks. As an example, the manual of one well-known device estimates longevity as about 6 years when the device is used only as a defibrillator and is required to deliver very few high-voltage shocks. On the other hand, the longevity estimate for this same device is only about 3.5 years if it is implanted in a patient who requires 100% pacing at nominal conditions and also undergoes a shock about once a month. This difference of a factor of two could be even greater if the patient required more tachyarrhythmia shocks or more extreme pacing parameters.

It is not unusual today for patients who require implantation of an ICD to either already have or need a bradycardia pacemaker. Three reports[26–28] have stated that 6% to 17% of patients require both bradycardia and tachycardia devices, whereas a fourth institution reported this figure as nearly 50%.[29] Having two devices also increases the complexity of programming for safe function.[30]

The ideal situation would be to have a single device that could act as both a dual-chamber defibrillator and a dual-chamber pacemaker or any combination of these functions that would last a long time. Such a device would allow the clinician to implant the minimum amount of hardware consistent with short-term and long-term patient safety. However, if adding dual-chamber pacing functions to a defibrillator for a patient who requires pacing 100% of the time markedly shortens the life of the defibrillator, the clinical balance for at least some patients might shift toward having independent devices. Even though technologic progress in pacing and defibrillation has been rapid and is continuing at an astounding pace,[15] no single combined device that does not involve some compromise in longevity or function is yet available.

Safety

Safety is a concern with high-power batteries because they contain a large amount of energy and are designed to deliver it quickly. If an internal short circuit occurs, the relatively large current traveling through the short can heat the cell contents and, in some rare cases, initiate a violent chemical reaction. Batteries for implantable defibrillators are designed and constructed with great care to ensure that the occurrence of such a hazardous condition is almost impossible. For example, a thicker layer of separator material is typically used in these batteries than in consumer lithium batteries of similar power capability. The polymeric separator materials chosen for this application are designed to melt at a relatively low temperature. This is useful if either an external or an internal short develops in the battery. If a short occurs, the separator melts, and the porous structure of the separator is lost. The dense polymer sheet that results from melting does not allow ions to pass through it, and the electrochemical reaction is stopped. These batteries also undergo extensive testing under other abuse conditions to ensure that they are safe even if a hazardous condition occurs.

Future Battery Chemistries for Pacemakers and Atrial Fibrillation Devices

Although the average power requirements of pacemakers have decreased in recent years as a result of advances in lead technology and efficient circuit operation, the short-term power requirements continue to increase. These requirements result, in part, from the introduction of microprocessor control of the pulse generator. The microprocessor typically operates (is powered on) only a small fraction of the time between pacing pulses, but the power demand during these intervals is high. As the algorithms executed by the microprocessor become more sophisticated with each new model, the microprocessor is required to operate either for longer times or at higher speeds. Both of these modes increase the power demand on the battery.

A second important influence is the trend to integrate more bradycardia and tachycardia therapies into a single device. New ICDs now incorporate not only ventricular pacing but also atrial pacing. Devices are now becoming available that manage both bradycardia and tachycardia in all chambers of the heart. In addition, new desirable features, such as very high-rate pacing used as an alternative antitachycardia therapy, also have much higher short-term power requirements. This is especially true for the growing number of devices designed specifically to treat atrial fibrillation.

These trends all increase the power demand on the battery and lessen the distinctions between bradycardia and tachycardia power sources that have existed up to this time. Thus, it is highly likely that there will be at least a partial transition from powering even bradycardia devices with lithium-iodine batteries, which are used almost exclusively in pacemakers today, to a battery chemistry with higher power capabilities. Such power sources will almost certainly be a battery (or batteries) with a liquid electrolyte. In some cases, manufacturers may even choose a single battery chemistry to power all of their implantable devices, and optimize each battery designed with this chemistry for the current requirements of the particular device it will power.

The changes the clinician will notice with the new battery chemistries are discharge curves and characteristics very different from those of the lithium-iodine battery. In fact, the new devices will have many of the characteristics that are found in the defibrillator power sources used today. The difficulty in designing these new power sources will be achievement of a high-energy density package without compromising safety and reliability.

■ CAPACITORS

ICDs defibrillate by delivering a high-energy, high-voltage shock to the heart, as has been described previously. The battery alone cannot deliver energy rapidly enough and does not have a high enough voltage to defibrillate the heart. High-voltage capacitors are used to store the charge and then deliver the shock. The use of these capacitors has important clinical implications. The capacitor is the largest component in an ICD, so it is mainly responsible for the larger size of ICDs as compared with cardiac pacemakers. Although this chapter focuses on ventricular defibrillators and cardioverters, the information also applies to atrial defibrillators that are capable of delivering a high-energy shock.

The Concept of Capacitance

In its simplest form, a capacitor consists of two conductors, separated in space and electrically insulated from each other. When the conductors are charged, each carries an equal and opposite amount of charge. In an ideal capacitor, the amount of charge (Q) on each conductor is proportional to the difference in voltage (V) between the two conductors. The proportionality constant, C, is called the *capacitance*.

$$(11) \quad Q = C \cdot V$$

Major Components of Capacitors

The simplest model of a capacitor is shown in Figure 6–12A. The conductors (or electrodes) consist of two parallel plates of area (A), separated by a distance (d). Figure 6–12A shows the plates, separated in a vacuum.

The capacitance, or ability to store charge as a function of voltage, is equal to A/d multiplied by a fundamental constant, ϵ_0, the permittivity of free space, which is a measure of the ability of a vacuum to separate charge. The value of the capacitance can be increased by inserting insulating materials, known as *dielectrics*, between the electrodes instead of a vacuum. The factor by which these materials increase the capacitance is called the *dielectric constant*, k, which is the ratio of the permittivity of the material to the permittivity of free space, e/e_0. A simple capacitor containing a dielectric material is shown in Figure 6–12B. A wide variety of materials are used as dielectrics, each with their own properties.

Energy Storage in Capacitors

Before a capacitor can deliver energy, it must store the energy because it is a passive device. The process of storing energy in a capacitor is called *charging*. The opposite terminals of the capacitors are connected to a voltage source, such as a battery, and they take on equal and opposite charges. The energy is stored in the separation of charge. The amount of energy that is stored in an ideal capacitor is proportional to the capacitance and to the square of the voltage. Thus, the energy stored increases much more quickly with an increase in voltage than with an increase in capacitance.

$$(12) \quad E = 1/2 \, C \cdot V^2$$

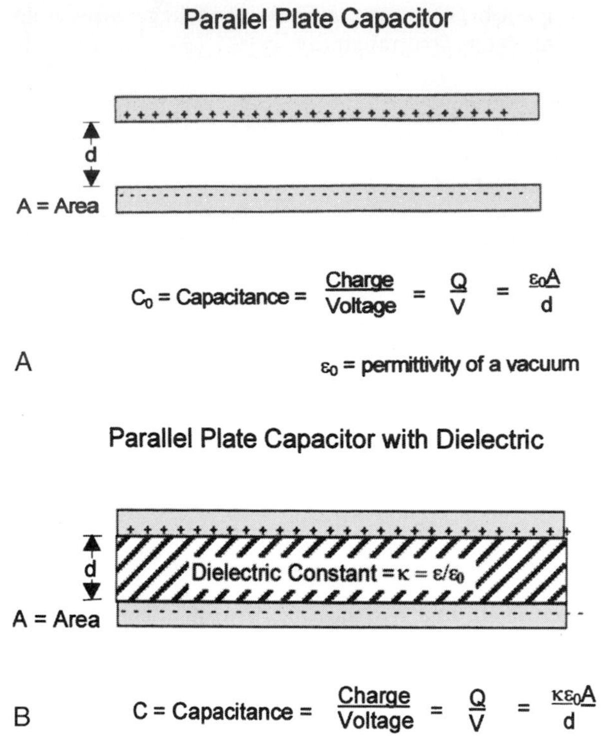

Parallel Plate Capacitor

$$C_0 = \text{Capacitance} = \frac{\text{Charge}}{\text{Voltage}} = \frac{Q}{V} = \frac{\varepsilon_0 A}{d}$$

A = Area

A

ε_0 = permittivity of a vacuum

Parallel Plate Capacitor with Dielectric

Dielectric Constant $= \kappa = \varepsilon/\varepsilon_0$

A = Area

B

$$C = \text{Capacitance} = \frac{\text{Charge}}{\text{Voltage}} = \frac{Q}{V} = \frac{\kappa \varepsilon_0 A}{d}$$

Figures 6–12. Schematic representation of a parallel plate capacitor with (A) a vacuum and (B) a dielectric between the capacitor plates. The capacitance is directly proportional to the area of the plates (A) and inversely proportional to the distance between the plates (d). The insertion of a dielectric between the plates increases the capacitance by a factor of κ, the dielectric constant, which is a characteristic of the particular insulating material.

Energy Delivery From Capacitors

The energy stored in the capacitor may be discharged (delivered to the heart) using leads to connect the heart in an electrical path between the opposing electrodes of the capacitor. This connection allows the separated charge to recombine by traveling through the leads and the heart. When an ideal capacitor is discharged through a constant resistance, R, the voltage decays with time in an exponential manner, as seen in Figure 6–13. The shape of the exponential decay depends on the capacitance, C, and the resistance of the electrical connection between the terminals of the capacitor, R. The exponential decay is characterized by a time constant, τ, which is simply R times C. When the capacitor has discharged for a period of time equal to τ, the voltage will have decayed to 37% of its initial value. For an ideal capacitor discharged to 0 V, the delivered energy is equal to the stored energy. In practical capacitors, losses of energy occur that reduce the amount of energy delivered to less than the stored amount. In an ICD, the discharge waveform is not allowed to decay all the way to 0 V before the pulse is terminated. This is done because a truncated waveform defibrillates the heart more effectively than if the voltage were allowed to decay all the way to zero, despite the fact that less energy is delivered to the heart and some is left in the capacitor.

Energy Density of Capacitors

Energy density is an important parameter for capacitors, just as for batteries, and is defined in the same manner. The volumetric energy density is typically expressed in joules per cubic centimeter (J/cm³). Because capacitors are the largest component in an ICD, and it is important for an ICD to be small, the capacitors used in them need to have a high energy density. This usually means they need to be made with an insulator that has a high dielectric constant that can also withstand high voltage.

Types of Capacitors
Electrostatic Capacitors

Electrostatic capacitors are conceptually the simplest capacitors, and they most closely resemble the idealized drawing in Figure 6–12B. They consist of thin sheets of dielectric material separating opposing metal electrodes. Typical dielectric materials used in these capacitors are polymer films and ceramics. Film capacitors use polymeric materials as the dielectric. They can be constructed either by coating a thin polymer film with a metallic electrode material or by using a discrete metal foil as the electrode. The film and electrode are usually wound into a cylindrical package, but they can also be fashioned into a flat stack cut from a large roll or sheet. Polymer film capacitors have high *dielectric strength*, which is defined as the ability to maintain a voltage over a given thickness of dielectric material. When the dielectric strength of a material is exceeded, the material fails, and a capacitor made using this material can no longer function properly. High dielectric strength has a favorable effect on energy density, but the dielectric constant of most polymers is relatively low, so the capacitance of film capacitors is usually low for a given volume. The energy density of polymer capacitors available today is not high enough for use in ICDs. However, a type of polymer film capacitor is used in external defibrillators, in which the requirement for small size is less important. If thinner, higher dielectric polymer films strong enough to fabricate into a capacitor become available, this type of capacitor may become competitive with other technologies.

A second type of electrostatic capacitor uses a ceramic

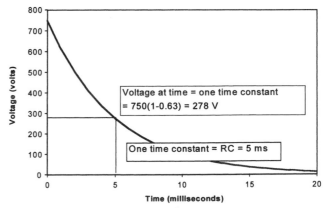

Figure 6–13. Waveform for the discharge of an ideal 100-microfarad capacitor, charged to 750 V, into a 50-Ω load. These parameters approximate those for an implantable defibrillator in use.

material rather than a polymer as a dielectric. Ceramic capacitors are constructed as stacked, alternating layers of the ceramic dielectric material and a layer of metal, which typically results in a rectangular prismatic shape. Ceramic dielectric materials typically have very high dielectric constants, but only at low voltages because the ceramic materials behave nonideally; their capacitance actually decreases as the applied voltage is increased. The result is that the energy density of ceramic capacitors available today is not high enough for use in ICDs. The high dielectric constant of these materials, however, is attractive enough that several groups are working to improve this type of capacitor for use in ICDs.

Double-Layer Capacitors

Double-layer capacitors are unusual because they do not contain a discrete dielectric material. These capacitors are sometimes called Supercaps or Ultracaps, which are actually trade names used by specific manufacturers. The separation of charge in these capacitors occurs at the interface of a solid electrode and an electrolyte. The electrolyte is typically a liquid, such as water, that contains dissolved salts to make it conductive. The solid electrode is usually a very high surface area carbon. When the electrode is charged, the salts in the electrolyte align with opposing charges close to the electrode. This is the same phenomenon that generates a capacitance at the pacing electrode–tissue interface in the body. The distance, d, which separates the charges is extremely small, on the order of angstroms, so the capacitance is extremely high. The maximum permissible voltage for these capacitors must be kept low (1 to 2 V) so that the electrolyte solvent is not electrochemically decomposed. To make an ICD capacitor, as many as 500 individual double-layer capacitors would have to be fabricated in a series arrangement to attain the 700 V needed for defibrillation. An equally serious drawback is that present-day double-layer capacitors have a high internal resistance and hence cannot deliver their charge quickly enough to defibrillate the heart effectively.

Electrolytic Capacitors

Electrolytic capacitors are based on either of two metals, aluminum or tantalum. The metal electrodes are fabricated in a manner so that they have a very high surface area, which results in a high capacitance. In the case of aluminum, the positive electrode (anode in a capacitor) consists of a thin foil that has been etched to create a huge number of tunnels that in some cases can go all the way through the foil. Figure 6–14 shows a scanning electron micrograph of a replica made from a cross-section of a highly etched anode foil. The long, tubular structures are the microscopic tunnels that have been etched into (and in some cases through) the aluminum from each side of the foil. There are more than 1 million tunnels per square centimeter in this foil, and they are responsible for the large surface area and high energy density of this type of capacitor. For tantalum capacitors, the anode is made from powdered tantalum metal that is pressed into a porous pellet and heated to a high enough temperature to make the powdered metal stick together (sinter) while remaining porous. For either metal, the anode is then formed, or anodized, to create an oxide on its surface. The oxide serves as the dielectric material. The forming is done using

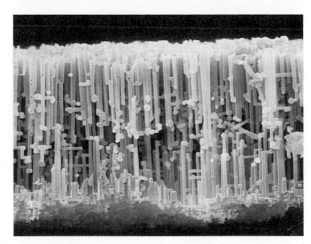

Figure 6–14. Photomicrograph of a replica made from the etched anode foil used in aluminum electrolytic capacitors. The long, linear structures are tunnels etched into the aluminum foil. In this example, some of the tunnels are etched completely through the foil to provide an electrical connection between the two sides. (Original magnification, about 800×.)

an electrochemical process during which a voltage is applied to the anode and a film of oxidized metal grows on the surface. This process, called *electrolysis*, gives rise to the name *electrolytic capacitor*. The thickness of the film increases with the voltage used to form it. The thicker the film, the lower the capacitance, but the higher the voltage the capacitor is able to attain. A dielectric oxide formed by electrolysis has a high dielectric strength because it is relatively free of defects. If any defects appear, they are healed the next time a voltage is applied to the capacitor because the dielectric regrows.

The dielectric, which coats the irregular anode surface, now needs to make contact with the opposing electrode, the cathode. Contact to the cathode is made by means of a conductive material called the *electrolyte*, just as in batteries. In the case of aluminum electrolytic capacitors, the electrolyte is usually a liquid containing dissolved salts to make it conductive. In aluminum electrolytic capacitors, the cathode is an aluminum foil that has been etched to create a very high surface area and then formed at a low voltage, so only a very thin layer of aluminum oxide forms. The capacitances of the anode and cathode are in series, so the total capacitance is calculated by adding the reciprocals of the capacitances of the anode and cathode. Because $C_{cathode}$ is much larger than C_{anode}, C_{anode} determines the overall capacitance of the capacitor.

$$(13) \quad \frac{1}{C_{total}} = \frac{1}{C_{anode}} + \frac{1}{C_{cathode}}$$

The voltage on the capacitor is divided between the anode and the cathode such that CV, the product of voltage and capacitance, is equal on each electrode. In other words, the charge on each electrode must be equal because charge (Q) equals C times V. Because the anode has a much lower capacitance than the cathode, most of the voltage is on the anode.

$$(14) \quad C_{anode} \cdot V_{anode} = C_{cathode} \cdot V_{cathode}$$

Aluminum electrolytic capacitors are the capacitors of choice for ICDs for several reasons. Because of the high capacitance and high dielectric strength, they have an energy density that may be more than 2.5 J/cm³. This means that 10 to 15 cm³ of the volume in an implantable defibrillator is taken up by the capacitors. They are able to operate at high voltage and have low internal resistance; hence, it is possible to deliver the energy quickly and efficiently. They have also been chosen for use in ICDs because aluminum electrolytic capacitors of about the right size, shape, and specifications had already been developed for photoflash applications in photography.

Tantalum capacitors operate on the same principles as aluminum electrolytic capacitors. Small tantalum capacitors are widely used in the electronics industry and have a long history of use in implantable devices for low-voltage circuits. The energy density of commercially available tantalum capacitors is too low for use in the high-voltage circuits of ICDs. However, a new type of tantalum capacitor with a high volumetric energy density has recently been developed for use in ICDs.

Aluminum Electrolytic Capacitors

Components of Aluminum Electrolytic Capacitors. The main components of an aluminum electrolytic capacitor are the anode, the cathode, the electrolyte, and the separator. The anode and cathode are aluminum foils that have been etched and formed, as described earlier. The electrolyte consists of a solvent, typically ethylene glycol with some dissolved salts that usually have a large organic cation and or anion. The electrolyte composition can vary widely depending on the manufacturer and the specific application. In a practical capacitor, the anode and cathode must be mechanically separated from each other to prevent a short circuit, just as with a battery. The dielectric material alone is not sufficient to keep the electrodes apart because it might easily wear through, resulting in direct metal-to-metal contact between the anode and cathode. Thus, a separator is employed. Whereas the lithium batteries used to power ICDs use a porous polymer as a separator material, aluminum electrolytic capacitors generally use porous paper as a separator. The porosity of the paper allows the electrolyte to pass through but does not allow the electrodes to touch each other.

Two nominal 380V capacitors are connected in series, doubling the maximum voltage to about 750 V. The choice of putting two 380V capacitors in series rather than using one 750V capacitor is made because high energy density 750V capacitors are not presently available.

Construction of Aluminum Electrolytic Capacitors. Most commercially available aluminum electrolytic capacitors are of a wound design constructed in a cylindrical shape. Long strips of anode and cathode foil, kept apart by a paper separator, are wound into a coil. Tabs of aluminum metal are connected to the ends of the electrodes. The coiled electrode assembly is saturated with electrolyte under vacuum (to remove entrapped air bubbles), then inserted into a cylindrical aluminum can. The tabs from each electrode are connected to terminals on the cover. The cover is usually then crimped to the can using a polymeric seal. Figure 6–15 shows a cut-away view of an aluminum electrolytic

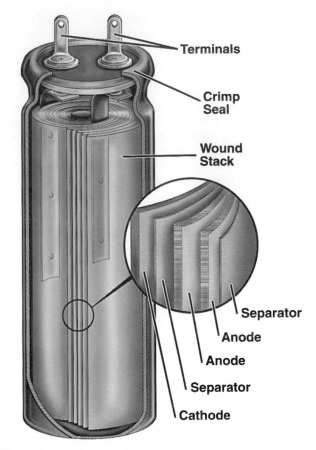

Figure 6–15. Cut-away view of a wound aluminum electrolytic capacitor used in many implantable defibrillators. In this capacitor, the anode and cathode connections are brought out of the capacitor using feedthroughs. The capacitor is closed with a crimp seal. Notice that two layers of anode material are used for each layer of cathode material in order to increase the energy density of the capacitor. The entire wound capacitor bundle is saturated with electrolyte, which is not shown.

photoflash capacitor of the type commonly used in the first few generations of ICDs.

Nonideal Behavior in Aluminum Electrolytic Capacitors. In an ideal capacitor, the amount of energy needed to charge the capacitor would be exactly equal to the energy delivered from the capacitor when it is discharged. Aluminum electrolytic capacitors deviate significantly from ideal behavior in ways that are sometimes clinically significant.

Deformation. The nonideal process that is most apparent to the clinician is called *deformation*. As explained previously, the dielectric material is created on the anode using an electrolytic process known as *forming* (anodization). Immediately after forming, the dielectric is nearly free of defects. Over time, however, defects such as small cracks or other imperfections appear in the dielectric. When the capacitor is charged to a high voltage after a long period of disuse, additional energy is required to reform the dielectric in these areas and heal the defects. This process is known as *reformation*. The additional energy needed to reform the dielectric is apparent to the clinician because of a longer than expected time required for charging. If an aluminum electrolytic capacitor has deformed, the charge time may increase by as much as 40%, depending on the capacitor design, manufacturer, and length of time between high-voltage charges. Deformation, however, disappears after the first charge of the capacitor following inactivity because the extra charge heals the dielectric defects. To prevent excessively long charge times after periods of inactivity, ICD manufacturers recommend charging the capacitors to a high voltage every 3 to 6 months if no high-voltage therapy has been delivered in that period. ICDs available today are capable of reforming the capacitors automatically.

Leakage Current. Leakage current is a nonideal process that occurs to some extent in all capacitors. After a capacitor is charged, it does not hold its charge indefinitely. The charge on the capacitor gradually decreases at a rate that can be stated in terms of a leakage current magnitude. Aluminum electrolytic capacitors have a relatively high leakage current compared with other types of capacitors. For example, an aluminum electrolytic capacitor may have a leakage current 1000 times higher than a good polymer film capacitor. If an aluminum electrolytic capacitor were charged to its maximum voltage and then left in an open-circuit condition, the voltage would decrease to a low level within a few minutes as a result of leakage current. Fortunately, there is little charge lost in the few moments between charging and delivery of the high-voltage shock, but this is the major reason that ICDs are charged only just before a shock is to be delivered.

Internal Resistance. Every capacitor has some internal resistance, just like batteries. For capacitors, this resistance is often referred to as *equivalent series resistance* (ESR). For aluminum electrolytic capacitors used in implantable defibrillators, the ESR is typically less than one ohm. ESR leads to some energy loss in the capacitor, but it is typically only about 2% of the energy delivered in the therapeutic pulse. Perhaps a more important aspect of ESR is its effect on the efficiency with which the capacitor can be charged. If ESR is too high, an appreciable amount of energy can be lost during the charging process.

Cycle Life. Aluminum electrolytic capacitors are designed to withstand a certain number of cycles, depending on the application. During repeated cycling, the oxide on the cathode may begin to grow thicker, thereby lowering the capacitance. If the cycle life is exceeded, the capacitance may decrease below a desirable level. Commercially available aluminum electrolytic capacitors used in ICDs are designed to withstand thousands of cycles because they were usually developed for photoflash applications. ICDs generally charge their capacitors only about 100 times before the battery is depleted, so the cycle life of these capacitors is more than adequate to maintain constant capacitance over the service life of the ICD.

Energy Output of an Implantable Cardioverter-Defibrillator

The energy output of an ICD is primarily defined by the capacitor, with some important contributions from the ICD itself. The internal circuitry of the ICD has some resistance that causes a drop in peak voltage according to Ohm's law.

ICD manufacturers sometimes define the energy of the device as the stored energy and sometimes as the actual delivered energy, and sometimes both values are given. The waveform of the defibrillation pulse is typically truncated at some voltage greater than zero to lower the defibrillation threshold. Depending on the specific device, the energy left on the capacitor varies. Because the situation is complicated, it is not straightforward to calculate the delivered energy from the voltage and capacitance alone, nor to accurately compare the output or comparative efficiency of two different devices, especially from different manufacturers. Many manufacturers provide tables in their technical manuals for conversion of energy to voltage.

Failure Modes for Capacitors

Short Circuit

When the electrodes at opposite polarity come into direct electrical contact, a short circuit occurs. In electrolytic and double-layer capacitors, a short circuit occurs when the anode and cathode come in direct contact. This may happen, for example, when the separator is punctured, torn, or not properly aligned. Short circuits can form in ceramic capacitors when the dielectric material breaks down because of the application of a voltage that is too high. Some polymer capacitors also form short circuits when their dielectric strength is exceeded. Other polymer capacitors are able to tolerate dielectric breakdown because of a self-healing process. The area of the capacitor in which the breakdown occurs vaporizes, and a small amount of capacitance is removed, but the capacitor still functions.

Electrolyte Dry-Out

Electrolytic and double-layer capacitors depend on a liquid electrolyte to function properly. If the capacitor is not well sealed, some evaporation of electrolyte might occur. Small amounts of the electrolyte may also be degraded over long periods of time by parasitic electrochemical reactions that occur inside the capacitor. It is also important that no electrolyte from the capacitor get outside the capacitor and onto the electronic circuits, where it might lead to conductive bridges between circuit traces. The capacitors used in today's ICDs are well sealed, but manufacturers do expect a very small amount of electrolyte solvent to be lost over the device's service life. To compensate, they add excess electrolyte, just as do manufacturers of nonaqueous lithium batteries. ICD and capacitor manufacturers perform accelerated testing to ensure that the amount of electrolyte lost is small and will not affect the function of the ICD over its expected service life.

Environmental Stress

Capacitors in ICDs are subject to a number of environmental stresses. Temperature excursions, vibration, and mechanical shock may occur during shipping and handling of the capacitors or assembled ICDs. If the capacitor is not robustly designed and manufactured well, these conditions may cause an open or short circuit, or they might degrade some chemical components, such as the electrolyte and polymeric seals. Manufacturers routinely design and qualify capacitors and ICDs to survive these environmental conditions with no loss of performance.

Clinical Implications of Capacitor Characteristics

The characteristics of the capacitor influence the charge time, longevity, and defibrillation waveform of an ICD.

Charge Time

The charge time is most strongly influenced by the battery design and the charging circuit; however, the capacitor also has an influence on the charge time. Some energy is lost during charging because of nonideal processes in the capacitor, such as leakage current, resistance, and deformation, which all lengthen charge time. The most important effect is caused by deformation (discussed previously) of the capacitor. The charge time of a completely deformed capacitor may be as much as 40% longer than that of a fully formed capacitor if the capacitor has not been charged for 6 months or more.

Device Longevity

Every time the capacitor is charged, some energy is drained from the battery, shortening the remaining longevity of the device. Because of the phenomenon of deformation, some of this energy is wasted, in the sense that it does not directly benefit the patient. Manufacturers recommend reforming the capacitors every 3 to 6 months to prevent the charge time from becoming unacceptably long. Each charge used for reforming the capacitor, however, may take as much as a few weeks off the service life of the ICD, which may add up to several months shorter longevity over the total life of the device. ICD longevity is very much influenced by the clinician's choice of programmed parameters in modern devices, which can be programmed in many complex ways.

Implantable Cardioverter-Defibrillator Shape and Size

The commercially available capacitors are cylindrical, which limits the choices of ICD shapes that are volume efficient. No suitable commercial, cylindrical electrolytic capacitor is smaller than 12 mm in diameter, which also limits the minimum thickness of these devices. Partly for this reason, some device manufacturers are starting to develop and use custom capacitors that are not based on a wound design. One manufacturer has developed and is using a flat, rather than cylindrical, aluminum electrolytic capacitor. This capacitor uses stacked, flat electrodes and has a higher energy density than commercially available capacitors. Its flat shape fits into an ICD more efficiently than a cylindrical shape and also makes it possible to make the entire device thinner.

Future Developments

In the near future, it appears that electrolytic capacitors will continue to be the type of choice. For the next couple of device generations, aluminum electrolytic capacitors will continue to be used. During this period, the energy density of aluminum electrolytic capacitors is expected to continue to increase incrementally as capacitor designers further hone this technology. This alone may remove 5 cm³ of volume from the ICD. Beyond that, a new type of tantalum electrolytic capacitor has promise for use in ICDs. This tantalum capacitor is in the late stages of development and is expected to have about twice the volumetric energy density of present cylindrical aluminum electrolytic capacitors. Besides the smaller size, another potential advantage of this type of capacitor is that it is not expected to deform like aluminum electrolytic capacitors when not used for an extended period of time. On the other side of the coin, the weight of this capacitor is a potential disadvantage. The density of tantalum is high, and although the capacitor may be half the size of the present aluminum electrolytic, it weighs twice as much.

Ceramic, polymer, and double-layer capacitors are all attractive for use in ICDs in the future, but all have significant technical barriers to overcome before they can be used. Ceramic capacitors need improved dielectric materials that can withstand higher electrical field strengths without their dielectric constant significantly decreasing. Polymer capacitors need polymer dielectric films with a much higher dielectric constant than is now available before they will be small enough for use in ICDs. Double-layer capacitors have very high energy density but too high a resistance. Because of this, they cannot release their energy fast enough to defibrillate the heart. It is also quite an engineering challenge to package enough of these nominal 1- to 2-V capacitors in series to form one 750-volt ICD capacitor.

REFERENCES

1. Brennen KR, Fester KE, Owens BB, Untereker DF: Pacemaker battery capacity: A consideration of the manufacturer's problem. Proceedings of the Sixth World Symposium on Cardiac Pacing. Montreal, Pacesymp, 1979.
2. Brennen KR, Fester KE, Owens, BB, Untereker DF: A capacity rating system for cardiac pacemaker batteries. J Power Sources 5:25, 1980.
3. Broadhead J: Electrochemical principles and reactions. In Linden D (ed): Handbook of Batteries and Fuel Cells, 2nd ed. New York, McGraw Hill, 1994, Chap. 2.
4. Visbisky M, Stinebring RC, Holmes CF: An approach to the reliability of implantable lithium batteries. J Power Sources 26:185, 1989.
5. Schmidt CL, Skarstad PM: Impedance behavior in lithium-iodine batteries. In Abraham KM, Solomon M (eds): Proceedings of the Symposium on Primary and Secondary Lithium Batteries. The Electrochemical Society, PV913, 1991, pp 75–85.
6. Schmidt CL, Skarstad PM: Development of a physically based model for the lithium-iodine battery. In Keily T, Baxter BW (eds): Power Sources 13. Leatherhead, England, International Power Sources Committee, 1991, pp 347–361.
7. Untereker DF, Owens BB: Microcalorimetry: A Tool for the Assessment of Self-discharge Processes in Batteries. Reliability Technology for Cardiac Pacemakers II. Gaithersburg, MD, National Bureau of Standards Workshop, October 1977.
8. Untereker DF: The use of a microcalorimeter for analysis of load dependent processes occurring in a primary battery. J Electrochem Soc 125:1907, 1978.
9. Abraham KM, Brummer SB: Secondary lithium cells. In Gabano JP (ed): Lithium Batteries. New York, Academic Press, 1983, pp 371–403.
10. Holleck GL: Rechargeable electrochemical cells as implantable power sources. In Owens BB (ed): Batteries for Implantable Biomedical Devices. New York, Plenum, 1986, pp 275–284.
11. Brummer SB: Ambient temperature lithium batteries. In Venkatasetty HV (ed): Lithium Battery Technology. New York, John Wiley, 1984, pp 159–177.
12. Lazzari M, Vincent CA: Metal-air batteries (section 3.7). In Vincent CA (ed): Modern Batteries. New York, John Wiley, 1997, pp 98–103.
13. Owens BB (ed): Batteries for Implantable Biomedical Devices. New York, Plenum, 1986.
14. Purdy DL: Nuclear batteries for implantable applications. In Owens BB (ed): Batteries for Implantable Biomedical Devices. New York, Plenum, 1986, pp 285–382.
15. Shepard RB, Epstein AE, Kay GN: Application of new pacemaker and defibrillator technology. Adv Card Surg 5:181, 1994.
16. Greatbatch W, Holmes CF: The lithium-iodine battery: A historical perspective. PACE 15:2034, 1992.
17. Antonioli G, Baggioni F, Consiglio F, et al: Stimulatore cardiac im-

plantible con nuova battaria a sato solido al litio. Minerva Med 64:2298, 1973.

18. Phillips GM, Untereker DF: Phase diagrams for poly-2-vinyl and 2-ethyl pyridine systems. Presented at the 156th National Electrochemical Society Meeting, Los Angeles, October 1979.

19. Phipps JB, Hayes TG, Skarstad PM, Untereker DF: Insitu formation of a solid-liquid composite electrolyte in Li-I$_2$ batteries. Solid State Ionics 18,19:1073, 1986.

20. Schmidt CL, Skarstad PM: Modeling the discharge behavior of the lithium-iodine battery. J Power Sources 43(1B3):111, 1993.

21. Walk CR: Lithium-vanadium pentoxide cells. *In* Gabano JP (ed): Lithium Batteries. London, Academic Press, 1983, pp 265–280.

22. Gabano JP, Broussely M, Grimm M: Lithium solid cathode batteries for biomedical implantable applications. *In* Owens BB (ed): Batteries for Implantable Biomedical Devices. New York, Plenum, 1986, pp 181–213.

23. Takeuchi ES, Quattrini JP: Batteries for implantable defibrillators. Med Electronics 119:114117, 1989.

24. Liang CC, Bolster E, Murphy RM: Metal oxide cathode material for high energy density batteries. US Patents 4,310,609 E1982 and 4,391,729 E1983.

25. Holmes CF, Keister P, Takeuchi E: High rate lithium solid cathode battery for implantable medical devices. Prog Batteries Solar Cells 6:64, 1987.

26. Sticherling C, Klingenheben T, Skupin M, et al: Combined therapy with transvenous cardioverter/defibrillator and anti-bradycardia pacemaker systems. Z Kardiol 86(2):105, 1997.

27. Brooks R, Garan H, McGovern BA, Ruskin JN: Implantation of transvenous nonthoracotomy cardioverter-defibrillator systems in patients with permanent endocardial pacemakers. Am Heart J 129(1):45, 1995.

28. Epstein AE, Kay GN, Plumb VJ, et al: Combined cardioverter-defibrillator and pacemaker systems: Implantation techniques and follow-up. J Am Coll Cardiol 13(1):121, 1989.

29. Geiger MJ, O'Neill P, Sharma A, et al: Interactions between transvenous nonthoracotomy defibrillator systems and permanent transvenous endocardial pacemakers. Pacing Clin Electrophysiol 20(3 Pt 1):624, 1997.

30. Epstein AE, Shepard RB: Permanent pacemakers and implantable cardioverter-defibrillators: potential interactions. *In* Estes NAM, Manolis AS, Wang PJ (eds): Automatic Implantable Cardioverter-Defibrillators: A Comprehensive Textbook. New York, Marcel Dekker, 1994, pp 479–494.

Chapter 7

Pacemaker and ICD Pulse Generator Circuitry

Jay A. Warren and James P. Nelson

The technology used in the development of pacemakers and implantable cardioverter-defibrillators (ICDs) has made impressive advances since the first pacemaker was implanted in 1959. These enhancements have translated into both patient and clinician benefit. For the patient, size reduction, improved longevity, noninvasive programmability, and improved therapy in the form of dual-chamber and rate-adaptive pacing are just a few of the benefits. For the clinician, enhanced therapeutics has improved patient outcomes, resulting in more effective care, and better diagnostics have led to more efficient care. The efficient delivery of care is particularly important in the environment of health care cost containment.

Design considerations play a fundamental role in device performance and operation, and device performance in turn plays an important role in clinical practice. For this reason, it is important for physicians and engineers to develop a common understanding of the role each plays in patient treatment. Engineers must understand the needs of the patient and the factors that drive clinical decisions in the care of patients. Physicians benefit from an understanding of the fundamentals of device technology and, with this knowledge, are able to make decisions that optimize device performance given inherent technical characteristics. Additionally, an understanding of device design allows the clinician to match the appropriate device to each patient more accurately.

The objective of this chapter is to provide an overview of the major technical issues that drive device design and performance. The material is presented as a description of the major functional blocks of a typical implantable device. A discussion of pacemaker technology is followed by an overview of the unique technology challenges faced in the design of ICDs. The chapter concludes with a discussion of

the impact of future technology on implantable device design.

The emphasis throughout this chapter is on highlighting the specific areas in which technology affects clinical performance and on providing guidance on how best to manage that impact. Rather than discussing the specifics of early device designs, we focus on how recent advances have altered and improved implantable device performance.

■ FUNCTIONAL DESIGN ELEMENTS OF PACEMAKERS

The major physical elements of a typical pacemaker are shown in Figure 7–1. This photograph shows the pacemaker can and header. Within the can, the lithium-iodine battery can be seen next to the hybrid substrate that carries the electronic components. Despite important advances in circuit design that have increased circuit density while reducing current drain, the ratio of battery volume to circuit board volume remained relatively constant since the mid-1980s. The potential for size reduction of pacemaker circuitry and batteries has been offset by a corresponding increase in pacemaker capability. This increased functionality translates into increased circuit complexity having power requirements similar to less capable devices of the past.

Major subsystems of the implanted pulse generator are shown in Figure 7–2. Functions of the various blocks are described briefly here:

Pace control: sense amplifiers, pacing output, and timing circuits to deliver pacing pulses to the heart when required; also tracks heart activity during an arrhythmia

Rate-adaptive circuitry: amplifiers, filters, and current sources for various types of sensors; this circuitry may be significantly different for each particular type of sensor

Microprocessor: controls overall system functions; an 8-bit design is sufficient for most systems; use of an industry

Portions reprinted, with permission, from Proceedings of the IEEE, Vol 84, No. 3, March 1996. © 1996.

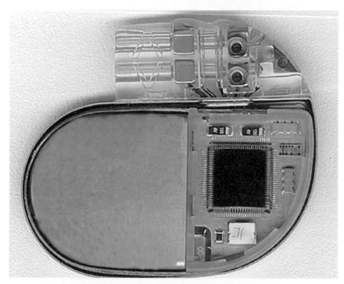

Figure 7–1. Cutaway view of DDDR pacemaker showing battery alongside the hybrid that contains integrated B circuits, accelerometer sensor, and electronic components.

requirements can be as large as 32 kilobytes in a pacemaker

RAM: used for additional program space, storage of operating parameters, and storage of lead electrogram data; storage of several minutes of electrograms requires a RAM of 16 to 512 kilobytes, depending on bandwidth, type of data compression used, and number of channels stored

Telemetry control: dedicated circuitry to control the specifics of communications protocol and telemetry schema

System control: contains support circuitry for the microprocessor, including the telemetry interface, typically implemented with a universal asynchronous receiver-transmitter (UART)–like interface, several general-purpose timers, and sleep–wake control

Voltage supply: supplies various current and voltage sources to the system. Digital circuits operate from 2.2 V or lower supplies; analog circuits typically require precision nanoampere current source inputs

Battery: one lithium-iodine battery supplies an open-circuit voltage of 2.8 V throughout life; high-energy density makes this chemistry appropriate for pacemaker applications; low-power density, acceptable in a pacing application, makes this chemistry inappropriate for defibrillation applications (see Chapter 6)

Pacing Output

The function of the output circuit is to translate the lithium-iodine battery voltage of 2.8 V into a programmable selection of pacing voltages that range from 0.1 V to more

standard design (6502, 8852, Z80, etc.) allows the use of standard development languages and tools and also facilitates integrated circuit implementation with a "megacell" or VHDL model

ROM: sufficient nonvolatile memory is available for system start-up tasks and some program space; program space

Figure 7–2. Block diagram of a DDDR pacemaker showing main functional elements.

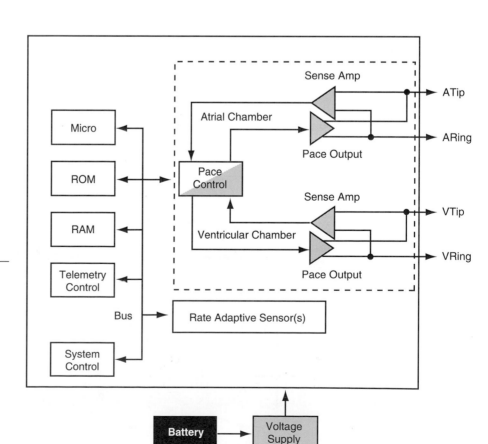

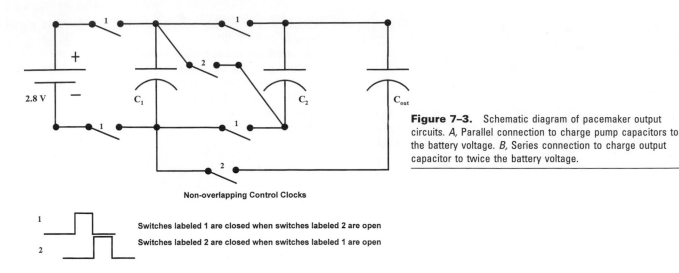

Figure 7–3. Schematic diagram of pacemaker output circuits. *A,* Parallel connection to charge pump capacitors to the battery voltage. *B,* Series connection to charge output capacitor to twice the battery voltage.

Non-overlapping Control Clocks

Switches labeled 1 are closed when switches labeled 2 are open

Switches labeled 2 are closed when switches labeled 1 are open

than 7 V. In the most simple situation, the output pulse is programmed to be identical to the voltage of the battery, 2.8 V for a lithium-iodine battery at beginning of life (BOL). In this case, the battery is used to charge a pacing capacitor, which itself is then discharged for a duration (t) to the myocardium, where t is the pulse width. Modern pacemakers, however, offer a variety of programmable stimulus amplitudes ranging from less than 2.8 V to more than 7.5 V. Increasing the stimulus amplitude to a value greater than the battery voltage requires that more than one capacitor be charged in parallel from the battery and then discharged in series to the myocardium.

Figure 7–3 is a schematic representation of an early pacing output circuit. This circuit, known as a *capacitive voltage doubler,* consists of a specific arrangement of switches and capacitors and operates in two distinct phases: one set of switches is closed during the first phase, and a second set of switches closes during the second phase. This clock circuit controls the two phases that are designed to be nonoverlapping, meaning that the switches controlled by each phase are never closed at the same time. Voltage doublers can be understood best by redrawing the circuit diagram to show the configuration of switches and capacitors during each phase. This is shown in Figure 7–4. The top panel is representative of when the switches labeled "1" are closed. During this first phase, capacitors C_1 and C_2 are connected in parallel with the battery, so that they charge to the battery voltage. In the second phase, these two capacitors are reconnected in series and their combined voltage is delivered to the heart, as shown in the bottom panel. The effect of this second phase is that the battery voltage is multiplied (in this case by a factor of 2), and the charge is transferred to the heart. In a similar manner, battery voltage can be tripled by making the same connecting scheme with three charging capacitors rather than two.

A limitation of this technique is that the voltage output is limited to three settings: $1\times$, $2\times$, $3\times$; corresponding to pacing voltages of 2.8, 5.6, and 8.4 V. The result is that the current drain due to a particular pacing output selection is often higher than necessary given the actual pacing thresh-

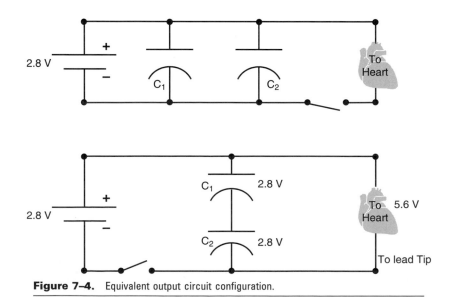

Figure 7–4. Equivalent output circuit configuration.

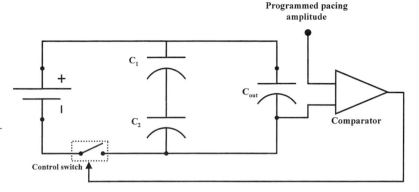

Figure 7–5. Schematic diagram of advanced pacemaker output circuit. A comparator circuit is added to the pacing output capacitor to allow programming to a range of output voltages between one and two times the battery voltage.

old. For example, consider a patient with a pacing threshold of 1.5 V. Providing for a pacing safety margin of 2:1 would require an output voltage selection of 3 V. Given 2.8, 5.6, and 8.4 V as the only choices, 5.6 V becomes the only reasonable selection. This 5.6-V selection results in substantially more current required by the pacing circuitry and an attendant reduction in longevity of the pulse generator.

Modern pacemakers overcome this limitation by adding additional circuitry, as depicted in Figure 7–5, which shows the addition of a voltage comparator and an output capacitor to the pacing output circuit. This circuit works in a like manner to the voltage doubler circuit, except that during phase two, the smaller doubler capacitors are reconnected in series and placed across a larger pacing output capacitor. Because the doubler capacitors in this configuration are smaller than the output capacitor, it takes a number of cycles of charging in parallel and then discharging in series to fill the output capacitor completely. This action is sometimes called a *charge pump* because charge is being transferred in discrete amounts from the battery, through the small capacitors, to the larger output capacitor. Additionally, a comparator circuit interrupts the charge transfer process when the output capacitor reaches a programmed value. This enhancement allows for finer resolution in pacing output voltage selection. Using the patient data from the previous example, the voltage output setting of a modern pacemaker given a 1.5-V threshold and using a 2:1 safety margin could be reduced from 5.4 to 3 V. The benefit of this pacing output reduction can be translated into an improvement in longevity by decreasing the current requirements. The equation that approximates average pacing current is as follows:

$$(1) \quad I_p = \frac{\dfrac{V_p}{R_l} \times PW}{Interval} \times \frac{V_x}{V_{bat}},$$

where:

I_p is pacing current
V_p is pacing amplitude
R_l is lead impedance
PW is pulse width
Interval is pacing interval
V_x is pacing multiple ($1\times$, $2\times$, or $3\times$)
V_{bat} is battery voltage

A couple of points are worth noting in this equation. First, voltage appears twice in the numerator, as pacing voltage

V_p, and as a voltage multiplier V_x. As a result, increasing pacing voltage has a squared effect on pacing current. The second point to note is that pacing is affected by lead impedance. This effect is reflected in the R_l variable in the pacing equation. This helps explain the benefit of the new generation of high impedance pacing leads.

Continuing with the $2\times$ pacing example, current drain for the 5.4-V ($2\times$) and the 3-V outputs is calculated as 8.6 and 4.8 µA, respectively. These values are based on nominal values of 0.4 msec for PW, 500 Ω for R_l, 1000 msec for interval (60 PPM), and 2 for V_x. Assuming a quiescent current (the quiescent current is the current required to power the device electronics required to do the "housekeeping" tasks) of 11 µA for a typical VVIR, and with an available battery capacity of 1.2 ampere-hours, the pacemaker longevity can be calculated as follows:

$$(2) \quad L = \frac{C_a}{I_c} \times K$$

where:

L is the longevity of the pacemaker under nominal conditions measured in years
C_a is the capacity available in a particular battery cell after subtracting reductions to theoretical capacity, as noted previously. Capacity is measured in amp-hours.
K is a constant that converts hours to years
I_c is the average current drain for pacing, sensing, and circuit function
Ic is current drain by the pacemaker from the battery

The resultant longevity is 7 years for the 5.4-V setting and 8.7 years for the 3-V setting. An improvement of 1.7 years in longevity is achieved with the addition of the more flexible pacing output voltage settings. A more detailed discussion of longevity is provided in the section of this chapter on pacemaker batteries.

Automatic Capture

A potentially important advance in pacing output circuitry is the concept of automatic capture (or autocapture) verification and threshold tracking.[1] *Capture verification* refers to the ability of a pacemaker to detect automatically when a pacing stimulus captures the chamber being paced. Threshold tracking uses capture verification as a means to adjust the pacing pulse amplitude automatically to guarantee capture. For example, if capture is verified, the pacing stimulus amplitude remains unchanged. If capture is lost, however, a large-amplitude backup pacing stimulus is delivered (typically within 100 msec) to ensure capture of the heart and the amplitude of subsequent pacing stimuli is increased. This basic technique can be modified to track the pacing threshold continuously by algorithmically iterating the output to adjust the stimulus output to a level slightly higher than what is necessary for capture. Paradoxically, continuously adjusting the pacing output to a level that is too close to threshold can actually result in increased energy demand from the battery. For each missed beat, the device delivers a large-amplitude pacing pulse closely coupled to the ineffective stimulus, and this high-output backup pacing pulse can consume as much as 25 times more energy than a stimulus at threshold.

A number of companies have developed pacemakers with autocapture verification. These attempts have proved that capture detection is possible, although with several limitations. The most common technique used to accomplish autocapture is to measure the evoked response. The *evoked response* is the alteration of the intracardiac signal in response to the pacing stimulus when capture is achieved. In other words, if capture occurs, an evoked response will arise and can be detected. If capture does not occur, there will be no evoked response.

There are a number of technical challenges facing the designer in the implementation of autocapture verification and threshold tracking. The primary technical challenge involves the accurate assessment of the evoked response after a pacing stimulus. This challenge can be appreciated by considering that the pacing stimulus can be 350 times greater than the signal to be measured (3.5 V for pacing versus 10 mV for a ventricular evoked response). Remnants of the stimulus afterpotential (known as *polarization*) remain long after the pacing pulse is complete, owing to the capacitance at the lead–tissue interface. These stimulus remnants have forced some designs to require leads with low polarization characteristics to allow correct operation. When combined with a low polarization lead, autocapture detection has been proved possible for most patients. This afterpotential must be removed within 50 to 100 msec to delineate the evoked response accurately. The difficulty in distinguishing the evoked response, combined with the fact that the evoked response of the atrial chamber is smaller in magnitude, has limited the introduction of this feature to the ventricular chamber.

An additional challenge in the implementation of autocapture is the accurate assessment in the presence of fusion and pseudofusion beats.[2] Fusion beats can confuse the autocapture algorithm and produce false-negative results, such that a stimulus is determined to be subthreshold when in fact capture has occurred. False-negative results with fusion beats occasionally occur when the intrinsic cardiac signal obscures the evoked response, causing the evoked potential to go undetected. In contrast, pseudofusion beats can result in a false-positive classification. Pseudofusion occurs when a pacing stimulus occurs coincident with the intrinsic depolarization. With pseudofusion, however, the pacing pulse does not capture the heart but is detected as capture. A false-positive classification can occur when the intrinsic waveform is incorrectly classified as an evoked response.

The impact of inaccurately classified events on a threshold-tracking algorithm can be serious. For example, a false-positive classification might promote loss of capture as the algorithm mistakenly assumes that capture has occurred and reduces the amplitude of the pacing stimulus. After a sequence of these misclassified events, the pacing output might be reduced to a dangerously low level. A false-negative classification would result in high-output pacing, as the algorithm increases pacing output to guarantee capture. This would result in a measurable decrease in device longevity because of the elevated pacing current. A number of approaches have been developed to minimize the impact of fusion and pseudofusion beats. Most of these approaches involve controlling the pacing rate to prevent the possibility of fusion events. As an example, the pacing rate can be automatically increased during a threshold test, so that intrinsic activity is overdriven.

The specific benefits of autocapture and threshold tracking have likely been overstated. Conventional wisdom is that an autocapture–threshold tracking algorithm that provides beat-to-beat verification in the ventricle would be beneficial. The benefits ascribed to such an algorithm have been safety, improved longevity, and ease of use. The impact of autocapture on each of these stated benefits is limited, however. For example, the safety benefit of autocapture is limited to the maximum output of the device, which is typically 7 V or less. As a result, loss of capture due to lead dislodgment or gross lead failure (such as lead fracture) cannot be prevented. Additionally, improvements in lead design over the years have significantly reduced the incidence of exit block.

The longevity benefit of such a system is commonly overstated. This notion is perpetuated by the belief that the lower pacing amplitudes provided by a threshold-tracking device substantially reduce the overall current drawn from the battery. Consider the following scenario as an example. A dual-chamber, rate-responsive pacemaker is implanted with both the atrial and ventricular leads having thresholds of 1 V (common chronic thresholds for modern pacing lead systems). An appropriate pacing amplitude for a 1-V threshold might be between 2 and 3 V, depending on the specific patient situation and clinical guidelines that are followed. Assuming that a 2.5-V setting is used, the pacing current for each chamber would be about 2.9 μA, resulting in a total pacemaker current drain for a typical DDDR device of 17.6 μA. Now assume that the same patient scenario exists, except that a pacemaker with ventricular autocapture is available. In this case, the ventricular pacing amplitude could be lowered from 2.5 V to potentially 1.3 V. (*Note:* It would not be appropriate to lower the amplitude all the way down to the pacing threshold because diurnal and physiologic variations in threshold might cause intermittent loss of capture, requiring frequent backup pacing pulses.) The resulting current drain for ventricular pacing is about 1 μA. This represents a less than 2 μA reduction in current drain. This reduction is partially offset by the incremental current drain required to implement the autocapture feature. This current drain would vary depending on the implementation used, but it would likely be in the 1-μA range. The net effect on total pacemaker current drain is a reduction from 17.6 μA for the conventional device to 16.6 μA for the automatic device. This translates into an increase in longevity of roughly 6%, or 5 months, for a 7-year device. The benefit of autocapture on longevity is diminished as advances in lead technology result in lower pacing currents due to lower thresholds and higher lead impedance. For example, the prior scenario assumed 500-Ω lead impedance. Many leads today have an impedance in excess of 1000 Ω, reducing the longevity benefit to less than 3 months.

Ease of use will likely be the most demonstrable benefit of autocapture, providing the physician with pacing threshold values automatically at each follow-up. Having the device automatically report the threshold values to the clinician through the programmer removes the need for threshold tests to be manually performed at follow-up. The key success factors for broad acceptance of these technologies will be the development of algorithms that do not require any special programming and pacing systems that do not require any specific lead for reliable operation. To completely eliminate the need for performing manual threshold tests for dual-chamber pacemakers, autocapture in the atrial chamber will need to be perfected and commercialized.

Sense Amplifiers

A dual-chamber pacemaker has two separate sensing channels: one for the atrium and one for the ventricle. Each sense amplifier has five primary attributes: gain; dynamic range; sensitivity; signal-to-noise ratio; and filtering capability. Each of these characteristics is discussed in this section. To begin the discussion, a block diagram of a typical atrial or ventricular sense amplifier is shown in Figure 7–6.

Connection to the input of the amplifier is made to the tip and can for unipolar sensing and to the tip and ring for bipolar sensing. Each connection from the patient to the sense amplifier is made through a capacitor and resistor network. This network acts as a prefilter to reduce baseline wander, which results from variations in the electrode–tissue interface. This prefilter also eliminates high-frequency noise, which would cause signal distortion, known as *aliasing*, if not removed before entering the sense amplifier.

Sense amplifier gain is defined as follows:

(3) $\quad V_{out} = A \times V_{in}$

where:

V_{out} is the amplifier output
V_{in} is the amplifier input and
A is the amplifier gain

The role of the sense amplifier is to increase the magnitude of the cardiac-originated signal, which can be as low as 0.25 mV, to a value that is squarely within the range of subsequent analog circuits (these circuits typically have a maximum range of 700 mV). Modern pacemaker sense amplifiers have several programmable gain settings to maximize the effective dynamic range. Dynamic range is the amplitude over which the sense amplifier can faithfully reproduce the input signal.

Filtering presents one of the most complex challenges in sense amplifier design.[3–15] The specific filter characteristics used in pacemaker sense amplifiers are designed to allow signals originating in the heart to be detected, while at the same time attenuating unwanted cardiac signals or environmental noise. There are generally four types of unwanted signals that need to be reduced. Cardiac signals that must be attenuated include T waves and far-field activity; noncardiac physiologic signals that must be attenuated include skeletal myopotentials. A third type of undesirable signal includes electrical noise inherent to the pacemaker circuitry itself. A fourth type of unwanted signal includes environmental noise such as microwave ovens, electrical welding equipment, or cellular phones.[16–25] Filtering provides the most important, although not the only, method available to pacemaker design engineers to prevent these unwanted signals from causing false oversensing by the sense amplifiers. Figure 7–7 shows the effect of amplifier filtering on a typical ventricular endocardial electrogram. The top panel shows the unfiltered electrogram. Notice the prominent T wave present in this electrogram. The bottom panel shows the same electrogram after going through a typical pacemaker filter with a pass band of 20 to 80 Hz. Note that the T wave is greatly attenuated by the filter. Except for some attenuation in amplitude and some narrowing of duration, the QRS complex is not affected.

An understanding of sense amplifier specifics requires a brief discussion of frequency domain analysis. Engineers use a mathematical formula known as *fast Fourier transformation* (FFT) to convert signals from their time domain into their frequency domain. Signals represented in the time domain include ventricular electrograms like the one shown in Figure 7–7. Time domain signals can be represented in the frequency domain by using the FFT. The basic concept of FFT is that any signal can be reconstructed as the sum of multiple sinusoidal waveforms of various frequencies. A simple rule of thumb is instructive. Signals that move rapidly in time, such as a QRS complex, are composed of higher frequencies than signals that move slowly in time, such as T waves. Figure 7–8 shows the results of an FFT of the ventricular electrograms provided in Figure 7–7. The top panel is an FFT of the unfiltered electrogram. The frequency content ranges from 2 Hz to 100 Hz. There is a peak in the range of 6 to 9 Hz that is due to the T wave. There is a

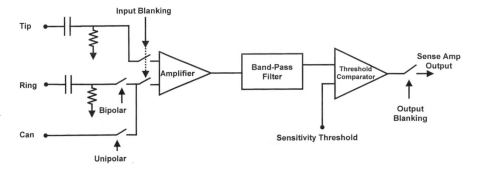

Figure 7–6. Block diagram of a pacemaker sense amplifier showing the main functional elements of a typical atrial or ventricular sense amplifier.

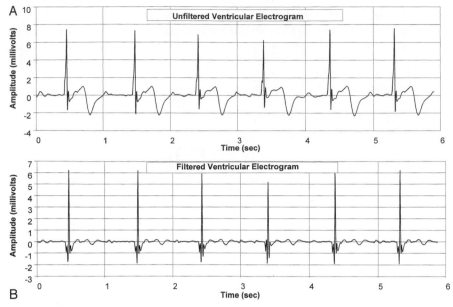

Figure 7–7. *A,* Unfiltered ventricular electrogram. Note the prominent T wave present. *B,* The same electrogram after filtering by a pacemaker sense amplifier. Note that the filtering has greatly reduced the amplitude of the T wave.

second peak between 10 and 11 Hz, with a gradual decline out to 40 Hz. This is caused by the QRS complex. The lower panel shows an FFT of the filtered electrogram. The filter has significantly reduced most frequency content less than 10 Hz. Most of the frequency content that remains after filtering is in the 10 to 80 Hz range.

Sense amplifier filters make use of the different frequency content of various signals. Specifically, the filter makes the amplifier most sensitive to frequencies that make up the signal of interest (such as QRS complexes) and less sensitive to frequencies that make up unwanted signals, such as T waves. The last component of the sense amplifier is the

threshold comparator. This circuit provides a reference voltage, such that signals above the programmed sensitivity are detected as P waves or R waves, whereas those below this amplitude are not detected. A curve representing how filtering and sensitivity are related is shown in Figure 7–9.

This figure shows sensitivity levels on the *y* axis and frequency on the *x* axis. As noted earlier, signals above the sensitivity level are detected by the sense amplifiers as P waves or R waves.

The concave shape of the curve is typical of a bandpass filter. Low-frequency signals require relatively large signal levels to be detected. This is due to the attenuation of these

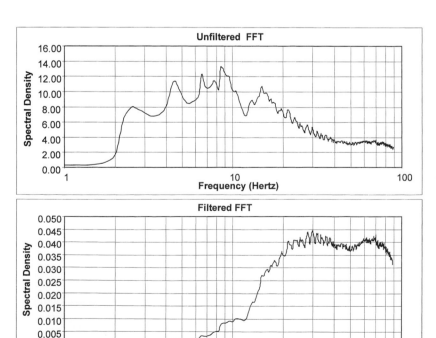

Figure 7–8. Frequency content of unfiltered and filtered ventricular electrogram. *Top,* Fast Fourier transformation of an unfiltered electrogram. Note the frequency content in the 2 to 10 Hz range caused by T waves; also note the frequency content between 10 and 40 Hz caused by R waves. *Bottom,* Fast Fourier transformation of filtered electrogram. Note that the frequency content from 2 to 10 Hz is removed by filtering.

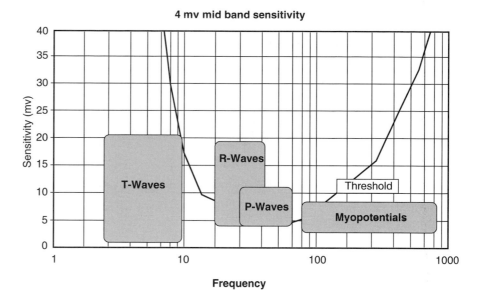

4 mv mid band sensitivity

Figure 7–9. Sense amplifier sensitivity versus frequency plot. Signals above the threshold (or sensitivity) line are sensed as P waves or R waves. Signals below the sensitivity line are not sensed. Frequencies of typical signals are superimposed on the plot.

signals by the bandpass filter. Signals in the mid-band or pass-band region of the filter are detected most easily because they require the smallest amplitude (i.e., minimal attenuation). As the frequency of the signal increases beyond the pass-band, they become harder to detect because of the higher signal levels required.

Various signals of interest are shown as shaded areas in the figure. The frequency content of typical QRS complexes is shown to be in the range of 25 to 40 Hz. Sense amplifiers are most sensitive to signals in this range and therefore easily detect R waves. T waves, on the other hand, are shown to be lower in frequency (3 to 10 Hz) and are more difficult to detect, as indicated by the fact that the shaded area lies mostly below the sensitivity line. Similar comments apply to myopotentials, which lay primarily below the sensitivity line in the 80 to 800 Hz range.

A limitation of sense amplifier filters is apparent from Figure 7–9. As shown in the figure, there is some overlap between unwanted signal frequencies and the sensitivity level corresponding to that frequency. For this reason, filtering alone is not sufficient to reject signals. Additional timing cycles are needed to complete the proper operation of sense amplifiers. The most straightforward example of timing cycles used to reject signals is the ventricular refractory period. The ventricular refractory period rejects T-wave signals that may still be present after filtering. This is accomplished as long as the refractory period covers the timing interval of a QRS to T wave.

A characteristic inherent to sense amplifiers is the signal-to-noise ratio. This is defined as the amplitude of the input signal divided by the amplitude of noise. Noise as used in this calculation is defined as extraneous signals that are inherent in the amplifier circuitry. All electronic circuits produce some amount of random noise because of physical properties of the components used in the design. One of the characteristics of circuit noise is that increasing the bias current used to power the sense amplifier can reduce it. This presents an interesting trade-off for engineers: noise performance can be improved by increasing current drain. This improvement in noise performance comes at the ex-

pense of pacemaker longevity. There is a relationship between signal-to-noise ratio, amplifier gain, sensitivity, and dynamic range. As sensitivity is set to smaller values, gain is increased to accommodate the sensitivity setting. Increased gain increases noise, which is also present at the input. The result is a lower signal-to-noise ratio, which makes the pacemaker more susceptible to over sensing.

It is valuable to understand the relationships among gain, sensitivity, and dynamic range when programming sensitivity settings in a pacemaker. A typical R wave of 6-mV amplitude is shown in Figure 7–10. The recommended sensitivity setting would be to provide a sensing margin of 2:1 or, in this case, 3 mV. If the programmed sensitivity is set at a level significantly less than this, for example, 0.25 mV, the gain of the amplifier will be increased to accommodate the low setting. The result is that the actual GmV R wave will be distorted (or clipped as shown in Figure 7–10 bottom panel) because it is beyond the dynamic range of the sense amplifier. The distortion of the signal can produce unexpected results, such as delayed recovery of the sense amplifier and oversensing of noncardiac signals. On the other hand, if the sensitivity is set too close to the actual measured R-wave, then undersensing may occur as a result of typical variations in R-wave amplitude.

Potential sensing complications, such as oversensing and undersensing, can be avoided with the following steps. Leads should be positioned such that a maximum signal amplitude and slew rate are obtained. This will minimize the risk for oversensing due to a low signal-to-noise ratio and to other noncardiac signals, such as myopotentials. The bipolar sensing configuration tends to minimize the amplitude of noncardiac signals. The programmed sensitivity setting should be kept in the range of 2:1 (measured amplitude–to–programmed setting ratio), with a 3:1 ratio at the maximum. Keeping a sensing margin of 2:1 is particularly important in the atrial channel. The smaller signal amplitude of P waves increases the potential for oversensing if a sensing margin greater than 2:1 is used. Some newer pacemakers provide automatic measurements of P-wave and R-wave amplitudes.[26] Devices that incorporate this feature rely on the

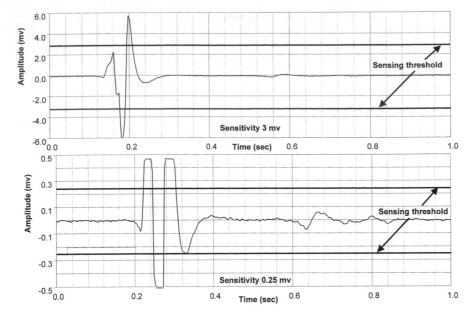

Figure 7–10. *Top,* Appropriate sensitivity setting of 3 mV for a 6-mV R wave. This 2:1 sensitivity margin is adequate for the typical variations in R waves. *Bottom,* Effect of setting the sensitivity setting too low (0.25 mV). Note the distortion of the R wave caused by sense amplifier clipping as a result of the increased gain; also note the increased noise.

programmed sensitivity (and gain) to make these automatic measurements. If the sensitivity margin is too great (such as 3:1), then the feature will in some cases give inaccurate results because of clipping, as shown in the lower panel of Figure 7–10. The use of automatic P-wave and R-wave measurements is yet another reason for programming an appropriate sensitivity margin.

An important consideration for sense amplifiers is rejection of environmental noise.[16–25] Environmental noise affects a pacemaker when the frequency content is in the pass-band of the amplifier. Noise can also affect a pacemaker if it is pulsed at a frequency similar to possible cardiac heart rates. Some digital cellular phones represent an example of pulsed noise. Several studies have been published that address this possible interaction. The following statements can be drawn from these studies. Interaction with cellular phones based on analog technology is uncommon and unlikely. This lack of interaction is due to the fact that the frequency content of the transmission is outside the pass-band of the implanted device amplifier. Interaction with digital cellular phones has been noted in some studies. This interaction occurs because some digital phones are pulsed at rates that are similar to heart rates. This causes the potential for interaction even though the carrier frequencies (at 900 MHz) are several orders of magnitude higher than the sense amplifier pass-band. The interaction is limited to cases in which cellular phones are placed well within 6 inches of the pacemaker. Simple precautions, such as not carrying a cellular phone in a pocket adjacent to an implanted device, can prevent interaction between a cellular phone and an implanted device.

Power Requirements of Pulse Generator Circuits

The capacity of the battery and the current drain of the pacemaker affect pacemaker longevity. Modern pacemakers use batteries that range in size from 3.5 to 4.5 cc and have capacities ranging from 1.2 to 1.5 ampere-hours. The ampere-hour is a unit of measure used by the battery industry to reflect capacity available in the cell. There are two capacity ratings that are of interest in pacemaker design: theoretical capacity and available capacity. Theoretical capacity measures the total capacity of the cell based on the electrochemical content. The available capacity, which is always less than the theoretical capacity, is the capacity available after taking into account practical limitations, such as minimum operating voltage of the circuits and reserve capacity needed to manage end of life (EOL).

Pacemaker longevity is calculated as follows:

$$\textbf{(4)} \quad L = \frac{C_a}{I_c} \times K$$

where:

L is the longevity of the pacemaker under nominal conditions measured in years

C_a is the capacity available in a particular battery cell after subtracting reductions to theoretical capacity, as noted previously. Capacity is measured in units of amp-hours.

I_c is the average current drain for pacing, sensing, and circuit function measured in amps

K is a constant, which converts hours to years

Table 7–1 provides a breakdown of pacing current for a typical dual-chamber rate-responsive pacemaker. Pacing

Table 7–1. **Peak and Average Current Drain Values for Pacemakers**

Function	Peak Current Drain	Average Current Drain	Average Current Drain as Percentage of Total
Pacing current	7 mA	8 μA	38%
Sense amplifiers	2 μA	2 μA	10%
Rate adaptive sensors	2 μA	2 μA	10%
Control	16 μA	8 μA	38%
Telemetry	60 μA	<1 μA	4%
Total	N/A	21 μA	100%

current is based on 100% pacing into a 500-ohm lead imped-ance at programmed settings of 3.5 V, 0.5 msec, and 60 bpm. As shown in Table 7–1, pacing current composes a significant percentage of the total current drain of the pace-maker. Proper attention to programming appropriate pacing amplitude is critical to maximizing pacemaker longevity. Another factor that significantly improves longevity is the use of high-impedance leads. Several companies have devel-oped leads that have a pacing impedance of more than 1000 Ω. This results in a substantial reduction in pacing current.

The current drain for both atrial and ventricular chamber sense amplifiers is just less than 1 μA each, for a total of 2 μA, as shown in Table 7–1. The current drain represents the energy required for the amplifiers and filters needed in a typical sense amplifier. As noted in the discussion of sense amplifiers, low-noise amplifiers needed for more sensitive settings require higher current drain from the battery.

The current drain shown for rate-adaptive sensors of 2 μA is typical of an accelerometer-based sensor. The type of sensor incorporated in the pacemaker can have a significant effect on current drain. Sensor current drain can range from less than 1 μA for activity-based sensors that do not use accelerometers to more than 4 μA for some of the physio-logic sensors, such as early devices using minute ventilation.

The control current of 8 μA includes the current to run microprocessor circuits as well as logic that supplements the operation of the microprocessor. The difference between the average current and the peak current for the control circuits is due to the fact that in most pacemakers, the microproces-sor is "halted" when it is not in use. When the microproces-sor is placed in stasis, the current drain is virtually zero.

The average telemetry circuit current drain of less than 1 μA reflects the fact that telemetry is only used during implantation and follow-up visits, a small fraction of the total operating life of a pacemaker. When telemetry is not in use, the only current drain required is for the telemetry receiver circuit. This circuit detects the presence of telemetry and powers up the remaining telemetry circuitry.

For pacing and telemetry, the peak current is significantly higher than the average current. This difference has a sig-nificant effect on the operation of the lithium-iodine battery used in pacemakers.

One of the unique aspects of lithium-iodine batteries is the discharge characteristic of the battery chemistry. As cell capacity is depleted, the internal series resistance of the cell increases. This is depicted in Figure 7–11, which shows a simplified model of a battery.

As shown in the figure, the series resistance can increase from about 100 Ω at BOL to as high as 10,000 Ω at EOL. This characteristic has significant implications for pacemaker design as well as patient management.

The effect on pacemaker design involves constraints that are imposed because of the high series resistance. The high resistance limits the peak current that can be drawn by pacemaker circuits such as telemetry, pacing output, and rate-adaptive sensing. This is seen in Table 7–1 by noting the significant difference in peak versus average current. Note that for telemetry, the average current is negligible because it is limited to short periods of time during patient follow-up visits. The peak current, however, is larger than for any other circuit. The peak current, combined with the high series resistance, reduces the voltage (according to Ohm's law) available to power the pacemaker electronics. As a result, peak telemetry currents must be limited to values at or below those shown in Table 7–1. This, in turn, limits the telemetry distance and telemetry speed. Greater telemetry distance would increase peak telemetry current because of the higher transmit current pulses needed. Faster telemetry speed would increase peak telemetry current because more pulses are delivered per second.

The high series resistance of lithium-iodine batteries also affects patient management near the end of the pacemaker's useful life (EOL). As the battery depletes and the series resistance increases, the variation in voltage increases. This fluctuation in battery voltage limits the ability of the pace-maker to predict remaining longevity with accuracy. Pace-makers provide a warning of approaching battery depletion. This indicator, known as Elective Replacement Indicator (ERT or ERI) is designed to provide 3 to 6 months' warning before EOL. To preserve remaining capacity and limit the voltage variations noted previously, most pacemakers limit functionality of the device at ERT by eliminating rate-adap-tive features and in some cases reverting to VVI mode. Because of the limitations in predicting actual battery EOL, as well as limited device functionality at ERT, it is important

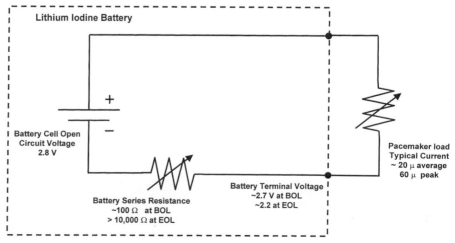

Figure 7–11. Simplified model of a lithium iodine battery. The open circuit voltage of 2.8 V is characteristic of lithium iodine chemistries. The series resistance increases from 100 Ω at beginning of life (BOL) to >10,000 Ω at end of life (EOL).

to schedule pacemaker replacement as soon as practical after ERT is set.

Lead Impedance Measurement

Modern pacemakers provide a number of diagnostic measurements that can aid in the evaluation of the pacing system. Measured lead impedance, one of the more clinically useful measurements, can provide important information regarding the integrity of the lead and the lead–pacemaker connection. This information, combined with pacing and sensing thresholds, can assist in troubleshooting lead-related issues.

The first step taken by an implanted device in reporting lead impedance is to measure the leading and trailing edge voltage of the pacing pulse, as shown in Figure 7–12. The difference between these two voltages (referred to as "droop" in the pacing pulse) is then used to calculate lead impedance. This impedance calculation is possible because the magnitude of the pacing droop is directly related to the lead impedance. Unfortunately, pacing pulse droop is also affected by components within in the pacemaker. As a result of variation in these component values internal to the implanted device, accuracy of lead impedance measurements is usually $\pm 20\%$. Although the precision of lead impedance measurements is relatively poor from device to device, the measurements taken from the same device are highly repeatable. Measurements from the same device can be as precise as $\pm 5\%$. Therefore, it is important to focus on relative trends in lead impedance rather than relying on absolute values when using this measurement for diagnostic purposes.

The method used in pacemakers to measure lead impedance might be different than the measurement method used in a pacing system analyzer (PSA). The different measurement methods used result in differences in the measured lead impedance. This difference is important to keep in mind, especially during implantation, when measurements taken from a PSA might differ from measurements of lead impedance taken moments later by the pacemaker.

Lead impedance measurements have traditionally been used only for diagnostic purposes. A relatively new application of lead impedance is the ability of the pacemaker to use lead impedance measurements to switch automatically to the appropriate pacing and sensing configuration. If, for example, a conductor within a bipolar pacing lead fractured, this system could automatically switch to a unipolar configuration using the remaining intact conductor. This ensures that the patient continues to receive pacing therapy until appropriate correction can be taken.

Another important use of automatic lead configuration switching occurs during device reset. Most pacemakers have a reset mode that is used to ensure proper device operation after disruption from external sources of energy, such as defibrillation shocks, electrocautery, or radiofrequency (RF) ablation. Some modern pacemaker models have incorporated an automatic lead configuration check as part of the reset routine, when, during reset, a lead impedance measurement is taken. If the measurement indicates that a bipolar lead is present, the device will configure pacing and sensing to the bipolar mode. This is an important feature of pacemakers that are implanted in combination with implantable defibrillators because unipolar pacing interferes with proper defibrillator sensing.

Another enhancement to pacemaker lead impedance measurements is the ability to measure impedance automatically on a periodic basis and store these results for analysis at follow-up. Because trends in lead impedance over time are the most meaningful indicator of lead integrity, this feature provides a valuable troubleshooting tool as well as a time saving tool during follow-up.

Adaptive Rate Sensors

Although a variety of sensors have been developed for rate-adaptive pacing, those detecting activity, acceleration, or minute ventilation have become dominant. The activity sensor has been the most commonly implanted adaptive rate sensor, and there are two basic types: motion sensors and accelerometers. The primary technical difference between a motion sensor and an accelerometer is that the accelerometer uses an isolated mass (known as a *proof mass*) as part of the sensor, whereas the motion sensor uses the pacemaker case as the mass. The effective mass that the pacemaker case presents to the sensor can vary considerably from patient to patient. Because force equals mass multiplied by acceleration ($F = ma$), using the constant mass in accelerometer sensors provides for a precise and repeatable measurement of acceleration.

Two material properties are exploited in the fabricating of activity sensors: piezoelectric and piezoresistive. Piezoelectric sensors redistribute charge when the material is deflected, which can be detected and converted to a voltage by the pacemaker circuitry. Piezoresistive sensors change

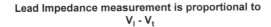

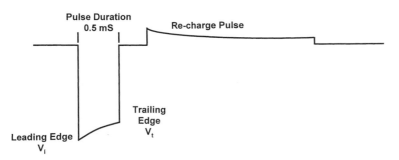

Figure 7–12. Pacemaker output pulse. The decrease in voltage between the leading edge and the trailing edge is measured and used to calculate lead impedance.

their resistance value when deflected, and this change in resistance is converted to voltage by driving the sensor with a constant current. The piezoelectric activity sensor requires less current than the piezoresistive sensors (about 1.5 μA for piezoelectric versus about 3 μA for piezoresistive).

Minute ventilation is another important adaptive rate sensor. There are several meaningful improvements that need to be addressed in the next generation of minute ventilation pacemakers. The most important improvement is the reduction of current drain required for measuring minute ventilation, which today ranges from 3 to 5 μA. Other technical issues include increasing the range of respiration rates from the 45 breaths per minute maximum (available in some current pacemaker models) to rates as high as 60 breaths per minute. The ability to measure higher respiration rates will allow the use of the minute ventilation sensor in a wider group of patients. The key technical challenge in extending the respiration rate will involve better rejection of the cardiac component of the impedance signal used to detect respiration.

The primary technical challenge for designing multiple sensor pacemakers will be reduction of current drain, so that device size and longevity are not adversely affected. An additional challenge will be integration of the individual sensor algorithms into an appropriate blend of the two.

Microprocessors

The microprocessor has affected the way digital design is accomplished more than any other innovation of the past 25 years. This technology has successfully been applied to the design of implantable devices. During this same period, circuit density has increased by more than 1,000,000 times, whereas the size of the circuitry and the current drain have decreased. These advances in circuit design have allowed implementation of more sophisticated algorithms, including those associated with rate-responsive pacing. These same advances in circuit size and current reduction have allowed greater memory for storing pacemaker software (sometimes called firmware) used to implement algorithms as well as increased diagnostic data storage.

Most early pacemakers were designed with discrete logic. The main attribute of these machines is that a specific combination of logic circuits is used to provide a specific function. For example, a group of logic circuits might be used to create a clock that keeps track of the ventricular pacing interval. Hundreds of logic circuits would need to be combined to provide control functions for a fairly simple VVI pacemaker. The primary advantage of these pacemakers is their extreme efficiency—every logic circuit has a specific function. This advantage was critical given the size and current constraints of pacemakers and the limitations of digital technology available at that time.

A microprocessor uses the same basic circuit elements as a discrete logic machine but adds the capability to change the specific function of the circuits by adding programming instructions. The programming instructions of a microprocessor make it possible to change the functionality of the device without the need to redesign the way the digital circuitry is interconnected. Instead, device functions can be changed by altering the contents of program memory. The benefits of this increased flexibility come at the expense of

decreased efficiency. Microprocessors require more circuits to implement a specific function than are required by a discrete logic machine, partly because of the memory requirements needed to store the firmware that controls the function of the circuits.

The result of the conflicting requirements for increased flexibility and the limited available circuit density was that several pacemaker companies developed custom microprocessors for use in their pacemakers. The goal was to balance the competing requirements by providing a microprocessor structure with instructions limited to the small set required by the pacemaker.

As the trend toward more complexity and improvements in digital circuits has continued to accelerate, some pacemaker companies have taken an additional step by replacing custom microprocessors with standard commercial microprocessors. The main advantage of using standard microprocessors rather than custom microprocessors developed by individual pacemaker companies is that standard microprocessors have more extensive design support tools. These support tools become increasingly important as the complexity of the pacemaker design application increases. Design support tools include hardware and software design support. The end result of the trade-offs between custom and standard microprocessors is that standard microprocessors have further increased the design flexibility, which, in turn, has increased the ability to implement increasingly complex pacing algorithms.

Memory

With the incorporation of microprocessors into pacemakers comes the requirement to store information in memory. There are two types of memory used in pacemakers: ROM and RAM. ROM, or read only memory, is used to store the software programs that the microprocessor uses to control pacemaker function. ROM is a type of nonvolatile memory, which means that once the memory is written during manufacture, it cannot be changed. This attribute limits the use of ROM to program storage (because diagnostic information will change over the life of the device). It does provide an advantage as well: it is immune to external interference sources, such as electrocautery and other electromagnetic interference sources, which can disrupt power. For this reason, critical pacemaker codes, such as those used for reset routines, are always stored in ROM.

The other type of memory used in implantable devices is RAM, or random access memory. The critical attribute of RAM is that the memory contents can be changed throughout the use of the device. RAM is a type of volatile memory. This attribute makes RAM uniquely suited for storing programmable parameters, such as pacing amplitude and diagnostic information.

Some pacemakers have used RAM to store software code as well as diagnostics. The use of RAM to store program code carries with it the potential risk that the code could be corrupted by external interference. This potential risk increases as memory density becomes greater with advances in digital fabrication technology. The minimum feature size used to manufacture digital circuits, including memory, continues to shrink to as small as 0.35 μM. The smaller feature size makes the circuits more susceptible to interference, such as interruptions in the power supply or interference from subatomic particle radiation from the atmosphere.

One of the important technologies available to help manage this risk is the use of error detection and error correction codes. Error detection codes are algorithms that can automatically detect if some event has caused a RAM location to be corrupted or changed. Error detection has been used in pacemakers for many years to ensure that data transmitted between the pacemaker and programmer during telemetry is intact. With increased memory density, these techniques will need to be incorporated into the use of RAM as well. The main technique used in error detection is the use of synthetic division, with the storage of the result in a different memory location. The division is performed using a number that results in a unique solution for each bit pattern being checked. Any result that is different from the stored result confirms an error in the memory. The same principles used for error detection can be extended to provide for error correction. Error correction routines can actually correct the memory location if an error is detected. This is accomplished with algorithms that have more complexity than those used for error detection only.

Error detection and error correction algorithms will become increasingly important as the size and density of memory continue to increase in pacemakers. These algorithms will allow more extensive use of RAM for program information as well as diagnostic storage, which will lead to the capability of pacemaker function to be changed or upgraded after implantation through the use of telemetry. This will someday provide for a functional upgrade years after implantation, with a new algorithm based on research completed during the years following the initial implantation.

Math Engine

The microprocessors used in most pacemakers are designed primarily to handle timing and control functions. Given the functional requirements of a modern pacemaker, this control architecture is ideal. As pacemaker complexity has expanded into the use of rate-adaptive algorithms and other more sophisticated features, however, the need for computational power has increased. The math engine augments the computational capability of the microprocessor by providing more complex math functions. This allows computations to be carried out by dedicated digital hardware, rather than by software code executed by the general-purpose hardware of the microprocessor. By using a math engine, several hundred lines of code that take several thousand clock cycles to execute can be replaced by a few lines of code that take only a dozen cycles to execute. This capability can dramatically reduce current drain.

As pacemaker complexity continues to increase with the use of more sophisticated sensors and automaticity, math engines will likely be replaced by *digital signal processors* (DSPs). DSPs are essentially microprocessors optimized for computational functions. Using a DSP, an engineer can change the computational function of an algorithm by modifying software, just as the engineer might change the control function with a microprocessor.

■ IMPLANTABLE CARDIOVERTER-DEFIBRILLATORS

The ICD was commercially introduced in 1985 after 3 years of clinical testing. The early devices were powered by a proprietary power source and fabricated without the modern microelectronics assembly technique of current implantable devices. Low-power analog functions were achieved with transistor arrays rather than custom integrated circuits, and logic functions were accomplished with surface-mounted complementary metal oxide semiconductor digital devices. High-power functions were achieved with discrete power transistors modified by hand to minimize their volume. Axial-lead resistors and capacitors were hand soldered on printed circuit boards. When the benefit of the implantable defibrillator was clinically accepted, the industry began to evolve rapidly, using advanced integrated circuit technology to reduce the size of these devices while enhancing their functionality.

A modern implantable defibrillator is an implanted computer that provides therapeutic options ranging from standard antibradycardia pacing to antitachycardia pacing and high-voltage defibrillation shocks. These devices store recordings of the intracardiac electrograms and collect extensive therapy history and diagnostic data files to aid the physician in individualizing device behavior for each patient. With a volume less than 50 cc and with more than 30 million transistors, these implantable devices draw about 15 μA (quiescent current) during years of constant monitoring of the cardiac status. Each device is hermetically sealed, biocompatible, able to survive an acceleration force of 500 Gs in all axes, and functional over a temperature range of −30°C to 60°C.

Evolution of the Implantable Defibrillator

The notion of an implantable defibrillator was conceived in the late 1960s by Mirowski[27] and reinforced later by Schuder.[28] Commercial development began in the basement of Sinai Hospital in Baltimore and was continued at Intec Systems in Pittsburgh in the mid-1970s. The defibrillator was first implanted in a human in February 1980.[29–32] The 1400 series defibrillators from Cardiac Pacemakers, Inc. (St. Paul, MN), were the first implantable defibrillators approved for widespread use by the U.S. Food and Drug Administration in 1985. An additional hardware-based, nonprogrammable version of the automatic implantable cardioverter-defibrillator was approved in 1986. These devices, the first using application-specific integrated circuits, became known as the first generation of devices.

A second generation of ICDs, which allowed the physician to program the therapy rate threshold noninvasively, instead of having to predetermine the appropriate rate threshold requirement before ordering the device from the manufacturer, was widely available in late 1988.[33] This second generation concluded with the addition of programmable shock therapy, available in 1991.

Devices available today are considered to be the third generation, combining a defibrillator to deliver high energy and a pacemaker to provide both antitachycardia and antibradycardia therapy.[34, 35] Other additions to the third-generation devices are more sophisticated algorithms for rhythm classification, storage of analog records of the patient's heart signals, and dual-chamber pacing.

System Components

Modern ICD systems contain three main system components: the ICD itself, the lead system, and the programmer recorder-monitor (PRM). The ICD is hermetically sealed in a biocompatible enclosure that houses the power source, sensing, defibrillation, pacing, and telemetric communications circuitry. The ICD lead system provides for the electrical connection between the ICD and the heart tissue. The PRM communicates with the implanted ICD and allows the physician to view status and diagnostic information and to modify the function and behavior of the device as necessary. This programming system is frequently the same as is used to program pacemaker products. Although each of these three constituent components of the system is crucial to appropriate system operation, the following discussion focuses on the implantable pulse generator.

Pulse Generator

The key design constraints of the modern implantable defibrillator are size and power.[36-44] Clinicians expect an ICD to be small enough for pectoral implantation. To reduce device size, circuitry must be contained in a compact space that is powered by a small battery. Functional requirements include the safe delivery of therapy on demand, a power supply system with a status indicator of the battery, and reliable monitoring of the heart rate. One of the challenges in the design of an implantable defibrillator is the large range of the voltages and currents being controlled in a very small physical package. The heart signal being monitored might be as small as 100 μV, whereas the therapeutic shocks approach 750 V with a leading edge current of 15 A and a pulse termination current spike of 210 A.

Safe delivery of therapy brings special problems to the designer of an implantable defibrillator. Because ICD batteries contain up to 20,000 J, a potential hazard exists if the charging and firing circuits were to "dump" all the energy either thermally or electrically to the patient in a brief time period. An implanted device might reach a temperature in excess of 85°C during a high-current state, such as a direct battery short or a component failure within the high-voltage circuit. Device designers may mitigate this thermal hazard by using both current and thermal fuses in the power supplies. The hazard of overapplication of therapy to a patient is partially mitigated by limiting the specific number of therapeutic shocks during any one episode (usually to a maximum five or six shocks per arrhythmia).

Although a device developed in the early 1990s required six or seven integrated circuits and two batteries, many current devices require as few as three integrated circuits and a single 3.2-V battery. Figure 7–13 shows the impressive progress in size reduction that has occurred in an extremely short time frame, during which functionality and longevity have both improved. To achieve an operating lifetime of about 5 years, the average current must be kept to about 15 μA for a single-cell, 3-V system. In a microprocessor-based device, these low average current drains can only be accomplished by minimizing the processor duty cycle. During charging for a high-voltage shock, this same cell must supply an average of 2 A for several seconds.

Major subsystems of dual-chamber, rate-responsive ICDs are shown in Figure 7–14. Functions of the various blocks that differ from an implantable pacemaker are described briefly here:

ROM: Sufficient nonvolatile memory is available for system start-up tasks and some program space. Program space requirements may be as large as 100 kilobytes in an ICD.

RAM: This memory is used for additional program space, storage of operating parameters, and storage of lead electrogram data. Storage of several minutes of electrograms from multiple lead sources requires a RAM of 128 to 512 kilobytes.

Battery: One or two cells with a high-power density are required. Lithium–silver vanadium oxide (SVO) batteries are the most widely used at present.

Low-voltage supply: This circuit supplies various current and voltage sources to the system. Digital circuits operate from 3-V or lower supplies. Separate voltage supplies are generated for pacing (about 5 V) and control of the charging circuits (10 to 15 V).

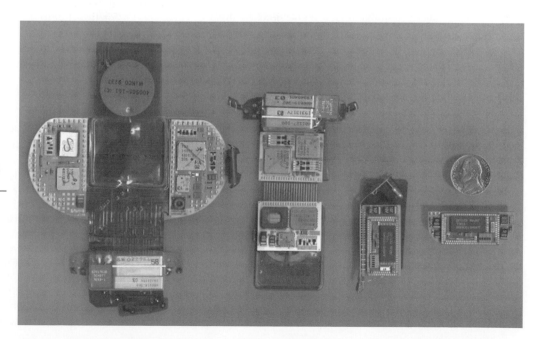

Figure 7–13. Size reduction in electronic defibrillator circuitry.

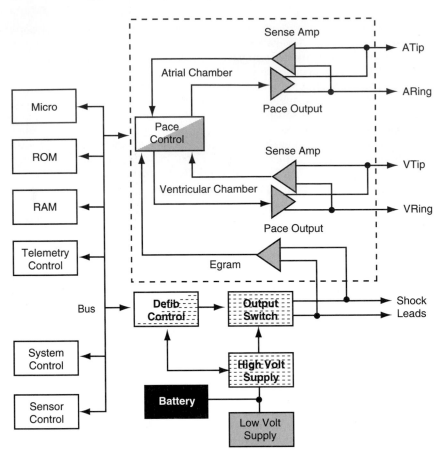

Figure 7–14. Block diagram of a dual-chamber rate-responsive implantable cardioverter-defibrillator.

High-voltage supply and output switch and defibrillation control: This circuit generates and controls the delivery of defibrillation energy.

Pacing control: Sense amplifiers are typically constructed using automatic gain controls. Sensitive input components must also be protected from the delivery of high-voltage defibrillation energies.

Within this general architecture, a wide range of design specifics may be employed. The ICD designer is faced with trade-offs between complexity and power consumption. A minimal system may employ simple interruptions to the microprocessor on each sensed cardiac event and require the microprocessor to determine the timing of all pacing impulses. In this manner, minimal overall circuitry is required, but the microprocessor must run several instructions for each cardiac event. Because the microprocessor system may need a few milliwatts of power when "awake," it is critical to its overall efficiency to keep it "asleep" as much as possible. Another approach is to integrate the pacing timing and control into support hardware, interrupting the microprocessor only when the heart rate exceeds a threshold, such as when an arrhythmia is suspected. Although it requires more support hardware, this design alternative requires far less intervention of the microprocessor, resulting in substantial power savings. Both alternatives have been employed successfully.

In general, when an algorithm is well defined and the circuitry to implement it can be contained on a single integrated circuit, it is advantageous to perform the function in

hardware. Newer or clinically unproved algorithms are best implemented under software control to maintain flexibility as late in the design as possible.

High-Power Circuits

Defibrillator high-power circuits convert the 3- to 6-V battery terminal voltage to the nearly 750 V necessary for a defibrillation pulse. The energy is stored in high-voltage capacitors for timed delivery and then finally is switched to deliver the high voltage to cardiac tissue, or to be discharged internally if the arrhythmia spontaneously terminates. These circuits are best understood by considering the major components: the battery; the DC-to-DC converter; the output storage capacitors; and the high-power output switches.

Battery

SVO is the dominant battery chemistry used in commercially available ICDs. Manganese dioxide (MnO_2) batteries have also been used by at least one ICD manufacturer. Some designs use a single cell producing about 3 V; others incorporate two cells in series to produce about 6 V. Unlike the 2.8-V lithium-iodine pacemaker cells, which develop high internal impedance as they discharge (up to 20,000 W over their useful life), SVO cells are characterized by low internal impedance (less than 1 W) over their useful life. The output voltage of SVO is higher than that of lithium-iodine, ranging from 3.2 V for a fresh cell to about 2.5 V when nearly depleted. The voltage discharge curve is unusual, having three distinct regions of roughly equal capacity (Fig. 7–15). Over the first region of the discharge curve, the voltage is

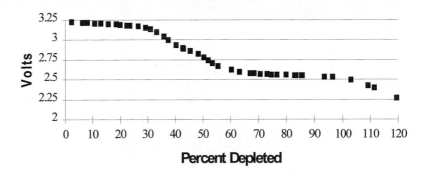

Figure 7–15. Cell voltage versus battery status.

relatively constant at 3.2 to 3.1 V. In the second region, the voltage falls from about 3.1 to 2.6 V. In the final region, the voltage is again relatively constant, falling from 2.6 to 2.5 V.

Although SVO cell chemistry has proved to be as reliable as the lithium-iodine technology used in pacemakers, there are a few idiosyncrasies that affect device design. The open circuit voltage (OCV) under a light load is a good indicator of remaining battery capacity, and there is little variation in OCV between SVO cells as a function of capacity delivered. This makes it tempting for the designer to use OCV exclusively to predict when device replacement is necessary, which would be a good plan if defibrillation therapy were not a factor. More important for the high-voltage circuit designer is the voltage under the heavy loads typical of DC-to-DC converter operation during charging. The battery terminal voltage under this load of several amperes is not well behaved, particularly during the last half of the useful life of the battery. When faced with the requirement of guaranteeing the time to charge for a defibrillation shock, the voltage under load is not the only important factor. Current products rely on a combination of charge time and OCV to predict when replacement is necessary. In defibrillator applications, the load on the battery varies from the continuous monitoring current (typically 15 μA), to the intermittent high-current demands of charging for a high-voltage defibrillation shock (up to 2 A for 10 to 15 seconds).

SVO cells combine the low self-discharge rate typical of pacemaker cells and the large effective electrode surface area typical of high-current delivery systems. An SVO cell meets the requirements for an implantable defibrillator but requires that high-current pulses be periodically drawn from the cell to maintain its characteristic low impedance. Perhaps the most significant peculiarity of SVO is a characteristic termed *voltage delay*. This has to do with the instantaneous resistance offered by the cell when switching from low- to high-current demands. Although dissipated quickly (a second or less in most applications), this transient impedance and the attendant droop in terminal voltage can surprise the unwary circuit designer who has made no allowance for the phenomenon. The effects of voltage delay are most pronounced at about the midlife point of the cell. Periodic high-current pulsing of the cell is the most effective way to minimize the effects of voltage delay, although making the circuitry tolerant of this aberrant behavior is clearly more energy efficient. Early defibrillators required that this periodic pulsing be accomplished manually by the physician during routine follow-up. Because the electrolytic capacitor used as storage elements for the high-current defibrillation pulse also require reforming periodically (to reform the oxide layer after significant periods of time absent applied voltage), the term *capform* has been applied to the need to exercise the charging circuitry periodically.

Modern defibrillators have automated this maintenance function by periodically charging and internally dumping the output capacitors. Of course, this comes at the expense of device longevity, with current products sacrificing about 1 to 3 weeks of longevity for each capform. During a period of 4 years, this consumes about 6 months worth of energy to maintain the cells and the capacitors.

DC-to-DC Converters

DC-to-DC converters are used in implantable defibrillators to convert the low voltage of the battery to the high voltages required for defibrillation. A number of unique issues confront the ICD designer:

- The sheer magnitude of the conversion from 3 to 750 V
- The intermittent nature of the charging operation
- The need to make the converter as small and lightweight as possible
- The high efficiency demanded
- The need to integrate the converter on a hybrid with circuitry that must sense intracardiac signals of 100 μV

The basic configuration, shown in Figure 7–16, includes a low-voltage, high-current switch (Q1) and fly-back transformer (T1), rectifying diode (D1), and capacitor storage elements (C2). Charging of the capacitors before a defibrillation shock requires closure of the low-voltage switch, causing a linear increase in primary current according to the following equation:

(5) $I = 1/L \int V dt$

The switch then opens, causing the energy stored in the fly-back transformer's magnetic field to be transferred to the secondary circuit. The energy stored in the transformer's magnetic field is proportional to the primary current squared. Diodes in the secondary circuit prevent current from flowing back into the secondary winding. In this way, the output storage capacitors are charged in small energy increments with each cycle until the desired voltage is reached. Roughly equal amounts of energy are delivered during each cycle and, because the energy stored in the capacitor is proportional to its voltage squared, the capacitor voltage pumps up as a function of the square root of elapsed time (Fig. 7–17).

Defibrillator DC-to-DC converters are operated at as high a frequency (typically, 30 to 60 kHz) as is practical to

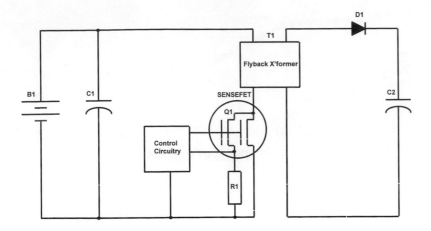

Figure 7–16. Functional diagram of a DC-to-DC converter.

facilitate the use of the smallest possible core. The design constraints are as follows: preventing core saturation, over-heating the core during the typical 10 to 15 seconds of operation, and hysteresis losses in the core itself. Efficiency rates on the order of 50% are typical when calculated as a percentage of the energy delivered to the heart versus the energy removed from the battery during charging. Primary currents average 2 A at a terminal voltage of 4 V (in a two-cell system), resulting in a 10-W converter. Considering a typical maximum energy charge (30 to 35 J) over a charging time of 8 seconds, this equates to 40 to 80 J of energy removed from the battery per charge.

Efficiencies are a function of the loaded battery terminal voltage and deteriorate gradually as the cell depletes. Peak primary currents can be 4 to 6 A and are supplied by a battery bypass capacitor (C1) with a capacitance in the range of 100 microfarads. The two basic designs used are the fixed-frequency design (mode B), which results in variable average primary current with battery terminal voltage, and the variable frequency design (mode A), which results in constant average primary current with battery voltage decay. The selection of charging circuit mode affects the time required to charge the output capacitors as the battery depletes as well as device longevity. In mode B operation, charge time is relatively constant over a wide range of battery voltages. Maintaining a constant charge time over the entire device lifetime, however, will result in reduced longevity. Mode A operation, on the other hand, results in a charge time that is inversely proportional to the battery

terminal voltage. Mode A implementations allow the designer to extract the maximum longevity from a battery, at the expense of increasing charge times as the battery is depleted.

Care must be taken to keep the resistance of all circuit connections to a minimum because even an additional 0.1 Ω in the primary circuit consumes 4 J of energy in a 10-second charge cycle. Minimizing the resistance of all circuit connections, wire bonds, die bonds, and circuit traces, while also minimizing crosstalk and high-voltage arcing in the secondary circuit, presents a formidable task for the hybrid circuit designer.

Capacitors

The storage capacitors are typically aluminum electrolytic because of the high volumetric efficiency and working voltage required. Most designs use at least two such capacitors in series to achieve a maximum of about 750 V for defibrillation. Although proven reliable in the implantable defibrillator application, the aluminum oxide on the surface of the anodal plate within the capacitor abates in the absence of applied voltage. As a result, aluminum electrolytic capacitors require periodic re-forming to minimize the leakage currents during charging. Although there remains some debate about the extent of the value of periodically reforming capacitors, the prevailing opinion is to provide some measure of periodic reformation to prevent leakage current from exceeding the capability of the DC-to-DC converter to charge the capacitors at low battery voltages. As mentioned earlier, the

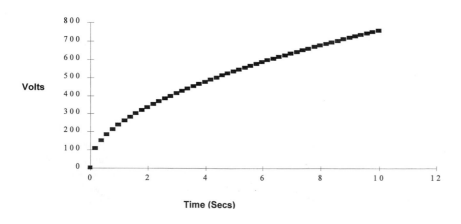

Figure 7–17. Charging profile of high-voltage capacitors in an implantable cardioverter-defibrillator system.

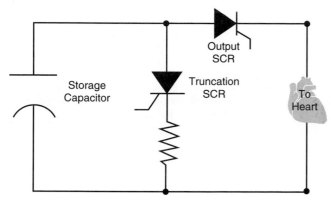

Figure 7–18. Simple monophasic output circuit (SCR).

periodic exercising of the charge circuitry is probably more important for operation of the battery than for the capacitors.

Output Switching

Defibrillation efficacy is affected by both the amplitude and pulse width of the defibrillation shock, and shocks of specific pulse widths are more effective in achieving defibrillation. Efficacy can be further improved by the delivery of a biphasic shock. Output switches have evolved from simple circuits employed in early models capable of delivering only monophasic pulses (SCR), to flexible output bridge circuitry capable of providing multiphasic output pulses. Because SCRs latch once they are triggered, to terminate a pulse, a truncation SCR is fired to clamp the output voltage to zero and reduce the current flow below the holding current required to keep the series SCR in the on state. A series resistor is included for limiting the current through the truncation SCR as shown in Figure 7–18.

To generate multiphasic output pulses, output bridge configurations (Fig. 7–19) with devices capable of turning on and off are required. SCRs are used in the monophasic devices, whereas *insulated gate bipolar transistors*, either alone or in conjunction with SCRs or Triacs, are used in the output bridge configurations capable of polarity switching. Because the load resistance associated with defibrillation is

in the range of 20 to 50 Ω, peak currents on the order of 40 A are common in output circuits.

To generate a conventional biphasic waveform, switches S1 and S4 are closed for either a predetermined time or until the output pulse reaches a predetermined voltage. During this phase, S2 and S3 must remain open. To follow phase one, switches S1 and S4 are opened, and S2 and S3 are closed. This second phase remains active until the completion of a certain time or until the output pulse reaches a predetermined voltage. All switches are then opened. Reversing the order of switch closure reverses the waveform polarity.

Timing of the output pulses is controlled by several methods, generally categorized as fixed-tilt or fixed-duration waveforms. With a fixed-tilt waveform, the output voltage is monitored during delivery, and the pulse is truncated or polarity reversed when a certain percentage of the initial voltage has been reached. For example, with 60% tilt, the output would be truncated or the polarity reversed when the voltage droops to 40% of the initial voltage (Fig. 7–20). This methodology delivers the selected energy independent of load impedance (Fig. 7–21). A fixed-duration waveform is generated by truncating or reversing polarity at a specific time. Apart from the basic configurations of monophasic and biphasic waveforms, there have been devices employing sequential pulse stimulation in a three-electrode system.

Sense Amplifiers

Proper sensing of electrical activity in the heart requires precise sensing and discrimination of each of the components that compose the intracardiac signal. An integrated or dedicated bipolar defibrillation lead in the right ventricular apex of the heart is the typical configuration of current ICD systems. These lead systems present the ICD with a signal that is composed of the near-field electrical events of ventricular depolarization and repolarization as well as the far-field effects of atrial depolarization and repolarization.

As discussed earlier, sensing ventricular electrical activity to determine heart rate in an implantable pacemaker is performed by using a comparator fixed to a given threshold and issuing a detection when that amplitude threshold is exceeded. Unfortunately, ventricular electrical activity may be polymorphic (varying in both amplitude and slew rate) in

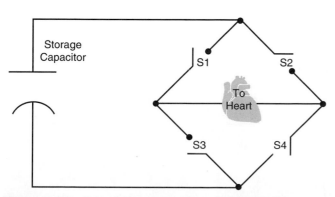

Figure 7–19. Output bridge circuit used to generate biphasic waveform.

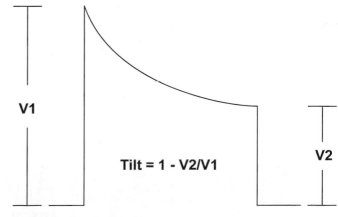

Figure 7–20. Definition of tilt.

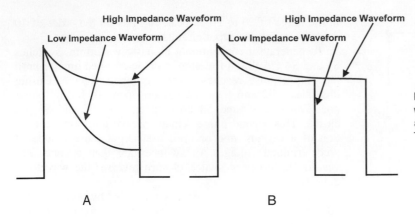

Figure 7–21. Fixed-duration *(A)* and fixed-tilt *(B)* waveforms. Effect of changing impedance on pulse duration and, as a consequence, energy content.

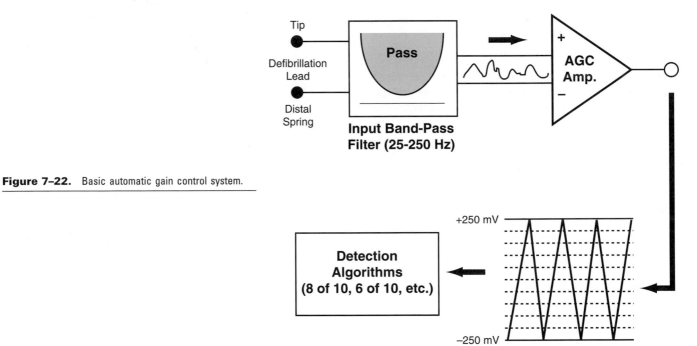

Figure 7–22. Basic automatic gain control system.

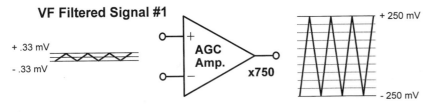

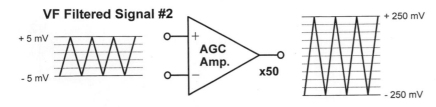

Figure 7–23. Analog automatic gain control operation.

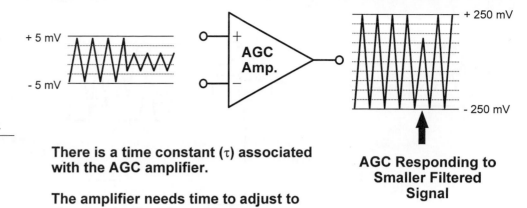

Figure 7–24. Automatic gain control operation and signal dropout.

There is a time constant (τ) associated with the AGC amplifier.

The amplifier needs time to adjust to changes to signal amplitudes.

AGC Responding to Smaller Filtered Signal

nature during tachyarrhythmia and fibrillation, and the amplitude of electrical activity may be an order of magnitude smaller than during normal sinus rhythm. Accordingly, a more robust sensing algorithm is required.

From an electrical standpoint, the sense amplifier must be able to operate properly over a rate range from 30 to 360 bpm or greater. Additionally, the amplifier must be able to respond quickly and accurately to the widely varying intracardiac signals presented during ventricular fibrillation. A number of sensing methods have been used to track these signals. An automatic gain control (AGC) and an AGC with a dynamic threshold are the only two techniques discussed here.

Sensing systems for defibrillators generally follow the basic configuration shown in Figure 7–22. Signals originating in the ventricles range from 100 μV to more than 20 mV and are amplified and filtered before being processed. After the preamplifier and filter, the signal enters the AGC amplifier, which processes the signal and feeds the processed signal to the computational circuitry for detection.

Early AGC implementations were primarily of the analog variety. An example of how these systems function is shown in Figure 7–23. The AGC amplifier normalizes the input signal and feeds the output to a fixed threshold comparator. In the top panel, the input signal post filtering is about 0.6 mV peak to peak, and the AGC amplifier automatically adjusts the gain to 750× to affect an output peak-to-peak voltage of 500 mV. In the lower panel, the input signal post filtering is about 10 mV peak to peak, and the AGC amplifier automatically adjusts the gain to 50× to normalize the output peak-to-peak voltage to the same 500 mV. This happens automatically without external intervention.

Figure 7–24 illustrates a more realistic situation. During fibrillation, the input signal to the endocardial lead is both time and frequency variant; hence, the magnitude of the output signal from the filter can vary widely. The AGC works to normalize the output by varying the gain and is generally successful. There is, however, a built-in time constant within the AGC that limits the rate at which the amplifier can respond to variations at the input. This time constant results in the occasional underamplification of some signals, which then go undetected. These undetected events are known as *dropout*.

The AGC time constant that caused undersensing in the

previous example is specifically added to the amplifier design to prevent oversensing. Figure 7–25 helps elucidate this apparent contradiction. Because the ventricular repolarization phase and ventricular fibrillation have similar frequency components, the designer cannot rely on filtering to distinguish between fibrillation and sinus rhythm. If the designer chooses an AGC time constant that aggressively follows the input signal (as shown by the *dashed line* labeled 3), the system will likely oversense the ventricular repolarization phase (T waves) during normal sinus rhythm. If the designer chooses an AGC time constant that is too conservative (as shown by the *dotted line* labeled 1), the device will likely undersense ventricular fibrillation, yet work extremely well during normal sinus rhythm. Therefore, the designer is forced to choose a time constant somewhere in the middle (as shown by the *solid line* labeled 2) that works reasonably well during normal sinus, but will unfortunately drop out occasionally during a wildly polymorphic rhythm. It is for this reason that all systems design some forgiveness into their detection algorithms. For example, if 8 of 10 or 12 of 16 intervals exceeded the ventricular rate detection criterion, an arrhythmia would be detected.

In some of the latest-generation ICD systems, digital

AGC Time Constant (τ)

● **Prevents T-wave oversensing**

✓ Filtering out T-waves also filters out VF because of common frequency components

✓ Proper value of τ is critically important

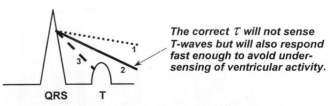

The correct τ will not sense T-waves but will also respond fast enough to avoid undersensing of ventricular activity.

Figure 7–25. Appropriate time constant selection is crucial in automatic gain control systems.

AGC amplifier keeps input to threshold detector within its operating range based on the maximum amplitude of the last 4 beats

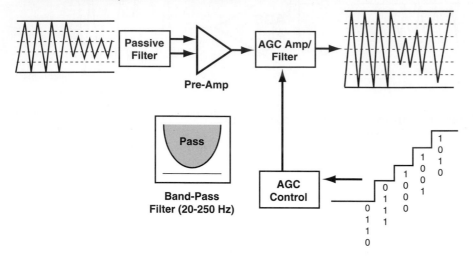

Figure 7–26. Digital automatic gain control system.

AGC designs have begun to appear. One example of such a design is shown in Figure 7–26. In this system, the system gain is slowly adjusted over time, such that the signal uses the maximum dynamic range of the sensing circuitry. If the signal being sensed drops suddenly in amplitude, as is common during fibrillation, the AGC increases the gain, so that the fibrillation signal continues to use the system's dynamic range. The fundamental difference between this newer design and prior designs is that the comparator threshold is dynamic and not fixed. This allows the computational circuitry to have complete control over the behavior of the system, allowing changing of system behavior dynamically. This performance attribute becomes particularly valuable to the rate-responsive ICD.

Choosing the right AGC time constant for a rate-responsive ICD can be difficult. Figure 7–27 shows a patient with both rates of 60 bpm and 120 bpm. If the AGC time constant optimized for rate 60 bpm is used when the patient's rate is being driven at 120 bpm, the pacemaker may undersense intrinsic activity and pace competitively in the face of varying amplitude intracardiac signals. If the AGC time constant optimized for rate 120 bpm is used when the patient's rate is being driven at 60 bpm, the pacemaker may oversense far-field atrial depolarizations (P waves) or ventricular repolarizations (T waves). Clearly, any one gain template is not appropriate for all rates. The digital AGC provides an opportunity for the ICD to have dozens of rate- and state-dependent templates, all controlled by the ICD dynamically.

Sensing circuitry is active throughout the entire life of an implantable defibrillator, and minimizing power consumption of these circuits has a significant and beneficial effect on device longevity. Typical sense amplifier current allowances for a 5-year device are less than 5 μA. In addition, the desired reduction of device sizes has strongly influenced the conversion from dual-cell to single-cell systems, resulting in typical system supply voltages of 2 to 3 V. For digital circuits operating at moderate speeds, these voltages are rarely a problem. On the other hand, analog circuits require some novel circuit design techniques.

Aside from accurately sensing R waves, which may have

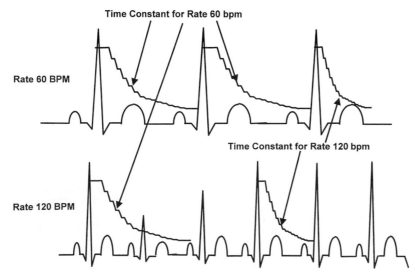

Figure 7–27. Rate-dependent templates. Improper match of automatic gain control template can result in both undersensing and oversensing.

amplitudes in the hundreds of microvolts range, the sense amplifier must be able to withstand defibrillation pulses from its own high-voltage output as well as external defibrillation. These defibrillation pulses, which may exceed 750 V, have rapid slew rates. Unless special precautions are taken in the design of the hybrid circuitry and integrated circuits, large in-rush currents will occur, resulting in latch-up conditions on the chip, system reset, system runaway, or permanent damage to the components.

■ FUTURE DIRECTIONS

Predicting the future of implantable technology is difficult at best; however, a few points regarding future directions are worth noting. The trend for increased device complexity will continue for both pacemakers and defibrillators. Combinations of adaptive-rate sensors will likely improve the performance of rate-responsive systems. Research will continue to identify more physiologically appropriate sensors. An example of this research is the development of a sensor that automatically determines the optimal maximum sensor rate for the patient at a given moment of time and level of exercise. This sensor will replace the need for physicians to program a maximum sensor rate based on nonspecific factors, such as age, gender, or lifestyle. Other important improvements will include increases in the pacemaker's ability to perform functions automatically, such as setting the sensitivity level and the pacing amplitude. Such automatic features will make implanted devices easier to use and less time-consuming for the clinician to follow. Improvements in diagnostic capability, such as automatic lead impedance trends, will aid in troubleshooting. Advances in diagnostics will expand into information that will assist in determining changes in the patient's physiology. For example, the use of minute ventilation sensors may identify progression of conditions such as congestive heart failure.

Advances in implantable defibrillators will focus on continued size reduction. In addition, advanced pacemaker features, such as adaptive-rate sensors, will continue to be incorporated into defibrillators. Research into pacing therapy for congestive heart failure represents a major opportunity in the coming years. This research will intensify the focus on sensors, lead technologies, and advanced algorithms.

All of the advances noted will need to be paralleled by continued advances in integrated circuit and component technologies. Smaller integrated circuit geometry will allow these new advances to be incorporated into devices while maintaining size and longevity. Research into new capacitor technologies for defibrillators will continue to be important. The capacitors in the current-generation ICDs require roughly 30% of the total device volume. New capacitor technologies, as well as advances in the high-power-density batteries, will be key to further size reduction.

REFERENCES

1. Sermasi S, Marconi M, Libero L, et al: Italian experience with Auto-Capture in conjunction with a membrane lead. Pacesetter Automatic Control of Energy and Membrane Automatic Threshold Evaluation (Pacemate) Study Group. PACE 19:1799–804, 1996.
2. Levine PA, Brodsky SJ: Fusion, pseudofusion, pseudopseudofusion, and confusion. Clin Prog Pacing Electrophysiol 1:70, 1983.
3. Irnich W: Intracardiac electrograms and sensing test signals: Electrophysiological, physical, and technical considerations. PACE 8:870, 1985.
4. Frohlig G, Schwendt H, Schieffer H, Bette L: Atrial signal variations and pacemaker malsensing during exercise: A study in the time and frequency domain. J Am Coll Cardiol 11:806, 1988.
5. Klitzner TS, Stevenson WG: Effects of filtering on right ventricular electrograms recorded from endocardial catheters in humans. PACE 13:69, 1990.
6. Steinhaus DM, Foley L, Knoll K, Markowitz T: Atrial sensing revisited: Do bandpass filters matter? PACE 16:946, 1993.
7. Fischler H: Polarization properties of small-surface-area pacemaker electrodes: Implications on reliability of sensing and pacing. PACE 2:403, 1979.
8. De Buitleir M, Kou WH, Schmaltz S, et al: Acute changes in pacing threshold and R- or P-wave amplitude during permanent pacemaker implantation. Am J Cardiol 65:999, 1990.
9. Schalhorn R, Markowitz T: Bipolar dual-chamber pacemakers: Is myopotential sensing still a problem? PACE 11:852, 1988.
10. Fetter J, Hall DM, Hoff GL, Reeder JT: The effect of myopotential interference on unipolar and bipolar dual-chamber pacemakers in the DDD mode. Clin Prog Electrophysiol Pacing 3:368, 1985.
11. Fetter J, Bobeldyk GL, Engman FJ: The clinical incidence and significance of myopotential sensing with unipolar pacemakers. PACE 7:871, 1984.
12. Lau CP, Linker NJ, Butrous GS, et al: Myopotential interference in unipolar rate-responsive pacemakers. PACE 12:1324, 1989.
13. Kleinert M, Elmqvist H, Strandberg H: Spectral properties of atrial and ventricular endocardial signals. PACE 2:11, 1979.
14. Brandt J, Fahraeus T, Schuller H: Farfield QRS complex sensing via the atrial pacemaker lead. II. Prevalence, clinical significance, and possibility of intraoperative prediction in DDD pacing. PACE 11:1546, 1988.
15. Hauser RG, Susmano A: Afterpotential oversensing by a programmable pulse generator. PACE 4:391, 1981.
16. Hayes DL, Wang PJ, Reynolds DW, et al: Interference with cardiac pacemakers by cellular telephones. N Engl J Med 336:1473–1479, 1997.
17. Joyner KH, Anderson V, Wood MP: Interference and energy deposition rates from digital mobile phones. *In* Frederick MD: Bioelectromagnetics 16th Annual Meeting Abstract Book. Frederick, Bioelectromagnetic Society, 1994, pp 67–68.
18. Hayes DL, VonFeldt L, Neubauer S, et al: Effect of digital cellular phones on permanent pacemakers [Abstract]. PACE 18(Pt II):863, 1995.
19. Hayes DL, VonFeldt LK, Neubauer SA, et al: Does cellular phone technology cause pacemaker or defibrillator interference? [Abstract] PACE 18(Pt II):842, 1995.
20. Carillo R, Saunkeah B, Pickels M, et al: Preliminary observations on cellular telephones and pacemakers [Abstract]. PACE 18(Pt II):863, 1995.
21. Carillo R, Saunkeah B, Traad E, et al: At what distance do cellular telephones interfere with pacemakers? [Abstract] PACE 18(Pt II):1777, 1995.
22. Ruggera PS, Witters DM, Bassen HI: In vitro testing of pacemakers for RF interference at fixed distances from U.S. type digital cellular phones [Poster]. Presented at the Annual Electromagnetic Compatibility Forum, Washington, DC, September 11, 1996.
23. Denny HW, Jenkins BM: EMC history of cardiac pacemakers. EMC Test Design 4:33–36, 1993.
24. Ziegler JF, Lanford WA: The effect of sea level cosmic rays on electronic devices. J Appl Physiol 52(6):4305–4312, 1981.
25. Gossett CA, Hughlock BW, Katoozi M, LaRue GS: Single event phenomena in atmospheric neutron environments. IEEE Trans Nucl Sci 40:1845–1852, 1993.
26. Castro A, Liebold A, Vincente J, et al: Evaluation of autosensing as an automatic means of maintaining a 2:1 sensing safety margin in an implanted pacemaker. Autosensing Investigation Team. PACE 19:1708–1713, 1996.
27. Mirowski M: Standby automatic defibrillator. Arch Intern Med 126:158, 1970.
28. Schuder JC, Stoeckie H, Gold JH, et al: Experimental ventricular defibrillation with an automatic and completely implanted system. Trans Am Soc Artif Int Organs 16:207, 1970.
29. Mower MM, Reid PR, Watkins L Jr, et al: Automatic implantable cardioverter defibrillator structural characteristics. PACE 7:1331–1337, 1984.
30. Thomas AC, Moser SA, Smutka ML, et al: Implantable defibrillation: Eight years of clinical experience. PACE 11:2053–2056, 1988.

31. Mirowski M, Reid PR, Mower MM, et al: Clinical performance of the implantable cardioverter-defibrillator. PACE 7:1345, 1984.

32. Mirowski M: Termination of malignant ventricular arrhythmias with an implanted automatic defibrillator in human beings. N Engl J Med 303:322, 1980.

33. Winkle RA, Mead H, Ruder MA, et al: Long-term outcome with the automatic implantable cardioverter-defibrillator. J Am Coll Cardiol 13:1353, 1989.

34. Winkle RA: The implantable defibrillator: Progression from first to third generation devices. *In* Zipes DP, Jaliffe J (eds): *Cardiac Electrophysiology: From Cell to Bedside.* Philadelphia, WB Saunders, 1990, p 963.

35. Mitchell JD, Lee R, Garan H, et al: Experience with an implantable tiered therapy device incorporating antitachycardia pacing and cardioverter/defibrillator therapy. J Thorac Cardiovasc Surg 105:453, 1993.

36. Horning RJ, Rhoback FW: New high rate lithium/vanadium pentoxide cell for implantable medical devices. Progress in Batteries & Solar Cells 4:97, 1982.

37. Takeuchi ES: Batteries for implantable defibrillators. Proceedings of the 3rd Annual Battery Conference on Applications and Advances, Section VI-3. Long Beach, CA, California State University, 1988.

38. Hnatec ER: Design of Solid-State Power Supplies, 2nd ed. New York, Van Nostrand Reinhold, 1981.

39. Schuder JC, Stoeckle H, West JA, et al: Transthoracic ventricular defibrillation in the dog with truncated and untruncated exponential stimuli. IEEE Trans Bio Med Eng 18:410–415, 1971.

40. Bach S: Engineering Aspects of Implantable Defibrillators: Electrical Therapy for Cardiac Arrhythmias. Philadelphia, WB Saunders, 1990.

41. Vittoz E: Micropower Techniques: Design of MIS VLSI Circuits for Telecommunications. New York, Prentice-Hall, 1985.

42. Gregorian R, Temes GC: Analog MOS Integrated Circuits for Signal Processing. New York, John Wiley & Sons, 1986.

43. Unbehauen R, Cichocki A: MOS Switched-Capacitor and Continuous Time Integrated Circuits and Systems. New York, Springer-Verlag, 1989.

44. Toumazou C, Hughes JB, Battersby NC (eds): Switched-Currents: An Analog Technique for Digital Technology. London, Peter Peregrinus, 1993.

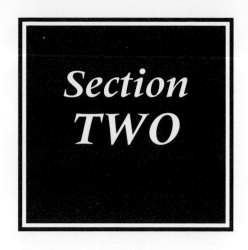

Section TWO

Artificial Sensors for Pacing, Defibrillators, and Hemodynamics

An Overview of Sensors: Ideal Characteristics, Sensor Combination, and Automaticity

Sum-Kin Leung, Chu-Pak Lau, and A. John Camm

The aims of physiologic pacing are to restore the rate and sequence of cardiac activation in the presence of abnormal cardiac automaticity and conduction. The atrial electrogram can be used for rate control when sinoatrial function is adequate. On the other hand, a high proportion of pacemaker recipients either have established or progressively develop abnormal sinoatrial function, occurring not only at rest but also during exercise. Such chronotropic incompetence commonly occurs as a result of medications or in association with intrinsically abnormal sinus node function. In addition, in patients whose right atrium is unreliable for sensing or pacing (such as during atrial fibrillation), an alternative means to simulate sinus node responsiveness is required.

These problems with the pacemaker function of the sinus node prompted the development of artificial implantable sensors for cardiac pacing. Although the optimal rate adaptation in a pacemaker recipient may be different from that of a healthy subject, it is assumed that these sensors should mimic the behavior of the healthy sinus node response to exercise and nonexercise needs. In addition, atrioventricular (AV) conduction is normally under the control of the autonomic nervous system, and a sensor may also contribute to adapting the AV interval to changes in atrial rate. The role of sensors has also been expanded to include functions other than rate augmentation—such as, for example, the detection of ventricular capture and the management of response to atrial arrhythmias.

In this chapter, the ability of sensors available for clinical and investigational purposes to match the ideal sinus node behavior is reviewed. The use of sensor combinations to overcome some of the shortcomings of a single artificial sensor is addressed. Finally, a sensor can be ideal only if correctly programmed and if capable of changing automatically according to changes in the patient's clinical or physical status.

■ HISTORICAL LANDMARKS OF RATE-ADAPTIVE PACING

The limitations of dual-chamber pacing in the setting of sinoatrial dysfunction led to the development of nonatrial sensors. This development was possible because of the recognition that during exercise an increase in heart rate, rather than the maintenance of AV synchrony, is the main determinant of increases in cardiac output.[1] Thus, in a single-chamber rate-adaptive pacemaker that varies the pacing rate with exercise according to a nonatrial sensor, near-normal exercise physiology in patients with bradycardia can be achieved.

Cammilli and associates[2, 3] implanted the first rate-variable single-chamber pacemaker, which sensed changes in blood pH during exercise. In 1981, a "physiologically adaptive" cardiac pacemaker responding to changes in the QT interval during exercise was described by Rickards and colleagues.[4] In the same year, Wirtzfeld and coworkers[5] reported the use of central venous oxygen saturation ($S\bar{v}O_2$) for the control of automatic rate-responsive pacing. Despite the fact that respiratory changes during exercise were proposed as a physiologic parameter to be sensed by a rate-adaptive pacemaker as early as 1975,[6] a rate-adaptive pacemaker that detected the respiratory rate was introduced by Rossi and colleagues[7] only in 1982. With continuing research, the number of sensors available for rate-adaptive pacing steadily increased. In particular, activity[8] and minute ventilation sensors[9, 10] have been used as sensors with extensive clinical application.

Although single-chamber ventricular rate-adaptive pacing was originally meant to replace dual-chamber pacing, the additional benefits of atrial sensing and pacing became well recognized. Thus, dual-chamber rate-adaptive pacing became available as early as 1986.[11] Since then, virtually all pacemaker companies have introduced their own versions of rate-adaptive dual-chamber devices. Technical improvement in the sensing of atrial electrograms with "floating" diagonally opposed atrial electrodes or closely spaced rings has enabled the use of a single-pass lead for VDD pacing. When combined with a rate-adaptive sensor, VDDR pacing with a single-pass lead has become a possibility.[12]

With the proliferation of sensor technology, it soon became apparent that none of the sensors could simulate the normal sinus node function in all aspects,[13] although different sensors were better in some areas of performance. Thus, it is logical to combine sensors for optimal rate adaptation. Although this idea is not new, investigational units only became available in 1988,[14] in the form of combining activity and QT interval sensing, and later activity and minute ventilation sensors.[15] The increasing sophistication of sensors and their combinations prompted the use of automatic sensor calibration for optimal programming.[16–18]

The increasing importance of rate-adaptive pacing in recent years and increasing pacemaker sophistication have led to the joint effort between the North American Society of Pacing and Electrophysiology Mode Code Committee and the British Pacing and Electrophysiology Group to revise the five-letter pacing code that was originally modified from the three-letter code for pacemaker mode proposed in 1974.[19–21] In this new code, the rate-adaptive function is denoted by the use of the letter *R* in the fourth position.

■ NORMAL HEART RATE AND RESPIRATORY RESPONSES TO EXERCISE AND NONEXERCISE NEEDS

Cardiac output is the product of heart rate and stroke volume. Stroke volume is enhanced during exercise when venous return increases cardiac filling, and cardiac contractility is augmented in response to sympathetic stimulation and a more vigorous pumping action of the skeletal muscles. Because of the difference in venous return, the changes in heart rate and cardiac hemodynamics are highly influenced by whether the exercise was carried out in the upright or supine posture.

Normal Heart Rate Response During Exercise

An anticipatory response of the heart rate occurs in many patients before exercise. With both supine and upright isotonic exercise, heart rate and cardiac output increase within 10 seconds of the onset of exercise.[22–24] This initial increase in heart rate is mediated by parasympathetic withdrawal rather than by sympathetic stimulation. The cardiac output may increase by as much as 40% within three heart beats after the onset of vigorous muscular exercise. Both cardiac output and sinus rate increase exponentially, with a half-time that ranges from 10 to 45 seconds (Fig. 8–1A), the rate of rise being proportional to the intensity of work[22] (see Fig.

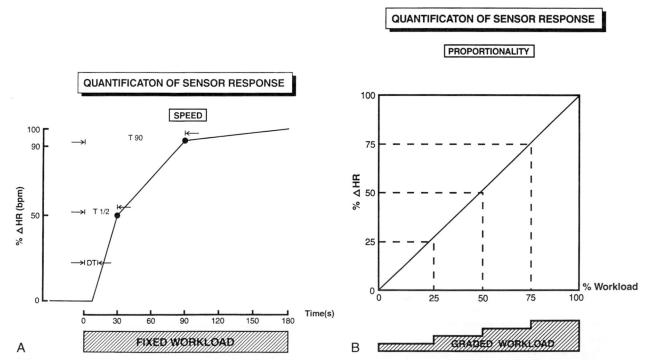

Figure 8–1. *A,* The speed of heart rate (HR) changes at the onset of exercise. The normal sinus rate responds almost immediately; half of the change is achieved in less than 30 seconds, and most of the change is achieved within 1 minute. This speed of response was quantified by the response times (DT, delay time; T½ and T90, times needed to reach 50% and 90% of maximum heart rate, respectively). *B,* Relationship between exercise workload and the heart rate increase during incremental exercise. The change in heart rate expressed as a percentage of the maximum increase in heart rate (%Δ HR) and the workload expressed as a percentage of the maximum work load (%Δ workload) at each quartile of exercise. The %Δ HR is linearly related to %Δ workload, with a slope that is nearly 1.

8–1*B*). At the termination of upright exercise, there is a delay of about 5 to 10 seconds before cardiac output starts to decrease, followed by an exponential fall with a half-time of 25 to 60 seconds. The recovery time is related to age, work intensity, total work performed, and physical condition of the patient.[25] Although the optimal rate onset and decay kinetics for patients with pacemakers have not been firmly established, artificial sensors for rate-adaptive pacing should probably simulate the onset and recovery kinetics of the normal sinus node as the ideal physiologic standard.

Respiratory Changes During Exercise

The change in heart rate during muscular exercise is linearly related to oxygen consumption and workload. Because of the relationship between oxygen uptake and ventilatory volume during aerobic metabolism, minute ventilation is closely related to heart rate during exercise. At rest, the respiratory rate is typically between 10 and 20 breaths/min. During low-intensity exercise, an increase in tidal volume is the primary respiratory adaptation.[26] At higher work levels, a further increase in tidal volume of up to 50% of the vital capacity occurs together with an increase in breathing frequency. The relationship between breathing rate and tidal volume varies considerably between individuals. In addition, the breathing rate is often synchronized with the work rhythm—for example, the walking pace. However, because respiration is carefully controlled to maintain the concentration of arterial carbon dioxide within a narrow physiologic range, compensatory adjustments in tidal volume ensure an appropriate minute ventilation and gas exchange.

Minute ventilation (the product of breathing rate and tidal volume) is linearly related to the rate of carbon dioxide production. At low- and medium-intensity workloads, minute ventilation is also linearly related to oxygen consumption during incremental exercise. Resting values for minute ventilation are about 6 L/min and can increase to 100 L/min during exercise for normal men and up to 200 L/min for trained athletes. Tidal volume may rise from a resting value of 0.5 L/min to 3 L/min at maximal exercise in normal individuals. The breathing rate may increase from a resting value of 12 to 16 breaths/min to 40 to 50 breaths/min during peak exercise. In normal children and some adults with restrictive lung disease, the respiratory rate may exceed 60 breaths/min.

At about 70% of the maximum oxygen uptake, the rate of tissue metabolism outstrips the rate of tissue oxygen delivery. Anaerobic metabolism of carbohydrate, fat, and protein is accelerated, resulting in an accumulation of lactic acid, the so-called anaerobic threshold. Acidosis is initially prevented by plasma buffers, but continuous lactate production eventually leads to excess production of carbon dioxide from plasma bicarbonate. This excess carbon dioxide stimulates the respiratory center, leading to respiratory compensation (increased minute ventilation). Hence, carbon dioxide production and minute ventilation increase in a manner that is disproportionate to the increase in oxygen consumption at workloads that surpass the anaerobic threshold. The anaerobic threshold is defined more clearly using a protocol in which the work intensity is increased more rapidly than with a more gradual exercise protocol.

It has been customary to use the heart rate–minute ventila-

tion slope as a measure of the appropriateness of rate adaptation by an artifical sensor, with the regression line at 1 to 2 bpm/L. In addition, this slope is said to be relatively independent of the functional class or the degree of left ventricular dysfunction.[27] At workloads that surpass the anaerobic threshold, however, oxygen consumption asymptotically reaches its maximum value, whereas carbon dioxide production and minute ventilation increase disproportionately to oxygen consumption. Because of the disproportionate increase in minute ventilation above the anaerobic threshold, the heart rate–minute ventilation slope is reduced when the anaerobic threshold is exceeded. The reduction in the heart rate–minute ventilation slope above compared with below the anaerobic threshold is an average of 29% for women and 26% for men.[28] This may be important both in assessment of rate adaptation and in the design of the minute ventilation–sensing algorithms.

Oxygen Uptake Kinetics

In healthy subjects, exercise-induced cardiac and respiratory changes occur simultaneously to provide blood flow commensurate with the increase in oxygen consumption in the skeletal muscles. Figure 8–2 shows the oxygen uptake curve during constant workload exercise. When exercise begins, oxygen uptake increases gradually, following an exponential time course because of the slow adjustment of respiration and circulation, until reaching a steady state when oxygen uptake corresponds to the demands of the tissues. Because oxygen uptake does not reach the required steady state immediately, the inadequate supply of energy from aerobic sources during the first 2 to 3 minutes must be met largely by use of creatine phosphate high-energy stores.[29] This inadequacy of oxygen use at the onset of exercise is described as the *oxygen deficit*. When exercise stops, replenishment of energy stores requires oxygen consumption in excess of the baseline recovery conditions before the oxygen uptake gradually decreases to the resting level. This elevated postexercise oxygen uptake repaid the initial deficit and was described as repaying the "oxygen debt."[30]

The oxygen debt includes a fast alactic phase during moderate exercise. Hence, the magnitude of the oxygen deficit is generally found to be about equivalent to that of the oxygen debt in submaximal exercise before the anaerobic threshold is reached.[31] If the level of exertion remains relatively modest, the oxygen deficit may be paid back during exercise, so that the debt measured after exercise is actually less than the deficit at the onset. In contrast, during more strenuous exercise, it has both a fast alactic and a slower lactic phase, and the oxygen debt exceeds the size of the deficit.[32] The rate-limiting step for the increase in oxygen uptake at the onset of exercise is the rate of oxygen transport and is primarily a cardiac function dependent on the change in the pulmonary blood flow.[33-34] Hence, an appropriate rate response behavior is the best way to ensure optimal oxygen delivery both at submaximal and maximal exercise. Because the oxygen debt may require a long period of time for repayment and may be affected by postexercise oxygen consumption for processes other than the simple deficit repayment,[35] and because of variability of the recovery baseline oxygen consumption,[36] the oxygen deficit is used to assess the contribution of rate response on oxygen transport.

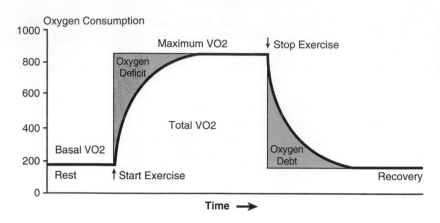

Figure 8–2. Oxygen kinetics during a steady-state exercise test. An oxygen deficit is incurred as the subject increases oxygen consumption (VO₂) to the steady state, which generally takes 3 to 5 minutes. The incurred deficit is repaid at the termination of exercise as the oxygen debt. The oxygen deficit is closely related to the alactic oxygen debt; hence, the oxygen debt, which includes the fast alactic and the slower lactic oxygen debt, is a better measurement of oxygen kinetics. (From Leung SK, Lau CP, Wu CW, et al: Quantitative comparison of rate response and oxygen uptake kinetics between different sensor modes in multisensor rate adaptive pacing. PACE 17:1920–1927, 1994).

By artificially increasing the rate response of a sensor beyond that expected of the sinus node, it has been shown that oxygen deficit is reduced compared to optimal sensor setting. The dependence on a quick initial response to minimize oxygen debt has been demonstrated in recent studies of minute ventilation and activity and dP/dt sensors,[37, 38] and oxygen uptake kinetics is often used as a sensitive indicator of appropriate rate-adaptive response at the submaximal workload.

Heart Rate Modulation for Nonexercise Needs

Exercise is but one of the many physiologic requirements for variation in heart rate (Table 8–1). Emotions such as anxiety may trigger a substantial change in heart rate. The sinus rate is higher when a person moves from the supine to the upright posture, and cardiac output decreases. Isometric exercise also results in an increase in cardiac output and heart rate in most people.[39] The changes in heart rate that occur during various physiologic maneuvers (e.g., Valsalva maneuver), baroreceptor reflexes, and anxiety reaction may also be potentially important. An appropriate compensatory heart rate response is especially important in pathophysiologic conditions such as anemia, acute blood loss, or other causes of hypovolemia.

Many physiologic processes demonstrate a rhythmic variation during the day. The normal resting heart rate peaks during the day and reaches a trough in the early morning hours during sleep. A sensor that is responsive only to exercise will increase the pacing rate during periods of physiologic stress, but the lower rate remains fixed at the programmed base rate. This faster programmed lower rate, which is normal for the day, may be too rapid during periods of rest. The lack of an ability to decrease the pacing rate in patients with VVI pacemakers during sleep may result in

palpitations and sleep disturbances.[40] By means of sensors that are always active in monitoring the level of metabolic demand, the appropriate lower rate can be calculated and adapted to individual need (see later). Heart rate increases during febrile episodes may be detected by a sensor that measures the central venous temperature.[41]

■ COMPONENTS OF A RATE-ADAPTIVE PACING SYSTEM

At least three aspects of a rate-adaptive pacing system influence its rate-modulating characteristics. First, a sensor (or a combination of sensors) must detect a physical or physiologic parameter that is related to metabolic demand either directly or indirectly. Each of the parameters used for control of pacing rate has its own intrinsic relation to exercise. Second, the rate-modulating circuit in the pulse generator must have an algorithm that relates changes in the sensed parameter to a change in pacing rate. The design of the rate-control algorithm may have a profound impact on the overall rate-response characteristics of a pacing system. Third, because the magnitude of the physical or physiologic changes that are monitored by a sensor differs between patients, physician input is usually necessary to adjust the "algorithm" (generally by programming one or more rate-responsive variables) to achieve the clinically desired rate response.[42]

Classification of Sensors
Physiologic Classification

One classification of sensors for rate-adaptive pacing is according to the physiologic "level" they sense.[43] A *primary* sensor is defined as one that detects the *physiologic factors* that control the normal sinus node during varying metabolic needs. Primary sensed parameters include circulating catecholamines and autonomic nervous system activities. Apparently, these parameters may be the most physiologically accurate indicators for use by a rate-adaptive pacing system. Actually, this system is inadequate because the sinus node is controlled simultaneously by many primary sensed parameters. Also, technical realization of a rate-adaptive pacemaker using a primary sensor has yet to be achieved. The bulk of rate-adaptive sensors that have been proposed belong to the class of *secondary* sensors, that is, those that detect physiologic parameters that are a *consequence* of exercise.

Table 8–1. Some Responses of the Sinus Node to Body Requirements

1. Exercise—isotonic and isometric, during and after exercise
2. Postural changes
3. Anxiety and stress
4. Postprandial changes
5. Vagal maneuvers
6. Circadian changes
7. Fever

Some of these parameters, such as the QT interval,[4] respiratory rate or minute ventilation,[9, 10, 44–46] average atrial rate,[47] central venous temperature,[41, 48, 49] venous blood pH,[2, 3] right ventricular stroke volume,[50] pre-ejection interval[51] or pressure,[52] $S\bar{v}O_2$,[5, 53] and ventricular inotropic indices (ventricular inotropic parameter[54, 55] and peak endocardial acceleration[56, 57]) have been developed for either clinical or investigational pacing systems. Each of these physiologic variables responds to the onset of exercise with its own kinetics and has a different proportionality to exercise workload. A third group of sensors, the *tertiary* sensors, detect *external changes* that result from exercise. An example of a tertiary sensor is body movement.[58] As expected, the relationship between exercise workload and these tertiary variables is less tightly linked, and there is often greater susceptibility to environmental influences, such as vibration. Other measures, such as the use of a 24-hour clock to vary the lower pacing rate, can be considered tertiary sensors. Likewise, in the most primitive rate-adaptive pacemaker, the pacing rate was changed by the patient using a hand-held programmer before beginning exercise.[59]

Technical Classification

Although conceptually attractive, the physiologic classification does not adequately separate the bulk of the so-called secondary sensors. A more practical classification is to categorize sensors according to the technical methods that are used to measure the sensed parameter (Table 8–2). During isotonic exercise, body movements (especially those produced by heel strike during walking) result in changes in acceleration forces that are transmitted to the pacemaker. Sensors that are capable of measuring the acceleration or vibration forces in the pulse generator are broadly referred to as activity sensors. The sensing of *body vibrations* is therefore a simple way to indicate the onset of exercise. Technically, detection of body movement can be achieved using a piezoelectric crystal, an accelerometer, a tilt switch, or an inductive sensor. Each of these devices transduces motion of the sensor either directly into voltage or indirectly into measurable changes in the electrical resistance of a piezoresistive crystal. Although a tertiary sensor, activity sensing is the most widely used control parameter in rate-adaptive pacing because of its ease of implementation and its compatibility with standard unipolar and bipolar pacing leads.

Impedance is a measure of all factors that oppose the flow of electric current and is derived by measuring resistivity to an injected electric current across a tissue. The impedance principle has been used extensively for measuring respiratory

Table 8–2. Major Classes of Sensors Used in Rate-Responsive Pacing, Classified According to Method of Technical Realization

Methods	Physiologic Parameters	Examples	
		Models	*Manufacturers**
Vibration sensing	Body movement	Activitrax, Legend, Thera, DX2, Kappa	Medtronic Inc.
		Sensolog, Sensorhythm, Trilogy	Pacesetter
		Relay, Dash, Marathon	Intermedics
		Excel	CPI
		Ergos	Biotronik
		Swing	Sorin
Impedance sensing	Respiratory rate	Biorate	Biotec
	Minute ventilation	Meta, Tempo	Telectronics
		Chorus RM	ELA Medical
		Legend Plus, DX2, Kappa	Medtronic Inc.
	Stroke volume, pre-ejection period, right ventricular ejection time	Precept	CPI
	Ventricular inotropic parameter	Diplos, Inos²	Biotronik
Ventricular evoked response	Evoked QT interval	TX, Quintech, Rhythmx	Vitatron
	Evoked R-wave area ("gradient")	Prism CL	Telectronics
Special sensors on pacing electrode	**Physical Parameters**		
	1. Central venous temperature	Kelvin 500	Cook Pacemakers
		Nova MR	Intermedics
		Thermos	Biotronik
	2. dP/dt	Deltatrax, Model 2503	Medtronic Inc.
	3. Right atrial pressure		
	4. Pulmonary arterial pressure		
	5. Peak endocardial acceleration	Best of living	Sorin
	Chemical Parameters		
	1. pH		
	2. Mixed venous oxygen saturation	OxyElite, OxyPace	Medtronic Inc.
			Siemens
	3. Catecholamine levels		

Manufacturers and their locations: Biotec, S.P.A., Bologna, Italy; Biotronik, GmbH & Co., Berlin, Germany; Cardiac Pacemakers Inc., St. Paul, MN; Cook Pacemakers Corporation, Leechburg, PA; ELA Medical, Rougemont, France; Intermedics Inc., Angleton, TX; Medtronic Inc., Minneapolis, MN; Siemens Pacesetter Ltd., Solna, Sweden; Sorin Biomedica, Saluggia, Italy; Telectronics Pacing Systems, Englewood, CO; Vitatron, Dieren, the Netherlands.

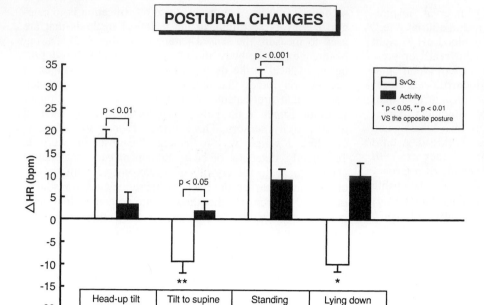

Figure 8–3. Feasibility of S$\bar{v}$O$_2$ and activity sensors to detect postural change. The S$\bar{v}$O$_2$ showed an increase in rate on upright posture (both passively or actively performed) over the rates during supine posture. An indiscriminate increase in rate was observed with the activity sensor, especially during active postural changes. (From Lau CP, Tai YT, Leung WH, et al: Rate adaptive cardiac pacing using right ventricular venous oxygen saturation: Quantification of chronotropic behavior during daily activities and maximal exercise. PACE 17:2236–2246, 1994.)

parameters[60, 61] and parameters associated with right ventricular contractility, such as relative stroke volume or the pre-ejection interval (PEI)[62] in situations involving invasive monitoring. The elegant simplicity of impedance has enabled it to be used with implant pacing leads, including both standard pacing leads and specialized multielectrode catheters. The pulse generator casing has been used as one electrode for the measurement of impedance in most of these pacing systems. Impedance can be used to detect relative changes in either ventilatory mechanics or right ventricular mechanical function or the combination of these parameters. Relative motions between electrodes for impedance sensing also lead to changes in impedance measured, and this is inversely related to the number of electrodes used to measure impedance.[63] In rate-adaptive pacemakers, motion artifacts are usually the result of arm movements that cause the pulse generator to move within the prepectoral pocket,[64, 65] thereby changing the relative electrode separation between the pacemaker and the intracardiac electrodes. Because arm movement accompanies normal walking, these artifacts in the impedance signal occur with both walking and upper limb exercises.

The *intracardiac ventricular electrogram* resulting from a suprathreshold pacing stimulus has been used to provide several parameters that can guide rate modulation. The area under the curve inscribed by the depolarization phase of the paced ventricular electrogram (the intracardiac R wave) has been termed the *ventricular depolarization gradient* or *paced depolarization integral* (PDI).[66] In addition to depolarization, the total duration of depolarization and repolarization can be estimated by the interval from the pacing stimulus to the intracardiac T wave (the QT or stimulus-T interval). Both of these parameters are sensitive to changes in heart rate and circulating catecholamines and can be derived from the paced intracardiac electrogram with conventional pacing electrodes. Because a large polarization effect occurs after a pacing stimulus, a modified waveform of the output pulse that compensates for afterpotentials is needed to eliminate

this effect, so that these parameters can be accurately measured. The interaction of the "square wave" output pulse with the endocardium of a ventricular pacemaker leads to a distortion of the pacing waveform,[67, 68] and the "shape" of the resultant output pulse has been proposed to be useful in estimating intracardiac volume.

The last group of sensors are those that are incorporated into the pacing lead. Examples of these specialized leads include thermistors (used to measure blood temperature), piezoelectric crystals (used to measure right ventricular pressure), optical sensors (used to measure S$\bar{v}$O$_2$), and accelerometers at the tip of pacing leads. Some of these sensors measure highly physiologic parameters. For example, S$\bar{v}$O$_2$ is closely related to oxygen consumption during exercise. Physical activities increase cardiac output and oxygen extraction from the blood, and a widening of the tissue arteriovenous oxygen difference occurs if the cardiac output does not match the requirements of increased tissue oxygen consumption.[53, 69, 70] However, S$\bar{v}$O$_2$ is not linearly related to the workload, and most of the drop in S$\bar{v}$O$_2$ occurs in the first minute of exercise, with less decrease in S$\bar{v}$O$_2$ with increased workload. The preliminary clinical experience with implanted S$\bar{v}$O$_2$ sensors showed a rate response proportional to exercise level.[71–73] In one study, the rate response of an S$\bar{v}$O$_2$ sensor (OxyElite, Medtronic Inc., Minneapolis) was compared with that of a conventional piezoelectric activity sensor during activities of daily living and non–exercise-related physiologic changes. The S$\bar{v}$O$_2$ sensor showed a better proportionality of rate response than the activity sensor and occurred at a comparable speed of onset[72, 73] (Fig. 8–3). The main concern with the S$\bar{v}$O$_2$ sensor is its long-term stability, which may be affected by fibrin coating on the sensor. Although to a certain extent this instability is reduced by using two different wavelengths for S$\bar{v}$O$_2$ measurements, the sensor's ability to function long-term remains an issue.[73]

Right ventricular pressure can be detected by a hermetically sealed pressure sensor containing a piezoelectric crystal and electronic circuitry incorporated into a pacing lead. The first derivative of the right ventricular pressure (dP/dt) is influenced by contractile state of the heart, the ventricular filling pressure, and the heart rate, with a positive correlation between maximum dP/dt and the sinus rate in healthy subjects.[74] Thus, the change in the maximum value of dP/dt is a sensitive indicator of the change in right ventricular contractility and is directly proportional to change in sympathetic tone.[75, 76] The dP/dt sensing principle is highly proportional to workload, as shown in a limited number of investigational implants (Deltatrax, DPDT, Medtronic). The pacing rate achieved with the dP/dt sensor was reported to correlate well with estimated oxygen consumption during exercise (r = 0.93).[13, 77, 78] The increases in pacing rate paralleled the heart rate that was expected from the metabolic reserve during treadmill testing in the VVIR mode. Exercise time was significantly prolonged in the VVIR mode compared with the VVI mode during paired exercise testing.[79]

Using an accelerometer incorporated at the tip of a unipolar ventricular electrode, the contractile state can be assessed indirectly from the endocardial vibration generated during isovolumic contraction of the heart, a parameter known as *peak endocardial acceleration* (PEA).[80, 81] This microaccelerometer is developed by Sorin Biomedica (Italy) and has a frequency response up to 1 kHz and a sensitivity of 5 mV/G (1G = 9.8 m/sec). In preliminary experience in sheep under basal conditions using an external system and an implantable radiotelemetry system, the PEA was not affected by heart rate but was significantly increased by emotional stress, exercise, and natural inotropic stimulation.[80] This parameter follows the changes in the maximum left ventricular dP/dt and apparently measures the global left ventricular contractile performance rather than the regional mechanical function of the right ventricle.[82, 83] In preliminary studies on the PEA-driven rate-adaptive pacemaker, there was a good correlation between the sinus rate and the PEA-indicated rate during activities of daily living and a submaximal stress test.[84, 85] A potential role of the PEA is its ability to optimize the AV interval automatically. Limitations with this sensor system are several. First, the effects of the relative contribution of valvular movement and change in preload to the myocardial vibrations and the measured peak endocardial acceleration are uncertain. Second, this system requires a dedicated lead with unproven long-term reliability and stability, although an initial study on sheep showed acceptable medium-term results.[81]

Closed-loop Versus Open-loop Sensors

A rate-adaptive pacing system can operate in either a *closed-loop* or an *open-loop* manner. In a completely closed-loop system (Fig. 8–4), the physiologic parameter that is monitored is used to effect a change in the pacing rate. In addition, changes in pacing rate in turn induce a physiologic change in the sensed parameter in the opposite direction. Thus, closed-loop pacing systems have *negative feedback,* such that the sensed physiologic variable tends to return toward its baseline value in the presence of an appropriately modulated pacing rate. A partial degree of closed-loop negative feedback control is observed with pacemakers that use $S\bar{v}O_2$ as the rate-control parameter.[53, 69, 70] Exercise in the absence of adequate cardiac output (as in a patient with a fixed-rate pacemaker) increases tissue oxygen extraction from arterial blood, thereby decreasing the content of oxygen in the returning venous blood. This decrease in $S\bar{v}O_2$ can be measured and used to increase the pacing rate, thereby increasing the cardiac output to a value that is optimal for the level of exercise workload, resulting in improved oxygen delivery to the tissues. Under conditions of equilibrium, the pacing rate is adjusted to maintain the maximum possible $S\bar{v}O_2$ for any level of metabolic demand. PDI was also advocated as a closed-loop sensor.[66] An increase in sympathetic activity decreases the PDI, whereas an increase in heart rate increases this parameter, thereby establishing a negative feedback loop that tends to maintain the sensed parameter at a relatively constant value during exercise. True closed loop performance, however, was not achieved in clinical trials with this sensor. Theoretically, the physician input required for a closed-loop system should be minimal because the system is designed to be fully automatic. In practice, a rate-adaptive algorithm is still necessary because the available pacing systems provide only partial closed-loop negative feedback. In an ideal closed-loop system, the sensor automatically takes into account any changes in the patient's cardiovascular condition. Apart from setting the lower and upper rate limits, the physician can indirectly control the rate changes in a closed-loop system by determin-

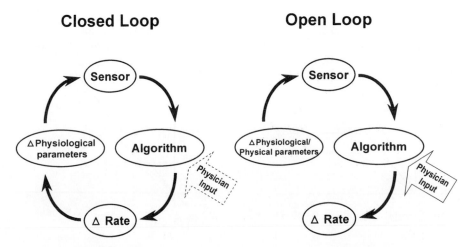

Figure 8–4. Design of a rate-adaptive system. *Open loop,* The physiologic-physical change detected by the sensor is converted to a change in rate using an algorithm. The resultant rate change does not have a negative feedback effect on the physiologic-physical parameter. *Closed loop,* The physiologic change detected by the sensor is converted to a change in rate using an algorithm. The resultant rate change induces a change in the physiologic parameter in the opposite direction, thus establishing a negative feedback loop. (Redrawn from Lau CP: The range of sensors and algorithms used in rate-adaptive pacing. PACE 15:1177–1211, 1992.)

Closed Loop   **Open Loop**

ing the speed at which the pacing rate adjusts to return the sensed parameter to its baseline value.

Although a closed-loop sensor is theoretically attractive, the practical application of this concept has been less than ideal. Normal control of heart rate involves multiple parameters and feedback measures, and it is unlikely that a single sensor can accurately control heart rate in all clinical circumstances. In addition, a closed-loop sensor involved in rate control may be affected by factors other than metabolic demand. Thus, at present, the potential of closed-loop sensors remains unrealized.

Open-loop logic is employed in most available sensors that measure either physiologic or biophysical parameters (see Fig. 8–4). In such open-loop systems, a change in the heart rate does not result in a negative feedback effect on the physiologic or physical parameter used to modulate pacing rate. Thus, open-loop algorithms require the physician to prescribe the relationship between the parameter monitored by the sensors and the desired change in pacing rate. An example of this is an activity-sensing pacing system that detects body movements. Physical exercise results in

acceleration forces on the pulse generator that can be used to increase the pacing rate.[8, 58] The resultant increases in pacing rate, however, usually have minimal effects on body movement.

In the extreme case, a positive feedback of heart rate on the rate-control parameter might occur, as exemplified by the old version of the QT interval sensing pacemaker. The QT interval shortens during exercise. An increase in the pacing rate itself, however, induces further shortening of the QT interval, especially when a linear slope is used to relate changes in the QT interval to changes in pacing rate. Increases in pacing rate during exercise could shorten the QT interval excessively, leading to an excessive increase in rate.[86] This type of "sensor feedback tachycardia"[87] has also been described with rate-adaptive pacemakers that detect minute ventilation[88] and body activity.[89] The mixed venous oxygen sensor also had the potential for positive feedback during exercise-induced myocardial ischemia. For example, the $S\bar{v}O_2$ decreases in response to either reduced cardiac output (such as might occur during ischemia) or increased oxygen consumption. If exercise-induced ischemia is the

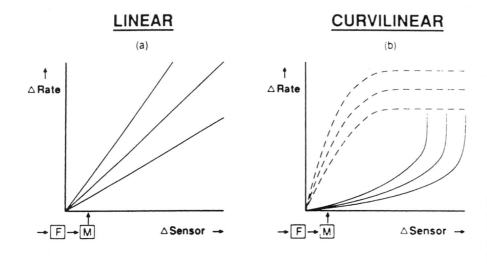

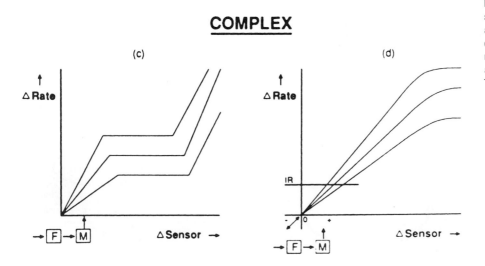

Figure 8–5. Types of rate-responsive curves used in rate-adaptive pacemakers employing a single sensor. An appropriate filter (F) eliminates unwanted raw signals (e.g., high- or low-pass frequency filters and thresholds). The filtered signals are then appropriately modified (M) (e.g., with gains and rectification) before being converted to a rate change. The curves can be linear, curvilinear, or complex. The physician can select an appropriate rate-responsive slope from a family of curves. See text for further discussion. IR, interim rate. (From Lau CP: The range of sensors and algorithms used in rate-adaptive pacing. PACE 15:1177–1211, 1992.)

cause, the resultant decrease in $S\bar{v}O_2$ might trigger a further increase in pacing rate, which may further exacerbate myocardial ischemia. Such a scenario has been observed with this sensor.

■ RATE-CONTROL ALGORITHMS AND RATE-RESPONSE CURVES

The term *algorithm* refers to the way in which the raw sensor data are converted to a change in pacing rate. Typically, sensor data are first filtered to exclude unwanted signals (e.g., signals outside the frequency range of the rate-control parameter). The changes of the sensor signal over an averaged baseline or, on rare occasions, the absolute sensor signals arc used for further processing. The filtered signals are then appropriately modified through rectification and gain control (Fig. 8–5). The processed signals are then used to modulate pacing rate through the use of a rate-control algorithm. The physician must determine the ultimate rate response that will be observed by choosing the lower pacing rate, the upper pacing rate, and a rate-response curve that determines the slope of the sensor-pacing rate relationship. In some pacemakers, the physician can also modify the rate response by changing the "filter" used to process the raw sensor signal. An example of such filtering is the threshold feature of activity-sensing pacemakers.

The relationship between the processed signals and pacing rate can be linear, curvilinear, or a more complex function (see Fig. 8–5). A linear relationship was first used to relate changes in minute ventilation to changes in pacing cycle length in the Meta MV pacemaker (Telectronics Pacing Systems, Lane Cove, Australia) (see Fig 8–5A). Although this algorithm is linear, because the pacing *cycle length* is inversely related to *pacing rate,* the net result is an exponential relationship between changes in minute ventilation and heart rate. Newer generations of minute ventilation–sensing, rate-adaptive pacemakers provide a linear relationship between minute ventilation and pacing rate. A power or logarithmic function is often used in curvilinear rate-responsive curves. A curvilinear relation can be parabolic (e.g., in the Activitrax, Medtronic) or hyperbolic (e.g., Meta MV) (see Fig. 8–5B). A complex triphasic rate-response curve is used in an accelerometer-based, activity-sensing pacemaker (e.g., Marathon, Intermedics Inc., Angleton, TX) (see Fig. 8–5C). This allows a steep relationship between the sensor output and the pacing rate at low and high levels of exercise and a stable rate during ordinary levels of exertion.

An example of an even more complex rate-response curve is the biphasic pattern of response of a more recent minute ventilation sensor. This algorithm provides a steeper slope of the pacing rate–minute ventilation relationship at the beginning of exercise than at the end of the exercise. The initial aggressive slope is made possible by a separately programmable "rate augmentation factor," such that different slopes control the first and second halves of the pacing range. Furthermore, a linear relationship is maintained within the aerobic range of exercise but a less aggressive slope is used above the anaerobic threshold when minute ventilation increases disproportionately to the heart rate change.

Perhaps the most sophisticated rate-response curves are those proposed for temperature sensing (see Fig. 8–5D). In one algorithm, a curvilinear relation is employed when the temperature increases. Because a temperature "dip" characteristically occurs at the beginning of exercise, this algorithm responds to a rapid decline in temperature with a rapid increase in the pacing rate to an interim value. Subsequent increases in temperature are used to modulate further increases in pacing rate. In addition to programming the rate-response curve, temperature-sensing pacing systems provide for a gradual decrease in the lower pacing rate in response to diurnal variation in blood temperature (*bidirectional arrow* in Fig 8–5D). Thus, the rate of change in the rate-control parameter (in this case, a slow decrease in temperature within predefined limits during periods of rest) is used to vary the lower rate limit. Although the rate-response curves discussed previously define the relationship between the sensor output and increases in pacing rate during exercise, many rate-adaptive pacemakers use a different set of curves to control decreases in pacing rate during the recovery phase.

Note that the rate-response curves that have been discussed relate changes in the sensed parameter to changes in the *desired* pacing rate. In addition to these sensor-desired pacing rate-response curves, other factors control the speed (or time constant) with which the sensor-indicated desired pacing rate is translated into a change in the *actual* pacing rate. Obviously, an abrupt change in the sensed parameter must be translated into a gradual increase (or decrease) in the pacing rate. For example, if the activity signal of a pacemaker were to double abruptly, the rate-response curve might indicate that the pacing rate should be increased from 70 to 100 bpm. The interval required for the pacing rate to increase from 70 to 100 bpm is a programmable feature in some rate-adaptive pacing systems and has a fixed time constant in others. Similarly, if the sensor indicates that the pacing rate should be decreased from 100 bpm to 70 bpm, a time constant is required to translate this desired change into an actual decline in pacing rate. Thus, these "attack" and "decay" constants can have a major effect on the chronotropic response characteristics of different rate-adaptive pacemakers.

■ CHARACTERISTICS OF AN IDEAL RATE-ADAPTIVE PACING SYSTEM

The normal human sinus node increases the rate of its spontaneous depolarization during exercise in a manner that is linearly related to VO_2. Because this response undoubtedly has evolutionary advantages, the goal of rate-adaptive pacemakers that modulate pacing rate by artificial sensors has been to simulate the chronotropic characteristics of the sinus node. It is uncertain, however, whether the sinus node provides the ideal rate response in patients who require permanent pacemakers. Nevertheless, until there is evidence indicating otherwise, rate-adaptive pacemakers will strive to reproduce this physiologic standard. Keeping these uncertainties in mind, the ideal rate-adaptive pacing system should provide pacing rates that are *proportional* to the level of metabolic demand. In addition, the change in pacing rate should occur with kinetics (or *speed of response*) similar to those of the sinus node. The artificial sensor should be *sensitive* enough to detect both exercise and nonexercise need for changes in heart rate and yet be *specific* enough not to be affected by unrelated signals arising from both the

Table 8–3. Characteristics of an Ideal Sensor for Rate-Responsive Pacing

Considerations	Examples and Remarks
Sensor Consideration	
Proportionality	Oxygen saturation sensing has good proportionality
Speed of response	Activity sensing has the best speed of response
Sensitivity	QT sensing can detect non–exercise-related changes, such as anxiety reaction
Specificity	Activity sensing is affected by environmental vibration
	Respiratory sensing is affected by voluntary hyperventilation
Technical Consideration	
Stability	Stability of early pH sensor was a problem
Size	Large size or requirement for additional electrodes may be a problem
	Energy consumption must not harm pacemaker longevity unduly
Biocompatibility	Important for sensor in direct contact with the bloodstream
Ease of programming	Difficult programming in early QT sensing pacemakers

internal and external environment. Although the ideal sensor should provide these functional characteristics, it must also be technically feasible to implement with a reliability that is acceptable with modern implantable pacemakers[89a] (Table 8–3).

■ SENSORS FOR PURPOSES OTHER THAN RATE MODULATION

Sensors may also be used for purposes other than modulation of pacing rate (Table 8–4). Several of the available sensors can be used to automate other diagnostic and therapeutic pacemaker functions. For example, the ability to detect the evoked intracardiac R wave may provide a means for capture

Table 8–4. Utility of Sensors for Purposes Other Than Rate Augmentation

Functions	Examples
1. Pacing lead	Sensing and pacing in atrium and ventricle (may extend to the left heart)
	Automatic switchable polarity
2. Basic pacemaker parameters	Autosensing and capture
	Automatic atrioventricular interval and PVARP
	Interference protection
	Upper rate behavior
3. Mode variability	Spontaneous mode changes
4. Tachycardia management	Pacemaker-mediated tachycardias
	Diagnosis and action (in conjunction with antitachycardia devices)
5. Monitoring	Rate
	Hemodynamics
	Hormonal and metabolic profiles
	Myocardial function
	Myocardial ischemia

detection and allow automatic regulation of the stimulus amplitude based on threshold measurements. In a DDDR pacemaker, sensors have been used to adapt the AV interval and the postventricular atrial refractory period (PVARP).[90] In these devices, an increase in the minute ventilation signal is translated into an increase in the "metabolic indicated rate." The AV interval and the PVARP decrease concomitantly as the metabolic indicated rate increases. A sensor can be used to monitor the atrial rate, and a disproportionate increase in the atrial rate compared with the sensor-indicated rate is interpreted by the pacemaker as an atrial tachyarrhythmia, which triggers a change in the pacing mode from DDDR to a nonatrial tracking mode. Thus, a rapid-paced ventricular response during atrial fibrillation can be avoided by an appropriate algorithm.[91]

AV interval optimization using PEA or stroke volume has also been proposed. These sensors may also allow the use of automatic features in implantable devices other than pacemakers. For example, hemodynamic sensors could be incorporated into implantable cardioverter-defibrillators to monitor the hemodynamics of arrhythmias, potentially increasing the specificity of tiered therapy, such as pacing or cardioversion shocks.

■ PRINCIPLES USED FOR COMPARING AND EVALUATING RATE-ADAPTIVE SYSTEMS

Proportionality of Rate Response

One of the best indicators of sensor proportionality is the correlation between the sensor-indicated pacing rate and the level of oxygen consumption during exercise.[13] In general, parameters such as minute ventilation and the paced QT interval are proportional sensors. Some sensors using specialized pacing leads are also highly proportional. For example, $S\bar{v}O_2$ is closely related to oxygen consumption during exercise.

To assess the proportionality of chronotropic response during exertion, the exercise workload should be increased gradually. Traditional treadmill exercise protocols used to evaluate coronary artery disease usually aim to reach maximum heart rate rapidly and tend to skip the lower workloads (3 to 5 Mets) that are performed normally by pacemaker recipients in their daily life. Thus, the use of exercise protocols with gradually increasing workloads, such as the Chronotropic Assessment Exercise Protocol, are probably more appropriate for assessing the rate response of a pacemaker over the wider range of workloads (and oxygen consumption) that are relevant to these patients.[92] Graded exercise testing to maximal tolerated workload may be impractical for some patients for assessing the function of a rate-adaptive pacemaker. Brief, submaximal ramp exercise tests are especially valuable for assessing the proportionality of current rate-adaptive pacing systems.[13] These tests can be "informal," for example, asking the patient to walk at different speeds or to ascend and descend stairs. In addition, monitoring of pacemaker function during activities of daily living may provide the most clinically relevant method of evaluating an elderly patient. Alternatively, submaximal exercises, such as treadmill tests at a low speed and grade, may be performed to assess the sensor response. These tests show that walking at a faster speed increases the pacing rate of

Figure 8–6. Brief activities are used to evaluate the proportionality of rate response of some common sensors. Maximum heart rate was derived from a 3-minute walking test done at different speeds (1.2 and 2.5 mph) and on different slopes (0% and 15%). There was no significant change in pacing rate when patients with the Sensolog pacemaker ascended an incline, whereas the pacing rate decreased significantly in patients with the Activitrax during the same activity. Bpm, beats per minute; NS, not significant; *, $P < .05$; **, $P < .01$; ***, $P < .001$; Tx, QT sensing pacemaker. (From Lau CP, Butrous GS, Ward DE, Camm AJ: Comparison of exercise performance of six rate-adaptive right ventricular cardiac pacemakers. Am J Cardiol 63:833–838, 1989.)

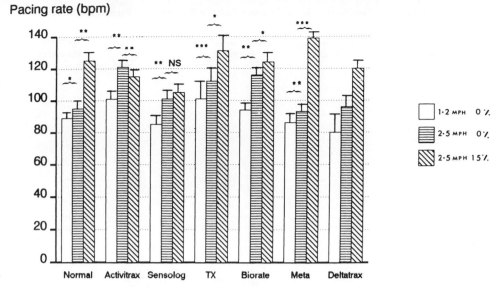

most rate-adaptive pacemakers (Fig. 8–6). However, the rate is not necessarily increased by walking up a slope in patients with activity-sensing pacemakers, which respond according to the pattern of body motion or vibration associated with each type of activity. For example, ascending stairs is associated with a lower pacing rate than is descending stairs with many activity-sensing pacemakers because the intensity of the heel strike is less walking upstairs than downstairs. These findings suggest that there is only a moderate correlation between the rate achieved by activity-sensing pacemakers and exercise workload.

These differences in chronotropic response may not be detected with graded treadmill exercise. Ambulatory electrocardiographic (ECG) monitoring, rate histograms, or stored rate trends may provide useful methods for evaluating the chronotropic response of rate-adaptive pacing systems in patients who are less active or who cannot exercise. Furthermore, very few patients with pacemakers (or, indeed, in the general population) exercise to maximal levels of workload on a regular basis. Thus, formal exercise testing may have little clinical relevance in these patients.

Speed of Onset of Rate Response and Recovery From Exercise

An appropriate speed of response of the pacing rate to the onset and recovery from exercise is an essential feature of a rate-adaptive pacing system. The onset kinetics are best assessed during treadmill exercise, such as walking at a fixed speed on the treadmill. From ECG monitoring, the *delay time* for the onset of rate response, the time to reach half of the maximum change in pacing rate during exercise (half-time), and 90% of the maximum response can be derived and used as a basis for comparison. The exercise responses of six different types of rate-adaptive pacemakers (with sensors for activity, QT interval, respiratory rate, minute ventilation, and right ventricular dP/dt) were compared with normal sinus rate in one study.[13] The results of this study demonstrated that the activity-sensing pacemakers best simu-

lated the normal speed of rate response at the start of exercise. The rate response of activity sensors is usually immediate (no delay time), and the time needed to attain half of the maximum change in rate occurred within 45 seconds from the onset of exercise (Fig. 8–7). The maximum change in pacing rate is reached within 2 minutes of beginning an ordinary activity, such as walking. The respiratory rate and the right ventricular dP/dt sensors had a longer

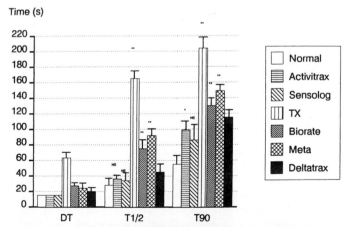

Figure 8–7. Speed of rate response of different pacemakers during walking at a nominal speed (2.5 mph at 0% gradient). The normal sinus rate responds almost immediately, half of the change being achieved in less than 30 seconds and most of the change within 1 minute. This speed of response was most closely simulated by the activity-sensing pacemakers. Significant differences were derived by comparing the response times of each pacemaker (T½ and T90) with those of the normal sinus response. Ninety percent of the maximum rate for this exercise was reached within the exercise period in all patients except those with the QT-sensing pacemaker (TX), who achieved this pacing rate only in the recovery phase. DT, delay time; T½ and T90, times needed to reach 50% and 90% of maximum heart rate. (From Lau CP, Butrous GS, Ward DE, Camm AJ: Comparison of exercise performance of six rate-adaptive right ventricular cardiac pacemakers. Am J Cardiol 63:833–838, 1989.)

Table 8–5. Physiologic Sensitivity of Some Currently Available Rate-Adaptive Pacemakers

Physiologic Measure	Exercise		Emotion	Valsalva Maneuver	Posture	Diurnal Variation
	Isotonic	Isometric				
Sinus	+	+	+	+	+	+
Activity	+					
Respiration	+			R		
QT	+		+			+
Gradient	+	+	+		R	
Temperature	+		±			+
PEI	+	+	+		V	
dP/dt	+	+	+	V	V	
S$\bar{v}$O$_2$	+	+				
PEA	+		+		+	
VIP	+		+			

S$\bar{v}$O$_2$, Mixed venous oxygen saturation; dP/dt, maximum first derivation of right ventricular pressure; PEI, pre-ejection interval; R, reversed response; V, variable.

delay time (about 30 seconds) and half-time (1 to 2 minutes), although the maximum change in rate was still attained within 2 to 3 minutes of exercise. The slowest sensor to respond to exercise was an early version of the QT-sensing pacemaker, which required up to 1 minute to initiate a rate response, and the maximum change in pacing rate was attained only in the recovery period following a short duration of exercise. The onset of rate response and proportionality to workload of the QT-sensing pacemaker was in sharp contrast to those of activity-sensing pacemakers.

The speed of onset of the QT-sensing pacemaker has been significantly improved by the use of a curvilinear rate-response slope that produces a larger change in pacing rate per unit change in QT interval at the onset of exercise (slow heart rates) than at higher workloads.[93] Similarly, the speed of rate response in an early minute ventilation–sensing pacemaker (Meta MV) was impeded by its curvilinear algorithm, which produced a lower slope at the lower range of minute ventilation (onset of exercise) than at higher ranges. This rate-response algorithm has been replaced by a linear slope, so that the rate of onset is significantly faster in the more recent models (e.g., Meta II and Meta III, Legend Plus [Medtronic], and Chorus RM [ELA Medical, Rougemont, France]). Thus, these minute ventilation–sensing pacemakers produce an increase in pacing rate that is linearly related to minute ventilation throughout exercise, providing the effect of shortening the rate-response half-time. Furthermore, the speed of onset of rate response is programmable in these newer generations of minute ventilation sensors.

After termination of exercise, body movement decreases, and the pacing rate of an activity-sensing pacemaker returns toward the resting level based on an arbitrary rate-decay curve.[94] If the rate decay is faster than is physiologically appropriate, adverse hemodynamic consequences may occur in the presence of a substantial decrease in heart rate. In one study in which pacing rate was reduced either abruptly or gradually after identical exercise, it was shown that an appropriately modulated rate recovery was associated with a higher cardiac output, lower sinus rate, and faster lactate clearance than with a nonphysiologic rate-recovery pattern.[95] Appropriate adjustment of the rate-recovery curve is important to enhance recovery from exercise.

Sensitivity of a Rate-Adaptive Pacing System to Changes in Exercise Workload and Other Physiologic Stresses

Table 8–5 shows the factors to which some rate-adaptive pacemakers are sensitive. Rate-adaptive pacemakers that are controlled by ventricular evoked response and intracardiac hemodynamic parameters are able to respond to emotional stresses. A reverse rate response has been observed during the Valsalva maneuver in patients with respiratory sensing pacing systems and some dP/dt sensing pacemakers. None of the available pacemakers reliably detects changes in posture, although several sensors, such as intracardiac impedance or temperature, have the potential to do so[73, 96] (see Fig. 8–3). A paradoxical decrease in heart rate may be observed during movement to the upright position with pacemakers that sense the ventricular depolarization gradient.[97] Although patients with rate-adaptive pacemakers that sense the pre-ejection interval (PEI) (Precept Cardiac Pacemakers Inc., St. Paul, MN) have had variable responses to posture, excessive tachycardia may occur with the adoption of upright posture. This response may require inactivation of the sensor in some patients.[98] A variable postural drop in heart rate has also been reported with a rate-adaptive pacemaker that detects the dP/dt.[77, 78] A diurnal rate variation is possible with temperature-sensing and QT-sensing pacemakers. The clinical implication of some of these rate changes to nonexercise stimuli remains to be determined.

Specificity of Rate-Adaptive Pacing Systems

One of the main limitations of activity-sensing pacemakers is their susceptibility to extraneous vibrations. This typically occurs during various forms of transport. The degree of susceptibility to extraneous vibrations may vary with different types of activity sensors. For example, an accelerometer using a tilt switch (Swing, Sorin Biomedica) may be one of the most susceptible. The QT interval and the PDI may be significantly affected by such factors as cardioactive medications and myocardial ischemia. Ischemia may result in shortening of the QT interval, leading to an increase in pacing rate and further myocardial ischemia.[99, 100] Sensors that use impedance to measure respiratory mechanics or the right ventricular PEI are susceptible to artifacts produced by arm movement, hyperventilation, and speech.[64, 65, 101] Electric diathermy is likely to cause inappropriate changes in pacing rate in pacemakers that measure impedance.[102] The same problem may be expected to occur during radiofrequency ablation in impedance-sensing pacemakers. In addition, external temperature change can significantly affect the pacing rate of temperature-sensing pacemakers.

■ CLINICAL CONTRAINDICATIONS TO SPECIFIC RATE-ADAPTIVE SENSORS

A number of clinical factors may preclude the use of some sensors for an individual patient (Table 8–6). When a parameter can be detected only at the ventricular level, the sensor cannot be used in an AAIR pacing system. The use of antiarrhythmic medications, the use of β-blockers, and the presence of myocardial ischemia may interfere with the detection of the QT and affect its duration. The QT system is sensitive to adrenergic stimulation and response to emotional stress.[103, 104] In patients with ischemic heart disease, this response to psychological stress may occasionally be excessive, with an undesirable rate increase, thereby precipitating angina. Excessive adrenergic tone may cause a QT pacemaker to pace at the upper rate limit in the setting of acute myocardial infarction, creating an undesirable and potentially harmful response.[99, 100] On the other hand, the dP/dt sensor does not appear to be adversely affected by myocardial ischemia.[105] The clinical impact of ischemia in patients with rate-adaptive pacemakers controlled by oxygen saturation remains to be determined.[72]

The minute ventilation–sensing pacemakers are best avoided in young children, who may have very rapid respiratory rates during exercise that may exceed the range detected by the pacemaker. Inappropriate tachycardia may occur in patients with advanced heart failure and the rapid breathing phase of Cheyne-Stokes dyspnea.[88] During cesarean section[106] and general anesthesia,[107] passive hyperventilation may induce pacemaker tachycardia; hence, the non–rate-adaptive mode is preferred when these patients are put under general anesthesia. Electrocautery in the thoracic area may affect impedance-sensing pacemakers and may lead to upper rate pacing; therefore, it is preferable to program the pacemaker to the non–rate-adaptive mode when electrocautery or radiofrequency ablation is used.[102]

Occupations associated with exposure to vibrations in the environment, such as horseback riding,[108] and various types of transportation that may cause rate acceleration are a relative contraindication to the use of an activity sensor. In patients with heart failure, the use of temperature sensors tends to be difficult because a prolonged temperature fall occurs at the onset of exercise in some of these patients.[109] In addition, replacing or upgrading a pulse generator requires that the sensor be compatible with the existing pacing lead. Thus, if one is to use a unipolar ventricular pacing lead, a minute ventilation pacemaker that requires a bipolar lead in the ventricle is not feasible.

■ SENSOR COMBINATIONS

Important issues concerning sensors have emerged. First, the only sensors used clinically are those that can be used with a standard lead. The instability of sensors requiring a special lead prevents their widespread use for rate adaptation. The surviving sensors include activity, minute ventilation, intracardiac impedance, and QT sensors (used only in combinations). Second, rate adaptation using combinations of clinical sensors is feasible and is superior to rate adaptation with a single sensor. Third, automatic programming of sensors is feasible and effective, making the complexity of multisensor pacemaker programming an insignificant issue.

Justification for Sensor Combinations

There has been significant improvement in instrumentation, and rate-adaptive algorithms have been incorporated in the "clinical sensors" to address the issues of speed of onset, proportionality, specificity, and sensitivity of sensor response. For example, piezoelectric crystals for activity sensing using a "peak counting" algorithm are limited by the relatively poor ability of the sensor to differentiate between different levels of workload[94] and their susceptibility to external vibration. Some of these aspects are improved by the

Table 8–6. Clinical Factors Contraindicating Use of Some Currently Available Rate-Adaptive Pacemakers

Factor	Atrial Pacing	Antiarrhythmic Drugs	Myocardial Ischemia	Young Children or Respiratory Disease	Standard Unipolar Lead	Exposure to High-Vibration Environment
Activity						−
Respiration				−	−	
QT interval	−	−	−			
Gradient	−	−	−		−	
Temperature	±				−	
PEI	−	−	−		−	
dP/dt	−	±	−		−	
SⱱO₂	±			−	−	
PEA	−	±	±		−	±
VIP	−	±	−			

PEA, peak endocardial acceleration; PEI, pre-ejection interval; dP/dt, maximum first derivation of right ventricular pressure; SⱱO₂, mixed venous oxygen saturation; −, unsuitable; ±, feasibility remains to be validated.

Table 8–7. Components of a Multisensor System for Rate-Adaptive Pacing (Only Sensors Using Standard Leads are Used for Examples)

Speed of Response	Proportionality	Sensitivity	Specificity	"Energy Saver"
Activity	Minute ventilation	Diurnal variation: 24-hour clock	Minute ventilation QT	Detection of capture: Evoked QRS Stroke volume
Gradient	Pre-ejection interval QT	Emotional response: QT Gradient	Activity	Rate reduction during sleep Minimize myocardial oxygen consumption

use of an accelerometer and an algorithm that integrates the activity signals to determine the sensor-indicated rate.[110–112] Because body movement has no direct relationship to metabolic requirement, however, this sensor remains inadequate to detect isometric exercise, nonexercise needs, and exercises that do not result in significant vibration (such as bicycle riding).

Minute ventilation as measured by impedance delivers appropriate rate-adaptive therapy that is proportional to workload.[9, 10] Criticism has centered on the slower heart rate response of minute ventilation sensors to the onset of exercise as compared with activity sensors, with a 30-second delay when compared with the response of the sinus node.[113] This response is also potentially influenced by conditions that may not be directly relevant to cardiac output, such as talking or voluntary respiration.[114] The new faster algorithm with a programmable rate augmentation factor and speed of response has improved this slow response during the early stages of exercise.[115] This, however, leads to a more rapid recovery with a significantly shortened recovery time at the end of exercise.

The main limitation of the QT sensor is the relatively slow speed of onset of rate response[116] and the susceptibility of the QT interval to drugs and ischemia. With the use of curvilinear rate-responsive curves using a higher slope at the onset of exercise, the lag in the onset of rate response is reduced,[93] but the speed of rate response is still too slow during brief periods of exercise.[117] Thus, the new generation of clinical sensors remains imperfect, even when only speed and proportionality of rate response are considered. In addition, apart from the QT and the ventricular impedance sensors, which react to emotional changes,[118] none of the other clinical sensors are sensitive to nonexercise needs such as changes induced by postural, postprandial, and vagal maneuvers, fever, and circadian variations.

These limitations of the available sensors mean that none of them is suitable for every patient under all circumstances. Despite the fact that the response of a sensor can be significantly enhanced by fine-tuning the characteristics of the sensor and the algorithms used to translate sensor output into modulation of pacing rate, the "clinical" sensors are mainly limited because a fast-responding sensor is not proportional, whereas a proportional sensor is relatively slow (Table 8–7). In addition, an activity sensor is relatively insensitive to nonexercise stress and is nonspecific and liable to external interference. Because the sinus node behavior is the result of multiple stimulatory or inhibitory reflexes, a

combination of sensors may theoretically best replicate the response of the sinus node during a variety of physiologic needs. Therefore, further technical improvements will not be limited to refinement or development of single sensor systems but must inevitably lead to a combination of complementary systems.

Dual-sensor pacemaker technology has been available for several years using many different sensor combinations, but there has been a recent surge in interest regarding multisensor rate-adaptive pacemakers (Fig. 8–8). These combinations aim to create an integrated sensor that simulates the sinus node response of healthy individuals by combining the strong points and eliminating the weak points of the individual sensors (Table 8–8). The sensor combination aims to improve the speed of rate response, proportionality to work-

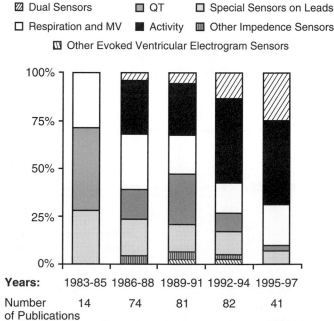

Figure 8–8. The popularity of the different sensors reflected by the quantity of publications expressed as the percentage of the total number of published articles in the past 15 years. Three sensors that can be used with a standard lead have emerged: the activity, minute ventilation, and QT sensors have become the most extensively reported rate-adaptive sensors. In the past 5 years, there is a surge in the publications in sensor combination.

Table 8–8. Relative Advantages of Clinical Sensors

	Speed	Proportionality	Specificity	Sensitivity
Activity	H	L	L	L
Minute ventilation	M	H	M	L
QT	L	M	H	M

H, high; L, low; M, moderate.

load, sensitivity to physiologic changes induced by exercise and nonexercise requirements, and specificity in rate adaptation (Fig. 8–9). A sensor that is more specific to the onset of exercise can be used to prevent false-positive rate acceleration by a more sensitive yet relatively nonspecific sensor. In the absence of the specific sensor indicating that exercise is occurring, the heart rate response of the other sensor can either be nullified or restrained.

Multisensor pacing may also offer the possibility of selecting an alternative sensor should one sensor fail or become inappropriate for an individual patient. In addition, an appropriate rate recovery can shorten repayment of oxygen debt and promote lactate clearance.[95] Therefore, it will be necessary to incorporate sensors that have more proportionality for this part of exercise. The potential for combining sensors for purposes other than rate modulation during exercise is a strong incentive for the development of multisensor pacemakers.

Principles for Integrating Rate-Adaptive Sensors

Algorithms for Combining Rate-Adaptive Sensors

Two basic methods for combining sensors to control chronotropic response during exercise have been used. The types

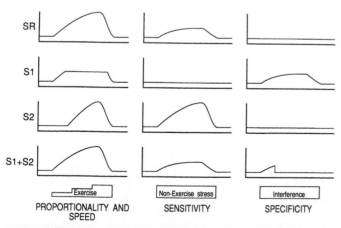

Figure 8–9. Different algorithms for sensor combinations needed to achieve better (1) proportionality and speed of response, (2) sensitivity, and (3) specificity. The graphs *(top to bottom)* depict the responses of the sinus node (SR), sensor 1 (S1), sensor 2 (S2), and combined rate profile of S1 and S2. SR shows ideal proportionality, speed of rate response, and freedom from interference. S1 is a rapidly responding sensor, although it is neither proportional nor sensitive and is susceptible to interference. S2 is a proportional and sensitive sensor, although it has a slow response. It is also specific to exercise. Note the improved ability of the combined sensor approach in simulating the sinus rate under different conditions. (From Lau CP: Rate-Adaptive Cardiac Pacing: Single- and Dual-Chamber. Mt. Kisco, NY, Futura, 1994.)

of sensor combination can be "faster-win" or "blending" (Fig. 8–10*A* and *B*). In the faster-win form, the inputs from two sensors are compared, and the sensor indicating the faster rate is chosen to regulate the pacing rate. A differential combination (blending) combines the input of two sensors, either as a fixed ratio of one sensor to the other or as a variable ratio that changes in relation to the heart rate. For example, a fast-responding sensor (such as activity) can be used to modulate pacing rate at the onset of exercise, and a second sensor (such as minute ventilation or QT) may modulate the pacing rate during more prolonged exercise. The pacing rate may increase to an "interim" or intermediate value when the faster sensor detects the onset of exercise, whereas a more proportional rate increase will occur when the slower, more proportional sensor "catches up." A variation of this approach is to calculate the output of each sensor in a relative proportion, so that the ultimate rate profile is a blend of both.

The pacing rate can be controlled by two sensors that have different sensitivities to exercise and nonexercise physiologic stresses, so that the system can respond to both exertional and emotional needs. It is conceivable that a separate rate-adaptive slope (or different upper and lower rates) can be programmed for modulation of rate in response to exertional and emotional needs. The algorithm can be designed to weigh the input of both sensors to diagnose a nonexercise physiologic stress and provide a different pattern of rate adaptation.

Sensor Cross-Checking—Algorithms for Enhancing Specificity

The response of one sensor can also be checked against the output from another sensor to improve the specificity of the chronotropic response (see Fig. 8–10*C*). A more specific sensor may be used to cross-check a nonspecific sensor, thereby avoiding an inappropriate rate acceleration. In this instrumentation, the rate adaptation of a less specific sensor is allowed to increase the pacing rate only over a restricted range of heart rates and for a limited duration. In the absence of the other sensor indicating exercise, a diagnosis of false-positive rate acceleration with the first sensor is made, and the pacing rate will return to the baseline, so that prolonged high rate pacing will be avoided. Such sensor cross-checking can be reciprocal between the two sensors, so that either sensor may limit the chronotropic response that results from the other. In practice, cross-checking is usually applied to limit the less specific of the sensors.

Possible Sensor Combinations

A number of possible sensor combinations have been suggested (see Table 8–7). These combinations are based on the chronotropic response characteristics of an ideal multisensor system as well as on the compatibility of these sensors with a standard unipolar or bipolar pacing lead. One of the simplest sensors is a 24-hour clock that is used to vary the lower pacing rate. The normal diurnal variation in heart rate is well recognized, and an automatic decrease in the lower rate during the hours of sleep is physiologically appropriate. Battery consumption can also be reduced by this reduction in average pacing rate. Because of its simplicity, reliability, and compatibility with any pacing lead, an activity sensor

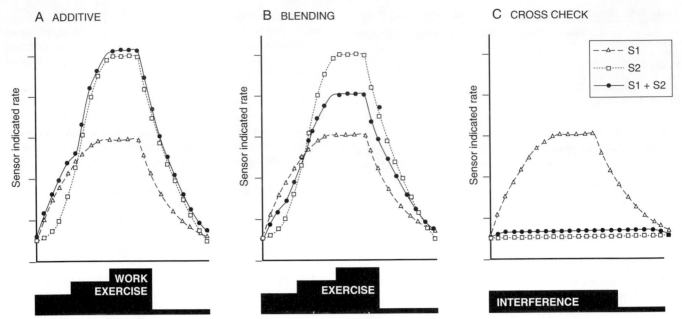

Figure 8–10. Algorithms to combine sensors. *A,* In the faster-win algorithm, the faster rate from sensor 1 (S1), sensor 2 (S2) is chosen. *B,* In the blending algorithm, the sensor rate responses from S1 and S2 are blended to give an intermediate rate. *C,* In the sensor cross-checking algorithm, the more specific sensor S2 cross-checks the less specific fast sensor S1 when S2 does not indicate the presence of exercise.

that has a fast onset of response to exercise is used as one sensor in combination with another sensor that provides a more proportional response to workload. An activity sensor can be easily added to the pulse generator. It requires minimal energy consumption to operate and is compatible with other sensors. Activity has been combined with central venous temperature,[119] a parameter that is more proportional to metabolic need during prolonged exertion than is activity. Similarly, the combination of the QT interval and activity enhances the speed of response compared with a QT sensor alone.[14, 120–122] An activity sensor has been combined with a minute ventilation sensor in a single- and dual-chamber pacemaker (Legend Plus and Kappa.400, Medtronic; Pulsar Max, Guidant, St. Paul, MN; and Talent, ELA Medical).

The sensing of intracardiac impedance is one of the simplest ways to combine sensors. Through the use of special filters, intracardiac impedance can be used to detect low-frequency respiratory signals and higher frequency cardiac signals, such as right ventricular stroke volume and PEI, simultaneously. Most sensors are limited by their inability to detect nonexercise needs, such as those occurring during changes in emotion, which can be detected by combining with the QT interval sensor. Because these parameters are easily measured using conventional pacing leads, their implementation may enable a pacing system to detect non–exercise-related changes in catecholamine concentrations. Despite the many possible sensor combinations, only three clinical sensors have been used clinically in sensor combination (activity, minute ventilation, and QT).

Finally, because many sensors require the consumption of energy to operate, it is desirable to minimize current drain by the use of electrodes that produce a very low chronic stimulation threshold. Algorithms for the automatic detection of ventricular capture may be necessary to minimize current drain further in case of borderline pacing threshold, so that

multiple sensors can be used without compromising longevity of the pulse generator.

Dual-sensor Rate-adaptive Pacemakers

QT and Activity

In the Topaz and Diamond pacemakers (Models 515 and 800, Vitatron Medical BV, Dieren, the Netherlands), a piezoelectric sensor is used for activity sensing. The algorithms for combining the activity and QT sensors are both blending and cross-checking. Activity and QT input can be programmed at different contributions: activity < QT, activity = QT, and activity > QT, representing ratios at 30%:70%, 50%:50%, and 70%:30%, respectively. To avoid false rate acceleration by the activity sensor, the pacemaker allows activity rate response for only a short duration unless confirmed by changes in QT sensor (sensor cross-checking).

The blending of the QT and activity sensors shows a quick rate response at exercise onset and a more proportional rate response during the latter part of exercise and during the recovery period.[120] The fast rate-adaptive response during the first stage of exercise is due primarily to the activity sensing, with a high correlation between the activity sensor counts and the mean pacing rate (r = 0.94), whereas the QT sensor predominates during higher levels of exertion, with a low correlation between activity sensor counts and the pacing rate (r = 0.14).[120] In a multicenter study of 79 patients with the Topaz pacemaker, exercise in the dual-sensor mode produced a more gradual rate response than did the activity mode alone. The rate profile during treadmill exercise testing with dual-sensor pacing was improved over that of single-sensor pacing.[38, 121] In one study, simultaneous recording and comparison of combined sensor and the sinus rate during daily life activities and standardized exercise testing were performed in 12 patients, and an improved correlation between the dual-sensor–indicated rate and the sinus rate during daily life activities and treadmill exercise was seen over that with either individual sensor (Fig. 8–11).[122] Furthermore, an inappropriate high rate response from the activity sensor due to external vibrations could be limited by sensor blending and cross-checking (Fig. 8–12).[123, 124] With a sensitive activity sensor setting, however, activity counts may be registered at rest when the QT sensor is inactive. This may result in the cross-checking of the activity sensor by the QT sensor at rest, and when exercise begins, this cross-checking can delay the speed of dual-sensor rate response.[124]

Minute Ventilation and Activity

A piezoelectric activity sensor has been combined with a minute ventilation sensor to improve the initial response time while allowing a proportional rate response to higher workload.

In the Legend-Plus VVIR pacemaker (Model 8446, Medtronic), an "additive" sensor combination algorithm is used. A sensor-indicated rate for each sensor is calculated, and the faster rate determines the sensor-driven pacing rate. The rate response settings for each sensor were determined by using a 3-minute walking test. Impedance values and the activity counts during the exercise were recorded, and the recommended activity and minute ventilation rate response settings were calculated.

A more sophisticated sensor combination algorithm is used in the Kappa.400 pacemaker. The pacing rate in this model is determined by automatic blending of the activity and minute ventilation sensors, using daily activities as a guide. Both sensors in the Kappa 400 contribute to the sensor-indicated rate between the lower and an interim rate limit, the so-called activity of daily living (ADL) rate.[125] The influence of the activity sensor diminishes and shifts toward the minute ventilation sensor as the integrated sensor-indicated rate increases toward the ADL rate. At heart rates above the ADL rate, the pacing rate is controlled by the minute ventilation sensor alone[125] (Fig. 8–13). The activity sensor will also cross-check against high minute ventilation–indicated pacing rates. Sensor cross-checking against the minute ventilation sensor is activated if the activity sensor counts are low, whereas the increase in the minute ventilation–indicated rate is limited. This minimizes the influence of nonphysiologic minute ventilation signals associated with upper body motion, such as arm movement, or during hyperventilation.[125]

During treadmill exercise and stair climbing, the combined sensor mode in the Legend-Plus was shown to be more proportional to low and high workload activities than the activity VVIR sensor mode but was similar to minute ventilation VVIR sensor mode.[15, 126] There was a faster speed of rate response with a shorter delay time, the time to 50% of the overall rate response, and the time to reach 90% of the rate response in the Kappa 400 pacemaker when compared with the minute ventilation sensor alone during submaximal exercise and activities of daily living. Although the sensor rate kinetics between the activity sensor and combined minute ventilation and activity sensor were similar,[125] the average maximal sensor rate was significantly higher for the dual-sensor mode than for either the activity or minute ventilation modes alone during daily activities (Fig. 8–14).

Automaticity

An appropriate rate-control algorithm or careful programming can overcome some intrinsic limitations of many sen-

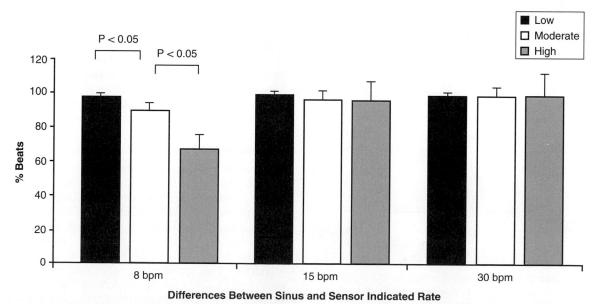

Figure 8–11. Sinus-sensor difference from 12 patients during daily activities, classified according to magnitude of differences (8, 15, and 30 bpm) and levels of activities, low (L), moderate (M), and heavy (H). At a low level of exercise, most of the sensor indicated rates were within 8 bpm of the sinus rate, although the sinus–sensor differences increased at higher exercise workload. The difference between the sensor-indicated rate and the sinus rate was almost always within 15 bpm at all rate ranges. (From Lau CP, Leung SK, Guerola M, et al: Efficacy of automatically optimized rate adaptive dual sensor to simulate sinus rhythm: Evaluation by continuous recording of sinus and sensor rates during exercise testing and daily activities. PACE 19:1672–1677, 1996.)

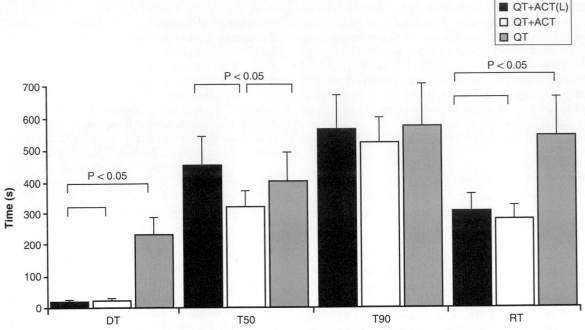

Figure 8–12. Rate-response kinetics of dual-sensor modes compared with QT-only VVIR pacing. DT, delay time; RT, recovery time; T50 and T90, time to reach 50% and 90% of rate response, respectively; QT + ACT, dual-sensor VVIR mode with optimally programmed activity sensor; QT + ACL (L), dual-sensor VVIR mode with an overprogrammed activity sensor (lowest threshold). (From Lau CP, Leung SK, Lee SFI: Delayed exercise rate response kinetics due to sensor cross-checking in a dual sensor rate adaptive pacing system: The importance of individual sensor programming. PACE 19:1021–1025, 1996.)

sors. In contrast, inappropriate programming of a pacing system can distort the chronotropic response of an otherwise ideal sensor. In addition, programming of rate-adaptive sensors is often time-consuming for clinicians. This may involve repeated exercise testing. The use of a dual-sensor pacemaker may more than double the effort required for appro-

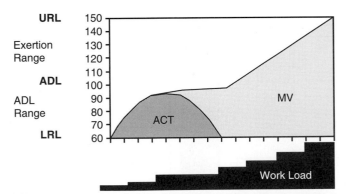

Figure 8–13. Sensor integration algorithm used by DX2 and Kappa combined minute ventilation (MV) + activity sensor (ACT) pacemaker. ACT contributes to the integrated sensor-indicated rate between the lower rate limit (LRL) and activity of daily living (ADL) rate. The influence shifts toward the MV sensor until the ADL rate is achieved; thereafter, MV determines the exertional rate up to the upper rate limit (URL). (From Leung SK, Lau CP, Tang MO, et al: New integrated sensor pacemaker: Comparison of rate responses between an integrated minute ventilation and activity sensor and single sensor modes during exercise and daily activities and nonphysiological interference. PACE 19:1664–1671, 1996.)

priate programming. There is no simple standard for programming one sensor, and often the sensor is programmed to achieve an output based on the physicians' "assessment" of the patients' overall physical state and activity level. For the patient, apart from the inconvenience of repeated reprogramming, the appropriate rate response may change over time as the patient's cardiac conditions change. Thus, the ability of a sensor to adjust itself automatically is not only a convenience for patients and physicians but also a clinical necessity. Automaticity can be achieved using a closed-loop sensor (theoretical only), semiautomatic adjustment, or autoprogramming.

Semiautomatic Programming

To simplify programming, many rate-adaptive pacemakers automatically determine the sensor output during a given workload and suggest the sensor threshold or slope settings that will provide a prescribed pacing rate. In the Sensolog and Synchrony activity-sensing pacemakers (Siemens-Elema AB, Solna, Sweden), sensor data were collected during casual and brisk walking to define two levels of exercise workload. The appropriate rate-adaptive parameters were then derived automatically to achieve the desired heart rate response.[127–129] The advantage of programming the activity sensor using walking as opposed to treadmill exercise testing is that the rate-response parameters determined by treadmill exercise tend to result in a higher than expected rate during activities of daily living and are highly dependent on the type of footwear worn.[127, 129, 130] In the accelerometer-based pacemakers (Dash, Relay, and Marathon [Intermedics]; Vigor, Meridian, and Discovery [Guidant]), acceleration data

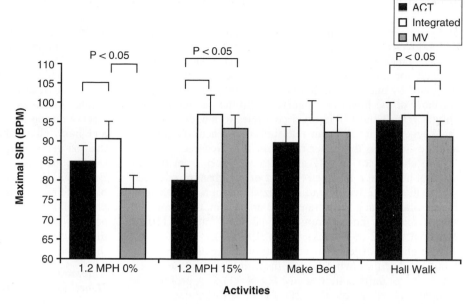

Figure 8-14. Comparison of the average maximal sensor-indicated rate (SIR) during submaximal exercise and activity of daily living (ADL). The minute ventilation (MV) + activity sensor (ACT) mode gave a better average maximal sensor rate during the submaximal exercise and hall walk than did the MV and ACT sensor modes. (From Leung SK, Lau CP, Tang MO, et al: New integrated sensor pacemaker: Comparison of rate responses between an integrated minute ventilation and activity sensor and single sensor modes during exercise and daily activities and nonphysiological interference. PACE 19:1664–1671, 1996.)

are collected during a 1- to 3-minute exercise test and automatically coupled to a programmable rate response, a feature known as "tailor to patient" for the Intermedics pacemakers. This is useful to achieve an appropriate rate response sufficient for most patients during daily activities. However, because the rate-adaptive slope uses a triphasic curve, which has a more aggressive slope at the lower and higher level of exercise, a formal exercise test may still be needed to assess the rate-response characteristics at the higher workloads.

In the minute ventilation–sensing pacemakers (Meta MV, Meta DDDR, and Tempo DR [St. Jude Medical]), the rate-response slope or the recommended rate response factor is determined automatically by matching the maximum pacing rate and the impedance changes at peak exercise. The recommended rate-response factor (RRF) is determined at peak exercise and by interrogation from the programmer.[9] Using this peak RRF to set the rate-responsive slope, the maximum pacing rate occurs when the impedance estimate of minute ventilation matches the impedance value determined during exercise testing. A more rapid adaptation to baseline minute ventilation is used in the newer versions of this sensor, and the rate-adaptive slope can be chosen using submaximal exercise tests.

Autoprogrammability

There are currently two methods of automatic programming for open loop sensors: one using sensor matching at upper and lower rate limits, the other using a target rate distribution approach.

Automatic Rate Adaptation by Matching Sensor Output at Upper and Lower Pacing Rate Limits. An automatic slope adaptation mechanism has been incorporated in the new version of the QT-sensing pacemaker (Rythmx, Vitatron),[16] and combined QT and activity-sensing pacemakers (Topaz VVIR and Diamond DDDR, Vitatron). This algorithm involves two different rate-adaptive slopes, one slope designed for low exercise workloads and the other for higher

workloads. The QT and activity slopes at the upper and lower rate limits are automatically adjusted by a daily learning process. The pacemaker monitors the dynamics of the QT interval and activity counts and continuously updates its maximum and minimum sensor values.[17] The self-learning process adjusts the rate-response slope at the upper rate and lower rate limits, respectively (Fig. 8–15). Each time the pacemaker reaches the upper rate limit, it continues to monitor the QT interval and the activity counts. Further shortening of the QT interval or increase in activity counts while

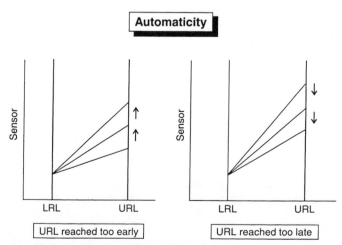

Figure 8-15. Automatic adjustment of the QT rate-response slope aims to pace at the lower rate limit (LRL) when the QT interval indicates no physical or mental stress and to pace at the upper rate limit (URL) when the QT interval indicates maximum workload. At the LRL, the QT–rate relationship is assessed once every night, and the slope is adjusted automatically one step in the direction of change. During maximum exercise at the URL, if further QT shortening occurs, the slope declining factor is advanced one step further, so that the URL will be attained later in a repeat exercise *(left panel)*. Conversely, if the upper rate is not attained in 8 days, the slope declining factor is reduced by one step *(right panel)*.

pacing at the upper rate limit indicates that the upper rate limit has been reached too soon, and the rate response slope at the upper rate is automatically decreased by one step, which gives a more gradual approach to the upper rate limit. On the other hand, if the upper rate limit has not been reached for more than 8 days, this slope is automatically increased by one step. Similarly, the QT interval is measured regularly at the lower rate interval, with the patient presumably at rest. If the QT interval continues to lengthen at rest, this suggests that the lower rate limit is reached too quickly, and the slope for the lower rate limit is decreased.

The changes of the QT and activity slopes from factory settings have been reported.[17] Most of the changes occurred within the first 2 weeks and stabilized within a 6-week time frame. Starting at a lower rate of 60 or 70 bpm, the combined sensor reached the programmed maximum rate of 110 or 120 bpm after 2 to 5 weeks (mean, 19 days).

The clinical efficacy of self-learning automatic programming has been shown to result in pacing rates close to the sinus rate for daily activities (see Fig. 8–11).[122] A prospective comparative study on the efficacy of self-learning versus manual programming was conducted in 12 patients with complete heart block and normal sinus node function who received a combined activity and QT DDDR pacemaker (Model 800, Diamond, Vitatron). Patients underwent treadmill exercise and 12 activities of daily living in the VDD mode. Sensor-indicated rates during these activities as derived from automatic programming and from manual optimization using a submaximal treadmill exercise were compared. The sensor rate determined by either method was close to sinus rhythm, although the rate-response profile and rate kinetics can be further improved by manual optimization.[131]

A similar automatic rate-adaptation algorithm matching sensor output at upper and lower pacing rate limits was also being used by the minute ventilation–sensing pacemaker and the combined accelerometer and minute ventilation–sensing DDDR pacemakers (Talent DR 213, ELA Medical). The pacemaker constantly monitors the minute ventilation signal at the upper and lower rates. The slope of the minute ventilation rate response decreased by one step every eight pacing cycles when the minute ventilation signals continue to rise while the pacemaker was pacing at the upper rate. The slope increased by 3% per day when the upper pacing rate was not reached in 24 hours. This automatic algorithm stabilized the rate response slope with the first month.[132] The pacing response by combining the acceleration sensor with the automatically calibrated minute ventilation sensor was shown to provide a good correlation to sinus rate during exercise.[133]

The main limitation of these self-learning approaches is that the algorithms assume every patient will exercise up to the programmed upper rate during their spontaneous activities. In practice, however, for those patients who perform maximum exertion infrequently or who have been confined to bed, the automatic optimization may potentially overadjust the rate-response slope at the upper rate range, resulting in inappropriately fast pacing rates when the patient resumes usual daily activities.

Automatic Rate Optimization by Target Rate Distribution. In healthy subjects, a characteristic rate distribution occurs over 24 hours, depending on the subject's sex, age, activity, and fitness level.[134, 135] Heart rate profiles have been recorded during 48-hour ambulatory ECG monitoring in healthy subjects while performing regular daily activities and seven upper and lower extremity exercises. In this study, the distribution of daily heart rates was mainly submaximal, but some transient heart rate increases exceeded 55% of the heart rate reserve.[135] The less physically fit subjects had greater increases in heart rate and used greater heart rate reserve during activities of daily living than did the average and more physically fit subjects. Patients who were older than 65 years of age also had a longer duration of heart rate increase to greater than 110 bpm during normal activities. Based on these data, a "nominal" target rate profile resembling the normal rate profile for the population with different physical fitness as determined by age, sex, and different activity levels was derived and used to adjust the desired distribution of pacing rate for an individual patient, using the following two approaches.

Automatic Slope Optimization by Target Distribution of Heart Rate Reserve. In this approach to automatic rate response adjustment, it is assumed that the heart rate of most individuals exceeds the 23rd percentile of the heart rate reserve only 1% of the day. The Triology DR+ (St. Jude Medical) activity-sensing pacemaker maintains a 7-day histogram of the sensor level and automatically adjusts the sensor slope once every 7 days, such that 99% of the sensor activity is within the initial 23% of the heart rate reserve (Fig. 8–16). The maximum adjustment is limited to two slopes, and the slope changes are not made if the patient is inactive (as defined by absence of activity sensor activities). In addition, offsets from −1 to +3 are available for fine titration of sensor response in individual patients. Positive offsets increase and negative offsets decrease the functional slope.

In 93 patients implanted with the Pacesetter Trilogy DR+ pacemaker, the sensor-indicated rate during a brisk walk after automatic slope optimization was compared with a desired sensor rate selected by the clinician. The automatic slope optimization provided the desired sensor rate in 75.6% of patients.[18] The rate modulation provided by the automatic slope optimization was appropriate in 76.3% of patients during follow-up. Despite the use of automatic slope optimization, about half of the patients required further programming of the slope offset to titrate the sensor rate response. Some of this reprogramming was necessary because of the relatively conservative upper rate programming used in this study. In this study, the desired sensor rate and the appropriateness of the rate modulation were decided subjectively at the discretion of the clinician rather than objectively evaluated.

Rate Profile Optimization by Target Rate Histogram. Based on the nominal rate histogram, another device was introduced to adjust the sensor setting automatically to match this target rate histogram. This device, the Kappa 400, is a combined activity- and minute ventilation–sensing DDDR pacemaker. In addition to sensor autoprogramming, the device initiates implant detection through the detection of lead impedance (Fig. 8–17) and lead polarity recognition.[136] After confirming implantation by measuring stable lead impedance for 6 hours, the device is automatically programmed to the DDDR mode, and the baseline minute ventilation is

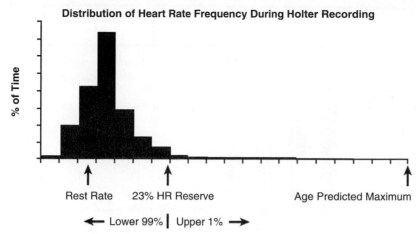

Figure 8–16. An illustration of the distribution of heart rate frequency on which the automatic rate adaptive algorithm of the Triology DR+ was based. The sensor is automatically adjusted, so that a rate response to occupy 23% heart rate (HR) reserve is attained. (From Gentzler RD, Lucus E, and the North American Trilogy DR+ Phase I Clinical Investigators: Automatic sensor adjustment in a rate modulated pacemaker. PACE 19:1809–1812, 1996.)

automatically measured.[125] An optimal heart rate profile based on the patients' activity level and frequency of exercise is programmed as the target rate histogram (Fig. 8–18). This template is used to adjust the submaximal rate response during both daily activities and more vigorous exercise. Once each day, the pacemaker evaluates the percentage of time spent pacing in both the submaximal and maximal rate ranges by comparing the sensor rate profile against the target rate histogram. From this comparison, the pacemaker

automatically controls how rapidly the sensor-indicated rate increases and decreases in these ranges.

The reliability of implant management in providing automatic detection of lead polarity and sensor initiation has been reported.[125] The efficacy of automatic optimization of the rate response was compared with that of manual programming in a prospective study measuring the rate kinetics during activities of daily living and maximal and submaximal treadmill exercise in seven patients who received this

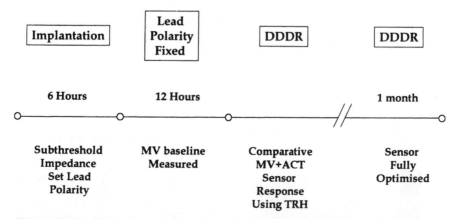

Figure 8–17. Automatic implant detection and sensor initiation algorithm used by DX2 and Kappa combined minute ventilation (MV) and activity (ACT) DDDR pacemaker. The first step is to detect lead implantation by continuous subthreshold current injection and impedance measurement by the pacemaker atrial and ventricular ports in the unipolar and bipolar fashion. Upon connection of the lead to the pacemaker port, the circuit is closed, and detection of implant and lead configuration and the lead polarity are set automatically. After stable lead impedance is measured for 6 hours, the MV and ACT sensors are initialized automatically, and operating baselines for the MV and ACT sensors are determined automatically by collecting MV and ACT sensor data while pacing at the programmed lower rate. After an additional 6 hours, the pacemaker automatically begins dual-sensor DDDR pacing, self-optimizing to achieve the programmed target rate histogram (TRH). (From Leung SK, Lau CP, Tang MO, et al: An integrated dual sensor system automatically optimized by target rate histogram. PACE [in press].)

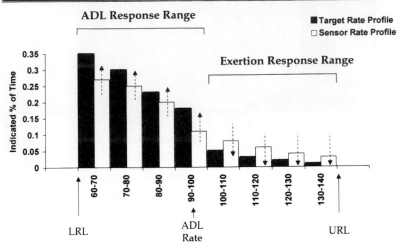

Figure 8–18. An illustration of the sensor rate profile matched against a target rate profile. The activity of daily living (ADL) range includes moderate pacing rates between the lower rate limit (LRL) and the ADL rate. The exertion rates are rates from the ADL rate to the upper rate limit (URL). By comparing the sensor rate profile with the target rate profile once each day, the pacemaker automatically controls how rapidly the sensor-indicated rate increases and decreases in these ranges. (From Leung SK, Lau CP, Tang MO, et al: An integrated dual sensor system automatically optimized by target rate histogram. PACE 21:1559–1566, 1998.)

device. The rate changes derived by automatic programming and by manual adjustment were compared. After automatic rate profile optimization, the pacing rate during a hall walk increased from 78 ± 3 bpm at predischarge to 90 ± 5 bpm at 2 weeks and 98 ± 3 bpm at 3 months of follow-up (Fig. 8–19). The pacing rate during maximal treadmill exercise increased from 89 ± 6 bpm to 115 ± 5 at 3 months after implantation, with a significant increase in exercise duration from 7.2 ± 1.0 minute to 9.6 ± 2.0 minutes. The accuracy of automatic programming versus manual programming was reassessed at 1 month, and the average maximal pacing rates attained and the speed of rate response for the dual-sensor mode after automatic and manual optimization did not differ significantly during maximal exercise, submaximal exercise, and activities of daily living between the two methods of programming[137] (Fig. 8–20).

The main limitation of the automatic rate optimization by the target rate distribution approach is that a nominal population standard for an individual patient still has to be programmed, and a wider patient population is necessary to

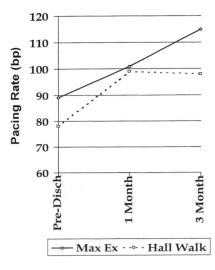

Figure 8–19. *Left,* Changes in the exercise duration during maximum exercise with the implant duration. There is an increase in exercise duration at 3 months, compared with a predischarged exercise test with automatic rate optimization. The exercise duration at 1 month did not differ significantly from the predischarged exercise. *Right,* Changes in sensor rate response to hall walk and maximal treadmill exercise with the duration of implant. The daily activity range has optimized by 1 month, but continuous adaptation of the sensor to achieve a higher rate response has occurred for up to 3 months after implantation. (From Leung SK, Lau CP, Tang MO, et al: An integrated dual sensor system automatically optimized by target rate histogram. PACE 21:1559–1566, 1998.)

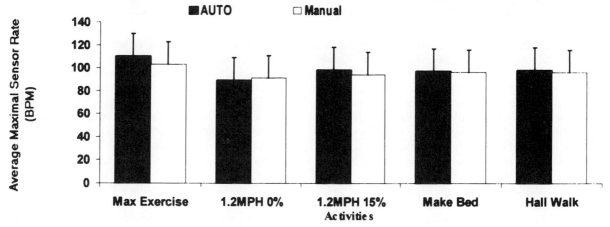

Figure 8–20. Comparison of the sensor rate response during hall walk, submaximal exercise, and maximal exercise between the manual and automatic rate optimization at 1 month. There was no significant difference in the average maximal sensor rate obtained after manual versus automatic programming of the rate-adaptive response. 1.2 mph 0%, submaximal exercise at 1.2 miles per hour at 0% gradient; 1.2 mph 15%, submaximal exercise at 1.2 miles per hour at 15% gradient; BPM, beats per minute. (From Leung SK, Lau CP, Tang MO, et al: New integrated sensor pacemaker: Comparison of rate responses between an integrated minute ventilation and activity sensor and single sensor modes during exercise and daily activities and nonphysiological interference. PACE 19:1664–1671, 1996.)

ascertain the safety of this approach. An inherent risk of using a histogram as the target for sensor setting is the uncertainty about whether the rate response that is recorded actually occurred at the appropriate time because only the rate distribution, rather than the rate profile, is used as the template. In addition, the onset and recovery patterns, which are important characteristics of the sensor rate response, are not addressed by the histogram approach.

Maximum and Minimum Sensor-Indicated Rates and Automaticity

In a rate-adaptive pacing system, apart from the sensitivity of the sensor and the rate-response slopes, a minimum and maximum pacing rate must also be programmed. In a VVI pacemaker, a lower rate must be programmed that is also the "average" pacing rate, which in most cases was arbitrarily programmed at about 60 to 80 bpm. Some authors have suggested that the optimum lower pacing rate can be adjusted to achieve the minimum atrial rate in patients who have complete AV block.[138] Unlike the VVI pacing mode, in which a single fixed pacing rate must be programmed to accommodate both rest and exercise, higher rates can be achieved during exercise by sensors in rate-adaptive pacemakers. Hence, the lower rate limit should be less crucial. Although the programmed lower rate does not affect the maximal pacing rate during exercise, it influences the rate response at the submaximal exercise levels.[139] In addition, it is clinically useful to program a lower pacing rate that is physiologically appropriate for the hours of sleep.[140] The lower resting heart rates also serve to improve the longevity of the pulse generator. On the other hand, in elderly patients who are generally limited in their ability to perform certain types of activities, a faster lower pacing rate could benefit the quality of life more than a lower heart rate.[141]

The variability of the lower and upper rate parameters is best addressed using automatic programming. The simplest of these programs is the use of a 24-hour clock to reduce the lower rate during sleep. This becomes difficult, however, when the patient changes the regular sleeping hours or travels to a different time zone. Hence, it is beneficial to have a sensor that varies the lower rate according to patient's need by directly monitoring the metabolic demand. This may also simulate the spontaneous circadian rhythm of the resting rate in healthy subjects. By using special software to memorize the 24-hour minute ventilation data, a minute ventilation–driven DDDR pacemaker (Chorus RM, ELA Medical) allows the continuous recording and analysis of the circadian variations in minute ventilation, which correlates well with the metabolic demand. This could be used to modify the minimum pacing rate automatically.[142, 143] Currently, however, full automaticity in lower rate programming still cannot be achieved because the "rate band" for the lower rate—the base rate and rest rate—needs to be programmed at the discretion of the physician.

Diurnal variation is also theoretically possible for the temperature-sensing,[144] pressure,[145] and QT sensing devices.[146] The QT signal showed a good correlation with the circadian sinus rate, with a correlation coefficient of more than 0.87.[147] The daily activity and heart rate trends showed a relatively high variation in the activity signals when awake and active and low variability during sleep. By measuring the variation of the activity signal (activity variance) by an activity-sensing pacemaker, the pacemaker can automatically adjust the lower rate during rest and sleep.[148] This circadian modulation based on accelerometer sensor signals was shown to match the normal sinus rate histogram.[149]

An appropriately programmed upper rate limit is important because it determines the hemodynamics at high exercise levels. The patient's age and activity level and the presence of structural heart disease should be taken into account when choosing the maximum sensor-driven rate. In general, a higher upper rate may benefit a young patient. In a review of nine studies of physiologic pacemakers, Nordlander and colleagues[150] found that the percentage of improvement in maximum exercise capacity was linearly related to the maximum heart rate achieved. An overly aggressive rate response, however, was associated with improved exercise performance as compared with no rate response, but produced the worst sense of well-being,[151] larger oxygen deficit, a worsened level of perceived exertion,[152] and deterioration in cardiac output and exercise performance.[153]

The proportion of time spent by these patients with heart rates near the upper rate limit must also be considered. A study using Holter monitor recordings of 44 patients with complete heart block who were treated with VDD pacemakers showed that only 5 of 39 patients with an upper rate of 150 bpm ever reached this limit during recording. The typical pacemaker recipient in this study (mean age, 68 years; range, 18 to 84 years) achieved a rate of 150 bpm for less than 0.5% of the day.[154] Using 12-minute walking distance as a measure of submaximal exercise capacity, the distance covered was longest in patients with an upper rate limit of 125 bpm and in those with a limit of 150 bpm[155] (Fig. 8–21). The exercise capacity was significantly reduced when the programmed rates were either higher or lower than these "optimal" rates. Thus, it appears that an upper rate of between 125 and 150 bpm can be chosen for most patients, except for young or athletic patients.

The effect of the upper programmed rate during submaximal exercise workloads and maximum exercise performance was recently assessed by oxygen kinetics in 11 patients with VVIR pacemakers implanted after AV nodal ablation for refractory atrial fibrillation.[156] By programming the upper rate limit of the VVIR pacemakers to either the maximum age-predicted heart rate or the nominal upper rate limit of 120 bpm, the patients were subjected to symptom-limited treadmill exercise. The exercise duration and maximum oxygen uptake during submaximal and maximal exercise were improved with an age-predicted upper rate. The oxygen deficit was also significantly lower during submaximal exercise with an age-predicted upper rate compared with the nominal upper rate. The mean Borg score was lower during both maximal and submaximal exercise with a higher upper rate. Although the results of this study may not be generally applied because of the younger age of the subjects and the use of only VVIR pacing, they do suggest the importance of upper rate adjustment not only for exercise capacity but also for avoiding myocardial ischemia.

In patients with angina pectoris, VVIR pacing may improve exercise tolerance by decreasing ventricular volume and wall stress compared with VVI pacing.[157] Nevertheless, an aggressively programmed rate-adaptive pacemaker may induce angina in some patients. Therefore, patients with angina pectoris may benefit from exercise testing to determine whether an appropriate chronotropic response can improve exercise capacity without exacerbating anginal symptoms.[157–159] A full clinical evaluation is required because myocardial ischemia is often subclinical. Provided that the upper rate is judiciously chosen, rate-adaptive pacing enhances cardiac efficiency compared with VVI pacing.

There is as yet no algorithm to vary the upper rate limit automatically. An attempt to maintain the rate profile at the daily activity level has been introduced in the new-generation minute ventilation pacemaker (Tempo DR, St. Jude Medical), in which the rate-adaptive slope is determined by the age-predicted anaerobic threshold level rather than by the rate chosen by the physician. A physiologic sensor that can truly monitor the patient's metabolic demand may be able to suggest the appropriate upper rate limit for that patient. For instance, it has been suggested that the degree

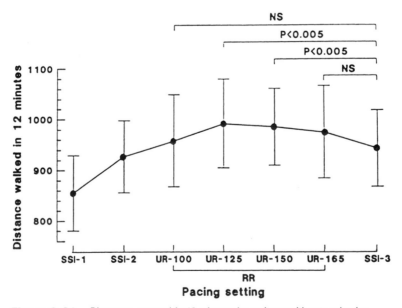

Figure 8–21. Distances covered in 12 minutes by patients with rate-adaptive pacemakers at different programmed settings. SSI-1 to SSI-3 represent repeated walking tests performed at a fixed rate, and SSI-3 is the distance covered after the "learning" effect resulting from SSI-1 and SSI-2. UR-100 to UR-165 represent the rate-adaptive pacing rates achieved during walking. The longest distance was covered with a maximum rate of 125 to 150 bpm. (From Lau CP, Leung WH, Wong CK, et al: Adaptive rate pacing at submaximal exercise: The importance of the programmed upper rate. J Electrophysiol 3:283–288, 1989.)

of slope decline factor in the QT-sensing pacemaker at the upper rate limit might indicate the patient's exercise tolerance as measured during daily life and be used to guide the appropriate upper rate limit programming.[160]

■ IS IDEAL BEHAVIOR NECESSARY?

This question can be addressed in terms of the need for rate response, accuracy of rate adaptation, physiologic benefit, and clinical benefit.[161]

The Need for Rate Response

In the broadest sense, a rate-adaptive pacemaker should be considered for all patients who require pacing. For patients with complete AV block, the VDD and DDD pacing modes provide both rate modulation and AV synchrony in the presence of normal sinoatrial nodal function. Thus, an artificial sensor is not a requirement for rate-adaptive pacing. On the other hand, patients with chronic atrial fibrillation or flutter with AV block cannot be managed with these dual-chamber pacing modes and are ideal candidates for VVIR pacing, especially if the ventricular rate is inappropriately slow during exercise. For patients in whom sinoatrial disease is the primary indication for pacing, the need for rate-adaptive pacing is more variable. Some patients with sinus node dysfunction may demonstrate normal chronotropic response to exercise and require AAI pacing only to prevent sinus pauses. In contrast, others with sinus node dysfunction may have little or no chronotropic response to exercise and are ideal candidates for AAIR or DDDR pacemakers, depending on the status of AV conduction.

The overall pattern of chronotropic response in an individual patient is variable and may evolve over time. Chronotropic incompetence tends to develop in patients with sick sinus syndrome; may be provoked by disease such as heart failure, cardiomyopathy, and ischemic heart disease; or may be induced by drugs. These conditions make the predictions unreliable regarding the ultimate need for rate-adaptive pacing. Furthermore, the frequency of chronotropic incompetence depends on the method of assessment and the definition that is chosen. In general, rate modulation and AV synchrony are provided whenever possible to all patients who require permanent pacemakers. The sinus node is given priority as the primary modulator of heart rate when its function is unimpaired. For patients with paroxysmal or chronic atrial arrhythmias, a rate-adaptive pacing system that incorporates an artificial sensor is usually preferred, and the choice of single- or dual-chamber pacing is dependent on the status of AV conduction and the frequency of atrial tachyarrhythmias.

Accuracy of Rate Adaptation

When programming in patients with rate-adaptive pacemakers is either above or below the optimum values, subjective well-being may be adversely affected.[162] Among 10 patients with activity-sensing, rate-adaptive pacemakers who were randomly programmed to the VVI mode, the VVIR mode with standard slope, or the VVIR mode with an excessively sensitive rate-adaptive slope, many requested early crossover from the VVI and the overprogrammed VVIR modes. Objec-

tive treadmill exercise tolerance was lowest in the VVI mode but there was no difference between the two VVIR modes. A similar decrease in general well-being was observed with the dual-chamber rate-adaptive modes, although objective differences in exercise tolerance were similar among a DDD, DDDR, and overprogrammed DDDR mode.

So far, none of the single sensors available has ideal rate-response characteristics. On the other hand, dual sensors show a more accurate rate response than do single sensors, especially activity sensors. For example, in the combined activity and minute ventilation sensor mode, the correlations between the pacing rate and the externally measured oxygen uptake for treadmill testing and bicycle testing are $r = 0.837$ and $r = 0.733$, respectively, as compared with $r = 0.620$ and 0.643 for the activity sensor alone.[126] There is no significant difference when compared with the minute ventilation sensor mode. In the combined QT and activity pacemakers, the activity sensor overpaced, the QT sensor underpaced, and the combination worked significantly better than the individual sensor.[38, 163] The effect of automaticity on fine tuning of sensors remains to be addressed. Thus, as far as proportionality and speed of rate response are concerned, the current sensor combination is an improvement over single-sensor pacing.

Physiologic Benefits

An accurate rate adaptation may lead to better cardiopulmonary physiology. At higher levels of exertion, the ability to increase rate is the most important determinant of cardiac output and exercise capacity. In pooled data, a positive linear correlation between improvement of exercise capacity and heart rate was also observed.[150] Because exercise capacity is a relatively insensitive measurement of functional benefit,[164] the total exercise duration and maximal exercise workload generally do not differ between the different sensors and the dual-sensor versus single-sensor rate-adaptive modes.[38, 163] Thus, the use of more sensitive and perhaps multiple indicators, such as cardiac output and respiratory gas exchanges, may be necessary to unmask sensor mode differences.

Application of oxygen kinetics to measure oxygen deficit at the onset of exercise may be an alternative indicator of an appropriate speed of rate response. When a minute ventilation–sensing pacemaker was programmed to two different rate-response slopes,[165] the anaerobic threshold was significantly enhanced by the higher slope (oxygen consumption at anaerobic threshold improved from 10.6 to 11.6 mL/kg per minute), with normalization of the minute ventilation–to–heart rate ratio compared with controls. Although both rate-adaptive settings were superior to fixed-rate pacing during exercise, the slight change in the rate-response slope significantly improved anaerobic threshold and chronotropic competence during submaximal exercise.

The heart rate–VO_2 relationship had been examined for dual-sensor and single-sensor modes in a combined minute ventilation and activity VVIR pacemaker.[15] The dual-sensor mode behaved similarly to that of minute ventilation mode, and both were superior to activity sensor mode alone. Anaerobic threshold and maximum exercise performance were also similar in the single-sensor mode compared with the dual-sensor mode.[15]

In the combined QT and activity pacemakers, it was

found that the activity sensor overpaced, the QT sensor underpaced, and the combined QT and activity sensors paced at an in-between rate. The activity sensor improved oxygen uptake kinetics compared with the QT sensor, although the dual-sensor device functioned at an intermediate level[38] (Fig. 8–22). Despite the marked difference in the pacing rate response among the three sensor modes, the different sensor response was not well reflected in the maximal oxygen uptake, the total exercise duration, or the anaerobic threshold. A similar finding was reported from the addition of activity to a minute ventilation sensor.[37]

It appears that sensor combination with an activity sensor to give a quick initial response significantly improves oxygen transport during daily life activity in patients with rate-adaptive pacemakers. The performance of single-sensor and combined QT and activity dual-sensor VVIR modes during submaximal and maximal treadmill exercise was compared using exercise cardiac output by carbon dioxide rebreathing method in eight patients.[163] Compared with the pacing rate response based on the change in metabolic workload, the activity-sensor mode overpaced, the QT-sensor mode underpaced, and the dual-sensor achieved the best approximation to normal. The increase in cardiac output at 1 minute after the exercise onset was higher in the activity-sensor mode and in the dual-sensor mode than in the QT-sensor mode (Fig. 8–23). The underpaced QT sensor mode uses the contractility reserve to compensate for the slower rate increase with a compensatory increase in stroke volume during submaximal exercise. The more rapid rate-dependent increase in cardiac output at the beginning of exercise may be related to the physiologic changes associated with the better heart rate and workload relationship in the dual-sensor pacing mode.

Clinical Benefit

The ultimate goal of pacemaker therapy is to improve symptoms and thus patient quality of life, and this has been used as a basis for comparing pacing modes. In terms of symptom improvement, VVIR pacing is superior to VVI pacing. The overall contribution, however, of improved control of symptoms to enhanced quality of life is probably small in the typical pacemaker recipient, in whom quality of life is already close to that of age-matched healthy subjects.[166] There is still no comparative study of different sensors in regard to their effect on symptoms or quality of life.

A randomized, double-blind crossover study was done on 10 patients using the combined activity and minute ventilation dual-sensor VVIR pacemaker for high-grade AV block and chronic or persistent paroxysmal atrial fibrillation. These patients performed 2 weeks of out-of-hospital activity in the activity-only, minute ventilation only, and dual-sensor VVIR and VVI modes.[167] Patients were assessed according to their perceived general well-being using the visual analog scale and Specific Activities Scale functional status questionnaire and on their objective improvement by standardized daily activity protocols and graded treadmill testing. Subjective perception of exercise capacity and functional status was significantly reduced in the VVI mode compared with the VVIR modes. There was no clear advantage, however, of dual-sensor VVIR pacing over activity-sensor pacing. Four of the 10 patients preferred the activity VVIR mode, 3 preferred the dual-sensor mode, and 3 had no preference. Three patients found dual-sensor VVIR least acceptable, 3 patients found minute ventilation least acceptable, and 1 patient found both dual-sensor and minute ventilation–sensor pacing unacceptable. There was no significant difference in the objective performance between the three VVIR modes. These not unexpected results suggest that there are no major differences between sensors and combinations of sensors in gross clinical terms.

The overall number of patients being studied is small, however, and does not have sufficient statistical power to unveil less than major differences, which may be important for the long-term effects of a pacing mode. In addition, the difficulty of multiple comparisons and the order of pacing modes studied are limitations. Lukl and colleagues[168] have also assessed patient quality of life with regard to cardiovascular symptoms, physical activity, psychosocial and emotional functioning, and self-perceived health during DDD and dual-sensor VVIR pacing. Significant improvement during DDD pacing was demonstrated in all subgroups of patients (patients with sick sinus syndrome, chronotropically competent and incompetent patients, and patients with high degree AV block). The overall result shows that DDD pacing offers better quality-of-life than dual-sensor VVIR pacing.

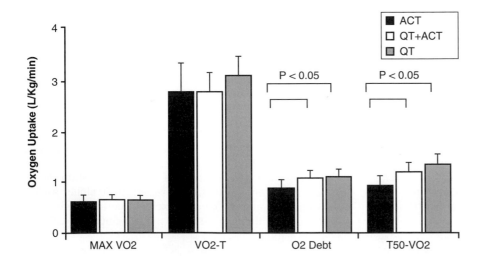

Figure 8–22. Oxygen kinetics in different VVIR sensor modes during constant submaximal exercise. Because the activity sensor is the fastest to respond, it incurs the minimum oxygen debt and time to achieve 50% of the maximal oxygen uptake (T50 − VO_2). There is no statistically significant difference in oxygen debt and T50 − VO_2 between the combine sensor mode and the QT sensor mode. The steady-state oxygen uptake (maximum VO_2) and the total oxygen uptake (VO_2 − T) were similar among the three sensor modes. (From Leung SK, Lau CP, Wu CW, et al: Quantitative comparison of rate response and oxygen uptake kinetics between different sensor modes in multisensor rate adaptive pacing. PACE 17:1920–1927, 1994.)

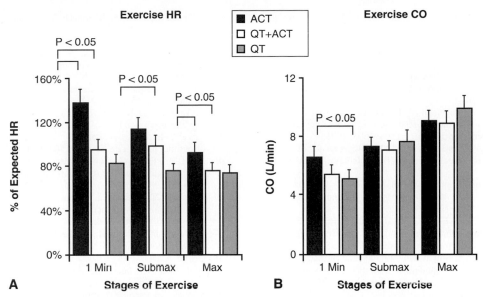

Figure 8–23. Heart rate (HR) and cardiac output (CO) in dual-sensor pacing. *Left,* Exercise HR response in the activity sensor (ACT), QT + ACT and QT VVIR modes expressed as a percentage of the HR predicted according to the metabolic workload. Overpacing is defined as actual HR ≥ 120% of the expected HR and underpacing ≤ 80% at each quartile of exercise. The ACT overpaced, especially in the first minute of exercise, whereas the QT sensor underpaced throughout exercise. The QT + ACT sensor gave a rate response close to the expected rate. *Right,* Exercise CO in the ACT, QT + ACT, and QT VVIR modes. The ACT VVIR sensor mode gave a significantly higher CO at 1 minute after the exercise began than did the QT VVIR sensor mode. The QT + ACT-VVIR sensor mode resulted in an intermediate response. There was no statistically significant difference in the CO between the three sensor modes at the submaximal and maximal exercise. (From Leung SK, Lau CP, Tang MO, et al: Cardiac output is a sensitive indicator of difference in exercise performance between single and dual sensor pacemakers. PACE 21:35–41, 1998.)

Thus, a dual-sensor VVIR pacing cannot compensate for the lack of AV synchrony. The only objective benefit of dual-sensor over single-sensor pacing identified so far was reported by Cowell and associates.[123] These investigators reported the benefit to a patient who had coronary artery disease. This patient had an inappropriately high rate response from the activity sensor as a result of external vibrations during car travel, which caused angina pectoris. The angina was prevented appropriately in the VVIR dual-sensor model by sensor cross-checking.

Summary

Significant advances in rate-adaptive pacing have occurred since its inception, with respect both to the number of sensors available and the pacing modes offered. Because of the simplicity and proven clinical efficacy of rate-adaptive pacing to improve cardiac output and exercise capacity over fixed-rate ventricular pacing, these devices are now the standard of practice in cardiac pacing. Dual-sensor pacemakers seek to exploit the advantages of each sensor to provide chronotropic modulation that more closely emulates that of the normal sinus node. The clinical benefits of dual-sensor pacemakers have yet to be proved in randomized trials. Nevertheless, the potential for automating rate response is an important advantage of combining rate-adaptive sensors.

REFERENCES

1. Karlof I: Haemodynamic effect of atrial triggered versus fixed rate pacing at rest and during exercise in complete heart block. Acta Med Scand 197:195–206, 1975.
2. Cammilli L, Alcidi L, Papeschi G: A new pacemaker autoregulating the rate of pacing in relation to metabolic needs. *In* Watanabe Y (ed): Proceedings of the Vth International Symposium, Tokyo. Amsterdam, Excerpta Medica, 1976, pp 414–419.
3. Cammilli L: Initial use of a PH triggered pacemaker. PACE 12:1000–1007, 1989.
4. Rickards AF, Norman J: Relation between QT interval and heart rate: New design of physiologically adaptive cardiac pacemaker. Br Heart J 45:56–61, 1981.
5. Wirtzfeld AL, Goedel-Meinen L, Bock T, et al: Central venous oxygen saturation for the control of automatic rate responsive pacing [Abstract]. Circulation 64(Suppl IV):299, 1981.
6. Funke HD: Ein Herschrittmacher mit belastung sabhangiger Frequenz-regulation. Biomed Tech 20:225–228, 1975.
7. Rossi P: The birth of the respiratory pacemaker. PACE 13:812–815, 1990.
8. Anderson KM, Moore AA: Sensors in pacing. PACE 9:954–959, 1986.
9. Lau CP, Antoniou A, Ward DE, Camm AJ: Initial clinical experience with a minute ventilation-sensing rate modulated pacemaker: Improvements in exercise capacity and symptomatology. PACE 11:1815–1822, 1988.
10. Mond H, Strathmore N, Kertes P, et al: Rate responsive pacing using a minute ventilation sensor. PACE 1988: 11:1866–1874.
11. Kappenberger LJ, Herpers L: Rate responsive dual chamber pacing. PACE 9:987–991, 1986.
12. Lau CP, Tai YT, Li JPS, et al: Initial clinical experience with a single pass VDDR pacing system. PACE 15:1504–1514, 1992.
13. Lau CP, Butrous GS, Ward DE, et al: Comparison of exercise perfor-

mance of six rate-adaptive right ventricular cardiac pacemakers. Am J Cardiol 63:833–838, 1989.

14. Landman MAJ, Senden PJ, van Pooijen, et al: Initial clinical experience with rate-adaptive cardiac pacing using two sensors simultaneously. PACE 13:1615–1622, 1990.

15. Ovsyshcher I, Guldal M, Karazguz R, et al: Evaluation of a new rate adaptive ventricular pacemaker controlled by double sensors. PACE 18:386–390, 1995.

16. Baig MW, Boute W, Begeman M, Perrins EJ: One-year follow-up of automatic adaptation of the rate response algorithm of the QT sensing, rate-adaptive pacemaker. PACE 14:1598–1605, 1991.

17. van Krieken FM, Perrins JP, Sigmund M: Clinical results of automatic slope adaptation in a dual sensor VVIR pacemaker. PACE 15:1815–1820, 1992.

18. Gentzler RD, Lucus E, and the North American Trilogy DR+ Phase I Clinical Investigators: Automatic sensor adjustment in a rate modulated pacemaker. PACE 19:1809–1812, 1996.

19. Bernstein AD, Camm AJ, Fletcher RD, et al: NAPSE/BPEG generic pacemaker code for antibradyarrhythmia and adaptive-rate pacing and antitachyarrhythmia devices. PACE 10:794–799, 1987.

20. Personnet V, Furman S, Smyth NPD: Implantable cardiac pacemakers: Status report and resource guidelines. Pacemaker Study Group, Intersociety Commission for Heart Disease Resources (ICHD). Circulation 50:a21, 1974.

21. Personnet V, Furman S, Smyth NDP: Revised code for pacemaker identification. PACE 4:400–403, 1981.

22. Loeppky JA, Greene ER, Hoekenga DE, et al: Beat-by-beat stroke volume assessment by pulsed Doppler in upright and supine exercise. J Appl Physiol 50:1173–1182, 1981.

23. Miyamoto Y: Transient changes in ventilation and cardiac output at the start and end of exercise. Jpn J Physiol 31:149–164, 1981.

24. Higginbotham MB, Morris KG, Williams RS, et al: Regulation of stroke volume during submaximal and maximal upright exercise in normal man. Circ Res 58:281–291, 1986.

25. Cardus D, Spenser WA: Recovery time of heart frequency in healthy men: Its relations to age and physical condition. Arch Phys Med 48:71–77, 1967.

26. Astrand P, Rodahl K: Textbook of Work Physiology: Physiological Basis of Exercise, 3rd ed. New York, McGraw-Hill, 1986, pp 260–261.

27. McElroy PA, Janicki JS, Weber KT: Physiological correlates of the heart rate response to upright isotonic exercise: Relevance to rate-responsive pacemakers. J Am Coll Cardiol 11:94–99, 1988.

28. Lewalter T, MacCarter D, Jung W, et al: The low intensity treadmill exercise protocol for appropriate rate adaptive programming of minute ventilation controlled pacemakers. PACE 18:1374–1387, 1995.

29. Margarta R, Edwards HT, Dill DB: The possible mechanism of contracting and paying the oxygen debt and the role of lactic acid in muscular contraction. Am J Physiol 106:689–714, 1933.

30. Astrand P, Rodahl K: Textbook of Work Physiology: Physiological Bases of Exercise, 3rd ed. New York, McGraw-Hill, pp 295–353.

31. Linnarsson D: Dynamics of pulmonary gas exchange and heart rate changes at start and end of exercise. Acta Physiol Scand 415(Suppl):1–68, 1974.

32. Cerretelli P, Rennie DW, Pendergast DP: Kinetics of metabolic transients during exercise. Int J Sports Med 1:171–180, 1980.

33. Jones PW: Ventilatory response to cardiac output changes in patients with pacemakers. J Appl Physiol 51:1103–1107, 1981.

34. Casaburi R, Spitzer S, Haskell R, et al: Effect of altering heart rate on oxygen uptake at exercise onset. Chest 95:6–12, 1989.

35. Brooks GA, Hittelman KJ, Faulkner JA, et al: Temperature, skeletal muscle mitochondrial functions and oxygen debt. Am J Physiol 220:1053–1059, 1971.

36. Stainsby WN, Barclay JK: Exercise metabolism: O_2 steady level O_2 uptake and O_2 uptake for recovery. Med Sci Sports 2:177–181, 1970.

37. Kay GN, Ashar MS, Bubien R, et al: Relationship between heart rate and oxygen kinetics during constant workload exercise. PACE 18:1853–1860, 1995.

38. Leung SK, Lau CP, Wu CW, et al: Quantitative comparison of rate response and oxygen uptake kinetics between different sensor modes in multisensor rate adaptive pacing. PACE 17:1920–1927, 1994.

39. Longhurst JC, Kelley AR, Gonyea WJ, et al: Cardiovascular responses to static exercise in distance runners and weight lifters. J Appl Physiol 49:676–683, 1980.

40. Neumann G, Grube E, Leschhorn JE, et al: Symptoms control and psychosocial rehabilitation of chronic pacemaker patients with differ-

ent pacing modes. *In* Steinback K, Glogar D, Laczkovics A (eds): Cardiac Pacing, Proceedings of the VIIth World Symposium on Cardiac Pacing. Darmstadt, Steinkopff Verlag, 1983, pp 455–461.

41. Alt E, Hirgstetter C, Heinz M, et al: Rate control of physiologic pacemakers by central venous blood temperature. Circulation 73:1206–1212, 1986.

42. Lau CP: The range of sensors and algorithms used in rate adaptive pacing. PACE 15:1177–1211, 1992.

43. Rickards AF, Donaldson RM: Rate-responsive pacing. Clin Prog Pacing Electrophysiol 1:12–19, 1983.

44. Rossi P, Plicchi G, Canducci G, et al: Respiratory rate as a determinant of optimal pacing rate. PACE 6:502–510, 1983.

45. Rossi P, Plicchi G, Canducci G, et al: Respiration as a reliable physiological sensor for the control of cardiac pacing rate. Br Heart J 51:7–14, 1984.

46. Nappholtz T, Valenta H, Maloney J, et al: Electrode configurations for respiratory impedance measurement suitable for rate-responsive pacing. PACE 9:960–964, 1986.

47. Goldreyer BN, Olive AL, Leslie J, et al: A new orthogonal lead for P synchronous pacing. PACE 4:638–644, 1981.

48. Griffin JC, Jutzy KR, Claude JP, et al: Central body temperature as a guide to optimal heart rate. PACE 6:498–501, 1983.

49. Fearnot NE, Smith HJ, Sellers D, et al: Evaluation of the temperature response to exercise testing in patients with single-chamber, rate-adaptive pacemakers: A multicentre study. PACE 12:1806–1815, 1989.

50. Salo RW, Pederson BD, Olive AL, et al: Continuous ventricular volume assessment for diagnosis and pacemaker control. PACE 7:1267–1272, 1984.

51. Chirife R: Physiological principles of a new method for rate responsive pacing using the presystolic interval. PACE 11:1545–1554, 1988.

52. Anderson KM, Moore AA: Sensors in pacing. PACE 9:954–959, 1986.

53. Wirtzfeld AL, Goedel-Meinen L, Bock T, et al: Central venous oxygen saturation for the control of automatic rate responsive pacing. PACE 5:829–835, 1982.

54. Schaldach M, Hutten H: Intracardiac impedance to determine sympathetic activity in rate responsive pacing. PACE 15:1778–1786, 1992.

55. Pichlmaier AM, Braile D, Ebner E, et al: Autonomic nervous system controlled closed loop cardiac pacing. PACE 15:1787–1791, 1992.

56. Occhetta E, Perucca A, Rognoni G, et al: Experience with a new myocardial acceleration sensor during dobutamine infusion and exercise test. Eur J Cardiac Pacing Electrophysiol 5:204–209, 1995.

57. Rickards AF, Bombardini T, Corbucci G, et al: An implantable intracardiac accelerometer for monitoring myocardial contractility. PACE 19:2066–2071, 1996.

58. Humen DP, Kostuk WJ, Klein GJ: Activity-sensing, rate-responsive pacing: Improvement in myocardial performance with exercise. PACE 8:52–59, 1985.

59. Palmer G, de Bellis F, Solinas A, et al: Sensor-free physiological pacing. *In* Behrenbeck DW, Sowton E, Fontaine G, Winter UJ (eds): Cardiac Pacemakers. Darmstadt, Steinkopff Verlag, 1985, pp 781–785.

60. Pacela AF: Impedance pneumography—a survey of instrumentation technique. Med Biol Eng 4:1–15, 1965.

61. Van de Water JM, Mount B, Barela JR, et al: Monitoring the chest with impedance. Chest 64:597–603, 1973.

62. Rushmer RF, Crystal DK, Wagner C, et al: Intracardiac impedance plethysmography. Am J Physiol 174:171–174, 1953.

63. Sahakian AV, Tompkins WJ, Webster JG: Electrode motion artifacts in electrical impedance pneumography. IEEE Trans Bio Med Eng 32:448–451, 1985.

64. Lau CP, Ritchie D, Butrous GS, et al: Rate modulation by arm movements of the respiratory-dependent rate-responsive pacemaker. PACE 11:744–752, 1988.

65. Webb SC, Lewis LM, Morris-Thurgood JA, et al: Respiratory-dependent pacing: A dual response from a single sensor. PACE 11:730–735, 1988.

66. Callaghan F, Vollmann W, Livingston A, et al: The ventricular depolarization gradient: Effects of exercise, pacing rate, epinephrine, and intrinsic heart rate control on the right ventricular evoked response. PACE 12:1115–1130, 1990.

67. Chirife R: Acquisition of hemodynamic data and sensor signals for rate control from standard pacing electrodes. PACE 14:1563–1565, 1991.

68. Chirife R: Sensor for right ventricular volumes using the trailing edge voltage of a pulse generator output. PACE 14:1821–1827, 1991.

69. Wirtzfeld A, Heinze R, Liess HD, et al: An active optical sensor for

monitoring mixed venous oxygen-saturation for an implantable rate-regulating pacing system. PACE 6:494–497, 1983.

70. Casaburi R, Daly J, Hansen JE, et al: Abrupt changes in mixed venous blood gas composition after the onset of exercise. J Appl Physiol 67:1106–1112, 1989.

71. Stangl K, Wirtzfeld A, Heinze R, et al: First clinical experience with an oxygen saturation controlled pacemaker in man. PACE 11:1882–1887, 1988.

72. Farerestrand S, Ohm OJ, Stangl K, et al: Long-term clinical performance of a central venous oxygen saturation sensor for rate adaptive cardiac pacing. PACE 17:1355–1372, 1994.

73. Lau CP, Tai YT, Leung WH, et al: Rate adaptive cardiac pacing using right ventricular venous oxygen saturation: Quantification of chronotropic behavior during daily activities and maximal exercise. PACE 17:2236–2246, 1994.

74. Stangl K, Wirtzfeld A, Heinze R, et al: A new multisensor pacing system using stroke volume, respiratory rate, mixed venous oxygen saturation and temperature, right atrial pressure, right ventricular pressure, and dP/dt. PACE 11:712–724, 1988.

75. Mason DT: Usefulness and limitations of the rate of rise of intraventricular pressure (dP/dt) in the evaluation of myocardial contractility in man. Am J Cardiol 23:516–527, 1969.

76. Gleason WL, Braunwald E: Studies of the first derivative of the ventricular pressure pulse in man. J Clin Invest 41:80–91, 1962.

77. Bennett T, Sharma A, Sutton R, et al: Development of a rate adaptive pacemaker based on the maximum rate of rise of right ventricular pressure (RV dP/dt max). PACE 15:219–234, 1992.

78. Ovsyshcher I, Guetta V, Bondy C, et al: First derivative of right ventricular pressure, dP/dt, as a sensor for a rate adaptive VVI pacemaker: Initial experience. PACE 15:211–218, 1992.

79. Kay GN, Philippon F, Bubien RS, et al: Rate modulated pacing based on right ventricular dP/dt: Quantitative analysis of chronotropic response. PACE 17:1344–1354, 1994.

80. Occhetta E, Perucca A, Rognoni G, et al: Experience with a new myocardial acceleration sensor during dobutamine infusion and exercise test. Eur J Cardiac Pacing Electrophysiol 5:204–209, 1995.

81. Rickards AF, Bombardini T, Corbucci G, et al: An implantable intracardiac accelerometer for monitoring myocardial contractility. PACE 19:2066–2071, 1996.

82. Wood JC, Fensten MP, Lim MJ, et al: Regional effects of myocardial ischemia on epicardially recorded canine first heart sound. J Appl Physiol 76:291–302, 1994.

83. Soldati E, Bongiorni MG, Arena G, et al: Endocardial acceleration signals detected by a transvenous pacing lead: Do they reflect local contractility? [Abstract] PACE 19:659, 1996.

84. Clementy J, Renesto F, Gillo L, et al: Stress test and 24 H Holter analysis of 79 patients implanted with a Peak Endocardial Acceleration (PEA) based DDDR pacemaker (Living 1) [Abstract]. PACE 20:1591, 1997.

85. Binner L, for the European PEA Clinical Investigation Group: One year follow-up of a new DDDR pacemaker based on contractility: A multicentric European study on Peak Endocardial Acceleration (PEA) [Abstract]. PACE 21:894, 1998.

86. Winter UJ, Behrenbeck DW, Candelon B, et al: Problems with the slope adjustment and rate adaptation in rate-responsive pacemakers: Oscillation phenomena and sudden rate jumps. In Behrenbeck DW, Sowton E, Fontaine G, Winter UJ (eds): Cardiac Pacemakers. Darmstadt, Steinkopff Verlag, 1985, pp 107–112.

87. Lau CP: Sensors and pacemaker mediated tachycardias. PACE 14:495–498, 1991.

88. Scanu P, Guilleman D, Grollier G, et al: Inappropriate rate response of the minute ventilation rate-responsive pacemaker in a patient with Cheyne-Stokes dyspnea [Letter]. PACE 12:1963, 1989.

89. Lau CP, Tai YT, Fong PC, et al: Pacemaker-mediated tachycardias in rate-responsive pacemaker. PACE 13:1575–1579, 1990.

89a. Wen HK: A review of implantable sensors. PACE 6:482–487, 1998.

90. Lau CP, Tai YT, Fong PC, et al: Atrial arrhythmia management with sensor controlled atrial refractory period and automatic mode switching in patients with minute ventilation-sensing, dual-chamber, rate-adaptive pacemakers. PACE 15:1504–1514, 1992.

91. Lau CP, Tai YT, Fong PC, et al: The use of implantable sensors for the control of pacemaker-mediated tachycardias: A comparative evaluation between minute ventilation-sensing and acceleration-sensing dual-chamber rate-adaptive pacemakers. PACE 15:34–44, 1992.

92. Wilkoff BL, Covey J, Blackburn G: A mathematical model of the

cardiac chronotropic response to exercise. J Electrophysiol 3:176–180, 1989.

93. Baig MW, Wilson J, Boute W, et al: Improved pattern of rate responsiveness with dynamic slope setting for the QT sensing pacemaker. PACE 12:311–320, 1989.

94. Lau CP, Mehtha D, Toff W, et al: Limitations of rate response of activity sensing rate responsive pacing to different forms of activity. PACE 11:141–150, 1988.

95. Lau CP, Wong CK, Cheng CH, et al: Importance of heart rate modulation on cardiac hemodynamics during post-exercise recovery. PACE 13:1277–1285, 1990.

96. Alt E, Matula M, Thilo R, et al: A new mechanical sensor for detecting body activity and posture, suitable for rate-responsive pacing. PACE 11:1875–1881, 1988.

97. Paul V, Garrett C, Ward DE, et al: Closed-loop control of rate-adaptive pacing: Clinical assessment of a system analysing the ventricular depolarization gradient. PACE 12:1896–1902, 1989.

98. Ruiter JH, Heemels JP, Kee D, et al: Adaptive rate pacing controlled by the right ventricular preejection interval: Clinical experience with a physiological pacing system. PACE 15:886–894, 1992.

99. Edelstam C, Hedman A, Nordlander R, Pehrsson SK: QT-sensing rate-responsive pacing and myocardial infarction. PACE 12:502–504, 1989.

100. Robbens EJ, Clement DL, Jordaens LJ: QT related rate-responsive pacing during acute myocardial infarction. PACE 11:339–342, 1988.

101. Lau CP, Ward DE, Camm AJ: Single-chamber cardiac pacing with two forms of respiration-controlled rate-responsive pacemakers. Chest 95:352–358, 1989.

102. Von Hemel NM, Hamerlijnck RPHM, Pronk KJ, et al: Upper limit ventricular stimulation in respiratory rate responsive pacing due to electrocautery. PACE 12:1720–1723, 1989.

103. Jordeans L, Backers J, Moerman E, et al: Catecholamine levels and pacing behavior of QT driven pacemakers during exercise. PACE 13:603–607, 1990.

104. Frais MA, Dowie A, McEwen B, et al: Response of the QT-sensing rate-adaptive ventricular pacemaker to mental stress. Am Heart J 126:1219–1222, 1993.

105. Candinas R, Mayer IV, Heywood JT, et al: Influence of exercise induced myocardial ischemia on right ventricular dP/dt: Potential implications for rate-responsive pacing. PACE 18:2121–2127, 1995.

106. Lau CP, Lee CP, Wong CK, et al: Rate responsive pacing with a minute ventilation sensing pacemaker during pregnancy and delivery. PACE 13:158–163, 1990.

107. Madsen GM, Anderson C: Pacemaker-induced tachycardia during general anaesthesia: A case report. Br J Anaesth 63:300–361, 1989.

108. Lamas GA, Keefe JM: The effects of equitation (horseback riding) on a motion responsive DDDR pacemaker. PACE 13:1371–1373, 1990.

109. Shellock FG, Rubin SA, Ellrodt AG, et al: Unusual core temperature decrease in exercising heart-failure patients. J Appl Physiol 52:544–550, 1983.

110. Lau CP, Stott JRR, Toff W, et al: Selective vibration sensing: A new concept for activity sensing rate responsive pacing. PACE 11:1299–1309, 1988.

111. Lau CP, Tai YT, Fong PC, et al: Clinical experience with an accelerometer based activity sensing dual chamber rate adaptive pacemaker. PACE 15:334–343, 1992.

112. Greenhut SE, Shreve EA, Lau CP: A comparative analysis of signal processing methods for motion-based rate responsive pacing. PACE 19:1230–1247, 1996.

113. Lau CP, Wong CK, Leung WH, et al: A comparative evaluation of a minute ventilation sensing and activity sensing adaptive-rate pacemakers during daily activities. PACE 12:1514–1521, 1989.

114. Lau CP, Antoniou A, Ward DE, et al: Reliablity of minute ventilation as a parameter for rate responsive pacing. PACE 12:321–330, 1989.

115. Slade AKB, Pee S, Jones S, et al: New algorithms to increase the initial rate response in a minute volume rate adaptive pacemaker. PACE 17:1960–1965, 1994.

116. Metha D, Lau CP, Ward DE, et al: Comparative evaluation of chronotropic response of activity sensing and QT sensing rate responsive pacemakers to different activities. PACE 11:1405–1414, 1988.

117. Roberts DH, Bellamy M, Hughes, et al: Limitations of rate response of new generation QT sensing (Rhythmx) pacemaker [Abstract]. PACE 13:1208, 1990.

118. Hedman A, Nordlander R: Changes in QT and Q-Ta intervals induced by mental and physical stress with fixed rate and atrial triggered ventricular inhibited cardiac pacing. PACE 11:1405–1414, 1988.

119. Alt E, Theres H, Heinz M, et al: A new rate-modulated pacemaker system optimized by combination of two sensors. PACE 11:1119–1129, 1988.

120. Provenier F, van Acker R, Backers J, et al: Clinical observations with a dual sensor rate adaptive single chamber pacemaker. PACE 15:1821–1825, 1992.

121. Connell DT, and the Topaz Study Group. Initial experience with a new single chamber dual sensor rate responsive pacemaker. PACE 16:1833–41, 1993.

122. Lau CP, Leung SK, Guerola M, et al: Efficacy of automatically optimized rate adaptive dual sensor to simulate sinus rhythm: Evaluation by continuous recording of sinus and sensor rates during exercise testing and daily activities. PACE 19:1672–1677, 1996.

123. Cowell R, Morris-Thurgood J, Paul V, et al: Are we being driven to two sensors? Clinical benefits of sensor cross checking. PACE 16:1441–1444, 1993.

124. Lau CP, Leung SK, Lee SFI: Delayed exercise rate response kinetics due to sensor cross-checking in a dual sensor rate adaptive pacing system: The importance of individual sensor programming. PACE 19:1021–1025, 1996.

125. Leung SK, Lau CP, Tang MO, et al: New integrated sensor pacemaker: Comparison of rate responses between an integrated minute ventilation and activity sensor and single sensor modes during exercise and daily activities and nonphysiological interference. PACE 19:1664–1671, 1996.

126. Alt E, Combs W, Fotuhi P, et al: Initial clinical experience with a new dual sensor SSIR pacemaker controlled by body activity and minute ventilation. PACE 18:1487–95, 1995.

127. Lau CP, Tse WS, Camm AJ: Clinical experience with Sensolog 703: A new activity-sensing, rate-responsive pacemaker. PACE 11:1444–1455, 1988.

128. Hayds DL, Higano ST: Utility of rate histograms in programming and follow up of a DDDR pacemaker. Mayo Clin Proc 64:495–502, 1989.

129. Mahaux V, Waleffe A, Kulbertus HE: Clinical experience with a new activity-sensing, rate-modulated pacemaker using autoprogrammability. PACE 12:1362–1368, 1989.

130. Lau CP: Sensolog 703 (Siemens-Elema, Solna, Sweden) activity-sensing rate-responsive pacing (Letter). PACE 3:819–820, 1990.

131. Leung SK, Lau CP, Tang MO: Appropriateness of automatic versus manual optimization in a dual sensor rate response pacemaker [Abstract]. Eur J Cardiac Pacing Electrophysiol 6(1):168, 1996.

132. Ritter P, Anselme F, Bonnet JL, et al: Clinical evaluation of an automatic slope calibration function in a minute ventilation controlled DDDR pacemaker [Abstract]. PACE 20:1173, 1997.

133. Geroux L, Bonnet JL, Cazeau, et al: Evaluation of a new principle of dual sensor. Archives des maladies du Coeur et des vaisseaux. Tome 91-N° special III: 40, 1998.

134. Mianulli M, Birchfield D, Yakimow K, et al: The relationship between fitness level and daily heart rate behavior in normal adults: Implication for rate-adaptive pacing [Abstract]. PACE 18:870, 1995.

135. Mianulli M, Birchfield D, Yakimow K, et al: Do elderly pacemaker patients need rate adaptation? Implications of daily heart rate behavior in normal adults [Abstract]. Eur J Cardiac Pacing Electrophysiol 6(1):182, 1996.

136. Lau CP, Pietersen A, Ohm O, et al: Automatic implant detection for initiating lead polarity programming and rate adaptive sensors: Multicentre study [Abstract]. PACE 19:592, 1996.

137. Leung SK, Lau CP, Tang MO, et al: An integrated dual sensor system automatically optimized by target rate histogram. PACE 21:1559–1566, 1998.

138. Mitsui T, Hori M, Suma K, Saigusa M: Optimal heart rate in cardiac pacing in coronary sclerosis and non-sclerosis. Ann N Y Acad Sci 167:745, 1969.

139. Leung SK, Lau CP, Choi YC, et al: Does the programmed lower rate affect the rate response in rate adaptive pacemakers? [Abstract] PACE 15:579, 1992.

140. Swinehart JM, Recker RR: Tachycardia and nightmares. Nebr Med J 58:314–315, 1973.

141. Zimerman L, Newby KH, Barold H, et al: Effects of the lower pacing rate on quality of life of elderly patients with a VVIR pacemaker implanted following AV node ablation for chronic atrial fibrillation [Abstract]. PACE 20:1191, 1997.

142. Morris-Thurgood, J, Chiang CM, Rochelle J, et al: A rate responsive pacemaker that physiologically reduces pacing rates at rest. PACE 17:1928–1932, 1994.

143. Bonnet JL, Vai F, Pioger G, et al: Circadian variations in minute ventilation can be reproduced by a pacemaker sensor. PACE 21:701–703, 1998.

144. Devyagina GP, Kraerskii YM: Circadian rhythm of body temperature, blood pressure and heart rate. Hum Physiol 9:133–140, 1983.

145. Jones RI, Cashman PMM, Hornung RS, et al: Ambulatory blood pressure and assessment of pacemaker function. Br Heart J 55:462–468, 1986.

146. Djordjevic M, Kocovic D, Pavlovic S, et al: Circadian variations of heart rate and stim-T interval: Adaptation for nighttime pacing. PACE 12:1757–1762, 1989.

147. Kocovic D, Velimirovic D, Djordjevic M, et al: Circadian variations of stim-T interval and their correlation with sinus rhythm [Abstract}. PACE 10:700, 1987.

148. Bornzin GA, Arambula ER, Florio J, et al: Adjusting heart rate during sleep using activity variance. PACE 17:1933–1938, 1994.

149. Park E, Gibb WJ, Bornzin GA, et al: Activity controlled circadian base rate. Archives des maladies du Coeur et des vaisseaux. Tome 91-N° special III: 144, 1998.

150. Nordlander R, Hedman A, Pehrsson JK: Rate-responsive pacing and exercise capacity [Editorial]. PACE 12:749–751, 1989.

151. Sulke N, Dritsas A, Chambers J, et al: Is accurate rate response programming necessary? PACE 13:1031–1044, 1990.

152. Kay GN, Bubien RS, Epstein AE, et al: Rate modulated pacing based on transthoracic impedance measurements of minute ventilation: Correlation with exercise gas exchange. J Am Coll Cardiol 15:1283–1288, 1989.

153. Payne G, Spinelli J, Garratt CJ, et al: The optimal pacing rate: An unpredictable parameter. PACE 20:866–873, 1997.

154. Kristensson B, Karlsson O, Rydén L: Holter-monitored heart rhythm during atrioventricular synchronous and fixed-rate ventricular pacing. PACE 9:511–518, 1986.

155. Lau CP, Leung WH, Wong CK, et al: Adaptive rate pacing at submaximal exercise: The importance of the programmed upper rate. J Electrophysiol 3:283–288, 1989.

156. Carmouche DG, Bubien RS, Neal Kay G: The effect of maximum heart rate on oxygen kinetics and exercise performance at low and high workload. PACE 21:679–686, 1998.

157. Kristensson BE, Arnman K, Ryden L: Atrial synchronous ventricular pacing in ischaemic heart disease. Eur Heart J 4:668–673, 1983.

158. De Cock CC, Panis JHC, Van Eenigl MJ, et al: Efficacy and safety of rate-responsive pacing in patients with coronary artery disease and angina pectoris. PACE 12:1405–1411, 1989.

159. Kenny RA, Ingram A, Mitsuoka T, et al: Optimum pacing mode for patients with angina. Br Heart J 56:463–468, 1986.

160. Stolwijk PWJ, Brants R, Hardeman J: Do self-learning algorithms of QT interval sensing rate responsive pacemakers provide an indication of the appropriateness of upper rate programming? Eur J Cardiac Pacing Electrophysiol 3:198–202, 1992.

161. Lau CP, Leung SK: Clinical usefulness of rate adaptive pacing systems; What should we assess? PACE 17:2233–2235, 1994.

162. Sulke N, Dritsas A, Chambers J, et al: Is accurate rate response programming necessary? PACE 13:1031–1044, 1990.

163. Leung SK, Lau CP, Tang MO, et al: Cardiac output is a sensitive indicator of difference in exercise performance between single and dual sensor pacemakers. PACE 21:35–41, 1998.

164. Jutzy RV, Florio J, Isaeff DM, et al: Comparative evaluation of rate modulated dual chamber and VVIR pacing. PACE 13:1838–1846, 1990.

165. Brachmann J, MacCarter DJ, Frees U, et al: The effects of pacemaker slope programming on chronotropic function and aerobic capacity [Abstract]. Circulation 84(III):158, 1990.

166. Lau CP, Rushby J, Leigh-Jones M, et al: Symptomatology and quality of life in patients with rate-responsive pacemakers: A double-blind crossover study. Clin Cardiol 12:505–512, 1989.

167. Sulke N, Tan K, Kamalvand K, et al: Dual sensor VVIR mode pacing: Is it worth it? PACE 19:1560–1567, 1996.

168. Lukl J, Doupal V, Heinc P: Quality of life during DDD and dual sensor VVIR pacing. PACE 17:1844–1848, 1994.

Chapter 9

Activity Sensing and Accelerometer-Based Pacemakers

Jay O. Millerhagen and William J. Combs

Activity sensing has achieved wide clinical acceptance as a rate-controlling parameter for implantable cardiac pacemakers. More than 300,000 adaptive-rate pacemakers incorporating sensors that monitor body activity have been implanted since the first implantation was performed in 1984. Activity-based pacemakers are theoretically and operationally simple and do not require a special sensor outside the pulse generator can. They work with virtually any type of pacing lead, have excellent long-term stability, and are highly reliable. Activity-guided pacemakers are easy to implant and, in general, react promptly to the start and end of physical exercise. The first activity sensors were piezoelectric crystals that responded mostly to the frequency of vibrations that were transmitted to the pulse generator. In 1987, the possibility of using accelerometer-based activity sensing for pacing rate control was reported for the first time.[1, 2, 3]

The use of sensed parameters other than the intrinsic atrial rate (i.e., artificial sensors) to adjust the pacing rate of implantable pulse generators was initially proposed by Krasner and colleagues[4] and later by Funke.[5] The specific use of an activity sensor for pacemaker rate augmentation was first described by Dahl[6] in 1979 (an accelerometer configuration) and later by Anderson and colleagues[7] in 1983 (a pressure-vibration configuration).

■ INITIAL ACTIVITY-SENSING, ADAPTIVE-RATE PACEMAKERS

Although a variety of techniques can be used to estimate the magnitude of body activity, piezoelectric devices have been the most widely applied. These pacing systems have also been highly effective clinically.[3, 8] Estimation of the intensity of physical activity by piezoelectric methods is an attractive concept for several reasons. First, because the concept of an activity sensor is easy to understand, it has been well accepted by physicians and patients alike. Second, the piezo-

electric principle has been widespread in both medical and nonmedical applications (e.g., ultrasonic imaging and phonographs). Consequently, application of this concept to cardiac pacemakers did not raise concerns about the reliability of a "new" technologic development. Third, the approach is both inexpensive to implement and robust. Additionally, the piezoelectric method consumes very little energy from the battery, can be hermetically sealed within the pulse generator, and is compatible with conventional pacing leads in either the atrium or ventricle.

Numerous clinical reports attest to the reliability and appropriateness of the heart rate response of activity-based pacing systems.[9–18] However, *physical activity is not a direct indicator of metabolic demand.* The potential for false activation of the sensor by environmental stresses unrelated to physical activity[18–20] and the inability of such systems to respond to metabolic stress not associated with physical movement are limitations of these devices.[17, 18, 21, 22]

Almost 14 years have passed since activity sensors were introduced clinically for controlling the pacing rate of cardiac pacemakers. During this period, several other adaptive-rate sensors have been introduced as well. Nevertheless, on a worldwide basis, the activity-based pacing systems have remained by far the most widely used. Furthermore, activity sensors not only have evolved in terms of clinical efficacy but also have been combined with other sensors in multisensor pacemaker applications.

Activity-sensing technology makes use of either piezoelectric or piezoresistive material properties. The piezoelectric effect was discovered and researched using natural crystals, such as tourmalines and quartz, by the Curie brothers more than 100 years ago. Today, piezoceramic materials with several characteristic properties are produced artificially. When a mechanical force is applied along the mechanical axis of a piezoelectric element, the shape of the element changes slightly, generating a voltage proportional to the

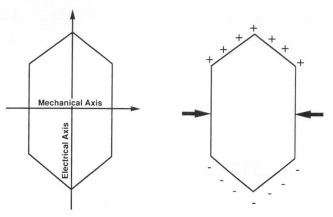

Figure 9–1. Piezoelectric effect. Pressure applied along the mechanical axis of materials with piezoelectric properties causes a voltage to be generated along the electric axis of the material.

force applied along the electric axis (Fig. 9–1). Similarly, application of a mechanical force on some materials with piezoresistive properties results in proportional changes in resistance of the material. These physical characteristics can be applied in the construction of mechanical-electric converters.

For pacing applications, the piezoelectric element in pressure-vibration configurations is typically a thin ceramic (approximate thickness, 0.010 to 0.012 inch) that is bonded to the inside surface of the pacemaker case (Fig. 9–2). The ceramic material is metal plated on both sides (nickel or gold) to provide a method for polarization of the crystal during manufacture and an electric connection to the monitoring electrodes. These electrodes are typically nickel wires

that electrically connect the piezoelectric element to the circuitry of the pacemaker. The total surface area of the crystal is relatively large (in the range of 0.08 square inch) to provide a signal of sufficient strength to the activity-sensing circuit of the pulse generator.

In current clinical practice, the pressure-vibration activity sensors have been by far the most commonly used (Fig. 9–3A). In this application, pressure waves initiated in the skeleton and soft body tissues by physical activity result in a physical deformation of the piezoelectric element.[2, 7–11, 23, 24] Because deformation of the piezoelectric sensor induces a voltage that is proportional to the degree of structural disturbance, measurement of these induced voltages permits estimation of the level of physical activity.

An alternative approach has been to place the piezoelectric element on the circuit board in a cantilevered manner to monitor accelerations in a single plane (see Fig. 9–3B) or, alternatively, to use a conductive ball within an enclosure with multiple contact points.[23, 24] In both of these configurations, the sensor functions as an accelerometer, measuring the forces resulting from body movement.

Because the piezoelectric element is usually attached to the posterior surface of the pulse generator can during manufacturing, it is typically positioned directly against the pectoralis major muscle to ensure good physical contact with the skeletal muscles. The pacemaker can be implanted with the sensor facing away from the muscle activity if the activity threshold or the rate response can be programmed to compensate for the reduced signal amplitude with this orientation. Vibrations of the piezoelectric element induce electric potentials that are processed by the pacemaker to determine the appropriate pacing rate. As the level of physical activity increases, the amplitude of body vibrations also increases (Fig. 9–4). This results in greater deformation of the sensor element and production of a higher voltage. Generally, the piezoelectric element produces potentials in the range of 5 to 50 mV during rest and as much as 200 mV during vigorous activity.[25] The range of frequencies to which these systems are most sensitive is generally about 10 Hz,[26] close to the typical resonant frequency of the human body.[27] Given these signal characteristics, activity-based pacemakers that

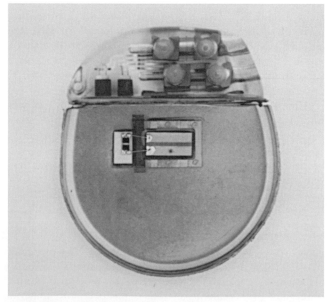

Figure 9–2. Cut-away view of a pulse generator case incorporating a piezoelectric activity sensor. The sensor is composed of a thin ceramic piezoelectric element that is bonded to the inside of the case. Two wires connect the sensor to the circuitry of the pulse generator.

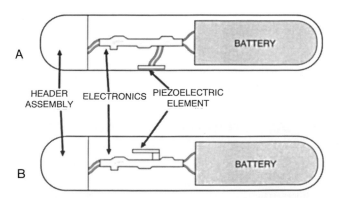

Figure 9–3. Alternative methods of positioning a piezoelectric sensor within a pulse generator. *A*, A traditional pressure-vibration sensor is bonded to the inside of the case. *B*, The piezoelectric element is bonded to the circuit board in a cantilevered fashion, so that it is more sensitive to acceleration within a single plane.

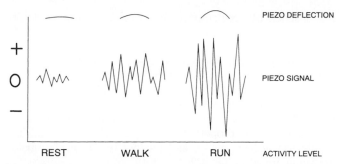

Figure 9–4. Electric signals generated by a piezoelectric sensor at rest, during walking, and during running. As the level of physical activity increases, the amplitude of body vibrations also increases. This results in greater flexion of the sensor element and production of a higher voltage. Potentials in the range of 5 to 50 mV may be recorded from an activity sensor during rest and may be as large as 200 mV during vigorous activity.

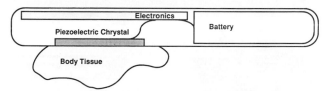

Figure 9–5. The piezoelectric sensor is bonded to the inside surface of the pacemaker case. Vibration is sensed through tissue contact. The mechanical forces are transmitted by the surrounding connective tissue, fatty tissue, and muscles. The extent of contact and the coupling mass of the mechanical forces can vary considerably.

use a piezoelectric element bonded to the inside of the pacemaker case appear to offer good correlation with upright physical movement involving walking or running.[9, 13–16, 22, 28]

■ BASIC CONCEPT OF ACCELEROMETER SENSORS

Another widely used activity-based sensor is the accelerometer. An accelerometer is a sensor designed to measure *acceleration*, defined as the rate of change in velocity. Accelerometers have widespread applications when accuracy in motion detection is important. Extremely sensitive accelerometers are used for navigational equipment in the aerospace industry. Other applications include sensors in automotive active-suspension systems, antilocking braking systems, and airbag deployment mechanisms.[29]

Accelerometers are ideally suited for pacemakers because they are compact and highly reliable and produce a sensor signal capable of being matched to body motion.

In an accelerometer-based pacemaker, the changes in movement of the body are detected by means of a miniature accelerometer situated on the hybrid electronic circuitry of the pulse generator. Physiologic studies have shown that rhythmic body motions, such as walking and riding a bicycle, fall within a narrow frequency range, typically 1 to 4 Hz,[30–33] in which accelerometers are most sensitive.

When an accelerometer device is implanted, no special orientation of the pulse generator is needed. It may be flipped over or rotated in the pocket, and excess lead may be coiled beneath it. The physician can use the simplest and most convenient surgical procedure without risk of sacrificing sensor response.

The main difference between an accelerometer and a piezoelectric crystal sensor that measures vibration is in the actual mass that, on activity, deforms the piezoelectric or piezoresistive material; this is referred to as the *coupling mass*. In the case of the vibration-measuring device, the crystal is bonded to the inside of the pulse generator can (Fig. 9–5). The coupling mass is the body tissue in close proximity to the sensor, which actually exerts a force on the pulse generator can during activity. This mass, consisting of

the connective tissue and muscles surrounding the pacemaker, may vary considerably among patients. Therefore, variation in rate response from patient to patient for the same level of activity can be expected from the vibrational piezoelectric crystal sensor.

In accelerometers, the coupling mass is a small seismic mass, typically weighing less than 100 mg, suspended on one or more levers (Fig. 9–6). The structure is mechanically insulated from the pulse generator can. On acceleration, this mass deflects the lever by an amount that is proportional to the change in velocity and the direction of acceleration. In accelerometers, this deflection can be translated into an electric signal by piezoelectric or piezoresistive material applied to the suspension levers. Because the pulse generator moves with the patient, the accelerometer detects acceleration or deceleration associated with body motion.

The main advantage can be found in the fact that the seismic mass of the accelerometer is constant. Equal acceleration forces induce equal sensor signals independent of the tissue mass surrounding the pacemaker or the physical characteristics of the patient, such as weight and height. This may be an improvement over the conventional piezoelectric crystal sensors because the constant coupling mass of the accelerometer provides a consistent and predictable rate response.

This concept can be rephrased using Newton's second law of motion:

$$F = m \cdot a,$$

where m is the seismic (coupling) mass of the device and F

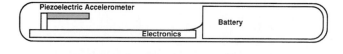

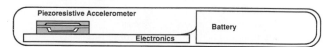

Figure 9–6. The accelerometer is mounted on the pacemaker's hybrid circuitry. The seismic mass of the accelerometer is fixed. Therefore, measured accelerations are independent of surrounding tissue and patient physical properties.

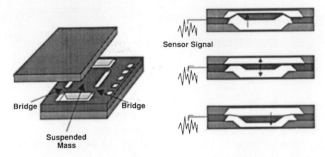

Figure 9–7. The silicon-based piezoresistive accelerometer consists of three layers of silicon bonded together to form a single integrated circuit chip.

is the force applied to the coupling mass as a result of body acceleration (a). Thus, the force acting on the coupling mass and hence on the suspension system depends only on the coupling mass and the acceleration being applied to the pulse generator. An advantage of accelerometer technology is that the sensor fits into the hybrid electronics of the pacemaker circuitry. Accelerometers currently used in clinical practice are very small (4.6 mm × 3.8 mm × 1.5 mm).

Piezoelectric and Piezoresistive Acceleration Sensors

In piezoelectric accelerometers, piezoelectric material is applied to the lever on which the seismic mass is suspended. On deflection, a voltage proportional to the amount of deflection is generated. This voltage is measured and used for rate modulation. This type of accelerometer does not require input current to generate a signal.

Another type of accelerometer is the silicon-based piezoresistive accelerometer. The piezoresistive accelerometer is contained entirely within a silicon chip. The silicon accelerometer consists of three layers of silicon wafers bonded together to form a sandwich. The center layer forms the mass and is suspended by silicon bridges within a cavity in the sandwich (Fig. 9–7). The silicon bridges suspending the mass act as springs. As the mass moves up and down or forward and backward in response to body motions, piezoresistors on each bridge are compressed or expanded. A constant current (3 to 4 mA) is applied to the resistors in the accelerometer. As the resistance changes with motion, the resultant voltage varies in direct proportion ($V = IR$). In

the absence of acceleration, the mass moves back to its resting location. Protective stops limit movement of the mass and guard against excessive shock or forces. This type of piezoresistive accelerometer is sensitive to low-frequency, low-amplitude signals. Both types of accelerometers have constant coupling masses, exhibit a linear frequency response, and are most sensitive in the lower-frequency range, below 8 Hz, which corresponds to typical body motions. The characteristic properties of the piezoelectric crystal, piezoelectric accelerometer, and piezoresistive accelerometer are summarized in Table 9–1.

Accelerometers Monitor the Anteroposterior Axis

The motion of the upper body in an anteroposterior direction mainly determines the energy expenditure.[34, 35] Figure 9–8 shows original recordings of acceleration signals in the three axes during treadmill exercise: vertical, lateral, and horizontal (anteroposterior). Note that treadmill exercise produces the most significant acceleration signals in the vertical and horizontal axes.

Figure 9–9 shows the orientation of the three axes. Although accelerations along the vertical axis generate a larger signal during walking or running, the anteroposterior axis generates signals that are more proportional to the exercise workload. In addition, other activities, such as cycling, gardening, and dishwashing, are best represented by acceleration signals in the horizontal plane. Because the orientation of a pulse generator in the pocket is likely to change somewhat after implantation, the vertical and lateral axes may change. For these reasons, accelerometer-based pacemakers are oriented along the anteroposterior horizontal axis.

Potential Clinical Benefits

Although algorithms for a conventional piezoelectric ceramic sensor bonded to the pacemaker housing can take into account both the frequency and the magnitude of the acceleration signal, they are not fully effective unless the coupling mass remains constant. As a result, nominal rate-response parameters for piezoelectric activity devices may not be appropriate for some patients. Because accelerometers have a constant coupling mass that is consistent for all devices, a narrow range of parameter settings or nominals may provide appropriate rate response for many patients.[36] Studies some years ago showed that, regardless of age, weight, and physi-

Table 9–1. Characteristics of Three Types of Activity Sensors Used for Adaptive-Rate Pacing

Characteristic	Piezoelectric	Piezoelectric	Piezoresistive
Activity sensor	Crystal bonded to can	Accelerometer	Accelerometer
Abbreviation	PZ	AC	AC
Indicator	Vibration	Body motion	Body motion
Mechanics	Bonded to pacemaker	Mounted on hybrid	Integrated chip
Coupling mass	Body tissue	85-mg seismic mass	12-mg seismic mass
Sensitivity	10–15 Hz	1–4 Hz	1–8 Hz
Current drain	0.0 mA	0.0 mA	3–4 mA
Signal analysis	Frequency dominant	Frequency and amplitude	Frequency and amplitude
Size	About 4 × 20 mm	4.6 × 3.8 × 1.5 mm	6.0 × 6.0 mm × 1.5 mm

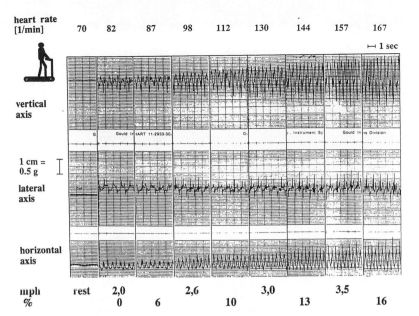

heart rate [1/min] 70 82 87 98 112 130 144 157 167

⊢⊣ 1 sec

vertical axis

1 cm = 0.5 g

lateral axis

horizontal axis

mph % rest 2,0 0 2,6 6 3,0 10 3,5 13 16

Figure 9–8. Acceleration signals in the vertical, lateral, and horizontal (anteroposterior) directions recorded from a healthy volunteer undergoing treadmill exercise. The protocol increased speed, starting with 2 mph and a 0% grade and ending with a maximum of 3.5 mph and a 16% grade. The heart rate of the volunteer increased from 70 bpm to 167 bpm in a linear manner. The frequency and amplitude of the acceleration signals provide a rather linear increase with increase in speed and slope. (From Alt E, Matula M: Comparison of two activity-controlled, rate-adaptive pacing principles: Acceleration vs. vibration. Cardiol Clin 10:635, 1992.)

cal condition, normal volunteers and pacemaker patients produced similar acceleration signals on performing the same kind of exercise.[32, 33] In addition, the accelerometer sensor may be able to detect smaller changes in activity levels than a conventional vibration sensor. Thus, this improved resolution may provide a more gradual increase in pacing rate that is more proportional to the exercise workload. Many pacemaker manufacturers now employ accelerometer-based pacing.

Signal Processing: Piezoelectric Vibration Sensors

The raw electric signal that has been generated by the piezoelectric sensor must be translated into an appropriate modulated pacing rate by an algorithm. Various characteristics of the signal may be measured and used for calculating an appropriate pacing rate. A simple measure, such as peak amplitude, may be used but may also be susceptible to overinterpretation of large transient signals caused by activi-

ties not related to increased metabolic demand for oxygen. Two methods of signal processing by piezoelectric sensor signals are in common use today. One group of devices counts the number of sensor signals that exceed a threshold per unit of time and provides an increase in the pacing rate that is proportional to the number of counts detected (peak counting method). The combination of threshold programming and a linear relationship between counts measured and pacing rate allow for patient-to-patient adjustments. An alternate method for signal processing integrates the area under the electric signal derived from the sensor element. This approach also uses a programmable threshold and slope of rate response. Both methods tend to be similar in their effectiveness for many exercise workloads.

A critical element of signal processing for all adaptive-rate sensors is the ability of the system to distinguish those signals that are associated with physical exertion from those that are not. Several methods are used to help detect appropriate sensor signals. First, because the frequencies of signals related to physical exercise are often different from the frequencies of signals related to environmental interference, the sensor can be designed to respond to a desired frequency range. The signal of interest for pacemakers is usually associated with walking. Measuring signals in the range of 1 to 20 Hz incorporates most signal energy related to walking or running. Excluding signals below 1 Hz excludes most signal energies related to respiration and cardiac activity. The second method for improving signal discrimination is the use of a signal threshold. Signals generated as a result of physical exercise are generally of greater amplitude than confounding noise signals, such as cardiac movement or vehicular vibration. Establishing threshold signal amplitude below which the pacemaker will not respond provides a relatively straightforward technique for separating signals that are associated with exercise from those that are not.

Peak Count Systems

The first adaptive-rate pacemakers to incorporate a piezoelectric sensor used the peak counting method.[6, 11] After

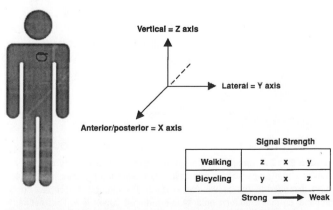

Vertical = Z axis

Lateral = Y axis

Anterior/posterior = X axis

	Signal Strength		
Walking	z	x	y
Bicycling	y	x	z

Strong ⟶ Weak

Figure 9–9. Orientation of the three axes: vertical, lateral, and anteroposterior. The accelerometer is oriented in the anteroposterior axis.

filtering and amplification of the raw signal, the signal was passed through a threshold discriminator.[2, 33, 37, 38] Three thresholds and 10 programmable slopes were available. Modern pacemakers that use the peak counting method have additional programmability, and the newest systems automatically adjust the rate-response parameters in response to a desired exercise test or desired sensor rate histogram profile. An algorithm that monitors the number of piezoelectric signals that exceed a programmable threshold (activity threshold) characterizes the peak counting method. As the intensity of physical activity increases, further increase in the amplitude of the piezoelectric signal does not affect the rate response if the peak has already crossed the threshold (Fig. 9–10). This results in a sensor that characteristically responds to exercise in a relatively "on" or "off" manner.[26, 37]

When a patient exercises, rate response occurs when the amplitude of the piezoelectric signal exceeds the threshold, and when passed, only increases in the number of signals counted will result in an increase in the paced rate. In clinical studies with this sensor, treadmill exercise testing with increased speed (increasing step frequency) resulted in an incremental increase in the pacing rate. On the other hand, tests of patients on a treadmill at a constant speed of 3.2 km/hr with a changing incline from 0% to 15% resulted in an initial increase in pacing rate that subsequently leveled off and did not increase with further increases in workload. This resulted in a weaker correlation between changes in pacing rate and changes in metabolic workload for this processing method (r = 0.2) compared with the integration method[26] (Fig. 9–11). On the other hand, Lau and associates[27] observed a more linear relation between oxygen consumption and pacing rate with the "peak count" method than with the integration approach in patients who exercised using the Bruce protocol (r = 0.70 vs. r = 0.47).

Integration Systems

The second technique for signal processing with a piezoelectric sensor is the integration method.[18, 23, 26, 37, 39] The raw

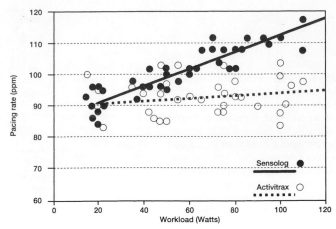

Figure 9–11. Comparison of the rate modulating provided by a peak counting algorithm (Activitrax) and an integration algorithm (Sensolog). Note that the pacing rate is relatively independent of workload for the peak counting device, whereas the integration method provides a pacing rate that is related to workload.

piezoelectric signal is integrated after the initial filtering, amplification, and rectification (Fig. 9–12). All signals are used to determine the level of rate response because there is no amplitude threshold that must be exceeded. By integrating the sensor signal, the sensor output is influenced by increasing both signal frequency (step frequency) and amplitude. A programmable threshold is used to determine the minimum sensor area that is required before the pacemaker responds with a rate increase (Fig. 9–13). When the sensor number (area) exceeds this programmable threshold, the programmed slope determines the desired pacing rate. Automatic threshold determination is also available with these pacemakers using a running average sensor value over a period of 18 hours. This value, which approximates the resting sensor level for most patients who are sedentary, in combination with a programmable offset, provides a means of reducing the responsiveness of the pacemaker system.

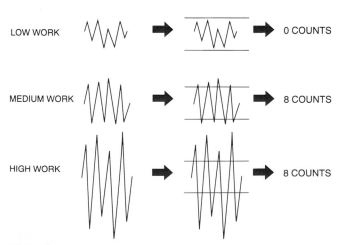

Figure 9–10. Peak counting method of signal processing. Note that at low levels of exertion, the amplitude of the sensor signals does not exceed the threshold amplitude, producing a sensor count of 0. At medium and high workloads, the amplitude of the sensor signals increases. Because this processing method counts only the number of threshold crossings, however, an identical sensor count is produced by medium and high workloads.

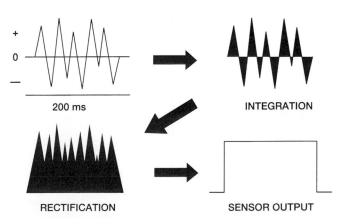

Figure 9–12. Integration method of signal processing. The raw activity signal (upper left) is processed by integrating the area under the curve inscribed by the sensor (upper right). The integrated area is then rectified, so that a uniform polarity is generated (lower left). The rectified sensor signal is then converted into a square wave that is directly related in duration to the area under the curve.

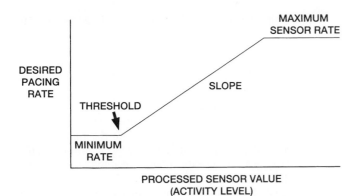

Figure 9–13. In the integration technique, the threshold is used in the software algorithm to determine the minimum processed sensor output that will produce an increase in pacing rate. When the sensor number exceeds this programmable threshold, the sensor output is converted to a desired pacing rate by a programmable slope.

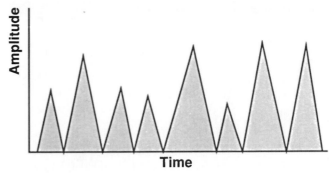

Figure 9–15. The signal processing of the accelerometer signal integrates the rectified signal to measure energy content.

Prior research has confirmed the ability of the integration processing method to provide a linear response of pacing rate to exercise workload.[26, 36] The integration system, however, also has the limitations inherent to all piezoelectric sensor systems, such as false activation due to environmental vibrations[18] and diminished responsiveness to lower body exercise (i.e., bicycling) or nonactivity physiologic stress.[17, 18, 39]

Signal Processing: Accelerometer Sensors

Studies have shown that measurement of acceleration provides a better correlation with the level of exertion than does measurement of the frequency of activity signals alone.[34, 35] Because the accelerometer measures acceleration continuously and instantaneously, there is no delay between the onset of acceleration and the moment at which sensor data are made available to the device's adaptive-rate algorithms. These adaptive-rate algorithms, controlled by programmable parameters, determine the actual speed of rate increase and decrease in response to exercise.

Figure 9–14 shows an example of the raw accelerometer signal recorded during the transition between slow walking and fast walking. Both the frequency and the amplitude of the accelerometer signal are evaluated during signal processing. The raw sensor signal is rectified and integrated by the pacemaker's analog circuits to yield the energy content of the motion associated with physical activity (Fig. 9–15).

The integrated result is available instantaneously for further algorithmic processing.

Signal processing is important to sensor performance. A key advantage of accelerometer technology is the ability to limit the sensor signal to frequencies that are associated with true body motion. Studies[32, 33, 40–44] have shown that the frequency content as determined by Fourier analysis of accelerometer signals during physical stress is in the low-frequency range (Fig. 9–16), with signals of maximum amplitude below 4 Hz. Signals originating from external noise sources, such as electric drills, reach maximum amplitude in the 10- to 50-Hz frequency range (Fig. 9–17). Note that accelerometers respond to frequencies that are typical of body motion, whereas conventional piezoelectric crystals are associated with a wider range of frequencies. The accelerometers currently used in accelerometer-based pacemakers are designed to be highly sensitive in the low-frequency ranges associated with body movements. Accelerometer-based pacemakers employ frequency ranges between 0.5 and 10 Hz. This selective filtering effectively discriminates between wanted and unwanted signals. The result is a pacing system that is less susceptible to external noise and more appropriately responsive to true physiologic activities. Piezoelectric crystals are highly sensitive in the 10- to 50-Hz frequency range.[45] Therefore, discrimination between noise signals and true physical signals is more difficult in vibrational pacemakers.

Reliability

The excellent sensing properties of accelerometers have been proved in epidemiologic studies conducted to track the activ-

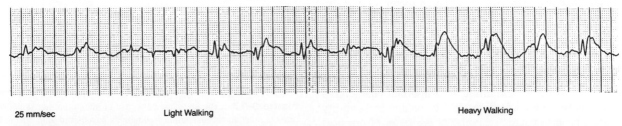

25 mm/sec   Light Walking   Heavy Walking

Figure 9–14. Telemetered Sensorgram as recorded from a VIGOR DR during the transition between light and heavy walking at about one step per second.

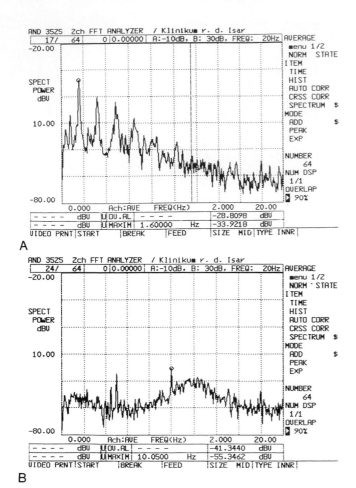

Figure 9–16. *A*, Fourier analysis of an accelerometer signal during walking (4.2 km/hr, 10% incline). The ordinate gives the power spectrum in a logarithmic manner, and the abscissa gives the frequency content from 0 to 20 Hz. The energy peak occurs at 1.6 Hz. *B*, Fourier analysis of signals from an accelerometer attached to a patient performing work with an electric drill. In the low-frequency range, little signal amplitude is present, whereas in the 10- to 12-Hz range, a signal of −55 dB can be detected.

determine the desired pacing rate according to the programmed threshold and slope settings. Although the *desired* pacing rate may change abruptly, there is a time delay between a change in the desired pacing rate and the change in the actual pacing rate. For example, if the onset of activity results in the device calculating a desired pacing rate of 100 ppm, the pacemaker must use algorithms to convert the activity sensor signal to a sensor-indicated paced rate. These vary from device to device depending on the manufacturer, but in general they have a similar purpose. Common sensor parameters typical of activity-motion systems are lower rate limit (LRL), maximum sensor rate (MSR), response factor, activity threshold reaction (or acceleration time), and recovery (or deceleration time). These are graphically described in Figure 9–18. These parameters are present in some form in most activity-based adaptive-rate pacemakers, and most are programmable. In newer pacemakers, several algorithms automatically regulate these parameters. Typically, automated devices monitor the history of activity for the patient and adjust the parameters according to the manufacturers' algorithms. The interested reader can refer to specific physicians' manuals for detailed operation.

Sensor-indicated rates are bounded at the lower end by an LRL, and they are bounded at the upper end by an MSR. Between these two boundaries, the activity sensor signal is converted to a sensor-indicated rate by the rate-response parameters. The paced rate may fluctuate over the entire range in response to varying physical activity. The response parameter determines the sensor-indicated rate that corresponds to a given activity level. Reaction determines how quickly the pacing rate will reach this rate. Recovery defines how slowly the rate will decrease at the conclusion of activity. LRL defines the slowest rate that a device will pace in the absence of intrinsic beats or detected activity. Rate modulation begins at the LRL for all programmed settings. An LRL should be selected that is typical of resting conditions but allows adequate cardiac output while the patient is awake (e.g., 50 to 80 ppm).

MSR defines the fastest rate at which the pacemaker will pace under sensor control. Together the LRL and the MSR

ity levels of patients. In one such study, subjects wore a modified accelerometer and a signal recorder during exercise testing.[46] Results confirmed that accelerometer measurements correlated more closely with oxygen consumption than did measurements taken with other types of activity sensors. In another study, continuous monitoring of subjects for several days showed that the accelerometer closely followed the motion of activities, such as walking, running, climbing stairs, and washing windows.[47] Accelerometer output increased in intensity with increased activity and effectively paralleled physiologic increases in heart rate.

■ ADAPTIVE-RATE ALGORITHMS

Perhaps the most useful and clinically important characteristic of an activity-based, adaptive-rate pacemaker is its ability to provide a prompt pacing response at the onset of physical activity. When physical activity begins, the device can identify the presence of the activity within one pacing cycle and

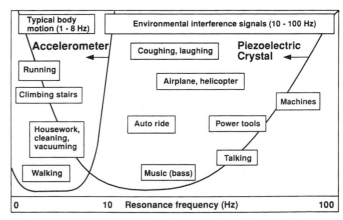

Figure 9–17. The low-filter bandpass of accelerometer technology detects mechanical resonance frequencies associated with typical body motion in the low-frequency range. Environmental signals greater than 8 Hz that can distort rate response are undetected.

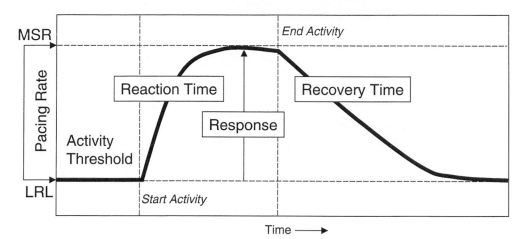

Figure 9–18. Typical adaptive-rate parameters of activity-based pacemakers. Not all activity will generate a paced response to the maximum sensor rate (MSR), but the parameters are referenced to the full range of rates between lower rate limit (LRL) and MSR.

determine the entire range of rate modulation prescribed for the patient. The choice of MSR is based on clinical judgment. The patient's typical activities, the desired heart rate for such activities, and the patient's age and condition are taken into consideration. The sensor drive rate is limited to the MSR setting. Pacing does not increase further, regardless of how strenuous the activity. An MSR is selected that is well tolerated by the patient.

Activity threshold defines the minimum level of detected activity (sensor signal) that must be exceeded before the pacing rate begins to increase above the LRL. In many respects, the activity threshold is analogous to the sensing threshold of conventional pacemakers; only in this case, it refers specifically to the activity sensor signal. An appropriate activity threshold "tunes out" unwanted background noise. Too high a threshold (undersensing) produces a response only to more vigorous body movement, indicated by delayed rate increase after activity begins. Conversely, too low a threshold setting (oversensing) causes the device to respond to minor body movements. This is indicated by inappropriate rate increases when the patient is sitting or standing. An activity threshold setting is used that allows a rate increase with minor activity (such as walking) but that is high enough so that background sources detected when the patient is inactive do not increase the pacing rate. A blunted rate response may indicate too high a threshold setting. In many of the newer devices, this feature automatically tracks typical sensor signals at rest and sets the threshold just above the most frequent vibrations.

Activity sensors typically provide a relatively rapid rate response. How quickly rate changes occur is determined by the reaction parameter. The reaction parameter allows smooth transitions from the current pacing rate to a new, higher, sensor-indicated rate. If the algorithm did not have a reaction factor, the pacing rate would simply parallel the sensor signal, resulting in abrupt rate changes. The parameter prescribes how quickly rate transitions will occur and implements those changes for several cycles until the sensor-indicated rate (or MSR) is achieved or until the detected activity level once again changes.

The response factor determines the sensor-indicated pacing rate that corresponds to the detected level of activity. The response factor acts as a "multiplier," translating the measured motion level into a prescribed pacing rate. The slope of the rate-response factor indicates how much activity is required to reach the higher rate. The physiologic relationship of heart rate to activity is linear, and most current activity devices use linear rate-response algorithms. Rate-response programming is used to provide a proportional response to a large range of activity levels. In some accelerometer-based devices, there is a linear relation between the rectified integrated accelerometer signal and the pacing rate (Fig. 9–19A). Nominal response slopes are provided, and optimal adjustments can be made easily. A sophisticated trending and replay feature allows sensor optimization using the data from a single exercise test. Another accelerometer-based device uses a three-stage relation between the acceleration signal and the pacing rate (see Fig. 9–19B).

The recovery parameter allows the paced rate to return to the lower rate limit at the conclusion of patient activity. To prevent a precipitous drop in pacing rate, recovery acts as a "cool-down" mechanism to mimic normal sinus rate recovery and allow patients to comfortably repay oxygen debt incurred from exercise. As rate decreases, cycle lengths are longer, resulting in a gradual, smooth slowing of heart rate. This process continues until the new lower, sensor-indicated rate, or the LRL if there is no activity, is reached.

When programmed to the VVIR or AAIR mode, the rate arbitration algorithm is simple. As shown in Figure 9–20, the pacing rate increases and decreases according to the output of the activity sensor and the reaction and recovery factors. The adaptive-rate performance of these pacemakers is analogous to continual reprogramming of the lower pacing rate up or down, depending on the activity level of the patient. The pacemaker continues to sense the intrinsic ventricular (or atrial) electrogram and is inhibited by the presence of an intrinsic beat that occurs at a rate faster than the sensor-indicated pacing rate. The minimum and maximum limits of the pacing rate are programmable.

When programmed to the DDDR mode, the adaptive-rate algorithm becomes more complicated (Fig. 9–21). Function in the DDDR mode is similar to that in the AAIR mode in regard to the lower pacing rate, which is continually adjusted by the activity sensor. As with the AAIR mode, sinus rates greater than the sensor-indicated lower rate inhibit the atrial pacing stimulus. As with the normal DDD pacing mode, the

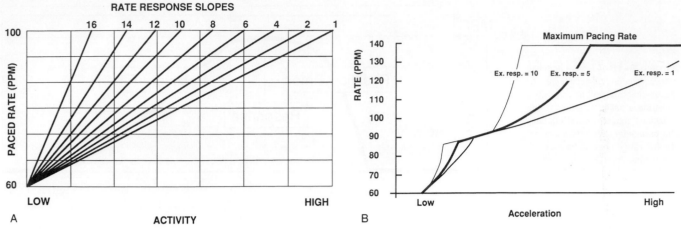

Figure 9–19. Different correlations between activity signals and pacing rate. *A,* A linear relation between activity and rate depending on rate-response slopes is established with Guidant/CPI's accelerometers. *B,* Intermedics' exercise rate-response curves have three stages corresponding to different levels of physical activity used in a "tailor to patient" protocol. (From Alt E, Matula M: Comparison of two activity-controlled, rate-adaptive pacing principles: Acceleration vs. vibration. Cardiol Clin 10:635, 1992.)

device can also pace the ventricle faster than the sensor-indicated lower rate (Fig. 9–22) by tracking intrinsic P waves (atrial synchronous operation). The presence or absence of intrinsic atrioventricular (AV) conduction within the programmed AV delay determines whether the ventricular pacing stimulus is delivered. Currently available DDDR devices can also be programmed to pace at different maximum P-wave tracking and sensor-indicated rates. When the programmed maximum sensor-indicated rate differs from the programmed maximum tracking rate, the device functions in the DDDR mode at rates below the upper tracking limit. At rates above the upper atrial tracking limit, the device functions in the DDIR mode up to the maximum sensor-indicated rate.

Programming the sensor maximum rate higher than the P-wave tracking rate (Fig. 9–23A) has been found to be useful for patients with intermittent atrial fibrillation or flutter to avoid tracking of these arrhythmias while still allowing an appropriately high MSR.[48] Alternatively, the MSR can be set below the maximum P-wave tracking rate (see Fig. 9–23B), which may be helpful for patients who typically have normal chronotropic response during exercise to avoid pacemaker Wenckebach or 2:1 block upper rate behavior. With this combination of settings, the upper sensor-indicated rate is limited, although the sensor can provide backup rate support should pacemaker Wenckebach or 2:1 block occur. The benefits of a DDDR pacemaker that provides this backup support at the upper P-wave tracking limit have been termed *sensor-driven rate smoothing.*[49, 50] Some pacemakers offer DDD rate smoothing with adaptive-rate sensor functions to manage upper rate behaviors. Most modern pacing systems also use mode switching to address atrial tracking automatically in the presence of sensed inappropriately high atrial rates.

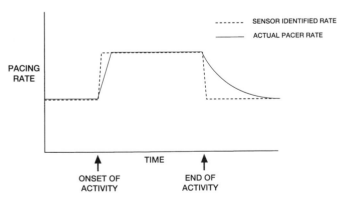

Figure 9–20. The relation between an instantaneously determined sensor rate *(dashed line)* and the actual pacing rate *(solid line)* of an activity sensor. Note that there is a lag between a change in the desired pacing rate and the achievement of an actual change in rate. Acceleration (also termed "reaction") and deceleration (also termed "recovery") time constants smooth the increase and decrease in sensor-indicated pacing rate.

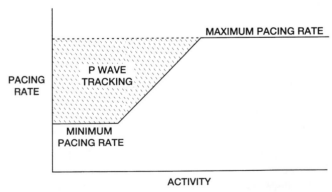

Figure 9–21. The relation between atrial pacing rate indicated by the activity sensor and normal P-wave tracking in a DDDR pacemaker. The lower pacing rate is effectively increased by the sensor up to the programmed maximum sensor-indicated rate. If the P-wave rate exceeds the lower pacing rate indicated by the sensor, normal tracking will occur.

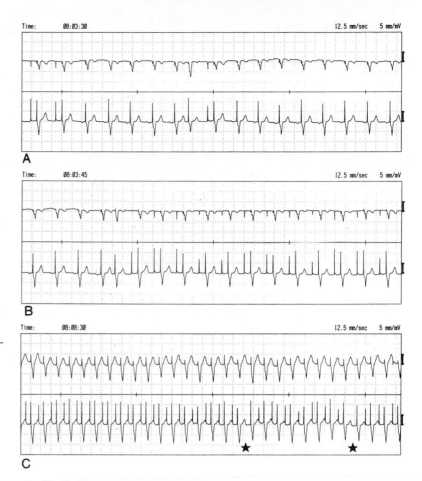

Figure 9–22. Normal DDDR pacemaker function over a range of atrial rates. As with a normal AAIR pacemaker, sinus rates greater than the sensor-indicated lower rate inhibit the atrial pacing stimulus. However, a DDD pacing system also paces the ventricle faster than the sensor-indicated lower rate *(A)* by tracking intrinsic P waves. Whether the ventricular pacing stimulus is delivered is determined by the presence or absence of intrinsic atrioventricular (AV) conduction within the programmed AV delay. When the activity sensor indicates that the lower pacing rate should be increased above the intrinsic atrial rate *(B)*, atrial pacing stimuli are delivered. At rates above the upper atrial tracking limit, the device functions in the DDIR mode up to the maximum sensor-indicated rate *(stars)*.

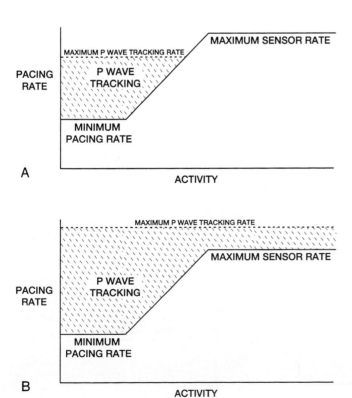

Figure 9–23. Separation of maximum sensor rate and maximum P-wave tracking rates. In *A*, the maximum sensor rate may exceed the maximum P-wave tracking rate. Such a programming scheme may prevent tracking of paroxysmal atrial tachyarrhythmias without limiting the maximum pacing rate that can be achieved with exercise. In *B*, the maximum P-wave tracking rate is programmed to a greater value than the maximum sensor rate. Such a programmed combination may be useful to avoid inappropriate sensor-indicated rates in patients with relatively intact sinus node function.

■ CLINICAL RESULTS

Piezoelectric Vibration

Several important clinical advantages of piezoelectric vibration-based, adaptive-rate pacemakers were enumerated earlier. From a physiologic perspective, however, their principal strength lies in the fact that they are inherently capable of providing a prompt response to activity signals of relatively low amplitude over a wide range of frequencies. On the other hand, piezoelectric-based pacemakers may be more susceptible to nonphysiologic vibrations, such as those accompanying riding in a motor vehicle or using heavy machinery. Additionally, these sensors may vary considerably in the chronotropic response observed with different types of physical activity despite comparable metabolic workloads.[27, 51] For example, walking on a soft surface may induce a lower increase in heart rate than would be observed with the same rate of walking on a hard surface. Finally, piezoelectric vibration-based pacemakers are not capable of physiologic rate adaptation in the presence of emotional upset or fever (in the absence of shivering) or in anticipation of physical exercise. On balance, however, clinical studies have convincingly demonstrated that piezoelectric vibration-based pacing systems offer the potential for greater exercise capacity and fewer exertionally related symptoms than do fixed-rate (VVI) pacemakers. The clearest evidence of this benefit has been provided by exercise laboratory studies measuring both cardiopulmonary indices and the perception of exertion.

In an early clinical study of a piezoelectric vibration-based, adaptive-rate pacemaker, Benditt and colleagues[52] compared exercise tolerance during fixed-rate VVI pacing with that in VVIR pacing using cardiopulmonary treadmill exercise. Adaptive-rate pacing prolonged exercise duration by 35% and led to similar improvements in peak observed oxygen consumption and oxygen consumption at anaerobic threshold (Fig. 9–24). Adaptive-rate pacing also reduced the patient's perception of exertion at comparable exercise levels[53] (Fig. 9–25). In a subset of the same patients, it was demonstrated that the improved performance with VVIR pacing was sustained when exercise testing was repeated after an average of 5 months of follow-up (Fig. 9–26).[54] Furthermore, at the time of follow-up exercise testing, reversion of the pacing system to a fixed rate (VVI) mode resulted in prompt deterioration of both observed oxygen consumption and exercise duration. Thus, the ability of a single-chamber piezoelectric vibration-based pacing system to provide immediate and long-term improvements in exercise tolerance was clearly demonstrated.

Others have also reported improved exercise capacity with adaptive-rate pacemakers based on activity sensors, although the results from studies using bicycle exercise have been less dramatic than those observed with treadmill exercise.[16, 55–57] For example, Smedgard and coworkers[16] reported a 10% improvement. Alt and associates[56] demonstrated a 6% improvement in exercise capacity with activity-based VVIR pacemakers compared with VVI pacing with bicycle exercise testing.

Buckingham and colleagues[57] used treadmill exercise testing to examine the impact of ventricular function on exercise responses of 16 patients with piezoelectric vibration-based, adaptive-rate pacemakers in the VVI and the VVIR modes. The findings clearly indicated that the provision of appropriate heart rate responsiveness by this technique resulted in a substantial increase in cardiac index that was independent of left ventricular systolic function (i.e., baseline ejection fraction). Whether diastolic function is helpful in predicting which patients might be more likely to benefit from chrono-

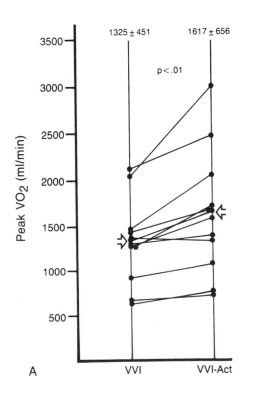

A

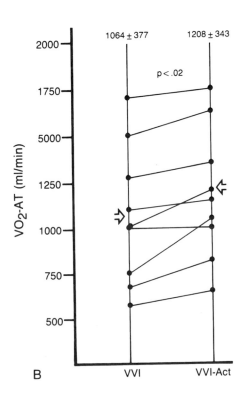

B

Figure 9–24. Effect of the VVIR pacing mode (labeled VVI-Act) on peak oxygen uptake ($\dot{V}O_2$) and oxygen uptake at anaerobic threshold ($\dot{V}O_2$-AT) with an activity-controlled pacing system. Note improvements in oxygen consumption with the VVIR pacing mode compared with the VVI mode. (From Benditt DG, Mianulli M, Fetter J, et al: Single-chamber cardiac pacing with activity-initiated chronotropic response: Evaluation by cardiopulmonary exercise testing. Circulation 75:184, 1987. Copyright © 1987 by the American Heart Association.)

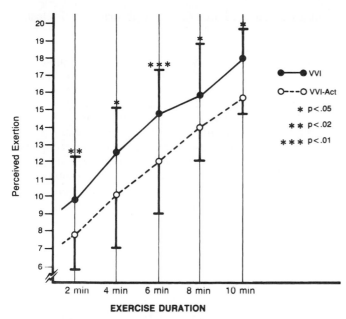

Figure 9–25. Effect of rate modulation provided by an activity-sensing VVIR pacing system on the perception of effort during exercise. Note that the perceived level of exertion was lower in the VVIR (VVI-Act) pacing mode than in the VVI mode at all stages of exercise. (From Benditt DG, Milstein S, Buetikofer J, et al: Sensor-triggered rate-variable cardiac pacing: Current technologies and clinical implications. Ann Intern Med 107:714–724, 1987.)

tropic responsiveness was not examined. However, Lau and Camm[58] were unable to predict the potential hemodynamic benefits of adaptive-rate pacing in 22 patients using echocardiographic techniques to estimate left ventricular systolic and diastolic function.

Although the benefits of activity-based VVIR pacing are well established compared with those of fixed-rate ventricu-

lar pacing, the VVIR pacing mode has also been compared with atrial-tracking, dual-chamber pacing modes (VDD, DDD). Menozzi and colleagues[59] compared the DDD and VVIR pacing modes in a crossover study using a dual-chamber, activity-based pacemaker that offered selection of both pacing modes. The pacemakers were programmed alternatively to VVIR or DDD for 6-week periods. Qualitative measures of symptomatic status, noninvasive estimates of cardiac output, and exercise capacity were evaluated. Not surprisingly, exercise tolerance was similar with the two modes (VVIR, 68 ± 15 W/min versus DDD, 70 ± 18 W/min). In this study, the DDD mode was clearly preferred from a symptom perspective, suggesting the importance of AV synchrony from a quality-of-life viewpoint.

In contrast to these results, Oldroyd and colleagues[60] found no significant difference between the DDD and VVIR modes with respect to symptom scores, maximal exercise performance (treadmill), or plasma concentrations of epinephrine, norepinephrine, and atrial natriuretic peptide (a finding disputed by Blanc and associates[61]). Furthermore, only one patient requested early reversion to the DDD mode from VVIR pacing, the only patient with intact retrograde conduction. Surprisingly, venous epinephrine and norepinephrine levels were not reported to be higher during exercise in the VVIR mode, as might have been expected given comparable exercise levels.

The findings of Oldroyd and colleagues[60] have been more recently echoed by those of Linde-Edelstam and associates.[62] In their study, two activity-based VVIR and DDDR pacemakers were used to compare the DDD and VVIR pacing modes. Cardiac output at rest tended to be higher with DDD than with VVIR pacing. However, right atrial and pulmonary capillary wedge pressures, coronary sinus blood flow, coronary sinus arteriovenous O_2 difference, and myocardial oxygen consumption did not differ between these pacing modes.

In summary, piezoelectric vibration-based VVIR pacemakers provide significant improvement in exercise capacity compared with fixed-rate VVI pacing. Additionally, exercise

Figure 9–26. In a subset of the same patients shown in Figure 9–25 at the time of follow-up exercise testing, reversion of the pacing system to the VVI mode resulted in prompt deterioration of observed oxygen consumption ($S\bar{V}O_2$) compared with VVIR pacing. (From Buetikofer J, Milstein S, Mianulli M, et al: Sustained improvement in exercise duration, rate pressure product and peak oxygen consumption with activity-initiated rate-variable pacing. In Belhassen B, Feldman S, Copperman Y [eds]: Cardiac Pacing and Electrophysiology: Proceedings of the VIIIth World Symposium on Cardiac Pacing and Electrophysiology. Tel Aviv, R & L Creative Communications, 1987, pp 53–59.)

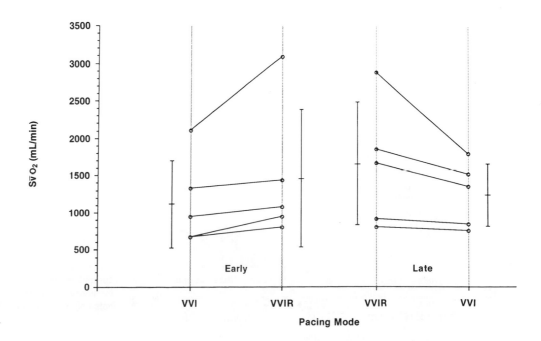

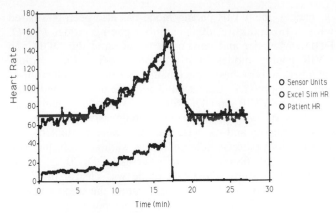

Figure 9–27. The results of treadmill testing an elderly subject according to the Chronotropic Assessment Exercise Protocol (CAEP). The piezoresistive accelerometer system strapped to the chest generated a paced rate that is comparable to the intrinsic rate for various speeds and elevations of the treadmill. The piezoresistive accelerometer shows a proportionately small rate response for small incremental levels of exercise.

tolerance with the VVIR mode is essentially equivalent to that with DDD pacing in many patients. In certain cases (particularly patients susceptible to "pacemaker syndrome"), however, dual-chamber pacemakers are clearly better tolerated. Additionally, dual-chamber pacing may offer other potential advantages, including preservation of atrial electric stability (i.e., a lower incidence of atrial fibrillation) and a lower incidence of congestive heart failure. Although the VVIR pacing mode offers similar exercise capacity compared with DDD pacing, the DDDR or AAIR pacing mode may be preferable for most patients with chronotropic incompetence who require a permanent pacemaker because of the inherent advantages of AV synchrony. Nevertheless, patients with chronic atrial fibrillation and impaired AV conduction remain excellent candidates for activity-based VVIR pacemakers.

Accelerometers

Because accelerometer-based adaptive-rate pacing systems have been clinically introduced only recently, fewer studies have been performed with them than with piezoelectric vibrational devices. Lau and colleagues[63] compared the behavior of accelerometer-based devices with that of piezoelectric crystal devices and reported that the accelerometer showed a better response to walking, jogging, and standing. They also observed that the subject's footwear had no significant effect on the results seen with the accelerometer, as opposed to the results obtained with vibrational piezoelectric devices. Increasing grade of the treadmill had a significant effect on pacing rate with the accelerometer device, whereas there was no change in pacing rate with the piezoelectric vibrational sensors. These investigators concluded that, compared with the vibrational device, the accelerometer sensor-controlled devices showed a more adequate rate response and were less susceptible to direct pressure or to tapping on the pulse generator. From visual inspection of the linear behavior of the sensor during exercise (see Fig. 9–8), it is evident that rate adaptation based on the accelerometer's signals provides an excellent basis for mimicking the natural heart rate response in many patients.

Figure 9–27 shows the results of treadmill testing an elderly subject according to the Chronotropic Assessment Exercise Protocol (CAEP). The CAEP test was designed to provide small incremental work rates that approximate typical daily activities of pacemaker patients. The piezoresistive accelerometer-based pacemaker strapped to the chest generated a paced rate that compared favorably to the subject's intrinsic rate for various speeds and grades of the treadmill.[64] The piezoresistive accelerometer also showed proportionately small changes in pacing rate for small incremental levels of exercise.

Bacharach and associates[36] (Fig. 9–28) found that the response of the accelerometer to graded treadmill testing was more strongly correlated with the patient's intrinsic heart rate ($r = 0.80$) than that of a vibrational adaptive-rate device ($r = 0.27$). They also compared the response of walking up and down stairs using a piezoresistive accelerometer device and a vibrational piezoelectric pacemaker (Fig. 9–29) with the intrinsic sinus rate in 10 elderly subjects. The accelerometer responded appropriately when subjects walked upstairs (103 ppm) and walked downstairs (98 ppm). The response of the vibrational devices was paradoxical, with a slower pacing rate when subjects walked upstairs (83 ppm) than when they walked downstairs (89 ppm).

Recent studies[34, 35] compared the response of an accelerometer with a vibrational device during treadmill exercises involving increasing and decreasing speed and grade. To avoid bias of the results by using different settings, the researchers calibrated the strapped-on pacemakers for six

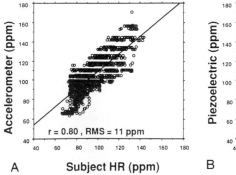

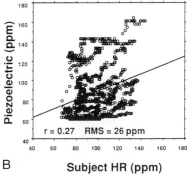

Figure 9–28. *A,* Clinical results obtained with CPI's Excel accelerometer-based adaptive-rate system. The heart rate of chronotropically competent patients was compared with the calculated pacing rate obtained from an externally strapped-on device. The correlation was found to be $r = 0.80$; the average rate variation noted by the root mean square (RMS) was 11 ppm. *B,* The performance of the vibrational device during treadmill testing was more variable. This variation depended on the individual subject. As a result, the correlation coefficient for the piezoelectric device rate and the intrinsic heart rate was 0.27; the average rate variation noted by the RMS was 26 bpm.

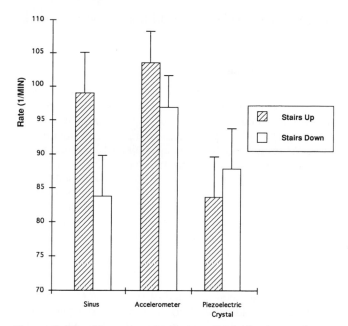

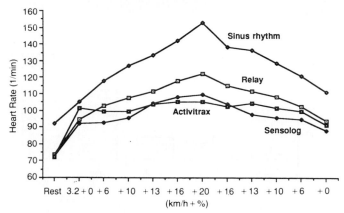

Figure 9–31. Response of accelerometer and vibrational devices to constant speed with increasing and decreasing slopes. The vibrational devices show little reaction to increasing workloads resulting from increasing slopes on a treadmill. The accelerometer corresponds more closely to the change in workload resulting from varied slopes. (From Alt E, Matula M: Comparison of two activity-controlled, rate-adaptive pacing principles: Acceleration vs. vibration. Cardiol Clin 10:635, 1992.)

Figure 9–29. Strap-on accelerometer and piezoelectric crystal vibrational sensor response to stair climbing. The accelerometer's response parallels the subject's intrinsic responses to stair climbing and descent, respectively. The piezoelectric crystal shows a paradoxical response to intrinsic rate, similar to clinical experience and published reports.

patients and six healthy subjects using identical methods. The basic pacing rate in each subject and patient was set to 70 ppm, and the individual systems were tailored to a response of 95 ppm with a treadmill speed of 2 mph and 0% grade. The sinus rate of the six subjects was recorded continuously as a reference. The treadmill protocol[65] represented a smooth and constant increase and decrease in the workload (Fig. 9–30). The accelerometer pacing rate correlated well with the natural sinus rhythm, responding not only to an increase in speed but also to an increase in grade during the entire protocol. In a second test, the effect of increasing and decreasing grade was studied at a constant

treadmill speed (Fig. 9–31). The accelerometer showed a more desirable behavior than that of vibrational devices. The correlation of sinus rate with treadmill grade was high (r = 0.97). The accelerometer device was close to this rate and produced a more appropriate response (r = 0.90) than the Activitrax (r = 0.52) or the Sensolog (r = 0.87).

Accelerometer systems typically demonstrate appropriate rate response with light changes in typical activities of daily living. In the European clinical evaluation of a piezoresistive accelerometer system (EXCEL VR, Guidant, St. Paul, MN), small changes in paced rate response were noted with postural changes: supine (3 ± 2 ppm), sitting (7 ± 3 ppm), standing (10 ± 5 ppm), slow walk (29 ± 9 ppm), and brisk walk (44 ± 11 ppm)[66] (Fig. 9–32).

In another study, Erdelitsch-Reiser and associates[67] administered a clinical protocol to observe the adaptive-rate response of an implanted piezoresistive accelerometer in seven patients during typical daily activities and incremental

Figure 9–30. Comparison of a strap-on accelerometer (Relay) with vibrational devices (Sensolog and Activitrax). All three devices were individually calibrated to the same basic conditions. The pacing rate at rest was set to 70 ppm, and the individual rate response was tailored to obtain a rate of 95 ppm with an initial treadmill walking speed of 2.0 mph at a 0% grade. The paced response of the accelerometer with increasing and decreasing work rate closely follows the natural sinus rhythm. At rest, the sinus rate was about 20 beats above the pacemaker-indicated resting rate of 70 ppm. This difference in paced to natural heart rate continued throughout the trial. (From Alt E, Matula M: Comparison of two activity-controlled, rate-adaptive pacing principles: Acceleration vs. vibration. Cardiol Clin 10:635, 1992.)

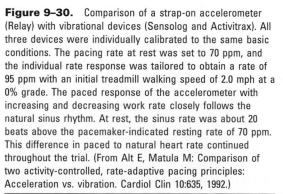

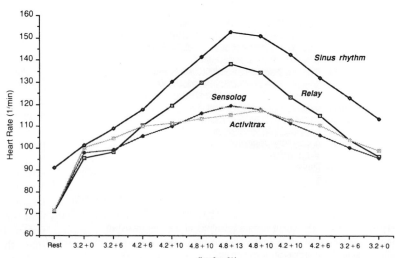

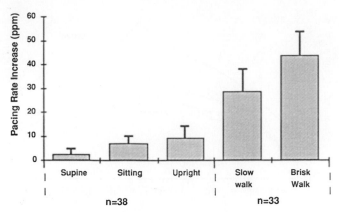

Figure 9–32. In the European clinical evaluation of patients with an implanted piezoresistive accelerometer system (CPI's Excel VR), appropriate changes in paced rate response were noted with postural changes and slow and brisk walks.

exercise on a treadmill. Mean pacing rates (Fig. 9–33) were 50 ppm (supine), 56 ppm (standing), 77 ppm (descending stairs), 81 ppm (slow walk), 83 ppm (slow stair climb), 91 ppm (fast walk), and 92 ppm (fast stair climb). When the arm proximal to the pulse generator was used for window washing, the rate rose to 87 ppm. When the opposite arm was used, the rate was 63 ppm. During treadmill testing, rates between 82 ppm (1.2 mph) and 104 ppm (3 mph) were observed. These investigators concluded that the device provided a proportional response to graded activities of treadmill exercise and daily living.

Clinical utility for an accelerometer-based system was demonstrated in several aspects of the VIGOR DR clinical trial for the US Food and Drug Administration. Analysis of paired cardiopulmonary exercise testing demonstrated that chronotropically incompetent patients are provided an important benefit with a statistically significant improvement in functional capacity (oxygen uptake and anaerobic threshold), heart rate, and exercise duration. These data were supplemented with activities of daily living, Holter monitoring data, and quality-of-life data that demonstrated the device to

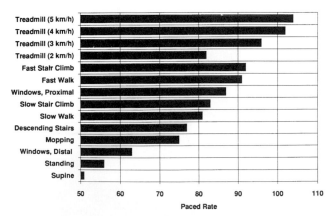

Figure 9–33. The adaptive-rate response of the piezoresistive accelerometer implanted in seven patients during typical daily activities and incremental exercise on a treadmill.

provide appropriate therapy, which positively affects patients' mental and physical well-being.[68]

Bicycle Exercise

Piezoelectric vibrational pacemakers typically are less responsive to bicycle exercise than to treadmill exercise because of the reduced upper body activity with bicycle ergometry, especially with stationary ergometers. Figure 9–34 shows the results with a strapped-on piezoelectric accelerometer-based pacemaker during stationary bicycle ergometry and compares the generated rate with the sinus rate seen in the same subjects with the same kind of activity. Bicycling on the street produced higher pacing rates than were observed on the stationary bicycle.

In a comparative evaluation[36] of the piezoresistive accelerometer system and a vibrational piezoelectric system during bicycle ergometry, rate responses of strapped-on devices were compared with the intrinsic response seen in 10 elderly subjects. The protocol consisted of two parts: (1) a progressively higher workload with constant revolutions per minute, and (2) a constant workload with progressively higher revolutions per minute. Although the accelerometer pacemaker did not achieve the intrinsic rate, it generated a significantly higher pacing rate than did the piezoelectric vibrational pacemaker during all stages of the cycling tasks (Fig. 9–35).

Potential for Atypical or Undesired Responses

In general, the peak counting and integration piezoelectric vibration configurations behave similarly in terms of their response to movement or vibration.[51] As a result, both may provide inappropriate heart rate responses when subjected to environmental vibrations, such as those induced by the movement of a motor vehicle over rough terrain or those resulting from air travel or the use of appliances or machinery. These pacemakers also respond to the application of static pressure on the pulse generator. Because static focal pressure on the posterior surface of the pacemaker case produces sensor deformation, an inappropriate pacing rate increase can occur in this situation. This can happen when a patient is sleeping or when the pulse generator is implanted directly over a rib. Respiratory movement of the rib cage can result in periodic pressure on the posterior surface of the pacemaker case, particularly in thin patients or when the device is implanted in a subpectoral location. This false-positive response to pressure is less of a problem with pacemakers that incorporate an accelerometer.[19]

Pacemaker-induced tachycardias caused by position are clearly undesirable in sleeping patients. On the other hand, in certain cases the heart rate increase associated with vehicular movement, rough air travel, or use of heavy machinery may prove to be appropriate despite the fact that nonphysiologic physical movement induces it rather than emotional stress. For instance, in a report by Matula and colleagues[69] the effects of various means of locomotion on pacing rate were assessed for different activity-based pacemakers. Three different activity-based pacing systems (peak detector, integration type, and accelerometer) were strapped to the chests of volunteers. Bicycling on the street resulted in higher pacing rates than did stationary bicycling for each type of pacemaker, although none of the pacemakers reached the heart

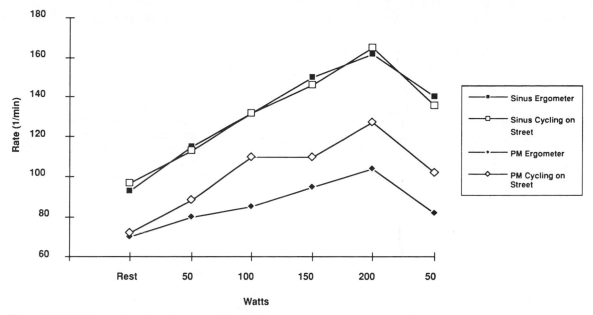

Figure 9–34. Comparison of pacing rate and intrinsic heart rate with bicycling on a stationary ergometer and on the street. Although the sinus rate of the subject with the strap-on device is the same with street cycling and bicycle ergometry, the accelerometer responds better to cycling on the street than to stationary ergometry; however, the paced rate is still below the sinus rate. PM, pacemaker. (From Alt E, Matula M: Comparison of two activity-controlled, rate-adaptive pacing principles: Acceleration vs. vibration. Cardiol Clin 10:635, 1992.)

rate achieved by the normal sinus node. During driving, the pacemakers increased the pacing rate, although the intrinsic sinus rate continued to be higher. In passively riding passengers, the pacemakers tended to produce a higher pacing rate than that of the normal sinus node. Of interest, the accelerometer-based system responded mainly to acceleration and curves, whereas vibration sensors responded primarily to vibrations and rough roads.

An additional category of potentially undesirable heart rate responses associated with piezoelectric vibration-based pacing systems may be the responses resulting from the particular characteristics of an exercise or the manner in which physical exertion is performed. As noted earlier, the responsiveness of the devices may be affected by factors such as the softness of the patient's shoes or the nature of the terrain. Additionally, piezoelectric vibration-based pace-

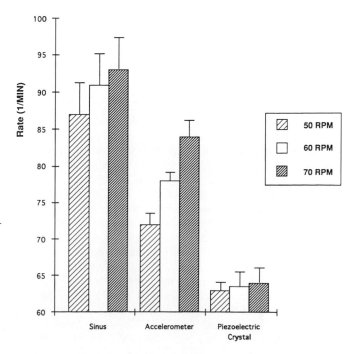

Figure 9–35. Comparison of pacing rate and intrinsic heart rate with bicycling on a stationary ergometer. Constant work rate with various pedaling speeds. In general, the piezoresistive accelerometer device generated about half the rate response of the intrinsic heart rate (HR), whereas the piezoelectric-based vibrational pacemaker provided only a moderate response in both cases.

makers have been shown to manifest paradoxically slower heart rates during walking uphill than during walking downhill. This appears to be related to the fact that activity sensors respond to heel strike frequency. Although the workload is higher walking uphill, the incline results in a slower walking rate and a lower heel strike frequency than walking downhill. The apparently poor performance of vibration-based systems during stationary bicycle exercise may be less important because when actual street bicycling is undertaken, additional vibrations associated with movement occur.[69]

Despite the potential for undesirable or nonphysiologic pacing responses, piezoelectric vibration-based, adaptive-rate pacemakers serve most patient well. For example, in a recent study involving everyday activities (such as walking, climbing stairs, and mental stress), piezoelectric vibration-based, adaptive-rate pacemakers proved sensitive during light physical exertion and compared favorably with respiratory-based and QT-based pacemakers.[70] When false-positive responses are detected, simple noninvasive programming steps usually alleviate the problem.[27]

Potential for Combination With Other Sensors

Despite the widespread popularity of activity sensors, there has been considerable interest in devising a more physiologic pacing system by combining two or more sensors. This strategy may balance the advantages and disadvantages of various technologies to optimize overall performance. In this regard, the sensitivity of activity sensors in detecting the onset of physical exertion and responding rapidly is unsurpassed. On the other hand, activity sensors are relatively unresponsive to many other conditions that call for increased heart rate, such as emotional stress, and may not be optimal for sustained physical activity. Consequently, the use of activity sensors in combination with more slowly responsive sensors has become the subject of both investigational interest and clinical application.

Informal Testing for Establishing Optimal Programming

Clinical experience with exercise testing for adjusting the rate-modulating parameters of piezoelectric and accelerometer-based pacemakers is extensive. In many cases, an informal approach is adequate. This may entail having the patient walk briefly at various rates on a flat surface and then proceed up and down several flights of stairs. During this evaluation, the pacing rate should be monitored by an attendant or through diagnostics of the device. After appropriate reprogramming, informal exercise can be repeated. The attendant can also assess the patient's level of fatigue and other symptoms. For patients with newer versions of piezoelectric or accelerometer-based pacemakers, rate histograms[71] or rate versus time recordings can be used effectively for the purpose of assessing rate response. The rate versus time, or "event recorder," feature monitors the rate response of the pacemaker during exercise testing (Fig. 9–36). With this feature, a beat-for-beat record of the pacing rate is documented through the programmer to assess sensor response during physical exercise. Newer systems allow input of a target rate and automatically determine the re-

quired rate-response settings to achieve the target. The attendant may then elect to program the recommended settings.

As an alternative to walking and stair climbing, a series of stationary exercises that are more suitable to the clinic environment can be used. Benditt and associates[72] compared the pacing rates of strapped-on and implanted adaptive-rate pacemakers during arm movement, walk-in-place exercise, and treadmill exercise. The findings indicated that the stationary exercise procedures could provide a useful assessment of rate response without the need to resort to formal exercise testing. Further studies have validated the use of strap-on piezoelectric or accelerometer-based adaptive-rate pacemakers to reproduce the pacing rate response of comparable implanted devices.[72a]

Moura and colleagues[73] also found such an approach useful in comparing the rate response of a piezoelectric sensor-based pacemaker with the response of the sinus node in control subjects. A crucial factor in selecting the appropriate programmed settings of an adaptive-rate pacemaker is an understanding of the range of heart rates that should be expected for a given form of exercise. Hayes and colleagues[71, 74] provided these data for normal subjects during casual or brisk walking. Mianulli and associates[75] have similarly examined the heart rate responses of normal subjects across a broad range of ages, based on ambulatory monitoring data during activities of daily living. As a result, the basic information with which to adjust pacemakers is now available in the clinic.[73, 76] This heart rate histogram data is the basis of an automatic-rate response algorithm that automatically adjusts rate-response parameters for a dual-sensor (piezoelectric and minute ventilation) pacemaker to achieve target histogram profiles.[76a]

Comparison of Activity Sensor Responses With Other Adaptive-Rate Pacing System Sensors

The basic goal of an optimal adaptive-rate pacing system is to provide a normal heart rate during a wide range of activities, from sleep to vigorous physical exercise. In this regard, the optimal adaptive-rate sensor should provide (1) a heart rate that is proportional to metabolic workload; (2) an appropriately rapid change in heart rate in response to a variable workload; (3) a high degree of sensitivity and specificity for exercise; and (4) an appropriate slowing of heart rate after exercise. McElroy and colleagues[77] have demonstrated a linear relationship between heart rate and oxygen consumption during exercise in normal volunteers and in patients with varying degrees of cardiac impairment.

Lau and associates[27] examined the heart rate–oxygen consumption relationship for six adaptive-rate pacing systems, including two with early activity sensors. They observed reasonable correlations between pacing rate and oxygen consumption for both activity-based pacing systems; thus, it can be concluded that these devices appear to perform well despite the reported perception of them as "nonphysiologic." It is true that piezoelectric vibration-based pacemakers appear to lack ideal proportionality with metabolic workload during treadmill exercise. Therefore, as pointed out by Lau and associates,[27] the Activitrax and the Sensolog failed to increase heart rate appropriately as treadmill *grade* was increased from 0% to 15% when the speed of walking

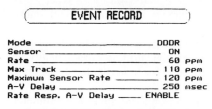

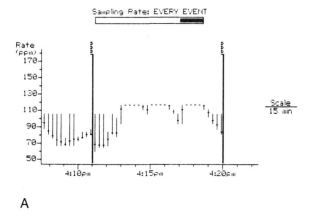

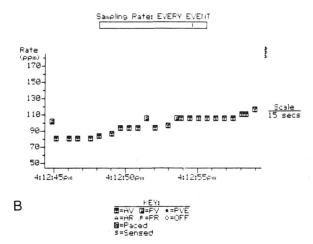

A

B

Figure 9–36. Examples of a rate trend *(A)* with a DDDR pacing system. Note that this device is programmed to log every pacing event, allowing the clinician to determine the pacing rate during a known period of time. In *B*, the pulse generator stores and displays the sequence of pacing and sensing over a brief period. AV, atrial pacing followed by ventricular pacing; PV, intrinsic P wave followed by ventricular pacing; AR, atrial pacing followed by intrinsic atrioventricular conduction; PR, intrinsic P wave followed by intrinsic atrioventricular conduction.

remained constant (2.5 miles/hr). In contrast, Stangl and colleagues[26] observed a better correlation between pacing rate and metabolic workload for the Sensolog. Whereas increments in treadmill speed (heel strike frequency) routinely increase the pacing rate in both piezoelectric-based systems, a steeper grade does not necessarily result in an appropriate chronotropic response. Attention to device programming can largely obviate this limitation of piezoelectric vibration-based sensors.

In addition to a proportional relationship between workload and heart rate, the speed of onset of a sensor may be important for maximizing exercise tolerance. Lau and colleagues[27] examined exercise responses during walking and found that piezoelectric vibrational pacemakers best corresponded with the rate of the sinus node in normal subjects. Not unexpectedly, the onset of an increased pacing rate was almost immediate in patients with activity-based systems and was considerably faster than that observed with adaptive-rate pacemakers based on minute ventilation, right ventricular pressure, or the QT interval.

In early piezoelectric vibration-based, adaptive-rate pacing systems, the heart rate decay after termination of exercise occurred more quickly than that observed with other sensors. This problem has been essentially eliminated, however, in the newer generations of these devices with the development of programmable recovery curves (see previous discussion). As a rule, physically active patients should have their pacemakers programmed to relatively long recovery times. These

values permit the heart rate to remain elevated for an extended time during exercise recovery, thereby accounting for needs associated with re-equilibration of thermoregulatory status after vigorous exercise.

The specificity and sensitivity of adaptive-rate pacing systems for detection of various physical or emotional maneuvers is variable. Activity-based sensors are probably best for rapid detection of physical activity. These sensors, however, are incapable of detecting emotional stress, such as that induced by mental arithmetic. In a direct comparison of an implanted minute ventilation sensor with an externally strapped-on, piezoelectric vibration-based pacemaker, Lau and associates[78] found that for relatively low levels of physical exercise, both pacemakers resulted in adequate heart rate responses. For more strenuous activities, however, the piezoelectric-based pacemaker appeared to be less adequate with respect to maximum pacing rate, although the onset of response with the activity sensor was clearly faster. These findings support the potential utility of combining activity-based systems with minute ventilation sensing.

■ ALTERNATE USES FOR ACCELEROMETER SENSORS

Piezoelectric and accelerometer-based sensors have potential uses beyond providing basic adaptive-rate pacing therapy. Studying the characteristics of sensor response over time will indicate patterns of response indicative of circadian rhythms and changes in general patient status. Bornzin and colleagues[79] explored the utility of monitoring accelerometer variance continuously as an indicator of diurnal variation and proposed an algorithm to automatically identify periods of time appropriate for lowering lower pacing rate coincident with sleep periods.

The utility of a uniaxial microaccelerometer within a lead indwelling within the right ventricle has been explored by Rickards and associates[80] as an indicator of myocardial function. Their study indicated a good correlation between peak endocardial acceleration and changes in right ventricular maximum change in pressure (dP/dt) as measured by a catheter-tip micromanometer. Dobutamine infusion was used as a means of changing myocardial contractility. These authors proposed that peak endocardial acceleration might be used to control adaptive-rate pacing therapy or offer potential diagnostic applications in the chronic monitoring of heart failure.

■ OTHER GENERAL BODY MOTION SENSORS

Several additional sensors that measure attributes of general body motion in a similar manner to piezoelectric crystals and accelerometer have been used clinically to implement adaptive-rate pacemaker systems. Clinical results have been reported for an adaptive-rate pacing system using the kinetic energy generated by a moving magnetic ball.[81] The sensor is composed of a magnetic ball surrounded by a copper wire coil within the metal housing of the pacemaker. Movement of the magnetic ball in any of three dimensions generates an electrical signal, which is converted into a cardiac pacing rate. The investigators noted improved patient response to treadmill exercise and improvements in exercise time, distance traveled, and $\dot{V}O_2$ maximum during adaptive-rate pacing when compared with fixed-rate pacing. Clinical results[82] have also been published for an adaptive-rate pacemaker system that uses a gravitational acceleration sensor to detect vertical movement of the center of gravity of a mercury ball. Displacement of the mercury ball during exercise modulates an electrical contact. The frequency of contact disturbance creates a signal; frequencies below 5 Hz have been shown to be specific for ambulatory motion. Five programmable slopes are available for rate increase and decrease.

Comparisons of various activity sensors have been studied recently. Candings and colleagues[83] compared adaptive-rate pacing in vibration-based, accelerometer-based, gravitational-based, and movement-based devices during a variety of activities. The gravitational sensor consists of a hermetically sealed cylinder containing a drop of mercury and a central switch. Detected movements of mercury measure "gravimeteric accelerations" that are used to determine rate-responsive pacing. The movement-based sensor mechanism is based on the movements of a magnetic ball within an ellipsoid housing. The authors report that accelerometer-based responsive pacemakers behaved more physiologically. They did not show a marked rate decline while walking uphill or over stimulation while walking downhill as compared to the first- (vibration based) or third-generation (body movement or gravitational based) devices. Overall, the accelerometer-based pacemaker simulated or paralleled sinus rate behavior the most closely.

Summary

Piezoelectric vibration-based sensors were used in the first clinically successful adaptive-rate pacemakers and have been the most thoroughly evaluated sensors in terms of patient benefit. These types of sensors have opened the door to a whole new aspect of "physiologic" cardiac pacing and remain the most widely used of all artificial sensors. They have advantages of simplicity, reliability, and compatibility with all standard pacing leads.

The new generation of accelerometer-based devices overcomes most of the limitations of vibrational piezoelectric devices. Because of their sensitivity to body movements in the anteroposterior direction and their constant coupling mass, their response to graded treadmill exercise and walking up and down stairs is more reflective of the true energy expenditure of these activities. The filter characteristics that limit the sensitivity of the accelerometer to signals below 8 Hz enable the device to discriminate more accurately between true physical activity and noise stemming from machines or from other environmental sources.[40]

Because the accelerometer is incorporated into the hybrid circuit board rather than attached to the pacemaker housing, susceptibility to direct pressure and tapping on the pacemaker is reduced significantly compared with that of piezoelectric crystal devices (Fig. 9–37). This is of practical importance for patients who lie on their chest during sleep, compressing the pacemaker case.

Although the accelerometer, like the piezoelectric vibration-based sensor, is a nonmetabolic sensor, the accurate detection of movement and proportional response of the accelerometer form the basis for simple, reliable algorithms that result in excellent chronotropic response and ease of use.

Truly metabolic adaptive-rate pacemakers of the future might incorporate a combination of an accelerometer with another sensor, such as minute ventilation, temperature, or QT interval, as suggested in earlier reports.[84–87] In addition, more sophisticated algorithms will help to create even better performance by activity-based pacemakers. With increased clinical use, the accelerometer may become the standard

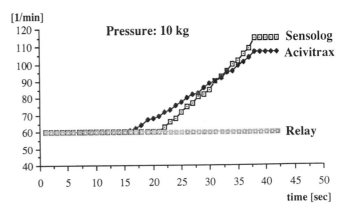

Figure 9–37. Application of 10 kg of pressure resulted in an increase in pacing rate with Activitrax and Sensolog in an in vitro laboratory trial. The accelerometer-based pacemaker (Relay) showed no sensitivity to externally applied pressure. (From Alt E, Matula M: Comparison of two activity-controlled, rate-adaptive pacing principles: Acceleration vs. vibration. Cardiol Clin 10:635, 1992.)

sensor for pacemakers and defibrillators offering accurate, reliable, and predictable rate adaptation as one of many programmable features within a multiprogrammable device.

ACKNOWLEDGMENTS

The authors wish to credit Eckhard Alt, Jan Pieter Heemels, Marcus Mianulli, David G. Benditt, and James L. Duncan for their contribution to the "Activity-Sensing, Rate-Adaptive Pacemakers" and "Accelerometers" chapters in preparation for publication of the first edition of this book.

REFERENCES

1. Rickards AF, Donaldson RM: Rate-responsive pacing. Clin Prog Pacing Electrophysiol 1:12, 1983.
2. Benditt DG, Milstein S, Buetikofer J, et al: Sensor-triggered, rate-variable cardiac pacing: Current technologies and clinical implications. Ann Intern Med 107:714, 1987.
3. Alt E, Matula M, Theres H, et al: The basis for activity controlled rate variable cardiac pacemakers: An analysis of mechanical forces on the human body induced by exercise and environment. PACE 12:1667, 1989.
4. Krasner JL, Voukidis PC, Nardella PC: A physiologically controlled cardiac pacemaker. J Assoc Advanced Med Instrument 1:14, 1966.
5. Funke HD: Ein Herzschrittmacher mit Belastungsabhängiger Frequenzregulation. Biomed Technik 20:225, 1975.
6. Dahl JD: Variable rate timer for a cardiac pacemaker. US Patent 4,140,132, Feb 20, 1979.
7. Anderson K, Humen D, Klein GJ, et al: A rate variable pacemaker which automatically adjusts for physical activity. PACE 6:12, 1983.
8. Benditt DG, Milstein S, Buetikofer J, et al: Sensor-triggered, rate-variable cardiac pacing: Current technologies and clinical implications. Ann Intern Med 107:714, 1987.
9. Lindemans FW, Rankin IR, Murtaugh R, et al: Clinical experience with an activity-sensing pacemaker. PACE 9:978, 1986.
10. Benditt DG, Mianulli M, Fetter J, et al: Single-chamber cardiac pacing with activity-initiated chronotropic response: Evaluation by cardiopulmonary exercise testing. Circulation 75:184, 1987.
11. Humen DP, Kostuk WJ, Klein GJ: Activity-sensing, rate-responsive pacing: Improvement in myocardial performance with exercise. PACE 8:52, 1985.
12. Zeigler VL, Gillette PC, Kratz J: Is activity sensored pacing in children and young adults a feasible option? PACE 13:2104, 1990.
13. Perrins EJ, Morley CA, Chan SL, et al: Randomized controlled trial of physiological and ventricular pacing. Br Heart J 50:112, 1983.
14. Zegelman M, Cieslinski G, Kreuzer J: Rate response during submaximal exercise: Comparison of three different sensors. PACE 11:1888, 1988.
15. Lau CP, Rushby J, Leigh-Jones M, et al: Symptomatology and quality of life in patients with rate-responsive pacemakers: A double-blind cross-over study. Clin Cardiol 12:505, 1989.
16. Smedgard P, Kristensson BE, Kruse I, et al: Rate-responsive pacing by means of activity sensing versus single rate ventricular pacing: A double-blind cross-over study. PACE 10:902, 1987.
17. Sulke AN, Pipilis A, Henderson RA, et al: Comparison of the normal sinus node with seven types of rate-responsive pacemaker during everyday activity. Br Heart J 64:525, 1990.
18. Kubisch K, Peters W, Chiladakis I, et al: Clinical experience with the rate-responsive pacemaker Sensolog 703. PACE 11:1829, 1988.
19. Wilkoff BL, Shimokochi DD, Schaal SF: Pacing rate increase due to application of steady external pressure on an activity-sensing pacemaker. PACE 10:423, 1987.
20. Lau CP, Mehta D, Toff W, et al: Limitations of rate response of activity-sensing rate-responsive pacing to different forms of activity. PACE 11:141, 1988.
21. Mehta D, Lau CP, Ward DE, et al: Comparative evaluation of chronotropic response of activity-sensing and QT-sensing rate-responsive pacemakers to different activities. PACE 11:1405, 1988.
22. Zegelman M, Beyersdorf F, Kreuzer J, et al: Rate-responsive pacemakers: Assessment after two years. PACE 9:1005, 1986.
23. Alt E, Heinz M, Theres H, et al: Function and selection of sensors for optimum rate-modulated pacing. In Barold S, Mugica J (eds): New Perspectives in Cardiac Pacing 2. Mt. Kisco, NY, Futura, 1991, pp 163–202.
24. Alt E, Matula M, Thilo R, et al: A new mechanical sensor for detecting body activity and posture, suitable for rate-responsive pacing. PACE 11:1875, 1988.
25. Furman S: Rate-modulated pacing. Circulation 82:1081, 1990.
26. Stangl K, Wirtzfeld A, Lochschmidt O, et al: Physical movement-sensitive pacing: Comparison of two "activity"-triggered pacing systems. PACE 12:102, 1989.
27. Lau CP, Butrous GS, Ward DE, et al: Comparison of exercise performance of six rate-adaptive right ventricular cardiac pacemakers. Am J Cardiol 63:833, 1989.
28. Faerestrand S, Breivik K, Ohm O: Assessment of the work capacity and relationship between rate response and exercise tolerance associated with activity-sensing rate-responsive ventricular pacing. PACE 10:1277, 1987.
29. Howe RT, Muller RS, Gabriel KJ, Trimmer WSN: Silicon micromechanics: Sensors and actuators on a chip. IEEE Spectrum 7:29–30, 1990.
30. Alt E, Matula M, Theres H, et al: Grundlage Aktivitätsgesteuerter frequenzvariabler Herzschrittmacher: Analyse von belastungs- und umweltbedingten mechanischen Einflussen am menschlichen Korper. Z Kardiol 78:587, 1989.
31. Anderson KM: An activity sensor to control heart rate. In Ko WH (ed): Implantable Sensor for Closed-Loop Prosthetic Systems. Mt. Kisco, NY, Futura, 1985.
32. Lau CP, Stott JR, Toff WD, et al: Selective vibration sensing: A new concept for activity-sensing rate-responsive pacing. PACE 11:1299, 1988.
33. Alt E, Matula M, Theres H, et al: The basis for activity-controlled rate-variable cardiac pacemakers: An analysis of mechanical forces on the human body induced by exercise and environment. PACE 12:1667, 1989.
34. Matula M, Alt E, Schrepf R, et al: Response of activity pacemakers controlled by different motion sensors to treadmill testing with varied slopes. PACE 15:523, 1992.
35. Matula M, Alt E, Fotuhi P, et al: Influence of varied types of exercise to the rate adaption of activity pacemakers. PACE 15:578, 1992.
36. Bacharach DW, Hilden RS, Millerhagen JO, et al: Activity-based pacing: Comparison of a device using an accelerometer versus a piezoelectric crystal. PACE 15:188, 1992.
37. Lau CP: The range of sensors and algorithms used in rate-adaptive cardiac pacing. PACE 15:1177, 1992.
38. Anderson KM, Moore AA: Sensors in pacing. PACE 9:954, 1986.
39. Lau CP, Tse WS, Camm AJ: Clinical experience with Sensolog 703: A new activity-sensing rate-responsive pacemaker. PACE 11:1444, 1988.
40. Alt E, Heinz M, Theres H, et al: A new body motion activity-based rate-responsive pacing system. PACE 10:422, 1987.
41. Lau CP, Stott JR, Toff WD, et al: Vibration sensing: New design of activity-sensing rate-responsive pacemaker. PACE 10:1217, 1987.
42. Cardiac Pacemakers Inc: Recent Developments in Adaptive Rate Pacing Technology. St. Paul, MN, Cardiac Pacemakers Inc, 1991.
44. Matula M, Alt E, Theres H, et al: Rate-responsive pacing based on a new activity sensing principle. PACE 10:1220, 1987.
45. Stangl K, Wirtzfeld A, Lochschmidt O, et al: Moglichkeiten und Grenzen eines "aktivitatsgesteuerten" Schrittmachersystems. Herz/Kreislauf 19:351, 1987.
46. Wong TC, Webster JG, Montoye HJ, et al: Portable accelerometer device for measuring human energy expenditure. Trans Biomed Eng 6:467, 1981.
47. Servais SB, Webster JG, Montoye HJ: Estimating human energy expenditure using an accelerometer device. IEEE Frontiers of Engineering in Health 309–312, 1982.
48. Higano ST, Hayes DL: Advantage of discrepant upper rate limits in a DDDR pacemaker. Mayo Clin Proc 64:932, 1989.
49. Hanich RF, Midei MG, McElroy BP, et al: Circumvention of maximum tracking limitations with a rate-modulated dual-chamber pacemaker. PACE 12:392, 1989.
50. Higano ST, Hayes DL, Eisinger G: Sensor-driven rate smoothing in a DDDR pacemaker. PACE 12:922, 1989.
51. Lau CP: Clinical comparison of currently available sensor-based rate-adaptive pacing systems. In Benditt DG (ed): Rate-Adaptive Pacing. Boston, Blackwell Scientific, 1993, pp 199–214.
52. Benditt DG, Mianulli M, Fetter J, et al: Single-chamber cardiac pacing with activity-initiated chronotropic response: Evaluation by cardiopulmonary exercise testing. Circulation 75:183, 1987.
53. Borg G: Perceived exertion as indicator of somatic stress. Scand J Rehabil Med 2:92, 1970.

54. Buetikofer J, Milstein S, Mianulli M, et al: Sustained improvement in exercise duration, rate-pressure product and peak oxygen consumption with activity-initiated rate-variable pacing. *In* Belhassen B, Feldman S, Copperman Y (eds): Cardiac Pacing and Electrophysiology: Proceedings of the VIIIth World Symposium on Cardiac Pacing and Electrophysiology. Tel Aviv, R & L Creative Communications, 1987, pp 53–59.

55. Lau CP, Wong C-K, Leung W-H, et al: Superior cardiac hemodynamics of atrioventricular synchrony over rate-responsive pacing at submaximal exercise: Observations in activity-sensing DDDR pacemakers. PACE 13:1832, 1990.

56. Alt E, Theres H, Heinz M: Evaluation of temperature- and activity-controlled rate-adaptive cardiac pacemakers by spiroergometry. *In* Winter UJ, Wassermann K, Treese N, et al (eds): Computerized Cardiopulmonary Exercise Testing. Darmstadt, Germany, Steinkopff Verlag, 1991, pp 159–170.

57. Buckingham TA, Wodruf RC, Pennington G, et al: Effect of ventricular function on the exercise hemodynamics of variable rate pacing. J Am Coll Cardiol 11:169, 1988.

58. Lau CP, Camm AJ: Role of left ventricular function and Doppler derived variables in predicting hemodynamic benefits of rate-responsive pacing. Am J Cardiol 62:906, 1988.

59. Menozzi C, Brignole M, Moracchini PV, et al: Intrapatient comparison between chronic VVIR and DDD pacing in patients affected by high-degree AV block without heart failure. PACE 13:1816, 1990.

60. Oldroyd KG, Rae AP, Carter R, et al: Double-blind crossover comparison of the effects of dual-chamber pacing (DDD) and ventricular rate-adaptive (VVIR) pacing on neuroendocrine variables, exercise performance, and symptoms in complete heart block. Br Heart J 65:188, 1991.

61. Blanc JJ, Mansourati J, Ritter P, et al: Atrial natriuretic factor release during exercise in patients successively paced in DDD and rate-matched ventricular pacing. PACE 15:397, 1992.

62. Linde-Edelstam C, Hjemdahl P, Pehrsson SK, et al: Is DDD pacing superior to VVIR? A study on cardiac sympathetic nerve activity and myocardial oxygen consumption at rest and during exercise. PACE 15:425, 1992.

63. Lau CP, Tai YT, Fong PC, et al: Clinical experience with an activity-sensing DDDR pacemaker using an accelerometer sensor. PACE 15:334, 1992.

64. Millerhagen J, Bacharach D, Street G, et al: A comparison study of two activity pacemakers: An accelerometer versus piezoelectric crystal device. PACE 14:665, 1991.

65. Alt E: A protocol for treadmill and bicycle stress testing designed for pacemaker patients. Stimucoeur 15:33, 1987.

66. Charles RG, Heemels JP, Westrum BL, et al: Accelerometer-based pacing: A multi-center study. PACE 16:418, 1993.

67. Erdelitsch-Reiser E, Langenfeld H, Millerhagen J, Kochsiek K: New concept in activity-controlled pacemakers: Clinical results with an accelerometer-based adaptive ratepacing system. PACE 15:2245, 1992.

68. Guidant/CPI: Summary of safety and effectiveness for VIGOR® DR. US FDA PMA #P940031, September 1994.

69. Matula M, Alt E, Fotuhi P, et al: Rate adaptation of activity pacemakers under various types of means of locomotion. Eur J Cardiac Pacing Electrophysiol 2:49, 1992.

70. Hamon D, Clementy J, Dulhoste MN, et al: Evaluation of four VVIR pacing systems using standardized usual everyday activities. Eur J Cardiac Pacing Electrophysiol 2:50, 1992.

71. Hayes DL, Higano ST, et al: Utility of rate histograms in programming and follow-up of a DDDR pacemaker. Mayo Clin Proc 64:495, 1989.

72. Benditt DG, Mianulli M, Fetter J, et al: An office-based exercise protocol for predicting chronotropic response of activity-triggered, rate-variable pacemakers. Am J Cardiol 64:27, 1989.

72a. Roberts D, Baxter S, Brennan P, et al: Comparison of externally strapped versus implanted accelerometer or vibration-based rate adaptive pacemakers during various physical activities. PACE 9:65, 1995.

73. Moura PJ, Gessman LJ, Lai T, et al: Chronotropic response of an activity-detecting pacemaker compared with the normal sinus node. PACE 10:78, 1987.

74. Hayes DL, Von Feldt L, Higano ST: Standardized informal exercise testing for programming adaptive rate pacemakers. PACE 14:1772, 1991.

75. Mianulli M, Lundstrom R, Birchfield D, et al: A standardized activities of daily living protocol for assessment of chronotropic incompetence. PACE 16:926, 1993.

76. Mianulli M, Lundstrom R, Birchfield D, et al: Pacemaker rate response optimization using a standardized activities of daily living protocol. PACE 16:873, 1993.

76a. Leung S, Lau C, Tang M, et al: New integrated sensor pacemaker: Comparison of rate responses between an integrated minute ventilation and activity sensor and single sensor modes during exercise and daily activities and nonphysiological interference. PACE 19:1664, 1996.

77. McElroy TA, Janicki JS, Weber KT: Physiologic correlates of the heart rate response to upright isotonic exercise: Relevance to rate-responsive pacemakers. J Am Coll Cardiol 11:94, 1988.

78. Lau CP, Wong CK, Leung WH, et al: A comparative evaluation of minute ventilation-sensing and activity-sensing adaptive-rate pacemakers during daily activities. PACE 12:1514, 1989.

79. Bornzin, Arambala E, Floria J, et al: Adjusting heart rate during sleep. . . . . using activity variance. PACE 17:1933, 1994.

80. Rickards SA, Bombardini T, Corbucci G, et al: An implantable intracardiac accelerometer for monitoring myocardial contractility. PACE 9:2066, 1996.

81. Faerestrand S, Ohm O: Clinical study of a new activity sensor for rate adaptive pacing controlled by electrical signals generated by cinetic energy of a moving magnetic ball. PACE 17:1944, 1994.

82. Bongiorni M, Soldati E, Giuseppe A, et al: Multicenter clinical evaluation of a new SSIR pacemaker. PACE 15:1799, 1992.

83. Candinas R, Jakob M, Buckingham TA, et al: Vibration, acceleration, gravitation, and movement: Activity controlled rate adaptive pacing during treadmill exercise and daily life activities. PACE 20:1777–1786, 1997.

84. Alt E, Heinz M, Theres H, et al: Function and selection of sensors for optimum rate-modulated pacing. *In* Barold S, Mugica J (eds): New Perspectives in Cardiac Pacing. Mt. Kisco, NY, Futura, 1991, p 163.

85. Alt E, Theres H, Heinz M, et al: A new rate-modulated pacemaker system optimized by combination of two sensors. PACE 11:1119, 1988.

86. Mugica J, Barold S, Ripart A: The smart pacemaker. *In* Barold S, Mugica J (eds): New Perspectives in Cardiac Pacing. Mt. Kisco, NY, Futura, 1991, p 545.

87. Schroeppel EA: Current trends in cardiac pacing technology. I. Bradycardia pacing. Biomed Sci Tech 3:90, 1992.

Chapter 10

Rate-Adaptive Pacing Based on Impedance-Derived Minute Ventilation

Tibor Nappholz and G. Neal Kay

Rate adaptation is now well established as an integral part of cardiac pacing. In the very short list of physiologic parameters that have been found to be suitable to control the rate of pacemakers, respiratory parameters have a special place, because of both their intimate relationship to metabolic processes in the body and the simplicity of their measurement in a pacemaker. These special attributes were recognized early in the history of pacing, starting with the conceptual work of Krasner and colleagues in 1966[1] and the subsequent attempt by Krasner and Nardella to implement this concept into practice in 1967.[2] More than 200,000 pacemakers have been implanted, in which the pacing rate is controlled by respiratory parameters in the form of minute ventilation (MV). In general, these devices have had an exceptional record of success in providing rate adaptation, realizing the enormity of the task of emulating the complex control system of the healthy sinus mode.

■ BIOMEDICAL IMPEDANCE

The mechanics of respiration involve the cyclic expansion and contraction of the thoracic cavity. MV pacemakers, however, do not actually measure airflow through the lungs. Rather, associated with the mechanical movements of ventilation is a change in the electrical impedance across the human torso. It is the measurement of these changes in impedance that enables the respiratory process to be monitored by relatively simple means that are adaptable to an implantable pacemaker. The measurement of impedance in biomedical applications is commonly referred to as *plethysmography* and has its basis in Ohm's law. This law states that the ratio of the applied voltage (V) to the current (I) flowing is as follows:

$$R = V/I,$$

where R is the impedance. If the current (I) is kept constant,

then the voltage (V) that is measured will reflect changes in resistance. The value of R is related to the resistivity (ρ) of the medium (blood, tissue, and so forth), by the length of the path (L), and inversely by the cross-sectional area (A + DA) of the conducting medium, as indicated by the following equation:

$$R = \rho \ (L/A + \Delta A)$$

Note that the cross-sectional area is displayed as having two components, a constant component (A) and a dynamic component (ΔA) that changes with respiration (and other factors).

Placing any two electrodes subcutaneously across the human torso will result in the impedances shown in Figure 10–1. A measurement of this type is termed a *bipolar* measurement. The resistances, R_1 and R_2, and the capacitances, C_1 and C_2, are due to the effects of polarization at the electrode–electrolyte interface (polarization effects). The values of these parameters are dependent on the frequency of the measurement current. At frequencies above a few thousand cycles per second (Hz), their contribution becomes negligible. For this reason, as well as for the purposes of minimizing battery drain and maintaining patient safety, the measurements in implantable devices are performed with high frequencies or very narrow pulse widths. As an example, a current pulse used in one of the MV pacing systems is 0.015-msec wide, roughly equivalent to a frequency of 33 kHz. This frequency eliminates all polarization effects.

We can use a fluid-flow analogy to understand the bipolar impedance measurement further. Using this model, we see that impedance consists of three "conduits" that impede the flow of electric current. The narrow conduits (R_p) are related to contact resistance at the electrode–tissue interfaces and have a considerably larger impedance than the wider conduit R_m, which is related to resistance across the torso (both R_p values are shown as equal for convenience). The impedance

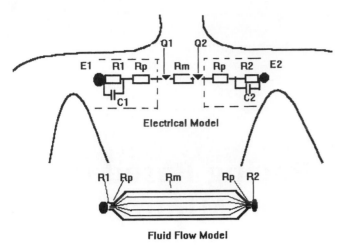

Figure 10–1. Constituents of impedance measurement across the human torso. When voltage is applied between electrodes E1 and E2, separate measurement points Q1 and Q2 give respiration changes independent of contact resistances. R_1, C_1, R_2, C_2, polarization elements; RP, contact resistance; RM, torso resistance containing respiration signal.

R_m contains the respiration signal that we want to measure to control the pacing rate of a rate-adaptive pacemaker. As a rule, the values of R_p are greater than those of R_m, especially for electrodes with a small surface area. This makes the regions around the electrodes prone to artifacts related to movement of the skin and underlying tissues. To eliminate this source of inaccuracy, normally either a four-electrode (quadripolar) system, as shown by the measurement points Q1 and Q2 in Figure 10–1, is used, or the electrodes are made large, thereby minimizing this funneling. It is important at the outset to understand these simple concepts as they relate to implanted pacemakers because the electrodes available are generally small and limited in number.

Magnitude of Impedance Signals

When considering how an MV pacemaker operates, it is instructive to look at the size of the signals that such an impedance measurement system must detect. The usual tip electrode–tissue impedance of a pacing lead is on the order of 400 Ω (the value of R_p in Fig. 10–1). For larger electrodes, such as those used subcutaneously, the impedance is about 200 Ω. The impedance around a pacemaker case depends on its size but is usually less than 20 Ω. The impedance across the torso (R_m in Fig. 10–1) is on the order of 50 Ω. The change in R_m that is related to respiration (the value that we want to measure) is in the vicinity of 1 Ω. To detect small changes in minute ventilation, we have to be able to distinguish changes of 0.06 Ω. This gives some indication of how sensitive the measurement system has to be.

▪ HISTORY OF DEVELOPMENT

As mentioned previously, respiration was recognized early in the history of pacing as the most likely candidate for monitoring metabolic demand by an implanted pacemaker. After the work of Krasner and associates,[1, 2] further work was done by Funke,[3] who used an intrapleural pressure

sensor, and by Ionescu.[4] The early work of Krasner and associates, however, formed the basis for the first production of a rate-responsive device by Rossi and colleagues in collaboration with Biotec, S.p.A. (Bologna, Italy) in April 1982.[5–7] This device, as prescribed by Krasner and associates, used a subcutaneous lead for sensing the respiratory rate. The measurement was made in a bipolar mode between the pulse generator case and an additional subcutaneous chest lead that had to be tunneled across the sternum. At about the same time (1983), Medtronic, Inc. (Minneapolis, MN) introduced a rate-responsive pacer based on activity, the Activitrax.[8] In a way, this device was also a byproduct of the respiration approach because it was during the search for a simple sensor to detect respiration by the measurement of chest wall movement that it was realized that the artifacts of motion are easier to measure than the signals associated with respiration.

Transvenous Approach to Measurement of Minute Ventilation

Krasner and associates, and subsequently Rossi and colleagues, measured respiration with the use of an auxiliary lead across the chest, as shown in Figure 10–2. In both of these configurations, the test current was delivered between the same electrodes (E1 and E2) that were used to measure the resultant voltage. Krasner's work never evolved into a reality, and it was actually Rossi and colleagues who made it into a practical concept. There were some disadvantages to Rossi's implementation from the perspective of conventional pacing therapy. First, the use of subcutaneous leads involved tunneling procedures during pacemaker implantation that are laborious and time-consuming and are an acquired skill. In addition, subcutaneous leads are prone to erosion and are generally an additional component that can fail. This was borne out by the experience with the Biotec devices,[7] which had a complication rate of 2%. Second, bipolar measurements taken subcutaneously are more prone to motion artifacts because of continued movement during normal activity, making accurate quantitative measurements of respiration more difficult. Third, respiratory rate is only one component of ventilation, the other being the depth of breathing (tidal volume).

With these disadvantages in mind, Nappholz, in collaboration with Maloney and Simmons of the Cleveland Clinic, carried out a series of studies to explore the use of transve-

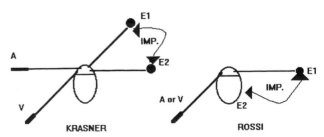

Figure 10–2. Subcutaneous bipolar transvenous approaches to the measurement of minute ventilation according to Krasner and Rossi. A and V, atrial and ventricular electrodes; E1 and E2, electrodes applying current and measuring impedance.

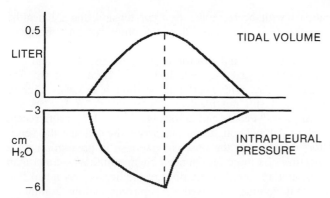

Figure 10–3. Tidal volume and intrapleural pressure relationships showing close relation and pressures similar to venous pressures; 6 cm of H₂0 translates roughly to 5 mm Hg.

nous electrodes to measure MV in exercising patients.[9–14] MV, the product of respiratory rate and tidal volume, was chosen because it was known to have excellent correlation with the rate of the normal sinus node and had a good dynamic range. These qualities had been demonstrated previously by Pearce and colleagues,[15, 16] and Whipp and Wasserman,[17] and more recently by the work of Weber[18] and McElroy,[19, 20] who emphasized studies in patients with cardiac disease. The other reason for selecting MV was the belief, on theoretical grounds, that the transvenous approach would be less prone to motion artifacts than the subcutaneous approach. Initial work on the transvenous system focused on plethysmographic measurements in the superior vena cava (SVC) because it was known from general clinical observation that this large vessel changes dimensions dramatically in response to changes in intrapleural pressure.

Figure 10–3 illustrates the relationship between intrapleural pressure and tidal volume, based on the work of Weber and Janicki.[21] Changes in intrapleural pressure are related in a monotonic manner to tidal volume. It is also apparent that the pressure range in the pleural cavity is comparable to pressures in the SVC, leading to dramatic changes in SVC volume during respiration. The impedance measurements at first were done using a quadripolar system in the SVC of dogs and subsequently in patients. The correlation of changes in impedance with actual changes in MV was excellent (r > 0.9).[9] It was noted in some of the subsequent experiments, however, that when the impedance measurements were extended through the innominate and subclavian veins to encompass some of the pectoral region, certain anomalies appeared. These anomalies could have been due to the nature of respiration, in that during inspiration, the thoracic cavity increases in volume during filling of the lungs, the greater volume of air leading to a higher impedance at the end of inspiration. As the chest expands in inspiration, the SVC initially decreases in blood volume and then increases in blood volume, leading to a decrease in impedance at the end of inspiration. These observations encouraged a departure from a pure venous approach and promoted a slightly modified configuration that was also more suitable for pacemaker implants.

Preclinical experiments used a cutaneous defibrillation pad that was placed over the prepectoral region (the site of the pacemaker case), and the measurement current was generated between the right ventricle and the cutaneous pad. The resultant voltage was sensed in the SVC.[10] The results confirmed that the use of a common electrode for both generating the current pulses and measuring the impedance was appropriate and that the impedance of a cutaneous pad was about the same as that for a pulse generator case (<20 Ω). At the same time, with this approach and with all subsequent approaches, the highest impedance was through the thoracic cavity, which dominated the measurement. This work was followed by a series of studies, first with dogs and then with patients, by Valenta and colleagues[11] and Fischer and associates,[12] using the configurations shown in Figure 10–4, which encompassed all the possibilities with standard pacemakers.

The results, specific to five exercising patients, are shown in Table 10–1. These experiments clearly show the good correlation between heart rate and MV that is obtained in the ventricle and the atrium.[22] Using these raw data, the algorithm for an implantable system was developed. A configuration in which the current pulse was generated between the pulse generator case and the ring electrode (A or V), with the measurement was taken between the tip electrode (A or V) and the case, was found to be the most suitable compromise. These measurements validated the application of this sensor for either atrial or ventricular pacemakers. In addition, this configuration is close to a quadripolar configuration, as shown in Figure 10–1, because the size of the pacemaker case overcomes the main disadvantages of the configuration, namely, that the pacemaker case is both the source of the measurement current and the reference for its measurement. The encouraging results from this work led to the use of right ventricular impedance for the measurement of stroke volume during arrhythmias by two biomedical engineers, Yeh[22] and Khoury.[23]

In more recent work, Pioger[24] and associates used implanted Chorus RM 7034 and Opus RM 4534 pacemakers (both from ELA Medical, Paris, France) to evaluate the

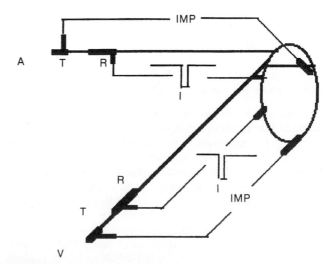

Figure 10–4. Measurements explored for conventional configurations. Measurements in both chambers of the heart are shown. A, V, atrium, ventricle; T, R, tip, ring; I, constant-current pulse; IMP, impedance measured.

Table 10–1. Respiration–Heart Rate Correlation

Patient	Lead	Respiration Parameter	Correlation
A01	SVC	Minute ventilation	0.681
		Respiration rate	0.861
A03	AB	Minute ventilation	0.908
		Respiration rate	0.896
		Tidal volume	0.867
A05	AB	Minute ventilation	0.959
		Respiration rate	0.867
		Tidal volume	0.347
	VE	Minute ventilation	0.956
		Respiration rate	0.852
		Tidal volume	0.309
A13	AB	Minute ventilation	0.921
		Respiration rate	0.621
		Tidal volume	0.761
	VE	Minute ventilation	0.898
		Respiration rate	0.609
		Tidal volume	0.736
A27	AB	Minute ventilation	0.965
		Respiration rate	0.670
		Tidal volume	0.904
	VE	Minute ventilation	0.767
		Respiration rate	0.585
		Tidal volume	0.547

Abbreviations: For atrium: AB, current from ring to case, measurement tip to case; For ventricle, VE, current from ring to case, measurement tip to case; For superior vena cava, current from ventricular ring to case, measurement in SVC.

effect of injecting current in the atrial or ventricular tip on the accuracy of MV measurement. In each of these cases, the MV was measured off the corresponding atrial and ventricular ring, except in the case of a single-pass lead, in which the MV was measured off the atrial sensing ring. In every case, the correlation with oxygen consumption ($\dot{V}O_2$) was better than 0.8.

■ APPROPRIATENESS OF RESPIRATORY PARAMETERS AS INDICATORS OF METABOLIC DEMAND

Relationship Between Heart Rate and Respiratory Parameters During Exercise

The process of aerobic metabolism requires the consumption of oxygen that is transported to the tissues by the heart. In fact, changes in heart rate during exercise are closely related to changes in $\dot{V}O_2$ at all levels of exertion. At metabolic workloads of less than anaerobic threshold, $\dot{V}O_2$ and heart rate are also directly proportional to MV. This is borne out by the work performed by several investigators.[18, 19, 25] The correlation coefficient for heart rate to MV has been found to be greater than 0.9 in most investigational work.[12, 22, 25]

The seminal work on rate response done by McElroy and associates[19, 20] and later confirmed by Vai and colleagues[25] showed that the correlation between respiratory rate and oxygen uptake during submaximal exercise was not particularly good, with both studies demonstrating correlation coefficients of less than 0.54. McElroy's study consisted of 81 patients with heart failure or hypertension and 27 healthy subjects. This study, more than any other, resolved the question of the effects of heart disease on the relationship between heart rate and respiratory parameters. Rossi and colleagues[5–7] reported a correlation coefficient of 0.7 for respiratory rate with heart rate. Although this was slightly better, it is still not ideal. The early work of Beaver and Wasserman,[26] Pearce and associates,[15, 17] and the more recent work of Alt and colleagues[27] clearly indicated that the ventilatory response at the onset of exercise is predominantly a reflection of a more pronounced change in tidal volume than in respiratory rate. In a number of studies, it was noted that the tidal volume increased to a plateau within 2 minutes after the onset of exercise. The relative speed of changes in respiratory rate and MV (the product of tidal volume and respiratory rate) during exertion is best illustrated by the study of Alt and colleagues[27] (Fig. 10–5). It is instructive to note from this study that the respiratory rate not only rises slowly during exercise but also declines faster than tidal volume at the cessation of exercise.

Anaerobic Threshold

In all patients, there comes a point during exercise when continued increases in oxygen demand cannot be matched by increases in oxygen delivery to the tissues by the cardiovascular system. When the heart is unable to meet the increased oxygen demand of the working muscles completely, anaerobic metabolism is initiated, resulting in an increased production of lactic acid. Lactic acid dissociates into lactate and H^+, which is buffered by bicarbonate, resulting in an abrupt increase in carbon dioxide production. Because MV is largely controlled by carbon dioxide production and blood pH rather than $\dot{V}O_2$, the increased rate of carbon dioxide production induces an increase in MV that is out of proportion to $\dot{V}O_2$. Because $\dot{V}O_2$ is linearly related to the normal sinus rate throughout exercise, at workloads above anaerobic threshold, MV increases disproportionately relative to $\dot{V}O_2$ and the sinus rate.

In a rate-responsive pacemaker that uses MV as the controller of pacing rate, if heart rate is made proportional to MV rather than $\dot{V}O_2$ as is normally the case, the onset of anaerobic metabolism may lead to an increase in the pacing rate in excess of true demand. The onset of anaerobic metabolism in patients with New York Heart Association (NYHA) class III and IV heart disease can become manifest by a drop in respiratory rate, but in all classes, MV increases disproportionately to oxygen demand.[18] This implies that in an MV-controlled pacemaker, the switch to anaerobic metabolism will lead to a drop in the correlation coefficient of $\dot{V}O_2$ to heart rate. Inattention to this break in the MV–heart rate relationship routinely leads to overpacing[28] and stresses the heart unnecessarily. Other studies[29, 30] clarified the relationship of MV to $\dot{V}O_2$ above and below anaerobic threshold and were used to guide the development of a more physiologic pacing algorithm, discussed later.

Sensitivity and Specificity of Minute Ventilation as a Metabolic Sensor

For a parameter to be appropriate for the control of heart rate, it must have good correlation with metabolic demand

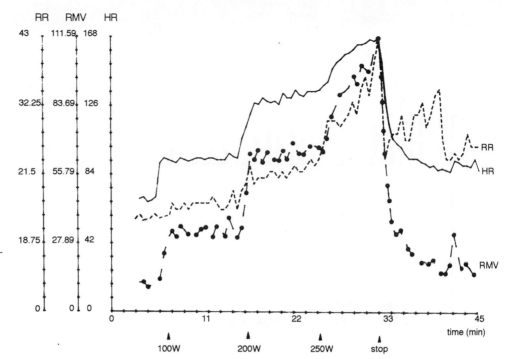

Figure 10–5. Study emphasizing the slower response of respiratory rate compared with minute ventilation. RR, respiratory rate (breaths per minute); RMV, minute ventilation (L/min); HR, heart rate (bpm). (From Alt A, Heinz M, Hirgestetter C, et al: Control of pacemaker rate by impedance-based respiratory minute ventilation. Chest 92:247, 1987.)

(i.e., $\dot{V}O_2$). In addition, it must have a dynamic range that allows reliable sensing of changes in the signal (sensitivity) and should not be prone to interference from various nonspecific sources (specificity). Based on the work of Pearce and Milhorn[15, 16] and others, the increase in the respiration rate from rest to the anaerobic threshold is variable among patients. The change in respiratory rate over this range tends to be on the order of 100% or less (e.g., 15 to 30 breaths/min). In the case of MV, typically about a 600% change occurs from rest to anaerobic threshold (e.g., 10 to 60 L/min). As a simple comparison, when temperature is monitored for the same range of metabolism, it often results in a change of about 3% from the baseline value.[20]

MV, however, is not directly measured to control the pacing rate. Rather, it is the byproduct of ventilatory mechanics that must be sensed, that is, changes in thoracic impedance. In the subcutaneous respiratory rate pacemaker RDP3 (Biotec), Rossi and colleagues[7] observed problems in sensing the respiration signal in about 10% of 143 implanted devices. The exact cause of this problem was not clear, but it implies insufficient size of the impedance signal.

The slope of the change in heart rate to change in MV (HR/MV) for patients with normal sinus node function is dependent on their functional status. McElroy and colleagues demonstrated that the HR/MV slope was steepest in patients with the greatest degree of functional cardiac impairment (Weber class D, $\dot{V}O_{2max} < 10$ mL O_2/kg/min). In patients with good functional capacity (Weber class A, $\dot{V}O_{2max} > 20$ mL O_2/kg/min), the HR/MV slope was the lowest. Because the HR/MV slope varies among patients, a pacemaker that controls heart rate based on changes in MV must have an algorithm that allows the HR/MV slope to be programmed. This is provided by all manufacturers of rate-adaptive MV pacemakers. For the first implantable MV pacemaker (Meta MV, model 1202, Telectronics Pacing Systems, Englewood,

CO), this slope relationship was provided by a programmable parameter, the *rate-response factor* (RRF).

In the transvenous MV system, early indications were that the changes in the impedance signal during respiration were very small. Figure 10–6 shows the values of the programmed RRF in the clinical study summary of the Meta MV.[31] This presentation highlights the relationship between RRF values and the actual impedance changes that were measured.

The RRF is the relationship between the change in MV and the corresponding change in pacing rate. The larger this value, the smaller the change in MV that is required to produce a desired change in heart rate. Among patients within any NYHA heart failure class, the relationship between heart rate and MV below the anaerobic threshold has been thoroughly characterized and lies between 1.4 bpm/L and 2.2 bpm/L.[20, 29, 30] The specific value for each patient is predominately influenced by body surface area (BSA).[29] The ratio of the slopes below anaerobic threshold to above anaerobic threshold appears to vary with the investigational group and tends to be in the range of 1.5 to 3.2. The range in the MV–heart rate relationship and the variation in the translation coefficient between true MV and impedance-derived MV require the individual programming of patients to different RRF values. Figure 10–6 shows a tight distribution for RRF values programmed. This distribution most likely bears close resemblance to the distribution of the BSA of the patients. The experimental data in the same figure highlight the difficulty of measuring such small impedances externally in a tripolar configuration.

Since the original work of Lau,[31, 32] there has been considerable focus on the specificity of MV signals in the presence of arm motion, coughing, talking, and various other maneuvers of everyday life. This has been extremely elusive to pin down quantitatively. A series of studies by Greenhut[33]

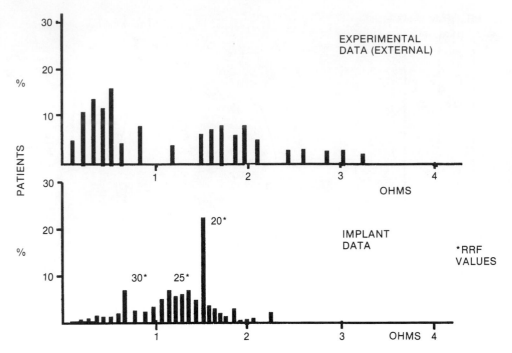

Figure 10–6. Early externally obtained experimental results and results of implanted device. RRF, rate response factor; Ohms, dynamic change of impedance due to minute ventilation.

attempted to do just that: truly measure the correlation of the impedance signal seen by the pacemaker with the actual MV measured by a calibrated metabolic chart. This addressed all the common suspected sources of interference. The results are shown in Table 10–2. Note that one patient (#5) had generally very poor correlation figures across the board. It is believed that this is due to either a faulty lead connection or fluid in the header.

In evaluating the results of this study, two simple conclusions could be made: (1) the overall correlation for a wide range of activities is actually very good, and (2) the two activities that stand out as having poor correlation are vigorous arm movement on the side of the pacer implant and bending over, particularly with dressing. The actual signals for these activities are shown in Figure 10–7A and B. As shown in the figure, only vigorous arm movements led to an unnecessarily large rate increase. It is questionable how well the addition of another sensor would minimize these inaccuracies, especially if the other sensor were also motion sensitive. The Legend Plus pacemaker (Medtronic) provides

a programmable feature known as the *MV range* that is designed to limit the influence of upper body motion and other artifacts on the MV impedance signal. These values clip the peak MV signal by a programmable percentage of the transthoracic impedance range. Four MV range settings, allowing a maximal change in impedance of 12.5%, 25%, 50%, and 100% of the MV signal range, are available.

Stroke volume is a potential problem in transvenous pacing systems that sense MV. An example of an early recording is shown in Figure 10–7C. As shown by the telemetered data (on an expanded time scale), the stroke volume component is effectively controlled by the design of the algorithm. Kay and associates[35] carried out studies to validate the ability of the system to reject stroke volume interference. Their conclusion that the algorithm effectively rejected stroke volume signals has been borne out by subsequent clinical data, which concurred with these findings. Mechanical ventilators create an artificially large variation in intrapleural pressure. All MV-based pacemakers sense these changes in transthoracic impedance, resulting in a large change in pacing rate.

Table 10–2. Correlation of Impedance and Actual MV During Activities

	Pt #1	Pt #2	Pt #3	Pt #4	Pt #5	Pt #6	Mean
Talking	0.87	0.87	0.95	0.85	0.57	0.95	0.84
16 bpm	0.83	0.91	0.91	0.90	0.53	0.96	0.84
OT shoulder	0.91	0.81	0.93	0.70	0.72	0.96	0.84
PM shoulder	0.28	0.46	0.87	0.48	0.19	0.57	0.48
Bend	0.34	0.43	0.60	0.18	0.28	0.31	0.36
CAEP3		0.54	0.91	0.77	0.51	0.94	0.73
CAEP Re		0.89	0.93	0.69	0.58	0.95	0.81
Mean	0.75	0.76	0.88	0.59	0.53	0.85	0.73

Regular breathing at 16 bpm; OT (other than) pacer shoulder, 30 rotations/min; PM shoulder, 30 rotations/min; Bend, bending over; CAEP3, stage 3 of exercise assessment protocol; CAEP Re, recovery from exercise protocol.

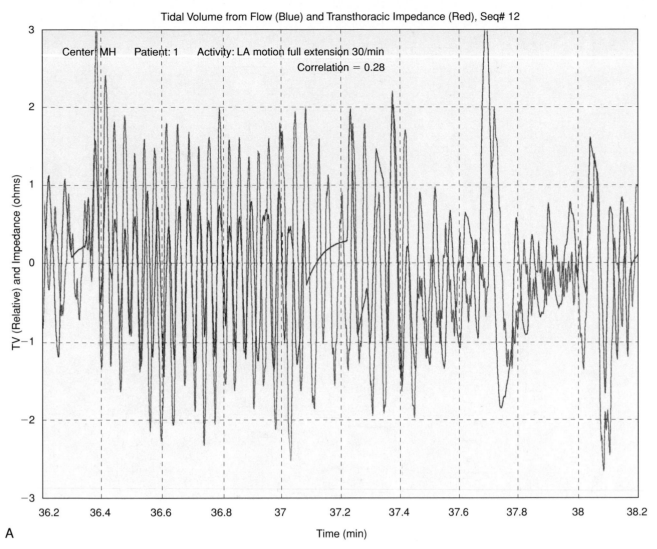

Figure 10–7. *A,* Tidal volumes signals telemetered from an implanted device. Patient is vigorously rotating the left arm, with pacer implanted in the left pectoral region. Flow measured with standard Medical Graphics CPX/D gas exchange system. *Illustration continued on following page*

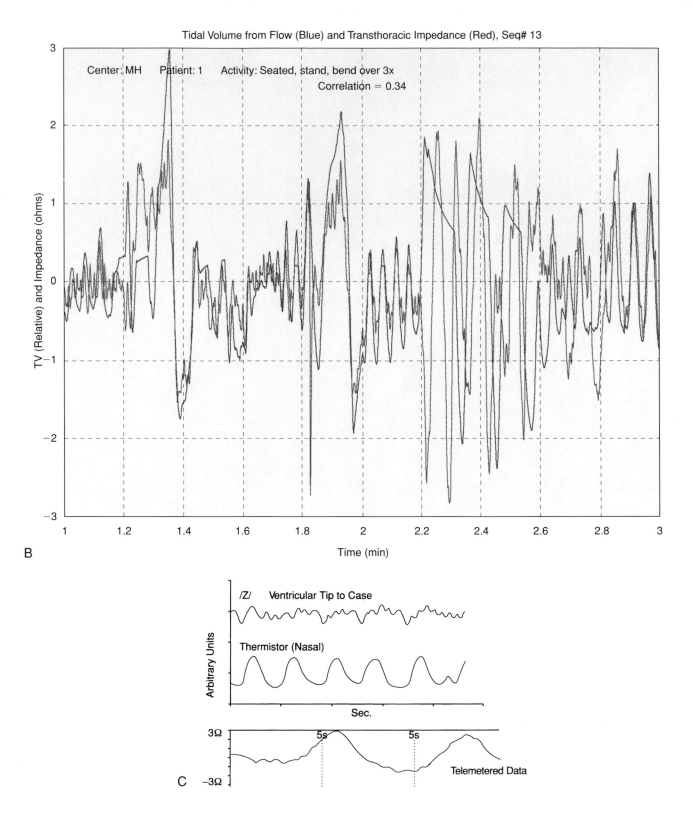

Figure 10–7, cont'd. *B,* Tidal volume measured with implanted device and compared with a Medical Graphics CPX/D flow measurement. Patient is bending over and dressing. *C,* Comparison of stroke volume on unprocessed and processed ventilation signals. Telemetered data are made on a different time scale and are shown only to illustrate results of processing of signal.

Consequently, when patients require mechanical ventilation, the rate-response function should always be turned off.

Changes in Minute Ventilation at the Onset and Cessation of Exercise

As discussed, the cardiac and pulmonary systems are closely integrated, their interdependency being modified only under conditions of anaerobic metabolism. Several careful studies[15-17] have shown that there is no loss in the coupling of MV to heart rate, either at the onset of exercise or at its cessation. Despite the known transient anaerobic metabolism (oxygen deficit) that occurs at the start of exercise, Pearce and Milhorn[16] found that the correlation coefficient between heart rate and MV was not significantly affected at the start or termination of exercise. Mond and Kertes,[36] working with the Meta MV pacing system, observed that the correlation coefficient between the actual MV and the pacing rate was more than 0.9 after the end of exercise. Hence, the linking of MV (as measured by thoracic impedance) is effective during this transition stage.

Not withstanding the previously mentioned physiologic arguments, the actual measurement of MV demands a certain amount of filtering to eliminate random noise. This filtering manifests as a delay in the rise or fall of the MV signal. From extensive observations with various products, a time constant of less than about 15 seconds (the time it takes for a step input to reach 67% of its final value) brings with it a noticeable increase in the randomness of the pacing rate.

Effect of Pulmonary Disease on Minute Ventilation Sensors

The effect of various pulmonary diseases on the relationship between heart rate and respiratory parameters as measured by thoracic impedance was unknown during the early development stage of an implantable rate-response pacing device. We now know that for patients with emphysema, chronic bronchitis, and restrictive lung disease, it is the pulmonary system that usually limits exercise, not the cardiovascular system. In a healthy patient at the end of exercise, MV is about 50% of the maximum voluntary ventilation. In a patient with pulmonary disease, this reserve is less and in many cases disappears before initiation of the anaerobic threshold, indicating that the patient will not reach this condition. The transthoracic estimate of MV is often higher for the same $\dot{V}O_2$ in patients with pulmonary disease, providing a strong signal for the implantable device to control heart rate, although often with a more limited range. To complicate matters, many patients requiring pacemakers have both cardiac and pulmonary disorders. This complex medical subject has been thoughtfully addressed by Weber and Janicki.[21]

How these issues affect the use of respiration as a rate-control parameter is best seen in reports of the results of implants of the Meta MV.[31, 37] The clinical study summary[31] included 35 patients with chronic lung disease who received this pacing system without reported complications. In addition, Kay and associates[37] reported on two patients with advanced pulmonary disease who demonstrated excellent rate response with this pacemaker during cardiopulmonary exercise testing. One study result is shown in Figure 10–8.

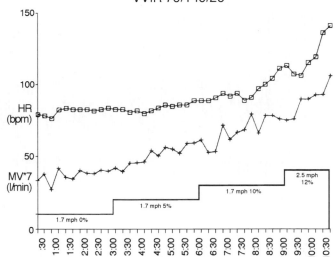

Figure 10–8. Patient with chronic obstructive pulmonary disease. Note small range of minute ventilation (MV) from about 5 L/min to 13 L/hmin. HR, heart rate.

The conclusion is that pulmonary disease does not present a problem in specificity and sensitivity of MV-sensing pacemakers. Unfortunately, the conclusions about the use of respiratory rate as a control parameter in patients with pulmonary disease are not as well defined.

Chronic Stability of Impedance Measurements

Early work by Li and colleagues[38] with implanted devices indicated that the selected RRF at implantation was appropriate for the patient over time. Since the first implantation of an MV-responsive pacemaker, a number of cases of sudden inappropriate pacemaker response were investigated, and most of them were traceable to mechanical contact or header problems. This still left a small number of cases in which the cause of the acceleration in pacing rate could not be identified. There was a strong correlation between sudden inexplicable rate increases and patients undergoing open heart surgery. Three carefully orchestrated animal studies were carried out to precipitate dramatic blood volume changes and pulmonary edema and to see its effect on the RRF value.[34] None of these studies yielded significant changes.

Unipolar and Epicardial Implants

In the early stages of development of an MV pacemaker, implementation for a unipolar pacing system using a bipolar impedance measurement from the pulse generator case to the tip electrode was rejected because of very large stroke volume components, a tendency toward erratic behavior,[13] and instabilities with intermittent pacing and sensing (Fig. 10–9A). This work has since been revisited, and a method of unipolar measurement has been developed.[39] From the previous discussion on unipolar impedance measurements,

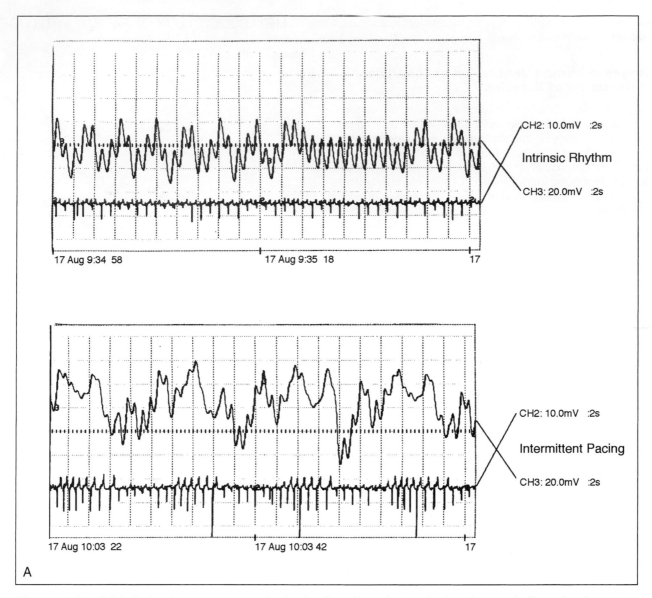

Figure 10–9. *A,* Unipolar impedance measurement showing the effect of intermittent pacing from the same tip. Top tracing shows ventilator turned off at about 9:35 for 8 seconds. Lower tracing shows pacing turned on and off with dramatic results.

the reason for the unpredictable nature of the signals was well understood. It was due to the dominance of the interface impedance between the small area tip electrode and the endocardial tissue. The answer lay in bypassing this bottleneck, and the one way to do it was to use a higher-frequency signal. This was achieved by narrowing the MV measurement pulse to 30 nsec (an increase in frequency by a factor of 500). With the pulse being this narrow, it became possible to monitor the return signal from the lead, just prior to it reaching the tip. In this manner, impedance modulations surrounding the lead could be sensed, which reflected the change in the volume of the thoracic cavity. Figure 10–9*B* shows how the sensed MV signal changes as a function of pulse width (delay). With a 50-nsec pulse width, we can clearly see the appearance of stroke volume, as the pulse

returns from the tip. Figure 10–9*C* shows that the signal is independent of the lead position in the heart.

Unipolar leads can, however, be accommodated with the existing pulse generators. Luttikhuis and Tuinstra,[40] as well as others, have shown that replacement of the ring electrode of a standard bipolar lead with a subcutaneous plate electrode in the prepectoral region allows accurate measurements of respiration using a transvenous unipolar pacing lead. The subcutaneous plate used in this study was about 2 cm[2] and was placed about 15 cm from the pulse generator.

With totally epicardial implants, the specificity of the MV system has not been proved to date. From the early developmental work, the stroke volume component of the impedance signal was found to be considerably greater with this approach. This problem can be alleviated to some extent

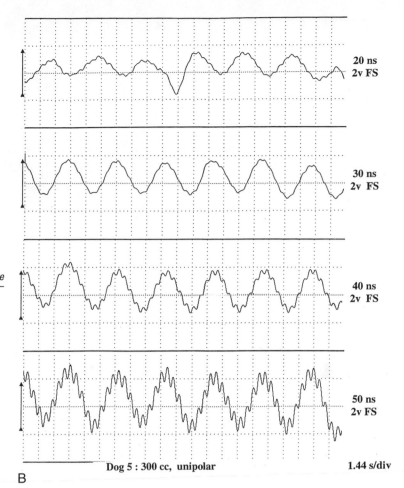

Figure 10–9 *Continued. B,* Unipolar impedance measurements, using time domain reflectometry (TDR). Stroke volume signal becomes more manifest as impedance signal travels beyond the tip of the lead. (Times are in 10^{-9} seconds.)

Illustration continued on following page

by separating the two epicardial electrodes as much as possible. To date, however, the clinical results from epicardial implants of MV pacing systems have been mixed.

■ IMPLANTABLE MINUTE VENTILATION PACING SYSTEMS

Ten years after the implantation of the first MV-controlled rate-responsive pacemaker, Telectronics released its fourth-generation product, Medtronic its third-generation product and second-generation dual-sensor (MV + activity) pacemaker, and ELA its second-generation product; Guidant (Minneapolis, MN) and Pacesetter (Sylmar, CA) have completed their first-generation products. All of these devices sense and process MV in fundamentally similar ways. The following description of the original Telectronics product, Meta MV, provides insight into the early algorithmic fundamentals.

Measurement Pulses

The measurement of transthoracic impedance using a standard pacing lead has to comply with two strict requirements: (1) it has to use very little energy to achieve its objective, and (2) it cannot in anyway jeopardize patient safety. The original Meta MV design achieved these objectives by using 1-mA current pulses, 15-μsec in duration and at a repetition rate of 20 pulses per second. This totals to a battery current of 0.3 μA, about 2% of the total current of a DDD pacemaker. From recent studies,[41, 42] a safe current pulse on a miniature tip, such as CapSure Z (Medtronic) or a model 1446T (Pacesetter), would be 85 μsec and 1.5 mA. This translates to a safety factor of about 500% at 1 mA.

Interference With Sensing

It is possible for some sense amplifiers to sense these small impedance pulses unless some preventive steps are taken. In some products, a blanking period of about 1 msec is applied to the amplifiers to "blind" them to these pulses. In other cases, special balancing of the pulse is carried out, achieving the same objective. Wilson and Lattner[43] reported an incident in which the sense amplifier did see the measurement pulse. This occurred in a patient with one of the early Meta MV pacemakers who was one of four patients noted to have this problem in the Meta MV clinical study summary.[31] The problem was traced to a residue of medical epoxy on the ring electrode of some Cordis-Telectronics pacing leads. This thin layer affected the impedance of the electrode during delivery of the 1-mA current pulses. Because the ring is a common electrode with the electrocardiographic (ECG) sense amplifier, this increase in impedance resulted in a sizable increase in the signal seen by the amplifier, enough to inhibit the pacing pulse under certain circumstances. In

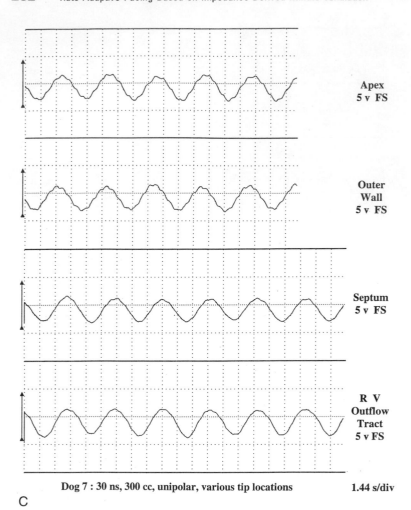

C

Dog 7 : 30 ns, 300 cc, unipolar, various tip locations   1.44 s/div

Apex
5 v FS

Outer
Wall
5 v FS

Septum
5 v FS

R V
Outflow
Tract
5 v FS

Figure 10–9 *Continued. C,* Unipolar TDR measurements at different locations in the heart, showing independence of positioning.

addition, the polarization of the ring also increased, thereby accentuating the problem during the blanking of the 15-msec impedance pulse. A multitude of leads have been used since then, with no reported problems.[31] The recent trend of generating these pulses off the tip of the leads instead of the ring electrode can make this self-inhibition more of a problem, especially in the atrium.

Interference With the Surface Electrocardiogram

Sensing of the impedance pulses by a surface ECG monitor is always a possibility and depends on the sensitivity of the ECG machine. The pulse width and the balancing of the impedance pulse influence this possibility. The clinical study summary for the Meta MV reported this phenomenon with some of the monitors and transtelephonic systems (those with pulse stretch capabilities). This could be minimized by repositioning the surface electrodes. In subsequent models of the Meta MV series, this problem has been almost eliminated, as shown in Figure 10–10. The problem was due to a balanced current pulse that was 7 msec in duration instead of 15 msec. The effect of decreasing the pulse width was not as noticeable as balancing it.

Interference From Electric Signals

As discussed previously, the monitoring of impedance involves the conversion of an impedance measurement into a voltage signal. This implies that other voltage signals can be mistaken for changes in impedance. The impedance is measured only for the duration of the narrow, 15-μsec pulse. So long as the electric signal does not change during this short interval, interference from underlying electric signals is rejected. This problem can be visualized by noting that a signal with a frequency of 60 Hz takes about 7000 msec to change from its minimum to its maximum value. In the 15 μsec required to make the impedance measurement, an intracardiac signal will obviously change very little. Hence, the effect of an intracardiac electrogram on the impedance pulse will be negligible. This type of filtering ensures that most common power frequencies, myopotentials, and endocardial signals do not affect the rate-response parameter measurement.

Frequencies above about a few kHz, however, could have some effect on the rate responsiveness of the device but become manifest only when the frequency is in specific ranges (at an exact multiple of the sampling frequency). Reports of electromagnetic interference (EMI) have been rare, but such incidents have been noted.[44, 45] The relevance of these recent reports is that the interference was observed

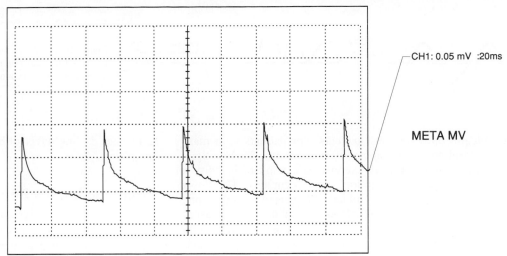

CH1: 0.05 mV :20ms

META MV

CH1: 0.05 mV :20ms

META II

Figure 10–10. Improvement in surface electrocardiograph display of artifact size due to balancing and narrowing of measurement pulse in META II. Top tracing was made with 15-msec pulse, no balancing. Bottom tracing was made with 7-msec pulse followed by 60-msec lower-amplitude balance pulse in reverse direction.

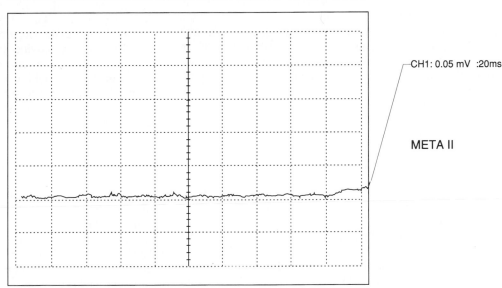

with external devices that are frequently in proximity of the pacemaker, such as the standard monitors of some manufacturers and the ubiquitous antitheft devices found in almost any shop. The Meta II, model 1206 (Telectronics), which was the device affected by the monitors, has an internal detector for EMI that can protect the patient from interference. This capability was, regrettably, never switched on because the initial field experience found no need for it. Electrocautery and electrosurgery generate high-energy, broad-band frequency interference. Because of their intensity and wide range of frequencies, these signals are detected by the rate-response circuitry and could drive the pacemaker to

its maximum rate. In fact, this was reported by Van Hemel and colleagues[46] and must be avoided at all times by turning the rate-response function off whenever electrosurgery is to be used.

Parameter Measurement

As discussed in the section on impedance measurement, respiration is sampled with constant-current pulses. These pulses are then reconstructed into the original respiration signal and processed (Fig. 10–11). The respiration signal contains all its relevant information under 1 Hz (under

Figure 10–11. Signal sampling with current pulse filtering and processing. Reconstructed signal on right shows polarity decisions. The offset would be a threshold set only in rate-respiration–based devices.

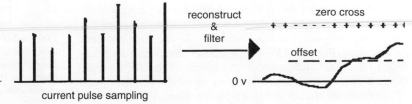

reconstruct & filter

zero cross

offset

0 v

current pulse sampling

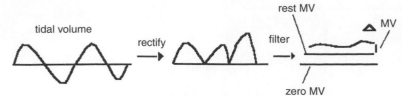

Figure 10–12. Processing of respiratory signal to obtain pacemaker rate driver (DMV). Tidal volume is as processed in Figure 10–11. DMV is change in minute ventilation and is converted to heart rate response factor. Filter step involves filtering and multiplication by respiration rate.

60 breaths/min) for most patients. For patients with maximum respiratory rates above 60 breaths/min, the MV signal may be degraded at peak exercise as a result of inability to measure very high respiratory rates accurately. The Pulsar Max DDDR pacemaker (Guidant, Minneapolis, MN), which measures MV, uses a rate-adaptive filter to allow measurement of respiratory rates above 60 breaths/min. Thus, after reconstruction from the impedance pulses, the signal is generally filtered for information between 0.1 and 1 Hz. In pacemakers controlled by respiratory rate (now obsolete), the physician had to program the "offset" of the signal (see Fig. 10–11) to allow adequate sensing of crossovers of the offset line from rest to heavy exercise. In a transvenous system, the objective is to measure the product of the respiratory rate and the tidal volume.

Each sample shown in Figure 10–11 is checked for the polarity of the signal. If 7 samples of 10 are of one polarity, the signal is considered to be of that polarity. Each time this polarity changes, it is registered and used to compute the respiratory rate. This mode of measurement makes allowances for considerable noise in the respiratory signal and allows accurate measurement of a tidal volume curve of any shape. Medtronic pacemakers do not determine the respiration rate but obtain MV by taking the derivative of the filtered respiration signal, which also gives the desired MV signal.

In addition to analog filtering, digital filtering is used to eliminate as much of the stroke volume as possible as well as any signal in excess of 60 breaths/min (Meta MV). The Legend Plus pacemaker (Medtronic) filters out impedance signals that occur faster than 48 per minute. The filtered respiration component is rectified, averaged, and then multiplied by the respiratory rate to give the MV value (called the delta MV), which controls pacing rate. This delta MV goes through a 30-minute filter to create the baseline shown in Figure 10–12, which acts as a reference for the short-term change in delta MV. The RRF value then converts this delta MV to pacing rate. If the delta MV is above an arbitrary threshold, with respect to the baseline, then it will not equilibrate to the baseline; if below this threshold, equilibration will occur. This is to minimize "rate hang-up" during operation.

The purpose of filtering the signal is to ensure, among other things, that the effect of random fluctuations is minimized. As a result, a step change in MV will not manifest as a step change in heart rate. Rather, the pacing rate will gradually rise from the present pacing rate to a new level dictated by the input of the sensor. The time required for this change in pacing rate is dependent on the time constant of the filter (Fig. 10–13), which allows the output to reach 66% of its final value in about 15 seconds. The RRF controls the size of the final value and hence can influence the speed of response, as shown in Figure 10–13. Use of RRF in such

a manner is not advised because it leads to overpacing the patient.

Programming the Rate-Response Slope

Programming of most MV-sensing, rate-adaptive pacemakers requires selection of a lower pacing rate, an upper pacing rate, and a slope that relates changes in MV to changes in pacing rate. For the Meta MV series of pacemakers, this slope parameter is known as the RRF. The RRF value is directly related to the slope of the rate-response curve. Thus, high RRF values provide very steep rate-response curves, whereas low values provide a more gradual rate response.

Accurate programming of the RRF is accomplished by the patient exercising to his or her symptomatic limit (usually past the anaerobic threshold). The programmer automatically uses the measured maximum value of MV that is stored in the pulse generator to calculate the RRF value that will give the maximum pacing rate for this level of MV. The relationship between MV change and these heart rate limits is shown in Figure 10–14A. In this representation, we see the relational modification from the patient attaining anaerobic metabolism, as discussed previously. Exercising patients to their symptomatic limit or to exhaustion has been replaced by either a short walk or a low-intensity treadmill exercise (LITE) routine.[46] The physician programs the anticipated rate for this level of exertion and the slope (RRF) is automatically extrapolated.

None of these techniques takes into consideration the nonlinearity due to the anaerobic threshold. To address this,

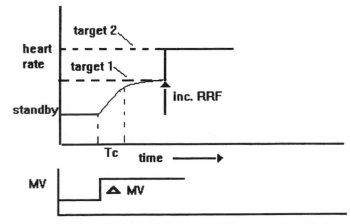

Figure 10–13. Diagram showing that changing rate response factor (RRF) changes only the target heart rate, not the time needed to reach target. RRF is the sensitivity that the controller needed to convert DMV to heart rate. TC, time constant of heart rate change to step change in minute ventilation; MV, minute ventilation.

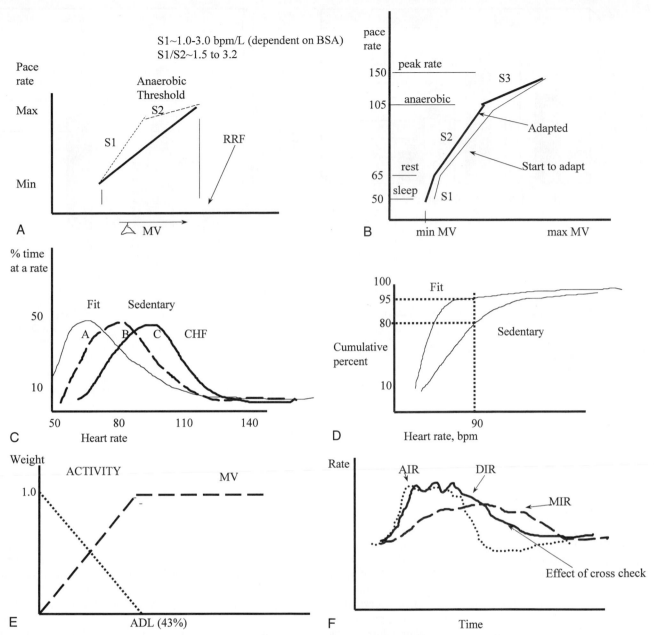

Figure 10–14. *A,* Various relationships between heart rate and minute ventilation change (DMV). The same change in minute ventilation (MV) can produce dramatically different heart rates. The standard relationship between change in MV (delta MV) and heart rate between minimum and maximum rate. In current devices, dual slopes S1 and S2 are used with relationships indicated. *B,* The comprehensive relationship between MV and heart rate in an automatic rate-adaptive pacemaker. The relationship adapts in time, as indicated, based on empirically derived rate profiles. *C,* Empirical rate profiles from patients of various levels of fitness. A, very fit; B, sedentary; C, with congestive heart failure (CHF). *D,* The relationship between heart rate and cumulative percentage of time spent below or above a specified rate. This concept is fundamental in automatically adapting a sensor's response to fit a specific rate profile. *E,* The weighting of activity and MV in a blended dual-sensor algorithm. The weight is rate dependent, hence requiring a recursive method of calculation. *F,* The actual response of a dual-sensor blended algorithm, in which activity is a weight of 1 up to 15%, and MV is only effective if activity is above a preset limit.

Illustration continued on following page

an interim refinement in the method of defining the RRF has been discussed by Brachmann and colleagues.[47] This revised method involves averaging the suggested RRF values at anaerobic threshold and at peak exercise to calculate the correct RRF. The Kappa.400 pacemaker (Medtronic) and the Pulsar Max pacemakers regulate rate response by comparing the sensor-indicated rate histograms to a reference value that

is indirectly programmed by the physician who chooses a fitness level of the patient (ranging from sedentary to athletic). The rate response is automatically adjusted to achieve a rate histogram that is within limits of the algorithm.

The Legend Plus pacemaker provides a programmable MV rate response that controls the relationship between changes in impedance and changes in pacing rate. There are

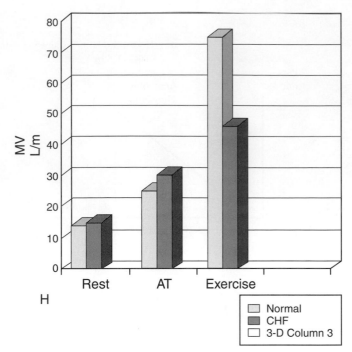

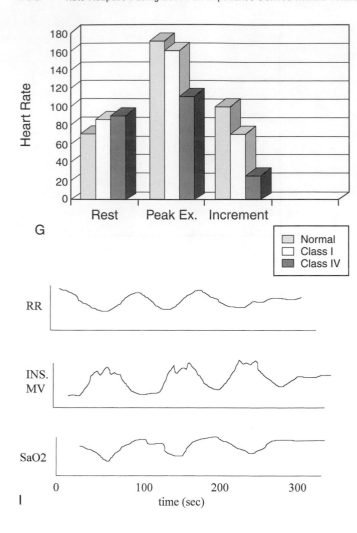

Figure 10–14 *Continued.* *G*, The effect of congestive heart disease on heart rate ranges in comparison with healthy subjects. *H*, The effect of CHF on MV ranges in comparison with healthy subjects. *I*, Typical modulation in heart rate (RR), instantaneous MV, and arterial oxygen saturation (SaO$_2$).

16 settings, with a value of 1 providing the smallest change in pacing rate in response to an increase in MV signal and a value of 16 providing the greatest change. All of these settings are linear and allow the pacing rate to increase to the maximum MV rate for most values. The programmer recommends a specific MV rate-response setting based on a low-level exercise protocol that involves exercising the patient for 2 minutes. The physician selects a target heart rate for the level of exercise. The programmer analyzes the MV signal to determine the appropriate MV rate-response curve that will provide the target heart rate. In addition to this programmable setting, acceleration and deceleration times can be programmed. These values control the interval required for a change in the MV-indicated pacing rate to be converted into a change in the actual pacing rate. The possible acceleration times are 0.25, 0.5, and 1 minute. The settings for deceleration times are 2.5, 5, and 10 minutes.

■ IMPROVEMENTS IN MINUTE VENTILATION PACING

The Ideal Response Curve

Soon after the first generation of MV rate-responsive pacemakers became available, it became clear that a simple linear relationship between MV and heart rate did not truly reflect the natural relationship between these two vital parameters. A more comprehensive relationship is shown in Figure 10–14B, in which the curve is segmented into three regions. S$_1$ is the segment controlling rate changes from sleep to daytime rest rates; S$_2$ determines the relationship for light exercise; and S$_3$ sets the relationship for anaerobic activity. The anaerobic threshold is set to about 75% of the maximum heart rate,[29, 48] which corresponds to about 40% of maximum MV. The actual value of S$_2$ can be set from the value of the patient's BSA, which will also be roughly the value of S$_1$. The value of S$_3$ is roughly half of this value.

Automatic Programming

It is evident from the previous discussion that ideal programming is not an easy affair. The approach that is gaining acceptance is the *rate profile matching* concept, or *rate profile optimization* (RPO), as called by Medtronic. The RPO concept simply states that a specific rate profile can be targeted and that, over time, the sensor response can be automatically adjusted to fit that rate profile. Representations of rate profiles are shown in Figure 10–14C, based on extensive studies,[49, 50] for a fit individual (A), for a sedentary individual (B), and for a typical patient suffering from congestive heart failure (CHF) (C). The physician decides what profile the patient fits best and programs the device to adapt to that profile. This adaptation process can best be demonstrated by Figure 10–14D, which shows much the same data that were presented with the rate profiles, but as cumulative percentages for each rate.

In simple terms, we say that on curve F (fit individual), 95% of the time is spent below 90 bpm. With a less fit subject, 80% is spent below the same rate. Because MV maintains a predictable relationship to metabolic demand (i.e., heart rate), a single point can be used to determine the RRF for the patient. This single point could be the activity of daily living (ADL) rate, and the stipulation for a sedentary patient would be that 80% of ADL rates should be below 90 bpm. Over a period of time (e.g., months), the values of S_2 and S_3 would gradually adjust to meet the stated target. The value of S_1 could also be automatically adapted to the patient's needs. By setting a rate for sleep, sometimes called *resting base rate* (RBR), and for a daytime rate, sometimes called *active base rate* (ABR), the boundary conditions would be defined that would equate to the sleep MV value and to the average MV value. The sleep MV value could be the value of MV below which MV goes only 10% of the time. In this manner, the sleep slope would adapt to meet these criteria. The Chorus 7234[51] and the original Sentri 1210 (Telectronics)[52] used these concepts with great success.

It is informative to look at the implementation of the automatic slope algorithm in the Chorus RM. The pacemaker determines the resting and maximum MV values on a daily basis and stores the mean values over the last 30 days. The MV signal is determined every 32nd respiratory cycle. The resting MV value is decreased by 6% if the mean value of MV calculated for the last 64 respiratory cycles is 6% or more below the present value. The resting MV is increased by 6% if more than 8 mean values for the MV signal (calculated every 64 respiratory cycles) are at least 6% above the present value. The maximal increase in the resting MV value is limited to 20% of the mean resting value the day before. The device calculates the exercise MV signal by looking for the maximal MV signal and recalculates this value every eighth cycle during which a change has occurred. The exercise MV value is increased or decreased in 6% intervals. The mean resting and exercise MV values are used to adjust the rate-response slope automatically over the range of values from 1 to 15 in steps of 0.1. By automatically adjusting the rate-response slope in this manner, the Chorus RM may be able to provide rate response that is individualized for each patient and can vary this as physiologic conditions evolve. In this description, two subtleties have to be noted: (1) because the maximum MV is continuously being adjusted in both positive and negative direction, the maximum MV is really the MV that is the largest value reached for a certain percentage of the time, usually less than 1%, and (2) the algorithm should have a faster adaptation for making the RRF smaller (more sensitive) than for making it large. This algorithm has now been tested extensively and found to be effective.[52–54]

In the case of the Kappa.400,[55] for automatic adaptation, two points have to be defined on the general curve: the ADL point and the exertion response range. The underlying concept of rate profile adaption with this product is also based on the cumulative percentage, over time, spent below a target rate. The target rates in question are about 95 bpm for ADL and an age-related maximum rate. In this product,

the two points will allow the calibration of both the MV and the activity sensors. The one drawback with using maximum exertion values for calibration is that most patients never reach these levels of exertion; hence, the system will automatically adapt to a sensitivity that is higher than appropriate. This is because it assumes that the maximum value of MV seen must correspond to the maximum rate.

Dual-Sensor Concepts

MV is recognized as being a parameter that is both reliable and correlated with the metabolic workload. These general qualities still leave certain inadequacies, such as insufficiently fast response to sudden metabolic demand, excessive artifacts from arm motion, EMI in certain higher-frequency bands, and in a small number of cases yet to be determined, rate-response anomalies. To eliminate or minimize these undesirable effects, it is natural to look at adding another sensor that could ameliorate these nonspecific responses. The currently accepted approach is to use an activity or accelerometer sensor in conjunction with the MV sensor to achieve the stated objectives. This combination is available in the Kappa.400, the Pulsar Max, and the ELA Talent pacemakers.[55–57] In these products, the combination of MV and activity is achieved by blending and cross-checking.

The basic concepts of blending for the Kappa.400 are shown in Figure 10–14E. This figure shows two weighting functions: one for activity and one for MV. Activity contributes to the resultant rate between lower rate limit (LRL) and ADL, which in this case correspond to 0% and 43% of rate range, respectively. MV contributes to gradual increases from LRL to ADL and then controls the rate exclusively at rates above the ADL rate. These blending concepts, sometimes going under the generic name of *fuzzy logic,* lend themselves well to this type of application.

In this example, which is the blend for the Kappa.400 pacemaker, the good correlation of the activity sensor to the sinus response at the onset of exercise and the good proportionality of MV to higher levels of workload are combined.[58] The algorithm also has a cross-check function, whereby the MV rate is limited to a certain value if the activity rate does not exceed a predesignated limit, usually below the ADL rate. The activity rate is not cross-checked because it can approach only ADL, not beyond. This particular implementation exploits the strong points of both sensors and, to a considerable extent, protects the patient from some bothersome interference artifacts that affect both sensors.

The response of a similar dual-sensor implementation to exercise is shown in Figure 10–14F. This figure shows the contribution from the activity sensor at onset and the decrease in rate due to cross-checking, when the activity rate goes below a certain value and the MV stays high.

There are, of course, many different methods of blending and cross-checking, and they all have the same drawbacks, including that the two sensors do not always respond correctly to metabolic demand or in a mutually exclusive manner to extraneous interference. This does not necessarily mean that the combination of these sensors can do harm, only that apart from improving the speed of onset, this particular combination will not achieve much more.

Utility of Minute Ventilation in Congestive Heart Failure

The close interdependence of the cardiovascular and pulmonary systems allows the data collected from one system (pulmonary) to give insight into the condition of the other (cardiac). There is considerable debate about whether patients in CHF are chronotropically incompetent because of their small range of heart rates and low maximum rates,[21] as shown in Figure 10–14G. This question remains perplexing because, in most cases, these patients have a functional sinus node and autonomic nervous system. The important observation is that the dynamics of ventilation, in these patients, mimics that of heart rate. Ventilation also has a higher resting rate and a lower maximum rate in patients with CHF.[59] This observation by McElroy and colleagues[19] in 64 CHF patients compared with 38 healthy subjects has been repeated in other studies with similar results.

In Figure 10–14H, based on data from Sullivan and associates,[59] the ratio of peak MV to resting MV in healthy patients is close to twice that in patients with CHF. It is immediately obvious that this ratio could be used in a pacemaker to limit the maximum rate and to guard against excessive sensitivity for rate response. This control must be applied with the knowledge that patients with severe obstructive lung disease would have similar ratios. These patients, however, would have a corresponding lower vital capacity.[21] When patients with CHF undergo a regimen of exercise training, their peak MV increases, as does their maximum heart rate. In the nine patients studied by Sullivan and associates,[59] peak MV increased by about 25% and maximum heart rate by 10%. These observations indicate that a pacemaker capable of monitoring MV could be used to evaluate the results of exercise training in patients with CHF.

The interdependence of the cardiac and pulmonary systems are best highlighted by a Cheyne-Stokes respiration pattern. Cheyne-Stokes respiration is a waxing and waning of tidal volume and respiratory rate with a periodicity of about 0.02 Hz. In excess of 60% of the patients with CHF show overt Cheyne-Stokes respiration or some form of pulsed breathing during sleep.[60] The periodicity of tidal volume modulation has been directly correlated with delayed circulation to the brain.[61] Manifestation of Cheyne-Stokes respiration during exercise[62] and ADL[63] tends to carry a poor prognosis. Appropriate treatment with diuretics and angiotensin-converting enzyme inhibitors may eliminate this respiratory pattern. Figure 10–14D shows the distinct tidal volume (shown as instantaneous MV) modulation and a corresponding heart rate modulation in a typical case of Cheyne-Stokes respiration. This heart rate modulation serves the important purpose of trying to augment circulation to maintain arterial oxygen saturation. Cheyne-Stokes respiration can be an effective index of CHF that a pacemaker, measuring MV, could monitor to guide therapy.

■ MINUTE VENTILATION MEASURED IN THE RIGHT ATRIUM

In the early developmental work on transvenous MV pacing systems (see Table 10–1) and in more current work by Pioger and colleagues,[24] the correlation coefficients for the relationship between heart rate and transthoracic impedance estimates of MV are comparable in the atrium and ventricle. These observations suggest that MV is feasible for AAIR and DDDR pacing and provides considerable flexibility. Thus, the same configuration for impedance measurement has been used in both the atrium and ventricle. A potential advantage of measuring MV in the right atrium is a lower stroke volume component in the transthoracic impedance signal. At present, there a number of MV controlled DDDR pacemakers, at least one from most of the major manufacturers.

The Meta DDDR pacemakers (models 1250, 1254, and 1256) process the impedance signal in a manner similar to that used in the Meta MV model 1202, with algorithmic improvements as the model numbers progress. All the products in this family continue to generate the current pulse off the ventricular ring and sense the impedance off the tip. In addition, they use MV to discriminate pathologic atrial arrhythmias from sinus tachycardia and use the same maximum rate for tracking the sinus node and the MV sensor.

The Chorus RM DDDR pacemaker was the second DDDR device to become available with MV as a rate controller. This device measures MV in the right atrium in fundamentally the same way with a similar rate-response algorithm and allows the use of a unipolar ventricular lead, a potential advantage in terms of lead reliability.

Automatic Mode Switching

All dual-chamber MV-sensing pacemakers that are presently marketed offer mode switching to avoid tracking pathologic atrial arrhythmias. The Meta DDDR model 1250 introduced the concept of automatic mode switching to DDDR pacing. The Telectronics devices used MV as the means of distinguishing pathologically high rates in the atrium from physiologically appropriate sinus tachycardia. This could be done only if there was strong confidence that the sensor would always respond to metabolic demand. Based on the extensive work in physiology and the establishment of impedance as a reliable indicator of respiration, the specificity of the transvenous MV sensor was thought to be very high. Thus, the Meta DDDR pacemaker was designed to track high atrial rates when the MV sensor indicates a high level of respiration but to revert to the VVIR pacing mode at the rate indicated by the sensor when the MV signal is not increased.

The *automatic mode switching* (AMS) operation of the Telectronics model 1250 DDDR pacemaker is explained in Figure 10–15. On the x-axis is plotted an increasing level of metabolic demand, as indicated by the MV impedance sensor. On the y-axis are the atrial pacing rates that the device is allowed to track, corresponding to the level of the MV signal. If the atrial rhythm is faster than the bounds set for it, the rhythm is judged to be inappropriately rapid, and AMS to the VVIR mode occurs. The device then continues in the VVIR mode until the atrial rate moves back into the "legal" limits indicated by the MV sensor, at which time reassociation occurs.

One of the main objectives of this approach was protection against pacemaker-mediated tachycardias by automatic modification of the atrioventricular (AV) delay and the postventricular atrial refractory period (PVARP) by input from the MV sensor. In the initial implementation, about 1% of patients still suffered symptoms of tachyarrhythmias because

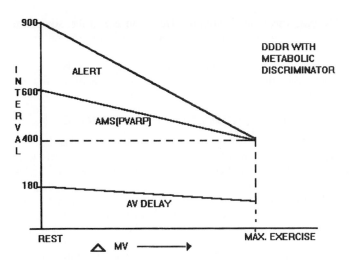

Figure 10–15. Response of DDDR timing parameters to metabolic demand. AMS, automatic mode switch zone in which atrial events contribute to decision to switch to ventricular control; Alert, atrial events in this zone trigger ventricular pacing after corresponding atrioventricular (AV) delay; PVARP, postventricular.

of dissociation after a single atrial premature beat.[64] Clinical experience with the initial implementation of AMS in the Meta DDDR device indicated that this concept had high sensitivity for detecting atrial fibrillation and flutter but suffered from low specificity. The model 1250 mode switched inappropriately during sinus rhythm, during premature atrial contractions, and from far-field sensing of the R wave.

These findings were substantially improved in the newer models, the Telectronics 1254 and 1256. In these newer models, a programmable number of atrial events must occur at a shorter preselected cycle length to trigger AMS (e.g., five of seven events). The problem of protecting the atrium from being paced with a very short interval between the last sensed complex within the vulnerable zone was addressed by introducing an *atrial protection interval* (API), which is always timed from a preceding atrial event. If the minimum rate is to be violated by the API, AV interval prolongation takes place instead. Whether the API actually reduces the induction of atrial arrhythmias is unknown.

The Chorus RM DDDR pacemaker offers the option of programming the device to a fallback mode with rate-adaptive pacing. This operation can be programmed to occur with the device in either the DDD or DDDR mode. When programmed in this manner, normal DDD or DDDR atrial tracking occurs at rates between the lower and upper rate limits. At rates above the upper rate limit, Wenckebach behavior occurs. The MV sensor is activated as soon as the pacemaker detects an atrial rate above the upper tracking rate. The Wenckebach upper rate behavior is allowed to function for a programmable number of cycles before the device changes modes to the VDIR mode (VVIR pacing with continued atrial sensing), with fallback to the sensor-indicated rate. As soon as the atrial rate decreases below the upper tracking limit, there is reassociation of the atria and ventricles with return to the DDD(R) mode.

The Chorus RM also offers the option of programming rate smoothing, a function that prevents abrupt changes in ventricular rate. Shortening of the AV delay also occurs with changes in the MV-indicated or intrinsic sinus rate with this device. The Pulsar Max DDDR pacemaker offers a similar mode-switching operation, with the advantage of a separately programmable atrial tachycardia response detection rate. The Kappa.400 pacemaker offers an improved mode switching algorithm that builds on the advantages of high specificity from the Thera family of pacemakers, with the addition of a more sensitive mode-switching detection criterion (4 of 7 beats greater than the programmed detection rate).

The Chorus RM 7234 DDDR has a more conservative approach, in which the two options are 28 of 32 cycles and 32 of 64 cycles.[65] This approach is claimed to be 100% reliable. The more conservative criteria mostly eliminate the AMS oscillations described by Ellenbogen and coauthors[66] in their study of the Meta 1254. The oscillations discussed in this study were due to the "blanking" times after the atrial and the ventricular events (manifest on the atrial sensing channel). The postventricular blanking time is particularly bothersome because it tends to cover a critical time from end of AV delay (about 150 msec) to about 300 msec. This problem was ameliorated in the study by shortening AV delay in six patients and lengthening it in one patient (with limited success). There were no problems with atrial sensing because the patients all had various forms of flutter, which produced large P waves. In the case of partial undersensing, similar AMS cycling has been known to take place.[67]

The original intent of using MV as a discriminator of pathological rhythms from physiological ones, has to some extent been overshadowed by the more pressing need for reliable sensing of the various atrial arrhythmias. With the resolution of this problem the need for sensor arbitration of various rhythms will again become relevant.

Clinical Experience With Minute Ventilation in DDDR Pacemakers

A good summary of the performance of MV in a dual-chamber device is available in the clinical study summary of the Meta DDDR, the first device to make use of this sensor.[64] The study included 782 patients, 63% of whom were male. Atrial or ventricular arrhythmias were reported in 43% of the patients. The most relevant findings of the study were that (1) 70% of patients had an RRF setting of between 20 and 24, (2) 90% of patients were in DDDR mode after 1 month, (3) 80% of patients had a PVARP setting of 360 msec or 400 msec, the lowest values that were programmable, and (4) 70% of patients were programmed to maximum rates between 120 and 140 ppm (55% at 120 ppm).

Of this patient group, 13 were selected to undergo cardiopulmonary exercise testing. These patients were judged to be chronotropically incompetent owing to a maximum attainable heart rate of less than 100 bpm or a maximum increase in heart rate that was less than 50% of their heart rate reserve. Each patient was exercised in the dual-chamber rate-responsive mode and the non–rate-responsive dual-chamber mode using the Chronotropic Assessment Exercise Protocol (CAEP).[68] The pacing modes were randomized, and the patients were blinded to the mode. Expired respiratory gases were analyzed continuously.

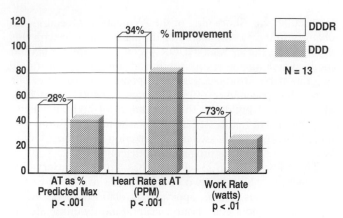

Figure 10–16. Improvements in DDDR versus DDD mode. Refer to text for discussion.

The key results of this study are shown in Figures 10–16 and 10–17. When programmed to the DDDR mode, these patients had a workload that increased by 85.2%, from 26 W to 50 W. Comparing the DDD with the DDDR modes, a statistically significant increase in oxygen uptake at an anaerobic threshold of 27% was observed in the DDDR mode (9.7 versus 12.1 mL/kg per minute). The anaerobic threshold occurred at 43.2% compared with 54.6% of the predicted $\dot{V}_{O_{2max}}$ in the DDD and DDDR modes, respectively. The time to anaerobic threshold (indicated by $\dot{V}_{O_{2max}}$) increased by 50% with DDDR pacing. The heart rate–$\dot{V}_{O_2}$ slope improvement indicates that there was a more prompt heart rate response in the DDDR mode with an increase in slope from 1.1 to 4.5. The heart rate slope $\Delta\frac{HR}{VE}$ increased to 1.9, which is the average predicted by McElroy and associates.[20] This pacing system has now been extensively reviewed in several publications.[69–71]

The Chorus RM pacemaker has proved to provide effective rate modulation with automatic regulation of rate response. This device allows rate modulation to be programmed in either a fixed or an automatic mode. In the automatic mode, the rate-responsive slope is reprogrammed based on the heart rates achieved in the previous 18 hours. The slope is updated conservatively to increase or decrease

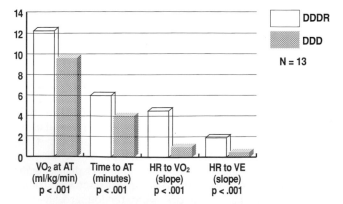

Figure 10–17. Improvements in DDDR versus DDD mode. Refer to text for discussion.

the pattern of rate response. This device has the advantage of not requiring a maximal exercise test for programming. The Kappa.400 pacemaker has proved to provide rate response that prevents gross underpacing or overpacing by continual adjustment of the MV slope to achieve the expected sensor-indicated rate histogram.

■ FUTURE IMPROVEMENTS IN MINUTE VENTILATION

Several improvements in the rate-adaptive algorithms must be introduced for MV to emulate the normal sinus node more closely. First, it is now well recognized that the HR/MV slope cannot be linear throughout exercise. Because the normal HR/MV slope decreases at workloads above anaerobic threshold, several manufacturers have suggested that an MV pacemaker should have a two-slope algorithm. Telectronics has demonstrated the utility of an MV algorithm that includes two HR/MV slopes that are designed to decrease the RRF by three settings at high heart rates. This feature, termed the *rate-augmentation factor,* sets up a breakpoint in the rate-response curve that may be set from 50% to 70% of the difference between the programmed lower and upper rate limits. For example, if a 60-year-old man had lower rate programmed to 60 bpm and an appropriately programmed upper rate of 160 bpm, the anaerobic threshold breakpoint at 50% of the heart rate reserve would occur at 110 bpm. For pacing rates below 110 bpm, the RRF might be programmed to a value of 20. Above the breakpoint, the RRF would be automatically decreased to 17. In this way, increases in MV above anaerobic threshold will not lead to an excessive increase in pacing rate. In addition, use of the rate-augmentation factor allows a more aggressive RRF to be programmed for lower levels of exercise while avoiding overpacing at higher levels of exercise. This improves the speed of response at the onset of exercise with the MV sensor.

A novel concept has been introduced by Kay and colleagues[67] in which a low level of exercise may be used to predict automatically the absolute MV value that will occur at anaerobic threshold and at peak exercise. If the MV at anaerobic threshold and peak exercise are known for a given patient, the correct heart rate can be calculated at any intermediate level of exercise. This concept is based on expired gas exchange analysis from patients with permanent pacemakers who performed both low-level, constant-workload exercise and maximal exercise testing. Measurement of the MV, tidal volume, and respiratory rate at rest and during low-level exercise was used to create a regression equation to predict the MV at anaerobic threshold and at peak exercise in a group of 10 patients with pacemakers. The regression equations were then prospectively applied to a test group of 10 patients. The predicted MV at anaerobic threshold and at peak exercise correlated with the actual values in the test group, with correlation coefficients of 0.96 and 0.95, respectively. This concept holds the promise that MV pacemakers may be able to calibrate themselves automatically for each patient and calculate the precise heart rate at any given level of exercise.

Summary

With more than 10 years of experience and thousands of implantations, MV measured by changes in transthoracic impedance has become a physiologic standard for rate-adaptive pacing. This sensor has the promise to become the dominant technology in rate-adaptive pacing as newer algorithms are introduced to correlate MV more closely with the function of the normal sinus node.

REFERENCES

1. Krasner JL, Voukydis PC, Nardella PC: A physiologically controlled cardiac pacemaker. J Assoc Adv Med Instrum 1:14, 1966.
2. Krasner JL, Nardella PC: US Patent No. 3,593,718. Filed 1967.
3. Funke HD: Ein Herzschrittmacher mit belastung abhanginger Frequenzregulation. Biomed Tech 20:225, 1975.
4. Ionescu VL: An on-demand pacemaker responsive to respiration rate. PACE 3:375, 1980.
5. Rossi P, Plicchi G, Canducci G, et al: Respiratory rate as a determinant of optimal pacing rate. PACE 6:502, 1983.
6. Rossi P, Plicchi G, Canducci G, et al: Respiration as a reliable physiological sensor for the control of cardiac pacing rate. Br Heart J 51:7, 1984.
7. Rossi P, Rognoni G, Occhetta E, et al: Respiration-dependent ventricular pacing compared with ventricular and atrial-ventricular synchronous pacing: Aerobic and hemodynamic variables. J Am Coll Cardiol 6:646, 1985.
8. Humen PP, Anderson K, Brunwell D, et al: A pacemaker which automatically increases its rate with physical activity. *In* Cardiac Pacing: Proceedings of the VIIth World Symposium on Cardiac Pacing, Vienna, 1983.
9. Nappholz TA, Lubin M, Maloney J, Simmons A: Measuring minute ventilation with a pacing catheter. Third Asian Pacific Symposium on Cardiac Pacing and Electrophysiology, Melbourne, Australia, October 1985.
10. Simmons A, Maloney J, Abi-Samra F, et al: Exercise-responsive intravascular impedance changes as a rate controller for cardiac pacing. PACE 9:285, 1986.
11. Valenta H, Maloney J, McElroy P: Correlation of heart rate with an intravenous impedance respiratory sensor. Instrumentation Society of America, No. 86–0002, 1986.
12. Fischer S, Nappholz TA, et al: Optimizing respiration as a parameter for rate-responsive pacing. Internal Document.
13. Nappholz TA, Valenta H, Maloney J, Simmons A: Electrode configurations for a respiratory impedance measurement suitable for rate-responsive pacing. PACE 9 (Pt. II):960, 1986.
14. Simmons TW, Valenta H, Masterson M, et al: Verification of a minute ventilation rate-responsive algorithm with a computer-based external pacing system [abstract]. PACE 11:505, 1988.
15. Pearce DH, Milhorn HT, Holloman GH, et al: Computer-based system for analysis of respiratory responses to exercise. J Appl Physiol 42(6):968, 1977.
16. Pearce DH, Milhorn HT: Dynamic and steady-state respiratory responses to bicycle exercise. J Appl Physiol 42(6):959, 1976.
17. Whipp BJ, Wasserman K: Oxygen uptake kinetics for various intensities of constant-load work. J Appl Physiol 33(3):351, 1972.
18. Weber KT, Kinasewitz GT, Janicki JS, Fishmann AP: Oxygen utilization and ventilation during exercise in patients with chronic cardiac failure. Circulation 65(6):1213, 1982.
19. McElroy P, Weber KT, Nappholz TA: Heart rate, ventilation, mixed venous temperature, pH, and oxygen saturation during incremental upright exercise. Third Asian Pacific Symposium on Cardiac Pacing and Electrophysiology, Melbourne, Australia, October 1985.
20. McElroy P, Janicki JS, Weber KT: Physiologic correlates of the heart rate response to upright isotonic exercise: Relevance to rate-responsive pacemakers. J Am Coll Cardiol 11(1):94, 1988.
21. Weber KT, Janicki JS: Cardiopulmonary Exercise Testing. Philadelphia, WB Saunders, 1986.
22. Fischer S: Internal document, Telectronics Pacing Systems, Inc., Denver, 1986.
22. Yeh E: The hemodynamic importance of atrio-ventricular synchrony during ventricular tachycardia in man. Thesis, Case Western Reserve University, Cleveland, OH, 1988.
23. Khoury DS: Continuous right ventricular volume assessment by catheter measurement of impedance for antitachycardia system control. Thesis, Case Western Reserve University, Cleveland, OH, 1989.
24. Pioger G, et al: Comparison of different electrode configurations in minute ventilation measurement. Eur J Cardiol Pacing 6(1), 1996.
25. Vai F, Bonnet JL, Ritter PH, Pioger G: Relationship between heart rate and minute ventilation, tidal volume and respiratory rate during brief and low level exercise. PACE 11(Pt. II):1860, 1988.
26. Beaver WL, Wasserman K: Tidal volume and respiratory rate change at start and end of exercise. J Appl Physiol 29(6):872, 1970.
27. Alt E, Heinz M, Hirgestetter C, et al: Control of pacemaker rate by impedance-based respiratory minute ventilation. Chest 92:247, 1987.
28. Glikson M, MacCarter DJ, Hopper DL, et al: Overpacing during moderate exercise reduces ventilatory efficiency. PACE 20:1521, 1997.
29. Soucie Luc, Carey C, Woodend AK, et al: Correlation of the heart rate-minute ventilation relationship with clinical data. PACE 20:1913, 1997.
30. Rickli H, MacCarter DJ, Maire R, et al: Age and sex related changes in heart rate in ventilation coupling. PACE 20:105, 1997.
31. Telectronics Pacing Systems: Meta MV, Clinical Study Summary. Document No. 130–2531, Rev 1, April 1989.
31. Lau CP, Antoniou A, Ward DE, Camm AJ: Reliability of minute ventilation as a parameter for rate-responsive pacing. PACE 12:321, 1989.
32. Lau CP, Ward DE, Camm AJ: Single-chamber cardiac pacing with two forms of respiration-controlled rate-responsive pacemaker. Chest 95:352, 1989.
33. Greenhut S: Comparison of Telectronics Meta transthoracic impedance signal to respiration flow. Internal Telectronics document, Denver, 1988.
35. Kay GN, Bubien R: Transthoracic impedance measurement with minute ventilation-sensing pacemakers: Discrimination of respiratory and stroke volume components. PACE 12:671, 1989.
36. Mond HG, Kertes PJ: Rate-Responsive Cardiac Pacing. Englewood, CO, Telectronics Pacing Systems, 1990.
37. Kay GN, Bubien SR, Epstein AE, Plumb VJ: Rate-modulated pacing based on transthoracic impedance measurements of minute ventilation: Correlation with exercise gas exchange. J Am Coll Cardiol 15:1283, 1989.
38. Li H, Neubauer SA, Hayes DL: Follow-up of a minute ventilation rate-adaptive pacemaker. PACE 15:1826, 1992.
39. Smith R: Time domain reflectometry (TDR) applied to sensing of respiratory signals. Telectronics internal document, Denver, 1992.
40. Luttikhuis HA, Tuinstra E: Unipolar pacemaker replacement—the option for minute ventilation rate response. Eur J Cardiac Pacing Electrophysiol Cardiostim 2:729, 1992.
41. Seger J, Mead RH, Nygaard G, et al: Safe amplitude and pulse width for minute ventilation pulses. PACE 20:1173, 1997.
42. Greenhut S: Animal experiments to examine the safety of measuring MV with high impedance lead. Telectronics internal document, Denver, 1997.
43. Wilson J, Lattner S: Apparent undersensing due to oversensing of low amplitude pulses in a thoracic impedance-sensing rate-responsive pacemaker. PACE 11:1479, 1988.
44. Chew EW, Troughear RH, Kuchar DL, et al: Inappropriate rate change in a minute ventilation rate responsive pacemaker due to interference by cardiac monitors. PACE 20:276, 1997.
45. Daryl D: Inappropriate rate rise in a Meta 1256 pulse generator due to proximity to anti-theft device. Telectronics internal document, Denver, 1995.
46. Gilliam FR, et al: Indicators of metabolic demand underscore the importance of adjusting rate response. Eur J Cardiac Pacing Electrophysiol 6:204, 1996.
46. Van Hemel N, Hamerlijnck RP, Pronk KJ, Van Der Veen EP: Upper limit ventricular stimulation in respiratory rate-responsive pacing due to electrocautery. PACE 12:1720, 1989.
47. Brachmann J, MacCarter DJ, Frees U, et al: Minimal algorithm changes in the rate-adaptive pacemaker slope cause significant differences in patient exercise capacity. ACC, March, 1991.
48. Anderson J: Ativa algorithm design and specification. Telectronics document, PS/002387, Denver.
49. Stimulation cardiaque et distribution des frequences cardiaques dans le nycthemere. Medtronic marketing publication.
50. Kristensson B-E, Karlsson D, Ryden L: Holtor monitored heart rhythm during atrioventricular synchronous and fixed-rate ventricular pacing. PACE 9:511, 1986.
51. Pioger G, Geroux L, Limousin M: Automatic basic rate variation algorithm driven by a minute ventilation sensor: Clinical results. PACE 20:1445, 1997.
52. Cornu L, et al: Sentri 1210: Final report. COM/000667. Internal Telectronics document.
53. Ritter P, Anselme F, Bonnet JL, et al: Clinical evaluation of an auto-

matic slope calibration function in a minute ventilation controlled DDDR pacemaker. PACE 20:1522, 1997.

54. Le Helloco A, et al: Optimal rate modulation slope provided by an automatic function in a DDDR pacemaker. Eur J Cardiac Pacing Electrophysiol 6:172, 1996.

55. Leung S-K, Lau C-P, Tang M-O, et al: New integrated sensor pacemaker. PACE 19:1664, 1996.

56. Greco EM, Arlotti M, Ricci R, et al: An automatic rate profile optimization algorithm: Clinical experience with a new rate adaptive dual sensor pacemaker. PACE 20:1446, 1997.

57. Schneider J, Lemke B, Lawo T, et al: Automatic rate profile optimization in a dual chamber pacemaker (DDDR) with a double sensor system. PACE 20:1523, 1997.

58. Lau C-P, Butrous GS, Ward DE, Camm AJ: Comparison of exercise performance of six rate-adaptive right ventricular cardiac pacemakers. Am J Cardiol 63:833, 1989.

59. Sullivan MJ, Higginbotham MB, Cobb FR: The anaerobic threshold in chronic heart failure. Circulation 81(Suppl II):II-47, 1990.

60. Mortara A, Sleight P, Pinna GD, et al: Abnormal awake respiratory patterns are common in chronic heart failure and may prevent evaluation of automatic tone by measures of heart rate variability. Circulation 96:246, 1997.

61. Millar TW, Hanley PJ, Hunt B, et al: The entrainment of low frequency breathing periodicity. Chest 98:1143, 1990.

62. Ben-Dov I, Sietsema KE, Casaburi R, and Wasserman K: Evidence that circulatory oscillations accompany ventilatory oscillations during exercise in patients with heart failure. Am Rev Respir Dis 145:776, 1992.

63. Andreas S, Hagenah G, Möller C, et al: Cheyne-Stokes respiration and prognosis in congestive heart failure. Am J Cardiol 78:1260, 1996.

64. Telectronics Pacing Systems: Meta DDDR, Clinical Study Summary. Document No. 130–3081, Rev 1, April 1992.

65. Bonnet J-L, Brusseau E, Limousin M, et al: Mode switching despite undersensing of atrial fibrillation in DDD pacing. PACE 19(Pt II):1724, 1996.

66. Ellenbogan KA, Mond HG, Wood MA, et al: Failure of automatic mode switching: Recognition and management. PACE 20:268, 1997.

67. Kay GN, Bubien RS, Hopper DL, et al: Tidal volume as a predictor of minute ventilation at anaerobic threshold and peak exercise: Automatic calculation of heart rate reserve for rate-adaptive pacing. Circulation 98(Suppl-I):714, 1998.

68. Wilkoff B, Corey J, Blackburn G: Mathematical model of the cardiac chronotropic response to exercise. J Electrophysiol 3:176, 1989.

69. Brinker J, MacCarter D, Shewmaker S, et al: Improved functional capacity with DDDR pacing in patients with chronotropic incompetence. PACE 14:684, 1991.

70. Lau CP, Tai Y-T, Fong P-C, et al: Atrial arrhythmia management with sensor-controlled atrial refractory period and automatic mode switching in patients with minute ventilation sensing dual chamber rate-adaptive pacemakers. PACE 15:1504, 1992.

71. Lemke B, Dryander B, Jager D, et al: Aerobic capacity in rate-modulated pacing. PACE 15:1914, 1992.

Chapter 11

Evoked QT Interval–Based and Intracardiac Impedance–Based Pacemakers

Wim Boute, Frederik Feith, Sum-Kin Leung, and Chu-Pak Lau

■ EVOKED QT INTERVAL–BASED PACEMAKERS

In 1920, Bazett[1] showed that changes in heart rate induced by exercise result in a progressive shortening of the QT interval on the surface electrocardiogram (ECG). The normal QT interval was found to be longer at relatively slow heart rates than at faster heart rates. Bazett proposed a nonlinear formula to correct the QT interval for changes in heart rate, a parameter known as the *corrected QT interval* (QTc). In 1981, Rickards and Norman[2, 3] found that QT interval shortening during exercise actually consisted of two components: an effect induced by exercise alone and an effect of an increased heart rate. They measured QT intervals during exercise in patients with normal sinus rhythm (in whom the QT interval was influenced by both factors), during atrial pacing at different rates with the patient at rest (a pure heart rate influence), and during exercise in patients with a VVI pacemaker (a pure exercise influence). These observations, which have been reproduced by other investigators,[4–7] led to the design of a cardiac pacemaker that uses the QT interval to modulate the pacing rate.

Shortening of the QT interval as a result of exercise is thought to be related to increasing catecholamine levels in the heart. Jordaens and associates[8] found a correlation coefficient of 0.963 (n = 8) between the mean pacing rate of a QT interval–driven, rate-responsive pacemaker and plasma noradrenaline levels.

In 1982, the first QT interval–driven, rate-responsive pacemaker was implanted (TX1, Vitatron Medical, Dieren, the Netherlands). Experience gained with this and later models has proved the clinical applicability of this concept and has led to a series of pacemakers characterized by progressive improvement in their rate-modulating behavior (Table 11–1).

The QT Interval as an Indicator of Metabolic Demand

During exercise, metabolically active tissues require an increased amount of oxygen and produce more carbon dioxide. The main task of the circulatory system is to provide sufficient blood flow to deliver oxygen to the tissues and to remove the carbon dioxide that is produced. The increased cardiac output needed to achieve the increased metabolic activity is mediated by an increase in both stroke volume and heart rate. During maximum exercise, the oxygen uptake may increase by 5-fold (in nonathletes) to up to 15-fold (in trained athletes). There is an almost linear relationship between oxygen consumption and heart rate during exercise, indicating that heart rate is the main factor in the increase in cardiac output during exercise. An ideal rate-adaptive sensor in a pacing system should probably provide the same linear relationship between heart rate and oxygen consumption.

Table 11–1. Improvements in QT Interval–Driven Rate-Responsive Pacemakers

Year	Vitatron Model	Improvement	Technology
1985	Quintech TX	T-wave detection	Fast recharge pulse
		T-wave detection	Dual fast recharge pulse
		Rate-response pattern	Nonlinear slope
1988	Rhythmyx	Slope programming	Automatic (daily learning)
		Onset of rate response	QT interval combined with activity
1992	Topaz	Sensor specificity	Sensor cross-checking

Autonomic Regulation

The neurohumoral control of the circulatory system allows the body to react properly to changes in metabolic demand. Different physiologic sensors send information to the autonomic centers in the central nervous system. These sensors collect information about arterial blood pressure, blood acidity, and the pressure of blood gases, such as oxygen and carbon dioxide. Higher brain centers also send information to the autonomic centers of the brainstem during stress. The information is processed in the autonomic centers of the brain stem and used to prepare the organism for changes in metabolic demand. The direct neural control, for example, on heart rate and peripheral vascular resistance is nearly instantaneous.

The autonomic nervous system also stimulates the adrenal glands to produce catecholamines (adrenaline and noradrenaline), thereby changing the concentration of these humoral transmitters in the blood. The effect of this humoral control on the different organs is similar to that of the neural control but with slower kinetics. The effect of circulating catecholamines on the contractile state of the myocardium, however, is long-lasting and important for the support of chronic stress situations, such as congestive heart failure.

At the onset or anticipation of exercise, the neural mechanisms are activated. Postural changes and higher centers in the brain influence heart rate through the balance of adrenergic and cholinergic neurotransmitters. At the onset of rate response, a decrease in vagal tone causes an immediate increase in heart rate. The second sustained mechanism is the influence of an increasing amount of circulating catecholamines on the blood vessels and metabolic status of the skeletal muscles. There is a direct vasodilatatory effect of these agents on the blood vessels, increasing their capacity to transport oxygenated blood to the metabolically active tissues. Also, catecholamines influence the mechanisms of contraction at the level of the muscle fibers. The combination of these mechanisms markedly increases the working capacity of muscle tissue. In the heart, this means an increase in contractility and work capacity for as long as the situation of increased neurohumoral stimulation exists.

Metabolic Demand and the QT Interval

With exercise or psychic stress, the metabolism of the myocardium and heart rate (sinus node) increase, mainly as a result of adrenergic stimulation. Available data indicate a relatively strong linear correlation between atrial rate and cardiac sympathetic activation.[9] The ionic currents responsible for cardiac depolarization and repolarization periods also change. These processes suggest that the cardiac parameters, such as the QT interval, are a reflection of autonomic regulation and therefore of the changing metabolic needs of the individual. At low levels of exercise, the catecholamine release is relatively low, and the cardiac acceleration is primarily due to vagal withdrawal. This implies that as a biosensor, the QT interval (catecholamine influence) may be slow to respond at the onset of exercise, although its major dependence on the sympathetic nervous system should result in it being a specific sensor.[9]

To study the influence of various factors (e.g., drugs, autonomic influence, heart rate) on cardiac repolarization,

investigators have looked for formulas to describe the QT-HR relationship under these different circumstances. Several studies[5, 10, 11] have shown that Bazett's formula is relatively accurate at heart rates between 60 and 100 bpm but is not correct in describing the relationship between the QT interval and heart rate over a wider range of rates. Several other formulas have been suggested to describe this relationship. These studies[5, 10, 11] on the influence of drugs that modify the sensitivity of the myocardium to catecholamines show a clear influence of the adrenergic system on the QT interval that is independent of the heart rate. In Figure 11–1, the atrium is paced at a constant rate of 130 bpm, and the QT interval is measured before and after the administration of isoproterenol. The QT interval clearly shortens after the administration of the drug, independently of the heart rate.

Figure 11–2 shows the influence of propranolol on the QT interval compared with the heart rate in the exercising subject. There is a clear shift of the curve, indicating the effects of this synthetic catecholamine on the heart. Alternative methods for studying autonomic effects on the QT interval during exercise that are independent of heart rate involve comparing the QT interval of patients (1) during pacing at different rates while at rest, and (2) during exercise at a constant heart rate. Between 1979 and 1982, Rickards and Norman[2] and Milne and colleagues[5] studied patients using these methods and came to the conclusion that the QT interval changed with stress independent of heart rate and that these effects could be used as a metabolic indicator for

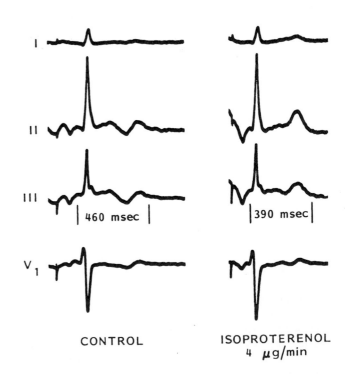

CONTROL   ISOPROTERENOL
4 μg/min

HIGH RIGHT ATRIAL PACING
PCL = 450 msec

Figure 11–1. Fixed rate atrial pacing at 130 bpm and the influence of a catecholamine mimicking drug, isoprenaline, on the length of the QT interval. (From Browne KF, Prystowsky E, Heger JJ, Zipes DP: Modulation of the Q-T interval by the autonomic nervous system. PACE 6(Pt II):1050–1056, 1983.)

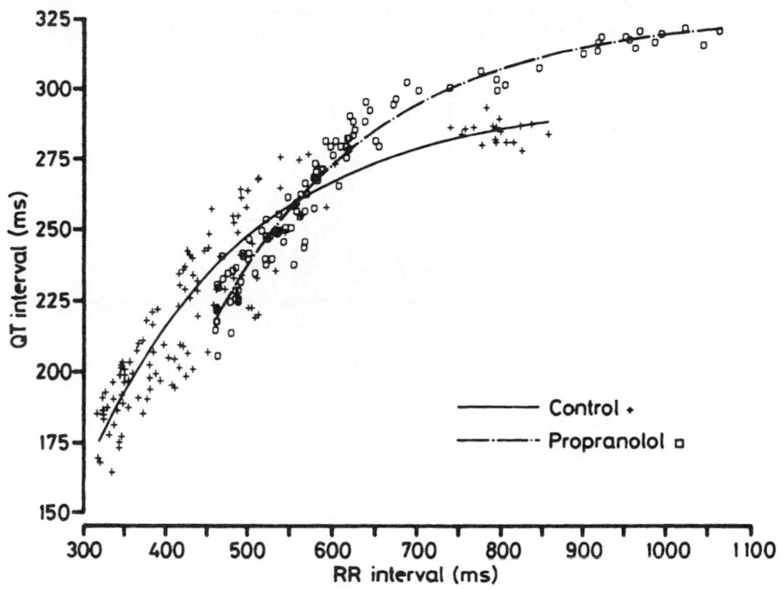

Figure 11–2. The influence of propranolol, a catecholamine effect–blocking agent, on the QT interval. A pronounced shift in the correlation line indicates the catecholamine component in the QT interval versus rate relationship during exercise. (From Sarma JSM, Venkataraman K, Samant DR, Gadgil UG: Effect of propranolol on the QT intervals of normal individuals during exercise: A new method for studying interventions. Br Heart J 60:434–439, 1988.)

a rate-adaptive pacing system. As previously described by Bazett, both Browne and associates[10] and Sarma and coworkers[11] found a large difference in the QT interval–heart rate relationship among individual patients. Therefore, it may not be appropriate to study a group of patients to derive a formula for predicting the QT interval–heart rate relationship from the combined set of data.[10] In 1988, Baig and associates[12] re-evaluated the rate-dependent QT interval changes in individual patients and confirmed that each patient had a different QT interval–heart rate relationship that was nonlinear. These findings had consequences for development of a rate-response algorithm based on the QT interval and resulted in an improved proportionality of the rate response based on automatic individualized slope programming (daily learning) by the pacemaker.

In summary, we can conclude from these studies the following:

1. The relationship between changes in the QT interval and changes in heart rate is a nonlinear function that is different for each individual.

2. The relationship between QT interval and heart rate during exercise consists of two components. One component is purely rate dependent and may be related to the hydromechanical changes necessary to allow optimal cardiac filling with increasing heart rate.[9] A second component is related to the neurohumoral influence on the myocardial tissues as a reflection of metabolic demand.

3. This catecholamine-induced QT interval change can be used as a modulator of pacing rate for a rate-adaptive pacemaker.

4. The resulting sensor will be specific to metabolic demand but will not have the ability to respond as fast as the sinus node, which responds directly to changes in the autonomic balance.

Measurement of the QT Interval

The QT interval in rate-adaptive pacemakers is defined as the interval between the pacing stimulus and the evoked endocardial T wave. Detection of the evoked T wave should occur by means of the same electrode that is used for pacing. As a consequence, accurate detection of the evoked T wave may be hampered by polarization afterpotentials at the electrode–tissue interface. After a conventional pacing stimulus, a slowly decaying voltage can be observed with an amplitude of several hundred millivolts that gradually dissipates over a period of more than 300 msec. These polarization afterpotentials can be minimized by using fast recharge techniques.[12] The recording shown in Figure 11–3 illustrates that the dual fast recharge technique, that is, a fast recharge just before and just after the stimulus, effectively eliminates these polarization afterpotentials, resulting in an almost undistorted recording of the paced evoked response.

The morphology of the unipolar endocardial evoked T wave was described by Rickards[2–4] and Brouwer.[13] T-wave sensing starts after an absolute blanking period of about 200 msec to avoid the detection of evoked R wave. Subsequently, the first derivative of the endocardial signal, that is, the speed of change of the signal, is obtained. This allows the pacemaker to sense the downslope of the evoked T wave (see Fig. 11–3). The reliability of evoked T-wave sensing has been evaluated using this method.[14] T-wave sensing was possible in 99.5% of patients (n = 368). Evoked T-wave amplitudes were 3.0 ± 1.3 mV at implantation and 2.2 ± 0.9 mV 3 months later, allowing for reliable sensing with a maximum T-wave sensitivity of 0.5 mV. Older, chronic leads tend to show slightly smaller T-wave amplitudes (1.6 ± 0.6 mV versus 2.3 ± 0.9 mV with newly implanted leads), mainly as a result of their electrode characteristics, such as a larger surface area and a nonporous surface structure.[15]

The QT Interval Rate-Adaptive Algorithm

From the initial data from Rickards and Norman,[2–4] a rate-adaptive pacemaker was designed with a linear QT interval–heart rate slope; that is, a QT interval shortening of 1 msec would result in the same pacing interval change over the entire rate range from lower to upper rate limit. These

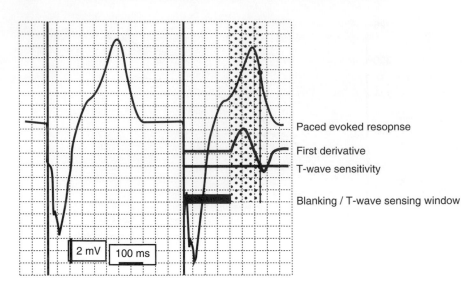

2 mV   100 ms

Paced evoked resopnse

First derivative

T-wave sensitivity

Blanking / T-wave sensing window

Figure 11–3. Recording of the paced evoked response from the pacing electrode using a dual fast recharge technique to eliminate polarization afterpotentials. The first derivative of the evoked T wave is compared with the programmed T-wave sensitivity.

pacemakers were designed to respond only to relative changes in the QT interval, making them insensitive to the absolute QT interval. This is necessary to eliminate the influence of individual differences in the QT interval response to exercise and of cardiovascular drug therapy,[16] many of which alter the absolute value of the QT interval. In addition, extremely slow variations in the QT interval, such as those caused by circadian influence, are filtered. Although the rate-adaptive behavior was found to be adequate for most patients, difficulties in optimal programming of the slope were reported.[17]

In 1987, Baig and colleagues[18, 19] conducted a reappraisal of the relationship between the evoked QT interval and ventricular pacing rate and found a nonlinear relationship between pacing and evoked QT intervals in individual patients. They found that the degree of QT interval shortening is least at low heart rates. This resulted in the development of a new rate-adaptive algorithm that featured a rate-dependent slope; that is, the slope is highest at low heart rates and decreases gradually as the heart rate increases.[20] This implies that a slope curve has to be programmed for each patient. To facilitate correct and easy programming of this slope curve, an automatic slope adjustment algorithm was implemented. The slope setting for low rates was adjusted automatically every night by measuring the QT interval at two different rates near the lower rate limit (daily learning). At the upper rate, the slope is adjusted in such a way that pacing at the upper rate occurs at the patient's shortest QT interval. Further shortening of the QT interval while pacing at the upper rate, an indication that the patient reached the upper rate at submaximal exercise levels, causes the slope at high rates to decrease.

Evaluation of the effectiveness of this new algorithm showed a faster initial acceleration of the pacing rate at the onset of exercise (a 10 bpm rate increase was obtained after 126 seconds, versus 255 seconds with the linear algorithm; n = 11; P = .02) and fewer instances of rate instability.[21, 22] Long-term stability of the automatic slope adjustments has also been evaluated by Baig and colleagues.[23] Slope settings were found to change considerably in the first 2 weeks, changing from relatively low settings initially to steeper values 2 weeks after implantation (n = 17; pacing cycle length–QT interval slope at lower rate limit changing from 3.7 msec/msec at implantation to 5.8 msec/msec after 2 weeks, P < .001). During the subsequent follow-up period of 1 year, only minor slope adjustments were found, resulting in satisfactory and reproducible rate modulation.

Combining the QT Interval With an Activity Sensor

After more than 10 years of experience with a variety of rate-adaptive sensors, it became clear that none of the available sensors could provide an optimal rate response under all circumstances.[24] To overcome these shortcomings, investigators indicated that pacemakers should be developed that derive their physiologic information from more than one source.[25–28] In general, this requires two sensors with complementary characteristics, thereby allowing one sensor to correct deficiencies of the other. Preferably, one sensor should be "physiologic" because such sensors tend to provide information that is more specific to the level of exercise, available during the recovery phase,[29] and responsive to mental stress and isometric exercise.

The second sensor should compensate for the major drawbacks of the physiologic sensor, which usually include slow response at the onset of exercise.[30–32] An activity sensor is perfectly suited to this purpose. A dual sensor algorithm should therefore initially respond to the activity sensor and automatically and gradually shift to the physiologic sensor if exercise continues. It should then continue to monitor the physiologic sensor during recovery to guide the rate decay.

After promising results with an experimental setup,[33] the Topaz dual-sensor VVIR pacemaker (Vitatron) was evaluated in a multicenter clinical study in 1992.[34] This study confirmed that the theoretical benefits could actually be achieved while maintaining a low level of complexity for programming procedures when compared with single-sensor systems. First, the pattern of the rate adaptation showed a rapid initial rate increase, driven by the activity sensor, followed by a more gradual increase guided by the QT interval. In addition, the pattern of the rate adaptation could be optimized for each patient by reprogramming only a single parameter, Sensor Blending, which determines the relative contribution of each sensor to the overall chronotropic response. Adding more influence of the activity sensor provides a more pronounced and faster rate increase at the onset of exercise, whereas adding more QT influence provides a less aggressive and more gradual pattern (Fig. 11–4).

In this study, Connelly and colleagues[34] investigated the influence of different Sensor Blending settings on the chronotropic response of the combined QT-activity sensor (see Fig. 11–4). A group of 45 patients were exercised using a modified chronotropic assessment exercise protocol (CAEP) (stage 1 was made identical to stage 2). Initially, all patients were programmed with QT = ACT blending. In 30 patients, the rate adaptation was judged to be appropriate; that is, heart rate increased after 1 minute of exercise between 25% and 50% of the rate range and after 2 minutes between 50% and 75% of the rate range. Twelve patients had an initial response that was too slow and were reprogrammed to a blending pattern of QT < ACT; in three other patients, however, the initial response was judged to be too aggressive. These patients were reprogrammed to QT > ACT. All patients in these two groups repeated an identical exercise test, and their chronotropic response met the expected criteria. This study demonstrated that Sensor Blending must be individualized in a subgroup of patients.

Sharp and coworkers[35] evaluated heart rate and oxygen uptake at rest and low exercise levels in patients with left ventricular dysfunction in whom an appropriate chronotropic response pattern is important because changes in stroke volume are less than normal during exercise. The fixed-rate VVI mode was compared with VVIR pacing based on the activity sensor only, the QT sensor only, and blending of both sensors. The dual-sensor chronotropic response reproduced the theoretical linear relationship among metabolic workload, heart rate, and oxygen uptake.

In addition to improving the pattern of rate adaptation, the overall sensor specificity can be improved by continuous cross-checking of the information from the two sensors. If the two sensors provide consistent information, either exercise or recovery is confirmed, and the pacing rate will increase or decrease respectively. If false-positive activity signals are received (increases in the activity counts without a change in the QT interval), the pacemaker will initially start to increase the pacing rate. If the QT interval still does not indicate an exercise condition after about 1 minute, Sensor Cross Checking is activated. This slowly decreases the pacing rate toward the QT-indicated rate. In case of false-positive activity sensing, the pacing rate gradually returns to the lower rate limit. Conversely, when the QT interval shortens while no activity is detected, mental stress or isometric exercise is most probable. Under these circumstances, the pacemaker is designed to increase the pacing rate, although its magnitude is limited.

In the same multicenter study, Connelly and colleagues[34] investigated the effectiveness of Sensor Cross Checking. They created three different, continuous levels of false-positive activity: gentle and vigorous tapping on the pacemaker case and applying massage equipment over the pacemaker, which created excessive activity signals. In all cases, Sensor Cross Checking prevented unphysiologic rate accelerations. The time taken for the pacing rate to decrease from its peak (85 ± 8 bpm) to about the lower rate limit was 2.7 ± 1.7 minutes with gentle tapping and 8.3 ± 2.4 minutes with the massage equipment. Staircase walking produced a satisfactory and appropriate chronotropic response, with maximum pacing rates being almost equal during ascending and descending.

Rognoni and associates[36] evaluated the effects of Sensor Cross Checking on subjective well-being and found clinical scores to be higher in QT-only and dual-sensor modes when compared with activity-only and VVI pacing (8.6 and 8.5 versus 8.0). While in the VVI mode, patients reported a higher symptom score (3.5) during moderate levels of exer-

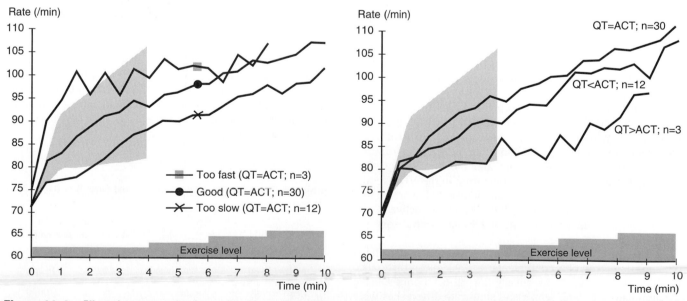

Figure 11–4. Effect of reprogramming Sensor Blending on the rate-response pattern. Initially, all patients exercised in the QT = ACT setting *(left)*. Two subgroups were reprogrammed because of a suboptimal rate response. A repeated exercise test *(right)* confirmed that the desired effect was actually obtained.

tion (mainly fatigue) than in the activity-only mode (1.8) (mainly palpitations), but they reported no symptoms in either the QT-only or dual-sensor mode.[36]

Dual-Chamber, Dual-Sensor Pacemakers Using the QT Interval

In 1993, the Diamond DDDR (Vitatron), a dual-chamber, dual-sensor pacemaker with beat-to-beat mode switching capabilities was introduced. The dual-sensor rate-adaptive algorithm was identical to that of the single-chamber version, with the Sensor Blending being the most important parameter used to control the pattern of rate adaptation. The dual-sensor rate was continuously compared with the sinus rate, and when the difference between the two exceeded 40 msec (to avoid atrial fusion pacing), atrial pacing commenced. To maintain a relatively stable ventricular rhythm at the onset of atrial tachyarrhythmias, beat-to-beat mode switching was introduced. This algorithm automatically switched to a non-tracking mode (DDIR) on detection of premature atrial activity, that is, a sensed atrial event occurring earlier than the average atrial rate plus 15 bpm. In such a case, the mode switched to DDIR, and the ventricular escape interval was determined by the sensors. This avoided tracking of even single premature atrial events, thereby maintaining a fairly constant ventricular rhythm, particularly if the sensor rate was close to the sinus rate just before the mode switch. Furthermore, while in the DDIR mode, the pacemaker automatically activated its Atrial Synchronization Pace (ASP) algorithm. This algorithm continuously attempted to insert an atrial stimulus before the ventricular stimulus while in the DDIR mode owing to mode switching, but only did so if the preceding atrial event occurred sufficiently earlier to prevent pacing in the atrial vulnerable zone. The length of this protection zone, the ASP interval, is programmable.

Figure 11–5 shows three examples of beat-to-beat mode switching: the response to a single premature atrial contraction, including the delivery of an ASP; the response to a sustained atrial tachyarrhythmia; and the response to the cessation of an atrial tachyarrhythmia. In all cases, an almost constant ventricular rhythm was maintained throughout the recorded period, whereas atrioventricular (AV) synchrony was restored as quickly as possible on cessation of the atrial tachyarrhythmia, whether it was a single event or a sustained arrhythmia.

Lau and coauthors[37] compared the dual-sensor–indicated pacing rate and sinus rate in 12 patients with normal sinus rhythm. They used a special downloadable software for the Diamond DDDR pacemaker that allowed continuous telemetry of both the sinus rate and the dual-sensor rate, even though the pacemaker was operating in the VDD mode. This special software contained an additional diagnostic feature that continuously stored the difference between the sensor and the sinus rate during a 1-month ambulatory period.

Sinus and dual-sensor rates were significantly correlated ($P < .001$; correlation coefficients > 0.90; mean difference throughout exercise and recovery 2.8 ± 6.1 bpm). During the ambulatory period, sensor and sinus rate differences were classified according to three activity levels (Table 11–2). Nearly 90% of the sensor-driven beats were within 8 bpm of the sinus rate at medium and low levels of exercise.

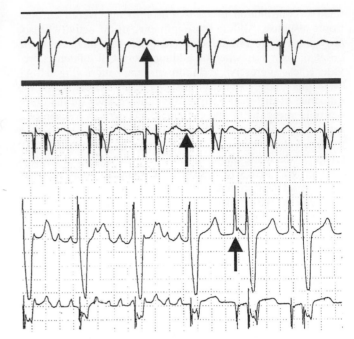

Figure 11–5. Three examples of beat-to-beat mode switching, illustrating the maintenance of a stable ventricular rate on detection of single premature atrial activity *(top)*, sustained atrial tachyarrhythmia *(middle)*, or cessation of atrial tachyarrhythmia *(bottom)*.

However, the difference increased at higher levels of exercise.

In modern dual-chamber pacemakers, the sensor information is used to drive the heart rate during both atrial bradyarrhythmias (DDDR mode) and atrial tachyarrhythmias in the DDIR pacing mode. A sensor-indicated rate close to the normal sinus rate not only avoids unnecessary pacing in the DDDR mode but also limits the ventricular rate variations on detection of an atrial tachyarrhythmia, assuming that the mode switch is instantaneous on detection of an unphysiologically rapid increase of the atrial rate. Kamalvand and associates[38] compared different mode switching algorithms in DDDR pacemakers and found that fast mode switching in combination with a physiologic sensor provided a more stable ventricular rate during episodes of atrial tachyarrhythmias. Therefore, patients with frequent, short-lived atrial arrhythmias preferred this type of device to those with slower mode-switching algorithms.

Table 11–2. Difference Between Sensor and Sinus Rate During Daily Life*

Activity Level	Sinus Rate (bpm)	Percentage of All Beats With Difference Less Than:	
		± 8/bpm	± 15/bpm
Low	<75	98	100
Medium	75–100	89	99
High	>100	66	95

*The sinus–sensor difference is dependent on the level of activities.

Other Applications of the Evoked QT Interval

The evoked QT interval is one of the few clinically available sensors that reflect cardiac metabolism. Several investigators have indicated other applications for the evoked QT interval.

Dynamic Pace Refractory Period

Because the T wave marks the end of cardiac refractoriness, it can be used to match automatically and dynamically the pacemaker's ventricular (pace) refractory period to cardiac refractoriness.[39] This behavior is implemented in the current pacemaker models and provides optimized detection of early premature ventricular contractions, especially during exercise. Under exercise conditions, the ventricular pace refractory period automatically shortens with the measured QT interval, thus allowing earlier ventricular sensing.

Optimal Atrioventricular Delay

Both Defaye and colleagues[40] and Sugano and coworkers[41] have shown that the evoked QT interval may have the potential to indicate the optimal AV delay. They varied the AV delay, while monitoring the evoked QT interval, in patients at rest and while pacing the atrium at a fixed rate, thus eliminating the effects of heart rate on the QT interval. Both groups of investigators found a positive correlation between the longest QT interval and highest cardiac output or cardiac index and the programmed AV delay. This information indicates that pacemakers could be developed that automatically adjust their AV delay based on a physiologic sensor.

Recognition of Ventricular Fusion Beats

Boute and colleagues[42] demonstrated that, in dogs, the amplitude of the evoked T wave significantly decreases during fusion. Recognition of ventricular fusion is important for reliable and effective operation of several future pacemaker functions. Automatic capture detection algorithms often mistake a fusion beat for a noncaptured beat, resulting in unnecessary increase of the output amplitude and subsequent battery drain. In patients with incomplete or intermittent AV block and a dual-chamber pacemaker, ventricular fusion may occur frequently. This not only negatively influences the ventricular contraction pattern but also drains unnecessary current from the pacemaker battery. On detection of fusion, a dual-chamber pacemaker could automatically extend its AV delay to allow the conducted R waves to prevail. Finally, in patients with hypertrophic obstructive cardiomyopathy, one would like to maintain ventricular pacing to obtain consistent septal preexcitation. In these patients, detection of ventricular fusion may shorten its AV delay, thereby providing an effective therapy through full ventricular capture.

Circadian Variations in the QT Interval

Browne and coworkers[43] and Djordjevic and colleagues[44] reported circadian variations in the QT interval. The difference in the QT interval at 60 bpm between being awake and sleep was 19 ± 7 msec,[43] reflecting increased vagal tone or sympathetic withdrawal. This difference could be used to decrease automatically the lower rate limit during those hours of the day that the patient is asleep. This would allow longer periods of sinus rhythm while at the same time conserving pacemaker battery energy.

Diagnosis of Cardiac Transplant Rejection

Grace and coauthors[45] monitored the evoked T-wave amplitude after transplantation using an external pacemaker with evoked T-wave sensing capabilities. A total of 13 patients were followed during the immediate post-transplantation period. In 11 patients, the initial biopsy that proved rejection was associated with a significant decrease in the evoked T-wave amplitude from 1.3 to 0.6 mV ($P < .005$), which began 1 to 4 days before the biopsy. These results suggest an alternative method for detecting cardiac transplant rejection.

Miscellaneous Applications

The paced evoked response can be used to evaluate drug-induced changes in myocardial repolarization.[46, 47] Furthermore, Donalson and colleagues[48, 49] showed that subendocardial ischemia can be detected using the paced evoked response. Res and associates[50, 51] found that the amplitude of the evoked T wave increased during exercise and suggested using the evoked T-wave amplitude as a second sensor in QT interval–driven rate-responsive pacemakers. Finally, den Dulk and coauthors[52] suggested using the T wave to identify the end of the absolute refractory period. Thus, a special algorithm in an antitachycardia pacing system could identify the earliest moment to deliver an effective stimulus.

Advantages and Limitations of Evoked QT Interval–Based Pacemakers

The evoked QT interval was the first commercially available rate-adaptive sensor. With more than 15 years of experience, this sensor is one of four survivors, the others being activity, minute ventilation, and intracardiac impedance. The drawbacks of the evoked QT interval as a rate-adaptive sensor (i.e., the delayed onset of rate adaptation and rate instability) have been overcome by adding a second, complementary sensor, namely activity. A wide range of these dual-sensor rate-adaptive pacemaker models are now in clinical use worldwide. Combining and cross-checking information from more than one sensor seems logical to attempt to obtain the benefits of both. In the dual-chamber versions, the dual-sensor rate is used both during atrial bradyarrhythmias (DDDR pacing mode) and during atrial tachyarrhythmias (DDIR pacing mode) to define the ventricular rate. These developments have brought rate-adaptive pacing closer to physiology and have reduced patient symptoms.[35–38]

■ INTRACARDIAC IMPEDANCE–BASED PACEMAKERS

In the absence of an increase in heart rate during exercise, cardiac contractility remains responsive to circulating catecholamines. Thus, cardiac contractility itself may be an alternative sensor for rate-adaptive pacing. In addition to the potential for being a rapidly responding sensor, detection of changes in contractility may also provide a means for responding to nonexercise stress. Because pacing rate may itself alter hemodynamics, a contractility sensor may present the possibility of either a negative or a positive feedback loop. Apart from their use in rate-adaptive pacemakers, implantable sensors for measurement of cardiac contractility may also be useful in an ICD to assess the hemodynamic consequences of ventricular tachyarrhythmias. The assessment of contractility may allow an ICD to apply antitachy-cardia pacing as therapy for hemodynamically stable ventric-ular tachycardia or to forego antitachycardia pacing in favor of immediate cardioversion-defibrillation for unstable ven-tricular tachycardia or ventricular fibrillation.

Cardiac contractility may be assessed by analysis of intra-cardiac impedance. A small amount of alternating current is injected across a tissue with measurement of the voltage difference generated, thereby allowing the resistance (or impedance) to be derived. Impedance is not a constant value but changes according to the timing of the cardiac and respiratory cycles. As compared with a minute ventilation sensor that uses changes in impedance related to respiration, a cardiac impedance sensor measures changes in impedance due to changes in right ventricular blood volume with car-diac contraction. Impedance can be easily incorporated into a permanent pacemaker using the pacing electrodes and pulse generator casing as the current source, and impedance is measured with the same configuration or by use of the pacing electrodes only. Because the cardiac and respiratory rates usually do not overlap, by appropriate filtering, either the intracardiac impedance or minute ventilation signals can be derived.

Figure 11–6 shows intracardiac impedance derived for the right ventricular cavity using a pair of electrodes incorpo-rated in a tripolar right ventricular lead (intracavitary imped-ance). The change in right ventricular dimensions during systole and diastole allows the stroke volume and the pre-ejection interval (PEI) to be determined. When current is injected and collected with the use of a unipolar ventricular lead, however, most of the impedance changes are due to regional changes in the myocardial and blood pool volume immediately surrounding the electrode (within 1 mL). This occurs because the current density is highest surrounding the ventricular pacing electrode (which has a very small surface area) as compared with the pulse generator case acting as the ground electrode (which has a very large surface area). The mechanical motion of the right ventricle in the region of the pacing electrode has been termed the *ventricular inotropic parameter* (VIP), which is thought to be related to cardiac contractility. Thus, both intracavitary and regional intracardiac impedance may have potential to detect changes in cardiac contractility for rate-adaptive pacing. The intracar-diac impedance–derived parameters that have been studied include relative stroke volume, PEI, and VIP.

Relative Stroke Volume

Principle

Cardiac output increases rapidly at the onset of exercise by a combination of increasing heart rate and stroke volume. Because of an initial decrease in venous return during supine exercise, stroke volume tends to decrease at the start of exercise and thereafter remains constant in healthy subjects.[53] On the other hand, upright exercise leads to an initial in-crease, followed by an almost constant stroke volume during continuous exercise. Thus, the sensing of stroke volume changes provides a crude sensor for exercise response. By increasing the pacing rate to keep the stroke volume constant during exercise, a negative feedback loop has been sug-gested.[54]

Impedance is the simplest method for determining stroke

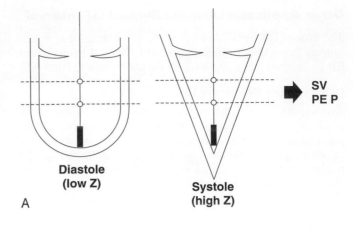

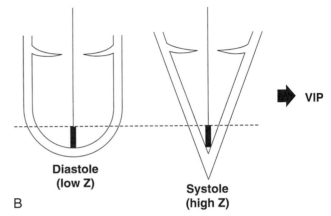

Figure 11–6. Schematic representation of intracardiac impedance sampling either the right ventricular cavity (cavity impedance) or a region of the right ventricular myocardium (regional impedance). In either case, the source current is injected between the pacemaker, and the right ventricular pace/sense electrode. The site of sampling and the filter characteristics determine the type of impedance signals. See text for details. PEP, pre-ejection period; SV, stroke volume; VIP, ventricular inotropic parameter.

volume (see Fig. 11–6). The basic impedance measurement technique has been described by Geddes and colleagues,[55] Baan and associates,[56] and McKay and coworkers.[57] In brief, a constant sinusoidal current is injected into the right ventric-ular cavity, and the change in resistivity is sampled between an electrode pair. A cylindrical volume of blood is assumed to encompass the electrode pair, and its change in resistivity reflects changes in stroke volume. With a number of assump-tions, right ventricular volume can be assessed by the follow-ing equation:

$$V = \rho L^2/R,$$

where:

V is the blood volume between sensing electrodes
ρ is the resistivity of blood
L is the distance between sensing electrodes
R is the magnitude of impedance between sensing electrodes

A number of electrode configurations have been proposed to measure intracavitary impedance, including octapolar,[56] hexapolar,[57] tripolar,[58] and bipolar designs.[59–61] A good correlation has been reported between changes in stroke volume measured by impedance and that directly measured by changes in ventricular volume. As the volume of blood sampled by this approach is variable, an absolute stroke volume cannot be determined. The change in stroke volume, however, is accurately reflected by the change in measured impedance.

Performance

Theoretically, stroke volume is a rapidly responding parameter.[60] During upright exercise with normal chronotropic response, stroke volume remains relatively unchanged after a small initial rise. If exercise is carried out at a fixed rate, stroke volume increases significantly. Thus, it was suggested that a closed-loop, rate-adaptive pacing system may be possible by maintaining stroke volume relatively constant.[54] An external system was devised that showed a delay of 2 minutes between the onset of exercise and a response of the heart rate. After this initial delay, the pacing rate increased appropriately.[54] Because the stroke volume remains relatively constant in the recovery period of upright exercise, stroke volume may also be a useful indicator for determining an appropriate recovery of heart rate after exercise.[62]

Despite theoretical advantages, the use of relative stroke volume as a rate-adaptive sensor has not found extensive application. Technical limitations have included the influence of respiratory changes on determination of stroke volume and bending of the catheter tip during ventricular contraction, which shortens the dipole for impedance sensing. More important, stroke volume changes tend to be variable during exercise, making reliable rate adaptation difficult. Because stroke volume increases when a subject lies down, a paradoxical rate response may be induced. Finally, the influence of a varying AV interval relationship and intrinsic conduction may further confound stroke volume measurement and the resulting rate adaptation. Thus, although relative stroke volume has been incorporated in a permanent rate-adaptive pacemaker (see later), it has not been used in clinical practice.

Pre-Ejection Interval

Principle

The systolic pre-ejection period is the time from the onset of ventricular contraction to the onset of ventricular ejection, the period of isovolumetric contraction. The pre-ejection period shortens in response to an increase in stroke volume or end diastolic volume.[63] In addition, it responds to factors that augment cardiac contractility, such as those occurring during exercise and emotional stress.[64–66] On the other hand, pre-ejection period has been reported to be unaffected by changes in heart rate,[67] atropine injection, and carotid sinus massage.[68] Thus, the pre-ejection period appears to be a possible sensor for rate-adaptive pacing.

The right ventricular pre-ejection period begins at the onset of the ECG QRS complex (or the ventricular pacing stimulus) and ends with the opening of the pulmonary valve. Because the motion of the pulmonary valve cannot be detected in by a pacing system with a standard lead, however, the PEI is used instead. PEI is defined as the time from the onset of electrical systole until detection of ventricular

ejection. The onset of electrical systole is determined at the initiation of a pacing stimulus or the detection of an intrinsic QRS complex. Mechanical systole is defined after electrical impedance has changed to a predetermined level. Thus, measured PEI also includes a portion of mechanical systole, which is longer than the conventionally defined pre-ejection period. It is assumed that these two intervals change in parallel during exercise and other stresses. In healthy subjects, the pre-ejection period is reported to be independent of the heart rate.[69] Less is known, however, about the effect of pacing rate on pre-ejection period in pacemaker-dependent patients. Because the ejection time is shortened when pacing rate is increased alone, the PEI is expected to shorten slightly. The net effect is that the PEI is a relatively rate-independent parameter. Using a temporary pacing system in 5 patients,[70] an increase in pacing rate from 70 to 130 bpm at rest did not significantly affect the PEI ($<8\%$ shortening). During exercise, however, shortening of the PEI could be up to 23%. A rapid onset of rate response was also reported with this temporary device during sudden strenuous exertion.

Pacemaker Description

The Precept pacemaker (CPI, Minneapolis, MN) used a tripolar ventricular pacing lead for ventricular pacing and sensing and for right ventricular impedance measurement. A 9F tripolar lead with the proximal two electrodes located 14.7 and 23 mm from the tip electrode was required. The Precept pacemakers were offered in both single-chamber (Model 1100) and dual-chamber (Model 1200) models.[71] A continuous, low-level, constant-amplitude (6 μA) alternating current (2700 Hz) was injected between the distal ventricular electrode and the pulse generator casing. Because the amplitude of the current was constant, the change in measured voltage between the proximal two ring electrodes was proportional to the change in impedance (see Fig. 11–6). PEI was measured from a ventricular pacing stimulus or sensed right ventricular apex electrogram to a point after a predetermined change in impedance. The impedance-derived PEI was measured as a count between 0 and 255 using a moving average of 16 cycles. In addition to PEI, the right ventricular volume was also monitored continuously, and the relative stroke volume was assessed by telemetry (the so-called sensorgram, Fig. 11–7).

The pacemaker allowed a selection of either PEI or relative stroke volume as the sensor for rate modulation. In the DDDR mode, the upper and lower P-wave tracking rates and a sensor-driven upper rate could be separately programmed. Eight different rate-response curves related the change in sensor parameter to a change in pacing rate. The baseline tracking function allowed continuous evaluation of the baseline PEI and relative stroke volume to account for changes in the sensors, such as those caused by diurnal variations or changes in medications or cardiac function.

Pacemaker Programming

Programming the Precept pacemaker involved setting a baseline PEI or stroke volume reference value. Rate-adaptive slopes were determined by appropriate exercise testing. In addition to the rate-adaptive slope, programming of other parameters, such as the upper and lower rates, the offset between paced and sensed ventricular beats, and baseline tracking, was required.

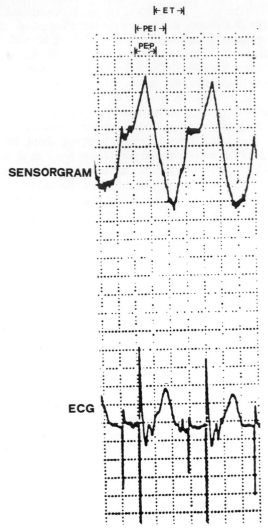

Figure 11–7. A telemetered right ventricular cavity impedance signal in the Precept pacemaker, which senses the pre-ejection interval (PEI) and relative stroke volume. The relative stroke volume is shown by the sensorgram. This allows the detection of PEI, which is measured from a ventricular paced event to the occurrence of a fixed change in impedance. The pre-ejection period (PEP) starts from the ventricular pacing spike to the beginning of ventricular ejection and cannot be directly obtained from the pacemaker because the start of ejection is not well defined. ET, ejection time.

Clinical Performance

The Precept-derived relative stroke volume was validated against Doppler-derived stroke volume in one study.[72] This study also showed the stability of the sensor-derived PEI and relative stroke volume over time, with these parameters achieving stable values within 2 days. Furthermore, PEI showed an appropriate decrease when patients adopted an upright posture as well as during incremental exercise. On the other hand, relative stroke volume decreased on adoption of an upright posture, resulting in a paradoxical rate reduction when the patient stands up. An increase in PEI or relative stroke volume detected during exercise successfully increased pacing rate in patients with an implanted Precept DDDR.

Rate-adaptive pacing with the PEI sensor was reported in detail for 10 patients in whom the Precept was implanted.[71] During symptom-limited cycle ergometry, PEI decreased from 138 ± 18 units to 103 ± 22 units ($P < .05$). This resulted in an increase in pacing rate from 97 bpm at an exercise workload of 100 W to 175 bpm at a workload of 175 W. When PEI was assessed during atrial pacing at a rate of 10 bpm above the intrinsic sinus rhythm, PEI shortened as compared with spontaneous rhythm. This is probably related to the more optimal AV interval and improved stroke volume during sinus rhythm as compared with "overdrive" atrial pacing. After 147 patient-months of follow-up, the measured resting PEI remained relatively constant. There was no consistent change in PEI as a result of postural change. Wide interindividual variability was observed, however, with 3 of 10 patients suffering from sensor-driven tachycardia as a result of changes in posture. This behavior was observed with both stroke volume and PEI as the rate-adaptive sensor and required either inactivation of the sensor (2 patients) or reprogramming to a suboptimal rate adaptive slope (1 patient). On the other hand, a case report[73] suggested that PEI may be helpful in patients who have orthostatic hypotension by providing an increase in pacing rate on upright tilt. In any case, the preload-dependent nature of PEI was demonstrated by these studies.

Advantages and Limitations

The PEI sensor is sensitive to both exercise and nonexercise requirements, and its response is proportional to workload. In addition, this system allows the detection of relative stroke volume as an alternative sensor for rate-adaptive pacing and provides information on the contractile state of the right ventricle. Its ability to determine relative stroke volume may be useful for automatic optimization of the AV interval. Because measurement of the PEI depends on the accurate determination of stroke volume, it may be affected by a variety of factors other than the contractility of the right ventricle. For example, stroke volume is affected by factors other than the sympathetic tone, such as right ventricular preload and afterload and the intrinsic contractile function of the right ventricle. Right ventricular preload is affected by the timing of atrial contraction (which is itself dependent on the AV interval and the conduction time through the AV node) as well as the posture of the patient. Although the pace/sense offset algorithm may correct for some of the differences between paced and sensed ventricular beats, it is expected that PEI will substantially vary with alternating sensed and paced events, intermittent bundle-branch block, and fusion beats.[71] To a certain extent, this problem may be reduced with the use of a 16-beat moving average in PEI. Further long-term study in a wider population is needed to confirm the efficacy of PEI as a stable sensor for rate-adaptive pacing.

VIP

Principle

VIP reflects the changes in regional impedance in the right ventricle induced by the contracting myocardium around a unipolar ventricular pacing electrode. Impedance is measured by injecting a 4-kHz square wave constant current of $40 \mu A$ through the tip of an implanted electrode, using the pulse generator casing as the indifferent electrode (see Fig. 11–6). The same electrode arrangement is used to sample impedance during cardiac contraction. A bandpass filter with corner frequencies between 0.3 and 40 Hz is used to exclude artifacts induced by ventilation and motion, with a sampling frequency of 8 msec.

Overall, impedance increases during the ejection phase because the right ventricular cavity becomes smaller during systole. During diastole, passive inflow of blood into the right ventricle gradually decreases the impedance value to the late diastolic value. To represent the ejection period, a critical "sampling window" is essential to detect the period of rising impedance. Several sampling windows have been tested.[74] An early window within the pre-ejection period was found to be unsatisfactory because of polarization artifact of the pacing stimulus. A late window during the rapid ejection phase of the ventricle does not provide adequate separation between rest and exercise. The most appropriate sampling window appears to be immediately after the pre-ejection period when the pulmonic valve opens.

Algorithm

Changes in impedance within the sampling window is defined as the *regional effective slope quantity,* or RQ (Fig. 11–8). The algorithm involves determination of the maximum RQ (RQ_{max}) during exercise and the resting RQ (RQ_{rest}). These two parameters are defined by the upper and lower rates that are programmed. Thus, an RQ during exercise ($RQ_{exercise}$) can be expressed as a fraction of the range of RQ, from which a pacing rate can be computed.

Clinical Results

Acute measurement of VIP was taken in 82 patients with chronically implanted unipolar ventricular leads at the time of pulse generator replacement.[74] A wide fluctuation of baseline impedance was observed (500 to 1500 Ω), whereas VIP fluctuated by about 4 to 25 Ω, with a good correlation between VIP and the baseline impedance. Using an investigational VVIR pacemaker with telemetry (Biotronik Neos-PEP, Biotronik, Lake Oswego, OR) in 158 patients, it was demonstrated that rate adaptation can be achieved with this sensor. In individual patients, it was reported that rate adaptation close to that of the sinus node was observed with this sensor during exercise, although it was necessary to adjust the VIP detection algorithm (Fig. 11–9). A delay in the onset of an increase in pacing rate was observed, as compared with that of the normal sinus rhythm in some patients. Because the increase in the normal sinus rate at the onset of exercise is due to parasympathetic withdrawal rather than sympathetic increase, a sensed parameter that responds to changes in sympathetic tone, such as the VIP, may not provide a rapid increase in pacing rate at the onset of exercise.

A clinical study involving 205 patients was performed to evaluate the VIP pacemaker.[75] A significant proportion of these patients were young subjects with complete AV block due to Chagas' disease. Calibration of the pacemaker at rest and during maximum exercise was required to determine the RQ_{rest} and RQ_{max}. Satisfactory rate modulation was reported in 93% of patients. In the remaining 7% of patients, rate adaptation could not be achieved because of such factors as poor exercise tolerance, severe myocardial dysfunction, or intermittent AV conduction.

The full report of a multicenter study on the VIP pacemaker has become available.[76] This study included 178 VVIR (Biotronik Neos-PEP) and 84 DDDR devices (Biotronik Diplos-PEP and Inos²DR). Physiologic rate adaptation

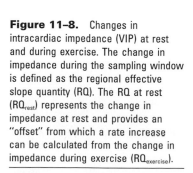

Figure 11–8. Changes in intracardiac impedance (VIP) at rest and during exercise. The change in impedance during the sampling window is defined as the regional effective slope quantity (RQ). The RQ at rest (RQ_{rest}) represents the change in impedance at rest and provides an "offset" from which a rate increase can be calculated from the change in impedance during exercise ($RQ_{exercise}$).

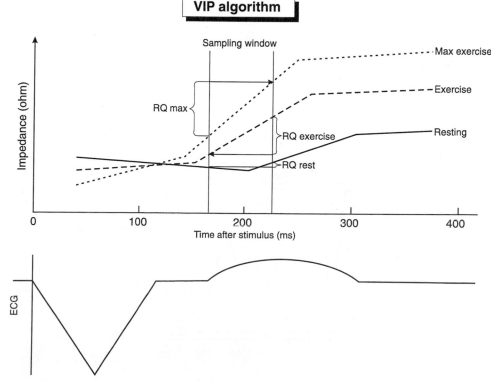

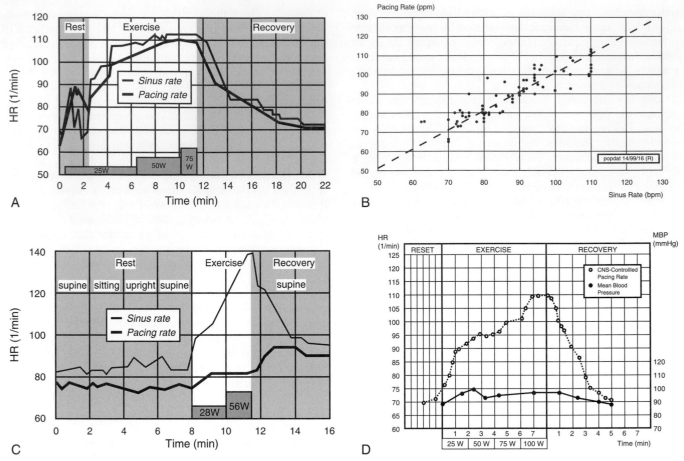

Figure 11–9. Simultaneous recording of the sinus- and VIP-derived pacing rates in a patient with atrioventricular block implanted with a Neos-VVIR pacemaker. *A,* Appropriate rate response during graded cycle ergometry. *B,* Good correlation of sinus rate and VIP-driven pacing rate. *C,* Inappropriately adjusted VIP detection with failure of rate response. *D,* Maintenance of constant mean arterial pressure during exercise with appropriate rate response. (From Schaldach M, Hutten H: Intracardiac impedance to determine sympathetic activity in rate responsive pacing. PACE 15:1778–1786, 1992.)

was possible in 93% and 96% of patients with these devices, respectively. Apart from exercise rate response, this study also involved mental stress testing using color-word matching (Fig. 11–10) and the infusion of inotropic agents. A moderate level of rate response was documented in some patients with VIP pacemakers during these nonexercise stresses.

In some patients with the VIP pacemaker undergoing

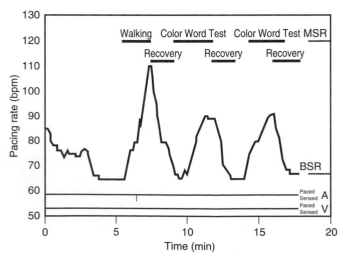

Figure 11–10. Response of the VIP pacemaker to walking and mental stress. BSR, baseline stimulation rate; MSR, maximum stimulation rate. (From Grubb BP, Wolfe DA, Samoil D, et al: Adaptive rate pacing controlled by the right ventricular preejection interval for severe refractory orthostatic hypotension. PACE 16:801, 1993.)

angioplasty, balloon inflation in the artery supplying the myocardium around the pacing electrode led to a decrease in VIP, suggesting that VIP reflected a change in local contractility of the myocardium. Within an increase in pacing rate from 70 to 90 bpm at rest, there was no change in VIP. This suggests that within the rate range studied, there is absence of a potential positive-feedback loop.

Advantages and Limitations

VIP appears to be an interesting sensor to measure contractility of the heart and can be achieved using a conventional ventricular pacing electrode. The demands on pacing energy are not excessive. As a contractility sensor, it is sensitive not only to exercise but also to nonexercise requirements, and it may therefore be used for monitoring cardiac contractility for non–rate augmentation purposes. Like the QT sensor, VIP can only be used in a pacing mode that incorporates a ventricular lead. The effects of pacing rate on VIP have not been completely studied, and the difference in VIP during pacing and intrinsic conduction may affect the resultant rate response. It is likely that VIP is affected by right ventricular ischemia or cardioactive medications, and these may influence rate adaptation with this sensor, requiring reprogramming for long-term function. A small proportion of patients are not suitable for the VIP pacemaker because of severely impaired right ventricular function, although it may be possible to identify such patients preoperatively.

Summary

Both evoked QT interval and contractility sensors have been successfully used for rate adaptation. These sensors respond to both exercise and nonexercise requirements. Because the initial part of exercise is mediated by parasympathetic withdrawal rather than an increase in sympathetic tone, some delay in the onset of rate response is expected with both the evoked QT interval and VIP sensors. This part of exercise can be complemented with an activity sensor, a combination that has been extensively used in dual-sensor pacemakers with good results.

REFERENCES

1. Bazett HC: An analysis of time relations of electrocardiograms. Heart 7:353, 1920.
2. Rickards AF, Norman J: Relation between QT interval and heart rate: New design of a physiologically adaptive cardiac pacemaker. Br Heart J 45:56, 1981.
3. Rickards AF, Norman J: The use of stimulus-T interval to determine cardiac pacing rate. Am J Cardiol 47:435, 1981.
4. Rickards AF: The use of stimulus-T interval to determine cardiac pacing rate [Abstract]. PACE 4(3):68, 1981.
5. Milne JR, Ward DE, Spurrel RAJ, Camm AJ: The ventricular paced QT interval: The effects of rate and exercise. PACE 5:352–358, 1982.
6. Hedman A, Nordlander R, Pehrsonn S: Changes in QT and QaT interval at rest and during exercise with different modes of cardiac pacing. PACE 8(6):825–831, 1985.
7. Donaldson RM, Rickards AF: Initial experience with a physiological, rate responsive pacemaker. Br Med J 286:667–671, 1983.
8. Jordaens L, Backers J, Moerman E, Clement D: Catecholamine levels and pacing behavior of QT-driven pacemakers during exercise. PACE 13(5):603–607, 1990.
9. Baig MW: The use of the paced endocardial QT interval in rate adaptive pacing. Thesis submitted to the University of London for the degree of Doctor of Medicine, 1993.
10. Browne KF, Prystowsky E, Heger JJ, Zipes DP: Modulation of the Q-T interval by the autonomic nervous system. PACE 6(Pt II):1050–1056, 1983.
11. Sarma JSM, Venkataraman K, Samant DR, Gadgil UG: Effect of propranolol on the QT intervals of normal individuals during exercise: A new method for studying interventions. Br Heart J 60:434–439, 1988.
12. Baig W, Walton C, Ecconomedes A, Perrins EJ: Quantification of improvement in electrode polarization reduction by single and dual fast reload techniques [Abstract 335]. Abstract from the 4th European Symposium on Cardiac Pacing, Stockholm, May 28–31, 1989.
13. Brouwer J, Nagelkerke D, De Jongste MJL, et al: Analysis of the morphology of the unipolar endocardial paced evoked response. PACE 13:302–313, 1990.
14. Boute W, Brunekreeft W, Albers BA: Reliability of T-wave sensing in 368 patients with QT interval sensing rate responsive pacemakers [Abstract]. Eur J Cardiac Pacing Electrophysiol 4(2):80, 1994.
15. Boute W, Derrien Y, Wittkampf FHM: Reliability of evoked endocardial T-wave sensing in 1,500 pacemaker patients. PACE 9(Pt II):948–953, 1986.
16. Zegelman M, Kreuzer J, Koch B: Effects of antiarrhythmic drugs on the stimulus-T interval and the rate response of QT-related pacemakers. Herzschrittmacher 7:191–195, 1987.
17. Winter UL, Behrenbeck DW, Möher M, et al: Probleme bei der Slope Einstellung und der Herzfrequenzanpassung in frequenz variabelen Schrittmachern: Oszillations Phanomene und plotzliche Frequenzeinbruche. Herzschrittmacher 5(2):50–60, 1985.
18. Baig MW, Perrins EJ: A reappraisal of the relationship between the evoked QT interval and ventricular pacing rate [Abstract]. PACE 10:1029, 1987.
19. Baig MW, Boute W, Begemann M, Perrins EJ: Nonlinear relationship between pacing and evoked QT intervals. PACE 11:753–759, 1988.
20. Boute W, Gebhardt U, Begemann MJS: Introduction of an automatic QT interval driven rate responsive pacemaker. PACE 11(Pt II):1804–1814, 1988.
21. Baig MW, Wilson J, Boute W, et al: Improved pattern of rate responsiveness with dynamic slope setting for the QT sensing pacemaker. PACE 12:311–320, 1989.
22. Baig MW, Green A, Wade G, et al: A randomized double-blind, crossover study of the linear and nonlinear algorithms for the QT sensing rate adaptive pacemaker. PACE 13:1802–1808, 1990.
23. Baig MW, Boute W, Begemann M, Perrins EJ: One-year follow-up of automatic adaptation of the rate response algorithm of the QT sensing, rate adaptive pacemaker. PACE 14(Pt I):1598–1605, 1991.
24. Lau CP: Rate adaptive cardiac pacing: Single and dual chamber. Mt. Kisco, NY, Futura, 1993.
25. Donaldson RM, Rickards AF: Towards multisensor pacing. Am Heart J 106:1454–57, 1983.
26. Benditt DG, Mianulli M, Lurie K, et al: Multiple-sensor for physiologic cardiac pacing. Ann Intern Med 121:960–968, 1994.
27. Sutton R: Dual sensor pacing technology [Editorial]. Eur Heart J 17:1136, 1996.
28. Camm AJ, Clifford G, Paul V: Single chamber rate adaptive pacing. J Electrophysiol 3(3):181, 1989.
29. Hamersma M, van Woersem RJ, Overdijk AD: Physical condition of patients reflected in the recovery time of the Quintech TX rate adaptive pacemaker. PACE 11:805, 1988.
30. Lau CP, Tse WS, Camm AJ: Clinical experience with Sensolog 703: A new activity sensing rate responsive pacemaker. PACE 11:1444–1455, 1988.
31. Lau C-P, Mehta D, Toff WD, et al: Limitations of rate response of an activity sensing rate responsive pacemaker to different forms of activity. PACE 11:141–150, 1988.
32. Matula M, Schlegl M, Alt E: Activity controlled cardiac pacemakers during stairwalking: A comparison of accelerometer with vibration guided devices and with sinus rate. PACE 19:1036, 1996.
33. Landman Ma, Senden PJ, van Rooijen H, van Hemel NM: Initial experience with rate adaptive cardiac pacing using two sensors simultaneously. PACE 13:1615, 1990.
34. Connelly DT and the Topaz Study Group: Initial experience with a new single chamber, dual sensor rate responsive pacemaker. PACE 16:1833–1841, 1993.
35. Sharp C, Busse E, Burgess J, Haennel R: Non-linearity of the oxygen uptake: Heart rate relationship in pacemaker patients with left ventricular dysfunction. *In* Vardas PE (ed): Proceedings of Europace 97. Athens, Monduzzi Editore, 1997, p 517.
36. Rognoni G, Ochetta E, Magnano V, et al: Multisensor rate responsive pacing: Cross checking improves quality of life. *In* Pozzi L (ed): How to Approach Cardiac Arrhythmias: Proceedings of the IVth Southern Symposium on Cardiac Pacing. Giardini Naxos–Taormina, Italy, 1994.

37. Lau CP, Leung SK, Guerola M, Crijns HJGM: Comparison of continuously recorded sensor and sinus rates during daily life activities and standard exercise testing: Efficacy of automatically optimized rate adaptive dual sensor pacing to simulate sinus rhythm. PACE 19(Pt II):1672, 1996.

38. Kamalvand K, Tan K, Kotsakis A, et al: Is mode switching beneficial? A randomized study in patients with paroxysmal atrial tachyarrhythmias. J Am Coll Cardiol 30(2):496–504, 1997.

39. Begemann MJS, Boute W: Automatic refractory period. PACE 11(Pt II):1684–1686, 1988.

40. Defaye P, Glace C, Ormezzano O, Denis B: Towards a new algorithm to optimize the AV delay by the QT? Eur J Cardiac Pacing Electrophysiol 6(1):198, 1996.

41. Sugano T, Ishikawa T, Ogawa H, et al: Relationship between atrioventricular delay and QT interval or cardiac function in patients with implanted DDD pacemakers. PACE 20(5 Pt II):1544, 1997.

42. Boute W, Cals GLM, den Heijer P, Wittkampf FHM: Morphology of endocardial T-waves of fusion beats. PACE 11(Pt II):1693, 1988.

43. Browne KF, Prystowsky E, Heger JJ, et al: Prolongation of the Q-T interval in man during sleep. Am J Cardiol 52:55–59, 1983.

44. Djordjevic M, Kocovic D, Pavlovic S, et al: Circadian variations of heart rate and stim-T interval: Adaptation of nighttime pacing. PACE 12:1757, 1989.

45. Grace AA, Newell SA, Cary NRB, et al: Diagnosis of early cardiac transplant rejection by fall in evoked T wave amplitude measured using an externalized QT driven rate responsive pacemaker. PACE 14:1024, 1991.

46. Donaldson RM, Rickards AF: Evaluation of drug-induced changes in myocardial repolarization using the paced evoked response. Br Heart J 48:381–387, 1982.

47. Furukawa T, Herscovici H, Desai T, et al: Rapid assessment of rate and antiarrhythmic drug effect on the myocardium using asymmetric biphasic pulse stimulation. PACE 12:52–64, 1989.

48. Donaldson RM, Taggart P, Swanton H, et al: Intracardiac electrode detection of early ischaemia in man. Br Heart J 50:213–221, 1983.

49. Donaldson RM, Taggart P, Rickards AF: Study of electrophysiological changes resulting from subendocardial ischaemia using the paced evoked response. PACE 6(2 Pt I):321, 1983.

50. Res J: The evoked T-wave amplitude during exercise [Abstract]. Eur J Cardiac Pacing Electrophysiol 6(1):179, 1996.

51. Res JC, Boute W: A dual sensor rate responsive pacemaker: The QT interval and the T-wave amplitude. Eur Heart J 11:199(a), 1990.

52. den Dulk K, Leerssen H, Vos M, et al: Applicability of the stimulus-T interval for antitachycardia pacing. PACE 14:1757, 1991.

53. Loeppky JA, Greene ER, Hoekenger DE, et al: Beat-by-beat stroke volume assessment by pulsed Doppler in upright and supine exercise. J Appl Physiol 50:1173–1182, 1981.

54. Salo RW, Pederson BD, Olive AL, et al: Continuous ventricular volume assessment for diagnosis and pacemaker control. PACE 7:1267–1272, 1984.

55. Geddes LA, Hoff HE, Mellow A: Continuous measurement of ventricular stroke volume by electrical impedance. Cardiac Research Centre Bulletin 4:118, 1966.

56. Baan J, Jong TT, Kerkhof PL, et al: Continuous stroke volume and cardiac output from intra-ventricular dimensions obtained with an impedance catheter. Cardiovasc Res 15:328–334, 1981.

57. McKay RG, Spears JR, Aroesty JM, et al: Instantaneous measurement of left and right ventricular stroke volume and pressure volume relationship with an impedance catheter. Circulation 69:703–710, 1984.

58. McGoon MD, Shapland E, Salo R, et al: The feasibility of utilizing the systolic pre-ejection interval as a determinant of pacing rate. J Am Coll Cardiol 14:1753–1758, 1989.

59. Neumann G, Bakels B, Niederau C: Intracardiac impedance as stroke volume sensor. In Behrenbeck DW, Sowton E, Fontaine G, Winter UJ (eds): Cardiac Pacemakers. Damstadt–New York, Springer Verlag, 1985, pp 803–809.

60. Stangl K, Wirtzfeld A, Heinze R, et al: A new multisensor pacing system using stroke volume, respiratory rate, mixed venous oxygen saturation and temperature, right atrial pressure, right ventricular pressure and dp/dt. PACE 11:712–724, 1988.

61. Alt E: Cardiac and pulmonary physiological analysis via intracardiac measurements with a single sensor. United States Patent No. 5,003,976. April 2, 1991.

62. Lau CP, Wong CK, Cheng CH, et al: Importance of heart rate modulation on cardiac hemodynamics during post-exercise recovery. PACE 13:1277–1285, 1990.

63. Wallace AC, Mitchell JH, Skinner NS, et al: Duration of the phases of left ventricular systole. Circ Res 12:611–619, 1963.

64. Spodick DH, Quarry-Pigoh VM: Effect of posture on exercise performance: Measurement by systolic time intervals. Circulation 48:74–78, 1973.

65. Whitest TL, Naughton J: The effect of exercise on systolic time intervals in sedentary and active individuals and rehabilitated patients with heart disease. Am J Cardiol 27:352–358, 1971.

66. Ponget JM, Harris WS, Mayron BR, et al: Abnormal responses of systolic time intervals to exercise in patients with angina pectoris. Circulation 43:289–298, 1971.

67. Harris WS, Schoenfield CD, Weissler AM: Effects of adrenergic receptor activation and blockade on the systolic pre-ejection period, heart rate, and arterial pressure in men. J Clin Invest 46:1704–1714, 1967.

68. Chirife R: Evaluation of systolic time interval as physiologic signals for rate responsive pacing [Abstract]. PACE 10:1209, 1987.

69. Spodick DH, Doi YL, Bishop RL, et al: Systolic time intervals reconsidered. Reevaluation of the preejection period: Absence of relation to heart rate. Am J Cardiol 53:1667, 1984.

70. McGoon MD, Shapland E, Salo R, et al: The feasibility of utilizing the systolic pre-ejection interval as a determinant of pacing rate. J Am Coll Cardiol 14:1753–1758, 1989.

71. Ruiter JH, Heemels JP, Kee D, et al: Adaptive rate pacing controlled by the right ventricular preejection interval: clinical experience with a physiological pacing system. PACE 15:886–894, 1992.

72. Burns CA, Sperry RE, Arrowood JA, et al: Doppler echocardiographic assessment of an impedance-based and dual-chamber rate-responsive pacemaker. Am J Cardiol 71:569–574, 1993.

73. Grubb BP, Wolfe DA, Samoil D, et al: Adaptive rate pacing controlled by the right ventricular preejection interval for severe refractory orthostatic hypotension. PACE 16:801, 1993.

74. Schaldach M, Hutten H: Intracardiac impedance to determine sympathetic activity in rate responsive pacing. PACE 15:1778–1786, 1992.

75. Pichlmaier AM, Braile D, Ebner E, et al: Autonomic nervous system controlled closed loop cardiac pacing. PACE 15:1787–1791, 1992.

76. Witte J, Reibis R, Pichlmaier AM, et al: ANS-controlled rate-adaptive pacing: Clinical evaluation. Eur J Cardiac Pacing Electrophysiol 6:53–59, 1996.

Chapter 12

Monitoring Applications of Pacemaker Sensors

Kenneth M. Riff

Sensors were originally developed for pacemakers in the 1980s to provide rate adaptation, and a wide variety of sensors have been developed and commercialized by different manufacturers for this purpose. Over time, these sensors have also found use in controlling other functions of the devices, such as discriminating atrial tachycardias from appropriate sinus tachycardia and modulating the mode-switching behavior of dual-chamber devices. The ability of chronically implanted sensors to provide long-term physiologic monitoring in patients with permanent rate-adaptive pacemakers has raised the possibility that these sensors could be used for diagnostic purposes other than modulation of the heart rate. Significant interest has been generated in using the information provided by implantable sensors to monitor the course of several clinical conditions, applications independent of a direct therapeutic role for these devices. This chapter reviews how pacemaker sensors have been adapted and used for long-term clinical monitoring applications, explores new monitoring applications for sensors currently under development, and looks forward to what the future may hold for the embryonic field of chronic implantable monitoring.

■ SENSOR TECHNOLOGIES AND POTENTIAL CLINICAL APPLICATIONS

A broad range of technologies have been used for chronic monitoring applications. They range at one extreme from the relatively simple task of sensing the intrinsic cardiac electrogram (EGM) to, at the other extreme, complex intracardiac sensors employing micropowered integrated circuits and micromachined microelectromechanical systems. The scope of potential clinical applications is equally expansive, including such diverse uses as heart transplant rejection monitoring, stratification of patients according to their risk for sudden cardiac death, determining the cause of syncope,

hemodynamic monitoring in heart failure, and evaluation of autonomic tone. There is no relationship between specific sensor technologies and clinical applications; rather, potential applications are driven by the inventiveness of how the sensed parameter can be used clinically. Some technologies have multiple potential applications, and some clinical applications have been approached through diverse technologies. Table 12–1 summarizes how various sensors have been used for potential clinical application and provides an overview of the material to be covered in this chapter. The chapter is organized by technology in a generally ascending order of technologic complexity, starting with the sensed intracardiac EGM and ending with a complex optical oxygen saturation sensor.

■ THE SENSED ELECTROGRAM

Physics

Perhaps the simplest sensor is the sensed EGM. The physics and characteristics of the near-field EGM have been studied for decades and are well-understood for pacemaker applications.[1, 2] However, some proposed clinical applications involve extracting information from the signal that reflects phenomena occurring farther from the electrode (e.g., left ventricular [LV] ischemia, transplant rejection), that is, the far-field signal, which is not as well characterized.[3, 4] In reviewing potential monitoring applications of the sensed EGM, it is important to identify the origin of the signal and determine whether the signal is known to reflect reliably the phenomena under investigation.

Rhythm Monitoring

The sensed EGM provides accurate and reliable timing information of atrial and ventricular electrical activity. Modern

Table 12–1. Potential Clinical Applications of Pacemaker Sensors That Have Been Used for Monitoring

	Potential Clinical Applications of Pacemaker Sensor Technologies								
	Disease/Clinical Application								
Sensor/Sensed Parameter	Cardiac Rhythm	Risk Stratification	Heart Transplant Rejection	Autonomic Tone	Etiology of Syncope	Stroke Volume	LV Contractility	RV and LV Filling Pressure	Cardiac Output
Sensed EGM									
Timing	X								
Heart rate variability		X		X					
Amplitude			X						
Ventricular Evoked Response (VER)									
Amplitude			X						
Stimulus–T Interval		X		X					
Subcutaneous ECG	X				X				
Intracardiac Impedance									
Absolute Value						X			
Change in Impedance				X					
Intracardiac Acceleration							X		
Intracardiac Pressure									
RV Absolute Pressure								X	
Mixed Venous Oxygen Saturation									X

The sensors are arranged in a generally increasing order of technical complexity from top to bottom.

devices provide a variety of functions and ever-increasing memory to store activation sequences, markers, and raw EGM signals that are finding increased utility not only in evaluating proper device performance but also in evaluating arrhythmias, transient symptoms, and antiarrhythmic drug efficacy.[5] In fact, the diagnostic information that can be obtained from storage of intracardiac EGMs is a critical part of ICD and pacemaker follow-up and is now considered to be an expected feature. Because the implanted device provides stable signals for up to a decade, these devices potentially provide better characterization of the frequency, type, and mode of onset of atrial arrhythmias than can be obtained by conventional 24-hour Holter recording.[6] The recent introduction of hand-held patient activators by several manufacturers expands these capabilities by allowing the patient to signal the implanted device that symptoms have occurred, thereby activating acquisition of markers and high-resolution data recording for later analysis.[7]

Heart Rate Variability

Heart rate variability (HRV), quantitated as the variation in R-R intervals on the surface electrocardiogram (ECG), has been studied for almost two decades as a sensitive indicator of autonomic influences on the heart. Abnormalities in HRV have been correlated with a variety of diseases and outcomes, including post–myocardial infarction risk stratification, worsening congestive heart failure, orthotopic heart transplant rejection, and risk for ventricular arrhythmia.[8] The sensed EGM provides accurate measurements of A-A or R-R intervals and has been proposed as a method of tracking long-term trends in HRV, although no clinical efficacy for this methodology has yet been demonstrated.

A practical concern with using the sensed EGM for quantitation of HRV relates to the problem of ectopic beats or frank arrhythmias, which must be excluded from the analysis.[9] These beats are identified and rejected on surface ECG recordings either by automated or manual morphologic analysis of the QRS complex, whereas the sensed EGM may not reliably discriminate normal from abnormal activation or rhythm. Reliable methods of identification and correction of ectopics and arrhythmias must be developed if the sensed EGM is to be used for long-term HRV monitoring.

Heart Transplant Rejection Monitoring

Before the use of cyclosporine in heart transplant immunosuppressive therapy, a reduced amplitude of the R wave on the surface ECG was used as a noninvasive indicator of organ rejection. With cyclosporine immunosuppression, however, monitoring of the R wave for rejection is unreliable. In an attempt to reduce the number and improve the specificity of endomyocardial biopsies, the amplitude of the ventricular EGM obtained from intramyocardial electrodes implanted epicardially at the time of surgery was investigated as a potential indicator of early rejection. The most commonly used measurement was the unipolar peak-to-peak amplitude (UPPA) obtained from several electrodes (typically four). In one study, a reduction in the mean UPPA of less than 8% from baseline was found to provide a 100% negative predictive value for biopsy-proven rejection.[10] As a result of less baseline variability in the paced ventricular evoked response (VER),[11] however, the use of the sensed spontaneous EGM in this application has been supplanted by the VER as described in the following section.

■ THE VENTRICULAR EVOKED RESPONSE

The local electrical signal resulting from a superthreshold pacing stimulus is termed the *evoked response* and consists of both depolarization and repolarization components, as shown in Figure 12–1. The unipolar VER has been the

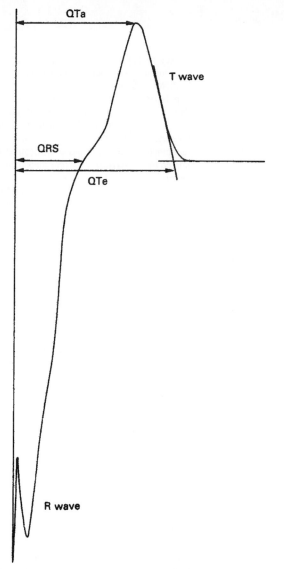

Figure 12-1. The unipolar ventricular paced evoked response. After the pacing stimulus, the initial deflection is negative due to the spread of the depolarization wavefront away from the electrode, followed by a positive evoked T wave. (From Baig WC, Cowan JC, Perrins EJ: Comparison of unipolar and bipolar ventricular paced evoked responses. Br Heart J 68:398–402, 1992.)

subject of intensive investigation since the early 1980s because it has been used to control various aspects of commercially released pacemakers. The signal can be difficult to detect because the amplitude of the evoked potential is several orders of magnitude smaller than the artifact generated by the pacing stimulus. The use of special low-polarization leads, triphasic charge-balancing output circuits, and special signal processing algorithms, however, has made detection of the signal feasible. Studies comparing the unipolar VER to the bipolar VER have demonstrated that the shapes and peak-to-peak amplitude of the unipolar VER are primarily influenced by distal excitation waves and therefore may reliably reflect global phenomena.[12]

One pacemaker (Prism-CL, Model 450A, Telectronics, Sydney, Australia) used the integral of the depolarization

waveform, termed the *ventricular depolarization integral,* as a rate controller. Since 1981, pacemakers from Vitatron (Vitatron BV, Dieren, the Netherlands) have used the time from the pace to a fiducial point on the evoked T wave, termed the *stimulus-T interval,* which approximates the local action potential duration, as a rate controller. Several manufacturers are using the evoked response as the basis of automatic capture detection algorithms. The VER is being investigated in two chronic monitoring applications: heart transplant rejection monitoring and evaluation of autonomic tone.

Amplitude and Heart Transplant Rejection Monitoring

Reliable noninvasive surveillance of rejection status of transplanted hearts could replace or reduce the number of costly and invasive endomyocardial biopsies. The VER obtained from epimyocardial leads and telemetrically transmitted from an implanted pacemaker to an external receiver appears to be a promising approach.

The Computerized Heart Acute Rejection Monitoring (CHARM) system[13] consists of special epimyocardial screw-in electrodes with a fractal surface structure designed to minimize poststimulus polarization artifact (ELC 54-UP, Biotronik, Lake Oswego, OR) implanted on the anterior wall of the right ventricle connected to a telemetric pacemaker (e.g., Mikros-Biogard, Physios CTM 01, Biotronik) that can transmit the VER to the appropriate receiver (CTM 1001, Biotronik). Data are recorded for 1 minute at standardized conditions, typically pacing at 100 bpm, and transferred to a workstation, which can be done through Internet file transfer. The signals are averaged, and relevant parameters are extracted from the averaged signal.[14] Parameters under investigation include the VER-depolarization amplitude (VERDA) and the VER-repolarization amplitude (VERRA), as shown in Figure 12–2, and the VER-amplitude (VERA), defined as follows:

$$\text{VERA} = \sqrt{(\text{VERDA}^2 + \text{VERRA}^2)}$$

Results from CHARM were first reported in 17 patients undergoing heart transplantation who underwent 439 VER recordings and 252 endomyocardial biopsies.[14] A VERA value of at least 90% of baseline yielded sensitivity and specificity of rejection compared with endomyocardial biopsy of 84% and 81%, respectively. Fourteen of 17 focal moderate (grade 2) rejection episodes and the two episodes of grade 3 rejection were correctly detected. Some false-positive results were noted to be associated with infection.

In subsequent trial, the VER was compared with endomyocardial biopsy in 30 patients from five transplantation centers with a total of 850 follow-up visits, resulting in 3515 EGM recordings and 307 endomyocardial biopsies.[15] A decrease in the maximum repolarization slew rate of the VER to 87% of baseline provided the highest diagnostic performance: sensitivity, 69%; specificity, 75%; negative predictive value, 96%; positive predictive, value 23%. The investigators noted that 71% of the biopsies could have been avoided if the VER had been used to indicate the need for biopsy.

Future research will likely focus on methods to increase both sensitivity and specificity as well as derivation of pa-

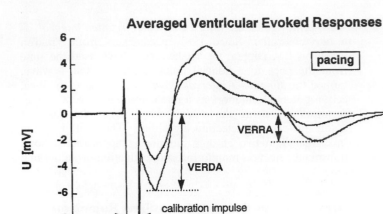

Figure 12–2. Two averaged ventricular evoked response signals from single patient, showing the derivations of the parameters VERDA (ventricular evoked response depolarization amplitude), and VERRA (ventricular evoked response repolarization amplitude). The curve with smaller amplitudes was associated with moderate rejection (endomyocardial biopsy grade 2) recorded on postoperative day 37; the larger amplitude curve indicated no rejection (endomyocardial biopsy grade 0) on postoperative day 42. (From Auer T, Schreier G, Hutten H, et al: Paced epimyocardial electrograms for noninvasive rejection monitoring after heart transplantation. J Heart Lung Transplantation 15:993–998, 1996.)

rameters that might better differentiate between rejection and infection. Larger-scale prospective trials are planned.

Stimulus-T Interval and Determination of Autonomic Tone

The complex influence of the autonomic nervous system (ANS) on the QT interval of the surface ECG has been known for many years.[16] The genetic abnormalities associated with the long-QT syndromes have provided opportunities for detailed understanding of the specific ion channels affecting the QT interval.[17] Abnormalities in the QT interval (e.g., QT dispersion, failure to adapt normally to changes in heart rate) have been postulated as predictors of risk for arrhythmias or sudden cardiac death, but their clinical utility is unknown.[18]

Measurement of the stimulus-T interval is a mature technology, and long-term monitoring is relatively easy to perform. This parameter is under investigation for potential utility in risk stratification, circadian variability, neurohormonal alterations in heart failure, and arrhythmia prediction.[19]

▪ THE SUBCUTANEOUS ELECTROCARDIOGRAM

The subcutaneous ECG is a new signal that has been used as a surrogate for the surface ECG for long-term implantable monitoring applications. In both canines[20] and humans,[21] bipolar subcutaneous electrodes with an interelectrode spacing of 2 to 3 cm placed in a precordial subcutaneous pocket generated signals of sufficient amplitude and signal-to-noise ratio for long-term recordings. The subcutaneous ECG is, as expected, greatly influenced by interelectrode spacing, orientation, and the precise position in the body. Positioning the electrodes facing superficially, away from the pectoralis muscle, significantly reduces electromyographic noise (Fig. 12–3).[21]

Compared with a surface ECG obtained with the same electrode system, in one series of 22 patients, the subcutane-

ous ECG R-wave amplitude was 4.6 times greater, with a mean amplitude of 831 ± 343 μV.[22] In another series of 18 patients followed longitudinally, the mean R-wave amplitude increased from 250 ± 124 μV at implantation to 353 ± 167 μV 4 to 6 months later.[23] Investigations continue in order to determine optimal device positioning and interelectrode spacing and orientation for the best electrical performance and reliable P-wave sensing.

Evaluation of Syncope

Syncope is a common medical problem in which determination of the cause can be difficult despite subjecting the patient to a diagnostic evaluation that is both time-consuming and expensive. Although data from the early 1980s documented that the cause remains unknown in up to half of patients despite intensive evaluation,[24] even data as recent as 1995 continue to demonstrate a diagnostic yield ranging from 22% for internists to 35% for cardiologists.[25] Although patients with syncope of unknown cause are said to have a "benign" long-term prognosis with respect to mortality,[26] their quality of life can be significantly affected. Syncope recurs in one third of patients in whom a diagnosis is not established, and quality of life is impaired to a degree similar to that with other serious chronic diseases, such as rheumatoid arthritis.[27]

Because cardiac arrhythmias are so frequently the cause of syncope, obtaining an ECG recording during a spontaneous syncopal episode is a high priority. Because of the limited period of time (typically days to weeks) that external monitors can be tolerated, however, only 25% of patients obtain diagnostically useful information from these devices,[28] typically in the first 4 weeks of monitoring.

For a subset of patients with recurrent undiagnosed syncope, it was therefore hypothesized that long-term ECG monitoring with an implanted device might provide diagnoses not obtainable by other means. This concept was first validated in a single-center feasibility study using commercially available devices.[29] Sixteen patients with recurrent

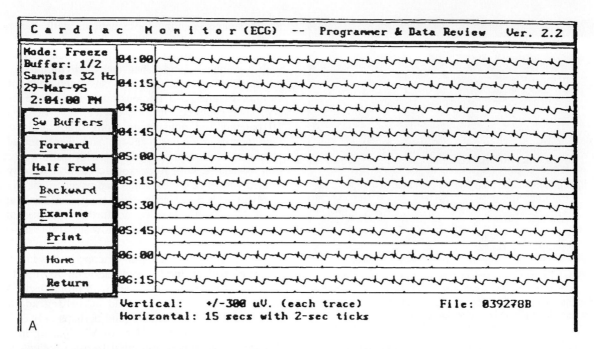

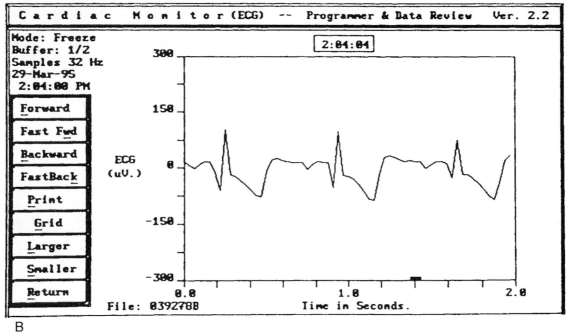

Figure 12–3. A typical subcutaneous ECG signal. *A*, 2.5-minute rhythm strip. *B*, Magnified rhythm strip demonstrating P waves. (From Krahn A, Klein G, Yee R: Recurrent syncope: Experience with an implantable loop recorder. Cardiol Clin 15:313–326, 1997.)

syncope of unknown cause (mean, 3.1 episodes during the previous 12 months) had pacemakers with a long-term monitoring function implanted. An event was captured in 10 patients at a mean interval of 4.9 ± 4.2 months after implantation; 6 patients had documented bradyarrhythmias, and 4 had no arrhythmia. Subsequent pacing therapy abolished recurrences in the 6 patients with bradyarrhythmias.

To extend this type of long-term monitoring to larger number of patients using a simpler implantation procedure and avoiding the necessity for intracardiac leads, devices employing subcutaneous ECG monitoring were developed.

Diagnosis of Syncope

The first device capable of chronic subcutaneous ECG monitoring was a research prototype (Implantable Syncope Monitor, Model 10339, Medtronic, Inc., Minneapolis) based on existing pacemaker technology and shown in Figure 12–4. It had two electrodes spaced 3.2 cm apart and continuously recorded a single-lead subcutaneous ECG, which was stored in a first-in, first-out looping memory. Positioning a magnet over the device would "freeze" the memory, which was capable of storing either one 15-minute or two 7.5-minute

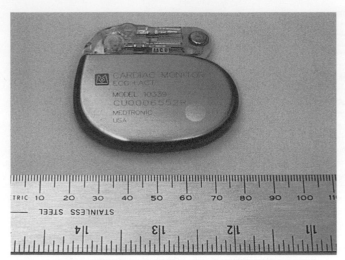

Figure 12–4. The prototype implantable syncope monitor. The pacemaker-size device recorded a subcutaneous ECG with one electrode at the end of the connector block and the second electrode as a hole in the parylene coating at the other end of the device.

rhythm episodes, which could be subsequently interrogated with standard pacemaker telemetry. It was implanted in a standard pacemaker pocket in the left pectoral region.

The device was evaluated in 24 patients with recurrent syncope of unknown cause despite extensive evaluation with a mean of 7.2 ± 6.0 syncopal episodes during the preceding 2 years.[30, 31] Syncope recurred in 20 patients 5.1 ± 3.8 months after device implantation. Syncope was arrhythmic in 10 patients. Among these patients with documented arrhythmias, 8 had bradyarrhythmias (5 sinus node dysfunction, 3 transient atrioventricular [AV] block) and were treated with pacemakers, and 2 had tachyarrhythmias (1 AV nodal reentrant tachycardia and 1 nonsustained ventricular tachycardia). Figure 12–5 demonstrates an episode of transient AV block captured with the device. Five of the remaining 10 patients had nonspecific sinus bradycardia compatible with neurocardiogenic syncope and were treated with β-blockers. Of the remaining 5, 1 had LV outflow tract obstruction associated with hypertrophic cardiomyopathy and was treated with β-blockers, and 1 had psychogenic syncope that resolved with psychiatric counseling. Further evaluation of these 17 patients revealed no further episodes of syncope during 26 ± 10 months of follow-up. Table 12–2 summarizes these results.

The diversity of causes of syncope in this highly selected group of patients provides a rationale for not treating all patients, as has been suggested, with prophylactic VVI pacemakers. Such a strategy would have been appropriate for only 8 of 24 (33%) patients (and perhaps only 3, because of questions regarding the safety of VVI pacing in sinus node disease), would have committed 16 other patients to inappropriate life-long pacing, and most likely would not have resolved symptoms in most patients.

As a result of the clinical utility demonstrated by this feasibility work, an insertable loop recorder (Reveal, Model 9525, Medtronic) has been developed and commercially released worldwide. This device, shown in Figure 12–6, is considerably smaller, requires only about 20 minutes to implant, and yet offers up to 42 minutes of memory, which is frozen with an external patient activator. Early reported

Table 12–2. Follow-Up in 20 Patients With Recurrent Syncope Diagnosed With an Implantable Loop Recorder

Patient	Months to Syncope	Cause	Treatment	Follow-Up After Treatment (mos)
1	1	Brady-tachy syndrome	Pacemaker	36
2	1	Complete atrioventricular block	Pacemaker	22
3	0.5	Nonarrhythmic*	β-blocker	44
4	4	Nonarrhythmic†	Counseling	38
5	2	Supraventricular tachycardia	RF Ablation	37
6	14	Ventricular tachycardia	Sotalol	33
7	15	Nonarrhythmic‡	None	38
8	0.25	Sinus arrest	Pacemaker	39
9	9	Atrioventricular block with torsades de pointes	Pacemaker	25
10	7	Vasodepressor	β-blocker	27
11	9	Brady-tachy syndrome	Pacemaker	23
12	3	Vasodepressor	β-blocker	13
13	4	Sinus arrest	Pacemaker	26
14	2	Vasodepressor	β-blocker	29
15	7	Vasodepressor	β-blocker	22
16	3	Nonarrhythmic‡	None	19
17	5	Brady-tachy syndrome	Pacemaker	19
18	0.25	Complete atrioventricular block	Pacemaker	24
19	1	Nonarrhythmic‡	None	18
23	14	Vasodepressor	β-blocker	4
Mean	5.1 ± 4.8			26 ± 10

* Presumed hemodynamic.

† Presumed psychogenic.

‡ Presumed neurologic.

From Krahn A, Klein G, Yee R: Recurrent syncope: Experience with an implantable loop recorder. Cardiol Clin 15(2):313–326, 1997.

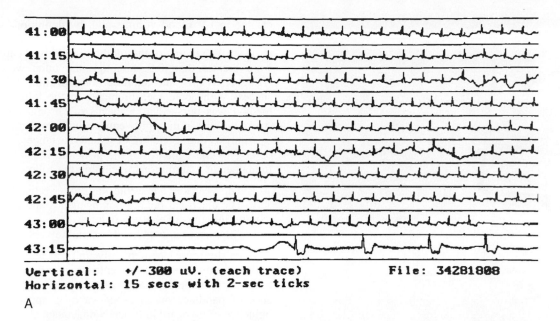

A

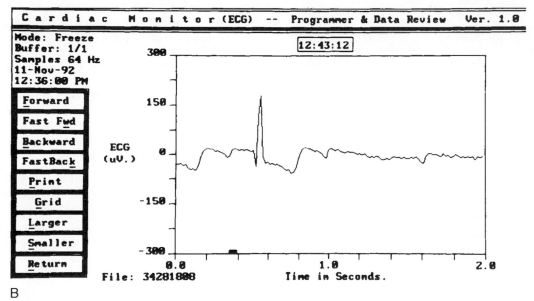

B

Figure 12–5. Monitor rhythm strip from a patient with previous cardiac transplantation. *A*, Sudden block in the atrioventricular (AV) node resulted in a syncopal episode with the rhythm captured by the device. *B*, Magnified view demonstrating complete AV block. (From Krahn A, Klein G, Yee R: Recurrent syncope: Experience with an implantable loop recorder. Cardiol Clin 15:313–326, 1997.)

clinical results[32, 33] are similar to those for the feasibility device, with about half of patients having an episode during the first 5 months of follow-up, of which about 40% were arrhythmic in cause and subsequently treated with either devices or drugs.

Future plans include device enhancements to provide more memory, automatic triggers with sophisticated arrhythmia detection algorithms, improved P-wave sensing, ECG morphology discrimination, and evaluation of use of the device earlier in the diagnostic workup of syncope.

■ INTRACARDIAC IMPEDANCE

Impedance reflects the resistance to electrical current flow and is easily measured by implantable electronic devices.

Using Ohm's law, which states that impedance equals voltage divided by current, a device may inject a known current between two electrodes and, by measuring the induced voltage across these electrodes, calculate the impedance (or its reciprocal, conductance) as the ratio of these two quantities. Because the impedance values of blood, tissue, and air are different, changes in blood or air volume between the two electrodes are reflected by changes in impedance. The technical simplicity of this approach has led to widespread use of impedance to track changes in blood volume and respiration in both external and implantable devices.

Because the same electrodes may be used for impedance measurements as are used for pacing, pacemaker manufacturers have used impedance for a variety of applications.

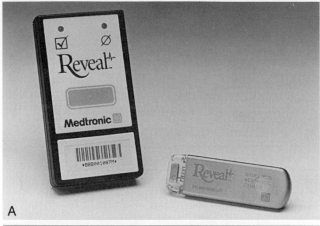

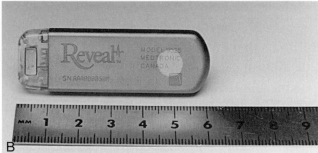

Figure 12–6. *A* and *B*, The Reveal Insertable Loop Recorder (Medtronic, Minneapolis, MN). The 2½ inch long device records up to 42 minutes of a looping subcutaneous ECG and can be interrogated with standard device telemetry.

Impedance measurements between an intracardiac electrode and the device housing are used as the basis for respiration-sensing, rate-adaptive pacemakers available from several manufacturers. Impedance has also been intensively investigated for physiologic monitoring applications. These measurements have been of two types: (1) absolute impedance (Z) between pairs of intracardiac electrodes serves as a surrogate for absolute or relative right ventricular (RV) blood volume, allowing calculation of either absolute or relative stroke volume and cardiac output; and (2) change of impedance (dZ/dt), as an indication of movement of the right ventricle as a surrogate for RV contractility.

Determination of Intraventricular Blood Volume

Impedance-based measurements of intracardiac volume were first investigated in the left ventricle of animals[34] and humans[35] in the early 1980s. Multipolar catheters, typically with 8 to 12 electrodes spaced 1 cm apart, were introduced in retrograde fashion across the aortic valve into the left ventricle. As shown in Figure 12–7, the ventricle was modeled as a set of stacked cylinders of blood, with each electrode defining a segmental boundary.

The conductance between adjacent pairs of electrodes defined the conductance of the segment, which was modeled as proportional to the blood volume contained in the segment. Summing the changes in conductance of all segments over a complete cardiac cycle was used as an indication of

change in LV blood volume and, by definition, stroke volume. Short-term correlations with either radionuclide-derived stroke volume or thermodilution-derived cardiac output were greater than 0.9, although the units were different (Ω^{-1} versus mL) and required normalization. Based on this success with acute measurements in the left ventricle, the method was pursued as a means of chronic monitoring of stroke volume in the right ventricle with implantable devices.

Analysis and modeling of the conductance catheter methodology[36] highlighted that the principle is based on certain fundamental assumptions, including the following:

1. The ventricle has a uniform cross-section.
2. The electrical field is homogeneous and parallel to the longitudinal axis of the ventricle.
3. All current is contained within the ventricular cavity.

Even the more geometrically uniform left ventricle does not satisfy these criteria. Eccentricity and variation of catheter position, underestimation of the apical segment, the presence of papillary muscles and valvular apparatus, and the influence of myocardial tissue conductance may all introduce significant errors. When these assumptions are tested against the more geometrically complex right ventricle, virtually none is valid. This is particularly true as the number of segments is reduced to accommodate the fewer electrodes available on chronically implantable pacemaker leads. These factors probably account for the failure of chronic RV conductance measurements to provide reliable estimates of stroke volume, as discussed in the next section.

Chronic Stroke Volume Measurements Using Right Ventricular Impedance

Early evaluations of the relationship between RV conductance using multipolar catheters similar to those used in the

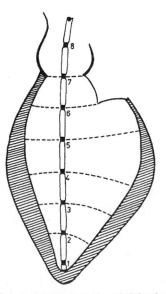

Figure 12–7. Schematic representation of eight-electrode catheter placed along the long axis of the left ventricle. Dashed lines indicate equipotential surfaces defining blood segments. (From Baan J, Jong T, Kerkhof P, et al: Continuous stroke volume and cardiac output from intraventricular dimensions obtained with impedance catheter. Cardiovasc Res 15:328–334, 1981.)

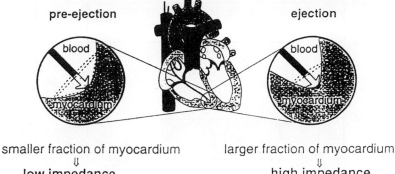

pre-ejection
ejection

blood
blood

smaller fraction of myocardium
⇓
low impedance

larger fraction of myocardium
⇓
high impedance

Figure 12–8. Change of the intracardiac impedance during the heart cycle. (From Schaldach M: Various methods of monitoring the autonomic nervous system using the pacing lead as a sensor. Clinical results and prospectives. *In* Oto A [ed]: Practice and Progress in Cardiac Pacing and Electrophysiology. Amsterdam, Kluwer Academic Publishers, 1996, pp 209–238.)

left ventricle and stroke volume determined by standardized methods of cardiac output demonstrated acute correlations in studies of a single human[37] or three canines[38] of greater than 0.9 between the two methods. Subsequently, a DDDR pacemaker (Precept DR, Guidant, St. Paul, MN) was developed that used a tripolar ventricular lead, with a tip electrode for pacing and two proximal ring electrodes for impedance measurements, effectively creating a single-segment model of the right ventricle. The device could telemeter the raw impedance signal ("sensorgram"), permitting evaluation of impedance as an estimate of stroke volume. A number of acute studies[39–41] demonstrated that the impedance signal qualitatively changed in the expected direction in response to various physiologic stimuli, such as postural change, Valsalva maneuver, handgrip, and lower-body negative pressure, as well as in response to various pharmacologic stimuli. However, evaluation of quantitative measurements of flow, as well as analysis of long-term trends, failed to demonstrate consistently reliable results with either bipolar or tripolar leads.

In six dogs fitted with pulmonary artery flow probes and impedance measurements from bipolar leads followed for up to 1 year, correlations between the stroke volumes ranged from 0.03 to 0.22.[42] In 10 patients with Precept devices evaluated by velocity-time integral (VTI) measurements of stroke volume, the correlations between the impedance signal and the VTI were not statistically significant.[41] Therefore, despite the attractiveness of the concept and the significant investment and experience with the Precept device, RV intracardiac impedance has yet to fulfill the initial promise as a method of chronically monitoring stroke volume.

Impedance-Based Measurements of Right Ventricular Wall Motion

RV wall motion can be detected by an impedance change if one electrode is within the right ventricle. The unipolar impedance signal is very sensitive to local effects within 1 cm of the electrode, and small changes in the geometry around the pacing tip electrode influence the percentage of blood in this region and have a large effect on the measured impedance.[43] This is illustrated in Figure 12–8.

During isovolumic contraction, the motion of the RV wall is unaffected by afterload and therefore primarily reflects local myocardial dynamics and ANS effects on the local myocardium. This principle has been used both as a pacemaker rate controller (Neos-PEP and Diplos-PEP, Biotronik) and as a monitor of ANS activity.

To the extent that local myocardial motion reflects the integrated "final common pathway" of complex ANS regulation, impedance-based quantitation of that motion may allow detection and trending of ANS activity.[44] In these devices, impedance is measured by injecting a 4096-Hz square-wave constant current of 40 μA from the lead tip to the pacemaker housing. Additional signal processing is required to remove the confounding effects of respiration. It has been claimed that evaluation of conductance during a time window of about 200 msec after a pacing stimulus (the *regional effective slope quantity*, or RQ) accurately reflects ANS influences on the heart, as shown in Figure 12–9.[45] In seven patients, injection of either 0.4 mg of digoxin or

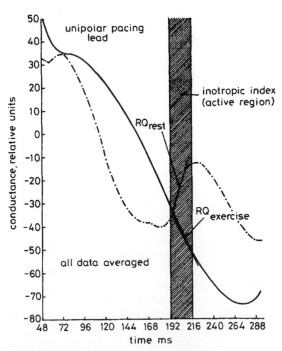

Figure 12–9. Typical shape of conductance curves measured with a unipolar electrode in the right-ventricular cavity against the pacemaker housing, during (--) rest and (-) exercise. The shaded area indicates the time interval for RQ-evaluation. (From Hutten H, Schaldach M: Rate-responsive pacing based on sympathetic activity. Med Biol Eng Computing 31:S108–S114, 1993.)

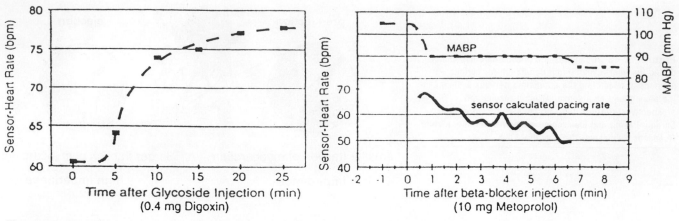

Figure 12–10. Effects of drugs on the RQ parameter, as reflected by the sensor-indicated heart rate. *Left*, Effect of glycoside injection. *Right*, Effect of β-blocker bolus injection on the blood pressure and the calculated pacing rate. (From Schaldach M: Various methods of monitoring the autonomic nervous system using the pacing lead as a sensor. Clinical results and prospectives. *In* Oto A [ed]: Practice and Progress in Cardiac Pacing and Electrophysiology. Amsterdam, Kluwer Academic Publishers, 1996, pp 209–238.)

10 mg of metoprolol produced the expected response in the RQ parameter, as reflected by the change in pacing rate shown in Figure 12–10.[43] In nine patients undergoing implantation of an Inos[2] (Biotronik) pacemaker, RV dP/dt and the RQ were measured at rest and during dobutamine infusion.[46] Correlations between RV dP/dt and RQ were between 0.8 and 0.96, suggesting that the RQ reflects RV contractility.

ANS monitoring using the RQ has been postulated to be a useful modality in evaluation of arrhythmia triggers, quantitation of mental stress, and potentially other applications.

■ INTRACARDIAC ACCELERATION

A novel chronically implantable intracardiac sensor has recently been developed (Sorin Biomedica, Saluggia, Italy) that allows quantitation of cardiac acceleration. It is being evaluated both for pacemaker rate control and for monitoring LV contractility.

The Intracardiac Acclerometer and Peak Endocardial Acceleration

The sensor (Biomechanical Endocardial Sorin Transducer, or BEST) is a micromass uniaxial acceleration sensor located in the pacing tip of a standard unipolar pacing lead, shown in Figure 12–11, which is implanted in the apex of the right ventricle.[47] Because the sensor capsule is nondeformable, the accelerometer is thought to be relatively insensitive to the potential effects of tissue encapsulation.

The sensor has a frequency response of DC to 1 kHz with a sensitivity of 5 mV/G (G = 9.81 m/sec²) and is linear to 10 G. The peak-to-peak amplitude of the peak endocardial acceleration (PEA) signal is detected during the isovolumic contraction phase and comprises the monitored parameter, as illustrated in Figure 12–12.

During isometric contraction, the myocardium generates vibrations, the audible component of which comprises the first heart sound, that can be detected by intracardiac acceler-ometry.[48] Because this occurs during isovolumic contraction,

the effect is independent of afterload and may reflect myocardial contractility. Because the LV musculature comprises most of the myocardium, the PEA was hypothesized to reflect primarily LV contractility. This hypothesis has been tested in a variety of studies.

The PEA signal was recorded with the sensor at the RV apex, coronary sinus, right atrial appendage, and floating in the right atrium in five patients undergoing cardiac catheterization, one of whom was in atrial fibrillation.[49] At each

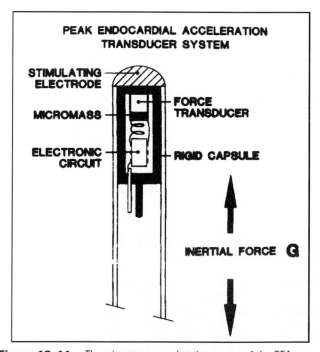

Figure 12–11. The micromass acceleration sensor of the PEA transducer system is located inside the stimulating tip of standard unipolar pacing lead. (From Occhetta E, Perucca A, Rognoni G, et al: Experience with a new myocardial acceleration sensor during dobutamine infusion and exercise test. Eur J Cardiac Pacing Electrophysiol 5:204–209, 1995.)

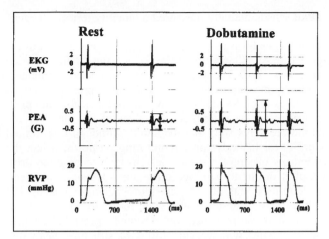

Figure 12-12. Typical endocavitary electrocardiograph (EKG, *upper panel*), endocardial accelerometer tracings (PEA, *middle panel*) and right ventricular pressure (RVP, *bottom panel*) at rest *(left)* and during dobutamine infusion *(right)*. (From Occhetta E, Perucca A, Rognoni G, et al: Experience with a new myocardial acceleration sensor during dobutamine infusion and exercise test. Eur J Cardiac Pacing Electrophysiol 5:204–209, 1995.)

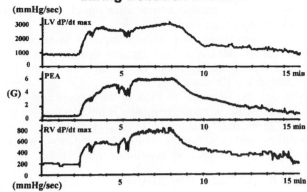

Figure 12-14. A 15-minute recording during dobutamine infusion in an anesthetized sheep. A close correlation is noted between acute changes of peak endocardial acceleration and both left and right ventricular dP/dt max. (From Rickards A, Bombardini T, Corbucci F and Plicchi G: An implantable intracardiac accelerometer for monitoring myocardial contractility. PACE 19:2066–2071, 1996.)

recording site, PEA signals with significant amplitude were always recorded during the isovolumic contraction phase independently of the recording site and the rhythm, although the signal was strongest in the RV apex. This behavior was interpreted as demonstrating that the PEA signal appears to be related to global ventricular contractility and not local myocardial motion. In 15 patients studied during AAI and VVI pacing at different rates, the PEA was not affected by pacing rate but did increase by a factor of three during dobutamine infusion, as depicted in Figure 12–13.[48] In anesthetized sheep, PEA was compared with RV and LV dP/dt during dobutamine infusion and during acute pulmonary

artery balloon occlusion.[48] PEA, RV dP/dt maximum (max), and LV dP/dt max all increased similarly during dobutamine infusion, as shown in Figure 12–14.

During pulmonary artery balloon occlusion, however, PEA tracked the fall in LV dP/dt max rather than the rise exhibited by RV dP/dt max, as shown in Figure 12–15.

PEA was found to track the LV dP/dt max during 13 5-minute episodes of acute left anterior descending coronary artery (LAD) occlusion in anesthetized pigs.[50] PEA was noted to increase before syncope in four of eight patients during tilt-induced syncope.[51] In six patients with chronic atrial fibrillation who had undergone AV node ablation, PEA

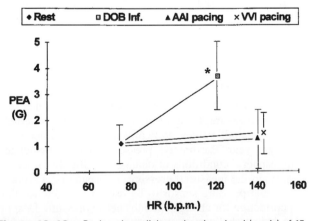

Figure 12-13. Peak endocardial acceleration signal (y axis) of 15 patients (mean values ± SD) in different study conditions listed on the x axis: rest (heart rate = 75 ± 14 beats/min), during AAI and VVI pacing (heart rate = 140 beats/min), and during dobutamine infusion up to 20 μg/kg per minute (heart rate = 121 ± 13 beats/min). (From Rickards A, Bombardini T, Corbucci F and Plicchi G: An implantable intracardiac accelerometer for monitoring myocardial contractility. PACE 19:2066–2071, 1996.)

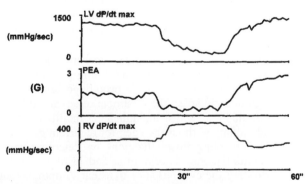

Figure 12-15. A 60-second recording during pulmonary artery balloon occlusion in an anesthetized sheep. Acute right ventricular (RV) pressure overload is associated with reduced left ventricular (LV) filling and a fall in peak endocardial acceleration, which follows directional changes in LV dP/dt max rather than RV dP/dt max. (From Rickards A, Bombardini T, Corbucci F and Plicchi G: An implantable intracardiac accelerometer for monitoring myocardial contractility. PACE 19:2066–2071, 1996.)

and cardiac output were measured at rest and exercise during ventricular pacing at either the RV apex or outflow tract. Both the PEA and cardiac output were significantly greater with RV outflow tract pacing.[52]

These observations have been interpreted as suggesting that PEA is an index of LV contractility that can be reliably measured by an accelerometer at the tip of a pacing lead implanted in the RV apex.

Although the behavior of PEA in the presence of structural heart disease or cardiomyopathy is unknown, it appears to be a promising method of chronic assessment of LV contractility and performance. Future investigations will assess its utility for long-term monitoring applications.

■ INTRACARDIAC PRESSURE

Monitoring of intracardiac and pulmonary artery pressures has been used routinely in the intensive care unit setting as a basis of clinical decision-making for more than two decades. Clear algorithms exist to guide therapy in a large number of disease processes.[53] The goal in chronic intracardiac pressure monitoring is to extend this type of sophisticated monitoring to the ambulatory setting. Although potential clinical applicability has been proposed in several diseases, including primary pulmonary hypertension and chronic obstructive pulmonary disease, the primary focus of investigation has been in the management of advanced congestive heart failure.

There is increasing awareness that the traditional methods of evaluating volume status and ventricular filling pressures, including physical signs as well as radiographic evaluation, are unreliable in chronic heart failure. In 50 patients with known chronic heart failure, pulmonary rales, edema, and elevated jugular venous pressure were absent in 18 of 43 patients with pulmonary capillary wedge pressures greater than or equal to 22 mm Hg.[54] Similarly, in a study of 52 patients, chest radiography failed to demonstrate congestion in 53% of patients with pulmonary capillary wedge pressures between 16 and 29 mm Hg and in 39% of patients with pulmonary capillary wedge pressures above 30 mm Hg.[55] At the same time, there has been increasing success in using hemodynamically directed therapy, termed *tailored medical therapy,* to improve outcomes in heart failure, which requires episodic invasive hemodynamic monitoring because of the inability to determine reliable filling pressures noninvasively.[56]

The use of implantable intracardiac pressure monitoring could extend reliable determinations of filling pressures into the chronic ambulatory setting. It has been hypothesized that this could significantly affect the treatment of advanced heart failure in a number of ways, including (1) facilitating tailored medical therapy without the need for recurrent catheterizations, (2) preventing hospitalizations by detecting early subclinical hemodynamic deterioration and instituting therapy, (3) permitting the evaluation of transient symptoms that occur in the outpatient setting and determining whether they are due to exacerbation of heart failure, and (4) allowing more precise evaluation of the hemodynamic effects of drugs.

Right Ventricular Dynamic Pressure

The first chronic RV pressure sensor (Model 6220 and subsequent generations, Medtronic), often (inappropriately) called a dP/dt sensor, actually measured a quantity termed *dynamic pressure,* or, more accurately, *relative pressure.* The RV pressure waveform was transduced with high fidelity, but the signal was AC coupled, and the mean value of the pressure signal was zero. The pressure waveform was maintained, permitting measurement of the RV pulse pressure and its derivatives (e.g., RV dP/dt); however, because absolute pressures were not measured, actual values of RV diastolic and systolic pressures were not available. Although this limited its utility for hemodynamic monitoring purposes, it had the advantages of simpler sensor design, lack of baseline drift, lack of error due to barometric pressure changes, and excellent long-term stability. A series of pacemakers using RV dP/dt max as a rate controller were found to provide excellent chronotropic responses proportional to metabolic workload in patients with varying forms of structural heart disease.[57]

Because of the technical advantages of this sensor, it underwent evaluation for chronic hemodynamic monitoring applications. In 12 patients with known coronary artery disease and exercise-induced ischemia and 10 control subjects without ischemia, RV dP/dt max increased similarly during exercise in both groups despite a decrease in LV ejection fraction from 63% to 51% in the ischemic patients.[58] Although this was interpreted as beneficial for a pacemaker rate controller, it implied that the signal is not useful for hemodynamic monitoring because it did not detect significant LV dysfunction. In 10 patients with known heart failure monitored acutely in the critical care unit, RV dP/dt max responded in the same direction as pulmonary artery diastolic pressure during nitroglycerin administration and during supine bicycle exercise, but in the opposite direction during pacing and dobutamine infusion.[59] In four patients with heart failure and one with chronic lung disease in whom a chronic dynamic pressure monitoring system was implanted and followed for more than 1 year, the pressure signal demonstrated significant chronobiologic variations and changes with activities of daily living, but no clear monitoring utility was reported.[60] Therefore, despite the relative simplicity and reliability of this sensor, no clear utility in chronic hemodynamic monitoring has been demonstrated, and efforts have shifted to absolute pressure monitoring, as described in the next section.

Absolute Pressure

Absolute pressure is significantly more difficult to measure than relative pressure. Long-term baseline drift must be held to extremely small values, typically several millimeters of mercury per year. Barometric pressure changes associated with atmospheric conditions or changes in altitude can cause large shifts in the measured pressure, necessitating a second, equally stable pressure sensor to be used as a reference that allows correction for changes in barometric pressure. Despite these technical challenges, absolute pressure monitoring has been evaluated in several different implantable systems.

Pulmonary Artery Absolute Pressure Monitoring

Chronic absolute pressure monitoring was first evaluated in the pulmonary artery. A specialized lead (Model 6229, Medtronic) with an end-mounted absolute pressure sensor was deployed in the pulmonary artery in 10 patients with severe LV dysfunction (ejection fraction 8 to 18%) and class III or IV heart failure.[61] The lead did not provide fixation; it floated freely in the pulmonary artery and was connected to a pacemaker capable of telemetering the absolute pressure waveform (Model 2507, Medtronic). Average pulmonary artery pressures at the time of implantation were 52 ± 16 mm Hg (systolic), 29 ± 11 mm Hg (diastolic), and 40 ± 12 mm Hg (mean). Patients were followed from 1 to 18 months and were evaluated every 2 weeks for the first 6 months with a variety of provocative maneuvers, including postural change, exercise, and administration of sublingual nitroglycerin. Pulmonary artery pressures determined with this sensor changed as expected, and variations in pressure correlated well with each patient's clinical course. In one patient, a significant rise in pulmonary artery pressure was noted just before sudden death. Data were useful in distinguishing exacerbations of pulmonary disease from worsening heart failure in two patients. During the course of the study, four patients underwent heart transplantation, three died from progressive heart failure, and one died suddenly. Four leads dislodged from the pulmonary artery position, two of which were successfully repositioned. Because of the problem of lead dislodgment and the unknown consequences of long-term pulmonary artery catheterization, subsequent systems were designed with the sensor in the right ventricle.

Right Ventricular Absolute Pressure and the Estimated Pulmonary Artery Diastolic Pressure: Acute and Chronic Evaluation

Positioning the sensor in the right ventricle provides a means of fixation, demonstrated long-term safety, and assessment of RV systolic and diastolic pressures. For chronic monitoring of heart failure, however, a parameter reflective of LV preload was thought to be required. In the absence of increased pulmonary vascular resistance, the pulmonary artery diastolic pressure (PADP) is normally only 1 to 4 mm Hg greater than the pulmonary capillary wedge pressure and can therefore serve as an indication of LV preload.[62] A method of estimating the PADP from the right ventricle was therefore pursued.

At the instant of pulmonic valve opening, RV and pulmonary artery pressures are equal, and the pulmonary artery pressure is near its minimum, corresponding to PADP. Therefore, RV pressure at the time of pulmonic valve opening approximates PADP. During isovolumic contraction, the RV dP/dt rises rapidly, reaching its maximum value at the time of pulmonic valve opening as pressure work converts to volume work and dP/dt begins to fall.[63] It was hypothesized that RV pressure at the time of RV dP/dt max could serve as an estimate of PADP ("ePAD"). This concept is illustrated in Figure 12–16. This hypothesis was tested in two acute studies,[64, 65] each with 10 patients who underwent right heart catheterization. RV and pulmonary artery pressures were measured simultaneously with high-fidelity micromanometer transducers and the ePAD was calculated and compared with the PADP during a variety of provocative maneuvers, including isometric work, Valsalva maneuver, supine bicycle exercise, and nitroglycerin and dobutamine infusion. Figure 12–17 shows the close relationship of ePAD to measured PADP during isometric exercise and Valsalva maneuver. The two values tracked very closely during all maneuvers except during dobutamine infusion, which is probably

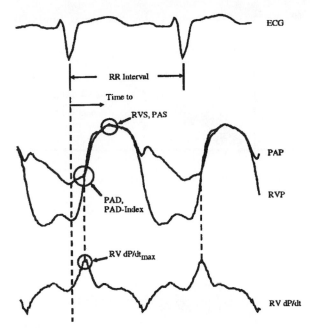

Figure 12–16. The ePAD concept. Data from one patient with tracings of the electrocardiogram (ECG), pulmonary arterial pressure (PAP), right ventricular pressure (RVP), and its rate of pressure development (RV dP/dt). Pulmonary arterial diastolic pressure (PAD) is defined as the minimal pressure in the pulmonary artery during the time period initiated by the QRS detection and lasting for 250 ms. The RV dP/dt$_{max}$ is calculated digitally based on a sampling frequency of 200 Hz, and the ePAD (noted in the figure as PAD-index) is the pressure in the right ventricle at this point. The two systolic pressures are simply defined as the maximum pressure observed during two consecutive beats (RVS, right ventricular systolic pressure; PAS, pulmonary artery systolic pressure). (From Ohlsson Å, Bennett T, Nordlander R, et al: Monitoring of pulmonary arterial diastolic pressure through a right ventricular pressure transducer. J Cardiac Failure 1:161–168, 1995.)

related to the change in RV pressure waveform morphology that occurs with dobutamine and can be seen in Figure 12–12.

Chronic monitoring of RV absolute and ePAD pressures was evaluated in 21 patients with clinical heart failure (New York Heart Association class 2 in 6 patients and class 3 in 15 patients; mean LV ejection fraction, 24%) in whom a specialized hemodynamic monitoring system was implanted and followed for up to 1 year.[66] The system consists of an implantable monitor with 32 kilobytes of RAM capable of telemetric interrogation (IHM-1, Model 10040, Medtronic); a special RV absolute pressure sensing lead (Model 4328, Medtronic), which was placed in the RV outflow tract; and an external pressure reference device (Model 2805, Medtronic), which the patient carried to provide compensation for ambient pressure. The device acquired pressure data on a beat-by-beat basis and stored it in memory in formats ranging from high-resolution, beat-by-beat data, containing about 4 hours of data, to lower-resolution, 17-minute mean and quartile values, containing about 2 weeks of data. Patients were seen at biweekly intervals for clinical evaluation and device memory acquisition. Sensor-derived pressures were compared with reference values obtained by catheterization at the time of implantation and after 2, 6, and

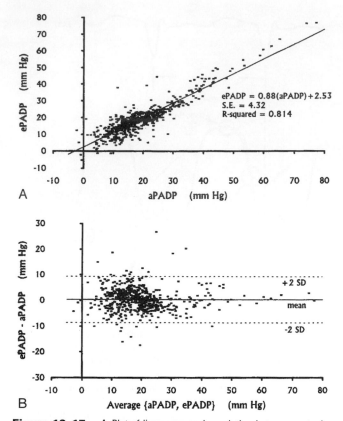

Figure 12–17. *A,* Plot of linear regression relation between actual (aPADP) and estimated (ePADP) pulmonary artery diastolic pressures in ten patients' responses to isometric exercise stress and Valsalva maneuvers. Data include beat-by-beat pulmonary artery diastolic pressure values from approximately 40 seconds of values, including baseline values before and after, as well as during, each stress. The regression equation, standard error of the estimate and multiple correlation coefficient are shown. *B,* Bland-Altman plot of difference between estimated and actual pulmonary artery diastolic pressures versus the mean value of their sum. Same data included as in regression plot. (From Reynolds D, Bartelt N, Taepke R, Bennett T: Measurement of pulmonary artery diastolic pressure from the right ventricle. J Am Coll Cardiol 25:1176–1182, 1995.)

11 months, during a variety of physiologic and pharmacologic interventions.

Two pressure sensors failed for mechanical reasons. In the remaining 19 sensors, correlations between sensor and reference pressures were greater than 0.9 for both systolic and diastolic pressures for the entire period of follow-up. The device demonstrated a systematic offset of −5 mm Hg in diastolic pressure compared with reference values, for unclear reasons, probably related to signal-processing circuitry. The device was not used for patient management, but correlations with clinical observations were tracked. Different patterns were observed, including (1) a pattern of gradual deterioration with a progressive rise in heart rate and rise in RV systolic, diastolic, and ePAD pressures; (2) a long period of clinical stability correlated with stable pressure readings; (3) severe pump failure correlated with falling RV systolic and rising RV diastolic pressures; and (4) pressure oscillations over several weeks associated with episodes of clinical deterioration.[67]

These studies have demonstrated that it is possible to build absolute pressure sensors with adequate long-term performance for chronic monitoring applications and that the ePAD appears to be a viable method of evaluating left-sided filling pressure from the right ventricle. Early observations suggest that there are patterns of hemodynamics that can predict or track decompensation in ambulatory patients with heart failure. Clinical trials are ongoing with a new device (Chronicle, Model 10440, Medtronic) containing 128 kilobytes of RAM and a redesigned absolute pressure sensor with 1- to 2-mm Hg accuracy, less than 2 mm Hg/year baseline drift, no baseline offset, and improved reliability. These trials are designed to assess the effects of chronic absolute pressure monitoring on clinical outcomes in advanced heart failure.

■ MIXED VENOUS OXYGEN SATURATION

Clinical Utility

Mixed venous oxygen saturation ($S\bar{v}O_2$) monitoring has been available for more than two decades and is a well-understood physiologic parameter.[68] A decrease in $S\bar{v}O_2$ indicates that at least one of the components of the oxygen delivery system has been compromised: hemoglobin concentration, cardiac output, or arterial oxygen saturation. $S\bar{v}O_2$ is superior to venous PO_2 as a measured parameter because of the steepness of the hemoglobin dissociation curve as well as other factors affecting the curve (e.g., temperature, pH, 2,3-DPG); hence, small errors in measured venous PO_2 can cause large errors in calculated $S\bar{v}O_2$. It also provides information beyond simple cardiac output because it directly indicates whether the body's metabolic needs are being met.

Measurement

Oxygen saturation is measured directly by reflectance oximetry, that is, essentially by measuring the color of blood. Red light (660 nm) and infrared light (880 nm) are emitted into blood, and the ratio of the reflectance of the two colors provides an indication of oxygen saturation. Figure 12–18 is a diagram of a dual-wavelength oxygen saturation sensor that has been used chronically on a RV pacing lead.

Classic teaching is that blood must be sampled from the pulmonary artery because complete mixing does not occur in the right ventricle. More recent data, however, have demonstrated both acutely and chronically that RV $S\bar{v}O_2$ provides an excellent approximation of pulmonary artery $S\bar{v}O_2$, implying that a pacemaker lead with a sensor in the right ventricle can be used to estimate mixed venous oxygen saturation.[69, 70]

During the past decade, more than 100 $S\bar{v}O_2$ sensors have been implanted in the right ventricle of patients, in various devices including VVI (CHF Pacemaker, Model 2507, Medtronic), VVIR (OxyTrax and OxyPace, Models 2505 and 2505A, Medtronic), and DDDR (OxyElite, Model 8007, Medtronic) pacemakers as well as several generations of monitors (Cardiac Function Status Monitor, Model 10343, and IHM-1, Model 10440, both Medtronic). There have been no known electrical or mechanical failures of the oxygen sensor. In some series, however, up to half of the sensors have delivered inaccurate measurements, either intermittently or chronically. It has been difficult to determine the

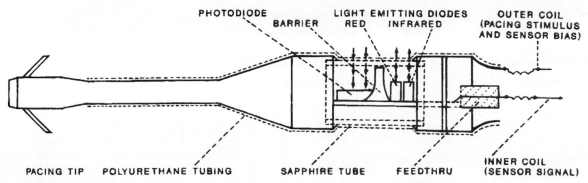

Figure 12–18. Distal tip of a unipolar ventricular pacing lead with an optical mixed venous oxygen sensor located 3.5 cm from the tip. The red and infrared light-emitting diodes emit light through the sapphire window into the blood pool, and the reflected light is detected by the photodiode on the other side of the internal light barrier. (From Faerstrand S, Skadberg BT, Ohm O-J: Long-term clinical performance of a central venous oxygen saturation sensor for rate adaptive cardiac pacing. PACE 17:1355–1372, 1994.)

exact mechanisms for these errors, owing to the inability to access the sensor in most patients. From extensive bench evaluations, animal studies, and some post-mortem examinations in humans, however, mechanisms appear to include acute thrombosis over the sensor window, entrapment of the sensor in the valvular apparatus or papillary muscles, or fibrous encapsulation of the sensor by the same mechanisms as those found with chronic pacing leads. As an optically based sensor, the emitted and reflected light must have access to the ventricular blood pool. The dual-wavelength approach, which allows normalization of the two wavelengths, does not appear to be robust enough to overcome the problems of thrombosis or fibrous encapsulation. It has been hypothesized that implantation of the sensor in the high-flow RV outflow tract, rather than in the low-flow RV apex, may protect against thrombosis, fibrosis, or obstruction, but this has not yet been verified experimentally.

Clinical Results

Although there have not been any long-term studies establishing the clinical utility of chronic $S\bar{v}O_2$ monitoring, a variety of chronic studies have evaluated potential applications.

Noninvasive Measurement of Cardiac Output

The Fick principle states that cardiac output can be determined if SaO_2, $S\bar{v}O_2$ oxygen consumption (V_{O_2}), and hemoglobin concentration are known, by the following formula:

$$C.O. = \frac{V_{O_2}}{(SaO_2\text{-}S\bar{v}O_2) \times 1.34 \times \text{Hemoglobin concentration}}$$

SaO_2 can be estimated noninvasively using a pulse oximeter, V_{O_2} can be determined with a breath-by-breath metabolic gas analyzer, and $S\bar{v}O_2$ can be obtained from the implanted sensor using standard device telemetry. Thus, if hemoglobin concentration is known or assumed to be stable, it is possible to obtain a continuous noninvasive measurement of cardiac output after an $S\bar{v}O_2$ sensor has been implanted. Figure 12–19 demonstrates this methodology and compares it with standard invasive measurements.

Measurements of cardiac output made in this manner were compared with cardiac outputs determined by continu-

ous wave Doppler of the ascending aorta under a variety of exercise provocations in eight patients in whom an OxyElite DDDR pacemaker was implanted.[71] These measurements, taken 1 month after implantation, demonstrated correlation in the cardiac outputs determined by the two methods of 0.8.

In a separate investigation, five patients were studied who had received a Medtronic Cardiac Function Status Monitor. Cardiac output under a variety of exercise and pharmacologic provocations was measured at device implantation and at 2-, 6-, and 11-month follow-up catheterizations. Cardiac output was determined by the Fick principle using simultaneous measurements of invasively and noninvasively obtained data. In the invasive reference measurements, SaO_2 was obtained by an arterial catheter and $S\bar{v}O_2$ by pulmonary artery catheterization. The noninvasive measurements were made using the methodology described previously. Cardiac outputs determined by the two methods were virtually identical, as shown in Figure 12–20.

Observational Clinical Studies

The chronic behavior of $S\bar{v}O_2$ in patients with significant heart failure has been studied in three observational longitudinal studies, using three different generations of implantable monitors. Although none of these studies was controlled or had sufficient patients enrolled to permit generalized conclusions to be drawn, they each have provided tantalizing clues to the potential utility of this parameter.

In the previously cited study of pulmonary artery absolute pressure monitoring, an RV $S\bar{v}O_2$ lead was also implanted with the device.[61] Resting $S\bar{v}O_2$ varied widely among patients, ranging from 25.7% to 69.4%, with changes noted during exercise and pharmacologic provocation as expected. During follow-up ranging from 5 weeks to 22 months, stability in $S\bar{v}O_2$ correlated with stability of clinical course, with marked reductions in $S\bar{v}O_2$ noted in one patient preceding clinical deterioration.

In the previously cited study of chronic RV dynamic pressure monitoring, RV oxygen saturation was also available from the device.[60] $S\bar{v}O_2$ demonstrated chronobiologic variability as expected, but no clinical correlations were reported during the 7- to 13-month follow-up period.

In the previously cited study of chronic RV absolute pressure monitoring,[66] RV oxygen saturation was also avail-

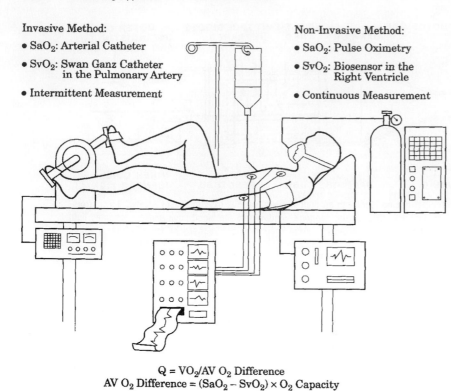

Invasive Method:

- SaO$_2$: Arterial Catheter
- SvO$_2$: Swan Ganz Catheter in the Pulmonary Artery
- Intermittent Measurement

Non-Invasive Method:

- SaO$_2$: Pulse Oximetry
- SvO$_2$: Biosensor in the Right Ventricle
- Continuous Measurement

Q = VO$_2$/AV O$_2$ Difference

AV O$_2$ Difference = (SaO$_2$ − SvO$_2$) × O$_2$ Capacity

Figure 12–19. Schematic presentation of the experimental set-up illustrating the Fick principle and the non-invasive and invasive data used for calculations. Q = cardiac output; VO$_2$ = oxygen uptake; AV O$_2$ difference = arteriovenous oxygen saturation difference; SaO$_2$ = arterial oxygen saturation; SvO$_2$ = mixed venous oxygen saturation. (From Olsson Å, Bennett T, Ottenhoff F, et al: Long-term recording of cardiac output via an implantable haemodynamic monitoring device. Eur Heart J 17:1902–1910, 1996.)

able.[66] Patterns consistent with both clinical stability and deterioration were noted. In one patient, lack of improvement in SvO$_2$ during dobutamine infusion despite clinical improvement predicted rapid clinical relapse.

In summary, a mixed venous oxygen sensor chronically implanted in the right ventricle has demonstrated the capability of providing accurate noninvasive measurement of cardiac output. The sensor is of unknown value in long-term ambulatory monitoring, and significant improvement in reliability and freedom from bio-interface interference is required before its widespread clinical use is possible. Active investigation of clinical utility and biostability are ongoing.

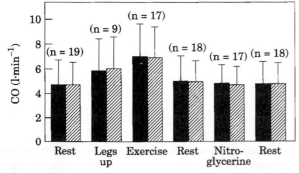

Figure 12–20. Pooled values for cardiac output determined by the invasive Fick method (▨) and non-invasively (■) by biosensor-derived data during different hemodynamic provocations at follow-up catheterizations. Mean ± standard deviation for the group (CO = cardiac output, n = number of observations). (From Olsson Å, Bennett T, Ottenhoff F, et al: Long-term recording of cardiac output via an implantable haemodynamic monitoring device. Eur Heart J 17:1902–1910, 1996.)

■ FUTURE DIRECTIONS

Future Technologies

Current monitoring is based on sensors that were developed for pacemaker applications. As the utility of chronic implantable monitoring becomes more firmly established, more complex sensors will be used. Possibilities include sonomicrometry for chamber dimensions and Doppler ultrasonic imaging for flow velocity. Two technologic revolutions, micromachined devices based on microfabrication technologies originally designed for integrated circuits and biologically based systems, have the potential of devising sensors capable of providing data currently available only in bench-top laboratory systems, such as electrolyte concentrations, enzyme assays, and glucose monitoring.[72] More powerful implantable power sources and advanced signal processing capabilities will be required to power and interpret data from these sensors. The hostile environment that the body presents to a chronically implanted sensor represents a major obstacle that must be overcome.

Clinical Acceptance and Utility

The drive to reduce health care costs has moved care from the inpatient to outpatient setting. The development of worldwide information transfer technology has made sophisticated remote ("telemedicine") and home-based care possible. The addition of sophisticated chronically implantable monitoring systems has given rise to the concept of the "virtual hospital," whereby large numbers of patients can be monitored and treated remotely while in their homes. Demonstration of decreased cost and health care use and improved clinical outcomes will be mandatory for this new paradigm to become a reality. These sensor technologies, combined with remote access and clinical information networking, have the potential to revolutionize the practice of medicine.

REFERENCES

1. Varriale P, Kwa R: The ventricular electrogram. *In* Barold S(ed): Modern Cardiac Pacing. Mt. Kisco, NY, Futura, 1985, pp 97–119.

2. Berbari E, Dyer J, Lander P, Geselowitz D. Simulation of intracardiac electrograms with a moving dipole source. J Electrocardiography 27(Suppl):146–50, 1994.

3. Damiano R, Blanchard S, Asano T, et al: Effects of distant potentials on unipolar electrograms in an animal model utilizing the right ventricular isolation procedure. J Am Coll Cardiol 11(5):1100–1109, 1988.

4. Anderson K, Walker R, Fuller M, et al: Criteria for local myocardial electrical activation: Effects of electrogram characteristics. IEEE Trans Biomed Eng 40(2):169–181, 1993.

5. Waktare J, Malik M: Holter, loop recorder, and event counter capabilities of implanted devices. PACE 20(Pt II):2658–2669, 1997.

6. Lascault G, Frank R, Himbert C, et al: Pacemaker Holter function and monitoring of atrial arrhythmias. Eur J Cardiac Pacing Electrophysiol 4:285–293, 1992.

7. Machado C, Johnson D, Thacker J, Duncan J: Pacemaker patient-triggered event recording: Accuracy, utility, and cost for the pacemaker follow-up clinic. PACE 19:1813–1818, 1996.

8. Malik M, and the Task Force of the European Society of Cardiology and the North American Society of Pacing and Electrophysiology: Heart rate variability. Circulation 93:1043–1065, 1996.

9. Kamath M, Fallen E: Correction of the heart rate variability signal for ectopics and missing beats. *In* Malik M, Camm J (eds): Heart Rate Variability. Mt. Kisco, NY, Futura, 1995, pp 75–85.

10. Warnecke H, Muller J, Cohnert T, et al: Clinical heart transplantation without routine endomyocardial biopsy. J Heart Lung Transplant 11:1093–1102, 1992.

11. Auer T, Schreier G, Hutten H, et al: Intramyocardial electrograms for the monitoring of allograft rejection after heart transplantation using spontaneous and paced beats. Transplant Proc 27(5):2621–2624, 1995.

12. Baig M, Cowan J, Perrins E: Comparison of unipolar and bipolar ventricular paced evoked responses. Br Heart J 68:398–402, 1992.

13. Grasser B, Schreier G, Iberer F, et al: Noninvasive monitoring of rejection therapy based on intramyocardial electrograms after orthotopic heart transplantation. Transplant Proc 28(6):3276–3277, 1996.

14. Auer T, Schreier G, Hutten H, et al: Paced epimyocardial electrograms for noninvasive rejection monitoring after heart transplantation. J Heart Lung Transplant 15:993–998, 1996.

15. Eisen J, Bourge R, Hershberger R, et al: Noninvasive rejection monitoring of heart transplants using high-resolution pacemaker telemetry: Initial US multicenter results [Abstract]. PACE 21(Pt II):814, 1998.

16. Browne K, Prystowsky E, Heger J, Zipes D: Modulation of the Q-T interval by the autonomic nervous system. PACE 6(5 Pt 2):1050–1056, 1983.

17. Ackerman M: The long QT syndrome: Ion channel diseases of the heart. Mayo Clin Proc 73(3):250–269, 1998.

18. Surawicz B: Will QT dispersion play a role in clinical decision-making? J Cardiovasc Electrophysiol 7(8):777–784, 1996.

19. Kocovic D, Velimirovic D, Djordjevic M, et al: Association between stimulated QT interval and ventricular rhythm disturbances: Influence of autonomic nervous system. PACE 11(2):1722–1731, 1988.

20. Lee B, Claxton M, Erickson M, Bennett T: Subcutaneous, bipolar "pseudo-ECG" recordings using an implantable monitoring system [Abstract]. PACE 15(2):588, 1992.

21. Leitch J, Klein G, Yee R, et al: Feasibility of an implantable arrhythmia monitor. PACE 15:2232–2235, 1992.

22. Krahn A, Klein G, Yee R, et al: Electrogram amplitude with a new minimally invasive insertable loop recorder: Surface mapping and implant electrograms [Abstract]. Circulation 96(Suppl 8):1–522, 1997.

23. Krahn A, Klein G, Yee R, Norris C: Maturation of the sensed electrogram amplitude over time in a new subcutaneous implantable loop recorder. PACE 20:1686–1690, 1997.

24. Kapoor W, Karpf M, Wieand S, et al: A prospective evaluation and follow-up of patients with syncope. N Engl J Med 309:197–204, 1983.

25. Mansoor M, AlKeylani A, Waters D, Kluger J: A comparison of success rates of internists and cardiologists in the investigation of

26. Silverstein M, Singer D, Mulley A, et al: Patients with syncope admitted to medical intensive care units. JAMA 248(10):1185–1189, 1982.

27. Linzer M, Pontinen M, Gold D, et al: Impairment of physical and psychosocial function in recurrent syncope. J Clin Epidemiol 44(10):1037–1043, 1991.

28. Hammill S. Value and limitations of noninvasive assessment of syncope. Cardiol Clin 15(2):195–218, 1997.

29. Murdoch C, Klein G, Yee R, et al: Feasibility of long-term electrocardiographic monitoring with an implanted device for syncope diagnosis. PACE 13:1374–1378, 1990.

30. Krahn A, Klein G, Norris C, Yee R: The etiology of syncope in patients with negative tilt table and electrophysiologic testing. Circulation 92:1819–1824, 1995.

31. Krahn A, Klein G, Yee R: Recurrent syncope: Experience with an implantable loop recorder. Cardiology Clinics 15(2):313–326, 1997.

32. Krahn A, Klein G, Yee R, Takle-Newhouse T: Symptom-rhythm correlation in patients with recurrent unexplained syncope: Results of a multicenter trial of the insertable loop recorder [Abstract]. PACE 21(Pt II):860, 1998.

33. Rosenbeck S, Geist M, Balkin J, et al: Initial Israeli experience with an insertable loop recorder [Abstract]. PACE 21(Pt II):860, 1998.

34. Baan J, Jong T, Kerkhof P, et al: Continuous stroke volume and cardiac output from intra-ventricular dimensions obtained with impedance catheter. Cardiovasc Res 15:328–334, 1981.

35. McKay R, Spears J, Aroesty J, et al: Instantaneous measurement of left and right ventricular stroke volume and pressure-volume relationships with an impedance catheter. Circulation 69(4):703–710, 1984.

36. Kun S, Peura R. Analysis of conductance volumetric measurement error sources. Med Biol Eng Computing 32:94–100, 1994.

37. Salo R, Pederson B, Olive A, et al: Continuous ventricular volume assessment for diagnosis and pacemaker control. PACE 7:1267–1272, 1984.

38. Woodard J, Bertram C, Gow B: Right ventricular volumetry by catheter measurement of conductance. PACE 10:862–870, 1987.

39. Wortel H, Ruiter J, de Boer J, et al: Impedance measurements in the human right ventricle using a new pacing system. PACE 14:1336–1342, 1991.

40. Chirife R, Ortega D, Salazar A: Feasibility of measuring relative right ventricular volumes and ejection fraction with implantable rhythm control devices. PACE 16:1673–1683, 1993.

41. Burns C, Sperry R, Arrowood J, et al: Doppler echocardiographic assessment of an impedance-based dual chamber rate-responsive pacemaker. Am J Cardiol 71(7):569–574, 1993.

42. Erickson M, Bennett T: Intracardiac impedance for chronic stroke volume measurement in paced and nonpaced dogs [Abstract]. Eur J Cardiac Pacing Electrophysiol 2(2):A22, 1992.

43. Schaldach M: Various methods of monitoring the autonomic nervous system using the pacing lead as a sensor: Clinical results and prospectives. *In* Oto A (ed): Practice and Progress in Cardiac Pacing and Electrophysiology. The Netherlands, Kluwer Academic Publishers, 1996, pp 209–238.

44. Schaldach M: New aspects in electrostimulation of the heart. Med Prog Technol 21:1–16, 1995.

45. Hutten H, Schaldach M: Rate-responsive pacing based on sympathetic activity. Med Biol Eng Computing 31:S108–S114, 1993.

46. Osswald S, Gradel C, Cron T, et al: New sensor technology: Correlation of intracardiac impedance and right ventricular contractility during dobutamine stress test [Abstract]. PACE 21:895, 1998.

47. Occhetta E, Perucca A, Rognoni G, et al: Experience with a new myocardial acceleration sensor during dobutamine infusion and exercise test. Eur J Cardiac Pacing Electrophysiol 5:204–209, 1995.

48. Rickards A, Bombardini T, Corbucci F, Plicchi G: An implantable intracardiac accelerometer for monitoring myocardial contractility. PACE 19:2066–2071, 1996.

49. Bongiorni M, Soldati E, Arena G, et al: Is local myocardial contractility related to endocardial acceleration detected by a transvenous pacing lead? PACE 19:1682–1688, 1996.

50. Padeletti L, Perna A, Michelucci A, et al: Contractility and peak endocardial acceleration (PEA) during temporary coronary occlusion in pigs [Abstract]. PACE 20:1464, 1997.

51. Brignole M, Menozzi C, Corbucci G, et al: Detecting incipient vasovagal syncope: Intraventricular acceleration. PACE 20:801–805, 1997.

52. Luttikhuis H, Gensini G, Padeletti L, Porciani M: Chronic comparison

of apical versus right ventricular outflow tract stimulation by peak endocardial acceleration assessment [Abstract]. PACE 21:894, 1998.

53. Connors A: Pulmonary artery catheterization: Role in clinical decision-making. *In* Tobin M (ed): Principles and Practice of Intensive Care Monitoring. New York, McGraw-Hill, 1998, pp 839–854.

54. Stevenson L, Perloff J: The limited reliability of physical signs for estimating hemodynamics in chronic heart failure. JAMA 261:884–888, 1989.

55. Chakko S, Woska D, Martinez H, et al: Clinical, radiographic, and hemodynamic correlations in chronic congestive heart failure: Conflicting results may lead to inappropriate care. Am J Med 90:353–359, 1991.

56. Stevenson L: Tailored therapy before transplantation for treatment of advanced heart failure: Effective use of vasodilators and diuretics. J Heart Lung Transplant 10:468–476, 1991.

57. Kay G, Philippon F, Bubien R, Plumb V: Rate modulated pacing based on right ventricular dP/dt: Quantitative analysis of chronotropic response. PACE 17:1344–1354, 1994.

58. Candinas R, Mayer I, Heywood J, et al: Influence of exercise induced myocardial ischemia on right ventricular dP/dt: Potential implications for rate responsive pacing. PACE 18:2121–2127, 1995.

59. Ohlsson A, Astrom H, Beck R, et al: Monitoring of right ventricular pressure and mixed venous oxygen saturation with a multisensor lead [Abstract]. PACE 16:885, 1993.

60. Ohlsson A, Nordlander R, Bennett T, et al: Continuous ambulatory haemodynamic monitoring with an implantable system: The feasibility of a new technique. Eur Heart J 19:174–184, 1998.

61. Steinhaus D, Lemery R, Bresnahan D, et al: Initial experience with an implantable hemodynamic monitor. Circulation 93:745–752, 1996.

62. Leatherman J, Marini J: Pulmonary artery catheterization: Interpretation of pressure recordings. *In* Tobin M (ed): Principles and Practice of Intensive Care Monitoring. New York, McGraw-Hill, 1998, pp 821–822.

63. Mason D. Usefulness and limitations of the rate of rise of intraventricular pressure (dp/dt) in the evaluation of myocardial contractility in man. Am J Cardiol 23:516–527, 1969.

64. Ohlsson A, Bennett T, Nordlander R, et al: Monitoring of pulmonary arterial diastolic pressure through a right ventricular pressure transducer. J Card Fail 1:161–168, 1995.

65. Reynolds D, Bartelt N, Taepke R, Bennett T: Measurement of pulmonary artery diastolic pressure from the right ventricle. J Am Coll Cardiol 25:1176–1182, 1995.

66. Kubo S, Ohlsson A, Steinhaus D, et al: Continuous ambulatory monitoring of absolute right ventricular pressure and mixed venous oxygen saturation in patients with heart failure using an implantable hemodynamic monitor: Results of a one year multicenter feasibility study. In press.

67. Connelly D, Steinhaus D, Kubo S, et al: Experience with an implantable hemodynamic monitor in the long-term assessment of congestive heart failure [Abstract]. J Am Coll Cardiol 29:504A, 1997.

68. Kandel G, Aberman A: Mixed venous oxygen saturation: Its role in the assessment of the critically ill patient. Arch Intern Med 143:1400–1402, 1983.

69. Ohlsson A, Beck R, Bennett T, et al: Monitoring of mixed venous oxygen saturation and pressure from biosensors in the right ventricle. Eur Heart J 16:1215–1222, 1995.

70. Ohlsson A, Bennett T, Ottenhoff F, et al: Long-term recording of cardiac output via an implantable hemodynamic monitoring device. Eur Heart J 17:1902–1910, 1996.

71. Lau C, Tai Y, Lee I, et al: Utility of an implantable right ventricular oxygen saturation-sensing pacemaker for ambulatory cardiopulmonary monitoring. Chest 107:1089–1094, 1995.

72. Kovacs G: Micromachined Transducers Sourcebook. New York, McGraw-Hill, 1998.

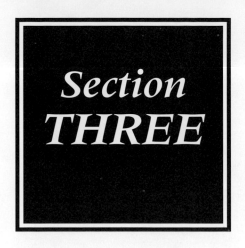

Section THREE

Clinical Concepts

Chapter 13

Pacemaker, Defibrillator, and Lead Codes

Alan D. Bernstein and Victor Parsonnet

The need for specialized symbols to describe pacemaker function has evolved along with pacemaker technology. Most pacemakers of the 1960s presented no problem in this regard because they were all essentially the same: they paced a single cardiac chamber, had no sensing capability (and thus no response to sensing that needed to be identified), and had no adjustable characteristics with settings that had to be readily communicated. With the subsequent development of atrial and ventricular pacemakers with outputs that were triggered or inhibited by spontaneous cardiac activity, awareness of the pacemaker's configuration and functional design became indispensable in verifying its proper operation or in identifying possible problems.

Two separate tasks needed to be addressed in designing a code to be used in describing cardiac-pacemaker function: first, identifying the information that needs to be conveyed and in what circumstances; and second, defining the appropriate symbols and code structure to convey that information. These considerations are central to the design of each of the pacemaker codes described in this chapter.

■ THE GENERIC CODES: HISTORICAL PERSPECTIVE

The Three-Position ICHD Code (1974)

In 1974, the Inter-Society Commission for Heart Disease Resources (ICHD) proposed a three-position "generic" or "conversational" pacemaker code to meet an increasingly apparent need for distinguishing different types of pacemakers according to three fundamental attributes: (1) the chamber or chambers paced, (2) the chamber or chambers in which native cardiac events were sensed, and (3) what the pacemaker did when a spontaneous depolarization was sensed. The 1974 code, which was based on an initial structure suggested several years previously by Smyth, is summa-

rized in Table 13-1,[1] and the existing pacing modes for which this code was formulated are listed in Table 13-2.

Position I represents the location of pacing (atrium, ventricle, or both), position II shows where spontaneous events are sensed (atrium, ventricle, or both), and position III denotes the pacemaker's response to sensing. Thus, a VVI pacemaker stimulates the ventricle (V), and whenever a spontaneous event is sensed in the ventricle (V), the pacemaker inhibits (I) a pending ventricular stimulus.

A certain degree of ambiguity is inherent in position III, although much of that ambiguity may be resolved by the context in which the code is used. For example, a VVT pacemaker is one that paces the ventricle, senses spontaneous ventricular depolarizations, and produces a triggered ventricular output immediately on ventricular sensing. In VAT pacing, on the other hand, triggering means something else: the production of a triggered ventricular output in response to atrial sensing after a delay intended to simulate the normal temporal pattern of atrioventricular (AV) conduction. The delay is assumed implicitly in this use of the code, as in other dual-chamber modes, such as DVI, DDD, and DDI.

Table 13-1. The 1974 Three-Position ICHD Code or Three-Letter Identification Code*

First Letter	Second Letter	Third Letter
Chambers paced	Chambers sensed	Mode of response

*Letters: V, ventricle; A, atrium; D, double-chamber; I, inhibited; T, triggered; O, not applicable.

Adapted from Parsonnet V, Furman S, Smyth NPD: Implantable cardiac pacemakers: Status report and resource guideline. Pacemaker Study Group, Inter-Society Commission for Heart Disease Resources (ICHD). Circulation 50:A-21, 1974. Copyright 1974 American Heart Association.

Table 13–2. Pacing Modes Described by the Three-Position ICHD Code

Mode	Description
VOO	Asynchronous ventricular pacing; no sensing function
AOO	Asynchronous atrial pacing; no sensing function
DOO	Dual-chamber (AV-sequential) asynchronous pacing; no sensing function
VVI	Ventricular pacing inhibited by ventricular sensing
VVT	Ventricular pacing triggered instantaneously by ventricular sensing
AAI	Atrial pacing inhibited by atrial sensing
AAT	Atrial pacing triggered instantaneously by atrial sensing
VAT	Ventricular pacing triggered after a delay by atrial sensing
DVI	Dual-chamber (AV-sequential) pacing inhibited by ventricular sensing

AV, atrioventricular.

Modified from Parsonnet V, Furman S, Smyth NPD: Implantable cardiac pacemakers: Status report and resource guidelines. Pacemaker Study Group, Inter-Society Commission for Heart Disease Resources (ICHD). Circulation 50:A21, 1974. Copyright 1974 American Heart Association.

Table 13–4. Pacing Modes Described by the Five-Position ICHD Code

Mode	Description
VDD,M (VDDM)	Ventricular antibradycardia pacing inhibited by ventricular sensing, triggered after a delay by atrial sensing. Multiprogrammable device. No antitachyarrhythmia function.
DDD,M (DDDM)	Dual-chamber (AV-sequential) antibradycardia pacing inhibited by sensing in either chamber, with ventricular pacing triggered after a delay by sensing in the atrium after a ventricular event. Multiprogrammable device. No antitachyarrhythmia function.
VVI,MB (VVIMB)	Ventricular antibradycardia pacing inhibited by ventricular sensing. Multiprogrammable device. Pacing bursts for ventricular tachyarrhythmia, means of activation unspecified.
AAR,ON (AARON)	No antibradycardia function. Nonprogrammable device. Normal-rate competition for termination of atrial tachycardia, activated by atrial sensing.
AOO,OE (AOOOE)	Asynchronous atrial antibradycardia pacing. Nonprogrammable device. Externally activated atrial antitachycardia pacing, nature unspecified.

Modified from Parsonnet V, Furman S, Smyth NPD: Revised code for pacemaker identification. PACE 4:400, 1981.

This was the first of the recognized generic or conversational codes. Its designers' identification of information priorities (the first task referred to previously) was so insightful and its design so convenient (the second task) that the code has been in continuous use worldwide since its publication and has served as the kernel of each of three successive generic codes that superseded it. Its forward compatibility stands as a tribute to its designers, particularly with respect to pacemakers that could sense in both chambers, which had not yet come into existence when the code was formulated.

The Five-Position ICHD Code (1981)

In 1981, a revised code was published by the same designers (Table 13–3).[2] Although it incorporated all of the features of the previous code, it was augmented by two additional positions to allow it to describe two major developments of the intervening 5 years: programmability and antitachyarrhythmia pacing.

With the advent of pacemakers, some of which had operating parameters that could be adjusted noninvasively by means of a programming device, it became important to know that the pacemaker's rate, output amplitude, mode, or

timing characteristics could be changed at will so that the reflections of such changes in the electrocardiogram would not be mistaken as evidence of a device malfunction. A fifth position was added to provide information about antitachyarrhythmia pacing functions and the means by which they were activated, whether automatically or by external command using a separate triggering device. The information about antibradycardia pacing modes represented by the five-position code remained in the first three positions and was expressed in the same manner as before, so that compatibility with the previous code was retained. Table 13–4 lists examples of pacing modes described by the five-position ICHD Code that did not exist at the time the original three-position code was designed.

In 1983, this code was amended once again, this time to include the option of the letter C (communicating) in position IV to denote any of three categories of *pacemaker telemetry*, defined as the ability of the implanted device to transmit (1) internally stored information, such as a serial

Table 13–3. The 1981 Five-Position ICHD Code

Position	I	II	III	IV	V
Category	Chambers paced	Chambers sensed	Modes of response	Programmable functions	Special antitachyarrhythmia functions
Letters used	V = ventricle	V = ventricle	T = triggered	P = programmable (rate and/or output)	B = bursts
	A = atrium	A = atrium	I = inhibited	M = multiprogrammable	N = normal rate competition
	D = double	D = double	D = double*	C = communicating	S = scanning
		O = none	O = one	O = none	E = external
			R = reverse		
Manufacturer's designation only	S = single chamber	S = single chamber		Comma optional here	

*Triggered and inhibited response.

Adapted from Parsonnet V, Furman S, Smyth NPD: Revised code for pacemaker identification. PACE 4:400, 1981.

Table 13–5. The NASPE/BPEG Generic Pacemaker Code

Position*	I	II	III	IV	V
Category	Chambers paced	Chambers sensed	Response to sensing	Programmability, rate modulation	Antitachyarrhythmia functions
Letters	O = none	O = none	O = none	O = none	O = none
	A = atrium	A = atrium	T = triggered	P = simple programmable	P = pacing (antitachyarrhythmia)
	V = ventricle	V = ventricle	I = inhibited	M = multiprogrammable	
	D = dual (A + V)	D = dual (A + V)	D = dual (T + I)	C = communicating	S = shock
				R = rate modulation	D = dual (P + S)
Manufacturer's designation only	S = single (A or V)	S = single (A or V)			

*Positions I to III are used exclusively for antibradyarrhythmia function.

Adapted from Bernstein AD, Camm AJ, Fletcher RD, et al: The NASPE/BPEG Generic Pacemaker Code for antibradyarrhythmia and adaptive-rate pacing and antitachyarrhythmia devices. PACE 10:794, 1987.

number; (2) device status information, such as the internal resistance of the battery; or (3) physiologic data, such as an intracardiac electrogram signal.[3] The presence of C in position IV of the revised ICHD Code was hierarchical in the sense that it implied that either simple programmability (usually rate and output) or multiprogrammability was present as well. For example, a VVI,C pacemaker would perform ventricular antibradycardia pacing inhibited by ventricular sensing and would be capable of pacemaker telemetry and some degree of programmability.

■ THE NASPE/BPEG GENERIC (NBG) PACEMAKER CODE

The pacemaker code in most common use at present was introduced in 1987 by the Mode Code Committee of the North American Society of Pacing and Electrophysiology (NASPE), together with the British Pacing and Electrophysiology Group (BPEG), in response to the continually growing need for a conversational code that could clearly signify the presence of device characteristics beyond basic antibradycardia pacing capabilities.[4] This newest generic code is summarized in Table 13–5.

This NASPE/BPEG Generic (NBG) Pacemaker Code retains all of the characteristics of the 1974 ICHD Code and some of those of the later five-position codes. To deal with the increasing complexity of later devices, however, it was considered necessary to clarify several features and to define more explicitly how the code was to be used.

The first three positions of the NBG Code are reserved exclusively for antibradycardia-pacing functions. As a result, the R in position III of the 1981 and 1983 ICHD Codes, which denoted reverse pacing, or pacing that was invoked only in the presence of tachycardia, is absent. O may be used in all five positions, to accommodate either antibradycardia or antitachycardia pacing without the other, although antibradycardia pacing is the intended focus of the code.

Position IV serves a dual purpose, describing two distinctly different device characteristics: the degree of programmability (P, M, or C), as in the revised ICHD Code, and the presence or absence of rate modulation (R). Like the C in the revised ICHD Code, the R is hierarchical in that it takes precedence over programmability; it is assumed that adaptive-rate pacemakers are multiprogrammable and

usually are capable of some degree of pacemaker telemetry. (All existing adaptive-rate pacemakers are multiprogrammable and incorporate telemetry capabilities.)

Position V indicates the presence of one or more *active* antitachyarrhythmia functions (i.e., excluding normal-rate competition or fixed-rate pacing to suppress a tachyarrhythmia), whether initiated automatically or by external command. A distinction is made between antitachycardia pacing (P) and shock (S) interventions for cardioversion (low en-

Table 13–6. Examples of the NASPE/BPEG Generic Code

Code	Meaning
VOOO or VOOOO	Asynchronous ventricular pacing; no adaptive rate control or antitachyarrhythmia functions (also VOO in clinical use but not in device labeling)
DDDM or DDDMO	Multiprogrammable physiologic dual-chamber pacing, no adaptive rate control or antitachyarrhythmia functions
VVIPP	Simple programmable VVI pacemaker with antitachyarrhythmia-pacing capability
DDDCP	DDD pacemaker with telemetry and antitachyarrhythmia-pacing capability
OOOPS	Simple-programmable cardioverter, defibrillator, or cardioverter-defibrillator
OOOPD	Simple-programmable cardioverter, defibrillator, or cardioverter-defibrillator with antitachyarrhythmia-pacing capability
VVIMD	Multiprogrammable VVI pacemaker with defibrillation (or cardioversion) and antitachyarrhythmia-pacing capabilities
VVIR or VVIRO	VVI Pacemaker with escape interval controlled adaptively by one or more unspecified variables
VVIRP	Programmable VVI pacemaker with escape interval controlled adaptively by one or more unspecified variables, also incorporating antitachyarrhythmia-pacing capability
DDDRD	Programmable DDD pacemaker with escape interval controlled adaptively by one or more unspecified variables, also incorporating antitachyarrhythmia-pacing capability and cardioversion (or defibrillation, or cardioversion and defibrillation) functions

Adapted from Bernstein AD, Brownlee RR, Fletcher RD, et al: Report of the NASPE Mode Code Committee. PACE 7:395, 1984.

Table 13–7. The NASPE Specific Code[5, 7]

Basic structure	Atrial-channel and ventricular-channel functions are described in the numerator and denominator, respectively, of a ratio-format code, or separated by a virgule (slash) or hyphen when restriction to a single line is unavoidable. Example:

$$DDD = \frac{PSIaIv}{PSIvTa} = PSIaIv/PSIvTa$$

Antibradycardia-pacing symbols

Function:	Pacing type:	Signal source:
O = none	T = triggered	a = atrium
P = pace	I = inhibited	v = ventricle
S = sense		
		Activation:
U = underdrive	X = extrastimulus	a = atrial sensing
B = burst	C = cardioversion	v = ventricular sensing
R = ramp	D = defibrillation	e = external

Antitachycardia-therapy symbols — Antitachycardia-therapy symbols are appended in parentheses as needed. Thus, a multiprogrammable DDD pacemaker with atrial-burst capability, either automatically or externally activated, plus automatic defibrillation, would be represented as follows:

$$DDDMD = \frac{PSIaIv(BaBe)}{PSIvTa(DV)} = PSIaIv(BaBe)/PSIvTa(DV)$$

ergy) or defibrillation (high energy) applied using cardiac electrodes. Position V is thus more general than the corresponding position of the 1981 and 1983 ICHD Codes. In designing the NBG Code, this modification was considered necessary, partly because of the increasing variety of antitachycardia pacing patterns and partly because the B, S, N, and E descriptors of the earlier codes were considered intrinsically restrictive, mixing function (B and N), timing (S), and means of activation (E) in a fashion that allowed only one of the three properties to be represented at a time.[4, 5]

To avoid possible confusion, it was also found necessary to identify the possible contexts in which the code could be used: to represent the maximal capabilities of a device (e.g., DDD), the mode to which the device is programmed (e.g., DVI), or the mode in which it is operating at a given moment (e.g., VAT).

The use of the NBG Code is illustrated in Table 13–6.

■ SPECIFIC CODES

Identifying high-priority information that needs to be conveyed quickly in clinical practice, although a prerequisite for designing a generic code, involves an inherent compromise because some information must be left out if the code is to be of practical value. Because this compromise inevitably generates ambiguity (as in the dual meaning of *triggered*), a need was identified in some situations for summarizing more

information than a generic code allows. One such situation is the task of determining whether an electrocardiographic rhythm strip reflects normal or abnormal operation of a complex dual-chamber pacemaker, particularly if instantaneous triggering is present in either chamber, a feature that cannot be conveyed by the NBG Code or its predecessors.

In 1981, a ratio-format code was described that provided separate descriptions of the pacing-mode elements operative in the atrial and ventricular channels of the pulse generator.[6] This code, with relatively few modifications, was adopted by NASPE a few years later as the NASPE Specific Code, which is summarized in Table 13–7.[5, 7]

Although inappropriate for conversational use, this code provides a means of summarizing pacing-mode characteristics, including antitachyarrhythmia-pacing features, in a concise but accurate manner that is, incidentally, convenient for computer processing. We have found it particularly useful in teaching and as shorthand when notation for an unusual mode is desired. For example, it clarifies the basic difference between the DDD and DDI modes:

$$DDD = \frac{PSIaIv}{PSIvTa} \qquad DDI = \frac{PSIaIv}{PSIv}$$

The difference lies in the ventricular-channel function: it may be seen that Ta is missing from the ventricular-channel descriptor (the denominator) of the DDI code. In the DDI mode, ventricular pacing is not triggered by atrial sensing as in DDD, but the other functions remain the same. In DDI,

Table 13–8. The NASPE/BPEG Defibrillator Code

Potential I	Potential II	Potential III	Potential IV
Shock Chamber	*Antitachycardia-Pacing Chamber*	*Tachycardia Detection*	*Antibradycardia-Pacing Chamber*
O = none	O = none	E = electrogram	O = none
A = atrium	A = atrium	H = hemodynamic	A = atrium
V = ventricle	V = ventricle		V = ventricle
D = dual (A + V)	D = dual (A + V)		D = dual (A + V)

Adapted from Bernstein AD, Camm AJ, Fisher JD, et al: The NASPE/BPEG Defibrillator Code. PACE 16:1776, 1993.

Table 13–9. The NASPE/BPEG Defibrillator Code, Short Form

ICD-S = ICD with shock capability only
ICD-B = ICD with bradycardia pacing as well as shock
ICD-T = ICD with tachycardia (and bradycardia) pacing as well as shock

ICD, implanted cardioverter-defibrillator.
Adapted from Bernstein AD, Camm AJ, Fisher JD, et al: The
 NASPE/BPEG Defibrillator Code. PACE 16:1776, 1993.

Table 13–11. Examples of the NASPE/BPEG Pacemaker-Lead (NBL) Code

Code	Meaning
UPSO	Unipolar passive-fixation lead with silicone-rubber insulation but without elution of an anti-inflammatory agent
BAPS	Bipolar active-fixation lead with polyurethane insulation and steroid elution

Adapted from Bernstein AD, Parsonnet V: The NASPE/BPEG
 Pacemaker-Lead Code. PACE 19:1535, 1996.

therefore, fast atrial rates are not tracked by ventricular pacing but merely inhibit pending atrial outputs, so that AV synchrony is not maintained when the spontaneous atrial rate exceeds the basic pacing rate.

Without the strict constraints on complexity that affect generic codes, the NASPE Specific Code is more amenable to amendment. For example, it has been suggested that adaptive functions, such as rate modulation and AV-interval hysteresis, could be represented by additional symbols appended in square brackets.

■ **THE NASPE/BPEG DEFIBRILLATOR (NBD) CODE**

On January 23, 1993, the NASPE Board of Trustees approved the adoption of the NASPE/BPEG Defibrillator (NBD) Code, which is summarized in Table 13–8.[8] It was developed by the NASPE Mode Code Committee, composed of members of NASPE and BPEG, and is intended for describing cardiac-defibrillator capabilities and operation in conversation, record keeping, and device labeling. The NBD Code is patterned after the NBG Code and is compatible with it. Like the NBG Code, it is a generic code; but whereas the NBG Code describes antibradycardia pacing functions in detail and indicates the presence of shock capability without providing specific information, the NBD Code gives more information about cardioversion and defibrillation capabilities and indicates the presence of antibradycardia pacing without providing details.

The NBD Code does not indicate shock-energy levels and thus does not distinguish between cardioversion and defibrillation. Positions I, II, and IV indicate only the location of shock, antitachycardia-pacing functions, and antibradycardia-pacing functions, respectively. Position III indicates the means of tachycardia detection and is hierarchical in the sense that a device that monitors hemodynamic variables is assumed to monitor the intracardiac electrogram signal as well. In this sense, H implies E.

In conversation, at least the first two positions are used, with others added as needed for clarity. In device labeling and record keeping, the first three positions are used, followed by a hyphen and the first four positions of the NBG

Code. For example, a ventricular defibrillator with adaptive-rate ventricular antibradycardia pacing would be labeled VOE-VVIR or VOH-VVIR, depending on its tachycardia-detection mechanism.

As an additional means of distinguishing concisely among devices limited to cardioversion or defibrillation and those that incorporate antitachycardia and antibradycardia pacing as well, a short-form code was defined, as summarized in Table 13–9. It is intended only for use in conversation.

■ **THE NASPE/BPEG PACEMAKER-LEAD (NBL) CODE**

In 1996, the NASPE Board of Trustees voted to adopt a generic code for pacemaker leads, to be known as the NASPE/BPEG Pacemaker-Lead (NBL) Code. The code was approved subsequently by BPEG, and its definition and usage conventions were published as a NASPE Policy Statement.[9]

The NBL Code is a four-position generic code intended for use in conversation, record keeping, writing, and labeling. All four positions, as defined in Table 13–10, are used in every circumstance (unlike the NBG Code, e.g., of which only three or four of the five positions often suffice).[4] Examples of the use of this simple code are shown in Table 13–11.

The NBL Code is designed so that it cannot be confused with the NBG or NBD Codes.[4,8] As is the case with those earlier codes, the characteristics considered are chosen in terms of clinical priority to describe characteristics with significant influence on the behavior of the device under consideration. For this reason, features such as connector design are not addressed.

Partly in view of the advent of multisite pacing, electrode location is not addressed by this code. Moreover, until the emergence of clearer patterns in the electrode configurations used for cardioversion and defibrillation, with and without the pulse-generator housing serving as part of the electrode system, it was thought that attempts to design a practical code encompassing leads used for cardioversion and defibrillation as well as pacing would be premature.

Table 13–10. The NASPE/BPEG Pacemaker-Lead (NBL) Code

Potential I	Potential II	Potential III	Potential IV
Electrode configuration	Fixation mechanism	Insulation material	Drug elution
U = Unipolar	A = Active	P = Polyurethane	S = Steroid
B = Bipolar	P = Passive	S = Silicone rubber	N = Nonsteroid
M = Multipolar	O = None	D = Dual (P + S)	O = None

Adapted from Bernstein AD, Parsonnet V: The NASPE/BPEG Pacemaker-Lead Code. PACE 19:1535, 1996.

■ CONCLUDING COMMENTS

In the context of clinical pacing, pacing education, and the development of pacing technology, additional symbolic representations not discussed in this chapter have been developed. These potentially useful resources, primarily diagrammatic, include pictorial mode codes,[7, 10] mechanisms for annotating electrocardiograms and other records with concise summaries of pacing mode and programmable parameter settings,[11] diagrammatic aids to interpreting paced electrocardiograms,[10] and state diagrams for illustrating pacemaker-timing design characteristics.[12]

Agreed-on symbols are a basic requirement of successful communication. Not surprisingly, therefore, the search for practical symbols for describing the function of increasingly versatile devices is an ongoing task that will continue as rhythm-management technology continues to evolve.

REFERENCES

1. Parsonnet V, Furman S, Smyth NPD: Implantable cardiac pacemakers: Status report and resource guidelines. Pacemaker Study Group, Inter-Society Commission for Heart Disease Resources (ICHD). Circulation 50:A21, 1974.
2. Parsonnet V, Furman S, Smyth NPD: Revised code for pacemaker identification. PACE 4:400, 1981.
3. Parsonnet V, Furman S, Smyth NPD, Bilitch M: Implantable cardiac pacemakers: Status report and resource guidelines, 1982. Pacemaker Study Group, Inter-Society Commission for Heart Disease Resources (ICHD). Circulation 68:227A, 1983.
4. Bernstein AD, Camm AJ, Fletcher RD, et al: The NASPE/BPEG Generic Pacemaker Code for antibradyarrhythmia and adaptive-rate pacing and antitachyarrhythmia devices. PACE 10:794, 1987.
5. Bernstein AD, Brownlee RR, Fletcher RD, et al: Report of the NASPE Mode Code Committee. PACE 7:395, 1984.
6. Brownlee RR, Shimmel JB, Del Marco CJ: A new code for pacemaker operating modes. PACE 4:396, 1981.
7. Bernstein AD, Brownlee RR, Fletcher RD, et al: Pacing Mode Codes. *In* Barold SS (ed.): Modern Cardiac Pacing. Mount Kisco, NY, Futura, 1985, pp 307–322.
8. Bernstein AD, Camm AJ, Fisher JD, et al: The NASPE/BPEG Defibrillator Code. PACE 16:1776, 1993.
9. Bernstein AD, Parsonnet V: The NASPE/BPEG Pacemaker-Lead Code. PACE 19:1535–1536, 1996.
10. Lindemans F: Diagrammatic representation of pacemaker function. *In* Barold SS (ed.): Modern Cardiac Pacing. Mount Kisco, NY, Futura, 1985, pp 323–353.
11. Parsonnet V, Bernstein AD: An annotation system for displaying operating-parameter values in dual-chamber pacing. Am Heart J 111:817, 1986.
12. Bernstein AD: Visualizing pacing modes. *In* Course Notebook, Cardiac Pacing 1988. Bethesda, MD, American College of Cardiology, 1988, pp C1–C24.

Chapter 14

Basic Physiology of Cardiac Pacing and Pacemaker Syndrome

Denise L. Janosik and Kenneth A. Ellenbogen

When permanent cardiac pacing was introduced in the late 1950s, the principal goal was to prevent death or syncope caused by ventricular asystole. Parallel advances in pacemaker technology and in our understanding of cardiac hemodynamics have expanded the indications for pacing and increased the expectations of patients and physicians[1-3] (Fig. 14–1). Today, in addition to relieving symptoms related to bradycardia, a major goal of pacing is to provide the most hemodynamically optimal pacing system for the individual patient.

Appreciation of the hemodynamic significance of atrial systole, along with improved pacemaker implantation techniques, resulted in the development of atrial synchronous ventricular pacemakers. Advances in atrial lead technology and programmability of pulse generators increased the utilization of dual-chamber pacemakers in the late 1970s. However, the ability of dual-chamber pacing systems to adapt to an individual's metabolic needs is dependent largely on normal sinus node function. In the early 1980s, it was demonstrated that heart rate was the primary means of augmenting cardiac output during exercise in paced subjects. This observation, along with the high prevalence of sinus node dysfunction in paced patients, encouraged the development of rate-adaptive pacemakers that increase the pacing rate in response to a metabolic sensor other than the sinus node. Evidence that ventricular rate-adaptive pacing yields exercise hemodynamics equivalent to those seen with dual-chamber pacing and involves the insertion of a single pacing lead contributed to the great popularity of VVIR pacemakers in the mid-1980s. A variety of metabolic sensors were introduced and clinically validated to improve exercise hemodynamics acutely. Before the availability of dual-chamber rate-responsive pacemakers in the late 1980s, there were heated debates regarding the relative importance of rate responsiveness and atrioventricular (AV) synchrony in the hemodynamics of cardiac pacing.

With the current availability of dual-chamber rate-responsive pacemakers, rate responsiveness and AV synchrony are no longer mutually exclusive features. It is now appreciated that a truly physiologic pacemaker will maintain the normal sequence and timing of atrial and ventricular activation over a wide range of heart rates, vary the heart rate in response to metabolic demands, and preserve the normal rapid synchronous sequence of ventricular activation when possible. The desire to achieve these requirements has led to increasingly sophisticated pacing systems. Recent technical advances include rate-adaptive AV delay algorithms to optimize AV synchrony, combined metabolic sensors designed to provide more physiologic rate responsiveness, and innovative multisite pacing devised to achieve more synchronous ventricular activation.

▪ HEMODYNAMIC IMPORTANCE OF ATRIOVENTRICULAR SYNCHRONY

Although the relative contribution of atrial systole to cardiac performance may vary among individuals, it has been demonstrated to be hemodynamically beneficial in those with normal hearts as well as those with diseased hearts, at rest and during exercise and in both acute and chronic interventions. An appropriately timed atrial systole maintains a low mean atrial pressure, thus facilitating venous return; maximizes preload and cardiac performance by means of the Starling mechanism; and closes the AV valves before ventricular systole, thereby minimizing AV valvular regurgitation (Fig. 14–2). In addition, it has been realized that important circulatory and neurohumoral reflexes originate in the atria and are regulated, in part, by atrial volume and filling pressure.

Animal Studies

Much of the early understanding of atrial function and its importance during cardiac pacing was derived from animal

Hemodynamics of Cardiac Pacing: A Historical Perspective

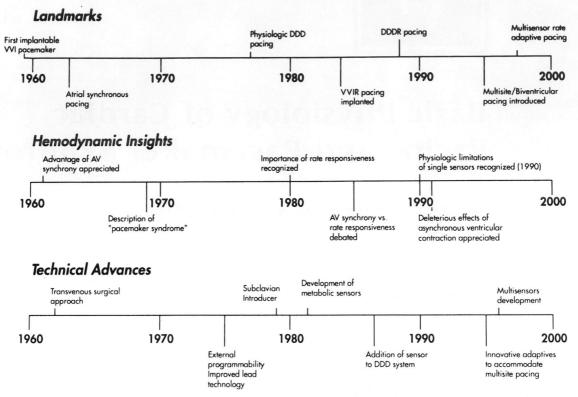

Figure 14–1. Historical perspective illustrating major landmarks in cardiac pacing and the parallel advances in hemodynamic insights and pacemaker technology.

Hemodynamic Effects of an Effective and Appropriately Timed Atrial Systole Concentration

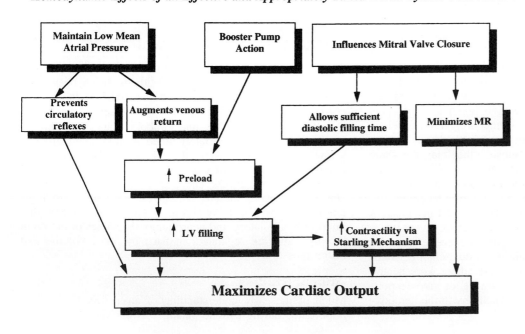

Figure 14–2. The hemodynamic importance of an effective and appropriately timed atrial contraction. LV, left ventricular; MR, mitral regurgitation.

models. Sir William Harvey[4] first observed the booster pump function of the atria in the 1600s in the excised frog heart: "when the auricles alone are beating, if you cut off the tip of the heart with a scissors, you will see blood gush out at each beat of the auricles." In 1910 Straub[5] described an early rapid phase of ventricular filling followed by a sudden increase in filling coincident in filling with atrial systole. Wiggers and Katz[6] further delineated and quantitated the phases of normal ventricular filling. They observed that early rapid inflow accounted for 30% to 50% of total filling and was followed by a phase of retarded filling (diastasis). The volume contributed by atrial systole was noted to vary under different conditions and accounted for 18% to 60% of total filling. In a series of experiments on dog preparations with heart block performed in the early 1900s, Gesell[7] demonstrated a 10% to 15% decrease in arterial blood pressure and an increase in venous pressure with loss of atrial systole and noted that the function of the atrium included "adequate filling of the ventricles with a comparatively low venous pressure, thus preventing continued strain upon the venous system." He also observed that the effectiveness of atrial systole varied, depending on its temporal relationship to ventricular systole, with auricular systoles completed 0.008 to 0.02 second before the initiation of ventricular systole being most advantageous. He later demonstrated that an appropriately timed atrial systole increased ventricular fiber length and intraventricular tension and optimized the surface–volume relation, thereby increasing ventricular efficiency and output by about 50% over that maintained by venous pressure alone.[8]

Subsequent investigations in animals confirmed that appropriately timed atrial contraction augments ventricular filling and cardiac output by 18% to 60%.[9-24] In addition, other factors altering the effectiveness of atrial systole were described, including the vigor of atrial contraction,[12, 14] heart rate,[12, 13] influence of the autonomic nervous system,[12, 14, 22, 23] left atrial volume[12, 17] and pressure,[12] left ventricular end-diastolic pressure–volume relationship,[9, 12, 18] and site of ventricular activation[11, 16, 19, 25-34] (Table 14–1). Using a canine heart block model, Mitchell and colleagues[12] demonstrated that cardiac output and left ventricular end-diastolic pressure were higher and mean left atrial pressure was lower with atrial pacing compared with ventricular pacing at the same rate (Fig. 14–3). For any given left ventricular end-diastolic pressure, the mean left atrial pressure was lower during atrial pacing than during ventricular pacing. They also demonstrated that heart rate and the vigor of atrial contraction

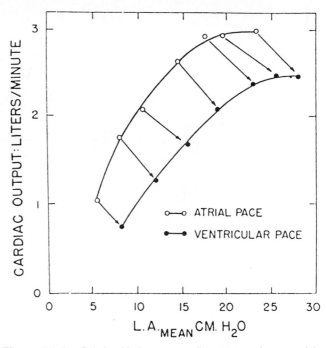

Figure 14–3. Relationship between cardiac output and mean atrial pressure (LA mean) during atrial pacing *(open circles)* compared with ventricular pacing *(solid circles)* in an intact dog model. For any given mean left atrial pressure, the cardiac output is higher with atrial pacing than with ventricular pacing. (From Mitchell JH, Gilmore JP, Sarnoff SJ: The transport function of the atrium: Factors influencing the relation between mean left atrial pressure and left ventricular end diastolic pressure. Am J Cardiol 9:237, 1962.)

exerted independent influences on the contribution of atrial function to cardiac performance and that both are affected by the autonomic nervous system.[12] Mean left atrial pressure was higher for any left ventricular end-diastolic pressure as heart rate increased and the relative period during which atrial emptying occurs decreased.[12] At a constant heart rate, left atrial pressure was higher at any given left ventricular end-diastolic pressure during efferent vagal stimulation because of a negative inotropic atrial effect and lower during sympathetic stimulation because of a positive inotropic effect on the atrium. In a subsequent study, Mitchell and associates[13] demonstrated that the atrial contribution to cardiac output remained significant over a wide range of heart rates, 60 to 210 bpm, and the percentage augmentation by atrial systole over ventricular pacing alone increased with increased rates of pacing at rest (Fig. 14–4). Investigations by Gilmore[11] and Kosowsky[16] and their colleagues suggested that the temporal relationship between atrial and ventricular contraction and the sequence of ventricular depolarization are independent and additive determinants of ventricular performance during pacing. Several subsequent investigators have demonstrated that the asynchronous ventricular contraction produced by right ventricular apical pacing is deleterious to systolic and diastolic ventricular function compared with more normal sequences of ventricular activation.[19, 25-34]

Normally, the atria function as a conduit that transfers blood to the ventricle when the AV valves are open, a reservoir to accept venous inflow during ventricular ejection,

Table 14–1. Factors Influencing Effectiveness of Atrial Contraction in Animal Models

Timing relative to ventricular contraction
Vigor of atrial contraction
Autonomic nervous system
Heart rate
Left atrial volume
Left atrial pressure
Presence of pericardium
Sequence of ventricular activation
Left ventricular end-diastolic pressure
Atrial compliance

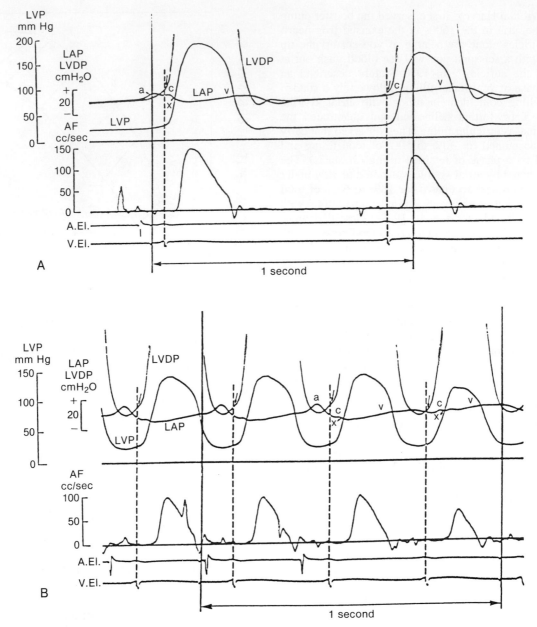

Figure 14–4. Hemodynamic effects of atrial systole at a low heart rate *(A)* and at a higher heart rate *(B)*. The a, v, and c waves and x descent are present in ejections in which ventricular systole is preceded by atrial systole. The a wave is absent, and there is no x descent when atrial systole is absent (last beat of each panel). The loss of atrial systole diminished effective left ventricular stroke volume by 25% at the low heart rate and by almost 50% at the higher heart rate. LVP, left ventricular pressure; LAP, left atrial pressure; LVDP, left ventricular diastolic pressure; AF, aortic flow; A.EL, left atrial bipolar electrogram; V.EL, left ventricular bipolar electrogram. Time lines are at 1-second intervals. (From Mitchell JH, Gupta DN, Payne RM: Influence of atrial systole on effective ventricular stroke volume. Circ Res 17:11, 1965).

and a booster pump during atrial systole. Payne and coworkers[17] investigated the effects of volume loading on left atrial contractile function in the intact dog model. They demonstrated that as left atrial diameter increased with volume loading, left atrial systolic shortening initially increased. However, the ascending limb of the function curve was short, and as volume further increased, the amplitude of atrial shortening decreased. Thus, at a critical level of distention, the optimal atrial end-diastolic diameter is exceeded,

the booster pump function of the atrium is diminished, and conduit function dominates. Studies of a circulatory analog model indicate that cardiac output is enhanced with increased atrial compliance in the presence of constant ventricular contractility.[35]

Linderer and associates[18] examined the influence of atrial systole on the left ventricular function curve in open-chest dogs with both intact and opened pericardia. When the pericardium was closed, withdrawal of atrial systole consistently shifted the relationship between left ventricular stroke volume and end-diastolic pressure downward. When the pericardium was opened, the entire curve shifted upward, and stroke volume was relatively independent of atrial contribution. Consistent with the Frank-Starling mechanism, the stroke volume increased with increased end-diastolic diameter regardless of the presence of atrial systole or an intact pericardium.

Animal studies have also defined the role of atrial systole in the initiation of mitral valve closure.[14, 15] The mitral valve closes as a result of the reversal of the AV pressure gradient before ventricular ejection. Sarnoff and colleagues[14] demonstrated in a heart block canine preparation that the timing and vigor of atrial contraction and relaxation contribute to the rate of rise of left ventricular end-diastolic pressure and the rate of decline of atrial pressure. By altering the timing of atrial contraction relative to ventricular contraction, they demonstrated that closure of the mitral valve could be induced solely as a result of atrial activity.[14] They further demonstrated that when atrial contraction and relaxation were able to promote mitral valve closure, this could be abolished by diminishing the contractility of the atrium through vagal stimulation and, conversely, enhanced by augmenting contractility by sympathetic stimulation. Using a similar animal model, Skinner and associates[15] demonstrated that with a very short AV contraction sequence or in the absence of atrial activity, the mitral valve was closed by the ventriculoatrial (VA) pressure gradient generated solely by ventricular systole, and mitral regurgitation was noted to occur. If the AV interval was excessively long, they demonstrated that the pressure generated by atrial systole occurred against a closed AV valve and, if too short, occurred simultaneously with ventricular contraction.[15] In more recent animal studies, Doppler echocardiography has demonstrated that diastolic filling is interrupted and cardiac output reduced by short (50-msec) AV delay intervals during AV sequential pacing.[24]

Observations in animal models have contributed to our understanding of the deleterious hemodynamic effects of ventricular pacing. In open-chest heart block dog models, ventricular pacing resulting in one-to-one retrograde VA conduction has been shown to cause significant decreases in cardiac output, left ventricular pressure, and systolic blood pressure and increases in right atrial and pulmonary venous pressures and left atrial size compared with ventricular pacing with complete retrograde VA block or random VA conduction.[19-21] An increase in left atrial size and elevation of atrial pressure during one-to-one VA conduction may be a stimulus for the abnormal atrial reflexes observed in the pacemaker syndrome in humans. Naito and associates[20, 21] evaluated the hemodynamic effects of abnormal AV sequencing in dog models of heart block by angiography and M-mode echocardiography. As the AV interval decreased from +100 to −100 msec, there was a progressive decrease in cardiac output, left ventricular and aortic pressure, and left ventricular dimension and an increase in left atrial pressure. At negative AV intervals, not only was there a loss of atrial contribution to ventricular filling but also pulmonary venous regurgitation or a "negative atrial kick" occurred, resulting in further hemodynamic deterioration. Varying the AV interval from +100 to −200 msec, Ogawa and coworkers[19]

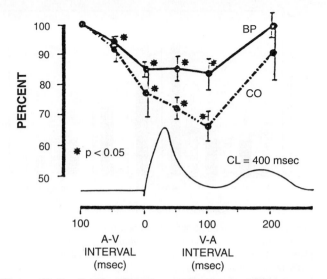

Figure 14–5. Relationship between atrioventricular (AV) and ventriculoatrial (VA) intervals and cardiac output (CO) and blood pressure (BP) in intact dogs. Cardiac output and blood pressure fall at AV intervals of less than 50 msec and are lowest at VA intervals of 100 msec. (From Ogawa S, Dreifus LS, Shenoy PN, et al: Hemodynamic consequences of atrioventricular and ventriculoatrial pacing. PACE 1:8, 1978.)

found the least favorable hemodynamics to occur at a VA interval of 100 msec (Fig. 14–5).

Hemodynamic Effects of Ventricular Pacing in Complete Heart Block

Initially, permanent ventricular pacemakers were implanted in the early 1960s to prevent death or syncope caused by ventricular asystole. Both the beneficial and the deleterious hemodynamic effects of ventricular pacing soon became known. In both animals and humans with acquired complete heart block and a slow ventricular escape, cardiac output is reduced compared with normal resting heart rates despite compensatory increases in sympathetic tone and end-diastolic ventricular volume that are manifested by increased atrial rates, enhanced ventricular contractility, and augmented stroke volume (Table 14–2). In patients with acquired complete heart block, ventricular pacing produces

Table 14–2. Hemodynamic Effects of Ventricular Pacing in Complete Heart Block

Hemodynamic Parameter	CHB with Slow Ventricular Response	Ventricular Pacing in CHB
Ventricular rate	↓	↑
Cardiac index	↓	↑
Stroke volume	↑	↓
Sympathetic tone	↑	↓
Ventricular contractility	↑	↓
Systemic vascular resistance	↑	↓
Atrial rate	↑	↓

CHB, complete heart block.

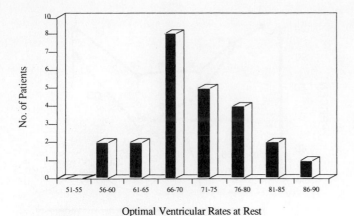

Figure 14–6. Histogram of optimal ventricular pacing rates at rest as defined by cardiac outputs determined by dye dilution in patients with complete heart block. (From Sowton E: Hemodynamic studies in patients with artificial pacemakers. Br Heart J 26:737, 1964.)

a more physiologically appropriate resting heart rate and increased cardiac output associated with decreased sympathetic tone and a reduction in end-diastolic ventricular volume that are reflected by decreased atrial rates, diminished stroke volume, and reduced ventricular contractility.[36–41] Brockman[36] described an immediate decrease in cardiac output and increase in left ventricular stroke volume after surgically induced heart block in dogs. The canine heart adapted to the increased diastolic volume produced by bradycardia acutely by dilation and chronically by hypertrophy. Despite compensatory mechanisms, animals remaining in heart block for more than 4 months tended to manifest signs of congestive heart failure. The frequency of congestive heart failure symptoms in patients with complete heart block correlates with the duration of heart block, suggesting that the ability

of ventricular dilation and hypertrophy to compensate for chronic bradycardia in humans is also limited.[37] Congestive heart failure has been described during chronic complete heart block even in patients with normal ventricular function. Brockman and Stoney[37] reported that in two thirds of patients with complete heart block and congestive heart failure, symptoms were relieved by ventricular pacing alone, and no additional medical therapy was required.

Early studies suggested that the maximal increase in cardiac output during ventricular pacing at rest occurs at rates between 70 and 90 bpm[38–41] (Fig. 14–6). Further increases in rates result in either no additional increase or a decrease in cardiac output accompanied by increased peripheral vascular resistance. Sowton[39] described two patterns of hemodynamic response to increased rates of ventricular pacing. In the flat response, after an initial increase, cardiac output remained relatively constant as stroke volume decreased with increasing heart rate (Fig. 14–7A). This response occurred most often in individuals with normal cardiac function and indicates that cardiac output is relatively independent of heart rate. In the peaked response, cardiac output increased progressively until the optimal pacing rate was achieved, and any further increase in rate resulted in a diminution in cardiac output (see Fig. 14–7B). The peaked response was more commonly observed in patients with myocardial disease, in whom cardiac output is more sensitive to changes in preload, afterload, myocardial contractility, and distensibility. The major factors limiting the increase in resting cardiac output that can be achieved by pacing rate alone are shortened diastolic filling time, reduced left ventricular compliance at higher rates of ventricular pacing, and increased systemic vascular resistance.[38–41]

Rowe and colleagues[42] examined cardiac output and coronary blood flow at low (47 bpm), intermediate (77 bpm), and high (117 bpm) ventricular pacing rates in subjects with complete heart block. Cardiac output increased from the low to the intermediate rate but decreased at the higher rate.

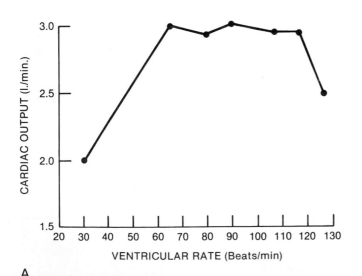

A

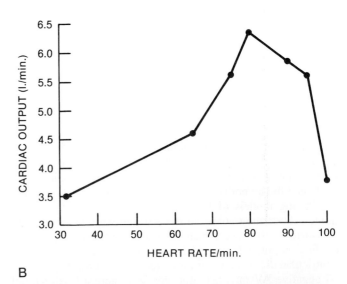

B

Figure 14–7. *A,* Example of flat response indicating a relatively constant cardiac output over a wide range of ventricular pacing rates. *B,* Example of a peaked response curve demonstrating progressive increase in cardiac output with heart rate until an optimal heart rate is achieved. After this optimal heart rate, a further increase in heart rate results in a decrease in cardiac output. (From Sowton E: Hemodynamic studies in patients with artificial pacemakers. Br Heart J 26:737, 1964.)

Table 14–3. Resting Cardiac Output During Physiologic Pacing Modes Compared With VVI Pacing

Reference	Method of Cardiac Output Measurement	Percentage Increment, DDD vs. VVI
Invasive studies		
Samet[52]	Dye dilution	19
Karlöf[57]	Thermodilution	10
Leinbach[58]	Dye dilution	24
Chamberlain[59]	Dye dilution	24
Hartzler[60]	Dye dilution	34
Greenberg[61]	Thermodilution	25
Reiter[63]	Thermodilution	17
Noninvasive studies		
Nanda[66]	Doppler	18
Zugibe[67]	Doppler	19.5
Boucher[69]	Radionuclide angiography	16
Nitsch[71]	Radionuclide angiography	10
Stewart[72]	Doppler	19
Labovitz[73]	Doppler	21
Faerestrand[74]	Doppler	21
Rediker[83]	Doppler	43
Janosik[85]	Doppler	33
Lascault[86]	Doppler	27
Masuyama[90]	Doppler	26

Hemodynamic Superiority of Atrioventricular Sequential Over Ventricular Pacing

Samet and associates[52, 53] demonstrated increased thermodilution cardiac output during temporary AV sequential pacing and atrial demand pacing compared with ventricular demand pacing at the same heart rate. Numerous subsequent studies have demonstrated 10% to 53% increments in resting cardiac output[54–90] with AV synchronous or sequential pacing compared with VVI pacing (Table 14–3). These studies have been performed using both invasive[52–64, 81, 82] and noninvasive[65–80, 83–90] (Fig. 14–8) assessment of cardiac output, during temporary pacing[47–58] as well as with acute reprogramming of permanent pacemakers,[64–89] and in patients with a diseased heart[55, 56, 58–63] and those with normal cardiac function.[53, 54, 75, 79] Higher left ventricular end-diastolic pressures[52, 62] and volumes,[62, 68, 69, 75, 76] higher systolic and mean blood pressures,[59, 64, 65] lower venous pressures, and lower pulmonary capillary wedge pressures[57, 61, 63] have been reported with modes of pacing that maintain AV synchrony compared with ventricular pacing. The significance of the atrial contribution to resting cardiac output persists over a wide range of paced heart rates in the upright position as well as in the supine position and in the presence of inotropic stimulation. At rest, the atrial contribution to cardiac output

Coronary blood flow and cardiac oxygen consumption increased progressively with increasing rates. They concluded that low and intermediate heart rates yield the most efficient systemic and coronary dynamics.

Fixed-rate ventricular pacing maintains a resting cardiac output adequate for the prevention of syncope in most individuals. However, VVI pacing is not physiologic in the sense of preserving an appropriate atrial-to-ventricular relationship or in terms of the ability to increase heart rate in response to metabolic demands. The importance of the atrial contribution to cardiac output has long been known. Loss of an effective atrial systole because of atrial fibrillation is recognized to cause symptoms of congestive heart failure even in some individuals with normal hearts and adequate control of the ventricular response of the atrial fibrillation.[43–46] During ventricular pacing for complete heart block, it was noted that QRS complexes preceded by P waves resulted in higher stroke volumes and systemic pressures than QRS complexes occurring in the absence of P waves.[47–51] Observations of the hemodynamic effects of randomly distributed AV coupling intervals during ventricular pacing suggested the importance of timing between atrial and ventricular contraction.[49–51] It was noted that very short or very long AV coupling intervals resulted in minimal hemodynamic improvement compared with ventricular pacing alone. An inverse relationship between the optimal PR interval and ventricular pacing rate was also described.[44] The relative contribution of a fortuitously timed P-wave to cardiac output during ventricular pacing for complete heart block has been reported to be greater at higher ventricular pacing rates.

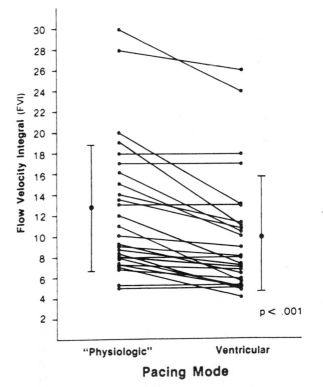

Figure 14–8. Comparison of Doppler flow velocity integrals in 26 patients during AV sequential physiologic pacing versus ventricular pacing at identical heart rates. A mean reduction in flow velocity integral of 21% occurred when programming from physiologic pacing mode to ventricular pacing. (From Labovitz AJ, Williams GA, Redd RM, Kennedy HL: Noninvasive assessment of pacemaker hemodynamics by Doppler echocardiography: Importance of left atrial size. J Am Coll Cardiol 6:196, 1985. Reprinted with permission of the American College of Cardiology.)

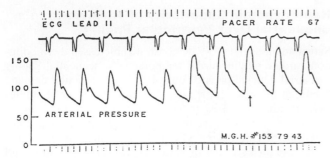

Figure 14–9. Radial artery pressure from a patient with complete A-V block during fixed-rate ventricular pacing. Peak systolic pressure is seen when the P-R interval is 270 msec *(arrow).*

Table 14–4. **Symptoms of Pacemaker Syndrome**

Mild
Pulsations in neck, abdomen
Palpitations
Fatigue, malaise, weakness
Cough
Apprehension
Chest fullness or pain, jaw pain
Headache
Moderate
Shortness of breath on exertion
Dizziness, tiredness, vertigo
Orthopnea, paroxysmal nocturnal dyspnea
Choking sensation
Confusion or alteration of mental state
Severe
Presyncope
Syncope
Shortness of breath at rest, pulmonary edema

and percentage augmentation in cardiac output with AV sequential pacing compared with ventricular pacing increases with increasing heart rate. Most radionuclide studies indicate higher cardiac outputs but no significant change in left ventricular ejection fraction (LVEF) with a dual-chamber pacing mode compared with VVI pacing at similar heart rates.[68–73, 75, 76] In fact, lower LVEFs have been reported in a few studies with DDD pacing than with VVI pacing. This may be explained by the fact that cardiac output is increased by augmenting ventricular filling with dual-chamber pacing and that relatively higher catecholamine levels and enhanced contractility are compensatory mechanisms for the lower volume with VVI pacing. In addition to the loss of the atrial contribution to cardiac output, ventricular pacing can result in significant tricuspid or mitral regurgitation in some patients because of asynchrony of atrial and ventricular contraction and poorly timed AV valve closure.[91, 92]

■ PACEMAKER SYNDROME

Diagnosis and Incidence

Most individuals can compensate for the reduction in cardiac output due to loss of atrial systole by activation of barorecep-

tor reflexes that increase peripheral resistance and maintain systemic blood pressure. In addition, during ventricular pacing in individuals without retrograde VA conduction, there is intermittent hemodynamic benefit from fortuitously timed P waves (Figs. 14–9 and 14–10). However, some individuals, particularly those with intact retrograde ventriculoatrial conduction, may tolerate ventricular pacing poorly and develop a variety of clinical signs and symptoms. The constellation of neurologic and cardiovascular signs and symptoms resulting from deleterious hemodynamics induced by ventricular pacing has been termed the *pacemaker syndrome.*[93, 94, 94a] The symptoms that have been associated with the pacemaker syndrome are listed in Table 14–4. The signs and symptoms arising from pacemaker syndrome are attributable to a decrease to cardiac output in arterial pressure because of loss of AV synchrony or to cardiovascular or humoral reflexes elicited by increases in pulmonary artery or pulmonary venous pressure. Symptoms may vary from mild to severe, and the onset of symptoms ranges from acute to chronic. A minority of patients present with acute severe symptoms,

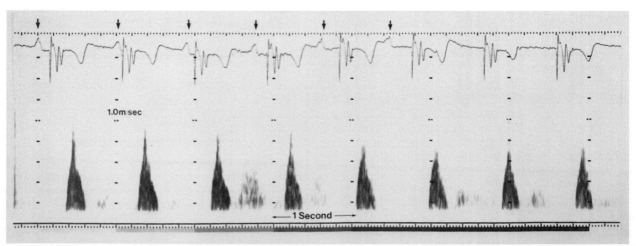

Figure 14–10. Doppler aortic flow velocity integrals during ventricular pacing in a patient with complete heart block. The effect of fortuitously timed P waves *(arrows)* on aortic flow is demonstrated.

such as syncope or pulmonary edema, which may require prompt discontinuation of ventricular pacing. More often, the onset is subacute or chronic, and the symptoms may be subtle and nonspecific. The pathophysiology of pacemaker syndrome results from a complex interplay among the cardiac conduction system, cardiovascular reflexes, autonomic nervous system, and humoral factors. Although most often associated with ventricular pacing, the pacemaker syndrome is not limited to this mode of pacing and may occur in any mode of pacing that results in permanent or temporary dyssynchrony of atrial and ventricular contraction.

In 1969, Mitsui and colleagues[95] first described a patient who was intolerant of ventricular pacing as manifested by complaints of chest pain, dizziness, shortness of breath, cold sweats, and facial flushing and referred to the condition as "pacemaking syndrome." The authors initially attributed these symptoms to a suboptimal cardiac output due to pacing rate rather than the mode of pacing. Subsequently, it was appreciated that symptoms were caused by the disruption of normal atrial and ventricular synchrony.[96–99] The exact incidence of pacemaker syndrome is unknown, but the most severe manifestations are estimated to occur in about 5% to 7% of ventricularly paced patients, whereas milder symptoms or substantial asymptomatic decreases in blood pressure and cardiac output may occur in more than 20%.[99] The incidence of more subtle forms of pacemaker syndrome may be even higher as defined by randomized crossover studies that compare the effects of single- and dual-chamber pacing modes on subjective and objective parameters.

In a study of 40 unselected patients with DDD pacemakers, Heldman and coauthors[100] reported that 83% of patients experienced new or worsened symptoms when programmed to VVI mode and that 42% were unable to tolerate ventricular pacing for the 1-week study period. In a randomized crossover study, Sulke and colleagues[101] compared the effects of DDDR, VVIR, DDD, and DDIR pacing modes on subjective criteria, including symptoms, functional class, health perception, and objective criteria, including exercise, treadmill time, and echocardiographic assessment. In patients with a preference, VVIR mode was the least acceptable pacing mode (73%), whereas DDDR was the most preferred (59%) mode of pacing (Fig. 14–11). In another investigation, the same authors[102] described a group of patients with VVI pacers who underwent atrial lead insertion and upgrade to a dual-chamber pacing system at the time of pulse generator replacement. Despite the fact that these patients had felt "generally well" for at least 3 years before upgrade, 75% of patients preferred the DDD mode, and their perceived general well-being, symptoms, scores, and exercise treadmill time were significantly better with dual-chamber pacing. The investigators suggested that "subclinical" pacemaker syndrome may be present in most patients with long-term VVI pacing, who do not complain of overt symptoms of pacemaker syndrome but will potentially derive symptomatic benefit from upgrading to a DDD pacing system.[102]

The diagnosis of pacemaker syndrome requires a high degree of suspicion and a willingness to evaluate all patient complaints thoroughly. Because the signs and symptoms may be identical to pacemaker malfunction, normal function of the pacemaker system must be verified. The diagnosis of pacemaker syndrome is best made by correlating the patient's symptoms with the cardiac rhythm. Various tech-

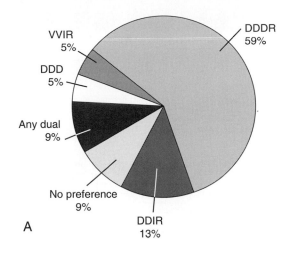

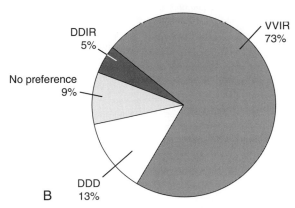

Figure 14–11. Preferred (A) and least acceptable (B) pacing modes based on symptom questionnaire. (From Sulke AN, Chambers J, Dritsas A, Sowton E: A randomized double-blind crossover comparison of four rate-responsive pacing modes. J Am Coll Cardiol 17:696, 1991. Reprinted with permission of the American College of Cardiology.)

niques may be used to document the cardiac rhythm during the patient's symptoms, including ambulatory electrocardiographic monitoring (Holter), transtelephonic monitoring, and patient-activated continuous-loop event recorders (Fig. 14–12). These techniques may demonstrate ventricular pacing with AV dissociation or the presence of retrograde VA conduction, echo beats or intermittent loss of AV synchrony due to "normal" (e.g., mode switching, rate smoothing) or abnormal pacemaker behavior (intermittent loss of atrial capture or sensing, nonphysiologic AV delay interval). In patients who are ventricularly paced most of the time, the presence of VA conduction increases the likelihood that pacemaker syndrome may be responsible for the patient's symptoms. Documentation of relief of the patient's symptoms with resumption of sinus rhythm or AV synchrony also strongly suggests a diagnosis of pacemaker syndrome.

On physical examination, the determination of arterial blood pressure during ventricular pacing in the supine and upright positions, compared with the blood pressure during sinus rhythm, may be helpful in making the diagnosis of pacemaker syndrome. A significant drop in systolic arterial pressure (usually greater than or equal to 20 mm Hg) implies that pacemaker syndrome is present. However, the absence

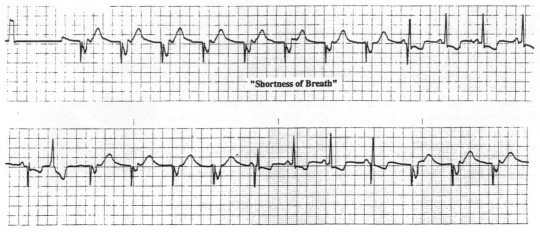

"Shortness of Breath"

Figure 14–12. Continuous rhythm strips recorded with a transtelephonic cardiac monitor in a 65-year-old farmer with pacemaker syndrome. This patient's underlying rhythm disorder was sick sinus syndrome with sinus bradycardia and multiple episodes of atrial fibrillation 1 year earlier. His sinus bradycardia was exacerbated by treatment with quinidine, verapamil, and digoxin. After implantation of a VVIR device, the patient returned to his physician complaining of fatigue, weakness, dizziness, malaise, and shortness of breath 1 month later. After documentation of this rhythm by a cardiac event monitor, he underwent further testing. During VVI pacing, ventriculoatrial (VA) dissociation occurred. During VVI pacing at 90 bpm, the patient's blood pressure dropped to 90/68 mm Hg, and during AAI pacing, it was 160/90 mm Hg (at 90 bpm). During sinus rhythm at 58 to 64 bpm, the blood pressure measured 136/70 mm Hg. A DDDR pacemaker was implanted, and within 48 hours, the patient's symptoms were abolished. He has returned to his active, vigorous lifestyle and has had no subsequent episodes of atrial fibrillation for 1 year. (From Ellenbogen KA, Wood MA, Strambler B: Pacemaker syndrome: Clinical, hemodynamic, and neurohumeral features. *In* Barold SS, Mujica J (eds): New Perspectives in Cardiac Pacing 3. Mt Kisco, NY, Futura, 1992.)

of a significant drop in arterial pressure does not exclude the possibility that pacemaker syndrome exists because retrograde VA conduction may be variable or symptoms may be secondary to an elevation in pulmonary pressure and adverse reflexes stimulated by elevated pulmonary pressures. Blood pressure should be checked immediately after institution of a new pacing mode, 30 seconds later, and several minutes after the pacing mode change. In some patients, blood pressure decreases 10 to 20 seconds after ventricular pacing is initiated. Other physical findings that support the diagnosis of pacemaker syndrome include cannon A waves in the jugular venous pulse, and palpable liver pulsations due to atrial contraction against a closed AV valve. Overt signs of congestive heart failure, such as elevated jugular venous pressure, S_3 gallop, pulmonary rales, and peripheral edema, may be present in moderate to severe cases of pacemaker syndrome.

Although the diagnosis of pacemaker syndrome is usually made clinically, other diagnostic testing may be necessary in patients with complicated symptomatology or required by insurers to justify pacemaker upgrade. Ocular pneumoplethysmography, Doppler echocardiography, and other noninvasive imaging techniques may be useful in documenting hemodynamic changes that occur during transition from sinus rhythm to ventricular pacing or pacing mode changes. Most of these studies consistently show that patients with the greatest decrease in stroke volume during ventricular pacing compared with AV sequential pacing or sinus rhythm are most likely to develop the symptoms of pacemaker syndrome.[72, 84, 101] In some cases, measurement of forearm vascular resistance with venous occlusion plethysmography may be performed to show a patient's failure to maintain forearm vascular resistance during ventricular pacing.[94]

Pathophysiology

Although the reduction in cardiac output due to the loss of atrial systole is an important component, the pathophysiology of pacemaker syndrome results from a complex interaction of hemodynamic, neurohumoral, and vascular changes induced by the loss of AV synchrony. Patients without retrograde VA conduction intermittently derive hemodynamic benefit from fortuitously timed P waves and, therefore, are less likely to develop pacemaker syndrome than are patients with 1:1 retrograde VA conduction who are in a state of constant AV dys-synchrony. During ventricular pacing in patients with intact VA conduction, the atria contract against closed AV valves, resulting in retrograde blood flow to the pulmonary and systemic veins, cannon A waves, and a marked increase in right and left atrial pressure (Fig. 14–13). In patients with retrograde VA conduction, compared with those in whom it is absent, there is a greater decrease in cardiac output and blood pressure as well as a greater increase in right atrial, pulmonary, and pulmonary capillary wedge pressures during ventricular pacing. The elevations in atrial pressure may be further transmitted to the jugular, hepatic, and pulmonary veins. Symptoms such as headaches, fullness in the head or neck, pulsations in the neck or abdomen, cough, and jaw pain may occur as a result of these pressure changes. Studies by Reynolds[103] and Ellenbogen[104] and their colleagues have demonstrated that simultaneous pacing of the ventricle and the atrium with a VA interval of 100 to 150 msec (simulating retrograde VA conduction) produces greater decreases in blood pressure and cardiac output and greater increases in right and left ventricular filling pressures than ventricular pacing alone

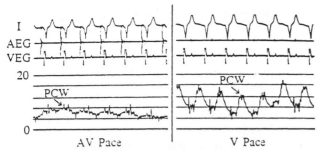

Figure 14–13. Surface electrocardiographic lead I, atrial electrogram (AEG), ventricular electrogram (VEG), and pulmonary capillary wedge pressure (PCW) recordings from a single patient during AV pacing (AV Pace) and ventricular pacing (V Pace) at 80 bpm with an AV interval of 150 msec. The cannon A wave is noted *(arrow)* on the PCW tracing. (From Reynolds DW: Hemodynamics of cardiac pacing. *In* Ellenbogen KA (ed): Clinical Cardiac Pacing. Cambridge, Blackwell Scientific, 1992, pp 120–161. Reprinted by permission of Blackwell Scientific Publications, Inc.)

when retrograde VA conduction is absent. Nishimura and associates[105] have reported that patients with intact VA conduction show a much greater decrease in systolic blood pressure with ventricular pacing (-24 ± 11 mm Hg) compared with those with VA dissociation (-4 ± 15 mm Hg; $P < .005$). Noninvasive imaging studies using Doppler echocardiography have demonstrated that patients with retrograde VA conduction experience the greatest decrease in stroke volume with ventricular pacing compared with AV synchrony and is predictive of the development of pacemaker syndrome.[72, 84, 101]

VA conduction occurs through the AV node and His-Purkinje system and cannot necessarily be predicted by the presence or absence of antegrade AV conduction. Retrograde VA conduction is present in about 15% of patients with complete antegrade AV block and in up to 67% of patients with intact antegrade AV conduction paced for sinus node disease.[106] In patients with intact AV conduction, VA intervals range from 100 to 400 msec and are dependent on the site of measurement of atrial and ventricular electrograms and autonomic tone.[107] Retrograde VA conduction is a dynamic phenomenon and may be absent during pacemaker implantation in the supine position but be present intermittently in the upright position or during exercise.[108] Facilitation of VA conduction may occur with catecholamines, increased heart rate, and appropriately timed ventricular contractions and after AV pacing due to facilitation of conduction in the AV node or His-Purkinje system. The presence of β-blockers, calcium-channel blockers, and type IA or IC or class III antiarrhythmic drugs may block VA conduction,[109] and subsequent withdrawal of these medications may allow retrograde VA conduction to appear.

In addition to the direct hemodynamic effects of loss of AV synchrony or 1:1 retrograde VA conduction, atrial and vascular reflexes initiated by atrial distention or elevated atrial pressures may also play a role in the pathophysiology of pacemaker syndrome. Atrial receptors and cardiopulmonary reflexes have been the subject of several in depth reviews.[110, 111] Briefly, the atria and pulmonary circulation are innervated by afferents from the vagus nerve. Myelinated

vagal afferents are present primarily at the venoatrial junction, and in animal models, their selective activation results in parasympathetic activation and diuresis.[111a] Nonmyelinated vagal afferents are also present throughout the cardiopulmonary circulation, posteriorly over both atria, pulmonary veins, and venoatrial junctions. In response to atrial distention, withdrawal of sympathetic tone occurs, resulting in a vasodepressor response and significant decrease in mean arterial blood pressure. The atrial and vascular responses to ventricular pacing have important hemodynamic consequences.

Erlebacher and associates[97] studied patients with and without retrograde VA conduction or cannon A waves and demonstrated that a significantly higher rise in total peripheral vascular resistance occurred during ventricular pacing in subjects without retrograde conduction compared with those with cannon A waves and retrograde VA conduction (22.8% versus 4.9%; $P < .002$). An increase in total peripheral vascular resistance maintains adequate systemic blood pressure and prevents symptoms attributable to cerebral hypoperfusion, such as lightheadedness, syncope, and near syncope. The protective vasoconstrictor reflex to ventricular pacing may be modified by inhibitory atrial reflexes, which are stimulated during increases in atrial pressure or stretch, as seen in patients with retrograde 1:1 VA conduction and cannon A waves. Data reported by Alicandri and colleagues[112] from the Cleveland Clinic support the importance of atrial reflexes in the pathogenesis of pacemaker syndrome. These investigators measured arterial pressure, cardiac output, right atrial pressure, and total peripheral resistance in three patients with hypotension and near syncope and compared these values to those in control patients without clinical manifestations of pacemaker syndrome. Both groups of patients developed similar decreases in cardiac output with ventricular pacing compared with sinus rhythm. However, the control patients increased their peripheral resistance by about 20%, compared with a failure of peripheral vascular resistance to increase in patients with pacemaker syndrome (Fig. 14–14).

Ellenbogen and colleagues[104] at the Medical College of Virginia measured forearm blood flow and vascular resistance, mean and phasic arterial pressure, cardiac output, and plasma nerve epinephrine, epinephrine, and dopamine during atrial, ventricular, and VA pacing with a VA interval of 100 to 150 msec. Forearm blood flow was measured by venous occlusion plethysmography, which provides an accurate measurement of changes in regional blood flow and reflects changes in regional vasomotor tone. Compared with atrial and ventricular pacing, there was a striking increase in vascular resistance and plasma norepinephrine levels during VA pacing, which occurred within 30 seconds. These changes were blocked by intra-arterial infusion of phentolamine, an α-sympathetic antagonist. The changes in forearm vascular resistance with VA pacing correlated significantly to systolic arterial blood pressure but not to changes in mean arterial pressure, pulse pressure, cardiac output, right atrial pressure, pulmonary artery pressure, or pulmonary capillary wedge pressure. These results suggest that changes in forearm vascular resistance in response to VA pacing are mediated by α-adrenergic receptors through arterial baroreflexes.

The same group of investigators[94] provided further evidence of these reflex changes using peroneal microneurogra-

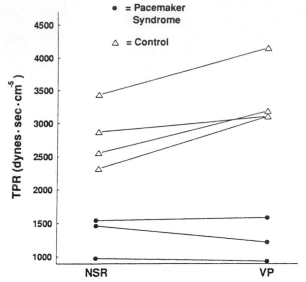

Figure 14–14. Changes in total peripheral vascular resistance (TPR) in dynes/sec/cm^{-5} during normal sinus rhythm (NSR) and ventricular pacing (VP) in four control patients and three patients with pacemaker syndrome. (Data from Alicandri C, Fouad FM, Tarazi RC, et al: Three cases of hypotension and syncope with ventricular pacing: Possible role of atrial reflexes. Am J Cardiol 42:137, 1978.)

phy, which allows measurement of local postganglionic muscle sympathetic nerve activity in the leg. A greater increase in local sympathetic nerve activity during ventricular pacing occurred compared with atrial pacing. The authors suggested that sympathetic nervous stimulation activation is a normal physiologic response in ventricular pacing, and inadequate sympathetic response may play a role in the genesis of pacemaker syndrome. When patients assume an upright position, blood is pooled in the lower extremities, and the arterial baroreceptors are activated to compensate for the decrease in cardiac output and systolic blood pressure. In some patients, pacemaker syndrome results from an inability to compensate further for the upright posture and augmentation of autonomic tone. In other patients, pacemaker syndrome may result from modification of these vascular responses by the effects of drugs, such as vasodilators and diuretics; underlying cardiac disease; volume status; and autonomic defects. In still other patients, pacemaker syndrome may result from the activation of inhibitory atrial and cardiopulmonary reflexes that counteract the protective vasoconstrictor reflex (Fig. 14–15). These responses may be further modified by the production of catecholamines and atrial natriuretic peptide (ANP).

Several studies have documented the humoral changes that take place during various modes of pacing.[113–115] These studies consistently show that plasma norepinephrine and epinephrine levels increase markedly in patients during shifts from sinus rhythm to ventricular pacing and that VVI pacing causes a greater increase in cardiac sympathetic nervous system activity than does AV synchronous pacing. Pehrsson and associates[115] found that coronary sinus norepinephrine was higher during VVI pacing at rest and exercise than during VAT or AV synchronous pacing. Other investigators have demonstrated that although only slight increases in plasma epinephrine levels occur during ventricular pacing without retrograde VA conduction, greater increases occur during ventricular pacing in the presence of retrograde VA conduction.[113]

It has been suggested that ANP, a regulatory hormone with the primary function of maintaining optimal circulating volume and arterial pressure, may play a role in pacemaker syndrome.[116–126] ANP is a 28–amino acid polypeptide produced primarily by granules located in the cardiac atria. ANP exerts a potent natriuretic effect, promoting excretion of water and sodium. It inhibits other volume-regulating hormones, such as the renin-angiotensin-aldosterone system and vasopressin. ANP is also a direct arterial and venous vasodilator, reducing both preload and arterial pressures. In animal models, it also results in vagally mediated inhibition in regional sympathetic nervous system activation.[116] The major stimuli for release of ANP is an increase in atrial pressure and stroke volume that occurs during tachycardia or volume overload. ANP levels correlate more closely with elevations in left atrial pressure than right atrial pressure. ANP is elevated in the presence of congestive heart failure, and its levels correlate with the severity of heart failure. ANP levels have been shown to be elevated in patients with complete heart block and bradycardia and reduced by AV sequential pacing but not by ventricular pacing alone.[117–120, 122, 123] Within minutes of acute reprogramming of permanent pacemakers from VVI to AV sequential pacing mode, decreases in ANP levels have been reported. The half-life is reported to be about 3 minutes, and levels steadily decrease for up to 20 minutes after change in pacing mode for VVI to DVI pacing.[123] Pacing rate and AV delay interval also influence ANP levels by altering atrial pressure and tension. Very short AV delay intervals result in high ANP levels, probably secondary to incomplete atrial filling. Elevation of ANP at long AV delays may be secondary to AV valvular regurgitation. The relative differences in ANP levels between DDD and VVI pacing decreases at faster pacing rates, suggesting that atrial contribution to cardiac output at higher rates may have less effect on cardiac hemodynamics than at lower rates.[120] Unlike cortisol and other hormones, ANP does not exhibit a circadian pattern of variation. In patients paced for 60 days in each mode, ANP levels were higher during VVI pacing than during DDD pacing throughout the 24-hour period. However, in patients paced in each mode for only 24 hours, the differences in ANP levels were only significant at certain times of the day.[126]

Strangl and colleagues[118] demonstrated that ANP levels rose by 3- to 3.5-fold during exercise in both VVI and DDD pacing modes but that ANP levels were 100% higher at rest and 70% higher during exercise with VVI compared with DDD pacing modes. ANP levels have been shown to be higher with rate-adaptive ventricular pacing as compared with DDD pacing at rest, during, and after exercise.[124] These studies confirm that AV synchrony leads to less atrial distention, producing lower atrial pressures and less ANP release both during exercise and at rest. A report on a small group of patients with pacemaker syndrome showed markedly elevated plasma concentrations of ANP during shifts from sinus rhythm to ventricular pacing compared with during shifts from sinus rhythm to DDD pacing.[121] The exact role of elevated ANP in the pacemaker syndrome is not clear, and it remains to be determined whether it is a causative factor

Figure 14–15. Diagrammatic representation of multiple reflex pathways involved in pacemaker syndrome. See text for discussion. The arterial baroreflexes detect a decrease in stroke volume when atrioventricular (AV) dys-synchrony occurs, leading to sympathetic activation and vasoconstriction. Conversely, AV dys-synchrony leads to increased atrial wall-tension and activation of reflex pathways leading to vagally mediated vasodilation as well as release of humoral substances, such as atrial natriuretic peptide (ANP), which further facilitate these reflexes (e.g., counteracting baroreflex-mediated vasoconstriction). LAP, left atrial pressure; PAP, pulmonary artery pressure; CO, cardiac output; SV, stroke volume; BP, blood pressure; EPI, epinephrine.

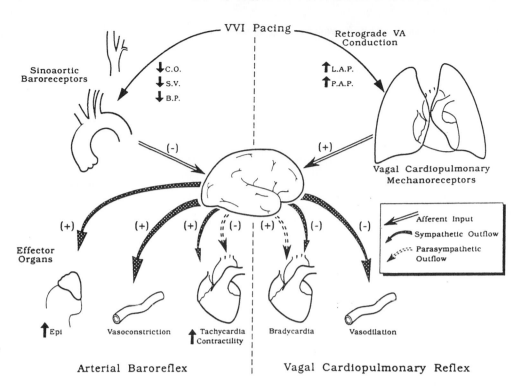

or a secondary result. It has been theorized that it may exert a protective effect by reducing atrial pressures and, therefore, the tendency for unfavorable atrial circulatory reflexes. Conversely, it may contribute to its severity by causing peripheral vasodilation in the setting of an already reduced cardiac output and hypotension. The role of ANP may differ depending on the underlying cardiac disease, the presence of cardiovascular drugs, baseline hemodynamics, the changes induced by pacing, and other undetermined factors.

Newer Forms of Pacemaker Syndrome

When pacemaker syndrome was first described, it was attributed to ventricular pacing and recognized primarily as a problem of single-chamber ventricular pacemakers. However, with the development of rate-responsive pacing and newer dual-chamber pacing modes, it has become apparent that pacemaker syndrome is not unique to ventricular pacing and should be more accurately termed *AV dys-synchrony syndrome*[127-134] (Table 14–5).

Pacemaker syndrome during AAI or AAIR pacing has been described and emphasizes the role of AV dys-synchrony in the pathogenesis of the syndrome. Patients originally paced for sick sinus syndrome may later develop AV conduction abnormalities, or AV nodal conduction may be impaired by drugs with AV nodal blocking properties (digoxin, β-blockers, calcium-channel blockers, antiarrhythmic drugs), leading to prolonged and hemodynamically unfavorable atrial–R wave (AR) intervals. AV dys-synchrony may also occur in patients with dual AV nodal pathway physiology during a shift in conduction from the fast pathway to the slow pathway with prolonged AV conduction time. Unfavorable sequencing of atrial and ventricular contraction may occur during AAIR pacing at high sensor-driven rates.[130] This most often results when the slope determining the

sensor-driven rate is programmed too aggressively and out of proportion to the exercise-induced increase in catecholamine levels. As the paced atrial rate progressively increases, the appropriate corresponding decrement in PR interval does not occur and may even lengthen, eventually resulting in a paced P wave occurring immediately after the preceding R wave (Fig. 14–16). This most frequently occurs in the earlier stages of exercise and, in some patients, corrects as the patient continues to exercise.

The VDD pacing mode functions like the DDD mode but without the capability of atrial pacing. The VDD mode, previously out of favor, has been revived by the development of single-pass leads specifically designed for VDD pacing. In the absence of sensed atrial activity, the VDD mode effectively becomes a VVI pacemaker at the lower rate. Pacemaker syndrome has been reported in a patient with VDD pacemaker when the sinus rate dropped below the lower rate limit and VVI pacing ensued.[127] Patients should be appropriately selected for this mode of pacing; carefully excluding chronotropic incompetence before implantation of this type of system is crucial. The increased popularity of VDD pacing requires heightened awareness of the possibility of pacemaker syndrome in patients who may be VVI paced at the lower rate limit a significant percentage of the time or who may subsequently require medications with negative chronotropic effects.

The DDI and DDIR pacing modes are used most often in patients with paroxysmal supraventricular or atrial tachycardia. Pacing and sensing ability is present in both chambers, but sensed atrial activity will only inhibit atrial output—it will not affect the timing of ventricular output. At the lower rate limit, AV sequential pacing occurs, but there is no tracking of P waves unless the atrial rate is identical to the programmed lower rate limit. When the atrial rate is above the lower rate limit, variable sensed P wave–paced ventricu-

Table 14–5. **Pacemaker Syndrome With Other Pacing Modes**

AAIR

Long AR intervals due to slow AV node conduction or dual AV nodal pathways

Inappropriately "aggressive" programming of rate response slope, leading to increased atrial rate before effect of catecholamines on AR interval is seen

Solution: Stop drugs with negative dromotropic effects; reprogram rate response slope; upgrade by implanting ventricular lead

VDDR

Pacemaker syndrome occurs only when atrial rate falls below lower rate

Solution: Stop drugs with negative chronotropic effects; program lower rate to a slower heart rate; begin trial of low-dose theophylline to increase atrial rate; implant atrial lead and upgrade to DDD(R) pacing

DDIR

Pacemaker syndrome occurs whenever spontaneous atrial rate exceeds lower rate or sensor-indicated rate

Solution: Program to DDDR and have separate upper rates for atrial tracking and sensor; begin antiarrhythmic drugs to suppress atrial arrhythmias, then reprogram to DDD or DDDR mode

Fallback and Rate-Smoothing in DDD or DDDR Mode, Conditional Ventricular Tracking Limit (CVTL) in DDDR Mode

Pacemaker syndrome occurs during paroxysmal tachycardias and abrupt heart rate changes or with divergence of information between sensor and sinus node

Solution: Program parameters so that fallback and rate-smoothing occurrences are limited and short in duration; use stress testing in patients to observe sensor response during rest and exercise; avoid CVTL behavior

Mode-Switching in DDDR

Pacemaker syndrome occurs with "inappropriate" mode switching

Solution: Use newer algorithms that allow greater programmability and avoid mode-switching for single PACs, sinus tachycardia, and PVCs with retrograde conduction; shorten PVARP; give antiarrhythmic drugs to suppress PACs, PVCs, and atrial tachyarrhythmias; reprogram to DDD mode if possible

DDD

Pacemaker-mediated or endless-loop tachycardia occurs; 2:1 AV block occurs during exercise

AV interval misprogramming is present

Repetitive nonreentrant ventriculoatrial synchrony

Solution: Reprogram pacemaker; use pacemaker algorithms to avoid endless-loop tachycardia (e.g., PVART extension after PVC), rate-responsive AV delay, and PVARP that allows tracking at higher rates. Intra-atrial conduction time may need to be measured and accounted for with AV interval programming

Miscellaneous

Reset from the DDD or DDDR mode to the VVI or VOO mode due to noise reversion or end-of-life generator behavior

---

PVARP, postventricular atrial refractory period; PVC, paroxysmal ventricular contractions; PAC, premature atrial contraction; AV, atrioventricular.

---

lar complex interval (PV) relationships occur, leading to dys-synchrony of the sensed atrium and paced ventricle (Fig. 14–17). In the DDIR pacing mode, the pacemaker increases its rate only in response to sensor input. If the atrial rate exceeds the sensor-driven ventricular pacing rate, atrial dissociation from ventricular paced events occurs.[132] With either DDI or DDIR pacing, AV dys-synchrony may result from ventricular pacing with retrograde VA conduction or antegrade P waves marching through the pacing cycles with variable PV relationships. In patients with DDI or DDIR pacemakers after AV nodal ablation for atrial fibrillation, DDI and DDIR pacing modes offer the advantage of

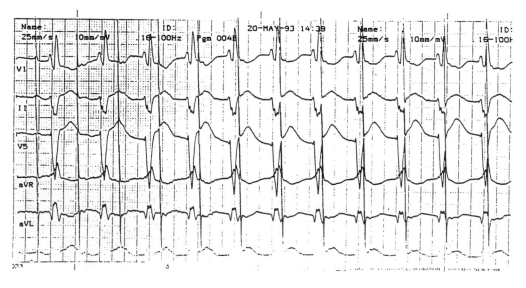

Figure 14–16. AAIR pacemaker recording in a patient receiving β-blockers who developed pacemaker syndrome while walking. His heart rate increased from 70 to 90 bpm, and his paced atrial–sensed QRS (AR) interval increased from 180 msec to more than 500 msec, resulting in shortness of breath. Discontinuing β-blockers and reprogramming the pacemaker to a less "aggressive" slope resulted in a much shorter prolongation of the AR interval with exercise.

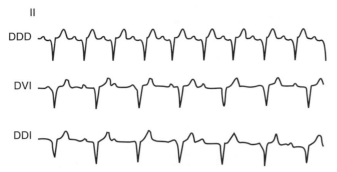

Figure 14–17. Demonstration of transient periods of AV dys-synchrony during DVI and DDI pacing in a patient whose atrial rate is above the programmed lower rate. AV dys-synchrony may be present for relatively long periods of time with this pacing mode. In the DVI pacing mode, there is no atrial sensing or tracking, whereas in the DDI mode, sensed P waves inhibit atrial pacing, but there is no tracking of P waves.

avoiding tracking of the atrial arrhythmias at the upper rate limit. When the patient is not in atrial fibrillation or flutter, however, relatively long periods of AV dissociation may result if the sinus rate exceeds the programmed lower or sensor-driven rate.

AV dys-synchrony and pacemaker syndrome may also occur during dual-chamber pacing as a result of inappropriate programming, prolonged atrial conduction time, or normal upper rate limit behavior.[128, 129, 134] In AV sequential pacing modes, selection of an inappropriate AV delay interval may result in an adverse AV sequencing and hemodynamics. Differential AV delay intervals for paced and sensed atrial events and rate-adaptive AV delay intervals may be useful in some patients in maintaining AV synchrony over a wide range of heart rates at rest and during exercise. The maximal ventricular tracking rate is determined by the total atrial refractory period (TARP), which is composed of the AV delay interval and postventricular atrial refractory period (PVARP). Long AV delay intervals are sometimes programmed to allow intrinsic conduction and conserve battery longevity, whereas long PVARPs are sometimes programmed to avoid pacemaker-mediated tachycardia. When the TARP is long, the maximal ventricular tracking rate is low. Patients may experience symptoms of pacemaker syndrome during exercise when their atrial rate exceeds the maximal ventricular tracking rate, resulting in 2:1 AV block and a sudden, marked decrease in cardiac output. This situation may be improved by reprogramming shorter AV delay or PVARP intervals to allow 1:1 ventricular tracking at higher atrial rates. Certain dual-chamber pacemakers have specific upper rate limit behavior designed to eliminate sudden changes in ventricular rate or prolonged periods of ventricular pacing at the upper rate limit, which may occur during pathologic atrial or supraventricular tachycardias (see Chapter 30 for details). These programmable features, which include rate fallback, rate smoothing, and the "conditional ventricular tracking limit," result in a period of AV dys-synchrony as the ventricular pacing rate is modified.

Some VDD, DDD, or DDDR pacemakers use an algorithm that allows mode switching from AV synchronous to VVIR pacing when successive atrial-sensed events fall within the PVARP but outside the 100-msec absolute atrial refractory period (Fig. 14–18). To avoid excessive mode switching, a minimum number of cycles without a P wave during the PVARP are required before the pacemaker switches back to AV synchronous pacing. The VVIR pacing mode is designed to be a temporary response to avoid dual-chamber pacing with ventricular tracking of rapid atrial rates during atrial fibrillation. Pacemaker syndrome has been described during inappropriate mode switching during sinus tachycardia, premature ectopic beats, far-field sensing of R or T waves in the atrial channel, and premature ventricular contractions (PVCs) with long retrograde VA conduction. Programming features that may predispose to inappropriate mode switching have been shown to be a low rate response factor, a low upper rate setting, a long base PVARP, and a long AV delay interval. In one study, some patients with pacemakers capable of automatic mode switching spent 50% of their time in VVIR pacing instead of DDDR pacing.[133]

Prevention and Treatment

Pacemaker syndrome is a preventable condition that can be avoided with selection of the correct type of pacemaker and appropriate programming of pacing parameters. In an important position paper on pacemaker and mode choice, the British Pacing Electrophysiology Group recommended that "the atrium be paced and sensed unless contraindicated."[135] The only indication for VVI and VVIR pacing modes is the presence of chronic atrial fibrillation or flutter and a slow ventricular response. Otherwise, dual-chamber or atrial pacing should be the mode of choice for permanent pacing in most patients. The pacemaker should be programmed carefully to avoid the development of AV dys-synchrony. With an increase in the complexity of pacemakers and pacing modes, there should be increased surveillance for detection of AV dys-synchrony and potential pacemaker syndrome during long-term clinical follow-up.

After the diagnosis of pacemaker syndrome is made, the treatment is straightforward (Table 14–6). Patients who are chronically ventricularly paced should be upgraded to dual-chamber AV synchronous pacing. Patients with VDD pacing systems and chronotropic incompetence may benefit from atrial lead implantation and upgrade to a DDD or DDDR pulse generator. In patients with AAI or AAIR pacing and long AR intervals, symptoms may be alleviated by implantation of a ventricular lead and upgrade to a dual-chamber pacemaker with physiologic AV delay intervals. Insurance companies may require documentation of pacemaker syndrome and hemodynamic benefit of dual-chamber pacing. This can be done by using Doppler measurements of cardiac output, occular plethysmography, pulmonary artery catheterization, or blood pressure measurement in supine upright position during ventricular pacing and sinus rhythm or dual-chamber pacing. Clearly, it is preferable to identify those patients at risk for developing pacemaker syndrome prospectively by carefully evaluating candidates for ventricular pacing before implantation.

In some patients with relatively mild pacemaker syndrome and sick sinus syndrome, other potential alternatives may be considered. First, the lower rate of a VVI pacemaker can be decreased to limit the amount of time spent on ventricular pacing. This can also be achieved by programming on rate hysteresis, which allows initiation of pacing

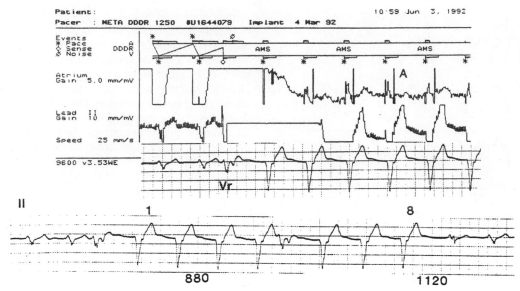

Figure 14–18. Automatic mode switching (AMS) and the retrograde sequence triggered by a ventricular extrasystole with the Meta DDDR device, programmed to the DDDR mode. There is bipolar atrial and ventricular sensing. The Telectronics 9600 programmer printout of the event recording demonstrates atrial pacing and the sensed ventricular extrasystole with retrograde conduction causing AMS, which continues because of retrograde atrial depolarization (A) following ventricular pacing. The symbol r denotes the sensing of noise or atrial electric activity within the PVARP; if this is appropriately timed, it will trigger AMS. There are three electrocardiographic (ECG) recordings, all of lead II. The top two are simultaneous recordings, one from the programmer and the other a high-quality surface recording. They demonstrate atrial and ventricular (fusion) pacing, the ventricular extrasystole (Vr), and ventricular pacing with retrograde P waves. The bottom nonsimultaneous ECG recording demonstrates the 8-beat sequence with the terminal 240 msec extension of the atrial escape or pacemaker VA interval. After the ventricular ectopic beat, AMS is triggered for 8 ventricular paced beats, provided that retrograde conduction occurs. Note that a sensed ventricular ectopic beat is included in the count because it too has retrograde conduction. After the eighth beat, the pacemaker VA interval is extended from 880 msec to 1120 msec, allowing atrial pacing (or atrial sensing) to occur and break the retrograde sequence. (From Mond H: Mode switching. *In* Barold SS, Mujica J (eds): New Perspectives in Cardiac Pacing 3. Mt Kisco, NY, Futura, 1992.)

only after a pause longer than the programmed lower rate limit (see Chapter 30). Another proposed strategy in these patients is to prescribe low-dose theophylline to increase sinus node automaticity, thereby leading to less ventricular pacing. Antiarrhythmic drugs have been used to block retro-

Table 14–6. Treatment of Pacemaker Syndrome

Avoid problem by ensuring appropriate selection of pacemaker and optimal programming.

Make diagnosis by maintaining a high level of suspicion.

Document symptoms of AV dys-synchrony by recording blood pressure measurements, transtelephonic event monitoring, Holter monitoring, Doppler measurement of stroke volume, or other objective testing.

Upgrade from VVIR to DDDR pacemaker by implanting atrial lead; ensure appropriate programming.

Decrease lower rate or program hysteresis to decrease frequency of VVI pacing if upgrade to DDD is not possible or is not selected.

Begin trial of antiarrhythmic drugs to eliminate retrograde conduction in selected cases.

Begin trial of theophylline to increase sinus rate and improve AV nodal conduction to decrease frequency and duration of ventricular pacing or AV dys-synchrony.

Schedule explantation if indications are unclear of if there are minimal symptoms from bradycardia.

grade VA conduction, which may lead to better tolerance of ventricular pacing. Both of these approaches are applicable only in patients with mild symptoms and in very elderly patients who may not wish to undergo another surgical intervention for pacemaker upgrade. These options may also be considered in patients in whom previous attempts at atrial lead placement or maintenance of atrial pacing and sensing have proved problematic. Finally, in rare patients with symptomatic pacemaker syndrome, the original indications for pacemaker implantation may be unclear or undocumented. It is conceivable that some of these patients might be best managed by pacemaker explantation.

In summary, pacemaker syndrome is an array of cardiovascular and neurologic signs and symptoms resulting from AV dys-synchrony due to a suboptimal mode of pacing, inappropriate programming of pacing parameters, or upper rate limit behavior of AV synchronous pacing systems. The pathogenesis of pacemaker syndrome is complex and involves atrial and vascular reflexes and the neurohumoral system as well as the direct hemodynamic consequences of loss of atrial systole. Patients most prone to the development of pacemaker syndrome are those with 1:1 retrograde VA conduction and those with low stroke volume during ventricular pacing compared with sinus rhythm or dual-chamber pacing. The syndrome is treatable by upgrading the patient to an appropriate pacing system or by reprogramming parameters to achieve optimal synchrony of atrial and ventricular contraction.

■ DIFFERENTIAL HEMODYNAMIC BENEFIT OF ATRIOVENTRICULAR SYNCHRONY

Although the hemodynamic superiority of dual-chamber pacing modes over VVI pacing has been demonstrated in a wide variety of clinical situations, it is clear that not all patients benefit equally from the maintenance of AV synchrony during cardiac pacing. Both invasive and noninvasive studies have attempted to identify factors predictive of the greatest relative benefit of AV synchrony during pacing (Table 14–7). Discrepancies in the results may be attributed partly to the small number of subjects in each study, heterogeneous populations of patients, and variable attempts to optimize the AV delay interval during pacing.

Benchimol and colleagues[56] compared invasive hemodynamic measurements during atrial and ventricular pacing in healthy subjects, patients with compensated nonvalvular heart disease, and patients with decompensated heart failure. In the healthy subjects, both atrial and ventricular pacing at increasing rates resulted in progressive and comparable increases in cardiac output and decreases in stroke volume. Thus, the contribution of atrial systole to cardiac output in the healthy subjects did not appear to be significant. However, in subjects with heart disease, incremental atrial pacing rates resulted in a progressive increase in cardiac output, whereas with ventricular pacing at increasing rates, there was a decrease in cardiac output and stroke volume. In patients with diseased hearts, the cardiac output and stroke volume were higher with atrial pacing than with ventricular pacing at the same heart rate.

Invasive studies directly measuring the atrial contribution to left ventricular filling and stroke volume support the concept that patients with the lowest baseline cardiac output and stroke volume derive the greatest benefit from maintenance of AV synchrony.[136–138] Braunwald and Frahm[136] studied a group of patients by means of trans-septal left heart catheterization and demonstrated that the duration of left

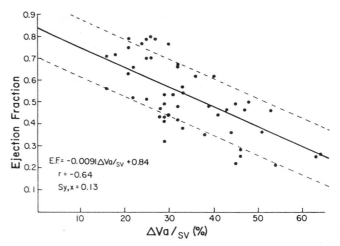

Figure 14–19. Relationship between left ventricular ejection fraction and atrial contribution to stroke volume (Va_{SV}) (%). Shown are the regression equation *(solid line)*, correlation coefficient (r), and one standard error of estimate (Sy,x, *dashed lines*). the percentage of atrial contribution to stroke volume and resting left ventricular ejection fraction are inversely correlated. (From Hamby RI, Noble WJ, Murphy DH, Hoffman I: Atrial transport function in coronary artery disease: Relation to left ventricular function. J Am Coll Cardiol 1:1011, 1983. Reprinted with permission of the American College of Cardiology.)

atrial contraction is longer and the magnitude of atrial kick is greater in patients with left ventricular hypertrophy than in healthy subjects. Matsuda and colleagues[137] evaluated left atrial function in healthy subjects and in patients with remote myocardial infarction and found that the ratio of active atrial emptying to left ventricular stroke volume and the amount of left atrial work were higher in patients with previous myocardial infarction than in the healthy subjects. Using simultaneous hemodynamic and angiographic volume studies, Hamby and coworkers[138] demonstrated a higher atrial contribution to stroke volume in patients with coronary artery disease than in healthy subjects (33% versus 20%; $P < .05$). They demonstrated significant negative correlations between the atrial contribution to stroke volume and baseline stroke volume and LVEF, and positive correlations with left ventricular end-diastolic pressure and left ventricular end-systolic volume (Fig. 14–19). The combination of congestive heart failure and cardiomegaly was the only clinical feature associated with a significantly higher atrial contribution to stroke volume in the subgroup of patients with coronary artery disease.

Greenberg and colleagues[61] performed ventricular and AV sequential pacing in a group of patients with diverse types of heart disease and demonstrated an inverse relationship between left ventricular filling pressure and the atrial contribution to cardiac output. In this study, the atrial contribution was less effective in augmenting cardiac output when the pulmonary capillary wedge pressure exceeded 20 mm Hg or the patient clinically manifested heart failure. The apparent conflict between the results of Greenberg and associates and the data indicating that the greatest relative benefit of atrial systole occurs in patients with diseased hearts may be partially explained by examining the left ventricular pressure–volume relationship (Fig. 14–20). Regardless of left ventric-

Table 14–7. Factors Associated With Increased Hemodynamic Benefit of Atrial Systole During Cardiac Pacing

Presence of clinical congestive heart failure[55]*
Absence of clinical congestive heart failure[61]*
Low baseline cardiac output and stroke volume[56,136–138]
Pulmonary capillary wedge pressure <20 mm Hg[61]
Cardiac index <2 L/m and normal LV volume[62]
Normal LV end-diastolic and systolic dimensions[81,86]
Retrograde VA conduction[72,84]
Normal LA size[73,86]
History of pacemaker syndrome[72]
Low stroke volume during VVI pacing[84]
Large increase in arterial pulse pressure from atrial systole[63]
Increased left ventricular wall thickness[86]
Presence of aortic valve disease[77]
High peak atrial to early rapid filling velocity[92]

LA, left ventricular; VA, ventriculoatrial.

*In independent investigations, both the presence and absence of clinical congestive heart failure have been reported to result in a relatively greater benefit of AV synchrony than ventricular pacing alone.

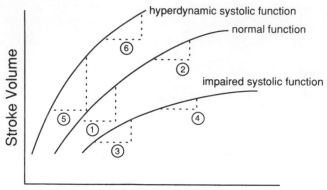

Figure 14–20. Left ventricular function curve indicating the relationship between left ventricular end-diastolic volume and stroke volume. In subjects with normal left ventricular systolic function on the ascending limb of the curve, increases in volume result in a substantial increase in stroke volume (1). If left ventricular filling pressures are higher (2), further increases in volume result in smaller increments in stroke volume. In subjects with impaired left ventricular systolic function on the ascending limb of the function curve (3), increases in end-diastolic volume result in an increase in stroke volume. Although the absolute increase in stroke volume may be less than that in the subject with normal systolic function (1), the relative increase in stroke volume may be greater in the subject with impaired systolic function. As left ventricular filling pressures increase in patients with impaired left ventricular systolic function, further increases in volume result in little further augmentation of the stroke volume. Cardiac output in patients with hyperdynamic systolic function is often critically dependent on preload. Similar increases (5 and 6) result in larger increments in stroke volume than are seen in subjects with normal function (1 and 2). (Adapted from Greenberg B, Chatterjee K, Parmley WW, et al: The influence of left ventricular filling pressure on atrial constriction to cardiac output. Am Heart J 98:742, 1979.)

ular function, patients functioning on the ascending limb of the Frank-Starling curve benefit from atrial contribution to the left ventricular volume and pressure, whereas those with high filling pressure derive little benefit because they already function on the plateau phase of the curve. Patients with systolic ventricular dysfunction may operate on a flatter curve, so that the absolute increase in stroke volume when filling pressures are optimized may be quantitatively less than in patients with normal hearts. However, this increase may represent a greater percentage increment and, therefore, result in a greater hemodynamic and clinical benefit than in individuals with normal ventricular function. Patients with diastolic dysfunction operate on a steeper function curve and may be especially dependent on volume to optimize cardiac performance. Patients with normal left ventricular function may be able to compensate for loss of atrial systole through increased ventricular contractility and stroke volume, whereas compensatory mechanisms are less effective in patients with impaired left ventricular function.

The validity of this postulation is supported by the finding of Rahimtoola and colleagues[62] that after myocardial infarction, the atrial contribution to stroke volume was significantly greater in patients with cardiac indices less than 2 L/min/m^2 compared with those with cardiac indices greater than 2 L/min/m^2 (56% versus 31%) and in those with normal left ventricular volumes compared with those with elevated left ventricular volumes (19% versus 10%). In other words, those deriving the greatest relative benefit were functioning on the ascending limb of a left ventricular function curve for a diseased heart. Using Doppler and M-mode echocardiographic assessment of hemodynamic responses to temporary pacing, Faerestrand and colleagues[80] demonstrated that the relative hemodynamic benefit of dual-chamber pacing over ventricular pacing diminishes as left ventricular end-diastolic and end-systolic dimension increases, placing function on the plateau phase of the left ventricular function curve. In patients with New York Heart Association (NYHA) functional class IIIB to IV failure, the increase in cardiac output with AV sequential temporary pacing compared with ventricular pacing correlated strongly with the increase in arterial pulse pressure observed when a dissociated atrial contraction preceded a ventricular paced beat by a physiologic AV interval during ventricular pacing.[63]

Noninvasive Doppler echocardiographic techniques have also been useful in identifying subgroups of patients who derive a relatively greater hemodynamic benefit from maintenance of AV synchrony during cardiac pacing. In patients with permanent dual-chamber pacemakers, Stewart and colleagues[72] reported a 19% increase in Doppler-derived cardiac output with reprogramming from VVI to DVI pacing mode for the overall group (Fig. 14–21). Patients with retrograde VA conduction or a history of the pacemaker syndrome derived the greatest increment in cardiac output (30.4% versus 14.4%; $P < .01$). This is consistent with the fact that patients without intact VA conduction receive intermittent benefit from fortuitously timed atrial contractions, whereas those with one-to-one VA conduction are in a constant state of AV dys-synchrony and have the highest susceptibility to adverse circulatory reflexes initiated by atrial receptors.

Labovitz and colleagues[73] reported a significantly greater decrement in Doppler cardiac output when AV sequential pacing was switched to ventricular pacing alone in patients with normal-sized left atria compared with those with enlarged left atria (32% versus 11%; $P < .01$). A negative correlation between left atrial dimension determined from M-mode echocardiograms and the percentage decrement in stroke volume with ventricular pacing was reported. The authors suggested that enlarged and abnormally compliant atria may be less capable of generating vigorous contraction and, therefore, less effective booster pumps than normal atria.[73] Other investigators have confirmed that patients with VA conduction and those with normal-sized left atria derive greater relative hemodynamic benefits from AV synchrony than patients lacking these factors.[84, 86] Additional factors that have been demonstrated by Doppler echocardiography to predict a relatively greater hemodynamic benefit of AV synchrony over VVI pacing include stroke volume less than 50 mL during VVI pacing independent of the presence of VA conduction,[84] normal end-systolic dimension,[86] increased left ventricular wall thickness and the presence of aortic valve disease,[77] and high peak atrial–to–rapid early filling velocity ratio on transmitral flow.[90] In noninvasive studies, there has been little correlation between measures of left ventricular systolic function and degree of benefit from AV synchrony. However, as is apparent from invasive studies, filling pressure plays an extremely important role in determining the relative benefit of atrial systole and cannot be measured reliably by noninvasive techniques.

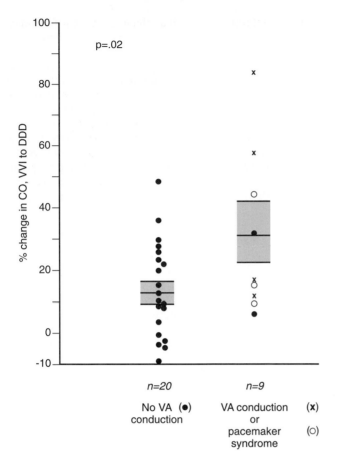

p=.02

% change in CO, VVI to DDD

n=20

No VA (●)
conduction

n=9

VA conduction (**x**)
or
pacemaker (○)
syndrome

Figure 14–21. Percentage change in cardiac output (CO) with DDD pacing according to the presence (x) or absence (●) of ventriculoatrial (VA) conduction or the presence of pacemaker syndrome (○). VA conduction is assessed at the time of pacemaker implant. (From Stewart WJ, Dicola VC, Hawthorne JW, et al: Doppler ultrasound measurement of cardiac output in patients with physiologic pacemakers. Am J Cardiol 54:308, 1984.)

In summary, it appears that the patients deriving the greatest benefit from maintenance of AV synchrony during cardiac pacing are those with poor hemodynamics with or without VA conduction during ventricular pacing alone, normal left atrial size, thick or noncompliant left ventricles that may be more dependent on atrial systole, and normal volume and filling pressure, thus placing their function on the ascending limb of the Frank-Starling left ventricular function curve. The relative importance of maintaining AV synchrony may be greatest in those with poor left ventricular function in whom compensatory hemodynamic mechanisms are impaired and in whom even a small increase in cardiac output may result in significant clinical improvement.

■ TIMING OF ATRIAL AND VENTRICULAR CONTRACTION DURING CARDIAC PACING

The mere presence of atrial systole is not sufficient to optimize cardiac performance. It is well established that the relative timing of atrial and ventricular contraction is crucial in maximizing hemodynamics during dual-chamber pacing. The appropriate timing of atrial contraction is necessary

to optimize left ventricular filling, minimize AV valvular regurgitation, maintain low mean atrial pressure, and prevent unfavorable circulatory and neurohumoral reflexes. An improperly timed atrial contraction may result in no hemodynamic benefit compared with ventricular pacing alone. In fact, a poorly timed atrial contraction may activate atrial reflexes, producing deleterious hemodynamic effects accompanied by symptoms of the pacemaker syndrome. Studies have demonstrated about a 25% increment in resting stroke volume, comparing the most advantageous to least advantageous AV delay interval during dual-chamber pacing.[84, 86]

Influence of Atrioventricular Delay Interval on Mitral Valve Closure and Left Ventricular Filling

Electrical and mechanical atrial activity plays an important role in the events of a normal cardiac cycle (Fig. 14–22). Atrial contraction followed by relaxation produces a negative

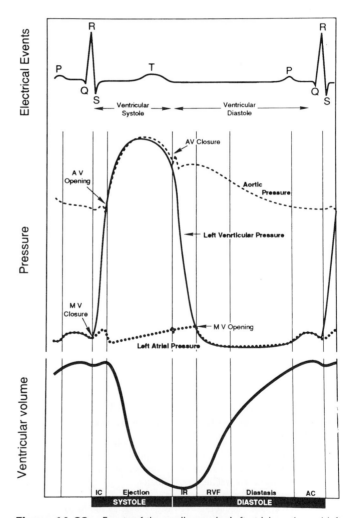

Figure 14–22. Events of the cardiac cycle. Left atrial, aortic, and left ventricular pressures are correlated with electric events and left ventricular volume. AC, atrial contraction; AV, aortic valve; MV, mitral valve; IC, isovolumetric contraction; IR, isovolumetric relaxation; RVF, rapid ventricular filling from 80 to 250 msec (*bottom on top*). (See text for description.)

pressure gradient, causing a surge of blood into the ventricle at the end of diastole. Reversal of the AV pressure gradient initiates mitral valve closure because of a rapid decrease in pressure between the AV valve cusps pulling them into apposition. A brief period of isovolumetric contraction exists after mitral valve closure and before aortic valve opening, during which the maximum rate of pressure change (peak dP/dt) occurs. Rapid ejection occurs during ventricular systole and is terminated when ventricular pressure falls below aortic pressure, thus closing the aortic valve. A brief period of isovolumic relaxation follows, during which the maximum rate of pressure decline (peak negative dP/dt) occurs. As left ventricular pressure continues to decline and fall below left atrial pressure, the mitral valve opens, and diastolic ventricular filling begins. Normally, diastolic filling is characterized by an initial rapid increase in ventricular filling during early diastole followed by a slow phase of filling during mid-diastole. A second rapid increase in ventricular filling occurs in late diastole as a result of atrial contraction.

The presence of atrial systole and its timing relative to ventricular systole can influence mitral valve closure and dramatically influence diastolic ventricular filling pattern and total diastolic filling time (Table 14–8). An atrial contraction, which occurs before the pre-ejection period of the ventricle, maximizes left ventricular filling and thus cardiac output by means of the Starling mechanism. An optimally timed atrial contraction occurs during late ventricular diastole and initiates AV valve closure before the onset of ventricular contraction. If the AV delay interval is too long, atrial contraction and relaxation occur too early in relation to ventricular contraction. This may result in atrial contraction before venous return is completed and may thus diminish ventricular volume and contractile force. Importantly, it may also initiate early mitral valve closure, thereby limiting ventricular diastolic filling time. AV valvular regurgitation may also occur with long AV delay intervals because once closed, valve cusps may separate again before ventricular contraction. If the AV delay interval is too short, there may be insufficient time for atrial ejection to occur, thus decreasing left ventricular filling and elevating left atrial pressure. With short AV delay intervals, preclosure of the mitral valve does not occur, and ventricular systole begins with the AV valves wide open, which may result in mitral or tricuspid regurgitation.

Several studies using M-mode echocardiography and Doppler echocardiography have clearly demonstrated the effects of AV delay intervals on left ventricular filling and

mitral valve closure during dual-chamber pacing. Freedman and colleagues,[139] using M-mode and Doppler echocardiography, demonstrated that mitral valve closure was closely related to the P wave, indicating an atriogenic mechanism of mitral valve closure at AV delay intervals of 100 msec or greater. At AV delays shorter than 100 msec, completion of mitral valve closure occurred earlier in relationship to the P wave, suggesting a ventriculogenic mechanism of mitral valve closure. These investigators suggested that both atrial and ventricular contraction may influence mitral valve closure and that the relative contribution of atrial and ventricular contraction to valve closure is dependent on the programmed AV delay interval. VonBibra and associates[140] reached similar conclusions using M-mode echocardiograms of the mitral valve and simultaneous apexcardiograms to define ventricular systole.

With long AV delay intervals, late diastolic mitral regurgitation can result because of reopening of the mitral valve before ventricular contraction. Ishikawa and associates[141] recorded mitral valve flow at varying AV delay intervals and found that diastolic mitral regurgitation could be induced in most patients with DDD pacemakers. The mean AV delay interval at which diastolic mitral regurgitation occurred was 230 msec, and the range was 140 to 260 msec. In patients with no clinical congestive heart failure, diastolic mitral regurgitation was observed only at PR intervals exceeding 200 msec but was observed even at physiologic AV intervals in patients with congestive heart failure. There was a significant negative correlation between the pulmonary capillary wedge pressure and the critical AV delay interval for inducing diastolic mitral regurgitation. Although the clinical significance of diastolic mitral regurgitation during dual-chamber pacing has not been defined, its presence at physiologic AV delay intervals may indicate elevated left ventricular end-diastolic pressure and thus be of prognostic significance. It has also been suggested that elimination of diastolic mitral regurgitation is one potential mechanism by which dual-chamber pacing with short AV delay benefits patients with dilated cardiomyopathy (discussed later).

Because of its influence on mitral valve closure, the timing of atrial contraction can markedly alter diastolic filling time. A strong negative correlation has been demonstrated between the AV delay interval during AV sequential (DVI) and atrial synchronous (VDD) pacing and the time to mitral valve closure and total diastolic filling time.[140–142] To understand the effects of AV delay on diastolic filling, the total diastolic filling time can be divided into the time period from mitral valve opening to the ventricular pacing spike and the period from the ventricular pacing spike to the time of mitral valve closure (Fig. 14–23). VonBibra[140] and Pearson[142] and their coworkers, in independent investigations, demonstrated that as the AV delay interval is increased during dual-chamber pacing, mitral valve closure occurs progressively earlier in relationship to the ventricular pacing spike. However, the time from mitral valve opening to the ventricular pacing spike is not significantly influenced by changes in the AV delay interval. Thus, the total diastolic filling time progressively shortens with increasing AV delay. This was noted during AV sequential pacing as well as during atrial synchronous pacing and at physiologic (mean, 69 bpm) heart rates as well as at high rates (97 bpm).[142]

In addition to its effects on mitral valve closure and

Table 14–8. Influence of Atrioventricular Delay on Left Ventricular Filling

Appropriately timed atrial systole (optimal AV delay)
   Closure of AV valve before ventricular systole
   Minimizes AV valvular regurgitation
   Optimizes diastolic filling
Atrial systole inappropriately early (AV delay too long)
   Incomplete venous return before atrial contraction
   Early mitral valve closure
   AV valvular regurgitation caused by reopening of cusps
Atrial systole inappropriately late (AV delay too short)
   Atrial ejection limited
   AV valvular regurgitation

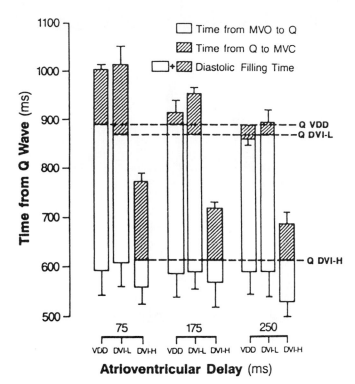

Figure 14–23. Effect of programmable AV delay interval on diastolic filling time. Time from the mitral valve opening (MVO) to the onset of the Q wave (Q) is represented by the white portion of the bars. The time from the Q wave to mitral valve closure (MVC) is represented by the hatched portion of the bar. The combined white and hatched segments represent the total diastolic filling time. These intervals are displayed at programmable AV delays of 75, 175, and 250 msec in the VDD, DVI low heart rate (DVI-L), and DVI high heart rate (DVI-H). Time on the ordinate represents time from the previous Q wave. *Horizontal dashed lines* indicate the time from the Q wave in the various modes. It is apparent that increasing the AV delay intervals results in abbreviated diastolic filling time regardless of mode and rate, primarily because of earlier mitral valve closure. (From Pearson AC, Janosik DL, Redd RM, et al: Doppler echocardiographic assessment of the effect of varying atrioventricular delay and pacemaker mode on left ventricular filling. Am Heart J 115:611, 1988.)

tion of early diastolic filling and that of atrial systole, including peak early and atrial velocities, the ratio of early to atrial velocity, the early and atrial flow velocity integral (area under the flow velocity curve), the ratio of early to atrial flow velocity integrals, and the amount of diastolic filling occurring in the first third of diastole (Fig. 14–24).

During ventricular pacing in the absence of atrial activity, mitral valve inflow recordings demonstrate only an early filling wave similar to that seen in patients with atrial fibrillation. During ventricular pacing in the presence of AV dissociation, the mitral valve inflow pattern varies from beat to beat, depending on the random timing of the dissociated P waves relative to paced ventricular contraction (Fig. 14–25A). During AV sequential pacing, mitral valve inflow recordings demonstrate early and atrial filling waves that vary in their relationship, depending on the rate of pacing and the AV delay interval (see Fig. 14–25B). If the AV delay interval increases, the atrial filling wave occurs progressively earlier and eventually becomes superimposed on the early rapid filling wave. Because the atrial filling wave receives a contribution from the early filling wave with long AV delay intervals, the peak atrial velocity and area under the A wave increase with increasing AV delay intervals.

We have demonstrated progressive decreases in early peak velocity integral and ratio of early to atrial flow velocity integrals with increasing AV delay intervals.[142] Rokey and colleagues[145] demonstrated an inverse relationship between the atrial filling wave and early diastolic filling wave with variance of AV delay interval. As the effectiveness of atrial contraction was increased by optimization of the AV delay interval, there was a significant decrease in early mitral valve inflow velocity and peak filling rate. The authors postulated that the changes in filling pattern were a reflection of changes in left atrial volume and pressure. At shorter AV delay intervals, there may be aborted emptying of the atria, resulting in larger residual volumes and higher pressure. During diastole, the left atrial volume and pressure continue to

left ventricular filling time, variance in AV delay has been demonstrated to change the left ventricular diastolic filling pattern markedly. The pattern of diastolic filling is a complex interaction between a multitude of passive and active properties of both the atria and the ventricles.[143–151] It is known to be influenced by heart rate, age, left ventricular relaxation and compliance, left ventricular and left atrial compliance and pressure, left ventricular radius to wall thickness, and, importantly, the temporal relationship between atrial and ventricular contraction. Pulsed Doppler echocardiography is a well-validated noninvasive method of recording beat-to-beat mitral valve inflow from which quantitative relationships between early and late atrial filling and indices of left ventricular diastolic compliance can be assessed.[146] The phases of diastolic filling include an initial rapid early filling phase, a slow filling phase during mid-diastole, and a second rapid filling phase in late diastole coincident with atrial contraction. Various measurements can be made from Doppler mitral valve inflow recordings to quantitate the contribu-

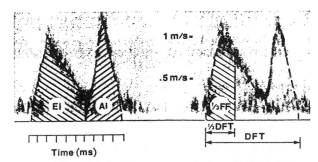

Figure 14–24. Pulsed Doppler recording of transmitral flow illustrating the technique used to measure various segments of the timed velocity integral and diastolic filling period. The relationship between early diastolic filling and that associated with atrial systole can be quantitated. Possible measurements include early and atrial velocities, the ratio of early to atrial velocity, the early (Ei) and atrial (Ai) flow velocity integral (area under the flow velocity curve), the ratio of early to atrial flow velocity integral, and the amount of diastolic filling occurring in the first one third of diastole (1/3 DFT). DFT, diastolic filling time. (From Pearson AC, Janosik DL, Redd RM, et al: Doppler echocardiographic assessment of the effect of varying atrioventricular delay and pacemaker mode on left ventricular filling. Am Heart J 115:611, 1988.)

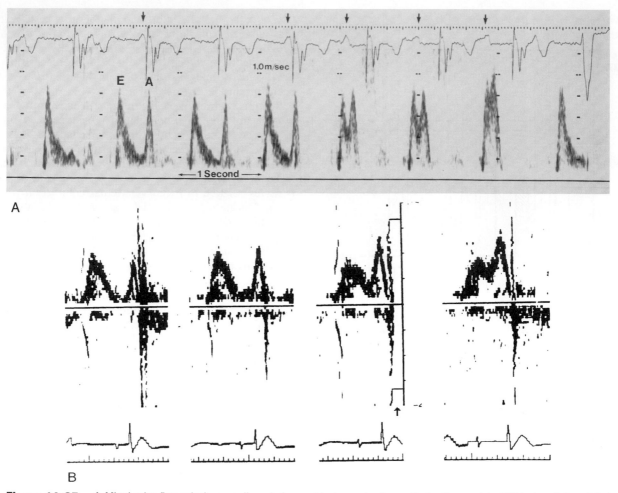

Figure 14–25. *A,* Mitral valve flow velocity recordings during ventricular pacing in a patient with complete AV block and dissociated atrial activity. Variation in the mitral flow pattern and duration of diastolic filling are evident, depending on the random occurrence of P waves. *B,* Mitral valve flow velocity pattern in a normal heart during AV sequential pacing. There is a marked variation in the temporal relationship between the A and the V waves and the magnitude of the A wave when the AV delay is modified. Note the abbreviation in total diastolic filling time and the increase in the magnitude of the A wave at longer AV delays (*right side* of panel) compared with the shortest AV delay (*left side* of panel). (*B,* From Lascault G, Bigonzi F, Frank R, et al: Noninvasive study of dual-chamber pacing by pulsed Doppler prediction of the haemodynamic response by echocardiographic measurements. Eur Heart J 10:525, 1989.)

increase, resulting in a higher AV gradient at the time of mitral valve opening and increased peak early inflow. At longer AV delay intervals, atrial emptying is completed, resulting in low left atrial pressure and, therefore, decreased peak early filling rate and increased atrial filling ratio.

This theory is supported by observations that early diastolic filling is increased in dilated cardiomyopathy, in which left atrial pressures are high and there is a relatively ineffective atrial contraction, whereas early diastolic filling is diminished in relation to atrial filling in conditions associated with reduced left ventricular compliance. Frienlingsdorf and colleagues[152] demonstrated normalization of left ventricular filling pattern and improvement in exercise capacity with manipulation of AV delay interval in a group of patients with normal LVEF but ventricular hypertrophy and diastolic dysfunction as evidenced by a reduced early-to-late peak velocity rate on mitral valve Doppler inflow tracing at a baseline AV delay interval of 200 msec. Shortening the AV delay interval to 100 msec resulted in normalization of the left ventricular filling pattern and improved exercise capac-

ity, anaerobic threshold, maximum minute ventilation, and maximum Vo_2 exercise testing.

In summary, the timing of atrial contraction relative to ventricular contraction influences mitral valve closure and has marked effects on total diastolic filling time and the pattern of diastolic filling. Excessively long AV delay intervals may cause early mitral valve closure, thus limiting diastolic filling time primarily through reduction in early diastolic filling. Excessively short AV delay intervals fail to close the mitral valve before left ventricular systole and may result in a diminished atrial contribution to left ventricular filling because of inadequate emptying. The pattern of left ventricular filling is influenced by the AV delay interval, with the relative contribution of the early filling compared with atrial filling phase decreasing with increasing AV delay interval. The clinical relevance of the AV delay interval to left ventricular filling would be expected to be most important in patients with baseline abnormalities in diastolic function and in those with increased dependence on atrial contribution to cardiac output.

Determination of Optimal Atrioventricular Delay Interval

Numerous investigations using invasive and noninvasive measurements of cardiac output have demonstrated that an optimal AV delay interval can be determined in most patients during dual-chamber pacing[67, 68, 71, 73–79, 81, 82, 84–89] (Fig. 14–26). Direct comparison of individual studies is difficult because most of the studies contain a relatively small number of patients with variable degrees of cardiac dysfunction and vary in the techniques used to measure cardiac output. In addition, most of the studies were conducted with patients at rest and in the supine position, thus limiting extrapolation of results to the clinical situation. Despite these limitations, the significance of AV delay intervals in optimizing resting hemodynamics is apparent. The AV delay interval that maximizes resting cardiac output during dual-chamber pacing varies widely among patients and in most studies is reported to be between 125 and 200 msec. The optimal AV delay interval determined by Doppler echocardiography correlates well with the optimal AV delay interval determined by radionuclide ventriculography.[153] The AV delay interval producing optimal hemodynamics at higher pacing rates is shorter than that which is optimal at lower rates.[154] Factors that may influence the optimal AV delay interval among patients include atrial capture and sensing latencies, interatrial conduction delay, ventricular capture latency, interventricular conduction delay, the presence or absence of myocardial disease, heart rate, and catecholamine levels[155–159] (Table 14–9). In addition to interpatient variability, important factors that may influence the optimal AV delay interval in the same patient include heart rate, paced versus sensed atrial event, catecholamine levels, drugs, and posture.[81, 85, 156, 158, 160]

It is extremely difficult to predict the optimal AV delay interval for a given patient. In some situations, AV delay intervals that are shorter than what is conventionally consid-

Table 14–9. Possible Factors Influencing Optimal Atrioventricular Delay Intervals

Interpatient Variables	Intrapatient Variables
Atrial capture latency	Heart rate
Atrial sensing latency	Paced or sensed atrial event
Intra-atrial conduction delay	Catecholamine levels
Ventricular capture latency	Drugs
Intraventricular conduction delay	
Underlying myocardial disease	
Heart rate	
Catecholamine levels	

ered physiologic may be advantageous. AV sequential pacing for complete heart block complicating an acute myocardial infarction[59] or following cardiac surgery[60] yields optimal hemodynamics at AV intervals of 100 msec or less. This may be secondary to elevated catecholamine levels and reduced left ventricular compliance in these acutely stressful situations. In patients with hypertrophic obstructive cardiomyopathy, shortening the AV delay interval so that a paced right ventricular contraction occurs has been demonstrated to decrease the intraventricular pressure gradient both acutely and chronically.[161, 162] It is believed that the altered sequence of ventricular contraction produced by right ventricular apical pacing alters septal motion, thus increasing left ventricular outflow tract diameter and reducing the obstruction and the subaortic pressure gradient.

Most studies have demonstrated no relationship between left ventricular function and optimal AV delay intervals, and the few that have reported such a relationship have yielded conflicting results. One small study using radionuclide assessment of acute changes in LVEF reported longer AV delay intervals to be more advantageous for patients with low LVEFs and suggested that these patients may require a longer atrial transport time.[76] In contrast, more recent clinical studies demonstrated significant acute and chronic hemodynamic improvement in patients with severe dilated cardiomyopathy who were physiologically paced with short AV delay intervals.[163–165] The discrepancy between studies may be explained by differences in interatrial and interventricular conduction times and the presence or absence of AV valvular regurgitation between the populations of patients studied.

Although the programmable AV delay settings regulate the timing of right atrial and ventricular contraction, left atrial and ventricular contraction is most important hemodynamically.[81, 82, 159] The physiologic left-sided AV delay interval is dependent on the programmed right-sided AV delay interval, latency in atrial capture and sensing, interatrial conduction time, latency in ventricular capture, and interventricular conduction time.[159] The relationship between right- and left-sided AV delay intervals during AV sequential, atrial synchronous, and atrial inhibited pacing is illustrated in Figure 14–27. It is apparent that with the same programmed right-sided AV delay interval, the left AV interval can vary by up to 200 msec, depending on whether atrial and ventricular events are paced or sensed. Wish and associates[81, 82] have demonstrated the effect of right-sided AV delay interval on the left atrial and left ventricular contraction sequence. They found a significant relationship between the optimal right-sided AV delay interval and the interatrial conduction time

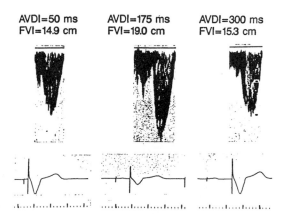

Figure 14–26. Left ventricular outflow recording at AV delay intervals of 50, 175, and 300 msec during AV sequential pacing at identical heart rates in the same patient. The largest flow velocity integral (FVI) reflecting ventricular stroke volume occurs at an AV delay interval of 175 msec. Significant decreases are noted in stroke volume at AV delay intervals of 50 and 300 msec. (From Janosik DL, Pearson AC, Buckingham TA, et al: The hemodynamic benefit of differential atrioventricular delay intervals for sensed and paced atrial events during physiologic pacing. J Am Coll Cardiol 14:499, 1989. Reprinted with permission of the American College of Cardiology.)

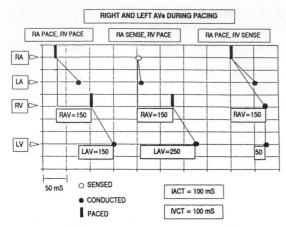

Figure 14–27. Effect of programmable right heart AV delay intervals on left heart AV delays during DDD pacing. RA, right atrium; LA, left atrium; RV, right ventricle; LV, left ventricle; IACT, intra-atrial conduction time; IVCT, intraventricular conduction time; RAV, right heart delay intervals; LAV, left heart delay intervals. (From Chirife R, Ortega DF, Salazar AI: Nonphysiological left heart AV intervals as a result of DDD and AAI "physiological" pacing. PACE 14:1752, 1991.)

as measured by the time from the atrial pacing spike to the atrial depolarization on the esophageal electrogram or to the A wave on an M-mode echocardiogram. Patients with short interatrial conduction times (90 msec) derived the greatest hemodynamic benefit from programmable AV delay intervals of 150 msec, and those with longer interatrial delay (120 msec) benefited most from programmed AV delays of 200 msec or more. Wish and colleagues[81] reported some patients with interatrial conduction delays that exceeded the programmed AV delay interval, resulting in left atrial depolarization following left ventricular activation. This negative left atrial-to-ventricular pacing sequence may produce hemodynamics equivalent to or less hemodynamically advantageous than those with VVI pacing alone.

Because of latency in atrial capture and sensing, the optimal programmable AV delay interval for sensed P waves and paced P waves may differ in an individual patient (Fig. 14–28). With a paced P wave, the programmed AV delay interval begins with the atrial pacing spike, and the physiologic PQ interval begins with atrial capture at the beginning of atrial depolarization. The physiologic PQ interval is therefore shorter than the programmed AV delay interval. The mean latency between atrial output and capture is reported to be 43 ± 10 msec; however, it may exceed 300 msec in some patients.[155–157] With a sensed P wave, the programmed AV delay interval begins when the native P wave is sensed in contrast to the physiologic PQ interval, which begins with the onset of the P wave. Thus, the physiologic PQ interval is longer than the programmed AV delay interval. In most studies, the latency from the beginning of the P wave to the time of atrial sensing is reported to be 30 to 50 msec.[156] The magnitude of atrial capture and sensing latencies varies among patients and may be affected by the lead and pacemaker circuitry characteristics, electrode position, tissue interface, amplitude and rate of stimulation, P-wave morphology, myocardial disease, electrolytes and other metabolic factors, and drugs. It is important to recognize that the

physiologic AV delay interval is never equivalent to the programmed AV delay interval for either a paced or a sensed atrial event.

Doppler echocardiography may be used to determine the difference in the timing of mechanical atrial systole when a paced compared with a sensed P wave occurs. We have found that in an individual patient, the peak A wave on the mitral valve inflow tracing occurs 40 ± 20 msec later with a paced than with a sensed P wave at similar heart rates.[89] Similarly, Alt and associates[160] have demonstrated that the peak A wave on the mitral valve M-mode recording occurs 46 ± 24 msec later with a paced P wave than with a sensed P wave and suggested that an automatic adjustment in AV delay interval may be hemodynamically beneficial. The same investigators reported that in patients with complete heart block, short AV delay intervals of 50 to 100 msec were most hemodynamically advantageous. This was attributed to the combination of atrial sensing latency and ventricular capture latency when a paced ventricular event follows a sensed P wave, thereby yielding a physiologic AV delay interval.

Wish and colleagues[81] demonstrated that when changing from atrial pacing (DVI mode) to atrial sensing (VDD mode), a change in the timing of the left atrial-to-ventricular sequence occurred and resulted a significant decrease in stroke volume (Fig. 14–29). Using Doppler-derived resting cardiac output in a group of patients with DDD pacemakers, we have demonstrated that the optimal AV delay for a sensed P wave was shorter than that for a paced P wave at similar heart rates in the same patient.[85] The mean difference between optimal AV delay intervals for a paced and a sensed P wave was 32 msec but was as great as 100 msec in some patients. At the respective optimal AV delay intervals for sensed and paced atrial events, there was no significant difference in the percentage increment over VVI pacing

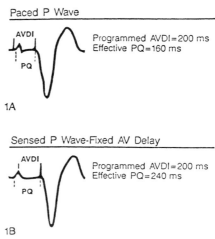

Figure 14–28. Programmed AV delay interval (AVDI) and effect of PQ intervals. When a paced P wave occurs *(top)*, the effective PQ interval is shorter than the programmed AV delay because of latency in atrial capture. When a sensed P wave occurs *(bottom)*, the effective PQ interval is longer than the programmed AV interval because of latency in atrial sensing. (From Janosik DL, Pearson AC, Buckingham TA, et al: The hemodynamic benefit of differential atrioventricular delay intervals for sensed and paced atrial events during physiologic pacing. J Am Coll Cardiol 14:499, 1989. Reprinted with permission of the American College of Cardiology.)

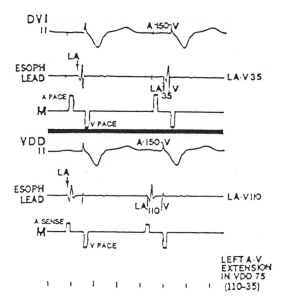

Figure 14–29. Interatrial conduction and change in the timing of left atrial (LA) depolarization with pacing mode change from DDD to VDD. The time delay between right atrial pacing artifact and left atrial depolarization is 115 msec, resulting in an LA-to-ventricular sequence of only 35 msec. With mode change to VDD *(bottom)*, the left LA-to-ventricular sequence extends by 75 msec, resulting in an LA-to-ventricular sequence of 110 msec. (From Wish M, Fletcher RD, Gottdiener JS, Cohen AI: Importance of left atrial timing in the programming of dual-chamber pacemakers. Am J Cardiol 60:566, 1987.)

left ventricular function, and had limited follow-up; hence, its applicability to other clinical situations is not clear.

In summary, the programmed right-sided AV delay interval differs significantly from the physiologic left-sided AV delay interval. The discrepancies between right-sided and left-sided delay intervals are dependent primarily on latencies in atrial capture and sensing, interatrial conduction delay, ventricular capture latency, and interventricular conduction delay. In an individual patient, the physiologic AV delay interval may vary, depending on whether a paced or a sensed atrial event and whether a paced ventricular depolarization or intrinsic ventricular depolarization follows atrial contraction. The optimal AV delay interval for a sensed P wave is about 30 to 40 msec shorter than the optimal AV delay interval for a paced P wave followed by a paced QRS at a similar heart rate. Although not practical or cost-effective for every patient, fine-tuning of the AV delay interval can be performed using Doppler-derived cardiac outputs at varying AV delay intervals. Alternatively, the interatrial conduction delay can be estimated noninvasively by measuring the time from the atrial pacing spike to the A wave on the M-mode echocardiogram or Doppler recording of the mitral valve and may be helpful in selecting hemodynamically advantageous AV delay intervals. These techniques may be beneficial in cases in which optimization of AV delay interval is critical to the patient's hemodynamics. Some newer dual-chamber pacemakers incorporate programmable features designed to adjust the AV delay interval automatically in response to paced versus sensed P waves and in response to the atrial rate.

Relative Sensitivity to Atrioventricular Delay Interval

Sensitivity to changes in the AV delay interval varies greatly among patients. Whereas changes in the AV delay interval of as little as 25 msec may result in significant changes in cardiac output in some patients, others are relatively insensitive to large alterations in AV delay.[60, 84, 86] We have investigated the relationship to Doppler and echocardiographic variables of systolic and diastolic ventricular function and sensitivity to variance in AV delay interval.[84] The augmentation of Doppler-derived cardiac output at the optimal AV delay interval compared with the least optimal AV delay interval was 25% during atrial synchronous pacing (VDD) and 26% during AV sequential pacing (DVI mode) (Fig. 14–30). The cardiac output at the least optimal AV delay interval was not significantly different from the cardiac output during VVI pacing. Patients with larger atrial contributions to left ventricular filling as measured from Doppler mitral valve inflow recordings derived the greatest benefit from the optimization of AV delay interval during VDD pacing. Iwase and colleagues[143] demonstrated a mean increase of 46% in mitral valve inflow from the least to the most optimal AV delay interval setting. The relative augmentation in left ventricular filling achieved by adjusting the AV delay interval correlated positively to the left atrial contribution to left ventricular filling as determined by Doppler mitral valve recordings. Thus, patients with significant atrial contributions to cardiac output, such as elderly patients and those with hypertrophied ventricles, may be particularly sensitive to changes in AV delay interval.

during AV sequential (DVI) or atrial synchronous (VDD) pacing. However, the cardiac output decreased significantly during VDD pacing at the optimal AV delay interval for a paced atrial event and during DVI pacing at the AV delay interval determined to be optimal for a sensed P wave. An additional 8% increment in cardiac output could be achieved by optimizing the AV delay interval for a sensed P wave rather than using that determined to be optimal for a paced P wave. This small increment may be clinically important in patients for whom it is vital to maximize resting cardiac output and supports the hemodynamic advantage of an automatic decrement in AV delay interval when a sensed rather than a paced P wave occurs (AV delay hysteresis) or the availability of separately programmable AV delay intervals for paced and sensed atrial events (differential AV delay intervals).

Although optimization of AV delay interval on resting hemodynamics is established, there are fewer data concerning the impact on functional capacity and quality of life. The effect of individually optimizing AV delay intervals on the patient's quality of life was investigated in a randomized double-blind study[153] of 13 patients with AV block. Patients were randomized to a 2-week period of dual-chamber pacing at the optimal AV delay interval or the "most unfavorable" AV delay and then switched to the alternate pacemaker settings. Although resting LVEF by radionuclide ventriculography was significantly higher at the optimal AV delay (51% versus 44%; $P < .0001$), functional capacity and quality of life did not differ between the two AV delay settings. The study was small, included patients with fairly well preserved

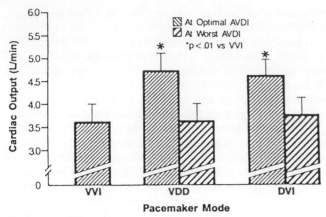

Figure 14–30. Doppler-derived output in VVI, VDD, and VDD mode at the optimal and worst AV delay intervals (AVDI). There was a 26% improvement in cardiac output from the least favorable to most favorable AV delay interval in both pacing modes. The cardiac output at the worst AV delay interval was not significantly different from that during VVI pacing in either pacing mode. (From Pearson AC, Janosik DL, Redd RM, et al: Hemodynamic benefit of atrioventricular synchrony: Prediction from baseline Doppler echocardiographic variables. J Am Coll Cardiol 13:1613, 1989. Reprinted with permission from the American College of Cardiology.)

The data regarding the effect of left ventricular systolic function on sensitivity to AV delay interval are conflicting. Lascault and colleagues[86] reported a 25% increment in Doppler-derived stroke volume in comparing the most hemodynamically advantageous AV delay interval to the least advantageous during DDD pacing at rest. In a linear discriminate analysis of multiple factors, only the left ventricular diastolic diameter on M-mode echocardiogram predicted sensitivity to AV delay interval. Patients with normal left ventricular diastolic dimension benefited more from optimization of AV delay interval than those with enlarged left ventricular end-diastolic dimensions. In contrast, Eugene and associates[88] used modified impedance plethysmography to assess changes in stroke volume at different AV delay intervals and suggested that patients with diseased left ventricles were more sensitive to changes in AV delay interval than those with normal left ventricular function. Patients temporarily paced during acute myocardial infarction or a postcardiac surgery have been reported to demonstrate marked sensitivity to changes in AV delay interval.[59, 60] The apparent discrepancy in these data may be related to the diverse populations of patients and their position on the Starling function curve. Regardless of baseline left ventricular function, patients functioning on the ascending limb of the curve would be expected to benefit most from optimizing the timing of atrial systole, and those on the plateau portion of the curve would derive little additional benefit.

■ EFFECT OF EXERCISE ON PACING HEMODYNAMICS

Effect of Posture on Pacing Hemodynamics

Most studies examining the hemodynamic importance of atrial contribution to cardiac output were performed with patients at rest in the supine position. It has been demon-strated by noninvasive and invasive hemodynamic techniques that assumption of an upright posture diminishes cardiac output by up to 30% because of venous pooling and a reduction in preload.[81, 87, 166] However, the relative hemodynamic benefit of dual-chamber pacing over ventricular pacing is similar in both the upright and the supine positions.[166] Wish and associates[81] found that more patients were sensitive to changes in AV delay interval in the upright position than in the supine position and suggested that timing of contraction relative to ventricular systole may be even more significant when preload and filling pressures are low. It appears that the same AV delay interval that maximizes cardiac output in the supine position is also usually optimal in the upright position in most patients.

Fixed-Rate Ventricular Compared With Atrial Synchronous Pacing

Healthy subjects are capable of increasing their resting cardiac output three- to five-fold during maximal exercise, depending on the level of physical fitness. In subjects with normal sinus node function, heart rate is the predominant means by which cardiac output increases during exercise, incrementing by as much as 200% to 300%. Stroke volume increases to a lesser degree, with maximal increments of about 60% occurring in healthy subjects at peak exercise[167] (Fig. 14–31). When comparing exercise hemodynamics during pacing modes capable of tracking atrial activity (VAT, VDD, or DDD) with fixed-rate ventricular pacing, physiologic pacing prolongs exercise duration, increases exercise cardiac output, reduces exercise-induced arrhythmias and hypotension, and decreases subjective complaints during exercise compared with ventricular pacing.[57, 63, 115, 168–174] The improvement in exercise capacity with acute changes from fixed-rate ventricular pacing to physiologic pacing has been reported to be 20% to 45%. The relative improvement persists and is even more marked after more prolonged periods in the two pacing modes.[64, 169] Baseline left ventricular function, patient age, and exercise capacity during VVI pacing do not predict the relative benefit of atrial synchronous pacing compared with fixed-rate ventricular pacing during exercise.[168]

The augmentation in exercise output with physiologic

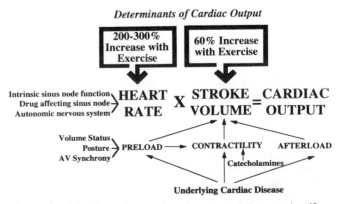

Figure 14–31. Determinants of cardiac output during exercise. (See text for discussion.)

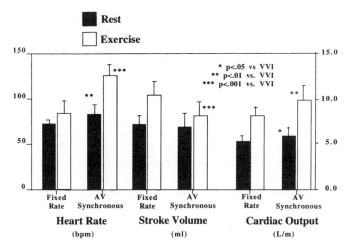

Figure 14–32. Comparison of exercise hemodynamics during fixed-rate ventricular pacing and atrial synchronous pacing. The exercise heart rate and cardiac output are significantly higher with atrial synchronous pacing than with fixed-rate ventricular pacing. The exercise heart rate is significantly higher with atrial synchronous pacing than with fixed-rate ventricular pacing, and the exercise stroke volume is significantly higher with fixed-rate ventricular pacing than with atrial synchronous pacing. The compensatory increase in exercise stroke volume, however, does not equal the benefit derived from the ability to increase heart rate; thus, the exercise cardiac output during atrial synchronous pacing is significantly higher than during fixed-rate ventricular pacing. (From Karlöf I: Haemodynamic effect of atrial triggered versus fixed rate pacing at rest and during exercise in complete heart block. Acta Med Scand 197:195, 1975.)

pacing is due primarily to the ability to increase heart rate in response to metabolic demands without significant increases in filling pressure or stroke volume. In contrast, fixed-rate VVI pacing results in higher end-diastolic volumes and stroke volumes and LVEF during exercise than does physiologic pacing. Although partially compensatory, the augmentations in end-diastolic volume and contractility fail to achieve the degree of hemodynamic benefit derived from rate responsiveness during exercise[57] (Fig. 14–32). At steady-state submaximal workloads, physiologic pacing results in a higher exercise cardiac output and increased exercise duration with similar expenditure of myocardial oxygen consumption and coronary artery blood flow compared with VVI pacing.[173] The increase in stroke volume during exercise that occurs with VVI pacing is due to enhanced preload from enhanced venous return during muscular contraction and, importantly, to heightened sympathetic nervous system activity resulting in greater ventricular contractility and ejection fraction.[172] Coronary sinus norepinephrine levels and arterial catecholamine levels are elevated at rest and during exercise during VVI pacing compared with physiologic pacing.[115] The heightened sympathetic activity and diminished cardiovascular reserve during fixed-rate pacing are evidenced by higher atrial rates and enhanced myocardial contractility compared with physiologic pacing at comparable workloads.

Relative Importance of Atrioventricular Synchrony Compared With Rate Responsiveness

The significance of the atrial contribution to cardiac output has been demonstrated over a wide range of resting heart

rates. Reiter and Hindman[63] reported that the atrial contribution to cardiac output and percentage augmentation in resting cardiac output with AV sequential compared with ventricular demand pacing increases with increasing pacing rate. However, it is now apparent that conclusions regarding the relative importance of atrial systole during pacing-induced tachycardia in the resting supine position cannot necessarily be extrapolated to tachycardia produced by upright exercise. Using Doppler assessment of left ventricular filling, Linde-Edelstam and associates[175] demonstrated that there is a significant difference in the kinetic energy of blood flow and left ventricular filling pattern with exercise-induced compared with pacing-induced increases in heart rate. Blood flow velocity and the ratio of early diastolic filling to late diastolic filling are increased during exercise-induced tachycardia compared with atrial pacing at equivalent heart rates. This suggests that an increase in the kinetic energy of blood flow is produced by sympathetic stimulation and enhanced contractility. This increase is accompanied by a decrease in atrial contribution to left ventricular filling, making the early rapid filling phase proportionally more important in exercise-induced tachycardia.[175]

Several studies have compared exercise capacity and hemodynamics during atrial tracking modes (VDD or VAT pacing) with those achieved during ventricular pacing, matched to the tracked atrial rate so that the peak heart rate in the two modes was equivalent.[57, 171, 176–179] The authors demonstrated similar exercise capacity and cardiac output with the two pacing modes and concluded that the major determinant of exercise cardiac output in paced patients is the ability of the pacing mode to augment heart rate. In addition, it has been demonstrated that there are no significant differences in right atrial pressure, pulmonary capillary wedge pressure, coronary sinus AV oxygen difference, or myocardial oxygen consumption between rate-matched ventricular pacing and atrial synchronous pacing during exercise.[179]

Ausubel and colleagues[178] demonstrated that atrial synchronous and ventricular rate-adaptive pacing augment cardiac output during exercise by different mechanisms. In a single-blind randomized crossover study using radionuclide ventriculography during exercise, the percentage changes in stroke volume and cardiac output at peak exercise were found to be similar in the two pacing modes (Fig. 14–33). The end-diastolic and end-systolic volumes were significantly higher during atrial synchronous pacing than during rate-matched ventricular pacing. Therefore, stroke volume increased mainly by means of the Frank-Starling mechanism, sparing myocardial contractile reserve. Conversely, rate-matched ventricular pacing was associated with lower end-diastolic volumes and end-systolic volumes but with higher levels of myocardial contractility and ejection fraction, thereby yielding stroke volumes similar to those achieved during atrial synchronous pacing.

Evidence that ventricular rate-adaptive pacing yields exercise hemodynamics equivalent to that with DDD pacing and involves the insertion of only one pacing lead contributed to the enthusiasm for VVIR pacemakers in the early and mid-1980s. Various sensors that regulate heart rate were introduced and found to improve exercise duration acutely compared with ventricular pacing. Sensors used have included activity, right ventricular blood temperature, respiratory rate

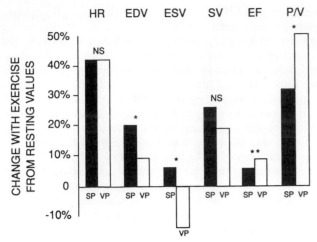

Figure 14–33. Percentage change in heart rate, left ventricular volume, and contractility with exercise during rate-adaptive ventricular pacing (VP) compared with atrial synchronous ventricular pacing (SP). The end-diastolic and end-systolic volumes were higher during atrial synchronous pacing, and the left ventricular ejection fraction was higher during ventricular pacing. HR, heart rate; EDV, end-diastolic volume; ESV, end-systolic volume; SV, stroke volume; EF, ejection fraction; P/V, peak systolic pressure/end-systolic volume ratio. *$P < .001$; **$P = .002$; NS, not significant. (From Linde-Edelstam CM, Juhlin-Dannfelt A, Nordlander R, Pehrsson SK: The hemodynamic importance of atrial systole: A function of the kinetic energy of blood flow? PACE 15:1740, 1992.)

and minute ventilation, stroke volume and pre-ejection period, and QT interval.[180–189] Buckingham and associates[186] demonstrated improved exercise duration and cardiac index with activity sensor rate-adaptive pacing compared with fixed-rate ventricular pacing using Doppler echocardiography during paired-symptom limited exercise tests (Fig. 14–34). The improvement in heart rate, cardiac index, and exercise duration with VVIR pacing did not correlate with resting baseline ejection fraction. In a similarly designed study, Lau and Camm[187] found a weak negative correlation between resting left ventricular fractional shortening on M-mode echocardiograms and the percentage increase in exercise duration with VVIR compared with fixed-rate VVI pacing. Both studies demonstrated that elderly and younger patients derived similar benefits from rate-adaptive pacing. Thus, it appears that poor left ventricular function and advanced age do not prevent rate-adaptive pacing from improving exercise capacity and cardiac output over fixed-rate ventricular pacing.

Before the availability of dual-chamber rate-responsive pacemakers in the late 1980s, the relative importance of rate responsiveness and AV synchrony during cardiac pacing was disputed.[190, 191] Most data indicate that AV synchrony is most important at rest and during lower levels of exercise, whereas rate responsiveness assumes the more important role at moderate and high levels of exertion.[180, 189] It is important to realize that the effectiveness of ventricular rate-responsive pacing has been demonstrated primarily by acute exercise studies. Obvious concerns exist regarding the long-term effects of asynchronous AV contraction on left ventricular function, AV valvular regurgitation, and even patient survival.[114, 192–203] The abnormal atrial reflexes that result in

pacemaker syndrome during fixed-rate ventricular pacing may also occur during ventricular rate-adaptive pacing, especially in patients with intact VA conduction. The increased incidence of atrial fibrillation and associated thromboembolic phenomena[195, 196, 198, 200–202] demonstrated with fixed-rate ventricular pacing compared with AAI or DDD pacing is also a potential problem with VVIR pacing. In addition, data suggest that there is improved survival with AV synchronous pacing compared with fixed-rate ventricular pacing (especially in patients with congestive heart failure), whereas no such survival benefit has been demonstrated with rate-adaptive ventricular pacing.[194, 197, 198–203]

Now that DDDR pacemakers are available, rate responsiveness and AV synchrony are no longer mutually exclusive features. Proctor and colleagues[204] demonstrated that DDDR pacing results in superior exercise hemodynamics compared with DDD or VVIR pacing in a group of patients with chronotropic incompetence. Importantly, only the DDDR pacing mode significantly increased exercise cardiac output compared with resting values, suggesting that a combination of AV synchrony and rate responsiveness is superior to either feature alone during exercise in patients with chronotropic incompetence. Other studies comparing DDDR and VVIR pacing showed increased exercise capacity and cardiac output with DDDR pacing compared with VVIR pacing as well as superior metabolic parameters, indicating improved left ventricular efficiency during dual-chamber rate-responsive pacing.[205, 206] Individual metabolic sensors are limited by their ability to replicate normal sinus node response to physiologic stress. The characteristics of metabolic sensors are discussed in detail elsewhere. Rate-adaptive pacing incorporating a self-optimizing dual sensor (activity and minute ventilation) has been shown to provide a better physiologic rate response than single-sensor rate-adaptive pacing.[207–212] However, the clinical significance in terms of improved

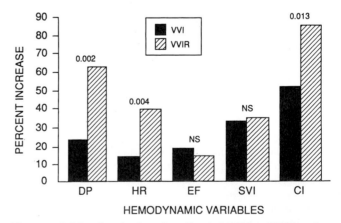

Figure 14–34. Exercise hemodynamics during VVI and VVIR pacing in 16 patients with activity-sensing rate-adaptive pacemakers. Percentage change in double product (DP), heart rate (HR), ejection fraction (EF), stroke volume index (SVI), and cardiac index (CI) during exercise in each pacing mode are displayed. HR, CI, and DP are significantly higher during exercise in the VVIR mode than with fixed-rate ventricular pacing. (From Buckingham TA, Woodruff RC, Pennington DG, et al: Effect of ventricular function on exercise hemodynamics of variable rate pacing. J Am Coll Cardiol 11:1269, 1988. Reprinted with permission of the American College of Cardiology.)

quality of life and reduction of symptoms is not clear. In patients with normal sinus node function and the ability to increase atrial rate with exercise, DDD pacing represents a physiologic pacing mode that preserves both AV synchrony and rate responsiveness. In patients with chronotropic incompetence, however, DDDR pacing has been shown to yield superior exercise hemodynamics compared with DDD pacing because of the ability to achieve higher rates.[213] These data, in combination with the well-accepted hemodynamic benefits of atrial systole at rest, strongly support preservation of AV synchrony during pacing whenever possible.

Atrioventricular Delay Interval During Exercise

The importance of variation in atrioventricular delay during exercise in physiologically paced patients is controversial. There are two theoretical reasons that a rate-adaptive AV delay interval would be hemodynamically beneficial. First, shortening of the AV delay interval with increasing atrial rates simulates normal physiologic PR shortening with exercise.[214, 215] With an increasing heart rate, there is disproportionate shortening of diastole, and therefore the timing of atrial and ventricular contraction may become even more crucial. Theoretically, shortening of the AV delay interval with increased rate of atrial sensed events would facilitate left ventricular filling and cardiac output during exercise. Second, shortening of the AV delay interval during exercise allows higher atrial tracking rates. Because the PR interval is part of the TARP, shortening of the AV delay interval with exercise allows higher atrial tracking rates before two-to-one block upper rate limit behavior occurs and therefore potentially increases exercise capacity.

The physiologic relationship between PR interval and heart rate in healthy individuals has been well characterized. Daubert and associates[214] demonstrated an inverse linear relationship between heart rate and PR interval that was independent of age and baseline PR interval. There is a mean decrease of 4 ± 2.1 msec in PR interval for a 10-bpm increase in heart rate. The normal PR shortening with exercise is caused by facilitation of AV nodal conduction because of increased sympathetic stimulation and diminished vagal tone. If the AV delay interval remained constant, atrial systole would occur early in diastole and result in a situation similar to that seen with unphysiologically long AV delay intervals at rest.

Initial data supporting the importance of rate-adaptive delay were obtained by examining the effects of various rates of AV sequential pacing at rest.[154] These data indicated that the most hemodynamically advantageous AV delay intervals at higher rates were shorter than that which was optimal at lower rates. Ritter and associates[154] demonstrated superior cardiac hemodynamics, including increased cardiac index and left ventricular stroke work index and decreased pulmonary capillary wedge pressure and systemic vascular resistance, with rate-adaptive AV delay compared with fixed AV delay intervals during AV sequential pacing at increasing rates. They further demonstrated that when comparing two fixed rates, the AV delay interval of 200 msec was more advantageous at lower pacing rates, whereas 150 msec was superior at higher heart rates. However, the hemodynamic

situation during pacing-induced tachycardia and exercise varies greatly.

Because the major determinant of augmentation of cardiac output during exercise is heart rate, the contribution of atrial systole and the relative timing of atrial and ventricular contraction may diminish in significance.

Studies analyzing the effects of variation in AV delay interval during exercise have yielded conflicting results.[217–223] During upright submaximal treadmill exercise in patients with complete heart block and normal left ventricular function, Mehta and colleagues[87] demonstrated that a fixed AV delay interval of 75 to 80 msec was optimal during exercise and significantly increased the Doppler-derived cardiac output compared with AV delay intervals of 150 and 200 msec. Comparing a physiologic AV delay interval (155 ± 10 msec) with a nonphysiologic AV delay interval (30 ± 29 msec) during exercise with DDD pacing, Landzberg and coworkers[219] reported a 16% increase in exercise duration, a 23% increase in time to anaerobic threshold, and a decreased level of perceived exertion with the physiologic AV delay. Lower ANP levels after maximal exercise with DDD pacing at shorter AV delay intervals suggest more physiologic hemodynamics than with longer AV delay intervals during exercise.[222] Using bicycle exercise and radionuclide ejection fractions, Leman and Kratz[75] found shorter AV delay intervals to result in larger stroke volumes. Haskell and French[78] reported that both short (66-msec) and long (160-msec) AV delay intervals during AV sequential pacing during maximum bicycle exercise were superior to VVI pacing; however, no hemodynamic advantage of short over long AV delay intervals was found. Ryden and colleagues[218] found that varying the fixed AV delay interval from 50 to 200 msec on serial exercise efforts had no effect on the maximum ventricular rate, maximum oxygen uptake, minute ventilation, or perceived level of exertion during upright exercise in patients with dual-chamber pacemakers and normal left ventricular function.

These studies, although varying the AV delay between exercise efforts, used a fixed AV delay interval during each exercise test. There is evidence that a rate-adaptive AV delay interval, which is automatically decremented in response to an increased atrial rate, is beneficial to cardiopulmonary performance during exercise. Ritter and associates[220] performed paired exercise tests, one with a fixed AV delay interval of 156 msec and one with an automatic AV delay interval ranging from 156 to 63 msec, in 23 patients with dual-chamber pacemakers implanted for high-degree AV block. Exercise duration to anaerobic threshold was significantly longer and V_{O_2} and V_{CO_2} at anaerobic threshold and peak exercise were significantly higher with an automatic AV delay interval. The mean automatic AV delay interval was 104 ± 24 msec at anaerobic threshold and 82 ± 28 msec at peak exercise. Lower plasma norepinephrine levels during exercise with autoadaptive AV delay than with fixed AV delay intervals have been reported and suggest more efficient cardiac hemodynamics.[222] In patients with chronotropic incompetence and high-degree AV block, Sulke and colleagues[221] performed randomized double-blind crossover assessment of rate-adaptive and different fixed AV delay settings during 2 weeks of normal activity and an exercise treadmill in DDDR mode. There was subjective improvement in the sense of general well-being and patients' prefer-

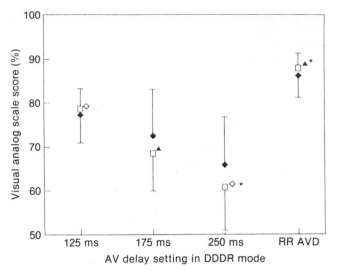

Figure 14–35. Exercise capacity (♦) and patient's perception of general well-being (□) during everyday activity at fixed AV delay settings of 125, 175, and 250 msec and rate-responsive AV delay (RR AVD) settings in DDDR mode. ◇, $P < .05$; ▲ m, $P < .03$; *$P < .01$. (Adapted from Sulke AN, Chambers JB, Sowton E: The effect of atrioventricular delay programming in patients with DDDR pacemakers. Eur Heart J 13:464, 1992.)

ence for rate-adaptive AV delay interval or fixed AV delay interval of 125 msec (Fig. 14–35). The longest AV delay interval (250 msec) was least preferred by patients and was associated with the highest symptom prevalence. Exercise duration was not significantly different in any setting in DDDR mode but was significantly reduced in DDD mode.[221]

Although the significance of an adaptive AV delay interval during DDD and DDDR exercise is controversial, it has been demonstrated that improper and deleterious sequencing of atrial and ventricular contraction can result during AAIR pacing for chronotropic incompetence. In some patients, the AV delay interval does not adapt normally with exercise and the stimulus–R interval and stimulus-to-R/RR ratio may actually increase. This may result in P waves occurring immediately after or even within the R wave of the preceding cycle. The paradoxical increase in stimulus–R interval and stimulus-to-R/RR ratio may be related to factors intrinsic to the patient, such as conduction disease, lead position, or drugs, or may represent overstimulation by the sensor-driven atrial pacemaker.[130, 224, 225] The overstimulation phenomenon occurs when the atrial sensor increases the atrial rate out of proportion to the sympathetic drive, so that no corresponding decrement in PR interval occurs. This is most frequently observed in early stages of exercise and in some patients is corrected as the patient continues to exercise. In other cases, implantation of a DDDR system with more physiologic AV sequencing alleviates symptoms.

■ IMPORTANCE OF VENTRICULAR ACTIVATION SEQUENCE

A normal cardiac contraction depends not only on the appropriate temporal sequence of atrial and ventricular events but also on the rapid synchronous depolarization of the ventri-

cles through the intrinsic specialized conduction system. Aberrant electric depolarization and mechanical contraction of the ventricle are produced by right ventricular pacing (VVI pacing) alone or in the presence of atrial systole, as in AV sequential (DVI) or atrial synchronous (VDD) pacing.[226] In patients capable of intrinsic AV conduction, a normal or paced ventricular depolarization may occur after a P wave, depending on the programmed AV delay interval and the effects of drugs, disease, and the autonomic nervous system on intrinsic AV conduction. Atrial inhibited (AAI) pacing in patients with intact AV conduction preserves both AV synchrony and the normal sequence of ventricular depolarization. With DDD and DDDR pacemakers representing most implants in the United States, defining the relative hemodynamic significance of ventricular activation sequence is clinically important.

As early as 1925, Wiggers[25] reported that in intact dog models, artificial stimulation of the right ventricle produced a less effective ventricular contraction than activation through the normal conduction system. The greater the amount of muscle activated before activation of the His-Purkinje system, the greater the degree of dys-synchrony and the weaker the contraction. Subsequent animal studies suggested that the loss of AV synchrony and asynchrony of ventricular contraction were independent and additive factors contributing to the hemodynamic deterioration observed with ventricular pacing compared with atrial or His bundle pacing.[11, 16, 28, 32–34] Comparing different endocardial pacing sites in the anesthetized dog, Grover and Glantz[32] demonstrated lower end-diastolic and stroke volumes with right ventricular apical pacing compared with right atrial pacing or left ventricular pacing. In isolated canine hearts, right ventricular epicardial pacing resulted in lower left ventricular end-diastolic pressure and a compensatory decrease in oxygen consumption compared with atrial pacing at the same heart rate.

The normal sequence of ventricular activation achieved with atrial pacing has been shown to be associated with superior cardiac energetics compared with the less energy efficient asynchronous contraction produced by ventricular pacing.[227] In a closed-chest dog study comparing the effects of right atrial, right ventricular apical, and AV sequential pacing on myocardial oxygen consumption and cardiac efficiency (defined as the ratio of oxygen equivalent of external work to MV_{O_2}), myocardial oxygen consumption was lowest and cardiac efficiency highest with right atrial pacing.[227]

Animal studies have demonstrated that regional changes in left ventricular mechanical performance induced by ventricular pacing may be detrimental to global left ventricular systolic function compared with atrial pacing. Badke and associates[228] performed pacing from the right atrium, right ventricular apex, left ventricular apex, and left ventricular base in open-chest dogs while assessing overall local ventricular function by ultrasonic crystal pairs. Ventricular pacing from all sites produced asynchrony of contraction with early shortening in ventricular regions close to the pacer site and then bulging (or lengthening) of these regions late in systole. There was a regional decrease in the percentage of shortening in early activated segments compared with atrial pacing. Segments removed from the pacing site were activated later and functionally least affected; some remote segments exhibited enhanced shortening compared with atrial pacing. Most important, there was an average

27% reduction in peak systolic function and left ventricular rate of pressure development (dP/dt), indicating impairment of global systolic function with ventricular as opposed to atrial pacing.

In addition to diminished systolic function, the inhomogeneity of ventricular contraction during right ventricular pacing may impair diastolic relaxation and, thus, filling of the ventricle. In open-chest dogs, Zile and colleagues[34] demonstrated a decrease in regional and global indices of relaxation (isovolumetric pressure decline and relaxation time constant) with right ventricular and AV sequential pacing compared with AAI pacing that was independent of loading conditions. Heyndrickx and colleagues[29] compared the effects of RV pacing and atrial pacing at similar heart rate on left ventricular contractile force and relaxation in conscious dogs at rest and during sympathetic stimulation produced by treadmill exercise. At rest, contractile strength was reduced as characterized by a decreased left ventricular rate of pressure development (dP/dt) with ventricular pacing compared with atrial pacing, whereas relaxation was not significantly altered. During exercise, however, there was a significant increase in the time constant of relaxation during ventricular pacing, indicating impaired relaxation.

Adomian and Beazell[229] demonstrated that in a majority of dogs with complete heart block and 3 months of ventricular pacing, there was histopathologic evidence of myocardial cellular derangement, including myofibrillar disarray, mitochondrial disorganization, prominent Purkinje cells, and dystrophic myocardial calcification not observed in control animals. Although there is no similar evidence in humans, the possibility that chronic asynchronous contraction with nonhomogenous workload and blood supply may lead to myocardial cellular changes must be considered.

Despite convincing evidence in animal models that the normal ventricular activation sequence is hemodynamically superior to asynchronous contraction, the clinical importance in humans is less clear. Comparing acute hemodynamic changes in humans during VVI, AV sequential, and AAI pacing, Samet and coworkers[55] concluded in the 1960s that asynchronicity of ventricular contraction was of minor importance compared with AV synchrony because AAI and AV sequential pacing yielded equivalent hemodynamic improvements compared with ventricular pacing. Greenberg and colleagues[61] reached similar conclusions, demonstrating that AAI and AV sequential pacings were equally beneficial and that both were superior to ventricular pacing alone. However, these acute studies were performed with selected groups of patients with significant cardiovascular and pulmonary disease at rest in an intensive care unit or postoperative setting and used temporary pacing modalities and invasive hemodynamic measurements.

Advances in noninvasive imaging techniques allow more sophisticated assessment of regional and global left ventricular systolic and diastolic function and suggest that the asynchronicity of ventricular contraction observed with a naturally occurring or pacing-induced left bundle-branch block electrocardiographic pattern may produce deleterious hemodynamic effects.[226, 230–236] Grines and colleagues[232] used a variety of noninvasive imaging techniques to compare left ventricular function at rest and during exercise in a group of patients with isolated left bundle-branch block and in a group of patients with a normal ventricular activation sequence. Patients with left bundle-branch block demonstrated a reduction in global LVEF both at rest and during exercise because of a regional decrease in interventricular septal ejection fraction. There was also a reduction in left ventricular diastolic filling time and an increase in the ratio of right to left ventricular filling time. Bramlet and colleagues[231] demonstrated an abrupt decrease in regional and global LVEF with the development of rate-dependent left bundle-branch block and no overall increase in exercise ejection fraction in a group of patients with no structural heart disease and no evidence of ischemia.

Using invasive hemodynamic measurements, Askenazi and colleagues[230] assessed the effects of AV sequential pacing and atrial-inhibited pacing at constant heart rates and preload conditions on left ventricular performance. There was no significant difference in end-diastolic volume between the two modes of pacing. However, there were a significant increase in end-systolic volume and a decrease in stroke volume and ejection fraction with AV sequential pacing compared with AAI pacing. Santomauro and coworkers[235] used radionuclide phase analysis during different pacing modes to quantitate the effects of the ventricular activation sequence on left ventricular performance. In modes resulting in a paced ventricular complex, temporal inhomogeneity of ventricular contraction and diminished global LVEF occurred, whereas with atrial pacing, ventricular contraction occurred through the intrinsic conduction system. There was an inverse correlation between the degree of temporal inhomogeneity and LVEF. Using resting radionuclide studies and rest and submaximal exercise Doppler studies during VVI, AAI, and AV sequential pacing, Rosenqvist and colleagues[226] investigated the relative hemodynamic importance of left ventricular activation sequence and AV synchrony. Ventricular pacing with or without atrial systole was associated with paradoxical septal motion, a 25% reduction in regional septal ejection fraction, and a significant reduction in global ejection fraction at rest (Fig. 14–36). In addition, peak diastolic early filling rate was decreased with AV sequential pacing compared with AAI pacing. The observed changes persisted during submaximal exercise, and Doppler-derived exercise cardiac output was higher during AAI pacing than during DDD or VVI pacing.

Leclercq and associates[236] reported a similar hemodynamic benefit of AAI pacing over AV sequential and ventricular pacing using invasive hemodynamic measurements and radionuclide ventriculography at rest and during exercise in patients with DDD pacemakers and normal intrinsic AV conduction. Cardiac output, left ventricular peak filling rates, and LVEF were higher and pulmonary capillary wedge pressures were lower with AAI pacing than with AV sequential and ventricular pacing both at rest and during exercise. As in Rosenqvist's study,[226] the improvement of LVEF was primarily due to a regional increase in septal ejection fraction during AAI pacing. In contrast to Rosenqvist's study, there was a significantly higher LVEF with AV sequential pacing than with VVI pacing at rest and during exercise. The discrepancy between the two studies in the differential benefit of AV sequential over ventricular pacing may be explained by the small number of patients in each study and the differences in relative benefit of atrial synchrony between the two populations studied. Leclercq's study included a higher percentage of patients with 1:1 VA conduction who

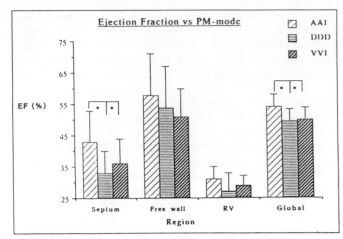

Figure 14–36. Regional and global ejection fractions (EF) during atrial demand pacing (AAI), synchronous atrioventricular pacing (DDD), and fixed-rate ventricular demand pacing (VVI). Septal and global ejection fractions are significantly reduced with both VVI and DDD pacing modes compared with AAI mode. (From Rosenqvist M, Isaaz K, Botvinick EH, et al: Relative importance of activation sequence compared to atrioventricular synchrony in left ventricular function. Am J Cardiol 67:148, 1991.)

may have been more prone to adverse hemodynamic effects from loss of AV synchrony (about 80% compared with 33% in Rosenqvist's study).

In addition to changes in left ventricular systolic function, there is evidence that the inhomogeneity of ventricular contraction induced by right ventricular pacing affects ventricular relaxation and diastolic function in humans. Askenazi and colleagues[230] demonstrated significant decreases in both peak dP/dt and peak negative dP/dt with a paced compared with an intrinsic ventricular contraction. They suggested that less effective contraction and relaxation occurred with asynchronously paced ventricular contractions and accounted for the diminished ejection fraction observed with AV sequential pacing compared with AAI pacing. Bedotto and associates[233] presented evidence that baseline ventricular function may influence the effects of asynchronous left ventricular contraction on left ventricular relaxation. The rate of positive dP/dt and negative dP/dt and the time constant of left ventricular relaxation were measured during atrial and AV sequential pacing in a group of healthy subjects and in a group of patients with impaired left ventricular systolic function. Whereas both groups demonstrated a decrease in positive dP/dt with AV sequential compared with AAI pacing, the relaxation time increased and peak negative dP/dt decreased only in patients with low baseline ejection fraction (Fig. 14–37). Impairment of left ventricular relaxation occurred independently of changes in systolic function and correlated with left ventricular wall thickness.[233]

Stojnic[237] and coworkers compared parameters of left ventricular relaxation in a group of patients with AAI pacing to those in a group with VDD pacing and similar heart rates, PR intervals, estimated preload, afterload, and ratio of late to early filling pressure by Doppler echocardiography. Compared with patients with AAI pacing, patients with VDD pacing demonstrated increased pre-ejection period, elevated

velocity of isovolumic relaxation flow, and prolonged isovolumic relaxation time. Paradoxical anterior systolic intraventricular septal motion occurred in 9 of 13 patients (about 70%) during VDD pacing and in none of the atrial-paced patients. Isovolumic relaxation flow indicating asynchronous left ventricular relaxation occurred in 100% of VDD-paced patients compared with 45% of AAI-paced patients.

The effects of asynchronous left ventricular contraction on parameters of systolic and diastolic ventricular function in patients with coronary artery disease, normal ventricular function, and stable angina were examined simultaneously with radionuclide angiography and cardiac catheterization during AAI and AV sequential pacing.[238] Compared with atrial pacing, AV sequential pacing resulted in a reduction in peak filling rate and cardiac index. The time constant of isovolumic relaxation increased, and the global diastolic pressure–volume curve shifted upward, indicating a reduction in left ventricular diastolic function. In another study comparing metabolic parameters during paired symptom-limited exercise stress tests, peak oxygen uptake and oxygen pulse were lower when a P wave was followed by a paced ventricular contraction than when it was followed by an intrinsic ventricular contraction, indicating a decrease in myocardial reserve.[234]

It has been shown in dog models that the asynchronous electrical activation produced by ventricular pacing results in a redistribution of mechanical work, oxygen demand, and blood supply. Delhaus and coauthors[239] demonstrated that pressure-sacromere length, myocardial blood flow, and oxygen uptake were significantly lower in early compared with late activated areas during left ventricular or right ventricular pacing. In another study,[240] epicardial fiber-strain and epicardial blood flow were compared during right atrial, right

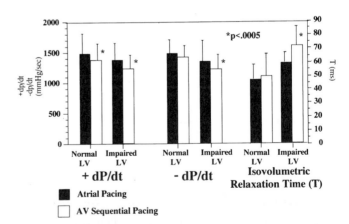

Figure 14–37. Hemodynamic effects of atrial and AV sequential pacing in patients with normal and impaired left ventricular (LV) systolic function. The positive dP/dt is significantly diminished in both groups of patients with AV sequential pacing compared with atrial pacing. However, the negative dP/dt is significantly lowered, and the isovolumetric relaxation time is significantly higher during AV sequential pacing compared with atrial pacing only in patients with impaired left ventricular systolic function. +dP/dt, maximal rate of rise in the left ventricular pressure; −dP/dt, maximal rate of decline in left ventricular pressure; T, isovolumetric relaxation time. *$P < .0005$. (From Bedotto JB, Grayburn PA, Black WH, et al: Alterations in left ventricular relaxation during atrioventricular pacing in humans. J Am Coll Cardiol 15:658, 1990. Reprinted with permission from the American College of Cardiology.)

ventricular outflow and left ventricular apical pacing in open-chest dogs. There was a homogenous distribution of fiber-strain and blood flow during atrial pacing. In contrast, during ventricular pacing, fiber-strain was reduced (as low as 13% of values during atrial pacing) in early activated ventricular regions and increased (as high as 268% of values during atrial pacing) in late activated areas. Similarly, there was a nonhomogenous pattern of epicardial blood flow during ventricular pacing, with early activated areas receiving about 80% blood flow measured during atrial pacing and late activated regions receiving up to 142% of blood flow during atrial pacing.

There is some evidence that changes in myocardial mass may occur in response to a nonhomogenous distribution of mechanical work, with thinning in early activated areas compared with later activated areas.[241] After 3 months of epicardial left ventricular pacing in dogs, there was a 20% decrease in echocardiographic thickness of the early activated anterior wall without an overall change in left ventricular cavity dimension or septal thickness. The reduction in wall thickness was observed in the segment in which the pacing electrode was located and to a lesser extent in adjacent areas activated slightly later. In the same publication, the investigators reported the results of 228 patients with left bundle-branch block and found that the early activated septum was significantly thinner than the later activated posterior wall, whereas no differences in regional thickness were observed in control patients. Although it is unclear whether these observations are relevant to patients undergoing chronic right ventricular pacing, there are clinical implications, especially for patients in whom a decrease in regional left ventricular mass may be beneficial (i.e., those with asymmetric septal or apical hypertrophy). Indeed, Fananapazir and associates[162] reported a reduction in the thickness of the ventricular septum by more than 4 mm in 23% of hypertrophic obstructive cardiomyopathy with long-term AV sequencial pacing. Early activation of the septum with a regional decrease in mechanical load and blood supply may play a role in the regional reduction of cardiac mass observed.

The potential adverse hemodynamic consequences of a ventricular contraction induced by right ventricular apical pacing are summarized in Figure 14–38. Although an intrinsic ventricular contraction appears to be necessary for optimal cardiac performance, the clinical significance as it applies to cardiac pacing remains controversial. Reports of patients experiencing symptoms related to the inhomogeneity of ventricular contraction during AV sequential pacing are rare. Some advocate programming a long AV delay interval to allow intrinsic conduction, but this must be weighed against the deleterious hemodynamic effects of a nonphysiologically long AV delay interval should intrinsic atrioventricular conduction fail. The relative importance of AV timing and synchronicity of ventricular contraction may vary among patients. The ability of either factor to affect pacemaker hemodynamics in the individual patient should be recognized. Although in many paced patients, these factors may be of minor clinical importance, one or the other factor may significantly influence hemodynamics and produce clinical symptoms in a given patient.

■ MULTISITE CARDIAC PACING

Reports have been made of temporary[242, 243] and permanent[244–246] multisite cardiac pacing devised to reduce the degree of atrial or ventricular electromechanical dys-synchrony (or both) by modifying the pathways of depolarization produced by conventional right atrial and right ventricular apical pacing. Multisite pacing includes techniques that involve pacing or sensing (or both) from more than one site in a given chamber or simultaneously in different chambers. Pacing from more than one site in the same chamber is termed *bifocal* or *multifocal* atrial or ventricular pacing, whereas pacing involving sites in both atria or both ventricles is referred to as *biatrial* or *biventricular* pacing. In most instances, the technical aspects of multisite pacing involve adaptations of traditional leads and pulse generators. The indications for multisite pacing are not yet clearly defined but may evolve into an important therapeutic option in specific subgroups of patients.

To date, multisite pacing has been described in a relatively small number of patients with a variety of conditions. Many reports exist in abstract form only, and the follow-up period is limited. Permanent multisite pacing has been used after cardiac transplantation to synchronize activity of the donor atrium with that of the recipient's intrinsic atrial activity.[247] Daubert and colleagues[248] introduced permanent bi-atrial pacing for the treatment of severe interatrial or intra-atrial conduction delay in patients with sick sinus syndrome. Simultaneous synchronous pacing from the right atrial appendage and left atrium through the coronary sinus improved hemodynamics by providing a more optimal mechanical AV delay on the left side of the heart. In addition, biatrial pacing was found to reduce the incidence of atrial tachyarrhythmias, especially type II atrial flutter. In patients with intact AV conduction, these investigators accomplished biatrial pacing with a single- or dual-chamber pulse generator programmed to the AAT mode. In patients with AV block, one atrial lead (the cathode) was connected to the other (the anode) by a Y connector to form a bipole and introduced into the atrial port

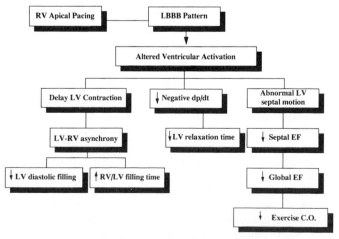

Figure 14–38. Potential deleterious hemodynamic consequences of a ventricular contraction induced by right ventricular apical pacing. (Adapted from Grines CL, Bashore TM, Boudoulas H, et al: Functional abnormalities in isolated left bundle branch block. The effect of interventricular asynchrony. Circulation, 79:845, 1989.)

of a conventional bipolar DDD pacemaker. A right ventricular apical lead was interfaced with the pacemaker to achieve "triple-chamber pacing." Saksena and coworkers[249] have described bifocal atrial pacing using a DDD pacemaker for control of paroxysmal atrial fibrillation.

Attempts to improve ventricular electromechanical synchronization have included bifocal ventricular pacing (from two right ventricular sites) and biventricular pacing in which the RV site is not necessarily the RV apex (i.e., right ventricle outflow–left ventricular pacing). Foster and colleagues[242] studied the acute hemodynamic effects of atriobiventricular pacing in postoperative patients who had epicardial electrodes placed in the right atrium and anterior paraseptal regions of the right ventricle and left ventricle at the time of coronary artery bypass grafting. Compared with atrial pacing, atrial–right ventricular pacing, or atrial–left ventricular pacing, atriobiventricular pacing increased the cardiac index and decreased systemic vascular resistance. A programmed AV delay interval of 150 msec was used for all modes of pacing. The investigators suggested that the hemodynamic advantage of atriobiventricular pacing may be due to a combination of factors, including more effective wall motion of the ventricular septum, more favorable timing between atrial and ventricular contraction, and neurohormonal or baroreceptor reflexes. The fact that atriobiventricular pacing was hemodynamically superior to atrial pacing with similar PR interval suggests that factors other than wall motion alone may be operative.

Saxon and colleagues[243] demonstrated improvement in left ventricular function and coordination of segmental ventricular contraction with temporary biventricular pacing in 11 patients with moderately severe left ventricular impairment undergoing coronary revascularization or valve surgery. Epicardial pacing wires were placed in the right ventricular apex (RVA), left ventricular apex (LVA), and right ventricular outflow tract (RVOT). The ventricle was paced in random order from the RVA, RVOT, LVA, LVA + RVA, and RVOT + LVA. The percentage of fractional area change as measured by transesophageal echocardiography improved significantly compared with baseline sinus rhythm with simultaneous RVA and LVA pacing but not with ventricular pacing from other sites (Fig. 14–39). The QRS duration produced by simultaneous RVA and LVA pacing was not significantly different from native QRS duration, whereas pacing from all other sites resulted in longer QRS intervals (Fig. 14–40). Phase analysis of transesophageal images revealed resequencing of segmental left ventricular activation and contraction compared with baseline ventricular activation. Although none of these patients had bundle-branch block, baseline activation may have been abnormal owing to myocardial scarring, hypertrophy, or fibrosis. The authors postulated that despite the lack of atrial synchrony in this acute temporary pacing study, ventricular activation improved with biventricular apical pacing as a result of a more coordinated and effective ventricular contraction. In this study, pacing the right ventricular outflow tract alone or in combination with left ventricular apical pacing resulted in a prolonged QRS interval and no improvement in global left ventricular function compared with baseline. The authors attributed the lack of improvement to the fact that with right ventricular outflow tract pacing, more ventricular activation occurs by spread through the myocardium than through the fascicles of

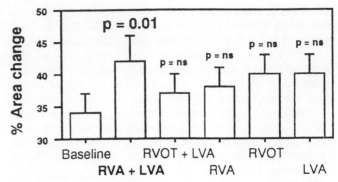

Figure 14–39. The percentage of left ventricular fractional shortening improved significantly with simultaneous right and left ventricular apical pacing when compared with baseline sinus rhythm, but not with other paced sites. RVA, right ventricular apex; RVOT, right ventricular outflow tract; LVA, left ventricular apex; RVA + LVA, simultaneous right and left ventricular apex. RVOT + LVA, simultaneous right ventricular outflow and left ventricular apex. (From Saxon LA, Kerwin WF, Cahalan MK: Acute effects of intraoperative multisite ventricular pacing on left ventricular function and activation/contraction sequence in patients with depressed ventricular function. J Cardiovasc Electrophysiol 9:13, 1998.)

the specialized conduction system. Conversely, biventricular apical pacing results in earlier activation of the fascicles, earlier recruitment of critical mass of myocardium on either side of the septum, and more rapid spread of depolarization through the myocardium.

In small, uncontrolled series, some authors have reported remarkable clinical improvements using permanent dual-chamber pacing with a short AV interval in patients with dilated cardiomyopathy and no traditional indication for pacing.[163–165, 250] Other subsequent studies have reported no significant hemodynamic or clinical improvement or even a deterioration in patients with a similar degree of heart failure.[251–253] One explanation for these conflicting results is that in some patients with severe left ventricular dysfunction, the altered mechanical activation sequence and delay in left ventricular contraction caused by right ventricular pacing may be deleterious and offset any potential benefit caused by improvement in AV timing, prolongation of the diastolic filling time, or reduction in diastolic mitral regurgitation. Case reports and small series have reported the technical feasibility of permanent atriobiventricular and biatrial-biventricular pacing in patients with dilated cardiomyopathy.[244, 246]

Cazeau and colleagues[245] reported the first prospective trial of atrial synchronous biventricular pacing in patients with end-stage dilated cardiomyopathy. All patients underwent acute hemodynamic studies comparing unifocal right ventricular pacing (from either the right ventricular apex or outflow tract) with biventricular pacing (from the left ventricular and right ventricular apex or from the left ventricle and right ventricular outflow tract). There was a significant acute hemodynamic improvement with biventricular pacing that was independent of AV delay optimization or the site of right ventricular pacing. The optimal right ventricular site was equally likely to be the right ventricular apex or the right ventricular outflow tract in combination with left ventricular pacing. Interestingly, most patients had the same

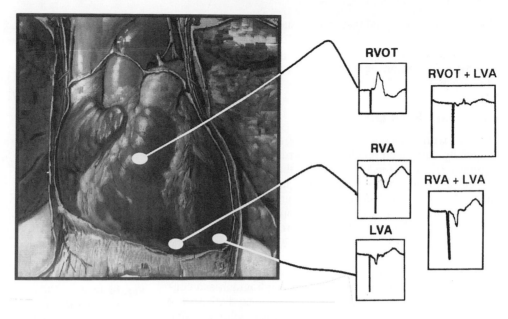

Figure 14–40. Illustration of the placement of epicardial pacing wires and the frontal plain QRS complex (lead II) resulting from pacing from various pacing sites. Abbreviations are the same as in Figure 14–39. (From Saxon LA, Kerwin WF, Cahalan MK: Acute effects of intraoperative multisite ventricular pacing on left ventricular function and activation/contraction sequence in patients with depressed ventricular function. J Cardiovasc Electrophysiol 9:13, 1988.)

optimal AV delay with standard dual-chamber pacing as with atrial synchronous biventricular pacing. The lack of difference is difficult to explain because it would be expected that biventricular pacing would shorten interventricular conduction compared with standard dual-chamber pacing delays, resulting in shorter optimal AV delay intervals. Based on the acute study results, the configuration of pre-existing pacemakers was modified or new systems implanted to achieve biventricular pacing that was atrial synchronous.[245] Biventricular pacing resulted in a mean 25% improvement in cardiac index, a mean 77% decrease in pulmonary capillary wedge pressure, and a 26% reduction in V-wave amplitude, suggesting a decrease in the amount of mitral regurgitation. In patients surviving longer than 4 months, their NYHA function class improved from class IV to class II. In long-term follow-up, cardiac index was shown to decrease by 15% when multisite pacing was temporarily discontinued, indicating a sustained hemodynamic advantage of this type of pacing. In patients undergoing scintigraphic evaluation, four of five showed abnormal activation sequence during standard pacing, which normalized with biventricular pacing. Systolic contraction times were shorter with biventricular compared with right ventricular stimulation, indicating enhanced inotropy.

In an attempt to clarify the mechanisms for hemodynamic improvement from standard dual-chamber pacing or biventricular pacing in congestive heart failure, Auricchio and Salo[250] performed acute pacing studies in patients with class II to IV congestive heart failure. Measurements of conduction time revealed normal intra-atrial conduction during sinus rhythm in all patients and wide variation between in the interventricular conduction times and left heart AV mechanical delays among patients. In most patients, the site of pacing significantly affected hemodynamics, although the optimal pacing site varied among patients. At the optimal pacing site, patients had an increase in mean pulse pressure compared with sinus rhythm. Maximum aortic pulse pressure was achieved when the atrium was sensed rather than paced owing to increased interatrial conduction times with atrial

pacing. Patients benefited acutely from individually optimizing pacing, with increased diastolic filling time, optimization of left ventricular mechanical atrial ventricular delay, and improvement of intraventricular activation all playing potentially important roles.

Multisite pacing poses a technical challenge with the current technology in pulse generators available.[246] In addition, our current technical terminology, including pacing modes and codes and description of polarity, does not adequately describe multisite pacing. Pacing between two widely separated intracardiac sites (cathode and anode) joined by a Y connector represents a hybrid system that cannot be accurately described by the traditional terminology of unipolar and bipolar. This type of pacing decreases pacemaker longevity because of high acute and chronic pacing thresholds. The future development of practical systems for multisite pacing will require refinement or advances in lead and pulse generator technology. Smaller leads with lower thresholds will be necessary to achieve reliable chronic stimulation from unconventional sites. A prototype dual-chamber device has already been designed that promotes ventricular resynchronization during pacing and sensing through the use of a dedicated triggered mode.[246] The ability to maximize the hemodynamic benefit of multisite pacing individually will require a wide range of programmable options in regard to AV timing intervals. Although the indications are not yet established, the potential applications of this new method of pacing, particularly in patients with congestive heart failure and intraventricular conduction abnormalities, is encouraging and warrants further investigation.

■ INFLUENCE OF UNDERLYING HEART DISEASE ON PACING HEMODYNAMICS

Underlying cardiac disease affects the hemodynamics of pacing and influences the relative benefit of pacing mode. In certain acute conditions, such as myocardial infarction or aortic insufficiency, and after cardiac surgery, temporary pacing may be critical in stabilizing hemodynamics. In addition, attention to special parameters, such as AV delay interval, rate, and the sequence of ventricular depolarization during temporary or permanent pacing, may be extremely important in optimizing hemodynamics in specific cardiac conditions.[59, 60, 161–165, 254–275]

Ischemic Heart Disease

Patients with ischemic heart disease who require pacing, especially those with previous myocardial infarction, benefit significantly from modes of pacing that maintain AV synchrony compared with VVI pacing alone.[59, 62, 79, 254–261] In angiographic volume studies, Hamby and colleagues[138] demonstrated that most patients with coronary artery disease have a higher atrial contribution to resting stroke volume than healthy subjects (33% versus 20%; $P < .05$). The highest atrial contribution to ventricular filling was noted in patients with the lowest stroke volume and ejection fraction. The presence of cardiomegaly on chest radiograph and congestive heart failure were clinical factors predictive of a relatively greater atrial contribution to stroke volume. Using a catheter tip micromanometer, Matsuda and colleagues[137] evaluated left atrial function in patients with and without remote myocardial infarction and determined that the ratio of active atrial emptying to left ventricular stroke volume and left atrial work was greater in patients with previous myocardial infarction.

Valero[254] reported clinical observations in acute myocardial infarction and noted that damaged hearts depend on atrial contribution to optimize end-diastolic volume and cardiac output. Unlike patients with normal left ventricular systolic function, who can compensate for effects of bradycardia and loss of AV synchrony by augmenting stroke volume and contractility, the loss of AV synchrony in acute myocardial infarction patients can result in severe hemodynamic impairment and systemic hypotension. This is particularly true in individuals suffering from a myocardial infarction with right ventricular involvement. The clinical syndrome of right ventricular infarction consists of electrocardiographic and echocardiographic evidence of right ventricular dysfunction associated with low cardiac output, hypotension, or shock.[255] The pathogenesis of the diminished cardiac output is attributed to diminished left ventricular filling resulting from right ventricular systolic dysfunction and the constraining effects of the pericardium. Maintenance of adequate cardiac output is critically dependent on maintaining adequate preload, and therapy includes aggressive administration of volume. Bradycardia and complete AV block caused by ischemia in the distribution of the right coronary artery are relatively common; temporary pacing is required in 45% to 75% of reported cases of right ventricular infarction.[256–258] Bradycardia, as well as the loss of atrial contribution to preload, further diminishes cardiac hemodynamics, and ventricular pacing alone is often insufficient in restoring systemic blood pressure. Temporary AV sequential pacing has been shown to reverse hypotension and shock in right ventricular infarction complicated by AV dissociation[257] (Fig. 14–41). The increases in systolic blood pressure, cardiac output, and stroke volume achieved with AV sequential pacing were significantly greater than with ventricular pacing. The relative timing of atrial and ventricular contraction is crucial in influencing left ventricular filling in right ven-

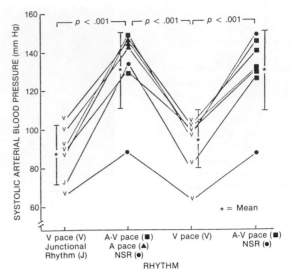

Figure 14–41. Effect of restoration of AV synchrony on systolic arterial blood pressure in patients with right ventricular infarction and complete heart block. The systolic blood pressure is significantly higher with AV sequential pacing compared with the underlying junctional rhythm or ventricular pacing. (From Love JC, Haffajee CI, Gore JM, Alpert JS: Reversibility of hypotension and shock by atrial or atrioventricular sequential pacing in patients with right ventricular infarction. Am Heart J 108:5, 1984.)

tricular infarction. With AV sequential pacing, atrial contraction during ventricular diastole increases the space in the pericardial cavity and enhances diastolic filling.[256] With AV dys-synchrony during ventricular pacing, left ventricular volume is impaired because of asynchronous atrial and ventricular contraction within a limited pericardial space.

Several studies have compared physiologic pacing modes to VVI pacing in patients requiring temporary pacing during acute left ventricular myocardial infarction and found AV sequential pacing to augment cardiac output by about 25% over that produced by VVI pacing alone.[59, 79, 259] In addition, Chamberlain and colleagues[59] demonstrated that a relatively short AV delay of 50 to 100 msec appears to be optimal during temporary pacing in acute myocardial infarction. This is possibly due to the relatively higher catecholamine levels and increased atrial rates during the acute infarction period. Murphy and colleagues[259] compared temporary dual-chamber pacing with fixed-rate ventricular pacing and ventricular pacing matched to the atrial rate that was tracked during DDD pacing in patients with acute myocardial infarction and high-degree AV block. Dual-chamber pacing resulted in enhanced cardiac output, increased systolic blood pressure, and reduced right atrial pressure compared with the patient's spontaneous escape rhythm, fixed-rate ventricular pacing, or ventricular pacing matched to the atrial tracked rate.

There is evidence that the hemodynamic superiority of AV sequential pacing to VVI pacing persists beyond the acute myocardial infarction period in patients with ischemic heart disease. Rahimtoola and coworkers[62] demonstrated that atrial systole made a larger contribution to left ventricular end-diastolic volume and pressure and left ventricular stroke volume in patients 3 to 6 weeks after myocardial infarction compared with healthy control subjects. Although the benefit of preserving AV synchrony was noted regardless of the degree of impairment in left ventricular function, the greatest relative benefit occurred in patients with low cardiac output and normal left ventricular end-diastolic volume. In comparing AOO, DVI, and VVI pacing modes in patients with ischemic heart disease, Shefer and coworkers[260] showed AOO mode to be associated with the highest and VVI pacing with the lowest radionuclide indices of left ventricular function. At rates exceeding 100 bpm, left ventricular function deteriorated, probably because of pacing-induced ischemia, and the authors cautioned against higher pacing rates in patients with coronary artery disease. Although in theory modes of pacing that allow physiologic increases in heart rate may increase myocardial oxygen consumption and exacerbate angina, most data indicate that DDD pacing is superior to fixed-rate ventricular pacing in alleviating angina.[173, 193, 261] This is probably because the improvement in cardiac output and augmentation of coronary artery blood flow outweigh the increased oxygen demand associated with the increase in heart rate (Fig. 14–42). Also, the compensatory mechanisms of increased contractility and left ventricular dilation associated with increasing cardiac output in VVI pacing may result in increased myocardial oxygen consumption and thus worsen angina.

Temporary Pacing Following Cardiac Surgery

Hartzler and coworkers[60] demonstrated that temporary AAI pacing and DVI pacing were superior to ventricular pacing alone in patients with and without postoperative heart block after cardiac surgery. They further demonstrated that this subgroup was extremely sensitive to changes in AV delay interval, and even small changes in AV delay interval resulted in significant changes in cardiac output. As with acute myocardial infarction patients, the optimal AV delay interval in patients after cardiac surgery was shorter than normally reported. In fact, in five of eight patients with intact AV conduction, an increase in cardiac output at AV delay intervals shorter than the patient's intrinsic AV delay interval was noted. Elevated catecholamines and changes in diastolic compliance induced by surgery may account for this observation.

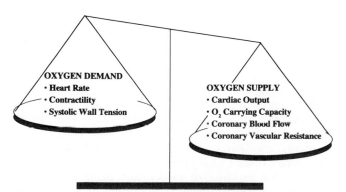

Figure 14–42. Factors affecting the balance of oxygen supply and demand in patients with coronary artery disease. Although physiologic pacing results in an increase in heart rate that raises oxygen demand, it is outweighed by the higher cardiac output and oxygen supply in most patients.

Acute Aortic Insufficiency

Acute severe aortic insufficiency is associated with a marked elevation in left ventricular diastolic pressure, which may exceed left atrial pressure and result in mitral valve closure during diastole. Rapid temporary AAI and AV sequential pacings have been reported as a method of stabilizing patients with acute aortic insufficiency until definitive intervention can be performed.[262, 263] The mechanism by which rapid pacing improves hemodynamics involves shortening of diastole and therefore regurgitation, without altering forward flow. Meyer and colleagues[263] measured thermodilution cardiac output during incremental atrial pacing at rates of 72 to 140 bpm in a group of patients with severe acute aortic insufficiency. They reported that atrial pacing at a mean of 120 bpm resulted in optimal hemodynamics with a 50% reduction in left ventricular end-diastolic pressure, 43% reduction in pulmonary capillary wedge pressure, and 12% increase in cardiac index. They further demonstrated that the interval from the R wave on the electrocardiogram to the diastolic mitral valve closure point on the M-mode echocardiogram closely correlated with optimal pacing interval, allowing prediction of the optimal pacing rate in individual patients with acute aortic insufficiency.

Dilated Cardiomyopathy

The role of cardiac pacing in the treatment of dilated cardiomyopathy patients without conventional indications for cardiac pacing is controversial.[264–266] Initial enthusiasm sparked by reports[163–165, 267] of impressive hemodynamic and clinical improvement in small series of patients with dilated cardiomyopathy has been diminished by the lack of convincing benefit in subsequent studies, including a recent randomized, double-blind, crossover study.[251–253] In the early 1990s, Hochleitner and associates[163] reported dramatic hemodynamic and clinical improvement in a group of 16 patients with severe, medically refractory idiopathic dilated cardiomyopathy treated with AV sequential pacing at an AV delay interval of 100 msec. Within 3 weeks of instituting pacing, LVEF increased significantly and was associated with an improvement in NYHA symptomology, diminished cardiothoracic ratio on chest radiograph, a decrease in right and left atrial size, and an increase in systolic and diastolic blood pressure. Normalization of heart rate occurred such that the heart rate increased in patients with baseline bradycardia and decreased in those with baseline tachycardia. Fractional shortening by M-mode echocardiography remained the same; thus, the striking improvement appeared to be related to factors influencing preload and afterload rather than changes in heart rate or contractility. The improvements in patients' symptoms persisted over the 1-year follow-up period. Although four patients died, none succumbed to cardiac pump failure. Limitations of the study included a small number of patients and the lack of a randomized controlled design.

Although the magnitude of pacing-induced improvement has not been duplicated in subsequent studies, the suggestion that artificial manipulation of the AV contraction sequence may improve the hemodynamics of dilated cardiomyopathy is provocative (Fig. 14–43). Due to dilated chambers and diffuse myocardial fibrosis, patients with dilated cardiomyopathy often have conduction abnormalities resulting in long

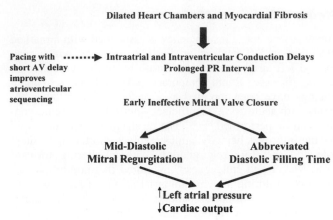

Figure 14–43. Proposed mechanism by which dual-chamber pacing with short AV delay interval improves hemodynamics in dilated cardiomyopathy. Myocardial fibrosis causes conduction abnormalities, which create unfavorable atrioventricular sequences. Early and ineffective mitral valve closure occurs, resulting in abbreviated diastolic filling time and mid-diastolic valvular regurgitation. Elevated left atrial pressure and decreased cardiac output result. Dual-chamber pacing with a short AV delay improves atrioventricular synchrony, abolishing mid-diastolic mitral regurgitation and prolonging diastolic filling.

PR intervals, intra-atrial conduction delays, and intraventricular conduction delays. Disturbances in the electromechanical AV contraction sequence may result in adverse hemodynamics, such as abbreviated diastolic filling times and mid-diastolic mitral regurgitation.[268, 269] Diastolic mitral regurgitation has been demonstrated by prolonging the PQ interval in patients with implanted DDD pacemakers, and an inverse correlation between the critical PQ interval that induces diastolic mitral regurgitation and the pulmonary capillary wedge pressure has been described.[270–272] Thus, patients with dilated cardiomyopathy and high pulmonary capillary wedge pressures may have significant amounts of diastolic mitral regurgitation at relatively short AV delay intervals. The concept of artificial shortening of the AV delay interval with dual-chamber pacing is, therefore, an attractive hypothesis explaining its apparent benefit in some patients.

Brecker and associates[164] evaluated ventricular filling and cardiac output by Doppler echocardiography during dual-chamber pacing at varying AV delay intervals in 12 patients with dilated cardiomyopathy and abbreviated diastolic filling times due to AV valvular regurgitation. The duration of presystolic mitral and tricuspid regurgitation was significantly diminished at shorter AV delay intervals, with accompanying increases in left ventricular and right ventricular filling times. For each 50-msec reduction in AV delay interval, the left ventricular filling time increased by 35 msec in patients with mitral regurgitation and right ventricular filling time by 30 msec in patients with tricuspid regurgitation. At short AV delay intervals, there was an increase in cardiac output, exercise duration, and maximum oxygen consumption and a decrease in subjective symptoms. In an acute pacing study, Auricchio and colleagues[250] optimized the pacing site and AV delay in nine patients with severe congestive heart failure. The optimal pacing site was equally likely to be the left ventricular apex as the right ventricular apex. The intraventricular conduction delay and right and left electrical

AV delay varied considerably within the patient population, as did the left heart mechanical AV delay interval. Because of long intra-atrial conduction delays with atrial pacing, modes in which the atrium was sensed rather than paced (VDD) appeared to be more hemodynamically beneficial than atrial pacing. Left ventricular atrial synchronous pacing at appropriately short AV delay intervals significantly increased mitral (by 102 msec) or tricuspid (by 34 msec) filling time compared with sinus rhythm.

The prolongation of diastolic filling time does not necessarily correlate with hemodynamic or clinical improvement in patients with dilated cardiomyopathy. Both acute[251] and long-term studies[252–253] using temporary and permanent pacing, respectively, have demonstrated no significant improvement, and even a hemodynamic deterioration in some dilated cardiomyopathy patients with DDD pacing despite significant lengthening of diastolic filling times. In an acute study using VDD pacing at short AV delay intervals of 100 msec and 60 msec in patients with severe cardiomyopathy, Innes and coworkers[251] reported a decrease in stroke volume in cardiac index despite prolongation of diastolic filling time. The most significant decrease occurred with VDD pacing at an AV delay interval of 60 msec, and the decrease in stroke volume was inversely related to baseline diastolic filling time. The authors emphasized that the difference between their results and those of previous studies reporting hemodynamic benefits may be secondary to patient selection. In the study by Innes and colleagues,[251] only 4 of 12 patients had abbreviated baseline diastolic filling times (less than 200 msec) during sinus rhythm. In contrast, the study by Brecker and colleagues[164] specifically selected patients with either right or left baseline diastolic filling times of less than 200 msec, thus increasing the likelihood that AV sequential pacing with short AV delay interval may improve hemodynamics.

Studies of chronic AV sequential pacing in patients with dilated cardiomyopathy have also failed to show a significant hemodynamic benefit. Linde and colleagues[253] found no significant improvement in NYHA functional class, stroke volume, cardiac output, ejection fraction, or quality of life assessed 1, 3, and 6 months after permanent dual-chamber pacing with Doppler-guided optimization of AV delay interval in a group of patients with severe dilated cardiomyopathy. The lack of benefit was noted despite a short-term improvement in stroke volume and cardiac output measured 1 day after pacemaker implantation and a significant sustained increase in diastolic filling time throughout the duration of the study. Although the study was nonrandomized and contained small numbers of patients, it suggests that acute hemodynamic improvement does not necessarily predict long-term benefit in this group of patients. It should be noted that the mean baseline diastolic filling time during sinus rhythm in this study was 278 ± 65 msec and therefore the results may not be applicable to patients with more abbreviated diastolic filling times.

In the first prospective randomized double-blind trial, Gold and associates[252] found no significant improvement in cardiac output, pulmonary capillary, wedge pressure, ejection fraction, or NYHA class during a 4- to 6-week period of VDD pacing with an AV delay interval of 100 msec compared with a crossover period of sinus rhythm with backup VVI pacing at 40 bpm in patients with dilated cardiomyopathy. The study did not report diastolic filling times, but the mean PR interval of the group was 214 msec, and 9 of 12 patients had an abnormally prolonged PR interval, suggesting that this patient population would potentially benefit from VDD pacing with short AV delay interval. As in all previous studies, the number of patients included was relatively small; in addition, the AV delay intervals were not individually optimized, and diastolic filling times were not reported. Despite these limitations, it does not appear that the routine use of atrial synchronous pacing with short AV delay interval as a primary therapy for congestive heart failure is justified. It is possible, however, that specific subgroups of patients with dilated cardiomyopathy may benefit from AV sequential pacing with a shortened AV delay.

In an acute hemodynamic study, Nishimura and associates[273] from the Mayo Clinic demonstrated a hemodynamic benefit in patients with dilated cardiomyopathy and prolonged PR intervals during sinus rhythm (mean, 283 ± 51 msec) but not in those with normal PR intervals (mean, 155 ± 36 msec). In the subgroup with long PR intervals, the cardiac output increased by a mean of 38% with AV sequential pacing compared with sinus rhythm, whereas the cardiac output decreased by 23% during AV sequential pacing in patients with normal PR intervals at baseline. In those with long PR intervals, the baseline diastolic filling time tended to be abbreviated, and it was increased significantly during AV sequential pacing at the optimal AV delay, which varied between 60 and 180 msec in individual patients (Fig. 14–44). There was a direct relationship between the percentage of change in cardiac output with AV sequential pacing and the percentage increase in diastolic filling time. Diastolic mitral

regurgitation, when present in the baseline state, was eliminated during AV sequential pacing (Fig. 14–45). In marked contrast, in the subgroup of patients with normal baseline PR intervals, there was a decrease in cardiac output with no significant change in diastolic filling time. None of the patients with normal PR intervals demonstrated diastolic mitral regurgitation at baseline or with pacing. Nishimura's study[273] may help to explain the apparent discrepancies between existing studies that examine the hemodynamic effects of AV sequential pacing in dilated cardiomyopathy. All studies reported to date contain a small number of patients; therefore, variation in the patient population studied in terms of underlying heart disease, baseline conduction abnormalities, and diastolic filling time may significantly contribute to conflicting results. Although not proved, it is possible that patients with dilated cardiomyopathy due to nonischemic causes derive deferential benefits from AV sequential pacing compared with those with an ischemic cause.

The original series by Hochleitner and associates[163] reporting a striking improvement with AV sequential pacing contained only idiopathic dilated cardiomyopathy patients. Subsequent studies have contained a mixture of patients with ischemic and nonischemic causes of dilated cardiomyopathy. Although it does not appear that AV sequential pacing with short AV delay intervals universally benefits all patients with dilated cardiomyopathy, some groups of patients with dilated cardiomyopathy and prolonged PR intervals, abbreviated diastolic filling times, or significant diastolic mitral regurgitation may benefit significantly. In patients who already have relatively normal PR intervals and diastolic filling times and no diastolic mitral regurgitation, further abbreviation of the

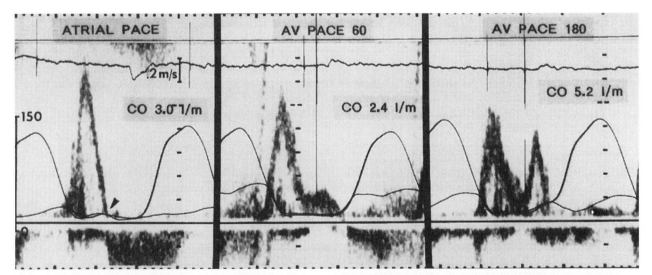

Figure 14–44. Mitral flow velocity curve and simultaneous left atrial and left ventricular pressure curves in a patient with severe left ventricular dysfunction and long PR interval. *A,* Atrial pacing with antegrade native conduction and long AV delay. There is an increase in left ventricular pressure above left atrial pressure during atrial relaxation and mid-diastole *(arrowhead),* resulting in a shortening of diastolic filling time and the onset of diastolic mitral regurgitation. The baseline cardiac output is 3 L/min. *B,* Atrial ventricular pacing at short AV delay interval of 60 msec. Diastolic filling occurs throughout all of diastole. Atrial contraction occurs simultaneous with left ventricular contraction resulting in a reduction in cardiac output and an increase in mean left atrial pressure compared to that seen in panel *A. C,* Atrioventricular pacing at the optimal AV delay interval of 180 msec. There is now an optimal relationship between the mechanical left atrial and left ventricular contraction, so that diastolic filling period is maximized and the mean left atrial pressure is maintained at a low level, resulting in an increase of left ventricular diastolic pressure and improvement in cardiac output to 5.2 L/min. (From Nishimura RA, Hayes DL, Holmes DR: Mechanism of hemodynamic improvement by dual chamber pacing for severe left ventricular dysfunction: An acute Doppler and catheterization hemodynamic study. J Am Coll Cardiol 25:281, 1995.)

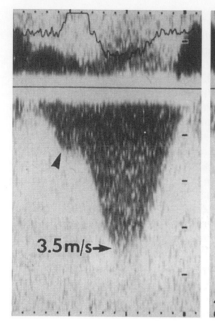
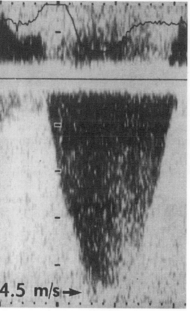

Figure 14–45. Continuous-wave Doppler recording from a patient with dilated cardiomyopathy and prolonged PR interval. *Left,* During native sinus rhythm, diastolic mitral regurgitation is indicated by the *arrowhead.* The peak velocity of mitral regurgitation is low, indicating an elevation of left atrial pressure. *Right,* Pacing in DDD mode at an AV delay interval of 100 msec. Diastolic mitral regurgitation has been abolished, and the peak velocity of mitral regurgitation has increased, indicating a reduction in left atrial pressure velocity, which suggests that dual-chamber pacing reduced the left atrial pressure. (From Glikson M, Espinosa RE, Hayes DL: Expanding indications for permanent pacemakers. Ann Intern Med 123:443, 1995.)

AV delay interval may be detrimental, or any potential benefit may be offset by the deleterious effects of asynchronous ventricular contraction produced by right ventricular pacing. It has been suggested that multisite or biventricular pacing may be of greater hemodynamic benefit in patients with dilated cardiomyopathy than conventional right ventricular pacing (see earlier).[242–246] Although it is too early to advocate the routine use of AV sequential or biventricular pacing in dilated cardiomyopathy, the prospect that the dismal prognosis of severe dilated cardiomyopathy may be favorably influenced by pacing therapy in some patients is promising and warrants further large-scale prospective trials.

Hypertrophic Obstructive Cardiomyopathy

It has long been known that patients with hypertrophic obstructive cardiomyopathy (HOCM) requiring pacing due to bradycardia benefit significantly from pacing modes that preserve AV synchrony compared with ventricular pacing.[274, 275] These patients are extremely sensitive to changes in preload and to conditions that diminish left ventricular filling, resulting in a decrease in left ventricular cavity size and an increase in intraventricular gradient. In addition, these patients have reduced left ventricular diastolic compliance and, therefore, derive proportionately more of their ventricular filling time from atrial systole than patients with normal hearts. The dependence on atrial contribution to cardiac output is manifested clinically by poor tolerance of atrial fibrillation and ventricular pacing in patients with HOCM.

It has been demonstrated that patients with HOCM in the absence of AV or sinus node disease may derive hemodynamic clinical benefits from the abnormal sequencing of ventricular contraction that is produced by right ventricular apical pacing.[161, 162, 276–279] In patients with HOCM, systolic anterior motion of the mitral valve toward the intraventricular septum is associated with left ventricular outflow tract obstruction and often significant mitral regurgitation. Right ventricular pacing causes the septum to move away from the free wall during systole and thus increases the left ventricular outflow tract diameter and reduces the intraventricular gradient (Fig. 14–46). In addition to widening of the left ventricular outflow gradient, apical pacing may also decrease the Venturi effect and decrease the systolic anterior motion of the mitral valve. Because the proposed mechanism of benefit results from the altered sequence of a paced ventricular contraction, AV sequential or atrial synchronous pacing must be performed with a short AV delay interval to ensure ventricular capture.

Uncontrolled studies with relatively small numbers of patients have reported marked decreases in the left ventricu-

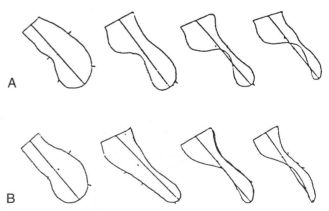

Figure 14–46. Schematic representation of a monoplane ventriculography in a patient with severe hypertrophic obstructive cardiomyopathy during AAI pacing at a rate of 90 bpm *(A)* and during DDD pacing at a rate of 90 bpm and AV delay interval of 50 msec *(B).* Note that the alteration in ventricular contraction pattern produced by right apical pacing results in less left ventricular outflow tract obstruction during systole. (From Jeanrenaud X, Goy JJ, Kappenberger LK: Effects of dual-chamber pacing in hypertrophic obstructive cardiomyopathy. Lancet 339:1318, 1992. © by The Lancet Ltd., 1992.)

lar outflow gradient during AV sequential or atrial synchronous pacing at short AV delay intervals when compared with sinus rhythm or AAI pacing in patients with HOCM.[161, 162, 276–278] All patients studied had significant resting or provocable gradients (or both) and symptoms refractory to medical therapy. In addition to the reduction in left ventricular outflow gradient, improvement in NYHA functional class and quality of life; prolongation of exercise duration; reduction in symptoms, including syncope and presyncope; and low overall and sudden-death 3-year mortality rates have been reported in AV sequentially paced HOCM patients. The reduction in left ventricular outflow tract pressure gradient has been reported to occur acutely when changing from sinus rhythm or AAI pacing to AV sequential pacing, and it persists chronically. The ventricular pacing site appears to be of crucial importance to the reduction of left ventricular outflow tract gradient in patients with HOCM. In one study,[280] temporary right ventricular apical pacing resulted in 60% decrease in outflow tract gradient in 15 patients with HOCM, while high septal pacing resulted in no change in the left ventricular outflow tract gradient. Although most of the improvement in symptoms and gradient is reported to occur in the first few months, Fananapazir and associates[162] have reported that further improvement may be seen in some patients up to 1 year later.

A significant correlation between the acute reduction in the outflow tract gradient by temporary AV sequential pacing before permanent pacemaker implantation and that observed in a long-term follow-up study has been reported.[162, 277] However, discordance between acute and chronic hemodynamic benefit have been observed in individual cases. There does not appear to be a correlation between the magnitude of gradient reduction and the degree of functional improvement.[277] The reduction in pressure gradient has been shown to persist even when AV sequential pacing is acutely discontinued after several months of pacing.[161] Although one study[162] reported a decrease in left ventricular wall thickness in a subset of HOCM patients receiving dual-chamber pacing, changes in left ventricular mass, septal thickness, and shortening faction have not been consistently observed. It is possible that the long-term improvement is due to changes in left ventricular contraction velocity and in metabolic, cellular, or molecular changes due to the altered pattern of ventricular activation or reduction in pressure gradient.

Although most studies have focused on the reduction in pressure gradient, a recent study[278] suggests that myocardial perfusion is altered by dual-chamber pacing in HOCM patients. Previous studies have demonstrated a reduced coronary flow reserve and demonstrable ischemia in patients with hypertrophic cardiomyopathy despite normal epicardial coronary arteries. The impairment in vasodilatory capacity may be related to regional abnormalities and autoregulation, small vessel disease, or reduced coronary artery perfusion due to impairment of relaxation of myocardium during isovolemic and rapid filling phases. Posma and colleagues[278] studied myocardial perfusion by means of nitrogen-13 ammonia and positron emission tomography before and during permanent dual-chamber pacing. During sinus rhythm, baseline perfusion was higher and perfusion reserve lower in hypertrophic cardiomyopathy patients compared with controls. During dual-chamber pacing, there was decreased perfusion at rest and with pharmacologic stress in HOCM patients, reflecting lower oxygen demand and left ventricular pressure. During sinus rhythm, stress perfusion and perfusion reserve were less evenly distributed in hypertrophic cardiomyopathy patients than in controls, and after AV synchronous pacing, stress perfusion and perfusion reserve became more homogenous. The clinical significance and the relationship of these findings to the change in intraventricular gradient is unknown.

Despite initial enthusiasm regarding the role of AV sequential pacing in hypertrophic cardiomyopathy, controversy exists regarding its efficacy and long-term safety, which have not yet been demonstrated in large randomized controlled studies.[279, 281, 282] In an acute hemodynamic study using Doppler echocardiography and high-fidelity pressure measurement during cardiac catheterization, Nishimura and colleagues[281] reported only a 15% reduction in left ventricular outflow tract gradient, with AV sequential pacing and adverse effects on both systolic and diastolic left ventricular function. The authors reported a decrease in cardiac output and peaked dP/dt, increase in mean atrial data pressure, and prolongation of left ventricular relaxation time. Although the most adverse hemodynamics were noted at the shortest AV delay interval, similar changes occurred even at the optimal AV delay interval. Whether these hemodynamic changes may result in long-term deterioration in systolic and or diastolic left ventricular function is not known.

In a double-blind, randomized study,[279] 21 patients with HOCM and dual-chamber pacemakers were randomized to 3 months of AAI or DDD pacing with short AV delay intervals and then crossed over to the alternate pacing mode. A significant reduction in left ventricular outflow tract gradient from baseline and in comparison with AAI pacing was observed in patients during dual-chamber pacing. The quality of life and exercise capacity improved with dual-chamber pacing as compared with baseline, however, were not significantly different than during AAI pacing. Although 63% of patients reported an improvement in symptoms during dual-chamber pacing, 42% reported improvement in symptoms during AAI pacing, suggesting that subjective improvement may partially be due to a placebo effect. In this study, 31% of patients reported no changes in symptoms with dual-chamber pacing, and 5% experienced a worsening of symptoms. The assessment of long-term improvement with dual-chamber pacing and hypertrophic cardiomyopathy may also be complicated by concomitant pharmacologic (calcium-channel blockers, β-blockers, or amiodarone to achieve sufficient slowing of AV conduction) or nonpharmacologic (AV nodal ablation or modification) interventions to ensure right ventricular pacing.

In summary, dual-chamber pacing with short AV delay interval reduces left ventricular outflow tract gradient acutely and chronically in a subset of patients with HOCM who have significant intraventricular gradients and symptoms despite medical treatment. Whether this reduction in gradient correlates with improvement in long-term outcome remains to be determined by large randomized trials. There is little information, but the few existing data suggest that pacing therapy is not beneficial in other subsets of patients, such as those with nonobstructive hypertrophic cardiomyopathy or those with minimal gradients.[283]

■ CHRONIC HEMODYNAMIC EFFECTS OF PACING

Although multiple studies have assessed the acute hemodynamic effects of various pacing modes and rates on left ventricular function and cardiac output, fewer data are available concerning the chronic effects of cardiac pacing. These studies indicate, however, that the hemodynamic advantage of dual-chamber pacing over ventricular pacing persists over long-term follow-up.[74, 83, 169] In a randomized crossover study, Kruse and colleagues[169] compared resting and exercise hemodynamics acutely and after 3 months of ventricular pacing and atrial VDD synchronous pacing. At the end of the period of VDD pacing, cardiac output was significantly higher both at rest and during exercise compared with acute reprogramming to VVI mode and after 3 months of VVI pacing. There was a mean 24% increase in working capacity with chronic VDD pacing compared with chronic VVI pacing. VDD pacing produced a higher exercise cardiac output because of the capacity to increase heart rate, which outweighed the compensatory augmentation in exercise stroke volume observed during chronic VVI pacing. The AV oxygen difference and lactate production were higher during exercise with VVI pacing, indicating less myocardial efficiency and reserve. The heart size as measured by left ventricular angiography was larger after 3 months of ventricular pacing than after 3 months of VDD pacing.

In a 6-week double-blind crossover study, Rediker and associates[83] demonstrated a 43% increase in resting cardiac output, a 25% increase in left ventricular shortening fraction, and a significant increase in exercise duration with physiologic pacing compared with VVI pacing. Faerestrand and Ohm[74] measured Doppler cardiac output during VVI and AV sequential pacing in patients with DDD pacemakers before implantation and at 1, 3, 6, and 12 months after implantation. The hemodynamic superiority of DDD pacing was demonstrated acutely and persisted over 12 months of follow-up. In both modes of pacing, there was a reduction in stroke volume over the first 6 months, which was stable after that time. The authors postulated that before implantation, patients were bradycardic and therefore had compensatory increases in stroke volume that became normal after several months of pacing at higher rates. The decrease in stroke volume and cardiac output with chronic pacing compared with acute hemodynamic measurements after initiation of pacing has been noted by others.

In a similarly designed study, Faerestrand and Ohm[192] assessed Doppler cardiac output as well as M-mode measurements of left ventricular end-diastolic and end-systolic dimension and shortening fraction before and at 1, 3, and 6 months after implantation of a rate-responsive ventricular pacing system. Stroke volume and end-diastolic dimension decreased progressively over the 6-month period, whereas end-systolic dimension remained constant. The shortening fraction decreased from 33% to 27% over the first 6 months, and the greatest reduction in end-diastolic volume and shortening fraction occurred in patients who were not previously paced. The authors suggested that these patients were now able to augment their cardiac output by increasing rate rather than by a compensatory increase in volume and shortening fraction. Thus, these observations may indicate a beneficial effect with increased contractile reserve rather than a deterioration in left ventricular function. Interestingly, the authors observed mitral regurgitation, tricuspid regurgitation, or a combination of mitral and tricuspid regurgitation to persist or develop in 9 of 13, or 69%, of the patients studied. The regurgitation was not quantitated, suggesting the need for further prospective studies assessing the effects of ventricular rate-responsive pacing on AV valvular regurgitation.

Studies assessing the symptoms and quality of life demonstrate the superiority of physiologic pacing over VVI pacing.[83, 193, 284–286] With the exception of prevention of syncope, DDD pacing was superior to fixed-rate VVI pacing in reducing symptoms of dizziness, low cardiac output, congestive heart failure, and angina and in overall sense of well-being.[193] In randomized crossover studies, patients expressing a mode preference invariably have chosen physiologic pacing over VVI pacing. More recently, DDD pacing has been shown to result in significant reduction in symptoms of shortness of breath, dizziness, and palpitations and improvement in cognitive function compared with VVIR pacing in randomized crossover studies assessing the two pacing modes in patients with complete heart block and preserved sinus node function.[287] In patients unable to receive dual-chamber pacing systems, VVIR pacing mode reduces symptoms and improves subjective sense of well-being compared with fixed-rate ventricular pacing.[288, 289]

An increasing amount of data suggest that physiologic pacing results in a lower incidence of permanent atrial fibrillation and thromboembolic complications, lower incidence of congestive heart failure, and lower overall mortality than with ventricular pacing alone.[193–201, 290] In a retrospective study of patients paced for sinus node disease, there was a 1.6 times higher incidence of atrial fibrillation, 2.5 times higher incidence of congestive heart failure, and 2.9-fold increase in mortality in patients paced in the VVI mode compared with the AAI mode.[199] The differences in cardiovascular morbidity and overall mortality between the groups tended to increase with time. In another study, Hesselson and colleagues[201] evaluated 950 patients paced for sick sinus syndrome as well as high-degree heart block and hypersensitive carotid sinus syndrome retrospectively over 12 years. The rate of development of atrial fibrillation was more than twice as high in patients with VVI pacing as in those with dual-chamber pacing. The incidence of atrial fibrillation was especially high in VVI-paced patients with sick sinus syndrome who were older than the age of 70 years. The mortal-

Table 14–10. Patient Characteristics to Consider in Selection of Pacing System

Mechanical and electrical atrial function or arrhythmias (intermittent supraventricular tachycardia, atrial fibrillation)
Presence of retrograde VA conduction
Sinus node function
AV conduction
Medications affecting sinus node and AV function
Possibility of future development of sinus and/or AV node disease
Underlying cardiac disease
    Systolic function
    Diastolic function
Age
Activity level
Concomitant illness

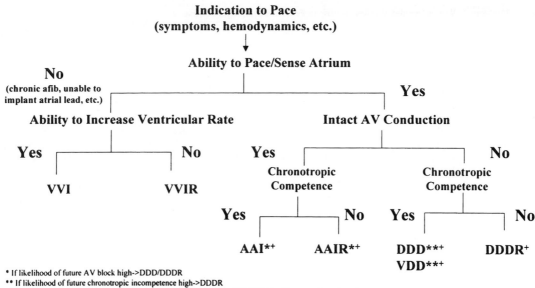

Indication to Pace
(symptoms, hemodynamics, etc.)

Ability to Pace/Sense Atrium

No
(chronic afib, unable to
implant atrial lead, etc.)

Yes

Ability to Increase Ventricular Rate

Intact AV Conduction

Yes   **No**   **Yes**   **No**

VVI   VVIR

Chronotropic
Competence

Chronotropic
Competence

Yes   **No**   **Yes**   **No**

AAI*+   AAIR*+   DDD**+ VDD**+   DDDR+

* If likelihood of future AV block high->DDD/DDDR
** If likelihood of future chronotropic incompetence high->DDDR
\+ If likelihood of intermittent atrial fibrillation high->DDDI mode, or DDD/DDDR with automatic mode switching

Figure 14–47. Algorithm demonstrating the selection of the hemodynamically optimal pacing system for an individual patient. (Adapted from Benditt DG, Milstein S, Beutikofer J, et al: Sensor-triggered, rate-variable cardiac pacing: Current technologies and clinical implications. Ann Intern Med 107:714, 1987.)

ity rate at 7 years was higher in the VVI group than in the DDD and DVI groups. Death occurred more frequently during VVI pacing than during DDD pacing regardless of age at pacemaker implantation or the initial indication for pacing. Although these data appear to show that physiologic pacing is preferable to VVI pacing in terms of mortality and cardiovascular morbidity, it must be emphasized that these studies were retrospective nonrandomized comparisons of the pacing modes.[291] Thus, a selective bias may have existed in terms of selecting VVI pacing mode for patients most prone to atrial fibrillation or those with a limited life expectancy.

OPTIMAL PACING MODE SELECTION

Numerous patient characteristics must be considered in the selection of the optimal pacing system (Table 14–10). The current status of the patient's sinus node and AV node function and the possibility of future development of sinus and AV node disease are important in selection of the most appropriate pacing system. Guidelines for the selection of the optimal pacing system are outlined in Figure 14–47. Although cost-effectiveness and the viability of the patient are important factors, they are not reflected in this algorithm, which illustrates optimal pacing mode selection. Once the decision has been made to implant a permanent pacemaker for symptomatic bradycardia, poor resting or exercise hemodynamics, or other indications, it should be determined whether the patient has intact mechanical and electrical atrial function. If the atrium cannot be reliably paced or sensed because of chronic atrial fibrillation, mechanically silent atrium, or technical difficulty prohibiting atrial lead placement, a ventricular pacing system should be implanted. If the patient is likely to benefit from rate responsiveness, a VVIR system would be preferable to a fixed-rate ventricular

pacing system. If the patient's heart rate increases adequately in response to metabolic stress or the patient has severe unstable angina making rate responsiveness undesirable, a fixed-rate ventricular pacing system may be preferable. If there is intact mechanical and electrical atrial activity and an atrial lead can be placed, implantation of a physiologic pacing system is recommended.[135, 292] If there is intact AV nodal conduction, an atrial pacing system may be placed. In chronotropically competent patients, a fixed-rate AAI system may be adequate; however, in those with chronotropic incompetence, an AAIR pacemaker would provide superior

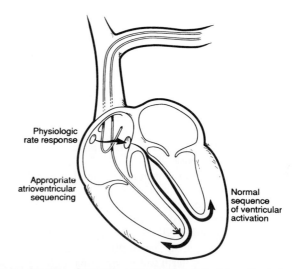

Physiologic
rate response

Appropriate
atrioventricular
sequencing

Normal
sequence
of ventricular
activation

Figure 14–48. Schematic representation of the interaction between the intrinsic conduction system and an implanted dual-chamber pacing pacemaker. The ability of the pacing system to optimize hemodynamics individually is dependent on this interaction. (See text for discussion.)

Table 14–11. Comparison of Various Modes in Their Ability to Provide Physiologic Pacing

Mode	AV Synchrony	Rate Responsiveness	Synchronous Ventricular Contraction
VVI	−	−	−
VVIR	−	+, Effectiveness dependent on sensor used	−
VDD	+, If atrial rate exceeds LRL	+, If sinus node normal	−
DDD	+, Effectiveness may depend on AVDI and URL response	+, If sinus node normal	±, Depends on AVDI and intrinsic PR interval
DDI	±, Only when atrial rate ≤ LRL, otherwise variable PV	−	±, Depends on AVDI and intrinsic PR interval
AAI	+, If AV conduction normal	−	+, Assuming intact AV conduction
AAIR	+, Effectiveness may depend on ability to shorten PR interval in response to atrial pacing rates	+, Effectiveness dependent on sensor used	+, Assuming intact AV conduction
DDDR	+, Effectiveness may depend on AVDI and URL response	+, Effectiveness dependent on sensor used	±, Depends on AVDI and intrinsic AV conduction

+, present; −, absent; AV, atrioventricular; AVDI, programmed atrioventricular delay interval; LRL, lower rate limit; PV, P-wave–V-paced interval; URL, upper rate limit.

hemodynamics. The new development of AV nodal disease in patients paced for sick sinus syndrome is reported to be 1% to 2.8% per year over follow-up periods ranging from 2 to 5 years.[196, 197, 200] If the decision is made to implant an atrial pacing system, the potential for future development of AV nodal disease should be considered. If the patient's disease process or need for medication suggests a future possibility of impaired AV conduction, a DDD or DDDR system would be recommended. If AV nodal conduction is absent or intermittently impaired at the time of the initial implantation, a dual-chamber pacing system should be implanted. In the presence of chronotropic incompetence or a high probability that the patient will develop chronotropic incompetence in the future, a DDDR pacing system may provide optimal hemodynamics compared with DDD pacing. If the patient has adequate sinus node function, a DDD pacing system may be sufficient.

In the decision to implant any physiologic pacing system, the past and future likelihood of intermittent atrial fibrillation or other supraventricular arrhythmias should be considered. If present, a DDDR or DDD system with VVIR mode, DDI mode, or automatic mode-switching capability may be preferable. However, the intermittent loss of AV synchrony with DDI pacing and mode switching must be considered. As a result of the development of single-pass leads with the capability of ventricular pacing from distal tip and atrial sensing from proximal electrodes, VDD pacing has regained popularity. This type of pacing system cannot provide atrial pacing and functions as a VVI unit if the atrial rate falls below the lower rate limit. Therefore, patients with a high likelihood of developing sinus node disease or requiring drugs with negative chronotropic potential are not appropriate candidates for this mode of pacing. In addition, the apparent long-term benefits of AV synchronous pacing in reducing the incidence of atrial fibrillation and embolic stroke have been observed only in dual-chamber systems incorporating atrial pacing capabilities. There are limited data regarding the long-term follow-up of patients with VDD pacing systems, but in one long-term study,[293] about 12% of patients had their pacemakers reprogrammed to VVI mode for supraventricular tachycardia or unsatisfactory atrial sensing over a mean follow-up period of 44 months.

The ability of any pacing system to optimize hemodynamics is dependent on factors related to the individual patient, programmed pacemaker parameters, and physiologic appropriateness of alternative rate sensors used in rate-adaptive pacing modes. The hemodynamic advantages and limitations of available pacing modes are displayed in Table 14–11. The ideal physiologic pacing system reproduces normal cardiac hemodynamics by replicating the rate responsiveness of a normal sinus node, maintaining appropriate AV sequencing over a wide spectrum of heart rates, and preserving rapid synchronous ventricular contraction when possible (Fig. 14–48). It is apparent that the ability of any pacing system to provide optimized hemodynamics is dependent on its interaction with the patient's intrinsic rhythm and conduction system. Our understanding of hemodynamics continues to evolve and lead to advances in pacemaker technology directed at providing even more sophisticated and physiologically appropriate pacing systems.

REFERENCES

1. Wirtzfeld A, Schmidt G, Himmler FC, Stangl K: Physiological pacing: Present status and future developments. PACE 10:41, 1987.
2. Baig MW, Perrins EJ: The hemodynamics of cardiac pacing: Clinical and physiological aspects. Prog Cardiovasc Dis 33:283, 1991.
3. Buckingham TA, Janosik DL, Pearson AC: Pacemaker hemodynamics: Clinical applications. Prog Cardiovasc Dis 34:347, 1992.
4. Harvey W: Movement of Heart and Blood in Animals. An Anatomical Essay (translated by D. Franklin). Oxford, England, Blackwell Scientific, 1957, p 34.
5. Straub H: The diastolic filling of the mammalian heart. J Physiol 40:387, 1910.
6. Wiggers CJ, Katz LN: The contour of the ventricular volume curves under different conditions. Am J Physiol 58:439, 1921–1922.
7. Gesell RA: Auricular systole and its relation to ventricular output. Am J Physiol 29:32, 1911.
8. Gesell RA: Cardiodynamics in heart block as affected by auricular systole, auricular fibrillation, and stimulation of the vagus nerve. Am J Physiol 40:267, 1916.
9. Linden RJ, Mitchell JH: Relation between left ventricular diastolic pressure and myocardial segment length and observations on the contribution of atrial systole. Circ Res 8:1092, 1960.
10. Brockman SK: Dynamic function of atrial contraction in regulation of cardiac performance. Am J Physiol 204:597, 1963.
11. Gilmore JP, Sarnoff SJ, Mitchell JH, Linden RJ: Synchronicity of ventricular contraction: Observations comparing hemodynamic effects of atrial and ventricular pacing. Br Heart J 25:299, 1963.
12. Mitchell JH, Gilmore JP, Sarnoff SJ: The transport function of the atrium: Factors influencing the relation between mean left atrial pres-

sure and left ventricular end diastolic pressure. Am J Cardiol 9:237, 1962.

13. Mitchell JH, Gupta DN, Payne RM: Influence of atrial systole on effective ventricular stroke volume. Circ Res 17:11, 1965.

14. Sarnoff SJ, Gilmore JP, Mitchell JH: Influence of atrial contraction and relaxation on closure of mitral valve: Observations on effects of autonomic nerve activity. Circulation 11:26, 1962.

15. Skinner NS, Mitchell JH, Wallace AG, Sarnoff SJ: Hemodynamic effects of altering the timing of atrial systole. Am J Physiol 205:499, 1963.

16. Kosowsky BD, Scherlag BJ, Damoto AN: Re-evaluation of the atrial contribution to ventricular function: Study using His bundle pacing. Am J Cardiol 21:518, 1968.

17. Payne RM, Stone HL, Engelken EJ: Atrial function during volume loading. J Appl Physiol 31:326, 1971.

18. Linderer T, Chatterjee K, Parmley WW, et al: Influence of atrial systole on the Frank-Starling relation and the end-diastolic pressure-diameter relation of the left ventricle. Circulation 67:1045, 1983.

19. Ogawa S, Dreifus LS, Shenoy PN, et al: Hemodynamic consequences of atrioventricular and ventriculoatrial pacing. PACE 1:8, 1978.

20. Naito M, Dreifus LS, Mardelli TJ, et al: Echocardiographic features of atrioventricular and ventriculoatrial conduction. Am J Cardiol 46:625, 1980.

21. Naito M, Dreifus LS, David B, et al: Reevaluation of the role of atrial systole to cardiac hemodynamics: Evidence for pulmonary venous regurgitation during abnormal atrioventricular sequencing. Am Heart J 105:295, 1983.

22. Williams JF, Sonnenblick EH, Braunwald E: Determinants of atrial contractile force in the intact heart. Am J Physiol 209:1061, 1965.

23. Wallick DW, Martin PJ, Masuda Y, Levy MN: Effects of autonomic activity and changes in heart rate on atrioventricular conduction. Am J Physiol 243:H523, 1982.

24. Ronaszeki A, Ector H, Denef B, et al: Effect of short atrioventricular delay on cardiac output. PACE 13:1728, 1990.

25. Wiggers CJ: The muscular reactions of the mammalian ventricles to artificial surface stimuli. Am J Physiol 73:346, 1925.

26. Fletcher FW, Theilen EO, Lawrence MS, Evans JW: Effect of pacemaker location on cardiac function in complete AV heart block. Am J Physiol 205:1232, 1963.

27. Lister JW, Klotz DH, Jomain SL, et al: Effect of pacemaker site on cardiac output and ventricular activities in dogs in complete heart block. Am J Cardiol 14:494, 1964.

28. Finney JO: Hemodynamic alterations in left ventricular function consequent to ventricular pacing. Am J Physiol 208:275, 1965.

29. Heyndrickx GR, Vantrimport PJ, Rousseau MF, Pouleur H: Effects of asynchrony on myocardial relaxation at rest and during exercise in conscious dogs. Am J Physiol 254:H817, 1988.

30. Walston A, Stair JW, Greenfield JC: Effect of different epicardial ventricular pacing sites on left ventricular function in awake dogs. Am J Cardiol 32:291, 1973.

31. Badke FR, Bolnay P, Covell JW: Effects of ventricular pacing on regional left ventricular performance in the dog. Am J Physiol 238:H858, 1980.

32. Grover M, Glantz SA: Endocardial pacing site affects left ventricular end diastolic volume and performance in intact anesthetized dog. Cir Res 53:72, 1983.

33. Burkhoff D, Oikawa RY, Sagawa K: Influence of pacing site on canine left ventricular contraction. Am J Physiol 251:H428, 1986.

34. Zile MR, Blaustein As, Shimizu G, Gaash WH: Right ventricular pacing reduces the rate of left ventricular relaxation and filling. J Am Coll Cardiol 10:702, 1987.

35. Suga H: Importance of atrial compliance in cardiac performance. Circ Res 35:39, 1974.

36. Brockman SK: Cardiodynamics of complete heart block. Am J Cardiol 16:72, 1965.

37. Brockman SK, Stoney WS: Congestive heart failure and cardiac output in heart block and during pacing. Ann N Y Acad Sci 167:534, 1969.

38. Benchimol A, Li Y, Dimond EG: Cardiovascular dynamics in complete heart block at various heart rates: Effect of exercise at a fixed heart rate. Circulation 30:542, 1964.

39. Sowton E: Hemodynamic studies in patients with artificial pacemakers. Br Heart J 26:737, 1964.

40. Karlöf I, Bevegård S, Ovenfors C: Adaption of the left ventricle to sudden changes in heart rate in patients with artificial pacemakers. Cardiovasc Res 7:322, 1973.

41. Samet P, Bernstein WH, Medow A, Nathan DA: Effect of alterations inventricular rate on cardiac output in complete heart block. Am J Cardiol 14:477, 1964.

42. Rowe GG, Stenlund RR, Thomsen JH, et al: Coronary and systemic hemodynamic effects of cardiac pacing in man with complete heart block. Circulation 40:839, 1969.

43. Mitchell JH, Shapiro W: Atrial function and the hemodynamic consequences of atrial fibrillation in man. Am J Cardiol 23:556, 1969.

44. Philips E, Levine SA: Auricular fibrillation without other evidence of heart disease: Cause of reversible heart failure. Am J Med 7:478, 1949.

45. Kory RC, Meneely GR: Cardiac output in auricular fibrillation with observations on the effects of conversion to normal sinus rhythm. J Clin Invest 30:653, 1951.

46. Shapiro W, Klein G: Alterations in cardiac function immediately following electrical conversion of atrial fibrillation to normal sinus rhythm. Circulation 38:1074, 1968.

47. Samet P, Bernstein W, Levin S: Significance of atrial contribution to ventricular filling. Am J Cardiol 15:195, 1965.

48. Benchimol A, Duenas A, Liggett MS, Dimond EG: Contribution of atrial systole to the cardiac function at a fixed rate and at a variable ventricular rate. Am J Cardiol 16:11, 1965.

49. Carleton RA, Passovoy M, Graettinger JS: The importance of the contribution and timing of left atrial systole. Clin Sci 30:151, 1966.

50. Benchimol A: Significance of the contribution of atrial systole to cardiac function in man. Am J Cardiol 23:568, 1969.

51. Ruskin J, McHale PA, Harley A, Greenfield JC: Pressure flow studies in man: Effect of atrial systole on left ventricular function. J Clin Invest 49:472, 1970.

52. Samet P, Bernstein WH, Nathan DA, Lopez A: Atrial contribution to cardiac output in complete heart block. Am J Cardiol 16:1, 1965.

53. Samet P, Castillo C, Bernstein CWH: Hemodynamic consequences of atrial and ventricular pacing in subjects with normal hearts. Am J Cardiol 18:522, 1966.

54. Samet P, Castillo C, Bernstein WH: Hemodynamic consequences of sequential atrioventricular pacing: Subjects with normal hearts. Am J Cardiol 21:207, 1968.

55. Samet P, Castillo C, Bernstein WH: Hemodynamic sequelae of atrial, ventricular and sequential atrioventricular pacing in cardiac patients. Am Heart J 72:725, 1966.

56. Benchimol A, Ellis JC, Dimond EG: Hemodynamic consequences of atrial and ventricular pacing in patients with normal and abnormal hearts. Am J Med 39:911, 1965.

57. Karlöf I: Hemodynamic effect of atrial triggered versus fixed rate pacing at rest and during exercise in complete heart block. Acta Med Scand 197:195, 1975.

58. Leinbach RC, Chamberlain DA, Kastor JA, et al: A comparison of the hemodynamic effects of ventricular and sequential A-V pacing in patients with heart block. Am Heart J 78:502, 1969.

59. Chamberlain DA, Leinbach RC, Vassaux CE, et al: Sequential atrioventricular pacing in heart block complicating acute myocardial infarction. N Engl J Med 282:577, 1970.

60. Hartzler GO, Maloney JD, Curtis JJ, Barnhorst DA: Hemodynamic benefits of atrioventricular sequential pacing after cardiac surgery. Am J Cardiol 40:232, 1977.

61. Greenberg B, Chatterjee K, Parmley WW, et al: The influence of left ventricular filling pressure on atrial contribution to cardiac output. Am Heart J 98:742, 1979.

62. Rahimtoola SH, Ehsani A, Sinno MZ, et al: Left atrial transport function in myocardial infarction: Importance of its booster pump function. Am J Med 59:686, 1975.

63. Reiter MJ, Hindman MC: Hemodynamic effects of acute atrioventricular sequential pacing in patients with left ventricular dysfunction. Am J Cardiol 49:687, 1982.

64. Fananapazir L, Srinivas V, Bennett DH: Comparison of resting hemodynamic indices and exercise performance during atrial synchronized and asynchronous ventricular pacing. PACE 6:202, 1983.

65. Schuster AH, Nanda NC: Doppler echocardiography and cardiac pacing. PACE 5:607, 1982.

66. Nanda NC, Bhandari A, Barold SS, Falkoff M: Doppler echocardiographic studies in sequential atrioventricular pacing. PACE 6:811, 1983.

67. Zugibe FT, Nanda NC, Barold SS, Akiyama T: Usefulness of Doppler echocardiography in cardiac pacing: Assessment of mitral regurgitation, peak aortic flow velocity and atrial capture. PACE 6:1350, 1983.

68. Coskey RL, Feit TS, Plaia R, Zicari T: AV pacing and LV performance. PACE 6:631, 1983.

69. Boucher CA, Pohost GM, Okada RD, et al: Effect of ventricular pacing on left ventricular function assessed by radionuclide angiography. Am Heart J 106:1105, 1983.

70. Romero LR, Haffajee CI, Levin W, et al: Noninvasive evaluation of ventricular function and volumes during atrioventricular sequential and ventricular pacing. PACE 7:10, 1984.

71. Nitsch J, Seiderer M, Bull U, Luderitz B: Evaluation of left ventricular performance by radionuclide ventriculography in patients with atrioventricular versus ventricular demand pacemakers. Am Heart J 107:906, 1984.

72. Stewart WJ, Dicola VC, Harthorne JW, et al: Doppler ultrasound measurement of cardiac output in patients with physiologic pacemakers: Effects of left ventricular function and retrograde ventriculoatrial conduction. Am J Cardiol 54:308, 1984.

73. Labovitz AJ, Williams GA, Redd RM, Kennedy HL: Noninvasive assessment of pacemaker hemodynamics by Doppler echocardiography: Importance of left atrial size. J Am Coll Cardiol 6:196, 1985.

74. Faerestrand S, Ohm OJ: A time-related study of the hemodynamic benefit of atrioventricular synchronous pacing evaluated by Doppler echocardiography. PACE 8:838, 1985.

75. Leman RB, Kratz JM: Radionuclide evaluation of dual-chamber pacing: Comparison between variable AV intervals and ventricular pacing. PACE 8:408, 1985.

76. Videen JS, Huang SK, Bazgan ID, et al: Hemodynamic comparison of ventricular pacing, atrioventricular sequential pacing, and atrial synchronous ventricular pacing using radionuclide ventriculography. Am J Cardiol 57:1305, 1986.

77. Forfang K, Otterstad JE, Ihlen H: Optimal atrioventricular delay in physiologic pacing determined by Doppler echocardiography. PACE 9:17–20, 1986.

78. Haskell RJ, French WJ: Optimum AV interval in dual-chamber pacemakers. PACE 9:670, 1986.

79. DiCarlo LA, Morady F, Krol RB, et al: The hemodynamic effects of ventricular pacing with and without atrioventricular synchrony in patients with normal and diminished left ventricular function. Am Heart J 114:746, 1987.

80. Faerestrand S, Qie B, Ohm OJ: Noninvasive assessment by Doppler and M-mode echocardiography of hemodynamic responses to temporary pacing and ventriculoatrial conduction. PACE 10:871, 1987.

81. Wish M, Fletcher RD, Gottdiener, JS, Cohen AI: Importance of left atrial timing in the programming of dual-chamber pacemakers. Am J Cardiol 60:566, 1987.

82. Wish M, Gottdiener JS, Cohen AJ, Fletcher RD: M-mode echocardiograms for determination of optimal left atrial timing in patients with dual-chamber pacemakers. Am J Cardiol 61:317, 1988.

83. Rediker DE, Eagle KA, Homma S, et al: Clinical and hemodynamic comparison of VVI versus DDD pacing in patients with DDD pacemakers. Am J Cardiol 61:323, 1988.

84. Pearson AC, Janosik DL, Redd RM, et al: Doppler echocardiographic assessment of the effect of varying atrioventricular delay and pacemaker mode on left ventricular filling. Am Heart J 115:611, 1988.

85. Janosik DL, Pearson AC, Buckingham TA, et al: The hemodynamic benefit of differential atrioventricular delay intervals for sensed and paced atrial events during physiologic pacing. J Am Coll Cardiol 14:499, 1989.

86. Lascault G, Bigonzi F, Frank R, et al: Noninvasive study of dual-chamber pacing by pulsed Doppler: Prediction of the haemodynamic response by echocardiographic measurements. Eur Heart J 10:525, 1989.

87. Mehta D, Gilmour S, Ward DE, Camm AJ: Optimal atrioventricular delay at rest and during exercise in patients with dual-chamber pacemakers: A noninvasive assessment by continuous wave Doppler. Br Heart J 61:161, 1989.

88. Eugene M, Lascault G, Frank R, et al: Assessment of the optimal atrioventricular delay in DDD paced patients by impedance plethysmography. Eur Heart J 10:250, 1989.

89. Janosik DL, Pearson AC, Labovitz AJ: Applications of Doppler echocardiography in cardiac pacing. Echocardiography 8:45, 1991.

90. Masuyama T, Kodama K, Vematsu M, et al: Beneficial effects of atrioventricular sequential pacing on cardiac output and left ventricular filling assessed with pulsed Doppler echocardiography. Jpn Circ J 50:799, 1986.

91. Morgan DE, Norman R, West RO, Burggraf G: Echocardiographic assessment of tricuspid regurgitation during ventricular demand pacing. Am J Cardiol 58:1025, 1986.

92. Mark JB, Chetham PM: Ventricular pacing can induce hemodynamically significant mitral valve regurgitation. Anesthesiology 74:375, 1991.

93. Ausubel K, Furman S: The pacemaker syndrome. Ann Intern Med 103:420, 1985.

94. Ellenbogen KA, Wood MA, Strambler B: Clinical, hemodynamic, and neurohumeral features. *In* Barold SS, Mugia J (eds): New Perspectives in Cardiac Pacing: 3. Mt Kisco, NY, Futura, 1992.

95. Mitsui T, Hori M, Suma K, et al: The "pacemaking syndrome." *In* Jacobs JE (ed): Proceedings of the Eighth Annual International Conference on Medical and Biological Engineering. Chicago Association for Advancement of Medical Instrumentation, 1969, pp 29–33.

96. Johnson AD, Laiken SL, Engler RL: Hemodynamic compromise associated with ventriculoatrial conduction following transvenous pacemaker placement. Am J Med 65:75, 1978.

97. Erlebacher JA, Danner RL, Stelzer PE: Hypotension with ventricular pacing: An atrial vasodepressor reflex in human beings. J Am Coll Cardiol 4:550, 1984.

98. Witte J, Bundke H, Mullers S: The pacemaker syndrome: A hemodynamic complication of ventricular pacing. Cor Vasa 30:393, 1988.

99. Travill CM, Sutton R: Pacemaker syndrome: An iatrogenic condition. Br Heart J 68:163, 1992.

100. Heldman D, Mulvihill D, Nguyen H, et al: True incidence of pacemaker syndrome. PACE 13:1742, 1990.

101. Sulke N, Chambers J, Dritsas A, Sowton E: A randomized double-blind crossover comparison of four rate-responsive pacing modes. J Am Coll Cardiol 17:696, 1991.

102. Sulke N, Dritsas A, Bostock J, et al: "Subclinical" pacemaker syndrome: A randomized study of symptom free patients with ventricular demand (VVI) pacemakers up-graded to dual chamber devices. Br Heart J 67:57, 1992.

103. Reynolds DW, Wilson MF, Burow RD, et al: Hemodynamic evaluation of atrioventricular sequential versus ventricular pacing in patients with normal and poor ventricular function at variable heart rates and posture. J Am Coll Cardiol 1:636, 1983.

104. Ellenbogen KA, Thames MD, Moharity PK: New insights into pacemaker syndrome gained from hemodynamic, humoral and vascular responses during ventriculo-atrial pacing. Am J Cardiol 65:53, 1990.

105. Nishimura RN, Gersh BJ, Vliestra RE, et al: Hemodynamic consequences of ventricular pacing. PACE 5:903, 1982.

106. Akhtar M: Retrograde conduction in man. PACE 4:548, 1981.

107. Hayes DL, Furman S: Atrio-ventricular and ventriculo-atrial conduction times in patients undergoing pacemaker implant. PACE 6:38, 1983.

108. Webb CK, Spielman SR, Greenspan AM, et al: Improved method for evaluating ventriculoatrial conduction before implantation of atrial-sensing dual chamber pacemakers. J Am Coll Cardiol 5:1395, 1985.

109. Akhtar M, Gilbert C, Mahmud R, et al: Pacemaker mediated tachycardia: Underlying mechanisms, relationship to ventriculoatrial conduction, characteristics, and management. Clin Prog 3:90, 1985.

110. Mary DASG: Electrophysiology of atrial receptors. *In* Hainsworth R, McGregor KH, Mary DASG (eds): Cardiogenic Reflexes. Oxford, Oxford Scientific, 1987, p 3.

111. Hainsworth R: Atrial receptors in reflex control of the circulation. *In* Zucker IH, Gilmore JP (eds): Reflex Control of the Circulation. Boca Raton, FL, CRC Press, 1991, p 273.

111a. Edis AJ, Donald DE, Shepherd JT: Cardiovascular reflexes from stretch of pulmonary vein-atrial junctions in the dog. Circ Res 27:1091, 1970.

112. Alicandri C, Fouad FM, Tarazi RC, et al: Three cases of hypotension and syncope with ventricular pacing: Possible role of atrial reflexes. Am J Cardiol 42:137, 1978.

113. Oldroyd KG, Rae AD, Carter R, et al: Double blind crossover comparison of the effects of dual chamber pacing (DDD) and ventricular rate adaptive (VVIR) pacing on neuroendocrine variables exercise performance and symptoms in complete heart block. Br Heart J 65:188, 1991.

114. Hull RW, Smow F, Herre J, Ellenbogen KA: The plasma catecholamine responses to ventricular pacing: Implications for rate responsive pacing. PACE 13:1408, 1990.

115. Pehrsson SK, Hjemdahl O, Nordlander R, Astram H: A comparison of sympatho-adversal activity and cardiac performance at rest and

during exercise in patients with ventricular demand or atrial synchronous pacing. Br Heart J 60:212, 1988.

116. Bishop VS, Haywood HR: Hormonal control of cardiovascular reflexes. *In* Zucker IH, Gilmore JP (eds): Reflex Control of the Circulation. Boca Raton, FL, CRC Press, 1989 p 253.

117. Vardas PE, Travill CM, Williams TDM, et al: Effect of dual chamber pacing on raised plasma atrial natriuretic peptide concentrations in complete atrioventricular block. Br Med J 296:94, 1988.

118. Strangl K, Weil J, Seitz K, et al: Influence of AV synchrony on the plasma levels of atrial natriuretic peptide (ANP) in patients with total AV block. PACE 11:1176, 1988.

119. Ellenbogen KA, Kapudia K, Walsh M, Mohanty PK: Increase in plasma atrial natriuretic factor during ventriculoatrial pacing. Am J Cardiol 64:236, 1989.

120. Noll B, Krappe J, Goke B, Maisch B: Influence of pacing mode and rate on peripheral levels of atrial natriuretic peptide (ANP). PACE 12:1763, 1989.

121. Travail CM, Williams TDW, Vardas P, et al: Pacemaker syndrome is associated with very high plasma concentrations of atrial natriuretic peptide (ANP). J Am Coll Cardiol 13:111, 1989.

122. Barotto MT, Berti S, Clerico A, et al: Atrial natriuretic peptide during different pacing modes in comparison with hemodynamic changes. PACE 13:432, 1990.

123. Wong CK, Lau CP, Cheng CH, et al: Delayed decline in plasma atrial natriuretic peptide levels after an abrupt reduction in atrial pressures: Observation in patients with dual chamber pacing. Am Heart J 120:882, 1990.

124. Blanc JJ, Mansourah J, Ritter P, et al: Atrial natriuretic factor release during exercise in patients successively paced in DDD and rate matched ventricular pacing. PACE 15:397, 1992.

125. Clemo HF, Baumgarten CM, Stranbler BS, et al: Atrial natriuretic factor implications for cardiac pacing and electrophysiology. PACE 17:70, 1994.

126. Vardas PE, Markianos M, Skalidis E, et al: Twenty-four hour variation in plasma atrial natriuretic factor during VVI and DDD pacing. Heart 75:620, 1996.

127. Levine PA, Seltzer JP, Pirzada FA: The "pacemaker syndrome" in a properly functioning physiologic pacing system. PACE 6:279, 1983.

128. Torresani J, Ebagost A, Alland-Latour G: Pacemaker syndrome with DDD pacing. PACE 7:1148, 1984.

129. Pierantozzi A, Bocconcelli P, Syarbi E: DDD pacemaker syndrome and atrial conduction time. PACE 17:374, 1994.

130. den Dulk K, Lindemans FW, Brugada P, et al: Pacemaker syndrome with AAI rate variable pacing: Importance of atrioventricular conduction properties, medication and pacemaker programmability. PACE 11:1226, 1988.

131. Liebert HP, O'Donoghue S, Tullner WF, et al: Pacemaker syndrome in activity-responsive VVI pacing. Am J Cardiol 64:124, 1989.

132. Cunningham TM: Pacemaker syndrome due to retrograde conduction in a DDI pacemaker. Am Heart J 115:478, 1988.

133. Pitney MR, May CD, Davis MJ: Undesirable mode switching with a dual chamber rate responsive pacemaker. PACE 16:729, 1993.

134. Pieterse MGC, den Dulk K, van Gelder BM, et al: Programming a long paced atrioventricular interval may be risky in DDDR pacing. PACE 17:252, 1994.

135. Clarke M, Sutton R, Ward D, et al: Working Party Report: Recommendations for pacemaker prescription for symptomatic bradycardia. Br Heart J 66:185, 1991.

136. Braunwald E, Frahm CJ: Studies on Starling's law of the heart. IV. Observations on the hemodynamic functions of the left atrium in man. Circulation 24:633, 1961.

137. Matsuda Y, Toma Y, Ogawa H, et al: Importance of left atrial function in patients with myocardial infarction. Circulation 67:566, 1983.

138. Hamby RI, Noble WJ, Murphy DH, Hoffman I: Atrial transport function in coronary artery disease: Relation to left ventricular function. J Am Coll Cardiol 1:1011, 1983.

139. Freedman RA, Yock PG, Echt DS, Popp RL: Effect of variation in PQ interval on patterns of atrioventricular valve motion and flow in patients with normal ventricular function. J Am Coll Cardiol 7:595, 1986.

140. VonBibra H, Witzfeld A, Hall R, et al: Mitral valve closure and left ventricular filling time in patients with VDD pacemakers: Assessment of the onset of left ventricular systole and the end of diastole. Br Heart J 55:355, 1986.

141. Ishikawa T, Kimura K, Nihei T, et al: Relationship between diastolic

mitral regurgitation and PQ intervals on cardiac function in patients implanted with DDD pacemakers. PACE 14:1797, 1991.

142. Pearson AC, Janosik, DL, Redd RM, et al: Doppler echocardiographic assessment of the effect of varying atrioventricular delay and pacemaker mode on left ventricular filling. Am Heart J 115:611, 1988.

143. Iwase M, Sotobata I, Yokota M, et al: Evaluation by pulsed Doppler echocardiography of the atrial contribution to left ventricular filling in patients with DDD pacemakers. Am J Cardiol 58:104, 1986.

144. Pauletti M, Raugi M, Bini G, et al: Pulsed Doppler verification of atrial contribution to ventricular filling in sequential pacing. PACE 10:333, 1987.

145. Rokey R, Quinones MA, Zoghbi WA, et al: Influence of left atrial systolic emptying on left ventricular early filling dynamics by Doppler in patients with sequential atrioventricular pacemakers. Am J Cardiol 62:968, 1988.

146. Rokey R, Kuo LC, Zoghbi WA: Determination of parameters of left ventricular filling with pulsed Doppler echocardiography: Comparison with cineangiography. Circulation 71:543, 1985.

147. Bahler RC, Vrobel TR, Martin P: The relation of heart rate and shortening fraction to echocardiographic indexes of left ventricular relaxation in normal subjects. J Am Coll Cardiol 2:926, 1983.

148. Arora RR, Machac J, Goldman ME, et al: Atrial kinetics and left ventricular diastolic filling in the healthy elderly. J Am Coll Cardiol 9:1255, 1987.

149. Pearson A, Labovitz A, Mrosek D, et al: Assessment of diastolic function in normal and hypertrophied hearts: Comparison of Doppler echocardiography and M-mode echocardiography. Am heart J 113:1417, 1987.

150. Thomas JD, Weyman AE: Echocardiographic Doppler evaluation of left ventricular diastolic function. Circulation 84:977, 1991.

151. Ishidu Y, Meisner JS, Tsujioka K, et al: Left ventricular filling dynamics: Influence of left ventricular relaxation and left atrial pressure. Circulation 74:187, 1986.

152. Frienlingsdorf J, Deseo T, Gerber NE, Bertel O: A comparison of quality-of-life in patients with dual chamber pacemakers and individually programmed atrioventricular delays. PACE 19:1147, 1996.

153. Moden MG, Rossi R, Carcangni A, et al: The importance of different atrioventricular delay for left ventricular filling in sequential pacing: Clinical implications. PACE 19:1595, 1996.

154. Ritter P, Daubert C, Mabo P, et al: Hemodynamic benefit of a rate-adapted AV delay in dual chamber pacing. Eur Heart J 10:637, 1989.

155. Ausubel K, Klementowicz P, Furman S: Interatrial conduction during cardiac pacing. PACE 9:1026, 1986.

156. Catania SL, Maue-Dickson W: AV delay latency compensation. J Electrophysiol 3:242, 1987.

157. Grant SCD, Bennett DH: Atrial latency in a dual chambered pacing system causing inappropriate sequence of cardiac chamber activation. PACE 15:116, 1992.

158. Sutton R: The atrioventricular interval: What considerations influence its programming? Eur J CPE 3:169, 1992.

159. Chirife R, Ortega DF, Salazar AI: Nonphysiological left heart AV intervals as a result of DDD and AAI "physiological" pacing. PACE 14:1752, 1991.

160. Alt EU, VonBribra H, Blömer H: Different beneficial AV intervals with DDD pacing after sensed or paced atrial events. J Electrophysiol 1:250, 1987.

161. Fananapazir L, Cannon RO, Tripodi D, Panza JA: Impact of dual-chamber permanent pacing in patients with obstructive hypertrophic cardiomyopathy with symptoms refractory to verapamil and β-adrenergic blocker therapy. Circulation 85:2149, 1992.

162. Fananapazir LF, Epstein ND, Curiel RV, et al: Long-term results of dual chamber (DDD) pacing in obstructive hypertrophic cardiomyopathy. Circulation 90:2731, 1994.

163. Hochleitner MH, Hörtnagl H, Ng CK, et al: Usefulness of physiologic dual-chamber pacing in drug-resistant idiopathic dilated cardiomyopathy. Am J Cardiol 66:198, 1990.

164. Brecker SJD, Xiao HB, Sparrow J, Gibson DG: Effects of dual-chamber pacing with short atrioventricular delay in dilated cardiomyopathy. Lancet 340:1308, 1992.

165. Hochleitner M, Hörtnagl H, Fridrich L, Geschnitzer G: Long-term efficacy of physiologic dual chamber pacing in the treatment of end-stage idiopathic dilated cardiomyopathy. Am J Cardiol 70:1320, 1992.

166. Hoeschen RJ, Reimold SC, Lee RT, et al: Effect of posture on response to atrioventricular synchronous pacing in patients with underlying cardiovascular disease. PACE 14:756, 1991.

167. Epstein SE, Beiser D, Stampfer M, et al: Characterization of the circulatory response to maximal upright exercise in normal subjects and patients with heart disease. Circulation 35:1049, 1967.
168. Kruse IB, Ryden L: Comparison of physical work capacity and systolic time intervals with ventricular inhibited and atrial synchronous ventricular inhibited pacing. Br Heart J 46:129, 1981.
169. Kruse I, Arnman K, Conradson TB, Ryden L: A comparison of the acute and long-term hemodynamic effects of ventricular inhibited and atrial synchronous ventricular inhibited pacing. Circulation 65:846, 1982.
170. Kappenberger L, Gloor HO, Babotai I, et al: Hemodynamic effects of atrial synchronization in acute and long-term ventricular pacing. PACE 5:639, 1982.
171. Pehrsson SK: Influence of heart rate and atrioventricular synchronization on maximal work tolerance in patients treated with artificial pacemakers. Acta Med Scand 214:311, 1983.
172. Pehrsson SK, Aström H, Bone D: Left ventricular volumes with ventricular inhibited and atrial triggered ventricular pacing. Acta Med Scand 214:305, 1983.
173. Nordlander R, Pehrsson SK, Aström H, Karlsson J: Myocardial demands of atrial-triggered versus fixed-rate ventricular pacing in patients with complete heart block. PACE 10:1154, 1987.
174. Karpawich PP, Perry BL, Farooki ZQ, et al: Pacing in children and young adults with nonsurgical atrioventricular block: Comparison of single-rate ventricular and dual-chamber modes. Am Heart J 113:316, 1987.
175. Linde-Edelstam CM, Juhlin-Dannfelt A, Nordlander R, Pehrsson SK: The hemodynamic importance of atrial systole: A function of the kinetic energy of blood flow? PACE 15:1740, 1992.
176. Fananapazir L, Bennett DH, Monks P: Atrial synchronized ventricular pacing: Contribution of the chronotropic response to improved exercise performance. PACE 6:601, 1983.
177. Kristensson BE, Arnman K, Ryden L: The hemodynamic importance of atrioventricular synchrony and rate increase at rest and during exercise. Eur Heart J 6:773, 1985.
178. Ausubel K, Steingart RM, Shimshi M, et al: Maintenance of exercise stroke volume during ventricular versus atrial synchronous pacing: Role of contractility. Circulation 72:1037, 1985.
179. Linde-Edelstam C, Hjemdahl P, Pehrsson SK, et al: Is DDD pacing superior to VVIR? A study on cardiac sympathetic nerve activity and myocardial oxygen consumption at rest and during exercise. PACE 15:425, 1992.
180. Benditt DG, Milstein S, Buetikofer J, et al: Sensor-triggered, rate-variable cardiac pacing: Current technologies and clinical implications. Ann Intern Med 107:714, 1987.
181. Lau CP: The range of sensors and algorithms used in rate-adaptive cardiac pacing. PACE 15:1177, 1992.
182. Donaldson RM, Rickards AF: Rate-responsive pacing using the evoked QT principle: A physiological alternative to atrial synchronous pacemakers. PACE 6:1344, 1983.
183. Alt E, Hirgstetter C, Heinz M, Blömer H: Rate control of physiologic pacemakers by central venous blood temperature. Circulation 73:1206, 1986.
184. Benditt DG, Mianulli M, Fetter J, et al: Single-chamber cardiac pacing with activity initiated chronotropic response: Evaluation by cardiopulmonary exercise testing. Circulation 75:184, 1987.
185. Faerestrand SF, Breivik K, Ohm OJ: Assessment of the work capacity and relationship between rate response and exercise tolerance associated with activity-sensing rate-responsive ventricular pacing. PACE 10:1277, 1987.
186. Buckingham TA, Woodruff RC, Pennington DG, et al: Effect of ventricular function on the exercise hemodynamics of variable rate pacing. J Am Coll Cardiol 11:1269, 1988.
187. Lau CP, Camm J: Role of left ventricular function and Doppler-derived variables in predicting hemodynamic benefits of rate-responsive pacing. Am J Cardiol 62:906, 1988.
188. Iwase M, Hatano K, Saito F, et al: Evaluation by exercise Doppler echocardiography of maintenance of cardiac output during ventricular pacing with or without chronotropic response. Am J Cardiol 63:934, 1989.
189. Gammage M, Schofield S, Rankin I, et al: Benefit of single-setting rate-responsive ventricular pacing compared with fixed-rate demand pacing in elderly patients. PACE 14:174, 1991.
190. Wish M, Fletcher RD, Cohen A: Hemodynamics of AV synchrony and rate. J Electrophysiol 3:170, 1989.

191. Markewitz A, Hemmer W: What's the price to be paid for rate response: AV sequential versus ventricular pacing? PACE 14:1782, 1991.
192. Faerestrand S, Ohm OJ: A time-related study by Doppler and M-mode echocardiography of hemodynamics, heart rate, and AV valvular function during activity-sensing rate-responsive ventricular pacing. PACE 10:507, 1987.
193. Stone JM, Bhakla RD, Lutgen J: Dual-chamber sequential pacing management of sinus node dysfunction: Advantages over single-chamber pacing. Am Heart J 104:1319, 1982.
194. Alpert MA, Curtis JJ, Sanfelippo JF, et al: Comparative survival after permanent ventricular and dual-chamber pacing for patients with chronic high degree atrioventricular block with and without preexistent congestive heart failure. J Am Coll Cardiol 7:925, 1986.
195. Sgarbossa EB, Pinski SL, Maloney JD: The rule of pacing modality in determining long-term survival in sick sinus syndrome. Ann Intern Med 119:359, 1993.
196. Sutton R, Kenny RA: The natural history of sick sinus syndrome. PACE 9:1110, 1986.
197. Rosenqvist M, Brandt J, Schuller H: Atrial versus ventricular pacing in sinus node disease: A treatment comparison study. Am Heart J 111:292, 1986.
198. Byrd CL, Schwartz SJ, Gonzales M, et al: DDD pacemakers maximize hemodynamic benefits and minimize complications for most patients. PACE 11:1911, 1988.
199. Rosenqvist M, Brandt J, Schuller H: Long-term pacing in sinus node disease: Effects of stimulation mode on cardiovascular morbidity and mortality. Am Heart J 116:16, 1988.
200. Santini M, Alexidou G, Ansalone G, et al: Relation of prognosis in sick sinus syndrome to age, conduction defects, and modes of permanent cardiac pacing. Am J Cardiol 65:729, 1990.
201. Hesselson AB, Parsonnet V, Bernstein AD, Bonavita GJ: Deleterious effects of long-term single-chamber ventricular pacing in patients with sick sinus syndrome: The hidden benefits of dual-chamber pacing. J Am Coll Cardiol 19:1542, 1992.
202. Kubica J, Stolarczyk L, Krzyminska E, et al: Left atrial size and wall motion in patients with permanent ventricular and atrial pacing. PACE 13:1737, 1990.
203. Lau CP, Wong CK, Leung WH, Liu WX: Superior cardiac hemodynamics of atrioventricular synchrony over rate-responsive pacing at submaximal exercise: Observations in activity-sensing DDDR pacemakers. PACE 13:1832, 1990.
204. Proctor EE, Leman RB, Mann DL, et al: Single-versus dual-chamber sensor-driven pacing: Comparison of cardiac outputs. Am Heart J 122:728, 1991.
205. Vogt P, Goy J, Kuhn M, et al: Single- versus double-chamber rate-responsive cardiac pacing: Comparison by cardiopulmonary noninvasive exercise testing. PACE 11:1896, 1988.
206. Jutzy RV, Florio J, Isaeff DM, et al: Limitations of testing methods for evaluation of dual-chamber versus single-chamber adaptive rate pacing. Am J Cardiol 68:1715, 1991.
207. Sulke N, Tan K, Kamaluand K, et al: Dual sensor VVIR mode pacing: Is it worth it? PACE 19:1560, 1996.
208. Leung SK, Lau CP, Tang MO, Leung Z: New integrated sensor pacemaker: Comparison of rate responses between an integrated minute ventilation and activity sensor and single sensor modes during exercise and daily activities and nonphysiological interference. PACE 19:1664, 1996.
209. Leung SK, Lau CP, Lam CT: Smart pacing. J H K Coll Cardiol 4:104, 1996.
210. Barold SS, Clementry J: The promise of improved exercise performance by dual sensor rate adaptive pacemakers. PACE 20:607, 1997.
211. Benditt DG, Mianulli M, Lurie K, et al: Multiple sensor systems for physiologic cardiac pacing. Ann Intern Med 121:960, 1994.
212. Deharo JC, Badier M, Thirien X, et al: A randomized, single-blind crossover comparison of the effects of chronic DDD and dual sensor VVIR pacing mode on quality-of-life and cardiopulmonary performance in complete heart block. PACE 19:1320, 1996.
213. Capucci A, Boriani G, Specchia S, et al: Evaluation by cardiopulmonary exercise test of DDDR versus DDD pacing. PACE 15:1908, 1992.
214. Daubert C, Ritter P, Mabo P, et al: Physiological relationship between AV interval and heart rate in healthy subjects: Applications to dual-chamber pacing. PACE 9:1032, 1986.
215. Luceri RM, Brownstein SL, Vardeman L, Goldstein S: PR interval behavior during exercise: Implications for physiological pacemakers. PACE 13:1719, 1990.

216. Barbieri D, Percoco GF, Toselli T, et al: AV delay and exercise stress tests: Behavior in normal subjects. PACE 13:1724, 1990.
217. Haskell RJ, French WJ: Physiological importance of different atrioventricular intervals to improve exercise performance in patients with dual-chamber pacemakers. Br Heart J 61:46, 1989.
218. Ryden L, Karlsson O, Kristensson BE: The importance of different atrioventricular intervals for exercise capacity. PACE 11:1051, 1988.
219. Landzberg JS, Franklin JO, Mahawar SK, et al: Benefits of physiologic atrioventricular synchronization for pacing with an exercise rate response. Am J Cardiol 66:193, 1990.
220. Ritter PH, Vai F, Bonnet JL, et al: Rate-adaptive atrioventricular delay improves cardiopulmonary performance in patients implanted with a dual-chamber pacemaker for complete heart block. Eur J CPE 1:31, 1991.
221. Sulke AN, Chambers JB, Sowton E: The effect of atrioventricular delay programming in patients with DDDR pacemakers. Eur Heart J 13:464, 1992.
222. Theodorakis GN, Kremastinos D, Markianos M, et al: Total sympathetic activity and atrial natriuretic factor levels in VVI and DDD pacing with different atrioventricular delays during daily activity and exercise. Eur Heart J 13:1477, 1992.
223. Igawa O, Tomokuni T, Saitoh M, et al: Sympathetic nervous system response to dynamic exercise in complete AV block patients treated with AV synchronous pacing with fixed AV delay or auto-AV delay. PACE 13:1766, 1990.
224. Irnich W, Conrady J: A new principle of rate-adaptive pacing in patients with sick sinus syndrome. PACE 11:1823, 1988.
225. Mabo P, Pouillot C, Kermarrec A, et al: Lack of physiological adaptation of the atrioventricular interval to heart rate in patients chronically paced in the AAIR mode. PACE 14:2133, 1991.
226. Rosenqvist M, Isaaz K, Botvinick EH, et al: Relative importance of activation sequence compared to atrioventricular synchrony in left ventricular function. Am J Cardiol 67:148, 1991.
227. Buller D, Wolpers HG, Zipfel J, et al: Comparison of the effects of right atrial, right ventricular apex and atrioventricular sequential pacing on myocardial oxygen consumption and cardiac efficiency: A laboratory investigation. PACE 11:394, 1988.
228. Badke FR, Boinay P, Covell JW: Effects of ventricular pacing on regional left ventricular performance in the dog. Am J Physiol 238:H258, 1980.
229. Adomian GE, Beazell J: Myofibrillar disarray produced in normal hearts by chronic electrical pacing. Am Heart J 112:79, 1986.
230. Askenazi J, Alexander JH, Koenigsberg DI, et al: Alternation of left ventricular performance by left bundle branch block simulated with atrioventricular sequential pacing. Am J Cardiol 53:99, 1984.
231. Bramlet DA, Morris KG, Coleman RE, et al: Effects of rate-dependent left bundle branch block on global and regional left ventricular function. Circulation 67:1059, 1983.
232. Grines CL, Bashore TM, Boudoulas H, et al: Functional abnormalities in isolated left bundle branch block: The effect of interventricular asynchrony. Circulation 79:845, 1989.
233. Bedotto JB, Grayburn PA, Black WH, et al: Alterations in left ventricular relaxation during atrioventricular pacing in humans. J Am Coll Cardiol 15:658, 1990.
234. Harper GR, Pina IL, Kutalek SP: Intrinsic conduction maximizes cardiopulmonary performance in patients with dual-chamber pacemakers. PACE 14:1787, 1992.
235. Santomauro M, Fazio S, Ferraro S, et al: Fourier analysis in patients with different pacing modes. PACE 14:1351, 1991.
236. Leclercq C, Gras D, Le Helloco A, et al: Hemodynamic importance of preserving the normal sequence of ventricular activation in permanent cardiac pacing. Am Heart J 129:1133, 1995.
237. Stojnić BB, Stojanov PL, Angelkov L, et al: Evaluation of asynchronous left ventricular relaxation by Doppler echocardiography during ventricular pacing with AV synchrony (VDD): Comparison with atrial pacing (AAI). PACE 19:940, 1996.
238. Betocchi S, Piscione F, Villari B, et al: Effects of induced asynchrony on left ventricular diastolic function in patients with coronary artery disease. J Am Coll Cardiol 21:1124, 1993.
239. Delhaus T, Arrs T, Prinzen F, Reneman RS: Regional fibre stress fibre strain area as an estimate of regional blood flow and oxygen demand in the canine heart. J Physiol 477:481, 1994.
240. Prinzen FW, Augustijn CH, Arrs T, et al: Redistribution of myocardial fiber strain and blood flow by asynchronous activation. Am J Physiol 259:H300, 1990.
241. Prinzen FW, Cheriex EC, Delhaas, T, Van Oosterhout MF, et al: Asymmetric thickness of left ventricular wall resulting from asynchronous electric activation: A study in dogs with ventricular pacing and in patients with left bundle branch block. Am Heart J 130:145, 1995.
242. Foster AH, Geld MR, McLaughlin JS: Acute hemodynamic effects of atrio-biventricular pacing in humans. Ann Thorac Surg 59:294, 1995.
243. Saxon LA, Kerwin WF, Cahalan MK, Kalman JM, et al: Acute effects of intraoperative multisite ventricular pacing on left ventricular function and activation/contraction sequence in patients with depressed ventricular function. J Cardiovasc Electrophysiol 9:13, 1998.
244. Cazeau S, Ritter P, Bakduch S, et al: Four chamber pacing in dilated cardiomyopathy. PACE 17:1974, 1994.
245. Cazeau S, Ritter P, Lazarus A, et al: Multisite pacing for end-stage heart failure: Early experience. PACE 19:1748, 1996.
246. Barold SS, Cazeau S, Mugica J, et al: Permanent multisite cardiac pacing. PACE 20:2725, 1997.
247. Barold SS: Cardiac pacing in special and complex situations. Cardiol Clin 4:573, 1992.
248. Daubert C, Gras D, Berder V, et al: Resynchronization article permanente par la stimulation biatriale synchrone pour le traitement preventif du flutter auriculaire associe a un bloc inter-auriculaire de haut degree. Arch Mal Coeur 87:1535, 1994.
249. Saksena S, Prakush A, Hill M, et al: Prevention of atrial fibrillation with dual-site right atrial pacing. J Am Coll Cardiol 28:687, 1996.
250. Auricchio A, Salo RW: Acute hemodynamic improvement by pacing in patients with severe congestive heart failure. PACE 20:313, 1997.
251. Innes D, Leitch JW, Fletcher PJ: VDD pacing at short atrioventricular intervals does not improve cardiac output in patients with dilated heart failure. PACE 17:959, 1994.
252. Gold MR, Feliciano Z, Gottlieb SS, et al: Dual-chamber pacing with short atrioventricular delay in congestive heart failure: A randomized study. J Am Coll Cardiol 26:967, 1995.
253. Linde C, Gerdler F, Ednor M, et al: Results of atrioventricular synchronous pacing with optimized delay in patients with severe congestive heart failure. Am J Cardiol 75:919, 1995.
254. Valero A: Atrial transport dysfunction in acute myocardial infarction. Am J Cardiol 16:22, 1965.
255. Cohn JN, Guitia NJ, Broder MI, Limas CJ: Right ventricular infarction: Clinical and hemodynamic features. Am J Cardiol 33:204, 1974.
256. Topol EJ, Goldschlager N, Ports TA, et al: Hemodynamic benefit of atrial pacing in right ventricular myocardial infarction. Ann Intern Med 96:594, 1982.
257. Love JC, Haffajee CI, Gore JM, Alpert JS: Reversibility of hypotension and shock by atrial or atrioventricular sequential pacing in patients with right ventricular infarction. Am Heart J 108:5, 1984.
258. Matangi MF: Temporary physiologic pacing in inferior wall acute myocardial infarction with right ventricular damage. Am J Cardiol 59:1207, 1987.
259. Murphy P, Morton P, Murtagh JG, et al: Hemodynamic effects of different temporary pacing modes for management of bradycardias complicating acute myocardial infarction. PACE 15:391, 1992.
260. Shefer A, Rozenman Y, Ben David Y, et al: Left ventricular function during physiological cardiac pacing: Relation to rate, pacing mode, and underlying myocardial disease. PACE 10:315, 1987.
261. Kenny RA, Ingram A, Mitsuoka T, et al: Optimum pacing mode for patients with angina pectoris. Br Heart J 56:463, 1986.
262. Laniado S, Yellin EL, Yoran C, et al: Physiologic mechanisms in aortic insufficiency. I. The effect of changing heart rate on flow dynamics II. Determinants of Austin Flint murmur. Circulation 66:226, 1982.
263. Meyer TE, Sareli P, Marcus RH, et al: Beneficial effect of atrial pacing in severe acute aortic regurgitation and role of M-mode echocardiography in determining the optimal pacing interval. Am J Cardiol 67:398, 1991.
264. Gliksch M, Itayes DL, Nishimura RA: Newer clinical applications of pacing. J Cardiovasc Electrophysiol 8:1190, 1997.
265. Symansla JD, Nishimura RA: The use of pacemakers in the treatment of cardiomyopathies. Curr Probl Cardiol 21:387, 1996.
266. Gliksen M, Epinosa RE, Hayes DL: Expanding indications for permanent pacemakers. Ann Intern Med 123:443, 1995.
267. Auricchio A, Scmmanra L, Salo RW, et al: Improvement of cardiac function with severe congestive heart failure and coronary artery disease with shortened AV delay. PACE 16:2034, 1993.
268. Ng K, Gibson DG: Improvement of diastolic function by shortened

filling period in severe left ventricular disease. Br Heart J 62:246, 1989.

269. Clements JP, Brown ML, Zinsmelster AR, et al: Influence of left ventricular diastolic filling on symptoms and survival in patients with decreased left ventricular systolic function. Am J Cardiol 61:1245, 1991.

270. Ishikana T, Sumita S, Kimura K, et al: Critical pulse generator interval for the appearance of diastolic mitral regurgitation and optimal pulse generator interval in patients implanted with DDD pacemakers. PACE 17:1989, 1994.

271. Guardigli G, Ansani L, Percoco GF: AV delay optimization and management of DDD paced patients with dilated cardiomyopathy. PACE 17:1984, 1994.

272. Postaci W, Yesil M, Susam I, et al: The influence of difference AV delays on left ventricular diastolic functions and on incidence of diastolic mitral regurgitation. Angiology 47:895, 1996.

273. Nishimura RA, Hayes DL, Holmes DR: Mechanism of hemodynamic improvement by dual-chamber pacing for severe left ventricular dysfunction: An acute Doppler and catheterization hemodynamic study. J Am Coll Cardiol 25:281, 1995.

274. Shemin RJ, Scott WC, Kastl DG, Morrow AG: Hemodynamic effects of various modes of cardiac pacing after operation for idiopathic hypertrophic subaortic stenosis. Ann Thorac Surg 27:137, 1979.

275. Gross JN, Keltz TN, Cooper JA, et al: Profound "pacemaker syndrome" in hypertrophic cardiomyopathy. Am J Cardiol 70:1507, 1992.

276. Jeanrenaud X, Goy JJ, Kappenberger LK: Effects of dual-chamber pacing in hypertrophic obstructive cardiomyopathy. Lancet 339:1318, 1992.

277. Slude A, Sadoul N, Shapiro L, et al: DDD pacing in hypertrophic cardiomyopathy: A multicentre clinical experience. Heart 75:44, 1996.

278. Posma JL, Blanksma PK, Vanberwall EF, et al: Heart 76:358, 1996.

279. Nishimura RA, Trusty JM, Hayes DL: Dual-chamber pacing for hypertrophic cardiomyopathy: A randomized, double-blind, crossover trial. J Am Coll Cardiol 29:435, 1997.

280. Gadler F, Linde C, Juhlin-Dannfeldt A, et al: Influence of right ventricular pacing site on left ventricular outflow tract obstruction in patients with hypertrophic obstructive cardiomyopathy. J Am Coll Cardiol 27:1219, 1996.

281. Nishimura RA, Hayes DL, Olstrup DM: Effect of dual-chamber pacing on systolic and diastolic function in patients with hypertrophic cardiomyopathy. J Am Coll Cardiol 27:241, 1996.

282. Marcin BJ: Appraisal of dual-chamber pacing therapy in hypertrophic cardiomyopathy: Too soon for a rush to judgement? J Am Coll Cardiol 27:431, 1996.

283. Cannon RO, Tripod D, Dilsizlan VT, et al: Results of permanent dual-chamber pacing in symptomatic on obstructive hypertrophic cardiomyopathy. Am J Cardiol 73:571, 1994.

284. Perrins EJ, Merley CA, Chan SL: Randomized controlled trial of physiological and ventricular pacing. Br Heart J 50:112, 1983.

285. Pehrsson SK, Aström H, Bone D: Left ventricular volumes with ventricular inhibited and atrial triggered ventricular pacing. Acta Med Scand 214:305, 1983.

286. Kristensson BE, Arnman K, Smedgård P, Ryden L: Physiological versus single-rate ventricular pacing: A double-blind cross-over study. PACE 8:73, 1985.

287. Linde-Edelstam C, Nordlander R, Unden AL, et al: Quality of life in patients treated with atrioventricular synchronous pacing compared to rate modulated ventricular pacing: A long-term, double-blind, cross-over study. PACE 15:1467, 1992.

288. Lipkin DP, Buller N, Freeneaux M, et al: Randomized crossover trial of rate responsive Activitrax and conventional fixed-rate ventricular pacing. Br Heart J 58:613, 1987.

289. Candinas RA, Gloor HO, Amann FW, et al: Activity-sensing rate responsive versus conventional fixed-rate pacing: A comparison of rate behavior and patient well-being during routine daily exercise. PACE 14:204, 1991.

290. Malticli AN, Castellani ET, Vivol D, et al: Prevalence of atrial fibrillation and stroke in paced patients without prior atrial fibrillation: A prospective study. Clin Cardiol 21:117, 1998.

291. Connolly SJ, Kerr C, Gent M, et al: Dual-chamber versus ventricular pacing: Critical appraisal of current data. Circulation 94:578, 1996.

292. Gregoratos G, Cheitlin MD, Conill A, Epstein AZ, et al: ACC/AHA Guidelines for implantation of cardiac pacemakers and antiarrhythmia devices. J Am Coll Cardiol 31:1175, 1998.

293. Curzio G, and the Multicenter Study Group: A multicenter evaluation of a single-pass lead VDD pacing system. PACE 14:434, 1991.

Chapter 15

Survival, Quality of Life, and Clinical Trials in Pacemaker Patients

Malcolm A. Barlow, Charles R. Kerr, Stuart J. Connolly

This chapter reviews studies that have reported on outcome events in patients who have pacemakers. The material is divided into the three sections suggested in the chapter title: survival, quality of life, and clinical trials.

The first section, on survival, is divided into discussions of studies dealing with atrioventricular block and those dealing with sick sinus syndrome. Each section begins with a review of the natural history of the nonpaced condition, followed by more detailed discussions on survival in paced patients and on the factors that modify survival in these patients. The impact of pacemaker mode on survival is also addressed. The section on quality of life is largely concerned with comparisons among the various pacemaker modes. Reference is also made to the effect of pacemaker mode on exercise capacity, as this assessment was often combined with the quality of life assessment. The final section, on clinical trials, deals with the randomized prospective trials on pacemaker mode selection, many of which are ongoing. Results of two of the smaller trials, the Danish study and the Pacemaker Selection in the Elderly (PASE) trial, have been published elsewhere and are discussed in this section.

In addition to providing a general review of the major outcome events in patients who have pacemakers, we hope that this chapter will serve as a critical review of the relative benefits of physiologic pacing compared with ventricular-based pacing, an area of current particular interest.

■ SURVIVAL IN PATIENTS WHO HAVE PACEMAKERS

Atrioventricular Block

Natural History
Complete Heart Block

A small number of observational studies have reported on the natural history of patients with complete atrioventricular

block. These studies have often been limited by incomplete follow-up and use of selected patients, but despite their limitations they have clearly demonstrated that complete heart block is associated with significant morbidity and mortality. The largest, most comprehensive, and most credible of these studies was conducted by Johansson.[1]

The Malmö Experience. In Johansson's study,[1] all 193 patients with electrocardiograms demonstrating complete heart block in the years 1950 to 1964 from the town of Malmö, Sweden were included. No patient was lost to follow-up and, because the town was served by only one general hospital, there was a high probability of including virtually all of the patients who had complete heart block from the area.

In the first year, 97 of the 193 patients died, 62 (64%) within the first 4 weeks after documentation. The mode of death was sudden in 33%, nonsudden cardiac in 47%, and noncardiac in 20%. The highest 1-year mortality rate was found in those with digitalis intoxication (presumably reflecting the increased use of digitalis to treat steadily worsening congestive heart failure), with the next highest in those with acute myocardial infarction. Advanced age, presence of syncope, and permanent (as opposed to transient or intermittent) block predicted a higher mortality. This poorer outlook for patients with syncope has been corroborated by a number of other studies.[2–8]

The overall 1-year survival rate from this study is 50%. Excluding those cases related to digitalis intoxication and acute myocardial infarction (and only one patient of this latter group with constant heart block survived more than 1 week), the 1-year survival is 60% (72 of 119 patients). This figure is comparable to the results from other series reporting on survival in patients with conservatively treated complete heart block [2–6, 9–11] (Table 15–1) and serves as a useful reference point for comparison with survival rates in patients with pacemaker-treated complete heart block.

Table 15–1. Survival Rates in Patients with Conservatively Treated Complete Heart Block*

Author(s)	No of Patients	Survival Time				
		6 mo	*1 yr*	*2 yr*	*5 yr*	*10 yr*
Campbell[2]	50	—	0.80	0.62	0.31	—
Cosby et al.[3]	36	—	0.56	—	0.28	0.15
Curd et al.[9]	113	0.65	0.57	0.47	—	—
Edhag and Swahn[4]	68	—	0.68	—	0.37	—
Friedberg et al.[5]	80	0.66	0.62	—	0.20	—
Johansson[1]	119	0.67	0.61	—	—	—
Ohm and Breivik[6]	52	—	0.62	0.49	0.29	—
Pader and Levy[10]	73	0.86	0.81	0.53	0.45	—
Siddons[11]	113	—	0.78	0.64	—	—
Weighted mean	**704**	**—**	**0.67**	**0.55**	**0.32**	**0.15**

*When possible, patients with complete heart block complicating acute myocardial infarction and digitalis intoxication were excluded.

Johansson's study[1] also suggests that much of the increased risk of death in patients with complete heart block is attributable to the underlying disease processes (Fig. 15–1). This relationship between underlying cardiac disease and survival has been a consistent finding in *every* other study reporting on the subject.[3–5, 9, 12, 13] Generally, patients with overt coronary disease have the worst outcome, those with rheumatic or valvular heart disease have an intermediate prognosis,[5, 12, 13] and those with congenital heart block (as opposed to heart block complicating congenital heart disease) have the best outlook.[4, 7, 9]

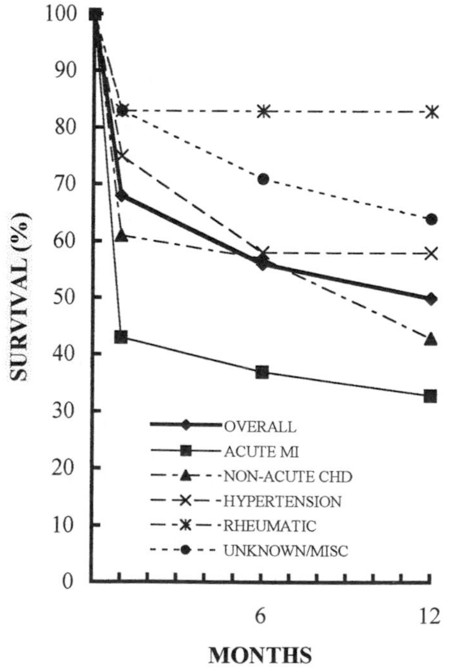

Comparison of Survival in Paced and Unpaced Patients. No prospective trials have compared survival in pacemaker-treated and conservatively treated patients with complete heart block. Two retrospective studies have directly compared outcomes between the two groups, and these demonstrated a substantial improvement in survival with pacing.[6, 11] In addition, a large number of observational studies have reported solely on survival in patients with heart block treated with pacemakers[11, 14–38] (Table 15–2). In all of these studies, the survival rates have been considerably greater than the rate reported previously for patients treated conservatively. Taken together, these retrospective analyses provide reasonable evidence that pacemaker therapy for complete heart block leads to a substantial reduction in mortality (Fig. 15–2).

Second-Degree Heart Block

The most detailed study on the natural history of second-degree heart block was reported by Shaw and colleagues in 1985.[39] This prospective study enrolled 214 patients with chronic second-degree atrioventricular block from the Devon area in England between 1968 and 1982. The patients were divided into 3 groups: group 1 had Mobitz type I atrioventricular block; group 2 had Mobitz type II atrioventricular block; and group 3 had persistent 2:1 or 3:1 atrioventricular block. Pacemakers were implanted in 103 patients. There was no difference in overall survival among the three groups. This was a little surprising as it was anticipated, on the basis of a greater likelihood of a more proximal block in the atrioventricular conducting system in patients with Mobitz type I block,[40–42] that survival would be better in group 1 than in groups 2 or 3. On the other hand, the difference in survival between the paced and unpaced patients was striking: a 5-year survival rate of 41% in the unpaced patients versus 78% in the paced group (P<.0001). When adjustment was made for the age differences in these groups, the improvement in the 5-year survival rate with pacing remained significant (49% in the unpaced and 72% in the paced patients; P<.015) (Fig. 15–3). In addition, patients with Stokes-Adams attacks who were not paced were found to

Figure 15–1. Survival rates for the different subgroups of patients from Johansson's series according to the underlying disease process. The group with digitalis intoxication was not included in the diagram but has been included in the calculation of overall survival rates. It can be appreciated that survival differs greatly depending on the underlying cardiac disease. CHD, coronary heart disease. (Modified from Johansson BW: Complete heart block: A clinical, hemodynamic and pharmacological study in patients with and without an artificial pacemaker. Acta Med Scand 180(Suppl 451):1–127, 1966.)

Table 15–2. Survival Rates From the Observational Studies in Patients Paced for Heart Block*

Author(s)	Study Year	Implantation Years	Mean Age (yr)	No. of Patients	Survival Time			
					1 yr	2 yr	5 yr	10 yr
Chardack et al.[14]	1965	1960–61	—	100	0.93	0.78	0.50	—
Edhag[15]	1969	1962–68	66	248	0.86	0.81	0.63	—
Harthorne et al.[16]	1969	1965–68	74	130	0.84	0.63	—	—
Torresani et al.[17]	1969	1962–68	69	372	0.92	0.83	0.48	—
Inberg et al.[18]	1971	1961–69	66	49	0.90	0.69	0.38	—
Sowton and Fiores[19]	1971	1964–70	65	161	0.93	0.84	0.65	—
Davidson et al.[20]	1972	1961–68	66	150	0.86	0.76	0.49	—
Van der Heide et al.[21]	1973	1961–73	67	285	0.86	0.76	0.58	0.40
Zion et al.[22]	1973	1963–72	63	48	0.81	0.71	0.58	—
Amikam et al.[25]	1974	1965–74	—	150	0.90	0.82	0.67	—
Fischer Hansen and Meibom[23]	1974	1962–70	69	164	0.87	0.76	0.50	—
Siddons[11]	1974	1960–72	68	649	0.88	0.80	0.65	—
Svendsen et al.[24]	1974	1960–73	72	188	0.83	0.77	0.53	—
Amikam et al.[25]	1976	1965–74	75	80	0.90	0.82	0.58	—
Yokoyama et al.[26]	1976	1967–71	50	59	0.85	0.81	—	—
Forsberg[27]	1978	1963 73	71	140	0.86	0.73	—	—
Simon and Zloto[28]	1978	1961–74	66	246	0.88	0.81	0.61	0.49
Fitzgerald et al.[29]	1979	1967–77	68	427	0.90	0.83	0.65	0.37
Alpert and Katti[30]	1982	1966–76	71	120	0.91	0.83	0.63	0.41
Kyle et al.[31]	1982	1961–77	71	352	0.85	0.78	0.59	0.35
Simon and Janz[32]	1982	1961–79	67	312	0.88	0.79	0.60	0.49
Hauser et al.[33]	1983	—	63	314	0.90	—	0.71	0.58
Alt et al.[34]	1985	1965–84	70	1049	0.86	0.78	0.56	0.34
Alpert et al.[35]	1986	1966–84	68	180	0.91	0.84	0.65	—
Zanini et al.[36]	1989	1968–86	70	962	0.84	0.77	0.58	0.33
Jelíc et al.[37]	1992	1967–85	63	1431	0.94	—	0.83	0.75
Shen et al.[38]	1994	1964–88	80	154	0.80	0.69	0.41	0.18
Weighted mean	—	—	**68**	**8194**	**0.88**	**0.79**	**0.64**	**0.47**

*Most of these studies have dealt solely with complete heart block; however, in some of the latter reports, a small number of patients with lesser degrees of atrioventricular block were included. The results from Amikam et al. (1976)[25] Simon and Zloto (1978)[28] and Alpert and Katti (1982)[30] are presented but have not been used in the calculation of the weighted means because these patients are included in larger series by the same authors elsewhere in this table.

have a much poorer outcome than those without these attacks (5-year survival rate of 25% versus 51%, respectively; $P<.01$).

In an earlier study,[43] the only other one on second-degree heart block containing more than a handful of patients, a poor overall survival in patients with chronic Mobitz type I atrioventricular block was also found (mortality rate of 8.7% per year in 56 patients, mean age 57 years), although only 3 of the 16 deaths were sudden.

The most serious limitation of Shaw's study is that, because a significant proportion (almost 50%) of the patients received pacemakers, the natural history of the disease has been influenced. Consequently, the true death rate in conservatively treated patients with second-degree atrioventricular block and the true impact of pacing on this death rate may have been underestimated or overestimated, depending on whether there was a consistent selection bias to implant pacemakers in the sickest or healthiest patients, respectively.

Survival in Patients Paced for Atrioventricular Block

The survival rates from studies reporting on patients treated with pacemakers for atrioventricular block of varying degrees are presented in Table 15–2 and Figure 15–2. All of the studies are retrospective and report on a highly selected group of patients (i.e., those who were selected to receive pacemakers as opposed to those who were not).

Factors Influencing Survival

Age and Underlying Disease. As with unpaced patients, most studies have shown that in patients paced for atrioventricular block, age and the type and severity of any underlying disease have a major influence on survival.

In only a small number of the studies was overall survival found to be comparable to that of the general population[29, 37]; in all others, survival fell far short of what would be expected. Most, if not all, of this increase in mortality can be attributed to the adverse impact of the underlying disease processes seen commonly in patients with atrioventricular block.[23, 38, 44] For instance, in a follow-up study on 164 patients with complete heart block receiving pacemakers between 1962 and 1970,[23] Hansen and Meibom found that survival rates in patients without coexisting diseases and without heart failure (40% of the cohort) were equal to those of an age-matched and sex-matched population, even though the survival rate of the entire group was well below that of the matched population. The lower-than-expected survival for the entire group could be explained by the excess mortality in those with coexisting diseases or heart failure

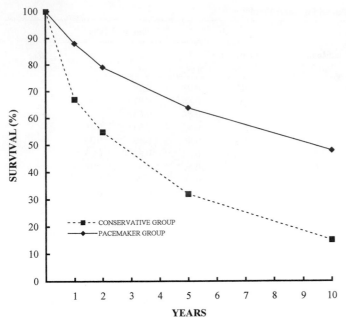

Figure 15–2. Survival rates in patients with in complete heart block who received pacemakers compared with those treated conservatively in the pre-pacing era. Data points are the weighted mean survival rates from Tables 15–1 and 15–2. Even allowing for the general improvement in cardiac care that has taken place in the pacing era, the improvement in survival with pacing is striking. Mortality in the conservatively treated patients is about double that seen in the pacemaker-treated patients.

(Fig. 15–4). Many other studies have also demonstrated that survival is adversely affected by the presence of underlying diseases, particularly congestive heart failure[23, 30, 32, 33, 35, 38, 45–47] or coronary heart disease.[28–30, 32, 33, 38, 48]

Preimplantation and Postimplantation Symptoms. In contrast to the studies reporting on the natural history of atrioventricular block, few of the studies on paced patients have specifically addressed the issue of the relation of symptoms to survival. In one such study,[47] which reported on 2256 patients who received pacemakers for a variety of indications, including atrioventricular block, those presenting with Stokes-Adams equivalents (i.e., dizziness) had significantly better survival rates than those presenting with Stokes-Adams attacks or heart failure (P<.0001). Other studies have also shown that syncope, both preimplantation and postimplantation, is an independent risk factor predictive of a poorer outcome.[37, 38, 45] In one study examining 1431 patients,[37] multivariate analysis also identified generalized fatigue as an independent predictor of subsequent mortality. Postimplantation generalized fatigue was the strongest predictor of an adverse outcome, more significant even than increased age or the presence of heart failure or myocardial infarction.

Pacing Mode. In virtually all studies previously discussed, only ventricular-based pacemakers were used. More recent studies have also employed dual-chamber pacemakers, and a small number of these studies have specifically examined the impact of pacing mode on survival. Alpert and col-

leagues[35] analyzed survival in 180 patients who had received pacemakers for high-degree atrioventricular block. Dual-chamber units (DVI or DDD) had been implanted in 48, and 132 had received VVI units. There was no difference in overall mortality between the groups, but in patients with congestive heart failure, survival was significantly greater in the dual-chamber group. Linde-Edelstam and colleagues[49] also compared survival in relation to pacing mode in 148 patients with atrioventricular block (74 receiving VVI and 74 VDD pacemakers) in a case-control study. Again, total mortality did not differ between the groups, but in those with heart failure, mortality in the VVI group was twice as great as that in the VDD group (P<.04).

There are cogent theoretical reasons for poorer survival rates with fixed-rate ventricular pacing in patients with congestive heart failure. Loss of atrioventricular synchrony means loss of the atrial contribution to ventricular filling and loss of ability to increase the heart rate. Loss of the atrial component to ventricular filling is associated with a decrease in cardiac output, most noticeable at rest.[50–52] Loss of the ability to increase the heart rate greatly limits exercise capacity because most of the increase in cardiac output accompanying exercise is due to a two-fold to three-fold increase in the heart rate.[52–54] Thus, for patients with a fixed-rate ventricular pacemaker, the only way to maintain and increase cardiac output is by means of an increase in stroke volume. This can be achieved only by an increase in myocardial contractility or an increase in ventricular dimension.[51] The increase in contractility is thought to be mediated primarily by an increase in cardiac sympathetic nervous activity,[55, 56] although there may be a contribution from myocardial hypertrophy in the long term. These changes are much less likely

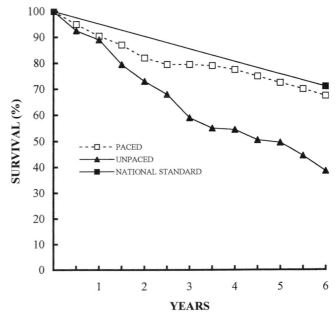

Figure 15–3. Survival rates in 103 paced and 111 unpaced patients with second-degree atrioventricular block compared with the national standard. Survival in the paced patients is significantly better than in the unpaced group and approximates that in the general population. (Modified from Shaw DB, Kekwick CA, Veale D, et al: Survival in second degree atrioventricular block. Br Heart J 53:589–593, 1985.)

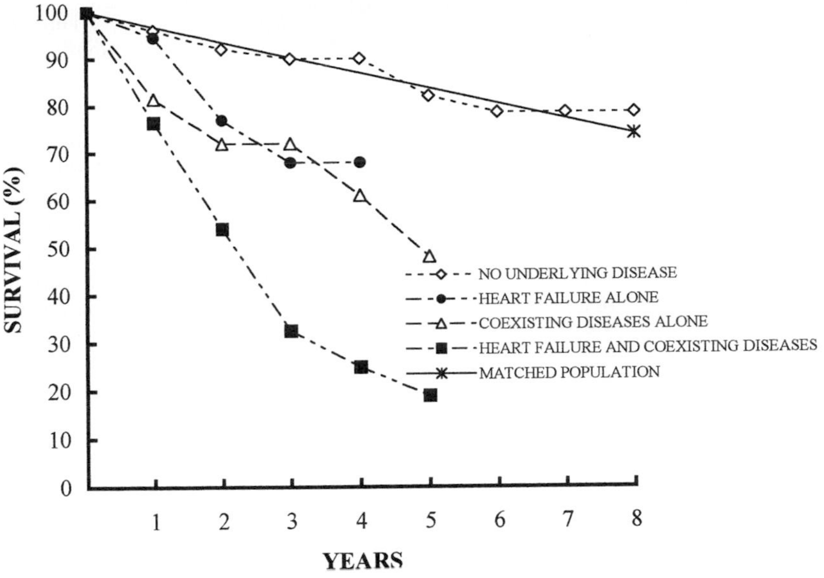

Figure 15–4. Survival rates in relation to the presence or absence of underlying disease in patients paced for atrioventricular block. See text for discussion. Survival for the matched population is taken from Figure 1 in the original article. (Modified from Fischer Hansen J, Meibom J: The prognosis for patients with complete heart block treated with permanent pacemaker. Acta Med Scand 195:385–389, 1974.)

to be tolerated in the person with compromised cardiac function. Activation of the sympathetic nervous system leads to an increase in myocardial metabolic demands and peripheral vascular resistance,[57] as well as bringing about activation of other potentially harmful neurohumoral systems, such as the renin-angiotensin system.[58] Cardiac dilation leads to an increase in wall tension (according to the Laplace relationship), which further stresses the failing heart unless compensated by myocardial hypertrophy, which in itself may hasten the deterioration and death of the cardiac cells.[59] Mechanisms such as these may explain why patients with heart failure and fixed-rate ventricular pacemakers fare worse than those receiving physiologic systems. Whether those receiving rate-adaptive ventricular units would fare better is unclear.

Although a survival benefit is likely with dual-chamber versus VVI pacing in patients with heart failure, there is little evidence at this stage to support any increase in survival in those without congestive heart failure. The only possible indication to the contrary comes from two fairly limited retrospective studies. In the first study of 1245 patients (77% with atrioventricular block, ventricular pacing in 97%, and dual-chamber pacing in only 3%), the authors stated that multivariate analysis demonstrated that survival was related to the mode of pacemaker therapy.[36] In a second study of 950 patients, 391 were paced for atrioventricular block or carotid sinus hypersensitivity.[60] DDD pacing was used in 273 patients and VVI pacing in 92, and the remaining 26 patients had DVI pacing. The survival rates at 7 years were 54% in the DDD group and 33% in the VVI group ($P<.05$).

Conclusions

1. Conservatively treated complete heart block has a poor prognosis, with 1- and 5-year survival rates of 60% and 30%, respectively. About one third of patients die suddenly. The prognosis is worse in those who are older, those who have associated cardiac diseases (particularly coronary heart disease), those with syncope, and those with constant (as opposed to transient or intermittent) complete heart block.

2. Conservatively treated chronic second-degree atrioven-

tricular block, independent of the type of second-degree block, is also associated with a reduced life expectancy, especially when associated with syncope.

3. There is a marked improvement in survival in those who are paced for complete and chronic second-degree atrioventricular block, but overall survival is still less than that of age-matched and sex-matched populations. Coexisting disease is common, and survival is adversely affected by these diseases, especially congestive heart failure and coronary heart disease. In the absence of these conditions, survival appears to be similar to that in the general population.

4. When compared with fixed-rate ventricular pacing, dual-chamber pacing appears to have a positive impact on survival in patients with congestive heart failure and atrioventricular block. At this stage, however, there is no firm evidence that this pacing mode has any impact on overall survival in patients without congestive heart failure.

Sick Sinus Syndrome

Natural History

The natural history of patients with sinus node dysfunction is not as clear as that in patients with atrioventricular block. This is partly related to the fact that the terms *sinus node dysfunction*, and especially *sick sinus syndrome*, encompass a heterogeneous spectrum of electrocardiographic abnormalities.[61–63] The clinical trials have tended to be restricted to inappropriate sinus bradycardia, sinoatrial block and sinus pauses, and the bradycardia-tachycardia syndrome. The major reason, however, for the scarcity of information on the natural history of sick sinus syndrome is that widespread interest in this condition began only after pacing had already been established as an effective treatment for atrioventricular block. Consequently, from the outset, pacemakers were implanted in symptomatic patients identified with the sick sinus syndrome. In 1989, it was estimated that the proportion of pacemaker implantations performed for sick sinus syndrome in the United States had risen to about 50%.[64]

The best study on the natural history of sick sinus syndrome is by Shaw and colleagues,[65] who followed 381 pa-

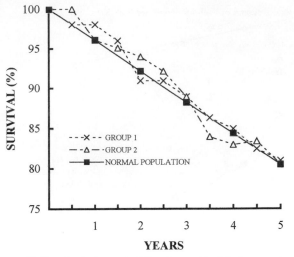

Figure 15–5. Survival rates in 381 patients with sick sinus syndrome. See text for discussion. (Modified from Shaw DB, Holman RR, Gowers JI: Survival in sinoatrial syndrome (sick-sinus syndrome). Br Med J 280:139–141, 1980.)

tients with sinus node dysfunction for up to 10 years (median, 5 years). All patients had persistent sinus bradycardia, defined as a heart rate of less than 56 bpm. The patients were divided into two groups: group 1, with "established sinus node dysfunction," had additional evidence of sinus node dysfunction documented on *routine* electrocardiogram, or associated tachyarrhythmias, and group 2, with "potential sinus node dysfunction," had only the sinus bradycardia. Pacemakers were implanted in 61 of the 381 patients. Survival in the two groups was identical, and similar to that of an age-matched and sex-matched normal population (Fig. 15–5). Furthermore, survival did not differ between the paced and unpaced patients. The two strongest predictors of mortality were syncope and a history of myocardial infarction. The authors concluded that sinus node dysfunction was "a relatively benign condition" and that "pacing should probably not be adopted as a routine measure but be reserved for patients with troublesome symptoms."[65] This conclusion has been widely accepted.[66]

This study has the same limitations as the publication by Shaw and colleagues on survival in second-degree atrioventricular block[39] (see above), which was also generated from the Devon Heart Block and Bradycardia Survey. By implanting pacemakers in a significant number of patients (16% of this group), those most at risk of succumbing may have been removed from the analysis, thus overestimating survival in conservatively-treated sick sinus syndrome. Unfortunately, given the ease and safety of pacemaker implantation, it is unlikely that any better information on the natural history of this disorder will ever be available.

Survival in Patients Paced for Sinus Node Dysfunction

Several studies have examined outcome in patients paced for sick sinus syndrome. Of the earlier trials, those that included more than 20 patients and allowed calculation of follow-up in patient-years are listed in Table 15–3.[67–77] In all of these reports, only fixed-rate ventricular-based pacing modes were employed (VOO or VVI). The studies were consistent in reporting a lower-than-expected survival rate in the paced patients compared with control populations.

Subsequent larger studies measured survival rates in the paced patients and usually compared these with those seen in age-matched and sex-matched control populations (Table 15–4).[31–34, 37, 76–84] Most have reported survival rates similar to those seen in the general population. In common with the earlier trials, many of these studies have employed only fixed-rate ventricular-inhibited pacing, although in the latest reports, physiologically based pacing modes have been used.

Factors Influencing Survival

Age and Underlying Disease. Various authors have reported that any excess in mortality in patients paced for the sick sinus syndrome over that seen in the general population can be accounted for by the presence of serious coexisting diseases, and that the presence of sick sinus syndrome per se is not accompanied by a reduced survival rate.[32, 71, 75, 77–78, 79, 84] More recent studies have also included multivariate analyses to determine which factors are independent predictors of mortality. In general, the strongest predictors have been advanced age and the presence of congestive heart failure, followed by coronary heart disease.[32, 33, 77, 80, 82–84] Valvular[33, 83, 84] or congenital[33] heart disease, peripheral vas-

Table 15–3. Early Studies of Survival in Patients Paced for Sick Sinus Syndrome*

Author(s)	Study Year	No. of Patients	Mean Age (yr)	Follow-Up (patient-years)	Death (%/yr)
Aroesty et al.[67]	1974	28	76	47	19.3
Radford and Julian[68]	1974	21	62	39	15.6
Härtel and Talvensaari[69]	1975	90	68	173	11.0
Krishnaswami and Geraci[70]	1975	33	69	49	22.4
Fruehan et al.[71]	1976	42	66	74	19.0
Wohl et al.[72]	1976	39	66	81	19.7
Amikam and Riss[73]	1977	25	—	60	9.9
Gould et al.[74]	1978	50	71	79	11.4
Breivik et al.[75]	1979	109	67	313	9.3
Simon and Zloto[76]	1979	59	65	246	7.3
Alpert and Katti[77]	1982	71	67	450	4.9

*Only those studies that included more than 20 patients and allowed calculation of follow-up in patient-years have been included. There appears to have been a steady improvement in survival with time, but this may simply reflect the changing criteria used in the selection of patients; that is, only the sicker and more symptomatic patients were selected in the earliest trials.

Table 15–4. Survival Rates From the Later Observational Studies Reporting on the Outcome of Patients Paced for Sick Sinus Syndrome

Author(s)	Study Year	Implantation Years	Mean Age (yr)	No. of Patients	Survival Time			
					1 yr	2 yr	5 yr	10 yr
Skagen et al.[78]	1975	1962–73	67	50	0.94	0.85	0.64	—
Simon and Zloto[76]*	1979	1965–78	65	59	0.86	0.86	0.73	—
Van Hemel et al.[79]	1981	1973–76	70	74	0.80	0.70	0.47	—
Alpert and Katti[77]	1982	1966–76	67	71	0.88	0.85	0.75	0.70
Kyle et al.[31]	1982	1961–76	71	34	0.82	0.64	0.44	—
Simon and Janz[32]	1982	1965–79	65	75	0.85	0.79	0.65	—
Hauser et al.[33]	1983	—	72	400	0.85	—	0.62	0.47
Alt et al.[34]	1985	1965–84	68	592	0.91	0.82	0.68	0.55
Lemke et al.[80]	1989	1972–87	65	100	0.99	0.95	0.85	0.61
Zanini et al.[81]	1989	1968–86	68	283	0.87	—	0.60	0.42
Brandt et al.[82]	1992	1979–89	68	213	0.97	0.96	0.89	0.72
Jelíc et al.[37]	1992	1967–85	63	173	0.94	—	0.86	0.82
Sgarbossa et al.[83]	1993	1980–89	66	507	0.95	0.92	0.80	0.61
Tung et al.[84]	1994	1969–91	76	148	0.84	0.77	0.57	0.29
Weighted mean	—	—	**68**	**2779**	**0.90**	**0.86**	**0.71**	**0.56**

*The results from Simon and Zloto (1979)[76] are presented but have not been used in the calculation of the weighted means because these patients were included in a later study by Simon and Janz[32] also contained in the table.

cular disease,[83] cerebrovascular disease,[84] and bundle-branch block[82, 83] have also been found to be significant.

Electrocardiographic Manifestations of Sick Sinus Syndrome. As discussed previously, sick sinus syndrome comprises a number of different electrocardiographic subtypes. The most obvious distinction is between patients with sinus node dysfunction alone (e.g., sinus bradycardia, sinus pauses) and those with added atrial tachyarrhythmias, in particular atrial fibrillation. It is well known that atrial fibrillation is a marker for increased mortality in general, and that it greatly increases the risk of stroke and thromboembolism.[85, 86] Consequently, a difference in survival between patients with isolated sinus bradycardia or sinus pauses or arrest and those with the bradycardia-tachycardia syndrome would not be surprising.

Although some studies have failed to show any difference in outcome between patients with sinus node dysfunction alone and those with added atrial tachyarrhythmias,[32, 33, 75, 77] a number have found a poorer survival in those with the bradycardia-tachycardia syndrome,[70, 73, 82] whereas none have suggested the opposite. Overall, these studies support the hypothesis of a more favorable prognosis with sinus node dysfunction alone. Confirmation of this hypothesis has been provided by a prospective randomized trial comparing atrial-based and ventricular-based pacing in patients with sick sinus syndrome,[87, 88] the results of which are presented later in the section discussing clinical trials. In this trial, multivariate analysis confirmed that the bradycardia-tachycardia syndrome is significantly associated with an increased risk of death, embolic events, and chronic atrial fibrillation (respective relative risks and probability values: 1.56, $P<.05$; 2.08, $P<.05$; and 3.92, $P=.001$).

Pacing Mode. In contrast to the small number of studies comparing outcome between the physiologically based and the fixed-rate ventricular-inhibited (VVI) pacing modes in patients with atrioventricular block, a considerable number

have done so in patients with sick sinus syndrome. Those studies in which sufficient data have been presented to enable calculation of death rates are presented in Table 15–5.[60, 81, 83, 84, 89–94] All of these reports are subject to the limitations common to retrospective studies on selected patient groups, and hence the results should be viewed as hypothesis generating rather than as definitive proof.

The studies have been unanimous in finding a lower mortality rate in patients receiving physiologically based pacing. Overall, the death rate in the physiologic group was about 5% per year, compared with 10% per year in the ventricular group. In many of the reports, this difference has achieved statistical significance.[89, 91–94] One of the better earlier studies reported on 168 patients with sick sinus syndrome from two separate institutions.[89] At one of these institutions, atrial pacing was the preferred mode, whereas at the other, the ventricular mode was preferred, thus giving rise to 89 patients with AAI and 79 patients with VVI pacemakers. The baseline characteristics of the two groups were similar, but the patients in atrial group were slightly younger and had less heart enlargement than those in the ventricular group. Also, the exclusion of patients with coexisting atrioventricular block from the atrial pacing group undoubtedly excluded some of the sicker patients. After 4 years, the group receiving atrial pacing had a significantly lower incidence of chronic atrial fibrillation, congestive heart failure, and death than was seen in the ventricular pacing group. There was no difference, however, in the incidence of stroke between the two groups.

In one of the more recent and larger studies, Sgarbossa and colleagues[83] compared outcome in 395 patients receiving physiologic pacing and 112 receiving VVI pacing who were followed for a mean of 5.5 years. On univariate analysis, VVI pacing was associated with a greater than 40% increase in risk of total and cardiovascular mortality, and this difference almost achieved statistical significance for total mortality ($P=.053$). With multivariate analysis, however, ventricular pacing was not found to be an independent risk factor.

Table 15–5. Survival Rates in Patients With Sick Sinus Syndrome in Relation to the Mode of Pacing, From Retrospective Observational Studies

| Author(s) | Study Year | Physiologic Mode | | Ventricular Mode | | Death (%/yr) | | |
		No. of Patients	Follow-Up (mo)	No. of Patients	Follow-Up (mo)	Phys.	Vent.	RR (%)
Rosenqvist et al.[89]	1988	89	44	79	47	2.1	5.9	−64*
Sasaki et al.[90]	1988	19	20	25	35	7.6	8.2	−7
Bianconi et al.[91]	1989	153	44	150	59	3.8	6.3	−40
Santini et al.[92]	1990	214	61	125	47	2.8	7.7	−64*
Stangl et al.[93]	1990	110	52	112	54	4.0	6.2	−35
Zanini et al.[81]	1990	53	45	57	40	2.5	5.3	−53
Nürnberg et al.[94]	1991	37	41	93	41	7.1	13.8	−49*
Hesselson et al.[60]	1992	308	30	193	44	8.3	12.8	−35*
Sgarbossa et al.[83]	1993	395	66	112	66	3.9	7.5	−48†
Tung et al.[84]	1994	36	44	112	44	8.3	16.5	−50†
Weighted mean	—	**1414**	**50**	**1058**	**49**	**4.8**	**9.4**	**−49**

RR, risk reduction.
*P < .05.
†P = .05.

The ventricular pacing mode was also identified as an independent predictor of chronic atrial fibrillation[95] (hazard ratio, 1.98; $P = .003$) and stroke[95] (hazard ratio, 2.61; $P = .008$), but not of congestive heart failure[96] (odds ratio, 0.86; $P = .603$).

The fact that all of these retrospective studies have shown a survival benefit in favor of physiologically based pacing over VVI pacing in patients with sick sinus syndrome is very suggestive. The results from a recent prospective, randomized trial have supported the findings from the retrospective studies, but it too has failed to provide definitive proof of a survival benefit (see later discussion of clinical trials for a more detailed presentation).[87, 88]

There are two likely mechanisms that could result in a higher mortality rate with the ventricular-based pacing mode in sick sinus syndrome. The first is through promotion of congestive heart failure through the same process as discussed previously in the section on atrioventricular block.[97] The second is through promotion of atrial fibrillation, which, even in the absence of pacing, occurs commonly in sick sinus syndrome.[98] A large number of retrospective[60, 81, 89–95, 98–102] and prospective[87, 88, 103, 104] trials have demonstrated an increase in the occurrence of atrial fibrillation and stroke in patients with sick sinus syndrome accompanying VVI pacing. The ventricular-based pacing modes may promote atrial fibrillation through several mechanisms:

1. Retrograde conduction through the atrioventricular node causes atrial contraction at a time when the atrioventricular valves are closed, resulting in high transient atrial pressures. This may eventually lead to atrial stretch and hypertrophy, which are known precursors of atrial fibrillation.[105]

2. Asynchronous atrial activation can trigger atrial fibrillation when retrograde premature atrial activation encroaches on the relative refractory period of the atrium.

3. Unrelieved sinus bradycardia may predispose to the development of atrial fibrillation through an increase in the dispersion of refractoriness of the atrial tissue.[106, 107] On the other hand, it is also possible that the atrial pacing–based physiologic modes may reduce the occurrence of atrial

fibrillation through overdrive suppression of atrial premature beats.[108]

Once atrial fibrillation develops, patients are exposed to a significant risk of stroke and systemic embolism. Numerous randomized clinical trials, which have included thousands of patients with atrial fibrillation, have established that these patients face a 4% to 8% annual risk of stroke.[109–113] Even with anticoagulant therapy the risk remains substantial at 1% to 3% per year.[109–115] Moreover, atrial fibrillation may easily be overlooked in patients with associated atrioventricular block. The patient may notice no change in heart rate or rhythm, and the physician may have difficulty in recognizing it on the electrocardiogram because of the regular ventricular pacing.

Conclusions

1. Sick sinus syndrome associated with minor symptoms carries a favorable prognosis, and survival appears equal to that of the general population. Death in such patients is more likely related to the presence of associated underlying disease (cardiovascular or otherwise) than to the electrophysiologic anomaly per se. In those with advanced symptoms due to the sinus node dysfunction (e.g., syncope), however, survival may be reduced.

2. Patients who are paced for sick sinus syndrome have a normal survival time. Those with the bradycardia-tachycardia syndrome, however, appear to have a slightly worse outlook than those with isolated sinus node dysfunction.

3. There is good evidence to suggest that physiologic pacing in sick sinus syndrome is associated with a reduced incidence of death, stroke, and atrial fibrillation when compared with single-chamber ventricular pacing.

Atrioventricular Block Versus Sick Sinus Syndrome

Survival

Several studies have compared survival in patients paced for sick sinus syndrome with that of patients paced for atrioventricular block.[31–33, 36, 37, 46, 116] All but two[31, 33] have shown better survival in the sick sinus syndrome group, but this difference achieved statistical significance in only one study.[34] When the pooled results from the studies presented in Tables 15–2 and 15–4 are compared, they too suggest a poorer overall survival in the heart block group (Fig. 15–6). Given that survival in paced patients without major associated diseases approximates that in the general population, it is likely that the difference in survival between those with atrioventricular block and those with sick sinus syndrome can be accounted for by differences in the prevalence or severity of the underlying diseases.

Causes of Death

Atrioventricular Block. Causes of death have been pooled from a number of the studies.[6, 11, 14, 17, 19, 22, 25, 26, 28, 30, 32, 35, 37, 38, 46, 49, 117] The total number of deaths from these studies is 1314. Not surprisingly, many patients who die after pacemaker treatment for heart block do so as a result of cardiac diseases. Overall, about 15% die suddenly; 30% die from cardiac conditions such as congestive heart failure and acute myocardial infarction; about 10% die from strokes; and another 30% die from noncardiac diseases, such as malignancy, renal failure, respiratory failure, and infections. Most of the sudden deaths are related to ventricular tachyarrhythmias.[47, 118] Some, however, particularly from the earlier days of pacing, have been a result of pacemaker failure. In contrast, the number of known pacemaker-related deaths in the later studies has been extremely small, generally less than 1%. A significant perioperative mortality in the early years of pacing,[17, 21, 22, 119] when a thoracotomy was required to attach the epicardial electrodes, is a problem that has all but disappeared.

Sick Sinus syndrome. The causes of death in patients paced for sick sinus syndrome have also been pooled.[32, 46, 69,]

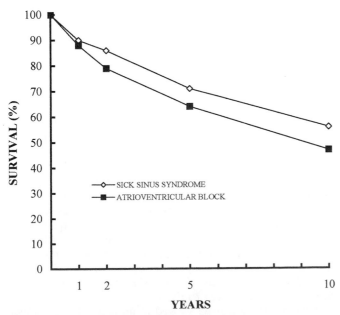

Figure 15–6. Survival rates in patients paced for atrioventricular block and sick sinus syndrome. Data are combined from Tables 15–2 and 15–4.

[70, 72, 75–77, 82–84, 88–90, 93]* The total number of deaths is 509. Overall, the proportions of patients dying from the various causes is remarkably similar to that seen in atrioventricular block: about 15% die suddenly; 35% die from cardiac causes; 10% die from stroke or systemic embolism; and 30% die from noncardiac diseases. Given the higher incidence of atrial fibrillation in patients with sick sinus syndrome, it is a little surprising that mortality due to stroke or embolism was no different from that in the heart block patients. The number of pacemaker-related and perioperative deaths is much less than 1%, in keeping with the fact that these studies are predominantly dealing with a group paced after 1970.

■ QUALITY OF LIFE IN PATIENTS WHO HAVE PACEMAKERS

Introductory Considerations

Why Quality of Life?

When the pacemaker was first introduced in 1960, the focus was on improving survival in patients with complete heart block and Stokes-Adams attacks. The benefit was obvious and justified the inconvenience of the early pacing systems and the relatively high perioperative mortality.[12] With the introduction of endocardial leads and the improvement in design, longevity, and reliability of the pacemaker, the indications for pacemaker treatment have gradually widened. Guidelines outlining the generally accepted indications for this therapy have been introduced on the basis of whether treatment has been associated with an improvement in symptoms or survival.[66]

With the introduction of newer pacing modalities and features, however, the question has shifted from whether patients with a certain condition should receive a pacemaker to which kind of pacemaker they should receive. Comparison among these alternatives, principally between the physiologically based pacing modes and the ventricular-based modes, has been the subject of recent research. The physiologically based pacing modes have been consistently shown to produce superior central hemodynamic parameters compared with the ventricular-based modes.[50, 121] Numerous crossover trials comparing exercise performance between the various modes have also been conducted[51, 52, 122–143] (Table 15–6). Here too, the physiologic modes have been demonstrated to provide a significant advantage, at least when compared with the VVI mode. There has been no benefit when the physiologic modes have been compared with the VVIR mode, and this is probably because most of the increase in cardiac output during exercise is dependent on an appropriate increase in heart rate rather than on the maintenance of atrioventricular synchrony.[52–54]

The clinical relevance of these findings, however, is questionable. Do differences in central hemodynamics or in exercise capacity translate into a noticeable difference in everyday activities, and do the patients *feel* any better? Because most pacemakers are implanted in people who are older and more sedentary, any potential hemodynamic benefit may go completely unnoticed. Furthermore, even if an improvement in hemodynamics might make the patient feel better, such an effect may be overwhelmed by the effects of other disease

---

*Reference No. 120 has been omitted.

Table 15–6. Results of the Crossover Studies Comparing Maximum Exercise Duration and Work Achieved Using Different Pacing Modalities*

Author(s)	Study Year	Indication for Pacing	No. of Patients	Study Period (wk)	Comparison	Percentage Increase in Exercise
					VDD/DDD vs. VVI	
Kruse et al.[51]	1982	AVB	16	12	VDD vs. VVI	24†
Fananapazir et al.[124]	1983	AVB	14	0	VAT vs. VOO	44†
Kristensson et al.[125]	1983	AVB	13	0	VDD vs. VVI	18†
Pehrsson and Åström[57]	1983	AVB	14	1	VAT vs. VVI	25†
Perrins et al.[126]	1983	AVB	13	4	VDD vs. VVI	28†
Yee et al.[127]	1984	AVB	8	12	VDD vs. VVI	30
Kristensson et al.[128]	1985	AVB	44	3	VDD vs. VVI	14†
Mitsuoka et al.[129]	1988	AVB	8	4	DDD vs. VVI	23†
Mitsuoka et al.[129]	1988	SSS	8	4	DDD vs. VVI	3‡
Rediker et al.[131]	1988	AVB/SSS	19	6	DDD vs. VVI	12†
Sulke et al.[132]	1992	AVB/SSS	16	4	DDD vs. VVI	21†
					VVIR vs. VVI	
Fananapazir et al.[124]	1983	AVB	14	0	VVIR§ vs. VOO	40†
Pehrsson and Åström[57]	1983	AVB	14	1	VVIR§ vs. VVI	20†
Benditt et al.[133]	1987	AVB/SSS	12	0	VVIR vs. VVI	33†
Lipkin et al.[134]	1987	AVB	10	4	VVIR vs. VVI	14‖
Smedgård et al.[135]	1987	AVB	15	1	VVIR vs. VVI	19†
Hedman and Nordlander[136]	1989	AVB	18	4	VVIR vs. VVI	9†
Lau et al.[137]	1989	AVB/SSS	16	4	VVIR vs. VVI	30†
Oto et al.[138]	1991	AVB	11	3	VVIR vs. VVI	35†
					DDD vs. VVIR	
Fananapazir et al.[124]	1983	AVB	14	0	VAT vs. VVIR§	−1
Pehrsson and Åström[57]	1983	AVB	14	1	VAT vs. VVIR§	4
Bubien and Kay[139]	1990	AVB	8	6	DDD vs. VVIR	2
Menozzi et al.[123]	1990	AVB	14	6	DDD vs. VVIR	3
Oldroyd et al.[122]	1991	AVB	10	4	DDD vs. VVIR	3
Sulke et al.[141]	1991	AVB + SSS	22	4	DDD vs. VVIR	−2
Linde-Edelstam et al.[142]	1992	AVB	17	8	DDD vs. VVIR	−4
Deharo et al.[143]	1996	AVB	15	4	DDD vs. VVIR	0
					DDDR vs. VVIR	
Vogt et al.[130]	1988	AVB/SSS	6	0	DDDR vs. VVIR	16
Jutzy et al.[140]	1990	AVB/SSS	14	0	DDDR vs. VVIR	10
Sulke et al.[141]	1991	AVB + SSS	22	4	DDDR vs. VVIR	11†

AVB, atrioventricular block; SSS, sick sinus syndrome.

*There is a significant increase in exercise capacity with the physiologic and ventricular rate-adaptive modes over that seen in the ventricular fixed-rate mode. There is no improvement in exercise capacity with the DDD mode over the VVIR mode, but there is with the DDDR mode, although this benefit is only of borderline statistical significance.

†$P < .05$.

‡All but one patient was in sinus rhythm (i.e., nonpaced rhythm) for the exercise tests.

§The ventricular pacing rate was increased to match the underlying atrial rate without allowing for atrioventricular synchronization.

‖The comparison was with maximum oxygen consumption rather than total exercise duration and work.

processes, which are common in this age group. Thus, when assessing the overall benefit of any particular pacing mode over another, particularly when one of the modes happens to be more costly and complicated (as is the case with dual-chamber pacing), it is not enough to point to an improvement in "laboratory" tests. One must show that the hemodynamic advantage actually translates into a real-life advantage, either making the patient's life more tolerable or affecting positively some major clinical outcome, such as mortality. Thus, assessment of quality of life has become an important area in modern pacing research.

Concepts and Definitions

Quality of life is difficult to define. The World Health Organization (WHO) defines *health* as "a state of complete physical, mental and social well-being and not merely the absence of disease or infirmity."[144] Similarly, quality of life

can be conceived of as "an individual's overall satisfaction with life, and one's general sense of personal well-being."[145]

As far as quality of life in clinical trials is concerned however, the definition, though still broad in its outlook, is necessarily more limited. Here, the investigator is primarily interested in the "health-related quality of life." In this setting, the definition of quality of life may be restricted to "the functional effect of an illness and its consequent therapy upon a patient, as perceived by the patient."[146] Although the definition is limited in comparison with the WHO definition, it is important to appreciate that "*it is this increased breadth of mission which distinguishes quality-of-life studies from traditional clinical trials.*"[147]

Quality of life can be viewed in an hierarchical manner. At the top is the unifying concept of the overall sense of well-being. This can be thought of as being composed of a number of broad areas (referred to as *domains* or *dimen-*

sions), which themselves can be further subdivided into *components*. The simplest subdivision of quality of life is into the three divisions contained in the WHO definition: physical, mental, and social. The latter domain is often further broken down into *social interactions* and *economic factors*[148] and other authors include further divisions. When considering health-related quality of life specifically, multiple surveys of patients and of the public have consistently demonstrated five key dimensions essential to quality-of-life considerations: death (the desire to live as long as possible), disability (the desire to function normally), discomfort (the desire to be free of symptoms), side effects (the desire to be free of iatrogenic problems), and economic factors (the desire to be financially solvent).[147]

Instruments and Measures

The quality-of-life measures, or *instruments*, can be used to discriminate among individual patients, to predict outcome or prognosis, or to evaluate change in a particular patient over a period of time.[149] Most quality-of-life trials in paced patients have been concerned with discrimination and evaluation. A quality-of-life instrument must be reliable (repeated administration to a stable population of patients gives the same results); valid (established by comparison with known standards); and sensitive (able to detect changes in a particular condition over the course of time).

Quality-of-life instruments are of two general types: generic instruments "designed to sample the complete spectrum of function, disability and distress that is related to quality-of-life,"[149] and specific instruments. The generic instruments consist of *health profiles* and *utility measures*. Health profiles are a single comprehensive measure that yields a number of category scores or a single overall score (in which case they are referred to as an *index*). Many validated health profiles are available, such as the Sickness Impact Profile, the Nottingham Health Profile, the McMaster Health Index, and the 36-item Medical Outcomes Study Short-Form General Health Survey (SF-36).[150] Health profiles allow the use of one global questionnaire as opposed to multiple smaller ones and have well-established reliability and validity. Their main disadvantage is that they may not focus on the major area of interest (a particular problem with arrhythmias) and thus can be insensitive in discriminating between treatments.

The specific instruments can be disease specific, population specific, or function specific. Their main advantage is their increased sensitivity, but they lack comprehensiveness and are often unvalidated. The use and limitations of the various instruments in paced patients has been reviewed by Linde.[151]

The Quality-of-Life Trials

Before examining the trials, it should be noted that they share a number of limitations necessitating that the results be interpreted cautiously. In the first place, the trials are small. Second, the trials often contain mixed groups of patients, that is, patients with atrioventricular block, sick sinus syndrome, or both. These groups do not necessarily respond in the same manner to different pacing modes. For instance, DDD pacing in the patient with persistent sinus bradycardia is not truly comparable to DDD pacing in the patient with intact sinus function and atrioventricular block. Third, in crossover studies, especially in those using devices like pacemakers, the potential for patient and investigator unblinding is relatively high. Finally, there is the problem of the quality-of-life instruments themselves. On the one hand, many of the trials have failed to use properly tested and validated instruments. On the other hand, most of the validated instruments have not been specifically designed with pacemaker patients in mind and thus may be insensitive. Even those measures designed for use in patients with cardiovascular disease, such as the Specific Activity Scale,[152] have proved relatively insensitive (at least in the crossover trials). Bearing these limitations in mind, the results of some of the quality-of-life trials are discussed next.

Comparison of Pacing Modes

The earliest studies compared the physiologic pacing modes to fixed-rate ventricular-inhibited pacing. More recent studies have compared the rate-adaptive and fixed-rate ventricular-inhibited pacing modes, and the most recent have contrasted dual-chamber pacing with rate-adaptive ventricular pacing. These studies are summarized in Table 15–7.[51, 122, 123, 126–133, 135–141, 143, 153–159]

DDD Versus VVI

In keeping with the findings from the hemodynamic investigations and the studies examining exercise capacity, the quality-of-life trials have shown a fairly consistent benefit of physiologic pacing over fixed-rate ventricular-inhibited pacing. Rediker and associates[131] reported on 19 patients who had DDD pacemakers implanted for atrioventricular block or sick sinus syndrome. The patients had been paced in the DDD mode for at least 2 months before randomization. Each patient completed a number of questionnaires (which included validated quality-of-life instruments) and an exercise test before randomization and after each of the 6-week pacing periods. During the study, 8 patients requested early crossover from VVI to DDD because of intolerable symptoms, whereas the other 11 completed the pacing protocols as planned. The group's perception of daily activity performance and health status favored the DDD mode, as did their ratings for fatigue, shortness of breath, and palpitations. This favoring of the DDD mode, however, was accounted for entirely by the 8 patients requesting early crossover; there was no difference in the subjective scores for the two modes in the 11 patients not requesting crossover.

This study is interesting because it demonstrates two distinct responses to VVI pacing. One group was unable to tolerate VVI pacing because of symptoms suggestive of pacemaker syndrome, whereas the other group was apparently able to tolerate the mode. It is not surprising that those patients with pacemaker syndrome showed a significant difference in subjective scores for the two pacing modes. Despite significant improvements in hemodynamic indices and in exercise tolerance, however, there was no difference in quality-of-life scores for the second group. When asked to indicate their preferred mode, only 4 of the latter group chose the DDD mode, whereas the other 7 expressed no preference. One other well-designed crossover comparison of these modes also failed to show any subjective benefit with the DDD mode.[127]

Sulke and colleagues,[132] however, in a study designed to

Table 15–7. Quality-of-Life Scores and Patient Preference in Crossover Comparisons of Pacing Modes*

Author(s)	Study Year	Indication for Pacing	No. of Patients	Study Period (wk)	Comparison	Instruments	Best Mode*	Preferred Mode†		
					VDD/DDD vs. VVI			DDD	VVI	None
Kruse et al.[51]	1982	AVB	16	12	VDD vs. VVI	Symptom score	?VDD	14	0	None
Perrins et al.[126]	1983	AVB	13	4	VDD vs. VVI	Symptom score	VDD	—	—	2
Yee et al.[127]	1984	AVB	8	12	VDD vs. VVI	Symptom score	None	1	0	7
Kristensson et al.[128]	1985	AVB	44	3	VDD vs. VVI	Symptom score	VDD	29	6	9
Boon et al.[153]	1987	AVB/SSS	15	4	DDD vs. VVI	Symptom score	DDD	12	1	2
Mitsuoka et al.[129]	1988	AVB/SSS	16	4	DDD vs. VVI	Symptom score	DDD	—	—	—
Rediker et al.[131]	1988	AVB/SSS	19	6	DDD vs. VVI	Symptom score; Functional Status Questionnaire; Specific Activity Scale§	DDD	12	0	7
Heldman et al.[154]	1990	AVB/SSS	40	1	DDD‡ vs. VVI	Symptom score	DDD	—	—	—
Sulke et al.[132]	1992	ABV/SSS	16	4	DDD vs. VVI	Symptom and General Well-Being scores; Specific Activity Scale§	DDD	12	2‖	2
					VVIR vs. VVI			VVIR	VVI	None
Lipkin et al[134]	1987	AVB	10	4	VVIR vs. VVI	McMaster Health Index§	VVIR	—	—	None
Smedgård et al.[135]	1987	AVB	15	1	VVIR vs. VVI	Symptom score	None	13	0	2
Hedman and Nordlander[136]	1989	AVB	18	4	VVIR vs. VVI	Symptom and General Well-Being scores	VVIR	11	2	5
Lau et al.[137]	1989	AVB/SSS	16	4	VVIR vs. VVI	Symptom score; Nottingham Health Profile§	None	—	—	—
Oto et al.[138]	1991	AVB/SSS	11	3	VVIR vs. VVI	Hacettepe Quality-of-Life Questionnaire§	VVIR	—	—	—
					DDD vs. VVIR			DDD	VVIR	None
Bubien and Kay[139]	1990	AVB	8	6	DDD vs. VVIR	Symptom Frequency and Distress score;§ Psychological General Well-Being Index; McMaster Health Index§	None	7	0	1
Menozzi et al.[123]	1990	AVB	14	6	DDD vs. VVIR	Symptom score	DDD	8	0	6
Oldroyd et al.[122]	1991	AVB	10	4	DDD vs. VVIR	McMaster Health Index§	None	1	0	9
Sulke et al.[141]	1991	AVB + SSS	22	4	DDD vs. VVIR	As per above, ref. 132	DDD	9	3	5
Linde-Edelstam et al.[142]	1992	AVB	17	8	DDD vs. VVIR	Karolinska Questionnaire§	DDD	—	—	—
Lau et al.[157]	1994	AVB/SSS	33	8	DDD vs. VVIR	Modified Bradford Somatic Inventory§; Illness Perception score; Oveall Quality-of-Life Score; Specific Activity Scale§	DDD	—	—	—
Lukl et al.[156]	1994	AVB/SSS	21	2	DDD vs. VVIR	Symptom score	DDD	18	1	2
Deharo et al.[143]	1996	AVB	15	4	DDD vs. VVIR	Symptom score; Specific Activity Scale§	None	—	—	—
					DDDR vs. VVIR			DDDR	VVIR	None
Hummel et al.[159]	1990	SSS	8	2	DDDR vs. VVIR	Symptom and General Well-Being scores	DDDR	—	—	None
Sulke et al.[141]	1991	AVB + SSS	22	4	DDDR vs. VVIR	As per above, ref. 132	DDDR	19	2	—
Lau et al.[157]	1994	AVB/SSS	33	8	DDDR vs. VVIR	As per above, ref. 157	DDDR	—	—	—
Lau et al.[158]	1994	SSS	15	4	DDR/AAIR vs. VVIR	Basically, as per above, ref. 157	DDDR/AAIR	—	—	—

AVB, atrioventricular block; SSS, sick sinus syndrome.

*Best mode indicates the results of the quality-of-life evaluation only if the difference between modes was statistically significant in one or more of the scores.

†Preferred mode indicates the patient's preference irrespective of the results of the quality-of-life evaluation.

§Validated quality-of-life instrument.

‡Ten of the 40 were actually programmed to DDI.

§Validated quality-of-life instrument.

‖The two patients who preferred the DDI mode; the study compared DDD, DDI, and VVI and found no difference between DDI and VVI.

look specifically at those patients able to tolerate long-term VVI pacing, did find a significant difference favoring DDD pacing. They evaluated 16 patients with long-standing VVI pacemakers who had no symptoms suggestive of pacemaker syndrome having their devices upgraded to DDD at the time of elective generator replacement. Postoperatively, all pacemakers were programmed to three modes (DDD, DDI, and VVI) in a random sequence. Subjective assessment consisted of three self-administered questionnaires: the first used a visual analog scale (the subjects placed a mark along a 15-cm line) to assess general well-being and exercise capacity; the second assessed functional capacity using the Specific Activity Scale; and the third, using a scale of 0 to 5, assessed specific symptoms suggestive of the pacemaker syndrome or mild cardiac failure. Objective assessments with exercise testing and echocardiography were also performed. Comparisons were made among the three postoperative modes and also with the preoperative VVI mode. The patients' perceptions of general well-being and exercise capacity were significantly better in the DDD mode than both the pre-replacement and post-replacement VVI mode. There was no significant difference in the perceived functional status using the Specific Activity Scale. The specific symptom scores were significantly better in the DDD mode than in the other modes. Overall, when asked to indicate their preferred mode, 11 patients chose the DDD mode, 1 chose either DDD or VVI, 2 chose DDI, and 2 had no preference (both were non-pacemaker independent). Despite toleration of the VVI mode preoperatively, three patients demanded early crossover from the postoperative VVI or DDI mode. All three had spent 4 weeks in the DDD mode before moving on to the VVI or DDI modes. The authors specifically commented that the patients' choice of least acceptable mode was highly dependent on programming sequence, so that if VVI was the first postoperative mode, subjective scores were better than if the VVI mode followed the DDD mode. Both subjectively and objectively, the DDI mode was no different from the VVI mode.

The authors interpreted these findings to indicate the presence of a "subclinical pacemaker syndrome," even in apparently well patients tolerating VVI pacing. Thus, on the basis of this study, along with the other studies listed in Table 15–7, DDD pacing appears to be subjectively superior to VVI pacing.

VVIR Versus VVI

Despite the clear improvement in exercise tolerance with rate-adaptive pacing, the studies comparing VVIR pacing to VVI pacing have not shown a consistent quality-of-life benefit with rate adaption.[134–138] In the two trials that specifically recorded patient preference, however, patients favored the VVIR mode. Such an unexpectedly modest response to the institution of rate-adaptive pacing may have a number of possible explanations:

1. Most elderly patients with pacemakers are relatively inactive and consequently are likely to derive only a limited benefit from rate adaption in the first place.

2. Those with near-normal cardiac function can presumably increase stroke volume sufficiently to cope with normal daily activities and thus may notice no benefit.

3. The rate-response programming may have been suboptimal.

4. Any benefit from the ability to vary the heart rate may have been counterbalanced by the persistence of any negative symptoms accompanying the loss of atrioventricular synchrony.

Smedgård and colleagues[135] studied 15 patients in a randomized crossover study of one week each of VVI and VVIR pacing. Subjective assessment included questions pertaining to specific symptoms, exercise tolerance, and general feeling of well-being. The total mean symptom score per day was lower (i.e., better) in the VVIR group (165 versus 194), but the difference was not significant. On the other hand, when questioned about their preferred mode, 13 of the 15 patients indicated a preference for the VVIR mode, and only 2 indicated no preference. This failure of the questionnaires to detect a significant difference between the two modes when most patients appeared to prefer the VVIR mode possibly indicates a lack of sensitivity of the questionnaires.

Using a quality-of-life instrument designed specifically for pacemaker patients, Oto and colleagues[138] performed a study in which 11 patients were randomized to either the VVIR or VVI modes for 3 weeks. At the end of each study period, an exercise test was performed, and quality of life was evaluated using the Hacettepe Quality-of-Life Questionnaire (reproduced in their publication). In addition to confirming a significant improvement in exercise duration with the VVIR mode, they also demonstrated a significant improvement in quality-of-life scores.

DDD Versus VVIR

On the basis of the studies presented so far, DDD pacing appears clearly superior to VVI pacing, both objectively and subjectively. There is less certainty, however, about whether the DDD mode, which provides atrioventricular synchronization and appropriate rate response (in the absence of sinus node disease), is better than the VVIR mode, which allows for appropriate rate response without providing atrioventricular synchrony. The studies looking at exercise duration suggest that there is *no* difference between the two modes. As discussed earlier, however, maximum exercise duration may be a poor predictor of overall quality of life.

In contrast to studies in which DDD pacing was compared with VVI pacing, virtually all of the studies comparing DDD with VVIR have included validated quality-of-life instruments. Results have varied, however, and may depend in part on the particular quality-of-life instrument chosen. Two studies showed no difference between these pacing modes, both using the McMaster Health Index.[122, 139] Another study (comparing VVIR and VVI), however, showed a significant difference in subjective scores using this instrument.[133]

Linde-Edelstam and associates[155] compared quality of life between the DDD and VVIR modes in 17 patients with high-degree atrioventricular block and preserved sinus function. The patients were randomized to each mode for a period of 8 weeks, after which a questionnaire was completed. This questionnaire, the Karolinska Questionnaire, was derived from a number of different validated instruments. Significant reduction of shortness of breath, dizziness, palpitations, and improvement in cognitive functioning were observed during DDD pacing. There was no significant difference in mood, sleep, physical and social ability, or self-perceived health. Nine of the patients expressed a preference for the DDD mode, 3 preferred the VVIR mode, and 5 had no preference. One patient insisted on early crossover from the VVIR mode because of shortness of breath.

In a triple crossover study of the DDDR, DDD, and VVIR modes, Lau and colleagues[158] compared quality of life in 33 patients with either atrioventricular block or sick sinus syndrome. Quality of life was evaluated using the Specific Activity Scale to assess functional class, a modification of the Bradford Somatic Inventory to assess physical malaise, a questionnaire designed to assess illness perception, and an overall quality-of-life score based on an interview with a clinical psychologist. As with many of the studies,[131, 132] no significant difference in the mean functional class for the three pacing modes was found using the Specific Activity Scale. There was no difference between the DDD and VVIR modes in any of the 41 physical malaise inventory items, and in only 1 of the 43 illness perception categories (contentment) was there a significant difference favoring the DDD mode. The overall quality-of-life score, however, was significantly better in the DDD group than in the VVIR group.

The remaining three studies comparing DDD with VVIR pacing used questionnaires designed to assess disease-related symptoms. All 3 favored the DDD mode. In summary, although most of the quality-of-life trials comparing these two particular modes have demonstrated a benefit in favor of the dual-chamber mode, the difference has been small, and given the methodologic limitations of most of these studies, it is difficult to draw definite conclusions.

DDDR Versus VVIR

Only a few studies have reported on quality of life in DDDR compared with VVIR pacing. Sulke and associates[141] performed a randomized crossover study of 4 pacing modes (DDDR, DDIR, DDD, and VVIR) in 22 patients with combined atrioventricular block and sick sinus syndrome. They reported significantly lower perception of general well-being, exercise tolerance, Specific Activity Scale score, and specific symptom score in the VVIR mode than in the other three modes, among which there was no difference.

Lau and colleagues[157] performed a triple crossover study of three rate-responsive pacing modes (DDDR, AAIR, and VVIR) in 15 patients with sick sinus syndrome. A number of objective assessments were performed along with a quality-of-life assessment. There were no significant differences in any of the specific symptoms assessed by questionnaire, except palpitations, which occurred more frequently during the VVIR mode. There was no difference in overall functional class as assessed by the Specific Activity Scale. Overall quality-of-life scores were no different for the 3 modes. The only difference was in general well-being, which was rated significantly lower in the VVIR mode than in either the AAIR or DDDR modes.

A randomized, prospective trial comparing quality of life with DDDR and VVIR pacing has been published. The results of this trial (the PASE trial) are discussed in detail in the next section on clinical trials and are presented only briefly at this stage. A total of 407 patients were enrolled; 201 had atrioventricular block, and 175 had sick sinus syndrome as the cause of their bradycardia. Overall, there was no substantial difference in quality of life between the two groups, although 26% of the VVIR group crossed over

to DDDR because of symptoms suggestive of pacemaker syndrome. In the subgroup with atrioventricular block, there was no difference in overall quality-of-life scores; however, in the patients with sick sinus syndrome, there were modest and statistically significant differences in quality of life, favoring the DDDR group, and it is likely that these differences would have been even more impressive had not more than 50% of the VVIR group (with sick sinus syndrome) crossed over to DDDR pacing.

Other Quality-of-Life Trials

A small number of trials have examined the effect of changes in atrioventricular delay on quality of life. Atrioventricular delay can be individually optimized to provide the greatest hemodynamic benefit at rest. Studies have shown that this hemodynamic benefit can be maintained during exercise,[160–162] but this does not necessarily translate into an improvement in maximum exercise duration.[163–165] Sulke and coworkers[165] found a significant difference in subjective scores favoring a fixed atrioventricular delay of 125 msec and a rate-adaptive atrioventricular delay over the longer fixed atrioventricular delays of 175 or 250 msec. Linde and colleagues[166] assessed quality-of-life and hemodynamic parameters in 10 patients with severe congestive heart failure who received dual-chamber pacing with individual optimization of atrioventricular delay. Despite lack of sustained improvement in hemodynamic parameters over the long term, there was a significant improvement in quality-of-life scores, which persisted for the entire 6-month observation period. As the authors point out, however, there was no blinding of the patients, and a placebo effect could well explain this apparent improvement, especially given the lack of sustained hemodynamic benefit. A third study failed to demonstrate any significant improvement in quality of life with individual optimization of atrioventricular delay.[167]

The effect of mode switching was evaluated in 48 patients with paroxysmal atrial tachyarrhythmias and atrioventricular block.[168] DDDR, with and without mode switching, was compared with the VVIR mode. DDDR with mode switching resulted in a longer exercise time and better quality-of-life than VVIR. DDDR with mode switching also resulted in a better quality of life than DDDR without mode switching, but no difference in exercise time.

Conclusions

1. Most patients appear to find the DDD mode preferable to the VVI mode.

2. The VVIR mode appears preferable to the VVI mode in most patients, but this benefit is not as obvious as would be expected based on the significant improvement in effort tolerance accompanying VVIR pacing.

3. At this stage, there is little evidence to support the hypothesis that the DDD or DDDR mode provides a superior quality of life to the VVIR mode in patients with atrioventricular block. In those with sick sinus syndrome, however, DDDR pacing appears to provide a modest improvement in quality of life over the VVIR mode.

4. There is too little information available to draw any conclusions regarding the potential subjective benefit of individual optimization of the atrioventricular delay in patients with dual-chamber devices.

■ CLINICAL TRIALS IN PACEMAKER PATIENTS: THE PROSPECTIVE RANDOMIZED TRIALS OF PACEMAKER MODE SELECTION

Intuitively, one would expect a benefit from the closer approximation of the normal cardiac activation sequence provided by physiologic pacing systems. Such systems, however, are more expensive and more complicated than ventricular-based devices. As discussed previously, a number of studies have demonstrated the hemodynamic advantages of the physiologic pacing modes, and other studies confirmed that this translated into a significant improvement in exercise capacity when compared with the fixed-rate ventricular mode, but not when compared with the rate-adaptive ventricular pacing mode.

A minority of patients develop symptoms in association with ventricular pacing as a result of the loss of atrioventricular synchrony,[169] and these symptoms can be alleviated by dual-chamber pacing.[170, 171] Additionally, as presented in the previous discussion, many small crossover studies have specifically examined the impact of pacing mode on quality of life. These trials have confirmed that, even when they do not have pacemaker syndrome, patients generally feel better when paced in a physiologic mode than in either of the ventricular-based modes.

Finally, a number of observational studies have also compared outcome between the physiologic and ventricular-based pacing modes. These studies (presented in Table 15–8[49, 60, 81, 83, 84, 89–96, 98, 99, 101, 102] and Fig. 15–7) have been consistent in suggesting that physiologic pacing is associated with less atrial fibrillation, stroke, congestive heart failure, and death than is ventricular pacing. Dual-chamber pacemaker selection was also found to be an independent predictor of increased survival in a large observational study of pacing practices in the United States.[172] If these findings are correct, this would more than justify the increased expense of the dual-chamber systems. To address these issues more conclusively, several prospective, randomized trials comparing the effects of physiologic and ventricular pacing modes on clinical outcomes and quality of life have been initiated. These trials are the focus of the final section of this chapter.

The Danish Study

Andersen and colleagues[87, 88] evaluated 225 patients with sick sinus syndrome who were enrolled in a prospective, randomized study comparing outcome in atrial versus ventricular pacing. Patients with chronic atrial fibrillation or evidence of atrioventricular conduction abnormalities were excluded. The end points were total mortality, atrial fibrillation, thromboembolism, and heart failure. Follow-up was for up to 8 years after implantation, with a mean duration of 5.5 years. Analysis was by intention-to-treat. The results from the two publications are presented in Table 15–9 and Figure 15–8.

In the first report from this study,[87] there were no significant differences in any of the primary end points, except for that of thromboembolism, which was more common in the ventricular pacing group. In the later publication,[88] however, atrial pacing was associated with a significant reduction in the incidence of atrial fibrillation, thromboembolism, and cardiovascular mortality and with a smaller reduction in overall mortality of borderline statistical significance. There also appeared to be a significant difference in the incidence and severity of heart failure between the two groups as assessed by average New York Heart Association functional class and use of diuretics, also favoring the atrial group. It should be borne in mind, however, when interpreting the findings reported in the second paper, that the second look at the data was not preplanned, nor was there any statistical power associated with this look—thus, the results of the long-term follow-up cannot be conclusive, but instead only hypothesis generating.

This study is important because it was the first randomized prospective trial examining the effect of pacing mode on patient outcome. Although the study was relatively small, the results support the observations from the retrospective studies suggesting a reduction in outcome events with physiologic pacing in patients with sick sinus syndrome.

The Pacemaker Selection in the Elderly Trial

The PASE trial was a single-blind, randomized, controlled comparison of DDDR and VVIR pacing in patients aged 65 years or older who required pacing therapy for the prevention or treatment of bradycardia.[173] Twenty-nine centers across the United States were involved. The primary end point was health-related quality of life, assessed using SF-36[150] and the Specific Activity Scale.[152] The prespecified secondary end points were: death from all causes; first nonfatal stroke or death; first hospitalization for heart failure, first nonfatal stroke, or death; development of atrial fibrillation; and development of the pacemaker syndrome. DDDR pacemakers were implanted in all patients. Randomization to either of the modes with appropriate programming of the device took place just before generator implant. Reprogramming from VVIR to DDDR was allowed when symptoms consistent with the pacemaker syndrome developed. Follow-up interviews took place at 3, 9, and 18 months after pacemaker implantation. Analysis was by intention-to-treat.

A total of 407 patients were enrolled, 203 randomized to

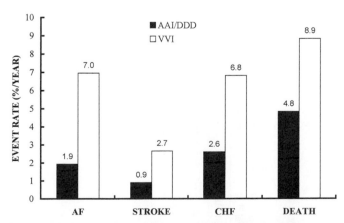

Figure 15–7. Graphical presentation of the combined results from the nonrandomized observational studies presented in Table 15–8. There is a substantial reduction in all of the outcome events with physiologic pacing compared with fixed-rate ventricular pacing. AF, atrial fibrillation; CHF, congestive heart failure.

Table 15–8. Association Between Pacing Mode and the Rate of Atrial Fibrillation, Stroke or Embolism, Congestive Heart Failure and Death in Nonrandomized Observational Studies

Author(s)	Study Year	Follow-Up		Atrial Fibrillation (%/yr)			Stroke or Embolus (%/yr)			Congestive Heart Failure (%/yr)			Death (%/yr)		
		Phys.	VVI	Phys.	VVI	RR (%)	Phys.	VVI	RR (%)	Phys.	VVI	RR (%)	Phys.	VVI	RR (%)
Sutton and Kenny[98]	1986	1121	2118	1.4	6.8	−85*									
Markewitz et al.[100]	1986	360	232	3.1	10.0	−69									−27
Ebagosti et al.[101]	1988	198	210	2.0	5.2	−62*	0	1.4	−100				3.5	4.8	
Langenfeld et al.[102]	1988	115	1150	0.9	5.4	−83									
Rosenqvist et al.[89]	1988	329	307	1.8	12.1	−85*	3.3	3.9	−15	3.9	9.4	−59*	2.1	5.9	−64*
Sasaki et al.[90]	1988	39	73	0.0	12.3	−100*	0	6.8	−100*	2.6	9.6	−73	7.6	8.2	−7
Bianconi et al.[91]	1989	558	743	4.8	7.9	−39*	1.2	2.1	−43				3.8	6.3	−40
Feuer et al.[99]	1989	367	440	2.5	4.5	−44*							2.2	3.9	−44
Santini et al.[92]	1990	1091	491	1.4	11.8	−88*	0.5	2.6	−81*				2.8	7.0	−64*
Stangl et al.[93]	1990	477	504	1.5	4.2	−64							4.0	6.2	−35
Zanini et al.[81]	1990	199	190	1.0	5.3	−81*	0	2.1	−100	0.5	1.6	−69	2.5	5.3	−53
Nürnberg et al.[94]	1991	126	318	4.8	11.0	−56	0	3.1	−100				7.1	13.8	−49*
Hesselson et al.[60]	1992	1453	1045	1.4	5.3	−74							9.0	13.6	−34
Linde-Edelstam et al.[49]	1992	414	385										5.8	7.0	−17
Sgarbossa et al.[83, 95, 96]	1993	2173	616			†			†			†	3.9	7.5	−48
Tung et al.[84]	1994	132	411										8.3	16.5	−50
Weighted mean	—	**9152**	**9233**	**1.9**	**7.0**	**−72**	**0.9**	**2.7**	**−66**	**2.6**	**6.8**	**−62**	**4.8**	**8.9**	**−45**

Phys., physiologic mode (ie, AAI[R], or VDD); RR, risk reduction.

*P<.05.

†Multivariate analysis identified the ventricular pacing mode as an independent predictor of chronic atrial fibrillation and stroke but not of congestive heart failure.

Table 15–9. **Results of the Danish Study***

Variable	First Report[87]			Second Report[88]		
	AAI	VVI	Probability Value	AAI	VVI	Probability Value
No. of Patients	110	115	—	110	115	—
Mean age (yr)	76	75	—	76	75	—
Mean follow-up (yr)	3.3	3.2	—	5.7	5.3	—
PPM mode change	12	3	—	16	6	—
Total mortality (%/yr)	21 (5.7)	25 (6.9)	0.74	39 (6.2)	57 (9.4)	0.045
Cardiovascular mortality (%/yr)	11 (3.0)	20 (5.5)	0.16	19 (3.0)	39 (6.4)	0.0065
AF at ≥ 1 follow-up visit (%/yr)	15 (4.1)	26 (3.6)	0.12	26 (4.1)	40 (6.6)	0.012
Chronic AF (%/yr)	7 (1.9)	13 (3.6)	0.24	9 (1.4)	22 (3.6)	0.004
Thromboembolism (%/yr)	6 (1.6)	20 (5.5)	0.008	13 (2.1)	26 (4.3)	0.023
Average NYHA class at end of follow-up	—	—	—	1.25	1.43	0.010
Increase in dose of furosemide (mg/day)	—	—	—	8	21	0.033
AV block (%/yr)	2 (0.5)	—	—	4 (0.6)	—	—

AF, atrial fibrillation; AV, atrioventricular; PPM, pacemaker; NYHA, New York Heart Association.
*See references 87 and 88; and see text for comments.

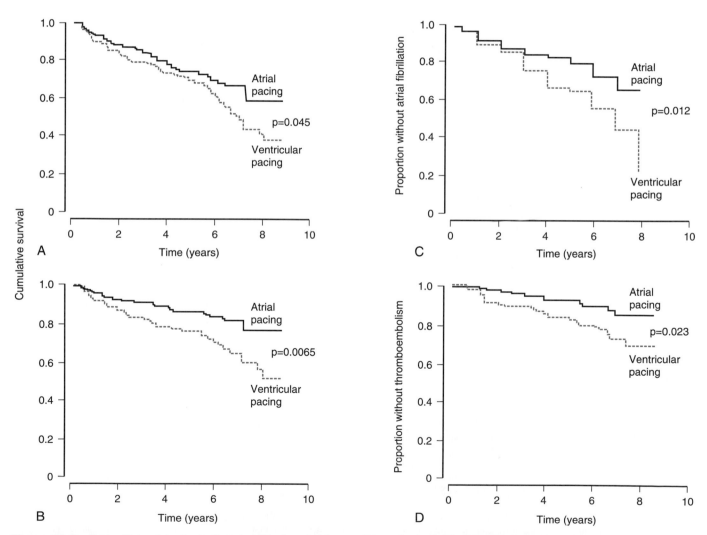

Figure 15–8. Kaplan-Meier plots of overall survival (*A*), of survival from cardiovascular death (*B*), of freedom from atrial fibrillation (*C*), and of freedom from thromboembolic events (stroke and peripheral arterial embolus) (*D*) from the Danish study. (Modified from Andersen HR, Nielsen JC, Thomsen PEB, et al: Long-term follow-up of patients from a randomised trial of atrial versus ventricular pacing for sick-sinus syndrome. Lancet 350:1210–1216, 1997.)

DDDR and 204 to the VVIR mode. The mean age was 76 years. There were no significant differences in the baseline characteristics of the two groups. Atrioventricular block was the cause of bradycardia in 201 patients (complete heart block in 119), and sick sinus syndrome was the cause in 175 patients. Symptoms consistent with the pacemaker syndrome and judged severe enough to warrant reprogramming to the DDDR mode were observed in 53 patients (26%) of the VVIR group. Of these 53 patients, 45 (85%) had sick sinus syndrome. Four patients crossed over from DDDR to VVIR because of chronic atrial fibrillation or supraventricular tachycardia.

There were no substantial differences in the SF-36 scores for the two groups. There were no differences in any of the prespecified secondary end points, other than that of suspected pacemaker syndrome. The only convincing difference was in the Specific Activity Scale, in which the score at 18 months and the longitudinal analysis demonstrated significant differences favoring the dual-chamber group. In the subgroup with atrioventricular block, there were no significant differences in *any* of the measured outcomes. On the other hand, in the group with sick sinus syndrome, significant differences favoring the DDDR group were detected in a number of the SF-36 subscales at 3 months and in the longitudinal analyses for the emotional-role and social-function subscales ($P = .001$ and 0.02, respectively) as well as for the Specific Activity Scale ($P = .02$). Furthermore, trends of borderline statistical significance favoring the DDDR group were also seen for the secondary outcomes of death ($P = .09$), atrial fibrillation ($P = .06$), and hospitalization for heart failure or nonfatal stroke or death ($P = .07$).

These results suggest that DDDR pacing, as compared with VVIR pacing, is accompanied by only a modest improvement in quality of life. Subgroup analysis detected significant differences in some of the quality-of-life scores, as well as suggesting a possible reduction in certain adverse clinical events in patients with sick sinus syndrome. It is possible that these differences may have been more conclusive had not more than 50% of the sick sinus group randomized to VVIR been crossed over to DDDR during follow-up. A significant number of patients appeared to develop symptoms consistent with pacemaker syndrome when paced in the ventricular mode. As the authors stated, however, crossovers occurred when symptoms *consistent* with pacemaker syndrome were judged sufficiently severe to warrant reprogramming, and because the trial was single-blind, there was considerable room for bias in this decision.

Ongoing Small Randomized Trials of Pacemaker Selection

PA[3]. Phase 2 of the Atrial Pacing Peri-Ablation for Paroxysmal Atrial Fibrillation (PA[3]) trial compared the effect of DDDR versus VDD pacing on time to first recurrence of paroxysmal atrial fibrillation, intervals between successive episodes of atrial fibrillation, and frequency and duration of atrial fibrillation after complete atrioventricular node ablation. Seventy-six patients have been enrolled (personal communication, Dr. A.M. Gillis).

Pac-A-Tach. The Pacemaker Atrial Tachycardia (Pac-A-Tach) trial has been designed to compare the effect of DDDR and VVIR pacing on atrial fibrillation recurrence in patients with the bradycardia-tachycardia syndrome. Secondary outcomes include total mortality, strokes and embolic events, heart failure, pacemaker syndrome, and quality of life. A secondary randomization will examine the effect of antiarrhythmic drugs. Two hundred and two patients have been enrolled for a 2-year follow-up (personal communication, Dr. J.M. Wharton).

RAMP. Another quality-of-life trial, the Rate-Modulated Pacing (RAMP) trial, has enrolled 404 patients to test whether an initial strategy to implant DDDR pacemakers in all dual-chamber pacemaker recipients will lead to a superior quality of life when compared with DDD pacing. Final results are expected in 1999 (personal communication, Dr. G.A. Lamas).

STOP-AF. The Systematic Trial of Pacing in Atrial Fibrillation (Stop-AF) trial has been designed to compare the effects of physiologic and ventricular pacing on the development of established atrial fibrillation (defined as resistant or recurrent atrial fibrillation after DC cardioversion) in patients with sinus node disease. Secondary end points include congestive heart failure, pacemaker syndrome, lead problems, and death. Follow-up is for 24 months (principal investigator, Dr. R. Charles).

Ongoing Large Randomized Trials of Pacemaker Selection

Three large multicenter randomized trials of pacemaker selection are underway. One is nearing completion, and the results should be available late in 1998. The other two will

Table 15–10. Salient Features of the Pending Multicenter Randomized Clinical Trials of Pacemaker Mode

	CTOPP	UKPACE	MOST
Age (yr)	>18	>70	>21
Pacing Indication	AVB and SSS	AVB	SSS
Mode comparison	DDR[R]/AAI[R] vs. VVI[R]	DDD vs. VVI/VVIR	DDDR vs. VVIR
Primary end point	Cardiovascular mortality and stroke	All-cause mortality	All-cause mortality and stroke
No. of patients	2550	2000	2000
Completion date	July 1998	August 2000	April 2000

CTOPP, the Canadian Trial of Physiologic Pacing, UKPACE, the United Kingdom Pacing and Cardiovascular Events study; MOST, the Mode Selection Trial; AVB, atrioventricular block; SSS, sick sinus syndrome.

not be completed until mid-2000. The primary features of these trials are summarized in Table 15–10.

CTOPP. The Canadian Trial of Physiologic Pacing (CTOPP) was designed to determine whether physiologic pacing reduces the risk of cardiovascular death or stroke compared with ventricular pacing. Patients requiring a first pacemaker for sick sinus syndrome or atrioventricular block, who are older than 18 years and do not have chronic atrial fibrillation were eligible for enrollment. There have been 2550 patients from 30 centers randomized to receive either a physiologic (DDD[R]/AAI[R]) or a VVI[R] pacemaker. Randomization involved device choice to minimize the tendency to program VVI[R]-randomized patients to physiologic modes. The primary outcome event is the first occurrence of either cardiovascular death or stroke. Secondary outcome events are overall mortality, chronic atrial fibrillation or paroxysmal atrial fibrillation, hospitalization for congestive heart failure, systemic thromboembolism, change of pacing mode, functional capacity and quality of life, and cost. The study was powered to have more than a 90% chance of detecting a 28% reduction in the primary end point. The mean duration of follow-up will be 3.5 years, and follow-up was completed in July 1998. Results will be published in late 1999.

UKPACE. The United Kingdom Pacing and Cardiovascular Events (UKPACE) study was designed to evaluate the long-term clinical and cost implications of DDD, VVI, and VVIR pacing in patients 70 years of age or older with high-grade atrioventricular block. It is a prospective, open, multicenter trial. Fifty percent of the patients will be randomized to receive DDD pacing, 25% to VVI, and 25% to VVIR. About 2000 patients will be enrolled by 40 centers and followed for a minimum of 3 years and a mean of 4 years. The primary outcome is all-cause mortality. The secondary outcome measures include cardiovascular events, such as thromboembolism, atrial fibrillation, heart failure, pacemaker upgrade, angina and myocardial infarction, and exercise capacity, quality of life, and cost. The study is designed to have a more than 90% power in detecting a 25% reduction in mortality with DDD pacing (personal communication, Dr. J.D. Skehan).

MOST. The Mode Selection Trial (MOST) has been designed to determine whether dual-chamber, rate-modulated pacing in patients with sick sinus syndrome improves event-free survival when compared with rate-modulated ventricular pacing, whether patients randomized to the DDDR mode have a better quality of life, and whether DDDR pacing is more cost-effective than VVIR pacing. Two thousand patients with sick sinus syndrome, enrolled from about 100 centers in the United States, will receive a dual-chamber, rate-responsive pacemaker and have the pacing mode randomized between DDDR and VVIR. The planned duration of follow-up is 2 to 4.5 years. The primary outcomes measured will be death and stroke. The secondary outcomes include quality of life and cost-effectiveness, total mortality, cardiovascular mortality, total mortality or stroke or heart failure requiring hospitalization, heart failure score, health status in women and the elderly, and occurrence of the pacemaker syndrome. The study is designed to have a more

than 90% power to detect a 25% reduction in the primary end point in the DDDR group. The trial is expected to be completed by April 2000 (personal communication, Dr. G.A. Lamas).

The patient populations of the three studies are complementary: elderly patients with atrioventricular block in UK-PACE, patients with sick sinus syndrome in MOST, and both groups in CTOPP. The independent and combined analyses of these studies will clarify the role of dual-chamber pacing in selected subpopulations. The studies should not only provide definitive information on the effect of pacing mode on mortality, atrial fibrillation, stroke, and heart failure but also should give a greater understanding of the effect of pacing mode on quality of life, functional capacity, and health-related costs.

REFERENCES

1. Johansson BW: Complete heart block: A clinical, hemodynamic and pharmacological study in patients with and without an artificial pacemaker. Acta Med Scand 180(Suppl 451):1–127, 1966.
2. Campbell M: Complete heart block. Br Heart J 6:69–92, 1944.
3. Cosby RS, Lau F, Rhode R, et al: Complete heart block: Prognostic value of electrocardiographic features and clinical complications. Am J Cardiol 17:190–193, 1966.
4. Edhag O, Swahn Å: Prognosis of patients with complete heart block or arrhythmic syncope who were not treated with artificial pacemakers. Acta Med Scand 200:457–463, 1976.
5. Friedberg CK, Donoso F, Stein WG: Nonsurgical acquired heart block. Ann N Y Acad Sci 111:835–847, 1964.
6. Ohm O-J, Breivik K: Patients with high-grade atrioventricular block treated and not treated with a pacemaker. Acta Med Scand 203:521–528, 1978.
7. Michaëlson M, Jonzon A, Riesenfeld T: Isolated congenital complete atrioventricular block in adult life: A prospective study. Circulation 92:442–449, 1995.
8. Zion MM, Bradlow BA: Atrioventricular block: A clinical study. S Afr Med J 38:144–148, 1964.
9. Curd GW Jr, Dennis EW, Jordan J, et al: Etiology of atrioventricular heart block: A study of its relevance to prognosis and pacemaker therapy. Cardiovasc Res Cent Bull 1:63–70, 1963.
10. Pader E, Levy H: Clinical and electrocardiographic studies in complete heart block. J Chron Dis 19:1101–1112, 1966.
11. Siddons H: Deaths in long-term paced patients. Br Heart J 36:1201–1209, 1974.
12. Penton GB, Miller H, Levine SA: Some clinical features of complete heart block. Circulation 13:801–824, 1956.
13. Rowe JC, White PD: Complete heart block: A follow-up study. Ann Intern Med 49:260–269, 1958.
14. Chardack WM, Gage AA, Federico AJ, et al: Five years' clinical experience with an implantable pacemaker: an appraisal. Surgery 58:915–922, 1965.
15. Edhag O: Long-term cardiac pacing: Experience of fixed-rate pacing with an endocardial electrode in 260 patients. Acta Med Scand 186(Suppl 502):1–110, 1969.
16. Harthorne JW, Leinbach RC, Sanders CA, et al: Clinical results of transvenous pacing. Ann N Y Acad Sci 167:1008–1015, 1969.
17. Torresani J, Bernard Y, Monties JR, et al: Clinical experience in transvenous and myocardial pacing. Ann N Y Acad Sci 167:996–1007, 1969.
18. Inberg MV, Kallio V, Linna MI, et al: Permanent endocardial pacing: Seven years' experience. Acta Med Scand 189:87–91, 1971.
19. Sowton E, Flores J: Natural history of pacemaker patients. Bull N Y Acad Med 47:999–1010, 1971.
20. Davidson DM, Braak CA, Preston TA, et al: Permanent ventricular pacing: Effect on long-term survival, congestive heart failure, and subsequent myocardial infarction and stroke. Ann Intern Med 77:345–351, 1972.
21. Van der Heide JNH, Bosma GJ, Kleine JW, et al: Results with pacemaker implantations: Is the transthoracic approach and implantation of intramural electrodes still justified? In Thalen HJTh (ed): Cardiac Pacing: Proceedings of the Fourth International Symposium

on Cardiac Pacing. Groningen, The Netherlands, Van Gorcum, 1973; pp 253–267.

22. Zion MM, Marchand PE, Obel IWP: Long-term prognosis after cardiac pacing in atrioventricular block. Br Heart J 35:359–364, 1973.

23. Fisher Hansen J, Meibom J: The prognosis for patients with complete heart block treated with permanent pacemaker. Acta Med Scand 195:385–389, 1974.

24. Svendsen V, Hyldebrandt N, Thygesen K: Long-term survival of patients with permanent implanted cardiac pacemaker. Dan Med Bull 21:158–160, 1974.

25. Amikam S, Lemer I, Roguin N, et al: Long-term survival of elderly patients after pacemaker implantation. Am Heart J 91:445–449, 1976.

26. Yokoyama M, Endo M, Sekiguchi M, et al: A 4-year survival rate after cardiac pacing in A-V block in the Heart Institute of Japan. Jpn Heart J 17:133–138, 1976.

27. Forsberg SÅ: Quantitation of the gain in mortality and life-time after pacemaker treatment. Acta Med Scand 204:11–15, 1978.

28. Simon AB, Zloto AE: Atrioventricular block: Natural history after permanent ventricular pacing. Am J Cardiol 41:500–507, 1978.

29. Fitzgerald WR, Graham IM, Cole T, et al: Age, sex, and ischaemic heart disease as prognostic indicators in long-term cardiac pacing. Br Heart J 42:57–60, 1979.

30. Alpert MA, Katti SK: Natural history of high-grade atrioventricular block following permanent pacemaker implantation. J Chron Dis 35:341–349, 1982.

31. Kyle J, Traugh CH, Krall J, et al: Long-term survival with ventricular pacemaking: initial 15-year experience. Am Surg 48:98–102, 1982.

32. Simon AB, Janz N: Symptomatic bradyarrhythmias in the adult: Natural history following ventricular pacemaker implantation. PACE 5:372–383, 1982.

33. Hauser RG, Jones J, Edwards LM, et al: Prognosis of patients paced for atrioventricular block or sino-atrial disease in the absence of ventricular tachycardia [Abstract]. PACE 6:123A, 1983.

34. Alt E, Völker R, Wirtzfeld A, et al: Survival and follow-up after pacemaker implantation: A comparison of patients with sick sinus syndrome, complete heart block, and atrial fibrillation. PACE 8:849–855, 1985.

35. Alpert MA, Curtis JJ, Sanfelippo JF, et al: Comparative survival after permanent ventricular and dual chamber pacing for patients with chronic high degree atrioventricular block with and without preexistent congestive heart failure. J Am Coll Cardiol 7:925–932, 1986.

36. Zanini R, Facchinetti A, Gallo G, et al: Survival rates after pacemaker implantation: A study of patients paced for sick sinus syndrome and atrioventricular block. PACE 12:1065–1069, 1989.

37. Jelíc V, Belkic K, Djordjevíc M, et al: Survival in 1,431 pacemaker patients: Prognostic factors and comparison with the general population. PACE 15:141–147, 1992.

38. Shen WK, Hammill SC, Hayes DL, et al: Long-term survival after pacemaker implantation for heart block in patients ≥65 years. Am J Cardiol 74:560–564, 1994.

39. Shaw DB, Kekwick CA, Veale D, et al: Survival in second degree atrioventricular block. Br Heart J 53:587–593, 1985.

40. Langendorf R, Pick A: Atrioventricular block, type II (Mobitz): Its nature and clinical significance. Circulation 38:819–821, 1968.

41. Puech P, Grolleau R, Guimond C: Incidence of different types of A-V block and their localization by His bundle recordings. In Wellens HJJ, Lie KI, Janse MJ (eds): The Conduction System of the Heart: Structure, Function and Clinical Implications. Philadelphia, Lea & Febiger, 1976; pp 467–484.

42. Narula OS: Atrioventricular block. In Narula OS (ed): Cardiac Arrhythmias: Electrophysiology, Diagnosis and Management. Baltimore, Williams & Wilkins 1979; pp 85–113.

43. Strasberg B, Amat-Y-Leon F, Dhingra RC, et al: Natural history of chronic second-degree atrioventricular nodal block. Circulation 63:1043–1049, 1981.

44. Nolan SP, Crampton RS, McGuire LB, et al: Factors influencing survival of patients with permanent cardiac pacemakers. Ann Surg 185:122–127, 1977.

45. Stoney WS, Finger FE, Alford WC, et al: The natural history of long-term cardiac pacing. Ann Thorac Sur 23:550–554, 1977.

46. Otterstad JE, Selmer R, Strom O: Prognosis in cardiac pacing. Acta Med Scand 210:47–52, 1981.

47. Müller CH, Cernin J, Glogar D, et al: Survival rate and causes of death in patients with pacemakers: Dependence on symptoms leading to pacemaker implantation. Eur Heart J 9:1003–1009, 1988.

48. Ginks W, Leatham A, Siddons H: Prognosis of patients paced for chronic atrioventricular block. Br Heart J 41:633–636, 1979.

49. Linde-Edelstam C, Gullberg B, Norlander R, et al: Longevity in patients with high degree atrioventricular block paced in the atrial synchronous or the fixed rate ventricular inhibited mode. PACE 15:304–313, 1992.

50. Karlöf I: Haemodynamic effect of atrial triggered versus fixed rate pacing at rest and during exercise in complete heart block. Acta Med Scand 197:195–206, 1975.

51. Kruse I, Arnman K, Conradson T-B, et al: A comparison of the acute and long-term hemodynamic effects of ventricular inhibited and atrial synchronous ventricular inhibited pacing. Circulation 65:846–855, 1982.

52. Pehrsson SK: Influence of heart rate and atrioventricular synchronization on maximal work tolerance in patients treated with artificial pacemakers. Acta Med Scand 214:311–315, 1983.

53. Kristensson B-E, Arnman K, Rydén L: The haemodynamic importance of atrioventricular synchrony and rate increase at rest and during exercise. Eur Heart J 6:773–778, 1985.

54. Benditt DG, Milstein S, Buetikoffer J, et al: Sensor-triggered, rate-variable cardiac pacing: Current technologies and clinical implications. Ann Intern Med 107:714–724, 1987.

55. Pehrsson SK, Hjemdahl P, Nordlander R, et al: A comparison of sympathoadrenal activity and cardiac performance at rest and during exercise in patients with ventricular demand or atrial synchronous pacing. Br Heart J 60:212–220, 1988.

56. Hedman A, Hjemdahl P, Nordlander R, et al: Effects of mental and physical stress on central haemodynamics and cardiac sympathetic nerve activity during QT interval-sensing rate-responsive and fixed rate ventricular inhibited pacing. Eur Heart J 11:903–915, 1990.

57. Pehrsson SK, Åström H: Left ventricular function after long term treatment with ventricular inhibited pacing compared to atrial triggered ventricular pacing. Acta Med Scand 214:295–304, 1983.

58. Katz AM: Cardiomyopathy of overload: A major determinant of prognosis in congestive heart failure. N Eng J Med 322:100–110, 1990.

59. Colucci WS, Braunwald E: Pathophysiology of heart failure. In Braunwald E (ed): Heart Disease: A Textbook of Cardiovascular Medicine (5th ed). Philadelphia, WB Saunders, 1997; pp 394–420.

60. Hesselson AB, Parsonnet V, Bernstein AD, et al: Deleterious effects of long-term single-chamber ventricular pacing in patients with sick sinus syndrome: The hidden benefits of dual chamber pacing. J Am Coll Cardiol 19:1542–1549, 1992.

61. Ferrer MI: The sick sinus syndrome in atrial disease. JAMA 206:645–664, 1968.

62. Ferrer MI: The sick sinus syndrome. Circulation 47:635–641, 1973.

63. Benditt DG, Sakaguchi S, Goldstein MA, et al: Sinus node dysfunction: Pathophysiology, clinical features, evaluation, and treatment. In Zipes DP, Jalife J (eds): Cardiac Electrophysiology: From Cell to Bedside (2nd ed.) Philadelphia, WB Saunders, 1995; pp 1215–1247.

64. Bernstein AD, Parsonnet V: Survey of cardiac pacing in the United States in 1989. Am J Cardiol 69:331–338, 1992.

65. Shaw DB, Holman RR, Gowers JI: Survival in sinoatrial syndrome (sick-sinus syndrome). Br Med J 280:139–141, 1980.

66. Gregoratos G, Cheitlin MD, Conill A, et al: Guidelines for implantation of cardiac pacemakers and antiarrhythmia devices: A report of the American College of Cardiology/American Heart Association Task Force on assessment of diagnostic and therapeutic cardiovascular procedures (Committee on Pacemaker Implantation). J Am Coll Cardiol 31:1175–1206, 1998.

67. Aroesty JM, Cohen SI, Morkin E: Bradycardia-tachycardia syndrome: Results in twenty-eight patients treated by combined pharmacologic therapy and pacemaker implantation. Chest 66:257–263, 1974.

68. Radford DJ, Julian DG: Sick sinus syndrome: Experience of a cardiac pacemaker clinic. Br Med J 3:504–507, 1974.

69. Härtel G, Talvensaari T: Treatment of sinoatrial syndrome with permanent cardiac pacing in 90 patients. Acta Med Scand 198:341–347, 1975.

70. Krishnaswami V, Geraci AR: Permanent pacing in disorders of sinus node function. Am Heart J 89:579–585, 1975.

71. Fruehan CT, Heneghan WF, Eich RH: Late mortality of patients with sick sinus syndrome [Abstract]. Circulation 53–54 (Suppl II):77A, 1976.

72. Wohl AJ, Laborde NJ, Atkins JM, et al: Prognosis of patients permanently paced for sick sinus syndrome. Arch Inlern Med 136:406–408, 1976.

73. Amikam S, Riss E: The natural history of sick sinus syndrome following permanent pacemaker implantation [Abstract]. Circulation 55–56 (Suppl III):155A, 1977.

74. Gould L, Reddy CVR, Becker WH: The sick sinus syndrome: A study of 50 cases. J Electrocardiol 11:11–14, 1978.

75. Breivik K, Ohm O-J, Segedal L: Sick sinus syndrome treated with permanent pacemaker in 109 patients: A follow-up study. Acta Med Scand 206:153–159, 1979.

76. Simon AB, Zloto AE: Symptomatic sinus node disease: Natural history after permanent ventricular pacing. PACE 2:305–314, 1979.

77. Alpert MA, Katti SK: Natural history of sinus node dysfunction after permanent pacemaker implantation. South Med J 75:1182–1188, 1982.

78. Skagen K, Fischer Hansen J: The long-term prognosis for patients with sinoatrial block treated with permanent pacemaker. Acta Med Scand 199:13–15, 1975.

79. Van Hemel NM, Schaepkens van Riempst ALE, Bakema H, et al: Long-term follow-up after pacemaker implantation in sick sinus syndrome. PACE 4:8–13, 1981.

80. Lemke B, Höltman BJ, Selbach H, et al: The atrial pacemaker: Retrospective analysis of complications and life expectancy in patients with sinus node dysfunction. Int J Cardiol 22:185–193, 1989.

81. Zanini R, Facchinetti AI, Gallo G, et al: Morbidity and mortality of patients with sinus node disease: Comparative effects of atrial and ventricular pacing. PACE 13:2076–2079, 1990.

82. Brandt J, Anderson H, Fåhraeus T, et al: Natural history of sinus node disease treated with atrial pacing in 213 patients: Implications for selection of stimulation mode. J Am Coll Cardiol 20:633–639, 1992.

83. Sgarbossa EB, Pinski SL, Maloney JD: The role of pacing modality in determining long-term survival in the sick sinus syndrome. Ann Intern Med 119:359–365, 1993.

84. Tung RT, Shen W-K, Hayes DL, et al: Long-term survival after permanent pacemaker implantation for sick sinus syndrome. Am J Cardiol 74:1016–1020, 1994.

85. Wolf PA, Dawber TR, Emerson Thomas H Jr, et al: Epidemiologic assessment of chronic atrial fibrillation and risk of stroke: The Framingham study. Neurology 28:973–977, 1978.

86. Flegel KM, Shipley MJ, Rose G: Risk of stroke in non-rheumatic atrial fibrillation. Lancet 1(8532):526–529, 1987.

87. Andersen HR, Thuesen L, Bagger JP, et al: Prospective randomised trial of atrial versus ventricular pacing in sick-sinus syndrome. Lancet 344:1523–1528, 1994.

88. Andersen HR, Nielsen JC, Thomsen PEB, et al: Long-term follow-up of patients from a randomised trial of atrial versus ventricular pacing for sick-sinus syndrome. Lancet 350:1210–1216, 1997.

89. Rosenqvist M, Brandt J, Schüller H: Long-term pacing in sinus node disease: Effects of stimulation mode on cardiovascular morbidity and mortality. Am Heart J 116:16–22, 1988.

90. Sasaki Y, Shimotori M, Akahane K, et al: Long-term follow-up of patients with sick sinus syndrome: A comparison of clinical aspects among unpaced, ventricular inhibited paced, and physiologically paced groups. PACE 11:1575–1583, 1988.

91. Bianconi L, Boccademo R, Di Florio A, et al: Atrial versus ventricular stimulation in sick sinus syndrome: Effects on morbidity and mortality, [Abstract]. PACE 12:1236A, 1989.

92. Santini M, Alexidou G, Ansalone G, et al: Relation of prognosis in sick sinus syndrome to age, conduction defects and mode of permanent cardiac pacing. Am J Cardiol 65:729–735, 1990.

93. Stangl K, Seitz K, Wirtzfeld A, et al: Differences between atrial single chamber pacing (AAI) and ventricular single chamber pacing (VVI) with respect to prognosis and antiarrhythmic effect in patients with sick sinus syndrome. PACE 13:2080–2085, 1990.

94. Nürnberg M, Frohner K, Podczeck A, et al: Is VVI pacing more dangerous than AV-sequential pacing in patients with sick sinus syndrome? [Abstract]. PACE 14:674A, 1991.

95. Sgarbossa EB, Pinski SL, Maloney JD, et al: Chronic atrial fibrillation and stroke in paced patients with sick sinus syndrome: Relevance of clinical characteristics and pacing modalities. Circulation 88:1045–1053, 1993.

96. Sgarbossa EB, Pinski SL, Trohman RG, et al: Single-chamber ventricular pacing is not associated with worsening heart failure in sick sinus syndrome. Am J Cardiol 73:693–697, 1994.

97. Alpert MA, Curtis JJ, Sanfelippo JF, et al: Comparative survival following permanent ventricular and dual-chamber pacing for patients with chronic symptomatic sinus node dysfunction with and without congestive heart failure. Am Heart J 113:958–965, 1987.

98. Sutton R, Kenny R-A: The natural history of sick sinus syndrome. PACE 9:1110–1114, 1986.

99. Feuer JM, Shandling AH, Messenger JC, et al: Influence of cardiac pacing mode on the long-term development of atrial fibrillation. Am J Cardiol 64:1376–1379, 1989.

100. Markewitz A, Schad N, Hemmer W, et al: What is the most appropriate stimulation mode in patients with sinus node dysfunction? PACE 9:1115–1120, 1986.

101. Ebagosti A, Gueunoun M, Saadjian A, et al: Long-term follow-up of patients treated with VVI pacing and sequential pacing with special reference to VA retrograde conduction. PACE 11:1929–1934, 1988.

102. Langenfeld H, Grimm W, Maisch B, Kochsiek K: Atrial fibrillation and embolic complications in paced patients. PACE 11:1667–1672, 1988.

103. Schrepf R, Koller B, Pache J, et al: Results of the randomized prospective DDD vs. VVI trial in patients with paroxysmal atrial fibrillation [Abstract]. PACE 20:1152A, 1997.

104. Mattioli AV, Castellani ET, Vivoli D, et al: Prevalence of atrial fibrillation and stroke in paced patients without prior atrial fibrillation: A prospective study. Clin Cardiol 21:117–122, 1998.

105. Davies MJ, Pomerance A: Pathology of atrial fibrillation in man. Br Heart J 34:520–525, 1972.

106. Han J, Millet D, Chizonnitti B, et al: Temporal dispersion of recovery of excitability in atrium and ventricle as a function of heart rate. Am Heart J 71:481–487, 1966.

107. Moe GK: Evidence for reentry as a mechanism of cardiac arrhythmias. Rev Physiol Biochem Pharmacol 72:56–81, 1975.

108. Saksena S, Giorgberidze I, Delfaut P, et al: Pacing in atrial fibrillation. *In* Rosenqvist M, (ed): Cardiac Pacing: New Advances. London, WB Saunders Company Ltd, 1997; pp 39–59.

109. Connolly SJ, Laupacis A, Gent M, et al: Canadian Atrial Fibrillation Anticoagulation (CAFA) study. J Am Coll Cardiol 18:349–355, 1991.

110. Petersen P, Boysen G, Godtfredsen J, et al: Placebo-controlled, randomised trial of warfarin and aspirin for prevention of thromboembolic complications in chronic atrial fibrillation: The Copenhagen AFASAK study. Lancet 1(8631):175–179, 1989.

111. Stroke Prevention in Atrial Fibrillation investigators: Stroke Prevention in Atrial Fibrillation study: Final results. Circulation 84:527–539, 1991.

112. The Boston Area Anticoagulation Trial for Atrial Fibrillation investigators: The effect of low-dose warfarin on the risk of stroke in patients with nonrheumatic atrial fibrillation. N Engl J Med 323:1505–1511, 1990.

113. Ezekowitz MD, Bridgers SL, James KE, et al: Warfarin in the prevention of stroke associated with nonrheumatic atrial fibrillation. N Engl J Med 327:1406–1412, 1992.

114. Stroke Prevention in Atrial Fibrillation investigators: Warfarin versus aspirin for prevention of thromboembolism in atrial fibrillation: Stroke Prevention in Atrial Fibrillation II study. Lancet 343:687–691, 1994.

115. Stroke Prevention in Atrial Fibrillation investigators: Adjusted-dose warfarin versus low-intensity, fixed-dose warfarin plus aspirin for high-risk patients with atrial fibrillation: Stroke Prevention in Atrial Fibrillation III randomised clinical trial. Lancet 348:633–638, 1996.

116. Hanson JS, Grant ME: Nine-year experience during 1973–1982 with 1,060 pacemakers in 805 patients. PACE 7:51–62, 1984.

117. Lagergren H, Johansson L, Schüller H, et al: 305 Cases of permanent intravenous pacemaker-treatment for Adams-Stokes syndrome. Surgery 59:494–497, 1966.

118. Zehender M, Büchner C, Meinertz T, et al: Prevalence, circumstances, mechanisms, and risk stratification of sudden cardiac death in unipolar single-chamber ventricular pacing. Circulation 85:596–605, 1992.

119. Seremetis MG, deGuzman VC, Lyons WS, et al: Cardiac pacemakers: Clinical experience with 289 patients. Am Heart J 85:739–748, 1973.

120. Reference 120 has been omitted.

121. Frielingsdorf J, Gerber AE, Hess OM: Importance of maintained atrio-ventricular synchrony in patients with pacemakers. Eur Heart J 15:1431–1440, 1994.

122. Oldroyd KG, Rae AP, Carter R, et al: Double blind crossover comparison of the effects of dual chamber pacing (DDD) and ventricular rate adaptive (VVIR) pacing on neuroendocrine variables, exercise performance, and symptoms in complete heart block. Br Heart J 65:188–193, 1991.

123. Menozzi C, Brignole M, Moracchini PV, et al: Intrapatient comparison between chronic VVIR and DDD pacing in patients affected by high degree atrioventricular block without heart failure. PACE 13:1816–1822, 1990.

124. Fananapazir L, Bennett DH, Monks P: Atrial synchronized ventricular pacing: Contribution of the chronotropic response to improved exercise performance. PACE 6:601–608, 1983.

125. Kristensson B-E, Arnman K, Rydén L: Atrial synchronous ventricular pacing in ischaemic heart disease. Eur Heart J 4:668–673, 1983.

126. Perrins EJ, Morley CA, Chan SL, et al: Randomised controlled trial of physiological and ventricular pacing. Br Heart J 50:112–117, 1983.

127. Yee R, Benditt DG, Kostuk WJ, et al: Comparative functional effects of chronic ventricular demand and atrial synchronous ventricular inhibited pacing. PACE 7:23–28, 1984.

128. Kristensson B-E, Arnman K, Smedgård P, et al: Physiological versus single-rate ventricular pacing: A double-blind cross-over study. PACE 8:73–84, 1985.

129. Mitsuoka T, Kenny RA, Yeung TA, et al: Benefits of dual chamber pacing in sick sinus syndrome. Br Heart J 60:338–347, 1988.

130. Vogt P, Goy JJ, Kuhn M, et al: Single versus double chamber rate responsive cardiac pacing: Comparison by cardiopulmonary noninvasive exercise testing. PACE 11:1896–1901, 1988.

131. Rediker DE, Eagle KA, Homma S, et al: Clinical and hemodynamic comparison of VVI versus DDD pacing in patients with DDD pacemakers. Am J Cardiol 61:323–329, 1988.

132. Sulke N, Dritsas A, Bostock J, et al: "Subclinical" pacemaker syndrome: A randomised study of symptom free patients with ventricular demand (VVI) pacemakers upgraded to dual chamber devices. Br Heart J 67:57–64, 1992.

133. Benditt DG, Mianulli M, Fetter J, et al: Single-chamber cardiac pacing with activity-initiated chronotropic response: Evaluation by cardiopulmonary exercise testing. Circulation 75:184–191, 1987.

134. Lipkin DP, Buller N, Frenneaux M, et al: Randomised crossover trial of rate responsive Activitrax and conventional fixed rate ventricular pacing. Br Heart J 58:613–616, 1987.

135. Smedgård P, Kristensson B-E, Kruse I, et al: Rate-responsive pacing by means of activity sensing versus single rate ventricular pacing: A double-blind cross-over study. PACE 10:902–915, 1987.

136. Hedman A, Nordlander R: QT sensing rate responsive pacing compared to fixed rate ventricular inhibited pacing: A controlled clinical study. PACE 12:374–385, 1989.

137. Lau C-P, Rushby J, Leigh-Jones M, et al: Symptomatology and quality of life in patients with rate-responsive pacemakers: A double-blind, randomized, crossover study. Clin Cardiol 12:505–512, 1989.

138. Oto MA, Müderrisoglu H, Ozin MB, et al: Quality of life in patients with rate responsive pacemakers: A randomized, cross-over study. PACE 14:800–806, 1991.

139. Bubien RS, Kay GN: A randomized comparison of quality of life and exercise capacity with DDD and VVIR pacing modes [Abstract]. PACE 13:524A, 1990.

140. Jutzy RV, Florio J, Isaeff DM, et al: Comparative evaluation of rate modulated dual chamber and VVIR pacing. PACE 13:1838–1846, 1990.

141. Sulke N, Chambers J, Dritsas A, et al: A randomised double-blind crossover comparison of four rate-responsive pacing modes. J Am Coll Cardiol 17:696–706, 1991.

142. Linde-Edelstam C, Nordlander R, Pehrsson SK, et al: A double-blind study of submaximal exercise tolerance and variation in paced rate in atrial synchronous compared to activity sensor modulated ventricular pacing. PACE 15:905–915, 1992.

143. Deharo J-C, Badier M, Thiron X, et al: A randomized, single-blind crossover comparison of the effects of chronic DDD and dual-sensor VVIR pacing mode on quality-of-life and cardiopulmonary performance in complete heart block. PACE 19:1320–1326, 1996.

144. World Health Organization: The first ten years of the World Health Organization. Geneva, WHO, 1958.

145. Shumaker SA, Anderson RT, Czajkowski SM: Psychological Tests and Scales. In Spilker B (ed): Quality of Life Assessments in Clinical Trials. New York, Raven Press, 1990, pp 95–114.

146. Schipper H, Clinch J, Powell V: Definitions and conceptual issues. In Spilker B, (ed): Quality of Life Assessments in Clinical Trials. New York, Raven Press, 1990, pp 11–24.

147. Fries JF, Spitz PW: The hierarchy of patient outcomes. In Spilker B (ed): Quality of Life Assessments in Clinical Trials. New York, Raven Press, 1990, pp 25–35.

148. Spilker B: Introduction. In Spilker B (ed): Quality of Life Assessments in Clinical Trials. New York, Raven Press, 1990, pp 3–9.

149. Guyatt GH, Jaeschke R: Measurements in clinical trials: choosing the appropriate approach. In Spilker B (ed): Quality of Life Assessments in Clinical Trials. New York, Raven Press, 1990, pp 37–46.

150. Ware JE Jr, Sherbourne CD: The MOS 36-item short-form health survey (SF-36). I. Conceptual framework and item selection. Med Care 30:473–483, 1992.

151. Linde C: How to evaluate quality-of-life in pacemaker patients: Problems and pitfalls. PACE 19:391–397, 1996.

152. Goldman L, Hashimoto B, Cook EF, et al: Comparative reproducibility and validity of systems for assessing cardiovascular functional class: Advantages of a new Specific Activity Scale. Circulation 64:1227–1234, 1981.

153. Boon NA, Frew AJ, Johnston JA, et al: A comparison of symptoms and intra-arterial ambulatory blood pressure during long term dual chamber atrioventricular synchronous (DDD) and ventricular demand (VVI) pacing. Br Heart J 58:34–39, 1987.

154. Heldman D, Mulvihill D, Nguyen H, et al: True incidence of pacemaker syndrome. PACE 13:1742–1750, 1990.

155. Linde-Edelstam C, Nordlander R, Undén A-L, et al: Quality-of-life in patients treated with atrioventricular synchronous pacing compared to rate modulated ventricular pacing: A long-term, double-blind, cross-over study. PACE 15:1467–1476, 1992.

156. Lukl J, Doupal V, Heinc P: Quality-of-life during DDD and dual sensor VVIR pacing. PACE 17:1844–1848, 1994.

157. Lau C-P, Tai Y-T, Leung W-H, et al: Rate adaptive pacing in sick sinus syndrome: Effects of pacing modes and intrinsic conduction on physiological responses, arrhythmias, symptomatology and quality of life. Eur Heart J 15:1445–1455, 1994.

158. Lau C-P, Tai Y-T, Lee PWH, et al: Quality-of-life in DDDR pacing: Atrioventricular synchrony or rate adaption? PACE 17:1838–1843, 1994.

159. Hummel J, Barr E, Hanich R, et al: DDDR pacing is better tolerated than VVIR in patients with sinus node disease [Abstract]. PACE 13:504A, 1990.

160. Leman RB, Kratz JM: Radionuclide evaluation of dual chamber pacing: Comparison between variable AV intervals and ventricular pacing. PACE 8:408–414, 1985.

161. Ritter P, Daubert C, Mabo P, et al: Haemodynamic benefit of a rate-adapted A-V delay in dual chamber pacing. Eur Heart J 10:637–646, 1989.

162. Mehta D, Gilmour S, Ward DE, et al: Optimal atrioventricular delay at rest and during exercise in patients with dual chamber pacemakers: A non-invasive assessment by continuous wave Doppler. Br Heart J 61:161–166, 1989.

163. Rydén L, Karlsson Ö, Kristensson B-E: The importance of different atrioventricular intervals for exercise capacity. PACE 11:1051–1062, 1988.

164. Haskell RJ, French WJ: Physiological importance of different atrioventricular intervals to improved exercise performance in patient with dual chamber pacemakers. Br Heart J 61:46–51, 1989.

165. Sulke AN, Chambers JB, Sowton E: The effect of atrio-ventricular delay programming in patients with DDDR pacemakers. Eur Heart J 13:464–472, 1992.

166. Linde C, Gadler F, Edner M, et al: Results of atrioventricular synchronous pacing with optimized delay in patients with severe congestive heart failure. Am J Cardiol 75:919–923, 1995.

167. Frielingsdorf J, Deseö T, Gerber AE, et al: A comparison of quality-of-life in patients with dual chamber pacemakers and individually programmed atrioventricular delays. PACE 19:1147–1154, 1996.

168. Kamalvand K, Tan K, Kotsakis A, et al: Is mode switching beneficial? A randomized study in patients with paroxysmal atrial tachyarrhythmias. J Am Coll Cardiol 30:496–504, 1997.

169. Mitsui T, Hori M, Suma K, et al: The "pacemaking syndrome." In Jacobs JE (ed): Proceedings of the Eighth Annual International Conference on Medical and Biological Engineering. Chicago, Association for the Advancement of Medical Instrumentation, 1969, pp 29–33.

170. Cohen SI, Frank HA: Preservation of active atrial transport: An important clinical consideration in cardiac pacing. Chest 81:51–54, 1982.

171. Nishimura RA, Gersh BJ, Holmes DR, et al: Outcome of dual-chamber pacing for the pacemaker syndrome. Mayo Clin Proc 58:452–456, 1983.

172. Lamas GA, Pashos CL, Normand S-LT, et al: Permanent pacemaker selection and subsequent survival in elderly Medicare pacemaker recipients. Circulation 91:1063–1069, 1995.

173. Lamas GA, Orav EJ, Stambler BS, et al: Quality of life and clinical outcomes in elderly patients treated with ventricular pacing as compared with dual-chamber pacing. N Engl J Med 338:1097–1104, 1998.

Chapter 16

Sinus Node Disease

Anne M. Gillis

Sinus node disease (SND) is a common clinical syndrome.[1–5] Indeed, in North America, SND is the most common indication for a cardiac pacing system.[6, 7] SND is characterized by electrophysiologic abnormalities of the sinus node and atria, including disturbances of impulse generation and exit from the sinus node to atrial tissue, impaired impulse transmission within the atria or specialized cardiac conduction system, failure of subsidiary pacemaker activity, and paroxysmal or chronic atrial tachycardias, including atrial fibrillation.[1–5, 8–11] The electrocardiographic (ECG) manifestations of SND are summarized in Table 16–1 and include (1) sinus bradycardia, (2) sinus pauses or sinus arrest, (3) sinoatrial exit block, (4) atrial tachycardia, (5) atrial fibrillation that is initially paroxysmal in nature, and (6) sinus node chronotropic incompetence.[12–20] Bradyarrhythmias, alternating with paroxysmal atrial flutter or fibrillation, are common in SND. This disorder has also been termed the *sick sinus syndrome,* the *tachycardia-bradycardia syndrome, sinus node dysfunction, sinoatrial disease,* and *sinoatrial dysfunction.*

■ ANATOMY AND PHYSIOLOGY OF THE SINUS NODE

Cardiac excitation usually originates in the sinoatrial node, which is located in the high right atrium at the junction of

Table 16–1. Electrocardiographic Manifestations of Sinus Node Disease

Sinus bradycardia
Sinus pauses or sinus arrest
Sinoatrial exit block
Atrial tachycardia
Paroxysmal atrial flutter or fibrillation

the superior vena cava and the base of the right atrial appendage.[21–25] The lateral boundaries of the sinus node are created by the crista terminalis and the interatrial septum.[3, 26] The sinus node consists of an ovoid collection of specialized cells about 5 mm wide, 15 mm long, and 1 to 1.5 mm thick. This region is richly innervated by both sympathetic and parasympathetic fibers.[27] The sinus node is not a uniform structure. There is more collagen in the sinus node than in other parts of the atria, and this amount increases with age.[28] Three different cell types encased in this framework of collagen have been described[3, 29]:

1. *P cells* are believed to be the primary pacemaker cells. They are round or ovoid, contain few mitochondria and myofibrils, and are seen only by electron microscopy. There are estimated to be about 5000 of these cells localized to the compact region of the sinus node.
2. *Transitional cells* are slender, elongated cells containing more myofibrils than P cells.
3. *Atrial myocytes* are also present and are believed to communicate with transitional cells but are not in contact with P cells.

Cardiac pacemaker activity originates in the specialized myocytes that are usually restricted to the sinus node or other specialized conducting tissue. It is thought that transitional cells conduct impulses from the P cells to the atrial myocytes, which are in contact with the atrial myocardium and specialized atrial conduction pathways. Spontaneous electrical activity arises as a result of a characteristic phase of the action potential: slow diastolic depolarization.[30–33] Sinoatrial node cells have a low maximum diastolic potential, ranging from -50 to -60 mV, which produces spontaneous action potentials over a broad range of rates as a result of the slow depolarization of the resting membrane potential. Although the dominant pacemaker cells are believed to be the specialized P cells that are located in the compact region of the sinus node, other cells in this region are capable of impulse initiation.

The ionic mechanisms of diastolic depolarization are not completely understood. It is thought that multiple ionic currents are activated at some point during diastolic depolarization[30, 31] (Fig. 16–1). Three current systems probably initiate the process of depolarization: (1) I_{Kr}, the delayed rectifier current that decays during diastole[34]; (2) the hyperpolarization-activated current I_f[35]; and (3) the sodium-calcium exchanger background current.[36] The T-type calcium current, $I_{Ca(T)}$, is activated midway through phase 4 of the action potential,[37] followed by the L-type calcium current, $I_{Ca(L)}$, which brings the membrane potential to the threshold potential.[38, 39] In some regions or under some conditions, the sodium current may also be important in bringing the membrane potential to threshold.[30, 40] The sodium current may be responsible for the phenomenon of pacemaker shift because it should be activated only when cells are hyperpolarized. The roles of specific currents in depolarization may also vary in different regions of the sinus node, with I_{Ca} being more important in the compact node and I_{Na} and I_f being more important in the periphery of the node.[41, 42] The roles of these currents in the depolarization process may be modulated by vagal or sympathetic stimuli.[24, 25, 43, 44]

Although each sinus node cell has a slightly different natural rate of depolarization, the rhythm is coordinated to produce a single impulse that is propagated to the rest of the heart.[31] Sinus node cells are coupled electrically by means of gap junctions with a high membrane resistance.[45, 46] It is believed that electrotonic, phase-dependent interactions between the specialized cells in the sinus node mediate synchronization of electrical activity of the pacemaker cells within the sinus node. The concept of a single pacemaker site within the sinus node is not supported by experimental and human data.[24, 25] Elegant mapping studies of activation in the atrium have demonstrated that the focus of origin of depolarization varies within the sinus node and may be

determined in part by heart rate and autonomic tone (Fig. 16–2).

■ PATHOPHYSIOLOGY

Disorders of sinus node function may be *intrinsic* (i.e., caused by processes that directly alter the anatomy and physiology of the sinus node or the surrounding atrial tissue)[1–5] or *extrinsic* (i.e., caused by processes that alter sinus node function in the absence of structural abnormalities, such as disturbances of autonomic neural regulation or drug effects, e.g., β-adrenoceptor blocking agents or class I and III antiarrhythmic agents).[47–50]

The pathology of SND must be interpreted in the context of age-related changes that occur in the structure of the sinus node. Aging is associated with loss of atrial myocytes in the approaches to the sinus node as well as within the sinus node, increased adipose tissue in internodal pathways, and increased deposition of amyloid in atrial myocytes.[28, 29] Indeed, only 10% of the nodal tissue may consist of muscle fibers in patients older than 70 years of age without documented symptomatic SND.

Detailed histopathologic evaluation of the sinus node and atria in patients with SND have identified four patterns[29, 51, 52]:

1. Amyloid deposition within the node and adjacent atrial muscle.

2. Marked loss of nodal cells exceeding the normal degree expected for age but with a node of normal size. Viral myocarditis and autoimmune processes have been hypothesized to contribute to these changes particularly because many patients with SND have coexistent loss of conduction fibers in the more distal conduction system and because autoantibodies to proteins isolated from sinus node cells have been identified in patients with this disorder.[53, 54] Apoptosis might be the cellular mechanism of premature cell death in sinus node tissue, but the triggers initiating such a response are presently unknown.[55, 56]

3. An atrophic or hypoplastic sinus node. Congenital anomalies may be involved.[57] Rarely, SND has been reported in families.[58]

4. Idiopathic SND without any detectable morphologic abnormality. In these cases, abnormalities of neural innervation or neural regulation are likely involved in the manifestations of SND.[47–50]

■ EPIDEMIOLOGY

The incidence of SND increases with age. More than half of patients with SND are older than 50 years of age at the time of diagnosis.[17, 59] In children and adolescents, the cause is likely congenital or secondary to trauma related to previous atrial surgery.[60–64] In the middle age group, acquired heart disease, most commonly coronary heart disease, is an important etiologic factor.[3–5] In most of these patients, however, significant stenosis of the sinoatrial artery is not present.[65, 66] Sinus bradycardia, atrial tachyarrhythmias, and less frequently, sinus arrest may be observed in the setting of acute myocardial infarction.[67, 68] Abnormal neural reflexes, however, may be more important than direct sinoatrial injury in mediating these effects.[69, 70] In the elderly, degenerative

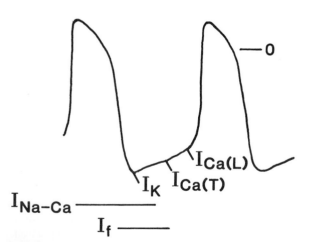

Figure 16–1. Ionic currents involved in diastolic depolarization of pacemaker cells in the sinus node. Representative action potentials from the sinus node and the activation of different ionic currents during diastole are shown. (Modified from Irisawa H, Hagiwara N: *In* Mazgalev T, et al [eds]: Electrophysiology of the Sinoatrial and Atrioventricular Nodes. New York, Allan R Liss, 1988, pp 33–52.)

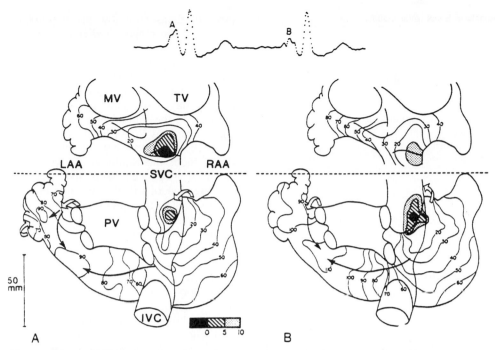

Figure 16–2. Shifting pacemaker sites in the region of the sinus node. The electrocardiogram is recorded in lead aVF. A and B indicate two different P-wave morphologies. The sites of impulse origin and resulting patterns of global atrial activation associated with each P wave are shown in the A and B isochrone maps; the anterior region of the atrium is shown on the top and the posterior region on the bottom. In A, the earliest area of activation occurred in the anterior region of the right atrial wall near the junction of the superior vena cava (SVC), which depolarizes 5 msec before the posterior site. During the next cycle shown in B, dominance of the posterior wall of the right atrium near the junction of the SVC, with later depolarization of the previously dominant anterior site, is now observed. Differences in activation within the sinus node lead to changes in atrial activation sequences and P-wave morphology and may explain the changing P-wave morphologies observed in sinus arrhythmia and other atrial rhythms. LAA, left atrial appendage; RAA, right atrial appendage; IVC, inferior vena cava; PV, pulmonary veins; MV, mitral valve; TV, tricuspid valve. The isochrone lines are 10-msec intervals. (From Boineau JP, Canavan TE, Scheussler RB, et al: Demonstration of a widely distributed atrial pacemaker complex in the human heart. Circulation 77:1221, 1988. By permission of the American Heart Association, Inc.)

changes within the sinus node or the nervous system innervating the sinus node are the most important factors leading to the development of SND.

Drugs may alter sinus node function by direct pharmacologic effects on nodal tissue or indirectly by neurally mediated effects. Drugs most commonly recognized to alter sinus node function include digitalis, sympatholytic agents used for treating hypertension, β-adrenoceptor blocking agents, calcium-channel blockers, and membrane active drugs, including class I and III antiarrhythmic agents, tricyclic antidepressants, and phenothiazines.[48–50, 71–80]

SND is the most common indication for cardiac pacemakers in North America, accounting for 40% to 60% of new pacemaker implants.[6, 7] About 150 to 250 patients per 1 million population receive pacemakers per year for the treatment of SND. The proportion of patients with SND as an indication for pacing varies between countries.[6, 7, 81, 82] This may reflect economic constraints, therapeutic conservatism (less likely to implant a pacing system for asymptomatic or minimally symptomatic bradycardia or borderline sinus pauses), or differences in therapeutic strategies (less aggressive use of class I and III agents to maintain sinus rhythm or less frequent use of β-adrenergic blocking agents or

potent calcium-channel blockers for rate control of atrial fibrillation in patients with paroxysmal atrial fibrillation). As the population ages, it is predicted that the incidence of SND will increase and, accordingly, that the number of pacemaker system implants per 1 million population per year will increase.

■ CLINICAL PRESENTATION

The most common symptoms for which patients with SND seek medical attention include presyncope, syncope, palpitations, decreased exercise tolerance, and fatigue (Table 16–2). Many patients with ECG evidence of SND do not have symptoms. Confusion and symptomatic congestive heart failure that can be attributed directly to the arrhythmias associated with this syndrome are observed less frequently. Symptoms secondary to systemic thromboembolism may also be observed. Symptoms are usually intermittent and may be of variable duration. Syncope may be secondary to bradycardia, asystole, or tachycardia. Syncope may occur without warning or may be heralded by dizziness or palpitations. The physical examination is frequently unremarkable, although sinus bradycardia or atrial fibrillation should raise suspicion

Table 16–2. Symptoms of Sinus Node Disease

Major
Syncope
Presyncope
Congestive heart failure
Less Specific
Fatigue
Decreased exercise tolerance
Palpitations
Confusion
Memory loss

of this disorder. Sinus bradycardia, however, is frequently observed in healthy people of all age ranges.[83–85] Sinus bradycardia with rates of less than 40 bpm in the absence of sleep or superb physical conditioning should raise suspicion about sinus node dysfunction. Clinical correlation with symptoms is important.

■ DIAGNOSIS

The diagnostic tools presently available for diagnosing SND are summarized in Table 16–3.

Noninvasive Tests

Electrocardiographic Monitoring

Because of the intermittent nature of this syndrome, the diagnosis is often time-consuming and frustrating. Ambulatory ECG monitoring or the use of event recorders to establish the rhythm associated with the patient's symptoms are valuable tools. Because symptoms are sporadic, event recorders with memory storage capabilities are generally more helpful than serial ambulatory ECGs.[86, 87] Symptomatic episodes can be stored in the device and the information transmitted to the monitoring center by telephone. Exercise testing to determine whether there is evidence of chronotropic incompetence may be valuable in some patients, although ambulatory ECG monitoring should also provide valuable insights concerning chronotropic function.[88–91] Specific exercise protocols, such as the Chronotropic Assessment Exercise Protocol, have been developed for this purpose.[92] This

Table 16–3. Diagnostic Evaluation of Sinus Node Function

Electrocardiographic (ECG)
12-Lead ECG, including carotid sinus massage
Ambulatory ECG monitoring
Event recorders (patient activated, memory storage capability)
Implantable loop recorder
Exercise Treadmill Testing
Autonomic Testing
Tilt table testing
Pharmacologic interventions
Invasive Electrophysiologic Assessment
Sinus node recovery time (SNRT)
Sinoatrial conduction time (SACT)
Sinus node effective refractory period (SNERP)
Direct recording of sinoatrial electrogram
Effect of autonomic blockade on SNRT, SACT, SNERP

protocol focuses on low and intermediate exercise levels, which are the ranges predicted for activities of daily living for most patients with SND. It must be emphasized that many patients with SND may achieve peak heart rates that are similar to matched control subjects, but the time course of heart rate acceleration during activity or deceleration after activity may be markedly abnormal.[93] Low-amplitude signals detected in the initial component of the filtered P wave on signal-averaged ECGs have been reported to be diagnostic of SND, with a sensitivity of 76% and a specificity of 91%.[94] In addition, the duration of the signal-averaged P wave is longer in patients with SND than in control subjects.[95] Prolongation of the P wave duration measured by signal-averaged ECG may predict the predisposition to paroxysmal atrial fibrillation. At this time, signal-averaged ECG for the diagnosis of SND is not widely employed.

An ECG example of sinus arrest is shown in Figure 16–3. Asymptomatic sinus pauses of longer than 2 seconds have been reported to occur in up to 11% of subjects during ambulatory ECG monitoring and are more commonly observed in trained athletes. Sinus pauses of longer than 3 seconds, however, are rare and are more frequently associated with symptoms.[83–85, 96] Associated atrioventricular (AV) node disease is common in patients with SND and may be characterized by slow ventricular rates during atrial fibrillation or flutter[97–99] (Fig. 16–4). Atrial tachycardias or atrial fibrillation with a rapid ventricular response followed by termination with a pause may also be observed (Fig. 16–5).

Assessment of Autonomic Tone

Abnormalities of autonomic regulation alone or in association with structural abnormalities of the sinus node may cause some of the electrophysiologic features and clinical symptoms of SND.[100–103] Assessment of neural reflexes on sinus node function might include assessment of the heart rhythm response to carotid sinus massage or Valsalva maneuver, assessment of heart rate response to upright tilt, or assessment of heart rate response to pharmacologic interventions.[102–110] Pharmacologic assessment of sinus node function can be made using atropine, isoproterenol, and β-blockers. Atropine, 1 to 3 mg (0.04 mg/kg), should increase or accelerate the heart rate over the basal rate by 20% to 50% and generally to more than 90 bpm. Many patients with symptomatic SND manifest a blunted response to atropine. Isoproterenol, 1 to 3 μg/min, should increase the resting heart rate by at least 25%. A blunted heart rate response to isoproterenol correlates with a blunted response during exercise. The intrinsic heart rate (IHR) can be determined after administration of combined atropine (0.04 mg/kg) and propranolol (0.2 mg/kg) using the following regression equation:

$$IHR = 117.2 - (0.53 \times age) \text{ bpm}^{108, 111}$$

A decreased intrinsic heart rate is a positive predictive marker of SND.

A number of patients with clinical and ECG evidence of SND have abnormal vasodepressor reflexes as assessed by tilt table testing.[102, 103] This abnormal reflex may account for many of the symptoms of presyncope and syncope in this population. See Chapter 18 for a more detailed review.

Invasive Electrophysiologic Assessment
Sinus Node Recovery Time

The sinus node recovery time (SNRT), an index of sinus node automaticity, measures the degree of prolongation of

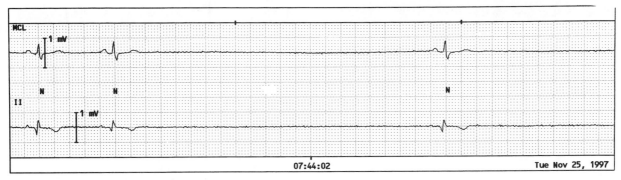

Figure 16–3. Example of sinus arrest of 4.4 seconds duration in a patient with recurrent syncope in the setting of hypertension. Recurrent episodes of sinus arrest were documented during monitoring in the hospital.

postpacing cycles compared with the control cycle lengths after prolonged (30 to 60 sec) overdrive pacing.[9–11, 111–113] The SNRT is dependent on the time required for the atrial impulse to enter the sinus node and the time required for the resulting sinus impulse to exit the node and enter the atrial tissue. The number of impulses entering the sinus node during the overdrive pacing train depends on the pacing rate as well as the conduction properties into and exiting the sinus node. Accordingly, SNRT should be assessed over a wide range of heart rates. Stimulation of the right atrium near the sinus node is initiated at progressively shorter pacing cycle lengths, commencing with a cycle length just below the spontaneous sinus cycle length.[111] The SNRT is measured as the longest pause from the last paced atrial depolarization to the first sinus depolarization at any pacing cycle length (Fig. 16–6). Sinus node recovery times of shorter than 1400 msec are considered normal.[111] Because the resting sinus cycle length may influence the sinus node recovery time, adjustments for the sinus cycle length are often made.[111, 115] The corrected sinus node recovery time (CSNRT) is calculated as the difference between sinus node recovery time and the sinus cycle length. A CSNRT of shorter than 550 msec is considered normal.[111]

Secondary pauses have been observed after termination of

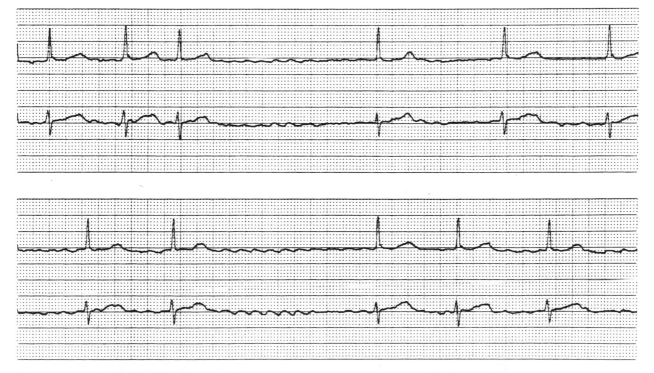

Figure 16–4. Atrial fibrillation with a slow ventricular response and pauses up to 2.2 seconds' duration in a patient who was not on antiarrhythmic therapy. The slow ventricular response in the absence of atrioventricular node blocking drugs is consistent with associated conduction system disease.

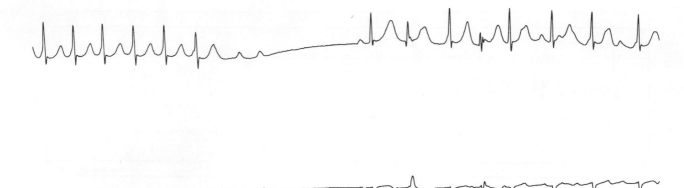

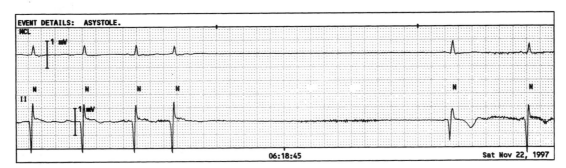

Figure 16–5. *Upper panel,* Paroxysmal atrial tachycardia that terminates with block in the atrioventricular node and a prolonged pause before restoration of sinus rhythm with frequent supraventricular premature beats. The ECG leads II *(top)* and V₁ were recorded during ambulatory monitoring. *Lower panel,* An episode of atrial fibrillation in a second patient terminates with a 4-second pause.

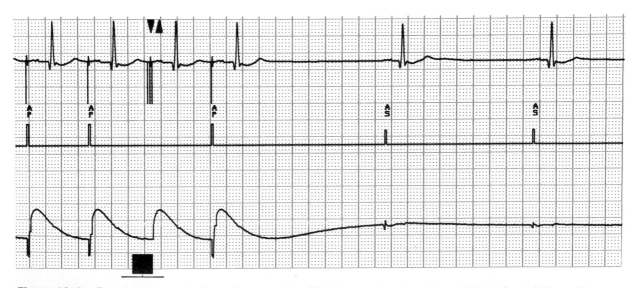

Figure 16–6. Example of prolonged sinus node recovery time (SNRT) in a patient after atrial overdrive pacing at 80 bpm using an implanted AAIR pacemaker. Lead II of the electrocardiogram, the Marker channel, and the atrial electrogram are shown. The SNRT is 1900 msec. The initial recovery beats are slow, with an AA interval of 1500 msec. The resting intrinsic cycle length was 1200 msec. Thus, the corrected SNRT is 700 msec.

rapid atrial pacing trains in patients with SND.[116] Secondary pauses that exceed the mean of the prepacing sinus cycle length by 2 standard deviations are considered abnormal.

Sinoatrial Conduction Time

Sinoatrial conduction time (SACT) is a measure of the interval from depolarization within the sinus node to activation of atrial muscle. Two methods can be used to estimate the SACT.[111, 117, 118] The Strauss method inserts a series of increasingly premature atrial extrastimuli.[111, 117] Four types of responses may be observed: interference, resetting, interpolation, and sinus node echoes. Resetting occurs when an atrial extrastimulus is premature enough to penetrate and depolarize the sinus node before the next spontaneous sinus depolarization would occur. Therefore, the resulting sinus pause is not fully compensatory, and the resulting recovery interval should include the sinus cycle length and the total time taken for the premature impulse to enter and exit the sinus node–that is, the SACT. Once resetting of the sinus node has been demonstrated, the SACT is calculated as the difference between the return cycle length and the spontaneous cycle length, which is usually divided by 2 (Fig. 16–7). This method assumes that the premature beat does not alter sinus node automaticity or conduction of the next beat from the node and that antegrade and retrograde conduction are equal.

The Narula method employs constant pacing for 8 beats at a rate 5 to 10 bpm faster than the sinus rate.[111, 118] The SACT is calculated as the difference between the first return cycle and the mean spontaneous sinus cycle length (see Fig. 16–7). An average of several determinations is usually calculated. Slight differences in SACT measurements may be calculated using these two methods.[119]

Some investigators have directly recorded sinus node electrograms by amplifying signals recorded in the sinus node region using standard electrode catheters.[120–125] Direct measurement of the SACT is defined as the interval from the onset of depolarization to the initial rapid deflection of the high right atrial electrogram. This technique is time-consuming and consequently is not frequently employed during diagnostic electrophysiologic studies. Direct SACT measurements tend to be slightly longer than indirect measures. Values of 120 msec or less are considered normal.

Sinus Node Refractory Period

Investigators have postulated that interpolation occurs as atrial premature beats encounter the refractory period of the preceding sinus impulse.[126, 127] Kerr and colleagues[127] showed that the transition from reset to interpolated responses after the introduction of atrial premature beats coincided with a fall in the amplitude of the action potential in the primary pacemaker site of the sinus node, which they interpreted to reflect sinus node refractoriness. These investigators extended this concept to define the sinus node effective refractory period (SNERP) in humans as the longest premature interval following a steady-state drive train that resulted in interpolation of the premature beat.[128] Using this technique, the SNERP was demonstrated to be significantly longer in patients with SND (522 ± 20 msec) than in patients without SND (325 ± 39 msec; P < 0.001; Fig. 16–8). SNERP lengthens with increasing pacing rate, is shortened by atropine, and tends to be prolonged by β-blockers.[129]

Role of Electrophysiologic Assessment

The utility of invasive electrophysiologic tests to confirm the diagnosis of suspected sinus node dysfunction is variable.[130–133] This is not surprising since a gold standard for making the diagnosis is lacking and the study populations evaluated in the literature were variable. The predictive value of SNRT, CSNRT, and SACT in the assessment of sinus node function reported by Reiffel and associates[133] are summarized in Table 16–4. The usefulness of electrophysiologic studies to identify SND as a potential cause of syncope is low (4% to 16%), although this investigation is probably superior to ambulatory ECG monitoring.[134–140]

Implantable loop recorders have become available as a diagnostic tool for patients with infrequent symptoms that might be due to cardiac arrhythmias.[141, 142] Studies in a limited group of patients with syncope undiagnosed by traditional means identified some abnormality of sinus node func-

Figure 16–7. Examples of determination of sinoatrial conduction time using the Strauss method in the upper panel and the Narula method in the lower panel. (From Josephson M: Sinus node function. *In* Josephson ME [ed]: Clinical Cardiac Electrophysiology: Technique and Interpretations. Philadelphia, Lea & Febiger, 1993, p 78.)

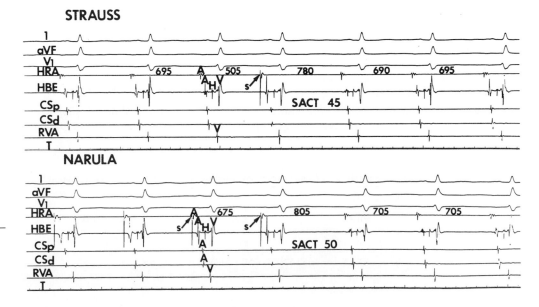

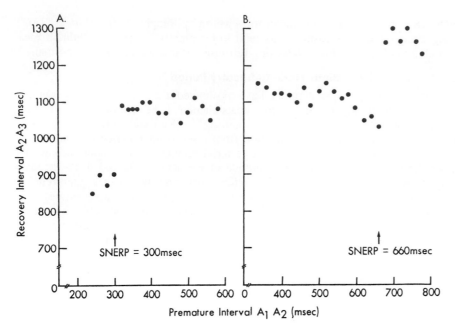

Figure 16–8. Examples of the measurement of the sinus node effective refractory period (SNERP) in a control subject *(left panel)* and in a patient with sinus node disease *(right panel).* (From Kerr CR, Strauss HC: The measurement of sinus node refractoriness in man. Circulation 68:1234, 1983. By permission of the American Heart Association, Inc.)

tion in 7 of 84 patients followed for a mean of 3 months.[143] An example of the information that can be retrieved from such a device is shown in Figure 16–9. The definitive role of this device in the investigation of patients with suspected SND remains to be determined.

■ NATURAL HISTORY

The course of SND is unpredictable; periods of symptomatic sinus node dysfunction may be separated by long periods of normal sinus node function.[1–5] Longitudinal follow-up studies in untreated patients are lacking, but the disease is believed to evolve over 10 to 15 years, commencing with an asymptomatic phase and ultimately progressing to complete failure of sinus node activity and the emergence of subsidiary pacemaker escape rhythms or the development of chronic atrial fibrillation (Fig. 16–10).

Syncope

In patients with symptomatic SND, including documented bradycardia and paroxysmal tachycardias, syncope tends to recur in patients presenting with this symptom, and pacing reduces the frequency of syncope.[144, 145] In a prospective clinical trial, the THEOPACE study investigators reported that dual-chamber pacing but not the chronotropic agent theophylline reduced the risk of recurrent syncope, as com-

pared with no treatment, in patients with ECG findings consistent with moderate sinus node dysfunction[145] (Fig. 16–11).

Atrioventricular Conduction Abnormalities

Sutton and Kenny[99] reviewed 37 studies and reported that concomitant AV conduction abnormalities were observed in 17% of 1808 patients at the time of diagnosis of SND. AV block was defined as a PR interval longer than 240 msec, complete bundle-branch block, Wenckebach block of 120 bpm or less, His–ventricular (HV) interval prolongation, and second-degree or third-degree AV block. High-grade AV block was observed in only 5% to 10% of cases at the time of diagnosis, and the probability of new AV block developing over time was reported to be less than 2.7% per year. Other investigators have reported that the risk of new AV block developing in symptomatic patients with SND is less than 1% per year if patients are younger than 70 years old and if there is no evidence of an intraventricular conduction delay on the surface ECG.[146–148] Progression of AV block over time may be related to the use of antiarrhythmic drugs.[149–154]

Atrial Fibrillation

At the time of diagnosis of SND, atrial fibrillation was reported in 8% of patients based on the review by Kenny

Table 16–4. Sensitivity and Specificity of Electrophysiologic Studies in Patients With Electrocardiographic Features of Sinus Node Disease

Sensitivity (%)			Specificity (%)		
SNRT/CSNRT	SACT	Either	SNRT/CSNRT	SACT	Either
56	54	69	88	88	88

SNRT, sinus node recovery time; CSNRT, corrected SNRT; SACT, sinoatrial conduction time.
Adapted from Reiffel JA, Kerrick K, Zimmerman J, Bigger JT Jr: Electrophysiologic studies of the sinus node and atria. *In* Brest AN (ed): Cardiovascular Clinics. Philadelphia, FA Davis, 1985, pp 37–59.

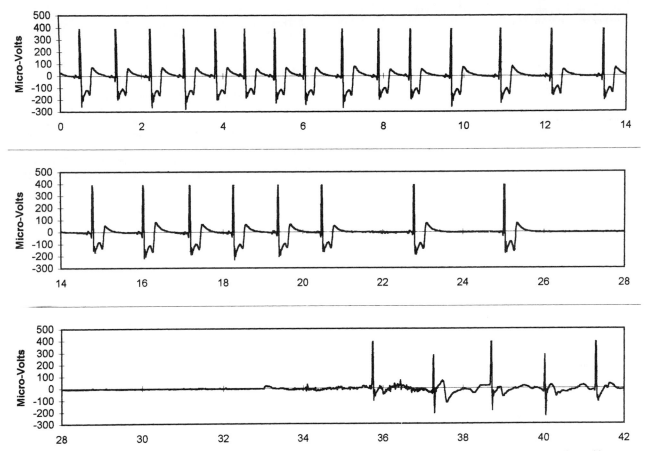

Figure 16–9. Prolonged sinus arrest of 10 seconds' duration, recorded using an implantable loop recorder in a young patient with recurrent syncope, a normal electrocardiogram, and negative tilt table test. The sinus arrest is preceded by gradual sinus bradycardia and junctional escape rhythm.

and Sutton[99] of 21 published studies reporting on 958 patients. The likelihood of atrial fibrillation developing in this population was about 5% per year. Atrial fibrillation was less likely to occur in patients treated with AAI pacemakers (3.9%) than in patients treated with VVI pacemakers (22.3%, over 33 months of follow-up).

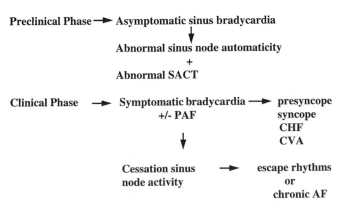

Figure 16–10. The natural history of sinus node disease. SACT, sinoatrial conduction time; PAF, paroxysmal atrial fibrillation; CHF, congestive heart failure; CVA, cerebrovascular accident; AF, atrial fibrillation.

A number of retrospective studies have suggested that atrial-based pacing prevents the development of chronic atrial fibrillation compared with VVI pacing.[155–163] The greatest benefit of atrial pacing for the prevention of the development of chronic atrial fibrillation has been reported in patients with a past history of atrial tachyarrhythmias at the time of pacemaker implantation[162] (Fig. 16–12). Furthermore, the purported benefits of atrial-based pacing in preventing the development of chronic atrial fibrillation continue to be observed in patients older than 70 years of age.[160] Only one prospective study to date has evaluated the effects of pacing modality on the development of atrial fibrillation over time in patients with SND.[148, 164] Andersen and colleagues[148] recently reported on the long-term follow-up of 225 patients with SND who were randomized to AAI or VVI pacing and followed for a mean of 5.5 years.[148] In the atrial pacing group, 9 patients developed chronic atrial fibrillation, compared with 22 patients in the VVI group ($P = 0.011$). The benefits of atrial pacing for the prevention of atrial fibrillation were seen only after 3 years of follow-up or longer. A multivariate analysis identified the bradycardia-tachycardia syndrome and left ventricular end-diastolic diameter at the time of randomization, but not atrial pacing mode, as the only independent predictors of the development of chronic atrial fibrillation during follow-up. Thus, although these data support the benefits of AAI pacing for patients

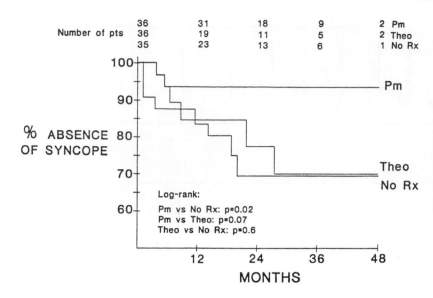

Figure 16–11. Event-free survival from recurrent syncope in patients with sinus node disease who were untreated, treated with theophylline, or treated with a dual-chamber pacemaker. (From Alboni P, Menozzi C, Brignole M, et al: Effect of permanent pacemaker and oral theophylline in sick sinus syndrome. The THEOPACE study: A randomized controlled trial. Circulation 96:263, 1997. By permission of the American Heart Association, Inc.)

with symptomatic SND, the results of larger multicenter trials comparing the effects of physiologic pacing to ventricular pacing on the natural history of atrial fibrillation in SND are eagerly awaited.

Thromboembolism

Patients with SND, particularly those with a history of paroxysmal atrial fibrillation, are at risk of thromboembolism.[165] Sutton and Kenny[99] in their review of 21 studies reported the overall incidence of thromboembolism to be 15% in unpaced patients, 13% in ventricular paced patients, and 1.6% in atrially paced patients. Santini and colleagues[160] reported that stroke mortality was higher in VVI-treated patients (8%) with SND compared with DDD treated patients (2.5%), but the difference in mortality was only statistically significant when compared with AAI-treated patients (2.2%; P <0.01). Moreover, this effect was observed only in patients older than 70 years of age (Fig. 16–13). Sgarbossa

and associates[162] reported that a history of cerebrovascular disease, ventricular pacing mode, and a history of paroxysmal atrial fibrillation were independent predictors of stroke after pacemaker implantation in patients with SND. Andersen and coauthors,[164] in the only prospective trial to date, reported that systemic thromboembolic events occurred in 17% of patients with SND randomized to VVI pacing, compared with 5% of patients randomized to AAI pacing (P < 0.01). The magnitude of this effect increased over time, plateauing 4 years after pacemaker implantation. During longer-term follow-up, the decreased risk of thromboembolism continued to be observed in patients treated with AAI pacemakers compared with VVI pacemakers.[148]

In this study, less than half of the patients who developed chronic atrial fibrillation were treated with warfarin, and we are not provided with information on warfarin use in other patients at risk for systemic thromboembolism. Although chronic atrial fibrillation was not observed to be an independent predictor of stroke, one has to wonder whether in-

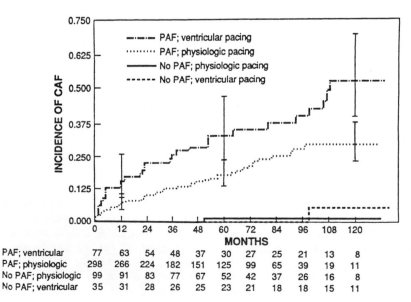

Figure 16–12. Incidence of chronic atrial fibrillation (CAF) developing over time after ventricular or physiologic pacing. CAF was significantly more likely to develop after ventricular pacing than after physiologic pacing in patients with a prior history of paroxysmal atrial fibrillation (PAF). Pacing modality did not influence the development of CAF in patients who had no prior history of atrial fibrillation. (From Sgarbossa EB, Pinski SL, Maloney JD, et al: Chronic atrial fibrillation and stroke in paced patients with sick sinus syndrome: Relevance of clinical characteristics and pacing modalities. Circulation 88:1049, 1993. By permission of the American Heart Association, Inc.)

	0	12	24	36	48	60	72	84	96	108	120
PAF; ventricular	77	63	54	48	37	30	27	25	21	13	8
PAF; physiologic	298	266	224	182	151	125	99	65	39	19	11
No PAF; physiologic	99	91	83	77	67	52	42	37	26	16	8
No PAF; ventricular	35	31	28	26	25	23	21	18	18	15	11

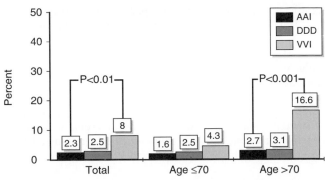

Figure 16–13. Stroke mortality rates in 135 patients treated with AAI pacing, in 79 patients treated with DDD pacing, and in 125 patients treated with VVI pacing who were followed for a mean of 5 years. Stroke mortality was significantly lower in AAI-paced patients than in VVI-paced patients; this effect was significant in patients older than 70 years of age. (From Santini M, Alexidou G, Ansalone G, et al: Relation of prognosis in sick sinus syndrome to age, conduction defects and modes of permanent cardiac pacing. Am J Cardiol 65:733, 1990.)

creased use of warfarin in high-risk patients based on current guidelines for anticoagulation would have altered the risk of thromboembolism in patients with SND independent of the pacing mode selected.[166–168] Unfortunately, none of these studies has reported on appropriate use of anticoagulation therapy, and thus it is unknown whether this intervention would reduce the differences in stroke mortality that have been reported in patients treated with AAI compared with VVI pacing systems.

Congestive Heart Failure

The THEOPACE study investigators reported that both theophylline therapy and dual-chamber pacing therapy reduced the occurrence of symptomatic heart failure over 48 months compared with no treatment in patients with SND ($P = 0.05$).[145] It is uncertain whether the mode of pacing influences the development of congestive heart failure. In a retrospective study, Rosenqvist and colleagues[155] reported that the incidence of congestive heart failure was higher in patients with SND who were treated with VVI pacemakers (37%) than in those treated with AAI pacemakers (15%; $P < 0.005$). In the only prospective study to date, Andersen and coauthors[148] reported that the New York Heart Association functional class was significantly higher in the VVI group than in the AAI group at each follow-up visit from 3 months to 7 years and that the use of diuretics was significantly higher in the VVI group than in the AAI group at the 5-year to 8-year follow-up visits. The development of congestive heart failure in patients with SND who are treated with VVI pacing may be secondary, in part, to the asynchronous contraction pattern,[169, 170] to the loss of the atrial contribution to cardiac filling or, in some, to a tachycardia-induced cardiomyopathy related to frequent paroxysmal atrial fibrillation with a poorly controlled ventricular rate.[171, 172] Whether atrial pacing is superior to dual-chamber pacing for the prevention of heart failure in patients with SND is unknown.

Chronotropic Incompetence

Sinus node chronotropic incompetence is the inability of the sinus node to achieve at least 80% of the predicted heart rate.[173] This may be secondary to intrinsic SND or to negative chronotropic drugs. Chronotropic incompetence is estimated to be present in 20% to 60% of patients with SND.[174, 175] Chronotropic incompetence probably progresses over time and more rapidly in patients with electrophysiologic abnormalities of sinus node function.[175] This may also be aggravated by drugs prescribed to control heart rate responses during paroxysmal atrial flutter or fibrillation or for maintenance of sinus rhythm. Several types of chronotropic incompetence have been described (Fig. 16–14)[93]:

1. Patients with complete chronotropic incompetence do not experience any increase in heart rate during exercise.
2. Patients with exercise-induced chronotropic incompetence may experience a normal heart rate increase initially, which then plateaus or decreases; some patients may not experience any heart rate increase until midway through exercise.
3. Some patients may experience frequent and unpredictable fluctuations in heart rate during activity.

All-Cause Mortality

Although cardiac pacing alleviates symptoms in patients with SND, the effect of pacing on the long-term survival of this population has been controversial. Some studies suggest that survival in patients with SND after pacemaker implantation is comparable to the expected survival of an age-matched population,[176–180] whereas other investigators have observed a poorer survival after permanent pacemaker implantation compared with an age-matched population that could be related to the underlying cardiac disease.[181] In our pacemaker population of 2418 patients followed since 1979, the diagnosis of SND as an indication for pacing is an independent predictor of survival (Fig. 16–15).[182] About half of patients with SND requiring cardiac pacing therapy do not have significant structural heart disease. Thus, it is not surprising that survival in this population might be better than that in patients receiving pacing therapy for conduction

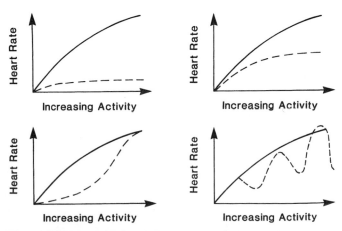

Figure 16–14. Examples of different types of chronotropic incompetence.

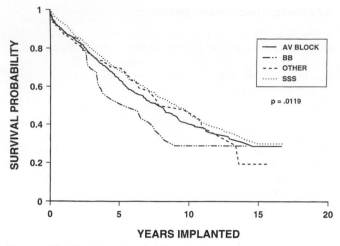

Figure 16–15. Survival probability rates in our pacemaker population based on the indication for pacing. Sinus node disease was an independent predictor of survival in our population of 2417 patients followed since 1979. AV, atrioventricular; BB, bundle branch block; SSS, sick sinus syndrome.

significantly lower in the atrial pacing group (Fig. 16–16; $P < 0.05$). By multivariate analysis, atrial pacing was significantly associated with survival from cardiovascular death ($P = 0.022$). This study was not powered at the outset to evaluate mortality as the primary study end point. Because this study evaluated outcomes only in the small subgroup of patients with SND who are candidates for atrial pacing, the results cannot be immediately extrapolated to the majority of patients with SND who receive dual-chamber pacing systems. The results of larger multicenter randomized trials to confirm this observation are awaited.[163, 183–187]

■ TREATMENT OF SINUS NODE DISEASE

Pharmacologic Treatment

Several drugs have been used to treat symptomatic bradycardia. Theophylline has been used with some success for the treatment of bradycardia.[187–189] A recent prospective trial compared theophylline or DDD pacing to no treatment in patients with mild to moderate symptoms of SND. Patients with sinus pauses of longer than 3 seconds' duration were excluded. Theophylline did not prevent recurrent syncope. β-Adrenergic receptor agonists have also been used to treat symptomatic bradycardia and have been reported to reduce the duration of sinus pauses.[190]

Digoxin, calcium-channel antagonists, and β-adrenergic blocking agents are used for heart rate control in patients with SND and paroxysmal atrial fibrillation. These drugs may exacerbate the abnormalities of sinus node function in some patients; hence patients should be monitored carefully. Experimental and clinical data have been reported demonstrating that electrical remodeling of the atria occurs during atrial fibrillation, which is characterized by shortening of atrial action potential durations and refractory periods.[191–193] The magnitude of this effect is dependent on the duration of atrial fibrillation, and these electrophysiologic changes predispose to the recurrence of atrial fibrillation. The shortening of the atrial action potential during atrial fibrillation is

abnormalities associated with structural heart disease and left ventricular dysfunction.

Major prospective randomized clinical trials evaluating the effect of pacing modality on overall cardiac mortality are under way (see Chapter 15).[163, 183–186] Several retrospective trials have suggested that atrial-based pacing reduces cardiac mortality compared with ventricular-based pacing in patients with SND (Table 16–5). The retrospective studies, however, may overestimate a beneficial effect of atrial-based pacing due to treatment bias–that is, sicker patients with a worse prognosis were more likely to receive a VVI pacemaker than an AAI pacemaker. Andersen and coauthors[164] recently reported their long-term follow-up results in patients prospectively randomized to AAI or VVI pacing and observed that total mortality and cardiovascular mortality were

Table 16–5. Mortality: Atrial-Based Pacing Versus Ventricular-Based Pacing in Patients With Sinus Node Disease

| Investigators | Atrial-Based Pacing | | | | Ventricular-Based Pacing | | | |
	Mode	No. of Patients	Mean Follow-Up (mo)	Mortality (%)	Mode	No. of Patients	Mean Follow-Up (mo)	Mortality (%)
Rosenqvist et al, 1988[155]	AAI	79	47	6	VVI	89	47	10
Santini et al, 1990[160]	AAI	135	60	13	VVI	125	60	30
	DDD	79	60	16				
Stangl et al, 1990[159]	AAI	110	40	17	VVI	112	33	27
Hesselson et al, 1992[161]	DDD	308	7-yr actuarial	40	VVI	193	7-yr actuarial	63
Sgarbossa et al, 1993[162]	DDD	395	66	21	VVI	112	66	41
Andersen et al, 1994[164]	AAI	110	40	19	VVI	115	38	22

AAI, atrial pacing; VVI, ventricular pacing; DDD, atrioventricular sequential pacing.

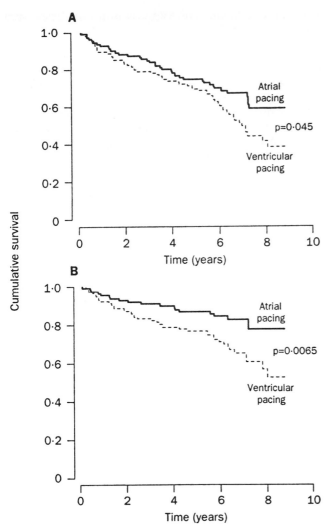

Figure 16–16. Overall survival and survival from cardiovascular death in 225 patients with sick sinus syndrome who were randomized to AAI (n = 110) or VVI (n = 115) pacing and followed for a mean of 5.5 years. (From Andersen HR, Nielsen JC, Thomsen PE, et al: Long-term follow-up of patients from a randomized trial of atrial versus ventricular pacing for sick-sinus syndrome. Lancet 350:1212, 1997 © by The Lancet Ltd., 1997.)

Table 16–6. **Indications for Pacing in Sinus Node Disease**

Class I
Sinus node dysfunction with documented symptomatic bradycardia
Class II
Sinus node dysfunction with heart rates <40 bpm without documented symptomatic bradycardia
Class III
Sinus node dysfunction in asymptomatic patients
Sinus node dysfunction in patients with symptoms suggestive of bradycardia documented not to be associated with bradycardia

Class I, general consensus that pacing is indicated; Class II, divergence of opinion on need for pacing; Class III, general consensus that pacing is not indicated.

Pacing in Sinus Node Disease

The indications for pacing in the setting of SND are shown in Table 16–6. Pacing therapy in SND should provide atrial pacing and chronotropic responsiveness whenever possible.[196–198] My approach to pacing mode selection for SND is shown in Figure 16–17. A VVIR system is prescribed if the atrium is electrically silent or if the patient is in chronic atrial fibrillation. If AV conduction is only intermittently impaired, then a VVI system may be sufficient. For patients in sinus rhythm, an AAIR system should be considered if the patient has intact AV conduction.[199, 200] If AV conduction is impaired, a DDDR system should be implanted.[201]

AAIR Pacing

About 5% to 10% of patients with symptomatic SND are candidates for AAI pacing systems.[146, 147] A rate-adaptive pulse generator should be considered because of the high incidence of chronotropic incompetence in patients with SND.[198–200] Although this is the most economical approach to providing physiologic pacing in this population, this modality is used for less than 1% of implants in North America.[6, 7] Concerns about progression of AV block and the development of chronic atrial fibrillation may explain the low utilization of the AAIR modality in SND. These concerns appear to be unfounded, however, when patients are carefully selected.[146–148] The risk of progression to AV block is less than

likely mediated by reduced density of $I_{Ca(L)}$.[194] Intracellular calcium overload has been postulated to cause these electrophysiologic abnormalities because this effect is blocked by verapamil.[193] Because digoxin may cause intracellular calcium overload, this drug might actually predispose to the recurrence of atrial fibrillation as suggested in experimental models.[195] As our knowledge of the cellular electrophysiology and molecular biology of ionic channels in atrial fibrillation expands, more rational approaches to the treatment of this arrhythmia in the setting of SND should evolve.

Class I and III antiarrhythmic drugs are frequently prescribed for the prevention of recurrent paroxysmal atrial fibrillation or flutter in patients with SND. These drugs may further suppress sinus node automaticity and exacerbate bradycardia or increase the frequency or duration of sinus pauses. Thus, antiarrhythmic drug therapy may increase or precipitate symptoms of SND; hence pacing therapy is often indicated because of the need to use such drugs.

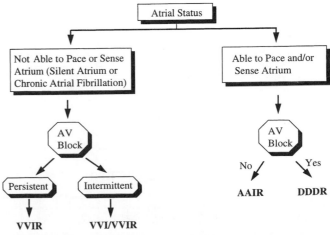

Figure 16–17. Optimal pacing modes in sinus node disease.

Table 16–7. Contraindications to AAI/AAIR Pacing

Absolute
AV block documented except during sleep
AV block during CSM
PR interval >220 msec
IVCD on electrocardiogram
Relative
Age >70 yr
Wenckebach block during atrial pacing <120 bpm
HV interval >75 msec
Infrahisian block during atrial pacing

AV, atrioventricular; CSM, carotid sinus massage; IVCD, intraventricular conduction delay; HV, His–ventricular interval.

1% per year if patients have normal AV conduction and no intraventricular conduction delays on the surface ECG at the time of implantation. The likelihood of developing chronic atrial fibrillation is small (less than 1.5% per year) when patients are younger than 70 years of age at the time of implantation and when there is no history of paroxysmal atrial fibrillation before implantation. Furthermore, improvements in lead technology and improved sense amplifiers in modern pulse generators have significantly reduced problems with atrial sense failure over time. At our institution we routinely assess the Wenckebach cycle length during atrial pacing at the time of implantation. If this is more than 120 bpm, we implant an AAIR system. There is some controversy, however, about the value of this parameter for pre-dicting the development of AV block over time. The contraindications to AAIR pacing are shown in Table 16–7.

DDDR Pacing

Because most patients with SND manifest some form of abnormal chronotropic response, a rate-adaptive dual-chamber pacing system should be considered for all patients with abnormal AV conduction. The improvements in cardiac hemodynamics and exercise tolerance associated with rate-adaptive pacing systems are well documented.[202–206] Rate-adaptive AV delays have improved exercise tolerance in some patients by allowing achievement of target heart rates during maximal activity.[207, 208] Mode-switching devices have become available, and this feature should be available in the device implanted because many of these patients have or will develop paroxysmal atrial fibrillation over time.[209–212] Mode switching permits the patient with SND to enjoy the benefits of physiologic pacing yet prevents atrial tracking at inappropriately high rates if the patient develops atrial tachyarrhythmia (Fig. 16–18). Improvements in atrial lead technology and atrial sense amplifiers have reduced atrial sense problems previously observed with earlier generations of dual-chamber pacemakers.[213–215]

The ideal rate sensor is the one that best mimics sinus node function (see Chapters 8 to 12). Activity and accelerometer sensors are the most popular because they are simple to program, consume relatively little energy, and initiate a rapid heart rate response at the onset of activity.[217] However, they may not be as physiologic as the minute ventilation sensor,[218] the QT sensor,[219] or the right ventricular pressure

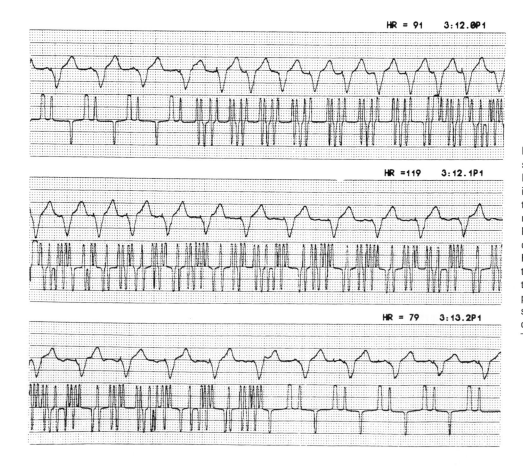

Figure 16–18. Example of mode switching from the DDDR mode to the DDIR mode after onset of atrial fibrillation in a patient with a history of the tachycardia-bradycardia syndrome who received a Medtronic Thera DR. The Marker channel was downloaded to one of the Holter channels during monitoring. High-rate atrial events are detected, and the mode switching rate occurs when the mean atrial rate reaches the programmed mode switch rate. Mode switching back to the DDDR mode occurs on termination of atrial fibrillation.

Table 16–8. Symptoms of Pacemaker Syndrome

Severe	Mild
Syncope	Venous pulsation in neck
Presyncope	Fatigue
Moderate	Weakness
Dizziness	Palpitations
Dyspnea	Fullness in chest
Chest pain	
Jaw pain	
Confusion	

sensor.[220] The minute ventilation sensor consumes considerable current and hence can reduce pulse generator longevity. Dual-sensor devices have become available that blend the best features of activity and minute ventilation or QT to optimize rate response.[221] Whether this approach improves clinical outcomes significantly is uncertain.

Pacemaker Syndrome

The pacemaker syndrome includes a constellation of symptoms associated with ventricular pacing (Table 16–8). Mild to severe symptoms attributed to pacemaker syndrome have been reported in 20% to 65% of patients during ventricular pacing.[222–229] The mechanisms include (1) detrimental hemodynamic effects associated with asynchronous atrial and ventricular contraction, including valvular regurgitation and ventricular contraction against a closed AV valve; and (2) neurohumoral mechanisms, including increased sympathetic activation and increased circulating atrial natriuretic peptide secondary to retrograde VA conduction associated with ventricular pacing.[229–231] Pacemaker syndrome has even been observed in patients with AAIR systems when the AV conduction has been excessively prolonged.[232] The magnitude of pacemaker syndrome in this population is difficult to quantitate because many of these patients are elderly, have concomitant medical problems, and are taking medications that might contribute to some of these symptoms. Studies comparing symptoms in patients during ventricular pacing and dual-chamber pacing have suggested that a subclinical pacemaker syndrome may exist. Sulke and associates[224] compared ventricular pacing to dual-chamber pacing in patients who had been upgraded to a dual-chamber pacing system at the time of pulse generator replacement. Dual-chamber pacing was preferred by 75% of patients, whereas no patient preferred ventricular pacing. Heldman and colleagues[222] also observed that 83% of patients experienced fewer symptoms during dual-chamber pacing compared with ventricular pacing. The absolute magnitude of pacemaker syndrome secondary to ventricular pacing and its impact on quality of life in patients with SND are unknown.

Detrimental Effects of Ventricular Pacing in Sinus Node Disease

A conceptual model illustrating the potential detrimental effects of ventricular-based pacing is shown in Figure 16–19. An asynchronous contraction pattern and loss of the contribution of atrial contraction to cardiac filling may alter cardiac hemodynamics and contribute to the development of cardiac dysfunction over time. Ventricular pacing may be proarrhythmic. Ventricular pacing causes asynchronous acti-

vation of the ventricles and is associated with increased valvular regurgitation. This and contraction of the atrium when the AV valves are closed may cause stretch-induced changes in atrial repolarization, which may provide the substrate for paroxysmal atrial fibrillation. Chronic or persistent atrial fibrillation may further contribute to the development of left ventricular dysfunction and ultimately the development of congestive heart failure. Whether this is due to altered myocardial mechanics or to inadequate rate control that leads to the development of tachycardia-induced myopathy is unclear. Thromboembolism secondary to atrial fibrillation and atrial venous stasis may contribute substantially to morbidity and mortality.

Does Atrial Pacing Prevent Atrial Fibrillation?

Atrial pacing might prevent atrial fibrillation by (1) prevention of bradycardia-induced dispersion of atrial repolarization that might predispose to atrial fibrillation[233, 234]; (2) overdrive suppression of supraventricular premature beats that trigger atrial fibrillation[233–240]; (3) preservation of an optimal atrial activation sequence, which minimizes areas of slow conduction in the atria[233, 241, 242]; and (4) maintenance of optimal hemodynamics through preservation of AV synchrony and normal ventricular activation.[164] Many studies are evaluating the effects of atrial pacing for the prevention of atrial fibrillation. Some researchers are investigating various atrial pacing sites,[243, 244] and some are investigating dual atrial pacing modalities.[245] Some studies evaluate different atrial overdrive pacing strategies.[240, 246] Some studies are being conducted in patients with the tachycardia-bradycardia syndrome,[247] and others are being conducted in patients with atrial fibrillation in the absence of documented bradycardia.[246] The outcome of these studies will have important implications for the design and application of future pacing systems. Final analysis of the results of the Atrial Pacing Peri-Ablation for Paroxysmal Atrial Fibrillation (PA³) Study are under way.[246] In this study, patients with a history of antiarrhythmic drug-refractory paroxysmal atrial fibrillation were randomized to a trial of atrial rate-adaptive pacing or no pacing and followed for 3 months before a planned AV node ablation. During this follow-up period, atrial pacing

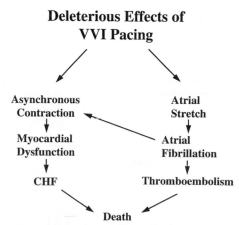

Figure 16–19. The potential detrimental effects of ventricular pacing in sinus node disease. See text for discussion. CHF, congestive heart failure.

did not prolong the time to the first recurrence of sustained atrial fibrillation, nor did it alter the frequency or duration of paroxysmal atrial fibrillation. This study, however, did *not* include patients with symptomatic sinus bradycardia, and thus the results cannot be directly extrapolated to patients with SND and paroxysmal atrial fibrillation.

Ablation and Pacing

Total AV node ablation and permanent pacemaker implantation are options frequently considered for patients with paroxysmal atrial fibrillation refractory to or intolerant of antiarrhythmic drug therapy.[248] At this time, the optimal pacing modality for these patients is unknown. DDDR pulse generators are implanted in many patients with paroxysmal atrial fibrillation in an effort to preserve the hemodynamic benefits of sinus rhythm after ablation. The natural history of paroxysmal atrial fibrillation after ablation is being actively studied by several investigators. Because antiarrhythmic drugs are often discontinued after AV node ablation, persistent or chronic atrial fibrillation is likely to develop over time in some patients. However, the predictors of the development of chronic atrial fibrillation and the time course of the evolution of chronic atrial fibrillation are not completely understood. Brignole and colleagues[248] reported that chronic atrial fibrillation had developed in 24% of patients within 6 months after a total AV node ablation. Gribbin and associates[249] reported that chronic atrial fibrillation had developed in 42% of patients 30 months after ablation. Age, underlying structural heart disease, and the need for prior cardioversion are some factors that might predict this risk. Phase II of the PA[3] Study compares the impact of atrial overdrive pacing with maintenance of AV synchrony alone on the time course of recurrence of paroxysmal atrial fibrillation.[236] Patients are randomized to DDDR or VDD pacing after AV node ablation. Final data analysis will be presented in 1999. Preliminary analysis shows that atrial fibrillation recurs soon after total AV node ablation and is not modified by DDDR or VDD pacing. Many patients (28%) develop persistent atrial fibrillation within 6 months of ablation.

Optimal Programming of Pacing Systems in SND

Many features of newer pacing systems may be used to optimize the management of the patient with SND. Pulse generators should be considered as diagnostic tools in addition to therapeutic devices. For instance, information on the frequency and temporal patterns of episodes of paroxysmal atrial fibrillation can be retrieved by programming on the high rate atrial episode diagnostic feature of some pulse generators. Review of episode trends over time may provide information about the efficacy of antiarrhythmic therapy (Table 16–9). If such an option is not available, use of heart rate histogram features in some devices may provide clues about the presence of atrial tachyarrhythmias.

In patients who have a history of paroxysmal atrial fibrillation, programming on the mode-switching feature should be considered.[209–212] This feature, however, may limit the range of programmability of the AV delay and thus increase the frequency of ventricular pacing. Because preservation of the normal ventricular activation pattern appears to be highly desirable in patients with SND, routine programming on of the mode-switching function is not recommended in patients without a history of atrial tachyarrhythmias.[250–253] Optimal programming of the AV delay in patients without complete heart block to promote intrinsic conduction also increases the longevity of the device.

A new feature of search AV hysteresis, which is designed to promote intrinsic conduction, is available in some pulse generators and is desirable in patients with SND in the absence of significant AV conduction abnormalities. Another feature that attempts to promote intrinsic sinus rhythm instead of atrial pacing might be beneficial if patients have an initial lag in heart rate response to activity (see Fig. 16–14) or if the intrinsic sinus rate just lags behind the sensor rate. In addition, this feature might be beneficial if prolongation of atrial conduction occurs secondary to the pacing site, for example, right atrial appendage pacing, which might cause detrimental hemodynamic effects or promote the development of atrial fibrillation. However, the benefits of this feature have not been proved.

Future Pacing Therapies

The goal of future device development is to design an intuitive pacing system that can automatically adjust most pacing system functions to optimize pacing system performance, thereby reducing time-consuming programming. The next generations of pulse generators will have greater data storage capabilities; hence, more diagnostic information will be retrieved about the patient and the pacing system performance. Trend reports of arrhythmia frequency, patient activity levels, and perhaps even cardiac function by some form of hemodynamic monitor (e.g., cardiac impedance), which should enhance patient management, will be available to the clinician. Future pulse generators will have antitachycardia pacing therapies, including perhaps some pacing therapies for atrial fibrillation or atypical atrial flutter. Such devices may also include preventive treatment algorithms for atrial fibrillation (e.g., overdrive pacing after termination of paroxysmal atrial fibrillation, overdrive pacing after detection of short runs of atrial tachyarrhythmias, or overdrive pacing after periods of increased supraventricular premature beat frequency). Such interventions in combination with selective atrial site pacing (septal, coronary sinus, or left atrial sites)

Table 16–9. Monitoring Antiarrhythmic Therapy

Drug	Sotalol, 80 mg bid	Sotalol, 80 mg tid	Sotalol, 160 mg bid
Date	Aug 25–Oct 8	Oct 8–Oct 22	Oct 22–Nov 19
VPBs (day^{-1})	174	46	19
NSVT (day^{-1})	1.1	0.5	1.2
Afib (episodes wk^{-1})	>42	9	3.5
Duration of Afib	6 sec–2 hr	11 sec–5 hr	6 sec–2 hr

VPBs, ventricular premature beats; NSVT, nonsustained ventricular tachycardia; Afib, atrial fibrillation.

may be proved to prevent paroxysmal atrial fibrillation in patients with the tachycardia-bradycardia syndrome. Algorithms to promote ventricular rate regularization during atrial fibrillation may become more widely applied if these features are proved beneficial.

Cost-Effective Pacing in Sinus Node Disease

Retrospective analyses suggest that the cost differential of a dual-chamber rate-adaptive pacing system for the management of SND is offset by the reduction in health care costs projected as a result of the reduction in the consumption of health care resources for the management of atrial fibrillation, stroke, and congestive heart failure.[254, 255] This issue is being addressed in the prospective clinical trials comparing atrial-based with ventricular pacing that are under way.

REFERENCES

1. Ferrer MI: The sick sinus syndrome in atrial disease. JAMA 206:645, 1968.
2. Ferrer MI: The sick sinus syndrome. Circulation 47:635, 1973.
3. Ferrer MI: The Sick Sinus Syndrome. Mt Kisco, NY, Futura, 1974.
4. Moss AJ, Davis RJ: Brady-tachy syndrome. Prog Cardiovasc Dis 16:439,197.
5. Kerr CR, Grant AO, Wenger TL, et al: Sinus node dysfunction. Cardiol Clin 1:181, 1983.
6. Bernstein AD, Parsonnet V: Survey of cardiac pacing and defibrillation in the United States in 1993. Am J Cardiol 78:187, 1996.
7. Goldman BS, Nishimura S, Lau C: Survey of cardiac pacing in Canada (1993). Can J Cardiol 12:573, 1996.
8. Short DS: The syndrome of alternating bradycardia and tachycardia. Br Heart J 16:208, 1954.
9. Mandel WJ, Hayakawa H, Allen HN, et al: Assessment of sinus node function in patients with sick sinus syndrome. Circulation 46:761, 1972.
10. Jordan J, Yamaguchi I, Mandel W: Studies on the mechanism of sinus node dysfunction in the sick sinus syndrome. Circulation 57:217, 1978.
11. Strauss HC, Bigger JT Jr, Saroff AL, et al: Electrophysiologic evaluation of sinus node function in patients with sinus node dysfunction. Circulation 53:763, 1976.
12. Strauss HC, Prystowsky EN, Sheinmann MM: Sino-atrial and atrial electrogenesis. Prog Cardiovasc Dis 19:385, 1977.
13. Lown B: Electrical reversion of cardiac arrhythmias. Br Heart J 29:469, 1967.
14. Laslett EE: Syncopal attacks associated with prolonged arrest of the whole heart. Q J Med 2:347, 1909.
15. Levine SA: Observations on sino-atrial heart block. Arch Intern Med 17:153, 1916.
16. Levander-Lindgren M, Lantz BO: Bradyarrhythmia profile and associated disease in 1,265 patients with cardiac pacing. PACE 11:2207, 1988.
17. Rubinstein JJ, Schulman CL, Yurchak PM, et al: Clinical spectrum of the sick sinus syndrome. Circulation 46:5, 1972.
18. Vardas P, Fitzpatrick A, Ingram A, et al: Natural history of sinus node chronotropy in paced patients. PACE 14:155, 1991.
19. Gwinn N, Lemen R, Kratz J, et al: Chronotropic incompetence: A common and progressive finding in pacemaker patients. Am Heart J 123:1216, 1992.
20. Chin C-F, Messenger JC, Greenberg PS, Ellestad MH: Chronotropic incompetence in exercise testing. Clin Cardiol 2:12, 1979.
21. Keith A, Flack M: The form and nature of the muscular connections between the primary divisions of the vertebrate heart. J Anat Physiol 41:172, 1906–1907.
22. Flack M: An investigation of the sinoatrial node of the mammalian heart. J Physiol 41:64, 1910–1911.
23. McWilliam JA: On the rhythm of the mammalian heart. J Physiol (Lond) 9:167, 1888.
24. Boineau JP, Miller CB, Scheussler RB, et al: Activation sequence and potential distribution maps demonstrating multicentric atrial impulse origin in dogs. Circ Res 54:322, 1984.
25. Boineau JP, Canavan TE, Schuessler RB, et al: Demonstration of a widely distributed atrial pacemaker complex in the human heart. Circulation 77:1221, 1988.
26. James TN: Cardiac conduction system, fetal and postnatal development. Am J Cardiol 25:213, 1970.
27. James TN: The sinus node as a servomechanism. Circ Res 32:307, 1973.
28. Davies MJ, Pomerance A: Quantitative studies of ageing changes in the human sinoatrial node and internodal tracts. Br Heart J 34:150, 1972.
29. Davies MJ, Ward DE: The pathology of arrhythmias, conduction disturbances, and sudden death. In Julian DG, Camm AJ, Fox KM, et al (eds): Diseases of the Heart. London, Balliere Tindall, 1989, pp 486–508.
30. Giles WR: Generation of pacemaker activity in mammalian sinoatrial node. In Huzinga JD (eds): Pacemaker Activity and Intercellular Communication. Boca Raton, CRC Press, 1995, pp 15–35.
31. Anumonwo JMB, Jalife J: Cellular and subcellular mechanisms of pacemaker activity initiation and synchronization in the heart. In Zipes DP, Jalife J (eds): Cardiac Electrophysiology from Cell to Bedside. Philadelphia, WB Saunders, 1995, pp 151–164.
32. Hoffman BF: Electrophysiology of single cardiac cells. Bull N Y Acad Med 35:689, 1959.
33. West TC: Ultramicroelectrode recording from the cardiac pacemaker. J Pharmacol Exp Ther 115:283, 1955.
34. Noma A, Irisawa H: Potassium current during the pacemaker depolarization in rabbit sinoatrial node cell. Pflugers Arch 388:255, 1980.
35. DiFrancesco D, Ducouret P, Robinson RB: Muscarinic modulation of cardiac rate at low acetylcholine concentration. Science 243:669, 1989.
36. Noma A, Irisawa H: Contribution of an electrogenic sodium pump to the membrane potential in rabbit sinoatrial node cells. Pflugers Arch 358:289, 1975.
37. Irisawa H, Brown HF, Giles W: Cardiac pacemaking in the sinoatrial node. Physiol Rev 73:197, 1993.
38. Doerr T, Denger R, Trautwein W: Calcium currents in single SA nodal cells of the rabbit heart studied with action potential clamp. Pflugers Arch 413:599, 1989.
39. Hagiwara N, Irisawa H, Kameyama M: Contribution of two types of calcium currents to pacemaker potentials of rabbit sinoatrial node cells. J Physiol (Lond) 395:233, 1988.
40. Muramatsu H, Berkowitz GA, Nathan RD: A characterization of a tetrodotoxin-sensitive Na+ current in pacemaker cells isolated from rabbit sinoatrial node. Am J Physiol 270:H2108, 1996.
41. Nikmaram MR, Boyett MR, Kodama I, et al: Variation in effects of Cs+, UL-FS-49, and 7D-7288 within sinoatrial node. Am J Physiol 272:H2782, 1997.
42. Kodama I, Nikmaram MR, Boyett MR, et al: Regional differences in the role of the Ca²⁺ and Na⁺ currents in pacemaker activity in the sinoatrial node. Am J Physiol 272:H2793, 1997.
43. Bouman LN, Gerlings ED, Bierstekerpa PA, et al: Pacemaker shift in the sinoatrial node during vagal stimulation. Pfluger Arch 302:255, 1968.
44. Goldberg JM: Intra-SA-nodal pacemaker shifts induced by autonomic nerve stimulation in the dog. Am J Physiol 229:1116, 1975.
45. Amumonwo JMB, Wang HZ, Trabka-Janik E, et al: Gap junctional channels in adult mammalian sinus nodal cells: Immunolocalization and electrophysiology. Circ Res 71:229, 1992.
46. Delmar M, Jalife J, Michaels D: Effect of changes in excitability and intercellular coupling on synchronization in the rabbit sinoatrial node. J Physiol (Lond) 370:127, 1986.
47. Strauss HC, Scheinmann MM, Labarre A, et al: Review of the significance of drugs in the sick sinus syndrome. In Bonke FIM (ed): The Sinus Node: Structure, Function, and Clinical Relevance. The Hague, Netherlands, Martinus Nijhoff, 1978, pp 103–111.
48. Scheinman MM, Strauss HC, Evans GT, et al: Adverse effects of sympatholytic agents in patients with hypertension and sinus node dysfunction. Am J Med 64:1013, 1978.
49. Desai JM, Sheinmann MM, Strauss HC, et al: Electrophysiologic effects of combined autonomic blockade in patients with sinus node disease. Circulation 63:953, 1981.
50. Linker NJ, Camm AJ: Drug effects on the sinus node: A clinical perspective. Cardiovasc Drug Ther 2:165, 1988.
51. Evans R, Shaw DB: Pathological studies in sino-atrial disorder (sick sinus syndrome). Br Heart J 39:778, 1977.
52. Thery C, Gosselin B, Lekieffre J, Warembourg H: Pathology of the

sinoatrial node: Correlation with electrocardiographic findings in 111 patients. Am Heart J 93:735, 1977.

53. Bergfeldt L: HLA-B27-associated rheumatic diseases with severe cardiac bradyarrhythmias: Clinical features in 223 men with permanent pacemakers. Am J Med 75:210, 1983.

54. Maisch B, Lotze U, Schneider J, et al: Antibodies to human sinus node in sick sinus syndrome. PACE 9:1101, 1986.

55. James TN: Normal and abnormal consequences of apoptosis in the human heart: From postnatal morphogenesis to paroxysmal arrhythmias. Circulation 90:556, 1994.

56. Davies MJ: Apoptosis in cardiovascular disease. Heart 77:498, 1997.

57. Bharati S, Nordenberg A, Bauerfiend R, et al: The anatomic substrate for the sick sinus syndrome in the adolescent. Am J Cardiol 46:163, 1980.

58. Lorber A, Maisuls E, Palant A: Autosomal dominant inheritance of sinus node disease. Int J Cardiol 15:252, 1987.

59. Hartel G, Talvensaari T: Treatment of sinoatrial syndrome with permanent cardiac pacing in 90 patients. Acta Med Scand 198:341,1975.

60. Sasaki R, Theilen EO, January LE, Ehrenhoft JL: Cardiac arrhythmias associated with the repair of atrial and ventricular septal defects. Circulation 18:909, 1958.

61. Greenwood RD, Rosenthal A, Sloss LJ, et al: Sick sinus syndrome after surgery for congenital heart disease. Circulation 52:208, 1975.

62. Yabek YM, Jarmakani JM: Sinus node dysfunction in children, adolescents and young adults. Pediatrics 61: 593, 1978.

63. Beder SD, Gillette PC, Garson A Jr, et al: Symptomatic sick sinus syndrome in children and adolescents as the only manifestation of cardiac abnormality or associated with unoperated congenital heart disease. Am J Cardiol 51:1133, 1983.

64. Marcus B, Gillette PC, Garson A Jr: Electrophysiologic evaluation of sinus node dysfunction in postoperative children and young adults utilizing combined autonomic blockade. Clin Cardiol 14:33, 1991.

65. Engel TR, Meister SG, Feitusa GS, et al: Appraisal of sinus node artery disease. Circulation 52:86, 1975.

66. Shaw DB, Linker NJ, Heaver PA, et al: Chronic sinoatrial disorder (sick sinus syndrome): A possible result of cardiac ischemia. Br Heart J 58:598, 1987.

67. Rokseth R, Hatle L: Sinus arrest in myocardial infarction. Br Heart J 33:639, 1971.

68. Fluck DC, Olsen E, Pentecost BL, et al: Natural history and clinical significance of arrhythmias after acute cardiac infarction. Br Heart J 29:170, 1967.

69. Headrick J, Willis RJ: Mediation by adenosine of bradycardia in rat heart during graded global ischaemia. Pflugers Arch 412:618, 1988.

70. Watts AH: Sick sinus syndrome: An adenosine-mediated disease. Lancet 1:786, 1985.

71. Engel TR, Schaal SF: Digitalis in the sick sinus syndrome: The effects of digitalis on sinoatrial automaticity and atrioventricular conduction. Circulation 48:1201, 1973.

72. Margolis JR, Strauss HC, Miller HC: Digitalis and the sick sinus syndrome: Clinical and electrophysiologic documentation of a severe toxic effect on sinus node function. Circulation 52:162, 1975.

73. Strauss HC, Gilbert M, Svenson RH, et al: Electrophysiologic effects of propranolol on sinus node function in patients with sinus node dysfunction. Circulation 54:452, 1976.

74. Grayzel J, Angeles J: Sino-atrial block in man provoked by quinidine. J Electrocardiol 5:289, 1972.

75. Josephson ME, Caracta AR, Lau SH, et al: Electrophysiologic properties of procainamide in man. Am J Cardiol 33:596–603, 1974.

76. Dhingra RC, Deedwania PC, Cummings JM, et al: Electrophysiologic effects of lidocaine on sinus node and atrium in patients with and without sinoatrial dysfunction. Circulation 57:448, 1978.

77. Vik-Mo H, Ohm OH, Lund-Johanen P: Electrophysiological effects of flecainide acetate in patients with sinus nodal dysfunction. Am J Cardiol 50:1090, 1982.

78. LaBarre A, Strauss HC, Scheinman MM, et al: Electrophysiologic effects of disopyramide phosphate on sinus node function in patients with sinus node dysfunction. Circulation 59:226, 1979.

79. Touboul P, Atallah G, Gressard A, Kirkorian G: Effects of amiodarone on sinus node in man. Br Heart J 42:573, 1979.

80. Wellens HJJ, Cats V, Duren DR: Symptomatic sinus node abnormalities following lithium carbonate therapy. Am J Med 59: 285, 1975.

81. Petch MC: Who needs dual chamber pacing? Br Med J 307:215, 1993.

82. Aggarwal RK, Roy SG, Connolly DT, et al: Trends in pacemaker mode prescription 1984–1994: A single centre study of 3710 patients. Heart 75:518, 1996.

83. Brodsky M, Wu D, Denes P, et al: Arrhythmias documented by 24-hour continuous electrocardiographic monitoring in 50 male students without apparent heart disease. Am J Cardiol 39:390, 1977.

84. Bjerregaard P: Mean 24-hour heart rate, minimal heart rate, and pauses in healthy subjects 40–79 years of age. Eur Heart J 4:44, 1983.

85. Talan DA, Bauernfiend RA, Ashley WW, et al: Twenty-four-hour continuous ECG recordings in long-distance runners. Chest 32:622, 1982.

86. Crook BRM, Cashman PMM, Stott FD, Raftery EB: Tape monitoring of the electrocardiogram in ambulant patients with sinoatrial disease. Br Heart J 35:1009, 1973.

87. Grodman RS, Capone RJ, Most AS: Arrhythmia surveillance by transtelephonic monitoring: Comparison with Holter monitoring in symptomatic ambulatory patients. Am Heart J 98:459, 1979.

88. Abbott JA, Hirschfield DS, Kunkel FW, et al: Graded exercise testing in patients with sinus node dysfunction. Am J Med 62:330, 1977.

89. Holden W, McAnulty JH, Rahimtoola SH: Characterization of heart rate response to exercise in the sick sinus syndrome. Br Heart J 20:923, 1978.

90. Valin HO, Edhag KO: Heart rate responses in patients with sinus node disease compared to controls: Physiological implications and diagnostic possibilities. Clin Cardiol 3:391, 1980.

91. Johnston FA, Robinson JF, Fyfe T: Exercise testing in the diagnosis of sick sinus syndrome in the elderly: Implications for treatment. PACE 10:831, 1987.

92. Wilkoff BL, Covey J, Blackburn G: A mathematical model of the cardiac chronotropic response to exercise. J Electrophysiol 3:176, 1989.

93. Forbath P, Darling D, Quimet S: Adapting the rate-modulation to the type of chronotropic incompetence. PACE 14:685, 1991.

94. Yamada T, Fukunami M, Kugagai K, et al: Detection of patients with sick sinus syndrome by use of low amplitude potentials early in the fitted P wave. J Am Coll Cardiol 28:738, 1996.

95. Keane D, Stafford P, Baker S, et al: Signal-averaged electrocardiography of the sinus and paced P wave in sinus node disease. PACE 18:1346, 1995.

96. Guilleminault C, Pool P, Motta J, Gillis AM: Sinus arrest during REM sleep in young adults. N Engl J Med 311: 1006, 1984.

97. Rosen KM, Loeb HS, Sinno MZ, et al: Cardiac conduction in patients with symptomatic sinus node disease. Circulation 43:836, 1971.

98. Narula OS: Atrioventricular conduction defects in patients with sinus bradycardia. Circulation 44:1096, 1971.

99. Sutton R, Kenny RA: The natural history of sick sinus syndrome. PACE 9:1110, 1986.

100. Leatham A: Carotid sinus syncope. Br Heart J 47:409, 1981.

101. Morley CA, Sutton R: Carotid sinus syncope. Int J Cardiol 6:287, 1984.

102. Brignole M, Menozzi C, Gianfranchi L, et al: Neurally mediated syncope detected by carotid sinus massage and head-up tilt test in sick sinus syndrome. Am J Cardiol 68:1032, 1991.

103. Alboni P, Menozzi C, Brignole M, et al: An abnormal neural reflex plays a role in causing syncope in sinus bradycardia. J Am Coll Cardiol 22:1130, 1993.

104. Jose AD: Effect of combined sympathetic and parasympathetic blockade on heart rate and cardiac function in man. Am J Cardiol 18:476, 1966.

105. Desai J, Scheinmann MM, Strauss HC, et al: Electrophysiological effects of combined autonomic blockade in patients with sinus node disease. Circulation 63:953, 1981.

106. Kang PS, Gomes JAC, El Sheriff N: Differential effects of functional autonomic blockade on the variables of sinus node automaticity in sick sinus syndrome. Am J Cardiol 49:273, 1982.

107. Sethi KK, Jaishanker S, Balachander J, et al: Sinus node function after autonomic blockade in normals and in sick sinus syndrome. Int J Cardiol 5:707, 1984.

108. Jose AD, Collison D: The normal range and determinants of the intrinsic heart rate in man. Cardiovasc Res 4:160, 1970.

109. Fitzpatrick A, Sutton R: Tilting towards a diagnosis in unexplained recurrent syncope. Lancet 1:658, 1989.

110. Almqvist A, Goldenberg JF, Milstein S, et al: Provocation of bradycardia and hypotension by isoproterenol and upright posture in patients with unexplained syncope. N Engl J Med 329:346, 1989.

111. Josephson ME: Sinus node function. In Josephson ME (ed): Clinical Cardiac Electrophysiology: Techniques and Interpretations. Philadelphia, Lea & Febiger, 1993, pp 71–94.

112. Mandel W, Hayakawa H, Danzig R, et al: Evaluation of sinoatrial node function in man by overdrive suppression. Circulation 44:59, 1971.

113. Narula OS, Samet P, Javier RP: Significance of the sinus-node recovery time. Circulation 45:140, 1972.

114. Pop T, Fleischmann D: Measurement of sinus node recovery time after atrial pacing. *In* Bonke FIM (ed): The Sinus Node: Structure, Function, and Clinical Relevance. The Hague, Netherlands, Martinus Nijhoff, 1978, pp 23–25.

115. Reiffel JA, Gang E, Bigger JT Jr, et al: Sinus node recovery time related to paced cycle length in normals and in patients with sinoatrial dysfunction. Am Heart J 104:746, 1982.

116. Benditt DG, Strauss HC, Scheinmann MM, et al: Analysis of secondary pauses following termination of rapid atrial pacing in man. Circulation 54:436, 1976.

117. Strauss HC, Saroff AJ, Bigger JT Jr, et al: Premature atrial stimulation as a key to the understanding of sinoatrial conduction in man: Presentation of data and critical review of the literature. Circulation 47:86, 1973.

118. Narula OS, Shantha N, Vasquez M, et al: A new method for measurement of sinoatrial conduction time. Circulation 58:706, 1978.

119. Breithardt G, Seipel L: Comparative study of two methods of estimating sinoatrial conduction time in man. Am J Cardiol 42:965, 1978.

120. Hariman RJ, Krongrad E, Boxer RA, et al: Method for recording electrical activity of the sinoatrial node and automatic atrial foci during cardiac catheterization in human subjects. Am J Cardiol 45:775, 1980.

121. Reiffel JA, Gang E, Gliklich J, et al: The human sinus node electrogram: A transvenous catheter technique and a comparison of directly measured and indirectly estimated sinoatrial conduction time in adults. Circulation 62:1324, 1980.

122. Gomes JA, Kang PS, El-Sherif N: The sinus node electrogram in patients with and without sick sinus syndrome: Technique and correlation between directly measured and indirectly estimated sinoatrial conduction time. Circulation 66:864, 1982.

123. Haberl R, Steinbeck G, Luderitz B, et al: Comparison between intracellular and extracellular direct current recordings of sinus node activity for evaluation of sinoatrial conduction time. Circulation 70:760, 1984.

124. Juillard A, Guillerm F, Chuong HV, et al: Sinus node electrogram recording in 59 patients: Comparison with simulation. Br Heart J 50:75, 1983.

125. Bethge C, Gebhardt-Seehausen U, Mullges W: The human sinus nodal electrogram: Techniques and clinical results of intra-atrial recordings in patients with and without sick sinus syndrome. Am Heart J 112:1074, 1986.

126. Narula OS: Sinus-node reentry: A mechanism for supraventricular tachycardia. Circulation 50:1114, 1974.

127. Kerr CR, Prystowsky EN, Browning DJ, et al: Characterization of refractoriness in the sinus node of the rabbit. Circ Res 47:742, 1980.

128. Kerr CR, Strauss HC: The measurement of sinus node refractoriness in man. Circulation 68:1231, 1984.

129. Kerr CR: Effect of pacing cycle length and autonomic tone on sinus node refractoriness in man. Am J Cardiol 62:1192, 1988.

130. Luderitz B, Steinbeck G, Naumann d'Alnoncourt C, Roenberger W: Relevance of diagnostic atrial stimulation for pacemaker treatment in sinoatrial disease. *In* Bonke F (ed): The Sinus Node: Structure, Function and Clinical Relevance. The Hague, Martinus Nijhoff, 1978, pp 77–88.

131. Breithardt G, Seipel L, Loogen F: Sinus node recovery time and calculated sinoatrial conduction time in normal subjects and patients with sinus node dysfunction. Circulation 56:43, 1977.

132. Scheinman MM, Strauss HC, Abbott JA, et al: Electrophysiologic testing in patients with sinus pauses and/or sinoatrial exit block. Eur J Cardiol 8:51, 1978.

133. Reiffel JA, Kerrick K, Zimmerman J, Bigger JT Jr: Electrophysiologic studies of the sinus node and atria. *In* Brest AW (ed): Cardiovascular Clinics: Philadelphia, FA Davis, 1985, pp 37–59.

134. DiMarco JP, Garan H, Hawthorne JW, Ruskin JN: Intracardiac electrophysiologic techniques in recurrent syncope of unknown cause. Ann Intern Med 95:542, 1981.

135. Gulamhusein S, Naccarelli GV, Ko PT, et al: Value and limitations of clinical electrophysiologic study in assessment of patients with unexplained syncope. Am J Med 73:700, 1982.

136. Hess DS, Morady F, Scheinman MM: Electrophysiologic testing in the evaluation of patients with syncope of undetermined origin. Am J Cardiol 50:1309, 1982.

137. Akhtar M, Shenasa M, Denker S, et al: Role of cardiac electrophysiologic studies in patients with unexplained recurrent syncope. PACE 6:192, 1983.

138. Benditt DG, Gurnick CC, Dunbar D, et al: Indications for electrophysiological testing in the diagnosis and assessment of sinus node dysfunction. Circulation 75(Suppl III):93, 1987.

139. Gann D, Tolentino R, Samet P: Electrophysiologic evaluation of elderly patients with sinus bradycardia: A long-term follow-up study. Ann Intern Med 90:24, 1979.

140. Fijimara O, Yee R, Klein GJ, et al: The diagnostic sensitivity of electrophysiologic testing in patients with syncope caused by transient bradycardia. N Engl J Med 321:1703, 1989.

141. Krahn AD, Klein GJ, Norris C, Yee R: The etiology of syncope in patients with negative tilt table and electrophysiologic testing. Circulation 92:1819, 1985.

142. Krahn AD, Klein GJ, Yee R: Recurrent unexplained syncope: Diagnostic and therapeutic approach. Can J Cardiol 12:989, 1996.

143. Medtronic Interim Report. Minneapolis, MN, Medtronic, Inc., July 1997.

144. Sgarbossa EB, Pinski SL, Jaeger FJ, et al: Incidence and predictors of syncope in paced patients with sick sinus syndrome. Pacing Clin Electrophysiol 15:1055, 1992.

145. Alboni P, Menozzi C, Brignole M, et al: Effects of permanent pacemaker and oral theophylline in sick sinus syndrome. The THEOPACE Study: A randomized controlled trial. Circulation 96:260, 1997.

146. Rosenqvist M, Obel IWP: Atrial pacing and the risk of AV block: Is there a time for change in attitude? PACE 12:97, 1989.

147. Brandt J, Anderson H, Fåahraeus T, Shueller H: Natural history of sinus node disease treated with atrial pacing in 213 patients: Implications for stimulation mode selection. J Am Coll Cardiol 20:633, 1992.

148. Andersen HR, Nielsen JC, Thomsen PEB, et al: Long-term follow-up of patients from a randomized trial of atrial versus ventricular pacing for sick-sinus syndrome. Lancet 350:1210, 1997.

149. Tonkin AM, Heddle WF, Tornos P: Intermittent atrioventricular block: Procainamide administration as a provocative test. Aust N Z J Med 8:594, 1978.

150. Puglisi A, Rica R, Angrisani G: The Ajmaline test in identifying patients at high risk for developing paroxysmal AV block. Ital Cardiol 12:866, 1982.

151. Bergfeldt L, Rosenqvist M, Vallin H, et al: Disopyramide-induced atrioventricular block in patients with bifascicular block: An acute stress test to predict atrioventricular block progression. Br Heart J 53:328, 1985.

152. Chamberlain-Webber R, Petersen MEV, Ahmed R, et al: Diagnosis of sick sinus syndrome with flecainide in patients with normal sinus node recovery times investigated for unexplained syncope. Eur J Cardiac Pacing Electrophysiol 2:106, 1992.

153. Vardas P, Ingram A, Theodorakis G, et al: Long-term results of disopyramide provocative test in syncopal patients with latent sinus node and atrioventricular conduction defects. PACE 16:1130, 1993.

154. Vardas PE, Kalogeropoulos CK, Kenny-Creedon RA, et al: Verapamil as a challenge to the conduction system in syncopal patients. PACE 10:A512, 1987.

155. Rosenqvist M, Brandt J, Schüller H: Long-term pacing in sinus node disease: Effects of stimulation mode on cardiovascular morbidity and mortality. Am Heart J 117:16, 1988.

156. Alpert MA, Curtiss JJ, Sanfelippo JF, et al: Comparative survival following permanent ventricular and dual-chamber pacing for patients with chronic symptomatic sinus node dysfunction with and without congestive heart failure. Am Heart J 113:958, 1987.

157. Sasaki Y, Shimotori M, Akahane K, et al: Long-term follow-up of patients with sick sinus syndrome: A comparison of clinical aspects among unpaced, ventricular inhibited paced, and physiologically paced groups. PACE 11:1575, 1988.

158. Feuer J, Shandling A, Messenger J, et al: Influence of cardiac pacing mode on the long term development of atrial fibrillation. Am J Cardiol 64:1376, 1989.

159. Stangl K, Seitz K, Wirtzfeld A, et al: Differences between atrial single chamber (AAI) and ventricular single chamber pacing (VVI) with respect to prognosis and antiarrhythmic effect in patients with sick sinus syndrome. Pacing Clin Electrophysiol 13:2080, 1990.

160. Santini M, Alexidou G, Ansalone G, et al: Relation of prognosis in sick sinus syndrome to age, conduction defects, and modes of permanent cardiac pacing. Am J Cardiol 65:729, 1990.

161. Hesselson AB, Parsonnet V, Bernstein AD, et al: Deleterious effects

of long-term single-chamber ventricular pacing in patients with sick sinus syndrome: The hidden benefits of dual-chamber pacing. J Am Coll Cardiol 19:1542, 1992.

162. Sgarbossa EB, Pinski SL, Maloney JD, et al: Chronic atrial fibrillation and stroke in paced patients with sick sinus syndrome: Relevance of clinical characteristics and pacing modalities. Circulation 88:1045, 1993.

163. Connolly SJ, Kerr C, Gent M, Yusuf S: Dual-chamber versus ventricular pacing: Critical appraisal of current data. Circulation 94:578, 1996.

164. Andersen HR, Thuesen L, Bagger JP, et al: Prospective randomized trial of atrial versus ventricular pacing in sick sinus syndrome. Lancet 344:1523, 1994.

165. Fairfax AJ, Lambert CD, Leatham A: Systemic embolism in chronic sinoatrial disorder. N Engl J Med 295:190, 1976.

166. Petersen P, Boysen G, Godtfredsen J, et al: Placebo-controlled randomised trial of warfarin and aspirin prevention of thrombo-embolic complications in chronic atrial fibrillation: The Copenhagen AFASAK Study. Lancet 1:175, 1989.

167. Stroke Prevention in Atrial Fibrillation Investigators: Stroke prevention in atrial fibrillation (SPAF). Circulation 84:527, 1991.

168. Boston Area Anticoagulation Trial for Atrial Fibrillation Investigators: The effect of low-dose warfarin on the risk of stroke in non-rheumatic atrial fibrillation. N Engl J Med 323:1505, 1990.

169. Rosenqvist M, Isaaz K, Botvinick EH, et al: The importance of a normal pattern of ventricular depolarization: A comparison between atrial, AV-sequential and ventricular pacing. Am J Cardiol 67:148, 1991.

170. Lee MA, Dae MW, Langberg JJ, et al: Effects of long-term right ventricular apical pacing on left ventricular perfusion, innervation, function and histology. J Am Coll Cardiol 24:225, 1994.

171. Redfield MM, Kay GN, Martin RC, et al: Tachycardia related cardiomyopathy: A common and reversible cause of ventricular dysfunction in patients with atrial fibrillation. Circulation 94:I-21, 1996.

172. Deshmukh P, Golyan FD, Anderson K, Zehr RD: AV nodal ablation in conjunction with direct His bundle pacing improves ventricular function in patients with atrial fibrillation and cardiomyopathy. Circulation 94:I-21, 1996.

173. Katritis D, Camm AJ: Chronotropic incompetence: A proposal for definition and diagnosis. Br Heart J 70:400, 1993.

174. Gwinn N, Leman R, Kratz J, et al: Chronotropic incompetence: A common and progressive finding in pacemaker patients. Am Heart J 123:1216, 1992.

175. Vardas PE, Fitzpatrick A, Ingram A, et al: Natural history of sinus node chronotropy in paced patients. PACE 14:155, 1991.

176. Simon AB, Janz N: Symptomatic bradyarrhythmias in the adult: Natural history following ventricular pacemaker implantation. PACE 5:372, 1982.

177. Alt E, Volker R, Wirtzfeld A, Ulm K: Survival and follow-up after pacemaker implantation: A comparison of patients with sick sinus syndrome, complete heart block and atrial fibrillation. PACE 8:849, 1985.

178. Skagen K, Hansen JF: The long-term prognosis for patients with sinoatrial block treated with permanent pacemaker. Acta Med Scand 199:13, 1975.

179. Shaw DB, Holman RR, Gowers JI: Survival in sinoatrial disorder (sick sinus syndrome). Br Med J 280:139, 1980.

180. Sgarbossa EB, Pinski SL, Maloney JD: The role of pacing modality in determining long-term survival in the sick sinus syndrome. Ann Intern Med 119:359, 1993.

181. Tung RT, Shen W-K, Hayes DL, et al: Long-term survival after permanent pacemaker implantation for sick sinus syndrome. Am J Cardiol 74:1016, 1994.

182. Gillis AM, Mattson L, Benson J, et al: Survival analysis of pacemaker patients [Abstract]. Can J Cardiol 13:120C, 1997.

183. Lamas GA: Pacemaker mode selection and survival: A plea to apply the principles of evidence based medicine to cardiac pacing practice. Heart 78:218, 1997.

184. Lammas GA, Estes NM, III, Schneller S, et al: Does dual-chamber or atrial pacing prevent atrial fibrillation? The need for a randomized controlled trial. PACE 15:1109, 1992.

185. Ovsyhcher IE: Matching optimal pacemaker to patient: Do we need a large scale clinical trial of pacemaker mode selection? PACE 18:1845, 1995.

186. Toff WD, Skehan JD, de Bono DP, Camm AJ: The United Kingdom pacing and cardiovascular events (UKPACE) trial. Heart 78:221, 1997.

187. Benditt DG, Benson W Jr, Kreitt J, et al: Electrophysiologic effects of theophylline in young patients with recurrent symptomatic bradyarrhythmias. Am J Cardiol 52:1223, 1983.

188. Alboni P, Ratto B, Cappato R, et al: Clinical effects of oral theophylline in sick sinus syndrome. Am Heart J 122:1361, 1991.

189. Saito A, Matsubara K, Yamanori H, et al: Effects of oral theophylline on sick sinus syndrome. J Am Coll Cardiol 21:199, 1993.

190. Avery PG, Small J, Shaw DB: Xamoterol in sinus node disease. Int J Cardiol 40:45,1993.

191. Wijffels MCEF, Kirchhof EJHJ, Dorland R, Allessie MA: Atrial fibrillation begets atrial fibrillation: A study in awake chronically instrumented goats. Circulation 92:1954, 1995.

192. Daoud EG, Bogun F, Goyal R, et al: Effect of atrial fibrillation on atrial refractoriness in humans. Circulation 94:1600, 1996.

193. Goette A, Honeycutt C, Langberg JJ: Electrical remodelling in atrial fibrillation: Time course and mechanisms. Circulation 94:2968, 1996.

194. Yue L, Feng J, Gaspo R, et al: Ionic remodelling underlying action potential changes in a canine model of atrial fibrillation. Circ Res 81:512, 1997.

195. Tieleman RG, van Gelder IC, Blaauw Y, et al: Digoxin delays recovery from electrical remodelling of the atria in goats. Circulation 96:I-235, 1997.

196. Dreifus LS, Fisch C, Griffin JC, et al: Guidelines for implantation of cardiac pacemakers and antiarrhythmia devices: A report of the ACC/AHA task force on assessment of diagnostic and cardiovascular procedures (Committee on Pacemaker Implantation). Circulation 84:455, 1991.

197. Clark M, Sutton R, Ward D, et al: Recommendations for pacemaker prescription for symptomatic bradycardia: Report of a working party of the British Pacing and Electrophysiology Group. Br Heart J 66:185, 1991.

198. Simonsen E: Assessment of the need for rate-responsive pacing in patients with sinus node dysfunction: A prospective study of heart rate response during daily activities and exercise testing. PACE 10:1229, 1987.

199. Rosenqvist M, Aren C, Kristensson BE, et al: Atrial rate-responsive pacing in sinus node disease. Eur Heart J 11:537, 1990.

200. Haywood GA, Katritsis D, Ward J, et al: Atrial adaptive rate pacing in sick sinus syndrome: Effects on exercise capacity and arrhythmias. Br Heart J 69:174, 1993.

201. Stone JM, Bhakta RD, Lutgen J: Dual-chamber sequential pacing management of sinus node dysfunction: Advantages over single-chamber pacing. Am Heart J 104:1319, 1982.

202. Lau CP, Rushby J, Leigh-Jones M, et al: Symptomatology and quality of life in patients with rate-responsive pacemakers: A double-blind randomized cross-over study. Clin Cardiol 12:505, 1989.

203. Linde-Eldelstam C, Nordlander R, Undén A-L, et al: Quality of life in patients treated with atrio-ventricular synchronous pacing compared to rate-modulated ventricular pacing: A long-term double-blind cross-over study. PACE 15:1467, 1992.

204. Mitsuoka T, Kenny R-A, Au Yeung T, et al: Benefits of dual-chamber pacing in sick sinus syndrome. Br Heart J 60:338, 1988.

205. Sulke N, Chambers J, Dritsas A, et al: A randomized double-blind crossover comparison of four rate-responsive pacing modes. J Am Coll Cardiol 17:696, 1991.

206. Benditt DG, Mianulli M, Fetter J, et al: Single-chamber cardiac pacing with activity-initiated chronotropic response: Evaluation by cardiopulmonary exercise testing. Circulation 75:184, 1987.

207. Ritter P, Vai F, Bonnet JL, et al: Rate-adaptive atrioventricular delay improves cardiopulmonary performance in patients implanted with a dual-chamber pacemaker for complete heart block. Eur J Cardiac Pacing Electrophysiol 1:31, 1991.

208. Mabo P, Pouillot C, Kermarrec A, et al: Lack of physiological adaptation of the atrioventricular interval to heart rate in patients chronically paced in the AAIR mode. PACE 14:2133, 1991.

209. Provenier F, Jordaens L, Verstraeten T, Clement DL: The "automatic mode switch" function in successive generations of minute ventilation sensing dual chamber rate responsive pacemakers. PACE 17:1913, 1994.

210. Ovsyshcher IE, Katz A, Bondy C: Initial experience with a new algorithm for automatic mode switching from DDDR to DDIR mode. PACE 17:1908, 1994.

211. Sutton R: Mode-switching in DDDR pacing. *In* Aubert AE, Ector H, Stroobandt R (eds): Cardiac Pacing and Electrophysiology: A Bridge to the 21st Century. Dordrecht, Netherlands, Kluwer Academic Publishers, 1994, pp 363–370.

212. Ricci R, Puglisi A, Azzolini P, et al: Reliability of a new algorithm for automatic mode switching from DDDR to DDIR pacing mode in sinus node disease patients with chronotropic incompetence and recurrent paroxysmal atrial fibrillation. PACE 19:1719, 1996.

213. Gross JN, Moser S, Benedek ZM, et al: DDD pacing mode survival in patients with a dual-chamber pacemaker. J Am Coll Cardiol 19:1536, 1992.

214. Ibrahim B, Sanderson JE, Wright B, Palmar R: Dual chamber pacing: How many remain in the DDD mode over the long term? Br Heart J 74:76, 1995.

215. Irwin M, Carbol B, Senaratine M, Gulamhusein S: Long-term survival of chosen atrial-based pacing modalities. PACE 19:1796, 1996.

216. Moura PJ, Gessman LJ, Lai T, et al: Chronotropic response of an activity-detecting pacemaker compared with the normal sinus node. PACE 10:78, 1987.

217. Humen DP, Kostuk WJ, Klein GJ: Activity-sensing rate-responsive pacing: Improvement in myocardial performance with exercise. PACE 8:52, 1985.

218. Lau CP, Antoniou A, Ward DE, Camm AJ: Initial clinical experience with a minute ventilation-sensing rate modulated pacemaker: Improvements in exercise capacity and symptomatology. PACE 11:1815, 1988.

219. Baig MW, Wilson J, Boute W, et al: Improved pattern of rate responsiveness with dynamic slope setting for the QT sensing pacemaker. PACE 12:311, 1989.

220. Hayman H, Sharma A, Sutton R, et al: Clinical experience with VVIR pacing based on right ventricular dP/dt. Eur J Pacing Electrophysiol 1:138, 1991.

221. Leung S-K, Lau C-P, Tang M-O, Leung Z: New integrated sensor pacemaker: Comparison of rate responses between an integrated minute ventilation and activity sensor and single sensor modes during exercise and daily activities and nonphysiologic interference. PACE 19:1664, 1996.

222. Heldman D, Mulvihill D, Nguyen H, et al: True incidence of pacemaker syndrome. PACE 13:1742, 1990.

223. Morgan DE, Norman R, West RU, Burgaff G: Echocardiographic assessment of tricuspid regurgitation during ventricular demand pacing. Am J Cardiol 58:1025, 1986.

224. Sulke N, Dritsas A, Bostock J, et al: "Subclinical" pacemaker syndrome: A randomized study of symptom free patients with ventricular demand (VVI) pacemakers upgraded to dual chamber devices. Br Heart J 69:57, 1992.

225. Ogawa S, Drufus LS, Shenoy PN, et al: Hemodynamic consequences of atrioventricular and ventriculoatrial pacing. PACE 1:18, 1978.

226. Alicandri C, Fouad FM, Tarazi RC, et al: Three cases of hypotension and syncope with ventricular pacing: Possible role of atrial reflexes. Am J Cardiol 42:137, 1978.

227. Leibert HP, O'Donoghue S, Tullner WF, et al: Pacemaker syndrome in activity-responsive VVI pacing. Am J Cardiol 64:124, 1989.

228. Wish M, Cohen A, Swartz J: Pacemaker syndrome due to a rate-responsive ventricular pacemaker. J Electrophysiol 2:504, 1988.

229. Erlebacher JA, Danner EL, Stelzer PE: Hypotension with ventricular pacing: An atrial vasodepressor reflex in human beings. J Am Coll Cardiol 4:550, 1984.

230. Ellenbogen KA, Thames MD, Mohanty PK, et al: New insights gained from hemodynamic, humoral, and vascular responses during ventriculoatrial pacing. Am J Cardiol 65:53, 1990.

231. Travill CM, Williams TDM, Vardas P, et al: Hypotension in pacemaker syndrome is associated with marked atrial natriuretic peptide (ANP) release. PACE 12:93, 1989.

232. Den Dulk K, Lindemans F, Brugada P, et al: Pacemaker syndrome with AAI rate-variable pacing: Importance of atrioventricular conduction properties, medication, and pacemaker programmability. PACE 11:1226, 1988.

233. Mehra R, Hill MRS: Prevention of atrial fibrillation/flutter by pacing techniques, In Saksena S, Luderitz B (eds): Interventional Electrophysiology: A Textbook, 2nd ed. Armonk, NY: Futura, 1996, pp 521–539.

234. Attuel P, Pellerin D, Mujica J, Coumel P: DDD pacing: An effective treatment modality for recurrent atrial arrhythmias. PACE 11:1647, 1988.

235. Garrigue S, Cazeau S, Gencel L, et al: Prevention of atrial arrhythmias during DDD pacing by atrial overdriving. PACE 20:1092, 1997.

236. Wyse DG: Current trials in the management of atrial fibrillation: Atrial pacing trial and investigation of rhythm management trial. In Murgatroyd FD, Camm AJ (eds): Nonpharmacological Management of Atrial Fibrillation. Armonk, NY, Futura, 1997, pp 133–138.

237. Lamas G, Stambler B, Mittelman R, et al: Clinical events following DDDR versus VVIR pacing: Results of a prospective trial. PACE 19:619, 1996.

238. Bellocci F, Nobile A, Spampinato A, et al: Antiarrhythmic effects of DDD rate-responsive pacing. PACE 14:622, 1991.

239. Spencer III WH, Markowitz T, Alagona P: Rate augmentation and atrial arrhythmias in DDDR pacing. PACE 13:1847, 1990.

240. Murgatroyd FD, Nitzsche R, Salde AKB, et al: New pacing algorithm for overdrive suppression of atrial fibrillation. PACE 17:1966, 1994.

241. Mabo P, Berder V, Ritter P, et al: Prevention of atrial tachyarrhythmias related to advanced interatrial block by permanent atrial resynchronization. PACE 14:648, 1991.

242. Daubert C, Mabo PN, Berder V, et al: Atrial tachyarrhythmias associated with high degree interatrial conduction block: Prevention by permanent atrial resynchronisation. Eur J Cardiac Pacing Electrophysiol 4:35, 1994.

243. Bailin SJ, Johnson WB, Hoyt R: A prospective randomized trial of Bachmann's bundle pacing for the prevention of atrial fibrillation. J Am Coll Cardiol 29:74A, 1997.

244. Spencer WH, Shu DWX, Markowitz T, et al: Atrial septal pacing: A method of pacing the atria simultaneously. PACE 20:1053, 1997.

245. Sakseena S, Prakash A, Hill M, et al: Prevention of recurrent atrial fibrillation with chronic dual-site right atrial pacing. J Am Coll Cardiol 28:687, 1996.

246. Gillis AM, Connolly SJ, Yee R, et al: Atrial pacing peri-ablation for paroxysmal atrial fibrillation: Phase I. Can J Cardiol 13:87C, 1997.

247. Charles RG, McComb JM: Systematic trial of pacing to prevent atrial fibrillation. (STOP-AF). Heart 78:224, 1997.

248. Brignole M, Gianfranchi L, Menozzi C, et al: Assessment of atrioventricular junction ablation and DDDR mode-switching pacemaker versus pharmacological treatment in patients with severely symptomatic paroxysmal atrial fibrillation: A randomized controlled study. Circulation 96:2617, 1997.

248a. Gillis AM, Connolly SJ, Dubuc M, et al for the PA³ investigators: Comparison of DDDR versus NDD pacing post total AV node ablation for prevention of atrial fibrillation. PACE (abstract, in press).

249. Gribbin GM, Bourque JP, McComb JM: Dual versus single chamber pacemakers in patients with paroxysmal atrial fibrillation treated with AV node ablation. PACE 20:1592,1997.

250. Gallik DM, Guidry GW, Mahmarian JJ, et al: Comparison of ventricular function in atrial rate adaptive versus dual chamber rate adaptive pacing during exercise. PACE 17:179, 1994.

251. Le Clercq C, Gras D, LeHellaco A, et al: Hemodynamic importance of preserving the normal sequence of ventricular activation in permanent cardiac pacing. Am Heart J 129:1133, 1995.

252. Karpawich PP, Mital S: Comparative left ventricular function following atrial, septal, and apical single chamber heart pacing in the young. PACE 20:1984, 1997.

253. Vardas PE, Simantirakis EN, Parthonakis F, et al: AAIR versus DDDR pacing in patients with impaired sinus node chronotrophy: An echocardiographic and cardiopulmonary study. PACE 20:1762, 1997.

254. Sutton R, Bourgeois J: Cost benefit analysis of single and dual chamber pacing for sick sinus syndrome and atrioventricular block: An economic analysis of the literature. Eur Heart J 17:574, 1996.

255. Mahoney CB: Pacing and outcomes: Economic implications. In Geisler E, Heller O (eds): Managing Technology in Healthcare. Boston, Kluwer Academic Publishers, 1996, pp 609–102.

Chapter 17

Pacing for Acute and Chronic Atrioventricular Conduction System Disease

Kenneth A. Ellenbogen, Maria de Guzman, David T. Kawanishi, and Shahbudin H. Rahimtoola

■ ANATOMY AND PATHOPHYSIOLOGY

The sinus node lies near the junction of the superior vena cava and the right atrium. It is supplied by the sinus nodal artery, which originates from the proximal few centimeters of the right coronary artery (RCA) in about 55% of patients and from the proximal few centimeters of the left circumflex artery (LCX) in the remainder (Fig. 17–1).[1–4]

The atrioventricular (AV) node lies directly above the insertion of the septal leaflet of the tricuspid valve just beneath the right atrial endocardium.[2–4] The AV junction is a structure encompassing the AV node with its posterior, septal, and left atrial approaches as well as the His bundle and its bifurcation. The AV node is a small subendocardial structure located within the interatrial septum at the distal convergence of the preferential internodal conduction pathways that course through the atria from the sinus node.[1] Like the sinus node, the AV node has an extensive autonomic innervation and an abundant blood supply.

Three regions, the transitional cell zone, the compact node, and the penetrating bundle, compose the AV node and are distinguished by functional and histologic differences. The transitional cell zone consists of cells composing the atrial approaches to the compact AV node and has the highest rate of spontaneous diastolic depolarization. The compact node is composed of groups of cells that have extensions into the central fibrous body and the annulus of the mitral and tricuspid valves. These cells appear to be the site of most of the conduction delay through the AV node.[5–7] The penetrating bundle consists of cells that lead directly into the His bundle and its branching portion.

Van der Hauwaert and associates[4] showed that only the proximal two thirds of the AV node is supplied by the AV nodal artery; the distal segment of the AV node has a dual blood supply in 80% of human hearts from the same AV nodal artery and the left anterior descending (LAD) artery. In 90% of patients, the AV nodal artery originates from the RCA. During acute myocardial infarction (AMI), conduction disturbances in the AV node are usually the consequence of an occlusion proximal to the origin of the AV nodal artery. The conduction abnormalities, therefore, are usually associated with inferior myocardial infarction. The AV nodal tissue merges with the His bundle, which runs through the inferior portion of the membranous interventricular septum and then,

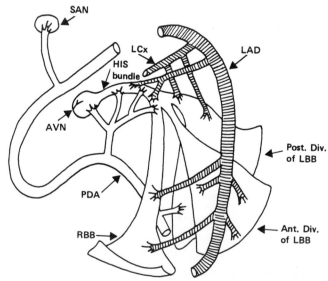

Figure 17–1. A diagrammatic representation of the conduction system and its blood supply. SAN, sinoatrial node; AVN, atrioventricular node, LAD, left anterior descending artery; LCX, left circumflex artery; PDA, posterior descending artery; RBB, right bundle branch; LBB, left bundle branch. (From de Guzman M, Rahimtoola SH: What is the role of pacemakers in patients with coronary artery disease and conduction abnormalities? *In* Rahimtoola SH: Controversies in Coronary Artery Disease. Philadelphia, FA Davis, 1983.)

in most instances, continues along the left side of the crest of the muscular interventricular septum. The His bundle usually receives a dual blood supply from both the AV nodal artery and branches of the LAD.[6]

The right bundle branch originates from the His bundle. It is a narrow structure that crosses to the right side of the interventricular septum and extends along the right ventricular endocardial surface to the region of the anterolateral papillary muscle of the right ventricle, where it divides to supply the papillary muscle, the parietal surface of the right ventricle, and the lower part of the right ventricular surface.[7] The proximal portion of the right bundle branch is supplied by branches from the AV nodal artery or the LAD artery, whereas the more distal portion is supplied mainly by branches of the LAD artery.

The left bundle branch is anatomically much less discrete than the right bundle branch. It may divide immediately as it originates from the bundle of His or continue for 1 to 2 cm before doing so.[4, 7] It is clinically useful to consider the left bundle as dividing into an anterior branch or fascicle and a larger and broader posterior branch or fascicle, both of which radiate toward the anterior and posterior papillary muscles of the left ventricle, respectively, even though there are many subendocardial interconnections that resemble a syncytium rather than two discrete fascicles.[7, 8] The left bundle branch and its anterior fascicle have a blood supply similar to that of the proximal portion of the right bundle branch; the left posterior fascicle is supplied by branches of the AV nodal artery, the posterior descending artery, and the circumflex coronary artery.

Clinicopathologic studies indicate that there is a relationship between the location of the infarct and the involvement of the conduction system.[8, 9] In most patients who develop AV block in AMI, there is usually no major structural damage of the conduction system; pathologic studies have shown that significant histologic degenerative changes in the conduction system are absent in most cases.[8–10] Several mechanisms have been proposed for AV block in the presence of inferior AMI. These include Bezold-Jarisch reflex, reversible ischemia or injury of the conduction system, local accumulation of adenosine or its metabolites, and local AV nodal hyperkalemia.

Bezold-Jarisch Reflex. Stimulation of this reflex causes an abnormally increased output of vagal nerve traffic; it is initiated by ischemia of the afferent nerves in the area of the inferoposterior left ventricle. Some studies, however, show that reperfusion of the RCA with thrombolytic agents is a strong stimulus for the Bezold-Jarisch reflex.[11, 12] Despite this, the TIMI II study[13] did not show an increase in AV block in patients with inferior AMI who received thrombolytic therapy and had a patent infarct-related artery.

Reversible Ischemia or Injury of the Conduction System. In inferior or posterior AMI, obstruction of the RCA produces reversible ischemia of the AV node. In patients who develop AV block, pathologic studies have demonstrated little or no necrosis in the conduction system.[10] Bilbao and colleagues,[14] however, identified a subgroup of patients with fatal inferior or posterior AMI and AV block who had necrosis of the prenodal atrial myocardial fibers. These necrotic fibers were absent in the patients without AV block.

Clinically, the transient nature of the AV block supports the concept that the injury to the AV node is reversible.[15] The anatomic data of Bassan and associates[16] support the concept that the blood supply of the AV node is dual. In their prospective study, 11 of 51 patients who survived an inferior AMI developed some degree of transient AV block, and about 90% of the patients with AV block had simultaneous obstruction of the RCA (or LCA when it was dominant) and the proximal segment of the LAD artery. Moreover, patients with inferior AMI and LAD obstruction had a six-fold higher risk of developing AV block compared with those without LAD obstruction. The TIMI II data do *not* support this finding; in these patients with inferior AMI and AV block, the incidence of disease in the LAD was low and was similar to that in patients with inferior AMI without AV block.[13] The TAMI study group also showed no increased incidence of LAD disease in patients with inferior AMI and complete AV block.[17]

Local AV Nodal Hyperkalemia. An increased level of potassium was found experimentally in the lymph draining from the infarcted inferior and posterior cardiac wall of dogs after RCA occlusion.[18] Sugiura and colleagues[19] found that serum potassium was an independent predictor of the occurrence of fascicular blocks in anteroseptal AMI.

Anterior or anteroseptal AMI results from obstruction of the LAD artery. Occurrence of AV block and bundle-branch block (BBB) is usually the result of necrosis of the septum and the conduction system below the AV node.[10, 20, 21] Wilber and colleagues,[22] however, reported on two patients with anterior AMI and complete AV block in whom 1:1 conduction returned within minutes after late reperfusion (over 40 hours) with angioplasty. Their experience suggests that reversible ischemia rather than necrosis of the conduction system occurs in some patients. Some experimental studies in dogs with anterior AMI suggest that extensive but reversible ischemia of the infranodal conduction tissue occurs, as evidenced by recovery from complete AV block. Several clinical observations[23–27] also showed that most patients with anterior AMI and high-grade AV block who are discharged from the hospital have returned to 1:1 conduction.

■ ACUTE MYOCARDIAL INFARCTION

Atrioventricular Block Without Bundle-Branch Block

Incidence

AV block occurs in 12% to 25% of all patients with AMI; first-degree AV block occurs in 2% to 12%, second-degree block in 3% to 10%, and third-degree block in 3% to 7%.[16, 28, 29] The onset of AV block usually occurs 2 to 3 days after the infarction but has a range of a few hours to 10 days. Its mean duration is usually 2 to 3 days and ranges from 12 hours to 16 days. In the series of 684 consecutive patients with AMI admitted to the Los Angeles County-University of Southern California Medical Center (LAC-USCMC) Coronary Care Unit (CCU) from October 1966 to July 1970, 110 developed AV block (16%)[30]; 79 of 110 patients (72%) with AV block did not have BBB. The total percentages of patients who had first-, second-, or third-degree AV block at some time were 6%, 7%, and 4%, respectively (Table 17–1).

Table 17–1. Atrioventricular Block in Acute Myocardial Infarction Without Bundle-Branch Block*

Incidence	(79/684 patients)	12%
First-degree AV block	(44/684 patients)	6%
Second-degree AV block	(50/684 patients)	7%
Third-degree AV block	(29/684 patients)	4%
Site of infarction		
Inferior		79%
Anterior		18%
Combined		6%
Progression		
First-degree AB block to second- or third-degree AV block		59%
Second-degree AB block to third-degree AV block		36%
Outcome		
Hospital mortality		29%
Return to 1 : 1 conduction in survivors		95%

*Data from 684 consecutive AMI patients at LAC-USCMC, Los Angeles, CA.
Adapted from de Guzman M, Rahimtoola SH: What is the role of pacemakers in patients with coronary artery disease and conduction abnormalities?
In Rahimtoola SH (ed): Controversies in Coronary Artery Disease. Philadelphia, FA Davis, 1983, pp 191–207.

Site of Infarction

Of the 79 patients, 60 (76%) had an inferior infarction, 14 (18%) an anterior infarction, and 5 (6%) a combined infarction. AV block is frequently associated with inferior infarction, and in those who develop second- and third-degree block, inferior AMI is present two to four times as often as anterior AMI. The site of block in inferior infarction is above the His bundle in about 90% of patients, whereas in anterior infarction, the conduction abnormality is usually localized below the His bundle in the distal conducting system[31] (Table 17–2).

Progression of Atrioventricular Block

In patients with inferior AMI, progression of AV block commonly occurs in stages, whereas in those with anterior AMI, it may occur in stages, or third-degree AV block or ventricular asystole may develop suddenly[15] (Fig. 17–2).

Outcome

AV block complicating AMI is associated with a high mortality rate (24% to 48%), two to three times that of patients without AV block (9% to 16%). The major cause of death is pump failure.[30, 32] Tans and coworkers,[29] however, reported that in their patients with inferior AMI, even those with high-degree AV block and no severe pump failure had a higher mortality rate (17%) than those without high-degree AV block (9%). In our series, the hospital mortality rate was 29% (32 of 110 patients); 29 of the 32 deaths (91%) were due to pump failure. Survival, therefore, is greatly influenced by the severity of the hemodynamic disturbance and is partly independent of the degree of heart block. Currently, use of AV sequential pacing may be expected to have some beneficial effect on the hemodynamic disturbance and therefore on the short-term mortality. Although death is primarily related to extensive myocardial damage, in an important minority of patients, it can be attributed to sudden ventricular asystole or severe bradycardia. In these cases, control of the cardiac rhythm by drugs or pacing may be life-saving.

Atrioventricular Block With Bundle-Branch Block

Incidence

BBB is present during hospitalization in 8% to 15% of patients with AMI.[33–38] Of 2779 patients with AMI admitted to our CCU from October 1966 to March 1977, 257 (9%) had BBB. Of the 257 patients, 83 (32%) had left bundle-branch block (LBBB), 80 (31%) had right bundle-branch block (RBBB), 72 (28%) had RBBB plus left-axis deviation, 21 (9%) had RBBB plus right-axis deviation, and one had alternating (alt) BBB. The conduction abnormality was "new" in 60%; that is, the BBB developed during the infarction and was documented by serial electrocardiograms (ECGs) (definitely new) or was present on admission and was not seen on previous ECGs or reverted to normal conduction later as documented by serial ECGs (probably new). Of the 257 BBB patients, 75 (29%) had AV block (Table 17–3).

Table 17–2. Atrioventricular Block in Inferior-Posterior and Anterior Acute Myocardial Infarction

	Anterior	Inferior-Posterior
Pathophysiology	Extensive necrosis of septum	Reversible ischemia, injury of conduction system
Site of block	Infranodal	Intranodal
Frequency	Less frequent	Two to four times more frequent
Progression to complete AV block	Sudden	Gradual
Intraventricular conduction defect	Common	Rare
Escape focus	Ventricular	Junctional
Escape rate	20–40 per minute	40–60 per minute
Prognosis	High mortality	Lower mortality

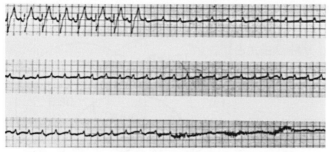

Figure 17–2. Lead II. Sudden ventricular asystole in a patient with acute myocardial infarction complicated by right bundle-branch block and LAD. (From de Guzman M, Rahimtoola SH: What is the role of pacemakers in patients with coronary artery disease and conduction abnormalities? *In* Rahimtoola SH: Controversies in Coronary Artery Disease. Philadelphia, FA Davis, 1983.)

Site of Infarction

When the site of infarction was not obscured by the BBB, the block was associated with anterior AMI about three times as often as it was with inferior AMI. In the presence of persistent LBBB, the diagnosis of myocardial infarction is difficult and was usually made by the history and serial changes in the cardiac enzymes.

Progression of Atrioventricular Block

Progression of AV block occurred in 75 of our 257 patients (29%) with AMI and BBB.

Initially Normal PR Interval. Of the 28 patients with AV block and BBB who initially had a normal PR interval, 13 (46%) developed first-degree AV block. Nine of the 13 (69%) stayed in first-degree block, 2 (15%) progressed to second-degree block type II only, 1 (8%) had type II second-degree block that progressed to third-degree AV block, and 1 developed third-degree block without having second-degree block. Six patients had type II second-degree block without initially having first-degree AV block; 4 of the 6 (67%) developed third-degree AV block.

First-Degree AV Block. Of the total 41 patients who had first-degree AV block and BBB, 13 (32%) progressed to high-grade block. Twenty-eight (68%) were admitted in first-degree AV block. Sixteen of the 28 (57%) stayed in first-degree block; 3 (11%) progressed to type II second-degree AV block, 1 of whom went on to third-degree block;

Table 17–3. Bundle-Branch Block in Acute Myocardial Infarction

Incidence	(257/2779 patients)*	9%
LBBB	(83/257 patients)	32%
RBBB	(80/257 patients)	31%
RBBB + LAD	(72/257 patients)	28%
RBBB + RAD	(21/257 patients)	9%
Onset of BBB		60%
New		40%
Old		21%
Site of infarction		
Inferior		
Anterior		52%
Combined		4%
Indeterminate		18%
Nontransmural		5%
Incidence of AV block	(75/257 patients)	29%
First-degree	(25/257 patients)	10%
Second-degree	(13/257 patients)	5%
Third-degree	(37/257 patients)	14%
Progression of AV block		32%
First-degree AV block to second- or third-degree AB block		46%
Second-degree AV block to third-degree AV block		18%
Progression of high-grade AB block	(46/257 patients)	50%
Bilateral BBB + first-degree AV block		43%
New *bilateral* BBB + first-degree AV block		30%
First-degree AV block		29%
New BBB + first-degree AV block		18%
Bilateral BBB		16%
New BBB		15%
New bilateral BBB		
Outcome		20%
Hospital mortality		89%
Return to 1:1 conduction in survivors		

*Data from 2779 AMI patients seen from October 1966 to March 1977 at LAC-USCMC, Los Angeles, CA.

Adapted from de Guzman M, Rahimtoola SH: What is the role of pacemakers in patients with coronary artery disease and conduction abnormalities? *In* Rahimtoola SH (ed): Controversies in Coronary Artery Disease. Philadelphia, FA Davis, 1983, pp 191–207.

5 (18%) progressed to type I second-degree block, 2 of whom went on to third-degree block; and 4 (14%) patients developed third-degree block without preceding second-degree AV block.

Second-Degree AV Block. Of the total 24 patients who had second-degree AV block and BBB, 11 (46%) progressed to third-degree block. Six had second-degree AV block on admission; of these, type II block occurred in 4, 1 of whom progressed to third-degree block, and type I occurred in 2, 1 of whom progressed to third-degree block.

Third-Degree AV Block. There were 37 patients with third-degree AV block and BBB, 13 (35%) of whom were admitted in third-degree block. Of the 24 who progressed to third-degree block, 11 (46%) had demonstrated second-degree block; 7 of the 11 had type II second-degree block.

Progression to High-Grade AV Block. AV block occurs in about one third of patients with AMI and BBB.[39-43] Two large studies have developed a data bank on patients with BBB in association with myocardial infarction. One is a large collaborative multicenter study involving five centers,[27] and the other is a study conducted at LAC-USC Medical Center.[43] Both studies have limitations because the data were obtained retrospectively, and no protocols existed to guide decisions pertaining to pacemaker insertion, which was performed at the physician's discretion in all cases. Furthermore, the number of patients admitted to the hospital but not included in the study was not evaluated. Thus, the studies are unable to answer conclusively and definitively questions about the natural history of BBB in association with AMI. Nevertheless, very valuable clinical information is available from both.

In the *multicenter study*, reported by Hindman and co-workers,[28] high-grade AV block (third- or second-degree block with a type II pattern) occurred in 55 of 432 patients (22%). To determine which patients were at considerable risk of developing high-grade AV block while hospitalized with AMI, several variables were analyzed. Combinations of three ECG findings of first-degree AV block, bilateral BBB (if both bundle branches were involved [e.g., RBBB plus left- or right-axis deviation] or alternating RBBB and LBBB), and "new" BBB identified high-risk patients. The absence of all variables or the presence of only one of the three defined variables was associated with a relatively low risk (10% to 13%) of developing high-grade AV block during hospitalization. The risk was moderate for patients with first-degree AV block with either new BBB or bilateral BBB (19% to 20%), and highest (31% to 38%) for new bilateral BBB regardless of the PR interval (Fig. 17–3).

In the LAC-USCMC study,[43] high-grade AV block occurred in 46 of 257 patients (18%). The absence of the three variables or the presence of either bilateral BBB or new BBB or new bilateral BBB was associated with a relatively low risk (10% to 18%) of developing high-grade AV block during hospitalization with AMI. The risk was moderate for first-degree AV block with or without new BBB (29% to 30%) and highest (50%) for bilateral BBB plus first-degree AV block regardless of whether the BBB was old or new (Fig. 17–4).

Despite some differences in the findings between the two

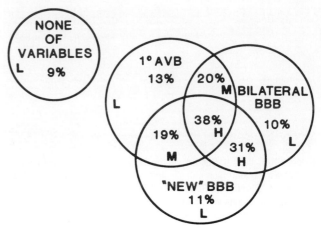

Figure 17–3. Venn diagram of 432 patients in the multicenter study depicting the risk for high-grade atrioventricular block (AVB) in patients with acute myocardial infarction (AMI) and bundle-branch block (BBB). (From Hindman MC, Wagner GS, JaRo M, et al: The clinical significance of bundle branch block complicating acute myocardial infarction. 2. Indications for temporary and permanent pacemakers. Circulation 58:689, 1978. Copyright 1978, American Heart Association.)

studies, both studies found that the following subgroups of patients were at *high risk* for high-grade AV block: (1) new bilateral BBB plus first-degree AV block (*risks*, 38% and 43% in the multicenter and LAC-USCMC studies, respectively); (2) bilateral BBB plus first-degree AV block (*risks*, 20% and 50%); and (3) new BBB plus first-degree AV block (*risks*, 19% and 29%). Thus, these subgroups of patients should be considered *mandatory* recipients of temporary prophylactic pacemakers during AMI. Subgroups in whom the findings of the two studies show different risks can be considered to be at *moderate risk* for high-grade AV block. These subgroups include patients with: (1) new bilateral

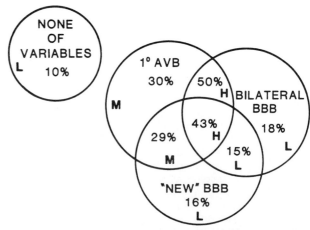

Figure 17–4. Venn diagram of 257 patients in the LAC-USCMC study depicting the risk for high-grade atrioventricular block (AVB) in patients with acute myocardial infarction (AMI) and bundle-branch block (BBB). (From de Guzman M, Rahimtoola SH: What is the role of pacemakers in patients with coronary artery disease and conduction abnormalities? *In* Rahimtoola SH: Controversies in Coronary Artery Disease. Philadelphia, FA Davis, 1983.)

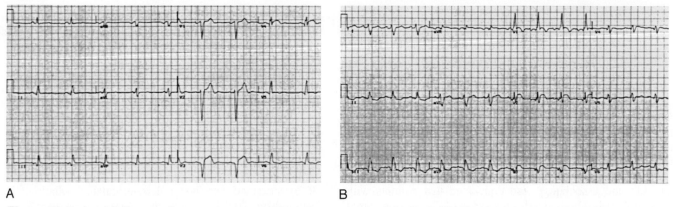

A   B

Figure 17–5. *A* and *B*, Electrocardiograms of a patient with anterior acute myocardial infarction (AMI) and development of "new" bilateral bundle-branch block (LBBB and RBBB with right-axis deviation). This patient had sudden ventricular asystole.

BBB (*risks,* 31% and 15%) (Fig. 17–5); (2) first-degree AV block (*risks,* 13% and 30%); and (3) bilateral BBB (*risks,* 10% and 18%). Thus, these subgroups of patients can be considered as probable or possible recipients of temporary prophylactic pacemakers during AMI. The rest of the patients can be considered to have a relatively low risk (about 10%) of high-grade AV block and therefore should probably not require prophylactic temporary pacemakers during AMI. The actual clinical decision about whether to institute temporary pacing should be individualized depending on the patient-related risk factors and on the available personnel and equipment at each institution.

The database assembled by the Multicenter Investigation of the Limitation of Infarct Size (MILIS) was used to develop a simplified method of predicting the occurrence of complete heart block. Data from 698 patients with a proven myocardial infarction were analyzed, and the presence or absence of ECG abnormalities of AV or intraventricular conduction was determined for each patient. The risk factors for the development of complete heart block were as follows: first-degree AV block, Mobitz type I AV block, Mobitz type II AV block, left anterior hemiblock, left posterior hemiblock, RBBB, and LBBB. A risk score for the development of complete heart block was devised that consisted of the sum of each patient's individual risk factors. An incidence of complete heart block of 1.2%, 7.8%, 25%, and 36% was associated with a risk score of 0, 1, 2, or 3 or more, respectively (Fig. 17–6). The risk score was subsequently tested on the published results of six studies for a combined total of 2151 patients.[44] The limitations of this scoring system include the lack of differentiation between newly appearing or old BBB, a factor that has been shown to be of predictive value. It is likely that consideration of such factors would further improve the accuracy of the scoring system, but it would also add to its complexity. Another criticism of the scoring system is that it would assign a risk score of only 1 to a patient with isolated Mobitz type II AV block, a disorder usually believed to be highly predictive of progression to complete heart block. Isolated Mobitz type II AV block is, however, relatively rare.

Outcome

The mortality rate in patients with AMI and BBB is higher (25% to 50%) than in those without BBB (15%).[29, 33–36, 40–42, 45]

When the infarction is extensive and produces diffuse conduction system abnormalities progressing to high-grade AV block, it is also extensive enough to damage a large amount of myocardial muscle. Therefore, these patients often die from pump failure and from ventricular tachyarrhythmias. Nevertheless, a substantial number of patients do *not* die from heart failure, and in these patients, the conduction abnormality may be contributory and can be the major cause of death. For example, sudden third-degree AV block or asystole may be abrupt and fatal (see Fig. 17–2). It is interesting that in our study, 75% of patients with BBB and AMI had either no heart failure or, at worst, mild heart failure. Our results, as well as those of the multicenter study, showed that high-degree AV block influenced hospital mortality independently of pump failure.

Intracardiac electrophysiologic studies have also been evaluated as a means of predicting which patients with myocardial infarction and BBB are likely to die. Harper and associates[46] reported on 72 patients with AMI complicated by AV block or BBB, or both, who underwent His bundle recording or electrophysiologic (HBE) studies during their

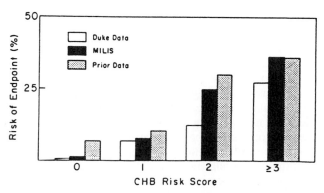

Figure 17–6. Comparison of the incidence of complete heart block (CHB) predicted by the CHB risk score method *(solid bars),* the observed incidence of CHB in the Duke University myocardial infarction database *(open bars),* and the observed incidence of CHB or CHB and Mobitz II in six reported studies *(screened bars).* MILIS, Multicenter Investigation of the Limitation of Infarct Size. (From Lamas GA, Muller JE, Turi AG, et al: A simplified method to predict occurrence of complete heart block during acute myocardial infarction. Am J Cardiol 57:1213, 1986.)

CCU stay. Thirty of 32 patients (94%) with AV block and narrow QRS complexes had a proximal block. Hospital mortality was low (13%), and HBE studies provided no additional information that was not obtained from the surface ECG. Of 18 patients with BBB and a normal PR interval, 9 had distal block, but there were no hospital deaths in this group of patients. Of 22 patients with BBB and AV block, 5 had proximal block, 14 distal, and 3 proximal and distal block. Hospital mortality in these patients, who progressed to second- or third-degree AV block, was higher (9 of 12 patients, 75%) than in those who remained in first-degree AV block (2 of 10 patients, 20%). Lichstein and colleagues[47] and Lie and associates[26] also concluded that patients with BBB and AMI who had a distal block by HBE had increased hospital mortality (73% and 81%, respectively) compared with those with normal HV (or HQ) intervals (25% and 47%, respectively). Gould and coworkers,[48] on the other hand, showed that the presence or absence of a prolonged HV interval did not affect mortality. Further studies are clearly needed to determine if electrophysiology studies are of help for further risk stratification of this patient population.

Bundle-Branch Block After Recovery From Acute Myocardial Infarction

It is now recognized that one major problem of patients who survive an AMI and are discharged from the hospital is late sudden death. It is also recognized that most sudden deaths are likely to result from ventricular tachyarrhythmias. An important question is whether patients with coronary artery disease and persistent BBB plus transient AV block during the acute infarction have a higher risk of dying suddenly as a result of complete heart block. If so, to maximize the therapeutic benefit of permanently implanting a pacemaker in this subset of patients, those at highest risk of late sudden death resulting from AV block should be identified.

The multicenter study[27] supports the previous reports of Atkins and Ritter and their colleagues,[49, 50] who found that the subset of patients with chronic BBB and transient high-degree AV block during AMI are at increased risk of late sudden death, presumably from a bradyarrhythmia. Their data were included in the data compiled by the multicenter study. These data showed that patients who were not paced continuously had a higher incidence of sudden death or recurrent high-degree AV block during follow-up (65%) compared with those who were paced continuously (10%). These investigators suggested that implantation of a permanent pacemaker protected against sudden death in these patients. Waugh and coworkers[51] also recommended the possible role of permanent pacemaker therapy in preventing syncope or sudden death in another group of high-risk patients: those with bilateral BBB plus transient high-grade AV block (type II progression).

Other studies suggest that these patients are not at high risk for sudden death from a bradyarrhythmia.[25, 42, 46, 52, 53] In the study by Nimetz and associates[42] of 13 survivors with BBB and second- or third-degree AV block, 4 (31%) had late sudden death; 14 of 41 survivors without AV block (34%) had late sudden death. In a study by Ginks and coworkers[25] of patients with anterior myocardial infarction complicated by complete heart block with return to normal sinus rhythm but with persistent BBB, 4 of 14 hospital survivors (29%) with anterior myocardial infarction, persistent BBB, and transient AV block died, and 2 of 4 (50%) with permanent pacemakers died during a follow-up period averaging 49 months. They concluded that long-term pacing was not justified in these patients. In a study by Murphy and associates[52] of patients surviving AMI complicated by BBB, none of the deaths resulted from heart block, even in those with transient AV block during the AMI. Lie and coworkers[53] reported on a group of 47 patients who had survived an anterior infarction complicated by BBB and who were kept for 6 weeks in the monitoring area; 17 of the 47 patients (36%) sustained late hospital ventricular fibrillation. The Birmingham Trial[54] of permanent pacing in patients with persistent intraventricular defects after AMI also showed no significant difference in survival during follow-up of up to 5 years. In a prospective long-term study by Talwar and colleagues[55] of 18 patients with anterior AMI, intraventricular defects, and transient complete AV block who were followed for a mean of 2 years, 8 had permanent pacemakers implanted, and 10 did not. There was one death in the unpaced group due to a cerebrovascular accident. Therefore, at the present time, one can conclude that it has not yet been proved that in most of these patients, sudden death is caused by heart block.

Role of Electrophysiologic Studies in Atrioventricular Block in Acute Myocardial Infarction

His bundle ECGs have been used to study the site of block, which has been shown to be either in the AV node (proximal block) or in the distal conduction system (distal block). The presence of a distal block may identify patients who may be at high risk for development of high-grade AV block.

It is generally accepted that in patients with inferior AMI, the block is usually proximal. Harper and colleagues[56] showed that 30 of 32 patients (94%) with inferior AMI and third-degree AV block had AV nodal block during HBE; the remaining two patients were in normal sinus rhythm during the study and had a normal PR interval and normal AH and HV intervals. Thus, in this group of patients, HBE offers no additional advantage over conventional ECG criteria in localizing the site of block.

In anterior AMI, the block is frequently in the distal conduction system. In Harper and colleagues' study, 50% of patients (9 of 18) with BBB and a normal PR interval on ECG had a prolonged HV interval.[56] Of their 22 patients who developed AV block and BBB, 5 had proximal block, 14 had distal block, and 3 had both proximal and distal blocks. Thus, in both groups of patients, HBE was the only means of localizing the block in the proximal or distal portion of the conduction system. Distal block indicates disease in either the His bundle or the remaining bundle branches, and clinically this is a common antecedent to sudden asystole and a poorer prognosis. Despite the fact that a prolonged HV interval could identify a group of patients who may be at high risk for high-grade AV block, several studies have shown that this does not help in assessing the short- or long-term prognosis of patients.[56, 57] Thus, the routine use of His bundle studies is probably not helpful; however, in individual cases, it may be useful.

■ INDICATIONS FOR PACING

Temporary Pacing in Acute Myocardial Infarction

Situations in which temporary pacing is recommended are listed in Table 17–4.

Atrioventricular Block Without Bundle-Branch Block

In patients with second-degree AV block, type I, those with inferior AMI and block above the His bundle (i.e., normal QRS width) normally do not require pacemaker insertion initially. These patients are not at risk for sudden asystole. However, it must be appreciated that a small number of patients with narrow QRS complexes have block in the His bundle and not in the AV node. Insertion of a pacemaker is recommended in patients with an anterior AMI or an inferior AMI with a wide QRS complex complicated by type I second-degree AV block in whom the block is presumed to be below the His bundle. This group of patients may be at risk for sudden asystole.

Regardless of the site of infarction, a temporary pacemaker should be placed whenever the AV block is associated with marked bradycardia (less than 40 to 50 bpm), hypotension, reduced cardiac output, heart failure, altered mental status, shock, and ventricular irritability.

Atrioventricular Block With Bundle-Branch Block

Prophylactic pacing is indicated for patients considered to be at high risk for developing high-grade AV block. In both the multicenter study and our study, such patients were recognized by (1) new bilateral BBB plus first-degree AV block; (2) bilateral BBB plus first-degree AV block; and (3) new BBB plus first-degree AV block. Those at moderate to high risk were identified by (1) new bilateral BBB, (2) first-degree AV block, and (3) bilateral BBB. These three subgroups of patients should probably receive a temporary pacemaker.

Permanent Pacing in Patients Recovering From the Acute Phase of Myocardial Infarction

Patients with persistent third-degree AV block or type II second-degree AV block, with or without BBB, should re-

Table 17–4. Temporary Pacing Recommendations in Patients with Acute Myocardial Infarction

I. Atrioventricular block without bundle-branch block
  A. Third-degree AV block
  B. Second-degree AV block, type II
    1. Patients with anterior AMI or with inferior AMI and wide QRS complex
    2. Patients with inferior AMI and narrow QRS complex if block recurs despite atropine administration
  C. Second-degree AV block, type I, and marked bradycardia
  D. AV block associated with marked bradycardia, hypotension, reduced cardiac output, heart failure, shock, or ventricular irritability
II. Atrioventricular block with bundle-branch block
  A. Third-degree AV block
  B. Second-degree AV block
  C. Prophylactic pacing for those at high risk for high-grade AV block

ceive a permanent pacemaker. This situation does not occur commonly, however. In patients who develop second- or third-degree block in the hospital, regardless of infarct or block location, our data show a return to 1:1 conduction in 95% of patients without BBB and in 89% of patients with BBB who survive the infarction and are discharged eventually from the hospital.

Permanent pacing is rarely needed in patients with an inferior wall acute myocardial infarction and narrow QRS. It may take up to 16 days for AV conduction to return. Some conservative clinicians recommend pacemaker implantation only after second- or third-degree AV block is present for more than 3 weeks after inferior wall myocardial infarction.[58]

A more difficult area of management pertains to patients who are survivors of an AMI complicated by persistent BBB and transient complete AV block during their hospitalization and may be at risk for serious bradyarrhythmias in the posthospitalization period. Should they be protected with a permanent pacemaker? Although some studies show that these patients have a higher incidence of late sudden death presumably caused by a bradycardia, such results must be viewed in the context of many other studies that show otherwise.

There are at least three possible ways of managing these patients: (1) all should receive permanent pacemakers; (2) only those with documented bradyarrhythmias should receive permanent pacemakers; or (3) patients should undergo left ventricular ejection fraction studies (by radionuclide study, two-dimensional echocardiography, or angiography), ambulatory 24-hour ECG monitoring, and possibly His bundle studies. Those with an ejection fraction equal to or less than 0.40, complex ventricular arrhythmias, and a greatly prolonged HV interval (65 msec or more) are at increased risk for death (including sudden death) from tachyarrhythmias, heart failure, and recurrent infarction. They should be closely followed, with performance of appropriate investigations, and therapy should be instituted accordingly. Other patients are at much lower risk for death and thus can be closely followed; insertion of permanent pacemakers may be considered in some patients.

Clearly, all patients with documented (symptomatic) bradyarrhythmias should receive a permanent pacemaker. The American College of Cardiology (ACC) and American Heart Association (AHA) current guidelines for permanent pacemaker implantation after acute myocardial infarction are listed in Table 17–5.[149]

■ SELECTION OF PACING MODE

The selection of pacing mode for patients with acute AV block usually takes into account many of the same considerations used for mode selection for chronic AV block. However, special clinical features of acute AV block include the following: (1) if the patient was in sinus rhythm, loss of chronotropic competence will have been recent and abrupt and (2) the loss of AV synchrony usually is associated with varying degrees of ventricular dysfunction, which may be severe. Restoration of chronotropic adaptation to activity may be achieved through VVIR and DDDR pacing, in which sensor detection of changes in various physiologic stimuli are used to adjust the pacing rate. Dual-chamber pacing with sensing of the native atrial complex and synchronous pacing

Table 17–5. Indications for Permanent Pacing after the Acute Phase of Myocardial Infarction

Class I

- Persistent second-degree AV block in the His-Purkinje system with bilateral bundle branch block or third-degree AV block within or below the His-Purkinje system after acute MI (Level of evidence: B)
- Transient advanced (second or third degree) infranodal AV block and associated bundle branch block. If the state of block is uncertain, an electropysiologic study may be indicated. (Level of evidence: B)
- Persistent and symptomatic second or third-degree AV block (Level of evidence: C)

Class IIa

- None

Class IIb

- Persistent second- or third-degree AV block at the AV node level. (Level of evidence: B)

Class III

- Transient AV block in the absence of intraventricular conduction defects. (Level of evidence: B).
- Transient AV block in the presence of isolated LAFB. (Level of evidence: B).
- Acquired LAFB in the absence of AV block (Level of evidence: B).
- Persistent first-degree AV block in the presence of bundle branch block that is old or of indeterminate age (Level of evidence: B).

From Gregoratos G, et al: ACC/AHA guidelines for implantation of cardiac pacemakers and antiarrhythmia devices: A report of the American College of Cardiology/American Heart Association Task Force on Practice Guidelines. J Am Coll Cardiol 31:1175, 1998. Reprinted with permission of the American College of Cardiology.

of the ventricle also restore both chronotropic response to activity (providing sinus node activity is normal) and AV synchrony. Multiple factors must be considered in choosing the appropriate pacing mode, including the status and activity level of the patient, the importance of AV synchrony, the presence of chronotropic incompetence, the underlying cardiac substrate, and the estimated likelihood of the frequency and duration of pacing. The importance of each of these factors varies from patient to patient.

For *temporary* pacing of patients with acute AV block, single-chamber right ventricular VVI pacing usually provides adequate rate correction of the bradyarrhythmia. If there is no or minimal hemodynamic compromise of cardiac function, this mode of pacing may be sufficient to tide the patient over what is usually a transient period of high-grade or complete AV block. If the underlying rhythm before acute AV block was atrial fibrillation, single-chamber ventricular pacing should provide a satisfactory rate, with no compromise of hemodynamic status because there was no pre-existing AV synchrony.

In the presence of sinus rhythm, or sinus bradycardia with or without chronotropic competence, restoration of AV synchrony even in the acute situation of temporary pacing may be a desirable therapeutic goal in patients with acute AV block. Restoration of AV synchrony may result in substantial hemodynamic improvement when correction of bradyarrhythmia by ventricular pacing alone fails to increase cardiac output in the presence of acute right ventricular infarction.[59] Similar benefit has been shown for AV sequential pacing in the presence of acute anterior infarction.[60] It is apparent, however, that optimization of the AV delay is also crucial because an excessively long AV interval may result in deteri-

oration with complete loss of the advantages of AV sequential pacing compared with ventricular pacing alone.[61, 62]

In patients with acute AV block who have indications for *permanent* pacing, the selection of pacing mode must take into account both the immediate condition of the patient and the possibility of future deterioration due to progression of the underlying disorder. Electrophysiologic and hemodynamic factors should be evaluated both in assessment of immediate needs and in anticipation of future problems.

There is no clear documentary proof that the occurrence of acute AV block as described earlier predisposes the patient to any different prognosis in regard to loss of sinus rhythm, loss of chronotropic competence, or development of paroxysmal supraventricular tachycardia. The selection of pacing mode in patients with acute AV block may also be strongly influenced by the nature and severity of the hemodynamic abnormalities due to the underlying cardiac pathology. Because most of these patients have had an acute myocardial ischemic event with varying extent of infarction, the impact of the pacemaker system on acute and long-term hemodynamic factors may be a relevant concern.

For permanent pacing, the benefit of restoring the patient's ability to increase heart rate with activity (chronotropic competence) must be considered. This may be accomplished through using the VVIR, DDD (with normal sinus node function), or DDDR modes. It is clear that in the absence of an ability to increase the heart rate with activity, the only remaining mechanism for increasing cardiac output is to increase stroke volume. The magnitude of increase achieved by this mechanism is small compared with that achieved by an increase in heart rate. Furthermore, the underlying myocardial dysfunction that is present in most patients with acute AV block limits even more the contribution of change in stroke volume to the adaptive response to activity. Therefore, at the least, a VVIR system appears to be advantageous for improving cardiac output and work capacity during activity in patients with acute AV block.[63]

If the indication for permanent pacing is transient advanced AV block and the patient is usually expected to be in sinus rhythm with normal AV conduction, a simple single-chamber VVI system may be adequate as a backup to provide a reasonable minimum heart rate. The selection of a VVIR unit in preference to a VVI unit may be appropriate for patients with more frequent dependence on the pacemaker and a higher projected activity level in the anticipation that increased cardiac output with activity is a desirable and reasonable therapeutic goal. If, for example, the patient has had an associated stroke and has minimal chance of regaining even modest levels of activity, there would be little to be gained by using the more expensive rate-adaptive VVIR mode. On the other hand, although rate-adaptive VVIR pacing can achieve increases in work performance and cardiac output, the maintenance of AV synchrony is desirable, particularly at slower heart rates and in patients with impaired ventricular function. Therefore, it has become accepted that in such patients, dual-chamber pacing is advantageous,[63] and the VVIR mode would appear to be appropriate only for patients with no pre-existing AV synchrony, such as those with permanent atrial fibrillation and those in whom the rate and hemodynamic demands on the pacemaker system are minimal even at rest.

In patients with acute complete persistent AV block and underlying intact sinus node function, dual-chamber pacing would maintain or restore AV synchrony at rest and would also allow the rate to increase with activity. If the sinus node is also diseased and chronotropically incompetent, the DDDR mode would restore both AV synchrony and rate response to activity, albeit with substitution of a physiologic parameter other than the P wave. Another consideration that might moderate the choice of pacing mode is the presence of concomitant paroxysmal supraventricular tachyarrhythmias. In such patients, an added benefit of the DDDR mode of pacing is the feature contained in several types of these units in which algorithms are used to detect and automatically change the pacing mode during such episodes. These units can automatically switch from the DDDR to VVI or VVIR mode and then, in some units, can automatically monitor the tachyarrhythmia and switch back to DDDR pacing when the supraventricular tachycardia terminates. Furthermore, the ability of many of the DDD and DDDR units to shorten the AV delay as pacing rate increases may increase the chances of providing maximum hemodynamic benefit during activity-induced rate increases.[62]

The long-term outcome of the minority of patients with acute AV block who require permanent pacing is usually most strongly affected by the extent of myocardial dysfunction or the severity of the underlying coronary disease and ischemia. In a 2-year follow-up study of 2021 permanently paced patients, the leading causes of the 249 recorded deaths were stroke (30%) and sudden cardiac death (22%).[64] The presence of BBB, which was seen predominantly in patients with AV block and myocardial infarction, was a predictor of sudden cardiac death because 28% of all patients with BBB and 35% of patients with bifascicular or trifascicular block died suddenly. In comparison, the prevalence of sudden death in the remaining 138 patients without such block was 18%. Undersensing of ectopic ventricular beats was reportedly more common in patients with BBB and uncommon in patients without BBB. In 21 of 220 (10%) of the undersensed ventricular ectopic beats, the subsequent pacing impulse was "effective" or was followed by spontaneous single or repetitive ventricular arrhythmias. The authors of this study postulated that atrial sensing of dual-chamber pacing might lessen the frequency of undersensing of ventricular ectopic beats or potentially life-threatening fusion beats. Critical analysis of the available data, however, suggests only that intercurrent ventricular tachycardia or ventricular fibrillation remains an important cause of mortality in permanently paced patients. Whether pacemaker malfunction or the mode of pacing contributes significantly to mortality higher than that due to the coexisting cardiac disease remains an unresolved issue.[65]

A final important consideration in selection of the mode of pacing is the recognition that the extent of myocardial dysfunction in patients with ischemic heart disease may not be a permanent condition. Stunning and hibernation of the myocardium, leading to apparent dysfunction, may resolve as the ischemia resolves and after adequate time has passed for recovery.[66, 67]

Therefore, the hemodynamic benefits achieved by various modes of permanent pacing should not be employed as a substitute for reperfusion therapy of myocardial ischemia but rather as an adjunct to maximize the performance of any residual permanently injured myocardium after recovery from ischemia has been allowed to take place.

■ IMPACT OF THROMBOLYTIC THERAPY

There have been two prospective trials involving thrombolytic therapy of AMI that provide data pertaining to the impact of such therapy on the development of high-grade second- and third-degree AV block.[13, 17] Both examined the impact of thrombolytic therapy for acute inferior myocardial infarction. In one, the study was designed to examine the effect of thrombolytic therapy and adjunctive angioplasty as a treatment strategy for AMI (TAMI trial).[17] All patients had treatment initiated with thrombolytic agents within 6 hours of symptom onset. There were 373 patients with an inferior AMI, of whom 50 (13%) had complete AV block; 54% of these patients had complete AV block on admission. In all but 2 patients, the block was manifest within 72 hours of onset of symptoms. The duration of block was less than 1 hour in 25% and less than 12 hours in 15%; the median duration of block was 2.5 hours. There was no difference in the rate of infarct vessel patency between those with and those without AV block (90% and 91%, respectively). A precipitating clinical event—vessel reperfusion, performance of percutaneous transluminal coronary angioplasty (PTCA)—or vessel reocclusion was identifiable in 38% of instances of complete AV block.

At the predischarge angiogram, the vessel patency rate was 11% lower in the AV block group than in the group without block (71% versus 82%, respectively). Those who developed AV block showed a decrease in ejection fraction between the early post-thrombolytic angiogram and the predischarge angiogram. Also, those who developed AV block had a higher in-hospital mortality, 10 of 50 (20%) versus 12 of 323 (4%, $P < .001$). When age, left ventricular ejection fraction in the acute phase, number of diseased vessels, and grade of blood flow through the culprit lesion were entered into a multivariate model, the development of complete AV block still contributed significantly to the risk for in-hospital mortality. After a median follow-up period of 22 months, hospital survivors had equivalent mortality rates (2%) in the groups with and without AV block. These data suggest that, compared with the prethrombolytic era, use of thrombolytics and angioplasty has not altered either the incidence of complete AV block or the associated greater ventricular dysfunction or in-hospital mortality.

In another study of 1786 patients with inferior AMI who received recombinant tissue–type plasminogen activator (rt-PA) within 4 hours of symptom onset, high-grade (second- or third-degree) AV block developed in 214 (12%) (TIMI II trial).[13] Of the group who had AV block, 113 (6.3% of the total, or 52% of those who ever had AV block) had this finding on admission. The remaining 101 patients (5.7%) developed heart block during the 24 hours after treatment with thrombolytics. Patients who already had high-grade AV block before receiving thrombolytic therapy tended to be older and had a higher prevalence of cardiogenic shock than those without heart block. Nevertheless, the presence of heart block did not carry an increased 21-day mortality independent of other variables such as shock, and the 1-year mortality rate was similar to that in the group without heart block.

In this study, patients were randomly assigned to coronary arteriography 18 to 48 hours after admission. Among those who developed heart block after admission, the infarct-related artery was less frequently patent than in those without heart block, 28 of 39 (72%) versus 611 of 723 (84.5%, P = .04). The RCA was the infarct-related artery more often in patients who developed heart block than in those who did not, 36 of 69 (92.3%) versus 542 of 723 (75.1%), respectively (P = .04). Among patients without heart block at the time of hospital admission, mortality occurred within 48 hours in 4 of 9 patients (44%) with new heart block and in 8 of 68 (12%) without new heart block at 24 hours. The 21-day mortality rate was higher in the group with AV block than the group without block, 10 of 101 (9.9%) versus 35 of 1572 (2.2%), respectively (P < .001), as was the 1-year mortality rate, 15 of 101 (14.9%) versus 65 of 1572 (4.2%), respectively (P = .001). A temporary pacemaker was inserted in about one third of patients with heart block on admission and in almost 30% of patients who developed heart block after institution of thrombolytic therapy, whereas only 6.5% of patients without heart block received temporary pacemakers. None of the patients who had heart block on admission or who developed heart block received a permanent pacemaker, but four patients without heart block at 24 hours went on to receive a permanent pacemaker. Heart block was not listed as a primary or contributing cause of death in any patient.

These data suggest that aggressive treatment with thrombolytic agents or thrombolytic therapy plus angioplasty is not associated with a lower incidence of high-grade or complete AV block in patients with inferior AMI compared with that seen in the prethrombolytic era; the incidence remains about 12% to 13%, with about half of cases appearing as new block during hospitalization. The infarct-related vessel is more often the RCA, and there is a lower vessel patency rate after thrombolysis among those who have AV block complicating their inferior AMI. In-hospital and early posthospitalization mortality is higher in patients with than in those without AV block among patients treated with thrombolytics, with or without angioplasty. It is not clear, however, that patients with acute AV block continue to be at greater risk for mortality if they survive the initial hospitalization. No causal relationship has been established between the presence of AV block and increased mortality. The presumption remains, as before the era of thrombolytic therapy, that the presence or development of AV block is associated with a higher mortality because it tends to indicate the presence of more extensive infarction or injury. The impact of permanent pacing on longevity in these patients remains unknown.

A more recent study[68] examined the significance of RBBB in AMI in the prethrombolytic era and compared it with the incidence and meaning of developing RBBB in the thrombolytic era. In a multicenter prospective study of 1238 patients with 1-year follow-up, the authors found a higher rate of new and transient RBBB and a lower rate of bifascicular block in patients receiving thrombolytic therapy. The overall meaning of RBBB, however, was unchanged and included a higher rate of heart failure, increased chance of needing a permanent pacemaker, and a higher 1-year mortality rate.[68] This study and a case report[69] highlight that the factors that govern the appearance and resolution of BBB are poorly understood. In the case report,[69] a patient with an acute anterior wall myocardial infarction developed bifascicular block just after the infusion of thrombolytic therapy. Catheterization revealed complete occlusion of the left ante-

rior descending artery; angioplasty restored flow to that artery and was associated with resolution of the bifascicular block. Complete heart block with ventricular asystole occurred abruptly 30 hours later despite persistent TIMI grade 3 flow in the left anterior descending artery.

■ CHRONIC AV BLOCK

Historically, chronic or acquired AV block with syncope was the first indication for cardiac pacing. Intermittent or chronic high-grade AV block still accounts for a large but variable number of permanent pacemaker implantations (e.g., between 30% and 70%), depending on the series. The site of AV block is important in that it determines to a great extent the rate and reliability of the underlying escape rhythm. Nevertheless, it is worth emphasizing that *symptomatic* AV block requires pacing regardless of the site, morphology, or rate of the escape rhythm.

Epidemiology

In complete heart block, there is either a transient or a chronic absence of AV conduction, with the atrial rhythm being independent of the escape rhythm. The escape rhythm may be generated by a pacemaker in the AV junction, His bundle, bundle branches, or distal conduction system. Rarely, the underlying rhythm may arise from the ventricular myocardium, or for all practical purposes, it may be absent. The ventricular rate depends on the site of the escape pacemaker.[70, 71] Complete AV block can be congenital or acquired. In patients with acquired complete AV block, the site of block is localized distal to the His bundle in about 70% to 90% of patients, in the His bundle in 15% to 20%, and within the AV node in 16% to 25%.[70] In patients with congenital heart block, the escape rhythm is more often found in the proximal His bundle or AV node.

Complete heart block can also be described as acute or chronic depending on its onset. Acute AV block associated with myocardial ischemia is rare but may occur and result in transient AV block. High-grade AV block is strictly defined as 3:1, 4:1, or higher AV ratios in which AV synchrony is intermittently present. As in complete AV block, block may be localized anywhere in the conduction system (Fig. 17–7). In some patients, block may be present at multiple

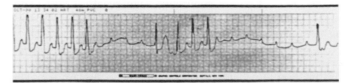

Figure 17–7. Rhythm strip of high-grade AV block. The baseline rhythm is sinus tachycardia in which the P wave occurs simultaneously with the T wave. After the fifth QRS complex, there is an abrupt, or paroxysmal, onset of AV block with four consecutive P waves that do not conduct to the ventricles. The sixth QRS complex probably represents a junctional escape rhythm followed by three conducted complexes and then a longer episode of high-grade AV block. Before both episodes of high-grade AV block, there is no obvious PR interval prolongation, nor is there slowing of the sinus rate to suggest hypervagotonia as a cause of this patient's block.

levels in the conduction system. Generically, the term *high-grade AV block* has been used to describe any form of AV block that suggests an increased risk for complete heart block or symptomatic bradycardia. This typically includes type II second-degree block, 2:1 AV block, strictly defined high-grade AV block, and complete heart block. The generic use of the term *high-grade AV block* should be avoided because the multiple forms of AV block included have variable pathogeneses and prognoses that blur the clinical utility of this term.

Paroxysmal AV block is defined as the sudden occurrence during a period of 1:1 AV conduction of block of the sequential atrial impulses resulting in a transient total interruption of AV conduction.[72, 73] It is thus the onset of a paroxysm of high-grade AV block usually associated with a period of ventricular asystole before conduction returns or a subsidiary pacemaker escapes. Paroxysmal AV block may occur in a variety of clinical conditions. Patients with neurally mediated syncopal syndromes may have transient heart block, typically with associated sinus slowing. It may occur in some patients with tachycardia-dependent AV block in the His-Purkinje system, during or after exertion, with the abrupt onset of bradycardia, and in type II second-degree AV block.

Acquired AV block may be secondary to a number of causes of generalized myocardial scarring (Table 17–6). Causes include atherosclerosis, dilated cardiomyopathy, hypertension, infiltrative cardiomyopathies, inflammatory disorders, and infectious diseases. An entity known as idiopathic bilateral bundle branch fibrosis, *Lev's disease*, is characterized by slowly progressive replacement of specialized conduction tissue by fibrosis, resulting in progressive fascicular and BBB.[74] Lev proposed that damage to the proximal left bundle branch and adjacent main bundle or main bundle alone is the result of an aging process exaggerated by hypertension and arteriosclerosis of the blood vessels supplying the conduction system. Another variant of idiopathic conduction system disorder is *Lenegre's disease*, which occurs in the younger population and is characterized by loss of conduction tissue, predominantly in the peripheral parts of the bundle branch.[75]

Patients with sick sinus syndrome are known to be at risk for concomitant symptomatic heart block.[76, 77] This may be due to progressive fibrodegenerative disease extending from the sinus node region to the AV conduction system. The relative frequency of this association varies between studies. Rosenqvist and Obel[78] pooled the data from 28 published studies and reported a mean incidence of development of second- or third-degree AV block to be 0.6% per year (range, 0% to 4.5% per year) in patients in whom permanent atrial pacemakers have been implanted for symptomatic sinus node dysfunction. The total prevalence of second- or third-degree AV block was 2.1% (range, 0% to 11%). In a retrospective review of 1395 patients with sick sinus syndrome who were followed for a mean of 34 months, Sutton and Kenny[79] estimated that the development of conduction system disease had an annual incidence of 3%; such conduction disease included significant first-degree AV block, BBB, HV prolongation, and a low Wenckebach heart rate. Thus, AV conduction system disease occurs relatively frequently in patients with sinus node dysfunction. Similarly, sinus node dysfunction, particularly chronotropic incompetence, may occur commonly in patients with acquired complete heart block.

Table 17–6. Causes of Acquired Complete Heart Block

Idiopathic Fibrodegenerative Disease

Lev's disease
Lenegre's disease

Ischemic Heart Disease

Myocardial infarction
Ischemic cardiomyopathy

Nonischemic Cardiomyopathies

Myocarditis
Idiopathic dilated cardiomyopathies
Hypertensive heart disease

Cardiac Surgery

Coronary artery bypass
Aortic, mitral, or tricuspid valve replacement
Ventricular septal defect repair
Septal myomectomy
Ablation of septal accessory pathways

Miscellaneous

Following radiofrequency and direct current His bundle ablation
Exercise-induced AV block

Infections

Endocarditis
Chagas' disease
Lyme disease
Multiple other infections: bacterial, viral, rickettsial, fungal

Neuromuscular Disease

Myotonic dystrophy
Fascioscapulohumeral dystrophy
Other muscular dystrophies
Kearns-Sayre syndrome
Friedreich's ataxia

Infiltrative Disease

Amyloidosis
Sarcoidosis
Hemochromatosis
Carcinoid

Neoplastic Disease

Postradiation therapy
Primary and metastatic tumors

Connective Tissue Disease

Rheumatoid arthritis
Systemic lupus erythematosus
Systemic scleroderma
Ankylosing spondylitis
Other connective tissue diseases

Complete AV block may occur in a variety of clinical situations. It may occur as a consequence of coronary artery bypass surgery with an incidence of less than 1% to 2%.[80] Complete heart block occurs more commonly after aortic, mitral, or tricuspid valve replacement, given the proximity of their annuli to the AV junction.[81] Complete heart block is more common after surgical procedures to repair ventricular septal defects, tetralogy of Fallot, AV canal defects, or subvalvular aortic stenosis.[82, 83] Heart block may also occur in patients undergoing septal myomectomy for hypertrophic cardiomyopathy.[84] Finally, heart block occurred in 1% to 10% of patients undergoing surgical ablation for the Wolff-

Parkinson-White syndrome when the accessory pathway was located in the anteroseptal, intermediate septal, or posteroseptal location, or after surgical modification of the AV node for treatment of AV nodal re-entrant tachycardia.[85] Heart block may also occur, although with a lower incidence, after radiofrequency ablation of septal accessory pathways.

After discontinuation of cardiopulmonary bypass, a variety of cardiac rhythm disturbances may be seen, including sinus arrest, junctional rhythm, BBB, AV block, and sinus bradycardia. Many of these rhythm disturbances are transient, resolving within 5 to 7 days. Transient BBB is quite common, occurring in 4% to 35% of patients and generally resolving within 12 to 24 hours.[80] Surgery for correction of valvular heart disease may also lead to conduction defects. Conduction disturbances are particularly common in patients with both aortic valve disease and after aortic valve replacement, with 5% to 30% of patients experiencing some conduction abnormality after valve replacement. Most of these abnormalities are transient; however, chronic complete heart block may occur. Intraoperative heart block does not predict the need for permanent pacing.[86] One study[87] showed that postoperative complete AV block was the most important predictor of subsequent pacemaker dependency. Based on these findings, the authors recommended earlier decisions on the timing of permanent pacemaker implantation, by the sixth postoperative day in patients with a wide QRS complex escape rhythm and by the ninth postoperative day in patients with a narrow QRS complex escape rhythm. Currently, pacing would be instituted earlier, probably by the fourth to sixth postoperative day.

The time course of conduction defects after bypass surgery was investigated in one study.[88] Operative technique consisted of cold, hyperkalemic cardioplegia, and conduction defects resolved partially or completely in 50% of patients. Patients with conduction defects generally had longer cardiopulmonary bypass times, longer aortic cross-clamp times, and more vessels requiring bypass. In three of the four patients with complete heart block, the heart block eventually resolved after discharge and implantation of a permanent pacemaker. Reasons for conduction abnormalities include ischemic injury to the conduction system, direct surgical manipulation or trauma to conduction tissue, traumatic disruption of the distal conduction system, or alterations in conduction caused by cardioplegia.

Complete heart block has been described in a large variety of infectious diseases. These include bacterial, viral, fungal, protozoan, and rickettsial infections. Heart block may occur with endocarditis and may be either transient or permanent. In most infectious diseases, heart block is transient and resolves with treatment of the underlying infection. In some cases, transient heart block may recur, and permanent pacing is required. This is particularly true in patients with entities such as endocarditis, in which a valve ring abscess may erode into the conduction system, and in those with infections such as Chagas' disease.[89–92]

Recently, much attention has been focused on Lyme disease. This systemic illness was first described in 1975 and was characterized later as an infection caused by a spirochete, *Borrelia burgdorferi*, transmitted to humans by a tick bite. This illness is often characterized by a skin rash, erythema chronicum migrans, followed by cardiac and neurologic abnormalities and then in some cases by an arthritis.[93]

Cardiac involvement may occur in 8% to 10% of patients, is generally transient, and may consist of a myocarditis or a myopericarditis.[94] Varying degrees of AV block are a common manifestation of carditis and occur in about 75% of patients. More than 50% of patients with AV block develop symptomatic high-grade or complete AV block that requires temporary pacing. Most often, the site of block is localized to the AV node, although occasional cases have been reported in which the site of block is intra-Hisian or infra-Hisian.[95, 96] Continuous cardiac monitoring is recommended in all patients with second-degree AV block and a prolonged PR interval of more than 0.30 seconds because of the risk of developing complete AV block. Complete AV block generally resolves within 1 to 2 weeks. Recurrent AV block has not been reported. Rarely, some patients may develop symptomatic AV block as the sole manifestation of Lyme disease.[97] Permanent pacing is rarely required except when complete heart block persists, which occurs uncommonly. Two important axioms worth repeating are that (1) heart block associated with infectious disease usually resolves with appropriate and prompt antibiotic treatment, and (2) rarely is conduction disease the only presenting feature of an infectious illness.

Heart block may occur after radiation therapy or chemotherapy. Heart block may occur after radiation therapy when radiation is directed at the mediastinum, as may be the case with Hodgkin's and some non-Hodgkin's lymphomas.[98] Rarely, tumors, including mesothelioma of the AV node and metastatic disease to the heart from breast, lung, or skin cancer, may involve the conduction system.[99] It is unusual for toxicity to antineoplastic drugs, such as doxorubicin (Adriamycin), to result in damage to the conduction system.

Certain neuromuscular diseases may also give rise to progressive and insidiously developing conduction system disease, including Duchenne's muscular dystrophy, fascioscapulohumeral muscular dystrophy, X-linked muscular dystrophy, myasthenia gravis, myotonic dystrophy, and Friedreich's ataxia.[100] Abnormalities of conduction manifest as infranodal conduction disturbances resulting in fascicular block or complete heart block. This has been noted particularly in Kearns-Sayre syndrome (progressive external ophthalmoplegia with pigmentary retinopathy), Guillain-Barré syndrome, myotonic muscular dystrophy, slowly progressive X-linked Becker's muscular dystrophy, and fascioscapulohumeral muscular dystrophy. It is worth noting that myotonic muscular dystrophy and Kearns-Sayre syndrome are both associated with a high incidence of conduction system disease that is frequently rapidly progressive and cannot be predicted by the ECG or isolated His bundle recordings. His-Purkinje disease can culminate in fatal Stokes-Adams attacks unless anticipated by pacemaker insertion.

Heart block may occur with amyloid and other infiltrative diseases, including hemochromatosis, porphyria, oxalosis, Refsum's disease, carcinoid, Hand-Schüller-Christian disease, and sarcoidosis.[101]

Connective tissue disorders giving rise to conduction system disease include periarteritis nodosa, rheumatoid arthritis, polymyositis, mixed connective tissue disorders, Reiter's syndrome, ulcerative colitis, scleroderma, Takayasu's aortitis, systemic lupus erythematosus, and ankylosing spondylitis.[102, 103] For example, in one study of 50 consecutive patients with scleroderma, invasive electrophysiologic studies revealed conduction abnormalities in up to 50% of patients, suggesting that a much higher degree of cardiac involvement may be present in patients than is readily apparent clinically. However, complete heart block is uncommon.[104] Most patients with AV conduction disorders have other clinical manifestations of their connective tissue disease.

Exercise-induced AV block is relatively rare, and studies have shown that the site of block is often in the His-Purkinje system (Fig. 17–8).[105] Donzeau and colleagues[106] reported 14 symptomatic patients with exercise-induced AV block, of whom 9 had block localized to an infranodal site. Other studies have also shown that exercise-induced AV block is primarily infra-Hisian.[107, 108] In these studies, about 25% to 75% of patients had underlying BBB. Permanent pacing is recommended in patients with exercise-induced AV block, even in the asymptomatic state, because of the high incidence of development of symptomatic AV block. Finally, several reports of patients with cardiac asystole following exertion have demonstrated postexercise sinus arrest with ventricular asystole.[109]

Vagally mediated AV block infrequently requires a permanent pacemaker. This form of AV block must be differentiated from type II second-degree AV block because these patients almost always require the implantation of a permanent pacemaker.[110] In most cases, vagally induced AV block occurs at the level of the AV node and is associated with a narrow QRS complex.[111] Rarely, vagal stimulation may precipitate phase IV or bradycardia-mediated block in the His-Purkinje system.[72] AV block may occur in the setting of increased vagal tone in response to various stimuli, such as carotid sinus hypersensitivity, coughing, swallowing, or visceral distention.[112–114] As a general rule, vagally mediated AV nodal block shows obvious heart rate slowing, even if only slight, before the onset of block, owing to the concomitant effect of increased vagal tone on the sinus node.

The prognosis and natural history of disease in patients with primary first-degree AV block and moderate PR prolongation has been shown to be benign.[115] Progression to complete heart block over time occurred in about 4% of patients in this study. Most of the patients (66%) had only mild to moderate PR prolongation, to about 0.22 to 0.23 second. In the great majority of subjects, the PR interval remained within a narrow range, changing by less than 0.04 second. These patients, however, may develop a pseudo-pacemaker syndrome due to AV dysynchrony. Zornosa and colleagues[116] described PR prolongation occurring after radiofrequency ablation due to injury of the fast pathway in patients with AV nodal re-entry undergoing ablation. Symptoms due to long PR intervals resolved after DDD pacing was performed. Kim and associates[117] also described a patient with intermittent failure of fast pathway conduction who developed lightheadedness, weakness, and chest fullness when the PR interval suddenly shifted from between 160 and 180 msec to 360 msec. This patient's condition also improved after pacing.[116, 117]

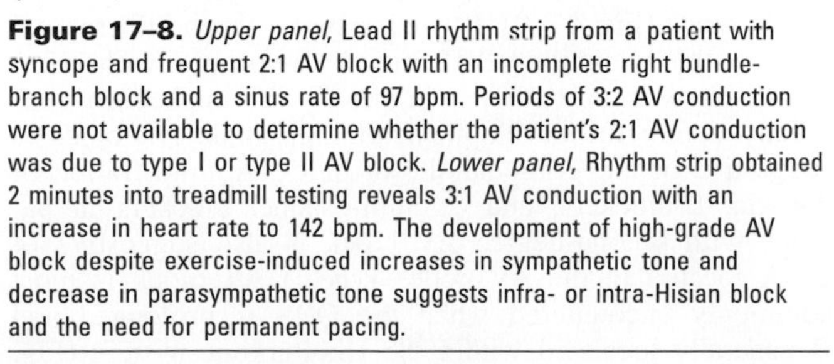

The natural history of 56 patients with second-degree AV block was described by Strasberg and colleagues.[118] They concluded that progression to complete heart block is also relatively uncommon. Their study is limited by the small number of subjects with structural heart disease studied. Many of their patients were younger than 35 years of age or were trained athletes. A more recent study by Shaw and coworkers[119] suggested that patients with type I second-degree AV block have a worse prognosis than age- and sex-matched individuals unless they had permanent pacemakers implanted. In patients with type I second-degree AV block and permanent pacemakers, survival was similar to that in the age- and sex-matched normal population.

Patients with BBB or bifascicular block are an important clinical problem. Not infrequently, a clinician is asked to evaluate a patient with BBB or bifascicular block and syncope. Most patients with chronic bifascicular block have underlying structural heart disease, the prevalence of which ranges from 50% to 80%.[120–123] Many studies have shown that chronic bifascicular block in this clinical situation is associated with substantial mortality.

Historically, it was thought that progression from chronic bifascicular block to trifascicular block was common. Retrospective studies in patients with chronic bifascicular block had suggested that the risk of progression to complete AV block was 5% to 10% per year. In the early 1980s, the results of several prospective studies questioned assumptions about the incidence and clinical implications of progression of conduction system disease in this patient population. Prospective studies of groups of symptom-free patients with bifascicular block and prolonged HV intervals at the time of electrophysiologic study revealed that these patients are at increased risk for complete heart block but that the absolute risk remains very low, about 1% to 2% per year.[120, 121] In the study by McAnulty and colleagues,[121] the risk of developing complete heart block was 5% in 5 years. A prolonged HV interval was associated with higher total cardiovascular mortality and mortality due to sudden death. It is likely that a prolonged HV interval is associated with more extensive structural heart disease. Furthermore, these studies demonstrated that routine His bundle recordings are of *limited* usefulness in patients with bifascicular block in the *absence* of symptoms.

On the other hand, patients with *syncope* and *bifascicular block* represent a *different* clinical problem. If a thorough clinical evaluation, including a history, physical examination, and ECG, do not uncover a cause of syncope, an electrophys-

Lead II at Rest

Lead II After 2 min. of Exercise

Figure 17–8. *Upper panel,* Lead II rhythm strip from a patient with syncope and frequent 2:1 AV block with an incomplete right bundle-branch block and a sinus rate of 97 bpm. Periods of 3:2 AV conduction were not available to determine whether the patient's 2:1 AV conduction was due to type I or type II AV block. *Lower panel,* Rhythm strip obtained 2 minutes into treadmill testing reveals 3:1 AV conduction with an increase in heart rate to 142 bpm. The development of high-grade AV block despite exercise-induced increases in sympathetic tone and decrease in parasympathetic tone suggests infra- or intra-Hisian block and the need for permanent pacing.

iologic study may be useful.[123, 124] Linzer and associates[125] found that the presence of first-degree AV block or BBB increased the odds ratio of finding abnormalities suggesting risk of bradyarrhythmia (predominantly heart block) by three- to eight-fold during electrophysiologic studies in patients with unexplained syncope (Table 17–7). Electrophysiologic studies may uncover other causes of syncope, such as sinus node dysfunction, rapid supraventricular tachycardias, or inducible monomorphic ventricular tachycardia. In some studies, a monomorphic ventricular tachycardia was discovered in 20% to 30% of patients with BBB and syncope.[123, 124] A minority of patients are found to have a markedly prolonged HV interval, abnormal or fragmented His bundle electrogram, or block distal to the His bundle with atrial pacing, suggesting the need for permanent pacemaker implantation.

Radiofrequency energy is now used to create complete AV block in patients with paroxysmal and chronic atrial fibrillation in whom the heart rate cannot be controlled by AV nodal blocking drugs or who are intolerant, unwilling, or unable to take drugs to maintain sinus rhythm or control the ventricular response during atrial fibrillation. Several studies have shown AV junction ablation with pacemaker therapy to be highly effective at controlling symptoms and to result in improved quality of life in patients with paroxysmal and chronic atrial fibrillation. In patients with depressed left ventricular function, significant improvements in ventricular function are measured after ablation and pacing in 20% to 40% of patients in some series.[126, 127]

Radiofrequency ablation of the AV junction is performed by placing an ablation catheter across the tricuspid valve and recording a His bundle potential or, less frequently, by placing the catheter in the left ventricle on the septum underneath the noncoronary cusp of the aortic valve to record a His bundle potential.[128] Radiofrequency current is delivered to create permanent complete AV block. In most studies, radiofrequency ablation can be accomplished in more than 90% of patients with a right-sided approach. Radiofrequency current ablation of the AV junction usually results in a junctional escape rhythm that has a rate generally ranging from 40 to 50 bpm.

In one study,[127] about 65% of patients had an escape rhythm with an average rate of 39 bpm, with a new RBBB in 24%, a new LBBB in 6%, and an idioventricular rhythm in 19%. In some cases, based on limited follow-up, this escape rhythm appears to be stable. On the other hand, a direct current shock delivered through a catheter to ablate the AV junction results in a fascicular or ventricular escape rhythm that has a rate of about 45 bpm or less, which may be unreliable.[129, 130] Overdrive pacing of the ventricle has led to prolonged ventricular asystole in these patients, and questions have been raised about the long-term stability of this escape rhythm. Until more information is available, *any patient* having either radiofrequency or direct current AV junction ablation *should undergo permanent pacemaker implantation.*

Some investigators perform AV nodal modification for patients with rapid atrial fibrillation by delivering radiofrequency energy in and around the slow AV nodal pathway and attempt to leave conduction intact over the fast pathway of the AV node. In some patients, the result is a slower ventricular response during atrial fibrillation, with a reduced likelihood of permanent pacemaker placement. The incidence of long-term AV block is quite variable in these patients as well as controversial, with estimates for late development of complete heart block ranging from 0% to greater than 20% in different studies.[131] This procedure is designed to avoid permanent pacemaker implantation, although some clinicians are concerned about the risk for sudden death due to unexpected late complete heart block.

Table 17–7. Odds Ratio for Abnormality on Electrophysiologic Testing in Patients with Syncope

Clinical Variables	Multivariable	95% Confidence Interval for Multivariable
Age	1.01	0.99–1.03
Duration (months)	1.00	0.98–1.02
Sex (male)	1.76	0.79–3.93
Organic heart disease	1.53	0.71–3.33
Sudden loss of consciousness	1.93	0.89–4.16
Left ventricular ejection fraction	0.99	
ECG variables		0.93–1.06
Bundle-branch block	2.97†	1.23–7.21
Sinus bradycardia	3.47†	1.12–10.71
First-degree heart block	7.89*	2.12–29.31
Premature ventricular contractions (PVCs)	1.47	
		0.37–5.82
Holter variables	0.68	0.21–2.23
Sinus bradycardia	1.04	0.26–4.23
Sinus pause	0.63	0.06–6.33
Mobitz IPVCs	0.87	0.35–2.13

*$p < .001$
†$p < .05$

Adapted from Linzer M, Prystowsky EN, Devine GW, et al: Predicting the outcomes of electrophysiologic studies of patients with unexplained syncope: Preliminary validation of a derived model. J Gen Intern Med 6:113, 1991.

Diagnosis

Electrocardiography

First-degree AV block is usually due to conduction delay within the AV node. Much less commonly, first-degree AV block is due to intra-atrial or infra-Hisian conduction delay.[70] Localization of the site of second-degree AV block to the AV node or His-Purkinje system can be obtained by His bundle recording during invasive electrophysiologic testing, but in most cases, careful analysis of the ECG and the effect of various pharmacologic agents on block may suffice.[132] Diagnosis of the site of block is particularly problematic with 2:1 AV block. As a general rule, type I second-degree AV block with a narrow QRS almost always occurs within the AV node (Fig. 17–9). However, type I second-degree AV block with concomitant BBB may be associated with infra-Hisian block in up to 30% of cases.[133–135] Wenckebach periodicity before the development of high-grade AV block is suggestive of an AV nodal site of block. Administration of digoxin, β-blockers, and calcium-channel blockers in patients with second-degree AV block is also suggestive of block located in the AV node. Type II AV block is most commonly encountered when the QRS is prolonged and is generally localized within the His-Purkinje system (Fig.

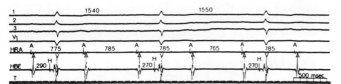

Figure 17–9. Spontaneous 2:1 (high-grade) AV block localized to the AV node. In this and subsequent figures, surface leads I, II, III, and V₁ are displayed with intracardiac electrograms recorded from the high right atrium (HRA), His bundle (HBE), and right ventricular apex (RV). Alternate atrial depolarizations (A) are not followed by either a His bundle or a ventricular depolarization. On the basis of a surface electrocardiogram (ECG), the finding of 2:1 AV block with a narrow QRS is compatible with a block at either the AV node or an infra-His site. The intracardiac recordings localize the site of block to the AV node. (From Josephson M: Clinical Cardiac Electrophysiology: Techniques and Interpretations. Philadelphia, Lea & Febiger, 1979, pp 79–101.)

17–10). Occasionally, type II AV block with a narrow QRS can be localized to the His bundle (i.e., intra-Hisian), but it may also be due to type I block with relatively long Wenckebach sequences and small increases in AV nodal conduction time.

In general, the response of block, particularly 2:1 AV block, to pharmacologic agents may help to determine the site of block. Atropine generally improves AV conduction in patients with AV nodal block; however, atropine is generally expected to worsen conduction in patients with block localized to the His-Purkinje system, owing to its effect on increasing sinus rates without improving His-Purkinje conduction (Fig. 17–11). Carotid sinus stimulation is expected to worsen block localized to the AV node, whereas it has no effect or improves conduction in patients with His-Purkinje system disease by causing sinus node slowing. The effect of any given drug, however, may be difficult to predict because its effect on the sinus node may be greater than its effect on the AV node. For example, atropine may improve AV node conduction, but if atropine causes excessive sinus node acceleration, AV conduction may improve marginally or not at all. The response to infusion of isoproterenol is less clear.

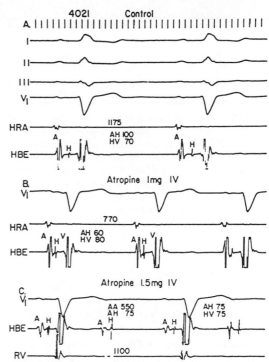

Figure 17–11. His-Purkinje AV block after an atropine-induced increase in sinus rate. *A,* Sinus rhythm at a cycle length of 1175 msec with 1:1 AV conduction. Left bundle-branch block is present, and the HV interval is slightly prolonged to 70 msec. *B,* After injection of 1 mg of atropine, the sinus rate speeds up to 770 msec and the HV interval increases to 80 msec, but 1:1 AV conduction is still present. The AH interval shortens despite the faster sinus rate because of the direct effect of atropine on AV nodal conduction. *C,* After injection of 1.5 mg of atropine the sinus cycle length decreases further to 550 msec, and 2:1 AV block occurs below the His bundle. Atropine worsens AV conduction in this patient, not through a direct drug effect but because the improvement in AV nodal conduction caused by atropine stresses the already abnormal His-Purkinje system. (From Miles WM, Klein LS: Sinus nodal dysfunction and atrioventricular conduction disturbances. *In* Naccarelli GV: Cardiac Arrhythmias: A Practical Approach. Mt Kisco, NY, Futura, 1991, pp 243–282.)

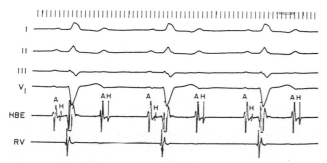

Figure 17–10. Intracardiac tracing of 2:1 second-degree AV block located in the His-Purkinje system. Sinus rhythm with left bundle-branch block is present. The AH intervals are constant, but every other atrial complex fails to activate the ventricle even though each atrial depolarization is followed by a His bundle deflection. This shows that the site of AV block is within the His-Purkinje system. (From Josephson ME: Clinical Cardiac Electrophysiology: Techniques and Interpretations. Philadelphia, Lea & Febiger, 1979, pp 79–101.)

Isoproterenol may improve conduction disorders localized in the AV node as well as occasionally in the His-Purkinje system.

Classic type I (Wenckebach) second-degree AV block has three characteristics: (1) progressive PR interval prolongation before the nonconducted beat, (2) progressive decrease in the increment of PR interval prolongation, and (3) progressive decrease in the RR interval, parallel to the progressive decrease in the increment of change in the PR interval.[133] All patterns of type I second-degree AV block not having this pattern are called *atypical* patterns, although in actuality, they may occur more commonly than the classic variety.[134, 135]

Lange and colleagues[136] reported on their experience with a large number of patients with transient second-degree AV block and narrow QRS complexes detected on ambulatory Holter monitoring. The authors emphasized the many ways in which second-degree AV block can be manifested. Classic type I AV block with progressive PR prolongation to more than 40 msec during at least three beats before the blocked

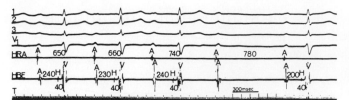

Figure 17–12. Example of atypical or uncommon type I second-degree AV block in the AV node. There is little alteration in the AH interval before the fourth atrial complex not conducting to the ventricle. The true nature of this arrhythmia is revealed by the first conducted P wave (A, atrial electrogram) after the pause, which is associated with substantial shortening of the AH interval from 230–240 msec to 200 msec. (From Josephson ME: Clinical Cardiac Electrophysiology: Techniques and Interpretations. Philadelphia, Lea & Febiger, 1979, pp 79–101.)

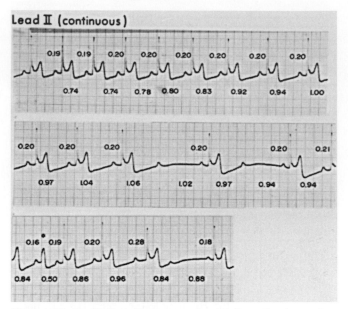

Figure 17–14. Rhythm strip demonstrating vagally mediated second-degree AV block. Note the progressive slowing of the heart rate before the first episode of block, although no change in PR interval can be discerned. During the second episode of block, there are both sinus slowing and PR interval prolongation, confirming the presence of type I second-degree AV block.

P waves was seen in only 50% of patients. Other patterns observed included a more subtle Wenckebach periodicity with minor PR prolongation of 20 to 40 msec before a blocked P wave in 29% of patients. Another pattern, seen in 8% of patients and termed *pseudo-Mobitz type II AV block*, demonstrated nearly constant PR intervals before the blocked P wave, followed by PR shortening on the subsequent conducted beat (Fig. 17–12). Classic Mobitz type II second-degree AV block with constant PR intervals for at least three beats before the blocked P wave followed by the same PR interval after the blocked P wave was seen in 4% of patients (Fig. 17–13). A mixed type I Wenckebach and pseudo–type II AV block were seen in 6% of all patients. Of all patients showing periods of pseudo-Mobitz type II block, 44% also demonstrated classic Wenckebach conduction patterns at some time.[136] Slowing of the sinus cycle length often preceded the blocked P wave in both classic and pseudo-Mobitz type II AV block (Fig. 17–14).

The diagnosis of complete heart block rests on demonstration of complete dissociation between atrial and ventricular activation. Care must be taken to distinguish transient AV dissociation due to competing atrial and junctional or ventricular rhythms with similar rates (so-called isorhythmic AV dissociation). If sufficiently long monitoring strips are available, intermittent conduction of appropriately timed atrial events is seen. Temporary atrial pacing can be performed to accelerate the atrial rate to overdrive the competing junctional or ventricular arrhythmia, demonstrating intact AV conduction. In the presence of atrial fibrillation, complete heart block can be inferred when the ventricular rate becomes regular rather than the typical irregular ventricular response (Fig. 17–15). Digoxin toxicity may be the cause of

heart block with atrial fibrillation, and this or other drug toxicity should be ruled out before assuming that structural AV conduction disease is present. In patients with atrial fibrillation, regular RR interval may on occasion be due to "concealed" sinus rhythm and not heart block.[137]

Electrophysiologic Study

Invasive electrophysiologic study (e.g., His bundle recording) can be a useful means of evaluating AV conduction in patients who have symptoms and in whom the need for permanent pacing is not obvious (Fig. 17–16). Electrophysiologic studies are *not indicated* in patients with symptomatic

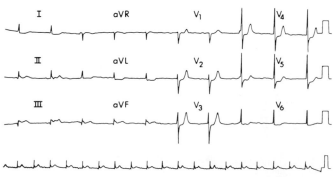

Figure 17–15. Twelve-lead electrocardiogram from a patient with recent aortic valve surgery and atrial fibrillation treated with digoxin. The QRS complexes are narrow and occur at a regular rate of 56 bpm, illustrating complete heart block with a junctional escape rhythm in the setting of atrial fibrillation. Despite discontinuation of digoxin, complete heart block persisted in this patient.

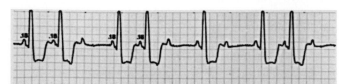

Figure 17–13. Example of type II second-degree AV block showing repeating episodes of block. Note that the PR interval is constant both before and after the nonconducted P wave and that there is associated bundle-branch block.

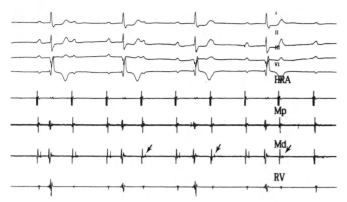

Figure 17–16. Surface leads I, II, III, and V₁ revealing sinus rhythm with 2:1 AV conduction, marked PR interval prolongation during conducted beats, and right bundle-branch block. Intracardiac electrograms from the high right atrium (HRA), proximal and distal poles of the His bundle catheter (M$_p$ and M$_d$, respectively), and the right ventricle (RV) are shown. The distal pole of the His bundle catheter registers a His bundle potential, which can be seen as a discrete sharp potential between the atrial and the ventricular electrograms on that channel. During nonconducted atrial complexes, spontaneous infra-Hisian block is apparent because the His bundle potential (arrow) is not followed by a ventricular electrogram.

high-grade or complete AV block recorded on surface ECG tracings, ambulatory Holter monitoring, or transtelephonic recordings because the need for permanent pacing has already been established, nor in patients whose symptoms are shown to be not associated with a conduction abnormality or block. In addition, patients without symptoms who have intermittent AV block associated with sinus slowing, gradual PR prolongation before a nonconducted P wave, and a narrow QRS complex should also not undergo electrophysiologic study given the benign prognosis of these findings.

As stated earlier, the incidence of progression of bifascicular block to complete heart block is variable, ranging from 1% to 6% per year. The method of patient selection affects this incidence, with patients who have asymptomatic bifascicular block progressing to complete heart block at a rate of 2% per year, and patients with symptoms (e.g., syncope or presyncope) progressing at a rate closer to 6% per year.[120, 122, 138] Many of these studies emphasize the high mortality associated with BBB and bifascicular block. It is worth emphasizing that the mortality associated with the presence of structural heart disease predominantly reflects death due to acute myocardial infarction, heart failure, or ventricular tachyarrhythmias rather than bradyarrhythmias.

Three large studies of patients with BBB have been performed to assess the role of His bundle conduction (e.g., HV interval) measurements in predicting progression to complete heart block. The measurement of the HV interval represents the conduction time through the His bundle and bundle branches until ventricular activation begins. Dhingra and colleagues[120] prospectively followed 517 patients with BBB and measured the time required for progression to second- and third-degree block. In their study, only 13% of patients presented with syncope; the remainder did not have symptoms. The cumulative 7-year incidence of progression to AV block was 10% in the group with a normal HV interval and 20% in the group with HV interval prolongation. The

cumulative mortality rate at 7 years was 48% in patients with a normal HV interval and 66% in patients with a prolonged HV interval.[120] This study emphasized that despite the high mortality associated with the presence of bifascicular block, there is only a low rate of progression to trifascicular block.

McAnulty and associates[121] studied 554 patients with "high-risk" BBB defined as LBBB, RBBB, and left- or right-axis RBBB, with alternating left and right axis, or alternating RBBB and LBBB. The cumulative incidence of AV block, either type II second-degree or complete heart block, was only 4.9%, or 1% per year, in patients with a prolonged HV interval and 1.9% in patients with a normal HV interval (difference not significant). HV interval prolongation did not predict a higher risk of development of complete heart block. In this study, 8.5% of patients developed syncope after entry into the study. The incidence of complete AV block was 17% in patients with syncope compared with 2% in patients without a history of syncope.

Scheinman and colleagues[122] studied 401 patients with chronic BBB for about 30 months. This study, in contrast to those of Dhingra[120] and McAnulty,[121] primarily included patients with symptoms referred for electrophysiology study. Patients with an HV interval of more than 70 msec had an incidence of 12% of progression to spontaneous second- or third-degree AV block. The incidence of complete AV block was 25% for those with an HV interval of 100 msec or greater. The yearly incidence of spontaneous AV block was 3% in those with a normal HV interval compared with 3.5% in those with a prolonged HV interval. In contrast, the study from Scheinman's group included the highest percentage of patients with a history of syncope, about 40%.[122]

Resolution of the *apparent* controversy about the clinical utility of His bundle recordings involves a realization that different patient populations are being studied. There does appear to be a relationship between a prolonged HV interval and the development of complete heart block during the ensuing years. It is also likely that this risk varies directly with the degree of HV prolongation. Demonstration of these relationships requires documentation of spontaneous high-grade complete heart block in enough patients because the absolute risk is very low overall. This can be done in one of two ways: by following a large number of patients for long periods of time, or by including patients with symptoms of unexplained syncope. Demonstration of this relationship in an unselected, symptom-free group of patients is difficult because the risk of complete heart block is so low. Current recommendations are therefore not to perform electrophysiologic studies in patients with asymptomatic BBB.[139]

Many studies have demonstrated the clinical utility of electrophysiologic testing in patients with *BBB* and *syncope*.[123] In one study, 112 patients with chronic BBB and syncope or near-syncope underwent electrophysiologic testing.[129] A normal electrophysiologic study result predicted a good long-term prognosis. About 25% of patients were found to have a significant conduction system disorder, underwent pacemaker implantation, and had symptoms recur at a rate of only 6%. In the study reported by Morady and associates,[124] 28% of patients (7 of 32) had sustained induced monomorphic ventricular tachycardia, whereas about 20% had conduction disturbances at electrophysiology study. Six of the 7 patients who received pacemakers had no recurrent symptoms. Thus, electrophysiologic studies are useful in patients with BBB or bifascicular block and syncope for several reasons. First, negative results of electrophysiologic studies identify a group of patients at low risk for cardiac events. More important, induction of sustained ventricular tachycardia during electrophysiologic testing identifies patients who are at risk for life-threatening ventricular arrhythmias and who require pharmacologic or other therapy (e.g., surgery or defibrillation). Finally, electrophysiologic testing also identifies those patients with advanced conduction system disease who require pacemaker implantation. Thus, current recommendations are to perform electrophysiologic testing in patients with syncope or near-syncope and BBB.

Methods Used to Identify Patients at Risk for AV Block

In addition to measurement of HV intervals, additional electrophysiologic testing has been suggested for use in patients with symptomatic BBB or bifascicular block. As stated previously, a *markedly* prolonged HV interval (100 msec or longer) is predictive of development of symptomatic heart block. HV intervals greater than 100 msec are uncommon; therefore, although marked HV prolongation is quite specific, it is also very insensitive.

The use of atrial pacing to stress the His-Purkinje system has been suggested by some to provide additional important information. Most healthy subjects do not develop second- or third-degree infra-Hisian block during atrial pacing in which the rate is gradually increased, as would occur spontaneously. However, certain pacing protocols with abrupt onset of pacing at rapid rates are more likely to induce infra-Hisian block, even in healthy subjects, but this rarely occurs at pacing rates below 150 bpm. Dhingra and colleagues[140] reported a 50% rate of progression to type II or complete AV block in patients who develop block distal to the His bundle at paced rates of less than 150 bpm. Because AV nodal dysfunction is frequently seen in patients with significant His-Purkinje system disease, AV nodal block may occur at lower pacing rates than those necessary to demonstrate infra-Hisian block. This "protective" effect of AV nodal dysfunction during resting states may lead to the incorrect conclusion that significant His-Purkinje disease is not present. Repeat atrial pacing, however, may demonstrate infra-Hisian block after administration of atropine or isoproterenol to facilitate AV nodal conduction.

Provocative drug tests have been suggested as another means of evaluating the distal conduction system (Fig. 17–17). There are only limited available data describing the experience with the intravenous type Ia antiarrhythmic drugs procainamide, ajmaline, and disopyramide and the type Ic agent flecainide.[141–144] Only intravenous procainamide is available in the United States. Administration of these agents may result in a doubling of the HV interval, a resultant HV interval greater than 100 msec, or precipitation of spontaneous type II second- or third-degree AV block, all of which indicate a higher risk of developing complete heart block. Tonkin and associates[144] administered procainamide at a dose of 10 mg/kg and produced intermittent second- or third-degree AV block in 5 of 12 patients. Progression to complete AV block over a period of 1 year was high in this group of patients with symptoms. Intravenous disopyramide has the potential benefit of facilitating AV nodal conduction by its anticholinergic properties while accentuating underlying infra-Hisian disease by its membrane-stabilizing effects.[143]

In patients with alternating BBB, electrophysiologic testing almost invariably demonstrates a high degree of His-Purkinje system disease. These patients typically have very long HV intervals and are at very high risk of progression to complete heart block in a short time span. Pacing in these patients is indicated on clinical grounds, and electrophysiologic testing is unnecessary.[142]

Although electrophysiologic testing has been considered the gold standard for identifying significant AV nodal or His-Purkinje dysfunction, it may have its limitations.[145] In a small study conducted by Fujimura and associates,[145] 13 patients with documented symptomatic transient second- or third-degree AV block referred for implantation of a permanent pacemaker underwent AV conduction testing at the time of pacemaker insertion. These tests included facilitation of AV nodal conduction with atropine and depression of His-Purkinje conduction with low doses of procainamide. Surprisingly, only 2 of the 13 patients showed significant abnormalities in the AV conduction system (inducible infra-Hisian block in both cases) during electrophysiologic testing, yielding a sensitivity of 15.4%. Two additional patients had moderately prolonged HV intervals, although much shorter than 100 msec. If these two patients are included as diagnostic, the sensitivity of electrophysiology testing is increased to 46%. Although the patient population was small in this study, the results raise serious questions about the sensitivity of electrophysiologic testing for identifying patients at risk of developing symptomatic AV block. Further data are clearly needed in this regard. Whether other pharmacologic stressors, as mentioned previously, would have improved the overall sensitivity awaits further investigation.

Indications

In 1984, a committee of the ACC-AHA put together a set of guidelines concerning the indications for permanent pacing.[146] These guidelines were revised in 1991 and again in 1998.[147, 148] Guidelines are categorized into three classes:

CLASS I. Conditions for which there is evidence or general agreement that a given procedure or treatment is beneficial, useful, and effective. There is general agreement among physicians that a permanent pacemaker should be implanted. This implies that the condition is chronic or recurrent but not due to drug toxicity, acute myocardial ischemia or infarction, or electrolyte imbalance.

CLASS II. Conditions for which cardiac pacemakers are generally found acceptable or necessary, but there is some divergence of opinion.

Class IIa: Weight of evidence and opinion is in favor of usefulness and efficacy.

Class IIb: Usefulness or efficacy is less well established by evidence and opinion.

CLASS III. Conditions considered insupportable by present evidence to benefit adequately from permanent pacemakers, and there is general agreement that a pacemaker is *not* indicated.

Recommendations supported by studies based on data derived from multiple randomized clinical trials with large

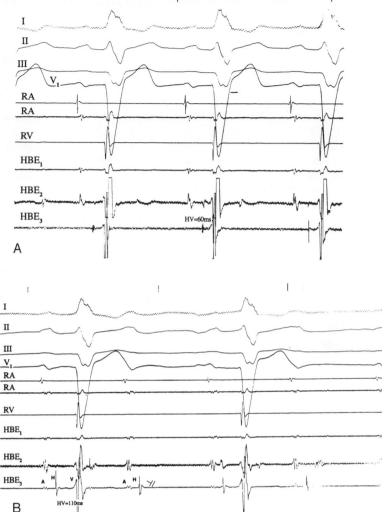

Figure 17–17. *A*, Electrophysiologic testing in the baseline state in a patient with syncope reveals a left bundle-branch block pattern during sinus rhythm. There is 1:1 AV conduction with an HV interval of 60 msec. *B*, After a loading dose of procainamide, 2:1 AV conduction develops. The first and third atrial activations are conducted to the ventricles with an HV interval of 110 msec. The third and fourth atrial activations conduct through the AV node to generate a His bundle potential without subsequent ventricular activation. Thus, this illustrates spontaneous infra-Hisian block induced by procainamide. RA, right atrial recordings; RV, right ventricular recording; HBE₁, HBE₂, HBE₃, proximal, middle, and distal His bundle catheter recordings, respectively.

numbers of patients are ranked "A," those based on a limited number of trials involving smaller numbers of patients from well-designed data analyses of nonrandomized studies or observational data registries are ranked "B," and those based on expert consensus and years of clinical experience are ranked "C."

Indications that are generally agreed on and included in the recent AHA-ACC guidelines are as follows[148]:

Pacing for Acquired AV Block in Adults

CLASS I

- Third-degree AV block at any anatomic level, associated with any one of the following conditions:
  - Bradycardia associated with symptoms presumed to be due to AV block including syncope or presyncope, congestive heart failure, mental confusion improving with temporary pacing, symptomatic ventricular ectopy, nonsustained or sustained ventricular tachycardia, or ventricular fibrillation related to an inadequate or slow escape rhythm (level of evidence: C)
  - Arrhythmias and other medical conditions that require drugs that result in symptomatic bradycardia (level of evidence: C)

- Documented periods of asystole lasting longer than 3 seconds or any escape rhythm less than 40 bpm in awake, symptom-free patients (level of evidence: B, C)
- After catheter ablation of the AV junction (level of evidence: B, C)
- Postoperative AV block that is not expected to resolve (level of evidence: C)
- Neuromuscular diseases with AV block, such as myotonic dystrophy, Kearns-Sayre syndrome, limb-girdle dystrophy of Erb, and peroneal muscular atrophy (level of evidence: C)
- Second-degree AV block regardless of the type or the site of block with associated symptomatic bradycardia (Level of evidence: B)

CLASS IIa

- Asymptomatic third-degree AV block with average, awake ventricular rates greater than 40 bpm (level of evidence: B, C)
- Asymptomatic type II second-degree AV block (level of evidence: B)
- Asymptomatic type I second-degree AV block at intra-His or infra-His level found incidentally at electrophysiologic study performed for other indications (level of evidence: B)

- First-degree AV block with symptoms suggestive of the pacemaker syndrome and documented alleviation of symptoms with temporary AV pacing. (level of evidence: B)

CLASS IIb
- Marked first-degree AV block of longer than 0.30 seconds in patients with left ventricular dysfunction and symptoms of congestive heart failure in whom a more physiologic AV interval results in hemodynamic improvement presumably by decreasing left atrial filling pressure (level of evidence: C)

CLASS III
- Asymptomatic first-degree AV block (level of evidence: B)
- Asymptomatic type I second-degree AV block at the supra-His (AV node) level (level of evidence: B, C)
- AV block that is expected to resolve and is unlikely to recur (e.g., drug toxicity, Lyme disease) (level of evidence: B)

Pacing in Bifascicular and Trifascicular Block (Chronic)

CLASS I
- Intermittent third-degree AV block (level of evidence: B)
- Type II second-degree AV block (level of evidence: B)

CLASS IIa
- Syncope not proved to be due to AV block when other likely causes have been excluded, specifically ventricular tachycardia (level of evidence: B)
- Incidental finding at electrophysiologic study of markedly prolonged HV (HV > 100 msec) interval in a symptom-free patient (level of evidence: B)
- Incidental finding at electrophysiologic study of atrial pacing–induced infra-Hisian block that is not physiologic (level of evidence: B)

CLASS IIb
- None

CLASS III
- Fascicular block without AV block or symptoms (level of evidence: B)
- Fascicular block with first-degree AV block without symptoms (level of evidence: B)

Barold has commented on earlier guidelines from 1984 and 1991 in an important editorial that has sparked many of the changes incorporated into the revised guidelines.[149] He emphasized the need for more precise definitions of second-degree AV block, particularly with 2:1 AV block. He noted that second-degree AV block classified as type I should be associated with progressive prolongation of PR intervals before a blocked beat and type II with constant PR intervals before and after a single blocked beat, usually in association with a wide QRS complex. *Trifascicular block* is a term that is also loosely applied. Barold argues that the use of the term trifascicular block to describe the combination of bifascicular block (RBBB plus left anterior hemiblock, RBBB plus left posterior hemiblock, or LBBB) and first-degree AV block is misleading because the site of block may be located in the AV node or His-Purkinje system. Trifascicular block should be used only to refer to alternating RBBB and LBBB, RBBB with a prolonged HV interval (regardless of the presence or absence of left anterior or posterior fascicular block), and LBBB with a prolonged HV interval. In addition, trifascicular block can refer to a patient with second- or third-degree AV block in the His-Purkinje system with permanent block

in all three fascicles, permanent block in two fascicles with intermittent conduction in the third, permanent block in one fascicle with intermittent block in the other two fascicles, and intermittent block in all three fascicles.

Patients who present with symptomatic first-, second-, or third-degree AV block usually have symptoms of syncope, dizziness, decreased energy, palpitations, or recurrent presyncope or dizziness. Other symptoms primarily reflect inadequate cardiac output or tissue perfusion and include fatigue, angina, or congestive heart failure. The most severe symptom is recurrent Stokes-Adams attacks with documented episodes of polymorphic ventricular tachycardia. Patients with long PR intervals may have symptoms suggestive of pacemaker syndrome and may demonstrate resolution of symptoms with institution of dual-chamber pacing. It is important to emphasize that symptoms can be subtle in some patients or may be of sufficiently long duration that temporary pacing may be indicated to document improvement or reversal of long-standing problems.

The *natural history* of spontaneously developing asymptomatic complete heart block in adult life dates back to the days before pacemaker therapy was available.[150–152] Today, almost all patients with complete heart block probably eventually develop symptoms and undergo pacemaker placement. Several studies published in the 1960s emphasized the poor prognosis of patients with complete heart block. The 1-year survival of patients who developed Stokes-Adams attacks due to complete heart block and were not paced was 50% to 75%, which is significantly less than that of a sex- and age-matched control population.[148, 151, 152] The "best" prognosis was in patients with an idiopathic or unknown cause. At least 33% of deaths were definitely related to complete heart block and Stokes-Adams attacks. These differences in survival persist even after 15 years of follow-up and appear to be related to the considerably higher incidence of sudden death.[152] There is some debate about whether the presence of syncope is associated with a worse prognosis. In contrast, the prognosis for transient complete heart block is better, with a 36% 1-year mortality.[151]

Edhag and Swahn[151, 152] reported on a mean 6.5-year follow-up of 248 patients, most of whom had high-grade AV block. The mean age at pacemaker implantation was 66 years, and the 1-year survival rate of paced patients was 86%, slightly lower than the 95% 1-year survival of an age- and sex-matched group of Swedish patients. After the first year, survival in the paced patients was similar to that in the general population. Edhag also compared survival among different age groups and found no difference in survival in elderly patients with heart block who underwent permanent pacing and the age- and sex-matched general population. In contrast, younger patients with heart block had an increased mortality even after pacing than sex- and age-matched controls from the general population (Fig. 17–18).[152] It is likely that this higher mortality is a reflection of the underlying structural heart disease that is responsible for high-grade AV block.

Alpert and colleagues[153] compared the prognoses of 132 patients with high-grade AV block and VVI pacemakers with those of 48 patients with DDD pacemakers for high-grade AV block during a 1- to 5-year follow-up period. They showed that permanent dual-chamber pacing enhanced survival to a greater extent than permanent VVI pacing in a

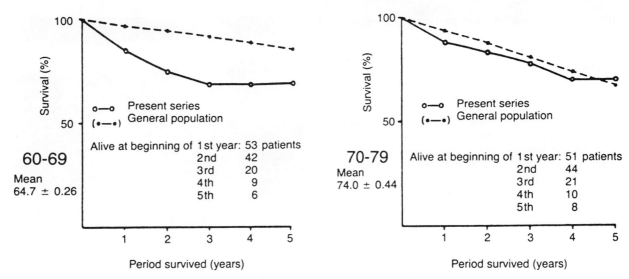

Figure 17–18. Survival after fixed-rate pacing in two different age groups in relation to the matched general Swedish population. (From Edhag O: Long-term cardiac pacing: Experience of fixed-rate pacing with an endocardial electrode in 260 patients. Acta Med Scand 502S:64, 1969.)

subgroup of patients with pre-existing congestive heart failure. The causes of congestive heart failure were variable; about 50% of patients had underlying ischemic heart disease, and the rest had hypertension, valvular heart disease, or idiopathic dilated cardiomyopathy. Most deaths in the patient group with VVI pacemakers were due to AMI or congestive heart failure.

Linde-Edelstam and associates[154] performed a case-controlled study comparing consecutive patients who received VDD pacemakers with the first available VVI patients who fulfilled certain "predetermined characteristics." The two groups were similar with respect to other concomitant diseases and severity of congestive heart failure. The investigators compared survival in 74 patients treated with VVI pacemakers with that in 74 patients with VDD pacemakers over a mean follow-up period of 5.4 years. The overall survival was different between the two pacing modes and was better with the VDD pacing mode than that of the age- and sex-matched general Swedish population (Fig. 17–19). Survival was no different between patients paced in the VVI and VDD modes if congestive heart failure was absent. There are several potential explanations for the negative effects on survival of VVI pacing in this population. These include progression of heart failure due to elevated catecholamines with ventricular pacing, absence of chronotropic competence, and increased myocardial oxygen demand from ventricular pacing.

The natural history of asymptomatic type II second-degree AV block has been addressed in only one study. In this study, from the University of Illinois, most patients were found to develop symptoms within a relatively short period of time.[155] These observations form the basis for the current recommendations to institute permanent pacing in all patients with type II second-degree AV block. A more recent study showed that patients with type I second-degree AV block also did poorly if left unpaced. Shaw and colleagues[119] reported on 214 patients with a mean age of 72 years who were followed over a 14-year time period. Their patient

population consisted of patients with permanent AV block, who were divided into three groups: type I block (77 patients), type II block (86 patients), and 2:1 or 3:1 block (51 patients). The 3- and 5-year survival times were similarly poor regardless of the type of block. Patients who received permanent pacemakers had a survival similar to that for a control population. Based on this study, elderly patients with type I AV block or 2:1 or 3:1 AV block with narrow QRS complexes should be followed closely because these ECG

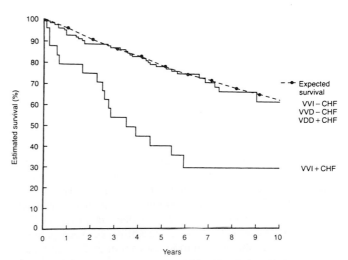

Figure 17–19. Expected survival rate for the general Swedish population and observed survival rates for patients with high-grade AV block and congestive heart failure (CHF) paced in fixed-rate ventricular (VVI) mode compared with (1) patients with high-grade AV block paced in atrial synchronous mode (VVD) with and without CHF and (2) patients without CHF paced in VVI mode. (From Linde-Edelstam C, Gullberg B, Nordlander R, et al: Longevity in patients with high-degree atrioventricular block paced in the atrial synchronous or fixed-rate ventricular inhibited mode. PACE 15:304, 1992.)

abnormalities may be markers for progressive conduction system disease.

■ VDDR PACING

The development of a single lead with a series of electrodes for atrial sensing and ventricular pacing and sensing occurred more than a decade ago to avoid the need for implanting two separate pacing leads. VDD or VAT pacing is an ideal mode of pacing for patients with complete heart block and normal sinus node function because it allows preservation of normal AV synchrony and rate responsiveness.[156, 157]

In the early 1970s, several groups studying different electrode configurations demonstrated clearly that a floating unipolar electrogram in the middle to high right atrium showed favorable characteristics for atrial sensing. In the 1980s, a bipolar configuration of atrial electrodes was developed to avoid sensing of myopotentials and electromagnetic interference as well as ventricular far-field signals. Various electrode configurations were studied, including bipolar leads with narrow and wide spacing and orthogonal and diagonal atrial electrodes. The optimal spacing of two poles of the floating bipolar lead was found to range between 0.5 and 1 cm. In addition, atrial amplifiers capable of reliably detecting the atrial signal were developed. Factors influencing atrial electrogram detection include electrode spacing, distance from the atrial wall, orientation of electrodes relative to atrial tissue, and electrode size.

Patient selection and programming are *crucial*. The ideal candidate for a single-lead VDD pacemaker is a patient with high-grade or complete AV block and normal sinus node function.[158, 159] Patients with retrograde VA conduction and sinus bradycardia may develop symptoms if their sinus rate frequently slows below the lower programmed rate, leading to VVI pacing at the lower rate. This problem is avoided by obtaining a 24-hour Holter monitor recording and programming the lower rate to a rate below the slowest sinus rate. Single-lead AV pacing is also best avoided if the atrial chamber diameter of the right atrium is greater than 3×3 cm and if the left atrium is larger than 4×3 cm in the echocardiographic apical four-chamber view. Patients with paroxysmal supraventricular tachycardia should also probably not receive VDD pacemakers.

The implant procedure for a VDD system consists of fixing the ventricular tip to allow the atrial electrodes to lie as close as possible to the high-middle location of the midlateral atrial wall (Fig. 17–20). An atrial signal should be measured at rest, during deep breathing, and during coughing as well as during arm and shoulder movements. The lowest acceptable atrial electrogram signal during any maneuver should be more than 0.5 mV during deep inspiration.[156, 157] In general, there is considerable variability between patients and within individuals from moment to moment with respect to atrial electrogram amplitude.

Pacemaker programming should take into account atrial sensitivity as well as programming of the postventricular atrial refractory period (PVARP), AV delay, and lower rate. Some generators allow programming of the bandwidth of the atrial amplifier. This may be very helpful and allows the implanter to attenuate interfering myopotentials as well as retrograde P waves in patients with ventricular ectopy.[160] VDDR generators with programmable atrial amplifier band-

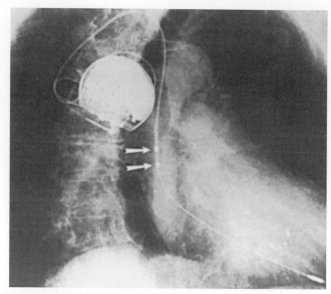

Figure 17–20. Lateral chest radiograph showing single AV lead with narrow-spaced AV ring electrodes connected to a LEM Biomedica/Cardiac Control Systems VDD pacemaker. The arrows denote atrial electrodes. (From Antonioli EG, Ansani L, Barbieri D, et al: Single-lead VDD pacing. *In* Barold SS, Mugica J: New Perspectives in Cardiac Pacing 3. Mt Kisco, NY, Futura, 1993, pp 359–381.)

widths allow the implanter to minimize the sensing of myopotentials and retrograde P waves, thus avoiding the need for programming long PVARPs. The PVARP should be programmed to contain retrograde P waves. The AV delay must take into account the delay in detecting atrial depolarization. The lower rate should be programmed to a value below the minimum sinus rate noted during the 24-hour Holter recording.

Clinical trials of different VDD pacing systems have shown overall good clinical performance. This technology has been successfully used in children and adolescents as well. Widespread application of this technology to children and adolescents should await longer mean follow-up times than the 1- to 2-year period reported in these studies.[161, 162] In one study, the mean maximum and minimum values of atrial electrogram characteristics within a whole respiratory cycle were 2.64 ± 1.05 mV and 1.65 ± 0.38 mV amplitude (maximum) and 0.31 ± 0.12 mV and 0.18 ± 0.09 mV (minimum).[157–160] Atrial oversensing during upper-body isometric exercises involving the pectoral muscles was not a clinical problem. Adequate P-wave amplitude was "easily" obtained at the time of implantation and remained stable during follow-up. P-wave amplitude was unaffected by maneuvers that simulated daily activities, such as coughing, hyperventilation, arm swinging, isometric exercises, and respiration. During a mean follow-up period of 36 months, 5 of 72 patients required conversion to the VVI mode, owing to complete loss of sensing (2 patients) and to chronic atrial fibrillation (3 patients). Ninety-three percent of patients remain paced in the VDD mode. Holter monitoring confirmed AV synchrony in most patients, with a few patients showing intermittent loss of atrial sensing lasting from 4 to 5 beats to up to 3% of the monitored period. Similar results have been achieved with other systems.

Ramsdale and Charles,[163] however, reported difficulty in obtaining an adequate P-wave amplitude at implantation, resulting in prolonged implantation times. In their series, almost 60% of patients showed intermittent failure of P-wave sensing. Marked fluctuations in the paced ventricular rate were noted especially during exercise, when intermittent failure to sense P waves occurred. Finally, in patients in whom sinus node dysfunction develops and a need for atrial pacing arises, upgrading to a DDDR pacing mode can be easily performed, as recently described.[164] Lau and associates[165] recently compared the clinical performance of two systems with different electrode configurations; one using a diagonally arranged bipole and one using closely spaced bipolar ring electrode. The clinical performance of atrial sensing was similar despite different electrode configurations.

One of the major advantages of the VDDR pacing mode is the use of the sensor to differentiate sinus tachycardia from the tracking of myopotentials. The implanted sensor can be used to judge the appropriateness of the atrial rate. In addition, the rate-adaptive sensor allows for rate smoothing of upper rate behavior.

Enthusiasm for the VDD pacing mode has diminished as the size and experience in manipulating the new atrial leads have increased. The additional risk and work of positioning an atrial lead outweigh the disadvantage of not having atrial pacing. Studies with earlier models of atrial leads reported a high incidence of atrial lead dislodgment as well as deterioration of atrial pacing and sensing characteristics over time. With the newer designs of atrial lead, including steroid-eluting atrial leads, as well as the redesign of bandpass filters for sensing atrial activity, technical stability of the atrial lead has improved. In some older series, atrial pacing and sensing are maintained for 5 years in almost 90% of patients.[166] The unpredictability in some patients of atrial chronotropic function over the long term has led some workers to favor implanting atrial leads in most patients with complete heart block who are undergoing pacemaker implantation. Ventricular pacing can arise when the atrial rate is slower than the programmed lower rate or during exercise in a patient with chronotropic incompetence if the patient has a VDDR pacemaker and the sensor rate exceeds the P-wave rate.

Several groups have talked about the possibility of pacing the atrium with a floating electrode. Naegeli and coworkers[167] reported on the feasibility of atrial pacing using a new quadripolar single-pass VDD lead with closely spaced cylindrical dipoles for atrial sensing and pacing. These authors were able to demonstrate continued atrial pacing and sensing during a 6-month follow-up period using a single-pass lead. Phrenic nerve pacing was not observed, and the atrial pacing threshold was 5.2 ± 1.4 V at a 0.5-msec pulse duration. Atrial pacing thresholds did not rise during follow-up. Presumably, newer pacing waveforms may result in lower atrial pacing thresholds with a floating atrial electrode.

Programming of the appropriate AV interval is discussed elsewhere. In brief, the optimal AV interval is one that provides the best timing of *left atrial* filling. There are many important factors to be considered, such as site of pacing, atrial size, ventricular function, intra-atrial and interatrial conduction times, and whether the atrial event is paced or sensed. The interatrial conduction time determines when the left atrial depolarization begins and therefore directly determines the important left atrial–left ventricular timing interval. It is important to note that about 25% of patients undergoing DDD pacemaker implantation have high-degree intra-atrial and interatrial conduction delays.[168] Many authors have suggested that the programming of differential AV intervals for sensing and pacing may give rise to small but significant increases in cardiac output in patients with left ventricular dysfunction.[168, 169] Not only will optimal AV synchrony optimize cardiac output by increasing ventricular preload, thus lowering mean atrial pressure, it will also minimize AV valvular regurgitation.

Optimal AV coupling intervals also depend on body position, catecholamine levels, interatrial conduction time, and left atrial electrical-mechanical coupling times. Practically speaking, these facts lead to programming the paced AV interval and allowing the sensed AV interval to be of shorter duration. The optimal AV interval varies from patient to patient, with shorter AV intervals possibly being more beneficial in patients with heart failure and valvular regurgitation and in those with hypertrophic cardiomyopathy.[170, 171] The optimal AV interval can vary considerably from patient to patient depending on many different factors and is difficult to predict a priori. The optimal AV interval can be determined by comparing the measured stroke volume at different AV intervals as measured by continuous-wave cardiac Doppler, right heart catheterization, or, more recently, impedance cardiography.

In a study using impedance cardiography to measure cardiac output at rest in patients with primarily AV block, the optimal AV delay at pacing rates of between 70 and 110 bpm was an average of less than 120 msec from the atrial stimulus to the ventricular stimulus.[170] In this study, the cardiac output in the DDD pacing mode was similar to that in the VVI pacing mode when the AV delay was more than 200 msec. The mean difference in cardiac index comparing the best with the worst AV interval setting was $34\% \pm 8\%$.

AV intervals may be shortened further during atrial tracking; when patients exercise and their heart rates increase, the sensed P wave to ventricular pacing stimulus can be shortened. This is termed *rate-adaptive AV interval shortening* or *automatic rate-adaptive AV delay* and is a programmable feature on several DDD pacemaker generators. This can be accomplished as one-step shortening or multistep shortening in discrete, nonprogrammable, or linear steps as the atrial rate increases. For example, in many Biotronik pulse generators, the sensed AV delay may be programmed to different values within a specified range of heart rates. In the Intermedics Cosmos II, the pacemaker adapts the AV delay after each sensed P wave to changes in the preceding sinus cycle length. For example, for a 20-msec shortening of the sinus cycle, the subsequent AV delay after a sensed P wave would be 2.5 msec shorter.

The minimum value below which the AV delay will not be shortened is calculated based on the programmed pacing rate and the upper ventricular rate limit and is set to a minimum of 75 msec. The Siemens-Pacesetter (St. Jude Medical, Sylmar, CA) models shorten the PV interval by 25-msec steps within the limit of 75 msec less than the programmed AV delay. In the DDDR mode, the paced AV delay shortens as the pacing rate increases in response to the sensor. The Vitatron (Dieren, The Netherlands) algorithm produces an exponential adaptation curve, whereas the ELA

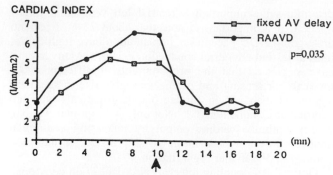

Figure 17–21. Comparison of an automatic rate-responsive AV delay (RAAVD) and a fixed but individually optimized (by Doppler echocardiography) AV delay in a patient with a chronically implanted DDD pacemaker for complete AV block. At each exercise level, and especially at peak exercise *(arrow)*, rate-responsive AV delay produced a significantly higher cardiac index (CI) compared with the fixed value. (From Daubert C, Ritter P, Mabo P, et al: AV delay optimization in DDD and DDDR pacing. *In* Barold SS, Mugica J: New Perspectives in Cardiac Pacing 3. Mt Kisco, NY, Futura, 1993, pp 259–287.)

Chorus (Plymouth, MN) algorithm mimics physiology by adapting the sensed AV delay to the atrial rate on a beat-by-beat basis, with linear shortening occurring between a maximal and a minimal value. The net result is a shortening of the total atrial refractory period, thereby allowing higher 1:1 tracking rates. The assumption behind the shortening of the PV or AV interval is that it maintains the proper timing of the atrial contraction and thereby optimizes stroke volume (Fig. 17–21). The shortened PV (or AV) intervals may result in a greater degree of ventricular pacing in patients with intermittent or catecholamine-sensitive AV conduction. If this results in fewer intrinsic beats and more ventricular pacing, there may be no improvement in hemodynamics and potentially even a worsening of hemodynamics in certain patients.

In rare patients with high-grade interatrial conduction slowing in the presence of atrial disease and either sick sinus syndrome or heart block, optimal AV synchrony may not occur with typical AV delays of 125 to 175 msec. AV intervals of 250 to 350 msec may be required to provide effective atrial systole. This has the disadvantage of necessitating long total atrial refractory periods and limiting the upper rate possible for exercise. Second, interatrial synchrony remains widely separated, and atrial arrhythmias may be triggered by atrial pacing during the vulnerable period. Daubert and colleagues[169] solved this problem by using two atrial leads, one placed in the right atrium and one placed in the coronary sinus to pace and sense the left atrium. This "triple-chamber" pacemaker provides simultaneous contraction of both the right and left atria and optimizes cardiac performance with traditional values for the AV interval and PVARP. This concept has been referred to as *permanent atrial resynchronization.*

Summary

It is likely that complete AV block will remain one of the major indications for cardiac pacing through the next decade. Most diagnoses can be made by careful analysis of the surface electrocardiogram, although electrophysiologic testing is a useful provocative tool, particularly in patients with unexplained syncope and BBB. Ultimately, in most cases, the decision to pace a patient is based on a correlation of symptoms with an abnormal ECG (rhythm). The causes of complete heart block may change, with radiofrequency ablation of the AV junction–His bundle accounting for an increasing fraction of patients with complete AV block. It is likely that DDD pacing with two separate leads will remain the major pacing modality for most patients with heart block if ongoing studies demonstrate its superiority over single-chamber ventricular pacing. Mode switching will be incorporated increasingly into DDD pacemakers, and separate programming of AV intervals based on P-wave sensing or atrial pacing as well as the use of rate-adaptive AV delays will become routine.

REFERENCES

1. James TN: Anatomy of the coronary arteries and veins: Anatomy of the conduction system of the heart. *In* Hurst JW (ed): The Heart. New York, McGraw-Hill, 1978, pp 33–56.
2. James TN: Anatomy of the coronary arteries in health and disease. Circulation 32:1020, 1965.
3. Lev M, Bharati S: Anatomic basis for impulse generation and atrioventricular transmission. *In* Narula OS (ed): His Bundle Electrocardiography and Clinical Electrophysiology. Philadelphia, FA Davis, 1975, p 1.
4. Van der Hauwaert LG, Stroobandt R, Verhaeghe L: Arterial blood supply of the atrioventricular node and main bundle. Br Heart J 34:1045, 1972.
5. Frink RJ, James TN: Normal blood supply to the human His bundle and proximal bundle branches. Circulation 47:8, 1973.
6. Massing GK, James TN: Anatomical configuration of the His bundle and bundle branches in the human heart. Circulation 53:609, 1976.
7. Pruitt RD, Essex HE, Burchell BH: Studies on the spread of excitation through the ventricular myocardium. Circulation 3:418, 1951.
8. Hunt D, Lie JT, Vihru J, et al: Histopathology of heart block complicating acute myocardial infarction: Correlation with the His bundle electrogram. Circulation 48:1252, 1973.
9. Sutton R, Davies M: The conduction system in acute myocardial infarction complicated by heart block. Circulation 38:987, 1968.
10. Blondeau M, Maurice P, Reverdy, et al: Troubles du rythme et de la conduction auriculo-ventriculaire dans l'infarctus du myocarde récent: Considérations anatomiques. Arch Mal Coeur 60:1733, 1967.
11. Wei JY, Markis JE, Malagold M, et al: Cardiovascular reflexes stimulated by reperfusion of ischemic myocardium in acute myocardial infarction. Circulation 67:796, 1983.
12. Koren G, Weiss AT, Ben-David Y, et al: Bradycardia and hypotension following reperfusion with streptokinase (Bezold-Jarisch reflex): A sign of coronary thrombolysis and myocardial salvage. Am Heart J 112:468, 1986.
13. Berger PB, Ruocco NA, Ryan TJ, et al, and the TIMI II Investigators: Incidence and prognostic implications of heart block complicating inferior myocardial infarction treated with thrombolytic therapy: Results from TIMI II. J Am Coll Cardiol 20:533, 1992.
14. Bilbao FJ, Zabalza IE, Vilanova JR, et al: Atrioventricular block in posterior acute myocardial infarction: A clinicopathologic correlation. Circulation 75:733, 1987.
15. Rosen KM, Ehrsani A, Rahimtoola SH: Myocardial infarction complicated by conduction defect. Med Clin North Am 57:155, 1973.
16. Bassan R, Maia IG, Bozza A, et al: Atrioventricular block in acute inferior wall myocardial infarction: Harbinger of associated obstruction of the left anterior descending coronary artery. J Am Coll Cardiol 8:773, 1986.
17. Clemmensen P, Bates ER, Califf RM, et al, and the TAMI Study Group: Complete atrioventricular block complicating inferior wall acute myocardial infarction treated with reperfusion therapy. Am J Cardiol 67:225, 1991.
18. Cohen HC, Gozo EG Jr, Pick A: The nature and type of arrhythmias in acute experimental hyperkalemia in the intact dog. Am Heart J 82:777, 1971.

19. Sugiura T, Iwasaka T, Takayama Y, et al: The factors associated with fascicular block in acute anteroseptal infarction. Arch Intern Med 148:529, 1988.
20. Rotman M, Wagner GS, Wallace AG: Bradyarrhythmias in acute myocardial infarction. Circulation 45:703, 1972.
21. Hunt D, Lie JY, Vohra J, et al: Histopathology of heart block complicating acute myocardial infarction. Circulation 48:1252, 1973.
22. Wilber D, Walton J, O'Neill W, et al: Effects of reperfusion on complete heart block complicating anterior myocardial infarction. J Am Coll Cardiol 4:1315, 1984.
23. Norris RM: Heart block in posterior and anterior myocardial infarction. Br Heart J 31:352, 1969.
24. Brown RW, Hunt D, Sloman JG: The natural history of atrioventricular conduction defects in acute myocardial infarction. Am Heart J 78:460, 1969.
25. Ginks WR, Sutton R, Winston DH, et al: Long-term prognosis after acute myocardial infarction with atrioventricular block. Br Heart J 39:186, 1977.
26. Lie KI, Wellens HJ, Schuilenburg RM, et al: Factors influencing prognosis of bundle branch block complicating acute antero-septal infarction. Circulation 50:935, 1974.
27. Hindman MC, Wagner GS, JaRo H, et al: The clinical significance of bundle branch block complicating acute myocardial infarction. 2. Indications for temporary and permanent pacemakers. Circulation 58:689, 1978.
28. Forsberg SA, Juul-Moller S: Myocardial infarction complicated by heart block: Treatment and long-term prognosis. Acta Med Scand 206:483, 1979.
29. Tans AC, Lie KI, Durrer D: Clinical setting and prognostic significance of high degree atrioventricular block in acute inferior myocardial infarction: A study of 144 patients. Am Heart J 99:4, 1980.
30. Greenfield L, DeGuzman M, Haywood LJ: Atrioventricular block and acute myocardial infarction: Factors influencing morbidity and mortality. Unpublished data, 1994.
31. Rosen KM, Loeb HS, Chiquimia R, et al: Site of heart block in acute inferior myocardial infarction. Circulation 42:925, 1970.
32. Kostuk WJ, Beanlands DS: Complete heart block with acute myocardial infarction. Am J Cardiol 26:380, 1970.
33. Bigger JT, Dresdale RJ, Heissenbuttal RH, et al: Ventricular arrhythmias in ischemic heart disease: Mechanism, prevalence, significance, and management. Prog Cardiovasc Dis 19:255, 1977.
34. Mullins CB, Atkins JM: Prognoses and management of ventricular conduction blocks in acute myocardial infarction. Mod Concepts Cardiovasc Dis 45:129, 1976.
35. Hindman MC, Wagner GS, JaRo H, et al: The clinical significance of bundle branch block complicating acute myocardial infarction. 1. Clinical characteristics, hospital mortality, and one-year follow-up. Circulation 58:679, 1978.
36. Norris RM, Croxson MS: Bundle branch block in acute myocardial infarction. Am Heart J 79:728, 1970.
37. Scheinman M, Brenman B: Clinical and anatomic implication of intraventricular conduction blocks in acute myocardial infarction. Circulation 46:753, 1972.
38. Lie KI, Wellens HJ, Schuilenburg RM: Bundle branch block and acute myocardial infarction. *In* Wellens HJ, Lie KI, Janse MI (eds): The Conduction System of the Heart: Structure, Function, and Clinical Implications. Philadelphia, Lea & Febiger, 1976, pp 662–672.
39. Godman MJ, Lassers BW, Julian DG: Complete bundle branch block complicating acute myocardial infarction. N Engl J Med 282:237, 1970.
40. Scanlon PJ, Pryor R, Blount G: Right bundle branch block associated with left superior or inferior intraventricular block. Circulation 42:1135, 1970.
41. Godman MJ, Alpert BA, Julian DG: Bilateral bundle branch block complicating acute myocardial infarction. Lancet 2:345, 1971.
42. Nimetz AA, Shubrooks SJ, Hutter AM, et al: The significance of bundle branch block during acute myocardial infarction. Am Heart J 90:439, 1975.
43. DeGuzman M, Ahmadpour H, Haywood LJ: Incidence, development, progression, and outcome of atrioventricular block in acute myocardial infarction with bundle branch block: A ten-year analysis. Circulation 64(Suppl IV):743, 1981.
44. Lamas GA, Muller JE, Turi AG, et al: A simplified method to predict occurrence of complete heart block during acute myocardial infarction. Am J Cardiol 57:1213, 1986.
45. Roos C, Dunning AJ: Right bundle branch block and left axis deviation in acute myocardial infarction. Br Heart J 32:847, 1970.
46. Harper R, Hunt D, Vohra J, et al: His bundle electrogram in patients with acute myocardial infarction complicated by atrioventricular or intraventricular conduction disturbances. Br Heart J 37:705, 1975.
47. Lichstein E, Gupta P, Liu MM, et al: Findings of prognostic value in patients with incomplete bilateral bundle branch block complicating acute myocardial infarction. Am J Cardiol 32:913, 1973.
48. Gould L, Reddy CV, Kim SG, et al: His bundle electrogram in patients with acute myocardial infarction. PACE 2:428, 1979.
49. Atkins J, Leshin S, Blomqvist CG, et al: Ventricular conduction blocks and sudden death in acute myocardial infarction. N Engl J Med 288:281, 1973.
50. Ritter WS, Atkins J, Blomqvist G, et al: Permanent pacing in patients with transient trifascicular block during acute myocardial infarction. Am J Cardiol 38:205, 1976.
51. Waugh RA, Wagner GS, Haney TL, et al: Immediate and remote prognostic significance of fascicular block during acute myocardial infarction. Circulation 47:765, 1973.
52. Murphy E, DeMots H, McAnulty J, et al: Prophylactic permanent pacemakers for transient heart block during myocardial infarction? Results of a prospective study. Am J Cardiol 49:952, 1982.
53. Lie K, Liem KL, Schuilenberg RM, et al: Early identification of patients developing late in-hospital ventricular fibrillation after discharge from the coronary care unit: A 5½-year retrospective and prospective study of 1,897 patients. Am J Cardiol 41:674, 1978.
54. Watson RDS, Glover DR, Page AJF, et al: The Birmingham Trial of permanent pacing in patients with intraventricular conduction disorders after acute myocardial infarction. Am Heart J 108:496, 1984.
55. Talwar KK, Kalra GS, Dogra B, et al: Prophylactic permanent pacemaker implantation in patients with anterior wall myocardial infarction complicated by bundle branch block and transient complete atrioventricular block: A prospective long-term study. Indian Heart J 39:22, 1987.
56. Harper R, Hunt D, Vohra J, et al: His bundle electrogram in patients with acute myocardial infarction complicated by atrioventricular or intraventricular conduction disturbances. Br Heart J 37:705, 1975.
57. Gould L, Reddy CVR, Kim SG, et al: His bundle electrogram in patients with acute myocardial infarction. PACE 2:428, 1979.
58. Barold SS: American College of Cardiology/American Heart Association guideline for pacemaker implantation after acute myocardial infarction: What is persistent advanced block at the atrioventricular node? Am J Cardiol 80:770–774, 1997.
59. Topol EJ, Goldschlager N, Ports TA, et al: Hemodynamic benefit of atrial pacing in right ventricular myocardial infarction. Ann Intern Med 96:594, 1982.
60. Chamberlain DA, Leinbach RC, Vassaux CE, et al: Sequential atrioventricular pacing in heart block complicating acute myocardial infarction. N Engl J Med 282:577, 1970.
61. Nordlander R, Hedman A, Pehrsson SK: Rate-responsive pacing and exercise capacity: A comment. PACE 12:749, 1989.
62. Luceri RM, Brownstein SL, Vardeman L, et al: PR interval behavior during exercise: Implications for physiological pacemakers. PACE 13:1719, 1990.
63. Dreifus LS, Fisch C, Griffin JC, et al: Guidelines for implantation of cardiac pacemaker and antiarrhythmia devices: A report of the American College of Cardiology/American Heart Association Task Force on Assessment of Diagnostic and Therapeutic Cardiovascular Procedures (Committee on Pacemaker Implantation). Circulation 84:455, 1991.
64. Zehender M, Buchner C, Meinertz T, et al: Prevalence, circumstances, mechanisms, and risk stratification of sudden cardiac death in unipolar single-chamber ventricular pacing. Circulation 85:596, 1992.
65. Furman S: Prevalence, circumstances, mechanisms, and risk stratification of sudden cardiac death in artificial ventricular pacing. Circulation 85:843, 1992.
66. Rahimtoola SH: The hibernating myocardium. Am Heart J 117:211, 1989.
67. Braunwald E, Rutherford JD: Reversible ischemic left ventricular dysfunction: Evidence for the "hibernating myocardium." J Am Coll Cardiol 8:1467, 1986.
68. Melgarejo-Moreno A, Galcera-Tomas J, Garcia-Alberola A, et al: Incidence, clinical characteristics, and prognostic significance of right bundle-branch block in acute myocardial infarction: A study in the thrombolytic area. Circulation 196:1139–114, 1997.
69. Wiseman A, Ohman EM, Wharton JM: Trasient reversal of bifascicu-

lar block during acute myocardial infarction with reperfusion therapy: A word of caution. Am Heart J 117:1381, 1989.

70. Josephson ME, Seides SF: Clinical Cardiac Electrophysiology. Philadelphia, Lea & Febiger, 1979, pp 79–101.

71. Puech P, Grolleau R, Guimond C: Incidence of different types of A-V block and their localization by His bundle recordings. In Wellens HJJ, Lie KI, Janse MJ (eds): The Conduction System of the Heart: Structure, Function, and Clinical Implications. Leiden, H.E. Stenfert Kroese BV, 1976, pp 467–484.

72. Sherif N, Scherlag BJ, Lazzara R, et al: The pathophysiology of tachycardia-dependent paroxysmal atrioventricular block after myocardial ischemia: Experimental and clinical observations. Circulation 50:515, 1974.

73. Rosenbaum MB, Elizari MV, Levi RJ, et al: Paroxysmal atrioventricular block related to hyperpolarization and spontaneous diastolic depolarization. Chest 63:678, 1973.

74. Lev M: The pathology of complete AV block. Prog Cardiovasc Dis 6:317, 1964.

75. Lenegre J: Etiology and pathology of bilateral bundle branch fibrosis in relation to complete heart block. Prog Cardiovasc Dis 6:409, 1964.

76. Narula OS: Atrioventricular conduction defects in patients with sinus bradycardia. Circulation 44:1096, 1971.

77. Evans R, Shaw DB: Pathological studies in sino-atrial disorder (sick sinus syndrome). Br Heart J 39:778, 1977.

78. Rosenqvist M, Obel IWP: Atrial pacing and the risk for AV block: Is there a time for change in attitude? PACE 12:97, 1989.

79. Sutton R, Kenny RA: The natural history of sick sinus syndrome. PACE 9:1110, 1986.

80. Caspi J, Amar R, Elami A, et al: Frequency and significance of complete atrioventricular block after coronary artery bypass grafting. Am J Cardiol 63:526, 1989.

81. Keefe DL, Griffin JC, Harrison DC, et al: Atrioventricular conduction abnormalities in patients undergoing isolated aortic or mitral valve replacement. PACE 8:393, 1985.

82. Rosenbaum MB, Corrado G, Oliveri R, et al: Right bundle branch block with left anterior hemiblock in surgically induced tetralogy of Fallot. Am J Cardiol 26:12, 1970.

83. Van Lier TA, Harinck E, Hitchcock JF: Complete right bundle branch block after surgical closure of permembranous ventricular septal defect. Eur Heart J 6:959, 1985.

84. Maron BJ, Merrill WH, Freier PA, et al: Long-term clinical course and symptomatic status of patients after operation for hypertrophic subaortic stenosis. Circulation 57:1205, 1978.

85. Ferguson TB Jr, Cox JL: Surgical treatment for the Wolff-Parkinson-White syndrome: The endocardial approach. In Zipes DP, Jalife J (eds): Cardiac Electrophysiology: From Cell to Bedside. Philadelphia, WB Saunders, 1990, pp 897–906.

86. Chu A, Califf RM, Pryor DB, et al: Prognostic effect of bundle branch block related to coronary artery bypass grafting. Am J Cardiol 59:798, 1987.

87. Glikson M, Dearani JA, Hyberger LK, et al: Indications, effectiveness, and long-term dependency in permanent pacing after cardiac surgery. Am J Cardiol 80:1309, 1997.

88. Baerman JM, Kirsh MM, de Buitleir M, et al: Natural history and determinants of conduction defects following coronary artery bypass surgery. Ann Thorac Surg 44:150, 1987.

89. Anderson DJ, Bulkley BH, Hutchins GM: A clinicopathologic study of prospective valve endocarditis in 22 patients: Morphologic basis for diagnosis and therapy. Am Heart J 94:325, 1977.

90. Maguire JH, Hoff R, Sherlock I, et al: Cardiac morbidity and mortality due to Chagas' disease: Prospective electrocardiographic study of a Brazilian community. Circulation 75:1140, 1987.

91. Hagar JM, Rahimtoola SH: Chagas' heart disease. Curr Probl Cardiol XX(12):825–928, 1995.

92. Hagar JM, Rahimtoola SH: Chagas' heart disease in the United States. N Engl J Med 325:763–768, 1991.

93. Steere AC: Lyme disease. N Engl J Med 321:586, 1989.

94. Steere AC, Batsford WP, Weinberg M, et al: Lyme carditis: Cardiac abnormalities of Lyme disease. Ann Intern Med 93(Pt 1):8, 1980.

95. VanderLinde MR, Crijns HJGM, DeKoning J, et al: Range of atrioventricular conduction disturbances in Lyme borreliosis: A report of four cases and review of other published reports. Br Heart J 131:162, 1990.

96. McAlister HF, Klementowicz PT, Andrews C, et al: Lyme carditis: An important cause of reversible heart block. Ann Intern Med 110:339, 1989.

97. Kimball SA, Janson PA, LaRaia PJ: Complete heart block as the sole presentation of Lyme disease. Arch Intern Med 149:1897, 1989.

98. Cohen IS, Bharati S, Glass J, et al: Radiotherapy as a cause of complete atrioventricular block in Hodgkin's disease. Arch Intern Med 141:676, 1981.

99. Almange C, Lebrestec T, Louvet M, et al: Bloc auriculo-ventriculaire complet par métastase cardiaque: A propos d'une observation. Sem Hôp Pans 54:1419, 1978.

100. Perloff JK: The heart in neuromuscular disease. In O'Rourke RA (ed): Current Problems in Cardiology. Chicago, Yearbook, 1986, pp 513–557.

101. Wynne J, Braunwald E: The cardiomyopathies and myocarditides. In Braunwald E (ed): Heart Disease: A Textbook of Cardiovascular Medicine, 4th ed. Philadelphia, WB Saunders, 1992, pp 1349–1450.

102. Hurd ER: Extraarticular manifestations of rheumatoid arthritis. Semin Arthritis Rheum 8:151, 1979.

103. Owen DS: Connective tissue diseases and the cardiovascular system: A review. Virginia Med 110:426, 1983.

104. Janosik DL, Osborn TG, Moore TL, et al: Heart in systemic sclerosis. Semin Arthritis Rheum 19:191, 1989.

105. Rozanski JJ, Castellanos A, Sheps D, et al: Paroxysmal second-degree AV block induced by exercise. Heart Lung 9:887, 1980.

106. Donzeau JP, Dechandol AM, Bergeal A, et al: Blocs auriculo-ventriculaires survenant à l'effort: Considerations générales à propos de 14 cas. Coeur 15:513, 1985.

107. Woelfel AK, Simpson RJ, Gettes LS, et al: Exercise-induced distal atrioventricular block. J Am Coll Cardiol 2:578, 1983.

108. Petrac J, Gjuroivič J, Vukoskovič D, et al: Clinical significance and natural history of exercise-induced atrioventricular block. In Belhassen B, Feldman S, Copperman Y (eds): Cardiac Pacing and Electrophysiology, Proceedings of the VIII World Symposium on Cardiac Pacing and Electrophysiology. Jerusalem, R & L Creative Communications, 1987, p 265.

109. Huycke EC, Card HG, Sobol SM, et al: Postexertional cardiac systole in a young man without organic heart disease. Ann Intern Med 106:844, 1987.

110. Strasberg B, Lam W, Swiryn S, et al: Symptomatic spontaneous paroxysmal AV nodal block due to localized hyperresponsiveness of the AV node to vagotonic reflexes. Am Heart J 103:795, 1982.

111. Zaman L, Moleiro F, Rozanski JJ, et al: Multiple electrophysiologic manifestations and clinical implications of vagally mediated AV block. Am Heart J 106:92, 1983.

112. Jonas EA, Kosowsky BD, Ramaswamy K: Complete His-Purkinje block produced by carotid massage. Circulation 50:192, 1974.

113. Hart G, Oldershaw PJ, Cull RE, et al: Syncope caused by cough-induced complete atrioventricular block. PACE 5:564, 1982.

114. Wik B, Hillestad L: Deglutition syncope. Br Med J 3:747, 1975.

115. Mymin D, Mathewson FAL, Tate RB, et al: The natural history of first-degree atrioventricular heart block. N Engl J Med 315:1183, 1986.

116. Zornosa JP, Crossley GH, Haisty WK Jr, et al: Pseudopacemaker syndrome: A complication of radiofrequency ablation of the AV junction [Abstract]. PACE 15:590, 1992.

117. Kim YH, O'Nunain S, Trouton T, et al: Pseudo-pacemaker syndrome following inadvertent fast pathway ablation for atrioventricular nodal reentrant tachycardia. J Cardiovasc Electrophysiol 4:178, 1993.

118. Strasberg B, Amat-Y-Leon F, Dhingra RC, et al: Natural history of second-degree atrioventricular nodal block. Circulation 63:1043, 1981.

119. Shaw DB, Kerwick CA, Veale D, et al: Survival in second-degree atrioventricular block. Br Heart J 53:587, 1985.

120. Dhingra RC, Palileo E, Strasberg B, et al: Significance of the HV interval in 517 patients with chronic bifascicular block. Circulation 64:1265, 1981.

121. McAnulty JH, Rahimtoola SH, Murphy E, et al: Natural history of "high risk" bundle branch block: Final report of a prospective study. N Engl J Med 307:137, 1982.

122. Scheinman MM, Peters RW, Morady F, et al: Electrophysiologic studies in patients with bundle branch block. PACE 6:1157, 1983.

123. Click RL, Gersh BJ, Sugrue DD, et al: Role of invasive electrophysiologic testing in patients with symptomatic bundle branch block. Am J Cardiol 59:817, 1987.

124. Morady F, Higgins J, Peters RW, et al: Electrophysiologic testing in bundle branch block and unexplained syncope. Am J Cardiol 54:587, 1984.

125. Linzer M, Prystowsky EN, Devine GW, et al: Predicting the outcomes of electrophysiologic studies of patients with unexplained syncope:

Preliminary validation of a derived model. J Gen Intern Med 6:113, 1991.

126. Brignole M, Giafranchi L, Menozzi C, et al: Assessment of atrioventricular junction ablation and DDDR mode-switching pacemaker versus pharmacological treatment in patients with severely symptomatic paroxysmal atrial fibrillation: A randomized controlled study. Circulation 96:2617, 1977.

127. Kay GN, Ellenbogen KA, Guidici M, et al: The Ablate and Pace Trial: A prospective study of catheter ablation of the AV conduction system and permanent pacemaker implantation for treatment of atrial fibrillation. J Intervent Cardiac Electrophysiol 2:121, 1998.

128. Jackman WM, Wang X, Friday KJ, et al: Catheter ablation of atrioventricular junction with radiofrequency current in 17 patients: Comparison of standard and large-tip catheter electrodes. Circulation 83:1562, 1991.

129. Olgin JE, Scheinman MM: Comparison of high-energy direct current and radiofrequency catheter ablation of the atrioventricular junction. J Am Coll Cardiol 21:557, 1993.

130. Morady F, Calkins H, Langberg J, et al: A prospective randomized comparison of direct current and radiofrequency ablation of the atrioventricular junction. J Am Coll Cardiol 21:102, 1993.

131. Garratt CJ, Skehan JD, Payne GE, Stafford PJ: Effect of sequential radiofrequency ablation lesions at fast and slow atrioventricular nodal pathway positions in patients with paroxysmal atrial fibrillation. Heart 75:502–508, 1996.

132. Zipes DP: Second-degree atrioventricular block. Circulation 60:465, 1979.

133. Cabeen WR, Roberts NK, Child JS: Recognition of the Wenckebach phenomenon. West J Med 129:521, 1978.

134. Denes P, Levy L, Pick A, Rosen KM: The incidence of typical and atypical A-V Wenckebach periodicity. Am Heart J 89:26, 1975.

135. Ursell S, Habbab MA, El-Sherif N: Atrioventricular and intraventricular conduction disorders: Clinical aspects. In El-Sherif N, Samet P (eds): Cardiac Pacing and Electrophysiology, 3rd ed. Philadelphia, WB Saunders, 1991, pp 140–169.

136. Lange HW, Ameisen O, Mack R, et al: Prevalence and clinical correlates on non-Wenckebach narrow complete second-degree atrioventricular block detected by ambulatory ECG. Am Heart J 115:114, 1988.

137. DeMotss H, Brodeur MTH, Rahimtoola SH: Concealed sinus rhythm: A cause of misdiagnosis of digitalis intoxication. Circulation 50:632–633, 1974.

138. Bauernfeind RA, Welch WJ, Brownstein SL: Distal atrioventricular conduction system function. Cardiol Clin 4:417, 1986.

139. Zipes DP, Gettes LS, Akhtar M, et al: Guidelines for clinical intracardiac electrophysiologic studies: A report of the American College of Cardiology/American Heart Association Task Force on Assessment of Diagnostic and Therapeutic Cardiovascular Procedures. J Am Coll Cardiol 14:1827, 1989.

140. Dhingra RC, Wyndham C, Bauernfeind R, et al: Significance of block distal to the His bundle induced by atrial pacing in patients with chronic bifascicular block. Circulation 60:1455, 1979.

141. Scheinman MM, Weiss AN, Shaffar A, et al: Electrophysiologic effects of procainamide in patients with interventricular conduction delay. Circulation 49:522, 1974.

142. Josephson ME: Clinical Cardiac Electrophysiology: Techniques and Interpretations, 2nd ed. Philadelphia, Lea & Febiger, 1992, pp 117–149.

143. Bergfeldt L, Rosenqvist M, Vallin H, et al: Disopyramide-induced second- and third-degree atrioventricular block in patients with bifascicular block: An acute stress test to predict atrioventricular block progression. Br Heart J 53:328, 1985.

144. Tonkin AM, Heddle WF, Tornos P: Intermittent atrioventricular block: Procainamide administration as a provocative test. Aust N Z J Med 8:594, 1978.

145. Fujimura O, Yee R, Klein GJ, et al: The diagnostic sensitivity of electrophysiologic testing in patients with syncope caused by transient bradycardia. N Engl J Med 321:1703, 1989.

146. Frye RL, Collins JJ, DeSanctis RW, et al: Guidelines for permanent cardiac pacemaker implantation, May 1984. A report of the Joint American College of Cardiology/American Heart Association Task Force on Assessment of Cardiovascular Procedures (Subcommittee on Pacemaker Implantation). Circulation 70:331A, 1984.

147. Dreifus LS, Fisch C, Griffin JC, et al: Guidelines for implantation of cardiac pacemakers and antiarrhythmia devices: A Report of the American College of Cardiology/American Heart Association Task Force on Assessment of Diagnostic and Therapeutic Cardiovascular Procedures (Subcommittee on Pacemaker Implantation). J Am Coll Cardiol 18:1, 1991.

148. Gregoratos G, Cheitlin MD, Conill A, et al. ACC/AHA guidelines for implantation of cardiac pacemakers and antiarrhythmia devices: A report of the American College of Cardiology/American Heart Association Task Force on Practice Guidelines. J Am Coll Cardiol 31:1175, 1998.

149. Barold SS: ACC/AHA guidelines for implantation of cardiac pacemakers: How accurate are the definitions of atrioventricular and intraventricular conduction blocks? PACE 16:1221, 1993.

150. Johansson BW: Complete heart block: A clinical hemodynamic and pharmacological study in patients with and without an artificial pacemaker. Acta Med Scand 180(Suppl 451):1, 1966.

151. Edhag O, Swahn A: Prognosis of patients with complete heart block or arrhythmic syncope who were not treated with artificial pacemakers. Acta Med Scand 200:457, 1976.

152. Edhag O: Long-term cardiac pacing: Experience of fixed-rate pacing with an endocardial electrode in 260 patients. Acta Med Scand 502(Suppl):64, 1969.

153. Alpert MA, Curtiss JJ, Sanfelippo JF, et al: Comparative survival after permanent ventricular and dual-chamber pacing for patients with chronic high-degree atrioventricular block with and without preexistent congestive heart failure. J Am Coll Cardiol 7:925, 1986.

154. Linde-Edelstam C, Gulberg B, Norlander R, et al: Longevity in patients with high-degree atrioventricular block paced in the atrial synchronous mode or the fixed-rate ventricular inhibited mode. PACE 15:304, 1992.

155. Dhingra RC, Denes P, Wu D, et al: The significance of second-degree atrioventricular block and bundle branch block: Observations regarding site and type of block. Circulation 49:638, 1974.

156. Lau CP: Rate-Adaptive Cardiac Pacing: Simple and Dual Chamber. Mt Kisco, NY, Futura, 1993, pp 249–264.

157. Antonioli GE, Anscani L, Barbieri D, et al: Single-lead VDD pacing. In Barold SS, Mugica J (eds): New Perspectives in Cardiac Pacing 3. Mt Kisco, NY, Futura, 1993, pp 359–381.

158. Lau CP, Tai YT, Li JPS, et al: Initial clinical experience with a single pass VDDR pacing system. PACE 15(Pt II):1894, 1992.

159. Antonioli GE, Ansani L, Barbieri D, et al: Italian multicenter study on a single-lead VDD pacing system using a narrow atrial dipole spacing. PACE 15(Pt II):1890, 1992.

160. Sermasi S, Marconi M: VDD single pass lead pacing: Sustained pacemaker-mediated tachycardias unrelated to retrograde atrial activation. PACE 15(Pt II):1902, 1992.

161. Rosenthal E, Bostock J, Qureshi SA, et al: Single pass VDD pacing in children and adolescents. PACE 20(Pt I):1975, 1997.

162. Rosenheck AS, Elami A, Amikam S, et al: Single pass VDD pacing in children and adolescents. PACE 20:1961, 1997.

163. Ramsdale DR, Charles RG: Rate-responsive ventricular pacing: Clinical experience with the RS4-SRT pacing system. PACE 8:378, 1985.

164. Nakata Y, Ogura S, Tokano T, et al: VDD pacing with a previously implanted single-lead system. PACE 15(Pt I):1425, 1992.

165. Lau CP, Leung S-K, Lee IS-F: Comparative evaluation of acute and long-term clinical performance of two single lead atrial synchronous ventricular (VDD) pacemakers. PACE 19(Pt. I):1574, 1996.

166. Gross JN, Moser S, Benedek ZM, et al: DDD pacing mode survival in patients with a dual-chamber pacemaker. J Am Coll Cardiol 19:1536, 1992.

167. Naegeli B, Straumann E, Gerber A, et al: A new approach for DDD(R) pacing using a single-pass DDD lead. Am J Cardiol 80:643, 1997.

168. Wish M, Fletcher RD, Gottdiener JS, et al: Importance of left atrial timing in the programming of dual-chamber pacemakers. Am J Cardiol 60:566, 1987.

169. Daubert C, Ritter P, Mabo P, et al: AV delay optimization in DDD and DDDR pacing. In Barold SS, Mugica J (eds): New Perspectives in Cardiac Pacing 3. Mt Kisco, NY, Futura, 1993, pp 259–287.

170. Ovsycher I, Zimlicheman R, Katz A, et al: Measurement of cardiac output by impedance cardiography in pacemaker patients at rest: Effects of various atrioventricular delays. J Am Coll Cardiol 21:761, 1993.

171. Haskell RJ, French WJ: Physiological importance of different atrioventricular intervals to improved exercise performance in patients with dual-chamber pacemakers. Br Heart J 61:46, 1989.

Chapter 18

Carotid Sinus Hypersensitivity and Neurally Mediated Syncope

Robert S. Sheldon and Fredrick J. Jaeger

The neurally mediated syncope syndromes constitute a complex collection of clinical disorders of heart rate and blood pressure regulation, all caused by exaggerated or overly compensating inherent autonomic reflexes[1-4] (Table 18–1). Many of these disorders include bradycardia as a crucial component; hence, permanent cardiac pacing has been promulgated as a therapy for some. In particular, permanent cardiac pacing has been under increasing scrutiny as a therapeutic intervention for carotid sinus syncope (CSS) and vasovagal syncope (VVS), the most common of the neurally mediated syncopes.

VVS generally has its onset at a much younger age, is usually associated with some warning (the "prodrome"), occurs in the absence of any underlying structural heart disease, and, if left untreated for rare or occasional episodes, usually results in spontaneous resolution. In contradistinction, CSS generally is a disease of the elderly occurring in the presence of underlying structural heart disease (usually coronary artery disease). In untreated cases, there may be progression and increased severity of symptoms until therapy is initiated, usually with permanent pacing.

Syncope, defined as the transient loss of consciousness with subsequent complete resolution and without focal neurologic deficits, occurs as a consequence of critical cerebral hypoperfusion, depriving the brain of sufficient oxygen to maintain function. Although significant strides have been made in establishing standardized nomenclature, many investigators are continuously trying to reinvent VVS and have applied a bewildering range of synonyms, including ventricular syncope, empty heart syndrome, neurocardiogenic syncope, neurally mediated hypotension bradycardia, and many other permutations. Several authors have used the term *neurally mediated syncope* interchangeably with VVS.[5, 6] We prefer the term VVS, partly in homage to Sir Thomas Lewis, and also to be consistent with its traditional usage.[7]

Although VVS and CSS reflect a relative hypersensitivity of a specific autonomic nervous system reflex, these disorders are distinct, with unique clinical characteristics, patient demographics, and pathophysiologic mechanisms. Both disorders can be diagnosed by relatively noninvasive and simple tests, which can be applied and interpreted with a fair amount of certainty. These tests, carotid sinus massage for carotid sinus hypersensitivity (CSH) and the head-up tilt table test (also called *upright tilt*) for VVS, are reviewed in detail later. These maneuvers are extremely valuable in the diagnosis of syncope of undetermined origin and should be incorporated fairly early in the diagnostic algorithm in patients with low probability of an arrhythmic cause of their syncope (i.e., lack of structural heart disease) (Fig. 18–1).

That two such divergent clinical entities as CSS and VVS shared common pathophysiologic etiologies was first suggested by Sir Thomas Lewis in 1932, in his intriguingly entitled paper, "Vasovagal syncope and carotid sinus mechanism," in which he first proposed the term *vasovagal syn-*

Table 18–1. Neurally Mediated Syncope

Vasovagal syncope
Carotid sinus syncope
Tussive syncope (may have multifactorial causes)
Glossopharyngeal neuralgia and deglutition syncope
Pallid breath-holding spells
Aortic stenosis
Hypertrophic obstructive cardiomyopathy
Pacemaker syncope
Syncope secondary to pulmonary hypertension
Micturition syncope
Mess trick (hyperventilation and Valsalva maneuver)
Diving reflex
Tachyarrhythmias (syncope from atrial fibrillation, supraventricular
   tachycardia, and ventricular tachycardia may have neurally mediated
   reflex component causing hypotension)

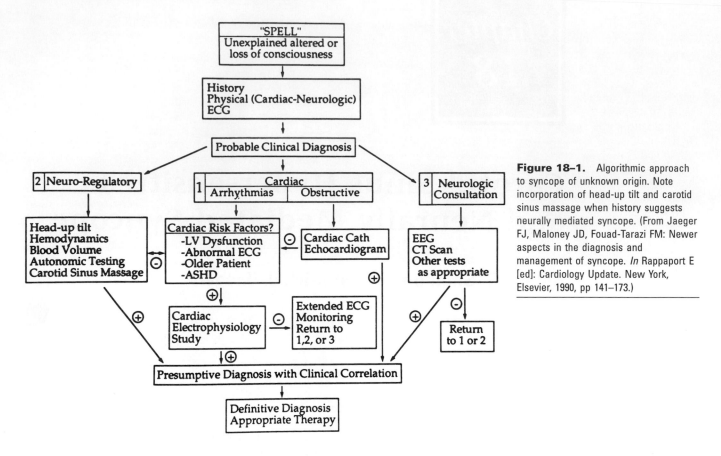

Figure 18–1. Algorithmic approach to syncope of unknown origin. Note incorporation of head-up tilt and carotid sinus massage when history suggests neurally mediated syncope. (From Jaeger FJ, Maloney JD, Fouad-Tarazi FM: Newer aspects in the diagnosis and management of syncope. *In* Rappaport E [ed]: Cardiology Update. New York, Elsevier, 1990, pp 141–173.)

cope.[7] The pathophysiologies of the two distinct disorders, CSS and VVS, are discussed separately in this chapter. In general, several statements can be made regarding the neurally mediated syncopes. All forms involve an abnormality in the reflex arc consisting of neural afferents, central nervous system (CNS) (especially the vasomotor regions of the medulla), and the neural efferents. The specific routes of these connections vary and are shown in Figure 18–2.[8]

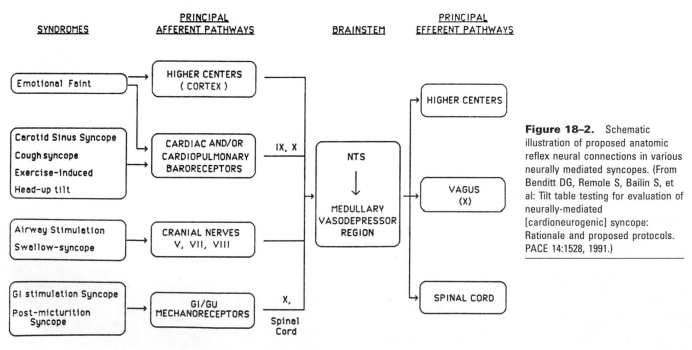

Figure 18–2. Schematic illustration of proposed anatomic reflex neural connections in various neurally mediated syncopes. (From Benditt DG, Remole S, Bailin S, et al: Tilt table testing for evaluation of neurally-mediated [cardioneurogenic] syncope: Rationale and proposed protocols. PACE 14:1528, 1991.)

Since the first edition of this text, many pathophysiologic, technical, and clinical advances have occurred in the neurally mediated syncopes, particularly in our understanding and approach to VVS. The past 5 years have seen the first consensus statements on head-up tilt table testing methodology, including indications for and standardization of interpretation of these tests. Similarly, expert panels on the topics of employment of and driving by patients with neurally mediated syncopes have convened. As discussed later, several ongoing multicenter prospective studies on permanent pacing for VVS have commenced. Finally, further indications that VVS no longer reflects the "lame child" of electrophysiologists are apparent by specific sessions dealing with VVS at meetings of the American Heart Association, the American College of Cardiology, and the North American Society of Pacing and Electrophysiology and by the fact that VVS has been recently added as a specific heading in MEDLINE.

■ CAROTID SINUS SYNCOPE

Definitions

In this chapter we use the term *carotid sinus hypersensitivity* (CSH) to denote the abnormal responses, either cardioinhibitory or vasodepressor or both, to carotid sinus massage (CSM). Pure cardioinhibitory response is the most common response in CSH, occurring in about 60% to 80% of cases.[9] Pure vasodepressor response, on the other hand, is relatively rare, occurring in only 5% to 10% of cases.[10] The remainder of the CSM responses are of the mixed variety. The incidence of the vasodepressor response, however, may actually be much higher. Underestimation of the vasodepressor component of CSS is a result of the previous difficulty in noninvasively documenting blood pressure decreases in an effective manner. Sphygmomanometer readings may miss the nadir of blood pressure during and after CSM. Also, the vasodepressor component may start even after CSM is completed and, hence, can demonstrate significant latency. Finally, because the hypotensive response during CSM may be missed with the patient supine, CSM should be performed not only with the patient supine but also with the patient in an upright posture, either sitting or, as many have done, during upright tilt. Finger plethysmography, and obviously an arterial line, can be used to overcome the limitations of the standard blood pressure cuff. McIntosh and colleagues[11] performed comprehensive CSM evaluations on patients with unexplained syncope, falls, and dizziness. They found the incidence of a predominantly vasodepressor component to be 37%, cardioinhibitory to be 29%, and the mixed type to be 34%. The term CSS, although used liberally by others, is reserved in this chapter for those patients with documented CSH and consistent clinical history, following elimination of all other potential causes of syncope. Historical features that strongly suggest CSS are syncope or near syncope occurring during carotid sinus stimulation, typical clinical spells reproduced during CSM, or fortuitous Holter monitoring or other documentation of asystole during syncope following maneuvers that could presumably stimulate the carotid sinus.[12–16] As discussed later, CSH is relatively common in healthy people and in patients without syncope, but true CSS is rare.

Pathophysiology of Carotid Sinus Hypersensitivity

The carotid sinus reflex has been recognized for many years as an integral component of the homeostatic mechanisms of blood pressure regulation.[17] Increases in intrasinus pressure stimulate mechanoreceptors, which exit the carotid sinus by Hering's nerve to join the glossopharyngeal (cranial nerve IX) and possibly vagus (cranial nerve X) nerves, terminating in the brain stem. These nerves then travel to peripheral end organs both through vagal efferents, which reflexly augment cardiac vagal input, slowing heart rate, and through the spinal cord to inhibit peripheral sympathetic activity in skeletal vasculature, resulting in peripheral vasodilation. The end result, in concert with other baroreceptors, is maintenance of blood pressure within a narrow range. The carotid sinus reflex may also suppress or decrease the rate and depth of respiration, although the clinical effect of this function is unknown.

The carotid sinus reflex may be abnormally heightened, causing exaggerated responses of heart rate and blood pressure. The exact site of the abnormality in the reflex loop is not fully understood. On the basis of several studies, however, it appears that the major defect may reside in the CNS component of the reflex arc. Evidence that the abnormality of the reflex arc does not reside in the carotid sinus or in its neural efferents includes the following:

1. The histology of intima and neural terminals of the carotid sinus is essentially normal in CSH.[18]
2. Patients with CSH and CSS may have the reflex activated by other independent vagal mechanisms, such as micturition, defecation, and so forth.[9]
3. The effects of CSM on blood pressure are prolonged and do not terminate abruptly with discontinuation of carotid pressure, although carotid sinus neural output does.[9]

The defect may reside in the afferent limb, although patients with CSS do not demonstrate increased sensitivity to cholinesterase inhibitors.[19] It has also been suggested that central neuropeptides may be involved in the genesis of CSS[18]; however, that is not to say that cardiac abnormalities are irrelevant. Certainly, superimposed abnormalities or disease of the sinoatrial (SA) or atrioventricular (AV) node may act synergistically with abnormal neural output to create the syndrome. It is believed, however, that the bulk of the abnormalities in CSS are present in the CNS, especially the brain stem and cardiovascular regulation centers.

This concept was recently challenged in a study by Tea and associates,[20] in which patients with overt CSS and controls underwent extensive neurophysiologic testing using evoked potentials and electromyography (EMG). Their hypothesis tested the prevailing notion that evoked potentials would uncover a defect in brain stem baroreflex centers (especially nucleus tractus solitarius). Contrary to what was expected, no indirect abnormalities in brain stem function could be found between patients and controls in brain stem somatosensory and auditory evoked potentials, blink reflexes, and sympathetic skin response. The EMG of the sternocleidomastoid muscle, however, was abnormal in most patients with CSS and rarely in control subjects. This suggested to the authors that neuromuscular structures surrounding the carotid sinus (i.e., the sternocleidomastoid muscle) may participate in the genesis of CSS.

From the same center, Blanc and coworkers[21] found similar results in 30 patients (none with known CSS, CSH, or syncope). Sternocleidomastoid EMG results demonstrated significant concordance with CSM responses; that is, abnormal EMGs were associated with abnormal response to CSM, and vice versa. These authors speculated that because denervation of the sternocleidomastoid muscle cannot provide or contribute information to the CNS baroreflex centers, any output from the carotid sinus is inappropriately interpreted as heightened blood pressure. The baroreflex centers then respond by withdrawing peripheral or sympathetic output, leading to slowing of heart rate and drop in blood pressure. Obviously, further studies are required in this area.

Clinical Characteristics

CSS, in contrast to VVS, tends to occur in older patients and demonstrates a male predominance, as does coronary artery disease (CAD). The incidence of CSS, although difficult to state with certainty, was calculated by one center to be 35 per 1 million population per year.[19] The presence of asymptomatic CSH, however, is quite common in adult populations. Brown and colleagues[22] found a positive cardioinhibitory response to CSM in 32% of patients undergoing coronary angiography. In addition, they found that the magnitude of the exaggerated response to CSM was proportional to the severity of the underlying coronary disease. The association of CSS and CSH to CAD has long been recognized. The demonstration of CSH in a patient without other symptoms may therefore suggest the diagnosis of concomitant CAD.

In contrast to CSH, which is quite common, CSS is probably relatively rare, occurring in only 11% to 19% of patients with syncope of undetermined cause.[23] Syncope in patients with CSS tends to occur abruptly, with little or no prodrome, and only half of patients may recognize a precipitating event. Many times no specific maneuver or action can be recalled to have preceded syncope. Historically, tight collars, shaving, head turning (as in looking to back up a car), coughing, heavy lifting, Valsalva maneuver, trumpet playing, and looking up (as in sitting in the front row of a theater) have been reported to initiate events. Syncope has also been described to result from seat belt pressure on the carotid sinus area.[24] It can also occur in the supine position and has been described with sleeping positions that put pressure on the carotid sinus.[25] Other physiologic activities that affect the autonomic milieu, especially vagal, can also precipitate a syncopal episode. These include swallowing, defecation, micturition, and eating.

Intrinsic anatomic distortion of the carotid sinus area, with internal carotid aneurysm, head and neck tumors, or lymphadenopathy, can predispose to CSS.[26, 27] Extrinsic deformation of the carotid sinus with episodic loss of consciousness has also been described with an orthodontic apparatus.[28] CSS may also be provoked during wrestling, although it is probably rare in children.[29] Another rare cause of CSS was reported in a study by Romano and coauthors,[30] in which a young patient with multiple symmetric lipomatosis had lipomatous involvement of the carotid sinus region, resulting in CSS. The coexistence of carotid artery stenosis and CSS has been reported. In these patients, transient ischemic attacks (TIAs) may be precipitated during

episodes of CSH.[31] These structural abnormalities, however, are unusual causes of CSS. In most cases, patients with CSS have essentially normal neck anatomy. Although rare, syncope associated with head flexion or extension can also occur with mechanical obstruction of the vertebral arteries.

Symptoms of CSS range from dizziness to profound loss of consciousness, occasionally with significant injuries. Episodes of syncope tend to occur abruptly with CSS; therefore, patients may sustain severe injuries (e.g., fractures, lacerations). Some patients may not recall losing consciousness and may present solely with unexplained falls. Kenny and Traynor[26] reported on patients with CSH who did not recall episodes of loss of consciousness during CSM, presumably because of retrograde amnesia. Of seven elderly patients who had previously suffered falls and developed loss of consciousness during CSM while undergoing upright tilt, five denied their loss of consciousness upon awakening. The assertion that CSS may be more common than previously thought is also supported by the observations from emergency rooms or from so-called "fits, falls, fractures, or syncope" clinics devoted to investigating these disorders, especially in the elderly. Reports from these types of clinics frequently describe a significant incidence of positive CSM responses, suggesting that this disorder is responsible for many unexplained or recurrent falls.[32] Therefore, frequent unexplained falls in the elderly should prompt evaluation for CSH.

The clinical spectrum of CSS may extend to patients with chronic atrial fibrillation and may be a cause of symptoms resulting from ventricular pauses or hypotension. CSM has not been previously studied extensively in patients with atrial fibrillation. Cicogna and coauthors[33] found abnormal responses to CSM and CSS and frequent pauses on Holter monitoring in 10 patients with atrial fibrillation complaining of shortness of breath, angina, syncope, and dizziness, compared with patients with asymptomatic chronic atrial fibrillation. Patients with CSH were given VVI pacemakers and had significant improvement in symptoms. Therefore, CSH may be an important contributor to symptoms of chronic atrial fibrillation, and comprehensive evaluation for CSS should be sought.

Treatment

Carotid Sinus Massage

Technique: CSM can be performed safely and easily at the bedside, ideally with continuous electrocardiographic (ECG) monitoring. Application of pressure to the carotid area is contraindicated in the presence of bruits or a history of cerebral vascular disease, TIAs, or endarterectomies. The carotid sinus is located high in the neck below the angle of the mandible. Sequential application of carotid massage to the left and right carotid arteries should be performed with at least 10 to 20 seconds in between. The duration of carotid massage should be 5 to 10 seconds, and it should be terminated with onset of characteristic asystole. In most series, the predominant responses to CSM were obtained on the right.[12]

In patients undergoing CSM for syncope of undetermined cause, comprehensive evaluation for CSH includes CSM while the patient is both supine and upright. This can be accomplished by having the patient stand erect or elevating the patient on a tilt table during CSM. This postural evaluation during CSM is necessary to unmask an otherwise covert vasodepressor component of CSH. Occasionally, the response to CSM can be augmented or accentuated by simultaneous Valsalva maneuver. This has been particularly helpful in the termination of supraventricular tachycardia (SVT) with CSM.

Responses to CSM that define CSH include cardioinhibitory and vasodepressor responses. A previously described "primary cerebral type" of CSH has now been disproved. The cause of syncope during CSM with this type was probably due to overly aggressive occlusion of the carotid artery, probably in the presence of contralateral vascular disease. This resulted in significantly decreased cerebral blood flow, with loss of consciousness, not caused by a reflex mechanism.

Cardioinhibitory CSH is defined as 3 seconds or greater of ventricular standstill or asystole during CSM. Ventricular asystole usually occurs as a consequence of a sinus pause but can be secondary to AV block as well. Using continuous sinus node electrogram recordings, it has been demonstrated that CSM produces sinus pauses by initiating sinus node exit block.[34] Although the most obvious effect of CSH during asystole is on the sinus node, the profound influence of the autonomic nervous system—particularly the vagus—can be pancardiac and can prevent other lower escape pacemaker foci from discharging.

Typically, in patients with true CSH, the onset of asystole is rapid and may produce prolonged asystolic responses with dramatic loss of consciousness. Invariably, complete recovery is also rapid after cessation of CSM.

A vasodepressor response to CSM is defined as a drop in systolic blood pressure of 50 mm Hg or more during CSM (Fig. 18–3). In patients who have a significant concomitant cardioinhibitory component to CSM, it may be more difficult to demonstrate the vasodepressor response. Various techniques to prevent asystole have been described and include pretreatment with intravenous atropine or temporary ventricular or AV sequential pacing during CSM.[10] Obviously, these techniques are best reserved for the electrophysiology laboratory. If temporary pacing is to be tested, it is necessary to first determine if ventricular pacing results in hypotension

due to ventriculoatrial (VA) conduction and the pacemaker syndrome.

In contrast to the induced cardioinhibitory component of CSH, which starts abruptly and resolves quickly with the discontinuation of CSM, the vasodepressor response may have a more insidious, slower onset and demonstrate a more prolonged resolution (Fig. 18–4). It may be difficult to demonstrate the drop in blood pressure with standard sphygmomanometer methods, and an arterial line can be placed if necessary. Other investigators have used continuous digital plethysmography or the more sophisticated Finipress (Ohmeda, Madison, WI). Either way, simple palpation of the radial or brachial arteries may occasionally be sufficient to confirm suspected hypotension.

The mixed type of CSH consists of varying proportions of vasodepressor and cardioinhibitory components. The mixed type of CSS can be subdivided on the basis of the magnitude of the vasodepressor component.[35] Type I appears to be the predominant cardioinhibitory response, but symptoms persist after atropine. In type II, symptoms are late in onset and continue after abolition of asystole with atropine, indicating a predominant vasodepressor component. Investigators found this subclassification useful in deciding between DVI/DDD and VVI pacemaker modes.[35] Patients with type I CSS and without evidence of orthostatic hypotension, pacemaker syndrome, or VA conduction could receive VVI pacing. Patients with mixed type II CSS should always receive DVI/DDD pacing.

Role of the Electrophysiologic Study: Although the demonstration of a hypersensitive carotid sinus with or without symptoms can be suggestive in a patient with syncope of undetermined cause, it cannot be relied on to be wholly diagnostic. As previously mentioned, CSH is common, particularly in patients with CAD and hypertension. This is exactly the same patient population who may have ventricular tachycardia as a cause of syncope. In 28 patients with syncope who were found to have CSH, 5 of 15 with CAD were found to have sustained monomorphic ventricular tachycardia provoked at comprehensive electrophysiology study.[36] Therefore, the demonstration of CSH in patients afflicted with syncope should not preclude the performance

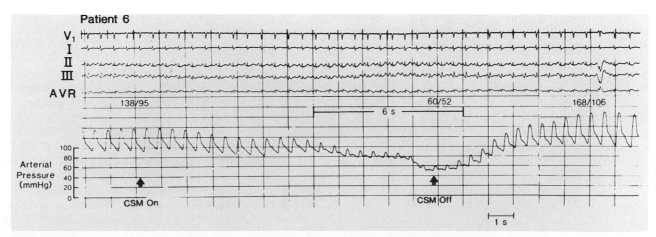

Figure 18–3. Pure vasodepressor response during carotid sinus massage. (From Almquist A, Gornick C, Benson W, et al: Carotid sinus hypersensitivity: Evaluation of the vasodepressor component. Circulation 71:927, 1985. Copyright 1985 American Heart Association.)

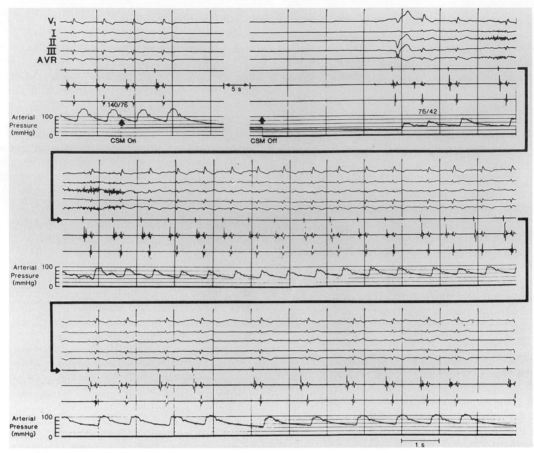

Figure 18–4. Combined cardioinhibitory and vasodepressor response to carotid sinus massage. Note slow return of blood pressure despite resolution of asystole. (From Almquist A, Gornick C, Benson W, et al: Carotid sinus hypersensitivity: Evaluation of the vasodepressor component. Circulation 71:927, 1985. Copyright 1985 American Heart Association.)

of electrophysiology study, particularly in those patients with risk factors for ventricular tachycardia, previous myocardial infarction, cardiomyopathy (dilated or hypertrophic), positive signal-averaged ECGs, or left ventricular dysfunction.

In addition to excluding more potentially lethal causes, such as ventricular tachycardia, in patients with CSH, the electrophysiology study can provide information on sinus node and AV node function. It is presumed that intrinsic abnormalities of these structures can be synergistic, with a tendency toward increased parasympathetic activity, and promote bradycardia and pauses. Also, electrophysiology studies can be used to assess the vasodepressor component of CSH during temporary pacing of the atrium, ventricle, or both sequentially during CSM. Finally, in patients in whom a permanent pacemaker is appropriate therapy, the electrophysiology study can be used to determine the optimal pacing mode. Ideally, as previously mentioned, VVI pacing should be reserved for patients in whom no potential for pacemaker syndrome can be demonstrated or who have chronic atrial fibrillation (in which cardioversion is not a consideration).

Complications: In general, CSM is safe when applied in appropriate circumstances. Rare complications include cerebrovascular accident and TIA, and CSM is contraindi-

cated in patients with a history of these or carotid bruits. Arrhythmic complications have been reported and include asystole and ventricular fibrillation.[37] In a review of 3100 episodes of CSM performed on 1600 patients, there were seven complications (0.14%), all of which were neurologic (e.g., hemiparesis, visual disturbance, TIA) and transient.[38] Therefore, CSM is relatively safe considering the potential benefit when appropriately performed in the evaluation of patients with syncope.

Medical Therapy

When CSS is the likely cause of syncopal episodes, the initial treatment recommendation should be simple elimination of any recognized maneuvers that may precipitate an event. Discontinuation of wearing tight collars and ties and shaving more carefully may be beneficial. If possible, medications (calcium-channel blockers, digoxin, and β-blockers) that may predispose the patient to CSH should be discontinued. Hypovolemia, secondary to diuretics or other causes, may exacerbate the vasodepressor component of CSH and should be corrected. Elimination of diuretics or addition of volume expanders such as Florinef[39] or high salt intake may be helpful.

Given the proven efficacy of pacemaker technology in ameliorating symptoms of CSS, other medical therapy has largely been adjuvant, reserved for cases in which the vasodepressor component of CSS predominates. Analogous to their use in preventing VVS, serotonin reuptake inhibitors (sertraline [Zoloft], paroxetine [Paxil], fluoxetine [Prozac]) may be useful in CSS. In uncontrolled case reports, these medications have been used as ancillary therapy in patients with CSS refractory to permanent pacing.[40] It has also been suggested that these medications can be used as primary therapy in similar cases.[41] Presumably, serotonin reuptake inhibitors work on the baroreflex centers of the brain stem. Serotonin surges in the brain stem can produce sympathetic withdrawal, mimicking the hypotension and bradycardia of neurally mediated syncope. Prolonged treatment with these medications can therefore lead to a downregulation of postsynaptic serotonin receptor density, lessening the response during serotonin surges. Other medications and combinations have also been used in CSS. Proposed combinations include sympathomimetics, such as ephedrine, and β-blockers,[42] although results of these medications generally remain disappointing.

In the prepacemaker era, recalcitrant cases of CSS were treated with carotid sinus denervation by surgical technique.[43] This practice has been largely abandoned owing to the development of hypertensive crisis after carotid sinus denervation. Surgery currently is reserved for CSS that is secondary to head or neck tumors or lymphadenopathy, or is performed in conjunction with carotid endarterectomy or in patients with severe refractory CSS of the pure vasodepressor variety. An additional antiquated treatment of CSS was localized radiation therapy to both carotid sinus regions.

Pacing

For cases of recurrent, frequent, or severe CSS, permanent pacemaker implantation is the conventional therapy, particularly for CSS of the predominant cardioinhibitory type.[44, 45] Although permanent pacing for such cases is almost universally accepted, some controversy exists regarding the pacing mode and the role of pacing for mixed forms of CSS. Even though CSS may have a substantial effect on quality of life, it has not been shown to significantly affect mortality, and patients with CSS who receive therapy do not appear to have worse prognoses than the general population. In a long-term (mean, 44 months) follow-up study by Brignole and colleagues,[46] survival in patients with CSS was not significantly different from that in control patients with syncope of other causes. As expected, mortality was dependent on age, sex, and associated underlying cardiac disease (congestive heart failure, abnormal ECG).[46] Factors relating to CSS, such as the hemodynamic type, severity, and abnormalities of the SA or AV node, were not predictive of prognosis. The overall predicted 5-year survival rate was 73%. Treatment of CSS in these patients was nonrandomized and heterogeneous; therefore, results of therapy could not be interpreted in terms of best treatment modality or effect on mortality.

A comprehensive summary of recent studies of pacing for CSS is shown in Table 18–2.[47–52] It is clear from these

Table 18–2. Pacemaker Therapy for Carotid Sinus Syndrome

Investigators	No. of Patients	No. of Patients Symptom Free at Follow-up (%)	No. of Patients With No Syncope (%)	Mean Follow-up (mo)	Comments
Sugrue et al, 1986					
No treatment	11	7 (64)	3 (73)	39	About 77% of patients had cardiac inhibition only
Pacing	23	16 (69)	21 (91)	23	About 83% of patients had cardiac inhibition only
VVI pacing	11	8 (73)			A total of 26 patients required pacing
DVI pacing	15	13 (87)			All recurrent syncopes in patients with mixed carotid sinus syncope
Anticholinergic drugs	19	15 (79)	15 (79)	41	About 90% of patients had cardiac inhibition only
Huang et al, 1988					
VVI pacing	9		9 (100)	42	All patients but one had cardiac inhibition only
DDD pacing	4		4 (100)	42	
No treatment	8		7 (88)	42	
Morley et al, 1982					
VVI pacing	54	48 (89)		18	5 patients with AAI converted to DDD/DVI and VVI pacing
DVI pacing	13	12 (92)		18	4 patients with VVI converted to DVI pacing
DDD pacing	3	2 (66)		18	
Brignole et al, 1988					
No treatment	19	6 (32)	10 (53)	8.4	63% of patients had cardiac inhibition
Pacing	16	13 (81)	16 (100)	7.2	69% of patients had cardiac inhibition only
VVI pacing	11		11 (100)	7.2	
DDD pacing	5		5 (100)	7.2	

Randomized study: Differences between pacing and no treatment statistically significant.

Brignole et al, 1991					
VVI pacing	26	7 (27)	24 (92)	2	73% of patients had mixed carotid sinus syncope
DDD pacing	26	18 (69)	26 (100)	2	

Crossover study: Differences between VVI and DDD statistically significant for general symptoms but not for syncope.

From Katritsis D, Ward DE, Camm AJ: Can we treat carotid sinus syndrome? PACE 14:1367, 1991.

and many other studies that pacemaker implantation should be reserved for patients with recurrent symptoms and a predominant cardioinhibitory response. Several additional points need to be emphasized. Earlier studies tended to be retrospective reports of pacing practices for CSS and therefore were inherently biased toward patients with a clear diagnosis of CSS who would truly benefit from pacing. More recently, prospective and randomized trials have been performed that examine outcome on the basis of presence of pacing and mode. It is clear that in all cases of CSS, AAI pacing is contraindicated because many patients may eventually demonstrate associated reflex AV block.[53] In general, patients benefit most from AV sequential pacing, even when a significant component of vasodepressor CSS is present. When VVI pacing is to be employed, it is crucial to ascertain susceptibility to pacemaker syndrome. Pacemaker syndrome, a form of neurally mediated vasodepression secondary to an atrial reflex, is frequently accompanied by intact VA conduction.[54] Lack of VA conduction may, therefore, suggest that patients with CSS could receive VVI pacemakers. Lack of VA conduction at a given point in time, however, does not ensure against its future development. Therefore, we again strongly recommend DDD pacemakers for patients with CSS and normal sinus rhythm.

Few studies have examined the role of rate-responsive pacing (DDDR) in CSS. As previously mentioned, many patients with CSS demonstrate evidence of sick sinus syndrome or chronotropic incompetence, either intrinsic or secondary to medications. Therefore, rate-responsive pacing could be beneficial. Also, few studies have prospectively examined pacing with additional rate-drop or hysteresis capabilities. This pacing mode has the theoretical advantage, as is being pursued in VVS, of providing more rapid, higher rate, AV sequential pacing to counteract the vasodepressor component during attacks of CSS.

No large prospective study has evaluated "rate-drop" in CSS thus far; however, the rate-drop investigators group reported on eight patients with CSS and four patients with CSS and VVS who received Thera DR pulse generator (Medtronic, Minneapolis, Minnesota).[55] During follow-up, there was significant reduction in syncopal recurrence. Although there was no control group receiving conventional DDD pacemakers, this certainly suggests a role for rate-drop in CSS. Programmed parameters used for rate-drop in CSS were similar to those used in VVS and are discussed later. This technology is available in several pacemaker models, including Thera DR (Medtronic), Relay and Marathon (Intermedics, Angleton, Texas), and Kappa (Medtronic).

Ultimately, the sine qua non for the diagnosis of CSS is the elimination of symptoms after pacemaker implantation. Predictors of success with permanent pacing include (1) multiple episodes before implantation, (2) episodes that occur while upright or sitting, and (3) episodes that are preceded by a recognized stimulus.[56] In cases of mixed CSH, pacing is frequently used for the bradycardia component and the previously described medications for the vasodepressor component.

When syncope recurs after implantation of a permanent pacemaker, its recurrence is attributed to persistence of the vasodepressor component. This component can be assessed and syncope recurrence predicted or explained with a positive response to head-up tilt table testing.[57]

Natural History

Previously published reports on the natural history of untreated or only medically treated patients with CSS indicated a low incidence of syncope recurrence of up to 25%.[48, 58] These studies, however, were primarily based on retrospective analyses, consisting of nonpaced patients with less severe symptoms of CSS or those in whom the diagnosis was in doubt. Whether there is a significant "spontaneous resolution" of CSS, as is frequently seen in VVS, is uncertain. At least, the persistence of a positive response to CSM in limited numbers of patients has been confirmed.[59] A prospective randomized trial from the group at Hospital of Reggio, Italy, reaffirmed the important role of permanent pacing for CSS.[58] In this study, 60 patients with CSS were randomized to pacing (32 patients) and nonpacing (28 patients) therapy. During follow-up of about 3 years, syncope recurred in 16 patients of the nonpaced group (51%) and in 3 (9%) of the paced group ($P = .002$). This observation confirms the efficiency of pacing for the prevention of syncope due to CSS.

Dangers Associated With Driving

Several panels of experts were convened to address the increasingly important issue of driving, both commercial and private, of patients afflicted with cardiac arrhythmias.[60] Significant portions of their discussions and recommendations were directed at patients with neurally mediated syncope and presyncope. Based on existing data and employing statistics, one panel was able to make preliminary recommendations of symptom-free "probationary periods" before the patient is allowed to return to unrestricted driving (Table 18–3). Obviously, each patient is unique, and the recommendations need to be modified by specific circumstances.

Table 18–3. Driving Recommendations for Patients with Neurally Mediated Syncope and Presyncope*

Type of Syncope	Private	Commercial
VVS—mild	A	B_1
VVS—severe		
Treated	B_3	B_6
Untreated	C	C
CSS—mild	A	A
CSS—severe		
Treated with control	B_1	B_1
Treated with uncertain control	B_3	B_6
Untreated	C	C

VVS, vasovagal syncope or presyncope; CSS, carotid sinus syncope or presyncope; Control was a pause of less than 3 sec with decrease in systolic blood pressure ≤10 mm Hg with carotid sinus massage after therapy.

*A, no driving restrictions; B, driving permitted after controlled arrhythmia is documented for a specified period of time (subscript indicates period of time in months driving is restricted) and an adequate pacemaker follow-up regimen is followed; C, driving completely prohibited.

From Epstein AE, Miles WM, Benditt DG, et al: Personal and public safety issues related to arrhythmias that may affect consciousness: Implications for regulation and physician recommendations. Circulation 94:1147, 1996.

■ VASOVAGAL SYNCOPE

VVS is by far the most common form of all the neurally mediated syncopes. Most who faint probably do not seek medical attention for rare, isolated events, instead ascribing them to environmental, nutritional, or other conditions. Prolonged standing, sight of blood, pain, and fear have been the traditional precipitating stimuli for the "common faint" (Table 18–4). Patients develop nausea, diaphoresis, and subsequent loss of consciousness due to hypotension with or without significant bradycardia or asystole. Return of consciousness after several seconds is the norm, and patients invariably recover fully.

In contrast to these benign forms of VVS, we and others have used the term *malignant VVS* to describe VVS with either little or no prodrome, no recognized precipitating stimulus, or marked bradycardia and asystole accompanying the VVS.[61–65] It is this syndrome that has generated extensive interest in the electrophysiology field. Most patients evaluated for VVS probably fall somewhere between these two extremes.

We prefer the term VVS to signify fainting due to bradycardia and hypotension. Pure vasodepressor reactions, which are much less common, involve only hypotension. Other synonyms for VVS include emotional faint, reflex syncope, empty heart syndrome, neurally mediated syncope, situational syncope, vasomotor syncope, ventricular syncope, neurocardiogenic syncope, hypotension-bradycardia syndrome, and autonomic syncope. In addition, the terms *convulsive syncope* and *venipuncture fits* have been used to describe those patients with VVS who develop generalized muscle movements that may mistakenly resemble epilepsy.[66, 67] The tilt table has been particularly useful in differentiating the diagnosis of these disorders.

The clinical scenario of syncope with documented intermittent sinus pauses or AV block with subsequent demonstration of normal AV node function on electrophysiology study may have several causes, including medication effects, ischemia, and early intrinsic disease of the conduction system but may also be due to abnormal autonomic input to the cardiac conduction system, the so-called extrinsic sick sinus syndrome. In a study by Fujimura and colleagues,[68] 21 patients with syncope and abnormal Holter monitoring findings (e.g., showing sinus pauses on intermittent AV block) underwent comprehensive electrophysiology testing. Abnormalities that could explain the syncope and Holter monitoring findings were demonstrated in only 24% of patients. Head-up tilt table testing was not performed in this patient population and may have identified VVS as the cause of their syncope.

Pathophysiology

It has been about 5 years since the first edition of this text, and thus far, no unified hypothesis encompassing and explaining all the aspects of the pathophysiology of VVS has yet emerged. Although it has been extensively studied, multiple questions still abound.[69–71] It has been proposed that VVS occurring from pain, fear, or emotion ("flight or fight") originates from corticohypothalamic centers, and this has been termed *central type* VVS,[72] presumably arising independent of cardiac receptors. The potential to develop this reflex is present in all humans and in many other mammals. The "conservation-withdrawal" or "playing dead" reactions may be analogous processes.

A second type of vasovagal response, called *peripheral type* VVS, results from stimulation of cardiac receptors. The classic explanation of this type of response is based on animal models that demonstrated left ventricular mechanoceptors and chemoreceptors that responded to intravenous nicotine or deformation from excessive contractions.[73] These receptors, called C fibers, are located primarily in the inferior and posterior portions of the left ventricle and carry impulses from the heart, through vagal afferents, to terminate in the medulla. Once stimulated, these connections reflexly decrease sympathetic output to the peripheral arteriolar vasculature, resulting in vasodilation and hypotension.

Withdrawal of sympathetic innervation to the heart leaves parasympathetic, "vagal" input unopposed, causing bradycardia. This reflex, called the *Bezold-Jarisch* reflex, would thus serve as a brake on an excessively active myocardium.[74] Stated another way, a relatively hypovolemic, vigorously contracting ventricle is the presumed trigger of the reflex. This reflex may also be an important contributor to syncope due to aortic stenosis, hypertrophic obstructive cardiomyopathy, or the hypotension-bradycardia syndrome observed in inferior myocardial infarction and during right coronary artery angiography.[74]

An alternative anatomic trigger to left ventricular mechanoreceptors has also been proposed. Dickinson[75] suggested that sudden deformation or "invagination" of the atria and great veins from hypovolemia may be responsible in a process called *collapse firing*.

The end results of the reflex, once activated, are profound hypotension, bradycardia, and loss of muscle tone with subsequent collapse. Although all humans are capable of initiating the vasovagal response under certain circumstances, it is unclear which defects in the autonomic nervous system can make some persons more susceptible and, hence, can cause a clinical problem. Grubb and associates[76] reported that during VVS episodes, marked paradoxical vasoconstriction of the CNS vasculature can occur that, when combined with other adverse hemodynamic effects, may act synergistically to promote syncope. It has been suggested that presyncopal hyperventilation may cause significant arterial hypocapnia,

Table 18–4. Situations That Provoke Vasovagal Syncope

Fear, anxiety, "flight or fight" response
Pain
Venipuncture
Pregnancy
Prolonged standing "at attention"
Hypovolemia
Anemia
Hemorrhage
Prolonged bedrest
Prolonged head-down tilt
Microgravity
Head-up tilt
Lower-body negative pressure
"First-dose phenomena"
Nitrates
β-Blocker withdrawal

which may produce cerebral vasoconstriction; however, these authors found no evidence of this. Others confirmed the paradoxical presence of cerebral vasoconstriction during orthostatic stress simulated by lower-body negative pressure, but not of a sufficient magnitude to lead to loss of consciousness.[77]

The observation of isolated cerebral vasoconstriction without systemic hypotension or bradycardia has led to the description of a new syndrome called *cerebral syncope*. In this disorder, intense cerebral vasoconstriction (measured by transcranial Doppler ultrasonography) results in syncope in the absence of systemic hypotension.[78] The incidence of this variant of neurally mediated syncope is unknown, but is probably rare, and may explain some cases previously thought to be psychogenic syncope.

Astronauts exposed to microgravity or patients undergoing prolonged head-down tilt (-50 degrees) may be susceptible to a vasovagal-like reaction during upright posture.[79, 80] Attenuation of cardiopulmonary baroreceptors due to sustained central hypervolemia, as seen in space or in the head-down tilt position, with subsequent decrease in blood volume, may be responsible.

Evidence supporting the above physiologic and autonomic changes during VVS can be obtained from a variety of studies. Wallin and Sundlöf[81] demonstrated withdrawal of sympathetic stimulation of the peripheral muscular vasculature (recorded using microneurographic techniques of the peroneal nerve) associated with the onset of VVS, consistent with the hypothesis that neurally mediated vasodilation in the musculature occurs secondarily to sympathetic inhibition. Shalev and coauthors[82] have demonstrated that left ventricular echocardiographic dimensions decrease significantly before onset of VVS during head-up tilt, implying that a hypovolemic ventricle may induce the reaction. Similar findings were reported by Fitzpatrick and associates,[83] who demonstrated decreased left ventricular dimensions and an increase in fractional shortening during echocardiography in patients who develop VVS during head-up tilt.[83]

Neuroendocrine and neurohormonal aspects of the vasovagal syndrome have also been extensively investigated. Serum epinephrine has been observed to significantly increase at the time of VVS induced by head-up tilt,[84] termed the so-called *epinephrine surge*. This increase may be secondary to ensuing hypotension or may be a primary event that precipitates the reflex. This observation tends to further support the beneficial effects of β-blockade in preventing syncope. Evidence that elevated epinephrine was not a primary effect was reported by Calkins and colleagues.[85] Administration of intravenous epinephrine was found to be not as effective as intravenous isoproterenol in initiating vasodepressor responses in susceptible patients. Patients who developed VVS on head-up tilt were also shown to have lower resting norepinephrine levels, which may reflect a relatively heightened vagal state or simply be secondary to their young age.[86]

Various other neuropeptide, neurohumoral, and hormonal agents, such as vasopressin, endorphins, adrenocorticotropic hormone, growth hormone, cortisol, prolactin, and the ubiquitous nitric oxide, have also been implicated as possible mediators in the genesis and expression of VVS.[72, 87–91] It is an interesting historical observation that urine output following a VVS episode is minimal for several hours. This is due

to the release (surge) of antidiuretic hormone (vasopressin) during the spell.[72, 89] Vasopressin may also be responsible for the prolonged pallor following a VVS episode.[89]

That the absence of appropriate vasoconstriction of the peripheral skeletal vasculature is an important component to the vasovagal response has been well established. Whether failure of vasoconstriction mechanism is a primary event or is secondary to the Bezold-Jarisch reflex, however, was examined by Sneddon and colleagues.[92] Patients who eventually developed a positive tilt test (i.e., vasovagal response) were found to demonstrate significantly reduced forearm vascular resistance almost immediately after assuming an upright position on the tilt table, as compared with those who demonstrated a normal tilt response. These data suggest that a heretofore unobserved abnormality in primary vasoconstriction responses may be involved in the pathophysiology of VVS.

Additional insight was provided by Manyari and coauthors.[93] In response to mental stress, patients susceptible to VVS were also found to have abnormal vasomotor responses. During arithmetic challenges, controls demonstrated appropriate forearm vasoconstriction (measured by radionuclide plethysmography). Of patients with a positive tilt test, 52% had abnormal responses, showing either venodilation or no increases in venous tone. Therefore, a potential component of VVS initiation may lie in abnormal reflex venomotor control.

Although Thomson and colleagues[94] could not demonstrate abnormal venoconstriction in the forearm in patients with VVS during low-grade, lower-body negative pressure, they did demonstrate that splenic capacitance vessels failed to venoconstrict during exercise in VVS patients. Again, these findings suggest alternative mechanisms that can precipitate the vasovagal response. Thomson and associates[95] also demonstrated that there is impairment of reflex vasoconstriction and occasional paradoxical vasodilation during lower-body negative pressure in patients with VVS, supporting their hypothesis that patients with VVS have decreased cardiopulmonary baroreceptor sensitivity. These investigations also point out, however, that deficits in the afferent limb of the cardiopulmonary reflex arc may not be the only operative factor in VVS and that this syndrome may result from a variety of heterogeneous mechanisms.

In contrast, postischemic reactive hyperemia–derived measurements of forearm vascular resistance have been shown to be similar in patients with VVS and in controls. Patients with VVS, however, demonstrated paradoxical decreases of brachial artery diameter despite elevated blood pressure, suggesting accentuated adrenergic nervous system response.[96]

The vasovagal reflex may have an important role in the genesis of hypotension and syncope in some supraventricular and ventricular tachycardias. Leitch and coworkers[97] performed the head-up tilt table test in patients with SVT and found no significant differences in tachycardia cycle length between those who developed syncope with SVT and those who did not. This suggested that syncope due to decreased blood pressure was not related to tachycardia rate and may have been related to vasomotor factors. Huikuri and colleagues[98] demonstrated that some patients develop significant slowing of sinus rate during unstable ventricular tachycardia. Although there were several possible explanations for this observation (sinus slowing was due to heightened vagal activity), it does suggest that in some patients the hemodynamic instability of the ventricular tachycardia may be mediated by a reflex mechanism, causing hypotension from vasodepression. It is also interesting to note that atrial fibrillation can occur as a consequence of vasovagal syncope.

Leitch and associates[99] reported on three patients in whom VVS, clinical syncope, and atrial fibrillation were all closely related. During head-up tilt–induced VVS, atrial fibrillation occurred spontaneously in two patients. The third patient demonstrated clinical atrial fibrillation after syncope and had a positive head-up tilt table test without atrial fibrillation. Brignole and colleagues[100] explored this phenomenon in detail and found a high incidence of positive CSM and head-up tilt responses in patients with paroxysmal atrial fibrillation (PAF) and syncope, suggesting a common causality. They proposed two possibilities: that VVS can occur shortly after a paroxysm of atrial fibrillation, or that VVS can actually precipitate atrial fibrillation. We call this "Brignole's syndrome." These scenarios have important clinical implications in evaluating patients with PAF and suggest the possibility of treating at least some patients who have this variant with antiarrhythmics with vagolytic properties, such as disopyramide (a medication that has also been used to treat VVS; see later section, Medical Treatment). It is speculated that atrial fibrillation develops during VVS from marked vagally induced alteration and nonuniformity of atrial refractoriness.

Another important potential contributor in the pathogenesis of VVS is adenosine. Adenosine, an endogenous nucleoside, demonstrates both significant excitatory and inhibitory effects at various levels of the autonomic nervous system, particularly cardiac and vasculature control. Specifically, adenosine has been demonstrated to augment certain cardiac sympathetic afferents, increasing heart rate and blood pressure. This effect, coupled with its direct vasodilatory effect, is reminiscent of augmented sympathetic nervous system tone observed before the onset of VVS.

This observation led the investigators at the Mayo Clinic to explore adenosine's potential as a trigger for VVS.[101] Patients with syncope and negative electrophysiologic studies were given intravenous adenosine during upright posture. Patients then also underwent head-up tilt table testing. Both interventions yielded a similar incidence of induction of a vasovagal response. These observations not only add further understanding to vasovagal pathophysiology but also suggest an alternative to tilt table testing in testing susceptibility to VVS.

In another study using adenosine, the 5′-triphosphate form (which has a pronounced cardiac vagal effect) was given to patients with syncope and presyncope. Those who demonstrated prolonged asystolic responses (longer than 10 seconds) as a consequence of the intravenous medication were presumed to be more susceptible to predominantly cardioinhibitory VVS.[102] They were then offered permanent pacemakers. During follow-up, those patients who received pacemakers had significantly fewer syncopal recurrences than those who refused pacemakers. The adenosine triphosphate test has not yet been adequately compared to conventional tilt table testing, but it suggests an intriguing alternative with therapeutic implications.

Further insight into the altered autonomic milieu encom-

passing the VVS response is the relatively preserved QT interval seen in the ECGs of patients experiencing VVS. These paradoxical short QT intervals can be seen even after patients have had prolonged asystole or prolonged bradycardia. This suggests intense persistent sympathetic stimulation of the heart at the cellular level, possibly from heightened circulating catecholamines (epinephrine). This observation suggests the possibility of using this phenomenon of relatively shortened QT intervals as a trigger for initiating pacing in patients with VVS.[103]

Despite these and many other studies, the previously proposed ventricular mechanism for provocation of the VVS reflex was significantly challenged by the seminal report of Scherrer and colleagues.[104] These investigators reported a cardiac transplant recipient who had an apparent VVS reaction while being infused with intravenous nitroprusside (Fig. 18–5). Theoretically, cardiac denervation after transplantation should have prevented the induction of VVS by eliminating left ventricular mechanoreceptors from the reflex arc. Certainly, higher CNS centers could have precipitated VVS through pain or fear, but this patient had neither. Similar results were recently reported by Fitzpatrick and colleagues.[105] In their study, 7 of 10 cardiac transplant recipients developed vasovagal reactions while undergoing head-up tilt with saddle support. Three of these 7 patients demonstrated donor heart bradycardia during VVS, suggesting cardiac vagal efferent reinnervation. These observations have yet to be explained and suggest alternate activation mechanisms for VVS.

Diagnosis

Most patients with vasovagal syncope can be diagnosed at the bedside (Table 18–5). Calkins and associates[106] reported that a careful history could diagnose VVS, contrasted with syncope due to ventricular tachycardia or complete heart

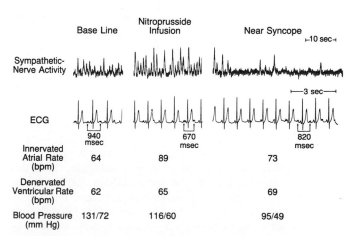

Figure 18–5. Electrocardiogram, vital signs, and sympathetic nerve activity (SNA) recording of 41-year-old heart transplant recipient who demonstrated vasovagal response during infusion of vasodilator. Note significant attenuation of SNA during near syncope and hypotension, challenging the concept that vasovagal syncope induction requires intact neural connections to left ventricular mechanoreceptors. (From Scherrer V, Vissing S, Morgan BJ, et al: Vasovagal syncope after infusion of a vasodilator in a heart transplant recipient. N Engl J Med 322:602, 1990. Copyright 1990 Massachusetts Medical Society.)

Table 18–5. Diagnostic Clues to the Cause of Syncope

Factors Favoring Vasovagal Syncope	Factors Against Vasovagal Syncope
Many spells	Only 1 or 2 spells
Associated presyncopal spells	No presyncopal spells
Prolonged presyncopal prodrome	No presyncopal prodrome
Associated nausea, vomiting, warmth, epigastric sensations	No associated symptoms
Provocative factors—stress, warm rooms, postexercise, prolonged sitting or standing	No provocative factors
Fatigue following syncope	No symptoms after syncope
Young patient	Older patient
Normal heart	Electrical or structural heart disease
Syncope following standing up	Syncope any time

block. Two analyses were performed. The first analysis, involving demographic data, showed that young women (younger than age 55) with a prolonged postsyncopal recovery period that included fatigue were much more likely to have VVS than ventricular tachycardia or complete heart block. The second analysis, which omitted demographic data, showed that patients with VVS could be identified if they had clear precipitating factors, diaphoresis and palpitations preceding syncope, and severe fatigue following syncope. This approach is complicated by the factor of patients in whom an arrhythmia provokes VVS, but once it is validated, it will probably lead to diagnostic criteria in a similar manner as that used for rheumatologic diseases.

Although the most important diagnostic maneuver is a thorough history, occasionally this does not help. There are also several tests that may prove useful in the diagnosis of patients with presumed VVS. These include Holter monitors, event recorders, and head-up tilt table testing. The latter provides the highest likelihood of making a diagnosis quickly and will probably prove to be the most cost-effective step in the investigation of syncope. Therefore, tilt table testing should be considered early in the assessment of syncope of unknown cause.

Tilt Table Testing

It became apparent in the early 1980s that many syncope patients remained undiagnosed despite invasive and aggressive diagnostic testing.[107] Tilt table tests had long been a research tool for the investigation of hemodynamic reflexes,[108] pacemaker syndrome,[54] high-speed flight,[109] and the effects of upright posture on tachyarrhythmias.[110] During these studies the occasional subject fainted, and this led to the development in a number of centers of tilt table testing for the assessment of presumed VVS. It is now an integral component in the evaluation of syncope.

Patients are usually considered for tilt table testing for one or more of several reasons.[3, 111] First, many patients with VVS do not have classic vagal symptoms associated with their syncope. Factors that would lead to the choice of tilt table testing include frequent syncope, syncope with no provocative factor, syncope not associated with vagal symptoms, syncope causing significant bodily trauma, and patients with a high level of anxiety. Second, many physicians are

more comfortable treating patients if a diagnosis can be established with a tilt table test. The American College of Cardiology Consensus document[111] recommended tilt table testing in the patients just listed, particularly when VVS is presumed to be the cause. Patients at risk of other causes of syncope, such as those with structural heart disease, should first have the appropriate investigations for those causes. There is uncertainty whether tilt table tests should be used to evaluate patients with a single uncomplicated syncopal spell, patients with dizziness or unexplained falls, patients with dysautonomias, and patients being treated for syncope. Tilt table tests are contraindicated in patients with severe aortic or mitral stenosis and in those with critical coronary or cerebral artery stenosis.

Methodology: In the 1990s, tilt table tests, like Darwin's finches, underwent divergent evolution as many centers developed their own protocols. There is a large literature devoted to the nuances of this technique, and the reference list of this chapter contains review articles that will serve as a portal to an in-depth review.[3, 112–114] Despite this, a tilt table test is simply a method of subjecting a patient to sustained orthostatic stress under somewhat controlled circumstances, with or without provocative agents. Patients should be tested after a fast of 4 to 8 hours and should be drug free. Discontinuation of β-blockers and α-adrenergic receptor agonists is strongly suggested. The basic principle of tilt table testing is simple: the patient is gently restrained on a bed, then passively tilted head up at an angle of 60 to 80 degrees for up to 60 minutes in the presence or absence of agents such as isoproterenol or nitroglycerin. This provokes hypotension, bradycardia, and presyncope or syncope in a variable proportion of syncope patients and in a smaller proportion of control subjects who have not fainted (Fig. 18–6). Patients should be instructed to remain still and to minimize leg movement. Use of a footboard is universal because a tilt table with saddle support has poor specificity.[115] Noninvasive blood pressure and heart rate measurements are obtained every 1 to 3 minutes throughout the test. Arterial cannulation and central venous access are not routinely performed be-

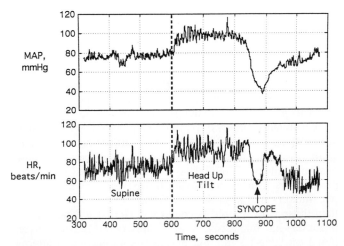

Figure 18–6. Hemodynamic changes during a positive drug-free passive tilt table test.

cause they may decrease the specificity of the test.[116] During the tilt table test, lighting in the room is dimmed, and extraneous talking and movement are minimized. Talking by the patient is discouraged except to report symptoms. Although there are many different tilt table test protocols, they can be grouped in two major categories: passive and provocative (Table 18–6).

Passive Tilt: This technique was developed in London[115, 117, 118] and Cleveland, based on the observation of syncope induced by head-up tilt in physiologic experiments. The patient is tilted with the head up for 20 to 60 minutes at an angle of 60 to 80 degrees. With this method,[109, 115, 117–127] about 30% to 40% of patients with syncope of unknown origin faint or become markedly lightheaded, and the specificity is about 90%. This type of test probably has a high specificity at the expense of reduced sensitivity. The proportion of positive responses in patients is higher[128] at 80 degrees than at 60 degrees, and the specificities are about equivalent. Angles of less than 60 degrees are less effective at inducing syncope. The proportion of positive tests rises in a sigmoidal manner to approach an asymptote[128] at about 45 minutes. Briefer durations of tilt, such as 20 minutes, miss patients who would have fainted in the absence of provocative factors. Children may behave differently in this protocol; they develop syncope rapidly, with most tests being completed within 20 minutes.[129]

Provocative Tilt: These techniques were first developed in Toronto,[130] Minneapolis,[131] and Maestre-Venice,[132] based partly on the Sharpey-Schafer hypothesis[133] of the genesis of VVS and partly on an older nitrate tilt table test literature.[134] During provocative tilt table testing, the patient undergoes head-up tilting at the same angle for shorter periods of time but while receiving oral or intravenous provocative agents such as isoproterenol,[130, 131] edrophonium,[135] or nitroglycerin.[121, 132] The positive diagnostic yield of the provocative tilt tends to be higher than that of the passive tilt, in the range of 60% to 85%. Although isoproterenol tilt table testing was developed in the United States and continues to be widely used there, nitroglycerin tilt table tests originated in Italy and appear likely to grow in popularity given their safety and reasonable diagnostic yield. Since 1995, a hybrid method first developed by Morillo and colleagues[136] has grown in use. In this method, patients first undergo passive

head-up tilt for 20 to 45 minutes, then receive an infusion of low-dose isoproterenol in the range of 1 to 2 μg/min. This protocol has a reported positive yield of about 60% and a specificity of about 90%. It resembles the protocol recommended by the consensus conference of the American College of Cardiology.[111]

There are several distinct isoproterenol tilt test protocols. The first and now largely abandoned method involved administering incremental boluses of isoproterenol to patients during head-up tilt.[130] This was soon superseded by a method that was in widespread use for several years,[131, 137] in which the patients were subjected to cycles of head-up tilt, with an increased dose of infused isoproterenol at each stage. Patients were supine between each head-up cycle. This protocol culminated with syncope, presyncope, or 5 μg/min of isoproterenol, and often lasted longer than 2 hours. A randomized crossover trial showed that a single brief tilt with 5 μg/min of isoproterenol was equally effective in provoking syncope.[138]

Although early estimates of specificity were high, there soon surfaced concerns that isoproterenol tilts might be nonspecific. Several groups first reported acceptably high specificities in the range of 80% in patients with other established causes of syncope, such as ventricular tachycardia.[120, 131, 137, 139, 140] These estimates have been challenged by two reports. Kapoor and Brant[141] showed that a protocol with up to 5 μg/min of isoproterenol and a tilt angle of 80 degrees had a specificity of 55% in young healthy subjects with no history of syncope and a mean age of 25 years. Although this is an unacceptably low specificity for a diagnostic test, it is noteworthy that half the outcomes occurred in the absence of isoproterenol. This is higher than estimates from most other institutions and may reflect some subtle selection bias, such as the young age of the patients. A second well-crafted study by Natale and associates[142] examined the effects of isoproterenol dose, tilt angle, and tilt duration on isoproterenol tilt table test specificity. The patients had a mean age of about 40 years. The specificities under most conditions were acceptably high, in the range of 90%, but exposure to isoproterenol and tilt at 80 degrees for more than 10 minutes, or to high doses of isoproterenol, led to a reduction in the specificity. Unfortunately, the positive yield of this type of isoproterenol tilt table test is proportional to the dose of isoproterenol, and increased specificity comes at the expense of reduced sensitivity.

These findings led to the development of the hybrid tilt table test.[136] Patients are subjected to an initial drug-free tilt for 15 to 60 minutes, which, if necessary, is followed by an infusion of low-dose isoproterenol, in the range of 1 to 2 μg/min. This method has a positive yield[34] of about 60% to 70% and a specificity[122, 136] of about 90%. It has numerous advantages, which include its high specificity, the ability to collect hemodynamic data in the absence of isoproterenol, and a reasonable yield. The American College of Cardiology, recognizing these advantages, recommended its use in their consensus statement.[111]

Nitroglycerin Tilt: Nitroglycerin is a potent venodilator, and its ability to induce syncope in patients with CAD has long been recognized.[134] This has led to the development of tilt table tests that use nitroglycerin as a provocative agent. Raviele and associates[132] gave incremental low-dose intrave-

Table 18–6. Comparison of Passive and Provocative Tilt Table Tests

Factor	Passive Tilt Tests	Provocative Tilt Tests
Provocative drugs	None	Isoproterenol, nitroglycerin, edrophonium
Duration	Up to 60 min	Variable, depending on duration of passive tilt
Sensitivity	Low, perhaps 35%	High, perhaps 75%
Specificity	High, perhaps >90%	Variable, 50%–90%
Reproducibility	About 70%	70%–85%
Advantages	Specific; drug-free observations	Sensitive; often faster
Disadvantages	Insensitive, lengthy	Nonspecific, isoproterenol side effects

nous infusions of nitroglycerin to syncope patients during head-up tilt. The doses were the equivalent of about 2 to 5 μg/min of nitroglycerin. Under these conditions, the positive yield and specificity were about 53% and 92%, respectively. The investigators then modified this protocol such that patients were tilted for an initial 20 to 45 minutes, then received 0.3 mg of sublingual nitroglycerin.[121] The specificity remained higher than 90%, and the positive yield was about 55%. Half of positive responses occurred during drug-free tilt and half after nitroglycerin administration. This benign and simple protocol therefore has about the same diagnostic performance as the hybrid isoproterenol tilt test.

The truth is that we simply do not know which tilt table test protocol is the best. It does appear likely that increased sensitivity is gained at the expense of decreased specificity (Table 18–7). The same factors that increase sensitivity, such as higher angles of tilt, higher doses of isoproterenol, and longer durations of head-up tilt, all decrease the specificity of tilt table testing. Indeed, we do not even know the meaning of specificity in a syndrome that affects such a large part of the population and that has its onset at any age. Some of the control subjects with positive tilt tests may simply be syncope patients who have not yet fainted.[122] Some authorities believe that the predilection to VVS may be a part of normal physiology, in which case the concern about specificity may be less.

Outcome Definitions: The purpose of a diagnostic tilt table test is to induce VVS. A positive test, therefore, is one that reproduces the patient's symptoms. This usually involves a comparison of the presyncopal and postsyncopal symptoms induced by the test with those that occur clinically. Not all positive tests do or can end with patients in frank syncope. Almost all positive passive drug-free tilt table tests end in syncope, but up to half of isoproterenol tilt table tests end with severe presyncope, regardless of the duration of exposure to the drug during head-up tilt. Using symptomatic criteria is a satisfactory approach most of the time, but occasionally patients are assessed with few or no remembered symptoms that preceded their syncope, or are uncertain if the test reproduced their symptoms. To help with this uncertainty, most centers also have objective outcome criteria based on a relative or absolute decrease in heart rate, blood pressure, or both. In general, hypotension, which is universally present during a positive response, precedes bradycardia. The bradycardia may be due to atrial standstill or arrest, sinus bradycardia, or AV block or may be superseded by a junctional escape rhythm. Although these data are useful descriptively, most patients who develop significant hypotension, bradycardia, or both on a tilt table test also have significant symptoms.

Can specific patient subgroups be identified based on tilt table responses? The European VASIS (Vasovagal Syncope International Study) investigators proposed a classification[143] based on whether patients become hypotensive, bradycardic, or both. This classification might prove useful in guiding therapy. For example, patients with profound bradycardia on tilt table testing might be good candidates for pacemaker therapy, whereas those who develop tachycardia before syncope might be good candidates for β-blocker treatment. This interesting proposal may prove to be fertile soil for future studies.

Other abnormalities can be detected with this test. Orthostatic hypotension, although not part of the vasovagal process, is defined by a *gradual* drop in systolic blood pressure of 30 mm Hg or more or by a diastolic drop of 10 mm Hg or more. The psychosomatic response[144] is an apparent loss of consciousness during the tilt table test with an adequate blood pressure and heart rate, and normal electroencephalogram and cerebral blood flow as determined by transcranial Doppler ultrasonography.

Positive Yield and Sensitivity: The sensitivity of tilt table testing is less than perfect, although the magnitude of this lack of sensitivity can only be estimated. This is because, with a single exception, tilt table test outcomes have not been studied in "gold standard" populations. Waxman and coauthors[130] found that only about 75% of patients who had definitely diagnosed VVS fainted on a tilt table test that included incremental boluses of isoproterenol. Drug-free passive tilt table tests are particularly insensitive.

Many centers use a passive tilt at 60 degrees for 20 to 45 minutes, yet Sexton and colleagues[128] showed that 60 degrees is significantly less sensitive than 80 degrees, and as many patients fainted with a subsequent low dose of isoproterenol as fainted drug free. A drug-free tilt at 60 degrees, therefore, is quite insensitive. A third piece of evidence is that tilt tests are only about 80% reproducible; that is, some patients have an initial negative test, then faint on a second one. Finally, patients with negative and positive isoproterenol tilt table test results have similar pretest clinical characteristics and similar post-test outcomes. In addition, similar clinical variables in both populations before the test predict syncope recurrence after the tilt test.[145, 146] This suggests that they may be part of the same population (Fig. 18–7). This supports the idea that even isoproterenol tilt table tests are incompletely sensitive. The positive diagnostic yields of drug-free and isoproterenol tilt table tests are about 30% to 40% and 65% to 80%, respectively, which sets the lower limit of their sensitivities.

Reproducibility: The reproducibility of tilt table tests is important in judging the long-term stability of the underlying pathophysiologic milieu, in determining the potential usefulness of the tests in evaluating therapies, and in designing acute studies of the physiology of syncope. Accordingly, much effort has been devoted to defining tilt table test reproducibility over various time periods. The most important issue is whether the same diagnostic outcome occurs in consecutive tests; this is the test concordance. Isoproterenol tilt table tests performed about 1 hour apart have a positive outcome concordance[147–149] of about 70% and a negative outcome concordance at least that high. Tilt table

Table 18–7. Factors That Affect the Diagnostic Performance of Tilt Table Tests

Increased Sensitivity	Increased Specificity
Lengthy head-up tilt	Brief duration of tilt
Isoproterenol, nitroglycerin, edrophonium	Drug-free tilt test
Steeper angles of tilt	Shallow angles of tilt
Volume-depleted patient	Volume-loaded patient
Pain or stressful instrumentation	Benign instrumentation

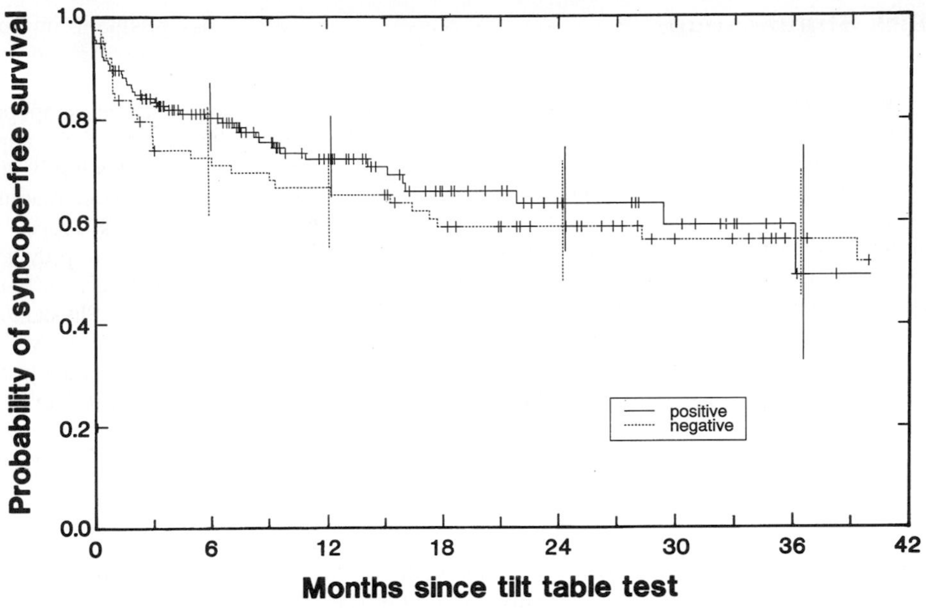

Figure 18–7. Probability of remaining free of syncope in 153 patients with a positive tilt table test result (*solid line*) and 74 patients with a negative tilt table test result (*broken line*). The bars are the 95% confidence intervals at 6, 12, 24, and 36 months. (From Sheldon RS, Rose S, Koshman ML: Comparison of patients with syncope of unknown cause having negative or positive tilt table tests. Am J Cardiol 80:581, 1997.)

tests performed over several days appear to perform equally well. The positive concordance of passive tilt tests performed over periods up to 1 week is about 65%, but the negative concordance is unknown.[150–152] The positive and negative concordances of isoproterenol tilt tests performed over periods ranging from a few days to several weeks[152] are each about 85%. In a study that has clear implications for our understanding of the persistence of the physiologic milieu, Petersen and associates reported a 64% positive concordance over 4 years.[153]

Reproducibility may be lower when patients receive placebos in placebo-controlled trials. Two studies, one evaluating disopyramide[154] and one evaluating etilefrine,[155] found a high proportion of patients with initially positive tests who subsequently had negative tests while receiving placebo. Both reports concluded that serial tests lacked the reproducibility to be an easily used tool for evaluating the response of patients to drugs.[154–156]

The degree of bradycardia seen during presyncope and syncope induced on isoproterenol tilt table tests may be reproducible,[147, 148, 152] although not all authors agree.[151] Although this might suggest that each patient has his or her own degree of bradycardia during syncope, it is possible that this simply reflects the rate of the patient's junctional escape rhythm induced by isoproterenol. The magnitude of hypotension during syncope is not reproducible.

These findings set the parameters for the use of serial tilt table tests in clinical investigative studies. For example, if the positive concordance is 80%, serial studies inexorably lead to patients converting from positive to negative outcomes, even in the absence of interventions. Serial test protocols need placebo-controlled arms and may need to be larger than was initially anticipated. These results will also enable power calculations for future studies. Finally, the imperfect concordance should lead to a healthy skepticism about the meaning of a tilt table test outcome.

Safety: Overall, the worldwide experience attests to the remarkable safety of tilt table testing, with no published

deaths. Occasionally, patients have prolonged asystole, but they invariably recover without any permanent sequelae. Patients with angina probably should not receive isoproterenol. There is legitimate concern that isoproterenol might increase the risk. In one study, 9% of patients with syncope and structural heart disease who underwent high-dose isoproterenol tilt table testing had poorly tolerated tachyarrhythmias, none died. Our current practice is to exclude inducible ventricular tachycardia first, then to apply defibrillator pads before testing in patients with structural heart disease. Finally, a variety of generally benign supraventricular arrhythmias can be provoked with head-up tilt and isoproterenol.[99, 140]

Other Tests

Ocular compression and carotid sinus massage (CSM) during head-up tilt have undergone assessment as diagnostic tools for VVS.[157, 158] Both these tests provoke hypotension, bradycardia, and syncope more often in syncope patients than in control subjects. There is concern, however, about the safety of ocular compression as a widespread screening test and uncertainty about whether head-up CSM may be either nonspecific or provoke CSS. Neither test has undergone widespread assessment.

The well-known ability of intravenous adenosine to provoke hypotension and bradycardia has led to the assessment of adenosine triphosphate as a diagnostic tool for VVS.[102, 159] It appears to provoke syncope more often in syncope patients than in control subjects. Whether it provokes VVS or a novel form of purine-sensitive syncope is unknown.

Holter monitor ECG analysis is of little use in the diagnosis of VVS. Syncope is sporadic and almost always too infrequent to be detected on a Holter monitor. To overcome this problem, a novel implantable digital event recorder has been developed (Reveal; Medtronic). Its memory can be frozen with application of an external magnet, and a tracing closely resembling a surface ECG is retrieved. Early results are promising, and it is now entering the clinical domain.[160]

Risk Stratification

Mortality

Although patients who faint may appear to be close to death while unconscious, VVS in itself is not life-threatening. The evidence for this is gathered from both community-based and hospital-based studies. The Framingham study[161] reported that the risk of death was no different in fainting subjects from that in nonfainting subjects. With the benefit of hindsight, it seems likely that almost all of the fainting subjects may have had VVS, suggesting that VVS does not pose a mortal risk to most patients.

Kapoor and colleagues[107] followed 97 syncope patients with no diagnostic cause despite aggressive investigations. The actuarial risk of sudden death in 1 year was only 3%. Almost all sudden deaths had a clearly arrhythmic, ischemic, or mechanical cause. If we assume that most of these patients had VVS, then hospitalized patients with VVS appear to have a low risk of sudden death. Similarly, Kushner and associates[162] followed 99 patients with unexplained syncope and a negative electrophysiologic study. Structural heart disease was present in 47 patients. During an average 20 months of follow-up, only 2 patients died suddenly. One had moderately severe left ventricular systolic dysfunction, and one had sustained polymorphic ventricular tachycardia induced by programmed ventricular stimulation with triple extrastimuli. Although none of these patients had undergone a tilt table test, this study is consistent with an overall benign outcome of patients with VVS. Thus, most patients with VVS are not at risk for sudden death.

Interestingly, patients have been reported to appear to have been resuscitated from sudden cardiac death and then found to have a positive tilt table test with no other abnormalities.[5] One case involved a patient who fainted while swimming and was resuscitated from drowning, and several resuscitated patients were health care personnel at work, spouses of health care personnel, or patients who fortuitously fainted while being monitored. Given the alarming and death-like appearance of patients who faint, it is reasonable that an attempt at resuscitation be made. Whether spontaneous recovery would have ensued is open to question.

One conjectured marker of sudden death is the development of asystole during tilt table testing. Brignole and co-workers[163] and Dhala and associates[164] followed 47 patients with recurrent syncope and asystole on a tilt table test for about 2 years, and none died. Thus, asystole on tilt table testing does not predict sudden death.

Natural History

Most people faint only once in a lifetime, but for some, VVS is a chronic, recurring, troublesome disorder. There is a wide range of symptom burden, from a few to thousands of spells over days to decades. The typical syncope patient, seen in syncope or arrhythmia clinics, has fainted several times over several years, but some are much more severely afflicted. Even most patients with moderate symptoms do surprisingly well after assessment. The average likelihood of recurrent syncope in the first 1 to 2 years after tilt table testing is only about 25% to 30% in patients who receive neither drugs nor pacemakers.[154, 165–169] Clearly, patients with a moderate number of syncopal spells in their history have a low risk of recurrence after tilt table testing. Some of this

may be due to improvement in clinical status. This decrease in syncope frequency may be as high as 90% after tilt table testing. This may be because all patients improve equally or because one subpopulation improves but another does not. The cause of this apparently great reduction in syncope after tilt table testing is unknown, but it may be due to spontaneous remission, reassurance, counseling about the pathophysiology of syncope, and coaching on appropriate postural maneuvers to prevent progression of presyncope to syncope. Unfortunately, at least 30% to 40% of patients continue to faint.[167–169] Physicians need to know how to predict which patients will do well and which patients will do poorly to counsel them about their prognosis, decide who to treat, and select appropriate subjects for clinical trials.

Pretest Risk Factors for Frequent Syncope

Several pretest factors predict the likelihood of a patient having recurrences of syncope after tilt table testing.[167, 168] Multivariate analyses showed that the frequency and number of syncopal spells preceding positive tilt table tests were independent risk factors that predicted an early recurrence of syncope after the test (Table 18–8). A multivariate model[168] was constructed that accurately stratified patients into groups with less than 25%, 25% to 50%, 50% to 75%, and more than 75% risk of syncope in the year following tilt table testing. For example, patients with greater than six syncopal spells over any duration of time have a more than 50% risk of at least one syncopal spell in the next 2 years, whereas patients with six spells or fewer have a less than 50% chance of a syncope recurrence in the next 2 years.

Tilt Table Test Results and Frequent Syncope

Can observations made during tilt table testing predict patient outcome after the test? Generally, the results of studies addressing this question have been disappointing. Univariate and multivariate analyses of tilt table tests and syncope in follow-up showed that otherwise similar syncope patients with either negative or positive tilt table tests had similar outcomes.[145, 146] The outcome of the tilt table test (negative versus positive) did not predict subsequent clinical outcome. Similarly, the lowest heart rate (including asystole) during tilt table testing does not predict the eventual likelihood of syncope in clinical follow-up.[145, 163, 164, 168] Menozzi and colleagues[170] found that asystolic events of a few seconds' duration were common, but only 0.7% of episodes 3 to 6 seconds in duration and 43% of episodes lasting longer than 6 seconds resulted in presyncope or syncope. Although asystole is common, it is rarely symptomatic unless it lasts

Table 18–8. Factors That Predict Early and Frequent Syncope After a Tilt Table Test

Factors That Predict Syncope Recurrences	Factors That Do Not Predict Syncope Recurrences
High number of syncopal spells ($\geq$6)	Tilt test diagnostic outcome (positive or negative)
High frequency of syncopal spells ($\geq$1 spell/year)	Lowest heart rate during tilt test
Early recurrence of syncope after tilt (within 1 yr)	Blood pressure during tilt test
Duration of history of syncope	Age or sex

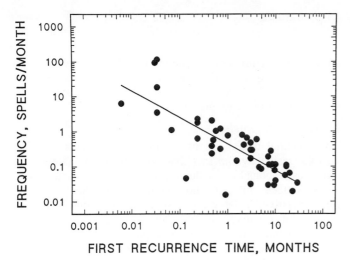

Figure 18–8. Relationship between the time of first syncope recurrence after a positive tilt table test result and the eventual frequency of syncope. (From Malik P, Koshman ML, Sheldon RS. Timing of first syncope recurrence predicts syncope frequency following a positive tilt table test. Preprinted by permission of the American College of Cardiology. J Am Coll Cardiol 29:1284–1289, 1997.)

more than 6 seconds. Thus, neither symptoms occurring at tilt table testing nor hemodynamic outcomes predict patient outcome.

Does the degree of bradycardia during tilt table testing predict which patients are most likely to benefit from pacing? Although this appealing concept was used by the investigators of the Vasovagal Pacemaker Study,[171] there is no evidence that heart rate during tilt table testing predicts either heart rate during clinical syncope or a beneficial response to permanent pacing.

Post-Test Prediction of Frequent Syncope

The use of a multivariate predictive model demands a reasonably accurate assessment of the duration and number of syncopal spells in the patient's history and is partly based on specific test protocols which involved the use of isoproterenol. Furthermore, many patients have a marked improvement in their symptoms after tilt table testing. A simple, practical, individualized measure of the eventual frequency of syncope is the interval to the first recurrence of syncope after testing.[172] Generally, the earlier the recurrence, the higher the eventual frequency of syncope (Fig. 18–8; see Table 18–8).

The first recurrence time has a number of potential uses. It can be used to risk-stratify patients. Patients whose VVS recurs within 1 year continue to faint frequently. Given that many patients stop fainting, the clinician may suggest that patients first be followed without specific therapy, returning for reassessment after the first recurrence of syncope. Patients at low risk for frequent recurrent fainting spells would therefore be spared the potential adverse effects and cost of treatment, and patients at high risk would gain a better estimate of their future course. Similarly, patients who do not have a recurrence within a specific follow-up period may be allowed to resume driving. Finally, the first recurrence

time can also be used as a study outcome measure, as was done in the Vasovagal Pacemaker Study.[171]

Medical Treatment

Most patients with VVS do not require specific therapy. They should be reassured and instructed to avoid situations that precipitate fainting. The use of support stockings or increased salt intake may be helpful. They should be taught to recognize an impending episode of fainting and to sit down or lie down quickly. For some patients, this is not enough, and other treatment options may be necessary.

Pathophysiology

Candidate therapeutic modalities are best understood in light of the current pathophysiologic model of VVS. This model has many limitations, and we present it only to put into perspective the use of the various drugs. The initial event is orthostatic stress, which reduces left ventricular volumes and elevates sympathetic tone. This causes either increased contractility or increased gain of the ventricular baroreceptors. This in turn causes paradoxically increased firing of the baroreceptors, which triggers a bradycardic and hypotensive response. This might be mediated by central serotonin and opiate receptors. Bradycardia is caused by increased vagal tone, and hypotension is caused by withdrawal of α-adrenergic tone. This paradigm has led to preliminary assessments of salt loading, disopyramide, and verapamil to reduce contractility, β-adrenergic receptor antagonists, serotonin reuptake inhibitors, α-adrenergic receptor agonists, anticholinergics, and permanent pacing.

Use of Tilt Tests as Surrogates for Clinical Trials

One of the uses of tilt table testing may be to select effective treatment, in the same way that electrophysiologic studies were used to select antiarrhythmic drugs in the 1980s and 1990s. Some of the same problems confound this use of tilt table testing as confounded the use of electrophysiologic studies. The assumption that tilt table testing physiology resembles clinical physiology has not been studied. To be useful, tilt table tests must be highly reproducible. Unfortunately, their reproducibility over days to weeks is probably only 75% to 80%, and their immediate reproducibility over a few hours may be less. Treatments that have some effect on preventing syncope during tilt table testing include pacing, β-blockers, α-adrenergic receptor agonists, disopyramide, and serotonin reuptake inhibitors.

Finally, initial attempts to show that tilt table tests can be used to select effective treatment have been unsuccessful. Morillo and colleagues[154] showed in a small placebo-controlled study that the response to intravenous disopyramide during tilt did not predict the response to chronic oral therapy with the drug. Brignole and coauthors[166] randomized patients to placebo or to drugs selected on the basis of tilt table tests. These authors were unable to demonstrate that treatment affected outcome and therefore were unable to demonstrate the usefulness of tilt table tests to guide therapy. Moya and associates[155] found tilt tests to be of limited effectiveness in predicting the response to etilefrine. Although all three studies were small, and at least two were unable to show any beneficial response to treatment, they do illustrate the lack of evidence for this approach.[156]

Clinical Trials

The effectiveness of drugs in preventing recurrent syncope is unproven. Studies were either not randomized or placebo-controlled, and the patients often had only a few historical syncopal spells. They might be predicted to do well regardless of whether or not they received treatment. Truly randomized controlled trials have generally been negative but often underpowered.

β-Blockers

β-Blockers show promise in the prevention of VVS for several reasons. β Stimulation is central to the theoretical pathophysiologic cascade of VVS, and plasma epinephrine and norepinephrine levels rise before patients faint on tilt table tests. The β-agonist isoproterenol provokes syncope or presyncope in about 75% of syncope patients during head-up tilt of such limited duration that the tilt alone is unlikely to cause the symptoms.[137, 138] About 40% of patients do not faint with prolonged tilt alone but do faint with adjunctive isoproterenol.[128] Finally, β-blockers block the development of syncope during isoproterenol tilt table tests.[173]

Three recent controlled studies have provided conflicting information about the usefulness of empiric β-blockade in preventing syncope recurrence. Cox and colleagues[174] administered a variety of β-blockers to 118 patients who had fainted a median of three times and who had a positive tilt table test response. Control groups included patients who either refused or discontinued β-blocker treatment. After about 2 years, the proportion of patients who experienced recurrence of syncope was 10% to 23% in the persistently treated group and 42% to 58% in the partially or completely untreated group, with a relative risk reduction of 68%.

Mahanonda and coauthors[175] studied a group of 42 patients with a history of presyncope or syncope and a positive tilt table test response, who then were randomized to atenolol or placebo. After 1 month, the frequencies of presyncopal and syncopal events in the treated and untreated populations were 1±2 and 6±9 episodes per week, respectively, with a relative risk reduction of 83%. Sheldon and associates[169] studied a cohort of 153 syncope patients with a positive tilt table test response, of whom 52 then received β-blockers. Syncope recurred in the same proportion of treated and untreated patients, and the actuarial probability of remaining free of syncope was similar in both groups. There remains uncertainty about the efficacy of chronic β-blockade in the prevention of syncope.

Some of the uncertainty about the efficacy of β-blockers may be due to patient selection. Three retrospective studies have suggested that older patients are more likely to respond to β-blockers.[169, 176, 177] Two groups reported that patients who developed sinus tachycardia during tilt table testing were more likely to respond to β-blockers as chronic treatment.[176, 178] Finally, the need for isoproterenol to induce syncope predicted a favorable clinical outcome on β-blockers.[176, 177] These data suggest that some form of drug-free and isoproterenol tilt table testing might select patients who subsequently respond to β-blockers.

Disopyramide

Disopyramide may work because it is both an anticholinergic and negative inotropic drug. An initial open-label study showed that it prevented syncope on tilt table testing, and patients subsequently did not faint.[179] A later placebo-controlled study had negative results. Both studies involved small numbers of patients.[154]

Adrenergic Agonists

The potential usefulness of α-adrenergic receptor agonists was suggested by the fact that withdrawal of sympathetic tone was responsible for the vasodepression associated with VVS. Sixteen children who had recurrent syncope and an initial positive tilt table test response were found to have a subsequent negative tilt table test response after they received an intravenous infusion of phenylephrine.[180] All but one were subsequently symptom free for about 1 year while taking oral pseudoephedrine. The adrenergic agonist midodrine[181] also showed early promise in an open-label series. These initially promising results were tempered by a later negative placebo-controlled study of etilefrine in the prevention of syncope on tilt table testing.[155] In late 1997, the European VASIS study group reported that a large multicenter, prospective, placebo-controlled trial found that etilefrine was no better than placebo in preventing the recurrence of syncope. Therefore, there is only mixed evidence for the role of α-agonists in preventing VVS.[181a]

Specific Serotonin Reuptake Inhibitors

Serotonin is involved in a number of cardiovascular reflexes and responses, generally at the brain stem level. This led Grubb and colleagues[182] to administer the serotonin reuptake inhibitor sertraline to adolescent syncope patients. Half of the patients subsequently had a negative tilt table test response, and all were symptom free during a 1-year follow-up. Similar results were noted with the related drug fluoxetine.[183] A dissenting note, however, is an apparent increase in the frequency of syncope when serotonin reuptake inhibitors were given to three syncope patients by a different investigator.[184]

Theophylline

Theophylline may exert its effects by adenosine receptor blockade. Oral theophylline suppressed syncope and bradycardias in children in an open-label study.[185] A similar study in adults with VVS also showed a suppression of inducible syncope on tilt table testing.[186] Although many patients taking oral theophylline remained syncope free during follow-up, half of the patients discontinued the medication in a subsequent clinical study because of side effects.

Salt and Fluid Loading

Salt loading increases plasma volume and therefore may improve orthostatic tolerance and prevent syncope. Simple salt loading increases orthostatic tolerance,[187, 188] and salt loading with or without the use of the mineralocorticoid fludrocortisone reduces the probability of a positive tilt table test response and of syncope in follow-up of young patients.[188–191]

Pacemakers

Both the American College of Cardiology/American Heart Association Task Force[192] and the British Pacing and Electro-

Table 18–9. Uncontrolled Trials of Pacemaker Therapy for Vasovagal Syncope

Investigators	Pacing Mode	No. of Patients Without Syncope (%)	Follow-Up Duration
Acute Studies			
Fitzpatrick et al, 1991[195]	DDD	5/6 (83)	Acute study
Samoil et al, 1993[196]	DDD	3/6 (50)	Acute study
Sra et al, 1993[197]	DDD	15/20 (75)	Acute study
El-Bedawi et al, 1994[198]	DDD	1/9 (11)	Acute study
Chronic Studies			
Sapire et al, 1983[199]	VVI	4/4 (100)	Not reported
Petersen et al, 1994[200]	DDD with rate hysteresis	23/37 (62); 89% of patients improved	50 mo
Benditt et al, 1997[55]	DDD with rate-drop response	30/36 (83); 59% of patients asymptomatic	6 mo
Sheldon et al, 1998[201]	DDD with rate-drop response	6/12 (50); 93% drop in syncope frequency	12 mo

physiology Group[193] cite pacing for VVS as either equivocal or a firm recommendation.[194] Both groups required preimplantation confirmation of benefit during a repeated tilt table test with temporary pacing. What is the evidence for these recommendations?

Bradycardia Rationale: Most physicians remember graphic cases of patients with syncope and profound hypotension and bradycardia, but whether recurrent VVS is always or often characterized by profound bradycardia is unknown. The only prospective study of asystole showed that syncope patients who developed asystole had numerous asystolic episodes, but that almost none of them had symptoms.[170] That bradycardia might be important is also suggested by the development during tilt table testing of asystole, sinus bradycardia, or an inappropriately low chronotropic response for the degree of hypotension.

Acute Pacing Studies: Three studies have shown that temporary transvenous pacing is partially effective in reducing the proportion of patients who faint during tilt table testing (Table 18–9). Fitzpatrick and colleagues[195] showed that acute dual-chamber pacing with rate hysteresis prevented syncope in five of six patients who had experienced syncope in a previous, unpaced tilt table test, but all five conscious patients remained presyncopal. Tilt table test results were irreproducible in another four patients. Samoil and associates[196] showed that dual-chamber pacing prevented syncope in three of six patients on tilt table testing; single-chamber ventricular pacing was unhelpful in all patients. Sra and coworkers[197] reported that acute dual-chamber pacing in 20 patients who previously had developed profound bradycardia and syncope during diagnostic tilt table testing prevented syncope in 15 of 20 patients. All 15 conscious patients developed presyncope. In a dissenting report, El-Bedawi and coauthors[198] found no benefit of dual-chamber pacing in nine patients with VVS. Taken together, temporary dual-chamber pacing prevented the development of syncope in 24 of 41 subjects (57%), although most conscious subjects were lightheaded. These acute pacing studies suggested that permanent pacing might be helpful.

Chronic Pacing Studies: Two early reports suggested the usefulness of permanent pacing in a small number of children and adults with VVS.[111, 199] Both studies used pacemakers that had conventional bradycardia support with a fixed

bradycardia detection rate. Because of the increased attention focused on the hemodynamics of syncope induced by tilt table testing, workers began the search for physiologic syncope sensors. The two pacemakers that have shown the most promise continuously scan heart rate trends and declare the onset of syncope when heart rate decreases abruptly by a small amount (Figs. 18–9 and 18–10). They then pace near or above the ambient rate for up to 2 minutes, with the intent of compensating for the presumed hypotension that also accompanies VVS.

Petersen and associates[200] reported the results of dual-chamber pacing with rate hysteresis in 37 syncope patients (see Table 18–9). These patients had experienced a median of two syncopal spells per year and had a positive tilt table test response, ending in a heart rate of less than 60 bpm. During a mean follow-up of 50 months, 62% of the patients remained free of syncope, and 89% reported symptomatic improvement. The number of syncopal spells in the total population decreased from 136 to 11. Although these results are encouraging, they resemble the improvement seen in counseled but otherwise untreated patients. Benditt and colleagues[55] reported equally encouraging results in a study of 28 patients with a mean syncope frequency of one spell per month. After receiving a pacemaker with automatic rate-drop sensing, the patients were followed for a mean of 6

```
MEDTRONIC 9790   PROGRAMMER  9886A320        1/13/98 10:19
Copyright (c) Medtronic, Inc. 1993
-------------- PARAMETER VALUES REPORT -------------- Page 4 of 4

Pacemaker Model: Thera DR 7962i          Serial Number: PDD400443

Parameter          Present   Saved
-----------------  --------  --------
-ADDITIONAL FEATURES-
V. Safe Pace          On        On


Trans Tele           Off       Off
Extend. Telem        Off       Off
Sleep Funct.         Off       Off


Rate Drop            On        On
   Top Rate          75        75    ppm
   Bottom Rate       60        60    ppm
   Confir-Beats       2         2    beats
   Width-Beats       20        20    beats
   Intervn Rate     110       110    ppm
   Intervn Dur.       2         2    min
```

Figure 18–9. Programming characteristics of the rate-drop response of the Medtronic Thera DR.

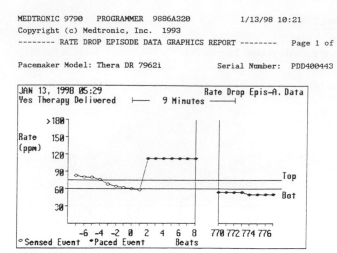

```
MEDTRONIC 9790   PROGRAMMER  9886A320        1/13/98 10:21
Copyright (c) Medtronic, Inc.  1993
-------- RATE DROP EPISODE DATA GRAPHICS REPORT --------  Page 1 of 1

Pacemaker Model: Thera DR 7962i          Serial Number:  PDD400443
```

Figure 18–10. Depiction of the various parameters of the rate-drop response in the Medtronic Thera DR.

months. During this time, syncope recurred in only six patients, and the mean syncope frequency decreased to 0.3 spell per month. Finally, Sheldon and coworkers[201] studied 12 patients who had experienced a median frequency of three spells per month. After implantation of a dual-chamber pacemaker with automatic rate-drop sensing, the actuarial syncope-free survival increased 20-fold, the syncope frequency decreased by 93%, and the patients' quality of life improved markedly (Fig. 18–11). Taken together (see Table 18–9), these studies provide hope that pacemaker therapy will reduce the number of syncopal spells in patients with frequent syncope.

A randomized clinical trial of permanent pacemakers in

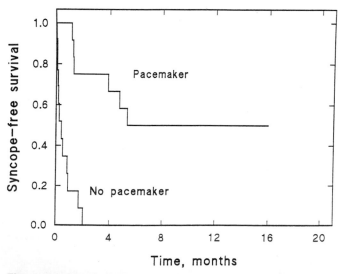

Figure 18–11. Probabilities of remaining free of syncope in 12 patients in the interval between tilt table testing and pacemaker implantation (no pacemaker) and following pacemaker implantation (pacemaker). (From Sheldon RS, Koshman ML, Wilson W, et al: Effect of dual chamber pacing with automatic rate-drop sensing on recurrent neurally mediated syncope. Am J Cardiol 81:158, 1998.)

patients with frequently recurring VVS has been completed.[171] Patients in the pacing arm had an 80% reduction in the likelihood of a recurrence of syncope. Thus, permanent dual-chamber pacing with automatic rate-drop sensing shows early promise of being a useful treatment of highly recurrent VVS. Permanent pacing is expensive and invasive, however, and although effective, is unlikely to be an initial therapy for most patients.

Dangers Associated With Driving

Unpredictable loss of consciousness poses clear risks for patients in unprotected environments. Syncope patients should avoid situations and vocations that increase the consequences of fainting. They should avoid jobs such as roofing, working on scaffolds, working around dangerous equipment, piloting, tightrope walking, and so on. Motor vehicle regulators have taken a particular interest in the field, and the Canadian Cardiovascular Society[202] and the American Heart Association/North American Society for Pacing and Cardiac Electrophysiology (AHA/NASPE)[60] have prepared expert consensus recommendations as guidelines (see Table 18–3). The Canadian guidelines aim to reduce the risk of death to the patient and bystander to less than 1 per 20,000 population per year. Using published data about the likelihood of syncope and that of syncope causing an accident,[203] they recommend that patients refrain from driving small vehicles for 1 month after each faint if they faint once per year or less, and for 3 months if they faint more than once per year. Commercial drivers should refrain from driving for 3 and 12 months, respectively, under the same conditions.

The AHA/NASPE guidelines distinguish between patients with mild and severe VVS.[60] Patients with mild syncope have only presyncope or a prolonged prodrome and faint rarely, only while standing, or in response to specific precipitating causes. Patients with severe syncope faint frequently, without warning, without clear precipitating causes, and in any position. Patients with untreated severe syncope are prohibited from driving. Patients with treated severe syncope may drive a private vehicle after 3 months of effective treatment and may drive a commercial vehicle after 6 months of effective treatment (see Table 18–3). Patients with mild syncope can continue to drive private vehicles and can resume driving commercial vehicles after 1 month of effective treatment.

Summary

The understanding of the pathophysiology of CSS and VVS has continued to advance, but much remains to be explained. Permanent pacing remains the conventional therapy for CSS and is yet unchallenged. The role of pharmacologic therapy, either adjunctive or primary, is evolving. Permanent pacing for VVS has been placed under intense scrutiny and shows promise as newer pacemaker technologies emerge. The pharmacologic therapies for VVS are largely empiric, and ideal medical therapy will require a better understanding of the autonomic reflex.

REFERENCES

1. Benditt DG, Remole S, Milstein S, et al: Syncope: Causes, clinical evaluation and current therapy. Annu Rev Med 43:283, 1992.

2. Schaal SF, Nelson SD, Boudoulas H, et al: Syncope. Curr Probl Cardiol 17:205, 1992.
3. Kapoor WN: Diagnostic evaluation of syncope. Am J Med 90:91, 1991.
4. Jaeger FJ, Maloney JD, Fouad-Tarazi FM: Newer aspects in the diagnosis and management of syncope. In Rappaport E (ed): Cardiology Update. New York, Elsevier, 1990, pp 141–173.
5. Milstein S, Buetikofer J, Lesser J, et al: Cardiac asystole: A manifestation of neurally mediated hypotension bradycardia. J Am Coll Cardiol 14:1626, 1989.
6. Chen MY, Goldenberg IF, Milstein S, et al: Cardiac electrophysiologic and hemodynamic correlates of neurally mediated syncope. Am J Cardiol 63:66, 1989.
7. Lewis T: A lecture on vasovagal syncope and the carotid sinus mechanism. Br Med J 1:873, 932.
8. Benditt DG, Remole S, Bailin S, et al: Tilt table testing for evaluation of neurally-mediated (cardioneurogenic) syncope: Rationale and proposed protocols. PACE 14:1528, 1991.
9. Strasburg B, Sagie A, Erdman S, et al: Carotid sinus hypersensitivity and the carotid sinus syndrome. Prog Cardiovasc Dis 31:376, 1989.
10. Almquist A, Gornick C, Benson W, et al: Carotid sinus hypersensitivity: Evaluation of the vasodepressor component. Circulation 71:927, 1985.
11. McIntosh SJ, Lawson J, Kenny RA: Clinical characteristics of vasodepressor, cardioinhibitory, and mixed carotid sinus syndrome in the elderly [see comments]. Am J Med 95:203, 1993.
12. Thomas JE: Hyperactive carotid sinus reflex and carotid sinus syncope. Mayo Clin Proc 44:127, 1969.
13. Volkmann H, Schnerch B, Kühnert H: Diagnostic value of carotid sinus hypersensitivity. PACE 13:2065, 1990.
14. Hartzler GO, Maloney JD: Cardioinhibitory carotid sinus hypersensitivity. Arch Intern Med 137:727, 1977.
15. Weiss S, Baker JP: The carotid sinus reflex in health and disease: Its role in the causation of fainting and convulsions. Medicine 12:297, 1933.
16. Zee-Cheng CS, Gibbs HR: Pure vasodepressor carotid sinus hypersensitivity. Am J Med 81:1095, 1986.
17. Lown B, Levine SA: The carotid sinus: Clinical value of its stimulation. Circulation 23:766, 1961.
18. Baig MW, Kaye GC, Perrins EJ, et al: Can central neuropeptides be implicated in carotid sinus reflex hypersensitivity? Med Hypotheses 28:255, 1989.
19. Morley CA, Sutton R: Carotid sinus syncope. Int J Cardiol 6:287, 1984.
20. Tea SH, Mansourati J, L'Heveder G, et al: New insights into the pathophysiology of carotid sinus syndrome. Circulation 93:1411, 1996.
21. Blanc JJ, L'Heveder G, Mansourati J, et al: Assessment of a newly recognized association, carotid sinus hypersensitivity and denervation of sternocleidomastoid muscles. Circulation 95:2548, 1997.
22. Brown KA, Maloney JD, Smith HC, et al: Carotid sinus reflex in patients undergoing coronary angiography: Relationship of degree and location of coronary artery disease to response to carotid sinus massage. Circulation 62:697, 1980.
23. Teichman SL, Felder SD, Matos JA, et al: The value of electrophysiologic studies in syncope of undetermined origin: Report of 150 cases. Am Heart J 110:469, 1985.
24. Iyer RP: Seat-belt syncope [Letter]. Lancet 346:1044, 1995.
25. Wiebe S: An unusual mechanism of recumbent syncope [Letter]. Lancet 347:1769, 1996.
26. Kenny RA, Traynor G: Carotid sinus sydrome: Clinical characteristics in elderly patients. Age Ageing 20:449, 1991.
27. Tulchinsky M, Krasnow SH: Carotid sinus syndrome associated with an occult primary nasopharyngeal carcinoma. Arch Intern Med 148:1217, 1988.
28. Achiron A, Reger A: Carotid sinus syncope induced by an orthodontic appliance. Lancet 2:1339, 1989.
29. Berger TM, Porter CJ: Carotid sinus syndrome and wrestling. Mayo Clin Proc 68:366, 1993.
30. Romano M, Spinelli A, Feller S, et al: An unusual cause of carotid sinus syndrome: Multiple symmetric lipomatosis. PACE 15:128, 1992.
31. Solti F, Mogan ST, Renyi-Vamos F, et al: The association of carotid artery stenosis with carotid sinus hypersensitivity. J Cardiovasc Surg 31:693, 1990.
32. Richardson DA, Bexton RS, Shaw FE, Kenny RA: Prevalence of cardioinhibitory carotid sinus hypersensitivity in patients 50 years or over presenting to the accident and emergency department with "unexplained" or "recurrent" falls. PACE 15:820, 1997.
33. Cicogna R, Mascioli G, Bonomi F, et al: Carotid sinus hypersensitivity and syndrome in patients with chronic atrial fibrillation. PACE 17:1635, 1994.
34. Gang ES, Oseran DS, Mandel WJ, et al: Sinus node electrogram in patients with the hypersensitive carotid syndrome. J Am Coll Cardiol 5:1484, 1985.
35. Brignole M, Sartore B, Barra M, et al: Ventricular and dual chamber pacing for treatment of carotid sinus syndrome. PACE 12:582, 1989.
36. Nelson SD, Kou WH, DeBuitter M, et al: Value of programmed ventricular stimulation in presumed carotid sinus syndrome. Am J Cardiol 60:1073, 1987.
37. Alexander S, Ding WC: Fatal ventricular fibrillation during carotid sinus stimulation. Am J Cardiol 18:289, 1966.
38. Munro NC, McIntosh S, Lawson J, et al: Incidence of complications after carotid sinus massage in older patients with syncope. J Am Geriatr Soc 42:1248, 1994.
39. daCosta D, McIntosh S, Kenny RA: Benefits of fludrocortisone in the treatment of symptomatic vasodepressor carotid sinus syndrome. Br Heart J 69:308, 1993.
40. Grubb BP, Samoil D, Kosinski D, et al: The use of serotonin reuptake inhibitors for the treatment of recurrent syncope due to carotid sinus hypersensitivity unresponsive to dual chamber cardiac pacing. PACE 17:1434, 1994.
41. Dan D, Grubb BP, Mouhaaffel AH, Kosinski DJ: Use of serotonin reuptake inhibitors as primary therapy for carotid sinus hypersensitivity. PACE 20:1633, 1997.
42. Keating EC, Burks JM, Calder JR: Mixed carotid sinus hypersensitivity: Successful therapy with pacing, ephedrine, and propranolol. PACE 8:356, 1985.
43. Trout HH, Brown LL, Thompson JE: Carotid sinus syndrome: Treatment by carotid sinus denervation. Ann Surg 189:575, 1979.
44. Madigan NP, Flaker GC, Curtis JJ, et al: Carotid sinus hypersensitivity: Beneficial effects of dual-chamber pacing. Am J Cardiol 53:1034, 1984.
45. Stryjer D, Friedensohn A, Schlesinger Z: Ventricular pacing as the preferable mode for long-term pacing in patients with carotid sinus syncope of the cardio inhibitory type. PACE 9:705, 1986.
46. Brignole M, Oddone D, Cogorno S, et al: Long-term outcome in symptomatic carotid sinus hypersensitivity. Am Heart J 123:687, 1992.
47. Katritsis D, Ward DE, Camm AJ: Can we treat carotid sinus syndrome? PACE 14:1367, 1991.
48. Huang SKS, Ezri MD, Hauser RG, et al: Carotid sinus hypersensitivity in patients with unexplained syncope: Clinical, electrophysiologic, and long term follow-up observations. Am Heart J 116:989, 1988.
49. Sugrue DD, Gersh BJ, Holmes DR, et al: Symptomatic "isolated" carotid sinus hypersensitivity: Natural history and results of treatment with anticholinergic drugs or pacemaker. J Am Coll Cardiol 7:158, 1986.
50. Morley CA, Perrins EJ, Grant P, et al: Carotid sinus syncope treated by pacing. Br Heart J 47:411, 1982.
51. Brignole M, Menozzi C, Lolli G, et al: Validation of a method for choice of pacing mode in carotid sinus syndrome with or without sinus bradycardia. PACE 14:196, 1991.
52. Brignole M, Menozzi C, Lolli G, et al: Natural and unnatural history of patients with severe carotid sinus hypersensitivity: A preliminary study. PACE 11:1678, 1988.
53. Probst P, Muhlberger V, Lederbauer M, et al: Electrophysiologic findings in carotid sinus massage. PACE 6:689, 1983.
54. Alicandri C, Fouad FM, Tarazi RC, et al: Three cases of hypotension and syncope with ventricular pacing: Possible role of atrial reflexes. Am J Cardiol 42:137, 1978.
55. Benditt DG, Sutton R, Gammage MD, et al: Clinical experience with Thera DR rate-drop response pacing algorithm in carotid sinus syndrome and vasovagal syncope. PACE 20:832, 1997.
56. Walter F, Crawley IS, Dorney ER: Carotid sinus hypersensitivity and syncope. Am J Cardiol 42:396, 1978.
57. Gaggioli G, Brignole M, Menozzi C, et al: A positive response to head-up tilt testing predicts syncopal recurrence in carotid sinus syndrome patients with permanent pacemakers. Am J Cardiol 76:720, 1995.
58. Brignole M, Menozzi C, Lolli G, et al: Long-term outcome of paced and non-paced patients with severe carotid sinus syndrome. Am J Cardiol 69:1039, 1992.

59. Nishizaki M, Arita M, Sakurada H, et al: Long-term follow-up of reproducibility in carotid sinus hypersensitivity in patients with carotid sinus syndrome. Jpn Circ J 59:33, 1995.

60. Epstein AE, Miles WM, Benditt DG, et al: Personal and public safety issues related to arrhythmias that may affect consciousness: Implications for regulation and physician recommendations. Circulation 94:1147, 1996.

61. Maloney JD, Jaeger FJ, Fouad-Tarazi FM, et al: Malignant vasovagal syncope: Prolonged asystole provoked by head-up tilt. Case report and review of diagnosis, pathophysiology and therapy. Cleve Clin J Med 55:543, 1988.

62. Sutton R: Vasovagal syncope: Could it be malignant? Eur J Cardiac Pacing Electrophysiol 2:89, 1992.

63. Fitzpatrick AP, Ahmed R, Williams S, et al: A randomized trial of medical therapy in "malignant vasovagal syndrome" or "neurally-mediated bradycardia/hypotension syndrome." Eur J Cardiac Pacing Electrophysiol 2:99, 1991.

64. Fitzpatrick A, Sutton R: Tilting toward a diagnosis in recurrent unexplained syncope. Lancet 1:658, 1989.

65. Grubb BP, Temesy-Armos P, Moore J, et al: Head-upright tilt-table testing in the evaluation and management of the malignant vasovagal syndrome. Am J Cardiol 69:904, 1990.

66. Jaeger FJ, Schneider L, Maloney JD, et al: Vasovagal syncope: Diagnostic role of head-up tilt test in patients with positive ocular compression test. PACE 13:1416, 1990.

67. Grubb BP, Gerard JG, Roush K, et al: Differentiation of convulsive syncope and epilepsy with head-up tilt testing. Ann Intern Med 115:871, 1991.

68. Fujimura O, Yee R, Klein GJ, et al: The diagnostic sensitivity of electrophysiologic testing in patients with syncope caused by transient bradycardia. N Engl J Med 321:1703, 1989.

69. Weissler AM, Warren JV, Estes EH, et al: Vasodepressor syncope: Factors influencing cardiac output. Circulation 15:875, 1957.

70. Goldstein DS, Spanarkel M, Pitterman A, et al: Circulatory control mechanisms in vasodepressor syncope. Am Heart J 104:1071, 1982.

71. Glick G, Yu PN: Hemodynamic changes during spontaneous vasovagal reactions. Am J Med 34:42, 1963.

72. Van Lieshout JJ, Wieling W, Karemakar JM, et al: The vasovagal response. Clin Sci 81:575, 1991.

73. Oberg B, Thoren P: Increased activity in left A ventricular receptors during hemorrhage or occlusion of caval veins in the cat: A possible cause of the vaso-vagal reaction. Acta Physiol Scand 85:164, 1972.

74. Mark AL: The Bezold-Jarisch reflex revisited: Clinical implications of inhibitory reflexes originating in the heart. J Am Coll Cardiol 1:90, 1983.

75. Dickinson CJ: Fainting precipitated by collapse-firing of venous baroreceptors. Lancet 342:970, 1993.

76. Grubb BP, Gerard G, Roush K, et al: Cerebral vasoconstriction during head-upright tilt induced vasovagal syncope. Circulation 84:1157, 1991.

77. Levine BD, Giller CA, Lane LD, et al: Cerebral versus systemic hemodynamics during graded orthostatic stress in humans. Circulation 90:298, 1994.

78. Grubb BP, Samoil D, Kosinski D, et al: Cerebral syncope: Loss of consciousness associated with cerebral vasoconstriction in the absence of systemic hypotension. PACE 20:1058, 1997.

79. Gaffney FA, Nixon JU, Karlsson ES, et al: Cardiovascular deconditioning produced by 20 hours of bedrest with head-down tilt ($-5°$) in middle-aged healthy men. Am J Cardiol 56:634, 1985.

80. Smith ML: Mechanisms of vasovagal syncope: Relevance to postflight orthostatic intolerance. J Clin Pharmacol 34:460, 1994.

81. Wallin BG, Sundlöf G: Sympathetic outflow to muscles during vasovagal syncope. J Auton Nerv Syst 6:287, 1982.

82. Shalev Y, Gal R, Tchou PJ, et al: Echocardiographic demonstration of decreased left ventricular dimensions and vigorous myocardial contraction during syncope induced by head-up tilt. J Am Coll Cardiol 18:746, 1991.

83. Fitzpatrick A, Williams T, Ahmed R, et al: Echocardiographic and endocrine changes during vasovagal syncope induced by prolonged head-up tilt. Eur J Cardiac Pacing Electrophysiol 2:121, 1992.

84. Benditt DG, Betloff B, Bailin S, et al: Exaggerated circulating epinephrine levels during neurally mediated hypotension-bradycardia syndrome: A causal factor or secondary event. PACE 14:661, 1991.

85. Calkins H, Kadish A, Sousa J, et al: Comparison of responses to isoproterenol and epinephrine during head-up tilt in suspected vasodepressor syncope. Am J Cardiol 67:207, 1991.

86. Jaeger FJ, Fouad-Tarazi FM, Bravo EL, et al: Supine norepinephrine levels and vasovagal response during head-up tilt. Circulation 80:II-90, 1989.

87. Waxman MB, Cameron DA, Wald RW: Role of ventricular vagal afferents in the vasovagal reaction. J Am Coll Cardiol 21:1138, 1993.

88. Abboud FM: Neurocardiogenic syncope. N Engl J Med 328:1117, 1993.

89. Semple PF, Thoren P, Lever AF: Vasovagal reactions to cardiovascular drugs: The first dose effect. J Hypertens 6:601, 1988.

90. Theodorakis GN, Markianos M, Livanis EG, et al: Hormonal responses during tilt-table test in neurally mediated syncope. Am J Cardiol 79:1692, 1997.

91. Jardine DL, Melton IC, Crozier IG, et al: Neurohormonal response to head-up tilt and its role in vasovagal syncope. Am J Cardiol 79:1302, 1997.

92. Sneddon JF, Counihan PJ, Bashir Y, et al: Impaired immediate vasoconstrictor responses in patients with recurrent neurally mediated syncope. Am J Cardiol 71:72, 1993.

93. Manyari DE, Rose S, Tyberg JV, Sheldon RS: Abnormal reflex venous function in patients with neuromediated syncope. J Am Coll Cardiol 27:1730, 1996.

94. Thomson HL, Atherton JJ, Khafagi FA, Frenneaux MP: Failure of reflex venoconstriction during exercise in patients with vasovagal syncope. Circulation 93:953, 1996.

95. Thomson HL, Wright K, Frenneaux M: Baroreflex sensitivity in patients with vasovagal syncope. Circulation 95:395, 1997.

96. Okabe M, Gross-Sawicka EM, Fouad FM: Vascular reactivity in patients with vasovagal syncope. Circulation 86:I-460, 1992.

97. Leitch JW, Klein GJ, Yee R, et al: Syncope associated with supraventricular tachycardia: An expression of tachycardia rate or vasomotor response? Circulation 85:1064, 1992.

98. Huikuri HV, Zaman L, Castellanos A, et al: Changes in spontaneous sinus node rate as an estimate of cardiac autonomic tone during stable and unstable ventricular tachycardia. J Am Coll Cardiol 13:646, 1989.

99. Leitch J, Klein G, Yee R, et al: Neurally mediated syncope and atrial fibrillation. N Engl J Med 324:495, 1991.

100. Brignole M, Gianfranchi L, Menozzi C, et al: Role of autonomic reflexes in syncope associated with paroxysmal atrial fibrillation. J Am Coll Cardiol 22:1123, 1993.

101. Shen WK, Hammill SC, Munger TM, et al: Adenosine: Potential modulator for vasovagal syncope. J Am Coll Cardiol 28:146, 1996.

102. Flamming D, Church T, Waynberger M, et al: Can adenosine 5'-triphosphate be used to select treatment in severe vasovagal syndrome? Circulation 96:1201, 1997.

103. Jaeger FJ, Pinski SL, Trohman RG, Fouad-Tarazi FM: Paradoxical failure of QT prolongation during cardioinhibitory neurocardiogenic syncope. Am J Cardiol 79:100, 1997.

104. Scherrer V, Vissing S, Morgan BJ, et al: Vasovagal syncope after infusion of a vasodilator in a heart transplant recipient. N Engl J Med 322:602, 1990.

105. Fitzpatrick AP, Banner N, Cheng A, et al: Vasovagal reactions may occur after orthotopic heart transplantation. J Am Coll Cardiol 21:1132, 1993.

106. Calkins H, Shyr Y, Frumin H, et al: The value of the clinical history in the differentiation of syncope due to ventricular tachycardia, atrio-ventricular block, and neurocardiogenic syncope. Am J Med 98:365, 1995.

107. Kapoor W, Karpf M, Wieland S, et al: A prospective evaluation and follow-up of patients with syncope. N Engl J Med 309:197, 1983.

108. Tarazi RC, Melsher HJ, Dustan HD, Frolich ED: Plasma volume changes with upright tilt: Studies in hypotension and syncope. J Appl Physiol 28:121, 1970.

109. Shvartz E, Meyerstein N: Tilt tolerance of young men and young women. Aerospace Med 3:253, 1970.

110. Hammill SC, Holmes DR, Wood DL, et al: Electrophysiologic testing in the upright position: Improved evaluation of patients with rhythm disturbances using a tilt table. J Am Coll Cardiol 4:65, 1984.

111. Benditt DG, Ferguson Dw, Grubb BP, et al: Tilt table testing for assessing syncope [Review]. J Am Coll Cardiol 28:263, 1996.

112. Sheldon R: Tilt table testing in the diagnosis and treatment of syncope [Review]. Cardiovasc Rev Rep 15:8, 1994.

113. Kapoor WN, Smith MA, Miller NL: Upright tilt testing in evaluation of syncope: A comprehensive literature review [review]. Am J Med 97:78, 1994.

114. Landau WM, Nelson DA: Clinical neuromythology. XV. Fainting

science: Neurocardiogenic syncope and collateral vasovagal confusion [review]. Neurology 46:609, 1996.

115. Fitzpatrick AP, Theodorakis G, Vardas P, et al: Methodology of head-up tilt testing in patients with unexplained syncope. J Am Coll Cardiol 17:125, 1991.

116. Stevens PM: Cardiovascular dynamics during orthostasis and the influence of intravascular instrumentation. Am J Cardiol 17:211, 1966.

117. Kenny RA, Ingram A, Bayliss J, et al: Head-up tilt: A useful test for investigating unexplained syncope. Lancet 1:1352, 1986.

118. Fitzpatrick A, Sutton R: Tilting toward a diagnosis in recurrent unexplained syncope. Lancet 1:658, 1989.

119. Abi-Samra F, Maloney JD, Fouad-Tarazi FM, Castle LW: The usefulness of head-up tilt testing and hemodynamic investigations in the work-up of syncope of unknown origin. PACE 11:1202, 1988.

120. Grubb BP, Temesy-Armos P, Hahn H, et al: Utility of upright tilt-table testing in the evaluation and management of syncope of unknown origin. Am J Med 90:6, 1991.

121. Raviele A, Menozzi C, Brignole M, et al: Value of head-up tilt testing potentiated with sublingual nitroglycerin to assess the origin of unexplained syncope. Am J Cardiol 76:267, 1995.

122. Grubb BP, Kosinski D, Temesy-Armos P, Brewster P: Responses of normal subjects during 80° head upright tilt table testing with and without low dose isoproterenol infusion. PACE 20:2019, 1997.

123. Raviele A, Gasparini G, DiPede F, et al: Usefulness of head-up tilt test in evaluating patients with syncope of unknown origin and negative electrophysiology study. Am J Cardiol 65:1322, 1990.

124. Strasberg B, Rechavia E, Sagic A, et al: The head up tilt table test in patients with syncope of unknown origin. Am Heart J 118:923, 1989.

125. Alehan D, Lenk M, Ozme S, et al: Comparison of sensitivity and specificity of tilt protocols with and without isoproterenol in children with unexplained syncope. PACE 20:1769, 1997.

126. Fouad FM, Sitthisook S, Vanerio G, et al: Sensitivity and specificity of the tilt table test in young patients with unexplained syncope. PACE 16:394, 1993.

127. Lipsitz LA, Marks ER, Koestner J, et al: Reduced susceptibility to syncope during postural tilt in old age: Is beta-blockade protective? Arch Intern Med 149:2709, 1989.

128. Sexton E, Koshman ML, Sheldon RS: Randomized trial of tilt angle, and contribution of tilt duration, isoproterenol, and nitroglycerin to the diagnosis of neurally mediated syncope [Abstract]. Circulation 96:I-265, 1997.

129. Ross BA, Hughes S, Anderson E, Gillette PC: Abnormal responses to orthostatic testing in children and adolescents with recurrent unexplained syncope. Am Heart J 122:748, 1991.

130. Waxman MB, Yao L, Cameron DA, et al: Isoproterenol induction of vasodepressor-type reaction in vasodepressor-prone persons. Am J Cardiol 63:58, 1989.

131. Almquist A, Goldenberg IF, Milstein S, et al: Provocation of bradycardia and hypotension by isoproterenol and upright posture in patients with unexplained syncope. N Engl J Med 320:346, 1989.

132. Raviele A, Gasparini G, Di Pede F: Nitroglycerine infusion during upright tilt: A new test for the diagnosis of vasovagal syncope. Am Heart J 127:103, 1994.

133. Sharpey-Schafer EP, Hayter CJ, Barlow ED: Mechanism of acute hypotension from fear or nausea. Br Med J 2:878, 1958.

134. Karp HR, Weissler AM, Heyman A: Vasodepressor syncope: EEG and circulatory changes. Arch Neurol 5:106, 1961.

135. Lurie KG, Dutton J, Mangat R, et al: Evaluation of edrophonium as a provocative agent for vasovagal syncope during head-up tilt-table testing. Am J Cardiol 72:1286, 1993.

136. Morillo CA, Klein GJ, Zandri S, Yee R: Diagnostic accuracy of a low-dose isoproterenol head-up tilt protocol. Am Heart J 129:901, 1995.

137. Sheldon R, Killam S: Methodology of isoproterenol tilt table testing in patients with syncope. J Am Coll Cardiol 19:773, 1992.

138. Sheldon R: Evaluation of a single-stage isoproterenol-tilt table test in patients with syncope. J Am Coll Cardiol 22:114, 1993.

139. Brignole M, Menozzi C, Gianfranchi L, et al: Carotid sinus massage, eyeball compression, and head-up tilt tests in patients with syncope of uncertain origin and in healthy control subjects. Am Heart J 122:1644, 1991.

140. Sheldon RS, Rose S, Koshman ML: Isoproterenol tilt-table testing in patients with syncope and structural heart disease. Am J Cardiol 78:700, 1996.

141. Kapoor W, Brant N: Evaluation of syncope by upright tilt testing with isoproterenol: A nonspecific test. Ann Intern Med 116:358, 1992.

142. Natale A, Akhtar M, Jazayeri M, et al: Provocation of hypotension during head-up tilt testing in subjects with no history of syncope or presyncope. Circulation 92:54, 1995.

143. Sutton R, Peterson M, Brignole M, et al: Proposed classification for tilt induced vasovagal syncope. Eur J Cardiac Pacing Electrophysiol 3:180, 1992.

144. Linzer M, Varia I, Pontinen M, et al: Medically unexplained syncope: Relationship to psychiatric illness. Am J Med 92:18(S), 1992.

145. Sheldon RS, Rose S, Koshman ML: Comparison of patients with syncope of unknown cause having negative or positive tilt table tests. Am J Cardiol 80:581, 1997.

146. Grimm W, Degenhardt M, Hoffmann J, et al: Syncope recurrence can be better predicted by history than by head-up tilt testing in untreated patients with suspected neurally mediated syncope. Eur Heart J 18:1465, 1997.

147. Chen XC, Chen MY, Remole S, et al: Reproducibility of head-up tilt table testing for eliciting susceptibility to neurally mediated syncope in patients without structural heart disease. Am J Cardiol 69:755, 1992.

148. Fish FA, Strasburger JF, Benson DW: Reproducibility of a symptomatic response to upright tilt in young patients with unexplained syncope. Am J Cardiol 70:605, 1992.

149. De Buitleir M, Grogan W, Picone MF, et al: Immediate reproducibility of the tilt table test in adults with unexplained syncope. Am J Cardiol 71:304, 1993.

150. Grubb BP, Wolfe D, Temesy-Armos P, et al: Reproducibility of head upright tilt table test in patients with syncope. PACE 15:1477, 1992.

151. Blanc JJ, Mansourati J, Maheu B, et al: Reproducibility of a positive passive tilt test at a seven-day interval in patients with syncope. Am J Cardiol 72:469, 1993.

152. Sheldon R, Splawinski J, Killam S: Reproducibility of isoproterenol tilt-table tests in patients with syncope. Am J Cardiol 69:1300, 1992.

153. Petersen MEV, Price D, Williams T, et al: Short AV interval VDD pacing does not prevent tilt induced vasovagal syncope in patients with cardioinhibitory vasovagal syndrome. PACE 17:882, 1994.

154. Morillo CA, Leitch JW, Yee R, Klein GJ: A placebo-controlled trial of intravenous and oral disopyramide for prevention of neurally mediated syncope induced by head-up tilt. J Am Coll Cardiol 22:1843, 1993.

155. Moya A, Permanyer-Miraldo G, Sagrista-Savleda J, et al: Limitations of head-up tilt test for evaluating the efficacy of therapeutic interventions in patients with vasovagal syncope: Results of a controlled study of etilefrine versus placebo. J Am Coll Cardiol 25:65, 1995.

156. Morillo C, Klein GJ, Gersh BJ: Can serial tilt testing be used to evaluate therapy in neurally mediated syncope? Am J Cardiol 77:521, 1996.

157. Jaeger FJ, Schneider L, Maloney JD, et al: Vasovagal syncope: Diagnostic role of head-up tilt test in patients with positive ocular compression test. PACE 13:1416, 1990.

158. Brignole M, Menozzi C, Gianfranchi L, et al: Neurally mediated syncope detected by carotid sinus massage and head-up tilt test in sick sinus syndrome. Am J Cardiol 68:1032, 1991.

159. Brignole M, Gaggioli G, Menozzi C, et al: Adenosine-induced paroxysmal atrioventricular block: A new possible cause of unexplained syncope? In Raviele A (ed): Cardiac Arrhythmias. Milano, Italy, Springer, 1997, pp 363–367.

160. Krahn AD, Klein GJ, Norris C, Yee R: The etiology of syncope in patients with negative tilt table and electrophysiological testing. Circulation 92:1819, 1995.

161. Savage DD, Corwin L, McGee DL, et al: Epidemiologic features of isolated syncope: The Framingham study. Stroke 16:626, 1985.

162. Kushner JA, Kou WH, Kadish AH, Morady F: Natural history of patients with unexplained syncope and a nondiagnostic electrophysiologic study. J Am Coll Cardiol 14:391, 1989.

163. Brignole M, Menozzi C, Gianfranchi L, et al: The clinical and prognostic significance of the asystolic response during the head-up tilt test. Eur J Cardiac Pacing Electrophysiol 2:109, 1992.

164. Dhala A, Natale A, Sra J, et al: Relevance of asystole during head-up tilt testing. Am J Cardiol 75:251, 1995.

165. Sheldon RS: Outcome of patients with neurally mediated syncope following tilt table testing [Review]. Cardiologia 42:795, 1997.

166. Brignole M, Menozzi C, Gianfranchi L, et al: A controlled trial of acute and long-term medical therapy in tilt-induced neurally mediated syncope. Am J Cardiol 70:339, 1992.

167. Natale A, Geiger MJ, Maglio C, et al: Recurrence of neurocardiogenic syncope without pharmacologic interventions. Am J Cardiol 77:1001, 1996.

168. Sheldon RS, Rose S, Flanagan P, et al: Multivariate predictors of syncope recurrence in drug-free patients following a positive tilt table test. Circulation 93:973, 1996.

169. Sheldon RS, Rose S, Flanagan P, et al: Effect of beta blockers on the clinical outcome of patients after a positive isoproterenol-tilt table test. Am J Cardiol 78:536, 1997.

170. Menozzi C, Brignole M, Lolli G, et al: Follow-up of asystolic episodes in patients with cardioinhibitory, neurally mediated syncope and VVI pacemaker. Am J Cardiol 72:1152, 1993.

171. Connolly SJ, Sheldon R, Roberts RS, et al: The North American Vasovagal Pacemaker Study (VPS): A randomized trial of permanent cardiac pacing for the prevention of vasovagal syncope. J Am Coll Cardiol 33:16, 1999.

172. Malik P, Koshman ML, Sheldon R, et al: Timing of first syncope recurrence predicts syncope frequency following a positive tilt table test. J Am Coll Cardiol 29:1284, 1997.

173. Sra JS, Murthy V, Jazayeri MR, et al: Use of intravenous esmolol to predict efficacy of oral beta-adrenergic therapy in patients with neurocardiogenic syncope. J Am Coll Cardiol 19:402, 1992.

174. Cox MM, Perlman BA, Mayor MR, et al: Acute and long-term beta-adrenergic blockade for patients with neurocardiogenic syncope. J Am Coll Cardiol 26:1293, 1995.

175. Mahanonda N, Bhuripanyo K, Kangkagate C, et al: Randomized double-blind, placebo-controlled trial of oral atenolol in patients with unexplained syncope and positive upright tilt table test results. Am Heart J 130:1250, 1995.

176. Leor J, Rotstein Z, Vered Z, et al: Absence of tachycardia during tilt test predicts failure of β-blocker therapy in patients with neurocardiogenic syncope. Am Heart J 127:1539, 1994.

177. Natale A, Newby KH, Dhala A, et al: Response to beta blockers in patients with neurocardiogenic syncope: How to predict beneficial effects. J Cardiovasc Electrophysiol 7:1154, 1996.

178. Klingenheben T, Kalusche D, Li Y, et al: Changes in plasma epinephrine concentration and in heart rate during head-up tilt testing in patients with neurocardiogenic syncope: Correlation with successful therapy with β-receptor antagonists. J Cardiovasc Electrophysiol 7:802, 1996.

179. Milstein S, Buetikofer J, Dunnigan A, et al: Usefulness of disopyramide for prevention of upright tilt-induced hypotension-bradycardia. Am J Cardiol 65:1339, 1990.

180. Strieper MJ, Campbell RM: Efficacy of alpha-adrenergic agonist therapy for prevention of pediatric neurocardiogenic syncope. J Am Coll Cardiol 22:591, 1993.

181. Sra J, Maglio C, Dhala A, et al: Efficacy of midodrine hydrochloride in neurocardiogenic syncope refractory to standard therapy. J Cardiovasc Electrophysiol 8:42, 1997.

181a. Raviele A, Brignole M, Sutton R, et al: Effect of etilefrine in preventing syncopal recurrence in patients with vasovagal syncope: A double-blind, randomized, placebo-controlled trial. J Am Coll Cardiol 99:1452, 1999.

182. Grubb BP, Samoil D, Kosinski D, et al: Use of sertraline hydrochloride in the treatment of refractory neurocardiogenic syncope in children and adolescents. J Am Coll Cardiol 24:490, 1994.

183. Grubb BP, Wolfe DA, Samoil D, et al: Usefulness of fluoxetine hydrochloride for prevention of resistant upright tilt induced syncope. PACE 16:458, 1993.

184. Tandan T, Guiffre M, Sheldon RS: Exacerbation of neurally mediated syncope associated with sertraline treatment. Lancet 349:1145, 1997.

185. Benditt DG, Benson W, Kreitt J, et al: Electrophysiologic effects of theophylline in young patients with recurrent symptomatic bradyarrhythmias. Am J Cardiol 52:1223, 1983.

186. Nelson SD, Stanley M, Love CJ, et al: The autonomic and hemodynamic effects of oral theophylline in patients with vasodepressor syncope. Arch Intern Med 151:2425, 1991.

187. El-Sayed H, Hainsworth R: Salt supplement increases plasma volume and orthostatic tolerance in patients with unexplained syncope. Heart 75:134, 1996.

188. Mangru NN, Young ML, Mas MS, et al: Usefulness of tilt table test with normal saline infusion in management of neurocardiogenic syncope in children. Am Heart J 131:953, 1996.

189. Scott WA, Giacomo P, Bromberg BI, et al: Randomized comparison of atenolol and fludrocortisone acetate in the treatment of pediatric neurally mediated syncope. Am J Cardiol 76:400, 1995.

190. Grubb BP, Temesy-Armos P, Moore J, et al: The use of head-upright tilt table testing in the evaluation and management of syncope in children and adolescents. PACE 15:742, 1992.

191. Balaji S, Oslizlok PC, Allen MC, et al: Neurocardiogenic syncope in children with a normal heart. J Am Coll Cardiol 23:779, 1994.

192. Dreifus LS, Fisch C, Griffin JC: Guidelines for implantation of cardiac pacemakers and antiarrhythmia devices: A report of the American College of Cardiology/American Heart Association Task Force on Assessment of Diagnostic and Therapeutic Procedures (Committee on Pacemaker Implantation). J Am Coll Cardiol 18:1, 1991.

193. Clarke M, Sutton R, Ward D, et al: Recommendations for pacemaker prescriptions for symptomatic bradycardia: British Pacing and Electrophysiology Group Working Party Report. Br Heart J 66:185, 1991.

194. Benditt DG, Petersen M, Lurie KG, et al: Cardiac pacing for prevention of recurrent vasovagal syncope [Review]. Ann Intern Med 122:204, 1995.

195. Fitzpatrick A, Theodorakis G, Ahmed R, et al: Dual chamber pacing aborts vasovagal syncope induced by head-up 60° tilt. PACE 4:13, 1991.

196. Samoil D, Grubb BP, Brewster P, et al: Comparison of single and dual chamber pacing techniques in prevention of upright tilt induced vasovagal syncope. Eur J Cardiac Pacing Electrophysiol 1:36, 1993.

197. Sra JS, Jazayeri MR, Avitall BA, et al: Comparison of cardiac pacing with drug therapy in the treatment of neurocardiogenic (vasovagal) syncope with bradycardia or asystole. N Engl J Med 328:1085, 1993.

198. El-Bedawi ICM, Wahbha MA, Hainsworth R: Cardiac pacing does not improve orthostatic tolerance in patients with vasovagal syncope. Clin Auton Res 4:233, 1994.

199. Sapire DW, Casta A, Safley W, et al: Vasovagal syncope in children requiring pacemaker implantation. Am Heart J 106:1406, 1983.

200. Petersen MEV, Chamberlain-Webber R, Fitzpatrick AP, et al: Permanent pacing for cardioinhibitory malignant vasovagal syndrome. Br Heart J 71:274, 1994.

201. Sheldon RS, Koshman ML, Wilson W, et al: Effect of dual chamber pacing with automatic rate-drop sensing on recurrent neurally mediated syncope. Am J Cardiol 81:158, 1998.

202. Brennan JF, Mitchell LB, Sheldon RS, et al: Assessment of the cardiac patient for fitness to drive: 1996 Update. Can J Cardiol 12:1164, 1996.

203. Sheldon RS, Koshman ML: Can patients with neuromediated syncope safely drive motor vehicles? Am J Cardiol 75:955, 1995.

Chapter 19

Pacing for Prevention of Tachyarrhythmias

Sanjeev Saksena, Rahul Mehra, and Kenneth A. Ellenbogen

It should be borne in mind that the condition is the outcome of a series of changes that have been going on for years, and it is foolish to suppose that we can remove the diseased processes . . . Attempts, therefore, to cure the condition are futile. What we have to do is, not to waste time in a hopeless quest, but to make the best of an irremediable condition. . .

Sir James Mackenzie, *Diseases of the Heart,* 1908

■ PACING FOR PREVENTION OF AF

The challenges associated with reestablishing rhythm control in patients with atrial fibrillation (AF) have long been recognized. One long-standing tenet in clinical medicine, as noted by the distinguished scholar above, has been the perceived irreversible nature of drug-refractory and chronic AF.[1] Thus, early hopeful efforts designed to restore sinus rhythm with direct current cardioversion were dampened by the frequent recurrences of AF.[2] Antiarrhythmic drug therapy was initially instituted at the turn of the 20th century to prevent atrial arrhythmias.[3] Current experience suggests that there is a high relapse rate with this modality during long-term follow-up.[4] Alternative nonpharmacologic methods for prevention of recurrent AF have been investigated. These include direct atrial surgery, catheter-based atrial ablation, internal atrial defibrillation, and atrial pacing.

Internal atrial defibrillation has also demonstrated limitations with respect to recurrent AF similar to transthoracic direct current cardioversion.[5–7] In retrospective analyses of patients with sick sinus syndrome, atrial-based pacing reduced the incidence and frequency of recurrence of AF in patients without and with manifest AF, respectively.[8–12] More recently, prospective study data have also supported this conclusion in specific subgroups.[13, 14] A recently published study, however, was unable to document a benefit to DDIR

pacing at 70 bpm in patients with drug-resistant frequent PAF.[146] Furthermore, clinical experience in populations with bradycardia or vagally mediated AF has also been similar.[15, 16] Development of more sophisticated pacing algorithms and pacing methods, such as dual-site atrial pacing, have recently been examined.[17, 18] Pacing techniques for prevention of reentrant supraventricular tachycardias and common atrial flutter were widely discussed in the 1970's and 80's but have largely been replaced by catheter ablation. For a detailed discussion, the reader is referred elsewhere.

It is the purpose of this chapter to examine the experimental basis for the use of atrial pacing methods in the prevention of AF, their individual clinical electrophysiologic effects, current clinical techniques, and the outcome of this therapy. On the basis of these data, new clinical trials and directions in device development are in progress and are also briefly examined. Also, the principles and techniques used in AF prevention are being considered for prevention of other arrhythmias, paroxysmal supraventricular tachycardias, and atrial flutter.

■ RATIONALE AND MECHANISMS OF ATRIAL FIBRILLATION PREVENTION WITH PACING METHODS

Most mapping data from experimental studies indicate that AF is sustained by a reentrant mechanism with multiple wavelets. AF, however, is initiated by an atrial premature beat that can be ectopic in origin owing to either abnormal automaticity or afterdepolarizations. Premature beats can also be reentrant in origin, occurring as a result of acceleration of the atrial rate. To prevent AF or atrial flutter, pacing must suppress these ectopic beats or prevent these ectopic beats from initiating sustained AF. The third mechanism by which pacing may prevent AF is by altering the atrial substrate such that even if AF is initiated by premature beats, it remains unsustained. Sustainability can be affected by electrical remodeling or changes caused by electromechanical feedback in the atrium. Each of these three mechanisms is discussed subsequently.

Overdrive Suppression of Ectopic Beats

It is hypothesized that suppression of premature beats can reduce the incidence of a sustained atrial or ventricular tachyarrhythmia. This association, however, was not observed in the Cardiac Arrhythmia Suppression Trial (CAST), in which sustained ventricular tachyarrhythmias were not suppressed despite a reduction in ventricular ectopy. One key factor was that the antiarrhythmic drugs not only suppressed ectopy but also could compromise the electrophysiologic substrate and increase its propensity to sustain tachyarrhythmias. With atrial pacing, one preventive effect would be on suppression of atrial ectopy, although changes in the electrophysiologic substrate also can occur. It has been observed that increasing the atrial pacing rate can suppress atrial ectopy.[19] This effect is due to direct overdrive suppression of atrial ectopy or to changes in the mechanical function that can modulate electrical activity (mechanoelectric feedback).[20] Electrocardiogram (ECG) tracings of onset of AF in patients with vagally mediated AF indicate that premature beats that initiate AF are frequently preceded by bradycardia.[15, 16] In these patients, increasing the pacing rate suppresses ectopy and therefore the induction of AF.[16, 21]

The relationship between atrial rate and frequency of atrial premature beats has not been investigated, whereas this relationship has been well studied for ventricular ectopy. Data indicate that in many patients the ventricular premature contraction frequency decreases with increasing rate, and then at higher rates ventricular ectopy increases again.[22] This relationship is altered with antiarrhythmic drugs as well as autonomic modulation. If the same effect occurs in the atrium, there will be a critical rate range within which atrial premature beats will be suppressed, and this critical rate will be dependent on the antiarrhythmic drugs as well as autonomic function. Clinically, there is an upper limit on this critical rate to avoid eliciting undesirable symptoms.

One method of avoiding continuous high rate pacing is to increase the pacing rate temporarily, only in the presence of ectopic atrial premature beats. Such an algorithm was tested in patients, and this "Consistent Atrial Pacing" algorithm increased the percentage of paced beats from 65% to 96%; however, a significant difference in the total number of symptomatic AF episodes or mode switches per day was not observed.[23] In another algorithm, sensed atrial premature beats increased the pacing rate by 12.5%, and this rate was maintained for 20 beats if no further atrial premature beats were sensed.[19] Subsequently, the pacing cycle length was increased by 63 msec until sinus rhythm or the lower pacing rate was reached. In this study, there was also no statistical reduction in AF episodes despite a reduction in premature beats. The authors noted that this may be due to the fact that the algorithm deactivated when two or more atrial premature beats were observed in succession. It is important to note that these algorithms not only increase atrial rate but also change the activation sequence of the atria. Reduction in ectopy would be expected with an increase in rate, but a change in the activation sequence by pacing from an undesirable site could negate the antiarrhythmic effect.

Pacing the atrium at a high rate can also theoretically suppress AF by suppressing ventricular premature beats. Csapo[24] showed that critically timed ventricular premature beats that conduct retrogradely can initiate atrial premature beats in the vulnerable period, resulting in AF. He observed that in animals after acetylcholine infusion, asynchronous ventricular pacing was able to elicit AF by initiating retrograde P waves. Therefore, overdrive atrial pacing may also prevent AF by suppressing ventricular ectopy.

Effect of Pacing Site on Prematurity of Ectopic Beats in the Arrhythmia Substrate

The most significant effect of pacing is a change in the activation sequence and its associated effects on induction of atrial tachyarrhythmias. It is well established that to induce atrial tachyarrhythmias, the coupling interval of the premature beat needs to be short.[25, 26] This has also been well investigated in canine models, in which induction of AF from multiple sites was studied.[27, 28] In the study by Wang and associates,[27] AF could be induced only from atrial sites with short effective refractory periods and only with extrastimuli delivered at close coupling intervals. Differences in local effective refractory periods largely accounted for site-dependent variations in AF induction. This closely coupled premature beat encounters conduction delay or block or both in the abnormal substrate, resulting in reentrant activation. Therefore, for reentry to be initiated, the coupling interval of the ectopic beat in the abnormal substrate must have a critical and short value.

Atrial pacing can alter the activation sequence in such a manner that the same premature beat results in a longer coupling interval in the abnormal substrate, preventing the initiation of reentry.[29] This can be achieved by pacing within the abnormal substrate or by pacing at a site such that it creates an activation that is antidromic to the activation of the abnormal substrate by the premature beat. This tends to "preexcite" the abnormal substrate, a concept that is discussed in more detail later. It is assumed that the site of origin of the premature beat is not altered with an alteration in the pacing site. Clinically, there may be several sites of origin for sinus and premature atrial beats as a result of alterations in autonomic tone as well as regional distribution of diseased tissue. Certain combinations of sinus and premature activation sequences could be proarrhythmic. If pacing is performed from an atrial site such that the coupling interval of the premature beats in the abnormal substrate is longer than under control conditions, it could reduce the incidence of atrial tachyarrhythmias.

Pacing Within the Abnormal Arrhythmia Substrate

The abnormal substrate is often the tissue where reentry is initiated because of its prolonged refractory periods, large refractory period gradients, or significant anisotropic properties. Figure 19–1 illustrates the concept of pacing from an abnormal substrate to prevent reentrant activation. In Figure 19–1A, the S1 and S2 stimulation sites are identical, and both triggered wavefronts conduct to the abnormal substrate such that the A1–A2 coupling interval is short enough to initiate reentry. If the location of this abnormal region is known and pacing is performed from within it, then the A1

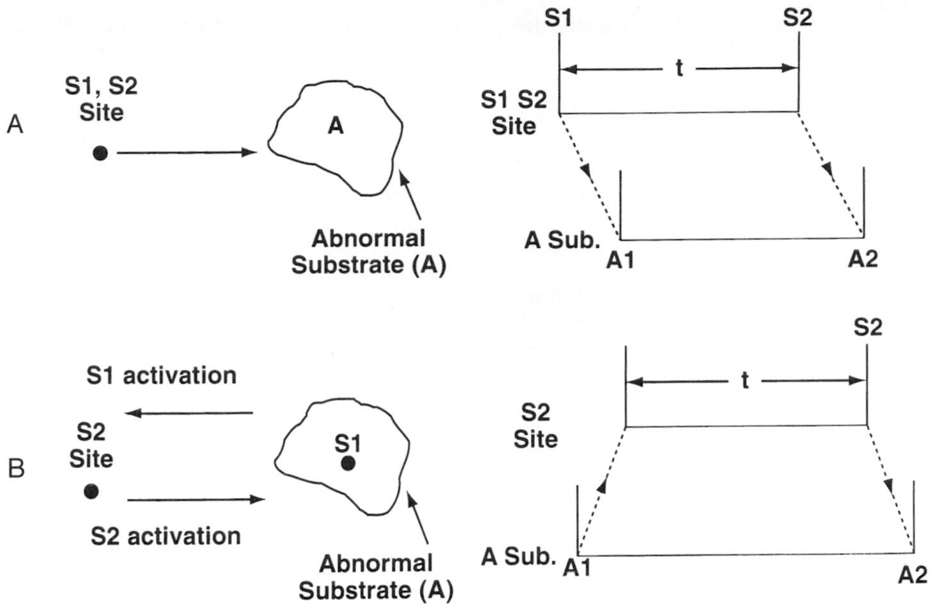

Figure 19–1. *A*, The site of pacing S1 and premature beat S2 are orthodromic to each other. The coupling interval of the premature beat at the site of stimulation is t. This results in activation of the abnormal substrate at a coupling of A1–A2, which is not significantly prolonged. *B*, The S1 stimulation is from the abnormal substrate, and neither the site nor the coupling interval of S2 changes. Now the activation of the S1 and S2 beats are antidromic to each other, resulting in a long A1–A2 coupling in the abnormal substrate.

beat conducts antidromic to the premature beat in such a manner that the A1–A2 interval in the abnormal substrate is prolonged. This can prevent initiation of reentry. This concept assumes that the coupling interval, as well as the site of the S2 premature beat, is not altered. This concept has been well documented with mapping for induction of ventricular tachyarrhythmias, but not in the atrium.[30–32] In these ventricular studies, the region of reentry was defined and when this tissue was preexcited, reentry could be prevented. Arrhythmias could not be prevented when pacing was done from two sites, if neither were within the abnormal substrate.

Determining the location of the abnormal substrate in patients makes practical implementation of this concept challenging. Some of the abnormal regions that have been suggested are the high right atrium, triangle of Koch region, isthmus between the inferior vena cava and tricuspid annulus, pulmonary vein inflow, coronary sinus ostium, or crista terminalis, although detailed information regarding conduction in these regions in humans is not available. Mapping of the initiation of typical flutter in patients indicates that initial block occurs in the low septal region between the tricuspid annulus and the coronary sinus and inferior vena caval region.[33] In animal models, the regions of conduction block vary with the model. In models using vagal stimulation, the region of conduction delay was in the vicinity of regions with a long refractory period in the left atrium, resulting in a single macroreentrant circuit.[27] These results are similar to those reported by Boineau and coworkers,[26] who observed slow conduction and block in the region of long refractory periods. In a right atrial enlargement model of atrial flutter, Schoels and colleagues[34] observed "islands" of short or long refractory periods, resulting in a high gradient of refractoriness. The average dispersion of refractory periods was similar in normal and enlarged hearts, but the spatial distribution was different. These investigators concluded that it was the spatial dispersion of refractory periods rather than the absolute degree of dispersion that produced the induction of stable atrial arrhythmias. The

ability of extrastimuli to induce AF varied with the stimulation site, and it was more difficult to induce AF from regions of long refractory periods, primarily because closely coupled premature beats could not be induced from those sites.

In the studies by Schuessler and associates[35] on isolated right atrial tissue perfused with acetylcholine, the initial site of conduction block frequently occurred close to the crista terminalis despite the site of the initial premature beats. Although the refractory periods were not measured in the preparations, this is known to be a region of large anisotropy. In the sterile pericarditis model of atrial flutter, reentry occurs in the same region of the right atrium, irrespective of the site of stimulation.[36] In chronic models of AF, macroreentry is generally not observed, and the site of initial reentrant activation frequently occurs in close proximity to the site of the premature stimulus.[37] It is possible that in atria with such heterogeneous electrophysiologic properties, multiple regions within the left and right atrium may be capable of initiating reentry. Conceptually, all these sites would need to be paced simultaneously to reduce the probability of initiating AF, and this is technically difficult.

Pacing Antidromic to the Activation of the Premature Beat

In most clinical situations, the location of the abnormal substrate may not be precisely known. If the location is known globally, however, one can still preexcite that region by pacing at an opposing site, so that the abnormal substrate is activated antidromic to its activation by the premature beat. This is illustrated in Figure 19–2. It is important to note that this requires that the site of origin of the premature beats be identified. Clinical studies indicate that apart from the sinus node, the superior aspect of the crista terminalis and the ostia of the pulmonary veins may be the most likely sites for their origin. Therefore, by pacing in the inferior atrial locations, one would create an activation wavefront antidromic to that of the premature beat.

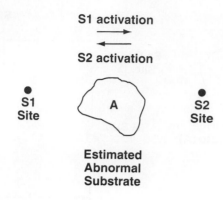

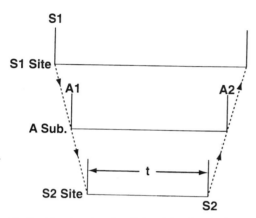

Figure 19–2. The site of pacing (S1) and the site of origin of the premature beat are on the opposite sides of the abnormal substrate. The S1 beat activates the abnormal substrate and then the site of origin of the premature beat. Because the coupling interval of the premature beats is t, its antidromic activation results in a significantly longer A1–A2 coupling interval in the abnormal substrate. (From Mehra R, Hill MRS: Prevention of atrial fibrillation/flutter by pacing techniques. *In* Saksena S, Luderitz B (eds): Interventional Electrophysiology: A Textbook, 2nd ed. Armonk, NY, Futura, 1996, p 533.)

Effect of Atrial Pacing on the Electrophysiologic Substrate

Although the factors discussed previously prevent initiation of AF, pacing may prevent AF by altering its sustainability. A change in the atrial pacing rate can alter the electrophysiologic substrate and prevent sustenance of AF. For example, it has been well documented that increasing the pacing rate reduces the dispersion of refractory periods. This decreases the likelihood of a premature beat experiencing conduction block and reentry for initiation of AF. The effect of pacing rate on dispersion has been documented in animal experiment, but not as well in clinical studies.[38] Preventing initiation of AF can have a cumulative effect on its sustenance. Animal studies by Wijffels and associates[39] indicate that when animals with chronic AF are maintained in sinus rhythm, it is much more difficult to sustain AF. This suggests that "sinus rhythm begets sinus rhythm" in a manner similar to "AF begets AF."[39] It was suggested that this effect is primarily related to a blunting of the rate adaptation of refractory periods.

The mechanism by which an alteration in the rate adaptation of refractory periods can affect AF sustenance was investigated in a computer simulation using a "cell automata" model.[40] In this model, reentry was initiated in a matrix of 900 units representing an aggregate of atrial cells. Each cell underwent time-dependent changes in excitability, and the refractory periods were dependent on the cycle length of the previous beat. The slope of the curve that defines the relationship between refractory period and cycle length was varied between 0.15 and 0.8, with the low slope representing almost constant refractory periods. It was observed that reentry was more stable and sustained at slopes of less than 0.6, whereas at higher slopes, the induced reentrant tachycardias were often unstable and terminated spontaneously.

Atrial pacing rate may also affect arrhythmogenesis by its indirect effect on atrial pressure and stretch. The association between large dilated atria and AF has long been recognized. Animal and clinical studies indicate that an increase in right atrial pressure increases the ability to sustain as well as initiate AF. Sideris and coworkers[41] showed in canine experiments that elevation of atrial pressure by venous transfusion facilitated induction of short duration AF. The increase in atrial pressure was also associated with an increase in atrial ectopy. This could be a result of localized early afterdepolarizations.[20] Satoh and Zipes[42] observed that increased atrial vulnerability in animals was associated with an increase in the effective refractory periods as well as the dispersion of effective refractory periods between the thin and the thick regions of the atria. Although all studies consistently show a greater vulnerability to atrial arrhythmias, the electrophysiologic effects of increasing atrial pressure have been more controversial.

In isolated animal studies[43] and in one clinical study,[44] an increase in pressure was associated with a decrease in refractory periods. In this clinical study, the atrial pressure was increased by shortening the paced atrioventricular (AV) interval from 120 to 0 msec. This resulted in a 7.3-msec shortening of the effective refractory period. These study results are in contrast to the findings of another clinical study, in which an increase in atrial pressure was associated with a marked increase in the atrial effective refractory periods.[45] One factor that could explain the contradictory results is that the changes in the refractory periods depends on the rate of change of the atrial pressure, a variable that was not controlled. In isolated tissues, gradual changes in load have little effect on the action potential, whereas abrupt changes result in shortening of the action potential duration.[46–50] In clinical pacing, a change in atrial pressure can be facilitated by a change in the AV interval, pacing rate, or site of stimulation.[51–53] During right ventricular apical pacing, changing the mode of pacing can also alter the right atrial pressures. In one study, right atrial pressures with AAIR and DDDR pacing at a mean AV delay of 142 msec were similar and significantly lower than during VVIR pacing at rest. During exercise, however, the atrial pressures with the three modes were significantly different, with the lowest pressures being seen in AAIR pacing and the highest pressures with VVIR pacing.

Dual-Site Pacing for Prevention of Atrial Fibrillation

A key question relates to the possible mechanisms by which dual-site atrial pacing may be more antiarrhythmic with respect to AF prevention than single-site pacing. The differential effect between these modes is primarily related to the activation sequence and electrophysiologic changes in the substrate associated with single-site and dual-site atrial pacing. Under certain conditions, dual-site atrial pacing can change the atrial activation sequence and prolong coupling intervals for premature beats to a greater extent than can single-site pacing. For example, if there is one atrial substrate for reentrant activation to occur, then single-site pacing from within it is preventative. If there are at least two anatomically distinct substrates, however, pacing from both of them is needed. Second, dual-site pacing may be more antiarrhythmic if the location of the abnormal substrate or the location of the sites of premature beats is unknown. In this case, pacing from two sites may increase the probability of preexciting the abnormal substrates, prolonging coupling intervals for premature beats, and reducing the chance of eliciting conduction block and reentrant activation. For example, in the mapping studies conducted by Schoels and colleagues[34, 54] in an animal mode of AF, reentrant circuits were most frequently observed in the inferior right atrium or the superior left or right atrium, and it would be desirable to pace from an inferior and superior location to preexcite both regions. However, if the location of the abnormal substrate is known and pacing was performed from this site, it could conceptually be more antiarrhythmic than dual-site pacing. Finally, dual-site atrial pacing can also alter the hemodynamics of atrial contraction so as to improve atrial emptying and facilitate a greater antiarrhythmic effect. Daubert and associates[55–57] showed that in patients with significant interatrial conduction delays, pacing from the left and the right atrium reduced pulmonary capillary wedge pressure significantly as compared with right atrial pacing alone. Biatrial pacing was associated with prevention of atypical atrial flutter in these patients.

The effect of dual-site pacing has been evaluated in animals who were chronically conditioned for AF by pacing them at high atrial rates for more than 2 months.[28] In these animals, the coupling window for induction of AF with a single premature stimulus was compared with single-site and dual-site right atrial pacing. The coupling window for premature beats from the atrial appendage was shorter with dual-site pacing from the right atrial appendage and the coronary sinus as compared with single-site pacing from the right atrial appendage alone. However, when premature beats were delivered from the coronary sinus, there was no reduction in the coupling window with dual-site pacing. This indicates that the antiarrhythmic effect of dual-site pacing may be dependent on the site of origin of the premature beats. The results indicate that in this model, the abnormal substrate may have been close to the coronary sinus, and its preexcitation helped prevent AF. Similar observations were also made in clinical studies in which a similar protocol was conducted.[58, 59] In one study, suppression of reproducibly inducible atrial arrhythmias with dual-site pacing was observed in 8 of 15 patients (Fig. 19–3). In the other study, in 17 of 25 patients with clinically documented AF, AF was induced with single atrial extrastimulus from the high right atrium.[59] AF could not be induced in 11 of these 17 patients, however, after dual-site atrial pacing from the high right atrium and the coronary sinus employing the same coupling of the extrastimulus from the high right atrium.[59] In a recently published study, 61 post-CABG patients were randomized to no atrial pacing, right atrial pacing, or biatrial pacing at 100 bpm for 96 hours or until the onset of atrial fibrillation in the postoperative period.[59a] The investigators concluded that continuous right or biatrial pacing was safe and well tolerated but did not prevent atrial fibrillation.

■ CLINICAL ELECTROPHYSIOLOGY OF SINGLE-SITE AND DUAL-SITE ATRIAL PACING

The clinical electrophysiologic effects of atrial pacing at various single atrial sites and using dual atrial pacing methods have been studied in our laboratory using catheter endocardial mapping.[60, 61] Regional atrial activation patterns vary greatly with different single-site atrial pacing methods. High right atrial pacing has been well studied in electrophysiology laboratories and has been shown to excite the crista terminalis and interatrial septum significantly earlier than inferior right and left atrial sites. In contrast, coronary sinus ostial pacing advances activation at the right AV junction near the His bundle as well in the inferolateral left atrium at the distal coronary sinus. However, it produces delayed activation of the interatrial septum. In contrast, distal coronary sinus pacing advances superior left atrial and coronary sinus ostial activation but delays activation at the septum and crista terminalis. Because of these offsetting effects, the overall P-wave duration is not seriously reduced by pacing at these sites as compared with sinus rhythm. Figure 19–4A summarizes mean activation times at different right and left atrial regions with single-site and dual-site atrial pacing methods. Dual-site right atrial pacing advances both right and left atrial activation in most sites, such as the septum, crista, coronary sinus, and left atrium. Biatrial pacing produces similar effects. Global P-wave duration is significantly reduced.

The sites of earlier activation recover excitability earlier and facilitate conduction of atrial premature beats. Thus, closely coupled high right atrial premature beats encounter less conduction delay with decrease in P-wave duration and earlier activation of septal, coronary sinus, and left atrial sites (see Fig. 19–4B). This reduces the opportunity for conduction delay, a crucial element in interatrial reentry. This would, as mentioned previously, reduce the window for AF initiation by premature beats. Initiation of AF or atrial flutter that can be induced reproducibly with programmed atrial stimulation can be suppressed by dual-site right atrial pacing in 56% of patients.[58]

Table 19–1 summarizes the important clinical electrophysiologic effects of dual-site right atrial pacing that can contribute to prevention of recurrent AF. Biatrial pacing has similar effects. Our data currently suggest that dual-site right atrial pacing can attenuate up to 25% of the incremental delay encountered by closely coupled atrial premature beats from the high right atrium. Figure 19–3 is an example of

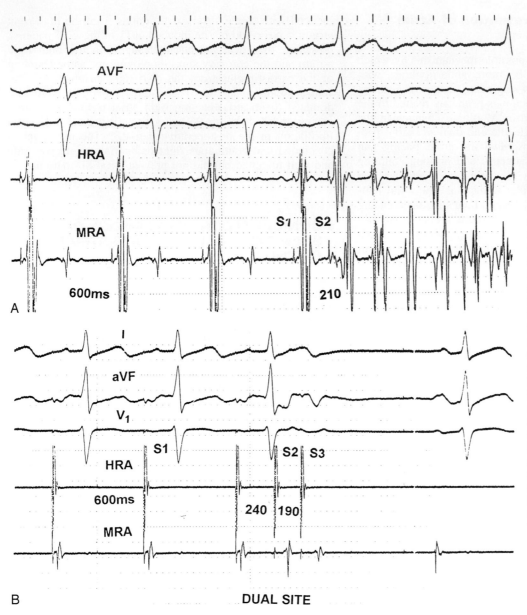

Figure 19–3. Effect of acute dual-site right atrial pacing on inducible atrial fibrillation (AF) in patients with spontaneous AF. *A,* Programmed atrial stimulation is performed using a single-site high right atrial drive with a single atrial extrastimulus delivered from the same site coupled at 210 msec. The atrial extrastimulus could reproducibly induce AF. *B,* Acute dual-site right atrial pacing is performed with simultaneous stimulation of the high right atrium and coronary sinus ostium for 8 beats, followed by delivery of two high right atrial extrastimuli coupled at 240 and 190 msec. Note the change in P-wave morphology during the drive with biphasic P wave in lead aVF. Two extrastimuli failed to induce atrial flutter or fibrillation. On withdrawal of the dual-site right atrial pacing drive, AF could again be reinduced with a single atrial extrastimulus. (From Prakash A, Saksena S, Hill M, et al: Acute effects of dual-site right atrial pacing in patients with spontaneous and inducible atrial flutter and fibrillation. J Am Coll Cardiol 29:1007–1014, 1997.)

suppression of induced AF with dual-site right atrial pacing in a patient with reproducibly inducible AF.

The interaction of each of these pacing modes with extrastimuli from other right and left atrial sites is still under

Table 19–1. Electrophysiologic Basis of Multisite Pacing in Atrial Fibrillation

Mechanisms of Atrial Fibrillation Prevention by Multisite Pacing

Substrate modification
  Reduction of atrial activation times during continuous overdrive pacing
  Reduction of conduction delays induced by APB
Reduction of APBs
Prevention of bradycardia
Reduction of dispersion of refractoriness
Reduction of the window for atrial fibrillation initiation
Possibly mechanical, hormonal, autonomic mechanisms

APB, atrial premature beat.

study. Using catheter endocardial mapping techniques in patients with spontaneous AF, we examined the conduction of atrial premature beats from different sites (Fig. 19–5). Atrial premature beats from a contralateral location to the pacing site fail to achieve similar prematurity to ipsilateral sites of origin owing to the interatrial conduction intervals. Figure 19–5 shows the propagation of a high right atrial extrastimulus coupled moderately closely at 300 msec during high right atrial site pacing, distal coronary sinus pacing, and dual-site right atrial pacing. There is incremental conduction delay with distal coronary sinus pacing and alleviation of this with dual-site right atrial pacing. Thus, if the critical site for slow conduction is near the pacing site, sufficient conduction delay for reentrant activation may not be possible because of two mechanisms: earlier recovery of excitability and inability to achieve close coupling for premature beats. Ideally, single-site stimulation at the site of critical conduction delay would maximize the benefit. Unfortunately, current data suggest that more than one site of delayed conduc-

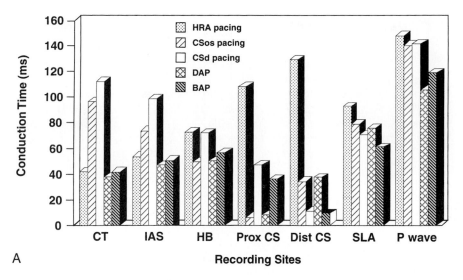

A

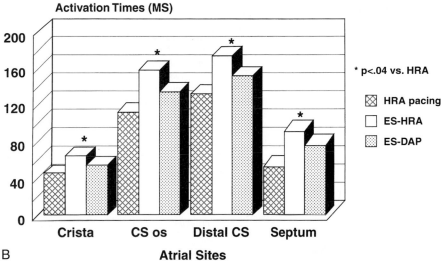

B

Figure 19–4. *A*, Regional atrial activation during single-site and dual-site atrial pacing in patients with atrial tachyarrhythmias. Note the wide variability in regional atrial activation times with single-site atrial pacing from high right atrium (HRA), coronary sinus ostium (CSos), and distal coronary sinus pacing (CSd). Also note, however, that the regional atrial activation times are uniformly shortened or at the lowest possible measured value with dual-site pacing modes during either dual right atrial pacing (DAP) or biatrial pacing (BAP). This overall reduction in atrial conduction manifests as a reduction in global P-wave duration with the dual-site pacing modes but not with the single-site pacing modes. CT, crista terminalis; Dist CS, distal coronary sinus at the lateral and inferior left atrium; HB, right atrioventricular junction at the His bundle region; IAS, interatrial septum; MS, milliseconds; Prox CS, proximal coronary sinus at the ostium; SLA, superior left atrium. *B*, Atrial activation times in milliseconds at different right and left atrial regions for atrial premature beats delivered during high right atrial pacing and dual-site atrial pacing. The baseline conduction time for a high right atrial drive is shown on the left bar in each grouping, the conduction time for coupled extrastimulus delivered from the high right atrium at 250 msec in the middle bar, and for an extrastimulus delivered after dual-site atrial pacing in the right bar. Note that there is a significant increase in conduction delay for extrastimuli from the high right atrium delivered after high right atrial pacing but not after dual-site right atrial pacing. ES-DAP, extrastimulus delivered from the high right atrium after dual site pacing; ES-HRA, extrastimulus delivered from the high right atrium after high right atrial pacing; HRA, high right atrial pacing drive. (*A* Modified from Prakash A, Delfaut P, Krol SB, Saksena S: Regional right and left atrial activation patterns with atrial fibrillation. Am J Cardiol 82:1197, 1998.)

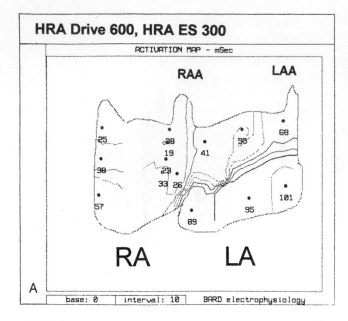

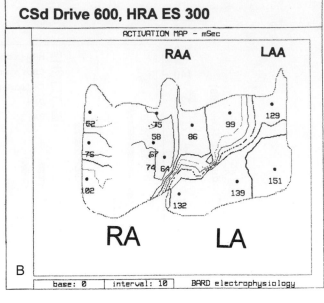

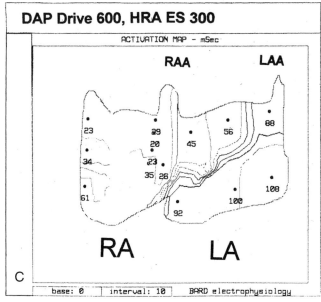

Figure 19–5. Effect of pacing drive locations and mode on propagation of moderately closely coupled high right atrial extrastimulus at 300 msec. *A*, Global right and left atrial activation after a high right atrial pacing drive is achieved by the premature beat in 101 msec with inferior left atrial activation occurring at the terminal end of the wavefront. *B*, Global activation is achieved in 151 msec by the same premature beat as in panel *A* after a distal coronary sinus pacing drive. Significant delays in multiple right and left atrial sites are noted. These delays may be functional and anatomic in nature (see text for details). *C*, Global atrial activation is achieved in 108 msec after a dual-site right atrial pacing drive for the same premature beat as in panel *A*. Note that the conduction delays seen in panel *B* are largely alleviated at most right and left atrial sites. CSd, distal coronary sinus pacing; DAP, dual-site right atrial pacing; ES, extrastimulus; HRA, high right atrium; MS, milliseconds.

tion is possible, and this may be best achieved with multisite pacing methods.

■ CLINICAL APPLICATION OF DUAL-SITE ATRIAL PACING

Patient Selection

A variety of patient groups have been identified on the basis of our experience and that of others. These have uniformly included patients with recurrent and frequent drug-refractory AF. An average frequency has been patients with two or more recurrences in the 3-month period preceding pacing system implantation. With longer-term experience, this criterion may be further relaxed. However, most patients have failed one or more antiarrhythmic drugs (type 1 or 3) and desire rhythm control. The ineffective antiarrhythmic drug

is often continued along with the pacing prescription. Patient groups that have been enrolled and for which outcome data are now available in small to moderate numbers include the following:

- Patients with paroxysmal or persistent and recurrent AF with moderate left atrial enlargement with or without P-wave duration prolongation
- Patients with recurrent atrial flutter (atypical form). In patients with incisional atrial flutter after congenital heart disease repair or hypertrophic cardiomyopathy, this technique has proved useful.
- Selected patients with chronic drug-refractory AF

In our opinion, contraindications to this technique include presence of NYHA class IV congestive heart failure, severe mitral regurgitation, or presence of a prosthetic tricuspid valve. Caution is necessary in using this approach in patients with previously implanted cardioverter-defibrillators, although this has been successfully performed.[62]

Technology for Dual-Site Right Atrial Pacing

Several technical issues arise with development of systems for dual-site pacing. Dual-site pacing can be conducted by three methods: (1) by having two separate bipolar pacing and sensing channels in the atrium, (2) by having one bipolar output that is bifurcated into two separate bipolar leads, or (3) by having the single bipolar output feed two separate unipolar leads. There are relative advantages and disadvantages of each technique. Providing two separate output channels in the atrium increases device complexity while providing the greatest flexibility. The longevity of such a system would be compromised because of an increase in the static current drain as well as the current drain that results from having two output circuits. In dual-chamber systems, it could reduce device longevity by about 15%. The advantage of such a system is that the two atrial pacing outputs can be programmed for simultaneous or sequential output if that is required to increase the efficacy of dual-site pacing.

If one output is bifurcated to feed two separate leads, the hardware design is simplified, but flexibility is compromised. Compared with a single-lead atrial pacing device, the longevity would be reduced by about 10% to 15% because each lead would draw current based on its impedance (voltage/resistance). Because the two outputs are in parallel, the change in impedance of one lead would not affect the current drain in the second lead system. However, if the voltage pacing threshold at one of the leads were to increase, the atrial pacing output would have to be increased accordingly, resulting in pacing at a higher value than necessary at the other lead. Also, the two pacing outputs would always occur simultaneously with no opportunity to alter the delay between the two stimuli. In this configuration, although sensing should not be affected normally, there is a potential for sensing at double the rate of the intrinsic rhythm. Typically, in most pacemakers, there is an atrial blanking period of about 80 to 100 msec following an atrial sensed or paced event, and unless the conduction delay between the two is greater than that, double sensing should not be observed. With leads in the right atrial appendage and the coronary sinus ostium, the average conduction delay is about 50 msec. If the conduction delay were to exceed this blanking period because of distal placement of the coronary sinus lead or long interatrial conduction delay, the device could classify sinus tachycardia as a pathologic atrial tachyarrhythmia and mode-switch inappropriately. Therefore, such systems are contraindicated in patients with long atrial conduction delays.

The third technique is unipolar pacing from two sites. The key advantage of this technique is that device longevity is not affected because the impedance of such a system is not significantly different than that of a standard bipolar lead. The disadvantage is that, owing to the wide dipolar spacing, one can frequently record a far-field QRS signal that can interfere with appropriate atrial sensing. Placing the two atrial leads such that the recording vector is orthogonal to the QRS vector minimizes the extent of far-field sensing. Sometimes this can be difficult. The published studies by the authors used this mode for dual-site atrial pacing. Minimal problems in pacing and sensing were observed and resolved by appropriate reprogramming. At one of the sites anodal stimulation occurs, and this is associated with higher thresholds. Therefore, the output must be increased enough to facilitate anodal stimulation. Such a pacemaker may need to be programmed at a higher output than those previously discussed, negating some of the advantage in longevity. With this dual-site pacing system, one can evaluate only that dual-site right atrial pacing is occurring by noting a change in the P-wave morphology to a biphasic waveform in leads II or III.

Clinical Technique

Dual-site right atrial pacing requires insertion of two atrial leads and, in many patients, additional insertion of a ventricular pacing lead for ventricular pacing.[63] It is accomplished by positioning one of the pacing electrodes in the high right atrium, preferably in the right atrial appendage, in patients who have not had an appendage resection. The electrode can also be located in the high lateral right atrium near the sinoatrial node complex in patients after cardiac surgery or when a satisfactory appendage location is not achieved. The other lead is placed at the ostium of the coronary sinus. To locate the latter precisely, the pacing lead is passed preferably from the left subclavian vein or cephalic vein. The configuring stylet is curved manually to provide the large sweeping curve along the lateral wall of the right atrium. The last 1 cm of the stylet is hooked and fashioned into a sharp perpendicular hook at the end of the stylet. For right subclavian or cephalic vein insertions, the stylet curve may have to be reduced for the main curve, but the distal anchoring hook is similar. The lead is passed under fluroscopic control into the right atrium until the tricuspid valve annulus is reached. The atrial and ventricular ectopy elicited by catheter movement can assist in defining the region of the AV annulus. Once in proximity to the AV annulus, the catheter tip exhibits a characteristic pattern of motion.[62] Upon approaching the coronary sinus ostium, the stylet is withdrawn 1 to 2 cm to make the tip more vertical and softer. The tip is then buckled against the inferior atrial wall and prolapsed into the coronary sinus. Upon entering the coronary sinus, atrial pacing is performed to demonstrate the typical inferosuperior P-wave vector with an inverted P wave and short PR interval in the inferior ECG leads. The catheter is then withdrawn gently, simultaneously as the stylet is advanced to its tip. The coronary sinus ostium is located by the site of angulation of the lead. The tip of the catheter is withdrawn to the ostium, and the stylet is withdrawn 1 cm. The lead is then popped out of the ostium, and the tip is allowed to hang below it. The lead is advanced 0.5 to 1 cm, and the stylet is passed to the tip. The assembly is then advanced so that the lead pointing medially engages just below the coronary sinus ostium. Typically, this is posterior to the ostium of the coronary sinus. It is then screwed into place. P-wave morphology for the distinctive inverted P wave is sought. In addition, atrial sensing is evaluated for double sensing and ventricular potentials. An evaluation of lead stability is performed after removal of the stylet.

The right atrial lead is then passed under fluoroscopic control using standard techniques for placement in the right atrial appendage. In patients in whom a ventricular lead is deemed appropriate for AV conduction disorders or the future development of the same, a ventricular lead is inserted under fluoroscopic control to the right ventricular apex. Bipolar and unipolar thresholds are obtained for the high right atrial lead and the coronary sinus ostial lead. Bipolar pacing is preferred for the ventricular lead, and bipolar thresholds are obtained. To obtain dual-site right atrial pacing thresholds, the distal high right atrial and coronary sinus ostial electrodes are connected using a Y connector for bipolar pacing. Typically, the high right atrial electrode is used as the cathode, although the coronary sinus ostial electrode has also been used as the cathode in a large number of patients in our experience without difficulties. A biphasic P wave in the inferior ECG lead is recorded during dual-site atrial pacing. A choice of one of the sites as cathode also allows the possibility of single-site unipolar pacing in these patients at that site, if needed. In general, the atrial site with the lower pacing threshold could be preferred as cathode. However, until data are obtained on the efficacy of one site or the other, no definite recommendation can be made from the point of view of efficacy in AF prevention.

Implant pacing thresholds in the bipolar mode at the high right atrium and coronary sinus ostium are compared with those in the dual-site right atrial mode in Figure 19–6. Pacing thresholds at the coronary sinus ostium are closely comparable to those at the high right atrium and are well within accepted ranges for atrial pacing. Dual-site right atrial pacing, however, results in a 20% to 30% increase in atrial pacing thresholds in most patients as compared with bipolar single-site pacing. This pacing threshold increment is statistically significant but is still within acceptable values for long-term atrial pacing. The bipolar end of the Y connector is inserted into the atrial port of the pulse generator, and the ventricular lead is present in the ventricular port.

The pacemaker is programmed to either the AAIR or the

DDDR pacing mode based on the presence or absence of the need for ventricular pacing. The lower rate of the program should ensure continuous atrial capture in more than 95% of patients at rest. Typically, this is set at a minimal value of 80 bpm and rarely above 90 bpm. Individual variation of patient prescription can be expected. The rate response is programmed to ensure continuous overdrive atrial pacing during all types of activity and exercise. This may require performance of a walk test, a stress test, and telemetric or Holter monitoring over the next 24 hours with moderate activity levels. Continuous atrial pacing is often difficult to achieve. Our initial approach is to administer β-blocker therapy to reduce sinus rates during rest and exercise. β-Blocker therapy is effective in achieving this goal in these patients. Alternatives include the use of type 3 agents, such as sotalol or amiodarone.

In patients with frequent and highly symptomatic AF, administration of concomitant antiarrhythmic drug therapy should be considered. The choice of antiarrhythmic agents, although arbitrary, can be based on available clinical experience. Type 1A agents, although effective, are often associated with long-term intolerance and are currently not used as first-line drugs. First-line therapy may include a type 1C agent such as propafenone or a type 3 agent such as sotalol. Alternatively, secondary choices include amiodarone or type 1A agents. Type 1A and 1C drugs should typically be used in combination with an AV nodal blocking agent, such as a β-blocker. Titration of drug therapy before hospital discharge is an important and essential part of patient management. Proper optimization of a drug and pacing regimen should ensure continuous atrial pacing as well as freedom from recurrent AF at the time of hospital discharge. During follow-up, it can be anticipated that drug regimen changes will be necessary, usually for purposes of intolerance but occasionally for purposes of inefficacy, particularly if single-site atrial pacing is undertaken.[42] Before drug therapy alteration for inefficacy, evaluation of drug dose and dosing schedule should be undertaken. Occasional relapses due to drugs and drug levels and noncompliance should be excluded. In occasional patients simple alteration and dosing may be adequate to address concerns. In general, during long-term follow-up, switching from type 1A and 1C drugs to type 3 drugs may occur with modest frequency.

Long-Term Follow-Up

Long-term follow-up typically entails three monthly clinic visits, designed to ensure the following:

- Continued incidence of overdrive atrial pacing
- Assessment for efficacy of the drug and pacing regimen
- Evaluation of drug tolerance and safety
- Evaluation of pacing thresholds and device data logs

Assessment of continuous overdrive pacing can be performed by use of periodic ambulatory ECG monitoring or device data storage on this function or both. All attempts should be made to ensure more than 90% atrial pacing during rest and exercise. A follow-up exercise test may be necessary to verify this observation.

Efficacy of AF prevention can be assessed by three methods:

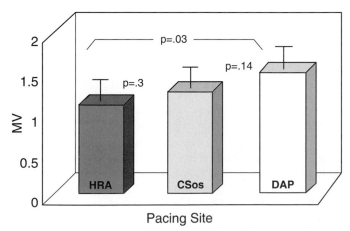

Figure 19–6. Pacing thresholds at the time of implantation of a dual-site right atrial pacing system. The atrial pacing site is in the high right atrium in the bipolar mode in the left bar and at the coronary sinus ostium in a bipolar mode in the middle bar; dual-site right atrial stimulation is simultaneously from the high right atrium and coronary sinus ostium in the right bar. The pacing threshold is measured in millivolts at a pulse width of 0.5 msec. Note that there is a small but significant increase in pacing threshold in the dual-site right atrial pacing mode (see text for details). CSos, coronary sinus ostium; DAP, dual-site atrial pacing; HRA, high right atrium.

Table 19–2. Pilot Observational Trials of Dual-Site Pacing

Investigators	No. of Patients	Follow-Up Time	Efficacy (%)	Mode	Drug Prescribed?
Daubert et al.[17, 65]	50	1–5 yr	80	Biatrial	Yes
Saksena[64]	100	2–5 yr (n = 30)	86 (n = 30)	Dual RA	Yes
Vardas[69]	10	1.5 yr	80	Dual RA	Yes
Friedman[82]	9	0.75 yr	50	Dual RA	No
Mirza[83]	16	1 yr	80	Biatrial	Yes
Prakash et al.[84]	19	2–18 mos	91	Dual RA	Yes
TOTAL	190	2–60 mos	50–87		

RA, right atrial.

1. Symptomatic AF episodes that have ECG documentation should be noted.

2. Patients who have previously demonstrated reliable symptom–arrhythmia correlation can often describe occurrence of explicit symptoms of AF. These should be considered tentative but often reasonable evidence of recurrence requiring further investigation. Further investigation should be performed using ambulatory ECG or event recorders for evaluation of device data logs. A correlation of the time of previous recurrences with device data logs or prospective use of ambulatory ECG or event monitors with future events after the clinic visit should be considered.

3. The device data logs should be interrogated to look for high rate atrial events above a preprogrammed rate threshold, typically 180 bpm. These episodes would allow assessment of asymptomatic AF recurrences.

Assessment of pacing thresholds is performed in the standard fashion (described later). P-wave morphology is an integral part of obtaining an accurate dual-site pacing threshold. The pacemaker output is programmed to ensure a safety margin of three times more than threshold in the pacing mode chosen. Pacemaker pulse width is maintained at the expense of reducing maximum output to the lowest acceptable stimulus output. Interrogation of device data logs is performed to seek high right atrial events with or without symptoms. A complete printout is obtained, and the event counter is cleared at each visit. Analysis of arrhythmia-free intervals for the time to first recurrence and time to subsequent recurrence should be undertaken. The duration of arrhythmic events should be recorded. Self-terminating brief episodes of AF may not prompt an immediate change in drug or pacing regimen.

Clinical Efficacy and Safety

The clinical efficacy of dual-site atrial pacing methods has been assessed in pilot prospective clinical studies of an observational nature. These were uncontrolled or used a prospective sequential design for comparison of single-site and dual-site pacing modes.[17, 18, 64] A variety of clinical centers in the United States, Europe, and Asia have now

undertaken this technique. A metaanalysis of the available reported and unreported data is presented in Table 19–2. In an early observational study of 30 patients, Daubert and coworkers reported an initial success rate for biatrial pacing for rhythm control of 50%, but with a significant inability (20%) to maintain biatrial pacing.[17, 65] This was due to dislodgment of a distal coronary sinus lead, and a more proximal lead position resulted in greater lead stability. Reestablishment of biatrial pacing after lead repositioning resulted in an overall 80% success rate in rhythm control. Belham and coworkers[66] compared the stability of lead positioning in the different segments of the coronary sinus and concluded that the proximal sites have greater lead stability and more effective long-term atrial pacing.

Using the dual-site right atrial pacing technique, we have performed 100 implantations of this pacing system. The clinical characteristics of the first 50 patients in our population are shown in Figure 19–7 and Table 19–3. In a prospective sequential clinical trial comparing dual-site and single-site right atrial pacing with a control pre-pacing period undertaken by our group, the study was designed to use each

- **50 patients, 27 male**
- **Mean age = 67 ± 12 yrs.**
- **Mean LA diameter = 39 ± 6 mm.**
- **Mean LVEF = 47 ± 12%.**

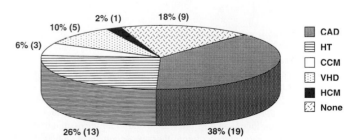

Figure 19–7. Clinical and arrhythmia characteristics of initial 50 patients undergoing dual-site right atrial pacing at the Atlantic Health Care System-Eastern Heart Institute (1994–1997).

Table 19–3. Comparison of Patients With Paroxysmal and Persistent/Permanent Atrial Fibrillation

Characteristics	Paroxysmal (n = 25)	Persistent/Permanent (n = 25)	P-value
Patient age (yr)	66 ± 14	68 ± 11	>.2
Disease duration (mos)	54 ± 48	68 ± 11	>.2
CAD (pts)	10 (40%)	9 (36%)	>.2
No heart disease (pts)	6 (24%)	3 (12%)	>.2
Primary bradycardia (pts)	15 (60%)	8 (32%)	.08
LVEF (%)	47 ± 12	45 ± 13	.2
LAD (mm)	38 ± 6	40 ± 6	>.2

CAD, coronary artery disease; LVEF, left ventricular ejection fraction.

pacing mode sequentially for a total of 9 months in two paired phases of 3 and 6 months (Fig. 19–8). The study enrolled a larger proportion of patients with paroxysmal or persistent than chronic AF, although both groups were represented. The mean arrhythmia-free interval for symptomatic AF recurrences before pacing system insertion was 9 ± 10 days. Atrial pacing used alone or in combination with drug therapy in most patients prolonged arrhythmia-free intervals. However, we noted significantly longer arrhythmia-free intervals and improved rhythm control with dual-site right atrial pacing. The mean time to first arrhythmia recurrence with dual-site right atrial pacing was 195 ± 96 days versus 143 ± 110 days (Fig. 19–9A). In addition, the frequency of recurrences was 0.23 AF events per patient for dual-site right atrial pacing and 0.54 AF events per patient for single-site right atrial pacing in the first 6 months. In a nonrandomized comparison, coronary sinus ostial pacing alone was not found to be superior to high right atrial pacing for single-site atrial pacing.

Patients in the study continued with dual-site right atrial pacing after the crossover phases. This long-term study provided insights into the ability to achieve rhythm control in refractory AF (see Fig. 19–9B). During a follow-up period of 18 to 44 months, 55% of all patients had no further recurrences of AF.[64] The mean arrhythmia-free interval increased to 513 ± 360 days. Thus, rhythm control was established after optimization of the drug and pacing prescription in the perioperative period and was maintained over the long term. Anticoagulation therapy could be and was often withdrawn in about one third of these patients. In the remaining patients, the total frequency of symptomatic AF recurrences varied from one to four events in the entire follow-up. Recurrences were often self-terminating and were somewhat more frequent in the first 6 months than later in the study.[64] This was accounted for by the need for drug and pacing therapy optimization in the first 6 months and the use of a single-site pacing mode in all patients by study design for half of this period. The frequency of recurrence in the first 6 months was estimated at less than 0.5 per patient, declining to about 0.3 symptomatic AF events per patient during any 6-month follow-up period after this period.[64] The need for cardioversion therapy was even lower because many of the recurrences were self-terminating or associated with a self-limiting intercurrent illness or intolerance to a type 1 drug, with cessation of drug therapy awaiting a replacement. Thus, even in patients with occasional recurrent AF, cardioversion therapy was required annually or biannually on average. Rhythm control was maintained during long-term management in fully 87% of all patients.

These pilot data clearly suggest that a significant (55%) subgroup of patients with drug-refractory AF can achieve full rhythm control with dual-site right atrial pacing. Most of the remaining patients also maintain rhythm control, with an occasional need for cardioversion. This can be accomplished with external methods or with an implantable defibrillator with dual-site pacing capabilities. Antitachycardia pacing using burst or high-frequency pacing methods has been shown to be effective in atypical flutter or short duration–induced AF, further reducing the need for shock therapy for AF cardioversion.[67, 68]

Other individual center reports have substantiated the efficacy of dual-site right atrial pacing as well. In a pilot study of 10 patients, Vardas and coworkers[69] demonstrated

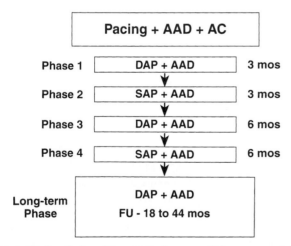

Figure 19–8. Design of the prospective sequential crossover pilot study, followed by the long-term dual-site right atrial pacing study described in reference 64. Note that the initial crossover period was preceded by a drug and pacing optimization period. This was followed by sequential crossover between dual-site pacing with continuation of previously ineffective drug therapy followed by single-site pacing with continuation of drug therapy in equal periods for a maximum of 18 months. Long-term follow-up was then continued in the dual-site atrial pacing mode with continuation of drug therapy. Anticoagulation was withdrawn in patients who were arrhythmia free for 1 year or more. AAD, antiarrhythmic drug therapy; AC, anticoagulation; DAP, dual-site right atrial pacing; FU, follow-up.

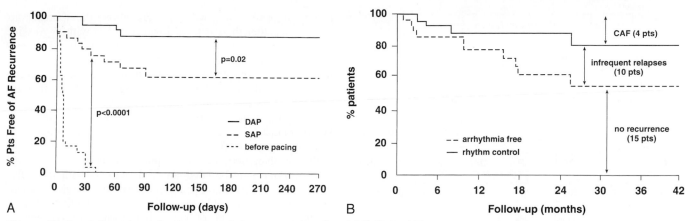

Figure 19–9. *A*, Percentage of patients free of recurrent symptomatic atrial fibrillation (AF) after insertion of a dual-site pacing system in the crossover pilot study as described in reference 64. Note that both atrial pacing modes result in a significant prolongation in arrhythmia-free intervals, which, by study design, are a maximum of 270 days. However, there is a significant increase during dual-site right atrial pacing over single-site right atrial pacing during long-term follow-up. *B*, Long-term results during dual-site right atrial pacing in the same study (reference 64) are shown here. More than half (56%) of patients were free of recurrent symptomatic AF at long-term follow-up. A smaller group have infrequent relapses (see text for details). Four patients (13%) remained in or developed chronic AF. (Modified from Delfaut P, Saksena S, Prakash A, Krol RB: Long-term outcome of patients with drug-refractory atrial flutter and fibrillation after single and dual site right atrial pacing for arrhythmia prevention. J Am Coll Cardiol 32:1900, 1998.)

an 80% efficacy rate of dual-site atrial pacing when combined with β-blocker drug therapy. Failure to use drug therapy lowered efficacy rates in this study. Early experiences from other centers suggest a 50% to 60% efficacy rate when drug therapy is not used in patients with refractory AF (see Table 19–2).

The safety of dual-site right atrial pacing can now also be assessed. Table 19–4 lists the complications with this technique during perioperative and long-term evaluation. Lead dislodgment rates are well within estimates for any type of atrial pacing, and long-term dislodgment has been obviated by the dual right atrial lead technique. The remaining complications have been largely similar to any pacemaker implantation procedure. Precipitation of angina in a patient with advanced coronary disease and exertional angina occurred in one patient. The major issue has been late intolerance to antiarrhythmic drugs with frequent replacement of type 1 agents with type 3 drugs. In two patients, right atrial ablation at multiple sites has been undertaken to avoid or replace the need for drug therapy. The outcome of this approach is still under evaluation.

Table 19–4. **Clinical Experience With Dual-Site Right Atrial Pacing***

Complication	No. of Patients
Coronary sinus lead dislodgment	
Intraoperative	1 (0.9%)
Late	0
High right atrial lead dislodgment (perioperative)	1 (0.9%)
Right ventricular threshold rise	2 (1.8%)
Pneumothorax	1 (0.9%)
Lead pocket late infection	1 (0.9%)
Pocket complications	2 (1.8%)
Clinical observations	
Angina with overdrive pacing	1

*Data are based on 55 implantations performed between 1994 and 1997.

Clinical Trials in Dual-Site Atrial Pacing

At the time of formulation of this chapter, two multicenter clinical trials assessing dual-site atrial pacing in comparison with other atrial pacing modes were in progress. The SYNBIAPACE trial has a randomized three-armed crossover design. Each arm consists of 3-month periods and compares biatrial pacing in the triggered atrial pacing mode with demand DDD pacing at 40 bpm and with standard DDD pacing at a lower rate of 70 bpm. It enrolls patients with two more episodes of paroxysmal AF in the past 3 months and either a P-wave duration of more than 120 msec or another standard indication for pacing. The initial pilot study required a P-wave duration of 180 msec, which was subsequently modified. Preliminary results indicate reduction in AF events in selected patients, but this was not statistically significant for the population. Drug therapy was not standardized, and the observation period was limited in this trial (J. Daubert, personal communication).

The DAPPAF (Dual Site Atrial Pacing for Prevention of Atrial Fibrillation) study is a North American multicenter prospective randomized trial comparing the efficacy of support pacing, high right atrial DDDR pacing, and dual-site right atrial pacing in the DDDR mode.[63] Support pacing is performed in the DDI or VVI mode. Figure 19–10 outlines the study design for the trial. Patients aged 21 to 80 years are enrolled in the trial. They have had symptomatic and drug-refractory AF with at least two episodes in the 3 months before pacing system implantation, and have a standard indication for cardiac pacing. This may include a primary bradyarrhythmia or bradycardia secondary to drug therapy for AF. Written informed consent is obtained for insertion of two atrial leads; randomized study design and study follow-up procedures are required, including periodic clinic visits, maintenance of log books, symptomatic event monitoring, quality-of-life assessments, and echocardiograms in each pacing phase. After dual-site right atrial pacing system implantation, optimization of drug and pacing therapies is performed. Pacing is performed at a relatively high lower

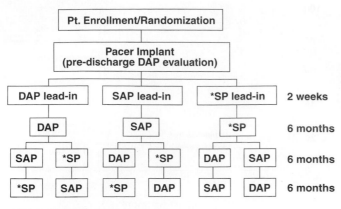

Figure 19–10. Flow diagram for the DAPPAF clinical trial. DAP, dual-site atrial pacing; SAP, single-site atrial pacing; SP, support pacing (includes both VDI and DDI). (From Fitts SM, Hill MRS, Mehra R, et al, for the DAPPAF Phase I Investigators: Design and Implementation of the Dual Site Atrial Pacing to Prevent Atrial Fibrillation (DAPPAF) clinical trial. J Intervent Card Electrophysiol 2:139–144, 1998.)

rate of 80 or 90 bpm in the DDDR mode to ensure continuous atrial pacing for 80% to 90% of all events. Antiarrhythmic drug therapy with a previously ineffective drug is undertaken to reduce the number and frequency of AF events. The three modes of pacing are then randomly selected for 6-month periods. The pacing modes are switched at the end of this period or earlier if two symptomatic AF recurrences are documented in a given mode. Device-based electrograms, ECG recordings from event recorders, or clinical evaluation of symptomatic AF events is required for endpoint documentation. The trial commenced in 1996 and has currently enrolled 120 patients with a follow-up of 18 months for each patient. The primary end point for the trial includes the time interval to first symptomatic AF recurrence in each mode, with secondary end points being quality of life, total AF event rates, and echocardiographic parameters of atrial and ventricular function. Other multicenter or single center trials are focused on other patient populations with AF. These include patients with lone AF and AF without bradyarrhythmias (the NIPP-AF study). This study has shown a significant increase in arrhythmia-free intervals with dual-site atrial pacing (C.P. Lau, personal communication).

■ FUTURE DEVELOPMENTS

Pilot clinical trial experience suggests that dual-site atrial pacing alone or most often in combination with antiarrhythmic drugs may provide effective prevention from recurrent AF during a 3- to 4-year follow-up period in 50% to 60% of unselected patients with drug-refractory AF. A significant proportion of the remainder are sufficiently improved, with rare arrhythmia recurrences, to achieve long-term rhythm control, whereas a distinct minority (10% to 20%) require infrequent but periodic cardioversion. Less than 15% experience no benefit from this therapy. For the initial group with effective prevention, future directions will involve simplification of the pacing therapy and substitution of drug therapy. Single-site atrial pacing may be adequate to maintain response in many patients, and these individuals have to be defined. Continuous atrial pacing may be achieved with new

pacing algorithms that will pace just above the spontaneous sinus rate rather than at fixed lower rates or with aggressive DDDR responses. Experience with drug therapy suggests that type 3 agents are preferable for purposes of efficacy, tolerance, and long-term administration. Alternatives to drug therapy include focal AF or partial right atrial ablative approaches to achieve hybrid therapy.

Some patients will continue to require therapy to revert symptomatic AF recurrences. Choices in their treatment will be defined by the frequency of recurrent AF. For patients with less than one recurrence per year, access to external cardioversion may be adequate. For patients with more frequent AF, a combination pacing-defibrillation device implantation may offer flexible long-term management. Antitachycardia pacing may be of value at the onset of AF events, when more organized rhythms may be in progress, and may be amenable to pace termination with burst, ramp, or high-frequency pacing. The latter pacing mode is most valuable in atypical atrial flutter or AF of short duration.[67]

Finally, internal atrial shocks may revert atrial flutter or AF recurrences at prespecified intervals or at patient demand. For this function, ventricular defibrillation therapy should be available for shock-induced proarrhythmia reversion. The first prototype device with these features is the Arrhythmia Management Device model 7250 (Medtronic, Minneapolis, MN). This device was first implanted in a patient with only recurrent and refractory AF in our center in November 1997

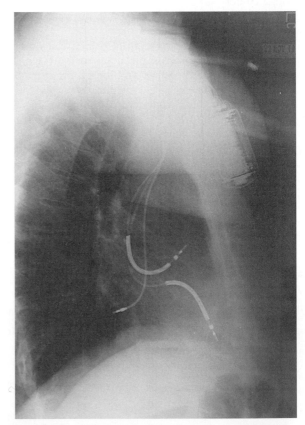

Figure 19–11. Lateral chest radiograph showing insertion of a Medtronic 7250 Jewel AF atrial pacemaker-defibrillator with two atrial pacing and defibrillation leads placed in the high right atrial appendage and right ventricular apex. Screw-in electrodes are clearly seen. An additional pacing lead is fixed at the coronary sinus ostium for temporary and, in future, permanent dual-site right atrial pacing if needed.

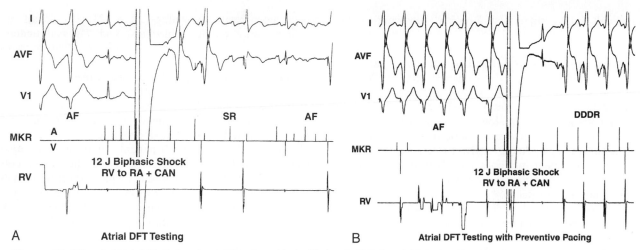

Figure 19–12. *A,* Atrial defibrillation threshold testing with the Medtronic 7250 Jewel AF device. Note the successful conversion of atrial fibrillation (AF) with a 12-J biphasic shock using two anodes (right atrial defibrillation electrode and the can of the defibrillator) due to a single cathode in the right ventricle. Successful conversion to sinus rhythm is noted with immediate early recurrence of AF. *B,* Atrial defibrillation threshold testing using exactly the same shock output as in panel *A* with immediate institution of DDDR pacing after shock delivery. Note that the early relapse into AF is prevented by this pacing method.

(Fig. 19–11). Two pacing and defibrillation electrodes were placed in the right atrial appendage and right ventricular apex, respectively. An additional pacing lead was placed at the coronary sinus ostium for dual-site atrial pacing for AF prevention if needed. Figure 19–12 is an example of atrial defibrillation followed by DDD pacing in this patient. Panel *A* shows atrial defibrillation with immediate recurrence of AF. Panel *B* shows that the institution of atrial pacing eliminated the recurrence of AF after successful atrial defibrillation.

■ CONCLUSIONS

The high density of arrhythmia events in patients with AF demands a major preventive strategy for device management of AF. The role of atrial pacing in this regard appears to be crystallizing as a major element of such a device. Further studies can define patients in whom prevention can eliminate the need for additional therapies or complex device therapies. These studies are in progress and can be expected to advance electrical therapy for AF rapidly in the near future.

■ PACING FOR PREVENTION OF VENTRICULAR TACHYARRHYTHMIAS

The principles discussed earlier in this chapter also apply to the prevention of ventricular tachyarrhythmias by cardiac pacing. Overdrive ventricular pacing has been studied by Fisher and associates[70] for evaluation of suppression of premature ventricular contractions (PVCs) and nonsustained ventricular tachycardia. In a crossover controlled study in 18 patients undergoing electrophysiologic evaluation, the investigators paced the ventricle at a rate 10 to 15 bpm above the patient's average heart rate.[70] Catheters were left in place, and the patients were monitored for a total of 720 hours: 346 hours paced and 374 hours unpaced. The frequency of ventricular ectopic activity (PVCs), couplets, and runs of nonsustained ventricular tachycardia was decreased. Ventricular pacing had a greater effect on suppressing PVCs

in patients who had a higher baseline frequency of PVCs. In another study, Winter and coworkers[71] increased the ventricular pacing rate only when PVCs were observed. The pacing rate was gradually slowed until sinus rhythm reemerged or another PVC was sensed. In this study, half of patients experienced an 80% reduction in frequency of ventricular premature beats. Overdrive suppression of ventricular tachycardia has had limited value in the clinical setting because of its unpredictable long-term efficacy and the frequent need to increase pacing rate. The increased pacing rates may eventually be quite fast and result in hemodynamic instability coupled with loss of AV synchrony.

Electrical stimulation with high current strength pacing at the left ventricular site of origin of ventricular tachycardia has been shown to have a marked effect on suppressing ventricular tachycardia initiation.[72] On a more basic level, however, ventricular pacing has been effective in preventing the initiation of tachycardia that is believed to be promoted by bradycardia or torsades de pointes in the long QT interval, in which a long short sequence is often a common trigger.[73] The role of pacing in patients with a long QT interval has been extensively studied.[74–81]

The long QT interval syndrome is an uncommon disorder in which affected patients demonstrate an abnormality of ventricular repolarization manifested as a prolonged QT or QT-U interval. Patients with this syndrome have an increased risk of syncope caused by polymorphic ventricular tachycardia. The syndrome is a genetic disorder and may be inherited as an autosomal dominant or autosomal recessive pattern. New cases may occur sporadically without obvious familiar inheritance patterns. New information has become available about the molecular biology of this syndrome, including isolation of several genetic defects that may cause the syndrome.

Early reports of the efficacy of cardiac pacing in this syndrome are problematic. Many patients undergoing pacemaker implantation also often have the dosage of their β-adrenergic agent (e.g., β-blockers) increased or have recently undergone left cardiac sympathetic nerve denervation. It is thus difficult to be certain about a positive therapeutic effect of pacemaker implantation alone.

The rationale for the use of pacemakers in this syndrome comes from several sources. Garson and colleagues[75] reported a 5% incidence of AV conduction block in a series of 287 children with long QT syndrome. Kugler[76] reported a high incidence of sinus bradycardia (20% to 25%) in a series of patients with the long QT syndrome that was believed to be secondary to sinus node dysfunction as well as β-blocker therapy. Additionally, evidence from Holter monitor recordings in patients with long QT syndrome shows that the onset of torsades de pointes in these patients is often preceded by a pause.[73]

The role of permanent cardiac pacing in patients with the long QT syndrome was first reported by Eldar and associates.[77] These investigators reported on a series of eight patients with long QT syndrome who underwent pacemaker implantation for recurrent syncope or seizure. Three patients were treated unsuccessfully with both β-blockers and cardiac sympathectomy. Two were refractory or intolerant to β-blockers, and three had pacemakers implanted (for AV block in one, for aborted sudden death in one, and according to patient preference in another). Six patients had episodes with documented polymorphic ventricular tachycardia. Pacing was instituted at a rate of 70 to 85 bpm with AAI pacing in four, VVI pacing in two, and DDD pacing in two. Only one patient had recurrent cardiac events and syncope.

Five years later, Eldar and associates[78] reported on an additional 13 patients with long QT syndrome. The most common indication for pacemaker implantation was aborted cardiac arrest or recurrent syncope. These investigators proposed setting the pacing rate to the level at which a clearcut shortening of QT interval occurs. In adults, paced rates between 70 and 85 bpm generally cause a significant QT shortening of about 100 msec. The extent of QT shortening in response to AAI, VVI, and DDD pacing appears to be similar.

The efficacy of permanent pacing in the management of patients was also studied by Moss and colleagues[79] in 30 patients culled from the international prospective registry of long QT syndrome. The average age at pacemaker implantation was 19 ± 13 years, the mean QT_c was 0.55 ± 0.08 seconds, and 87% of the patients were female. The median cardiac event was significantly reduced by pacing. Twenty-one of 30 patients experienced no cardiac events during an average follow-up of 49 months. Four of the other 9 patients had a decrease in the yearly cardiac event rate. In this study, 43% of patients received AAI pacemakers, 37% received VVI pacemakers, and 13% received DDD pacemakers. The mode of pacing was unknown in 7% of patients. It should be noted that 57% of patients were receiving β-blockers, and 10% had previously undergone cervicothoracic sympathetic denervation.

In a recently published monograph on the long QT syndrome, Schwartz[74] reviewed the outcome of 122 patients who were enrolled in the international prospective registry and had a pacemaker implanted. Thirty-one percent of patients had an AAI pacemaker implanted, 29% had a VVI pacemaker implanted, and 26% had a DDD pacemaker implanted. This likely represents an increase in the DDD pacemaker implantation rate for this syndrome compared with Moss' earlier report in 1991.[79] The age at implantation was once again relatively young (28 ± 21 years), half of the patients were taking β-blockers, and 7% had undergone cervicothoracic sympathetic denervation. The pacemaker was implanted before it was determined whether β-blockers would be sufficient to prevent cardiac arrest or syncope. The overall data suggest about a 50% reduction in the incidence of cardiac events following pacemaker implantation during a follow-up period averaging 9 years before pacemaker implantation and 5 years after implantation.

Schwartz[74] identified 30 patients in whom a pacemaker was implanted after β-blocker failure. In this patient cohort, β-blockers were *not* increased after pacemaker implantation. Pacemaker implantation was associated with a dramatic reduction in the number of syncopal spells, from an average of 4 to 0.4 over a 2-year follow-up period. Another subgroup consisted of 10 patients in whom β-blockers were withdrawn after pacemaker implantation. The follow-up in these patients was 2 years before and 2 years after implantation. The yearly incidence of cardiac events in this group did not change. However, three of these patients died suddenly. Additionally, another seven patients died after pacemaker implantation. The follow-up in these patients was 4 years before and 5 years after pacemaker implantation. The number of cardiac events in this subgroup of patients increased markedly in the period after pacemaker implantation. Four of the seven patients were not taking β-blockers, and one of them also had previously undergone left cervicothoracic sympathectomy.

Summary

In young patients undergoing pacemaker implantation, multiple lead and pulse generator replacements may be necessary during their lifetime. Rapid ventricular pacing, especially in very young patients not taking β-blockers, may lead to the development of tachycardia-induced cardiomyopathy.[80] It is generally recommended that all patients undergoing pacemaker implantation should also be taking β-blockers to facilitate a pacing rate that is not too fast. Patients with recurrent syncope should have their pacing system immediately evaluated to rule out a pacing lead fracture, which can lead to bradycardia and can trigger episodes of polymorphic ventricular tachycardia. Occasionally, T-wave oversensing is a problem that can be managed by pacemaker reprogramming (e.g., prolongation of the ventricular refractory period). Evaluation of appropriate pacemaker function can be confirmed by Holter monitoring.

The indications for permanent pacing in the long QT syndrome remain somewhat controversial. Clearly, any patient who has the long QT syndrome and evidence of spontaneous or treatment-induced bradycardia or 2:1 AV block should undergo pacemaker implantation. Additionally, patients with recurrent cardiac events, such as syncope, while taking β-blockers may be candidates for pacemaker implantation. Generally, DDD pacing is recommended, particularly in older patients because AV block may develop later. In younger patients, dual-chamber pacemaker programming is more difficult because a high upper tracking rate may need to be programmed to allow fast heart rates during exercise. A long QT interval, however, may lead to T-wave oversensing and thus pacing at a slower rate. Pacing therapy is not recommended as sole therapy for the long QT syndrome.

Based on recent data with the long-term recurrences of symptoms or sudden cardiac death, back-up defibrillator therapy is increasingly preferred. Finally, the recent availability of dual-chamber defibrillators may make these devices an alternative to dual-chamber pacing in these patients, especially those with a family history of sudden cardiac death.

Increased understanding of the molecular basis for this condition may lead to a better use of cardiac pacing. For example, patients with long QT (LQT3) linked to the third chromosome have a mutant gene that results in delayed or incomplete sodium channel inactivation. These patients often have a peaked T wave that begins late. Pause-dependent mechanisms may play an important role in these patients, and they may have cardiac events at rest and during sleep.[81] It is thought that some of these patients may benefit particularly from pacing, which can prevent sudden pauses likely to induce further QT prolongation. In contrast, LQT2 patients have a mutant gene coding for the cardiac potassium channel, which results in abnormal function of the delayed inward potassium rectifier current. These patients are at risk for arrhythmias in all conditions of adrenergic activation and would probably benefit from cardiac pacing in a less specific fashion, primarily when β-blockers cause extreme bradycardia.

REFERENCES

1. MacKenzie J: Disorders of the Heartbeat. London, Oxford University 1908, p 165.
2. Lown B, Perlroth MG, Bey SK, Abe T: "Cardioversion" of atrial fibrillation: A report on the treatment of 65 episodes in 50 patients. N Engl J Med 269:325–331, 1963.
3. Wenckebach K: Arrhythmia of the Heart. Groningen, Austria; 1903, p 581.
4. Crijns HJ, Van Gelder IC, Van Gilst WH, et al: Serial antiarrhythmic drug treatment to maintain sinus rhythm after electrical cardioversion for chronic atrial fibrillation or atrial flutter. Am J Cardiol 68:335–341, 1991.
5. Tse H-F, Lau C-P: Is there a role for cardioversion of very chronic atrial fibrillation by transvenous atrial defibrillation? [Abstract] J Am Coll Cardiol 31(Suppl A):332A, 1998.
6. Saksena S, Prakash A, Mongeon L, et al: Clinical efficacy and safety of atrial defibrillation using biphasic shocks and current nonthoracotomy endocardial lead configurations. Am J Cardiol 76:913–921, 1995.
7. Prakash A, Saksena S, Mathew P, Krol RB: Internal atrial defibrillation: Effect on sinus and atrioventricular nodal function and implanted cardiac pacemakers. PACE 20:2434–2441, 1997.
8. Rosenqvist M, Brandt J, Schuller H: Long-term pacing in sinus node disease: Effect of stimulation mode on cardiovascular mortality and morbidity. Am Heart J 116:16–22, 1988.
9. Boccadamo R, Toscano S: Prevention and interruption of supraventricular tachycardia by antitachycardia pacing. In Luderitz B, Saksena S (eds): Interventional Electrophysiology. Mt Kisco, NY, Futura, 1991, pp 213–223.
10. Sgarbossa EB, Pinski SL, Maloney JD, et al: Chronic atrial fibrillation and stroke in paced patients with sick sinus syndrome: Relevance of clinical characteristics and pacing modalities. Circulation 88:1045–1053, 1993.
11. Reimold SC, Lamas GA, Cantillon CO, Antman EM: Risk factors for the development of recurrent atrial fibrillation: Role of pacing and clinical variables. Am Heart J 129:1127–1132, 1995.
12. Hesselson AB, Parsonnet V, Bernstein AD, Bonavita G: Deleterious effect of long term single chamber ventricular pacing in patients with sick sinus syndrome: The hidden benefits of dual chamber pacing. J Am Coll Cardiol 19:1542–1549, 1992.
13. Andersen HR, Nielsen JC, Thomsen PEB, et al: Long-term follow-up of patients from a randomised trial of atrial versus ventricular pacing for sick-sinus syndrome: Lancet 305:1210–1216, 1997.
14. Lamas GA, Orav EJ, Stambler BS, et al, for the Pacemaker Selection in the Elderly Investigators: Quality of life and clinical outcomes in elderly patients treated with ventricular pacing as compared with dual-chamber pacing. N Engl Med 338:1097–1104, 1998.
14a. Gillis AM, Wyse DG, Connolly SJ, et al. Atrial pacing periablation for prevention of paroxysmal atrial fibrillation. Circulation 99:2253, 1999.
15. Attuel P, Pellerin D, Mugica J, Coumel P: DDD pacing: An effective treatment modality for recurrent atrial arrhythmias. PACE 11:1647–1654, 1988.
16. Coumel P, Friocourt P, Mugica J, et al: Long-term prevention of vagal atrial arrhythmias by atrial pacing at 90/minute: Experience with 6 cases. PACE 6:552–560, 1983.
17. Daubert C, Mabo PH, Berder V, et al: Atrial tachyarrhythmias associated with high degree interatrial conduction block: Prevention by permanent atrial resynchronisation. Eur JCPE 1:35–44, 1994.
18. Saksena S, Prakash A, Hill M, et al: Prevention of recurrent atrial fibrillation with chronic dual site right atrial pacing. J Am Coll Cardiol 1996;28:687–694, 1996.
19. Murgatroyd FD, Nitzsche R, Slade AKB, et al: A new pacing algorithm for overdrive suppression of atrial fibrillation. PACE 17:1966–1973, 1994.
20. Nazir SA, Lab MJ: Mechanoelectric feedback and atrial arrhythmias. Cardiovasc Res 32:52–61, 1996.
21. Coumel P: Anatomic influences in atrial tachyarrhythmias. J Cardiovasc Electrophysiol 7:999–1007, 1996.
22. Winkle RA: The relationship between ventricular ectopic beat frequency and heart rate. Circulation 66:439–446, 1982.
23. Ricci R, Puglisi A, Azzolini P, et al: Consistent atrial pacing algorithm to suppress recurrent paroxysmal atrial fibrillation: A randomized prospective cross over study [Abstract]. PACE 21(II):798, 1998.
24. Csapo G: Role of ventricular premature beats in initiation and termination of atrial arrhythmias. Br Heart J 33:105–110, 1971.
25. Capucci A, Santarelli A, Boriani G, et al: Atrial premature beats coupling interval determines lone paroxysmal atrial fibrillation onset. Int J Cardiol 36:87–93, 1992.
26. Boineau JP, Schuessler RB, Mooney CR, et al: Natural and evoked atrial flutter due to circus movement in dogs: Role of abnormal atrial pathways, slow conduction, nonuniform refractory period distribution and premature beats. Am J Cardiol 45:1167–1181, 1980.
27. Wang J, Liu J, Feng J, et al: Regional and functional factors determining induction and maintenance of atrial fibrillation in dogs. Am J Physiol 71:H148–H158, 1996.
28. Hill M, Mongeon L, Mehra R: Prevention of atrial fibrillation: Dual site atrial pacing reduces the coupling window of induction of atrial fibrillation [Abstract]. PACE 19(II):630, 1996.
29. Mehra R: How might pacing prevent atrial fibrillation? In Murgatroyd FD, Camm AJ (eds): Nonpharmacological Management of Atrial Fibrillation. Armonk, NY, Futura, 1997.
30. Mehra R, Gough WB, Zeiler R, et al: Dual ventricular stimulation for prevention of reentrant ventricular tachyarrhythmias. J Am Coll Cardiol 2:272, 1984.
31. Mehra R, Santel D: Electrical preexcitation if ischemic tissue for prevention of ventricular tachyarrhythmias. PACE 9:282, 1986.
32. Restivo M, Gough WB, El-Sherif N: Reentrant ventricular rhythms in the late myocardial infarction period: Prevention of reentry by dual stimulation during basic rhythm. Circulation 77:429–444, 1988.
33. Cosio FB, Lopez-Gil M, Aribas F, Gonzalez HD: Mechanisms of induction of typical and reversed atrial flutter. J Cardiovasc Electrophysiol 9:281–291, 1998.
34. Schoels W, Kubler W, Yang H, et al: A unified functional/anatomic substrate for circus movement atrial flutter: Activation and refractory patterns in the canine right atrial enlargement model. J Am Coll Cardiol 21:73–84, 1993.
35. Schuessler RB, Grayson TM, Bromberg BI, et al: Cholinergically mediated tachyarrhythmias induced by a single extrastimulus in the isolated canine right atrium. Circ Res 71:1254–1267, 1992.
36. Shimizu A, Nozaki A, Rudy Y, et al: Onset of induced atrial flutter in the canine pericarditis model. J Am Coll Cardiol 17:1223–1236, 1991.
37. Hill RS, Mongeon LR, Keen PJ, Mehra R: Epicardial mapping of the induction of atrial fibrillation in a canine model of chronic atrial fibrillation [Abstract]. PACE 20(II):1215, 1997.
38. Han J, Millet D, Chizzonitti B, et al: Temporal dispersion of recovery of excitability in atrium and ventricle as a function of heart rate. Am Heart J 71:481, 1966.
39. Wijffels M, Kirchhof C, Dorland R, et al: Atrial fibrillation begets atrial fibrillation: A study in awake chronically instrumented goats. Circulation 92:1954–1968, 1995.

40. Mehra R, Ruetz L: Effect of refractory period changes with cycle length on stability of a reentrant tachycardia [Abstract]. PACE 19(II):560, 1996.

41. Sideris DA, Toumanidis ST, Tselepatiotis E, et al: Atrial pressure and experimental atrial fibrillation. PACE 18:1679–1685, 1995.

42. Satoh T, Zipes D: Unequal atrial stretch in dogs increases dispersion of refractoriness conducive to developing atrial fibrillation. J Cardiovasc Electrophysiol 7:833–842, 1996.

43. Ravelli F, Allessie MA: Atrial stretch decreases refractoriness and induces atrial fibrillation in the isolated rabbit heart. Circulation 92:1754–1755, 1995.

44. Calkins J, El-Atassi R, Leon AN: Effect of the atrioventricular relationship on atrial refractoriness in humans. PACE 15:771–778, 1992.

45. Klein LS, Miles WM, Zipes DP: Effect of atrioventricular interval during pacing or reciprocating tachycardia on atrial size, pressure, and refractory period. Circulation 82:60–68, 1990.

46. Lab MJ: Transient depolarization and action potential alterations following mechanical changes in isolated myocardiium. Cardiovasc Res 14:624–637, 1980.

47. Sanders R, Myerburg RJ, Gelband J, et al: Dissimilar length-tension relations of canine ventricular muscle and false tendon: Electrophysiologic alterations accompanying deformation. J Mol Cell Cardiol 11:209–219, 1979.

48. Dominquez G, Fozzard HA: Effect of stretch on conduction velocity and cable properties of cardiac Purkinje fibers. Am J Physiol 237:C119–C124, 1979.

49. Hennekes R, Kaufman R, Lab M, et al: Feedback loops involved in cardiac excitation-contraction coupling: Evidence for two different pathways. J Mol Cell Cardiol 9:699–713, 1977.

50. Yamashita T, Oikawa N, Murakawa Y, et al: Contraction-excitation feedback in atrial reentry: Role of velocity of mechanical stretch. Am J Physiol 267:H1254–H1262, 1994.

51. Leclercq C, Gras D, Le Helloco A, et al: Hemodynamic importance of preserving the normal sequence of ventricular activation in permanent cardiac pacing. Am Heart J 129:1133–1141, 1995.

52. Sideris DA, Kontoyannis DA, Michalis L, et al: Acute changes in blood pressure as a cause of cardiac arrhythmias. Eur Heart J 8:45–52, 1987.

53. Sideris DA, Toumanidis ST, Tselepatiotis E, et al: Atrial pressure and experimental atrial fibrillation. PACE 18:1679–1685, 1995.

54. Schoels W, Gough WB, Restivo M, et al: Circus movement atrial flutter in the canine sterile pericarditis model: Activation patterns during initiation, termination, and sustained reentry in vivo. Circ Res 67:35–50, 1990.

55. Daubert C, Berder V, De Place C, et al: Hemodynamic benefits of permanent atrial resynchronization in patients with advanced interatrial blocks, paced DDD mode [Abstract]. PACE 14(II):650, 1991.

56. Daubert C, Mabo P, Berder V: Arrhythmias prevention by permanent atrial resynchronization in advanced interatrial block. Eur Heart J 11:237, 1990.

57. Daubert C, Mabo P, Berder V, et al: Atrial tachyarrhythmias associated with high degree interatrial conduction block: Prevention by permanent atrial resynchronization. Eur JCPE 4:35–44, 1994.

58. Prakash A, Saksena S, Hill M, et al: Acute effects of dual-site right atrial pacing in patients with spontaneous and inducible atrial flutter and fibrillation. J Am Coll Cardiol 29:1007–1014, 1997.

59. Yu WC, Chen SA, Tai CT, et al: Effects of different atrial pacing modes on atrial electrophysiology. Circulation 96:2992–2996, 1987.

59a. Gerstenfeld EP, Hill MRS, French SN, et al: Evaluation of right atrial and biatrial temporary pacing for the prevention of atrial fibrillation after coronary artery bypass surgery. J Am Coll Cardiol 33:1981, 1999.

60. Munsif AN, Prakash A, Krol RB, et al: Crista terminalis, atrial septal and coronary sinus activation during single and dual site atrial pacing. PACE 19(II):578, 1996.

61. Prakash A, Delfaut P, Krol RB, Saksena S: Regional right and left atrial activation patterns during single and dual site atrial pacing in patients with atrial fibrillation. Am J Cardiol 82:1197, 1998.

62. Prakash A, Delfaut P, Giorgberidze I, et al: Interventional therapeutic procedures in patients with preexisting dual site right atrial pacing

63. Fitts SM, Hill MRS, Mehra R, et al, for the DAPPAF Phase 1 Investigators: Design and implementation of the Dual Site Atrial Pacing to Prevent Atrial Fibrillation (DAPPAF) clinical trial. J Intervent Card Electrophysiol 2:139–144, 1998.

64. Delfaut P, Saksena S, Prakash A, Krol RB: Long-term outcome of patients with drug-refractory atrial flutter and fibrillation after single and dual site right atrial pacing for arrhythmia prevention. J Am Coll Cardiol 32:1900, 1998.

65. Daubert JC, Leclercq C, Pavin D, Mabo P: Biatrial synchronous pacing: A new approach to prevent arrhythmias in patients with atrial conduction block. In Daubert JC, Prystowsky EN, Ripart A (eds): Prevention of Tachyarrhythmias with Cardiac Pacing. Armonk, NY, Futura, 1997, pp 99–119.

66. Belham M, Bostock J, Bucknall C, et al: Bi-atrial pacing for atrial fibrillation: Where is the optimal site for left atrial pacing? [Abstract] PACE 20(II):1074, 1997.

67. Giorgberidze I, Saksena S, Mongeon L, et al: Effects of high frequency atrial pacing in atypical atrial flutter and atrial fibrillation. J Intervent Card Electrophysiol 1:111–123, 1997.

68. Haffajee C, Stevens S, Mongeon L, et al: High frequency atrial burst pacing for termination of atrial fibrillation [Abstract]. PACE 18(Suppl II):804, 1995.

69. Vardas PE, Simantirakis EM, Manios EG, et al: Acute and chronic hemodynamic effects of bifocal vs. unifocal right atrial pacing [Abstract]. J Am Coll Cardiol 27:74A, 1996.

70. Fisher JD, Teichman S, Ferrick A, et al: Antiarrhythmic effects of VVI pacing at physiologic rates: A crossover controlled evaluation. PACE 10:822–830, 1987.

71. Winter UJ, Behrenbeck DW, Brill TH, et al: Hemodynamic and antiectopic effects of long term dynamic overdrive pacing in implanted VVI pacemakers. In Behrenbeck DW, Sowton E, Fontaine G, Winters UJ (eds): Cardiac Pacemakers. New York, Springer-Verlag, 1985.

72. Marchlinski FE, Buxton AE, Miller JM, Josephson ME: Prevention of ventricular tachycardia induction during right ventricular programmed stimulation by high current strength pacing at the site of origin. Circulation 76:332–342, 1987.

73. Viskin S, Alla SR, Barron HV, et al: Mode of onset of torsades de pointes in congenital long QT syndrome. J Am Coll Cardiol 28:1262–1268, 1996.

74. Schwartz PJ: The Long QT syndrome. Armonk, NY, Futura, 1997.

75. Garson A, Dick MD, Fournier A, et al: The long QT syndrome in children: An international study of 287 patients. Circulation 87:1866–1872, 1993.

76. Kugler JD: Sinus nodal dysfunction in young patients with long QT syndrome. Am Heart J 121:1132–1136, 1991.

77. Eldar M, Griffin JC, Abbott JA, et al: Permanent cardiac pacing in patients with the long QT syndrome. J Am Coll Cardiol 10:600, 1987.

78. Eldar M, Griggin JC, Van Hare GF, et al: Combined use of beta-adrenergic blocking agents and long-term cardiac pacing in patients with the long QT syndrome. J Am Coll Cardiol 20:830–837, 1992.

79. Moss AJ, Liu JE, Gottlieb S, et al: Efficacy of permanent pacing in the management of high risk patients with long QT syndrome. Circulation 84:1530, 1991.

80. Klein HO, Levi A, Kaplinsky E, et al: Congenital long QT syndrome: Deleterious effect of long term high-rate ventricular pacing and definite treatment by cardiac transplantation. Am Heart J 132:1079–1081, 1996.

81. Zareba W, Moss AJ: Pacing in the long-QT syndrome. In Rosenqvist M (ed): Cardiac Pacing: New Advances. Philadelphia, WB Saunders, 1997, pp 173–188.

82. Friedman PA, Hill MR, Hammill SC, et al: Randomized prospective pilot study of long-term dual site atrial pacing for prevention of atrial fibrillation. Mayo Clinic Proc 73(9):1848, 1998.

83. Mirza I, Gill J, Bucknall P, et al: Biatrial pacing in non-brady atrial fibrillation: Interatrial conduction as a selection criterion for successful prevention. PACE 22:503, 1999. (abstract)

84. Prakash A, Boccadamo R, DiBelardino R, et al: Multicenter experience with dual site atrial pacing using different pacemaker generator systems. Long term results (submitted for publication).

system for refractory atrial fibrillation. Am J Cardiol 81:1274–1277, 1998.

Chapter 20

Pacing in Patients With Heart Failure

Michael R. Gold and Robert W. Peters

During the past 40 years, permanent pacemakers have become standard therapy for patients with symptomatic sinus node disease and documented or suspected high-grade atrioventricular (AV) block. In addition, the role of pacing as adjunctive therapy in patients with various types of tachyarrhythmia is well appreciated. Although the hemodynamic effects of both single-chamber and dual-chamber pacing have been well described previously, there has been a recent increase in interest in the use of permanent pacing techniques as a primary means of improving hemodynamic function. This interest has focused on patients with heart muscle disease, specifically dilated and hypertrophic cardiomyopathies.

Despite important therapeutic advances, patients with symptomatic dilated cardiomyopathies continue to have a relatively poor prognosis, especially when their disease is accompanied by signs and symptoms of congestive heart failure. In addition to the high prevalence of disabling symptoms, survival rates have remained disappointingly low, with about half of the deaths occurring suddenly.[1, 2] In the setting of severe heart disease, it has been assumed that most of these sudden deaths were the result of malignant ventricular arrhythmias.[3] Studies involving relatively small numbers of patients have suggested, however, that a substantial proportion of sudden deaths that occur in heart failure patients may actually be due to bradyarrhythmias.[4] In addition, some medications (e.g., β-blockers, amiodarone) that may be beneficial in the setting of heart failure have negative chronotropic properties, which may cause or exacerbate bradycardia.[5, 6] This information and the availability of new and improved pacing techniques have triggered a burst of interest in the use of permanent pacemakers in this patient population. The potential added benefit of improving hemodynamic function in heart failure has been the focus of much recent study.

Similarly, patients with hypertrophic cardiomyopathy may be faced with a variety of disabling symptoms as well as an increased risk of sudden cardiac death. Pharmacologic therapy for this disorder is of limited help, whereas more definitive measures, such as surgical myomectomy of the ventricular septum, chemical septal ablation, or mitral valve replacement, may be associated with considerable morbidity and some mortality. As in dilated cardiomyopathy, there is evidence to suggest that permanent pacing may be of benefit to patients with symptomatic hypertrophic cardiomyopathy. In this chapter, we briefly review the hemodynamic aspects of cardiac pacing and explore the possible mechanisms by which pacing may benefit patients with dilated or hypertrophic cardiomyopathy. In addition, we review the major clinical studies that have been performed in these areas.

■ HEMODYNAMIC EFFECTS OF CARDIAC PACING

In healthy subjects, atrial contraction generally contributes about 15% to 30% to the cardiac output at rest.[7] This figure may vary considerably, however, depending on the heart rate, the functional integrity of the atria and ventricles, the state of activity of the person, the intracardiac pressures and volumes, autonomic influences, and other factors. With the advent of permanent cardiac pacing in the early 1960s, it became clear that certain patients were intolerant of ventricular demand pacing, and the resulting symptom complex (e.g., hypotension, near syncope) was termed the *pacemaker syndrome*.[8] Although the full-blown symptom complex is relatively uncommon, it has become apparent that many patients experience some symptoms or discomfort associated with ventricular pacing. Because organic heart disease with significant left ventricular dysfunction tends to occur frequently in a population with permanent pacemakers, the effects of permanent pacing in patients with heart failure is a clinically important issue. Although the atrial contribution to cardiac output may be relatively small in patients with heart failure and a markedly elevated left ventricular filling pressure, medical therapy may decrease the filling pressure and restore the importance of atrial systole. Patients with a component of diastolic dysfunction, in particular, are dependent on a properly timed atrial contraction for maintenance of cardiac output. Other problems associated with ventricular pacing in heart failure include systolic mitral (and tricuspid) valve incompetence due to interference with the valvular apparatus, diastolic incompetence associated with delayed mitral valve closure, systemic and pulmonary venous congestion associated with atrial contraction against closed AV valves, and the activation of autonomic reflexes associated with atrial distention that produce inappropriate diminution in peripheral vascular resistance in the face of reduced cardiac output.

Several studies have helped to elucidate some of the mechanisms involved in the pathogenesis of the symptom complex produced by ventricular demand pacing. Jutzy and coworkers[9] studied 9 patients with permanent dual-chamber pacemakers who had intact AV conduction with first-degree AV block. They found that there was a significant improvement in cardiac output and stroke volume in patients with PR intervals longer than 220 msec and little change in those with shorter AV conduction times. The incidence of congestive heart failure in their group was not specified. Ishikawa and associates[10] correlated AV delay with hemodynamics and the appearance of diastolic mitral regurgitation in 11 patients undergoing permanent pacemaker implantation, 10 of whom had preserved left ventricular function. They found that cardiac output was highest at an AV delay of 0.18 ± 0.04 seconds, which was 0.02 ± 0.02 seconds shorter than the AV interval at which diastolic mitral regurgitation began to be observed. Further increase in the AV delay resulted in a marked increase in mitral regurgitation and hemodynamic deterioration. Modena and associates[11] studied 30 patients with permanent dual-chamber pacemakers and normal left ventricular ejection fractions using Doppler echocardiography and graded exercise testing. They found that the 18 patients with left ventricular hypertrophy and abnormal diastolic relaxation patterns benefited from AV interval shortening with normalization of the filling pattern when the AV delay was programmed to 100 msec. In contrast, in those without diastolic relaxation abnormalities, changes in AV delay caused no consistent variation in filling pattern. Also of note is a study by Mukharji and coworkers[12] that compared the importance of the atrial contribution to cardiac function in two patient groups: 10 patients with severe congestive heart failure and 10 patients with normal ventricular function. Both groups demonstrated improved hemodynamics with dual-chamber pacing (compared with VVI pacing), but interestingly, the improvement was similar in the two groups (Fig. 20–1).

Thus, it is likely that the timing of atrial systole can have an important effect on hemodynamics, at least in some patients. The optimal AV delay and the population of patients that most benefit from adjustment of the AV interval have not been completely elucidated. It appears, however, that patients with prolonged PR intervals and diastolic dysfunction are most likely to show improved hemodynamic function with dual-chamber pacing. Other factors, such as intraatrial conduction times and the presence of diastolic mitral

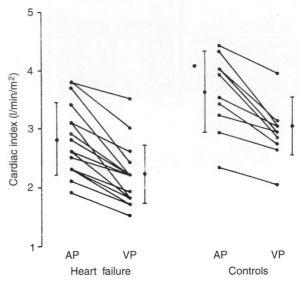

Figure 20–1. Comparison of cardiac index between right atrial pacing and pacing from the right ventricular apex. P < 0.01. AP, atrial pacing; VP, ventricular pacing. (From Mukharji J, Rehr RB, Hastillo A, et al: Comparison of atrial contribution to cardiac hemodynamics in patients with normal and severely compromised cardiac function. Clin Cardiol 13:639, 1990.)

regurgitation, may also be important because they may affect the relationship between programmed right-sided AV delay and optimal left atrial to left ventricle activation times. Nevertheless, as experience with permanent pacing has grown, it has become apparent that dual-chamber pacing is preferable in most patients and obviates many of the problems encountered with single-chamber ventricular stimulation.

Similarly, it has been found that the loss of the normal activation sequence of the atria and ventricles associated with pacing may interfere with normal cardiac function.[7] Thus, although dual-chamber pacing has been designated "physiologic," the loss of simultaneous contraction of the right and left heart chambers and alteration of the pattern of ventricular activation may have important hemodynamic consequences. For example, Rosenqvist and associates[13] examined the hemodynamic effects of both single-chamber and dual-chamber pacing in 12 patients with chronotropic incompetence and intact AV conduction. They found that left ventricular systolic performance was more dependent on normal ventricular activation (during AAI pacing) than on AV synchrony. Similar results were reported by Askenazi and colleagues.[14] These and other observations have stimulated interest in the use of pacing techniques to improve cardiac performance in patients with dilated cardiomyopathies and heart failure.

The goals of permanent pacing are somewhat different in patients with hypertrophic cardiomyopathy. Unlike the dilated cardiomyopathies, which are a heterogeneous group of disorders of diverse etiologies with severe left ventricular systolic dysfunction as the common denominator, hypertrophic cardiomyopathy is a genetically determined condition characterized by massive thickening of the ventricular walls. There is diminution of the left ventricular cavity with variable degrees of outflow tract obstruction, either in the baseline state or provoked by changing preload or by catecholamine infusion. The goal of therapy in hypertrophic cardiomyopathy is aimed at depressing myocardial contractile function, inducing some degree of ventricular dilation, reducing outflow tract obstruction, when present, and improving diastolic relaxation of the ventricles, in part by reducing heart rate. Specifically, reducing contractility and inducing AV and interventricular dyssynchrony can produce ventricular dilation and has the potential for improving hemodynamics and relieving symptoms in patients with outflow tract obstruction. This could conceivably be accomplished by shortening the AV delay to the point that the ventricular septum is preexcited maximally (producing the widest QRS complex possible); the resultant alteration in the contraction sequence of the interventricular septum widens the left ventricular outflow tract.[15]

■ CLINICAL STUDIES

Dilated Cardiomyopathies

Optimization of Atrioventricular Delay

The observations described previously have stimulated investigators to explore the role of manipulation of the AV delay as a means of improving hemodynamic parameters in patients with impaired left ventricular function (Table 20–1). The work of Hochleitner and associates[16] was probably the first to demonstrate a beneficial effect of dual-chamber pacing in heart failure. In 16 patients with end-stage idiopathic dilated cardiomyopathy, dual-chamber pacing with an AV delay of 100 msec produced a striking improvement in left ventricular ejection fraction and pulmonary congestive symptoms. The authors postulated that the improvement in cardiac function was due to a decrease in mitral regurgitation and preservation of atrial systole. A follow-up study by the same group[17] showed that the symptomatic improvement persisted for up to 5 years. Subsequent case reports of patients with dilated or ischemic cardiomyopathy also noted marked functional improvements after dual-chamber pacing with a 100-msec AV delay.[18, 19]

These initial studies of short AV delay pacing for the primary treatment of congestive heart failure were uncontrolled. Thus, some of the benefit observed may have been due to factors other than pacing, such as persistent effects of intravenous inotropic therapy that many patients were receiving at the time of pacemaker implantation, spontaneous improvement of the underlying disease process, better medical management through participation in a study, changes in drug therapy, or a placebo effect of undergoing an intervention. In addition, these studies did not assess the possible mechanisms of clinical benefit. Nevertheless, these early experiences stimulated many further trials.

Brecker and associates[20] measured ventricular filling time and cardiac output with Doppler echocardiography and exercise treadmill time with varying AV delays in 12 patients with dilated cardiomyopathies and short ventricular filling times due to mitral regurgitation. They found that right and left ventricular filling times, cardiac output, and exercise duration increased simultaneously with decreases in the duration of mitral and tricuspid regurgitation when the AV delay was shortened. In an acute study of 15 patients with ejection fractions of 30% or less, Nishimura and colleagues[21] found a significant hemodynamic improvement in the 8 patients with PR intervals longer than 200 msec. In contrast, the conditions of those with normal PR intervals were unchanged. Similarly, Guardigli and colleagues[22] used Doppler echocardiography to evaluate the optimal AV delay in 10 patients with dilated cardiomyopathies (New York Heart Association [NYHA] functional class III or IV) and permanent dual-chamber pacemakers. They found that an AV delay of 100 msec was associated with the best diastolic filling and systolic function; and during acute testing shortening the AV delay further, to 80 msec, caused deterioration in systolic performance. They also found that the improvement in left ventricular function persisted for 2 months and was associated with a similar improvement in NYHA functional class.

In an acute study, Auricchio and Salo[23] found that atrial pacing with an optimal AV delay improved mean pulse pressure in 6 of 9 patients with class II–IV heart failure.[23] Of particular note is that they found that atrial pacing was inferior to atrial sensed modes (VDD pacing). They postulated that the increase in interatrial conduction time associ-

Table 20–1. Studies of Short Atrioventricular Delay Pacing for Congestive Heart Failure

Investigators	No. of Subjects	EF (%) (NYHA)	AV Delay (msec)	Duration	Clinical Results
Hochleitner et al, 1990[16]	16	16 (III–IV)	100	<15 days	Major improvements
Hochleitner et al, 1992[16]	17	—(III–IV)	100	Up to 5 yr	Symptoms improved, but 10 patients died and 4 had transplantations
Nishimura et al, 1995[21]	15	—(II–IV)	Optimum	Acute	Hemodynamics improved in 8 patients with long PR intervals but not in those with normal PR intervals
Brecker et al, 1992[20]	12	Not specified	Optimum	Acute	Hemodynamics improved with decreased MR & TR
Guardigli et al, 1994[22]	10	40 (III or IV)	Optimum	2 mo	Symptoms and left ventricular function improved
Gold et al, 1995[24]	12	20 (III or IV)	100	12 wk	Symptoms and left ventricular function unimproved*
Innes et al, 1994[25]	12	21 (II or IV)	60, 100	Acute	Hemodynamics unimproved
Linde et al, 1994[26]	10	21 (III or IV)	Optimum	6 mo	Symptoms and left ventricular function unimproved
Auricchio & Salo, 1997[23]	9	—(II to IV)	Optimum	Acute	VDD superior (hemodynamically) to DDD pacing
Gilligan et al, 1998[27]	17	25 (—)	Optimum	12 wk	Symptoms unimproved*

EF, mean ejection fraction; NYHA, New York Heart Association class; MR, mitral regurgitation; TR, tricuspid regurgitation.
*Randomized, double-blind trial.

ated with atrial pacing shortened left heart AV delay and interfered with left ventricular filling, with resultant depression of left ventricular function.

Several controlled studies have failed to confirm the benefit of short AV delay pacing in this patient population. Gold and coworkers[24] were unable to demonstrate any benefit, either acutely or chronically, in a double-blind, randomized, crossover trial in 12 patients with class III or IV (by the NYHA functional classification) chronic congestive heart failure refractory to medical management (Fig. 20–2). VDD pacing with a 100-msec delay was compared with VVI pacing using a crossover design with each patient serving as his or her own control. The AV delay (100 msec) was chosen empirically for the chronic study, although in acute hemodynamic measurements obtained after pacemaker implantation, the AV delay was systematically and randomly varied without effect on pulmonary artery wedge or mean right atrial pressures. Of note is that 9 of the 12 subjects had pre-existing first-degree AV block. Similarly, Innes and associates[25] found that dual-chamber pacing with a short AV delay did not acutely improve hemodynamic function in 12 patients with heart failure despite a significant increase in left ventricular filling time.

Linde and associates[26] were unable to demonstrate significant clinical improvement during a 3-month follow-up period in a group of 10 patients with NYHA class III or IV congestive heart failure. The AV delay was programmed at an interval (between 50 and 120 msec) that optimized stroke volume and cardiac output at the initiation of the study. These authors concluded that VDD pacing did not improve this patient population. Gilligan and colleagues[27] similarly failed to demonstrate improvement of quality of life or

exercise duration in a randomized double-blind crossover trial of 17 patients with symptomatic left ventricular dysfunction (mean ejection fraction, $25 \pm 9\%$) in whom an optimal AV delay (chosen during an acute hemodynamic study) was compared with a nominal setting.

In summary, dual-chamber pacing with a short or optimal AV delay has produced mixed results in patients with congestive heart failure and has been the subject of some controversy in the medical literature.[28] Controlled trials have not confirmed the promising results reported in early studies. Because beneficial effects appear to occur in at least some patients, however, larger trials are needed that allow subgroup analysis, before the issue can be settled.

Alternative Pacing Sites

All of the studies described used ventricular pacing at the right ventricular apex for evaluation of short AV delay pacing on hemodynamics and functional status. When endocardial leads first became available for permanent pacing, the right ventricular apex was chosen as the position of choice, primarily because it was relatively easy to obtain a stable position with good pacing and sensing characteristics and an acceptable incidence of lead dislodgment. There have been many important advances in lead design in the intervening years (e.g., tined leads, active fixation leads, steroid eluting leads), and pacing from other parts of the ventricles has become feasible. Atrial (AAIR) pacing with intact AV conduction is usually associated with a higher cardiac output than DDD pacing,[13] suggesting that the pattern of ventricular activation may be playing a role. In people with normal ventricular function, cardiac output with DDD pacing is usually adequate, so there is little impetus to explore alternative pacing sites. In the setting of congestive heart failure, however, improving cardiac output is a much higher priority (Table 20–2).

In a canine model, Karpawich and coauthors[29] used a long introducer and screw-in electrode lead to pace the His bundle consistently. The feasibility of pacing the His bundle chronically through an endocardial approach, however, has not yet been demonstrated. As a possible alternative, Karpawich and Vincent[30] performed endocardial pacing from the right ventricular apex and from the right ventricular septum, also in a canine model. They found that septal pacing improved left ventricular function and postulated that pacing adjacent to the conduction system normalized the pattern of ventricular activation with resulting improvement in hemodynamic parameters.

It has been demonstrated that permanent pacing from the right ventricular outflow tract is feasible in humans.[31] Giudici and coworkers[32] found that right ventricular outflow tract pacing improved cardiac output over pacing from the right ventricular apex in 89 patients undergoing dual-chamber pacemaker implantation for sinus node dysfunction. However, the pacing sites were not randomized, measurements were not blinded, VVI pacing was evaluated in patients with intact sinus node function, invasive hemodynamic measurements were not obtained, and the patient population was not restricted to those with congestive heart failure. In this regard, Victor and colleagues[33] evaluated 10 patients with preserved left ventricular function, complete heart block, and chronic atrial fibrillation. Each patient received a dual-

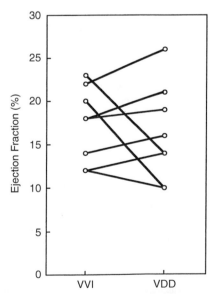

Figure 20–2. Effect of pacing on left ventricular ejection fraction as measured by radionuclide ventriculography after 4 to 6 weeks of dual-chamber pacing in VDD mode (100-msec atrioventricular delay) and after a similar period in backup mode (VVI). *Circles*, individual patient data. (From Gold MR, Feliciano Z, Gottlieb SS, et al: Dual chamber pacing with a short atrioventricular delay in congestive heart failure: A randomized study. J Am Coll Cardiol 26:967, 1995.)

Table 20-2. Studies of Effects of Alternative Pacing Sites on Hemodynamic and Functional Parameters

Investigators	No. of subjects	Pacing Site	EF (%) (NYHA)	Duration	Results
Gold et al, 1997[34]	13	RVOT	23 (III–IV)	Acute	No benefit of RVOT over RVA pacing
Giudici et al, 1997[32]	89	RVOT	Not specified	Acute	CO increased by RVOT pacing
Buckingham et al, 1997[37]	11	RVA and RVOT	10 patients had normal LV function; in 1, EF = 30%	Acute	Simultaneous RVA and RVOT pacing narrowed QRS and increased CO
Foster et al, 1995[38]	18	Epicardial BIV	Preoperative EF > 40% in 14 patients (all were NYHA class I)	12–36 hr after CABG	Atrial BIV pacing improved hemodynamics
Cazeau et al, 1994[41]	1	Four-chamber; LV epicardial, others transvenous	—(IV)	6 wk	Marked clinical improvement with four-chamber pacing
Bakker et al, 1994[39]	5	BIV (RV endocardial, LV epicardial)	5–23 (III–IV)	3 mo	All improved with BIV pacing
Cazeau et al, 1996[43]	8	Four-chamber or BIV; 5 patients had epicardial	22 (IV)	6 mo (mean)	4 patients died, 4 improved with BIV pacing
Maloney et al, 1996[44]	3	Four-chamber; all transvenous	End-stage heart failure	3 mo	Major clinical improvement with four-chamber pacing and all transvenous lead system
Brockman et al, 1998[35]	20	RVA, RVOT	21 (II–IV)	Acute	No benefit of DDD pacing from RVOT over RVA
Victor et al, 1997[33]	10	RVA, RVOT	40 (Not specified)	7 mo	No benefit of DDDR pacing from RVOT over RVA
Daubert et al, 1996[42]	13	BIV (transvenous)	End-stage heart failure	7.5 mo (mean)	Permanent LV pacing could be reliably performed through the left cardiac vein
Blanc et al, 1997[45]	23	BIV (transvenous)	27 (III–IV)	Acute	LV or BIV pacing superior to RVA or RVOT
Kass et al, 1997[46]	14	BIV (transvenous)	19 (III–IV)	Acute	LV preferable to RV or BIV pacing
Cowell et al, 1994[36]	15	RVA, RV septum	33 (Not specified)	Acute	RV septal preferable to RVA pacing
Auricchio et al, 1998[47]	16	BIV	22 (III–IV)	Acute	BIV preferable to either RV or LV pacing

EF, mean ejection fraction; NYHA, New York Heart Association class; RVOT, right ventricular outflow tract; RVA, right ventricular apex; CO, cardiac output; BIV, biventricular pacing; LV, left ventricular; RV, right ventricular; CABG, coronary artery bypass graft.

chamber pacemaker with one lead in the right ventricular apex and the other in the outflow tract. In a randomized study of pacing from these two sites, no effect on exercise parameters or hemodynamic measurements was observed.

Gold and associates,[34] in a prospective, randomized, double-blind study, found that VDD pacing from the septal wall of the right ventricular outflow tract conferred no hemodynamic benefit over intrinsic conduction using a wide range of AV delays. Their study population consisted of 13 patients with chronic NYHA class III or IV congestive heart failure undergoing dual-chamber pacemaker implantation for sinus node dysfunction or intermittent high-grade AV block. Subsequently, Brockman and colleagues,[35] in a prospective, randomized study of 20 patients with congestive heart failure, found that VVI overdrive pacing worsened hemodynamic parameters acutely (compared with AAI pacing) but that there was no significant difference between DDD pacing from the right ventricular apex and right ventricular outflow tract. In addition, DDD pacing from either right ventricular site provided no hemodynamic benefit over AAI pacing (Fig. 20–3). Thus, pacing mode, but not right ventricular pacing site, affected hemodynamic parameters in the setting of congestive heart failure.

Somewhat different results were obtained by Cowell and colleagues,[36] who found that temporary VDD pacing with a short AV delay from the right ventricular outflow pacing increased cardiac output compared with pacing from the right ventricular apex in 15 patients with impaired left ventricular systolic function (mean ejection fraction, 32.7 ± 11.6%). A rather unique approach was employed by Buckingham and associates[37] in 11 patients referred for electrophysiologic study for routine clinical indications. These investigators postulated that pacing simultaneously from two right ventricular sites would produce more rapid and uniform ventricular depolarization, narrow the QRS complex, and improve cardiac performance. Using pacing catheters in the right ventricular apex and outflow tract, they found that the mean QRS duration narrowed significantly (from 130 to 110 msec), although there was no significant improvement in cardiac output. The application of this technique to a patient population with heart failure has not, to our knowledge, been performed.

In theory, the use of pacing that allows for simultaneous contraction of *both* ventricles has the potential to narrow the QRS complex and improve cardiac output more than dual site-pacing from the right ventricle. Foster and associates[38] used temporary epicardial electrodes to pace the right atrium and paraseptal locations simultaneously on the right and left ventricles in 18 patients 1 to 2 days after elective coronary artery revascularization. Simultaneous biventricular activation was documented by fusion on the surface electrocardiogram and isochronal epicardial activation mapping. They

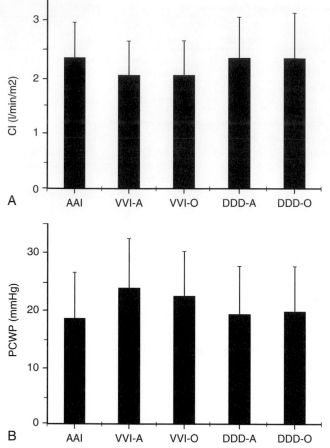

Figure 20–3. Effect of right ventricular pacing mode and site on hemodynamic function. Cardiac index (CI, *panel A*) and pulmonary capillary wedge pressure (PCWP, *panel B*) were measured with right atrial pacing (AAI), overdrive ventricular pacing from the right ventricular apex (VVI-A) and outflow tract (VVI-O), and DDD pacing from the apex (DDD-A) and outflow tract (DDD-O). Note that DDD pacing prevents the hemodynamic deterioration with VVI pacing, with no effect of pacing site.

found that atrial biventricular pacing was associated with a significantly higher cardiac output and lower systemic vascular resistance than either atrial, atrial right ventricular, or atrial left ventricular pacing. It is interesting that despite studying primarily patients with preserved left ventricular function and normal AV conduction, ventricular pacing was superior hemodynamically to normal ventricular activation with AAI pacing.

After the initial demonstration of the potential benefit of temporary biventricular pacing following cardiac surgery, modifications of this technique were applied to patients with congestive heart failure. Initially, endocardial right ventricular and epicardial left ventricular sites were evaluated.[39, 40] Pacing was performed by using one lead as the anode and the other as the cathode. Exit block developed in most patients, however, requiring lead modification to allow for dual cathode pacing.

Cazeau and coworkers[41] performed permanent four-chamber pacing in a 54-year-old man with alcoholic cardiomyopathy and end-stage heart failure refractory to intravenous dopamine and dobutamine. The patient's surface electrocar-

diogram revealed a left bundle-branch block, a PR interval of 200 msec, and an interatrial conduction delay. Of note is that echocardiography revealed a 250-msec delay between septal and posterior wall contractions. After an acute study of four-chamber pacing showed improvement in cardiac output and pulmonary capillary wedge pressure, a permanent pacemaker was implanted using endocardial right atrial and ventricular leads, a permanent coronary sinus lead (left atrial pacing), and an epicardial left ventricular lead. After 6 weeks of four-chamber pacing, the patient had a weight loss of 17 kg and had become functional class II by the NYHA criteria. Beneficial results of four-chamber pacing were also described by Bakker and associates[39] in five patients with end-stage dilated cardiomyopathy, left bundle-branch block, and PR interval prolongation.

The feasibility of a purely transvenous approach to four-chamber pacing was demonstrated by Daubert and associates[42] in a group of patients with drug-refractory heart failure. Chronic left ventricular stimulation was successful in 7 of 13 patients using a very thin unipolar lead that was introduced through the coronary sinus and advanced to a posterolateral or lateral vein of the left ventricular free wall. Dislodgment of the left ventricular leads was not encountered, and pacing and sensing characteristics remained stable for a mean follow-up interval of 7.5 months. Sustained hemodynamic improvement was described by Cazeau and coworkers[43] in 8 patients with a widened QRS complex and end-stage heart failure. In two of these patients, transvenous left ventricular leads were employed. It should be emphasized that the stimulation of separate chambers in a widely spaced bipolar manner ("extended bipole") may lead to a major rise in pacing threshold and compromise the efficacy of the system. Of particular interest is the study by Maloney and colleagues[44] using coronary sinus access for left ventricular pacing in three patients with congestive heart failure and widened QRS complexes. Pacing and sensing thresholds remained excellent in the three patients, all of whom experienced sustained hemodynamic improvement. Despite these encouraging findings, one of the major goals for allowing widespread use of biventricular pacing is the development of leads that can be routinely positioned in left ventricular branches of the coronary venous system with adequate long-term stability.

Blanc and colleagues[45] performed acute hemodynamic studies in 23 patients with severe heart failure and pulmonary capillary wedge pressures of greater than 15 mm Hg. Hemodynamic parameters were similar when pacing was performed from either the right ventricular apex or outflow tract but were markedly improved by left ventricular endocardial pacing, either alone or in combination with simultaneous stimulation from the right ventricle (Fig. 20–4). Similarly, Kass and associates[46] found a significant improvement in systolic function with left ventricular pacing (through the coronary sinus) in 18 patients with severe dilated cardiomyopathies (NYHA class III or IV; mean ejection fraction, 19.2 ± 7%).[46] Results with biventricular pacing or right ventricular pacing were worse than with single-site left ventricular pacing. Of particular note is that improvement in systolic function correlated with baseline QRS duration. In contrast, Auricchio and colleagues[47] found that biventricular pacing conferred hemodynamic benefit over univentricular

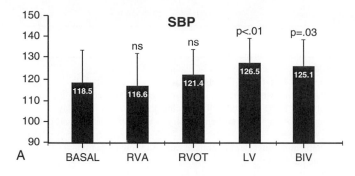

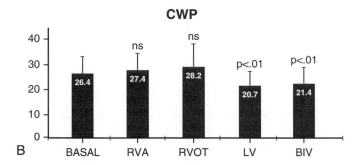

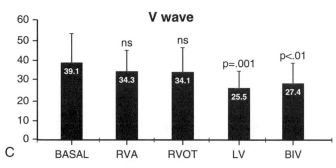

Figure 20–4. Changes in hemodynamic parameters induced by pacing at each ventricular site compared with baseline (basal). Values are mean ± SD: (*A*) systolic blood pressure (SBP); (*B*) capillary wedge pressure (CWP); (*C*) V-wave amplitude. RVA, right ventricular apex; RVOT, right ventricular outflow tract; LV, left ventricular free wall; BIV, biventricular. (From Blanc J-J, Etienne Y, Gilard M, et al: Evaluation of different ventricular pacing sites in patients with severe heart failure: Results of an acute hemodynamic study. Circulation 96:3273, 1997. Copyright 1997 by the American Heart Association.)

til further studies are completed that may identify subgroups who are likely to benefit (e.g., patients with PR interval prolongation, diastolic mitral regurgitation), the routine use of dual-chamber pacing with a short AV delay *cannot* be recommended for patients with heart failure. The use of multisite pacemakers, especially biventricular pacing, holds considerable promise. The techniques are still being refined, but positive results have been reported in animal models, in acute studies involving patients, and in relatively small chronic studies with limited follow-up. These promising results await confirmation by large, rigorously controlled clinical trials. In addition, a number of important clinical issues remain regarding the use of permanent pacing in patients with heart failure and dilated cardiomyopathy (Table 20–3).

Hypertrophic Cardiomyopathy

Interest in permanent pacing in hypertrophic cardiomyopathy began with a case report in 1975 that described symptomatic improvement in a patient receiving a pacemaker for high-grade AV block (Table 20–4).[48] In the same year, Hassenstein and colleagues[49] described four patients with the obstructive form of hypertrophic cardiomyopathy who had a 56% mean reduction in outflow tract gradient with VVI pacing associated with symptomatic improvement. The first large series was reported by Duck and associates,[50] who investigated various temporary pacing modes (VOO, VAT, and DOO) in 23 patients with hypertrophic cardiomyopathy and significant resting outflow tract gradients. They found an appreciable reduction in gradient in all but 1 patient regardless of the pacing mode employed. Objective evidence of symptomatic improvement was provided by McDonald and colleagues,[51] who performed serial exercise stress tests in 11 patients with hypertrophic cardiomyopathy in whom dual-chamber pacemakers had been implanted. Stress tests were performed during VDD pacing and also with the pacemakers inactivated (OOO mode) in a randomized double-blind manner. The investigators found that mean exercise time was prolonged by 31%.

In 1992, the results of two important studies were published that considerably heightened the enthusiasm for pacing in hypertrophic cardiomyopathy. Jeanrenaud and coauthors[52] performed acute hemodynamic studies in 13 patients with hypertrophic cardiomyopathy refractory to medical management. They observed that dual-chamber pacing with

pacing from *either* the left or right ventricle in 16 patients with severe congestive heart failure.

■ Summary: Pacing in Dilated Cardiomyopathies

There is considerable theoretic rationale for some of the previously mentioned pacing techniques to improve substantially the clinical status of patients with dilated cardiomyopathies and severe congestive heart failure. Despite early reports of dramatic success, the benefit of dual-chamber pacing with a short AV delay has not been substantiated by randomized controlled trials, although these follow-up studies have generally involved relatively small numbers of patients. Un-

Table 20–3. Pacing Issues in Patients With Dilated Cardiomyopathy

1. Is biatrial (i.e., four-chamber) pacing necessary with biventricular pacing?
2. What is the optimal stimulation site for right and left ventricular leads?
3. Does a single left ventricular lead provide sufficient hemodynamic benefit, or is it necessary to employ simultaneous right ventricular (i.e., biventricular) stimulation?
4. Does the etiology (i.e., ischemic versus dilated) or severity of heart failure predict clinical benefit?
5. What is the role of pacing in systolic versus diastolic dysfunction?
6. Are there subgroups of patients in whom right ventricular pacing with an optimum atrioventricular delay or right ventricular outflow tract pacing may be of benefit?

Table 20–4. Studies of Pacing in Patients With Hypertrophic Cardiomyopathy

Investigators	No. of Subjects	NYHA Class	Duration	Results
Duck et al, 1984[50]	23	Not specified	Acute	Reduced gradient regardless of pacing mode
McDonald et al, 1988[51]	11	Not specified	Up to 2 yr	Improved EST time with DDD pacing
Jeanrenaud et al, 1992[52]	13	III	Acute	DDD pacing with short AV delay; reduced LVOT gradient
Jeanrenaud et al, 1992[52]	8	III	Up to 62 mo	Improved symptoms with DDD pacing and optimum AV delay
Fananapazir et al, 1992[53]	44	III–IV	1.5–3 mo	Improved symptoms and hemodynamics with DDD pacing and optimum AV delay
Fananapazir et al, 1994[54]	84	III–IV	2.3 ± 0.8 yr	Symptom improvement continued during follow-up period; only 2 deaths
Nishimura et al, 1997[57]	19	II–IV	6 mo	No definitive improvement with optimal AV delay*
Slade et al, 1996[58]	56	II–IV	11 mo (mean)	Symptom improved but no correlation with gradient
Rishi et al, 1997[55]	10	Not specified	23 ± 4 mo (mean)	Symptoms and hemodynamics improved with DDD pacing
Kappenberger et al, 1997[56]	83	Not specified	6 mo	Symptoms improved and LVOT gradient decreased

NYHA, New York Heart Association; LVOT, left ventricular outflow tract; EST, exercise stress test.
*The only study with a randomized double-blind crossover design.

a short AV delay (50 to 90 msec) reduced the subaortic pressure gradient by a mean value of 43% without altering aortic pressure or cardiac output, whereas pacing with longer AV delays had little or no effect. In the second aspect of the study, 8 patients had permanent dual-chamber pacemakers implanted using the AV delay that provided the optimum hemodynamic response in the acute study. In a follow-up

period of up to 62 months, there was a marked improvement in chest pain and dyspnea despite a lack of change in septal wall thickness or left ventricular contractility. There was, however, a trend toward a spontaneous decrease in outflow tract obstruction.

Fananapazir and colleagues[53] studied 44 consecutive patients with obstructive hypertrophic cardiomyopathy refrac-

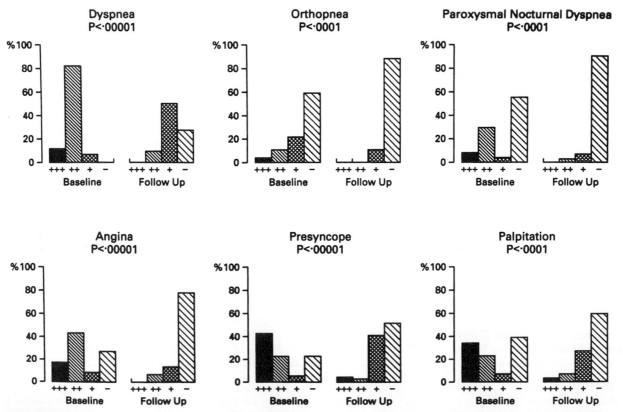

Figure 20–5. Bar graphs showing the prevalence and severity of individual cardiac symptoms before and after the institution of DDD pacing with a short AV interval in patients with obstructive hypertrophic cardiomyopathy. The severity of symptoms is shown as follows: −, symptoms absent; +, mild symptoms; ++, moderate symptoms; +++, severe symptoms. (From Fananapazir L, Cannon RO III, Tripodi D, et al: Impact of dual chamber permanent pacing in patients with obstructive hypertrophic cardiomyopathy with symptoms refractory to verapamil and β-adrenergic blocker therapy. Circulation 85:2149, 1992. Copyright 1992 by the American Heart Association.)

RA Pacing 120 bpm   A-V Sequential Pacing 120 bpm (A-V = 120ms)

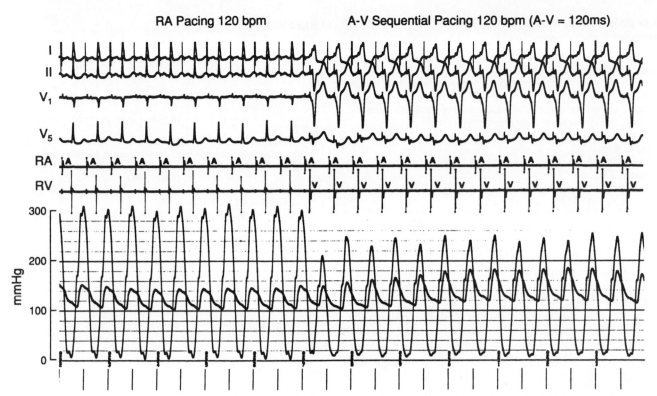

Figure 20–6. Tracing showing the impact of atrioventricular (AV) sequential pacing on left ventricular and femoral arterial pressure in an individual patient. On the left, during right atrial (RA) pacing at 120 bpm, the maximum left ventricular pressure is 330 mm Hg and the left ventricular outflow gradient is 170 mm Hg. On the right, an acute change in AV sequential pacing at the same rate is made with an AV interval of 120 msec to pre-excite the ventricular septum. The left ventricular systolic pressure is reduced to 250 mm Hg, and a left ventricular outflow tract gradient to 70 mm Hg is shown. These changes were accompanied by an improvement of the femoral arterial systolic and pulse pressure. Shown from top to bottom are surface electrocardiogram leads I, II, III, V_1 and V_5; RA, right atrial intracardiac recording, A and V, atrial and ventricular intracardiac electrograms. (From Fananapazir L, Cannon RO III, Tripodi D, et al: Impact of dual chamber permanent pacing in patients with obstructive hypertrophic cardiomyopathy and symptoms refractory to verapamil and β-adrenergic blocker therapy. Circulation 85:2149, 1992. Copyright 1992 by the American Heart Association.)

tory to medical management before and 1.5 to 3 months after implantation of a DDD pacemaker (Figs. 20–5 and 20–6). All patients' pacemakers were programmed to short (75- to 125-msec) AV delays associated with maximal pre-excitation (widest QRS complex induced by pacing) and the patients were discharged from the hospital receiving no medication. At the time of the follow-up evaluation, symptoms, NYHA functional classification, and exercise treadmill duration were all improved and were accompanied by a significant increase in systemic arterial blood pressure and cardiac output and a decrease in mean left ventricular outflow tract gradient. Interestingly, these improvements persisted, in part, after pacing was temporarily discontinued and the measurements were repeated during normal sinus rhythm.

Long-term follow-up information was presented by Fananapazir's group[54] in 84 patients with hypertrophic cardiomyopathy. During the 2.3 ± 0.8 year (mean) follow-up, symptoms were eliminated or diminished in 89% of patients. Although there was no control population available for comparison, there were only two deaths, both sudden and both occurring in patients who had experienced symptomatic improvement. Particularly encouraging was the relatively benign outcome in patients who had a history of syncope, previously considered an ominous prognostic sign. Also of note is that, at least in some patients, maximal benefit was not observed immediately and required a year or more to become clinically manifest. In 23% of their patients, there was regional regression of left ventricular hypertrophy that was not accompanied by a deterioration of left ventricular function. This suggests that myocardial remodeling may be responsible for some of the persistent clinical benefit observed. The authors found no baseline parameters that predicted a favorable outcome with pacing and hence recommended that baseline studies need not be performed.

Similar beneficial effects of dual-chamber pacing in seven children with hypertrophic obstructive cardiomyopathy was reported by Rishi and colleagues.[55] Preliminary results of a randomized double-blind crossover study of DDD pacing with a short AV delay in 83 patients with hypertrophic cardiomyopathy were recently reported by Kappenberger and associates.[56] Significant improvement in angina and dyspnea were noted in most of these patients, along with a marked reduction in left ventricular outflow gradient, although there was no change in left ventricular function or septal wall thickness.

In contrast, more variable results were reported by Nishimura and colleagues[57] in a double-blind randomized comparison of DDD (with a short AV delay) and AAI pacing in 19 patients with obstructive hypertrophic cardiomyopathy.

Table 20–5. Pacing Issues in Patients With Hypertrophic Cardiomyopathy

1. Is an invasive hemodynamic study required to demonstrate benefit before implanting a permanent pacemaker?
2. Does an optimum atrioventricular delay need to be identified for each patient?
3. Is there a direct correlation between reduction of the outflow tract gradient and symptomatic improvement?
4. Can pacing prolong survival and reduce the incidence of sudden cardiac death?
5. Does pacing lead to permanent structural or biochemical changes in the ventricular septum?
6. What is the role of pacing in patients with symptomatic nonobstructive cardiomyopathy?

Although quality of life improved in 63% of patients during DDD pacing, 42% experienced improved quality of life during AAI pacing (P = NS). In addition, 31% had no change in symptoms, and 5% experienced deterioration during DDD pacing. Similarly, Slade and associates[58] described their experience with 56 patients with obstructive hypertrophic cardiomyopathy refractory to medical management. Although most of these patients reported symptomatic improvement after permanent pacemaker implantation programmed with a short AV delay, there was no correlation between the improvement in functional status and the reduction in outflow tract gradient, nor was there any decrease in pharmacologic therapy.

Summary: Pacing in Hypertrophic Cardiomyopathy

Despite promising early reports, the benefits of dual-chamber pacing in hypertrophic cardiomyopathy have only been conclusively documented in a randomized double-blind manner (by preliminary results) in one study. It is clear that pacing can reduce the outflow tract gradient in many patients, but the exact mechanism of this reduction is unclear.[15] Similarly, the relative importance of other suggested beneficial effects, such as improvement in ventricular diastolic function, depression of systolic function, reduction in mitral regurgitation, and improvement in coronary blood flow, will require further investigation. Importantly, permanent pacing has *not* been demonstrated to reduce mortality or the frequency of sudden cardiac death.[59] In addition, the role of pacing in patients with nonobstructive cardiomyopathy or in other populations, such as children and patients with concomitant atherosclerotic coronary artery disease, needs clarification. The observation that pacing-induced improvement may be sustained and demonstrable even during normal sinus rhythm is intriguing and suggests that the regression of left ventricular hypertrophy described by some investigators may be both real and clinically important. Further studies, especially clinical trials with sufficient power to address the issue of reduction in mortality and sudden cardiac death, are needed to elucidate better the role of pacing compared with medical therapy and with surgical myomectomy in patients with hypertrophic cardiomyopathy. These issues are summarized in Table 20–5.

REFERENCES

1. The SOLVD Investigators: Effect of enalapril on survival in patients with reduced ejection fractions and congestive heart failure. N Engl J Med 325:293, 1991.
2. Consensus Trial Study Group: Effects of enalapril in severe congestive heart failure: Results of the Cooperative North Scandinavian Survival Study. N Engl J Med 316:1429, 1987.
3. Linde C, Ryden L: Pacing in dilated cardiomyopathy. PACE 18:1341, 1995.
4. Luu M, Stevenson WG, Stevenson LW, et al: Ventricular tachycardia is not the predominant cause of monitored sudden death in heart failure. Circulation 80:1675, 1989.
5. Singh SN, Gross Fisher S, Fletcher RD, et al: Amiodarone in patients with congestive heart failure with asymptomatic ventricular arrhythmias. N Engl J Med 33:77, 1995.
6. Doval HC, Nul DR, Grancelli HO, et al: Randomized trial of low-dose amiodarone in severe congestive heart failure. Lancet 344:493, 1994.
7. Barold SS, Zipes DP: Cardiac pacemakers and antiarrhythmic devices. *In* Braunwald E (ed): Heart Disease: A Textbook of Cardiovascular Medicine, 5th ed. Philadelphia, WB Saunders, 1997, pp 705–741.
8. Reynolds DW: Hemodynamics of cardiac pacing. *In* Ellenbogen KA (ed): Cardiac Pacing, 2nd ed. Cambridge, Blackwell Scientific, 1996, pp 124–167.
9. Jutzy RV, Feenstra L, Pai R, et al: Comparison of intrinsic versus paced ventricular function. PACE 15:1919, 1992.
10. Ishikawa T, Sumita S, Kimura K, et al: Critical PQ interval for the appearance of diastolic mitral regurgitation and optimal PQ interval in patients implanted with DDD pacemakers. PACE 17:1989, 1994.
11. Modena MG, Rossi R, Carcagni A, et al: The importance of different atrioventricular delay for left ventricular filling in sequential pacing: Clinical implications. PACE 19:1595, 1996.
12. Mukharji J, Rehr RB, Thompson JA, et al. Comparison of atrial contribution to cardiac hemodynamics in patients with normal and severely compromised cardiac function. Clin Cardiol 13:639, 1990.
13. Rosenqvist M, Isaaz K, Botvinick EH, et al: Relative importance of activation sequence compared to atrioventricular synchrony in left ventricular function. Am J Cardiol 67:148, 1991.
14. Askenazi J, Alexander JH, Koenigsberg DI, et al: Alteration of left ventricular performance by left bundle branch block simulated with atrioventricular sequential pacing. Am J Cardiol 53:99, 1984.
15. Criley JM: Unobstructed thinking (and terminology) is called for in the understanding and management of hypertrophic cardiomyopathy. J Am Coll Cardiol 29:741, 1997.
16. Hochleitner M, Hortnagl H, Ng C-K, et al: Usefulness of physiologic dual-chamber pacing in drug-resistant idiopathic cardiomyopathy. Am J Cardiol 66:198, 1990.
17. Hochleitner M, Hortnagl H, Hortnagl H, et al: Long-term efficacy of physiologic dual-chamber pacing in the treatment of end-stage idiopathic dilated cardiomyopathy. Am J Cardiol 70:1320, 1992.
18. Kataoka H: Hemodynamic effect of physiological dual chamber pacing in a patient with end-stage dilated cardiomyopathy: A case report. PACE 14:1330, 1991.
19. Auricchio A, Sommariva S, Salo RW, et al: Improvement of cardiac function in patients with severe congestive heart failure and coronary artery disease by dual chamber pacing with shortened AV delay. PACE 16:2034, 1993.
20. Brecker SJD, Xiao HB, Sparrow J, et al: Effects of dual-chamber pacing with short atrioventricular delay in dilated cardiomyopathy. Lancet 340:1308, 1992.
21. Nishimura RA, Hayes DL, Holmes DR, et al: Mechanism of hemodynamic improvement by dual-chamber pacing for severe left ventricular dysfunction: An acute Doppler and catheterization hemodynamic study. J Am Coll Cardiol 25:281, 1995.
22. Guardigli G, Ansani L, Percoco GF, et al: AV delay optimization and management of DDD paced patients with dilated cardiomyopathy. PACE 17:1984, 1994.
23. Auricchio A, Salo RW: Acute hemodynamic improvement by pacing in patients with severe congestive heart failure PACE 20:313, 1997.
24. Gold MR, Feliciano Z, Gottlieb SS, et al: Dual-chamber pacing with a short atrioventricular delay in congestive heart failure: A randomized study. J Am Coll Cardiol 26:967, 1995.
25. Innes D, Leitch JW, Fletcher PJ: VDD pacing at short atrioventricular intervals does not improve cardiac output in patients with dilated heart failure. PACE 17:959, 1994.

26. Linde C, Gadler F, Edner M: Results of atrioventricular synchronous pacing with severe congestive heart failure. Am J Cardiol 75:919, 1995.

27. Gilligan DM, Sargent DA, Wood MA, et al: A double-blind, randomized, crossover trial of dual chamber pacing with an "optimized" versus a nominal atrio-ventricular delay in symptomatic left ventricular dysfunction [Abstract]. J Am Coll Cardiol 31:389A, 1998.

28. Leinbach RC: Dilated cardiomyopathy: To pace or not to pace. J Am Coll Cardiol 26:974, 1995.

29. Karpawich PP, Gates J, Stokes KB: Septal His-Purkinje ventricular pacing in canines: A new endocardial electrode approach. PACE 15:2011, 1992.

30. Karpawich PP, Vincent JA: Ventricular pacing site does make a difference: Improved left ventricular function with septal pacing. PACE 17:820, 1994.

31. Buckingham TA: Right ventricular outflow tract pacing. PACE 20:1237, 1997.

32. Giudici MC, Thornburg GA, Buck DL, et al: Comparison of right ventricular outflow tract and apical lead permanent pacing on cardiac output. Am J Cardiol 79:209, 1997.

33. Victor F, France R, Dupuis JM, et al: Comparative effects of permanent right ventricular pacing at the outflow tract and at the apex: A prospective crossover study [Abstract]. Circulation 98:I–707, 1997.

34. Gold MR, Shorofsky SR, Metcalf MD, et al: The acute hemodynamic effects of right ventricular septal pacing in patients with congestive heart failure secondary to ischemic or idiopathic dilated cardiomyopathy. Am J Cardiol 79:679, 1997.

35. Brockman RG, Olsovsky MR, Shorofsky SR, et al: The acute hemodynamic effects of pacing site and mode in congestive heart failure [Abstract]. J Am Coll Cardiol 31:389A, 1998.

36. Cowell R, Morris-Thurgood J, Ilsley C, et al: Septal short atrioventricular delay pacing: Additional hemodynamic improvements in heart failure. PACE 17:1980, 1994.

37. Buckingham TA, Candinas R, Schlapfer J, et al: Acute hemodynamic effects of atrioventricular pacing at differing sites in the right ventricle individually and simultaneously. PACE 20:909, 1997.

38. Foster AH, Gold MR, McLaughlin JS: Acute hemodynamic effects of atrio-biventricular pacing in humans. Ann Thorac Surg 59:294, 1995.

39. Bakker PF, Meijburg H, de Jonge N, et al: Beneficial effects of biventricular pacing in congestive heart failure [Abstract]. PACE 17:820, 1994.

40. Gold MR, Fisher ML, Gottlieb SS: Failure of short atrioventricular delay pacing to improve hemodynamic function in patients with congestive heart failure. Heart Web 2, 1996.

41. Cazeau S, Ritter P, Bakdach S, et al: Four chamber pacing in dilated cardiomyopathy. PACE 17:1974, 1994.

42. Daubert C, Ritter P, Cazeau S, et al: Permanent biventricular pacing in dilated cardiomyopathy: Is a totally endocardial approach technically feasible? [Abstract]. PACE 19:699, 1996.

43. Cazeau S, Ritter P, Lazarus A, et al: Multisite pacing for end-stage heart failure: Early experience. PACE 19:1748, 1996.

44. Maloney JD, Martin R, Chodinella V, et al: Transvenous bi-atrial and biventricular pacing is technically feasible for management of arrhythmias and end-stage heart failure [Abstract]. PACE 19:699, 1996.

45. Blanc J-J, Etienne Y, Mansourati J, et al: Evaluation of different ventricular pacing sites in patients with severe heart failure: Results of an acute hemodynamic study. Circulation 96:3273, 1997.

46. Kass DA, Chen-Huan C, Curry C, et al: Improved left ventricular mechanics from acute VDD pacing in patients with dilated cardiomyopathy and ventricular conduction delay. Circulation 99:1567, 1999.

47. Auricchio A, Stellbrink C, Block M, et al: Clinical and objective improvements in severe congestive heart failure using univentricular or biventricular pacing: Preliminary results of a randomized prospective study [Abstract]. J Am Coll Cardiol 31:31A, 1998.

48. Johnson AD, Daily PO: Hypertrophic subaortic stenosis complicated by high degree heart block: Successful treatment with an atrial synchronous ventricular pacemaker. Chest 67:491, 1975.

49. Hassenstein P, Walther H, Dittrich J: Haemodynamische Veranderungen durch Einfach-oder Gekoppelte Stimulation bei patienten mit obstruktiver Kardiomyopathie. Verh Dtsch Ges Inn Med 81:17, 1975.

50. Duck HJ, Hutschemeier W, Paneau H, et al: Atrioventricular stimulation with reduced AV-delay time as a therapeutic principle in hypertrophic obstructive cardiomyopathy. Z Gesamte Inn Med 39:437, 1984.

51. McDonald K, McWilliams E, O'Keefe BO, et al: Functional assessment of patients treated with permanent dual chamber pacing as primary treatment for hypertrophic cardiomyopathy. Eur Heart J 9:893, 1988.

52. Jeanrenaud X, Goy J-J, Kappenberger L: Effects of dual-chamber pacing in hypertrophic cardiomyopathy. Lancet 339:1318, 1992.

53. Fananapazir L, Cannon RO, Tripodi D, et al: Impact of dual-chamber permanent pacing in patients with obstructive hypertrophic cardiomyopathy with symptoms refractory to verapamil and β-adrenergic blocker therapy. Circulation 85:2149, 1992.

54. Fananapazir L, Epstein ND, Curiel RV, et al: Long-term results of dual-chamber (DDD) pacing in obstructive hypertrophic cardiomyopathy. Circulation 90:2731, 1994.

55. Rishi F, Hulse JE, Auld DO, et al: Effects of dual-chamber pacing for pediatric patients with hypertrophic obstructive cardiomyopathy. J Am Coll Cardiol 29:734, 1997.

56. Kappenberger L, Linde C, Daubert C, et al: Pacing in hypertrophic obstructive cardiomyopathy (PIC): A randomized crossover study [Abstract]. J Am Coll Cardiol 29:387A, 1997.

57. Nishimura RA, Trusty JM, Hayes DL, et al: Dual-chamber pacing for hypertrophic cardiomyopathy: A randomized, double-blind, crossover trial. J Am Coll Cardiol 29:435, 1997.

58. Slade AKB, Sadoul N, Shapiro L, et al: DDD pacing in hypertrophic cardiomyopathy: A multicentre clinical experience. Heart 75:44, 1996.

59. Maron BJ: Appraisal of dual-chamber pacing therapy in hypertrophic cardiomyopathy: Too soon for a rush to judgment? J Am Coll Cardiol 27:431, 1996.

Chapter 21

Cardiac Chronotropic Responsiveness

Bruce L. Wilkoff and Michael S. Firstenberg

The mandate to name and measure all that surrounded our first two ancestors is basic, a divine provision, and our most basic occupation—common to all humankind. Consequently we occupy ourselves with nomenclature, descriptions, and definitions of every type. Even so, description of the normal and pathologic cardiac chronotropic responses to exertion began only in the 20th century after the development of sensor-driven rate-modulated pacemakers. The advent of rate-modulated pacemakers continues to challenge our understanding of normal and dysfunctional cardiac physiology. This chapter provides the historical, physiologic, and practical context by which the concept of chronotropic responsiveness can be applied to patients with and under consideration for rate-modulated pacemakers.

■ HISTORY OF EXERCISE TESTING

Monitored exertion for the purpose of clinical or physiologic evaluation is a 20th-century phenomenon. In 1918 Bousfield[1] made the initial descriptions of electrocardiographic (ECG) changes during exercise. Ten years later, Feil and Siegel[2] produced a pivotal observation when they documented the fact that exertion could produce pain and ST changes that resolved with rest. Maximal stress testing by climbing stairs was first advocated by Missal in 1938[3] but was not widely accepted until 1955, when Master and coworkers[4] simplified the procedure. The Master's step test was the first protocol specifically proposed as a means of evaluating functional capacity, including measurements of heart rate and blood pressure.[4, 5] Further developments were necessary to overcome the limitations of low exercise intensity and the inability to observe the subject's heart rate and ECG during stress. In 1956, Bruce[6] described a treadmill stress test that categorized patients according to their New York Heart Association (NYHA) class.[6] During the same decade, Astrand and Rhyming[7] teamed up and established the progressive

exercise test as a tool for physiologic evaluation. They observed that maximal oxygen uptake, or aerobic capacity, is correlated with maximal heart rate during maximal exercise. This foundational concept has become the basis for the development and evaluation of rate-modulated pacemakers. Balke and Ware[8] added to these developments by producing a method of estimating oxygen uptake during treadmill exertion. At about the same time, Hellerstein and Hornsten[9] safely applied treadmill exercise to patients who had had a myocardial infarction. This initiated the concept of cardiac rehabilitation and sending cardiac patients back to work.

Since that time, coronary artery disease has clearly dominated the development of exercise testing. Exercise stress testing today continues to be used primarily in the screening and management of patients with coronary artery disease. Applications include the physiologic assessment of angiographic lesions, detection of postinterventional restenosis, response to medical therapy, postmyocardial infarction risk stratification, and guiding cardiac rehabilitation exercise prescriptions. Exercise stress testing has also become useful in the assessment of systolic and diastolic cardiac dysfunction, determining objective measures for interventions such as heart transplantation, cardiomyoplasty, left ventricular assist devices, and left ventricular reduction surgery as well as for cardiovascular fitness, dyspnea of unclear etiology, exercise-induced arrhythmias, cardiac disability, valvular heart diseases, aortic outflow tract obstruction in hypertrophic cardiomyopathy, and evaluation of chronotropic responsiveness.

■ HISTORY OF CHRONOTROPIC EVALUATION

Originally used for descriptive purposes in the study of exercise physiology, the recording of heart rate during clinical exercise testing has become a standard procedure. As an outgrowth of the work of Astrand and Rhyming[7] in the early 1950s, the maximal chronotropic exercise response was determined to be an age-related value. Although frequently calculated subtracting a subject's age from 220, the origin of this accurate formula for the maximal predicted heart rate (MPHR) is obscure. Others have produced similar but more technically complicated formulas for this relationship without evidence of improved clinical value.[10] This unquestionably useful calculation provides the most common measure of maximal exertional effort, reaching 85% of MPHR. Nevertheless, different authors sometimes employ different definitions of maximal heart rate response when evaluating rate-adaptive pacemakers or chronotropism.

The chronotropic response has also been viewed predominantly in terms of the patient's ability or inability to reach the MPHR during maximal exertion. Because patients rarely achieve maximal exertion, the relevance of reaching MPHR is debatable except in its relationship to heart rates achieved during activities of daily living. The ability to control chronotropic function with rate-modulated pacemaker technology provided the developmental impetus for techniques evaluating heart rate response during submaximal exertion. If a pacemaker is to respond at a specific rate with a certain amount of sensor stimulation, a predetermined rate must be specified as being appropriate for that amount of exertion.[11] Despite the attractiveness and relative simplicity of this approach, other factors, including patient symptoms, concurrent diseases, and effect on device longevity, also need to be included in the calculation. Until pacemaker sensors are able to detect the efficiency, quality, and magnitude of a patient's hemodynamic response to the chronotropic manipulations of the pacemaker, the techniques discussed in this chapter must be considered preliminary and descriptive rather than definitive.

■ RELATION OF HEART RATE TO HEMODYNAMICS

The delivery of oxygen for metabolism by the tissues in adequate quantity is the bottom-line principle in the evaluation of clinical hemodynamics. Factors affecting this process are multiple, including inspired F_{IO_2}, alveolar gas exchange, respiratory muscle mechanics, pulmonary vascular resistance, systemic regional blood flow shifts, and oxygen-carrying capacity, which in turn is affected by hemoglobin concentration, hemoglobinopathies, and local tissue factors.

(1) Arterial blood oxygen concentration (CaO_2) =
$$(1.34 \times Hgb \times SaO_2) + (0.003 \times PaO_2)$$

where Hgb = hemoglobin
SaO_2 = arterial oxygen saturation
PaO_2 = arterial oxygen pressure

For example, patients in the early postoperative period after coronary revascularization may exhibit multiple physiologic alterations limiting their ability to effectively delivery oxygen. Hemoglobin concentration may be depressed secondary to surgical blood loss, weakened chest wall and respiratory mechanics after sternotomy, pulmonary atelectasis, and decreased alveolar gas exchange from postcardiopulmonary bypass pulmonary edema. Overall, however, the heart's ability to generate cardiac output and the appropriate increase in cardiac output with exercise are central to the principle of oxygen delivery and constitute the core of this chapter.

Cardiac output is the product of heart rate and stroke volume. Augmentation of these two factors during exertion is produced by reduced parasympathetic and increased sympathetic activity, increased circulating catecholamines, the Bainbridge reflex (increased venous return producing right atrial distention), increased myocardial contractility, and probably also decreased left ventricular afterload. During low-intensity exercise, both a rise in stroke volume and a rise in heart rate contribute to the increase in cardiac output. Above heart rates of 110 to 120 bpm, there are no further increases in stroke volume. Therefore, heart rate alone contributes to further elevations in the cardiac output. Throughout exercise, heart rate increments are linearly related to increases in maximal ventilatory oxygen uptake ($\dot{V}O_2max$).[12] Near peak exercise, an increase in oxygen extraction provides the major adaptive mechanism. The heart rate increments continue but tend to level off. The anaerobic threshold is crossed when oxygen demand exceeds supply, and further activity is accomplished at the expense of lactate accumulation. In addition, increasing heart rate results in increasing myocardial oxygen demands.

When the ability to deliver oxygen to the myocardium is impaired independent of peripheral tissue oxygenation, such as in coronary artery disease, the transition from myocardial aerobic to anaerobic metabolism occurs at a lower workload. Sometimes, depending on the condition of the ventricles and valves, stroke volume decreases as heart rate increases. At elevated heart rates, the shorter RR interval can result in impaired ventricular filling and consequently compromise preload, which according to the Frank-Starling mechanism, reduces stroke volume. When decline in stroke volume occurs faster than the heart rate increases, cardiac output subsequently also decreases. The net result can be an undesirable reduction in cardiac output with increased heart rate and myocardial oxygen consumption.

The capacity to increase oxygen delivery is designated the *oxygen delivery reserve*. Although the affinity of oxygen to hemoglobin and the complex biochemical and cellular metabolism that occurs with changing physiology (most of which is beyond the scope of this chapter) play a crucial role in the ability to deliver and use oxygen (Fig. 21–1), most of the major compensatory changes with increased metabolic demand occur at the systemic level. To achieve this increase in oxygen delivery, the changes in cardiac output and oxygen extraction are multiplied. Normally, the cardiac output reserve is six times the baseline value. In an athletic subject, it rises from 5 to 6 L/min at baseline to about 36 L/min during maximal exercise. Arterial oxygen saturation is about 95%. As a result of oxygen consumption, this drops to a mixed venous oxygen saturation of 75% under resting conditions. During exertion, oxygen extraction triples and yields a mixed venous oxygen percentage saturation of 35%. Therefore, the total oxygen delivery reserve is the oxygen delivery reserve times the cardiac output reserve, or 3 times 6, which yields 18 times the baseline oxygen delivery, as expressed in the following equation:

(2) Oxygen delivery ($\dot{V}O_2$) =
$$(HR \times CO) \times 1.3 \times Hgb \times (SaO_2 - SvO_2)$$

where HR = heart rate
CO = cardiac output
Hgb = hemoglobin
SaO_2 = arterial oxygen saturation
SvO_2 = venous oxygen saturation

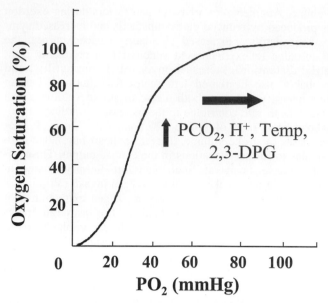

Figure 21–1. Oxyhemoglobin dissociation curve. The curve demonstrates the relationship between oxygen saturation and arterial oxygen pressure. Shifting of the curve to the left is a result of increasing arterial carbon dioxide pressure (Pco_2), acidosis (H^+), temperature (temp), and 2,3-diphosphoglycerate (2,3-DPG, a byproduct of anaerobic metabolism). Shifting of the curve to the left promotes tissue oxygen release but interferes with oxygen binding in the lung.

Because heart rate is only one factor in the equation governing exercise capacity, the role played by each factor in any given patient's symptoms can become confusing. Furthermore, resting cardiac output, ejection fraction, and left ventricular filling pressure do not correlate well with $\dot{V}o_2max$ and therefore fail to predict cardiac output reserve. Despite multiple equations and attempts to predict $\dot{V}o_2max$ (Table 21–1), most are just estimates, and their use in clinical practice is limited by large individual variability, particularly in patients with underlying coronary, pulmonary, or vascular disease. There are many important factors in the biochemical use of oxygen at the cellular level, many of which are beyond the scope of this chapter but nevertheless play an important role in cellular oxygen delivery and use. Estimates of heart size by chest radiograph and ECG also correlate poorly with cardiac output and thus with oxygen delivery reserve.[13]

■ MARKERS OF INCREASING METABOLIC DEMAND

With the increase in cardiac output that occurs with activity, there are additional systemic and cardiovascular responses that correlate with the need for increased oxygen demands. In the absence of a normal chronotropic response, these hemodynamic changes can serves as markers for increased metabolic demands. Sensors incorporated into rate-adaptive pacemakers have been designed to respond to or parallel these hemodynamic changes and increase the pacing rate (either atrial, ventricular, or both) *appropriately*. Despite advances in sensor technology and the incorporation of mul-

tiple sensors, the development of a method to determine accurately and reliably an appropriate heart rate response for a given person at a specific workload remains the "Holy Grail" of rate-adaptive pacing. Unfortunately, a major limitation is the ability to transform our understanding of the normal chronotropic response to apply to patients with chronic cardiac disease, and then to incorporate further this understanding into computer-based algorithms.

■ PROBLEMS AND ASSUMPTIONS

To assess adequately any patient's chronotropic response to the metabolic stress of exercise, the patient and testing environment must be free of confounding variables that may alter the heart rate response. The presence of fever, active infection, emotional stress, pain, metabolic derangements, severe anemia, dehydration, or a hot testing environment may contribute to a premature and excessive rise in chronotropic response for any given level of exercise. Likewise, the pharmacologic milieu, including the presence of β-blocking agents, blunts the intrinsic chronotropic response. Physiologic hormonal variations, both normal and abnormal, can also affect a chronotropic response. Varying levels in serum cortisol can result in lower morning heart rates, and abnormal thyroid hormone levels can alter not only heart rate but also metabolic parameters. Dietary changes can also affect metabolic results. Different energy substrates (i.e., fats, proteins, and carbohydrates) release different levels of CO_2 when metabolized and hence can alter the respiratory quo-

Table 21–1. Difference Estimates of $\dot{V}o_2max$

Age and Gender

$4.2 - (0.0032 \times Age)$ L/min for men
$2.6 - (0.014 \times Age)$ L/min for women

Age, Height, and Gender

$(5.41 \times Height) - (0.025 \times Age) - 5.66$ L/min for men
$(3.01 \times Height) - (0.017 \times Age) - 2.56$ L/min for women
$(0.83 \times Height^{2.7}) \times (1 - 0.007 \times Age)$ for men
$(0.62 \times Height^{2.7}) \times (1 - 0.007 \times Age)$ for women

Age, Height, Weight, and Gender

$(3.45 \times Height) - (0.028 \times Age) + (0.022 \times Weight) - 3.76$ L/min for men
$(2.49 \times Height) - (0.018 \times Age) + (0.010 \times Weight) - 2.26$ L/min for women

Height

$(4.36 \times Height) - 4.55$ L/min for boys
$(2.25 \times Height) - 1.84$ L/min for girls
$0.83 \times Height^{2.7}$ for men
$0.62 \times Height^{2.7}$ for women
$0.67 \times Height^{2.7}$ for boys
$0.48 \times Height^{2.7}$ for girls

Thigh Volume

$0.306 \times Thigh\ volume - 1.04$ L/min

Vital Capacity

$0.74 \times Vital\ capacity - 1.04$ L/min

Data from Jones NL: Clinical Exercise Testing, 4th ed. Philadelphia, WB Saunders, 1997, pp 129–135.

Table 21–2. **Exercise Testing Indications and Contraindications**

Absolute Contraindications in Exercise Testing	Absolute Indications for Termination of Exercise Testing
A recent signficant change in the resting ECG suggesting infarction or other acute cardiac event Recent complicated myocardial infarction (unless patient is stable and pain free) Unstable angina Uncontrolled atrial arrhythmia that compromises cardiac function Third-degree AV heart block without pacemaker Acute congestive heart failure Severe aortic stenosis Suspected or known dissecting aneurysm Active or suspected myocarditis or pericariditis Thrombophlebitis or intracardiac thrombi Recent systemic or pulmonary embolus Acute infections Significant emotional distress (psychosis)	Acute myocardial infarction or suspicion of a myocardial infarction Onset of moderate to severe angina Drop in systolic blood pressure with increasing workload accompanied by signs or symptoms or drop below standing resting pressure Serious arrhythmias Signs of poor perfusions (e.g., pallor, cyanosis, or cold and clammy skin) Unusual or severe shortness of breath Central nervous system symptoms (e.g., ataxia, vertigo, visual or gait abnormalities) Technical inability to monitor ECG or blood pressure Patient request
Relative Contraindications to Exercise Testing	**Relative Indications for Termination of Exercise Testing**
Resting diastolic BP >115 mm Hg or systolic BP >200 mm Hg Moderate valvular disease Known electrolyte abnormalities Fixed rate pacemaker Frequent or complex ventricular ectopy Ventricular aneurysm Uncontrolled metabolic disease (e.g., diabetes, thyrotoxicosis, myxedema) Chronic infectious disease Neuromuscular, musculoskeletal, or rheumatoid disorders exacerbated by exercise Advanced or complicated pregnancy	Significant ECG changes from baseline (>2 mm of horizontal or downsloping ST-segment depression, or >2 mm of ST-segment elevation—except in aVR) Any increasing chest pain Any manifestations of severe fatigue or shortness of breath Wheezing Leg cramps or intermittent claudication Hypertensive response (systolic BP >260 mm Hg or diastolic BP >115 mm Hg) Less serious arrhythmias Exercise-induced bundle-branch block that cannot be distinguished from ventricular tachycardia.

ECG, electrocardiogram; AV, atrioventricular; BP, blood pressure.
Adapted from American College of Sports Medicine: Guidelines for Exercise Testing and Prescription, 5th ed. Baltimore, Williams & Wilkins, 1995.

tient ($\dot{V}CO_2/\dot{V}O_2$), which may hinder metabolic exercise testing reproducibility. Rate-responsive pacemakers based on respiratory variables are also subject to the variations in CO_2 production that can accompany variations in fats, proteins, and carbohydrates consumed.

Absolute contraindications to chronotropic exercise testing are the same as those used for any exercise test and include the acute stage of myocardial infarction, unstable angina, severe aortic stenosis, severe hypertension, acute systemic illness, and uncompensated congestive heart failure (Table 21–2). Care should be taken to choose an exercise testing situation within the musculoskeletal ability of the patient. Strict attention should also be paid to the physical and hemodynamic responses to increasing exercise with regard to the indications for discontinuing the test (see Table 21–2). The quality of the testing environment affects the interpretability and reproducibility of the response.

Clinical end points for exercise testing usually assume a normal chronotropic response. However, achievement of a heart rate response above 85% of the maximally predicted heart rate for age at maximal exertion does not always indicate an appropriate chronotropic response. On the other hand, chronotropic abnormalities disqualify heart rate as the variable used to determine the end point of the exertional assessment. Unrealistic expectations by the observer can produce evaluations that result in misleading conclusions about the cardiopulmonary response.

The anaerobic threshold has been defined as the oxygen uptake before the systemic increase in the ventilatory equiva-lent for oxygen ($\dot{V}E/\dot{V}O_2$) without a concomitant increase in the ventilatory equivalent for carbon dioxide ($\dot{V}E/\dot{V}CO_2$).[14] More recent publications, however, have cast doubt on both the validity of this concept and the relationship between blood lactate levels and gas exchange indices of the anaerobic threshold.[15, 16] Because of this, it is preferable to call the oxygen uptake before the increase in $\dot{V}E/\dot{V}CO_2$ the *ventilatory threshold.*[17]

Simple exercise testing, which monitors only heart rate and blood pressure, does not detect when the patient's anaerobic threshold is crossed or measure the magnitude of the subject's effort. In every subject, there is a point at which oxygen delivery is outstripped. The crossing of the anaerobic threshold is the most reproducible indicator of this condition. Exercise testing without the collection and measurement of inspired and expired gases relies on estimated oxygen consumption, usually recorded as calculated metabolic equivalents (METs). One MET has been defined as 3.5 mL O_2/kg per minute, and using simple vector-based equations, individual exercise velocities and grades can be converted to approximate metabolic equivalents.[18] Despite representing a rough approximation, the MET has become the standard unit of metabolic work for which patient performance and improvement is based. This estimate assumes the presence of normal physiology and tends to overestimate the measured or actual METs achieved during metabolic stress testing, when it is used for testing patients with left ventricular dysfunction, valvular, pulmonary, or orthopedic disease, or ischemic heart disease.

Sinus Node: Is It the Best Pacemaker?

The normal sinus node response to increased workloads is considered the gold standard on which rate responsive pacemaker and studies of chronotropic incompetence are based. Although from a teleologic standpoint, it is logical to consider the heart rate response resulting from normal sinus node function as optimized to match oxygen delivery needs, there is some question about the validity of these assumptions.[19] If the ultimate goal of the cardiovascular system is to deliver sufficient levels of oxygen to meet tissue demands, there is evidence that change in cardiac output, primarily through an increase in heart rate, is inadequate in the early stages of activity in healthy subjects undergoing metabolic exercise testing. The exponential increase in oxygen consumption with changing activity levels results in a linear increase in heart rate. The inability for the change in cardiac output to match oxygen demand acutely results in an oxygen deficit. This oxygen deficit can result in a mixed aerobic and anaerobic metabolism, lactic acidosis, and an inappropriately greater level of perceived exertion, which continues until a physiologic steady state is achieved, with oxygen delivery matching oxygen demand.

The mechanisms contributing to the oxygen deficit are multifactorial and poorly understood. The slope of the chronotropic response may be a consequence of the physiologic milieu, or, alternatively, the initial lagging of venous return from changes in arteriovenous shunting may not provide an adequate preload to an increased stroke volume demand. In a controlled study of patients with dual-chamber rate-responsive pacemakers and normal sinus node function, Kay and colleagues[20] were able to demonstrate that a more rapid heart rate response to a predetermined submaximal exercise level resulted in a lower oxygen deficit and a lower level of perceived exertion than those measures in the same patients whose devices were programmed to a less steep heart rate response curve. The investigators further argued, and demonstrated, that overestimation of the heart rate response either as a result of an inappropriately rapid response (steeper heart rate–work curve) or an inappropriately elevated heart rate for a given workload (heart rate overshoot) can result in an increased perceived level of exertion, palpitations, or, in patients with ischemic heart disease, angina.

The clinical implications of these studies must be interpreted with caution. The activity levels and heart rate responses were based on a predetermined fixed level of submaximal exercise; consequently, an accelerated chronotropic response may not be appropriate for all patients despite an improvement in the oxygen deficit. In addition, the potential physiologic importance of an oxygen deficit needs to be considered. The physiologic consequences of an oxygen deficit during the initial stages of activity may be a crucial driving variable in determining an appropriate chronotropic, hemodynamic, and neurohormonal response. In addition, elevated perceived levels of activity may also represent an innate protective mechanism, limiting potentially harmful rapid increases in activity. Attempting to abolish the physiologic oxygen deficit may paradoxically result in an inappropriate, and possibly harmful, chronotropic or hemodynamic response. Further clinical studies should be pursued with this thought in mind.

Importance of Atrioventricular Synchrony

Although the primary focus of this chapter is on the chronotropic response to increasing workloads, another factor that needs to be included when evaluating for or attempting to correct chronotropic incompetence is the role of atrioventricular (AV) synchrony. Simple increases in the atrial or ventricular contraction rate with increasing work demands may not result in a physiologic beneficial response. An appropriate physiologic chronotropic response must also consider the timing intervals between atrial and ventricular contraction. This is less of an issue in patients with chronic atrial fibrillation or normal AV nodal function. As demonstrated by Lemke and associates[21] in a group of patients with sinus node dysfunction, changes in pacing mode can result in a significantly increased work rate and oxygen uptake. When pacing was programmed to a DDDR mode, patients were able to respond with a greater $\dot{V}o_2$, heart rate, and work level than when DDD or VVIR pacing modes were used.

The importance of AV synchrony is further demonstrated when evaluating the clinical role of AAIR pacing. Despite clinical evidence and the theoretical advantages of rate-responsive pacing (either DDDR or VVIR), there is some concern regarding the physiologic advantages of AAIR pacing. Haywood and colleagues[22] studied 30 patients with sick sinus syndrome who randomly received either a Medtronic Activitrax II (accelerometer sensor, Medtronic, Minneapolis, MN) or a Meta MV (minute ventilation, Telectronic, Sylmar, CA) rate-responsive pacemaker. Half of the patients evaluated were considered chronotropically incompetent as defined by the inability to obtain a peak heart rate of $0.8 \times (220 - \text{age in years})$. Each patient served as his or her own control; the pacemaker was programmed to the AAIR and AAI mode for exercise testing. Patients who were chronotropically incompetent were, despite being able to obtain a higher heart rate, unable to exercise longer when the rate responsive sensor was activated. Additionally, although metabolic evaluations were not performed, perceived levels of exertion were independent of pacing mode. Despite the fact that the benefits of AAIR pacing were questioned, a significant issue, which was not addressed but illustrated by atrial rate adaptive pacing without subsequent AV delay shortening, is the need for maintaining optimal AV synchrony in patients with known sinus and potential AV nodal conduction abnormalities.

The timing of atrial contractions in reference to the ventricle becomes even more important in patients with either severe ventricular dysfunction or other underlying structural disease. For example, the adverse hemodynamic effects of valvular disease, most particularly mitral regurgitation, can worsen with dysrhythmic AV contractions. With marginal baseline cardiac output, loss of AV synchrony with accompanying loss of part, if not all, of the up to 20% contribution from atrial contraction can easily offset any potential gains from improving the chronotropic response to augment cardiac output.

■ CARDIAC CHRONOTROPISM

Although there is a tremendous desire on the part of physicians, pacemaker manufacturers, and the Food and Drug Administration to define chronotropic incompetence, we must first be able to recognize chronotropic competence. This is a fundamental issue that is not easily solved. Although age-related MPHRs have been recognized since the 1950s, assessment of heart rate at submaximal exercise intensities is poorly defined. Until recently, chronotropic insufficiency has been defined mainly as an inability to achieve an age-specific MPHR. In 1991, the American College of Cardiology and the American Heart Association published a joint paper that indicated that rate-modulated pacemakers are used appropriately in patients who fail to achieve a heart rate of 100 bpm at maximal exertion.[23] In a later revision of the joint paper in 1998, the American College of Cardiology and the American Heart Association Task Force, recognizing that 83% of all pacemakers implanted in the United States had rate-responsive capabilities, implied that patients with chronotropic incompetence may benefit from their use.[24] The Task Force revised the definition of chronotropic incompetence to those patients who are "unable to increase sinus node rate appropriately with exercise" and suggested the use of rate-adaptive pacing in patients in whom a rate response was desirable. Although the original definition may be high in specificity, it is lacking in sensitivity, failing to account for age or other clinical characteristics. Limiting the use of rate-modulated pacemakers to this group of patients would prevent its effective use in many other patients with significant chronotropic incompetence, paroxysmal atrial arrhythmias, vasovagal syncope, and conditions with difficult to control upper–rate-limit programming situations. The revised definition recognizes that the broad definition of chronotropic incompetence may be overly simplistic, vague, and subjective.

Another reasonable method uses a statistical approach, defining age-specific and protocol-specific heart rate responses in terms of one and two standard deviations of the mean heart rate for each stage. Ellestad and Wan[25] used such an approach, defining mild chronotropic incompetence as one standard deviation below the mean heart rate and more severe chronotropic incompetence as two standard deviations below the mean heart rate. In doing so, they coined the term *chronotropic incompetence*. With further understanding of the many intricate complexities of the normal heart rate response to activity and pathologic abnormalities that may result from a breakdown of this complex mechanism, it is becoming clear that a single definition of chronotropic incompetence may not be applicable. As previously defined, there are many potential causes of chronotropic incompetence and many different manifestations. Traditional definitions have relied on the inability to achieved a lower-than-expected heart rate for a given level of activity. Chronotropic incompetence may also manifest itself by an erratic and sometimes unpredictable heart rate response during activity with or without eventual attainment of the predicted maximal heart rate. Alternatively, heart rate response slope at either the onset of or after termination of activity may be abnormal regardless of the ability to achieve the predicted maximum heart rate. Further complicating the evaluation for chronotropic incompetence, repeat exercise testing in some patients can produce different results, with some patients, in the absence of any intervention, demonstrating an improvement or acute deterioration in their heart rate response. Many others have proposed alternatives to produce a practical definition of chronotropic incompetence that can be applied in everyday practice.[26–30]

■ NORMAL CHRONOTROPIC RESPONSE

Cardiac output in a normally adaptive person varies directly in proportion to oxygen consumption ($\dot{V}o_2$). During exertion, this cardiac output response is produced by a cooperative rise in heart rate, sympathetic stimulation, and use of the Frank-Starling mechanism. Augmentation of cardiac output during low-intensity exercise is mediated through increases in both stroke volume and heart rate. The increase in stroke volume, however, soon levels off, and further increases are primarily mediated by heart rate. As the maximal heart rate is approached, the rate of increase of heart rate slows and levels off, producing a linear relationship between $\dot{V}o_2$max and heart rate, up to near maximum oxygen consumption.[7]

The trained athlete has a lower resting heart rate and, during progressive exercise testing, a decreased rate of change in heart rate as exercise intensity increases. This produces a lower heart rate at any given level of exercise as compared with matched untrained controls subjects. Circulating catecholamines are also lower at any given submaximal exercise load. Sinoatrial node responsiveness to catecholamine stimulation is unaffected by training.[31] The final result, despite relative bradycardia, is that the cardiac output response is preserved and augmented as a result of left ventricular hypertrophy and an increase in end-diastolic ventricular volume.

In the average 20-year-old, heart rate increases from about 65 bpm at rest to 200 bpm during maximal exercise. The difference between maximal age-predicted heart rate and resting heart rate can be expressed as the heart rate reserve (HRR). The maximal heart rate is age related and reproducible and decreases linearly with advancing age. The resting heart rate is variable, depending on various factors including autonomic tone, volume status, and environmental temperature. In our laboratory, the resting heart rate in 537 healthy subjects was 65 ± 10 bpm.[32] Another, more reproducible measure of a baseline heart rate is the *intrinsic heart rate*, defined as the resting heart rate during complete pharmacologic autonomic blockade. Total blockade is usually accomplished by administration of intravenous atropine (1 mg) and propranolol (10 mg) and not only is reproducible to within a few beats per minute but also declines linearly with age, similar to the maximal exercise heart rate.[33] Despite its reproducibility, intrinsic heart rate is elevated compared with the measured resting heart rate and therefore is an unattractive index of the "normal" resting heart rate.

At the onset of exercise, heart rate increases within 0.5 second, probably secondary to an abrupt withdrawal of vagal tone. A "sawtooth" effect has been observed in the first few seconds of exercise. This probably reflects a flux in the autonomic nervous system tone before steady state is again achieved.[34] Bates,[35] in studying cardiac output as a limiting factor on exercise, demonstrated that heart rate, cardiac output, and oxygen consumption increased in a linear fashion up to an oxygen uptake of 1500 mL/min. Above about 80% of maximal capacity, both heart rate and cardiac output tended to level off. Further increase in peripheral oxygen consumption was achieved through widening of the arteriovenous oxygen gradient. The overall effect is that submaximal exercise heart rates increase in a linear manner with $\dot{V}O_2$.

The oxygen uptake of a seated person is about 1 MET.[36] (The term *metabolic equivalent* was coined as the quantity of oxygen consumed by the body-inspired air under basal conditions and is equal, on average, to 3.5 mL of O_2/kg per minute.) Oxygen consumption ($\dot{V}O_2$) can be translated into METs by dividing by 3.5, thus providing a unitless, convenient, and accurate reference for exercise capacity. MET levels can be used for writing exercise prescriptions and for estimating levels of disability by using tables listing the demands of most common activities (Table 21–3).[37] The maximal MET value minus the baseline or resting MET value is defined as the metabolic reserve (MR). Using an identical approach, the predicted HRR is defined as the difference between the age-predicted maximal heart rate (220 − age in years) and the resting heart rate.

Wilkoff and colleagues[38] first described the mathematical relationship between heart rate and oxygen consumption termed the *metabolic–chronotropic relation*. This mathematical model has now been refined and defines the normal chronotropic response during exercise as being primarily dependent on age, resting heart rate, and peak functional capacity. Previously, it had been shown that heart rate is a linear function of oxygen consumption. This new model, however, demonstrates that the percentage of HRR achieved during exercise equals the percentage of metabolic reserve achieved when a normally functioning adult exercises on an exercise treadmill. Regardless of the exercise protocol, subjects exhibited a linear rise in the percentage of HRR equal to the percentage of MR. Therefore, the model suggests that when the percentage of HRR is plotted against the percentage of MR, a linear response with a slope of close to 1.0 and a y-intercept of 0.0 is to be expected (Fig. 21–2).

This physiologic concept was confirmed by exercising 537 normal adults on one of two exercise protocols. One was the standard Bruce protocol (n = 234), and the other was the chronotropic assessment exercise protocol (CAEP; n = 303). Each subject demonstrated this linear relationship despite varying ages, resting heart rates, and peak functional capacities. The mean slope of this relation was 1.058 ± 0.134, with an R^2 value of 0.982 ± 0.016 for the CAEP subjects, and 1.044 ± 0.112 with an R^2 value of 0.992 ± 0.012 for the Bruce protocol subjects. The mathematical expression of this metabolic chronotropic relation is expressed as follows:

$$(3) \quad HR_{stage} = \frac{(200 - age - HR_{rest}) \times (METS_{stage} - 1)}{(METS_{peak} - 1)} + HR_{rest}$$

Or, when simplified:

$$(4) \quad HR_{stage} = (HRR \times \%MR) + HR_{rest}$$

Table 21–3. Estimated Energy Requirements of Selective Activities

Mild	METs	Moderate *(Continued)*	METs
Baking	2.0	Sailing	3.0
Billiards	2.4	Swimming (slowly)	4.5
Canoeing (leisurely)	2.5	Walking (3 mph)	3.3
Dancing, ballroom (slow)	2.9	Walking (4 mph)	4.5
Golf (with cart)	2.5		
Horseback riding (walking)	2.3	**Vigorous**	
Playing a musical instrument		Chopping wood	4.9
Accordion	1.8	Climbing hills	
Cello	2.3	No load	6.9
Flute	2.0	With 5-kg load	7.4
Horn	1.7	Cycling (moderately)	5.7
Piano	2.3	Dancing	
Trumpet	1.8	Aerobic or ballet	6.0
Violin	2.6	Ballroom (fast) or square	5.5
Woodwind	1.8	Field hockey	7.7
Volleyball (noncompetitive)	2.9	Ice skating	5.5
Walking (2 mph)	2.5	Jogging (10-min mile)	10.2
Writing	1.7	Karate or judo	6.5
		Roller skating	6.5
Moderate		Rope skipping	12.0
Calisthenics (no weights)	4.0	Skiing (water or downhill)	6.8
Croquet	3.0	Squash	12.1
Cycling (leisurely)	3.5	Surfing	6.0
Gardening (no lifting)	4.4	Swimming (fast)	7.0
Golf (without cart)	4.9	Tennis (doubles)	6.0
Mowing lawn (power mower)	3.0		
Playing drums	3.8		

MET, metabolic equivalent (3.5 mL/kg^{-1}/min^{-1} oxygen uptake).

*These activities can often be done at variable intensities, assuming that the intensity is not excessive and that the courses are flat (no hills) unless so specified. Categories are based on experience of tolerance; if an activity is perceived to be more than indicated, it should be judged accordingly.

Modified from Fletcher FF, Froelicher VF, Hearley LH, et al: Exercise standards: A statement for health professionals from the American Heart Association. Circulation 82:2307, 1990. Copyright 1990 American Heart Association.

Metabolic – Chronotropic Relation

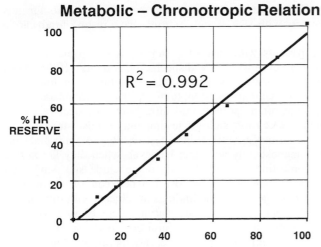

Figure 21–2. Data plotted from a healthy subject. The metabolic–chronotropic relation (MCR) plots normalized heart rate response (percentage heart rate reserve) versus normalized oxygen consumption (percentage metabolic reserve). The response is linear (R^2 = 0.992), with an MCR slope of 1.0 and a y-intercept of 0.0. This response is consistent regardless of age, peak functional capacity, resting heart rate, and exercise protocol for all healthy subjects.

By using this formula, the heart rate achieved at any point of exercise can be classified as consistent or inconsistent with normal chronotropic function. To classify the entire metabolic chronotropic response, the slope of this relation must be measured and classified as being within the 95% confidence intervals of the normal response (Fig. 21–3).

■ CHRONOTROPIC DYSFUNCTION

Abnormal Sinus Rhythm

When the sinus node is the controlling natural pacemaker, the presumption is that a homeostatic negative feedback loop mechanism metabolically couples cardiac output to need. Abnormal chronotropic function results in a heart rate that is too fast or too slow for the demands of the situation. As an example, tachycardia due to re-entrant or automatic focus mechanisms is clearly abnormal and represents a situation in which there is an uncoupling of oxygen demand and supply.

Recognition of chronotropic dysfunction is difficult because it inconsistently manifests as either intermittent or continuous bradycardia, tachycardia, or both. There may be a sinus pause, a conduction disturbance producing varying degrees of heart block, or a sinus mechanism that is firing too slowly because of intrinsic or extrinsic disease. In many patients, bradycardia may be present only at rest, whereas during exertion, the response reaches the age-predicted maximal heart rate. Other subjects with normal resting heart rates, however, demonstrate relative bradycardia during exercise and an inappropriately low maximal heart rate at peak exercise. Finally, some patients have symptoms of dyspnea on exertion and easy fatigability with early exercise, but as they warm up, they are able to perform prolonged exertional tasks without difficulty. This result may be due to an inappropriately slow chronotropic mechanism during early exercise that eventually "warms up."

To illustrate these phenomena, 52 subjects with symptomatic sinus node dysfunction that was severe enough to require a permanent pacemaker were tested by treadmill exercise in an effort to define the exertional chronotropic manifestations of this disease.[39] The data were compared with data compiled from 100 healthy subjects using the metabolic–chronotropic relation analysis described earlier in equations 3 and 4. Despite the need for permanent pacemakers, only 18 of the 52 patients (33%) failed to reach the maximum age-predicted heart rate (Fig. 21–4). These patients also lost the linear response described in healthy subjects (Fig. 21–5). Thus, abnormal sinus function can manifest periodically, sometimes requiring a pacemaker to prevent syncope, sometimes providing a normal linear heart rate response to exercise, and sometimes producing a nonlinear response to exercise.

Although *sinus bradycardia* can be defined as a sinus rate that is less than 60 bpm, it is not always apparent when a heart rate is inappropriately slow. For example, a well-trained athlete may be symptom free with a resting heart rate in the 40s, owing in part to an increase in stroke volume. An octogenarian may feel fatigued and washed out with a heart rate in the 50s. A significant problem is present when the "bradycardia" produces clinical symptoms.

Sick sinus syndrome, the major cause of a clinically inappropriate chronotropic response, is a collection of various clinical heart rate patterns.[40] These include persistent sinus bradycardia, sinus arrest, sinoatrial node exit block, and the tachycardia-bradycardia syndrome. *Carotid sinus hypersensitivity* (CSH) is usually defined as ventricular asystole lasting at least 3 seconds or a decrease in systolic blood pressure of at least 50 mm Hg after a 5-second carotid sinus massage.[41–43] *Carotid sinus syndrome* (CSS) refers to symptoms such as bradycardia, dizziness, presyncope, or syncope, resulting from hypersensitivity of the carotid sinus

Confidence Intervals

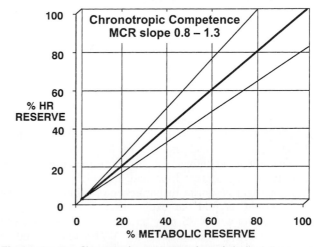

Figure 21–3. Chronotropic competence is statistically defined as the response to physical exertion that provides a metabolic–chronotropic relation (MCR) slope of between 0.8 and 1.3. The normal essential characteristic of the MCR is a y-intercept of 0.0 and a linear MCR slope of 1.0. Instead of calculating the heart rate achieved at a particular level of exertion, the MCR slope provides the best statistical method for identification of chronotropically incompetent patients.

Percent Maximal Predicted Heart Rate
Sinus Node Dysfunction

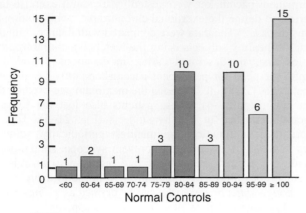

Normal Controls

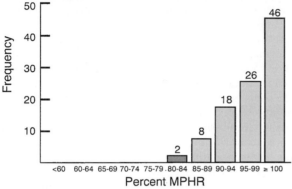

Percent MPHR

Figure 21–4. Histogram of the response to exercise of patients with a history of pacemaker implantation for the primary indication of sinus node dysfunction. Only 33% of these patients failed to achieved 85% of the age-predicted maximal heart rate (MPHR). Their response is compared with that of 100 control subjects.

in one patient, one or more may be evident. Although most patients with sick sinus syndrome have resting bradycardia, this is not always the case. There are many ways of evaluating patients with suspected sick sinus syndrome, but none has perfect sensitivity and specificity. Although Holter monitoring remains a key tool in correlating symptoms with rhythm disturbances, symptoms and Holter monitoring findings are often sporadic and infrequent. Provocative means, such as electrophysiologic testing and exercise stress testing, are often useful. When these test results are abnormal, they are diagnostically accurate; however, when they are normal or borderline normal, they do not exclude sick sinus syndrome. There is a large overlap between the findings in healthy subjects and the findings in subjects with this diagnosis. Furthermore, there are varying degrees of severity of sick sinus syndrome; the natural course is usually progression over time. Because of the various presentations of sick sinus syndrome, the different degrees of severity, and the lack of sensitivity of electrophysiologic testing, exercise stress testing can be a valuable instrument in the evaluation of this condition.

In 1978, Holden and colleagues[52] compared the heart rate response to exercise in seven subjects with sick sinus syndrome with the response in seven healthy age-matched controls and seven young athletically trained subjects. They found that the subjects with sick sinus syndrome had a lower maximal heart rate and a reduced rate of change of heart rate as exercise intensity increased as compared with age-matched controls. The sick sinus syndrome subjects did, however, reach a peak oxygen consumption ($\dot{V}O_2$max) that was equivalent to that of age-matched controls but much lower than that reached by well-trained subjects. When the

reflex.[44] This differentiation is of obvious clinical importance because hypersensitivity is a sign that is found in patients with asymptomatic disease.

CSH may be found in up to 30% of patients with hypertension or ischemic heart disease.[45] The incidence of CSS among patients investigated for syncope is unknown, and the reported numbers vary considerably, from 0.5% to 41%.[46, 47] There is rarely evidence of abnormalities of the sinus node or of chronotropic responsiveness in patients with a hypersensitive carotid sinus.[48] The pathophysiology of CSH is unclear, and the site of hypersensitivity with the reflex arc is unknown. Denervation-like acetylcholine sensitivity of the efferent limb and, especially, inappropriately high vagal response to baroreceptor stimulation have been proposed as possible explanations.[49] Because up to 70% of patients with CSS may have reflex AV block, AAI pacing is obviously contraindicated.[43] VVI pacing should be considered only if preimplantation assessment has confirmed the absence of retrograde ventriculoatrial (VA) conduction and symptoms of pacemaker syndrome.[50] If permanent pacing is chosen, a DDD pacemaker is indicated. If the patient has retrograde conduction with a long VA time, DDI or, ideally, DDIR pacing is advocated.[51]

Although all of these characteristics are seldom present

Sinus Node Dysfunction

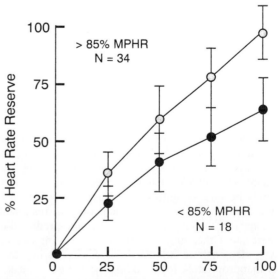

Figure 21–5. The metabolic–chronotropic relation (MCR) in patients with sinus node dysfunction and pacemakers has been plotted for 18 patients (*dark circles*) who failed to achieve and 34 patients (*shaded circles*) who achieved 85% of the age-predicted maximal heart rate (MPHR) during exercise testing. Note the nonlinear response of both groups.

velocity of HRR to exercise in the subjects with sick sinus syndrome was measured as the change in heart rate versus change in $\dot{V}O_2$ per kilogram, the HRR demonstrated a lower slope than that reached by age-matched controls but was equivalent to that seen in the younger, well-trained subjects. This suggests that patients with sick sinus syndrome may have circulatory adaptations similar to those seen in well-trained athletes, such as an exaggerated increase in stroke volume with exercise, a widening of the arteriovenous oxygen difference, and an increased efficiency of perfusion to the peripheral exercising muscles.[52] Similar responses have been seen in the denervated heart and in patients with AV block or during atrial pacing at a fixed rate, in whom the changes in cardiac output are mediated primarily through changes in stroke volume.[53, 54]

In a 1997 study of 16 subjects with sick sinus syndrome, Abbott and associates[55] demonstrated that patients with sick sinus syndrome are unable to achieve maximal heart rates comparable to those reached by age-matched and sex-matched controls. These patients, however, attained a lower $\dot{V}O_2$max than the controls, a finding different from the findings of Holden and colleagues.[52] This difference, according to Holden, is most likely attributable to the presence of coexisting heart disease as a confounding variable in 8 of the 16 subjects with sick sinus syndrome in the Abbott study.

Ischemic Heart Disease

Chronotropic incompetence in some patients is related to ischemic heart disease. These patients tend to have appropriate resting heart rates but during exercise fail to achieve an adequate heart rate response. Ellestad[56] described a subgroup of patients who, despite being deconditioned, had an inadequate heart rate response to stress testing. This has been associated with a poor prognosis.[25] Ellestad[56] also described a 51-year-old man with a similar heart rate response that became normal after successful coronary artery bypass revascularization, implicating ischemia as the major cause of his chronotropic insufficiency. Hinkle and colleagues[57] confirmed this concept when they reported an increased incidence of sudden death in middle-aged men who had "sustained relative bradycardia" in response to exercise and daily activities.

Chin and colleagues[58] retrospectively evaluated 25 patients with mild chronotropic insufficiency whose peak heart rate fell 1 standard deviation below the predicted mean for age and sex, and 28 patients with more severe chronotropic incompetence whose peak heart rate fell 2 standard deviations below the predicted mean for age and sex. There were 45 controls. Coronary angiograms were performed in all 98 patients after maximal treadmill exercise testing. Of note is the finding that 72% of the patients with chronotropic incompetence alone, without ST-segment depression, had significant coronary disease. A prospective study in which coronary angiograms are performed in all patients with chronotropic incompetence has yet to be done to demonstrate the true prevalence of significant coronary disease in this subgroup of patients.

In a study similar to the one done by Ellestad and colleagues relating chronotropic dysfunction to ischemia, the chronotropic responses of 48 normal controls was compared to those of 12 patients with severe ventricular dysfunction

and no ischemia.[59] These patients had an elevated resting heart rate, a depressed maximal heart rate, and a linear percentage HRR response to exercise (Fig. 21–6). In patients with both ischemia and severe ventricular dysfunction, there is a teleologic argument that the responses that occur are protective, minimizing the opportunity for ischemia and optimizing cardiac output. If this were so, then a rate-modulated pacemaker tuned to produce the "normal" chronotropic response would produce a maladaptive balance. In practice, it is rare to see a rate-modulated pacemaker produce angina despite the frequent coexistence of coronary artery disease in pacemaker patients older than the age of 65 years.

Brener and associates[60] also investigated the correlation between chronotropic incompetence and angiographically proven coronary artery disease. Despite a theoretical belief that compromised blood flow to the sinus node or other conductive tissues would contribute to chronotropic incompetence, no relationship between chronotropic incompetence and proximal right coronary artery lesions has been found. Of greater interest, even after correcting for age and gender, severity of proximal left anterior descending (LAD) stenosis strongly correlated with both peak heart rate (odds ratio, 1.23, 95% CI, 1.07–1.41 for each 10 bpm below predicted maximum) and percentage of peak maximal heart rate achieved (odds ratio, 1.44, 95% CI, 1.15–1.81 for each 10% below percentage of peak maximal heart rate). In addition, a direct correlation was observed between the number of diseased vessels and both peak maximal heart rate and percentage of target heart rate obtained during exercise testing (Fig. 21–7).

A subset of patients from the Framingham Heart Study who underwent exercise testing also showed a strong rela-

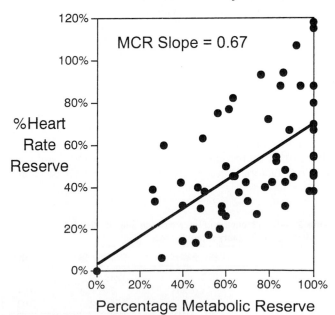

Figure 21–6. The metabolic chronotropic response (MCR) is plotted for 12 patients with left ventricular dysfunction who are being considered for cardiomyoplasty. The responses were linear, with a mean MCR slope of 0.67.

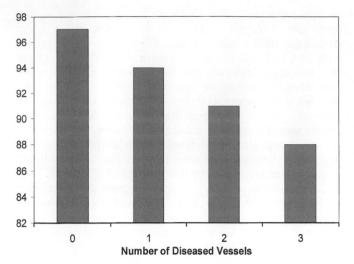

Figure 21–7. Association between percentage of predicted maximal heart rate achieved and number of angiographically documented diseased vessels. (From Brener SJ, Pashkow FJ, Harvey SA, et al: Chronotropic response to exercise predicts angiographic severity in patients with suspected or stable coronary artery disease. Am J Cardiol 76:1228–1232, 1995.)

tionship between chronotropic incompetence and coronary artery disease.[61] After following 1575 patients for almost 8 years, those patients who were initially unable to obtain 85% of the peak maximal heart rate experienced a greater incidence of complications from coronary artery disease than those who were able to achieve their target heart rates. This difference in morbidity and mortality remained significant even after correcting for smoking, age, and other major cardiovascular risk factors (Tables 21–4 and 5; Fig. 21–8).

Chronotropic incompetence has also been shown to correlate statistically with ECG evidence of wall motion abnormalities. Of 231 patients studied by Lauer and coworkers[62, 63] undergoing stress ECG, 18% were considered chronotropically incompetent. ECG evidence of myocardial ischemia was observed in 41%, as compared with 22% of patients with a normal chronotropic response (odds ratio, 2.48, 95% CI, 1.22–5.04). Thirty-three percent of patients with chronotropic incompetence had evidence of myocardial scarring, as compared with 19% who were able to achieve their peak maximal heart rate (odds ratio, 2.07, 95% CI, 0.96–4.32). After further correcting for potential confounding cardiovascular risk factors, chronotropic incompetence was associated

Table 21–4. Chronotropic Incompetence and the Risk for Complications of Coronary Artery Disease

	<85% PMHR	>85% PMHR	P-Value
No. of patients	327	1248	
Deaths (all causes)	21 (6%)	34 (3%)	0.04
Coronary event	44 (14%)	51 (4%)	0.02

PMHR, Predicted maximal heart rate.
Data from Lauer MS, Okin PM, Larson MG, et al: Impaired heart rate response to graded exercise: Prognostic implications of chronotropic incompetence in the Framingham Heart Study. Circulation 93:1502–1506, 1996.

with a much greater risk for an adverse coronary event after more than 3 years of follow-up (odds ratio, 2.20; 95% CI, 1.11–4.37). Additionally, the risk of adverse coronary events increased dramatically in patients who had wall motion abnormalities and were chronotropically incompetent (Table 21–6).

The relationship between adverse coronary events in patients with both coronary artery disease and chronotropic incompetence has raised the concern of precipitating ischemic complications after implantation of rate-responsive pacemakers. Although this represents a reasonable concern, there is little evidence to support it; on the contrary, there is evidence that patients with coronary artery disease, when closely monitored for complications, tolerate rate-adaptive pacing well and may actually benefit from its use. The aggressive approach to myocardial revascularization in the United States, however, has made studying patients with coronary artery disease undergoing implantation of rate-adaptive pacemakers difficult and potentially unethical.

Although the correlation between chronotropic incompetence and coronary artery disease is clear, the causal mechanisms are complex. Many have argued a neurohormonal or vagal compensatory mechanism secondary to underlying ischemia that is often correctable after revascularization.[64–66] The fact that chronotropic incompetence and significant coronary artery disease are often found independently, however, implies much more complex mechanisms than chronic ischemic or autonomic compensatory changes.

Atrial Fibrillation

Despite many similarities in the exertion-related response of patients with atrial fibrillation to that of patients with a sinus node abnormality, the chronotropic response is quite different. Some of the similarities include catecholamine release, autonomic response, and an increase in venous return. Each of these factors exerts its major chronotropic influence on the AV node in patients with atrial fibrillation, whereas the site of action is the sinus node in patients with a sinus mechanism. The sinus node usually functions as the primary natural pacemaker, generating depolarizations at its own autonomous rate and accelerating and decelerating as indicated. The AV node is also capable of functioning as a depolarization-initiating pacemaker but at a slower rate than the sinus node, resulting in a junctional escape rhythm if sinus pauses occur that are long enough.

In patients with atrial fibrillation, the AV node is not the primary initiator of depolarizations but rather the gatekeeper and conduit, controlling the frequency of depolarization entry into and the rate of transit through the AV node. The rate of repolarization and the effective refractory period are variables that help to determine the rate at which the AV node may conduct impulses to the His-Purkinje system. Furthermore, the pharmacologic milieu of the AV node, specifically AV node–depressing drugs, plays a large role in altering the chronotropic response. These drugs are usually present in patients with atrial fibrillation to prevent an inappropriately rapid ventricular response and may also occasionally influence sinoatrial node activity in patients with normal sinus rhythm and paroxysmal atrial fibrillation.

Early work in evaluating the heart rate response to exercise in atrial fibrillation was described by Knox in 1949.[67]

Table 21–5. Effect of Failure to Achieve Target Heart Rate on the Association of Smoking With Outcome: Results of Cox Proportional Hazards Analyses

	Events/ No. of Patients	8-Yr Kaplan-Meier Rate (%)	Hazard Ratio (95% CI)*
All-Cause Mortality (48 Events): Group			
Nonsmokers, reached THR	17/740	2	1.0 (reference group)
Nonsmokers, failed THR	4/128	3	0.71 (0.23–2.19)
Smokers, reached THR	15/446	3	1.96 (0.94–4.09)
Smokers, failed THR	12/152	8	2.45 (1.14–5.24)
Coronary Heart Disease (90 Events): Group			
Nonsmokers, reached THR	23/740	3	1.0 (reference group)
Nonsmokers, failed THR	11/128	9	1.44 (0.68–3.05)
Smokers, reached THR	25/446	6	2.40 (1.34–4.27)
Smokers, failed THR	31/152	21	4.92 (2.84–8.53)

THR, target heart rate.

*After adjustment for age, body mass index, blood pressure, antihypertensive medications, physical activity index, diabetes, ratio of total to high-density lipoprotein cholesterol, FEV_1-to-FVC ratio, and ST-segment response to exercise.

From Lauer MS, Pashkow FJ, Larson MG, et al. Association of Cigarette Smoking with Chronotropic Incompetence and Prognosis in the Framingham Heart Study. Circulation 96:897–903, 1997.

Using the step test as the mode of exercise, several important observations were made. At first, the heart rate decreases in comparison with the pretest value, unlike the normal anticipatory response to heart rate acceleration. Second, a delayed acceleration occurs in very early exercise, followed by an exaggerated heart rate response. Last, prolonged tachycardia persists well into the recovery period.

Corbelli and associates[68] described some additional patterns of chronotropic response in 19 patients with chronic atrial fibrillation, VVI demand permanent pacemakers, and medication-controlled ventricular responses. Heart rate and metabolic reserve were calculated as described previously in

the section on the normal cardiac chronotropic response (see equations 3 and 4). The percentage of HRR was tabulated for the end of each quartile of metabolic reserve. The metabolic–chronotropic relation plot for each patient with atrial fibrillation was compared with the averaged data from 100 healthy subjects. Subjects who had a percentage of HRR of more than 1 standard deviation above or below the mean of the control population were considered abnormal. The quartile heart rate response was divided into the early and late exercise responses. Early exercise response data were defined as the percentage of HRR observed at 25% and 50% of metabolic reserve. Late exercise response data were calculated at 75% and 100% of metabolic reserve. No patient in chronic atrial fibrillation had a normal heart rate response during both early and late exercise (Table 21–7). Three distinct patterns were established: relative tachycardia throughout exercise, relative bradycardia throughout exercise, and relative tachycardia early, with a plateauing of the heart rate response at either a normal or bradycardic rate (Fig. 21–9).

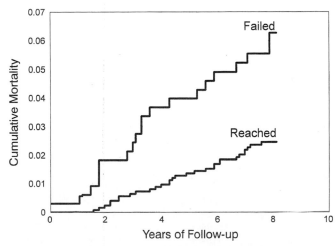

Figure 21–8. Kaplan-Meier plot of cumulative mortality according to ability to achieve target heart rate. Inability to achieve target heart rate includes effects of factors other than inherent chronotropic response (i.e., pulmonary disease). (From Lauer MS, Okin PM, Larson MG, et al: Impaired heart rate response to graded exercise: Prognostic implications of chronotropic incompetence in the Framingham Heart Study. Circulation 93:1502–1506, 1996.)

Table 21–6. Age-Adjusted Cox Proportional Hazards Analyses Relating Risk for Major Events to Failure to Reach 85% of the Age-Predicted Maximal Heart Rate and Echocardiographic Myocardial Ischemia

Subset	No. of Patients	Relative Risk (95% CI)	P-Value
Reached HR, no ischemia	147 (64%)	1.0 (—)	Reference
Failed to reach HR, no ischemia	25 (10%)	1.30 (0.42–4.03)	>0.6
Reached HR, ischemia	42 (18%)	3.26 (1.47–7.25)	0.004
Failed to reach HR, ischemia	17 (7%)	6.87 (2.91–16.18)	<0.0001

HR, heart rate.

From Lauer MS, Mehta R, Pashkow FJ, et al: Association of chronotropic incompetence with echocardiographic ischemia and prognosis. J Am Coll Cardiol 32:1280–1286, 1998.

Table 21-7. Chronotropic Abnormalities of Patients With Atrial Fibrillation During Exercise*

Response	Early Stage (%)	Late Stage (%)	Either Stage (%)	Both Stages (%)	Neither Stage (%)
Slow	21	53	58	16	42
Fast	74	32	74	32	26
Normal	5	16	21	0	79
Slow or fast	95	84	100	21	0

The chronotropic response of patients with pacemakers because of inadequate heart rate during atrial fibrillation is divided into quartiles. The early stage represents exercise at 25% and 50% of metabolic reserve. The late stage represents chronotropic responsiveness at 75% and 100% of metabolic reserve. All patients demonstrated inappropriate chronotropic responsiveness during exercise.

From Corbelli R, Masterson M, Wilkoff BL: Chronotropic response to exercise in patients with atrial fibrillation. PACE 13:179, 1990.

During early exercise, 95% of patients had an abnormal chronotropic response (21% slow, 74% fast), and during late exercise, 84% of patients had an abnormal chronotropic response (53% slow, 32% fast). In terms of maximal heart rate achieved, 16% exceeded 115% (2 standard deviations) of their age-predicted maximal heart rate, and 42% did not reach 85% (2 standard deviations) of their age-predicted maximal heart rate. Therefore, chronotropic incompetence in patients with chronic atrial fibrillation can be categorized as tachychronotropism, bradychronotropism, and a mixed chronotropic response.[68] From these data, it appears that

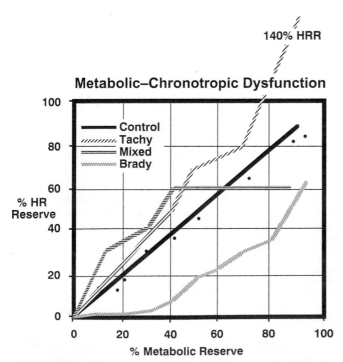

Figure 21-9. The metabolic–chronotropic relation (MCR) is plotted for 3 of 19 patients with atrial fibrillation and compared with the responses in 100 control subjects. All 19 patients demonstrated inappropriate bradycardia (Brady), inappropriate tachycardia (Tachy), or both tachycardia and bradycardia (Mixed) responses.

few patients with chronic atrial fibrillation have appropriate chronotropic responses throughout the entire spectrum from rest to maximal exertion.

Congestive Heart Failure

Patients with congestive heart failure have significant autonomic abnormalities that contribute to the heart rate variability as well as evidence of concomitant chronotropic incompetence. The limited exercise capacity in these patients has also been attributed, in part, to an abnormal heart rate response during exercise.[69] In a recent study by Fei and colleagues,[70] 41 patients with congestive heart failure from idiopathic dilated cardiomyopathy were evaluated with exercise testing with continuous $\dot{V}O_2$ monitoring. Twenty-four percent demonstrated chronotropic incompetence, as defined by the inability to achieve more than 80% of predicted maximal heart rate. Those patients with chronotropic incompetence also exhibited a diminished exercise capacity and other ECG abnormalities despite similarities in age, left ventricular ejection fraction, and use of angiotensin-converting enzyme inhibitors (Table 21–8).[70] Whether chronotropic incompetence contributes to an increased mortality from arrhythmic complications in patients with cardiomyopathy and whether these patients may benefit from rate-adaptive pacing remain to be thoroughly evaluated.

Cardiac Transplantation

Chronotropic incompetence after cardiac transplantation can also be common. Initial bradyarrhythmias after transplantation are common in the early postoperative period, and most are either asymptomatic or easily controlled pharmacologically or with temporary pacing. In two large transplantation series, less than 10% of patients required permanent pacemaker implantation for symptomatic sinus node or AV node dysfunction, and less than 60% of these patients still required pacemaker support at 1 year.[71, 72] Although the exact mecha-

Table 21–8. Characteristics of Patients With Congestive Heart Failure and Chronotropic Incompetence

	Normal Heart Rate Response	Chronotropic Incompetence	P-Value
Number	31	10	NS
Age (yr)	46 ± 13	53 ± 6	NS
LVEF (%)	24 ± 10	22 ± 10	NS
NYHA class			0.002
II	25	2	
III	6	8	
$\dot{V}O_2$max (ml/kg/min)	22.1 ± 8.5	13.3 ± 3.8	0.004
SBP$_{rest-exe}$ (mm Hg)	27 ± 21	6 ± 9	0.006
HR$_{rest}$ (bpm)	99 ± 15	91 ± 19	NS
HR$_{max}$ (bpm)	164 ± 16	122 ± 9	0.001

NYHA, New York Heart Association; SBP$_{rest-max}$, difference between resting systolic blood pressure and systolic blood pressure at peak exercise; LVEF, left ventricular ejection fraction; $\dot{V}O_2$max: maximum oxygen consumption obtained; HR$_{rest}$, heart rate at rest; HR$_{max}$, maximum heart rate obtained with exercise.

From Fei L, Keeling PJ, Sadoul N, et al: Decreased heart rate variability in patients with congestive heart failure and chronotropic incompetence. PACE 19 (Pt I):477–483, 1996.

nisms are unclear, several theories have been proposed. Iatrogenic surgical trauma or ischemia to the sinus node may be a primary, and potentially avoidable or time limited, cause. Autonomic denervation may, despite elevated levels of circulating catecholamines, contribute to post-transplantation chronotropic incompetence. The gradual decline in elevated levels of circulating catecholamines associated with end-stage heart disease after transplantation may contribute to the improvement in the chronotropic response observed. In addition, ischemic injury after prolonged or inadequate organ preservation may also damage conductive tissues.

Posttransplantation rejection has also been proposed, but remains unproved, as a potential mechanism of chronotropic incompetence. Kao and coworker[73] studied 30 patients up to 16 months after orthotropic cardiac transplantation and found that, despite surgical denervation, the chronotropic response, though limited, was similar to that in healthy control group. Despite having a 30% higher resting heart rate and a 30% lower maximal heart rate (to produce a 79% lower heart rate reserve), the transplant recipients were able to increase progressively, in a linear fashion, their heart rate, with increasing workloads. Although the exact incidence of post-transplantation chronotropic incompetence is unknown, Young and colleagues,[74] in the American College of Cardiology Task Force report on Cardiac Transplantation, conveyed the potential role of sinus node dysfunction in pathologic bradycardia, unexplained asystole, and death after transplantation. Transplant recipients, in either the early or late postoperative period, who exhibit evidence of exercise intolerance or symptomatic bradycardia should be evaluated for chronotropic incompetence and may benefit from rate-adaptive pacing. Even though the need for pacing may be temporary, it may facilitate hospital discharge and potentially prevent arrhythmia-related morbidity and mortality.

■ EXERCISE TESTING FOR CHRONOTROPIC ASSESSMENT

Goals

Exercise testing can be used as a diagnostic and therapeutic tool in the adjustment of rate-modulated pacers. The first step is to identify who might be an appropriate candidate for chronotropic exercise testing. For patients with symptoms, such as syncope, lightheadedness, dyspnea on exertion, or easy fatigability, exercise testing can be used as a diagnostic test. Although the range of indications for rate-adaptive pacing is broad and outside the scope of this chapter, it is important to consider that just as the 20-year-old patient with sinus node disease and symptomatic bradycardia during strenuous activity can benefit from rate-adaptive pacing, so too can the 80-year-old patient with severe left ventricular dysfunction who requires the increased heart rate response to perform simple activities of daily living.

The documented correlation of symptoms with an inadequate heart rate response to exercise should lead to implantation of a sensor-driven rate-modulated pacemaker in these patients. For other patients who have already demonstrated a need for pacing, exercise stress testing can be performed before a permanent pacemaker is implanted. This test can help to determine whether the sensor-driven pacing option,

with its added expense, would significantly improve the patient's quality of life.

Once a permanent pacemaker with rate-modulated pacing capacity has been implanted, exercise testing is useful for evaluating pacemaker behavior as well as for optimizing the pacemaker response. Each situation has its unique aspects, and an ability to simulate different activities is essential in comparing the responses of different sensors, pacemakers, programmed settings, and sensor algorithms. For example, because stationary bicycle exercise tends to underestimate the response of systems using piezoelectric activity sensors, the mode of exercise must be appropriate to both the patient and the pacing system. Exercise testing also helps to improve our understanding of the physiology of exercise and provides direction for future advance in the development of rate-modulated pacing.

Last, exercise testing is essential in documenting improvements in measurable end points with improved chronotropic responsiveness to exercise after placement of a rate-modulated pacemaker. The exercise test documents what degree of chronotropic insufficiency is present at baseline, and what magnitude of improvement the pulse generator provides. Even though the exercise response is an important index of rate-modulated pacemaker systems, the value of these systems is not completely described by exercise duration, oxygen uptake, anaerobic threshold, or achievement of a particular chronotropic goal. When a pacing system consistently meets all the present and future symptomatic and physiologic needs of the patient, the medical community will have succeeded. Even so, proper exercise evaluation tools are an essential component in producing the perfect pacing system.

Techniques

The major modality used for chronotropic testing in North America continues to be the treadmill exercise test. The wide range of protocols available makes this a convenient test for young and elderly, trained and untrained patients alike. Continuous ECG monitoring is extremely valuable for identifying tachyarrhythmias or bradyarrhythmias as well as the heart rate response during each stage of exercise. To obtain near steady-state heart rate data, the stage duration should be long enough or the increments in exercise intensity small enough to collect heart rate data that are representative of the subject's physiology. Heart rate is usually recorded during the last 15 seconds of each test stage. Steady-state heart rate is reached by 2 minutes in most people but is completely dependent on the appropriateness of the exercise protocol to the patient's degree of fitness, with the total test duration being between 15 and 20 minutes.

Obtaining multiple heart rate data points before exhaustion is advantageous in evaluating chronotropic response, especially in the range of activities of daily living. Blackburn and colleagues[75] developed the Chronotropic Assessment Exercise Protocol (CAEP) specifically with these points in mind (Table 21–9). This protocol allows formation of plots of heart rate versus exercise intensity, with multiple data points between rest and peak exertion. The resultant graph allows analysis of the heart rate response at rest, at submaximal exertion, and at maximal exertion. Selection of a proto-

Table 21–9. **Chronotropic Assessment Exercise Protocol***

Stage	Speed (mph)	Grade (%)	Time (min)	Cumulative Time	METs
Warmup: 0	1.0	0			1.5
1	1.0	2	2.0	2.0	2.0
2	1.5	3	2.0	4.0	2.8
3	2.0	4	2.0	6.0	3.6
4	2.5	5	2.0	8.0	4.6
5	3.0	6	2.0	10.0	5.8
6	3.5	8	2.0	12.0	7.5
7	4.0	10	2.0	14.0	9.6
8	5.0	10	2.0	16.0	12.1
9	6.0	10	2.0	18.0	14.3
10	7.0	10	2.0	20.0	16.5
11	7.0	15	2.0	22.0	19.0

METs, metabolic equivalent.

*This protocol was designed to test physiologic and chronotropic responses to exercise at submaximal and maximal exertional levels. Because the protocol incorporates gradual increases in elevation and treadmill velocity, subjects with rate-modulated pacemaker sensors that are sensitive to stepping frequency (i.e., activity sensors) can be compared with subjects with other sensor responses. This protocol is well suited for the evaluation of patients with limited functional capacity or mild orthopedic difficulties with treadmill exercise.

col with smaller work increments and shorter stages is ideal for producing more data points and a more complete chronotropic assessment (Fig. 21–10).

To evaluate maximal heart rate response exhaustion should be produced by an adequately large workload rather than by generalized fatigue or boredom from an excessively prolonged test. Therefore, selection of the protocol should be suited to the characteristics of the patient being tested.

Proper administration of the treadmill test is also im-

portant. If a subject is allowed to hold onto the front rail, the side arm rail, or the test supervisor during exercise, the estimated workload for that stage will be falsely elevated. The oxygen uptake and heart rate will also be reduced compared with a test performed without arm support. Furthermore, running rather than walking at the same speed and grade produces a higher oxygen uptake and a higher heart rate.[76]

Cycle Ergometry

Cycle ergometry has more frequently been used in Europe, during metabolic testing, and when a subject is unable to ambulate adequately on a treadmill. When physical impairment prevents a subject from ambulating, however, the use of alternative modalities, such as arm or leg ergometry, to test cardiac chronotropic responsiveness is probably a moot point. Heart rate response is not likely to be the most limiting factor for that subject.

For a cycle ergometer, the mechanical work rate, in oxygen consumption (in milliliters per minute), is relatively fixed, being dependent on cycle resistance and revolutions per minute. It is independent of body weight, except in extremely obese or frail subjects. When METs are calculated (in milliliters per kilogram per minute), however, the larger the subject the smaller the relative $\dot{V}O_2$ becomes. Oxygen consumption can be estimated relatively accurately for work rates between 50 and 200 W for leg ergometry and for work rates between 25 and 125 W for arm ergometry. When evaluating chronotropic response by cycle ergometry, it is important to remember that the heart rate response to arm ergometry is higher than the response to leg ergometry for the same submaximal work rate; however, the peak heart rate achieved with arm ergometry is lower than that achieved with leg ergometry. Untrained patients can obtain about a 10% greater maximum $\dot{V}O_2$ on treadmill than on leg cycle ergometers, yet patients using bicycles as their primary form of exercise are able to obtain higher maximum $\dot{V}O_2$ values than those using treadmills.[77] Cycle stages are typically 2 to 3 minutes long, and the heart rate is measured during the last 15 seconds of each stage. With each stage, workload can be progressively increased at an individualized rate. For example, 15-W increases per interval can be used for older, less fit patients, whereas 30-W intervals can be used for younger, more fit patients. The peak heart rate attained by a cycle ergometer is only 65% to 70% of the age-adjusted maximal heart rate, making the cycle stress test less optimal than the treadmill for chronotropic evaluation.[78]

Arm Ergometry

Arm ergometry is becoming a popular alternative to both treadmill and cycle ergometry testing. Its ease of performing and administrating, combined with reproducibility of results, make it a desirable exercise testing option. Similar to its bicycle counterpart, arm ergometry allows testing of specific calibrated workloads to determined a physiologic response. These workloads can be progressively increased with each successive stage, unlike treadmill testing, which relies on the somewhat unnatural incremental ramping in speed and grade. Balady and colleagues[79] sought to investigate the heart rate and calculated metabolic response to progressively increasing work loads on healthy volunteers. Despite producing what appears to be a linear chronotropic response with

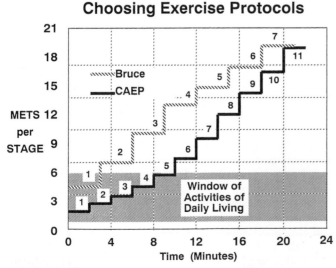

Choosing Exercise Protocols

Figure 21–10. The chronotropic assessment exercise protocol (CAEP) is compared with the most commonly employed Bruce protocol. The strength of the CAEP is demonstrated in this graph, which illustrates several stages of work intensities reflecting activities of daily living. Chronotropic and metabolic assessments of submaximal levels of work require this type of analysis whether or not the patient has a pacemaker.

each stage (Fig. 21–11), they did find a large heart rate variable (15% to 20%) at each stage among the subjects tested. A significant difference in chronotropic response was observed between men and women, only part of which may be explained by their differences in body weight (men, 79.5 ± 12 kg; women, 60.2 ± 10 kg, $P < .0001$), peak oxygen consumption (men, 20.7 ± 3.9 mL/kg per minute; women, 15.5 ± 3.1 mL/kg per minute; $P < .001$), and maximum power output (men, 95 ± 25 W; women, 56 ± 19 W; $P < .001$). Most important, the heart rate change per MET was lower in men at each stage ($P < .001$). Balady and colleagues also noticed a significant difference in METS utilized at each stage when adjusted for body weight. This difference was observed in both men and women. These differences demonstrate the significant role of lean body mass and amount of exercising, or working, muscle mass on metabolic efficiency and overall oxygen consumption—an important observation demonstrated by several investigators in comparing the gender or type of activity on chronotropic or metabolic response (discussed further later).

Although arm ergometry, because of the continuous arm movements and its lack of similarity to daily activities, may not represent the ideal exercise protocol for testing chronotropic incompetence or evaluating the appropriate response of rate-responsive pacemaker, the observations and clinical implications are important to consider. Because arm ergometry represents a non–weight-bearing activity that is not subjected to the limitations of exercising patients with lower extremity vascular insufficiency, it may represent a useful tool in the evaluation of cardiac chronotropism. Nevertheless, the significant metabolic and heart rate response differences that are observed in both men and women of varying body mass should be considered when evaluating patients for cardiac pathology.

Informal stress testing, such as walking in place, hallway walking, or climbing up and down flights of stairs, and individualized ramp treadmill tests may be useful for general screening but has many disadvantages.[80] These include lack of calibration in terms of work expenditure, lack of continuous monitoring, lack of hard-copy rhythm strips, lack of proper supervision, and lack of proper emergency equipment. However, the importance of these techniques increases in patients who need postimplantation adjustment of rate-modulated parameters in pacemakers. Protocols that measure how far patients can walk in a fixed interval of time (e.g., 6-minute walk test) or how long it takes to cover a fixed distance are important in documenting clinical improvement after interventions, but their reproducibility and correlation with known workloads make crucial decision-making impossible.[81] The advantages of these informal tests are their simplicity and their ability to reproduce the symptoms and activities that are similar to those experienced by the subject on a day-to-day basis.

In recent years, a call for "optimizing" exercise testing, including customizing the test given with respect to the specific conditions, patient, and test purpose, has been made. Other forms of exercise can be attempted. Formal tests, such as the Harvard step test or the Master's test, are not calibrated into stages to evaluate submaximal heart rates and workloads. Furthermore, maximal stress produced with step testing tends to produce lower oxygen consumption than treadmill testing. Some physicians have used these tests to evaluate how long a person can exercise at a single workload, but this can also be done on treadmills. Although these two tests were once popular, their use has rapidly declined, and they are scarcely used today because of the advantages of other modalities.

Exercise Protocols

The treadmill remains the most widely used instrument for exercise evaluation of chronotropic response. There are many treadmill protocols available, each varying in factors such as incline, treadmill velocity, and duration of each stage. In choosing an exercise protocol, important factors to consider are the maximal speed that can be reasonably achieved by the subject and whether the subject can be expected to trot or run. If treadmill speed is a limitation, incline increase should be the major variable for adjusting the treadmill work intensity.

Nagle and coworkers,[82] Naughton and associates,[83] and Fox and associates[84] advocate a constant speed with a gradual increase in grade (Fig. 21–12). The modified Astrand protocol also has a constant speed with progressive grade step increases, however, the speed selected is between 5 and 8.5 miles per hour based on the individual subject's ability to run.[85] The Bruce and Ellestad protocols have stepwise increases in both grade and speed, the modified Bruce (or Sheffield) protocol adding two lower-workload, 3-minute stages onto the beginning of the standard Bruce protocol.[86–88]

The CAEP protocol also has progressive stepwise increases in both grade and speed and was developed specifically with chronotropic evaluation in mind (Fig. 21–10). Its main advantage is the use of 2-minute stages, which produce multiple data points at low levels of exercise in the range of activities of daily living. This protocol also has one other valuable feature. Protocols for chronotropic assessment

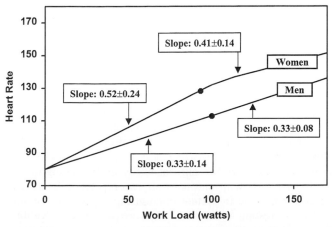

Figure 21–11. Heart Rate Response to Increasing Work Load: Gender Differences. These two curves demonstrate the gender difference in heart rate response to increasing workloads below and above anaerobic threshold (AT). Slopes (bpm per Watt) are significantly different ($P < 0.01$) through the entire work range. Women demonstrated a change ($P < 0.03$) in slope at AT, whereas men did not. AT is indicated by circles. (Data from Lewalter T, MacCarter D, Jung W, et al: Heart rate to work rate relation throughout peak exercise in normal subjects as a guideline for rate-adaptive pacemaker programming. Am J Cardiol 76:812–816, 1995.)

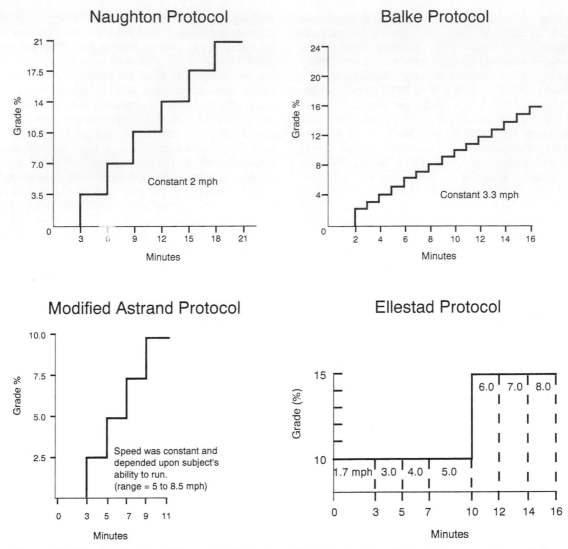

Figure 21–12. The Naughton, Balke, modified Astrand, and Ellestad protocols are illustrated to compare the treadmill elevations and velocities required by each. The protocols hold constant either the treadmill velocity or the treadmill elevation for large portions of the study. Sometimes, large increases in elevation or velocity require significant adjustments by the patient. This presents problems in making patient-to-patient comparisons of submaximal exercise unless the patient group is homogeneous.

should allow people with moderate functional aerobic impairment or orthopedic limitations an opportunity to produce data at several stages of exercise before the velocity of the treadmill requires the subject to jog. Comparison of the Balke, Bruce, Ellestad, and modified Astrand protocols by Pollock[89] demonstrated a linear rise in $\dot{V}o_2max$ and heart rate over time, although at different slopes, with similar peak $\dot{V}o_2$ attainment for each of these protocols. A similar result has been obtained with the CAEP protocol.[68] If the assumptions of the exercise protocol for steady-state measurements are met, any protocol that produces enough data points is acceptable for chronotropic assessment.

Lehmann and colleagues[90] in Munich have proposed a new protocol that is designed to cover activities ranging between 0 and 200 W in 25-W increments, with smaller gradations between each stage. The potential benefit, according to Lehmann and coauthors, is a greater applicability

in evaluating early response to exercise in patients with severe underlying cardiac or physical limitations, thus addressing a major limitation of the more commonly used Bruce and, to a lesser extent, CAEP and modified CAEP protocols. Although the clinical utility of evaluating or following patients with chronotropic incompetence has yet to be verified, some important relationships between treadmill and cycle testing were determined as part of the "calibration" of this protocol and involved a physiologic comparison to a bicycle protocol (Table 21–10). These investigators demonstrated that the overall relationships between workload, heart rate, and metabolic demands are similar between treadmill and bicycle testing. When regression analysis was performed, however, there was enough difference, although not statistically significant to illustrate the metabolic and chronotropic differences that must be taken into consideration when comparing the results of various exercise testing

Table 21–10. Munich Exercise Protocol: Physiologic Comparison Between Treadmill and Bicycle Exercise Testing

Physiologic Parameter	Bicycle	Treadmill	P-Value
Exercise duration (min)	14.3	15.5	$P < .05$
Max. power output (W)	180	197	$P < .05$
Heart rate (bpm)	$= 87.27 + 11.37 \times \text{Stage}$	$= 90.60 + 11.6 \times \text{Stage}$	NS
Oxygen uptake ($\dot{V}O_2$ mL/min)	$= 344.44 + 293.73 \times \text{Stage}$	$= 488.86 + 285.90 \times \text{Stage}$	$P < 0.5^*$
$\dot{V}O_2/\text{kg}$	$= 5.40 + 4.23 \times \text{Stage}$	$= 6.90 + 4.15 \times \text{Stage}$	NS
$\dot{V}CO_2$	$= 200.21 + 329.14 \times \text{Stage}$	$= 280.33 + 311.75 \times \text{Stage}$	NS
Minute ventilation ($\dot{V}E/\text{L/min}$)	$= 9.43 + 7.93 \times \text{Stage}$	$= 11.41 + 7.63 \times \text{Stage}$	NS

*At anaerobic threshold.

Adapted from Lehmann G, Schmid S, Ammer R, et al: Evaluation of a new treadmill exercise protocol. Chest 112:98–106, 1997.

Table 21–11. Minnesota Pacemaker Response Exercise Protocol*

Stage	Speed (mph)	Grade (%)	Time (min)	Cumulative Time	METs
1	1.5	0.0	2.0	2.0	2.0
2	2.0	2.0	2.0	4.0	3.0
3	2.5	3.0	2.0	6.0	4.0
4	3.0	4.0	2.0	8.0	5.0
5	3.5	5.0	2.0	10.0	6.0
6	4.0	5.0	2.0	12.0	7.0
7	4.5	3.5	2.0	14.0	8.0
8	5.0	2.0	2.0	16.0	9.0
9	5.5	1.5	2.0	18.0	10.0
10	6.0	2.5	2.0	20.0	11.0
11	6.5	2.5	2.0	22.0	12.0
12	7.0	3.0	2.0	24.0	13.0
13	7.0	5.0	2.0	26.0	14.0
14	7.0	7.0	2.0	28.0	15.0
15	7.0	9.0	2.0	30.0	16.0
16	7.0	11.0	2.0	32.0	17.0

*This protocol is specifically designed to evaluate the chronotropic response and rate-adaptive pacemaker function using a linear and constant increase in METs per stage.

From Mianulli MJ: Exercise physiology: Relation of physiologic pacing. *In* Benditt DG (ed): Rate Adaptive Pacing. Boston, Blackwell Scientific, 1993, pp 43–67.

modalities. Despite a strong correlation when linear regression analysis was performed on the entire data set, there was significant intrapatient variability that limits strict application of the linear equations in determining a heart rate to work load response in an individual patient.

A potential explanation for the physiologic differences is, as discussed previously, the greater overall and more efficient use of muscle mass during treadmill testing than during bicycle testing results in a prolonged time to exhaustion. The application of these results to areas of the world where bicycle riding is a common means of transportation or exercise is difficult. Muscle group adaptation to the demands of bicycle riding may produce metabolic results indicative of more efficient oxygen uptake and subsequently less cardiovascular demand for comparable workloads when compared with routine daily activities that stress alternative muscle groups, such as walking and climbing stairs.

Although the CAEP, modified CAEP, and Munich protocols have been specifically designed to evaluate for chronotropic incompetence, they have been criticized for their nonlinear workload changes between stages and difficulty in testing both activities of daily living and strenuous activity. To address these concerns, Mianulli and colleagues[91] at the University of Minnesota produced a useful incremental treadmill protocol. Treadmill inclination is increased or decreased with increasing velocity to achieve a consistent MET magnitude increase (Table 21–11). The protocol increases the MET level in a linear fashion that theoretically facilitates directly correlating heart rate response with a wide range of activity levels. Although scientifically appealing, widespread use of this protocol is hindered by broad familiarity with the Bruce and CAEP protocols.

Submaximal Exercise Testing

One of the major concerns of symptom-limiting maximal exercise testing is that the ramping protocols (speed and incline) and levels of activity are not representative of usual daily patient activities, and extrapolating results to pace-

maker programming may be inappropriate. Additionally, peak exercise testing is limited by patient motivation, arrhythmogenic consequences of pursuing elevated heart rates, and difficulty in reproducibility. To overcome these limitations, Lewalter and colleagues[92] developed a "Low Intensity Treadmill Exercise" (or LITE protocol) to attempt to correlate the minute ventilation slope during maximal activity to the slope obtained during low intensity activity (Fig. 21–13).

To validate the LITE protocol, 41 healthy subjects initially underwent exercise testing using a modified CAEP protocol ("RITE"—ramping incremental treadmill exercise). Metabolic analysis and heart rate to workload response data were obtained. The same patients underwent repeat metabolic exercise testing using the LITE protocol. The investigators were able to determine that the heart rate–minute ventilation (HR/MV) slope derived from rest to anaerobic threshold was comparable to the slope obtained from the

LOW INTENSITY TREADMILL EXERCISE ("LITE") PROTOCOL

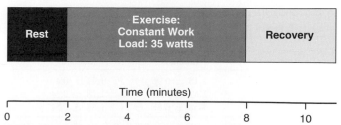

Time (minutes)

Figure 21–13. "LITE" protocol developed by Lewalter for submaximal exercise testing (see text). (Data from Lewalter T, MacCarter D, Jung W, et al: The "Low Intensity Treadmill Exercise" protocol for appropriate rate adaptive programming of minute ventilation controlled pacemakers. PACE 18:1374–1387, 1995.)

LITE protocol. Additionally, they observed a difference in the HR/MV slopes between men and women. Although not statistically significant, this difference once again illustrated the growing importance of a gender difference in chronotropic response (Table 21–12; see Fig. 21–11).

A major limitation to using these results is the assumption of the linear response between heart rate and minute ventilation; although there is a strong correlation, further evidence indicates that the response is more exponential. As workload increases, respiratory rate must increase at a faster rate to help eliminate the CO_2 that accumulates from buffering the increased production of anaerobic metabolic byproducts, such as lactate. The results of LITE protocol testing may not be applicable to patients with underlying pulmonary disease or to those whose activity level often exceeds 35 W. It is valuable, however, in that it provides, in a simple and time-efficient manner, information to guide clinicians to minute ventilation-based rate-adaptive pacemakers. Its overall utility in evaluating the chronotropic responsive has yet to be thoroughly determined.

Cycle ergometer protocols typically increase workload in 2- to 3-minute stages, increasing workload 25-to 50-W per stage. Alt[93] has proposed a cycle stress protocol designed for pacemaker patients that has 25-W incremental stages. This protocol allows multiple low MET points of assessment, which is ideally suited for pacemaker patients. In addition, a ramp cycle protocol increases workload slowly in a continuous manner and can be used for chronotropic assessment.[94] The advantage of the ramp approach, on either a bicycle or a treadmill, is a nearly continuous direct relationship between oxygen consumption, heart rate, and steady state. The assumption is that the ramp does not increase faster than the rate of the patient's adaptation to it.

Metabolic Stress Testing

There are certain situations in which a standard exercise test may be inadequate for full evaluation of a patient. For example, a patient with mixed pulmonary and cardiac pathology may have symptoms that are difficult to attribute to one specific disease process or another. Other patients may have vague, nonspecific symptoms, such as easy fatigability or dyspnea on exertion, that could be due to chronotropic incompetence, pulmonary disease, congestive heart failure, coronary artery disease, pericardial disease, pulmonary hypertension, anxiety with hyperventilation, malingering, or

Table 21–12. Heart Rate Increased per Liter of Oxygen Consumes ($\dot{V}o_2$): LITE Versus RITE Testing

	LITE (beats/L)	RITE (beats/L)
Men	1.15 ± 0.96	1.41 ± 0.43
Women	1.67 ± 0.80	1.78 ± 0.54
Overall	1.58 ± 0.88	1.58 ± 0.51

LITE, Low Intensity Treadmill Exercise; RITE, Ramping Incremental Treadmill Exercise.
Adapted from Lewalter T, MacCarter D, Jung W, et al: The "Low Intensity Treadmill Exercise" protocol for appropriate rate adaptive programming of minute ventilation controlled pacemakers. PACE 18:1374–1387, 1995.

other processes. The metabolic cart breath-by-breath analyzer is a useful instrument for assessing these difficult patients. It allows simultaneous measurement of exhaled oxygen and carbon dioxide, respiratory rate, and minute ventilation during exercise.

The patient with advanced pulmonary disease tends to develop oxygen desaturation during exercise, limiting peak oxygen consumption as a result of a premature anaerobic threshold. The respiratory quotient (RQ) is the ratio of carbon dioxide produced to oxygen consumed during metabolism. Healthy subjects have an RQ of about 0.85 at low levels of exertion. The quotient increases to more than 1.0 and usually to more than 1.2 at the termination of exercise. This ratio rises further in the postexercise period.[95] An RQ of greater than 1.0 indicates a near maximal effort; failure to reach an RQ of 1.0 indicates a submaximal exercise test, owing to inadequate effort, malingering, musculoskeletal limitation, claudication, or congestive heart failure.

In patients with heart failure the arterial blood gas values are not altered during exercise. Although healthy subjects reach a plateau in oxygen consumption, patients with heart failure rarely achieve this plateau because they stop exercising because of malaise or generalized fatigue.[96] Minute ventilation increases with maintenance of a normal carbon dioxide tension, whereas anaerobic metabolism leads to a progressive metabolic acidosis as a result of inadequate cardiac output.[97] Higginbotham and coworkers[98] demonstrated that patients with heart failure have a heart rate response similar to that of healthy subjects for a given workload; however, the patients with heart failure terminated exercise before achieving the age-predicted maximal heart rate response. Therefore, although it appeared that these patients had a significant heart rate response to exercise, they actually terminated exercise prematurely because of an inadequate rise in stroke volume and hence cardiac output, leading to increased metabolic acidosis.

Additional insights arise from the metabolic–chronotropic relation analysis described previously. The exercise data obtained from 12 patients with severe left ventricular dysfunction who were under consideration for cardiomyoplasty were evaluated and compared with the responses achieved by 48 healthy controls.[99] Compared with controls, the resting heart rate was elevated, and the peak heart rate was reduced. As in the control patients, the responses remained linear, but the average slope was reduced by one third (see Fig. 21–6). The question, which remains unanswered at this time, is whether this altered but apparently balanced chronotropic response is optimally adaptive. Perhaps the stroke volume would decrease if heart rate increased to the age-predicted maximal heart rate. Certainly, it is necessary to hold a different standard of chronotropic dysfunction for these patients than for people with normal ventricular function.

One of the major goals of exercise testing is to correlate work with physiologic parameters, including heart rate. Application of these complex relationships to clinical questions often requires obtaining metabolic data, including $\dot{V}co_2$ and $\dot{V}o_2$. The ability to quantify the slope of the heart rate–workload response curve would be invaluable in understanding both the normal and abnormal chronotropic response without having to perform complex metabolic, symptom-limiting exercise testing. Additional application of the heart rate–workload slope would be to evaluate for potential heart

Table 21–13. Gender Differences in Chronotropic Response*

	Men	Women	*P*-Value
V̇O₂max (mL/kg/min)	26.7 ± 4.7	20.9 ± 2.0	<.05
V̇O₂ at AT	15.4 ± 4.7	13.9 ± 2.3	NS
Peak HR at AT	109 ± 19	120 ± 21	NS
Peak HR	143 ± 22	150 ± 20	NS
HR to V̇O₂ slope (below AT)	2.60 ± 0.71	3.66 ± 1.34	<.05
HR to V̇O₂ slope (above AT)	3.24 ± 1.12	4.44 ± 1.43	<.05
HR to V̇E slope (below AT	1.59 ± 0.45	2.05 ± 0.90	<.05
HR to V̇E slope (above AT)	0.97 ± 0.35	1.27 ± 0.42	NS

V̇O₂max, maximum oxygen consumption; AT, anaerobic threshold; HR, heart rate.

*Gender differences in chronotropic response with regard to oxygen consumption above and below the anaerobic threshold.

Adapted from Treese N, MacCarter D, Akbulut O, et al: Ventilation and heart rate response during exercise in normals: Relevance for rate variable pacing. PACE 16:1693–1700, 1993.

rate over-response or underresponse programming in rate-adaptive pacemakers. Lewalter and associates,[100] performed metabolic treadmill testing in 41 healthy subjects (22 men and 19 women) and were able not only to quantify a normal chronotropic slope but also to observe a significant slope difference between men and women up to and after the anaerobic threshold (see Fig. 21–11).

The differences in chronotropic response between men and women must be considered when evaluating, comparing, and treating patients. Failure to do so may result in classifying a woman's exercise response as chronotropic incompetence as compared with standard on male responses, or vice versa. For example, in a study of 39 sedentary, otherwise healthy patients (23 men and 16 women), despite similar although slightly different overall peak heart rate and heart rate at anaerobic threshold, the heart rate–V̇O₂ and heart rate–tidal volume slopes were both different (Table 21–13).[101] According to the oxygen delivery equation (see equations 1 and 2), gender differences in hemoglobin have been

shown to play a significant but overall relatively small role in the metabolic and subsequent chronotropic responses of men and women.[102] Clearly, the gender differences are complex and warrant further investigation.

■ PRACTICAL ASPECTS OF CARDIAC CHRONOTROPISM

Programming Rate-Modulated Pacemakers

Despite the complexity of the descriptions in this chapter, once the rate-modulated pacemaker has been implanted, only three or four programming decisions need to be made to define the chronotropic responsiveness of the patient. These parameters are the lower rate, the upper rate, the sensor threshold to heart rate response, and the slope or incremental response desired for increased sensor activation. With the exception of sensor threshold, each of these parameters has a closely correlative physiologic parameter that is useful in programming the pacemaker response.

The sensor threshold should be conceived as the calibration parameter between the patient and the pacemaker. The smallest sensor response to an increase in activity or metabolic demand above the sensor threshold should initiate the chronotropic response. Ideally, the sensor threshold should be used to distinguish inactivity from minimal activity (Fig. 21–14). Another way of looking at the situation is that the sensor threshold is the parameter designed to distinguish false activity (noise) from true activity. "Noise" is the variation in sensor output intrinsic to the sensor and is not produced by a response to patient activity. Optimally, as incorporated in some of the current pacemakers, the pacemaker should recognize the noise sensor activity and automatically set the sensor threshold at just above that level. If the pacemaker algorithm is unable to distinguish rest from activity, then the sensor threshold should be set at the level that causes some heart rate response with a minimal amount of activity but no response when the subject is at complete rest.

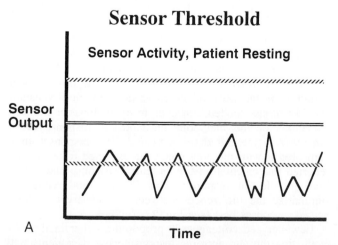

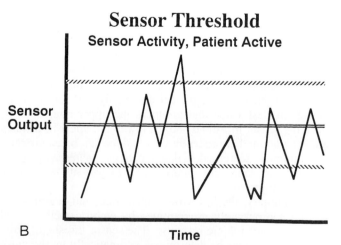

Figure 21–14. The sensor threshold with the patient resting should be set so that the sensor output fails to cross the threshold, but it should not be set so high that large increases in output are needed to cross the threshold. The middle horizontal line represents the appropriate choice for the activity shown in these graphs. If the lower threshold was chosen, the patient would experience sensor-driven rate increases during inactivity. If the higher threshold was chosen, the patient might not experience a rate increase during activities of daily living.

The other three parameters can be appropriately programmed only if the pacemaker expert understands chronotropic physiology. The lower rate of the pacemaker corresponds to the normal patients, desired resting heart rate of the patient. Of 537, the average resting heart rate was 65 ± 10 bpm. This is a good starting point, but adjustments should be made up or down to address the specific symptoms and issues facing the patient. If the patient is experiencing lightheadedness at rest or while standing still, then the lower heart rate should be increased by between 5 and 25 bpm. If all the patient's symptoms are related to significant exertion, however, reducing the lower rate to promote pacemaker longevity is advisable. Be careful to consider whether changing the lower rate will prevent or increase the incidence of atrial fibrillation.

The upper rate of the pacemaker should be programmed according to the age-predicted maximal heart rate. Subtracting the patient's age from 220 yields the expected sinus heart rate plus or minus standard deviations from the mean. Because a patient with a normal chronotropic response may be 2 standard deviations below the mean, calculating 85% of the predicted maximal heart rate (220 − age in years) and initially programming the upper rate to this value is appropriate. This relatively conservative upper rate value is significantly higher than the values in common use around the world. For every beat per minute below this value, however, there is a reduction in cardiac output in proportion to the stroke volume. For a 67-year-old person, the upper rate should be initially programmed to 130 bpm, and for a 50-year-old patient, it should be programmed to 145 bpm. If the patient has symptoms during significant exertion, the response should be increased by 15% to 20%. However, if the patient has symptoms related to angina or significant ventricular, pulmonary, or orthopedic dysfunction, the response should be reduced by about 10%.

The goal of the sensor slope, which is the parameter that determines the incremental heart rate response to a change in sensor activation, is to produce a linear heart rate increase with exercise that is directly related to the percentage of exercise capacity achieved. To simplify this description, the sensor slope should provide an appropriate change in heart rate from the lower to the upper rate over the entire range of patient activities. The more the patient can do, the smaller the desired slope. Patients with the smallest functional capacity should be given a very steep sensor slope (Fig. 21–15). Because the sensor threshold has been set to detect the smallest amount of activity, one way of setting the sensor slope is to exercise the patient maximally and set the slope at the smallest value that produces the upper rate. Usually, once the sensor threshold and the lower and upper heart rates are programmed, a moderate sensor slope can be empirically programmed, decreased in active patients, increased in inactive patients, and only finely tuned in patients who show further symptoms.

In summary, the lower rate, upper rate, and sensor slope can be appropriately programmed by empiric methods and produce a physiologic response. The sensor threshold, however, should either be determined automatically by the pulse generator or determined experimentally. An understanding of chronotropic physiology permits the physician to use a rational method for programming pacemaker rate responsiveness without intensive exercise testing.

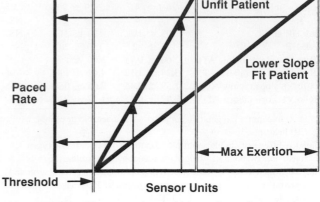

Figure 21–15. The sensor slope, which may be nonlinear, produces rate increases from the sensor threshold to maximal exertion when properly adjusted. The same level of exertion (sensor activation) provides different rate responses related to the sensor slope. Because resting heart rate and peak heart rate are not related to peak functional capacity, it is necessary to adjust for functional capacity by adjusting the sensor slope. The most unfit patient needs the highest (most aggressive) slope, whereas the most fit patient requires a more gentle sensor slope.

■ EVALUATING THE CHRONOTROPIC RESPONSE

Evaluation and optimization of a sensor-driven rate-modulated pacemaker response is the ultimate clinical goal of understanding chronotropic physiology. Knowing what to expect is the first step, but evaluating the actual response is critical in evaluating the relationship between the patient, the pacemaker, and the patient's activities. Kay[103] described three methods of evaluating the chronotropic response of rate-modulated pacemaker systems. Employing the concepts of heart rate and metabolic reserve, the metabolic–chronotropic response was plotted, and linear regression analysis provided a line with a y-intercept and slope. It was clear from the analysis of Kay's 10 patients that the response was not well described by linear regression (Fig. 21–16A). He then divided exercise into quartiles of exertion, calculating the difference between the expected and observed heart rate responses at the midpoint and end of each quartile (see Fig. 21–16B). This analysis allowed the possibility of variations in the slope of the curve during various stages of exercise. It also tended, however, to overemphasize transient deviations of the metabolic–chronotropic response curve. Finally, Kay integrated the area under the response curve, compared it with the area under the expected response, and reported this calculation for the entire response and for the four quartiles of response. This final method seemed to summarize the differences between the observed and expected responses best (see Fig. 21–16C).

Lewalter and colleagues[104] proposed another method for evaluating the chronotropic responsiveness of patients with pacemakers.[104] During low-intensity, fixed-workload treadmill exercise, oxygen consumption is measured. When steady-state $\dot{V}O_2max$ is obtained, the area between the actual and the ideal $\dot{V}O_2max$ response is integrated. The goal is to program the rate response to minimize the metabolic difference (O_2 deficit) (Fig. 21–17).

It is interesting to analyze the responses of Kay's 10 VVIR patients and compare their responses to the reported responses in healthy subjects, heart failure patients, and patients with atrial fibrillation. Healthy subjects provide the standard, which is a purely linear response ($R^2 = 0.95$) with a slope of 0.99. Similarly, the heart failure patients produced a linear response ($R^2 = 0.75$) with a slope of 0.67. In contrast, the atrial fibrillation patients produced responses that are extremely similar to the responses provided by rate-modulated pacemakers. Some of the responses were too slow throughout, others too fast, and some were too fast at low-intensity exertion but too slow at higher exertional intensities.

Device interrogation can also assist in documenting changes in the chronotropic response. The use of histograms can relay the amount of time the heart was being paced within defined intervals. If histogram reporting reveals a large percentage of time is spent at higher than baseline heart rate, the results may imply overaggressive activation of the rate response sensor. Conversely, if little time is spent at the upper rates, sensor underresponse or malfunction should be suspected. The caveat to histogram reporting is the lack of correlation with desired heart rate or activity. Histograms merely report that a given device was able to

pace at different heart rates, they do not convey information about the appropriateness of the pacing rate. Better reporting of both heart rate and simultaneous sensor activity would benefit follow-up, but unless the information can be correlated with actual activity levels or metabolic demand, their utility is limited. At this point, the best follow-up continues to be patient recording. Subjective reporting of symptoms during exertion can often provide the best clues about the appropriateness of the rate response and the potential need for more quantitative follow-up.

In summary, analysis of the metabolic–chronotropic responsiveness of a patient's pacemaker should include measurement of linearity and slope and quantification of the contribution of each quartile of response to expected behavior. Even so, heart rate reflects only one of the two components of cardiac output and fails to reflect the adequacy of the response in regard to oxygen consumption. However, expired gas analysis exercise testing, as described previously, validates the use of heart rate as the measure of a metabolically appropriate response.

Summary

Cardiac chronotropic analysis has just begun to develop into a clinically relevant science. In the past, formal exercise testing was usually reserved for assessment of ischemia or

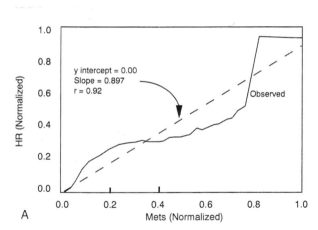

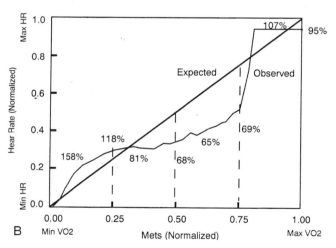

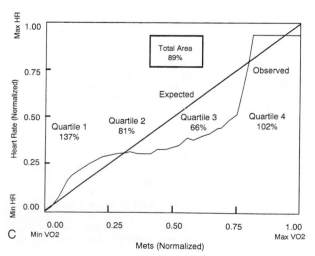

Figure 21–16. Kay uses normalized heart rate and normalized metabolic equivalents (Mets) instead of percentage heart rate and metabolic reserve, but the process is the same. *A,* Method 1 calculates the metabolic–chronotropic relation (MCR) slope of 0.897 (r = 0.92) but clearly incompletely describes the rate response of the pacemaker. *B,* Method 2 divides the exertion into four quartiles of response. The heart rate is measured at the midpoint and end of each quartile and is expressed as the percentage of the expected response. *C,* Method 3 compares the area under the expected and observed MCR curves during each quartile and for the entire exertion. The patient achieved only 89% of the expected heart rate area but, during early and late exercise, demonstrated excessive responses with a lag in response during the second and third quartiles. (From Kay GN: Quantitation of chronotropic response: Comparison of methods for rate-modulating permanent pacemakers. J Am Coll Cardiol 20:1534, 1992. Reprinted with permission from the American College of Cardiology.)

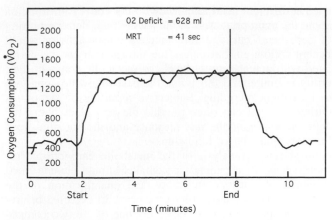

Figure 21–17. During low-intensity (35 W/min) but constant-intensity exercise, oxygen consumption (VO₂) is measured. During the plateau phase, a horizontal line is drawn, and the area is integrated between this line and the observed VO₂max from the initiation of exercise to the plateau. The mean response time (MRT) and O₂ deficit *(integrated area)* are calculated. (Courtesy of Dr. Thorsten Lewalter, University of Bonn, Bonn, Germany.)

cardiac rehabilitation. The establishment of rate-modulated pacemakers as a potentially effective treatment for chronotropic incompetence forced investigators to define cardiac chronotropism and assess the pacemaker response. Little is known about the normal chronotropic response, and less has been established about patients with ventricular dysfunction or ischemia, but standards are being set, and modern pacemakers have produced the ideal clinical laboratory for investigation. Advanced telemetry, including sensor and actual rate trends, histograms, and sensorgrams, produce previously unobtainable clinical data. Scientific inquiry now demands that chronotropic evaluations seek to match the pacemaker-augmented response of the chronotropically incompetent patient to the metabolic requirements of his or her body. Only with formal exercise testing will this goal be defined and achieved. Once the physiology has been completely defined, the lessons learned can be implemented with less formal techniques.

REFERENCES

1. Bousfield G: Angina pectoris: Changes in electrocardiogram during paroxysm. Lancet 2:457, 1918.
2. Feil H, Siegel M: Electrocardiographic changes during attacks of angina pectoris. Am J Med Sci 175:225, 1928.
3. Missal ME: Exercise tests and the electrocardiograph in the study of angina pectoris. Ann Intern Med 11:2018, 1938.
4. Master AM, Oppenheimer EJ: A simple exercise tolerance test for circulatory efficiency with standard tables for normal individuals. Am J Med Sci 177:223, 1929.
5. Master AM, Jafe HL: The electrocardiographic changes after exercise in angina pectoris. J Mt Sinai Hosp 7:629, 1941.
6. Bruce RA: Evaluation of functional capacity and exercise tolerance of cardiac patients. Mod Concepts Cardiovasc Dis 25:321, 1956.
7. Astrand PO, Rhyming I: Nomogram for calculation of aerobic capacity (physical fitness) from pulse rate during submaximal work. J Appl Physiol 7:218, 1954.
8. Balke B, Ware RW: An experimental study of physical fitness of Air Force personnel. US Armed Forces Med J 10:675, 1959.
9. Hellerstein HK, Hornsten TR: The coronary spectrum: Assessing and preparing a patient for return to a meaningful and productive life. J Rehabil 32:48, 1966.
10. Froelicher VF: Interpretation of hemodynamic response to the exercise Test. *In* Manual of Exercise Testing, 2nd ed. St Louis, CV Mosby, 1994.
11. Wilkoff BL: Criteria for optimal pacemaker function. J Cardiovasc Electrophysiol 2:416, 1991.
12. Astrand PO, Cuddy TE, Saltin B, et al: Cardiac output during submaximal and maximal work. J Appl Physiol 19:268, 1964.
13. Franciosa JS, Park M, Levine B: Lack of correlation between exercise capacity and indices of left ventricular performance in heart failure. Am J Cardiol 47:33, 1981.
14. Wasserman K, Whipp BJ: Exercise physiology in health and disease. Am Rev Respir Dis 112:219, 1975.
15. Green HJ, Hughson RL, Orr GW, Ranney DA: Anaerobic threshold, blood lactate, and muscle metabolites in progressive exercise. J Appl Physiol 54:1032, 1983.
16. Simon J, Young JL, Gutin B, et al: Lactate accumulation relative to the anaerobic and respiratory compensated threshold. J Appl Physiol 54:13, 1983.
17. Hughes EF, Turner SC, Brook GA: Effects of glycogen depletion and pedaling speed on anaerobic threshold. J Appl Physiol 53:58, 1982.
18. American College of Sports Medicine: ACSM's Guidelines for Exercise Testing and Prescription, 5th ed. Baltimore, Williams & Wilkins, 1995.
19. Dailey SM, Bubien RS, Kay GN: Effect of chronotropic response pattern on oxygen kinetics. PACE 17(Pt I):2307–2314, 1994.
20. Kay GN, Ashar MS, Bubien RS, Dailey SM: Relationship between heart rate and oxygen kinetics during constant workload exercise. PACE 18:1853–1860, 1995.
21. Lemke B, Dryander SV, Jager D, et al: Aerobic capacity in rate modulated pacing. PACE 15(Pt. II):1914–1918, 1992.
22. Haywood GA, Katritsis D, Ward J, et al: Atrial adaptive rate pacing in sick sinus syndrome: Effects on exercise capacity and arrhythmias. Br Heart J 69:174–178, 1993.
23. Dreifus LS, Fisch C, Griffin JC, et al (eds): Guidelines for implantation of cardiac pacemakers and antiarrhythmic devices: A report of the ACC/AHA task force on assessment of diagnostic and therapeutic cardiovascular procedures. Circulation 84:455, 1991.
24. Gregoratos G, Cheitlin MD, Conill A, et al: Guidelines for implantation of cardiac pacemakers and antiarrhythmia devices: A report of the American College of Cardiology/American Heart Association Task Force on Practice Guidelines (Committee on Pacemaker Implantation). J Am Coll Cardiol 31:1175–1209, 1998.
25. Ellestad MH, Wan M: Predictive implications of stress testing: Follow-up of 2700 subjects after maximum treadmill stress testing. Circulation 51:363, 1975.
26. Batey R, Sweesy M, Scala G, et al: Comparison of low rate dual chamber pacing to activity responsive rate variable ventricular pacing. PACE 13:646–652, 1990.
27. Isaeff DM, Jutzy RV, Florio J: Programming of rate responsive pacemakers. J Electrophysiol 3:2102–2116, 1989.
28. Gwinn N, Leman F, Zile M, et al: Pacemaker patients become chronotropic incompetent with time [Abstract]. PACE 13:535, 1990.
29. Rosenqvist M: Atrial pacing for sick sinus syndrome. Clin Cardiol 13:43–47, 1990.
30. Katritsis D, Camm AJ: Chronotropic incompetence: A proposal for definition and diagnosis. Br Heart J 70(5):400–402, 1993.
31. Blomqvist CG, Saltin B: Cardiovascular adaptations to physical training. Annu Rev Physiol 45:169, 1983.
32. Wilkoff BL, Beck G, Pashkow F, et al: Confidence interval calculation of chronotropic incompetence. PACE 13:1215, 1990.
33. Jose AD, Collison D: The normal range and determinants of the intrinsic heart rate in man. Cardiovasc Res 4:160, 1970.
34. Fagraeus L, Linnarsson D: Autonomic origin of heart rate fluctuations at the onset of muscular exercise. J Appl Physiol 40:679, 1976.
35. Bates DV: Commentary on cardiorespiratory determinants of cardiovascular fitness. Can Med Assoc J 96:704, 1967.
36. Jette M, Sidney K, Bluchen G: Metabolic equivalent (METS) in exercise testing, exercise prescription, and evaluation of functional capacity. Clin Cardiol 13:555, 1990.
37. Fletcher GF, Froelicher VF, Hartley LH, et al: Exercise standards: A statement for health professionals from the American Heart Association. Circulation 82:2286, 1990.
38. Wilkoff BL, Corey J, Blackburn G: A mathematical model of the cardiac chronotropic response to exercise. J Electrophysiol 3:176, 1989.

39. Wilkoff BL, Blackburn G, Pashkow F, et al: Exercise testing in the identification of sinus node dysfunction. Euro-pace 93: 6th European Symposium on Cardiac Pacing. Ostend, Belgium, 1993, pp 105–111.
40. Ferrer MI: The sick sinus syndrome in atrial disease. JAMA 206:645, 1968.
41. Sugrue DD, Gersh BJ, Holmes DR, et al: Symptomatic "isolated" carotid sinus hypersensitivity: Natural history and results of treatment with anticholinergic drugs or pacemaker. J Am Coll Cardiol 7:158, 1986.
42. Morley CA, Perrins EJ, Grant P, et al: Carotid sinus syndrome treated by pacing: Analysis of persistent symptoms and role of AV sequential pacing. Br Heart J 47:411, 1982.
43. Almquist A, Gornick C, Benson W, et al: Carotid sinus hypersensitivity: Evaluation of the vasodepressor component. Circulation 5:927, 1985.
44. Strasberg B, Sagie A, Erdman S, et al: Carotid sinus hypersensitivity and carotid sinus syndrome. Prog Cardiovasc Dis 5:379, 1989.
45. Thomas JE: Hyperactive carotid sinus reflex and carotid sinus syncope. Mayo Clin Proc 44:127, 1969.
46. Kapoor WN, Karpf M, Wieand S, et al: A prospective evaluation and follow-up of patients with syncope. N Engl J Med 309:197, 1983.
47. Volkmann H, Sehnerch B, Kuhnert H: Diagnostic value of carotid sinus hypersensitivity. PACE 13:2065, 1990.
48. Vardas PE, Fitzpatrick A, Ingram A, et al: Natural history of sinus node chronotropy in paced patients. PACE 14(2):155, 1991.
49. Gang ES, Oseran DS, Mandel WJ, et al: Sinus node electrogram in patients with the hypersensitive carotid sinus syndrome. J Am Coll Cardiol 5:1484, 1985.
50. Brignole M, Menozzi C, Lolli G, et al: Validation of a method for choice of pacing in carotid sinus syndrome with or without sinus bradycardia. PACE 14:186, 1991.
51. Ketritsis D, Ward DE, Camm AJ: Can we treat carotid sinus syndrome? PACE 14:1367, 1991.
52. Holden W, McAnulty JH, Rahimtoola SH: Characterization of heart rate response to exercise in the sick sinus syndrome. Br Heart J 40:923, 1978.
53. Donald DE, Shepherd JT: Response to exercise in dogs with cardiac denervation. Am J Physiol 205:293, 1963.
54. Ross JJ Jr, Linhart JW, Braunwald E: Effects of changing heart rate in man by electrical stimulation of the right atrium. Circulation 32:549, 1965.
55. Abbott JA, Hirshfeld DS, Kunkel FW, et al: Graded exercise testing in patients with sinus node dysfunction. Am J Med 62:330, 1977.
56. Ellestad MH: Parameters to be measured. In Stress Testing: Principles and Practice, 3rd ed. Philadelphia, FA Davis, 1986.
57. Hinkle LE, Carver ST, Plakun A: Slow heart rates and increased risk of cardiac death in middle-aged men. Arch Intern Med 129:732, 1972.
58. Chin CF, Messenger JC, Greenberg PS, et al: Chronotropic incompetence in exercise testing. Clin Cardiol 2:12, 1979.
59. Hamer DS, Wilkoff BL, Blackburn CG, et al: Chronotropic incompetence during exercise in patients with severe left ventricular dysfunction. J Am Coll Cardiol 2:329A, 1993.
60. Brener SJ, Pashkow FJ, Harvey SA, et al: Chronotropic response to exercise predicts angiographic severity in patients with suspected or stable coronary artery disease. Am J Cardiol 76:1228–1232, 1995.
61. Lauer MS, Okin PM, Larson MG, et al: Impaired heart rate response to graded exercise: Prognostic implications of chronotropic incompetence in the Framingham Heart Study. Circulation 93:1502–1506, 1996.
62. Lauer MS, Mehta R, Pashkow FJ, et al: Association of chronotropic incompetence with echocardiographic ischemia and prognosis. J Am Coll Cardiol 32:1280–1286, 1998.
63. Lauer MS, Pashkow FJ, Larson MG, et al: Association of cigarette smoking with chronotropic incompetence and prognosis in the Framingham Heart Study. Circulation 96:897–903, 1997.
64. Dyer AR, Persky V, Stamler, et al: Heart rate as a prognostic factor for coronary heart disease and mortality: Findings in three Chicago epidemiologic studies. Am J Epidemiol 112:736–749, 1980.
65. Hayano J, Yamada A, Mukai S, et al: Severity of coronary artherosclerosis correlated with the respiratory component of heart rate variability. Am Heart J 121:1070–1079, 1991.
66. Chin CF, Messenger JC, Greenberg PS, Ellestad MH: Chronotropic incompetence in exercise testing. Clin Cardiol 2:12–18, 1979.
67. Knox JAC: The heart rate with exercise in patients with auricular fibrillation. Br Heart J 11:119, 1949.
68. Corbelli R, Masterson M, Wilkoff BL: Chronotropic response to exercise in patients with atrial fibrillation. PACE 13:179, 1990.
69. Colucci WS, Ribeiro JP, Rocco MB, et al: Impaired chronotropic response to exercise in patients with congestive heart failure: Role of postsynaptic β-adrenergic desensitization. Circulation 80:314–323, 1989.
70. Fei L, Keeling PJ, Sadoul N, et al: Decreased heart rate variability in patients with congestive heart failure and chronotropic incompetence. PACE 19(Pt I):477–483, 1996.
71. Raghavan C, Maloney JD, Nitta J, et al: Long-term follow-up of heart transplant recipients requiring permanent pacemakers. J Heart Lung Transplant 14:1081–1089, 1995.
72. DiBiase A, Tse TM, Schnittger I, et al: Frequency and mechanism of brady cardia in cardiac transplant recipients and need for pacemakers. Am J Cardiol 67:1385–1389, 1991.
73. Kao AC, Trigt PV, Shaeffer-McCall GS, et al: Central and peripheral limitation to upright exercise in untrained cardiac transplant recipients. Circulation 89:2605–2615, 1994.
74. Young JB, Winters WL Jr, Bourge R, et al: 24th Bethesda conference: Cardiac transplantation. Task Force 4: Function of the heart transplant recipient. J Am Coll Cardiol 22(1):31–41, 1993.
75. Blackburn G, Harvey S, Wilkoff B: A chronotropic assessment exercise protocol to assess the need and efficacy of rate-responsive pacing. Med Sci Sports Exerc 20:S21, 1988.
76. Astrand PO: Principles in ergometry and their implications in sports practice. Sport Med 1:1, 1984.
77. Wasserman K: Diagnosing cardiovascular and lung pathophysiology from exercise gas exchange. Chest 112(4):1091–1101, 1997.
78. Hansen JE, Casaburi R, Cooper DM, Wasserman K: Oxygen uptake as related to work rate increment during cycle ergometer exercise. Eur J Appl Physiol 57:140, 1988.
79. Balady GJ, Weiner DA, Rose L, Ryan TJ: Physiologic response to arm ergometry relative to age and gender. J Am Coll Cardiol 16:130–135, 1990.
80. Myers J, Buchman N, Smith D, et al: Individualized ramp treadmill: Observations on a new protocol. Chest 101(5):236s, 1992.
81. Mianulli M, Crossley G, Wilkoff B, Benditt DG: Optimizing rate-adaptive pacemaker response: Are simple common tests accurate? [Abstract]. PACE 21(Pt II):914, 1998.
82. Nagle FJ, Balke B, Naughton JP: Graduation step tests for assessing work capacity. J Appl Physiol 20:745, 1965.
83. Naughton J, Balke B, Nagle F: Refinements in methods of evaluation and physical conditioning before and after myocardial infarction. Am J Cardiol 14:837, 1964.
84. Fox SM, Naughton JP, Haskell WL: Physical activity and the prevention of coronary artery disease. Ann Clin Res 3:404, 1971.
85. Astrand PO, Rodahl K: Textbook of Work Physiology. New York, McGraw-Hill, 1970.
86. Bruce RA, McDonough JR: Stress testing in screening for cardiovascular disease. Bull N Y Acad Med 45:1288, 1969.
87. Ellestad MH, Allen W, Wan M, et al: Maximal treadmill stress testing for cardiovascular evaluation. Circulation 39:517, 1969.
88. Sheffield LT, Roitman D: Stress testing methodology. Prog Cardiovasc Dis 19:33, 1976.
89. Pollock ML: A comparative analysis of 4 protocols for maximal exercise testing. Am Heart J 93:39, 1976.
90. Lehmann G, Schmid S, Ammer R, et al: Evaluation of a new treadmill exercise protocol. Chest 112:98–106, 1997.
91. Mianulli MJ: Exercise physiology: Relation of physiologic pacing. In Benditt DG (ed): Rate adaptive pacing. Boston, Blackwell Scientific, 1993, pp 43–67.
92. Lewalter T, MacCarter D, Jung W, et al: The "Low Intensity Treadmill Exercise" protocol for appropriate rate adaptive programming of minute ventilation controlled pacemakers. PACE 18:1374–1387, 1995.
93. Alt E: A protocol for treadmill and bicycle stress testing designed for pacemaker patients. Stimucoeur 15:33, 1987.
94. Whipp BJ, Davis JA, Torres F: A test to determine parameters of aerobic function during exercise. J Appl Physiol 50:217, 1981.
95. Jones NL, Campbell EJM: Physiology of exercise. In Clinical Exercise Testing, 2nd ed. Philadelphia, WB Saunders, 1982.
96. Poole-Wilson PA: Exercise as a means of assessing heart failure and its response to treatment. Cardiology 76:347, 1989.
97. Franciosa JA, Leddy CL, Wilen M, et al: Relation between hemodynamic and ventilatory responses in determining exercise capacity in severe congestive heart failure. Am J Cardiol 53:127, 1984.

98. Higginbotham MB, Morris KG, Conn EH, et al: Determinants of variable exercise performance among patients with severe left ventricular dysfunction. Am J Cardiol 51:52, 1983.

99. Hamer DS, Wilkoff BL, Blackburn GG, Alexander LA: Chronotropic incompetence during exercise in patients with severe left ventricular dysfunction. J Am Coll Cardiol 21:329A, 1993.

100. Lewalter T, MacCarter D, Jung W, et al: Heart rate to work rate relation throughout peak exercise in normal subjects as a guideline for rate-adaptive pacemaker programming. Am J Cardiol 76:812–816, 1995.

101. Treese N, MacCarter D, Akbulut O, et al: Ventilation and heart rate response during exercise in normals: Relevance for rate variable pacing. PACE 16:1693–1700, 1993.

102. Cureton K, Bishop P, Hutchinson P, et al: Sex difference in maximal oxygen uptake: Effect of equating haemoglobin concentration. Eur J Appl Physiol 54(6):656–660, 1986.

103. Kay GN: Quantitation of chronotropic response: Comparison of methods for rate-modulating permanent pacemakers. J Am Coll Cardiol 20:1533, 1992.

104. Lewalter T, Jung W, MacCarter D, et al: Heart rate and oxygen uptake kinetics: A goal of rate-adaptive pacemakers? PACE 16(Pt 2):852, 1993.

Chapter 22

Indications for Implantable Cardioverter Defibrillators: Clinical Trials

D. George Wyse and H. Leon Greene

■ INTRODUCTION TO THE CLINICAL PROBLEM OF SUDDEN CARDIAC DEATH

Sudden cardiac death is a major health problem throughout the developed countries of the world and is estimated to be the cause of 300,000 deaths annually in the United States.[1] Sudden cardiac death is the ultimate cause of demise for about half of all people who die from cardiac disease. Sudden cardiac death, however, is a clinical diagnosis that has a number of causes, rather than being a single and distinct entity. This concept is critical to the application of the implantable cardioverter defibrillator (ICD) to increase survival because this device is intended to treat a specific cause of sudden *arrhythmic* cardiac death, namely, hemodynamically unstable ventricular tachycardia (VT) or ventricular fibrillation (VF). Of course, those devices which provide backup pacing should also prevent death due to primary bradyarrhythmia.

Some sudden cardiac deaths are not arrhythmic, such as left ventricular rupture, aortic aneurysm dissection, or pulmonary embolus. Accordingly, the impact of the ICD on survival is through prevention of only a portion of sudden cardiac death. The size of that portion is not known with any certainty. The reason for this uncertainty begins with the definition of sudden arrhythmic cardiac death. In fact, there are several definitions, all of which are a variation on a theme. The usual elements in a definition of sudden cardiac death include, for example, death due to known or presumed cardiac cause; witnessed and instantaneous death; witnessed death within 1 hour of onset of new or worsening symptoms; and unwitnessed death but no other apparent cause. Many potential causes for death occur under such a definition.

On the basis of a few small series of patients who died while wearing an ambulatory electrocardiogram (ECG) and whose mode of death met such a definition for sudden cardiac death, it has been commonly stated that 80% to 90% of sudden cardiac death is due to VT or VF.[2] The accuracy of such estimates applied to the overall population who experience a sudden cardiac death is questionable. Patients wearing an ambulatory ECG monitor were doing so for a reason. Patients whose arrhythmias provided premonitory symptoms may be different from the general population of patients who die suddenly from an arrhythmia. Drugs taken during the Holter monitor recording may change the terminal arrhythmia. Furthermore, it is not known how many such episodes of VT, VF, or bradycardia occur in hearts that are not capable of extended survival even with successful resuscitation efforts. These gaps in our knowledge are important because the ICD can only be expected to prolong survival when VT, VF, or bradycardia is the cause of sudden cardiac death in a patient who would otherwise be likely to survive. Finally, ICDs may be implanted for hemodynamically stable VT, and in this role they may have little effect on survival. Obviously, patient selection becomes crucial in both clinical trials and patient care.

■ APPLICATION OF RANDOMIZED CLINICAL TRIAL SCIENCE TO IMPLANTABLE CARDIOVERTER-DEFIBRILLATOR THERAPY

Not every question in clinical medicine can or should be addressed in randomized clinical trials. However, important clinical questions should be examined in well-designed randomized clinical trials, particularly those questions that address frequent and devastating problems and that employ therapies for which the best application remains uncertain. Unquestionably, the use of the ICD to prevent sudden cardiac death falls within such a rubric. Although the execution of such trials cannot await the full temporal evolution of technology of the ICD and the refined capability for selection of the ideal patient, such studies also cannot be done in a setting of such primitiveness that there is little likelihood of demonstration of their true benefit. Although the concept of an ICD was first realized clinically in 1980, it was only in the early 1990s that the technical development of the device reached a point at which it was mature enough to be tested in a randomized clinical trial. Furthermore, device technology will continue to evolve. Such developments will lead to further refinements of the clinical questions, particularly if the costs can be decreased and patient selection improved.

Although there have been marked improvements in ICD technology in the 1980s and 1990s, the selection of the most appropriate patients to receive an ICD has not advanced at the same pace. Patient selection remains the Achilles' heel for both clinical application and planning of randomized clinical trials using the ICD. Patient selection is not so important when the therapy is inexpensive and free of risk. That is not the case for the ICD. To assess impact of the ICD on sudden cardiac death, the ideal patient for randomized clinical trials of the ICD is one who has a high likelihood of death from VT, VF, or bradycardia and low likelihood of death from other causes. The methodology for selection of such patients remains imperfect. A variety of measures have been proposed as markers of VT and VF, including frequency of ventricular arrhythmia, signal-averaged ECG, heart period variability, QT interval dispersion, and others. So far, none of these has been widely accepted as providing the ideal sensitivity and specificity. Left ventricular function is a powerful predictor of sudden cardiac death, but the capability of determining which of these patients will have VT, VF, or bradycardia but could survive with prompt cardioversion and defibrillation or pacing remains elusive. Accordingly, discussion of patient selection is crucial when considering the individual trials described later.

Furthermore, it is important to consider the end points of each of the trials carefully. There should be little dispute with respect to use of total mortality, as opposed to cause-specific mortality, as an end point. The considerations examined in a North American Society of Pacing and Electrophysiology Policy Conference[3] relegate most earlier observational studies (which used the surrogate end point of device shocks) into the "seriously flawed" category. Important secondary end points are cost and quality of life. Until recently, these issues have been understudied.

The limitations of nonrandomized trials have been discussed in a number of recent articles.[4] The major issue is that in the absence of randomization of therapy, important bias is introduced in assignment of therapy—bias that cannot be dispelled simply by consideration of measured variables. Bias may be present in relation to variables that were known to be important but not measured. For example, depression is a well-known factor influencing arrhythmic death,[5] but it is seldom measured. Furthermore, bias may be present in relation to variables that are totally unknown at this time, or even if known, may be unmeasurable. When the treatment effect is quantitatively indisputable, randomized clinical trials become less important (which is not the same as unnecessary). Nonrandomized studies, however, really usually only provide a basis from which randomized clinical trials can be planned.

■ RANDOMIZED CLINICAL TRIALS OF IMPLANTABLE CARDIOVERTER-DEFIBRILLATOR THERAPY

The following discussion will be divided into two major subcategories: (1) trials that have been completed and (2)

trials that are still in progress. Within each of these major subcategories we will look at *primary prevention* trials and *secondary prevention* trials.

Completed Studies

Only two completed randomized trials examine the role of the ICD in the primary prevention of sudden cardiac death. Unfortunately, the results of these two trials superficially appear to be in conflict. Resolution of this apparent paradox may be found in the differences in the two populations of patients studied.

The first study to be completed was the Multicenter Automatic Defibrillator Implantation Trial (MADIT).[6, 7] Patients were treated either with an ICD or with "conventional therapy." Patients qualified for MADIT by having documented episodes of unsustained ventricular tachycardia and poor left ventricular function (left ventricular ejection fraction of 0.35 or less), but in addition, they had to have inducible sustained VT or VF that was not suppressed by pharmacologic therapy with intravenous procainamide. MADIT showed a clear advantage of the ICD over standard pharmacologic therapy with respect to overall survival. The magnitude of the treatment effect was large (Fig. 22–1), possibly because this trial selected for study a population resistant to antiarrhythmic drugs. In addition, the large treatment advantage of the ICD in MADIT may have been partly due to lack of a clearly specified "conventional therapy" in the alternative treatment arm, although most of these patients were treated with amiodarone.[7] Whatever the reasons, MADIT was the first randomized clinical trial to show an advantage of the ICD for reduction of total mortality.

The Coronary Artery Bypass Graft Patch (CABG-Patch) trial[8, 9] was also a primary prevention trial that attempted to select patients with a high risk for sudden cardiac death due to VT or VF. All patients were scheduled to undergo coro-

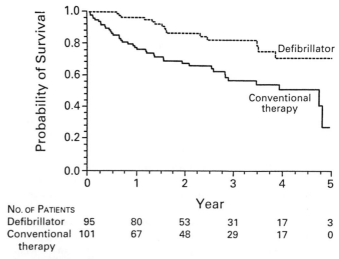

No. of Patients					
Defibrillator	95	80	53	31	17	3
Conventional therapy	101	67	48	29	17	0

Figure 22–1. Main results of the Multicenter Automatic Defibrillator Implantation Trial. Total mortality, defibrillator versus conventional therapy. (From Moss AJ, Hall WJ, Cannom DS, for the Multicenter Automatic Defibrillator Implantation Trial Investigators: Improved survival with an implanted defibrillator in patients with coronary disease at high risk for ventricular arrhythmia. N Engl J Med 335:1933–1940, 1996.)

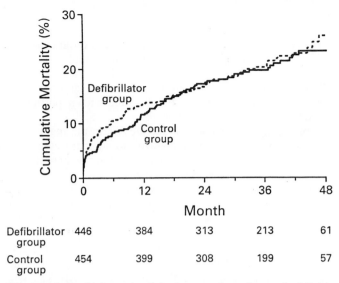

Figure 22–2. Main results of the Coronary Artery Bypass Graft Patch Trial. Total mortality, defibrillator group versus control group. (From Bigger JT Jr, for the Coronary Artery Bypass Graft [CABG] Patch Trial Investigators: Prophylactic use of implanted cardiac defibrillators in patients at high risk for ventricular arrhythmias after coronary-artery bypass graft surgery. N Engl J Med 337:1569–1575, 1997.)

nary artery bypass graft (CABG) surgery for obstructive coronary artery disease. Additional qualifications used to identify high risk for sudden cardiac death from VT or VF were reduced ventricular function (left ventricular ejection fraction of 0.35 or less) and an abnormal signal-averaged ECG.[8] Eligible and consenting patients had therapy randomized to CABG surgery alone or CABG surgery *and* an ICD with an epicardial lead system implanted at the time of CABG surgery. No other specific antiarrhythmic therapy was prescribed. The ICD did not affect overall survival in this patient population (Fig. 22–2). The CABG-Patch results were disappointing, particularly because the ICD was effective therapy in MADIT. The outcome may have been due to failure to select an appropriate group to treat. The signal-averaged ECG may not have been a powerful enough marker for risk of sustained VT or VF. Furthermore, the beneficial effect of revascularization in CABG-Patch may have been large enough to obscure any potential benefit from the ICD. Patient selection is thus crucial to successful application of the ICD.

At the time of this writing, only one of the several randomized clinical trials of the ICD for secondary prevention of sudden cardiac death has been completed and published in a peer-reviewed journal. Two other studies just completed have been presented briefly at major medical meetings[10] but have not yet been published in peer-reviewed journals. They will be discussed later. The Antiarrhythmics Versus Implantable Defibrillators (AVID) Trial[11, 12] has shown a clear advantage of the ICD over antiarrhythmic drug therapy, primarily using amiodarone. The AVID investigators selected patients in a simpler fashion than methods used in either of the completed primary prevention trials. Furthermore, the treatment in the alternative therapy arm was carefully specified. The AVID investigators selected patients who had survived a nearly fatal episode of ventricular arrhythmia,

either cardiac arrest from VF or hemodynamically important VT. These patients were randomly assigned to receive an ICD or the best available antiarrhythmic drug therapy. In the antiarrhythmic drug therapy arm of AVID, most patients (96%) were treated with amiodarone, and the remainder were treated with sotalol guided by the results of electrophysiologic testing or quantitative ambulatory ECG. In AVID, the ICD was significantly better than pharmacologic therapy for secondary prevention in patients who had a recent episode of nearly fatal VT or VF, using total mortality as the primary end point (Fig. 22–3).

An important feature of AVID is the AVID registry. All patients with VT or VF screened for AVID were entered into this registry. The noneligible patients and those eligible patients who declined randomization are followed through the National Death Index. Data analysis from the AVID Registry is just now in progress, and some data have appeared in abstract form. AVID will provide important observational data on a large cohort of VT or VF patients and help to provide a context for the results obtained in the randomized portion of AVID.

Two large trials that examined a secondary prevention strategy similar to the AVID design have been completed, and a summary of their results has been presented at a major meeting.[10] In fact, both of these studies began to enroll patients long before AVID. Yet they were not terminated early, despite the AVID results. The Cardiac Arrest Study: Hamburg (CASH) was conducted in Germany.[13] Like the other two secondary prevention trials, it selected patients who had survived a recent cardiac arrest. Originally, CASH randomized to four treatment arms: amiodarone, propafenone, metoprolol, or ICD. A published interim analysis, however, suggested excess mortality in the propafenone arm, and that arm was discontinued.[13] The number of randomized patients remaining in CASH was 349, about equally divided

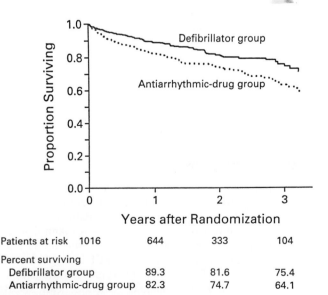

Patients at risk	1016	644	333	104

Percent surviving				
Defibrillator group		89.3	81.6	75.4
Antiarrhythmic-drug group		82.3	74.7	64.1

Figure 22–3. Main results of the Antiarrhythmics Versus Implantable Defibrillators Trial. Total mortality, defibrillator group versus antiarrhythmic drug group. (From AVID Investigators: A comparison of antiarrhythmic drug therapy with implantable defibrillators in patients resuscitated from near-fatal ventricular arrhythmia. N Engl J Med 337:1576–1583, 1997.)

among the three remaining treatment arms. The patients were followed for a minimum of 2 years. The 2-year mortality rate was 12.1% in the ICD arm and 19.6% in the two drug arms combined (P = .047).[10] The study does not have enough power to perform a three-way comparison, and although it is stated that there was no significant difference between the amiodarone arm and the metoprolol arm, there is limited power to detect even a moderate difference. The results of CASH support the findings of AVID but with a larger treatment effect of the ICD.

The other large secondary prevention trial that began before AVID is the Canadian Implantable Defibrillator Study (CIDS).[14] The patient population of CIDS was similar to the populations of CASH and AVID, with the exception that it included a small number of patients with syncope and inducible sustained VT or VF. The completed enrollment in CIDS included 659 randomized patients, and follow-up ended in January 1998. CIDS also followed all eligible patients who declined randomization, and this registry should provide yet another large observational cohort. As in AVID and CASH, the comparison in CIDS was between the ICD and antiarrhythmic drug therapy. In CIDS, patients were randomized to receive an ICD or empiric amiodarone. Once again, the mortality rate was lower in patients randomized to receive an ICD, but the treatment effect was smaller (about 20% decrease in mortality) and did not reach statistical significance.[10]

One other small randomized study of secondary prevention has been completed. The Netherlands study accepted patients who had experienced a cardiac arrest and had inducible VT or VF (4 to 12 weeks) after a myocardial infarction.[15] Patients were randomized to receive an ICD or antiarrhythmic drugs guided by the results of electrophysiologic testing. Although this study has a number of technical weaknesses,[16] primarily its small size, the main result was similar to that of AVID, suggesting a treatment advantage of the ICD. It is interesting to note the large treatment effect in this trial, which had many drug-resistant patients in the conventional treatment arm.

On the basis of the results of MADIT, AVID, CIDS, CASH, and the Netherlands study, the ICD appears to be superior to available antiarrhythmic drugs for reduction of mortality from VT or VF. It is noteworthy that these data from randomized trials affirm the findings of earlier nonrandomized studies, albeit with a smaller treatment effect. The exact size of the treatment effect may be more fully known as further trial results become published.

Studies in Progress

Other primary prevention trials are in progress or beginning. Of these, the Multicenter Unsustained Tachycardia Trial (MUSTT) is the closest to completion.[17] Patient enrollment in MUSTT has finished, and follow-up was planned to end in the latter part of 1998. Patient selection for MUSTT had some similarities to MADIT, and MUSTT is a substantially larger study than MADIT (about 700 versus 200 randomized patients). To qualify, patients had ischemic heart disease, reduced left ventricular function (left ventricular ejection fraction of 0.40 or less), unsustained ventricular tachycardia, and inducible, sustained ventricular tachycardia. It is at this point that similarities between MUSTT and MADIT end. Unlike MADIT, the MUSTT candidates who were noninduc-

ible are followed in the MUSTT follow-up study without any specific intervention. This study will provide the largest experience thus far collected concerning the prognostic significance of inducibility compared with noninducibility of VT or VF at invasive electrophysiologic testing. The MUSTT follow-up study will also provide a large observational cohort and a context for the randomized portion of the study.

Consenting patients with inducible VT in the main study portion of MUSTT were randomized to standard care or to intensive antiarrhythmic therapy. The intensive antiarrhythmic therapy arm of MUSTT is also different from that of MADIT in that the ICD is only part of a tiered therapy approach. The first tier of therapy is antiarrhythmic drugs guided by invasive electrophysiologic testing. Only after failure of at least one trial at suppressing VT or VF inducibility is an ICD implanted. Furthermore, the MUSTT patients who receive an ICD are resistant to antiarrhythmic drug therapy, as were those in MADIT. Accordingly, MUSTT will not be able to validate the MADIT results directly. However, the MUSTT "standard therapy" arm and the MADIT "conventional therapy" arm may be similar. The preliminary MUSTT results have recently been presented at a major medical meeting, but no written data are available to be cited as of this writing. In the randomized portion of MUSTT, intensive antiarrhythmic therapy resulted in improved survival. This benefit was largely achieved in patients receiving an ICD. The MUSTT results confirm the powerful treatment effect of the ICD seen in drug-resistant patients, as was also observed in MADIT.

Two other primary prevention trials are just beginning at the time of this writing. These are the Sudden Cardiac Death in Heart Failure (SCD-HeFT) Trial and the Multicenter Automatic Defibrillator Implantation Trial-II (MADIT-II). The protocols for these studies have not yet been published. Both trials intend to evaluate the role of the ICD in patients with heart failure, poor left ventricular function, or both. In SCD-HeFT, patients must have heart failure present for at least 3 months and have a left ventricular ejection fraction of 0.35 or less. In addition to conventional vasodilator heart failure therapy, SCD-HeFT has three randomized treatment arms: placebo, empiric amiodarone, or the ICD. MADIT-II requires a previous myocardial infarction and left ventricular ejection fraction of 0.30 or less. MADIT-II will randomize to an ICD or to conventional therapy with no ICD. One advantage of SCD-HeFT is that it may help to provide further information about the role of amiodarone in such patients.[18–20] Both of these studies will provide data on the role of the ICD in the setting of congestive heart failure or left ventricular dysfunction.

Other ongoing major studies with the ICD are: **De**fibrillators **i**n **N**on-**I**schemic Cardiomyopathy **T**reatment **E**valuation (DEFINITE), **Be**ta-blocker **St**rategy plus Implantable Cardioverter-Defibrillator Trial (BEST-ICD), and **D**efibrillator **in** **A**cute **M**yocardial **I**nfarction **T**rial (DINAMIT) (Table 22–1). These studies will further explore the role of the ICD in high-risk patients. In addition, other studies are evaluating the role of adding antiarrhythmic drugs (sotalol, dofetilide) to the ICD.

Soon, the appropriate place for the ICD in the management of VT and VF will be established by a rich and robust pool of data from randomized clinical trials. Furthermore,

Table 22–1. Major Ongoing Clinical Trials With the Implantable Cardioverter Defibrillator

Trial Name	Entry Criteria	Treatment	Projected Size	End Point
MUSTT	IHD MI >1 mo EF ≤0.40 NSVT Ind	EP-AAD/ICD None	704*	Total mortality
MADIT-II	IHD MI >1 mo EF ≤0.30 ≥10 VPDs/hr	ICD None	200	Total mortality
SCD-HeFT	CHF, II-III EF ≤0.35	ICD Placebo Amiodarone	2500	Total mortality
DEFINITE	CHF Nonischemic CM EF ≤0.35 NSVT, or >10 VPDs/hr	ICD None	440	Total mortality
BEST-ICD	Recent MI EF ≤0.35 ≥10 VPDs/hr or abn HRV, or abn SAECG	EP-AAD/ICD None	1500	Total mortality
DINAMIT	MI, 6–31 days EF ≤0.35 Abn HRV	ICD None	525	Total mortality

MUSTT, Multicenter Unsustained Tachycardia Trial; MADIT-II, Multicenter Automatic Defibrillator Implantation Trial II; SCD-HeFT, Suddent Cardiac Death in Heart Failure Trial; DEFINITE, Defibrilllators in Non-Ischemic Cardiomyopathy Treatment Evaluation; BEST-ICD, Beta-Blocker Strategy Plus Implantable Cardioverter-Defibrillator Trial; DINAMIT, Defibrillator in Acute Myocardial Infarction Trial; IHD, ischemic heart disease; EF, left ventricular ejection fraction; NSVT, nonsustained ventricular tachycardia; Ind, inducible sustained ventricular tachycardia; EP-AAD/ICD, electrophysiologic study-guided treatment with antiarrhythmic drugs or ICD; none, no specific antiarrhythmic therapy; ICD, implantable cardioverter defibrillator; MI, myocardial infarction; SAEGG, signal-averaged electrocardiogram; CM, cardiomyopathy; VPDs, ventricular premature depolarizations; CHF, congestive heart failure; HRV, heart rate variability; abn, abnormal.

there should be considerable opportunity to use meta-analysis and to pool some of these data to take advantage of the large sample sizes in these randomized clinical trials. A pooled analysis of the data of AVID, CASH, and CIDS is in progress and should give a more precise estimate of the ICD treatment effect and help to identify subgroups that can expect the greatest benefit. We have just begun to see the main results of these trials. We are also beginning to see the secondary end-point results that address issues such as cost and quality of life. These results will be nearly as crucial as the main study data because practicing physicians try to fulfill their complex dual role of patient advocate and gatekeeper, ensuring the best use of expensive and increasingly scarce health care resources.

Secondary End-Point Results

In the past decade, assessment of quality of life has been increasingly recognized as an important aspect of randomized clinical trials. Such measurements are included in several of the large randomized clinical trials of ICD therapy in progress or recently completed. Thus far, only fragmentary data have been reported. In AVID, there was no overall difference in quality of life in the two treatment arms, although quality of life did improve over time in both groups.[21] However, analysis of these quality of life data from AVID remains incomplete at this time. Many physicians have intuitively noted poor quality of life in ICD patients who receive frequent shock therapies, which commonly require addition of antiarrhythmic drug therapy. The clinical impression of reduced quality of life in some patients with an ICD has not yet been fully supported by rigorously evaluated data. Nevertheless, it is interesting to note that quality of life measured in the CABG-Patch trial was poorer in patients randomized to receive an ICD than in those who did not receive an ICD.[22] The ICDs in CABG-Patch were implanted prophylactically, however, rather than after an episode of nearly fatal VF or VF. Data are still too fragmentary to be interpreted as anything more than intriguing. If such results are confirmed, however, a limitation of quality of life may be a concomitant undersirable consequence of improved overall survival benefit in a subset of ICD patients.

Cost and the translation of cost and efficacy into cost-effectiveness are equally important secondary end points in randomized controlled trials of the ICD. The issues involved in consideration of cost and cost-effectiveness are complex. Partly because the ICD is perceived to be an expensive therapy, this issue has received much attention among the secondary end points. Thus far, however, the available analyses are largely based on hypothetical costs[23–27] and must be considered as only crude estimates. Furthermore, the data that have been generated in this fashion confirm that the ICD is a more expensive form of therapy than antiarrhythmic drug therapy. These estimates, however, are based on projected rather than measured efficacy. They suggest a cost-effectiveness for the ICD which is similar to that seen for several other widely accepted cardiac therapies. Substantial errors could be made using this approach.

MADIT was the first study to publish actual data concerning the cost of the ICD as compared with antiarrhythmic drug therapy.[28, 29] These data suggest that ICD therapy is cost-effective, but it is important to remember that MADIT found the greatest estimate of the average increase in life conferred by ICD therapy in comparison to antiarrhythmic drug therapy. Thus far, the AVID data with respect to this issue are preliminary, but they suggest that cost-effectiveness may be considerably less[30] than has been suggested by other estimates. The AVID financial data are based on charges, and this analysis is clearly not the same as that of "costs." How one deduces cost from charges can also be complex. Both MADIT and AVID data, however, suggest that in the short-term, the actual difference in costs between the two treatment alternatives is about the price of the device itself. Accordingly, the cost-effectiveness of the ICD is largely determined in any study by the size of the treatment effect. For the MADIT population, the treatment benefit of the ICD was more substantial than in AVID. Cost-effectiveness is closer to the accepted range for a useful therapy in MADIT. Furthermore, the duration of follow-up in both AVID and MADIT was brief, and there was little opportunity to account for the effect of device replacement. Nevertheless, cost-effectiveness of the ICD may turn out to be unfavorable unless the cost of devices decreases or their use is reserved for those who are most likely to receive a large treatment benefit. The problems are that (1) there has been little or no trend thus far for prices of ICDs to decrease, and (2) the means for selection of patients most likely to benefit are not well developed. Clearly, there is a need for further data collection and analysis in this area.

■ CURRENT RECOMMENDATIONS FOR IMPLANTABLE CARDIOVERTER-DEFIBRILLATOR THERAPY

With the current data available, any evidence-based recommendations (Table 22–2) must be considered preliminary.[31] The patient who has had an episode of cardiac arrest due to VT or VF, hemodynamically important VT (syncope or other serious symptoms and left ventricular ejection fraction of 0.40 or less), regardless of the nature of underlying heart disease, should be offered an ICD (class I recommendation supported by level A evidence). There are no other level A evidence recommendations that can be made. The patient who has had no previous episodes of VT or VF but who has coronary heart disease, reduced left ventricular function, unsustained ventricular tachycardia, and inducible sustained VT or VF that cannot be suppressed by procainamide should be offered an ICD (class I recommendation supported by level B evidence). For patients undergoing CABG surgery who have not yet had near-fatal VT or VF, there is no indication for treatment with an ICD (class III recommendation supported by level B evidence), even when the patient is thought to be at high risk because of reduced ventricular function and presence of late potentials.

Other than these recommendations, all other indications for implanting an ICD should be considered class II with levels of evidence B or C.

REFERENCES

1. Gillum RF: Sudden coronary death in the United States: 1980–1985. Circulation 79:756–765, 1989.
2. Bayes de Luna A, Coumel P, Leclercq JF: Ambulatory sudden cardiac death: Mechanisms of production of fatal arrhythmia on the basis of data from 157 cases. Am Heart J 117:151–159, 1989.
3. Kim SG, Fogoros RN, Furman S, et al: Standardized reporting of ICD patient outcome: The report of a North American Society of Pacing and Electrophysiology Policy Conference. PACE 16:1358–1362, 1993.
4. Connolly JF, Yusuf S: Evaluation of the implantable cardioverter defibrillator in survivors of cardiac arrest: The need for randomized trials. Am J Cardiol 69:959–962, 1992.
5. Ahern DK, Gorkin L, Anderson JL, et al, for the CAPS Investigators: Biobehavioral variables and mortality or cardiac arrest in the Cardiac Arrhythmia Pilot Study (CAPS). Am J Cardiol 66:59–62, 1990.
6. MADIT Executive Committee: Multicenter Automatic Defibrillator Implantation Trial (MADIT): Design and clinical protocol. PACE 14:920–927, 1991.
7. Moss AJ, Hall, WJ, Cannom DS, et al, for the Multicenter Automatic Defibrillator Implantation Trial Investigators: Improved survival with an implanted defibrillator in patients with coronary disease at high risk for ventricular arrhythmia. N Engl J Med 335:1933–1940, 1996.
8. The CABG Patch Trial Investigators and Coordinators: The Coronary Artery Bypass Graft (CABG) Patch Trial. Prog Cardiovasc Dis 36:97–114, 1993.
9. Bigger JT Jr, for the Coronary Artery Bypass Graft (CABG) Patch Trial Investigators: Prophylactic use of implanted cardiac defibrillators in patients at high risk for ventricular arrhythmias after coronary-artery bypass graft surgery. N Engl J Med 337:1569–1575, 1997.
10. Ferguson J: Meeting highlights. 47th Annual Scientific Sessions of the American College of Cardiology. Circulation 97:2377–2381, 1998.
11. AVID Investigators: Antiarrhythmics versus implantable defibrillators (AVID): Rationale, design, and methods. Am J Cardiol 75:470–475, 1995.
12. Antiarrhythmics Versus Implantable Defibrillators (AVID) Investigators: A comparison of antiarrhythmic-drug therapy with implantable defibrillators in patients resuscitated from near-fatal ventricular arrhythmias. N Engl J Med 337:1576–1583, 1997.
13. Siebels J, Kuck K-H: Implantable cardioverter defibrillator compared with antiarrhythmic drug treatment in cardiac arrest survivors (the Cardiac Arrest Study, Hamburg). Am Heart J 127:1139–1144, 1994.
14. Connolly SJ, Gent M, Roberts RS, et al: Canadian Implantable Defibrillator Study (CIDS): Study design and organization. Am J Cardiol 72:103F–108F, 1993.
15. Wever EF, Hauer RN, van Capelle FJ, et al: Randomized study of implantable defibrillator as first-choice therapy versus conventional strategy in postinfarct sudden death survivors. Circulation 91:2195–2203, 1995.
16. Zipes DP: Are implantable cardioverter-defibrillators better than conventional antiarrhythmic drugs for survivors of cardiac arrest? Circulation 91:2115–2117, 1995.
17. Buxton AE, Fisher JD, Josephson ME, et al, for the MUSTT Investiga-

Table 22–2. Evidence-Based Criteria as Modified for the American College of Cardiology and American Heart Association Task Forces

Strength of Evidence

Level A: Data from multiple randomized clinical trials
Level B: Data from single randomized clinical trial or nonrandomized studies
Level C: Consensus opinion of experts

Classification of Recommendations

Class I: Evidence and/or general agreement that treatment is useful and effective
Class II: Conflicting evidence and/or divergence of opinion about treatment usefulness and efficacy
    a. Evidence or opinion more in favor of usefulness and efficacy
    b. Evidence or opinion less in favor of usefulness and efficacy
Class III: Evidence and/or general agreement that treatment is not useful and effective, and in some cases harmful

tors: Prevention of sudden death in patients with coronary artery disease: The Multicenter Unsustained Tachycardia Trail (MUSTT). Prog Cardiovasc Dis 36:215–226, 1993.

18. Doval HC, Nul DR, Grancelli HO, et al, for the Grupo de Estudio de la Sobrevida en la Insuficienca Cardiaca en Argentina (GESICA): Randomised trial of low-dose amiodarone in severe congestive heart failure. Lancet 344:493–498, 1994.

19. Garguichevich JJ, Ramos JL, Gambarte A, et al, for the EPAMSA Investigators: Effect of amiodarone therapy on mortality in patients with left ventricular dysfunction and asymptomatic complex ventricular arrhythmias: Argentina Pilot Study of Sudden Death and Amiodarone (EPAMSA). Am Heart J 130:494–500, 1995.

20. Singh SN, Fletcher RD, Fisher SG, et al, for the Survival Trial of Antiarrhythmic Therapy in Congestive Heart Failure: Amiodarone in patients with congestive heart failure and asymptomatic ventricular arrhythmia. N Engl J Med 333:77–82, 1995.

21. Jenkins LS, Steinberg JS, Kutalek SP, et al, for the AVID Investigators: Quality of life in patients enrolled in the Antiarrhythmics Versus Implantable Defibrillators (AVID) Trial [Abstract]. Circulation 96:I-439, 1997.

22. Namerow PB, Firth B, Heywood GM, et al, for the CABG Patch Trial Coordinators & Investigators: Health-related quality of life six months post-CABG surgery in patients randomized to ICD versus no ICD therapy: Findings from the CABG Patch Trial [Abstract]. Circulation 96:I-439, 1997.

23. Kuppermann M, Luce BR, McGovern B, et al: An analysis of the cost effectiveness of the implantable defibrillator. Circulation 81:91–100, 1990.

24. O'Brien BJ, Buxton MJ, Rushby JA: Cost effectiveness of the implantable cardioverter defibrillator: A preliminary analysis. Br Heart J 68:241–245, 1992.

25. Wever EF, Hauer RN, Schrijvers G, et al: Cost-effectiveness of implantable defibrillator as first-choice therapy versus electrophysiologically guided, tiered strategy in postinfarct sudden death survivors. Circulation 93:489–496, 1996.

26. Larsen GC, Manolis AS, Sonnenberg FA, et al: Cost-effectiveness of the implantable cardioverter-defibrillator: Effect of improved battery life and comparison with amiodarone therapy. J Am Coll Cardiol 19:1323–1334, 1992.

27. Owens DK, Sanders GD, Harris RA, et al: Cost-effectiveness of implantable cardioverter defibrillators relative to amiodarone for prevention of sudden cardiac death. Ann Intern Med 126:1–12, 1997.

28. Mushlin AI, Zwanziger J, Gajary E, et al: Approach to cost-effectiveness assessment in the MADIT trial. Am J Cardiol 80:33F–41F, 1997.

29. Mushlin AL, Hall WJ, Zwanziger JU, et al, for the MADIT Investigators: The cost-effectiveness of automatic implantable cardiac defibrillators: Results from MADIT. Circulation 97:2129–2135, 1998.

30. Larsen GC, McAnulty JH, Hallstrom A, et al, for the AVID Investigators: Hospitalization charges in the Antiarrhythmics Versus Implantable Defibrillators (AVID) Trial: The AVID economic analysis study [Abstract]. Circulation 96:I-77, 1997.

31. Sackett DL: Rules of evidence and clinical recommendations for the management of patients. Can J Cardiol 9:487–489, 1993.

Chapter 23

Testing of Implantable Defibrillator Functions at Implantation

Mark W. Kroll and Patrick J. Tchou

Since the inception of clinical implantation of automatic defibrillators in the early 1980s, testing of the device function at implantation has been an integral part of the surgical procedure. Because implantable defibrillators serve to terminate life-threatening cardiac arrhythmias, it is imperative that the device be able to appropriately sense a tachyarrhythmia and terminate it successfully. Verification of these functions at implantation involves measurement of the detected ventricular and, more recently, atrial electrograms, during both the normal rhythm and during ventricular fibrillation and tachycardia. Testing of sensing is especially important during ventricular fibrillation, when the amplitudes of the recorded ventricular complexes can vary considerably from beat to beat. Such variation can cause dropout of detection owing to automatic adjustment of sensitivity in the recording amplifiers or detection thresholds. This dropout of detection may result in prolonged delays in device activation and termination of the ventricular fibrillation.

A measurement of defibrillation threshold (DFT) is important in ensuring that the implanted device has the shock strength to terminate ventricular fibrillation in a reliable manner. Although defibrillation shock energy measured in joules has been a common way of describing the DFT in the clinical setting, one must be cognizant of the fact that defibrillation, similar to pacing, has a strength–duration relationship (voltage/time, or current/time). Thus, higher delivered energies may not necessarily improve the probability of defibrillation. Although biphasic shocks and newer electrode systems have improved the reliability of defibrillation, occasionally one still encounters a patient in whom the defibrillation threshold is high. The physician performing implantation must be familiar with the means of lowering this threshold so that implantation of a device is feasible.

■ STRENGTH, DURATION, AND PROBABILISTIC NATURE OF SHOCK RESPONSE

The process of terminating ventricular fibrillation can best be described in a three-dimensional relationship of shock strength (voltage or current), shock duration (milliseconds), and the probability of success of such a shock. Conceptually, a defibrillation shock has certain similarities to a pacing impulse. The strength–duration relationship of pacing has been well defined. Similarly, there is a strength–duration relationship for defibrillation shocks.[1-7] In a rectangular monophasic shock waveform, there exists a rheobase voltage/current below which pulses will not defibrillate regardless of pulse duration. Shortening the pulse width increases the voltage/current required to defibrillate. This relationship of pulse width to voltage/current has been well established in experimental models. The slope of this curve rises as the pulse width shortens, such that the voltage/currents rises asymptotically when the pulse width approaches zero (Fig. 23–1).

For pacing, such a strength–duration curve gives a good description of myocardial capture because the threshold of myocardial capture is essentially an all-or-none phenomenon. That is, the probability of capture rises steeply as the parameters of a pacing impulse (strength and duration) traverse the strength–duration curve. Essentially 100% capture is found on one side of the curve and no capture on the other side of the curve.

Such is not the case for defibrillation. The probabilistic nature of defibrillation cannot be adequately described with a single strength–duration relationship of defibrillation is best described as a family of curves in which each curve has a particular probability of successful defibrillation. Thus, another manner of looking at the defibrillation phenomenon is described by the defibrillation success curve (Fig. 23–2).

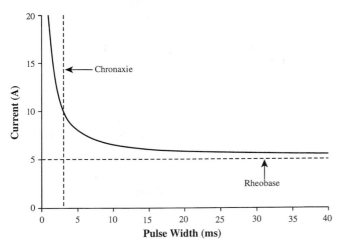

Figure 23–1. A generalized strength–duration curve for defibrillation. The rheobase current in the human heart is generally in the range of 2.3–5.6 A, whereas the chronaxie is about 2–4 msec. Measurements of transmembrane voltage change in response to defibrillation type of shock show that the time constant of this response is in the same range as that of the chronaxie.

This sigmoidal dose–response curve has been commonly described as a logistic regression curve.[8] In fact, this would suggest that at low levels, one could occasionally "get lucky" and defibrillate. However, recent studies and data analysis suggest that a more appropriate curve is one that rises steeply from a 0% probability and then asymptotically approaches 100%.[9, 10] The use of extremely high energies can also reduce the efficacy of a defibrillation shock as a result of the deleterious effects of high energies, as discussed later in this chapter.

The postulated mechanisms by which a shock terminates ventricular fibrillation (VF) have undergone modifications over the years. These have been reviewed, and a thorough

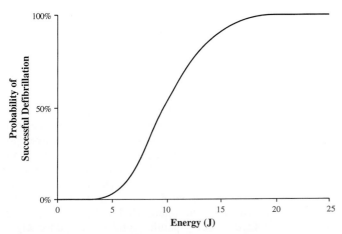

Figure 23–2. A typical defibrillation success curve showing the probability of successful defibrillation according to the amount of energy used. This type of percentage success curve can just as easily be described for the average current of the shock or the voltage. More effective defibrillation waveforms would shift this curve to the left and generate a steeper slope.

discussion is beyond the scope of this chapter.[11, 12] Although the defibrillation phenomenon and its probabilistic nature are still incompletely understood, several factors contribute to the difference between a pacing threshold and a defibrillation threshold. A pacing impulse is delivered at a time when the myocardium is at a relatively homogenous state, diastole. Furthermore, pacing capture occurs within a small volume of myocardium in the immediate vicinity of the pacing electrode. Thus, the electrical state of the myocardium within this small volume at the time of impulse delivery is highly homogenous. In contrast, defibrillation involves the influence of an electric shock across the entire myocardium. Studies have demonstrated that successful monophasic defibrillation shocks have to achieve minimum voltage gradients of about 5 V/cm at all myocardial sites.[13] This shock is delivered at a time when the myocardium is in a highly nonhomogenous state of activation and refractoriness. Furthermore, this nonhomogenous state is changing rapidly in time. This spatial as well as temporal inhomogeneity is the most likely explanation of the probabilistic nature of defibrillation.

■ WHY DO DEFIBRILLATION THRESHOLD TESTING?

Some form of testing to ensure that the implanted device is capable of accomplishing the task of defibrillation is needed at the time of implantation. This testing allows the physician to judge the efficacy of defibrillation and to ensure that the device can deliver a shock waveform of sufficient amplitude to provide reliable defibrillation. Because defibrillation is a probabilistic phenomenon, a single success at a shock strength near the maximum output of the device is not adequate assurance that the device will work well in clinical circumstances when defibrillation is needed. Furthermore, clinical circumstances may be complicated by additional variables that may alter defibrillation energy requirements. The variability of serum electrolytes, the changes in sympathetic stimulation, the rise and fall of serum antiarrhythmic drug levels, and the diastolic filling pressures of the heart are some of the factors that may change defibrillation energy requirements on a day-to-day-basis.

When testing demonstrates that defibrillation can be reproduced at relatively low shock strengths, one can program the device to deliver the first shock with a lower shock strength. This lower output would require a shorter capacitor charge time and shorten the time from the initiation of ventricular tachyarrhythmia to the delivery of the first shock. Such a shortened response of the device can mean the difference between maintenance or loss of consciousness. Sudden and unexpected loss of consciousness is always an undesirable occurrence because it can increase patient morbidity and even cause mortality. Lower shock strengths may also have the advantage of decreasing the probability of myocardial damage. This is especially true with circumstances that produce multiple shocks over a short period of time, such as a "storm" of ventricular arrhythmias, inappropriate device discharges in response to atrial fibrillation with rapid ventricular response or device malfunction. The use of lower shock strength accelerates postshock hemodynamic recovery and lengthens battery longevity. Another advantage of determining the actual DFT is that it can be monitored for increases. This could provide an early warning of lead problems or change in the substrate.

A thorough understanding of the defibrillation threshold requires multiple fibrillation and shock sequences during implantation testing. The value of an accurate DFT measurement is further diminished by the knowledge that this threshold can vary from day to day in response to clinical changes in a patient's physiologic status and medication levels. Patients who receive defibrillator implants frequently have markedly depressed ventricular function as a reflection of the underlying substrate that puts them at risk for clinical ventricular tachyarrhythmia. In such patients, multiple shocks for determining the DFT may cause deterioration of ventricular function during implantation and increase the procedure risk. Thus, during clinical implantation of a defibrillator, one needs to strike a balance between safety of the patient, adequate performance of the implanted device, and adequate understanding of the DFT to allow appropriate programming of the first shock strength.

The most common definition of DFT is the shock amplitude that provides a 50% chance of success. This is the definition we will use as the default. When there is danger of confusion, we will refer to this as DFT_{50}. Other useful definitions are DFT_{70}, DFT_{80}, and DFT_{90}. One can theoretically define a DFT_{95} or a DFT_{100}, but the number of shocks to establish a 95% success is excessive, and one can never guarantee 100% of anything. At implantation, testing can determine a DFT. Specific protocols are discussed later.

Alternatively, one can simply verify that the device, at its maximum output, has an adequate safety margin to defibrillate reliably. The role of verification is to confirm that the DFT is below a certain level and that the device can thus be safely implanted.[10, 14] The advantage of a verification approach is that one minimizes the number of shocks during the implantation and shortens its duration. If the device to be implanted is capable of maximum energy shocks at 30 J and a single shock at 15 J, or if two successive shocks at 20 J are successful in converting VF in the patient, then one could have a high degree of confidence that 30 J will be sufficient. The advantages of this approach are its simplicity and brevity. In patients in whom the amount of VF induction and shocks should be minimized, this approach would allow the implantation of a device with a minimal amount of testing. The disadvantages of using a verification approach are that the first shock energy may be set unnecessarily high and that there is no baseline DFT for tracking changes. There will also be no good DFT data for scientific comparisons.

The main method for determining the DFT is to induce VF in the patient, wait about 10 seconds, and deliver a shock of a given energy. If this shock is successful, VF is induced again, and a lower-energy shock is tried. If the shock was unsuccessful, a rescue shock is delivered, and a higher-energy shock is tried next. Various protocols, discussed later in this chapter, are used to determine the sequence of shocks, the number of shocks, and the calculation to determine the DFT.

Animal studies have shown that prolonged DFT testing with multiple inductions of VF can lead to hemodynamic compromise and decreased cardiac function.[15] Human results are mixed, and there is no clear consensus. One study showed no decrease in the mean ejection fraction but reported one patient whose ejection fraction decreased from 20% to 11%.[16] Two studies found that the only hemodynamic damage from VF testing was a significant impairment in diastolic filling.[17, 18] Another study found that, in the first hour after VF, there is no hemodynamic deterioration and, in fact, diastolic filling was *enhanced*.[19] Other studies have suggested that there is no morbidity from VF inductions for patients with left ventricular ejection fractions of more than (LVEF) 30%.[20] Patients with lower LVEFs, however, can have serious reductions in cardiac index, with reports of prolonged inotropic support being necessary in one case.

Another human study, which looked specifically at patients with LVEFs of 35% or less, found no deterioration, even with an average of nine inductions each.[21] In the Medtronic PCD trials, physicians were encouraged to find a combination of leads that would allow the implantation of the monophasic sequential shock device. Many of these patients received more than 50 shocks, with no reported trends in mortality and morbidity. Thus, there is considerable variation in the tolerance of repeated VF induction and defibrillation, even in patients with reduced ejection fractions. It is important to use clinical judgment at the time of implantation to assess the safety of repeated VF inductions. Patients with ejection fractions of less than 30% may need closer hemodynamic monitoring during and immediately after the implantation procedure. When defibrillation is followed by a prolonged episode of hypotension or marked bradycardia, it would be prudent to limit DFT testing to a verification protocol.

Initial electroencephalographic (EEG) data suggested that exceeding six inductions can cause, at least, transient cerebral dysfunction (defined as an increase in delta wave power on the EEG longer than 2.5 minutes).[22] More recent studies have shown that the duration of EEG changes is correlated with VF duration.[23, 24] These changes occur within 8 to 12 seconds of induction and last an average of about 1 minute.[23] A study of 36 patients with 286 inductions found that although EEG recovery time was correlated with VF duration, it was negatively correlated to the *number* of inductions.[25] Thus, there was no indication of a cumulative effect on the EEG of repeated induction of VF.

■ METHODS OF PERFORMING DEFIBRILLATION THRESHOLD DETERMINATION

Induction Methods

Before one can test a defibrillation shock, one must induce the fibrillation. There are four methods for inducing VF: (1) high-rate pacing, (2) delivering a shock on the T wave, (3) applying DC current across the defibrillation electrodes, and (4) delivering AC current across the defibrillation electrodes. The classic approach has been to use high-rate pacing. This was done with external control devices or through the implantable cardioverter-defibrillator (ICD). High-rate pacing has the advantage of being painless and using little energy. It has the disadvantage of being not uniformly successful, and it has significantly reduced effectiveness in patients taking amiodarone.

A popular method is shocking on the peak of the T wave (Fig. 23–3). This has the advantage of reliably inducing VF. It has an added advantage of providing a rough estimate of

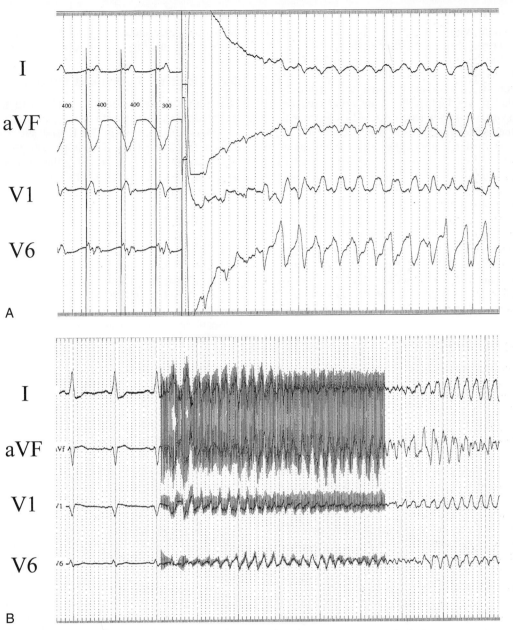

Figure 23–3. *A,* Induction of ventricular fibrillation with a shock on the T wave or with high-frequency stimulation. This method can reliably induce ventricular fibrillation in most clinical circumstances. Typically, a low-energy shock of 1 to 2 J, or about 100 to 200 V, is used. For a paced ventricular cycle length of 400 msec, the coupling interval of the shock is typically about 300 msec after the last paced beat. Such a shock likely generates one or more spiral waves in the myocardium. A polymorphic ventricular tachycardia or ventricular fibrillation is initiated immediately after the shock. The test shock for terminating the ventricular fibrillation is generally delivered for about 10 seconds. With device-based testing, however, the exact time of shock delivery is not controlled by the operator but rather depends on the time needed for device detection of the tachycardia and capacitor charge time. Thus, the duration of fibrillation may vary depending on the programmed strength of the shock. *B,* Induction of ventricular fibrillation with high-frequency pacing. The original style of accomplishing this used modulated AC current applied directly to the heart. With device based testing, however, this is usually accomplished with high-frequency pacing (20–30 msec cycle length) activated from the device at a high-voltage output.

the upper limit of vulnerability (ULV, discussed later in this chapter) to VF if the shock was unsuccessful in inducing fibrillation, provided that the timing of the shock in relationship to the T wave was correct. It has been suggested that an efficient strategy for inducing VF with this approach is to start with a 200-V shock about 10 msec before the peak of the T wave.[26] The T-wave shocking approach has three associated disadvantages. First, the shock generates pain, and thus the patient needs to be sedated more heavily than otherwise; however, the patient should generally be well sedated during DFT testing anyway. Second, the shock requires an alignment with the T wave. Third, the shock consumes some energy from the batteries of the ICD.

The third method is to apply a low-voltage DC current, about to 5 to 12 V, across the defibrillation electrodes. This has usually been done with an external test approach in which the leads are implanted, but then connected to an external test apparatus. A 9-V battery provides a convenient DC source. One advantage of this approach is the high success rate for induction without the need for alignment to a T wave. There is no energy drainage for the ICD batteries. The disadvantages are possible plating of electrodes and the need to have an external connection to the fibrillation leads.

The final method for induction is the use of low-voltage AC current coupled directly to the defibrillation leads. Either 50 or 60 Hz AC (depending on the continent) has proved to be extremely effective for this role.[27] Transformer reduction to a 3-V level provides sufficient current to induce VF within 2 to 4 seconds in almost any subject. A disadvantage is the tetanic contraction of skeletal muscle often seen for the period of AC current application.

Determining the Defibrillation Threshold

It is important to understand the DFT both for historical and clinical reasons. The DFT must be exceeded by the capability of the device. In addition, even when the DFT is not evaluated explicitly, it must be evaluated implicitly by assessing an upper bound to verify that the device has a shock of sufficient magnitude to reliably defibrillate. This is what Singer and Lang[14] referred to as a "verification" approach. Finally, an explicit DFT must be calculated for research purposes if one wishes to demonstrate that a certain waveform or lead system has advantages over others.

The definition of DFT is deceptively simple. It is the electrical dosage required for defibrillation of the heart. This definition has two major subtleties. The first is the choice of units for the dosage. This issue is dealt with later in the chapter under The Energy Crisis. Historically, energy has been chosen to compare efficiency when comparing the DFT obtained by two different defibrillation systems. Although the use of energy is acceptable as a means of comparing DFTs, one must be aware that merely increasing the "delivered" energy does not necessarily translate to a better safety margin for defibrillation. Because of the ease with which the shock energy is measured, the amount of literature tied into energy, and its common use for thresholds, it has become accepted practice to speak of the DFT in terms of energy and to discuss safety margins in terms of units of energy. Thus, the discussion in this chapter is focused on joules of energy for defibrillation.

The second subtlety in the definition of the DFT is the alleged probabilistic nature of the dose–response curve for defibrillation.[28] The probabilistic character of defibrillation efficacy inherent in this curve may be due to random variation in the size of the myocardial mass,[29] conductive properties of myocardial cells,[30] or systematic alteration of cellular or tissue electrophysiologic characteristics involved in the initiation and perpetuation of VF.[31] We say "allegedly probabilistic" because no one has been able to establish that the dose–response relationship is truly probabilistic on a level comparable to, for instance, electron position in quantum mechanics. In fact, evidence suggests that a large portion of the probabilistic nature of the shock response is actually a result of our inability to time the shock better.[32–34]

Defibrillation Threshold Protocols

The simplest protocol for the DFT is to reduce the shock amplitude until a shock fails to defibrillate. This is known as a *step-down protocol*. The lowest successful shock level is then called the DFT. This approach gives, on average, a DFT estimate that approximates the 70% success level.[35–37] However, given the probabilistic nature of a shock's success in converting VF, such a determination of DFT may have as low an overall success rate as 25%. Thus, one would need a device that has a maximum output of about twice the energy of the DFT to be confident that it would defibrillate reliably. For example, a DFT of 15 J would require that the device have a maximum output of 30 J. When the DFT measured in this manner is at 20 J, one does not have the confidence that this device would work properly. One means of reducing the need for such a large safety margin is to require two consecutive successful shocks at the lowest successful energy. This DFT has been referred to as a DFT+, indicating the two shock successes at this energy.[14] With a DFT+ determination, there is a greater likelihood that this DFT is at the upper end of the DFT curve. Thus, one can reduce the required safety margin. For a DFT+ of 20 J, one can implant a 30-J device. Similarly, with three consecutive successful shocks at 25 J (DFT++), one can implant a device with 30-J maximum output.

To arrive at a more accurate estimate of DFT, one could average a step-down and a step-up value.[38] The most popular method for determining a DFT has been the classic step-up and step-down method first popularized by the Purdue group.[2, 35] With this protocol, the attempted shock strength begins at a high level. It is then reduced with a fixed step until failure to defibrillate occurs. Typical fixed steps are 2 J or 100 V. After failure to defibrillate occurs, the direction is then reversed, and the shock strengths are increased by a finer step, such as 1 J or 50 V. This protocol is simple to perform, and the DFT is defined as the lowest amplitude for a successful shock. The disadvantage of this protocol is that it can require many shocks and is not extremely accurate. The mean estimate tends to overestimate the DFT_{50} with a fairly wide error band.

A variant on the step-up and step-down method is the three-reversal approach.[39] With this approach, the step sizes are kept fixed. After stepping down to failure, the steps are increased until success occurs. At this point, the steps are reversed again until failure occurs again. At this point, the third reversal is assumed on paper, which assumes that one more step up would result in success. All of the shock energies from the lowest-energy successful shock in the first step out to the final "paper" shock are then averaged. This approach has the advantage of giving a more accurate estimate of the DFT and has proved useful in research studies comparing the relative benefits of different waveforms.[40] The disadvantage of this reversal approach is that it requires numerous shocks.

An example of the three-reversal approach is as follows. Shock energies were reduced by 1 J at a time, with the lowest successful shock being 8 J. Reduction to 7 J found failure. The first reversal was then performed, and the shocks went up to 8 J (another failure) and to 9 J before success was seen again. The second reversal then occurred, the shock being reduced to 8 J, which found a failure. The final reversal then was the paper shock, which assumed that a 9-J shock would be successful. The DFT estimate then is the average of the shocks (in order) of 8, 7, 8, 9, 8, and 9 J, which is 8.16 J. The inclusion of the higher paper shock balances the downward bias from including the failure shocks and results in an accurate, unbiased estimation of DFT_{50}.

In practical clinical applications, it is typical to use a step-down method with coarse steps, such as 5 J. This allows for the determination of an approximate DFT while exposing the patient to the minimum number of shocks. In an attempt to achieve a high resolution DFT estimate by staying with a lower number of shocks, the binary search technique has been suggested. With this approach, the range of possible values for the DFT is continually cut in half to focus rapidly on the DFT. This approach is best explained by example. For a 32-J device, the first attempt at a shock would be 16 J. If that shock is successful, then the energy is cut in half to 8 J. Assuming that the shock was a failure, the next energy attempted is halfway between 8 and 16 J, or 12 J. If the 12-J shock was a failure, the energy is cut in half again, and 14 J is tried. The procedure is continued until the desired resolution is obtained. The advantage of a binary search is that it gives high resolution with few shocks. The disadvantage is that the high resolution may be misleading because is not necessarily associated with high accuracy.

Malkin has derived a unique approach, which would appear to combine the best features of all of the DFT protocol techniques in his Bayesian technique.[41] This has also proved useful in scientific studies.[42] Depending on the number of shocks one is willing to use, Malkin has published tables and formulas to give the exact sequence of shocks. Then, depending on the success and failure of each of the shocks, there is an optimal Bayesian estimate of the actual DFT. Malkin has published one version that combines this with the ULV approach.[43]

Upper Limit of Vulnerability

There is a time interval near the peak of the T wave (within 40 msec) known as the vulnerable period during which a shock of sufficient but not too great a magnitude will induce VF. When such a shock generates an electric field with its voltage gradient not parallel to a repolarizing wavefront, it initiates a spiraling wavefront around a critical point, which can initiate VF. As one increases the shock strength, there is a limit above which VF can no longer be induced. This ULV to VF has been demonstrated to correlated well with the DFT. That is, shocks with energies above the ULV should defibrillate the heart as well.[44] This concept can also explain the probabilistic nature of defibrillation. In the myocardial regions of relative low-voltage gradients, the exact orientation of a repolarizing wavefront with the local voltage gradient generated by a shock is a random phenomenon. Thus, the vulnerable zone of shock strengths for initiating (or reinitiating) VF in that region follows a probabilistic distribution.

The clinical attraction of the ULV approach is that one could perform implantation testing of the DFT with the use of only actual VF induction. That approach would work as follows. Shocks are delivered synchronized to the T wave (in a sinus or paced rhythm) at a high energy and decreased in a stepwise fashion with successive shocks. If the 20-J shock fails to induce VF, it must be greater than the ULV and hence greater than the DFT. Note that the patient was not put into fibrillation with that shock. The shock strength then is reduced successively until either a sufficiently weak shock does not induce VF (which means that there was no induction of VF) or the first VF occurs, which, in turn, has significance similar to a failed defibrillation shock.

The timing of the shock within the T wave is crucial. The peak ULV within the vulnerable zone is not necessarily at the peak of the T wave and can vary from patient to patient. In isolated rabbit hearts, accuracy with monophasic shocks appears to be optimized with a delivery in the up slope, whereas shocks at or after the peak are best for the biphasic waveforms.[45] Accuracy and repeatability are improved with multiple shock positions within the T wave. For example, the shock is delivered at the peak and 20 msec before.[46] One can also add a third shock position of 40 msec before the T-wave peak.[47, 48] This also results in a higher estimate of the probability of defibrillation success. To use this method as a reliable approach to predict successful defibrillation, one should apply this approach at varying intervals before the peak of the T wave, for example, 0, 20, and 40 msec.

Although there occasionally are significant differences between the ULV and DFT,[49] the two values correlate well regardless of the pacing site,[50] presence of ischemia,[51] whether testing is acute or chronic,[52] electrode polarity,[53] and waveform durations.[53] The disadvantage of the ULV approach is the high number of shocks that need to be delivered for a reliable determination of defibrillation efficacy. The advantage is that one can minimize the induction of VF. The ULV and DFT are both predictors of a shock strength that defibrillates with a given probability of success. The prediction of defibrillation efficacy is actually more important than the precise correlation between ULV and DFT.

Verification

The verification approach is used to ensure that the maximum output of the ICD is well above the DFT without actually determining a DFT. Singer and Lang[14] have provided a classification of various approaches to verification. Their one-shock verification protocol means that one low-energy shock was given that was successful in defibrillating the heart. This assumes that this shock was so low in strength that even though it was tested only once, there was a large margin between that low-energy shock and the much higher output of the device. For example, if the low-energy shock of 10 J terminated VF, then one can have reasonable confidence that a device with a maximum output of 27 J would defibrillate reliably. Similarly, one could use a two-shock protocol, in which two shocks of identical energy are used to defibrillate. With this protocol, one can reduce the amount of margin between that energy and the output of the device. For further detail, the reader is invited to read their book chapter and article.[14, 54]

Equipment for Defibrillation Threshold Testing

Classically, external implant support devices were used to generate fibrillation induction and defibrillation shocks. With the use of the unipolar approach, device-based testing has become more popular.[55, 56] However, one can certainly use a "dummy" can as a proxy and use an external support device for determining the threshold.

The advantages of performing device-based testing over using an external support device are numerous. First, the device operator can be confident that there is a perfect match between the waveform for the testing and the waveform that will be used for the therapy. The operator can also be confident that the measurements of the shock amplitude and impedance will match. A third advantage is that the lead connections are all being well exercised with each shock that is being used. A fourth advantage is that the exact same sensing circuit and algorithm are exercised. Finally, the storage and maintenance of the external device is avoided. Major disadvantages of the external devices are that they are not updated as frequently as the actual ICD and that the sensing amplifiers, filters, and sensing algorithms are rarely identical to those of the ICD. Thus, sensing performance is not adequately tested in many cases with the external system.

The advantages of using the external box are that shock energy is conserved for later therapies in the ICD. Second, higher-energy rescue shocks can be used if bailout becomes necessary. Third, the use of the external support device for defibrillation testing gives the physician the flexibility of choosing a lower-energy ICD (presumably much smaller) for the final implant. This can be done without breaking the sterility of the smaller device, which may be a risk if it is unable to perform the defibrillation.

Regardless of the device used for testing DFT, backup defibrillation is essential. The most common approach is to use a 360-J external defibrillator with flexible adhesive patches attached to the chest. These adhesive patch electrodes are relatively radiolucent and generally donot obstruct the view under fluoroscopy during the implantation procedure. A typical anteror posterior placement of these electrodes keeps them out of the operating field. It is important to verify the proper placement of the internal defibrillation leads and the absence of a pneumothorax before initiating VF for DFT testing. Occasionally, with a pneumothorax, even the external device will not successfully defibrillate the patient.[57] When implanting a device that has a lower maximum-energy output, it may be necessary to have an external defibrillation device ready to attach to the leads in case the implanted device does not defibrillate at its maximum output. The external device would generally provide a high-output rescue shock capability. One backup approach has been to use two external devices with skin patches applied close to each other. The shock is delivered from both in close succession by simultaneously pressing the discharging buttons on both devices. However, this approach may be an advantage only in large patients, in whom transcutaneous impedance may be high and the average current density in the heart may be low. In cases in which external defibrillation is difficult, intramyocardial current may be shunted in some manner. For example, if the RV apex electrode is shorted to

the ICD can or the SVC electrode in some manner, shunting of current through this path may decrease external defibrillation efficacy. If all external defibrillating attempts fail, extracorporeal cardiopulmonary bypass using peripheral vessel access can be tried if such equipment is readily available.

How Much Shock Energy Is Enough?

Two main questions remain on the issue of energy sufficiency. First, does the device have enough safety margin in its output over the DFT to ensure reliable therapy for the patient? Second, at what energy output should the first (and maybe second) shock amplitude be set? Although there is some overlap in the considerations for these two questions, they are actually quite different.

For the first question, we have presumably determined the DFT or an upper bound on it through a verification protocol. How much additional energy must the device have to give an adequate safety margin for implantation? Early systems occasionally had DFT shifts of more than 10 J, and patient deaths resulted or revisions occurred.[58, 59] The classic rule of thumb was that a 10-J safety margin was sufficient, and this rule has achieved the status of accepted medical practice. Others have championed a safety margin equal to the DFT.[79] In other words, the device maximum shock capability must be equal to *twice* the DFT for successful implantation. Originally, this was a significantly more conservative role than the 10-J safety margin. With thresholds now typically being single digit, however, this rule is actually more liberal than the 10-J safety margin.[60] With a DFT of less than 6 J, the setting of twice the DFT gave a 95% success rate, whereas using the classic DFT plus 10 J rule gave 99.5% successful conversions.[60] When the DFT is very low, such as 4 J or less, using twice the DFT energy may render only a 67% successful first shock.[61] Thus, when the DFT is below 5 J, it would be more reliable to set the first shock energy with a safety margin of at least 7 J to achieve a first shock defibrillation success rate of 96%.

Finally, one should not take excessive comfort in a low DFT because these numbers may have less stability (or confidence) associated with them. A shock of twice the energy had a success rate of 98% for patients with a DFT of more than 4 J but only a 67% success rate for those with a DFT of less than 4 J![61] The Malkin-Bayesian approach may be used to calculate the shock strength required to achieve a conversion rate of 95%.[62, 63]

The safety margin is needed to cover two basic problems—first, due to the probabilistic nature of the defibrillation dose–response curve, a shock must have higher energy than the DFT to give a reasonable confidence of defibrillation (i.e., the shock strength should be that which would suggest a near 100% probability of success). A more difficult number to estimate is the required level of "insurance" against long-term drift in the DFT. Chronic DFT rises have been reported with the early monophasic devices[64–67]; other reports found no increase even with monophasic devices.[68, 69] It is not clear that this is a problem with modern biphasic transvenous devices.[69–71] One study has reported a rise in chronic biphasic thresholds,[72] whereas the typical result is a rise over the first 1 or 2 months, followed by a gradual return to the implantation values. Although an earlier study of an animal model using epicardial patches suggested that rapid pacing–induced cardiomyopathy would elevate defibrillation threshold,[73] a more recent animal study of transvenous endocardial defibrillation has shown that progressive heart failure does not increase the DFT.[74]

Although the mean values of DFT in these studies using transvenous lead systems do not appear to show marked increases, clearly there are individual cases in which significant increases in DFT occur. The reasons for long-term changes in DFT are not well understood. One can imagine that fibrosis might tend to increase resistance, and it often does. However, these increases in resistance have not been correlated with the increases in DFTs that one might expect. Lead shifts can significantly affect the DFT, although confirmed cases of a chronic DFT being affected by a lead shift (short of a complete dislodgment) are relatively rare. There are also circadian changes in the DFT, with a somewhat higher value in the morning than in the afternoon, corresponding to the peak incidence of failed first shocks in response to clinical tachycardias.[75] The need for antiarrhythmic drug therapy could arise in patients who have an ICD either for the treatment of atrial arrhythmia or for suppression of frequent ventricular arrhythmias. These can also affect the DFT, as discussed later. A pneumothorax can lead to increased DFTs.[57, 76, 77] Thus, multiple factors can lead to changes in DFT after implantation that would make an adequate safety margin of the shock energy important.

Setting the First Shock Energy

Traditionally, it was believed that the shock energies for VF should all be set to the maximum output of the device because one "just couldn't take a chance." Now with typical threshold being in the single digits, however, this practice has come into question. There are several problems with using excessive shock energy. The first is that the charge time is directly proportional to the shock energy. Thus, the charge time to a 10-J shock is one third of that for the 30-J shock. This delayed therapy can increase thresholds, increase dysfunction, and increase the chance of accidental sequelae.

In addition, the idea that a maximum-energy shock has a better chance of success than low-energy shock is not universally true. The dose–response curve for defibrillation is not monotonic. Above a certain level, the success rate may begin to go down from near 100%. Although the voltage output of clinical devices does not typically generate this phenomenon, it is still seen clinically from time to time.[78] A report comparing the setting of the first shock to twice the DFT with the device maximum of 34 J demonstrated no significant difference in the incidence of first shock conversion of spontaneous ventricular tachyarrhythmia. The lower setting actually had a *higher* first shock conversion rate (98.5% versus 92%).[79]

The third problem with the use of maximum-energy shocks is that higher-energy shocks can temporarily cause depressed ventricular function. Although this is seen only occasionally, it may last for multiple seconds, delaying the hemodynamic recovery from the VF. Thus, if the goal is to have the patient regain good cardiac output and consciousness as soon as possible, the use of a maximum-energy shock could actually be counterproductive.

■ FACTORS THAT AFFECT THE DEFIBRILLATION THRESHOLD

Lead Systems

The current defibrillation leads typically have either a single shocking electrode located in the right ventricle or two shocking electrodes with the second one located on the proximal portion of the lead, positioning it in the superior vena cava. The advantage of the two-electrode lead is its ease of use. It has the pace/sense electrodes and both shocking electrodes on one lead, allowing for implantation with a single insertion (the single-pass lead). However, separate leads for the two shocking electrodes may allow for better positioning of the proximal electrode. Occasionally, better results are reported from placing the proximal electrode up in the innominate vein[80, 81] or the subclavian vein.[82] In general the left brachiocephalic vein does not appear to offer improved threshold.[83] Various patients have their lowest DFTs with this proximal lead in different locations.[84]

A more recent innovation has been the use of the device can itself as an electrode (the unipolar approach). With the device sizes now in the 45-cc range and further size reductions in progress, pectoral implantation of the ICD generator has become almost universally feasible. The can electrode has reduced defibrillation threshold by about 30% over previous transvenous lead systems.[85, 86] In fact, these so-called unipolar systems now offer thresholds that are comparable to those seen with monophasic shocks using epicardial patches. This is clearly the preferred system for minimizing the DFT. In most patients, using the right ventricular (RV) shocking electrode in conjunction with the can electrode provides adequate DFT for implantation of a device without the need for another electrode. This configuration can allow use of a thinner transvenous lead. Furthermore, such a unipolar lead may be more reliable because no high-voltage differences would exist within the lead body.

Adding a patch or subaxillary array can reduce thresholds as compared with a simple transvenous (i.e., cold can) system.[87, 88] A subcutaneous patch may actually be as effective as an epicardial patch.[89] Based on the evidence from the use of dual patches,[90, 91] this should help even with the use of a can electrode. The addition of such a patch electrode is helpful in reducing DFT through several potential mechanisms. The most direct one is that the overall system impedance decreases; therefore, for a given maximum voltage from the ICD, the current increases. In addition, there may be a shift of the higher intramyocardial voltage gradients toward the left ventricular apex. Finally, for a tilt-based waveform, by lowering the resistance, the extra patch electrode decreases the shock time constant, reduces the first-phase pulse width of a biphasic shock, making it closer to the human chronaxie, and improves the efficiency of the waveform.

The most important electrode in transvenous defibrillation systems is the one placed in the right ventricle, although it obviously cannot function in isolation. While this coil is typically placed in the RV apex, there is some evidence that even better DFTs can be obtained by placing it in the septum near the outflow tract.[92, 93]

Assuming a right ventricular coil and a can electrode in the left pectoral region, a natural question arises: To what extent will the addition of a superior vena cava (SVC) lead reduce thresholds? It probably makes no difference for most patients,[94] but, in some patients, it can lower thresholds.[95, 96] The reason for the lowering of threshold with the addition of an SVC electrode may be related to the decrease in shock impedance rather than the improved distribution of current in the myocardium. Again, although the vector may not be ideal, the simple act of lowering the resistance helps for two reasons—first, it allows more current to run through the septum, and second, by lowering the resistance, the waveform may be narrowed more closely to optimum durations.

A report confirms such an explanation by demonstrating that addition of an SVC electrode lowers DFT energy but *increases* the current at DFT.[96] Because an increased current is associated with higher tissue voltage gradients, the lower DFT energy was actually associated with a higher DFT in terms of tissue voltage gradient, implying a less efficient distribution of current through the myocardium. Because DFTs using the RV coil to pectoral can defibrillation pathway typically are 10 J or less, it is unclear whether using a single-pass lead has any significant advantage over using a lead with only one RV shocking electrode. Curiously, placing a second electrode in the coronary sinus does not appear to reduce DFT further in a left pectoral can to RV apex electrode system.[97]

In certain clinical circumstances, the right pectoral region is not available for implantation of an ICD generator. Infection, a pre-existing pacemaker, or other anatomic problems may prevent implantation in that region. Whereas a left-sided approach gives the best DFTs for the endocardial can electrode systems,[98] animal[99] and clinical data suggest that placement of the generator in the right side[100–102] or even over the abdomen[99, 103] allows achievement of reasonable DFTs. With the abdominal implantation site, the use of an SVC lead appears to offer significant advantage and should probably be used routinely even with a hot can.[99] With the downsizing of the generator that has occurred since the early 1990s, one may question whether reduction of the can electrode size may influence DFT. However, the can size, at least within the anticipated range of potential reductions, does not appear to have significant influence of DFT.[104, 105] Interestingly, the radius of the RV electrode[106] or the surface area of the RV electrode,[107] within reasonable bounds, has little effect on the DFT. One study found a small benefit in using an 11F versus a 7F SVC electrode.[108] The polarization of the RV electrode during shock delivery may contribute to increased impedance and affect the DFT. Niebauer and colleagues[109] reported a decrease in DFT in animal studies when using iridium oxide–coated electrodes and attributed this decrease to the reduced polarization associated with such coating.

Shock Waveforms

Because of the clearly demonstrated benefits of biphasic waveforms, all ICDs now harbor biphasic waveforms.[110] Several factors, however, affect the efficiency of biphasic waveforms.

Capacitance

The choice of defibrillation capacitance values ranges from 90 to 150 microfarad (μF). Defibrillation models all show that the optimal capacitance is inversely related to the inter-electrode resistance.[111–113] To be precise, the product of the resistance and the capacitance should be about 80% of the chronaxy value.[111] Thus, in a patient with a chronaxie of 5 msec[114] and a resistance of 50 Ω, the optimal capacitance is 80 μF. Numerous animal and clinical studies have shown the benefits of reductions in the capacitance value from the conventional values of 140 to 150 μF.[40, 115–118]

The benefit of the reduced capacitance values is, of course, more dramatic in patients with higher resistance.[119] The converse is also true. With extremely low resistance pathways, there is little or no benefit. For example, one study with an average resistance of 32 Ω found no difference between a 125-μF and a 450-μF capacitor—although the tilts and durations were not held constant.[120]

The benefit of the smaller capacitance values probably accrues from the shortening of the first phase so that its duration is closer to the defibrillation chronaxie. In addition, the second phase is closer to the passive time constant required for optimum membrane discharge as described by the so-called "burping hypothesis."[121] A simple example explains why this is so crucial for the patient with high resistance. Imagine a device with the classic capacitance of 140 μF, a patient with an impedance of 70 Ω, and an ICD of a 65% tilt for both phases. The first phase duration is 10 msec, and the second phase duration is also about 10 msec. Both these phases are significantly longer than the chronaxie (3 to 5 msec) and passive membrane time constant (2 to 4 msec), respectively. If in the same situation the output capacitance were 70 μF, these durations would be halved and much closer to optimal.

For the average patient, the best capacitance value is probably about 90 μF.[122] One concern about using lower capacitance values is that, even though they have lower-energy DFTs, they store less energy for a given fixed voltage level. With the limits of capacitor voltages using current technology, the maximum stored energy would be reduced in proportion to the capacitance. Thus, the resulting safety margin may not, in fact, be improved. However, if future technology would permit higher voltages in capacitors, smaller capacitors, in the 50 to 60 μF range, may be optimal. In addition, for patients with DFTs below 10 J, a maximum energy of 18 to 20 J can provide appropriate safety margins. With current and improving lead systems, most patients may fall into this category. Thus, for these patients, a smaller capacitance would allow the use of a smaller device. At present, outside of receiving shocks, the size of the device is still the most aggravating issue for most patients receiving an ICD. Thus, size reduction may have significant psychological benefit in improving patients' quality of life. Finally, smaller capacitance tends to improve the DFT in patients with high shock electrode impedance at implantation. Because the impedance stays relatively constant with implanted lead systems, smaller capacitance may be most helpful in these patients.[111, 122, 123]

Pulse Durations

Assume that the ICD already has the optimal capacitance for defibrillation. It is now well understood that a major function of the first phase is to act as a monophasic shock designed to synchronize most of the myocytes by extending their refractory periods.[121, 124] Thus, the first phase should be set at between 3 and 5 msec because this is the typical range for the human chronaxie.[114, 122] However, if one has a large capacitance value (i.e., more than 100 μF), a compromise is in order. A duration roughly equal to the average of the chronaxy and shock time constant is required. This is to achieve a balance between the chronaxie and the need to deliver a charge from the capacitor. Consider a 50-Ω electrode system with a 140-μF capacitor. This time constant is simply their product, which is 7 msec. Choosing a 4-msec chronaxie, the optimal first phase duration should then be the average of the 4 and the 7, or about 5.5 msec.

The second phase is far simpler. Regardless of the shock time constant or the impedance, the second phase duration should be set at slightly less than the passive membrane time constant to actively "burp" the cell membrane.[42, 121, 125] This duration should be in the order of 2.5 to 3 msec for optimal performance. Simply reducing the second (and first) phase duration from standard settings tends to lower the DFT in clinical studies.[126–128] The effect of optimizing the first and second phase durations is sometimes dramatic, as can be seen in studies using devices for which these durations are programmable.[129]

Some devices have their durations determined in terms of tilt instead of fixed times. This is an acceptable approach for the first phase duration, because some adjustment for the first phase duration is warranted for changes in resistance. On average, a tilt-based first phase performs no worse or no better than a fixed time period first phase. The fixed time duration has no means for adjustment, so the tilt-based system may overadjust. Imagine the case of a patient's impedance increasing to 100 Ω with a 140 μF capacitor and 65% tilt. This would result in a first phase duration of 14 msec. This is at least *triple* the chronaxie. For the second phase, use of the tilt-based duration is highly nonoptimal based on our present understanding of the operation of the biphasic waveform. The tilt approach would tend to make the second phase increase in proportion to impedance, while the burping theory suggests that the second phase duration should actually *decrease* slightly with increases in durations.[121, 125]

More complex waveforms under study may lower thresholds even further than those achieved by using lower capacitance. These so-called parallel-series waveforms achieve a more "square" first phase while leaving enough charge for a fully functioning second phase to operate. Such a waveform operates by running multiple capacitors in parallel for a few

milliseconds and then, after they have discharged sufficiently, switching them to series, which brings the upper voltage back up to near the initial voltage.[130, 131] Another improvement may occur with waveform approximations to the ascending ramp. Ascending-ramp waveforms theoretically outperform the conventional descending waveform because the ascending ramp more closely tracks the required charging of the cell membrane. The difficulty has been in generating an ascending ramp from an implantable device. The ramp may be approximated by sequentially "stacking" the capacitors on top of each other during the progress in the first phase. Thus, the first part of the first phase has just one capacitor delivering charge, whereas the second part has two capacitors in series, and the third part has three capacitors in series. Such an arrangement has the potential to reduce thresholds of biphasic waveforms by an additional 20% to 30%.

Shock Polarity

The defibrillating shock polarity may have some importance for the DFT. Because most ventricular pacing is done with the tip as a cathode, it was naturally assumed that this polarity was appropriate for defibrillation. However, it is clear that with monophasic waveforms, the use of anodal defibrillation significantly reduces thresholds over those found with cathodal defibrillation.[132, 133] The same changes have been found—although not as dramatic or as consistent—for biphasic waveforms. A listing of recent reports on the influence of first phase polarity of biphasic shocks on DFT is shown in Table 23–1.[134–138] These studies covered 110 patients and showed an average reduction in DFTs of 16% when the RV electrode started the shock as an anode. This was the best polarity for 46% of the patients, whereas 42% had equal DFTs with either polarity. It is interesting to note the varied findings. Natale and colleagues[136] and Keelan and associates[138] found the anodal configuration superior, Strickberger and coworkers[137] found no difference between the two polarities.

Animal studies with more optimal biphasic waveforms, those with a short phase 1 duration and a phase 2 duration closer to optimal burping, have shown no superiority of either polarity.[139] It may be that polarity makes no difference in optimal biphasic waveforms, and to the extent that the waveforms are suboptimal, they resemble monophasic waveforms in demonstrating lower DFTs in the anodal configuration. Observations by Efimov and colleagues[140] relating to

Table 23–1. Influence of Right Ventricular Electrode Polarity on Defibrillation Threshold

Investigators	No. of Patients	RF+ (J)	RV− (J)	Reduction in Mean (%)	Lower RV+	Lower RV−	Equal DFT
Schauerte et al, 1997[134]	27	11.1	13.3	17	10	3	14
Shorofsky and Gold, 1996[135]	26	11.1	12.2	9	—	—	—
Natale et al, 1995[136]	20	16.3	21.5	24	12	2	6
Strickberger et al, 1995[137]	15	9.9	9.5	−4	3	3	9
Keelan et al, 1997[138]	10	6.6	10.8	39	7	0	3
Keelan et al, 1997[138]	12	12	16.3	26	7	2	3
Merged	110			16	39	10	35
Percentage of patients					46	12	42

the presence of the "virtual electrode" effect surrounding the RV shock electrode may provide an explanation of these empiric observations. The virtual electrode effect induces regions of high transmembrane voltage gradient as well as points of phase singularity. This combination of high-voltage gradients near a point of phase singularity can generate re-entrant wavefronts.[141] Anodal shocks appear less able to induce re-entrant wavefronts that persist to reinitiate VF, probably because of propagation of these wavefronts from a surrounding area of depolarization toward a central area of hyperpolarization. On the other hand, cathodal shocks generate wavefronts that propagate away from a central area of depolarization, rendering wavefronts more likely to spread to the rest of the ventricle. Biphasic shocks, through the burping function, appear to counteract the persistence of the virtual electrode effect. If this were the primary mechanism by which biphasic shocks are superior to monophasic ones, optimized biphasic shocks would not demonstrate a polarity preference in defibrillation because they would eliminate or minimize the virtual electrode effect.

Timing of the Shock

Timing of the shock during ventricular fibrillation may be important. At present, a shock is synchronized to ventricular activation at the sensing electrode, usually located at the RV apex or sometimes in the RV outflow or mid-septum. In the future, however, this timing may change. Ventricular fibrillation may have periods of greater organization or susceptibility to shock termination. For example, timing the shock to large amplitude points on the electrocardiogram (ECG) may reduce the DFT.[142, 143] The absence of such timing in shock delivery during DFT determination and in current ICDs may contribute to the probabilistic nature of defibrillation.[33, 34, 144, 145]

Greater coherence of myocardial activation suggests fewer random wavefronts. Shocks delivered during periods of fibrillation with greater coherence of ventricular activation appear to have a better chance of success with equal energies than shocks delivered in other periods.[146] Timing the shock to activation as opposed to repolarization of left ventricular regions where the voltage gradient is the lowest, such as the left lateral portion of the ventricular free wall in a transvenous lead system, may also improve defibrillation. Presumably, shocks that occur during repolarization in those regions are more likely to induce spiral waves when the local voltage

gradient is below the threshold of the ULV—5 V/cm for monophasic waveforms.

The influence of VF duration on DFT is somewhat controversial. Many studies have shown that the DFT increases steadily for monophasic shocks.[147, 148] This can be shown for shocks delivered from 2 seconds to 9 minutes after induction of VF and has been attributed to increases in adenosine levels.[149, 150] The situation for biphasic waveforms, however, is much more controversial. Although early animal studies suggested that the DFT for biphasic waveforms also increased with time, more recent papers have challenged that notion, even suggesting that the threshold may dip to a minimum at about 20 seconds after VF initiation.[151] In the time interval between onset of VF and delivery of the first or even the second shock from an ICD, however, it is unlikely that VF duration would affect defibrillation efficacy.

Finally, the time of day affects the DFT, just as most human functions are affected by the human circadian rhythm. DFTs are higher in the morning,[75] which unfortunately is when the incidence of tachyarrhythmias also peaks.[152]

Drugs

Most antiarrhythmic and anesthetic drugs can affect the DFT. However, reports on these influences are mixed and may depend on whether a monophasic or a biphasic waveform was used in the study. These reports are listed in Table 23–2.[153–221] Pharmacologic therapy is often used in patients with ICDs to minimize the frequency of therapy delivery by the device. Because some antiarrhythmic drugs also affect the DFT, the effects of antiarrhythmic therapy on the DFT are important to consider when establishing safety margins during the ICD implantation or testing and when the pharmacologic therapy is modified.

Drugs That Increase the Defibrillation Threshold

Class IC drugs, such as encainide, can increase the DFT.[153] Fain and colleagues[190] reported on intravenous encainide and the two metabolites, o-dimethyl encainide (ODE) and 3-methoxy-ODE (MODE). Intravenous encainide and ODE increased the average DFT in dogs by 129% and 76%, respectively, from control values. The DFT returned to normal after washout. No significant increase in DFT was reported with MODE. Another Class 1C drug, flecainide, had widely divergent effects on DFT reported in different

Table 23–2. Antiarrhythmic Drug Effects on Defibrillation Threshold

Increase	No Change	Conflicting Reports	Decrease
Ajmaline[180]	Atenolol[193]	Amiodarone (acute)[182, 183, 198–200]	Clofilium[211]
Amiodarone (chronic)[181–187]	Disopyramide[194, 195, 215]	Bretylium[154, 166, 167, 192]	E-4031[212, 213]
Atropine[188]	MODE[190]	Flecainide[153–155, 195, 201, 212]	Ibutilide[214, 215]
Bidisomide[189]	Phenylephrine[193]	Isoproterenol[188, 193, 202]	LY-190147[216]
Diltiazem[180]	Phentolamine[193]	Lidocaine[180, 203–207]	MS-551[217]
Encainide[190]	Procainamide[196, 205, 206]	Moricizine[208–210]	Sotalol[218–220]
ODE[190]	Propafenone[197]	Mexiletine[163, 164, 204]	Tedisamil[221]
Recainam[191]		Quinidine[159, 161, 162]	
Verapamil[192]			

ODE, o-dimethyl encainide; MODE, 3-methoxy-ODE.

animal species. In dogs, it markedly raised the DFT, so that defibrillation was nearly impossible with the existing equipment.[201] Flecainide, however, was reported to have no effect on DFT in pigs.[154, 155] Recainam may increase the DFT.[191] Bidisomide (SC-40230), a class Ia/Ib agent, raises the DFT in dogs.[189]

Amiodarone, a class 3 drug, tends to elevate the DFT. Acutely, amiodarone may lower the DFT,[181, 182] but chronic oral administration of amiodarone may increase DFT.[184, 187, 198] Haberman and associates[181] reported two separate time dependencies: DFTs increased with longer exposure of an animal to the drug and also with longer VF duration.

Fogoros[184] reported on a case in which amiodarone increased the DFT, with return of the DFT to a baseline level after drug discontinuation. Guarnieri and coworkers[185] found larger increases in the DFT in patients taking amiodarone who were undergoing generator change. DFT increased from 10.9 ± 4.3 J to 20 ± 4.7 J. The mean DFT decreased in patients taking no antiarrhythmics or only class 1A agents. Epstein, and colleagues[186] found that 52% of patients with high DFTs (more than 25 J) at implantation were taking amiodarone. However, such elevated DFTs may reflect preselection of patients with poor prognosis rather than an intrinsic effect of amiodarone on the DFT. For example, one clinical study found no difference with chronic amiodarone use.[198] A rabbit study also found no chronic difference.[199] A canine study found an increase in DFT with chronic amiodarone use but no change with acute intravenous loading.[200] These differences may be caused by a metabolite and the total-body load of amiodarone.[156] Amiodarone and its metabolite, desethylamiodarone, are stored in cardiac tissue, which delays the drug's action on the myocardium and might explain the increase in DFTs for patients taking the drug long term.[157]

The selective potassium blocker, barium, lowers the DFT.[158] Ajmaline and calcium-channel blockers tend to increase the DFT.[192]

Drugs With Minimal Effects or With Conflicting Reports

Class 1A drugs have minimal effects on DFT. Dorian and associates[159] found no changes in DFT with quinidine infusion. In dogs and pigs, intravenous infusion of procainamide (15 mg/kg) had no significant influence on DFT.[160, 196] Procainamide generally has no effect on DFT in humans at the usual therapeutic doses.[205] Guarnieri and coworkers[185] reported that DFTs actually decreased in patients taking class 1A agents at the time of the generator replacement, compared with at the time of initial implantation. DFT increases were reported by Woolfolk and colleagues[161] and Babbs and associates[162] when using very high doses of quinidine in animal studies.

The class 1B drug mexiletine increased DFTs in a case report.[204] Animal studies, however, have shown little or no increase in the DFT using this drug.[163, 164] Moricizine does not affect DFTs in pigs[208] but increases the DFT in dogs,[209] especially in the presence of lidocaine.[210] One clinical report found a decrease in DFT, whereas another found an increase.[206, 208] Oral propafenone does not affect the human DFT.[197] Lidocaine raises the DFT in dogs,[203, 206] especially with monophasic waveforms.[165] One study in dogs found that lidocaine did not increase DFT when using chloralose

anesthesia, but a large increase in DFT was seen pentobarbital.[168]

Bretylium did not affect DFT in two animal studies.[159, 166] Interestingly, in another study, the DFT was reported to be lowered 15 to 90 minutes after intravenous bretylium tosylate (10 mg/kg) injection in dogs.[167] A study in pigs also showed a reduction in DFTs.[192]

Drugs that Decrease the Defibrillation Threshold

Potassium-channel blockers tend to decrease the DFT.[168] This effect is most likely a result of lengthening of the refractory period.[169] Clofilium blocks outward potassium current and can directly defibrillate. Tacker and coworkers[167] found that clofilium lowers the DFT in dogs, possibly as a result of its ability to increase the refractory period extension associated with a defibrillating shock.[170]

Ibutilide significantly lowers the DFT and occasionally causes spontaneous defibrillation.[214, 215] The research class III drug E-4031 cut the DFT in *half* in a dog study,[212] even in the presence of isoproterenol.[213] The experimental class III agent LY-190147 also lowers the DFT,[169] as does MS-551. Tedisamil increases the electrogram coherence and reduces the DFT.[221] D-Sotalol and DL-sotalol decrease the DFT in humans.[218–220]

What is the effect of β-adrenergic modulation? A dog study showed that isoproterenol decreased the DFT with a return to baseline after β-blockade.[171] However, others have reported a DFT increase with isoproterenol in dogs.[188, 202] and no change in pigs.[193] Aminophylline has been reported to decrease the DFT.[172] This effect, however, may be due to phosphodiesterase inhibition rather than its sympathomimetic effects.

Anesthetic Agents

Fentanyl reduces the DFT, as opposed to enflurane or pentobarbital.[173] The common inhalation agents and barbiturates, however, do not appear to have significant effects on measured DFTs in dog studies,[174] with the possible exception that they may interact with lidocaine to increase the DFT, as noted previously.

The Energy Crisis

Energy is used as the primary defibrillation dosage unit for unfortunate historical and nonscientific reasons. Although it is the dosage unit of common medical practice, energy simply does not defibrillate.

A simple *gedanken* experiment shows why this is the case. If merely delivering 70 J of energy to the heart would defibrillate, paramedics could save a lot of money by merely shooting a pistol into the heart of the patient. The 100 foot-pounds of energy from a .22 caliber pistol are equivalent to about 70 J—and this is "delivered" energy. If this example seems extreme, and one would like to limit the therapeutic universe to electrical energy, then we can still eliminate the ICD. One could merely turn on a pacer battery output of 3 V for 120 seconds. Assuming an impedance of 50 Ω, total energy delivered would be 3 V squared times 120 seconds divided by 100 Ω, which would be 21.6 J. This would eliminate the need for the bulky capacitors and inverter that drive the size of the present ICD. This is energy delivered directly to the heart, yet no one would ever imagine that that energy would defibrillate the heart.[175]

The confusion of energy with defibrillation has led to some accepted practices that are not justified. Scientifically, for example, the idea that energy defibrillated led to the corollary that the capacitance probably did not matter. As long as the capacitor stored enough energy, it did not matter if it was a smaller-value capacitance or a large-value capacitance. This delayed the arrival of the smaller-capacitance, higher-efficiency waveforms.

As unfortunate as the concept of energy for defibrillation is for understanding and optimization, the concept of "delivered" energy is even more damaging. This is the misconception that the more energy delivered to heart, the better the result. A related theme held that some systems are not subject to the vagaries of electrode impedance changes because they are able to "guarantee" a certain energy delivery. No ICD can actually determine exactly how much energy is delivered to the heart after the electrode–electrolyte interfaces and lung and muscle losses with, for example, an active can implant.

Simple reflection demonstrates that the concept of delivered energy has no scientific basis. It was demonstrated more than 20 years ago that truncating the shock with a monophasic waveform significantly decreases the DFT—in fact by up to 50%.[176] More recently, shortening of the exponential shock waveform by truncation did not demonstrate any deterioration in the DFT of delivered energy until the pulse width was shortened to the range of 5 to 6 msec. By truncating the shock, however, less energy is delivered, which violates the philosophy of delivered energy being the critical parameter for defibrillation.[111]

Transthoracic modeling studies have shown that current is far superior to an energy-based dosage parameter.[177] This has been confirmed in clinical studies.[178] Current, of course, has a direct relationship to tissue voltage gradient. That is, for a fixed electrode configuration, a higher current is associated with a higher tissue voltage gradient. In some situations, an increase in delivered energy may actually have a negative relationship to the average current of the pulse.

A more pernicious and damaging effect from the concept that more delivered energy would defibrillate better and provide greater safety margin is the example of increasing delivered energy by expanding the waveform. This approach, which has been blamed for patient deaths, can actually generate negative safety margins. There was a clinically studied device with higher-energy shocks of 21, 24, 28, and 33 J. While the voltage increased very slightly between the lowest and the highest of these four high-energy shocks, the pulse widths increased dramatically, from 4 out to 12 msec. Although the 33 J shock did in fact "deliver" the most energy, it had an as low or lower average current than any of the other shocks. Thus, patients whose DFT was found to be equal to one of the lower applied shocks (i.e., 21 J), could actually have a zero or negative safety margin when the device was set at the 33 J.

A further harmful effect comes from the attempt to apply the delivered energy concept to biphasic waveforms. By confusing the role of the second phase as just another means of delivering energy, some devices extend the second phase out proportionally to the resistance (by maintaining the same tilt) to guarantee the delivered energy of the whole waveform. This results in second phase durations that are significantly suboptimal, especially for patients with high resistance (see Table 23–1).

The final problem with this concept of delivered energy is that there is no consistent definition. Although marketing claims might suggest that some devices have magic eyes inside the heart to read this value, the truth is that different manufacturers simply take a different discount off of the stored energy (e.g., 11%) and label that as delivered energy. Other manufacturers, however, might use discounts of 2% and 5%, thus, there is no comparability between these numbers.

Despite the significant problems in the use of energy as the defibrillation dosage measurement, it is supported by a wealth of published literature and is given by every manufacturer. It has become accepted practice to measure thresholds in terms of joules. It is acceptable to use energy as a dosage measurement so long as the model of device, the lead resistance, the capacitance value, *and* the pulse duration are not changing.[179] If the model changes, one might assume that the capacitance values and durations are also changing. If any of those four items are changing and one needs to make a DFT comparison, then the average current should be calculated. Average current is very easy to calculate: it is simply equal to the capacitance times the peak voltage times the tilt divided by the pulse width in milliseconds. This calculation applies to the first phase.

Dosage calculations for the second phase are irrelevant and misleading. As recent literature would support, the small amount of charge delivered in a second phase merely functions as a counterbalance (albeit a very important one) to the deleterious actions of the first phase,[42, 121, 125] including the virtual electrode effects.[140, 141] If the pulse duration for phase 1 changes, ideally one would calculate the effective current, which corrects for changes in pulse duration. This is analogous to a rheobase value in pacing and defibrillation research. The effective current has a slightly modified formula from the average current. It is equal to the capacitance times the peak voltage times the tilt, all divided by the sum of the pulse duration and the chronaxie.

Table 23–3 lists the maximum outputs for several popular devices that are approved or in clinical trials. Phase 2 duration is shown next to the optimal adjusted phase two duration based on the charge burping model. The calculations are based on both a 40- and a 70-Ω impedance. The last column gives the theoretical effectiveness of the shock as it uses the phase 1 effective current adjusted for the action of the second phase as recommended or as a fixed duration.[42, 121] Note that the effectiveness does not always rank-correlate with the energy. That is, in many cases, a higher-energy device has lower effectiveness because of suboptimal capacitance values or durations. The effectiveness of the Contour ICD (St. Jude Medical, Sylmar, CA) can be increased significantly by reducing the pulse duration from the manufacturer's recommendations, as shown here.

■ APPROACH TO THE PATIENT WITH A HIGH DEFIBRILLATION THRESHOLD

Although certain clinical characteristics may be associated with high DFTs, the predictive value of these characteristics is generally not very accurate because of the wide variability of patients. A number of papers have attempted to predict the DFT from clinical data available before implantation. The results are mixed. Several studies have found no clinical

Table 23–3. Capacitance, Peak Voltage, and Current Output of Clinical Cardioverter-Defibrillators

Device	Capacitance	Phase 1 Tilt* (%)	Added Fixed Duration	Resistance	Phase 1 Duration (ms)	Resulting Tilt (%)	Peak Voltage	Stored Energy	Effective Current	Phase 2 Duration	Overall Efficacy
Mini I	140	60	0	40	5.1	60	700	34	6.4	3.4	6.4
	140	60	0	70	9.0	60	700	34	4.6	6.0	3.2
Mini II	115	60	0	40	4.2	60	700	28	5.9	2.8	5.9
	115	60	0	70	7.4	60	700	28	4.2	4.9	3.3
Sentinel	95	44	1.6	40	3.8	63	750	27	5.8	2.5	5.8
	95	44	1.6	70	5.5	56	750	27	4.2	2.5	4.2
Micro Jewel	120	65	0	40	5.0	65	750	34	6.5	5.0	4.9
	120	65	0	70	8.8	65	750	34	4.6	8.8	2.8
Contour II	150	65	0	40	6.3	66†	750	42	7.1	6.3	4.9
	150	65	0	70	11.0	67†	750	42	4.9	11.0	2.8
Angstrom II	110	65	0	40	4.6	68†	750	31	6.2	4.6	5.0
	110	65	0	70	8.1	65†	750	31	4.4	8.1	2.8

*Programmable to any duration to the nearest millisecond. The programmer-recommended durations are chosen to give approximately 65% tilts.
†Higher effective currents and higher overall efficacy obtained with shorter durations and tilts than those recommended and shown here.

predictors of high DFT, possibly because of limited sample size.[222–224] Other studies have found statistically significant predictors of a high DFT.[225–230] The most common predictors are male gender, large cardiac size, and large body size. Other predictors are wide QRS (more than 120 msec), high New York Heart Association (NYHA) class, VF as the presenting arrhythmia, and low ejection fraction. These characteristics are helpful in alerting the implanting physician to the potential for a higher DFT, but their predictive value in an individual patient is not good enough to be reliable. Thus, a large patient with an enlarged heart may not necessarily have a high DFT. Another and perhaps more reliable item to consider is the obvious one of the previously determined threshold. If DFTs at prior implantations were high, assuming that the electrodes were positioned in appropriate locations, then one should expect a high DFT at a device change-out, or when implanting a new system.

In a typical pectoral implantation of a hot can system, a patient with high DFTs is occasionally encountered. There are several approaches that can be used to lower the DFT. The first is to check that the RV electrode is in a reasonable position. Attempts can be made to reposition the RV electrode as far into the apex as possible. This may increase the voltage gradients in the area of low-voltage gradient located at the apical region of the left ventricular free wall. An alternative is to position the tip of the electrode in the high septum and RV outflow region while placing the proximal end of the electrode toward the apex. This configuration may also improve the DFT by bringing the main body of the electrode closer to the septum.

The addition of a right atrial and SVC lead can sometimes improve the DFT.[90, 96, 231] The mechanism of such lowering is primarily through the lowering of impedance, increasing the current of the shock and perhaps reducing pulse width. Fortuitously, this lowering of DFT is seen primarily in patients with higher DFTs without the SVC lead. Although pectoral device implantation is clearly becoming the standard, occasional clinical circumstances prevent the implantation of a pectoral device. Implantation of a device in the abdominal area may still be necessary in these patients. In the past, such implantation used a long single-pass lead containing both the RV electrode and an SVC electrode.

Incorporating the device canister into the shocking configuration by connecting the SVC and the abdominal can—as the same polarity can—significantly improves the DFT.[99] When an independent SVC electrode is available, one can consider positioning that electrode higher into the left inominate vein to attempt an improvement in the DFT.[81] Withdrawing the SVC electrode too far into the brachiocephalic region, however, may reduce any benefit of such an electrode because of higher impedance in this location.[83]

The addition of one or more subcutaneous patches in the left anterolateral or subaxillary parts of the chest may also improve the DFT.[232] Again, the mechanism may be lowering the impedance of the system, thus optimizing the pulse width and increasing the peak current for a particular shock energy.[90] The presence of epicardial patches from a prior ICD implantation may affect DFT. Animal studies have suggested that locating an inactive epicardial patch in low-voltage gradient areas of the apical left ventricular free wall, a not unusual area for such a patch, can markedly increase the DFT.[233, 234] However, a clinical study in patients in whom pectoral hot can systems were used did not demonstrate an unusually high DFT.[235] When encountering a high DFT of a newly implanted transvenous defibrillation system in which epicardial patches are present, consideration can be given to incorporating the existing left ventricular epicardial patch into the shocking configuration by connecting it to the RV electrode.[236]

For every trick to lower the patient's DFT, there are costs and benefits. Certainly a cost in terms of physician time exists, as do material costs. There are also patient costs with each trial of threshold lowering, resulting from additional time in VF and delivery of possibly unwanted additional shocks. Thus, the optimal path to getting the optimal DFT reduction should be followed. Additional leads bring additional potential complications.[237] Table 23–4 summarizes the various approaches to lowering the DFT in an order that could minimize these costs.

If all these maneuvers fail to provide an adequate safety margin for defibrillation, one can still consider implanting the device if defibrillation can be achieved on multiple testing with the highest output of the device. Clinical evidence suggests that these patients would nevertheless benefit

Table 23–4. Approaches to Reducing the Defibrillation Threshold in Patients Undergoing a Pectoral Device Implantation

Step	Percentage of Patients in Whom Benefit Is Possible	Negative Effects	Comments
Optimize durations	5–25	Not possible with MDT and CPI	Most helpful with high impedance
Try RV − polarity switch	An average of 16 (helps in 40% of patients)		May not help with optimized duration
Add atrial lead	0–15	More metal in the body	Benefit of the SVC lead is not well established with the active can[94, 184]
Disconnect SVC lead (if using a lead system that includes it)	0–15	Must cap off the lead pin unless using a system that allows switching off, such as Angeion	
Add subcutaneous lead	10–50	More metal in the body	

SVC, Superior vena cava; MDT, Medtronic, Minneapolis, MN; CPI, Cardiac Pacemakers Inc., St. Paul, MN.

from such an implant.[238] The alternative is to proceed to an epicardial or pericardial implant. A minimally invasive approach can incorporate a small patch over the apical portion of the left ventricular free wall into the shocking configuration by connecting it to the RV apex electrode of an active can pectoral system.

■ EVALUATION OF SENSING

The most crucial function for the ICD, of course, is to sense ventricular fibrillation. As opposed to ventricular electrograms during sinus rhythm, the electrograms during VF can vary widely in amplitude. In addition, the T wave may have sufficient amplitude during sinus rhythm to be sensed by the device. Various makes of ICDs have different engineering approaches to accomodate such variability. Thus, the best approach to assess VF detection is to induce VF and assess this function of the implanted device. The availability of annotation on the stored or telemetered real-time electrogram indicating detection of ventricular beats is helpful in analyzing the reliability of detection (Fig. 23–4). Because the variability of VF amplitude, some dropout of detection from

a beat-to-beat basis may be present in all devices. Such dropout, however, will not be long enough to divert the device from progressing to delivery of therapy in an expeditious manner.

Sensing of the T wave should be avoided, especially during nontachycardia rhythms, to avoid inappropriate activation of the device. The T wave may be large enough that it could be sensed as a ventricular event when the automatic gain control of the device is near its maximal amplitude. Although modern devices incorporate some form of automatic gain adjustment, some devices have means of adjusting the range of this adjustment. When feasible, ventricular sensing can be tested at maximal gains to see if the T wave would be sensed, and limits on such maximal gains may be programmable to avoid oversensing of the T wave. Some devices, for example, may maximize their gain after a paced event. Thus, the postpacing detection of the T wave would be an important test to perform.

A second sensing function that must be tested is interference from electrical pulses delivered from another device, typically a pacemaker. Although this problem may become less important as dual-chamber ICDs become more com-

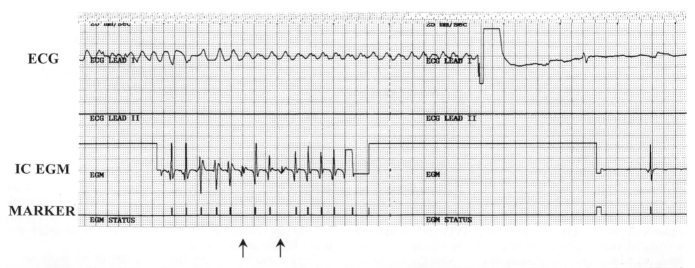

Figure 23–4. Telemetry of real-time ventricular electrogram detection markers during ventricular fibrillation. Most devices now have the capability of sending a marker signal by means of telemetry to an external programmer to indicate the exact timing of ventricular detection in relation to the recorded ventricular electrogram. This helps to confirm appropriate sensing and to document dropout of detection during ventricular fibrillation. Marked variation in ventricular electrogram amplitudes can generate dropout of detection *(arrows)* and delay initiation of therapy by the implantable cardioverter-defibrillator.

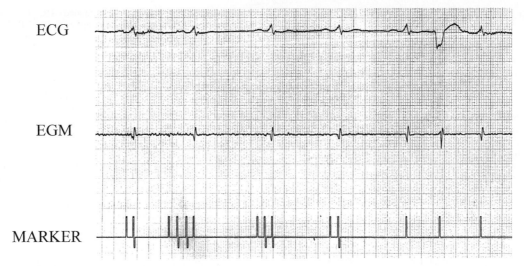

Figure 23–5. Detection of noncardiac muscle depolarizations in an implantable cardioverter-defibrillator (ICD). This tracing was obtained from a patient who received an ICD shock during sinus rhythm. Interrogation of the device showed multiple short detections intervals in the 117–150 msec range, as shown on the marker channel. These were thought to be nonphysiologic. Real-time electrograms, however, did not show any suspicious artifacts as a cause of abnormal sensing. With the presence of a marker channel, however, far-field sensing of low-amplitude fasciculation could be confirmed. This was thought to be coming from the intercostal muscles. The tip of the sensing lead was located anteriorly near the chest wall. Replacement of this lead to a different location eliminated the problem.

monly used, such testing must ensure that the pacemaker will not interfere with ICD detection of VF. Even with the availability of dual-chamber ICDs implantation of a separate pacemaker may be the desirable approach under particular patient circumstances. When implanting an ICD lead into the right ventricle where a previous pacemaker lead is already present, or when implanting a pacemaker lead with an existing ICD lead, it is ideal to separate the ICD lead from the pacemaker lead as much as possible and to their have their sense and pace electrodes oriented more or less perpendicular to each other.[192] In addition, choosing the pacemaker leads with the closest available bipolar interelectrode separation is important. With current lead technologies, this minimal separation is about 1 cm.

An additional improvement can be obtained by using ICD leads with dedicated bipolar sensing rather than the more common "integrated bipolar" sensing, which incorporates the RV shocking electrode into the sensing circuit.[240, 241] Dedicated bipolar sensing leads use two closely spaced electrodes at the lead tip for sensing, thus minimizing far-field sensing. The disadvantage of dedicated bipolar leads is that the RV shocking electrode is moved away from the tip of the lead to accomodate the sensing electrodes, which may reduce its efficacy. However, in most circumstances in which one wants to use this lead, there is a pacemaker lead in the RV apex, and the ICD lead should be placed higher on the septum. With such placement, the position of the shocking coil near the tip of the lead may not be important. A further advantage of dedicated bipolar ICD leads is that it may even be possible to implant the lead with a unipolar pacemaker, a circumstance generally considered a contraindication to ICD implantation. Because of dedicated bipolar sensing, unipolar pacing artifacts may be small enough to not interfere with VF sensing. Such a system, of course, should be thoroughly tested at implantation to ensure lack of interference by pro-

gramming the pacemaker to its maximal output in the VOO or DOO mode during VF induction. One must not forget about the potential sensing interference that the atrial lead may generate when a dual-chamber pacemaker is present in conjunction with the ICD. The output of the leads from both chambers should be maximized during VF testing to ensure that they would not interfere with ICD sensing of VF.

Finally, the pacemaker's ventricular sensing should be set as sensitive as possible while still avoiding oversensing. This approach to setting the ventricular sensing threshold in a pacemaker in which there is a coexisting ICD is somewhat different from the standard approach, in which a patient has only a pacemaker. The standard approach for setting ventricular sensitivity in a pacemaker is to set the sensing threshold as high as possible while providing adequate safety margin (usually half of the sensed ventricular electrogram amplitude). This would minimize the potential for ventricular pacing inhibition from oversensing of any noncardiac electronic interference. However, in a patient with an ICD, the goal is to minimize the potential that the pacemaker's pacing output may interfere with the ICD detection of VF. The best means of reducing this potential is for the pacemaker to be inhibited during VF. Thus, increasing the sensitivity of the pacemaker in the ventricular channel is important in rendering it inhibited during VF, when the electrogram amplitudes may be considerably smaller than during the patient's normal supraventricular rhythm. The rare inappropriate inhibition of the pacemaker from noncardiac electronic signals may not be as serious a problem in these patients because they have another backup ventricular pacing source in the ICD (Fig. 23–5).

With the advent of dual-chamber defibrillators, sensing in the atrium may also play a role in tachycardia detection and therapy delivery. Because automatic gain controls may amplify the atrial signals considerably, it is important to locate the atrial lead in an area in which there is minimal or no ventricular electrogram detectable even with high gain. This would avoid confounding the detection enhancements available with such devices that incorporate the sensing of atrial tachyarrhythmia as part of a detection algorithm.

REFERENCES

1. Koning G, Schneider H, Hoelen AJ, et al: Amplitude-duration relation for direct ventricular defibrillation with rectangular current pulses. Med Biol Eng 13:388–395, 1975.
2. Gold JH, Schuder JC, Stoeckle H, et al: Transthoracic ventricular defibrillation in the 100 kg calf with unidirectional rectangular pulses. Circulation 56:745–750, 1977.
3. Bourland JD, Tacker WA, Geddes LA: Strength duration curves for trapezoidal waveforms of various tilts for transchest defibrillation in animals. Med Instr 12:38–41, 1978.
4. Geddes LA, Bourland JD, Tacker WA: Energy and current requirements for ventricular defibrillation using trapezoidal waves. Am J Physiol 238:H231–H236, 1980.
5. Niebauer MJ, Babbs CF, Geddes LA, et al: Efficacy and safety of defibrillation with rectangular waves of 2- to 20-milliseconds duration. Crit Care Med 11:95–98, 1983.
6. Geddes LA, Niebauer MJ, Babbs CF, et al: Fundamental criteria underlying the efficacy and safety of defibrillating current waveforms. Med Biol Eng Comp 23:122–130, 1985.
7. Wessale JL, Bourland JD, Tacker WA, Geddes LA: Bipolar catheter defibrillation in dogs using trapezoidal waveforms of various tilts. J Electrocardiol 13(4):359–365, 1980.
8. Davy JM, Fain ES, Dorian P, Winkle RA: The relationship between successful defibrillation and delivered energy in open-chest dogs: reappraisal of the "defibrillation threshold" concept. Am Heart J 113(1):77–84, 1987.
9. Malkin RA, Souza JJ, Ideker RE: The ventricular defibrillation and upper limit of vulnerability dose-response curves. J Cardiovasc Electrophysiol 8(8):895–903, 1997.
10. Degroot PJ, Church TR, Mehra R, et al: Derivation of a defibrillator implant criterion based on probability of successful defibrillation. Pacing Clin Electrophysiol 20(8 Pt 1):1924–1935, 1997.
11. Dillon SM, Kwaku KF: Progressive depolarization: A unified hypothesis for defibrillation and fibrillation induction by shocks. J Cardiovasc Electrophysiol 9:529–552, 1998.
12. Chen PS, Swerdlow CD, Hwang C, Karacueuzian HS: Current concepts of ventricular defibrillation. J Cardiovasc Electrophysiol 9:552–562, 1998.
13. Zhou X, Daubert JP, Wolf PD, et al: Epicardial mapping of ventricular defibrillation with monophasic and biphasic shocks in dogs. Circ Res 72(1):145–160, 1993.
14. Singer I, Lang D: The defibrillation threshold. In Kroll M, Lehmann M (eds): Implantable Cardioverter Defibrillator Therapy: The Engineering-Clinical Interface. Boston, Kluwer Academic Publishers, 1996, pp 89–129.
15. Spotnitz HM: Does ventricular fibrillation cause myocardial stunning during defibrillator implantation? J Cardiac Surg 8(Suppl 2):249–256, 1993.
16. Antunes ML, Spotnitz HM, Livelli FD Jr, et al: Effect of electrophysiological testing on ejection fraction during cardioverter/defibrillator implantation. Ann Thorac Surg 45(3):315–318, 1988.
17. Poelaert J, Jordaens L, Visser CA, et al: Transoesophageal echocardiographic evaluation of ventricular function during transvenous defibrillator implantation. Acta Anaesthesiol Scand 40:913–918, 1996.
18. Runsio M, Bergfeldt L, Brodin LA, et al: Left ventricular function after repeated episodes of ventricular fibrillation and defibrillation assessed by transoesophageal echocardiography. Eur Heart J 18(1):124–131, 1997.
19. Stoddard MF, Redd RR, Buckingham TA, et al: Effects of electrophysiologic testing of the automatic implantable cardioverter-defibrillator on left ventricular systolic function and diastolic filling. Am Heart J 122(3 Pt 1):714–719, 1991.
20. Steinbeck G, Dorwarth U, Mattke S, et al: Hemodynamic deterioration during ICD implant: predictors of high-risk patients. Am Heart J 127(4 Pt 2):1064–1067, 1994.
21. Meyer J, Mollhoff T, Seifert T, et al: Cardiac output is not affected during intraoperative testing of the automatic implantable cardioverter defibrillator. J Cardiovasc Electrophysiol 7(3):211–216, 1996.
22. Singer I, van der Laken J, Edmonds HL Jr, et al: Is defibrillation testing safe? Pacing Clin Electrophysiol 14(11 Pt 2):1899–1904, 1991.
23. Behrens S, Spies C, Neumann U, et al: Cerebral ischemia during implantation of automatic defibrillators. Z Kardiol 84(10):798–807, 1995.
24. de Vries JW, Visser GH, Bakker PF: Neuromonitoring in defibrillation threshold testing: A comparison between EEG, near-infrared spectroscopy and jugular bulb oximetry. J Clin Monit 13(5):303–307, 1997.
25. Vriens EM, Bakker PF, Vries JW, et al: The impact of repeated short episodes of circulatory arrest on cerebral function: Reassuring electroencephalographic (EEG) findings during defibrillation threshold testing at defibrillation implantation. Electroencephalogr Clin Neurophysiol 98(4):236–242, 1996.
26. Swerdlow CD, Martin DJ, Kass RM, et al: The zone of vulnerability to T wave shocks in humans. J Cardiovascular Electrophysiol 8:145–154, 1997.
27. Cua M, Veltri EP: A comparison of ventricular arrhythmias induced with programmed stimulation versus alternating current. Pacing Clin Electrophysiol 16(3 Pt 1):382–386, 1993.
28. Rattes MF, Jones DL, Sharma AD, Klein GJ: Defibrillation threshold: A simple and quantitative estimate of the ability to defibrillate. Pacing Clin Electrophysiol 10(1 Pt 1):70–77, 1987.
29. Zipes DP, Fisher J, King RM, et al: Termination of ventricular fibrillation in dogs by depolarizing a critical amount of myocardium. Am J Cardiol 36:37–44, 1975.
30. Jones JL, Jones RE: Improved defibrillator waveform safety factor with biphasic waveforms. Am J Physiol 245:H60–65, 1983.
31. Mower MM, Mirowski M, Spear JF, et al: Patterns of ventricular activity during catheter defibrillation. Circulation 49:858–861, 1974.
32. Deale OC, Wesley RC Jr, Morgan D, Lerman BB: Nature of defibrillation: Determinism versus probabilism. Am J Physiol 259(5 Pt 2):H1544–H1550, 1990.
33. Province RA, Fishler MG, Thakor NV: Effects of defibrillation shock energy and timing on 3-D computer model of heart. Ann Biomed Eng 21(1):19–31, 1993.
34. Hsia PW, Mahmud R: Genesis of sigmoidal dose-response curve during defibrillation by random shock: A theoretical model based on experimental evidence for a vulnerable window during ventricular fibrillation. Pacing Clin Electrophysiol 13(10):1326–1342, 1990.
35. McDaniel WC, Schuder JC: The cardiac ventricular defibrillation threshold: Inherent limitations in its application and interpretation. Med Instrum 21:170–176, 1987.
36. Rattes MF, Jones DL, Sharma AD, et al: Defibrillation threshold: A simple and quantitative estimate of the ability to defibrillate. PACE 10:70–77, 1987.
37. Davy JM, Fain ES, Dorian P, et al: The relationship between successful defibrillation and delivered energy in open-chest dogs: Reappraisal of the "defibrillation threshold" concept. Am Heart J 113:77–84, 1987.
38. Church T, Martinson M, Kallok M, Watson W: A model to evaluate alternative methods of defibrillation threshold determination. Pacing Clin Electrophysiol 11(11 Pt 2):2002–2007, 1988.
39. Gill RM, Sweeney RJ, Reid PR: The defibrillation threshold: A comparison of anesthetics and measurement methods. Pacing Clin Electrophysiol 16(4 Pt 1):708–714, 1993.
40. Leonelli FM, Kroll MW, Brewer JE: Defibrillation thresholds are lower with smaller storage capacitors. Pacing Clin Electrophysiol 18(9 Pt 1):1661–1665, 1995.
41. Compos AT, Malkin RA, Ideker RE: An up-down Bayesian, defibrillation efficacy estimator. Pacing Clin Electrophysiol 20(5 Pt 1):1292–1300, 1997.
42. Swerdlow CD, Fan W, Brewer JE: Charge-burping theory correctly predicts optimal ratios of phase duration for biphasic defibrillation waveforms. Circulation 94(9):2278–2284, 1996.
43. Malkin RA, Pilkington TC, Ideker RE: Estimating defibrillation efficacy using combined upper limit of vulnerability and defibrillation testing. IEEE Trans Biomed Eng 43(1):69–78, 1996.
44. Chen PS, Feld GK, Kriett JM, et al: Relation between upper limit of vulnerability and defibrillation threshold in humans. Circulation 88(1):186–192, 1993.
45. Behrens S, Li C, Franz MR: Timing of the upper limit of vulnerability is different for monophasic and biphasic shocks: Implications for the determination of the defibrillation threshold. Pacing Clin Electrophysiol 20(9 Pt 1):2179–2187, 1997.
46. Hwang C, Swerdlow CD, Kass RM, et al: Upper limit of vulnerability

reliably predicts the defibrillation threshold in humans. Circulation 90(5):2308–2314, 1994.

47. Swerdlow CD, Ahern T, Kass RM, et al: Upper limit of vulnerability is a good estimator of shock strength associated with 90% probability of successful defibrillation in humans with transvenous implantable cardioverter-defibrillators. J Am Coll Cardiol 27(5):1112–1118, 1996.

48. Swerdlow CD, Davie S, Ahern T, Chen PS: Comparative reproducibility of defibrillation threshold and upper limit of vulnerability. Pacing Clin Electrophysiol 19(12 Pt 1):2103–2111, 1996.

49. Souza JJ, Malkin RA, Ideker RE: Comparison of upper limit of vulnerability and defibrillation probability of success curves using a nonthoracotomy lead system. Circulation 91(4):1247–1252, 1995.

50. Fan W, Gotoh M, Chen PS: Effects of the pacing site, procainamide, and lead configuration on the relationship between the upper limit of vulnerability and the defibrillation threshold. Pacing Clin Electrophysiol 18(6):1279–1284, 1995.

51. Behrens S, Li C, Franz MR: Effects of myocardial ischemia on ventricular fibrillation inducibility and defibrillation efficacy. J Am Coll Cardiol 29(4):817–824, 1997.

52. Martin DJ, Chen PS, Hwang C, et al: Upper limit of vulnerability predicts chronic defibrillation threshold for transvenous implantable defibrillators. J Cardiovasc Electrophysiol 8(3):241–248, 1997.

53. Huang J, KenKnight BH, Walcott GP, et al: Effects of transvenous electrode polarity and waveform duration on the relationship between defibrillation threshold and upper limit of vulnerability. Circulation 96(4):1351–1359, 1997.

54. Singer I, Lang D: Defibrillation threshold: Clinical utility and therapeutic implications. Pacing Clin Electrophysiol 15(6):932–949, 1992.

55. Grimm W, Timmann U, Menz V, et al: Simplified implantation of single lead pectoral cardioverter defibrillators using device based testing. Am J Cardiol 81:503–505, 1998.

56. Rugge FP, Savalle LH, Schalij MJ: Subcutaneous single-incision implantation of cardioverter defibrillators under local anesthesia by electrophysiologists in the electrophysiology laboratory. Am J Cardiol 81:302–305, 1998.

57. Schuchert A, Hoffman M, Steffgen F, Meinertz T: Several unsuccessful internal and external defibrillations during active can ICD implantation in a patient with pneumothorax. PACE 21:471–473, 1998.

58. Marchlinski FE, Flores B, Miller JM, et al: Relation of the intraoperative defibrillation threshold to successful postoperative defibrillation with an automatic implantable cardioverter defibrillator. Am J Cardiol 62(7):393–398, 1988.

59. Daoud EG, Man KC, Morady F, Strickberger SA: Rise in chronic defibrillation energy requirements necessitating implantable defibrillator lead system revision. Pacing Clin Electrophysiol 20(3 Pt 1):714–719, 1997.

60. Strickberger SA, Man KC, Souza J, et al: Prospective evaluation of two defibrillation safety margin techniques in patients with low defibrillation energy requirements. J Cardiovasc Electrophysiol 9(1):41–46, 1998.

61. Strickberger SA, Daoud EG, Davidson T, et al: Probability of successful defibrillation at multiples of the defibrillation energy requirement in patients with an implantable defibrillator. Circulation 96(4):1217–1223, 1997.

62. Compos AT, Malkin RA, Ideker RE: An up-down Bayesian, defibrillation efficacy estimator. Pacing Clin Electrophysiol 20(5 Pt 1):1292–1300, 1997.

63. Malkin RA, Burdick DS, Johnson EE, et al: Estimating the 95% effective defibrillation dose. IEEE Trans Biomed Eng 40(3):256–265, 1993.

64. Poole JE, Bardy GH, Dolack GL, et al: Serial defibrillation threshold measures in man: A prospective controlled study. J Cardiovasc Electrophysiol 6(1):19–25, 1995.

65. Higgins SL, Rich DH, Haygood JR, et al: ICD results: Results and potential benefit from routine predischarge and 2-month evaluation. PACE 21:410–417, 1998.

66. Tummala RV, Riggio DR, Peters RW, et al: Chronic rise in defibrillation threshold with a hybrid lead system. Am J Cardiol 78(3):309–312, 1996.

67. Venditti FJ Jr, Martin DT, Vassolas G, Bowen S: Rise in chronic defibrillation thresholds in nonthoracotomy implantable defibrillator. Circulation 89(1):216–223, 1994.

68. Hsia HH, Mitra RL, Flores BT, Marchlinski FE: Early postoperative increase in defibrillation threshold with nonthoracotomy system in humans. Pacing Clin Electrophysiol 17(6):1166–1173, 1994.

69. Neuzner J, Pitschner HF, Stohring R, et al: Implantable cardioverter/defibrillators with endocardial electrode systems: Long-term stability of the defibrillator's effectiveness. Z Kardiol 84(1):44–50, 1995.

70. Schwartzman D, Callans DJ, Gottlieb CD, et al: Early postoperative rise in defibrillation threshold in patients with nonthoracotomy defibrillation lead systems: Attenuation with biphasic shock waveforms. J Cardiovasc Electrophysiol 7(6):483–493, 1996.

71. Newman D, Barr A, Greene M, et al: A population-based method for the estimation of defibrillation energy requirements in humans: Assessment of time-dependent effects with a transvenous defibrillation system. Circulation 96(1):267–273, 1997.

72. Martin DT, John R, Venditti FJ Jr: Increase in defibrillation threshold in non-thoracotomy implantable defibrillators using a biphasic waveform. Am J Cardiol 76(4):263–266, 1995.

73. Lucy SD, Jones DL, Klein GJ: Pronounced increase in defibrillation threshold associated with pacing-induced cardiomyopathy in the dog. Am Heart J 127:366–376, 1994.

74. Friedman PA, Foley DA, Christian TF, Stanton MS: Stability of the defibrillation probability curve with the development of ventricular dysfunction in the canine rapid paced model. PACE 21:339–351, 1998.

75. Venditti FJ Jr, John RM, Hull M, et al: Circadian variation in defibrillation energy requirements. Circulation 94(7):1607–1612, 1996.

76. Luria D, Stanton MS, Eldar M, Glikson M: Pneumothorax: An unusual cause of ICD defibrillation failure. PACE 21:474–475, 1998.

77. Cohen TJ, Lowenkron DD: The effects of pneumothorax on defibrillation thresholds during pectoral Implantation of an active can implantable cardioverter defibrillator. PACE 21:468–470, 1998.

78. Winters SL, Casale AS, Inglesby TV, Curwin JH: Setting of relatively low energy outputs may permit implantation of a nonthoracotomy automatic cardioverter defibrillator system when high energy outputs prove ineffective. Pacing Clin Electrophysiol 19(10):1516–1518, 1996.

79. Neuzner J: Safety margins: Lessons from the Low Energy Endotak Trial (LEET). Am J Cardiol 78(5A):26–32, 1996.

80. Nitta J, Khoury DS: Role of proximal electrode position in transvenous ventricular defibrillation. Ann Biomed Eng 24(3):418–423, 1996.

81. Stajduhar KC, Ott GY, Kron J, et al: Optimal electrode position for transvenous defibrillation: A prospective randomized study. J Am Coll Cardiol 27(1):90–94, 1996.

82. Markewitz A, Kaulbach H, Mattke S, et al: Influence of anodal electrode position on transvenous defibrillation efficacy in humans: A prospective randomized comparison. Pacing Clin Electrophysiol 20(9 Pt 1):2193–2199, 1997.

83. Block M, Hammel D, Bocker D, et al: Bipolar transvenous defibrillation: Efficacy of two different positions of the anode. Pacing Clin Electrophysiol 18(11):1995–2000, 1995.

84. Trappe HJ, Pfitzner P, Fain E, et al: Transvenous defibrillation leads: Is there an ideal position of the defibrillation anode? Pacing Clin Electrophysiol 20(4 Pt 1):880–892, 1997.

85. Gold MR, Shorofsky SR: Transvenous defibrillation lead systems. J Cardiovasc Electrophysiol 7:570–580, 1996.

86. Bardy GH, Johnson G, Poole JE, et al: A simplified, single-lead unipolar transvenous cardioversion-defibrillation system. Circulation 88:543–547, 1993.

87. Kall JG, Kopp D, Lonchyna V, et al: Implantation of a subcutaneous lead array in combination with a transvenous defibrillation electrode via a single infraclavicular incision. Pacing Clin Electrophysiol 18(3 Pt 1):482–485, 1995.

88. Kuhlkamp V, Khalighi K, Dornberger V, Ziemer G: Single-incision and single-element array electrode to lower the defibrillation threshold. Ann Thorac Surg 64(4):1177–1179, 1997.

89. Obadia JF, Janier M, Chevalier P, et al: Defibrillation threshold and electrode configurations: An experimental study testing three configurations in twelve pigs. J Cardiovasc Surg (Torino) 38(5):495–499, 1997.

90. Solomon AJ, Swartz JF, Rodak DJ, et al: A second defibrillator chest patch electrode will increase implantation rates for nonthoracotomy defibrillators. Pacing Clin Electrophysiol 19(9):1304–1310, 1996.

91. Verdino RJ, Hannan RL, Tracy CM, Solomon AJ: Implantation of a nonthoracotomy defibrillator using a second defibrillator patch in the abdominal pocket. Pacing Clin Electrophysiol 19(10):1526–1527, 1996.

92. Tang AS, Hendry P, Goldstein W, et al: Nonthoracotomy implantation of cardioverter defibrillators: Preliminary experience with a defibrillation lead placed at the right ventricular outflow tract. Pacing Clin Electrophysiol 19(6):960–964, 1996.

93. Singer I, Goldsmith J, Maldonado C: Transseptal defibrillation is superior for transvenous defibrillation. Pacing Clin Electrophysiol 18(1 Pt 2):229–232, 1995.

94. Bardy GH, Dolack GL, Kudenchuk PJ, et al: Prospective, randomized comparison in humans of a unipolar defibrillation system with that using an additional superior vena cava electrode. Circulation 89(3):1090–1093, 1994.

95. Gold MR, Foster AH, Shorofsky SR: Effects of an active pectoral-pulse generator shell on defibrillation efficacy with a transvenous lead system. Am J Cardiol 78(5):540–543, 1996.

96. Gold MR, Foster AH, Shorofsky SR: Lead system optimization for transvenous defibrillation. Am J Cardiol 80(9):1163–1167, 1997.

97. Kudenchuk PJ, Bardy GH, Dolack GL, et al: Efficacy of a single-lead unipolar transvenous defibrillator compared with a system employing an additional coronary sinus electrode. Circulation 89:2641–2644, 1994.

98. Epstein AE, Kay GN, Plumb VJ, et al: Elevated defibrillation threshold when right-sided venous access is used for nonthoracotomy implantable defibrillator lead implantation: The Endotak Investigators. J Cardiovasc Electrophysiol 6(11):979–986, 1995.

99. Yamanouchi Y, Mowrey KA, Niebauer MJ, et al: Additional lead improves defibrillation efficacy with an abdominal 'hot can' electrode system. Circulation 96(12):4400–4407, 1997.

100. Natale A, Sra J, Geiger MJ, et al: Right side implant of the unipolar single lead defibrillation system. Pacing Clin Electrophysiol 20(8 Pt 1):1910–1912, 1997.

101. Jensen SM, Pietersen A, Chen X: Implantation of active can implantable defibrillators in the right pectoral region. PACE 21:476–477, 1998.

102. Flaker GC, Tummala R, Wilson J, et al: Comparison of right- and left-sided pectoral implantation parameters with the Jewel active can cardiodefibrillator. PACE 21:447–451, 1998.

103. Neuzner J, Schwarz T, Strasser R, et al: Effect of the addition of an abdominal hot can cardioverter/defibrillator pulse generator on the defibrillation energy requirements in a single-lead endocardial defibrillation system. Eur Heart J 18(10):1655–1658, 1997.

104. Jones GK, Poole JE, Kudenchuk PJ, et al: A prospective randomized evaluation of implantable cardioverter-defibrillator size on unipolar defibrillation system efficacy. Circulation 92(10):2940–2943, 1995.

105. Newby KH, Moredock L, Rembert J, et al: Impact of defibrillator-can size on defibrillation success with a single-lead unipolar system. Am Heart J 131(2):261–265, 1996.

106. Leonelli FM, Wright H, Latterell ST, et al: A long thin electrode is equivalent to a short thick electrode for defibrillation in the right ventricle. Pacing Clin Electrophysiol 18(1 Pt 2):221–224, 1995.

107. Tomassoni G, Pendekanti R, Dixon-Tulloch E, et al: Importance of electrode conductive surface area and edge effects on ventricular defibrillation efficacy. J Cardiovasc Electrophysiol 8(11):1246–1254, 1997.

108. Halperin BD, Reynolds B, Fain ES, et al: The effect of electrode size on transvenous defibrillation energy requirements: A prospective evaluation. Pacing Clin Electrophysiol 20(4 Pt 1):893–898, 1997.

109. Niebauer MJ, Wilkoff B, Yamanouchi Y, et al: Iridium oxide-coated defibrillation electrode: Reduced shock polarization and improved defibrillation efficacy. Circulation 96(10):3732–3736, 1997.

110. Kroll MW, Anderson KM, Supino CG, Adams TP: Decline in defibrillation thresholds. Pacing Clin Electrophysiol 16(1 Pt 2):213–217, 1993.

111. Kroll MW: A minimal model of the monophasic defibrillation pulse. Pacing Clin Electrophysiol 16(4 Pt 1):769–777, 1993.

112. Irnich W: Optimal truncation of defibrillation pulses. Pacing Clin Electrophysiol 18(4 Pt 1):673–688, 1995.

113. Cleland BG: A conceptual basis for defibrillation waveforms. Pacing Clin Electrophysiol 19(8):1186–1195, 1996.

114. Gold MR, Shorofsky SR: Strength-duration relationship for human transvenous defibrillation. Circulation 96(10):3517–3520, 1997.

115. Rist K, Tchou PJ, Mowrey K, et al: Smaller capacitors improve the biphasic waveform. J Cardiovasc Electrophysiol 5(9):771–776, 1994.

116. Bardy GH, Poole JE, Kudenchuk PJ, et al: A prospective randomized comparison in humans of biphasic waveform 60-microF and 120-microF capacitance pulses using a unipolar defibrillation system. Circulation 91(1):91–95, 1995.

117. Poole JE, Kudenchuk PJ, Dolack GL, et al: A prospective randomized comparison in humans of 90-mu F and 120-mu F biphasic pulse defibrillation using a unipolar defibrillation system. J Cardiovasc Electrophysiol 6(12):1097–1100, 1995.

118. Swerdlow CD, Kass RM, Davie S, et al: Short biphasic pulses from 90 microfarad capacitors lower defibrillation threshold. Pacing Clin Electrophysiol 19(7):1053–1060, 1996.

119. Swerdlow CD, Kass RM, Chen PS, et al: Effect of capacitor size and pathway resistance on defibrillation threshold for implantable defibrillators. Circulation 90(4):1840–1846, 1994.

120. Block M, Hammel D, Bocker D, et al: Biphasic defibrillation using a single capacitor with large capacitance: Reduction of peak voltages and ICD device size. Pacing Clin Electrophysiol 19(2):207–214, 1996.

121. Kroll MW: A minimal model of the single capacitor biphasic defibrillation waveform. Pacing Clin Electrophysiol 17(11 Pt 1):1782–1792, 1994.

122. Swerdlow CD, Brewer JE, Kass RM, Kroll MW: Application of models of defibrillation to human defibrillation data: Implications for optimizing implantable defibrillator capacitance. Circulation 96(9):2813–2822, 1997.

123. Kroll MW, Lehmann MH, Tchou PJ: Defining the defibrillation dosage. In Kroll M, Lehmann M (eds): Implantable Cardioverter Defibrillator Therapy: The Engineering-Clinical Interface, Boston, Kluwer Academic Publishers, 1996, pp 63–88.

124. Dillon SM: Synchronized repolarization after defibrillation shocks: A possible component of the defibrillation process demonstrated by optical recordings in rabbit heart. Circulation 85(5):1865–1878, 1992.

125. Walcott GP, Walker RG, Cates AW, et al: Choosing the optimal monophasic and biphasic waveforms for ventricular defibrillation. J Cardiovasc Electrophysiol 6(9):737–750, 1995.

126. Swartz JF, Fletcher RD, Karasik PE: Optimization of biphasic waveforms for human nonthoracotomy defibrillation. Circulation 88(6):2646–2654, 1993.

127. Natale A, Sra J, Krum D, et al: Relative efficacy of different tilts with biphasic defibrillation in humans. Pacing Clin Electrophysiol 19(2):197–206, 1996.

128. Schauerte P, Schondube FA, Grossmann M, et al: Influence of phase duration of biphasic waveforms on defibrillation energy requirements with a 70-microF capacitance. Circulation 97(20):2073–2078, 1998.

129. Tomassoni G, Newby K, Deshpande S, et al: Defibrillation efficacy of commercially available biphasic impulses in humans: Importance of negative-phase peak voltage. Circulation 95(7):1822–1826, 1997.

130. Yamanouchi Y, Brewer JE, Mowrey KA, et al: Sawtooth first phase biphasic defibrillation waveform: A comparison with standard waveform in clinical devices. J Cardiovasc Electrophysiol 8(5):517–528, 1997.

131. Yamanouchi Y, Mowrey KA, Nadzam GR, et al: Large change in voltage at phase reversal improves biphasic defibrillation thresholds: Parallel-series mode switching. Circulation 94(7):1768–1773, 1996.

132. Strickberger SA, Hummel JD, Horwood LE, et al: Effect of shock polarity on ventricular defibrillation threshold using a transvenous lead system. J Am Coll Cardiol 24(4):1069–1072, 1994.

133. Thakur RK, Souza JJ, Chapman PD, et al: Electrode polarity is an important determinant of defibrillation efficacy using a nonthoracotomy system. Pacing Clin Electrophysiol 17(5 Pt 1):919–923, 1994.

134. Schauerte P, Stellbrink C, Schondube FA, et al: Polarity reversal improves defibrillation efficacy in patients undergoing transvenous cardioverter defibrillator implantation with biphasic shocks. Pacing Clin Electrophysiol 20(2 Pt 1):301–306, 1997.

135. Shorofsky SR, Gold MR: Effects of waveform and polarity on defibrillation thresholds in humans using a transvenous lead system. Am J Cardiol 78(3):313–316, 1996.

136. Natale A, Sra J, Dhala A, et al: Effects of initial polarity on defibrillation threshold with biphasic pulses. Pacing Clin Electrophysiol 18(10):1889–1893, 1995.

137. Strickberger SA, Man KC, Daoud E, et al: Effect of first-phase polarity of biphasic shocks on defibrillation threshold with a single transvenous lead system. J Am Coll Cardiol 25(7):1605–1608, 1995.

138. Keelan ET, Sra JS, Axtell K, et al: The effect of polarity of the initial phase of a biphasic shock waveform on the defibrillation threshold of pectorally implanted defibrillators. Pacing Clin Electrophysiol 20(2 Pt 1):337–342, 1997.

139. Yamanouchi Y, Mowrey KA, Nadzam GR, et al: Effects of polarity on defibrillation thresholds using a biphasic waveform in a hot can electrode system. Pacing Clin Electrophysiol 20(12 Pt 1):2911–2916, 1997.

140. Efimov IR, Cheng YN, Biermann M, et al: Transmembrane voltage changes produced by real and virtual electrodes during monophasic defibrillation shock delivered by an implantable electrode. J Cardiovasc Electrophysiol 8(9):1031–1045, 1997.

141. Efimov IR, Cheng Y, Van Wagoner DR, et al: Virtual electrode-induced phase singularity: A basic mechanism of defibrillation failure. Circ Res 82:918–925, 1998.

142. Clayton RH, Murray A, Campbell RWF: Evidence for electrical organization during ventricular fibrillation in the human heart. J Cardiovasc Electrophysiol 6:616–624, 1995.

143. Hsia PW, Frerk S, Allen CA, et al: A critical period of ventricular fibrillation more susceptible to defibrillation: Real-time waveform analysis using a single ECG lead. Pacing Clin Electrophysiol 19(4 Pt 1):418–430, 1996.

144. Hsia PW, Frerk S, Allen CA, et al: A critical period of ventricular fibrillation more susceptible to defibrillation: Real-time waveform analysis using a single ECG lead. Pacing Clin Electrophysiol 19(4 Pt 1):418–430, 1996.

145. Murakawa Y, Yamashita T, Ajiki K, et al: Electrophysiological background of individual variability in electrical defibrillation efficacy. Am J Physiol 271(3 Pt 2):H1094–H1098, 1996.

146. Hsia PW, Fendelander L, Harrington G, Damiano RJ: Defibrillation success is associated with myocardial organization: Spatial coherence as a new method of quantifying the electrical organization of the heart. J Electrocardiol 29(Suppl):189–197.

147. Yakaitis RW, Ewy GA, Otto CW, et al: Influence of time and therapy on ventricular defibrillation in dogs. Crit Care Med 8(3):157–163, 1980.

148. Winkle RA, Mead RH, Ruder MA, et al: Effect of duration of ventricular fibrillation on defibrillation efficacy in humans. Circulation 81(5):1477–1481, 1990.

149. Lerman BB, Engelstein ED: Increased defibrillation threshold due to ventricular fibrillation duration: Potential mechanisms. J Electrocardiol 28(Suppl):21–24, 1995.

150. Lerman BB, Engelstein ED: Metabolic determinants of defibrillation: Role of adenosine. Circulation 91(3):838–844, 1995.

151. Windecker S, Kay GN, KenKnight BH, et al: The effects of ventricular fibrillation duration and a preceding unsuccessful shock on the probability of defibrillation success using biphasic waveforms in pigs. J Cardiovasc Electrophysiol 8(12):1386–1395, 1997.

152. Tofler GH, Gebara OCE, Mittleman MA, et al: Morning peak in ventricular tachyarrhythmias detected by time of implantable cardioverter defibrillator therapy. Circulation 92:1203–1208, 1995.

153. Reiffel JA, Coromilas J, Zimmerman JM, et al: Drug-device interactions: Clinical considerations. PACE 8:369–373, 1985.

154. Szabo TS, Jones DL, McQuinn RL, Klein GJ: Flecainide acetate does not alter the energy requirements for direct ventricular defibrillation using sequential pulse defibrillation in pigs. J Cardiovasc Pharmacol 12(4):377–383, 1988.

155. Natale A, Jones DL, Kleinstiver PW, et al: Effects of flecainide on defibrillation threshold in pigs. J Cardiovasc Pharmacol 21(4):573–577, 1993.

156. Holt DW, Tucker GT, Jackson PR, et al: Amiodarone pharmacokinetics. Am Heart J 106:840–847, 1983.

157. Barbieri E, Conti F, Zampieri P, et al: Amiodarone and desethylamiodarone distribution in the atrium and adipose tissue of patients undergoing short and long-term treatment with amiodarone. J Am Coll Cardiol 8:210–213, 1986.

158. Dorian P, Witkowski FX, Penkoske PA, Feder-Elituv RS: Barium decreases defibrillation energy requirements. J Cardiovasc Pharmacol 23(1):107–112, 1994.

159. Dorian P, Fain ES, Davy JM, et al: Effect of quinidine and bretylium on defibrillation energy requirements. Am Heart J 112:19–25, 1986.

160. Deeb GM, Hardesty RL, Griffith BP, et al: The effects of cardiovascular drugs on the defibrillation threshold and the pathological effects on the heart using an automatic implantable defibrillator. Am Thorac Surg 4:361–366, 1983.

161. Woolfolk DI, Chaffee WR, Cohen W, et al: The effect of quinidine on electrical energy required for ventricular defibrillation. Am Heart J 72:659, 1966.

162. Babbs CF, Yim GKW, Whistler SJ, et al: Elevation of ventricular defibrillation energy requirements. Am Heart J 112:19, 1986.

163. Sato S, Tsuji MH, Naito H: Mexiletine has no effect on defibrillation energy requirements in dogs. Pacing Clin Electrophysiol 17(12 Pt 1):2279–2284, 1994.

164. Murakawa Y, Inoue H, Kuo TT, et al: Prolongation of intraventricular conduction time associated with fatal [correction of fetal] impairment of defibrillation efficiency during treatment with class I antiarrhythmic agents. J Cardiovasc Pharmacol 25(2):194–199, 1995.

165. Ujhelyi MR, Schur M, Frede T, et al: Differential effects of lidocaine on defibrillation threshold with monophasic versus biphasic shock waveforms. Circulation 92:1644–1650, 1995.

166. Kerber RE, Pandian NG, Jensen SR, et al: Effect of lidocaine and bretylium on energy requirements for transthoracic defibrillation: Experimental studies. J Am Coll Cardiol 7:397–405, 1986.

167. Tacker WA, Niebauer MJ, Babbs CF, et al: The effect of newer antiarrhythmic drugs on defibrillation threshold. Crit Care Med 8:177–180, 1980.

168. Echt DS, Black JN, Barbey JT, et al: Evaluation of antiarrhythmic drugs on defibrillation energy requirements in dogs: Sodium channel block and action potential prolongation. Circulation 79:1106–1117, 1989.

169. Beatch GN, Dickenson DR, Tang AS: Effects of optical enantiomers CK-4000(S) and CK-4001(R) on defibrillation and enhancement of shock-induced extension of action potential duration. J Cardiovasc Electrophysiol 6(9):716–728, 1995.

170. Sweeney RJ, Gill RM, Steinberg MI, Reid PR: Effects of flecainide, encainide, and clofilium on ventricular refractory period extension by transcardiac shocks. Pacing Clin Electrophysiol 19(1):50–60, 1996.

171. Ruffy R, Schechtman K, Monje E, et al: β-Adrenergic modulation of direct defibrillation energy in anesthetized dog heart. Am J Physiol 248:H674–677, 1985.

172. Ruffy R, Monje E, Schechtman K: Facilitation of cardiac defibrillation by aminophylline in the conscious, closed-chest dog [Abstract]. J Electrophysiol 2:450, 1988.

173. Wang M, Dorian P: Defibrillation energy requirements differ between anesthetic agents. J Electrophysiol 3/2:86–94, 1989.

174. Gill RM, Sweeney RJ, Reid PR: The defibrillation threshold: A comparison of anesthetics and measurement methods. Pacing Clin Electrophysiol 16(4 Pt 1):708–714, 1993.

175. Valentinuzzi ME: Defibrillation, either in clinical practice or in basic and applied research, uses mainly energy (expressed by and large in joules) as the reference parameter to dose the discharge or to describe thresholds [Comment, Letter]. Pacing Clin Electrophysiol 18(7):1465–1466, 1995.

176. Schuder JC, Stoeckle H, West JA, Keskar PY: Transthoracic ventricular defibrillation in the dog with truncated and untruncated exponential stimuli. IEEE Trans Biomedical Eng 13(6):410–415, 1971.

177. Lehr JL, Ramirez IF, Karlon WJ, Eisenberg SR: Test of four defibrillation dosing strategies using a two-dimensional finite-element model. Med Biol Eng Comput 30(6):621–628, 1992.

178. Lerman BB, DiMarco JP, Haines DE: Current-based versus energy-based ventricular defibrillation: A prospective study. J Am Coll Cardiol 12(5):1259–1264, 1988.

179. Wesley RC Jr, Farkhani F, Porzio D, et al: Transepicardial defibrillation dose response: Current versus energy. Pacing Clin Electrophysiol 16(1 Pt 2):193–197, 1993.

180. Anvari A, Mast F, Schmidinger H, et al: Effects of lidocaine, ajmaline, and diltiazem on ventricular defibrillation energy requirements in isolated rabbit heart. J Cardiovasc Pharmacol 29(4):429–435, 1997.

181. Haberman RJ, Veltri, EP, Mower MM: The effect of amiodarone on defibrillation threshold [Abstract]. J Electrophysiol 2:415, 1988.

182. Fain ES, Lee JT, Winkle RA: Effects of acute intravenous and chronic oral amiodarone on defibrillation energy requirements. Am Heart J 114:8–17, 1987.

183. Kentsch M, Kunze KP, Bleifeld W: Effect of intravenous amiodarone on ventricular fibrillation during out-of-hospital cardiac arrest [Abstract]. J Am Coll Cardiol 7:82A, 1986.

184. Fogoros RN: Amiodarone-induced refractoriness to cardioversion. Am Intern Med 100:699–700, 1984.

185. Guarnieri T, Levine JH, Veltri EP: Success of chronic defibrillation and the role of antiarrhythmic drugs with the automatic implantable cardioverter/defibrillator. Am J Cardiol 60:1061–1064, 1987.

186. Epstein AE, Ellenbogen KA, Kirk K, et al: Clinical characteristics and outcome of patients with high defibrillation thresholds: A multicenter study. Circulation 86:1206–1216, 1992.

187. Jung W, Manz M, Pizzulli L, et al: Effects of chronic amiodarone therapy on defibrillation threshold. Am J Cardiol 70:1023–1027, 1992.

188. Wang M, Dorian P, Ogilvie RI: Isoproterenol increases defibrillation energy requirements in dogs. J Cardiovasc Pharmacol 19:201–208, 1992.

189. Hackett AM, Gardiner P, Garthwaite SM: The effect of bidisomide (SC-40230), a new class Ia/Ib antiarrhythmic agent, on defibrillation energy requirements in dogs with healed myocardial infarctions. Pacing Clin Electrophysiol 16(2):317–326, 1993.

190. Fain ES, Dorian P, Davy JM, et al: Effects of encainide and its metabolites on energy requirements for defibrillation. Circulation 73:1334–1341, 1986.

191. Frame LH, Sheldon JH: Effect of recainam on the energy required for ventricular defibrillation in dogs as assessed with implanted electrodes. J Am Coll Cardiol 12:746–752, 1988.

192. Jones DL, Kim YH, Natale A, et al: Bretylium decreases and verapamil increases defibrillation threshold in pigs. Pacing Clin Electrophysiol 17(8):1380–1390, 1994.

193. Rattes MF, Sharma AD, Klein GJ, et al: Adrenergic effects on internal cardiac defibrillation threshold. Am J Physiol 253:(3 Pt 2):H500–H506, 1987.

194. Murakawa Y, Sezaki K, Inoue H, et al: Shock-induced refractory period extension and pharmacologic modulation of defibrillation threshold. J Cardiovasc Pharmacol 23(5):822–825, 1994.

195. Murakawa Y, Inoue H, Kuo TT, et al: Prolongation of intraventricular conduction time associated with fatal [correction of fetal] impairment of defibrillation efficiency during treatment with class I antiarrhythmic agents. J Cardiovasc Pharmacol 25(2):194–199, 1995.

196. Echt DS, Black JN, Barbey JT, et al: Evaluation of antiarrhythmic drugs on defibrillation energy requirements in dogs: Sodium channel block and action potential prolongation. Circulation 79(5):1106–1117, 1989.

197. Stevens SK, Haffajee CI, Naccarelli GV, et al: Effects of oral propafenone on defibrillation and pacing thresholds in patients receiving implantable cardioverter-defibrillators: Propafenone Defibrillation Threshold Investigators. J Am Coll Cardiol 28(2):418–422, 1996.

198. Huang SK, Tan de Guzman WL, Chenarides JG, et al: Effects of long-term amiodarone therapy on the defibrillation threshold and the rate of shocks of the implantable cardioverter-defibrillator. Am Heart J 122(3 Pt 1):720–727, 1991.

199. Behrens S, Li C, Franz MR: Effects of long-term amiodarone treatment on ventricular-fibrillation vulnerability and defibrillation efficacy in response to monophasic and biphasic shocks. J Cardiovasc Pharmacol 30(4):412–418, 1997.

200. Frame LH: The effect of chronic oral and acute intravenous amiodarone administration on ventricular defibrillation threshold using implanted electrodes in dogs. Pacing Clin Electrophysiol 12(2):339–346, 1989.

201. Hernandez R, Mann DE, Breckinridge S, et al: Effects of flecainide on defibrillation thresholds in the anesthetized dog. J Am Coll Cardiol 14(3):777–781, 1989.

202. Wang M, Dorian P, Ogilvie RI: Isoproterenol increases defibrillation energy requirements in dogs. J Cardiovasc Pharmacol 19(2):201–208, 1992.

203. Dorian P, Fain ES, Davy JM, et al: Lidocaine causes a reversible, concentration-dependent increase in defibrillation energy requirements. J Am Coll Cardiol 8:327–332, 1986.

204. Marinchak RA, Friehling TD, Line RA, et al: Effect of antiarrhythmic drugs on defibrillation threshold: Case report of an adverse effect of mexiletine and review of the literature. PACE 11:7–12, 1988.

205. Echt DS, Gremillion ST, Lee JT, et al: Effects of procainamide and lidocaine on defibrillation energy requirements in patients receiving implantable cardioverter defibrillator devices. J Cardiovasc Electrophysiol 5:752–760, 1994.

206. Echt DS, Black JN, Barbey JT, et al: Evaluation of antiarrhythmic drugs on defibrillation energy requirements in dogs: Sodium channel block and action potential prolongation. Circulation 79(5):1106–1117, 1989.

207. Lake CL, Kron IL, Mentzer RM, Crampton RS: Lidocaine enhances intraoperative ventricular defibrillation. Anesth Analg 65(4):337–340, 1986.

208. Pharand C, Goldman R, Fan C, et al: Effect of chronic oral moricizine and intravenous epinephrine on ventricular fibrillation and defibrillation thresholds. Pacing Clin Electrophysiol 19(1):82–89, 1996.

209. Avitall B, Hare J, Zander G, et al: Cardioversion, defibrillation, and overdrive pacing of ventricular arrhythmias: The effect of moricizine in dogs with sustained monomorphic ventricular tachycardia. Pacing Clin Electrophysiol 16(11):2092–2097, 1993.

210. Ujhelyi MR, O'Rangers EA, Kluger J, et al: Defibrillation energy requirements during moricizine and moricizine-lidocaine therapy. J Cardiovasc Pharmacol 20(6):932–939, 1992.

211. Dorian P, Wang M, David I, et al: Oral clofilium produces sustained lowering of defibrillation energy requirements in a canine model. Circulation 83:614–621, 1991.

212. Murakawa Y, Sezaki K, Inoue H, et al: Shock-induced refractory period extension and pharmacologic modulation of defibrillation threshold. J Cardiovasc Pharmacol 23(5):822–825, 1994.

213. Sezaki K, Murakawa Y, Inoue H, et al: Effect of isoproterenol on facilitation of electrical defibrillation by E-4031. J Cardiovasc Pharmacol 25(3):393–396, 1995.

214. Wesley RC Jr, Farkhani F, Morgan D, Zimmerman D: Ibutilide: Enhanced defibrillation via plateau sodium current activation. Am J Physiol 264(4 Pt 2):H1269–H1274, 1993.

215. Labhasetwar V, Underwood T, Heil RW Jr, et al: Epicardial administration of ibutilide from polyurethane matrices: Effects on defibrillation threshold and electrophysiologic parameters. J Cardiovasc Pharmacol 24(5):826–840, 1994.

216. Beatch GN, Dickenson DR, Wood RH, Tang AS: Class III antiarrhythmic effects of LY-190147 on defibrillation threshold. J Cardiovasc Pharmacol 27(2):218–225, 1996.

217. Murakawa Y, Yamashita T, Kanese Y, Omata M: Can a class III antiarrhythmic drug improve electrical defibrillation efficacy during ventricular fibrillation? J Am Coll Cardiol 29(3):688–692, 1997.

218. Wang M, Dorian P: DL and D sotalol decrease defibrillation energy requirements. PACE 12:1522–1529, 1989.

219. Dorian P, Newman D: Effect of sotalol on ventricular fibrillation and defibrillation in humans. Am J Cardiol 72(4):72A–79A, 1993.

220. Dorian P, Newman D, Sheahan R, et al: D-Sotalol decreases defibrillation energy requirements in humans: A novel indication for drug therapy. J Cardiovasc Electrophysiol 7(10):952–961, 1996.

221. Dorian P, Newman D: Tedisamil increases coherence during ventricular fibrillation and decreases defibrillation energy requirements. Cardiovasc Res 33(2):485–494, 1997.

222. Neuzner J, Bahawar H, Berkowitsch A, et al: Clinical predictors of defibrillation energy requirements. Am J Cardiol 79(2):205–206, 1997.

223. Schwartzman D, Concato J, Ren JF, et al: Factors associated with successful implantation of nonthoracotomy defibrillation lead systems. Am Heart J 131(6):1127–1136, 1996.

224. Raitt MH, Johnson G, Dolack GL, et al: Clinical predictors of the defibrillation threshold with the unipolar implantable defibrillation system. J Am Coll Cardiol 25(7):1576–1583, 1995.

225. Brooks R, Garan H, Torchiana D, et al: Determinants of successful nonthoracotomy cardioverter-defibrillator implantation: Experience in 101 patients using two different lead systems. J Am Coll Cardiol 22(7):1835–1842, 1993.

226. Leitch JW, Yee R: Predictors of defibrillation efficacy in patients undergoing epicardial defibrillator implantation: The Multicenter Pacemaker-Cardioverter-Defibrillator (PCD) Investigators Group. J Am Coll Cardiol 21(7):1632–1637, 1993.

227. Strickberger SA, Brownstein SL, Wilkoff BL, Zinner AJ: Clinical predictors of defibrillation energy requirements in patients treated with a nonthoracotomy defibrillator system: The ResQ Investigators. Am Heart J 131(2):257–260, 1996.

228. Gold MR, Khalighi K, Kavesh NG, et al: Clinical predictors of transvenous biphasic defibrillation thresholds. Am J Cardiol 79(12):1623–1627, 1997.

229. Khalighi K, Daly B, Leino EV, et al: Clinical predictors of transvenous defibrillation energy requirements. Am J Cardiol 79(2):150–153, 1997.

230. Horton RP, Canby RC, Roman CA, et al: Determinants of nonthoracotomy biphasic defibrillation. PACE 20(Pt I):60–64, 1997.

231. Gold MR, Olsovsky MR, Pelini MA, et al: Comparison of single- and dual-coil active pectoral defibrillation lead systems. J Am Coll Cardiol 31(6):1391–1394, 1998.

232. Saksena S, Krol R, Kaushik R, et al: Endocardial defibrillation with dual, triple, and quadruple nonthorocotomy electrode systems using biphasic shocks [Abstract] PACE 17:743, 1994.

233. Callihan RL, Idriss SF, Dahl RW, et al: Comparison of defibrillation probability of success curves for an endocardial lead configuration with and without an inactive epicardial patch. J Am Coll Cardiol 25(6):1373–1379, 1995.

234. Fotuhi PC, Ideker RE, Idriss SF, et al: Influence of epicardial patches on defibrillation threshold with nonthoracotomy lead configurations. Circulation 92(10):3082–3088, 1995.

235. Nasir N Jr, Cedillo-Salazar FR, Doyle TK, Henry PD, Pacifico A. Effect of preexisting epicardial patch electrodes on defibrillation thresholds of unipolar defibrillators. Am J Cardiol 79(10):1408–1409, 1997.

236. Fotuhi PC, Ideker RE, Idriss SF, et al: Influence of epicardial patches on defibrillation threshold with nonthoracotomy lead configurations. Circulation 92(10):3082–3088, 1995.

237. Schwartzman D, Nallamothu N, Callans DJ, et al: Postoperative lead-related complications in patients with nonthoracotomy defibrillation lead systems. J Am Coll Cardiol 26(3):776–786, 1995.

238. Epstein AE, Ellenbogen KA, Kirk KA, et al: Clinical characteristics and outcome of patients with high defibrillation thresholds: A multicenter study. Circulation 86(4):1206–1216, 1992.

239. Spotnitz HM, Ott GY, Bigger JT, et al: Methods of implantable cardioverter-defibrillator: Pacemaker insertion to avoid interactions. Ann Thorac Surg 53:253–257, 1992.

240. Haffajee C, Casavant D, Desai P, et al: Combined third generation implantable cardioverter-defibrillator with dual-chamber pacemakers: Preliminary observations. PACE 19:136–142, 1996.

241. Brooks R, Garan H, McGovern BA, et al: Implantation of transvenous nonthoracotomy cardioverter-defibrillator systems in patients with permanent endocardial pacemakers. Am Heart J 129:45–53, 1995.

Chapter 24

The Implantable Atrial Defibrillator: Basic Development to Clinical Implementation

Randolph A. S. Cooper, David G. Reuter, and Gregory M. Ayers

Atrial fibrillation remains the most commonly encountered arrhythmia in clinical medicine, and a recent study suggests that previous estimates of atrial fibrillation incidence were too low.[1] With life expectancies increasing, the number of patients presenting with atrial fibrillation is expected to increase dramatically.[2] The health care costs associated with atrial fibrillation have motivated and will continue to motivate development of improved treatment strategies.[3]

The treatment of atrial fibrillation in the past was addressed largely through pharmacologic approaches that in general have proved inadequate.[4] This inadequacy has resulted in renewed research interest in the mechanism as well as in the development of newer treatment modalities for atrial fibrillation.[5, 6] These emerging atrial fibrillation treatment strategies are being evaluated and will require careful clinical trials to compare their safety and effectiveness to established treatment modalities. Their role in the clinical management of patients with recurrent atrial fibrillation is being debated.[7]

One of these novel therapies is the implantable atrial defibrillator. The clinical benefits of implanted devices capable of providing automatic or on-command atrial defibrillation therapy for recurrent episodes of atrial fibrillation have probably not yet been fully appreciated. It remains to be seen if repeated internal cardioversion has a clinical advantage over the more established therapies for atrial fibrillation. Clinical trials with the first generation of implantable atrial defibrillators are under way in patients with intermittent persistent atrial fibrillation.[8] These and future trials should compare device therapy with other, more established therapies for atrial fibrillation to evaluate the clinical utility of the implantable atrial defibrillator.

In this chapter, the basic science and clinical development of the implantable atrial defibrillator are discussed. The development of the electrode systems and shock waveforms used in the modern clinical devices are explained. We also address some of the safety issues raised in conjunction with a stand-alone atrial defibrillator as well as current research focusing on minimizing the pain associated with internal defibrillation shocks. Subsequent sections discuss the engineering aspects of the first implantable atrial defibrillator, including lead system, waveform, detection algorithms, and other capabilities. Finally, the preliminary results of the ongoing clinical trials of the first generation of implantable atrial defibrillators are presented.

■ DEFIBRILLATION ELECTRODES

Animal studies have demonstrated a close relationship between the extracellular potential gradient distribution produced throughout the ventricles by a shock and whether the shock will successfully terminate ventricular fibrillation.[9–14] For defibrillation to occur, it is thought that a minimal potential gradient must be generated by the shock throughout most or all of the ventricular myocardium.[12–14] The distribution of potential gradients in the heart after a shock is uneven for electrodes located on or in the heart. There are high-gradient areas near the electrodes and low-gradient areas farthest away from the electrodes.[12, 14, 15] These areas of low gradient are the regions in which earliest activation originates after unsuccessful defibrillation shocks.[12, 14] Furthermore, high potential gradients can have detrimental effects on the heart, including postshock arrhythmias,[16] conduction disturbances,[17, 18] myocardial dysfunction,[19] and myocardial necrosis.[20]

The potential gradient distribution created by a shock in the heart depends on several factors, including the electrode size and location.[21] The optimal electrode system for ventricular defibrillation minimizes the high-gradient areas near the electrodes and raises the critical amount of ventricular tissue above the minimum gradient to achieve defibrillation. Cooper and colleagues[22] tested multiple electrode configurations in a sheep model of atrial fibrillation. They demonstrated that the optimal single-current pathway found for internal atrial defibrillation employed electrodes that surrounded both atria. In this study, a right-to-left electrode configuration (e.g., right atrial appendage and distal coronary sinus) resulted in mean defibrillation thresholds of 1 to 2 J. In humans, a similar electrode configuration requires slightly higher shock energies for acute atrial fibrillation and significantly higher shock energies for chronic atrial fibrillation.[23–29] Alt and coworkers[30] showed that in patients with chronic atrial fibrillation, the thresholds were initially high but decreased over time as recurrent fibrillation episodes were treated more promptly.

Modeling studies of internal atrial defibrillation demonstrated that the efficacy of lead systems increase when larger amounts of atrial tissue are encompassed. Min and colleagues[31] performed computational simulations of atrial defibrillation using finite element methods in a three-dimensional model of the human thorax. Realistic tissue conductivities were assigned to isolated tissue volumes obtained from magnetic resonance image slices. Atrial defibrillation thresholds were computed by determining the peak voltage required to produce an electric field intensity of more than 5 V/cm throughout 95% of the atrial tissue. Several electrode configurations were evaluated. The authors concluded that the lowest atrial defibrillation thresholds were obtained for the configuration having electrodes in the right atrial appendage and the coronary sinus, similar to the in vivo results from both animal[22, 32] and human[33] experiments.

One way to reach the minimal gradient to achieve defibrillation throughout the heart and minimize the gradient near the electrodes is by giving two smaller shocks separated spatially and temporally instead of one large shock. Cooper and associates[34] demonstrated that the earliest sites of atrial activation after unsuccessful single-current pathway shocks in a sheep model of atrial fibrillation were dependent on electrode configuration and appeared to occur in regions where the potential gradient field produced by the shock would be predicted to be low. Cooper and coworkers[35, 36] developed and tested dual-electrode configurations that were designed to employ a second shock and current pathway that encompassed the areas where the previous mapping study had shown the earliest activations to occur. In animals studies,[35] they were able to show that delivered-energy atrial defibrillation thresholds were reduced 70% when sequential biphasic shocks were applied to dual-current pathways. The mean single-current pathway (right atrial appendage to distal coronary sinus) defibrillation threshold was 1.3 ± 0.3 J, whereas the mean sequential shock configuration (right atrial appendage to distal coronary sinus followed by proximal coronary sinus to pulmonary artery) defibrillation threshold was 0.36 ± 0.13 J.

These findings were confirmed in a clinical study in 12 patients with chronic atrial fibrillation (mean duration, 165 ± 187 days).[36] The atrial defibrillation threshold of a single-shock, single-current pathway configuration (right atrial appendage to distal coronary sinus) was compared with a sequential-shock, dual-current configuration (right atrial appendage to distal coronary sinus followed by proximal coronary sinus to left subclavian vein). In this study, the atrial defibrillation threshold for the single-shock, single-current system was significantly higher than that for the sequential-shock, dual-current configuration (5.1 ± 1.8 J versus 2.0 ± 0.4 J; $P < .05$).

In summary, previous studies have established that electrode size and location affect atrial defibrillation thresholds, and electrodes positioned to surround the atria have the lowest thresholds. Atrial defibrillation thresholds are higher in patients with chronic atrial fibrillation, and they decrease over time with prompt treatment of atrial fibrillation. Further decreases in atrial defibrillation thresholds may be achieved through innovative shocking strategies, including sequential pulse defibrillation.

■ IMPLANTABLE ATRIAL DEFIBRILLATOR LEAD SYSTEM

Having determined that a lead system that encompasses both atria is important for defibrillation, a prerequisite for an implantable atrial defibrillator is a coronary sinus lead that maintains a stable position over time. Initial animal studies by Ayers and coworkers[37] demonstrated that a coronary sinus defibrillation lead with a distal preformed spiral shape had improved positional stability as compared with leads without the spiral tip. Using a coronary sinus lead in which the spiral tip is deployed on stylet removal, they found that the mean atrial defibrillation threshold in a sheep model was less than 1 J over the 2 months the lead system was implanted. Jung and Lüderitz[38] evaluated the stability and chronic performance of the lead system to ensure successful defibrillation efficacy over time (Fig. 24–1). In the Metrix (InControl, Seattle, WA) clinical trial, atrial defibrillation thresholds were measured at implantation and at 3-month follow-up in 51 patients. Analysis using only the paired threshold voltage data showed no significant difference in threshold between implantation and 3 months ($P = .85$) with the ability to detect a 50-V difference. They concluded from the initial experience that the spiral-shaped coronary sinus lead (Fig. 24–2) produces a stable system with no significant acute to chronic changes in atrial defibrillation thresholds. The clinical experience to date in more than 140 patients has revealed no coronary sinus dislodgments.

There are several means to position a right atrial lead in such a way as to achieve reasonable defibrillation thresholds for a single-current pathway system. Lok and colleagues[39] noted in a study of 28 patients that the high right atrium (HRA) and anterolateral right atrial lead locations had higher conversion rates (89% and 81%, respectively) compared with the inferomedial location (50%), and the atrial defibril-

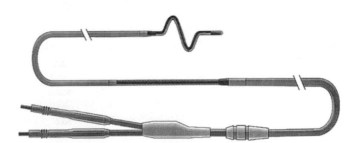

Figure 24–1. Schematic of leads with distal coronary sinus spiral shocking coil and proximal right atrial shocking coil.

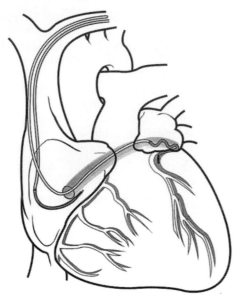

Figure 24–2. The three-lead system for the Metrix (InControl, Seattle, WA) atrial defibrillator includes a spiral coronary sinus lead, an active fixation right atrial lead, and a bipolar right ventricular lead (not shown) for synchronization.

lation threshold for the HRA was lower (3.9 ± 1.8 J) than the anterolateral position (4.6 ± 1.8 J). In an attempt to simplify the implantation procedures, a single lead is being developed with a distal electrode positioned in the coronary sinus in a spiral configuration and with a proximal electrode positioned in the right atrium near the superior vena cava (SVC). Sopher and coworkers[40] compared the defibrillation thresholds between a two-lead system and a single catheter with both coronary sinus and right atrial shocking coils see (Fig. 24–1).[40] They found that in three patients, the atrial defibrillation threshold using a single-pass catheter was lower than that using the two-lead system, whereas in one patient, a higher threshold was obtained with the single-pass system than with the two-lead system.

The benefit of having an implantable atrial defibrillator with leads in the coronary sinus and right atrium, as well as the right ventricle, is that it allows for sensing of atrial events across the right atrial–coronary sinus vector. Typical atrial bipolar electrodes have difficulty distinguishing sinus tachycardia, atrial flutter, and atrial fibrillation because the local activity, as viewed from the bipole, is similar for the different rhythms. Sensed atrial events from a right atrial–coronary sinus vector provide a comprehensive view of left-sided and right-sided atrial activity; this comprehensive field allows for more discriminate diagnostic possibilities.

■ DEFIBRILLATION WAVEFORMS

Defibrillation waveforms used in implantable ventricular and atrial defibrillators are created by charging a capacitor and then discharging it between electrodes at an exponential rate. In studies comparing the efficacy of various waveforms, the variables that have been assessed are the duration of the waveform, the type of waveform (i.e., monophasic or bipha-

sic), the tilt and shape of the waveform, and the number of shocks delivered. The duration of a waveform or a phase of a multiphase waveform is set by truncating or ending the discharge of the capacitor to the electrodes at a certain time. The type of waveform is determined by the switching mechanisms associated with the output of the capacitor discharge. By switching the polarity of the output to the electrodes at a certain time during a capacitor discharge, multiphase waveforms can be created. A biphasic waveform is created by reversing the polarity of the electrodes using a switching scheme to control phase duration, polarity, and trailing edge truncation point. The tilt of the waveform is determined by the slope of the voltage decay from the capacitor during discharge.

Tilt is also defined as a time constant, which is the time at which the capacitor voltage declines to $1/e$ (37%) of the starting voltage. The time constant is determined by the product of the capacitance (microfarads) of the capacitor and the impedance (ohms) of the electrode system during the shock. Thus, the shape of a truncated exponential capacitor discharged waveform is determined by the size of the capacitor as well as the impedance of the electrode system. Other methods can be used to change the shape, including the addition of an inductor in the defibrillation output circuit to "round" the waveform and lower the leading edge voltage/current. All of these variables are thought to be important for the development of the optimal atrial defibrillation waveform. The optimal atrial defibrillation waveform is believed to be one that minimizes the discomfort associated with the shocks and that minimizes the size of the device. It has been theorized that the pain associated with shocks in part is related to the intensity of the shock.

For internal ventricular[41, 49] and atrial[22, 23, 50] defibrillation in animals and humans, certain biphasic waveforms consisting of two phases of opposite polarity decrease the shock strength required for defibrillation compared with equal duration monophasic waveforms. Cooper and colleagues[22] demonstrated in a sheep model of atrial fibrillation that monophasic waveform durations of 1.5 to 6 msec were not significantly different in terms of threshold voltage; thus, the strength–duration curve was flat for durations of 1.5 to 6 msec. For symmetric biphasic waveforms, shorter (3 msec) and longer (12 msec) total pulse durations were associated with higher threshold voltages than with a total pulse width in the middle of this spectrum (6 msec). Thus, the strength–duration curve for biphasic waveforms for atrial defibrillation in sheep showed a relatively steep increase at shorter (3 msec) and longer (12 msec) total pulse durations, with a distinct nadir at 6 msec.

Johnson and coworkers[50] compared a biphasic waveform with a monophasic waveform of the same total duration for transcatheter internal cardioversion of atrial fibrillation in humans. They found that for a total duration of 6 msec a symmetric biphasic waveform (3/3 msec) had a significantly lower atrial defibrillation threshold than a monophasic (6 msec) waveform in 18 patients undergoing electrophysiologic procedures. In another clinical study, Cooper and colleagues[23] compared multiple monophasic and biphasic waveforms of the same total duration in 13 patients. They found that biphasic waveforms with total durations of 4 to 20 msec had significantly lower atrial defibrillation threshold than monophasic waveforms of the same total duration. There was no difference between symmetric biphasic waveforms of 4 to 20 msec. They also demonstrated that the individual phase durations of the biphasic waveform were important to defibrillation efficacy. An asymmetric biphasic waveform with the first phase longer than the second phase (7.5/2.5 msec) had a significantly lower atrial defibrillation threshold than an asymmetric biphasic waveform with the first phase shorter than the second phase (2.5/7.5 msec), a symmetric biphasic waveform with phases of equal duration (5/5 msec), and a monophasic waveform of the same total duration (10 msec). Ammer and associates[26] compared a longer biphasic (6/6 msec) waveform to a control waveform (3/3 msec) in 31 patients with a history of atrial fibrillation. They reported a significantly lower leading-edge voltage for the longer 6/6 msec biphasic waveform compared with the 3/3 msec biphasic waveform (254 ± 92 versus 355 ± 127 V) at the atrial defibrillation threshold, with no significant difference in energy (6.8 ± 2.8 versus 6.2 ± 1.5 Js) (Fig. 24–3). Tomassoni and coworkers[51] compared the effect of different capacitances on the atrial defibrillation threshold in humans. They found that a higher capacitance waveform (120 μF) was associated with a higher atrial defibrillation threshold energy requirement than was a lower capacitance waveform (50 μF). They found that the atrial defibrillation threshold for 120 μF shocks was 2.0 ± 1.0, compared with 1.4 ± 0.8 J for the 50-μF shocks. Heisel and coworkers[52] compared the efficacy of two biphasic waveforms with different capacitances (500 μF and 60 μF) in humans with acutely induced atrial fibrillation. They found that the atrial defibrillation threshold in terms of voltage was significantly lower for the 500-μF capacitance than for the 60-μF waveform (73 ± 23 versus 191 ± 46 V) without a significant difference in delivered energy (0.9 ± 0.6 versus 1.23 ± 0.6 J).

Peak voltage can also be reduced by including an inductor, used for many years in transthoracic defibrillation, in the discharge circuit. Newer integrated circuit technology allows for creation of rounding with transistor-switching technology. In animal studies, it has been reported that a rounded biphasic waveform had a lower atrial defibrillation threshold in terms of leading-edge voltage, current, and energy, com-

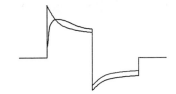

Shock Type	Mean DFT (V)	Mean DFT (J) (range)	Mean Shocks Tolerated (shocks/patient)
Rounded	136	0.63 (0.33-0.99)	2.8
Standard	100	0.44 (0.36-0.49)	1

Figure 24–4. Rounded waveform associated with decreased peak voltage and energy. DFT, defibrillation threshold.

pared with a conventional biphasic capacitor discharge waveform (Fig. 24–4).[53] Clinical studies are in progress to determine if a rounded biphasic waveform decreases the discomfort associated with internal atrial defibrillation shocks. This technology may prove valuable to improving patient tolerance. It has also been shown in both animal[35] and human[54] studies that sequential biphasic shocks delivered over a single-current pathway result in a significantly lower atrial defibrillation threshold leading-edge voltage without a significant difference in delivered energy. As previously discussed in this chapter, it has been demonstrated that delivered-energy atrial defibrillation thresholds were reduced 70% when sequential biphasic shocks were applied to dual-current pathways in both animal[35] and human[36] studies. Although these impressive reductions in atrial defibrillation threshold move us closer to "painless" atrial defibrillation, the clinical benefit of a more complex waveform generator or implanted lead system associated with these newer systems is not clear.

The Metrix implantable atrial defibrillator employs a 6/6 msec biphasic shock. Initial clinical studies revealed that the ED[50] (the voltage at which half the atrial fibrillation episodes could be successfully cardioverted) was about 180 V. The Jewel AF model 7250 (Medtronic, Minneapolis, MN) also uses a biphasic capacitor discharge waveform, although little data are available regarding thresholds for atrial defibrillation for this device. Certainly, future designs may benefit from optimizing the waveforms or developing systems that facilitate sequential pulse defibrillation.

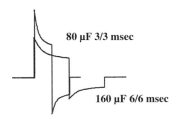

Shock Type	Mean DFT (V)	Mean DFT (J)	Mean Pain Score (1 - 10)
3/3 msec	355 ± 127	6.3 ± 1.5	4.5 ± 2.2
6/6 msec	258 ± 112	6.8 ± 1.8	1.8 ± 1.3

Figure 24–3. The 6/6-msec waveform associated with lower pain scores and sedation requirements as well as lower voltage. DFT, defibrillation threshold.

■ ATRIAL FIBRILLATION DETECTION ALGORITHMS

The approach to atrial fibrillation detection algorithms for an implantable atrial defibrillator is conceptually diametrically opposed to those algorithms required for a ventricular defibrillator. Because ventricular fibrillation is a fatal arrhythmia, the algorithms required by ventricular defibrillators must by necessity diagnose a rhythm rapidly, and must error on the side of shocking if the diagnosis is uncertain. By placing a greater importance on sensitivity than specificity, it is un-

First Stage Detection Algorithm: Quiet Intervals Analysis

━━━━ = "Quiet" Intervals

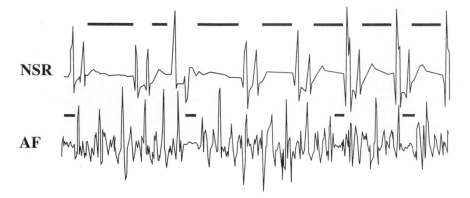

NSR

AF

Figure 24–5. Comparison of quiet interval analysis for normal sinus rhythm (NSR) and atrial defibrillation (AF).

likely that a patient with ventricular fibrillation will not be shocked; however, many patients with sinus tachycardia, considered a "noise signal," are at risk for receiving unwanted shocks.

Because atrial fibrillation is not a life-threatening arrhythmia, the detection algorithms have the luxury of "taking their time" in the diagnosis of atrial fibrillation, and in so doing they can emphasize specificity over sensitivity. In contrast to ventricular implantable cardioverter-defibrillators, (ICDs), which must quickly diagnose and treat an arrhythmia, an atrial defibrillator may withhold therapy until the diagnosis is confirmed. In fact, the current implantable atrial defibrillator can be programmed to allow the patient to activate the device and initiate therapy when the atrial fibrillation becomes clinically problematic.

For the Metrix atrial defibrillator, a Mirror Image detection algorithm uses a two-part analysis to diagnose atrial fibrillation. In the first part of the algorithm, termed the *Quiet*

Interval analysis, the device determines what percentage of the electrogram signal exists beyond certain sensitivity threshold limits (Fig. 24–5). During sinus rhythm, the baseline electrogram is quiet; thus, only the R and T waves would be detected by the algorithm as activity beyond the limits of threshold. During atrial fibrillation, however, the baseline electrogram, which is recording all the deflections characteristic of atrial fibrillation, crosses over the threshold values frequently. A percentage of quiet time is calculated over an 8-second segment by dividing accumulated quiet time by total sample duration and multiplying by 100%. If at least 10% to 30% of the time is void of activity (i.e., is quiet), the algorithm concludes that the rhythm is sinus. If, however, there is less than 10% to 30% of quiet activity, the algorithm concludes that there is a high likelihood that the rhythm is not sinus.

The second part of the Mirror Image detection algorithm, termed *Baseline Crossing Analysis,* would then be invoked.[55]

Second Stage Detection Algorithm: Baseline Crossings

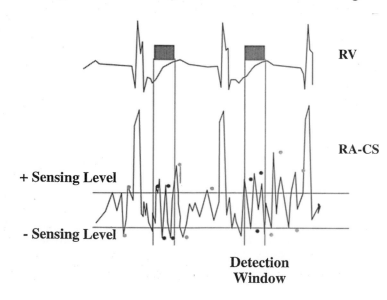

RV

RA-CS

+ Sensing Level

- Sensing Level

Detection Window

Figure 24–6. The baseline crossing algorithm is applied only to data samples with a low probability of sinus rhythm and a high probability of atrial defibrillation. By determining how frequently the signal crosses both the positive and negative sensing level, it maintains a high specificity for atrial defibrillation. RV, right ventricle; RA-CS, right atrium–coronary sinus.

The Baseline Crossing Analysis algorithm uses a detection window in the S-Q region, during which the number of times the signal crosses the sensitivity threshold are counted (Fig. 24–6). If the average Baseline Crossing count exceeds the programmed value (programmable from 1.6 to 3.0), the rhythm is considered atrial fibrillation.[55]

The combined benefit of these two algorithms is that the Quiet Interval analysis is sensitive for sinus rhythm, whereas the Baseline Crossing algorithm is specific for atrial fibrillation. Furthermore, if the device is not satisfied with the quality of the electrogram signal being analyzed, it simply collects a new rhythm strip to analyze. It is this freedom to analyze the recorded data that is the foundation of the safety and efficacy of the implantable atrial defibrillator.

In addition to the stand-alone atrial defibrillator, there is in development a ventricular defibrillator that has atrial tachyarrhythmia therapy abilities. This device, the Jewel AF model 7250, gives priority to the detection and treatment of ventricular tachyarrhythmias and thus would be indicated only for patients with concurrent ventricular and atrial arrhythmias. An example of its detection priorities is illustrated in Figure 24–7.[56]

The Jewel AMD 7250 also has a two-step atrial arrhythmia algorithm, termed *preliminary atrial fibrillation–atrial tachycardia detection,* and *sustained atrial fibrillation–atrial tachycardia detection.* The first algorithm determines whether the mean atrial cycle length falls within a programmed detection zone, and the atrial fibrillation–atrial tachycardia evidence counter has detected 32 ventricular events in which the P:R pattern supports the presence of an atrial tachyarrhythmia (i.e., greater than 1:1 A:V conduction, without far-field R-wave sensing). If the preliminary detection occurs, the second algorithm is invoked.

The sustained atrial fibrillation–atrial tachycardia detection algorithm programs a time interval (1 minute to 24 hours) after which, if the arrhythmia is still present, the device initiates therapy. Five different therapies for atrial arrhythmias may be initiated: (1) atrial burst pacing, (2) atrial ramp pacing, (3) atrial 50-Hz burst pacing, (4) automatic defibrillation, and (5) patient-activated atrial defibrillation.

▪ SAFETY OF INTERNAL ATRIAL DEFIBRILLATION

The safety of internal atrial defibrillation is absolutely imperative because in most cases, the arrhythmia is not life-threatening. The potential proarrhythmic risk of the shocks must be the first concern in the development of an automatic implantable atrial defibrillator without ventricular defibrillation backup capabilities. Several studies have shed some light on this risk. Cooper and coworkers[22] found that shock strengths even as low as 30 to 40 V delivered between the right atrial appendage and the distal coronary sinus in sheep could result in ventricular fibrillation with appropriate poor synchronization of the shock to ventricular activation. Also, they found that high-voltage shocks delivered with electrodes near the sinus or atrioventricular nodes resulted in temporary sinus or atrioventricular block, and the duration of block was related to the strength of the shock.

Ayers and colleagues[57] delivered 1870 synchronized shocks to sheep with induced atrial fibrillation and varied

Detection Priorities

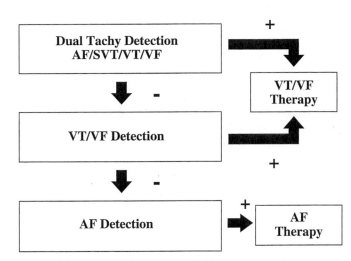

Figure 24–7. The dual-chamber defibrillator looks for evidence of arrhythmia in both atrial and ventricular channels, but gives priority to ventricular tachycardia/ventricular fibrillation (VT/VF) detection and therapy. AF, atrial fibrillation; SVT, supraventricular tachycardia.

the preshock ventricular cycle length. They found that a predictor of induction of ventricular tachyarrhythmias was a preshock ventricular cycle length of less than 300 msec. No ventricular tachyarrhythmias were induced with a preshock ventricular cycle length of greater than 300 msec. They also found that the risk of induction of ventricular tachyarrhythmias was extremely low (11 episodes, 0.6% overall; 0% for preshock ventricular cycle length of more than 300 msec, and 1.1% for preshock ventricular cycle length of less than 300 msec). This information has been used in the development of the shock-delivery algorithm for the current stand-alone implantable atrial defibrillator.[58]

Murgatroyd and associates[59] summarized the safety record of temporary transvenous atrial defibrillation from multiple centers. They found that in more than 3043 synchronized shocks given to 226 patients, there were no induced sustained ventricular tachyarrhythmias. There were two episodes of potential nonsustained ventricular arrhythmias (an alternative diagnosis was postshock aberrant conduction), both lasting less than 8 beats. A total of 39 unsynchronized shocks were delivered unintentionally, and 3 of these episodes resulted in ventricular fibrillation requiring external defibrillation. The authors found that postshock transient bradycardia, defined as less than 50 bpm (15.5%) or pauses of longer than 2000 msec (8.2%), was common after both successful and unsuccessful shocks without any clearcut predictors. No patient developed persistent postshock sinus or atrioventricular node conduction abnormalities. They concluded that the risk for proarrhythmia in terms of ventricular tachyarrhythmias from internal atrial defibrillation shocks is extremely low with appropriately synchronized shocks and that transient bradycardia with or without pauses is common but difficult to predict.

Having established that the risk for proarrhythmia is associated with short RR intervals and that no ventricular fibrillation could be induced with cycle lengths greater than

300 msec[60] an implantable atrial defibrillator must reliably identify R waves. The existence of multiple vectors (right ventricle bipolar, and right ventricle–coronary sinus) from which to analyze R-wave amplitude morphology is one benefit of the Metrix implanted lead system (Fig. 24–8). The orthogonal vectors offered with this system allow for improved R-wave identification independent of different R-wave axes. Second, the option of the implantable defibrillator to "discard" poor-quality R waves in favor of a rhythm with acceptable R waves is an opportunity afforded only an atrial defibrillator because there is no urgency to shock an abnormal rhythm. Hence, the implantable defibrillator can establish several criteria to identify optimal or acceptable R waves from which it can calculate the ventricular cycle length or defer shocks. For example, acceptable R-wave criteria could include R-wave width (to rule out premature ventricular contractions and T waves); acceptable morphology (high slew rate); and amplitude variability rejection (to facilitate automatic gain control and noise rejection).

Safety of internal atrial defibrillation is directly related to R-wave synchronization. Implantable stand-alone defibrillators employ a sophisticated algorithm to identify R waves, then invokes timing criteria to ensure that no shocks are delivered on short or long-short RR intervals. Both animal and clinical studies have shown that risk of proarrhythmia is extremely low, if not nonexistent, with appropriately timed and synchronized shocks.

■ TOLERANCE OF INTERNAL ATRIAL DEFIBRILLATION

The ability of patients to tolerate the shock associated with atrial defibrillation may be associated with several parameters, including shock intensity, shock waveform, sedation, patient characteristic and personality type, number of shocks received, and ability of the patient to control when the shock is delivered. In a study performed by Alt and colleagues,[61]

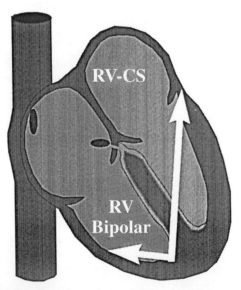

Figure 24–8. The orthogonal vectors (right ventricle [RV], bipolar, right ventricle–coronary sinus [RV-CS]) significantly enhance R-wave identification to ensure accuracy with the interval timing.

16 patients received either 3/3-msec or 6/6-msec biphasic shocks, and a pain score was recorded. Pain scores were significantly lower in the 6/6-msec shock group (1.3 ± 1.1 versus 4.0 ± 2.0), as was the voltage (251V versus 305V), implying that the energy determines the success of a shock, but voltage determines the pain perceived by the patient. They concluded that the use of waveforms that deliver greater energy at lower peak voltages offers the possibility of internal cardioversion with less sedation and greater patient tolerance.

Murgatroyd and coworkers[62] studied the efficacy and tolerability of low-energy internal cardioversion in 22 patients with paroxysmal atrial fibrillation. Using an atrial defibrillation threshold protocol that started at 10 to 20 V with a 40-V step-up, they noted that patients had a mean tolerance of 116 ± 51 V. They also noted that patients could tolerate three to four shocks per episode.[62] Expanding on the work of Murgatroyd, Lok and colleagues[39] determined the atrial defibrillation threshold of 28 patients with chronic atrial fibrillation with a protocol that started at 180 V and increased in 40-V increments. They found that, on average, patients were able to tolerate 3.4 ± 2 shocks with a tolerability threshold of 255 ± 60 V.

To evaluate further the tolerability of low-energy shocks, Steinhaus and coworkers[63] prospectively evaluated the discomfort and acceptance of low-energy shocks in 18 patients undergoing testing of their ventricular ICD. Two synchronized shocks of 0.4 and 2 J were delivered in random order without sedation while the patients were in sinus rhythm. Responses were quantified using a Visual Analogue Scale (VAS). The mean VAS for the first shock was 7.0 ± 2.1, and there was no difference between 0.4 and 2.0 J shocks (P = 0.55). There was, however, a significant difference based on order, with the second shock perceived as more uncomfortable than the first (6.9 versus 7.6, P = .03). Despite no clinical benefit to the patients, most patients were willing to accept similar shocks for non–life-threatening arrhythmia. Based on these studies, it appears that patients are willing to accept a limited number of shocks (about two to three) if it stops their non–life-threatening arrhythmia.

The understanding of patient tolerance has improved significantly as the number of patients implanted with defibrillators has increased. When patients were asked to describe what they think of the therapy, several of them have asked, "Don't you want to know first what it is like to be in atrial fibrillation?" Often, the shock is perceived as a jolt, or a punch, but it is tolerable because it is so quick and it immediately restores sinus rhythm without the need to visit the hospital for an external cardioversion. The visit to the hospital is time-consuming and can be associated with burns on the skin. Recognizing that an implantable atrial defibrillator affords the patient the opportunity to activate the device when atrial fibrillation is clinically symptomatic, several studies have started to evaluate whether patients tolerate therapy better if they are in control of the timing of the shock and their surroundings. The flexibility of patient-activated therapy would allow for a patient to self-treat immediately if desired, or to wait several hours as needed. An implantable device may not be able to cure atrial fibrillation, but it appears to give back to the patient the ability to manage the disease, which is perceived by many patients as tolerable. In summary, studies suggest that the number of shocks determines tolerability more than the absolute voltage, that tolerance can be improved with waveform modification, and that the tolerability of the shock must be put in the context of the tolerability of atrial fibrillation.

■ CLINICAL EXPERIENCE WITH ATRIAL DEFIBRILLATORS

More than 140 patients worldwide have undergone implantation of the Metrix atrial defibrillator and have been followed for an average of 9 months and as long as 2 years. In these patients at least three antiarrhythmic drugs had failed to provide relief because of poor efficacy or poor tolerability before implantation. The safety and efficacy of the device continues to be evaluated, as does the perceived patient benefit.

Several parameters are being evaluated to assess device safety. First, the atrial defibrillation detection algorithms (including Quiet Interval and Baseline Crossing Analyses) have included more than 3000 tests to detect atrial fibrillation, with a sensitivity of 90% and a specificity of 100%. Specifically, there have been no false-positive results, in which the detection algorithm diagnosed atrial fibrillation when in fact no atrial fibrillation was present. Once atrial fibrillation has been diagnosed, the device proceeds to evaluate specific R waves to determine a suitable time to deliver a shock. Almost 300,000 R waves have been analyzed, and roughly half were considered appropriate for shock. The synchronization accuracy has been 100%, with no inappropriate R waves or non–R waves being marked. There have been more than 6000 shocks delivered, with no proarrhythmia.

To proceed cautiously with novel device therapy and to optimize the algorithm programming for individual patients, any patient who has received the Metrix system must have the treatment of the atrial fibrillation episodes observed by the physician for the first 3 months. After the observation and device fine-tuning period, patients have the option to treat themselves by applying a hand-held therapy activator over the device to initiate the detection and shock algorithms if they experience symptoms of atrial fibrillation. During the observation period, more than 400 atrial fibrillation episodes have been treated. On average, 2.5 shocks per episode are required to achieve sinus rhythm. To date, 96% of episodes were converted to sinus rhythm as a result of the defibrillation, and 86% of conversions were associated with sustained sinus rhythm.

Previous experience with both internal and external cardioversion has documented the phenomenon whereby atrial fibrillation recurs soon after a successful conversion to sinus rhythm. The exact cause of this phenomenon has not been clearly elucidated, although it may be related to atrial premature contractions (APCs) occurring during the vulnerable window of a previous atrial beat. When early recurrence of atrial fibrillation (ERAF) is defined as the resumption of atrial fibrillation within 1 minute after a successful cardioversion that resulted in a return of confirmed sinoatrial nodal activation for at least 1 beat, 13% of patients have ERAF associated with cardioversion.[64] However, when ERAF is seen, it typically merely delays, but does not prevent, the return of sustained sinus rhythm. For example, if 100 atrial defibrillation episodes were treated, 30 might be associated

with ERAF, but eventually 86% could be converted to sustained sinus rhythm with an average of two to three shocks per episode. Pretreatment with antiarrhythmic drugs, such as procainamide, may further reduce the incidence of ERAF.

The real benefit of an implantable atrial defibrillator is that it gives back to a patient control of the disease. Specifically, by the patient's having the capability to treat the condition at home, at work, or while on vacation rather than having to return to the hospital to undergo external cardioversion, his or her life may be significantly less affected by the paroxysmal nature of atrial fibrillation. Thirty patients worldwide who have the Metrix system are able to provide patient-controlled therapy. So far, more than 150 episodes of atrial fibrillation have been treated in the ambulatory setting under patient control, and 87% of episodes were converted to sinus rhythm, with about 1.5 shocks per episode.

As with the Metrix, more than 150 patients have been implanted with the AMD 7250. The initial experience with the dual-chamber defibrillator was recently summarized by Jung and associates.[65] Seven of the patients had both ventricular and supraventricular tachycardias. A total of 105 tachycardia episodes were evaluated. High-frequency burst pacing (HFBP) was effective in terminating 56% (13 of 23) of the induced atrial fibrillation episodes, whereas atrial ramp or burst pacing was effective only in 31% (5 of 21) or 13% (2 of 16) of the induced episodes. The atrial defibrillation threshold was 1.8 ± 0.4 J for induced atrial fibrillation using a shock vector encompassing the right atrium, the right ventricle, and a left prepectoral defibrillator can. Ventricular tachycardia therapy was appropriately withheld in 90% (28 of 31) of the induced atrial fibrillation episodes with a rapid ventricular response.

Feasibility testing of the AMD 7250 dual-chamber defibrillator detection algorithm was summarized by Gillberg and colleagues.[56] The use of this algorithm prevented the inappropriate detection of ventricular tachycardia or fibrillation instead of supraventricular tachycardia. The dual-chamber algorithms failed to detect one potentially lethal ventricular tachycardia and ventricular fibrillation out of a total of 68 episodes, and incorrectly identified 17 of 60 episodes of atrial fibrillation and supraventricular tachycardia as ventricular tachycardia and ventricular fibrillation.

These results suggest that the AMD 7250 device is a viable alternative for patients with both ventricular and atrial tachyarrhythmias. Because 10% to 26% of atrial fibrillation episodes were interpreted as ventricular tachycardia and immediately shocked, however, this device may not be ideal for the lone atrial defibrillation patient.

■ CLINICAL UTILITY OF ATRIAL DEFIBRILLATORS

Innovative engineering has created a device that treats atrial fibrillation. The next challenge is to educate physicians and patients about the clinical effect that atrial fibrillation has on a patient's life. There is an emerging body of data regarding alternative electrical therapeutic options available to patients with atrial fibrillation. Internists, family practitioners, cardiologists, and electrophysiologists need to know that focal ablation can sometimes cure patients with a focal ectopic source of atrial fibrillation. In addition, some patients with presumed chronic atrial fibrillation may actually have paroxysmal atrial fibrillation when appropriate therapeutic modalities are employed to cardiovert their arrhythmia. Many patients prefer to be in sinus rhythm and are willing to cardiovert themselves electively to achieve that result. As continued data on the safety, efficacy, and quality of life associated with implantable atrial defibrillators become available, the dissemination of that information to physicians and their patients becomes an increasing priority. Proving clinical utility of these new technologies is a crucial step in their adoption.

The primary goals of treating a patient with atrial fibrillation focus on reducing the associated morbidity (e.g., stroke, congestive heart failure), and improving the patient's quality of life. It is difficult to assess accurately and comprehensively a patient's quality of life. However, there have been significant attempts to assess the effects of various therapies with validated questionnaires and test instruments. For example, the well-accepted SF-36 can be used to observe quality of life in patients with atrial fibrillation, and changes can be tracked over time to assess the adequacy of different therapies. Several quality of life studies are under way in the ongoing clinical trials of implantable defibrillators to evaluate the impact of device therapy over time and to try to understand which patients benefit most from this therapy.

Ideally, in addition to patient benefit, improved therapy for atrial fibrillation will also have a positive economic benefit. The cost of atrial fibrillation to the medical system is related to the frequency of emergency room visits, inpatient admissions, and outpatient procedures and can range from $6000 to $15,000 per year.[66] Wolf and coworkers[67] compared 12,625 patients with recent onset atrial fibrillation and cardiovascular disease with 13,809 patients with cardiovascular disease but without atrial fibrillation and found that mortality rates were 20% to 50% greater in the atrial fibrillation group. In addition, they found that costs were substantially higher in men and women with atrial fibrillation, over and above the mortality and costs associated with concomitant cardiovascular disease. They concluded that atrial fibrillation is a disease with a malignant medical and economic impact.

Invoking device therapy to treat atrial fibrillation obviously requires the up-front cost of the device; however, if this means the incidence of stroke, external cardioversions, and inpatient hospitalizations is reduced, the initial investment may pay off. As device therapy becomes more established, prospective analyses regarding the economic benefits of these therapy modalities will be needed.

The best data supporting the potential benefit of atrial ICD therapy for atrial fibrillation and quality of life were put forward by Timmermans and colleagues.[68] They analyzed the data from the first 51 patients in whom the Metrix device was implanted, with a mean follow-up of 259 ± 138 days. They focused on those patients who had more than three treated atrial fibrillation episodes, and divided the follow-up time into four parts, or quartiles. The time between atrial fibrillation episodes was calculated during each quartile of follow-up. Four Kaplan-Meier curves for the set of interepisode times corresponding to each quartile were calculated. The median interepisode durations were 7.3, 17, 21, and 35.3 days for the first, second, third, and fourth quartiles, respectively. The authors concluded that longer interepisode durations are more likely as time from implantation in-

creases. The implications of this analysis are powerful if, in fact, prompt treatment of atrial fibrillation episodes progressively decreases the chances that a patient will have a subsequent episode. Pathophysiologically, if atrial fibrillation begets atrial fibrillation, then the converse, that sinus begets sinus, may be equally true. Although preliminary, these data suggest that prompt treatment of atrial fibrillation is important and may be the best way to reduce the need for recurrent atrial defibrillation.

If prompt treatment of atrial defibrillation indeed reduces the frequency of recurrent episodes, perhaps leading to reverse remodeling, the future management of patients with atrial fibrillation should entail more aggressive measures to prevent the chronic changes associated with long-standing atrial fibrillation. This may reduce the remodeling associated with atrial fibrillation and allow for newer therapies to promote sustained sinus rhythm, further reducing the medical and socioeconomic burden of the disease.

Summary

Both animal and human studies have shown that atrial fibrillation can be internally defibrillated with relatively low energies. This is especially true for a single–current system if the electrodes are placed in the right atrial appendage and in the distal coronary sinus near the left atrial appendage so that they surround the atria. Biphasic waveforms are more efficacious for internal atrial defibrillation than monophasic waveforms of similar durations. The phase durations of the biphasic waveform are important determinants of defibrillation efficacy. Furthermore, both animal and human studies have demonstrated that marked reductions in the atrial defibrillation thresholds can be obtained with the use of sequential shocks and dual-current pathways. However, the amount of energy reduction may not warrant the added complexity of the dual-current system. Changing the shape of the defibrillation waveform using different capacitances or adding an inductor into the defibrillation output circuit can lower the leading-edge voltage/current of the shock. Whether this actually decreases the discomfort associated with shocks is unclear and will require further clinical evaluation.

The safety of internal atrial defibrillation has been analyzed in both animal and human studies. The risk of induction of tachyarrhythmias is low as long as the shock is appropriately synchronized to ventricular activation. This risk is even lower, if not nonexistent, if the shock is not delivered during periods of rapid ventricular response. Present studies have shown that modern devices appear to function well in patients with atrial fibrillation only (Metrix) or atrial fibrillation with ventricular tachycardia and ventricular fibrillation (AMD 7250). Positive enhancements in technology further the use of these devices. Despite good safety and efficacy records for these devices and anecdotal data demonstrating significant individual patient benefit, studies focusing on overall clinical utility are needed before this technology is widely adopted.

REFERENCES

1. Psaty BM, Manolio TA, Kuller LH, et al: Incidence of and risk factors for atrial fibrillation in older adults. Circulation 96:2455–2461, 1997.
2. Mackstaller LL, Alpert JS: Atrial fibrillation: A review of mechanism, etiology, and therapy. Clin Cardiol 20:640–650, 1997.
3. Gorelick PB: Stroke prevention: An opportunity for efficient utilization

of health care resources during the coming decade. Stroke 25:220–224, 1994.

4. Hohnloser S, Li Y: Drug treatment of atrial fibrillation: What have we learned? Curr Opin Cardiol 12:24–32, 1997.

5. Wellens HJJ: Atrial fibrillation: The last big hurdle in treating supraventricular tachycardia. N Engl J Med 331:944–945, 1994.

6. Murgatroyd FD, Camm AJ: Atrial fibrillation: The last challenge in interventional electrophysiology. Br Heart 74:209–211, 1995.

7. Lüderitz B, Pfeiffer D, Tebbenjohanns J, Jung W: Nonpharmacological strategies for treating atrial fibrillation. Am J Cardiol 77:45A–52A, 1996.

8. Lau CP, Tse HF, Lok NS, et al: Initial clinical experience of an implantable human atrial defibrillator. Pacing Clin Electrophysiol 20:220–225, 1996.

9. Krassowska W, Frazier DW, Pilkington TC, Ideker RE: Potential distribution in three-dimensional periodic myocardium. II. Application to extracellular stimulation. IEEE Trans Biomed Eng 37:267–284, 1990.

10. Lepeschkin E, Jones JL, Rush S, Jones RE: Local potential gradients as a unifying measure for thresholds of stimulation, standstill, tachyarrhythmia and fibrillation appearing after strong capacitor discharges. Adv Cardiol 21:268–278, 1978.

11. Frazier DW, Krassowska W, Chen P-S, et al: Extracellular field required for excitation in three-dimensional anisotropic canine myocardium. Circ Res 63:147–164, 1988.

12. Chen P-S, Wolf PD, Claydon FJ, III, et al: The potential gradient field created by epicardial defibrillation electrodes in dogs. Circulation 74:626–636, 1986.

13. Witkowski FX, Penkoske PA, Plonsey R: Mechanism of cardiac defibrillation in open-chest dogs with unipolar DC-coupled simultaneous activation and shock potential recordings. Circulation 82:244–260, 1990.

14. Wharton JM, Wolf PD, Smith WM, et al: Cardiac potential and potential gradient fields generated by single, combined, and sequential shocks during ventricular defibrillation. Circulation 85:1510–1523, 1992.

15. Tang ASL, Wolf PD, Claydon FJ III, et al: Measurement of defibrillation shock potential distributions and activation sequences of the heart in three-dimensions. IEEE Trans Biomed Eng 76:1176–1186, 1988.

16. Lesigne C, Levy B, Saumont R, et al: An energy-time analysis of ventricular fibrillation and defibrillation thresholds with internal electrodes. Med Biol Eng 14:617–622, 1976.

17. Yabe S, Smith WM, Daubert JP, et al: Conduction disturbances caused by high current density electric fields. Circ Res 66:1190–1203, 1990.

18. Jones JL, Lepeschkin E, Jones RE, Rush S: Response of cultured myocardial cells to countershock-type electric field stimulation. Am J Physiol 235:H214–H222, 1978.

19. Pansegrau DG, Abboud FM: Hemodynamic effects of ventricular defibrillation. J Clin Invest 49:282–297, 1970.

20. Dahl CF, Ewy GA, Warner ED, Thomas ED: Myocardial necrosis from direct current countershock: Effect of paddle size and time interval between discharge. Circulation 50:956–961, 1974.

21. Ideker RE, Wolf PD, Alferness CA, et al: Current concepts for selecting the location, size, and shape of defibrillation electrodes. Pacing Clin Electrophysiol 14:227–240, 1991.

22. Cooper RAS, Alferness CA, Smith WM, Ideker RE: Internal cardioversion of atrial fibrillation in sheep. Circulation 87:1673–1686, 1993.

23. Cooper RAS, Johnson EE, Wharton JM: Internal atrial defibrillation in humans: The improved efficacy of biphasic waveforms and the importance of phase duration. Circulation 95:1487–1496, 1997.

24. Levy S, Richard P, Lau CP, et al: Multicenter low energy transvenous atrial defibrillation (XAD) trial results in different subsets of atrial fibrillation. J Am Coll Cardiol 29:750–755, 1997.

25. Johnson E, Smith W, Yarger M, et al: Clinical predictors of low energy defibrillation thresholds in patients undergoing internal cardioversion of atrial fibrillation [Abstract]. Pacing Clin Electrophysiol 17:742–742, 1994.

26. Ammer R, Alt E, Ayers G, et al: Pain threshold for low energy intracardiac cardioversion of atrial fibrillation with low or no sedation. Pacing Clin Electrophysiol 20:230–236, 1997.

27. Alt E, Coenen M, Schmitt C, et al: Intracardiac electrical conversion of atrial fibrillation: Which energies should be used? Circulation 90:I-14, 1994.

28. Alt E, Schmitt C, Ammer R, et al: Effect of electrode position on outcome of low-energy intracardiac cardioversion of atrial fibrillation. J Am Coll Cardiol 79:621–625, 1997.

29. Heisel A, Jung J, Neuzner J, et al: Low-energy transvenous cardiover-

30. Alt E, Ammer R, Schmitt C, et al: Repeated internal low-energy cardioversion of atrial fibrillation. J Am Coll Cardiol 27:302A, 1996.

31. Min X, Mongeon LR, Mehra R: Low threshold non-CS electrode systems for atrial defibrillation and compared with CS-RA by finite element human thorax model [Abstract]. Circulation 96:I-529, 1997.

32. Cooper RAS, Smith WM, Ideker RE: Early activation sites after unsuccessful internal atrial defibrillation shocks: The effect of electrode configuration [Abstract]. Pacing Clin Electrophysiol 19:706, 1996.

33. Saksena S, Prakash A, Mangeon L, et al: Clinical efficacy and safety of atrial defibrillation using biphasic shocks and current nonthoracotomy endocardial lead configurations. Am J Cardiol 76:913–921, 1995.

34. Cooper RAS, Smith WM, Ideker RE: Early activation sites after unsuccessful internal atrial defibrillation shocks: The effect of electrode configuration. Pacing Clin Electrophysiol 19:706, 1996.

35. Cooper RAS, Smith WM, Ideker RE: Internal cardioversion of atrial defibrillation: Marked reduction in defibrillation threshold with dual current pathways. Circulation 96:2693–2700, 1997.

36. Cooper RAS, Plumb VJ, Epstein AE, et al: Marked reduction in internal atrial defibrillation thresholds with dual current pathways and sequential shocks in humans. Circulation 97:2527–2535, 1998.

37. Ayers GM, Helland JR, Kreyenhagen PE, et al: Defibrillation lead with pre-formed spiral shape enhances positional stability. Am Heart J 128:637, 1994.

38. Jung W, Lüderitz B: Performance of the lead system for the Metrix automatic implantable atrial defibrillator. J Am Coll Cardiol 31:2, 513A, 1998.

39. Lok NS, Lau CP, Tse HF, Ayers GM: Clinical shock tolerability and effect of different right atrial electrode locations on efficacy of low energy human transvenous atrial defibrillation using an implantable lead system. J Am Coll Cardiol 30(5):1324–1330, 1997.

40. Sopher SM, Ayers GM, Obel OA, et al: Atrial defibrillation in man by low energy biatrial shocks employing a single-pass transvenous catheter. Circulation 94:I-563, 1996.

41. Gurvich NL, Yuniev GS: Restoration of regular rhythm in the mammalian fibrillating heart. Bull Exp Biol Med 8:55–58, 1939.

42. Schuder JC, McDaniel WC, Stoeckle H: Defibrillation of 100-kg calves with asymmetrical, bidirectional, rectangular pulses. Cardiovasc Res 18:419–426, 1984.

43. Dixon EG, Tang ASL, Wolf PD, et al: Improved defibrillation thresholds with large contoured epicardial electrodes and biphasic waveforms. Circulation 76:1176–1184, 1987.

44. Tang ASL, Yabe S, Wharton JM, et al: Ventricular defibrillation using biphasic waveforms: The importance of phasic duration. J Am Coll Cardiol 13:207–214, 1989.

45. Chapman PD, Vetter JW, Souza JJ, et al: Comparative efficacy of monophasic and biphasic truncated exponential shocks for nonthoracotomy internal defibrillation in dogs. J Am Coll Cardiol 12:739–745, 1988.

46. Kavanagh KM, Tang ASL, Rollins DL, et al: Comparison of the internal defibrillation thresholds for monophasic and double and single capacitor biphasic waveforms. J Am Coll Cardiol 14:1343–1349, 1989.

47. Bardy GH, Ivey TD, Allen MD, et al: A prospective randomized evaluation of biphasic versus monophasic waveform pulses on defibrillation efficacy in humans. J Am Coll Cardiol 14:728–733, 1989.

48. Winkle RA, Mead RH, Ruder MA, et al: Improved low energy defibrillation efficacy in man with the use of a biphasic truncated exponential waveform. Am Heart J 117:122–127, 1989.

49. Saksena S, An H, Mehra R, et al: Prospective comparison of biphasic and monophasic shocks for implantable cardioverter-defibrillators using endocardial leads. Am J Cardiol 70:304–310, 1992.

50. Johnson EE, Yarger MD, Wharton JM: Monophasic and biphasic waveforms for low energy internal cardioversion of atrial fibrillation in humans [Abstract]. Circulation 88:I-592, 1993.

51. Tomassoni G, Newby KH, Kearney MM, et al: Testing different biphasic waveforms and capacitances: Effect on atrial defibrillation threshold and pain perception. J Am Coll Cardiol 28:695–699, 1996.

52. Heisel A, Jung J, Schubert BD: Evaluation of two new biphasic waveforms for internal cardioversion of atrial fibrillation [Abstract]. Circulation 96:I-207, 1997.

53. Harbinson MT, Allen JD, Imam Z, et al: Rounded biphasic waveform reduces energy requirements for transvenous catheter cardioversion of atrial fibrillation and flutter [Abstract]. Pacing Clin Electrophysiol 20:226–229, 1997.

54. Cooper RAS, Plumb VJ, Epstein AE, et al: Reduction in voltage and current requirements for internal atrial defibrillation with sequential shocks in humans. Pacing Clin Electrophysiol [Abstract]. Pacing Clin Electrophysiol 18:531, 1998.

55. Sra J, Maglio C, Chen V, et al: Atrial fibrillation detection in humans using the METRIX™ atrial defibrillation system. J Am Coll Cardiol 27:375A, 1996.

56. Gillberg JM, Brown ML, Olson WH, et al: Acute human testing of a prototype dual chamber defibrillator at Mayo Clinic. Circulation 94(8):I-562, 1998.

57. Ayers GM, Alferness CA, Ilina M, et al: Ventricular proarrhythmic effects of ventricular cycle length and shock strength in a sheep model of transvenous atrial defibrillation. Circulation 89:413–422, 1994.

58. Adams JM, Ayers GM, Infinger KR, et al: Preceding ventricular interval: A programmed criterion for an implantable atrial defibrillator [Abstract]. Am Heart J 128, A-38, 1994.

59. Murgatroyd FD, Johnson EE, Cooper RA, et al: Safety of low energy transvenous atrial defibrillation: World experience [Abstract]. Circulation 90:I-14, 1994.

60. Ayers GM, Alferness CA, Ilina M, et al: Ventricular proarrhythmic effects of ventricular cycle length and shock strength in a sheep model of transvenous atrial defibrillation. Circulation 89:413–422, 1994.

61. Alt E, Ammer R, Schmitt C, et al: Pain threshold for internal cardiove sion with low or no sedation. Pacing Clin Electrophysiol 19:737, 199c

62. Murgatroyd FD, Slade AKB, Sopher M, et al: Efficacy and tolerability of transvenous low energy cardioversion of paroxysmal atrial fibrillation in humans. J Am Col Cardiol 25(6):1347–1353, 1995.

63. Steinhaus DM, Cardinal D, Mongeon L, et al: Atrial defibrillation: Are low energy shocks acceptable to patients? Pacing Clin Electrophysiol 19:625, 1996.

64. Timmermans C, Rodriguez L-M, Lambert H, Ayers GM: Incidence and mechanism of immediate reinitiation of atrial fibrillation following internal atrial defibrillation. Circulation 96(8):I-208, 1997.

65. Jung W, Spehl S, Christian W, et al: Initial experience with a new dual-chamber defibrillator in humans. Circulation 96(8):I-208, 1997.

66. Maglio C, Ayers GM, Tidball EW, et al: Health care utilization and cost of care in patients with symptomatic atrial fibrillation. Circulation 94:1-169, 1996.

67. Wolf PA, Mitchell JB, Baker CS, et al: Mortality and hospital costs associated with atrial fibrillation. Circulation 92:I-140, 1995.

68. Timmermans C, Wellens HJJ: Effect of device-mediated therapy on symptomatic episodes of atrial fibrillation. J Am Coll Cardiol 31:331A, 1998.

Chapter 25

Permanent Pacemaker and Implantable Cardioverter-Defibrillator Implantation

Peter H. Belott and Dwight W. Reynolds

The approach to cardiac pacemaker implantation has evolved during the past half century.[1] From the initial epicardial implants of Senning[2] and transvenous implantation by Furman and Schwedel,[3] cardiac pacemaker implantation has seen radical change not only in the implanted hardware but also in the preoperative planning, anatomic approach, personnel, and implantation facilities. The early trend from the epicardial approach to the simpler transvenous cutdown has led the way to the percutaneous technique developed by Littleford and Spector.[4] Preoperative planning and in particular device selection, which once were simple, have become complex. The pacemaker system, both device and electrodes, must be individualized to the patient's particular clinical and anatomic situation. The implantation procedure, previously the exclusive domain of the cardiovascular surgeon, has also become the purview of the invasive cardiologist. Similarly, the procedure has undergone a transition from the operating room to the cardiac catheterization laboratory or special procedures room. The luxury of an anesthesiologist has, except in special instances, disappeared, with the implanting physician assuming additional responsibilities. Finally, because of concerns about cost containment, the usual in-hospital postoperative observation period has been dramatically reduced or replaced by an ambulatory approach to pacemaker implantation.

Similarly, since Mirowski and colleagues[5] implanted the first implantable cardioverter-defibrillator (ICD) in 1980, its evolution has been comparable to that of the cardiac pacemaker. The ICD that was initially placed epicardially with an abdominal pocket has given way to a transvenous approach and a pectoral pocket. The surgery initially performed in the operating room exclusively by a cardiovascular surgeon is now carried out by nonsurgeons in the catheterization or electrophysiology laboratory. Finally, protracted hospital stays have been replaced by much shorter hospital stays, even outpatient situations. The once-simple ICD device is

now much more complex, offering total arrhythmia control as well as backup dual-chamber rate-adaptive pacing. All of these changes have not been without a price: New techniques have brought new challenges as well as problems and concerns. This chapter attempts to explore all aspects of modern pacemaker and ICD implantations from a practical point of view. It also addresses these new challenges, problems, and concerns.

■ PACEMAKER IMPLANTATION

Personnel

Traditionally, pacemaker implantation procedures have been performed exclusively by a thoracic or cardiac surgeon. The skills were acquired during a residency or fellowship. Early pacemaker implantations involved more extensive surgery and, at times, an open-chest procedure for epicardial electrode placement. The pulse generator and electrodes were large, requiring considerable dissection and surgical skill. Since 1980, decreasing pacemaker size has limited the more extensive surgery previously required. Today, the knowledge and skills required for dual-chamber pacing are well suited for the physician trained in cardiac catheterization.

It has become generally well accepted that the implanting physician may be either a thoracic surgeon or an invasive cardiologist.[6] At times, the two may even act as a team, with the surgeon isolating the vein and the cardiologist positioning the electrodes. With the current reimbursement structure and the changing economic environment, however, this team approach is rapidly becoming burdensome; in any event, it is frequently unnecessary. Today, the credentialing for pacemaker implantation procedures poses a dilemma. The trainee in thoracic surgery has ever-diminishing exposure to pacemaker implantation as the procedure becomes more the responsibility of the cardiologist. At the same time, the cardiologist has little or no exposure to proper surgical technique, the use of surgical instruments, or preoperative and postoperative care.

Considerable controversy exists about what constitutes an appropriate implantation experience and how long that experience should extend. *One thing that appears certain is that physicians with limited training and ongoing experience have unacceptable complication rates.*[7] It has been suggested that to remain proficient, one must perform a minimum of 12 procedures per year.

There is a definite need for formal training programs specifically designed to teach cardiac pacing.[8-10] Such programs should be offered to both cardiologists and surgeons interested in cardiac pacing. The ideal program should be comprehensive and integrated, involving not only all implantations but also follow-up and troubleshooting. To be an effective implanter, one must understand the problems of follow-up and troubleshooting. A formal didactic experience and hands-on exposure are necessary. Although a formal, year-long, comprehensive, integrated training program is ideal, consideration of physicians who are out of formal training programs requires, at times, combining more intensive didactic programs with extended, supervised hands-on experience. Even this latter approach should require involvement in nonimplantation aspects of pacing. It has been our frequent experience that there is substantially less enthusiasm for mastering these aspects of pacing. We ardently believe such mastery is crucial to becoming an effective implanter.

Regardless of how one has become trained to implant pacemakers, careful review (by those responsible for credentialing in a given institution) of the training and experience of individuals in pacing will assist in preventing inadequately trained individuals from performing independent, unsupervised pacemaker implantation. Criteria for adequate training and experience should include a minimum number of pacemaker procedures, including single-chamber and dual-chamber implantations, lead replacements, pulse generator replacements, and upgrades to dual-chamber from single-chamber systems. Also, some documentable experience in an active pacemaker service clinic should be required.[11]

Support personnel are crucial to the success and safety of any pacemaker procedure. Historically, whether in a large medical center or a small community hospital, the procedure was performed in the operating room. This had its drawbacks because each case could be a first-time experience for the operating room staff. Pacemaker procedures were frequently added at the end of a busy operating room schedule and were assigned to the first available room with support personnel, who changed from procedure to procedure. Personnel not familiar with the procedure can interrupt the flow of the case. Even with the transition to the cardiac catheterization laboratory for pacing procedures, the same problems can exist. Conversely, depending on the volume of procedures in the operating room and the cardiac catheterization laboratories, there may be a greater opportunity for consistent, recurrent availability of cardiovascular technicians, nurses, and radiography personnel in the latter. These more focused staff members tend to have a certain appreciation for the procedure and are better equipped to deal with the unique problems that may be enountered during pacemaker implantation. Whether in the operating room or catheterization

laboratory, the minimal personnel required are the same and include a scrub nurse or technician familiar with each operator's surgical preferences, a circulating nurse to support the personnel who have scrubbed (with this generally involving delivering supplies and equipment to the sterile field as needed and patient monitoring and medication administration, although this is somewhat limited in the operating room when an anesthesiologist is present), and an individual responsible for the performance of electric testing. It is also useful to have access to an experienced cardiovascular radiology technician, which generally is more easily accomplished in the cardiac catheterization laboratory than in the operating room.

The presence of an anesthesiologist or nurse anesthetist is becoming something of a luxury. Initially an essential member of the implantation team, an anesthesiologist in many centers is now involved only in special situations requiring airway support in an unstable or otherwise problematic patient. Anesthesiology staff should always be available for emergency situations and consulted if problems are anticipated.

The participation of the pacemaker manufacturer's representative support personnel has always been a subject of debate. This person's role varies from center to center.[12] At one extreme, the representative merely delivers the pacemaker and leads to the hospital. At the other extreme, he or she is a vital member of the support team, retrieving threshold data, filling out registration forms, and at times, offering technical advice. The latter is particularly true in smaller institutions with less pacemaker activity. A well-trained, experienced pacemaker representative can be an important member of the support team. An experienced representative dedicated to cardiac pacing frequently has a broad experience and knowledge base in problems especially unique to his or her company's products. Although such a representative of industry can be helpful, such a person, no matter how experienced or knowledgeable, should not be considered an acceptable alternative to a knowledgeable, skilled, and experienced physician implanter. If an industrial representative is to be used during implantations for support, hospital approval is advisable.

When the support personnel requirements of the operating room and the catheterization laboratory are compared, there are the previously noted general advantages to the latter. There is one other important concern that relates to sterile technique. The regular operating room personnel tend to be more keenly aware of sterile technique and are scrupulous in this regard. In contrast, the cardiac catheterization laboratory personnel are not routinely trained in operating room and sterile technique, and if these procedures are not strongly reinforced, they can be disastrously neglected.

Implantation Facility and Equipment

The cardiac catheterization laboratory and special procedures room appear well suited for permanent pacemaker procedures.[13, 14] Early concerns about safety and sterility have been shown to be unfounded when these issues are appropriately addressed prospectively. The unique capabilities from a radiologic point of view are invaluable. High-resolution images, unlimited projections, and angiographic capabilities can be extremely helpful in venous access and electrode placement as well as in variable image magnification, digital image acquisition, and image imposition techniques and storage. In addition, these facilities tend to be equipped for ready access with all of the catheters, guide wires, sheaths, and angiographic materials that might be required for special situations. The implantation facility is also typically the location of the most sophisticated physiologic monitoring and recording equipment (Fig. 25–1), offering continuous surface and endocardial electric recordings as well as extensive hemodynamic monitoring capabilities. The importance of staffing with qualified cardiovascular nurses and technicians has already been mentioned.

Concerns about the potential for infection must be addressed. These facilities are designated as intermediate sterile areas. The sterile precautions tend to be less rigid than in the operating room. The cardiac catheterization laboratory also tends to be a high-traffic area. A rigid protocol for sterile technique must be established and the room sealed from traffic after it has been cleaned for the surgical procedure. All personnel entering this area must wear scrub clothing, a hat, and a mask. The ventilation system should also meet the standards for an intermediate sterile area.

The cardiac catheterization laboratory and special procedures room generally have another drawback. Most do not allow the patient to be placed in the Trendelenburg position, which can be important in the percutaneous approach to pacemaker implantation. This problem, however, can be obviated by use of a wedge under the legs early in the procedure.

Of course, the ideal is a room or suite dedicated to pacemaker procedures and containing all of the capabilities previously noted as well as skilled staffing as previously described. The ability to maintain sterility, as well as dedicated equipment and staff, in such a room is attractive, although it is clearly the exception at present. As growth occurs in the number of transvenously implantable defibril-lators, the establishment of rooms dedicated to pacemaker and defibrillator implantation will likely also increase.

The strongest arguments for implanting a pacemaker in the operating room are sterility and patient control. It is typically the area of best sterility and sterile technique. A pacemaker represents a foreign body; therefore, one prime concern is infection. A procedure in the operating room generally offers the maximum in protection from infection. In addition, patient control is better because most operating rooms, as a matter of policy, require that an anesthesiologist be available. This allows for more effective airway control and ventilation in the unstable or uncooperative patient. The anesthesiologist is available to intubate and even to administer general anesthesia if necessary. Another small advantage is the seemingly endless availability of surgical instruments and supplies. It can also be argued that if a catastrophe should occur requiring more extensive surgery, such as an open-chest procedure, the patient is already in the operating room. Conversely, in our independent experience, this is only a theoretical advantage.

The biggest pitfall of the operating room is the fluoroscopy equipment. It is usually of lesser quality and of limited capability when compared with that available in the catheterization laboratory. In addition, it is frequently shared with other services, such as orthopedics. Conflicts can occur when more than one service is trying to use it at the same time. The lack of immediate access to angiographic materials and catheterization equipment is another drawback to using the operating room for pacemaker procedures. Unless pacemaker implantation is given special consideration and is performed in a specific operating room with equipment and supplies under the control of a pacemaker physician and staff, there is a tendency to be unprepared technically. This disrupts the flow of the procedure and can adversely affect the outcome. This same caveat holds, however, for a busy catheterization laboratory.

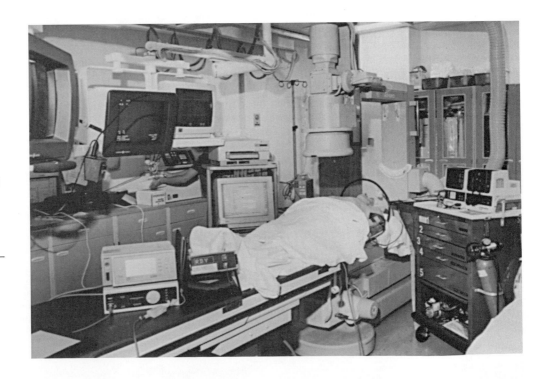

Figure 25–1. Cardiac catheterization laboratory. The patient is surrounded by sophisticated monitoring equipment that includes a pulse oximeter, a physiologic recorder, an external defibrillator, an automatic blood pressure cuff, and an emergency crash cart.

The monitoring equipment used for a pacemaker procedure is variable. A multichannel electrocardiogram (ECG) recording system is frequently recommended; such systems are able to monitor and record a minimum of three surface and one intracardiac ECGs.[15] From a more practical point of view, all that is absolutely required is continuous ECG monitoring on an oscilloscope. The ECG pattern need only be clear. ECG lead selection should demonstrate adequate atrial and ventricular morphology for defining underlying rhythm, arrhythmias, and atrial and ventricular capture. Threshold information can be obtained from the combined use of a pacing system analyzer (PSA) (see later) and an oscilloscope. Sensing data can be obtained from a reliable PSA alone. Multichannel recorders provide more thorough evaluation and documentation and occasionally are extremely valuable in discerning arrhythmias, capture, capture morphology, timing, and so on. The multichannel recorder also allows retrieval of intracardiac signals, precise waveform analysis, and assessment of ventriculoatrial conduction. High-quality hard copy for analysis is also generally available with these more sophisticated recording devices, which tend to be ubiquitous in the catheterization laboratory but uncommon in the operating room.

Patient monitoring should also include a reliable means for blood pressure and arterial oxygen saturation determinations. This can usually be accomplished adequately by use of an automatic noninvasive blood pressure cuff and a transcutaneous oxygen saturation monitor (some institutions place indwelling arterial lines for blood pressure monitoring, although this is generally not necessary and has some associated morbidity). These devices are of particular value when an anesthesiologist is not in attendance. Continuous oxygen saturation monitoring can detect hypoventilation from sedation, pneumothorax, and air embolization. A direct current (DC) defibrillator and complete emergency cart should be in the room where the pacemaker procedure is performed. The cart must include an Ambu bag and intubation equipment.

The surgical instruments for a pacemaker procedure usually call for something akin to a "minor surgical" setup (Fig. 25–2). At times, depending on the institution, the contents of a minor surgical setup can be rather overwhelming. This is particularly true for the nonsurgeon implanting physician. The rows of unnamed clamps and retractors would suggest that some major body cavity might have to be entered. Actually, a pacemaker procedure can be performed efficiently with only a few, well-selected instruments,[16] and there are many acceptable variations and personal preferences. Problems can occur, however, with the nonsurgeon implanting physician who is unfamiliar with the instruments and their appropriate uses. The contents of a basic acceptable surgical tray for pacemaker implantations are outlined in Table 25–1. There are several valuable retractors worthy of individual comment. The Gilpey or Weitlaner (see Fig. 25–2) retractor, or both, can be used throughout the procedure for improved visual exposure. The Senn retractor is used for more delicate retraction (see Fig. 25–2). One end is shaped in an L and the other has tiny claws. This instrument allows the more delicate lifting of tissue edges. Another useful retractor is the Goulet retractor (see Fig. 25–2), which can be replaced with a Richardson retractor. It is extremely helpful in retraction when creating the pacemaker pocket. Unlike other large retractors, the smooth, scalloped ends of

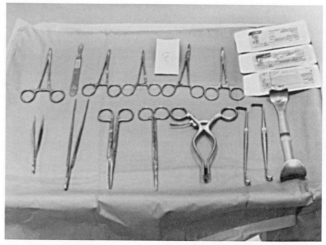

Figure 25–2. Minor surgical tray displaying the minimum required surgical instruments and supplies. From the top left and clockwise: needle holder, scalpel, four sizes of curved hemostats and clamps, Goulet retractor, two Senn retractors, Weitlaner self-retaining retractor, Metzenbaum scissors, suture scissors, nontoothed forceps, toothed forceps. The four packages include "free needles" and three packages of resorbable and nonresorbable suture.

these retractors are gentle to the tissues while affording a generous area of exposure. Army-Navy retractors can also be helpful for this purpose. Other instruments, such as forceps (with or without "teeth"), hemostats, scissors (tissue and other), needle holders, and clamps are a necessity, but their use does not require explanation here. It is important to add that proper use and care of the instruments is crucial, and replacement of worn-out instruments is mandatory in avoiding frustration, delays, and suboptimal work.

Pacemaker procedures performed in the operating room typically benefit from excellent lighting. Multiple high-inten-

Table 25–1. Pacemaker Surgical Instrument Tray

Two Adson forceps with teeth
One mouth-tooth forceps
One smooth forceps
One medium blunt Weitlaner retractor
One small Weitlaner retractor
Two Senn retractors
One Army-Navy retractor
Four baby towel clips
Five curved mosquito clamps
One Peers clamp
Two curved Kelly clamps
One small Metzenbaum scissors
One curved Mayo scissors
One No. 3 knife handle
Two small needle holders
One Goulet retractor
One Bozeman uterine dressing forceps
One package of 1-0 silk 18-inch suture material
One package of 2-0 polyglactin mesh nonabsorbable suture material
One package of 4-0 polyglactin mesh nonabsorbable suture material
No. 3 or 4 F eye needle
No. 10 scalpel blade

sity lamps light the surgical field. This is not the case for pacemaker procedures performed in the catheterization laboratory or special procedures room. Frequently, lighting is marginal at best. One solution to this problem is the use of a high-intensity head lamp (Fig. 25–3). A head lamp is extremely useful when creating the pocket and inspecting for bleeders, particularly when the operator's head blocks out other light. The use of the head lamp initially can be frustrating and requires practice. Once the operator is facile with its use, it will become the major light source for creating the pocket. Even in the operating room, despite all the lighting, the head lamp can be very helpful.

The final piece of equipment to be discussed is the electrocautery device. This device can be useful, and some experienced implanters consider it essential to any pacemaker procedure. Its use, however, has been the subject of controversy.[17–19] Historically, the use of electrocautery equipment for cutting or coagulation during a pacemaker procedure was considered taboo. Concerns have been raised with respect to its causing burns at the myocardium–electrode interface, destruction of the pulse generator, and damage to the pacemaker leads. There is a growing consensus that the use of an appropriately grounded electrocautery device is safe when precautions are taken. First, active cautery should never touch the exposed proximal pin of the electrode. Second, the use of all electrocautery should cease when the pulse generator is on the surgical field.

During pulse generator changes, electrocautery can be extremely useful. Cutting with electrocautery expedites the freeing up of the pulse generator and, at the same time, avoids the misfortune of cutting the lead. At times, even in the most experienced hands, a tedious dissection ends with the scalpel or scissors nicking or cutting the electrode insulation. Use of rapid strokes with cautery avoids the build-up of heat, preventing injury to leads.

Experience leads us to believe that there are no important untoward effects on the myocardium if the cautery touches the pulse generator. There is, however, a risk of causing a

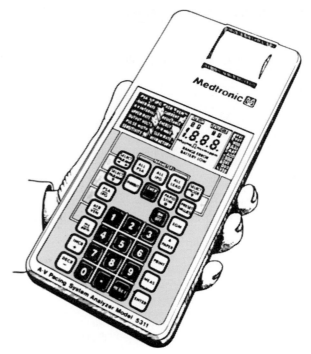

Figure 25–4. The multifunction hand-held Medtronic 5311 (Medtronic Inc., Minneapolis, MN) pacemaker system analyzer. This device determines the pacing and sensing functions of the electrode and the pulse generator as well as the electric integrity of the electrode. (From Barold S: Modern Cardiac Pacing. Mt Kisco, NY, Futura, 1985, p 444.)

permanent no-output situation by destroying the pulse generator. This appears to be particularly true in certain pulse generators. The risk to the patient of sudden lack of output can be prevented by placing a temporary pacemaker in patients who are pacemaker dependent. This is a consideration that is fundamental to all pacemaker procedures whether or not electrocautery is used.

The PSA is extremely valuable during pacemaker procedures. Even when stimulators and recorders are available, a PSA, the circuitry (especially sensing) of which mimics that of the planned pulse generator, will more accurately predict the performance of the pulse generator. In some institutions, the PSA is provided by the pacemaker manufacturer. The early PSAs were simple and were designed to measure the pacing and sensing thresholds for single-chamber ventricular pacing. They were unable to perform (or were cumbersome when performing) the tasks required for atrial and dual-chamber pacing.[20] Today's PSA should be able to perform all of the measurements required for any pacemaker procedure for both the pulse generator and the pacing electrode. At the same time, it should offer backup pacing support during parameter measurements. The modern PSA should be able to function in any mode and measure from either chamber, offering a clear digital display as well as extensive programmability. It should have emergency capabilities of high output and high rate. The capacity to generate a hard copy for analysis and record keeping is also desirable. An example of a PSA is the Medtronic 5311 (Medtronic, Inc., Minneapolis, MN) (Fig. 25–4). A summary of its desirable features is provided in Table 25–2. Some of the sensor-

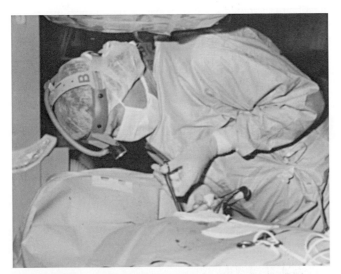

Figure 25–3. High-intensity head lamps optimize visualization in situations of limited lighting experienced frequently in the catheterization laboratory and sometimes in the operating room.

Table 25–2. 5311 PSA Operating Features

Programmable Parameters Mode	Adjustable Range (VVI/T/0, AAI/T/0, VDD, DDD, DVI, DOO)
Lower rate	30–180 ppm
AV interval	25–250 msec
Upper rate	100–180 ppm
Output volts	0.1–10 V
Pulse width	0.05–2 msec
Sensitivity	
Atrium	0.75–1 mv
Ventricle	1.0–10 mv

Measurable Pacing Electrode Parameters

Output volts	0.5–10.2 V
Output current	0.1–25 ma
Resistance	100–1900 ohms
Energy	1–1000 mJ
P-wave amplitude	0.5–25.4 mv
R-wave amplitude	0.5–25.4 mv
Slew rate	0.1–7.5 V/sec

Measurable Pulse Generator Parameters Mode

Lower rate	20–1999 ppm
AV interval	1–500 msec
Upper rate	100–180 ppm
Output volts	1–10 V
Pulse width	0.05–19.99 msec
Sensitivity	0.5–10 mv
Current	0.2–20 ma
Energy	1–1000 mJ
Refractory period	50–1000 msec

Special Features

Rapid stimulations— AOO, BOO, DOO modes	800 ppm
Rate	180–800 ppm
Nodes	AOO, VOO, DOO
Printout	All electrode programmed and measured data
	All pulse generator measured data
	Endocardial electrogram—VA conduction system atrium, ventricular

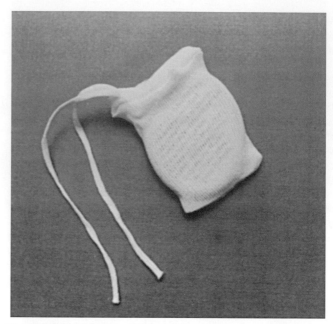

Figure 25–5. The polyester (Dacron) Parsonnet pouch is useful in patients with little subcutaneous tissue. The pouch is usually soaked in povidone-iodine (Betadine) before inserting the pacemaker into the pouch, and then into the pacemaker pocket.

driven pacemakers, for example, temperature and oxygen sensors, require special additional sensor analysis by a specialized PSA tool. Whether supplied by the institution or the manufacturer, a good PSA is a must.

It sometimes seems that there are never enough spare parts during a pacemaker procedure. It is certainly common that just when you need it, the key spare part is unavailable. Most manufacturers offer service kits containing splice kits, stylets, lead adapters, wrenches, lubricant, lead caps, wire cutters, and so on (Table 25–3). It is advisable to set up a pacemaker cart stocked with all the supplies you are likely to need. This cart should include (1) a temporary pacemaker tray that contains the materials for venous insertion as well as the temporary pulse generator and leads; (2) an assortment of sheath sets, dilators, and guide wires; (3) the service kits of the manufacturers most commonly used; (4) the equip-

ment for lead retrieval; and, if they are used, (5) a supply of polyester (Parsonnet) pouches (Fig. 25–5). Someone should be designated to make sure supplies are reordered and up to date.

There are other, rarely used supplies that can be obtained from the operating room or central supply facility. An example would include a Jackson-Pratt drain (Fig. 25–6) for managing hematomas and various sizes of Penrose drains that may be used for tunneling.

Preoperative Planning

The planning that goes into a pacemaker procedure is important if the case is to proceed smoothly. It starts with the evaluation of the patient. A history elucidating patient symptoms, medications the patient is taking, and associated conditions is essential. The physical examination may dem-

Table 25–3. Pacemaker Supplies and Spare Parts

Lead stylets
  Varying lengths
  Variable stiffness
Straight and variable J curve
Silicone oil
Helical coil adaptor with 5-mm pin
Sterile medical adhesive
Wire crimper-cutter
Lead connector caps, 3.2, VS-1, and 5-mm sizes
Step-up and step-down adapters
Adapter sleeves
Screwdriver kit and torque wrenches
One set of connecting cable introducer sets, 11 and 12F

onstrate the effects of bradycardia, including altered vital signs, evidence of cardiac decompensation, or neurologic deficits. Anatomic issues potentially affecting the implant can also be uncovered. One of the most important preoperative considerations is the documentation of the bradyarrhythmia. This can be accomplished with the 12-lead ECG, Holter monitor, event recordings, as well as inhospital critical care unit and telemetry unit monitoring. Supporting laboratory data, such as digitalis levels, thyroid panels, and chemistries, help document the nontransient nature of the problem. The workup of the patient should substantiate the indications outlined by the American College of Cardiology–American Heart Association joint task force.[21] The documentation should be readily available and is usually affixed to the patient's chart.

With all of the documentation obtained and indications met, the next step is the scheduling of the pacemaker procedure. The pacemaker surgery can be performed on either an inpatient or an outpatient basis.

Traditionally, pacemaker procedures have been performed on an inpatient basis, which involves formal admission of the patient to the hospital for the procedure. The preoperative evaluation (in most cases), the pacemaker procedure, and early postoperative care are carried out in the hospital. Generally, the patient has already been admitted to the hospital because of symptoms (e.g., syncope) and the diagnosis of a bradyarrhythmia subsequently established. The pacemaker procedure is then scheduled. Alternatively, some or most of the workup is completed before admission; and after the need for a pacemaker is determined, the patient is admitted for the pacemaker procedure and postoperative care. In some cases, this inpatient approach is inefficient and cost-ineffective.

The early pacing systems were large, had brief longevity, and were prone to catastrophic complications, such as lead dislodgment, perforation, and wound infection. Postoperatively, patients were managed with extreme caution because of these concerns, and an abbreviated hospital stay seemed radical, whereas the concept of an ambulatory procedure was unthinkable. Today, complications are rare, the pacemakers are small, venous access is easy and quick by the introducer technique, and the surgery is relatively minor. Refinements of the electrode systems with active and passive fixation have reduced the dislodgment rate to near zero. In addition, the indications have been expanded to include more patients who are less pacemaker dependent. Finally, and perhaps most directly, there is an increasing mandate for cost containment. The very technology that has made cardiac pacing physiologic, reliable, and safe has resulted in higher cost. For all these reasons, it seems logical that an ambulatory approach for pacemaker procedures could at once be safe and effective as well as less expensive.

There is a trend toward performing pacemaker procedures on an ambulatory basis. The experiences at several centers, both in Europe and the United States, have clearly supported the safety and efficacy of this approach.[22, 23] Concerns about potential complications continue to be expressed.[24–26] Questions about lead selection, the timing of discharge, and the intensity of follow-up are raised frequently. In addition, the economic impact has yet to be fully appreciated. We believe that more pacemaker procedures are being performed on an ambulatory basis, but this has not been reflected in the pacing literature. Since the original reports of Zegelman and colleagues[22] and Belott,[23] Haywood and associates[27] have reported a randomized, controlled study of the feasibility and safety of ambulatory pacemaker procedures. Although the study group was small (50 patients), the results were similar to the experience of one of us (PHB). There was good patient acceptance, no evidence of a higher complication rate, and cost savings of £540 (at that time, about $810).

Since the initial report of 181 new pacemaker implants in 1987, our own ambulatory experience continues to be gratifying. During a recent 13-year span, that experience included 1474 pacemaker procedures, 1043 (69%) of which were performed on an ambulatory basis.[28] That experience also included pulse generator changes, all of which have been performed on an outpatient basis since 1987. Based on this experience, it appears that between 60% and 75% of new pacemaker implantations can be successfully performed on an ambulatory basis (Table 25–4). There have been no additional ambulatory failures, pacemaker-related emergencies, or deaths. An ambulatory failure is a case that is initiated on an ambulatory basis but for which the hospital stay is extended to an admission because of a complication. The complications encountered in ambulatory cases included one hemothorax detected 2 weeks after discharge. This was successfully managed by hospitalization and chest tube drainage. Three hematomas were managed on an ambulatory basis by reoperation, control of bleeding, and drain placement. Two small pneumothoraces, not requiring chest tubes, occurred fortuitously in hospitalized patients not intended for an ambulatory procedure.

These experiences underscore the safety of the ambulatory approach. At present, one of us (PHB) approaches all elective pacemaker procedures (new implants, electrode repositioning, upgrade procedures, electrode extractions, and pulse generator changes) on an ambulatory basis. A simple protocol is used, and the patients often go home 1 to 2 hours after the procedure. They are seen the following day in the pacemaker clinic. A simple outpatient protocol is outlined in Table 25–5.

In most institutions, patients can remain in the hospital

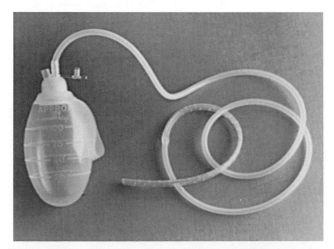

Figure 25–6. The Jackson-Pratt drainage system allows for sterile closed wound drainage. The negative-pressure squeeze bulb has a one-way valve that prevents drainage from returning to the wound.

Table 25–4. Ambulatory Pacemaker Procedure Analysis 1983–1995

Year	83	84	85	86	87	88	89	90	91	92	93	94	95	Total
TP	99	102	112	110	112	123	100	107	135	119	145	113	97	1474
TA	34	34	56	60	78	87	70	87	124	94	128	104	87	1043
TRUE	8	16	44	56	78	86	68	83	124	90	125	102	87	967
<24	26	18	12	4	0	1	2	4	0	4	3	2	0	76
% AMB	34	34	50	60	69	70	70	77	91	78	88	92	88	69

TP, Total patients; TA, total ambulatory; TRUE, cases discharged the same day of procedure; <24, cases discharged within 24 hours (overnight hospitalization); % AMB, percent ambulatory procedures.

overnight and still be considered outpatients. This conforms to the present Health Care Financing Administration definition of ambulatory surgery for reimbursement in the United States (Table 25–6). An important caveat of ambulatory pacemaker procedures is that if there is any doubt or concern about the patient's well-being, the stay can be extended.

For ambulatory procedures to become more widely practiced, reasonable and equitable reimbursement schedules will have to be instituted. As of this writing such schedules are lacking, and this fact may be contributing to a slower than optimal transition toward more ambulatory procedures.[29]

The preoperative patient assessment relates to the synthesis of all patient information, including history, physical examination, old records, rhythm strips, and laboratory data. With this information, appropriate decisions can be made pertaining to the pacemaker mode, leads, and general approach.

The first such decision is whether the patient requires a single-chamber or dual-chamber pacemaker. As a rule, if the patient has intact atrial function, every effort is made to preserve atrial and ventricular relationships. Single-chamber ventricular pacing is usually reserved for the patient with chronic atrial fibrillation or atrial paralysis. A device is selected with acceptable size, longevity, and programmability. If the heart is chronotropically incompetent, a device that offers some form of rate adaptation is considered. Just as important is the lead selection. The issue of lead selection is more completely addressed in Chapter 4. One necessary decision is whether to use passive-fixation or active-fixation leads. Generally, an active-fixation electrode is selected when problems of dislodgment are expected, such as in the patient with a dilated right ventricle or amputated atrial appendage. Active-fixation leads are one of several factors that enhance removability of the lead, if it is necessary in the future. Also important is the pacing configuration (unipolar versus bipolar). This decision relates to both electrodes

and the pulse generator. Although the use of bipolar pacing and sensing has definite advantages, bipolar leads have historically been more complicated and prone to problems. Bipolar leads are also larger in diameter. The compatibility of electrodes and the pulse generator is extremely important, particularly when using an older existing electrode with a modern new pulse generator. If incompatibility exists, an appropriate adapter must be obtained.

If an ambulatory approach is a consideration, the patient is assessed with respect to the risk of this approach. An unstable patient should always be admitted to the hospital. If the patient is critically ill, pacemaker dependent, or unstable, a temporary pacemaker is considered. It is frequently better to take the few extra minutes and place a temporary pacemaker. It can avoid moments of "terror" during the procedure if asystole occurs. This is particularly true in patients with complete atrioventricular (AV) block in whom an apparently stable escape rhythm can suddenly disappear, a common situation after initial pacing has been established.

The timing of the procedure usually relates to the stability of the patient. In the critically ill patient in whom there are concerns about the stability of the cardiac rhythm or temporary pacemaker, an early permanent procedure is in order. Conversely, in a patient whose survival is in doubt, one may appropriately decide to wait for stabilization. At times, the procedure is delayed because of systemic infection or sepsis. A permanent pacemaker implantation performed on a septic patient may lead to the seeding of bacteria on the pacemaker or electrode. It has been our approach that if there is active infection, the procedure is deferred until the patient is afebrile and no longer septic, to reduce the risk for pacemaker system infection.

Decisions with regard to the implantation site are not as important currently as they were when only large pulse generators were available. The currently available devices, weighing less than 30 g, make the site, in most situations, moot. They tend to be tolerated well in almost any location.

Table 25–5. Outpatient Protocol

Surgery scheduled as outpatient with outpatient number assigned
Preoperative blood work, ECG, and chest x-ray study performed on outpatient basis within 24 hours prior to admission
Patient instructed to fast after midnight of the evening prior to the procedure
Patient instructed to report to the outpatient department in the morning
Postoperative ECG and chest x-ray film
Discharged when fully awake and vital signs stable
Instructed to report to the pacemaker center the following morning

Table 25–6. Definition of Ambulatory Surgical Procedures

When a patient with a known diagnosis enters a hospital for a specific minor surgical procedure or treatment that is expected to keep him or her in a hospital for only a few hours (less than 24) and this expectation is realized, he or she will be considered an outpatient regardless of the hour of admission, whether or not he or she occupied a bed, and whether or not he or she remained in the hospital past midnight.

From Health Care Financing Administration; Hospital Manual, publication 10, section 210A.

There are, however, special circumstances that deserve mention. These are hobbies, recreational and occupational activities, cosmetic issues, and previous medical conditions. The hunter, for instance, should have the pacemaker placed on the side opposite where the rifle butt is placed. Similar considerations are appropriate for the tennis enthusiast or golfer (although, in our experience, it is variable for the golfer as to whether the backswing or follow-through side is better). In a young person, placement of the pacemaker under the breast (women) or in the axilla may be more desirable from a cosmetic point of view. Medical conditions, such as previous surgery, radiation therapy, and skeletal or other anatomic abnormalities, should be considered. In the patient who is small with little subcutaneous tissue, a subpectoral implantation may be required. This calls for the use of a bipolar system to avoid skeletal muscle stimulation.

The preoperative orders are generally simple. The patient fasts for at least 6 hours before the procedure. If the implantation is being performed on an ambulatory basis, the patient is instructed to report to the hospital on the day of the procedure, allowing enough time to obtain the necessary preoperative testing; generally, 2 hours is adequate. The preoperative procedures include posteroanterior (PA) and lateral chest radiographs, an ECG, a complete blood count, prothrombin time, partial thromboplastin time, and electrolytes, blood urea nitrogen, and creatinine determinations. Because the patient is fasting, adequate hydration is maintained with a stable intravenous (IV) line. Hydration is extremely important for subsequent venous access and prevention of air embolization during the procedure. It can be frustrating and dangerous to try to gain venous access in a patient who is dehydrated after prolonged fasting without IV hydration. We generally request that the IV line be started on the side of the planned procedure to facilitate venography during attempts at venous access if this becomes a problem.

The management of pacemaker surgery in the anticoagulated patient is controversial. There is a paucity of information throughout the literature with respect to the handling of a patient requiring anticoagulation. One thing is clear: The patient receiving anticoagulants, including heparin and platelet antagonists, is at risk for hematoma formation. It is commonly held that patients who require oral anticoagulants should have the prothrombin time brought to normal before implantation. Anticoagulants can be resumed between 24 and 48 hours after pacemaker implantation. Reducing the prothrombin time to normal in patients requiring anticoagulants, such as those with artificial heart valves, places these patients at grave risk for thromboembolic complications. Addressing this issue, many operators choose to admit the patient to the hospital and start intravenous heparin while the warfarin is withheld and the prothrombin time brought to normal values. This often takes several days. When the prothrombin time has reached control, the patient is scheduled for surgery. On the day of surgery, the heparin is stopped and, in some situations, the anticoagulation reversed and the surgery carried out. Several hours after surgery, the heparin is resumed. Then, after 24 to 48 hours with no evidence of significant hematoma, the warfarin is resumed; when therapeutic levels are reached, the heparin is stopped, and the patient is discharged on oral warfarin therapy.

In this day of cost control and managed care, this maneuver proves to be problematic. In addition, despite vigorous attempts at hemostasis, significant hematomas have resulted from the use of heparin. Although anecdotal, it is our general experience that the greatest risk for bleeding complications, hemorrhage, and hematoma occurs with the use of heparin or platelet antagonists, such as aspirin. Having experienced a devastating thromboembolic complication from withdrawal of warfarin, as well as multiple large hematomas from the use of heparin, one of us has chosen to perform pacemaker and ICD procedures with the patient anticoagulated on the oral agent warfarin. This policy has been in effect for at least 15 years. As a rule, patients taking oral anticoagulants have their INR reduced to about 2. There have been no devastating hematomas or thromboembolic events. It is our opinion that pacemaker and ICD procedures can be performed safely with the patient anticoagulated in this way. This approach has been supported by a 4-year experience reported by Goldstein and colleagues.[30] There was no difference in the incidental bleeding complications between patients receiving warfarin and those not anticoagulated. There were no wound hematomas, blood transfusions, or clinically significant bleeding in any patients receiving warfarin. The medicolegal risks from interrupting continuous anticoagulant therapy and a resultant thromboembolic event are not insignificant. Although there is a risk for hemorrhage during and after pacemaker procedures in patients with therapeutic levels of anticoagulation, the risk appears to be minimal. The bleeding can generally be treated by local measures, such as the placement of drains or reoperation. The risk for bleeding is greatly outweighed by the risk for thromboembolism after withdrawing anticoagulant therapy. The issue of pacemaker and ICD surgery in the anticoagulated patient is becoming more prevalent as more patients receive anticoagulant therapy for the common arrhythmia of atrial fibrillation.

The patient is instructed to continue maintenance oral medications, which may be taken with small sips of water. Patients taking hypoglycemic agents are instructed to reduce the preoperative dose by 50%. The administration of prophylactic antibiotics is controversial. Our individual preferences call for a broad-spectrum cephalosporin, such as cefazolin, to be given intraoperatively. Many others use vancomycin, which covers all the gram-positive potentially pathogenic organisms. We also have the patient scrub the chest, neck, shoulders, and supraclavicular fossae with a povidone-iodine (Betadine) sponge the evening and the morning before the procedure. In most instances, skin shaving is carried out in the procedure room. Finally, we ask the patient to void before coming to the procedure room.

Pacemaker Implantation: General Information

On arrival at the procedure room, the patient is transferred to a radiography table. In the catheterization laboratory or special procedures area, the table's radiolucent properties are expected. In the operating room, prior arrangements are made for a special radiolucent operating table. In this latter situation, it is advisable to test the fluoroscopy equipment's ability to penetrate the table. It is also helpful to establish proper x-ray tube orientation. Attention to these details can avoid considerable hassle later when it is discovered that the patient is on the wrong table, the radiographic equipment is inoperative, or the image is upside down, backward, or both.

Almost immediately, the patient is connected to physiologic monitoring (ECG, pulse oximetry, and automatic blood pressure cuff). If it has not already been accomplished, a reliable venous line is established, preferably on the side of the operative site. The circulating nurse must have easy access to the IV line for drug administration, introduction of radiographic materials, or both. Oxygen can be administered by nasal cannula or mask. If a temporary pacemaker is to be placed, the appropriate site is shaved and prepared, and the temporary pacemaker is placed using the Seldinger technique. It is important to secure the lead and sheath adequately to maintain accessibility, so that they can be easily removed at the end of the procedure.

When effective patient support has been established, focus turns to the operative site. If not already accomplished, skin shaving and cleansing are carried out, which should be generous in scope and include the neck, supraventricular fossae, shoulders, and chest. The operative site, shaved and cleansed, is now formally prepared and draped. There are several ways to accomplish this. One can use a povidone-iodine scrub, followed by alcohol, followed by povidone-iodine solution, with skin drying before the final povidone-iodine solution is applied. This older, more time-consuming, although effective, scrub can be replaced by the use of povidone-iodine solution gel, which is a gelatinous preparation of povidone-iodine. It is spread liberally over the operative site. Within 30 seconds, an optimal bactericidal effect is achieved. With this approach, scrubbing the area is not required. In the case of patients who are allergic to povidone-iodine, a chlorhexidine (Hibiclens) or hexachlorophene (pHisoHex) scrub can be carried out. The draping process is a matter of personal preference. One of us (DR) applies a sterile, see-through plastic adhesive drape (impregnated with an iodoform solution) over the entire operative area. The other (PB) uses one or more sterile plastic drapes with adhesive along one side (Fig. 25–7). The adhesive surface is applied from shoulder to shoulder at the level of the clavicle, which serves to create a sterile barrier from the shoulder level down. Depending on the situation, other barriers can be created. In both cases, the use of the plastic drape is to optimize sterility.

After establishing some form of sterile barrier, the operative site is draped with sterile towels, and one or more large sterile surgical sheets are applied. Care is taken to avoid smothering the patient or causing claustrophobia. This is best achieved by keeping the drapes off the patient's face and maintaining the cephalic aspect of the main drape perpendicular to the patient's neck. This allows unrestricted access to the patient's head and neck. The main drape is clipped to some form of support on both sides of the patient. This support can consist of IV poles placed on each side of the patient. This arrangement may not be possible in laboratories, where it interferes with radiographic equipment. In this case, the drape may be fixed to the C arm or image intensifier. This solution is less than optimal, because the drapes pull away every time the C arm or radiographic table is repositioned. This increases the risk for contamination and breaks in sterile technique. More recently, a simple, cost-effective solution to this problem has been developed. A length of common house wire (8/3-gauge Romex) is shaped into an arc over the patient's neck. The ends of the wire are bent at right angles to the arc and tucked under the x-ray table padding at the level of the patient's shoulders (Fig. 25–8). The weight of the patient's shoulders supports the wire arc. The wire can be shaped to fit any patient. The wire positioned under the shoulder is checked under fluoroscopy to avoid interference with the radiographic field of view. The Romex wire is strong enough to maintain its shape under the weight of the surgical drape. This offers optimal patient comfort and a reliable sterile barrier. There is no interference with the C arm, and claustrophobia is avoided. The traditional use of a Mayo stand over the patient's face

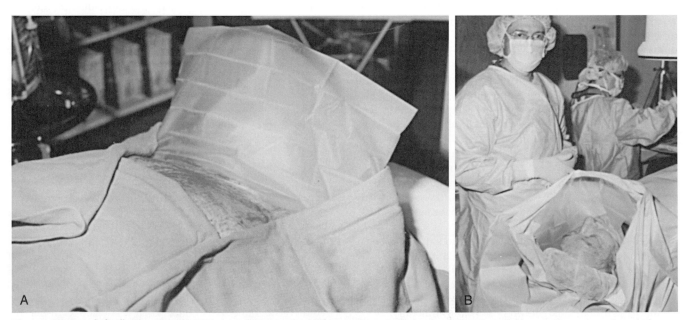

Figure 25–7. *A,* Application of a 3M 10/10 drape (Minneapolis, MN) to create a sterile barrier. *B,* The drape folds over the common house wire (Romex wire) support, creating an effective sterile barrier and preventing patient claustrophobia.

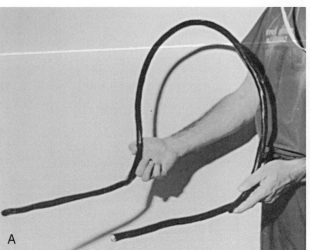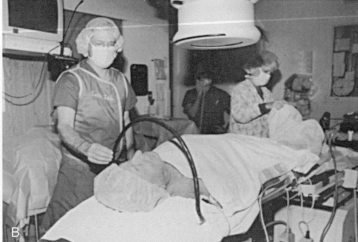

Figure 25–8. *A* and *B,* Romex wire shaped to form an arch over the patient's head is positioned under the patient's mattress and bent to accommodate differences in patients and circumstances.

is problematic in that it can cause claustrophobia, makes access to the patient's airway difficult in an emergency, and may interfere with the x-ray equipment.

From the moment the catheterization laboratory or special studies room is cleaned, it must be treated as a surgical suite. All personnel must wear surgical clothing, hats, and masks. There should be an attempt to seal the room, limiting traffic and restricting access to those participating in the procedure.

Most pacemaker procedures are performed with local anesthesia and the addition of some form of sedation and pain reliever.[31] Local anesthesia alone is inadequate for optimal patient comfort. Even in the best of circumstances, the effect of local anesthesia does not avoid the discomfort associated with the creation of the pacemaker pocket. For this reason, the additional combination of a narcotic and sedative is recommended. The use of sedation alone is frequently inadequate. The challenge to the physician in charge is the achievement of patient comfort without risking oversedation or respiratory depression. If an anesthesiologist or nurse anesthetist is part of the implantation team, patient comfort is usually achieved easily and safely. In this situation, if respiratory depression occurs, the patient can easily be ventilated. In the circumstance in which the implanting physician orders the sedation and narcotics, the patient must be carefully monitored by the circulating nurse. It is recommended that the medications be administered slowly.

The selection of the local anesthetic and the dose delivered are also important considerations. The use of a local agent in therapeutic concentration that provides rapid onset of action and sustained duration is desirable. Local agents can be used in combination to achieve the desired effect. An example is the use of lidocaine for its rapid onset and bupivacaine for its sustained action. There is also an upper limit of total local anesthetic dose that should not be exceeded. Toxic blood levels of commonly used local anesthetics can result in profound neurologic abnormalities, including obtundation and seizures. A number of local anesthetic agents are listed in Table 25–7.

The selection of sedative and narcotic is dependent on personal preference. We use midazolam and fentanyl. The operator should become familiar with one or more sedative agents as well as an analgesic, preferably a narcotic. There are many newer agents available. The selection of a benzodiazepine in combination with a semisynthetic narcotic can achieve ideal sedation, amnesia, and analgesia. A cooperative, relaxed, and pain-free patient is fundamental to the success of the procedure and the avoidance of complications. Pentothal and nitrous oxide have been used to effect brief periods of complete sedation at times of anticipated maximum discomfort, but the use of these drugs requires the expertise of an anesthetist because temporary respiratory support is frequently required.

In the United States, the Joint Commission of Hospital Accreditation mandates that institutions establish a policy and protocol for patients receiving conscious sedation. Pacemaker procedures would be included in such a protocol. In essence, the protocol requires formal patient assessment before sedation. The sedation and recovery areas must have resuscitation equipment present at all times, and patients

Table 25–7. Pharmacologic Properties of Commonly Used Local Anesthetic Agents

	Onset (min)	Duration (hr)	Protein Binding	Maximum Adult Dose
Esters				
Chloroprocaine (Nesacaine)	Slow (5–10)	Short (0.5–1.5)	5%	800 mg (11 μg/kg)
Procaine (Novocain)	Fast (5–15)	Short (0.5–1.5)		800 mg (11 μg/kg)
Tetracaine	Slow (20–30)	Long (3–5)	85%	200 mg
Amides				
Bupivacaine (Marcaine)	Moderate (10–20)	Long (3–5)	82–96%	100 mg
Lidocaine (Xylocaine)	Fast (5–15)	Moderate (1–3)	55–65%	300 mg (4 μg/kg)

Table 25–8. Conscious Sedation Drug Protocols

Drug name	Route of Administration	Dosage	Maximum	Comments
Meperidine	IM or IV	25–100 mg	100 mg	Long acting
Morphine	IM or IV	1.5–15 mg	20 mg	Long acting
Fentanyl	IM or IV	50–100 μg	100 mg	Short acting, very
Valium	IV	2–10 mg	10 mg	
Droperidol	IV	8–17 mg/kg	17 mg/kg	
Midazolam	IV	1–2.5 mg	5 mg	
Nitrous oxide	Inhalation	30–50%	50%	
Thiopental	IV	1–4 mg/kg		Temporary loss
Ketamine	IV	0.5 mg/kg	0.5 mg/kg	Temporary loss

Abbreviations: IM, intramuscular; IV, intravenous.

undergoing conscious sedation must be monitored with pulse oximetry, continuous ECG rhythm monitoring, and automatic blood pressure recordings. Monitoring of the patient should continue for at least 30 minutes after the last intravenous sedative drug administration and for at least 90 minutes after intramuscular sedative drug administration. There are also strict discharge criteria. A common conscious sedation drug protocol is shown in Table 25–8.

On May 3, 1995, a North American Society of Pacing Electrophysiology (NASPE) Policy Conference on IV sedation was held in Boston. A NASPE expert consensus document on the use of IV conscious sedation/analgesia by nonanesthesia personnel in patients undergoing arrhythmia-specific diagnostic, therapeutic, and surgical procedures was generated.[32] The policy conference (1) reviewed the current state of the art with respect to conscious sedation; (2) reviewed current position statements developed by other relevant health professional groups; (3) reviewed the legal and licensing applications of IV conscious sedation; (4) developed recommendations for the use of IV sedation; (5) specified the minimum training requirements for professionals administering IV sedation for arrhythmia-specific procedures; and (6) reviewed the cost-effectiveness and economic impact implications of IV conscious sedation.

The use of prophylactic antibiotics to reduce the incidence of postoperative wound infection in a pacemaker procedure is controversial.[33] It is important to point out that antibiotics are not a substitute for good infection control practices, an adequate surgical environment, and good surgical technique. The use of antibiotics in a pacemaker procedure follows the principle of prophylaxis in which the risk for infection is low but the monetary penalty or morbidity is high.[34–36] The selection of antibiotics is based on site-specific flora for wound infection and the spectrum, kinetics, and toxicity of the antimicrobial agent. The risk factors for infection have been well defined. The National Research Council for Wound Classification places the risk for infection from an elective procedure closed primarily at less than 2%. One important factor to be considered is the increased risk for infection in operations lasting longer than 2 hours. Although not formally studied, the use of prophylactic antibiotics in the low-risk, high-morbidity group, such as patients receiving pacemakers, appears justified. There are no specific references in the literature to antibiotic prophylaxis for pacemaker procedures, only for prosthetic devices. The spectrum of the antibiotic prophylaxis need only cover the gram-positive skin flora, primarily *Staphylococcus epidermidis* and *Staphylococcus aureus*. In the case of pacemakers and cardiac procedures, the cephalosporins appear ideal (i.e., 1 to 2 g cefazolin IV, preanesthesia). If an institution has a high incidence of methicillin-resistant *S. aureus* or *S. epidermidis*, vancomycin should be considered (i.e., 1 g vancomycin IV given slowly preoperatively). Postoperative doses are left to clinical judgment. Generally, 1 g of either drug may be given intravenously up to 8 hours postoperatively. Occasionally, the postoperative doses of cephalosporin are given orally for several days. These drug guidelines are also reflected in the *Medical Letter* of January 1992.[37] It is interesting to note that the *Medical Letter* specifically does not recommend antibiotic prophylaxis for pacemaker procedures.

An additional strategy in the prevention of infection is topical antibiotic prophylaxis or antibiotic wound irrigation.[38] Controlled trials evaluating the benefit of antibiotic irrigations are lacking. The concept of irrigation is to provide a high concentration of antibiotic at the site of potential infection at the time of contamination. The technique has proved most efficient in the absence of established infection. It calls for the use of nonabsorbable antibiotics. Historically, aminoglycosides and bacitracin combinations have been used, but there are many regimens that are varied in number, type, concentration, and duration of antibiotic use. Systemic toxicity with antibiotic irrigation is a major concern. When large volumes of irrigating solutions are used in combination with systemic antibiotics, the therapeutic range can be greatly exceeded. The superiority of irrigation over systemic antibiotic administration has never been proved, and given the potential toxicity, caution is recommended. Some popular antibiotic irrigation protocols are shown in Table 25–9.

Despite the controversial nature of prophylactic systemic

Table 25–9. Common Antimicrobial Irrigation Protocols

Agent	Concentration
Bacitracin	50,000 units in 200 mL of saline
Cephalothin	1 g/L of saline
Cefazolin	1 g/L of saline
Cefuroxime	750 mg/L of saline
Vancomycin	200–500 mg/L of saline
Povidone-iodine	Concentrated or diluted in aliquots of saline

antibiotics and topical irrigation, the E1 Cajon experience has been very gratifying. A protocol of intravenous antibiotics and wound irrigation has been followed since 1978. In each case, 1 g of cefazolin was given intraoperatively, followed by cefadroxil monohydrate, 500 mg, twice daily for 4 days. A sponge soaked in povidone-iodine is placed in the pacemaker pocket just after pocket formation and is removed at the time of wound closure. In more than 1500 pacemaker procedures, there have been two wound infections. A similar low incidence of infection has occurred at the University of Oklahoma where, since 1980, our regimen has included a preoperative dose of cefazolin, 1 g IV, followed by 1 g IV for one to five more doses every 8 hours (depending on length of stay), as well as pocket irrigation with a solution of bacitracin, gentamycin, and polymyxin. Although the issue is admittedly controversial, all one needs is one pacemaker infection with all of its problems to become convinced that infection should be avoided at all cost.

There are two basic anatomic approaches to the implantation of a permanent pacemaker.[39, 40] From a historical perspective, the first is the epicardial and the second is the transvenous approach. The epicardial approach calls for direct application of pacemaker electrodes on the heart. This requires general anesthesia and surgical access to the epicardial surface of the heart. The transvenous approach is usually performed with local anesthesia and IV sedation. Each approach can be accomplished by several unique techniques. Today, 95% of all pacemaker implantations are performed transvenously.

The epicardial approach is generally reserved for patients who cannot undergo safe or effective pacemaker implantation by the transvenous route. The epicardial techniques (Fig. 25–9) include applying the electrode or electrodes directly to a completely exposed heart or performing a limited thoracotomy through a subxiphoid incision. A third technique places the leads by mediastinoscopy. There is even a fourth technique that is a combination of epicardial and endocardial lead placement.

Several techniques are used for the transvenous approach. All involve a venous surgical cutdown, percutaneous venous access, or a combination of both (Table 25–10). The pros and cons of the various approaches and techniques are reviewed.

A thorough knowledge of the anatomic structure of the

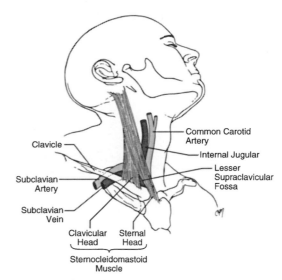

Figure 25–10. Anatomic relationship of the vascular structures in the neck and superior mediastinum.

neck, upper extremities, and thorax is essential for cardiac pacing (Fig. 25–10). The precise location and orientation of the internal jugular, innominate, subclavian, and cephalic veins is important for safe venous access.[41, 42] Their anatomic relation to other structures is crucial in avoiding complications.

The venous anatomy of interest from a cardiac pacing point of view starts peripherally with the axillary vein.[42] The axillary vein is a large venous structure that represents the continuation of the basilic vein. It starts at the lower border of the teres major tendon and latissimus dorsi. The axillary vein terminates immediately beneath the clavicle at the outer border of the first rib, where it becomes the subclavian vein. The axillary vein is covered anteriorly by the pectoralis minor and pectoralis major muscles and costocoracoid membrane. It is anterior and medial to the axillary artery, which it partially overlaps. At the level of the coracoid process, the axillary vein is covered only by the clavicular head of the pectoralis major (Fig. 25–11). At this juncture, the axillary vein receives the more superficial cephalic vein. The cephalic vein terminates in the deeper axillary vein at the level of the coracoid process beneath the pectoralis major muscle. The cephalic vein commonly used for pacemaker venous access is classified as a superficial vein of the upper extremity. This vein, which actually commences near the antecubital fossa, travels along the outer border of the biceps muscle and enters the deltopectoral groove. The deltopectoral groove

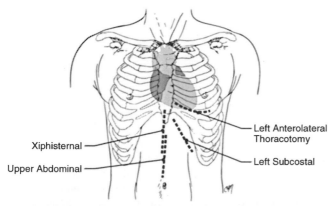

Figure 25–9. Location of surgical incisions for the placement of epimyocardial systems.

Table 25–10. Techniques for Axillary Venous Access

1. Blind percutaneous puncture using surface landmarks
2. Blind puncture through the pectoralis major muscle using deep landmarks
3. Direct cutdown on the axillary vein
4. Fluoroscopy: Needle the first rib for reference
5. Contrast venography
6. Doppler-guided
7. Ultrasound-guided

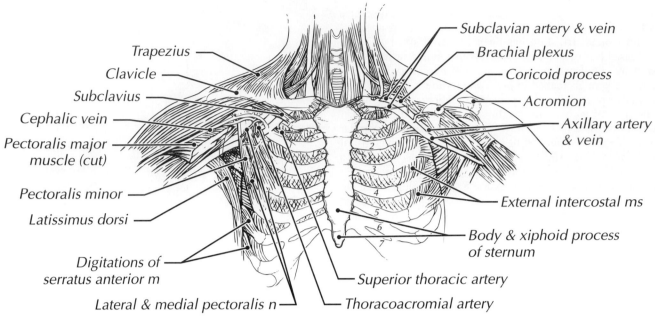

Trapezius

Clavicle

Subclavius

Cephalic vein

Pectoralis major
muscle (cut)

Pectoralis minor

Latissimus dorsi

Digitations of
serratus anterior m

Lateral & medial pectoralis n

Subclavian artery & vein

Brachial plexus

Coricoid process

Acromion

Axillary artery
& vein

External intercostal ms

Body & xiphoid process
of sternum

Superior thoracic artery

Thoracoacromial artery

Figure 25–11. Detailed anatomy of the anterolateral chest demonstrating the axillary vein with the pectoralis major and minor muscles removed.

is an anatomic structure formed by the deltoid muscle and clavicular head of the pectoralis major. The cephalic vein traverses the deltopectoral groove and superiorly pierces the costocoracoid membrane, crossing the axillary artery and terminating in the axillary vein just below the clavicle at the level of the coracoid process.

The subclavian vein is a continuation of the axillary vein. The subclavian vein extends from the outer border of the first rib to the inner end of the clavicle, where it joins with the internal jugular vein to form the brachiocephalic trunk or innominate vein. The subclavian vein is just inferior to the clavicle and subclavius muscle. The subclavian artery is located posterior and superior to the vein. These two structures are separated internally by the scalenus anticus muscle and phrenic nerve. Inferiorly, this vein is associated with a depression in the first rib and upon the pleura. The brachiocephalic trunks or innominate veins are two large venous trunks located on each side of the base of the neck. The right innominate vein is relatively short. It starts at the inner end of the clavicle and passes vertically downward to join with the left innominate vein just below the cartilage of the first rib. This junction forms the superior vena cava. The left innominate vein is larger and longer than the right, passing from left to right for approximately 2½ inches where it joins with the right innominate vein to form the superior vena cava. The left innominate vein is in the anterior and superior mediastinum.

The internal and external jugular veins have also been used for pacemaker venous access. The external jugular vein is a superficial vein of the neck receiving blood from the exterior cranium and face. This vein starts in the substance of the parotid gland at the angle of the jaw and runs perpendicular down the neck to the middle of the clavicle. In this course, it crosses the sternocleidomastoid muscle and runs parallel to its posterior border. At the attachment of the

sternocleidomastoid muscle to the clavicle, this vein perforates the deep fascia and terminates in the subclavian vein just anterior to the scalenus anticus muscle. The external jugular vein is separated from the sternocleidomastoid muscle by a layer of deep cervical fascia. Superficially, it is covered by the platysma muscle, superficial fascia, and skin. The external jugular vein can be variable in size and even duplicated. Because of its superficial orientation, the external jugular vein is less frequently used for cardiac pacing venous access (Fig. 25–12).

The internal jugular, although an unusual site for pacemaker venous access, is used more frequently than the external jugular vein. This is because of its larger size and deeper and more protected orientation. The internal jugular vein starts just external to the jugular foramen at the base of the skull. It drains blood from the interior of the cranium as well as superficial parts of the head and neck. This vein is oriented vertically as it runs down the side of the neck. Superiorly, it is lateral to the internal carotid and inferolateral to the common carotid. At the base of the neck, the internal jugular vein joins the subclavian vein to form the innominate vein. The internal jugular vein is large and lies in the cervical triangle defined by the lateral border of the omohyoid muscle and the inferior border of the digastric muscle and medial border of the sternocleidomastoid. The superficial cervical fascia and platysma muscle cover the vein. It is easily identified just lateral to the easily palpable external carotid artery.

From a venous access perspective, the location of the subclavian vein may vary from a normal lateral course to an extremely anterior or posterior orientation in elderly patients. Byrd[43] has described the subclavian venous anatomy of two distinct deformities. Both conditions make venous access more difficult and hazardous. The first deformity involves a posteriorly displaced clavicle (Fig. 25–13). This is com-

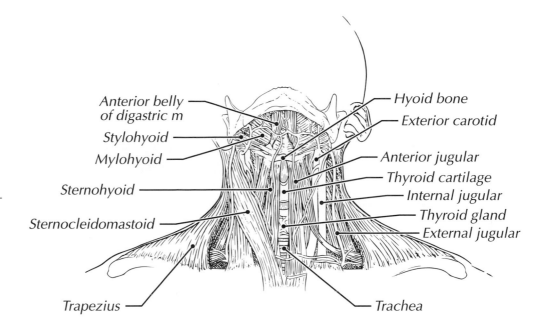

Figure 25–12. Detailed anatomy of the neck demonstrating the relationship of venous anatomy to the superficial and deep structures.

Anterior belly of digastric m
Stylohyoid
Mylohyoid
Sternohyoid
Sternocleidomastoid
Trapezius

Hyoid bone
Exterior carotid
Anterior jugular
Thyroid cartilage
Internal jugular
Thyroid gland
External jugular
Trachea

monly seen in patients with chronic lung disease with antero-posterior chest enlargement. These patients can be identified by a horizontal deltopectoral groove and the posteriorly displaced clavicle. The second deformity is an anteriorly displaced clavicle (Fig. 25–14), which is found occasionally, especially in elderly women. In this situation, the clavicle is anteriorly bowed or actually displaced anteriorly. It is important that these variations are recognized to avoid complications of pneumothorax and hemopneumothorax when approaching the patient percutaneously.

It is assumed that the implanting physician is also completely familiar with the anatomy of the heart and great vessels.[44] However, their spatial orientation is at times confusing. This is particularly true with respect to the right atrium and ventricle. It is recalled that in the frontal plane, the border of the right side of the heart is formed by the right atrium. The border of the left side of the heart is composed of the left ventricle. Importantly, the right ventricle is located anteriorly (Fig. 25–15) and is triangular. The

apex of the right ventricle is the generally accepted initial "target" for ventricular lead placement. Unfortunately, the location of the apex of the right ventricle can be variable. Its normal location, distinctly to the left of midline, depends on the rotation of the heart, which is affected by various pathologic and anatomic conditions. At times, it may be located directly anterior to or even to the right of midline. A lack of appreciation of these variances can lead to considerable difficulty in electrode placement.

The choice of site for pacemaker implantation is also occasionally important anatomically. This decision is typically made most appropriately based on the patient's dominant hand, occupation, recreational activities, and medical conditions. The decision should not be made based on the dominant hand of the implanting physician. There are, however, some fundamental differences between the anatomy of the right side and that of the left side. These differences can result in frustration when one is passing a pacemaker electrode. Although it seems to be easier for many right-handed

Figure 25–13. Posterior displacement of the clavicle, recognized by a horizontal rather than oblique position of the deltopectoral groove. (From Byrd CL: Current clinical applications of dual-chamber pacing. *In* Zipes DP [ed]: Proceedings of a Symposium. Minneapolis: Medtronic, Inc, 1981, p 71.)

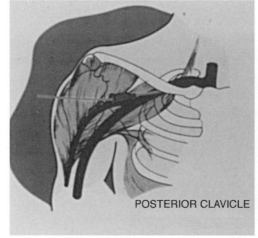

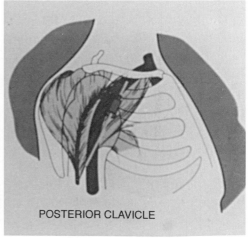

POSTERIOR CLAVICLE

POSTERIOR CLAVICLE

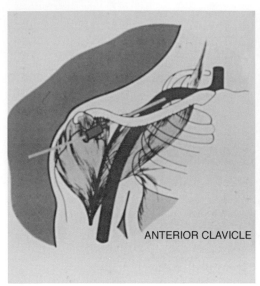

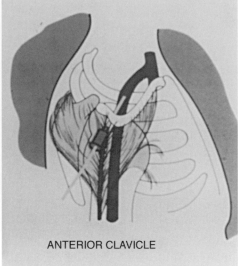

ANTERIOR CLAVICLE

ANTERIOR CLAVICLE

Figure 25–14. Anterior displacement of the clavicle. The deltopectoral groove is nearly vertical. (From Byrd CL: Current clinical applications of dual-chamber pacing. *In* Zipes DP [ed]: Proceedings of a Symposium. Minneapolis: Medtronic, Inc, 1981, p 71.)

implanters to work on the right side of the patient (and vice versa), from a surgical point of view, catheter manipulation from the right can be a frustrating experience. When entering the central venous circulation from the left upper limb, the pacemaker electrode tracks along a smooth arc to the right ventricle. There are generally no sharp angles or bends (Fig. 25–16A). Conversely, when approaching from the right, the electrode is forced to negotiate a sharp angle or bend at the junction of the right subclavian and internal jugular veins where the innominate vein is formed (see Fig. 25–16B). This acute angulation can make the manipulation of the pacemaker electrode difficult when a curved stylet is fully inserted. Another anatomic pitfall occurs when there is a persistent left superior vena cava, making passage to the heart from the left more difficult and, if there is no right

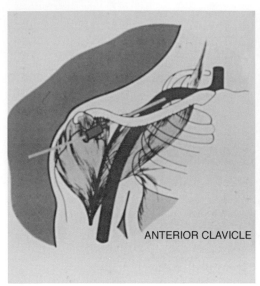

Right Atrium

Left Ventricle (posterior)

Right Ventricle (anterior)

Plane of Tricuspid Valve

Figure 25–15. The spatial orientation of the right ventricle as an anterior structure in relationship to the left or posterior ventricle or coronary sinus, which is also posterior.

superior vena cava, from the right impossible. These situations are considered when ventricular electrode placement is discussed later.

Transvenous Pacemaker Placement

The right or left cephalic vein is the most common vascular entry site for insertion of pacemaker electrodes by the cutdown technique.[45] The cephalic vein is located in the deltopectoral groove (Fig. 25–17). This is a groove formed by the reflections of the medial head of the deltoid and the lateral border of the greater pectoral muscles. It can be precisely located by palpating the coracoid process of the scapula. The dermis along the deltopectoral groove is infiltrated with local anesthetic, encompassing the anticipated length of the incision. A vertical incision is made adjacent to and at the level of the coracoid process. It is extended for about 2 to 5 cm. Care is taken to keep the scalpel blade perpendicular to the surface of the skin. Smooth skin edges are created by making an initial single stroke that carries through the dermis to each corner of the wound. The subcutaneous tissue is infiltrated with local anesthetic along the edges of the incision. The Weitlaner retractor is applied to the edges of the wound, and the subcutaneous tissue is placed under tension. The tension is released by light strokes of the scalpel from corner to corner of the wound in the midline. As the subcutaneous tissue falls away, tension is restored by reapplying the Weitlaner retractor. This process is continued down to the surface of the pectoral fascia. The fascia is left intact. At this level, the borders of the pectoral and deltoid muscles forming the deltopectoral groove are identified. A Metzenbaum scissors is used to dissect along the groove by separating the muscles' fibrous attachments. The Weitlaner retractor is reapplied deeper to retract the muscle. Gradual release of the fascial tissue between the two muscle bodies will expose the cephalic vein.

At times, the cephalic vein is diminutive or atretic and unable to accommodate a pacemaker lead. In this case, the cephalic vein can be dissected, centrally, to the axillary vein and this larger vein catheterized. Once the vein to be

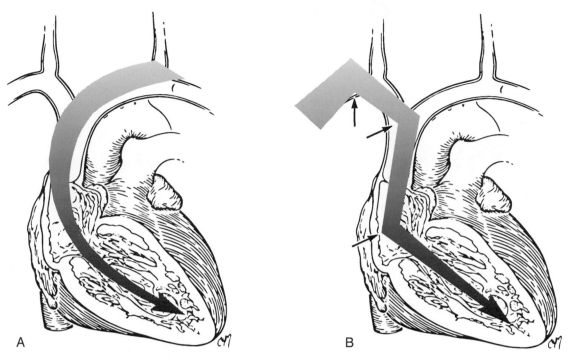

Figure 25–16. *A,* Smooth course of an electrode entering from the left side. *B,* Acute angulation of the catheter course when the lead enters the venous system from the right.

catheterized is localized, it is freed of all fibrous attachments. Ligatures are applied proximally and distally (Fig. 25–18*A*). The distal ligature is tied and held by a small clamp. The proximal ligature is not tied but is kept under tension with another clamp. An arbitrary entry site is chosen between the two ligatures. The anterior half of the vein at this site is grasped with a smooth forceps, and the vein is gently lifted. A small horizontal venotomy is made using iris scissors (see Fig. 25–18*B*) or a No. 11 scalpel blade. The vein is continuously supported by the forceps. The venotomy is held open by any of several means: a mosquito clamp, forceps,

or vein pick. Gentle traction is applied on the distal ligature while tension is released on the proximal ligature. With the venotomy held widely open, the electrode or electrodes are inserted and advanced into the central venous circulation (see Fig. 25–18*C*).

For many years, vascular access has been achieved for many purposes by use of the Seldinger technique. This simple approach calls for the percutaneous puncture of the vessel with a relatively long, large-bore needle; passage of a wire through the needle into the vessel; removal of the needle; and passage of a catheter or sheath over the wire into the vessel with removal of the wire. An 18-gauge thin-walled needle 5 cm in length is commonly used, although smaller needles are available. These needles come prepackaged with most introducer sets (Fig. 25–19), but an extra supply should be available. The historical problem limiting the use of this technique in cardiac pacing was the inability to remove the sheath from the pacemaker lead. The development of a peel-away sheath by Littleford solved this problem.[46–49]

Use of the percutaneous approach calls for a thorough knowledge of both normal and abnormal anatomy to avoid complications. The subclavian vein is generally the intended venous structure used for percutaneous venous access in cardiac pacing. Given the previously discussed anatomic variations, the subclavian vein puncture is typically made near the apex of the angle formed by the first rib and clavicle.[50] This defines the "subclavian window" (Fig. 25–20). At this puncture site (and following both skin infiltration with local anesthetic and a 1-cm incision at the site, which generally is 1 to 2 cm inferolateral to the point where the clavicle and first rib actually cross), the needle is aimed in a medial and cephalic direction. It is important to make the

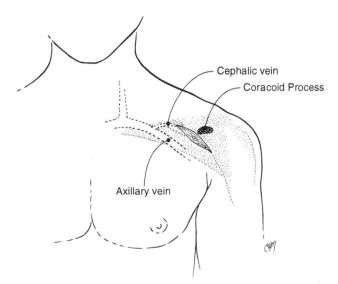

Figure 25–17. Anatomy of the deltopectoral groove.

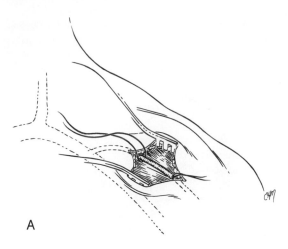

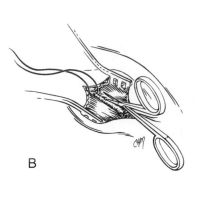

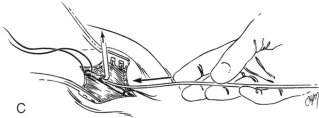

Figure 25–18. *A,* Introduction of a lead into the cephalic vein. The cephalic vein is isolated and tied off distally. *B,* Venotomy performed with iris scissors. *C,* Lead inserted while venotomy is held open with a vein pick.

puncture with the patient in a "normal" anatomic position. The infraclavicular space or costoclavicular angle should not be artificially opened by maneuvers such as extending the arm or placing a towel roll between the scapulae. These maneuvers can open a normally closed or tight space and result in undesirable puncture of the costoclavicular ligament or subclavius muscle, which can result in lead entrapment and crush. With the patient in the normal anatomic position, access to the subclavian window is medial yet usually avoids the costoclavicular ligament. The more medial puncture and needle trajectory of this approach vastly increases the suc-

cess rate and dramatically reduces the risks of pneumothorax and vascular injury compared with a more lateral approach. With this medial position, the vein is a much larger target and the apex of the lung is more lateral. This safer approach is a departure from the conventional subclavian venous punc-

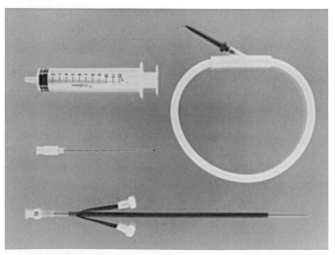

Figure 25–19. Prepackaged introducer set with 18-gauge needle, guide wire, and sheath with rubber dilator.

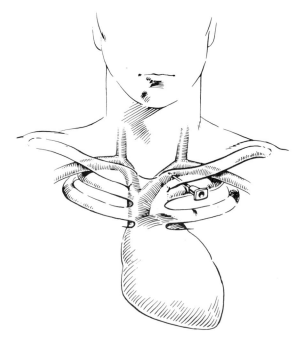

Figure 25–20. The subclavian window. (From Barold SS, Mugica J: New Perspectives in Cardiac Pacing 1. Mt Kisco, NY, Futura, 1988, p 257.)

ture, which calls for introduction of the needle in the middle third of the clavicle.

There are legitimate concerns that this medial approach, although safer, results in a later increase in the complication rate of failure from conductor fracture and insulation damage.[51] It is postulated that the extreme medial position results in a tight fit, subjecting the lead to compressive forces, causing binding between the first rib and the clavicle. Occasionally, this binding can even crush the lead and today is called the *subclavian crush phenomenon*. This phenomenon is more common in larger, complex leads of the in-line bipolar, coaxial design. Fortunately, the incidence of this complication is low. Fyke first reported insulation failure of two leads placed side by side using the percutaneous approach through the subclavian vein where there was a tight costoclavicular space.[52, 53] More recently, this issue has been addressed thoroughly by two independent groups. Jacobs and associates[54] analyzed a series of failed leads for the mechanism of failure. They correlated the anatomic relationship of lead position to compressive forces by autopsy study (Fig. 25–21). These autopsy data demonstrated a significant increase in pressure generated when leads were inserted in the costoclavicular angle as compared with that occurring

with a more lateral puncture. They concluded that the tight costoclavicular angle should be avoided. Magney and colleagues[55] derived similar data from cadaveric studies and suggested that lead damage is caused by soft tissue entrapment by the subclavius muscle rather than bony contact. This soft tissue entrapment causes a static load on the lead at that point, and repeated flexure around the point of entrapment may be responsible for the damage. Concern about this problem also has been communicated by pacemaker manufacturers in company literature.[56, 57] Reduction in lead diameter and, perhaps, modification of lead technology may be required to eliminate this problem. In the meantime, technique modification appears to be effective at reducing the occurrence of this problem. It has been our experience that if a pacemaker lead feels tight in the costoclavicular space, it is more susceptible to being crushed, and it has become our practice at the University of Oklahoma to remove the lead from the vein in this situation and repuncture the vein in a slightly different location with reintroduction of the lead. We believe that this has reduced the incidence of crush, although more substantial modifications in technique, described later, may be indicated.

Addressing this issue, along with other introducer- or

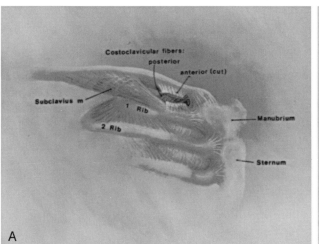

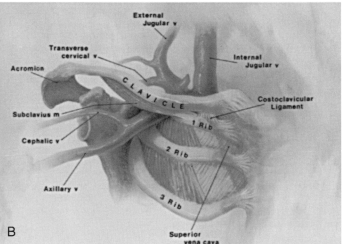

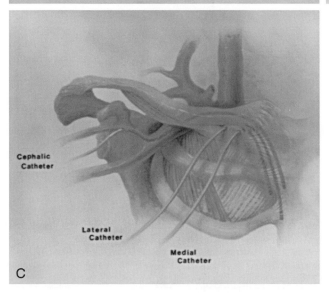

Figure 25–21. *A*, Musculoskeletal anatomy of the infraclavicular space. *B*, The relationship of the venous structures to clavicle, first rib, and costoclavicular ligaments. *C*, Course of leads through the venous structures demonstrating how the pacemaker electrode can become entrapped. (From Jacobs DM, Fink AS, Miller RP, et al: Anatomical and morphological evaluation of pacemaker lead compression. PACE 16:434, 1993.)

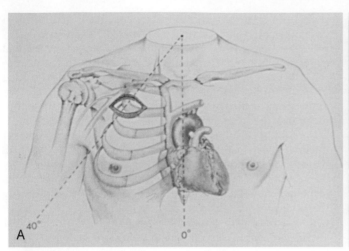
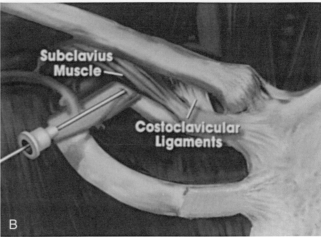

Figure 25–22. *A*, Anatomic orientation of the "safety zone" for intrathoracic subclavian vein puncture. *B*, Safe access to the extrathoracic portion of the subclavian vein as described by Byrd. (*A* from Barold SS, Mugica J: New Perspectives in Cardiac Pacing 2. Mt Kisco, NY, Futura, 1991, p 108. *B* from Byrd CL: Recent developments in pacemaker implantation and lead retrieval. PACE 16:1781, 1993.)

percutaneous-related complications, Byrd[58] has described a "safe introducer technique." This technique consists of a "safety zone" associated with precise conditions ensuring a safe puncture. Also described is a new technique for cannulating the axillary vein if this safety zone cannot be entered. Byrd's safety zone is defined as a region of venous access between the first rib and the clavicle, extending laterally from the sternum in an arc (Fig. 25–22*A*). As a condition for puncture, the site of access must be adequate for ease of insertion to avoid friction and puncture of bone, cartilage, or tendon. With this technique, subclavian vein puncture should never be made outside the safety zone or in violation of the preceding conditions. If the safety zone is inaccessible, or the preceding conditions are not met, an axillary vein puncture is recommended. As previously mentioned, the axillary vein is actually a continuation of the subclavian vein after it exits the superior mediastinum and crosses the first rib. It is also frequently referred to as the *extrathoracic portion* of the subclavian vein (Fig. 25–23).

The axillary vein approach is actually not new. In 1987, based on cadaveric studies that established reliable surface landmarks, Nichalls[59] and Taylor and Yellowlees[60] reported this approach as an alternative safe route of venous access for large central lines. The axillary vein has a completely infraclavicular course. The needle path must always be anterior to the thoracic cavity, avoiding risks of pneumothorax and hemothorax. The suggested landmarks for this infraclavicular course of the axillary vein (Fig. 25–24) are as follows:

- The axillary vein starts medially at a point below the aspect of the clavicle where the space between the first rib and clavicle becomes palpable.
- The vein extends laterally to a point about three fingerbreadths below the inferior aspect of the coracoid process.
- The skin is punctured along the medial border of the smaller pectoralis muscle at a point above the vein as it is defined by the surface landmarks.
- The axillary vein is punctured by passing the needle anterior to the first rib, maneuvering posteriorly and medially

corresponding to the lateral to medial course of the axillary vein.
- The needle never passes between the first rib and the clavicle, staying lateral to this juncture.

Some have found it useful to abduct the arm 45 degrees in using this approach.

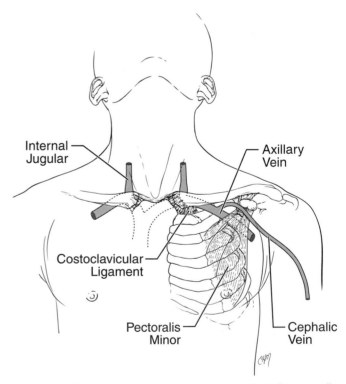

Figure 25–23. Anatomic relation of the axillary vein to the pectoralis minor muscle. The pectoralis major has been removed. Note the cephalic vein draining directly into the axillary vein at approximately the first intercostal space. (From Belott PH, et al. Unusual access sites for permanent cardiac pacing. *In* Barold S, Mugica J [eds]: Recent Advances in Pacing for the 21st Century. Armonk, NY, Futura, 1998, p 139.)

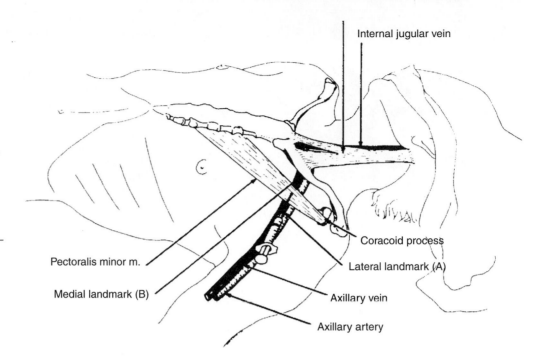

Figure 25–24. Nichalls' landmarks for axillary venipuncture. (From Belott PH, Byrd CL: Recent developments in pacemaker implantation and lead retrieval. *In* Barold S, Mugica J [eds]: New Perspectives in Cardiac Pacing. Armonk, NY, Futura, 1991.)

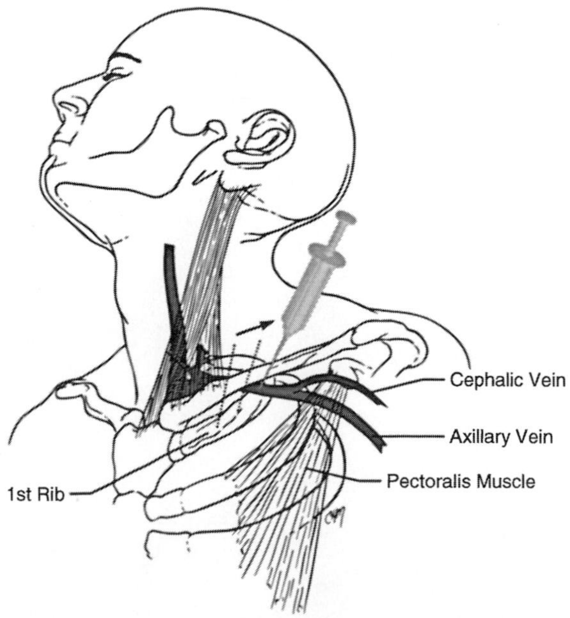

Figure 25–25. Byrd's technique for access to the extrathoracic portion of the subclavian vein. Sequential needle punctures are walked posterolateral along the first rib. (From Belott PH.)

In the technique described by Byrd, the axillary vein puncture is performed as a modification of the standard subclavian vein procedure without repositioning the patient (Fig. 25–25; see Fig. 25–20*B*). The introducer needle is guided by fluoroscopy directly to the medial portion of the first rib. The needle is held perpendicular to, and touches, the first rib. The needle, held perpendicular to the rib, is "walked" laterally and posteriorly, touching the rib with each change of position. Once the vein is punctured, as

indicated by aspiration of venous blood into the syringe, the guide wire and the introducer are inserted using standard technique. This approach essentially guarantees a successful and safe venipuncture without compromising the leads if the conditions for entering the safety zone are adhered to and if the first rib is touched to maintain orientation. The only complication not prevented by this approach is inadvertent puncture of the axillary artery.

Byrd[61] has reported success in a series of 213 consecutive cases in which the extrathoracic portion of the subclavian vein (axillary vein) was successfully cannulated as a primary approach. Magney and associates[62] subsequently reported a new approach to percutaneous subclavian venipuncture to avoid lead fracture. This technique is very similar to Byrd's. It uses extensive surface landmarks for venipuncture (Fig. 25–26). The technique involves puncture of the extrathoracic portion of the subclavian vein. Magney defines the location of the axillary vein as the intersection with a line drawn between the middle of the sternal angle and the tip of the coracoid process. This is generally near the lateral border of the first rib.

Belott[63] described blind axillary venous access using a modification of the Byrd and Magney recommendations. In this technique, the deltopectoral groove and coracoid process are primary landmarks. The deltopectoral groove and coracoid process are palpated, and the curvature of the chest wall is noted (Fig. 25–27). An incision is made at the level of the coracoid process. It is carried medially for about 2½ inches and is perpendicular to the deltopectoral groove (Fig. 25–28). The incision is carried to the surface of the pectoralis major muscle. The deltopectoral groove is visualized. The needle is inserted at an angle 45 degrees parallel to the deltopectoral groove and 1 to 2 cm medial (Fig. 25–29). If the vein is not entered, fluoroscopy is then used to define the first rib (Fig. 25–30). The needle is advanced and touches the first rib. Sequential needle punctures are walked laterally

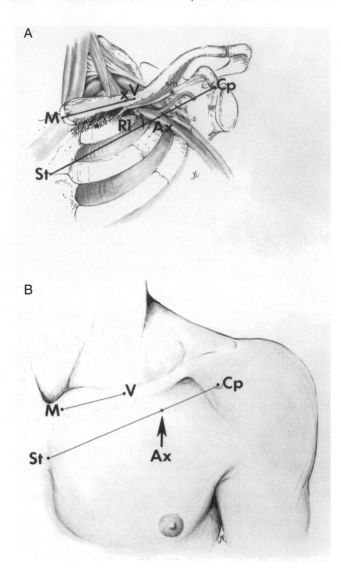

Figure 25–26. Deep *(A)* and superficial *(B)* anatomic relationships of the Magney approach to subclavian venipuncture. Point M indicates the medial end of the clavicle. X defines a point on the clavicle directly above the lateral edges of the clavicular/subclavius muscle (tendon complex) R1. Point D overlies the center of the subclavian vein as it crosses the first rib. St, center of the sternal angle; Cp, coracoid process; Ax, axillary vein; spar, costoclavicular ligament; open circle with closed circle inside, costoclavicular ligament; sm, subclavius muscle. The arrow points to Magney's ideal point for venous entry. (From Magney JE, Staplin DH, Flynn DM, et al: A new approach to percutaneous subclavian needle puncture to avoid lead fracture or central venous catheter occlusion. PACE 16:2133, 1993.)

and posteriorly until the vein is entered (Fig. 25–31). Because one cannot palpate the axillary pulse, it is not a reliable landmark. The axillary artery and brachial plexus are usually much deeper and more posterior structures. This simple technique using basic anatomic landmarks of the deltopectoral groove and a blind venous stick has been used successfully in 168 consecutive pacemaker and ICD procedures. There have only been three failures requiring an alternate approach. With a thorough knowledge of the regional anatomy, the axillary vein can be safely used as a primary site for venous access.

Access to the axillary vein may also be achieved by direct cutdown. Using the Metzenbaum scissors, fibers of the pectoralis major muscle are separated adjacent to the deltopectoral groove at the level of the coracoid process. This is just above the level of the superior border of the pectoralis minor. If the pectoralis major is split in this area and the fibers are gently teased apart in an axis parallel to the muscle bundle, the axillary vein will be found directly beneath the pectoralis major. A pursestring stitch is applied to the axillary vein, which can then be cannulated by a direct puncture or cutdown technique. The pursestring stitch will serve for hemostasis and ultimately assist in anchoring the electrodes after positioning.

A number of techniques can facilitate access to the axillary vein. Varnagy and coauthors[64] described a technique for isolating the cephalic and axillary veins by introducing a radiopaque J-tipped Teflon guide wire through a vein in the antecubital fossa under fluoroscopic control (Fig. 25–32). The metal guide wire is then palpated in the deltopectoral groove or identified by fluoroscopy. This guides the subsequent cutdown or puncture of the vessel by fluoroscopy. A cutdown can be performed on a vein and the intravascular guide wire pulled out of the venotomy to allow the application of an introducer. If a percutaneous approach is used, the puncture can always be extrathoracic, using fluoroscopy to guide the needle to the guide wire. This technique offers the benefit of rapid venous access while avoiding the risk for a pneumothorax by the percutaneous approach.

Contrast venography, described subsequently, can also be used for axillary venous access. The venous anatomy can be observed by contrast fluoroscopy in the pectoral area and, if possible, recorded for repeat viewing. The needle trajectory

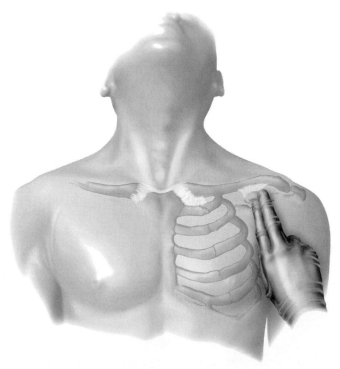

Figure 25–27. Superficial landmarks of the deltopectoral groove. Palpation of the deltopectoral groove and coracoid process.

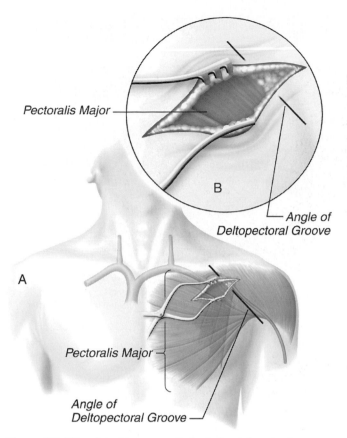

Figure 25–28. *A*, Incision perpendicular to the deltopectoral groove at the level of the coracoid process. *B*, Close-up view of incision demonstrating the plane of the deltopectoral angle and plane of the deltopectoral groove and pectoralis muscle.

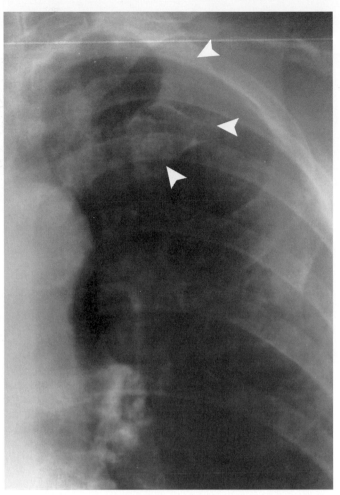

Figure 25–30. Radiograph demonstrating the location of the first rib.

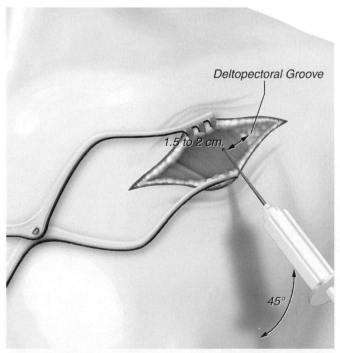

Figure 25–29. Needle and syringe trajectory and angle with respect to the deltopectoral groove and chest wall.

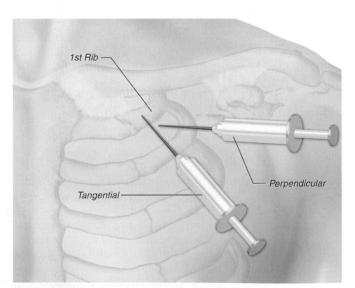

Figure 25–31. Needle trajectory in relationship to the first rib for axillary vein puncture. Note that when the needle is held tangential, there is little risk for pneumothorax and little risk of entering the intercostal space.

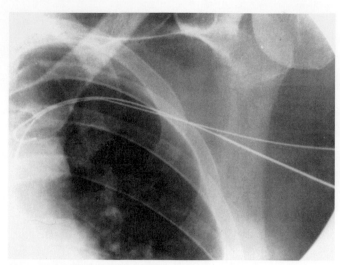

Figure 25–32. Percutaneous access to the axillary vein using a J wire introduced by means of the antecubital vein for reference.

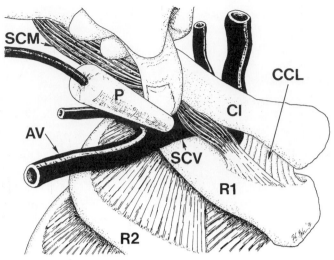

Figure 25–33. Doppler location of the axillary vein crossing the first rib. AV, axillary vein; CCL, costoclavicular ligament; CL, clavicle; P, Doppler; R, first rib; R2, second rib; SCM, subclavius muscle; SCV, subclavian vein.

and venipuncture are guided by the contrast material in the axillary vein. Once again, laboratories with sophisticated imaging capabilities can create an image "mask." Spencer and colleagues[65, 66] reported the use of contrast for localizing the axillary vein in 22 consecutive patients. Similarly, Ramza and associates[67] demonstrated the safety and efficacy of the axillary vein for placement of pacemaker and defibrillator leads when guided by contrast venography. Lead placement was successfully accomplished in 49 of 50 patients using this technique.

Venous access of the axillary vein can also be guided by Doppler and ultrasound techniques. Fyke[68] has described a Doppler-guided extrathoracic introducer insertion technique in 59 consecutive patients (total of 100 leads) with a simple Doppler flow detector. A sterile Doppler flow detector is moved along the clavicle. Once the vein is defined, the location and angulation of probe are noted, and the venipuncture is carried out (Fig. 25–33). Care is taken to avoid directing the Doppler beam beneath the clavicle. Gayle and coworkers[69, 70] have developed an ultrasound technique that directly visualizes the needle puncture of the axillary vein. A portable ultrasound device with sterile sleeve and needle holder are used. The ultrasound head is placed over the skin surface in the vicinity of the axillary vein. Once the vein is visualized, the puncture technique can be used. This technique has been used with considerable success for both pacing and defibrillator electrodes. There have been no reported pneumothoraces. This technique can be carried out transcutaneously or through the incision on the surface of the pectoralis muscle (Figs. 25–34 and 25–35).

In summary, the axillary vein is becoming a common venous access site for pacemaker and defibrillator implantations, given the concerns of the subclavian crush and the requirement for insertion of multiple electrodes for dual-chambered pacing and at least one large complex electrode for transvenous defibrillation. There are now a number of reliable techniques for axillary venous access (see Table 25–10). Given the recent interest in the axillary vein, it is recommended that the implanting physician become thor-

oughly familiar with the relevant anatomy. It is imperative that the interested physician visit the anatomic laboratory to refresh and review the regional anatomy and surface landmarks.

For a more conventional subclavian vein approach, Lamas and colleagues[71] have even recommended fluoroscopic observation of the needle trajectory for achieving a successful and safe subclavian vein puncture. They initially identify

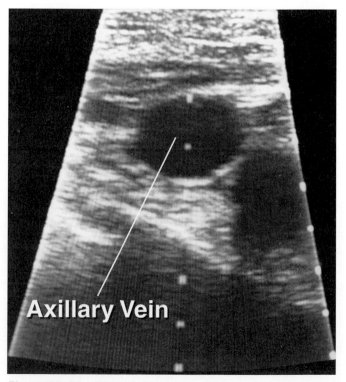

Figure 25–34. Ultrasonic image of the axillary vein.

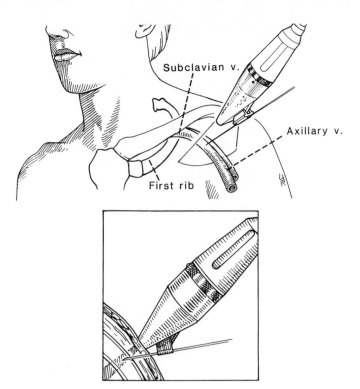

Figure 25–35. Ultrasound-guided puncture of the axillary vein using the Site-Rite device.

the clavicle on the side of puncture, noting its course and landmarks. The skin is entered about 2 cm inferior to the junction of the medial and lateral halves of the clavicle, aiming with fluoroscopic guidance for the caudal half of the clavicular head.

Whether using the techniques of the subclavian window, the safety zone, the axillary vein puncture, or fluoroscopic guidance, there are some common features. Needle orientation is always medial and cephalad, almost tangential to the chest wall. All needle probing should use a forward motion. Lateral needle probing should be avoided because it could cause laceration of important structures. Anatomic landmarks are defined, and the puncture is made, with rare exception, with the patient in the anatomic position. The costoclavicular angle is not artificially opened by maneuvers. Although the essence of the nonaxillary approaches is medial to avoid the lung, the undesirable puncture of the costoclavicular ligament should be avoided. In the obese patient, the tendency is to orient the needle more perpendicular to the chest wall in an attempt to pass between the clavicle and first rib. This perpendicular angle is to be avoided with the medial approaches because it is associated with a higher incidence of pneumothorax. In this circumstance, a more inferior skin puncture is recommended, allowing the needle to slip between the first rib and clavicle. The needle is, therefore, maintained almost tangential to the chest wall, avoiding the lung. Some implanters bend the needle in an attempt to slip under the clavicle. We do not recommend this because of a higher incidence of pneumothorax and vascular trauma. In the morbidly obese patient, it is recommended that the subclavian puncture be carried out after direct visualization of the pectoral muscle. This can be done

only by making an initial skin incision and carrying it down to the pectoral muscle. Once the anatomic landmarks are defined, the needle is slipped between the first rib and the clavicle with a trajectory that is nearly tangential to the chest wall directed cephalad and medial.

This raises the question of whether the skin incision should routinely be made first, with percutaneous venous access carried out through the incision, or whether an initial percutaneous venous puncture should be performed, followed by the incision. It is, arguably, better not to commit oneself with an initial pocket-length incision and subsequent venipuncture. This avoids the embarrassment of having to explain matching incisions if venous access could not be achieved through the initial incision and one is forced to move to the other side. It is difficult enough explaining multiple unsuccessful skin punctures. As an acceptable alternative, and one that we used regularly for some time at the University of Oklahoma, a 1 cm-long stab wound can be made initially, through which the venipunctures can be accomplished. This allows easy incorporation of the puncture sites (especially if two separate punctures are used for a dual-chamber pacing system) into a single incision that is extended after successful venipuncture. We use a full incision to the greater pectoral fascia before gaining venous access to the vein.

As with axillary vein access techniques, the subclavian puncture can also be facilitated by the use of contrast venography.[72] This is helpful in patients in whom venous access can be anticipated to be a problem. It should be considered before any puncture in which venous patency is in doubt or abnormal anatomy is suspected. The technique has been described by Hayes and colleagues.[72] A venous line is established in the arm on the side of planned pacemaker venous access. The line should be reliable and 20-gauge or larger. The patient should not have an allergy to radiographic contrast material. The contrast material injection is performed by a nonsterile assistant. Ten to 50 mL of contrast material (nonionic or ionic) is injected rapidly into the IV line in the forearm. This should be followed by a saline bolus flush. The contrast medium moves slowly in the peripheral venous system and can be moved along by massaging the arm through or under the sterile drapes. The venous anatomy is observed under fluoroscopy in the pectoral area and, if possible, recorded for repeated viewing (Fig. 25–36). The needle trajectory and venipuncture are guided by the contrast material in the subclavian vein. In more sophisticated radiologic laboratories, a mask or map can be made for guidance after the contrast medium has dissipated. The process can be repeated as necessary.

The actual percutaneous stick is carried out with a syringe attached to the 18-gauge needle. A common practice is to fill the syringe partially with saline. The theory behind this practice is that if a pneumothorax occurs, it will be detected by air bubbles aspirated through the saline. In addition, the saline can be used to flush out tissue plugs that may obstruct the needle and prevent aspiration. We avoid this practice because we believe that one does not need air bubbles to detect an inadvertent pneumothorax. More important, the syringe even partially filled with saline makes it difficult to differentiate between arterial and venous blood. This is because when blood (arterial or venous) mixes with the saline, it takes on the color of oxygenated blood. If saline is not

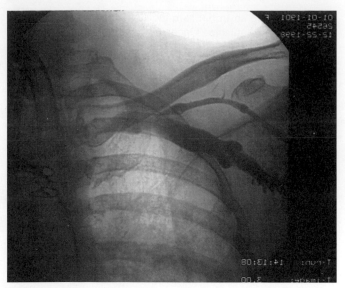

Figure 25–36. Contrast venography-guided venipuncture. With contrast material, the needle is guided under fluoroscopy directly to the vein.

used, which vascular structure has been entered is more readily apparent.

When proceeding with a percutaneous venipuncture, the syringe should be held in the palm of the hand with the dorsal aspect of the hand resting on the patient. This gives support and control as the needle is advanced. With the needle held this way, tactile sensation is enhanced, and one can frequently feel the needle enter the vein. Once the vessel is entered, the guide wire is inserted and the tip advanced to a position in the vicinity of the right atrium (Fig. 25–37). We prefer to use J or curved-tip guide wires for safety reasons. If resistance is encountered, the wire is withdrawn slightly and readvanced. If the resistance persists, the wire position is checked under fluoroscopy. If the wire just outside the tip of the needle is coiled, it is probably extravascular. In this case, the wire and needle are removed, and a new venous stick is carried out. Extremely rarely, one may not be able to re-enter the vein. This may be due to collapse of the vein by a resultant hematoma caused by a small tear in the vein from the misdirected guide wire. In this case, one should probably proceed to an alternative approach or site of venous access, avoiding an unnecessary waste of time and increasing the risk for pneumothorax with multiple subsequent unsuccessful percutaneous punctures. Occasionally the guide wire tracks up the internal jugular vein. By changing the angle of the needle slightly to a more medial and inferior direction while the guide wire is still in the internal jugular vein, withdrawing the guide wire back into the needle and then readvancing usually results in passage of the guide wire through the innominate vein and superior vena cava into the right atrium. At times, this maneuver has to be repeated several times with varying needle angulations. Care must be exercised to avoid tearing the vein. The application of a 5F or 6F dilator can sometimes help steer the guide wire in the right direction. In rare instances, the guide wire and needle must be removed and a new puncture site se-

lected. The key point is that once venous access has been achieved, every effort is made to retain it.

When air is withdrawn through the needle during attempted venipunctures, suggesting lung puncture and raising the possibility of a pneumothorax, our practice is to withdraw the needle, wait a moment or two to make certain that a rapid-onset, large, markedly symptomatic pneumothorax is not occurring, and then proceed (obviously with a different needle trajectory) with reattempts at venipuncture. In our experience, most lung punctures occurring with forward (not lateral!) needle motion do not result in a clinically apparent (by chest radiography) pneumothorax. If a pneumothorax does develop, it may do so in this setting over a matter of hours and may not even be apparent radiographically at the end of the procedure. If a lung puncture has occurred, repeating the postoperative upright chest radiograph 6 hours after completion of the procedure is advisable. If a pneumothorax has developed, a chest tube or catheter evacuation procedure may be necessary, although frequently, a small to moderate pneumothorax that is not expanding can be managed conservatively without evacuation.

Similarly, if an arterial puncture occurs inadvertently, removal of the needle, compression at the site of the puncture for 5 minutes or so, followed by repeated venipuncture attempts with a different needle path has been our approach. It is rare for such arterial punctures to result in a hemothorax, provided that no tearing of the artery has occurred (avoidance of lateral needle motion is crucial here also). Follow-up chest radiographs taken 6 to 18 hours after the procedure are advisable, and postoperative hemoglobin and hematocrit measurements are suggested. The most important problem to avoid if the artery has been punctured is nonrecognition and placement of a sheath into the artery. If there is any doubt about whether the artery has been punctured, a blood sample withdrawn through the needle and subjected to oximetric analysis should clarify the situation.

Once the wire is successfully in the vein, some implanters place a pursestring suture in the tissue around the point of entry of the wire into the tissue. Alternatively, a figure-of-eight stitch can be applied (Fig. 25–38). This can be helpful later for hemostasis.[73] These sutures require that an incision be made beginning at the needle and extending inferiorly to the depth of the pectoral fascia.

Once the guide wires are in the subclavian vein, it is usually a simple procedure to advance the appropriate-sized dilator and peel-away sheath over the wire into the venous circulation. Occasionally, there is substantial resistance to dilator-sheath advancement, and repetitive dilation with progressively larger dilators is necessary. Alternatively, a 15- to 20-degree bending of the tip of the full-sized introducer frequently facilitates advancement over the wire. If difficulty with advancement occurs, we generally remove the sheath from the dilator and use only the dilator initially to dilate the track into the vein. This protects these rather delicate sheaths from damage. After successfully advancing the dilator alone over the wire, the dilator can be withdrawn, the sheath added, and both then advanced over the wire. We have found that gentle back-pressure on the guide wire when advancing the dilator-sheath also facilitates advancement in difficult or tortuous vessel situations.

After the sheath has been successfully passed over the guide wire to the vicinity of the superior vena cava, the

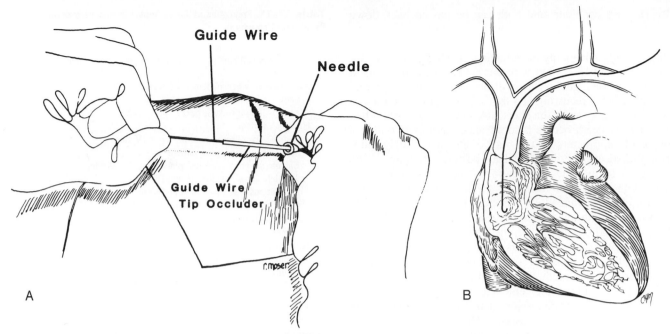

Figure 25–37. *A*, Once venous access is achieved, the needle is supported with one hand and the guide wire with tip occluder advanced with the other hand. *B*, Guide wire tip advanced to the middle right atrium. (*A* from Belott PH: Retained guide wire introducer technique, for unlimited access to the central circulation. Clin Prog Pacing Electrophysiol 1:59, 1983.)

dilator and guide wire can be removed and the lead advanced through the sheath. Problems can be encountered when passing the lead through the sheath. Occasionally, in the process of introduction, the sheath buckles at a point in the venous system where there is a bend (Fig. 25–39).[74] This usually occurs after the removal of the dilator. It can also occur if the sheath is advanced against the lateral wall of the superior vena cava. If a buckle occurs, the lead will not pass this point. Forcing the lead can result in damage to the cathode

and insulation. This kink can usually be observed on fluoroscopy. There are several solutions to this problem. If the guide wire and dilator have both been removed, both can be replaced down the sheath. The dilator with wire inside is now functioning not only as a way to stiffen the sheath but

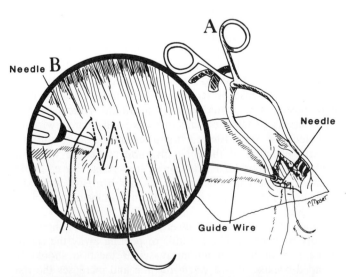

Figure 25–38. Placement of the figure-of-eight stitch to enhance hemostasis. (From Belott PH: Retained guide wire introducer technique, for unlimited access to the central circulation. Clin Prog Pacing Electrophysiol 1:59, 1983.)

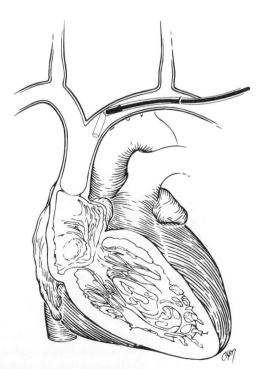

Figure 25–39. Buckling of the introducer sheath prevents the passage of the electrode.

also as a tip occluder, and both can be passed back down the sheath. The tapered tip of the dilator will straighten the buckle. The position of the buckle point can be changed by either slightly advancing or retracting the sheath. The dilator is removed but the guide wire can be retained. It is hoped that the retained guide wire will act as a stent, preventing the buckle from recurring and thus allowing the electrode to pass completely down the sheath. Another option when this buckling of sheath occurs is to advance the lead to within a couple of centimeters of the buckle and then slowly withdraw the sheath, holding the lead position stationary. The sheath, including the buckle point, may occasionally be easily withdrawn over the tip of the lead, and the lead can be cautiously advanced. In this situation, it is sometimes necessary to withdraw the stylet from the tip of the lead to allow easy advancement of the lead beyond the buckle point. Inexperienced implanters should be cautious with this technique because distal electrode damage can occur. If these maneuvers fail, the guide wire and dilator are reinserted and the sheath and dilator are removed, leaving the guide wire in the vein. Tissue compression or traction is applied to the pursestring suture for hemostasis. The sheath is inspected for buckling. At this point, the implanter should consider advancing the next larger-sized sheath over the retained guide wire. The application of the same-sized sheath usually results in recurrence of the same problem. Again, the important point is that despite this frustrating experience, one must be reluctant to relinquish the vein once it has been catheterized. Generally, the larger sheath is less likely to buckle, especially if the guide wire is retained to act as a stent. With successful electrode introduction, the sheath is briskly pulled back out of the circulation, and skin compression or traction is applied to the pursestring or figure-of-eight suture for hemostasis.

The risk for air embolization is substantial with the percutaneous approach. This issue has been addressed by the recommendation that the Trendelenburg position be used. With the shift of the pacemaker procedure to the cardiac catheterization laboratory or special procedures room, however, it is frequently impossible to place the patient in the Trendelenburg position. Consequently, the patient is at greater risk for air embolization if the percutaneous approach is used. It is most important that the implanting physician be aware of the danger and take steps necessary to avoid this potential catastrophe (Table 25–11). The physician must be aware that removal of the sheath dilator in a patient who is fasting and somewhat volume depleted can rapidly cause aspiration of large quantities of air. Because the luxury of the Trendelenburg position is unlikely to be available in the catheterization laboratory, other steps must be taken. Contrary to some practices, the preoperative pacemaker patient should be maintained in a euvolemic or even a relatively volume-overloaded state if there is no contraindication. Instead of administering intravenous fluids at a restricted rate, adequate hydration should be maintained. We routinely place a large wedge sponge under the patient's legs to enhance blood return and increase central venous pressure. An assessment of the state of hydration can be carried out during the procedure. With the sheath in the central venous circulation, by carefully withdrawing the dilator from the sheath, the state of hydration and venous pressure can be observed.

After the dilator is withdrawn in the hydrated patient with

Table 25–11. Prevention of Air Embolism During Permanent Pacemaker Procedures

Awareness of the potential problem
A well-hydrated patient, avoiding long periods of nothing by mouth
Awareness of when patient is at greatest risk, i.e., open sheath in vein
Assess hydration (take a peek)
High-risk patient
   Increase hydration, i.e., wide open IV lines
   An awake, cooperative patient
   Elevate lower extremities, place wedge under legs
   Trendelenburg position (if available)
   Expeditious lead placement and sheath removal
   Check for introduction of air
   Continuous monitoring (vital signs, oxygen saturation, blood pressure)
In an extremely high-risk, uncooperative patient, intubation and sedation causing temporary loss of consciousness may be required.

adequate venous pressure, there is continuous blood flow out of the sheath despite the cycle of respiration. In the case of the dehydrated patient, withdrawal of the dilator results in little or no flow of blood. The blood meniscus is barely visible. More important, on inspiration, the blood meniscus is observed to move substantially inward. If this is observed, the dilator can be rapidly advanced back into the sheath; alternatively, the sheath can be pinched and additional precautions taken to avoid air embolization. If a wedge has not been placed under the patient's legs, this can be done now and is frequently helpful. Also, at this point, it is most important to have the cooperation of the patient. If the patient is sleeping, he or she should be aroused. The patient should be coached to reduce the depth of respirations and avoid the sudden large inspiration that can result in the aspiration of a lethal volume of air. At the same time, administration of intravenous fluids is increased to enhance hydration. Having the patient hold the breath after maximal inspiration offers the greatest latitude in time because the patient will have to exhale before pulling negative intrathoracic pressure and aspirating air. This gives the implanter time to insert the lead. Pinching of the sheath with the lead going through it to avoid air embolization is ineffective and gives a false sense of security. A peel-away sheath with a nonrebleed valve would be useful. In the patient who is substantially sedated or uncooperative, adequate hydration and elevation of the lower extremities are the only solutions. Careful planning of the lead insertion procedure will also help. Expeditious lead insertion is important. For example, positioning the electrodes with the sheath in situ is unwise because it may result in air embolism or unnecessary blood loss.

Once the lead has been inserted, the introducer should be rapidly withdrawn. The practice of peeling away the sheath while part of it is in an intravascular location should be avoided because it is a waste of time and increases the risk for air embolization and blood loss. In this regard, the actual peeling away of the sheath is not even a necessity at this point so long as it is completely extravascular. It can be peeled away later at one's convenience. In fact, the tabs of

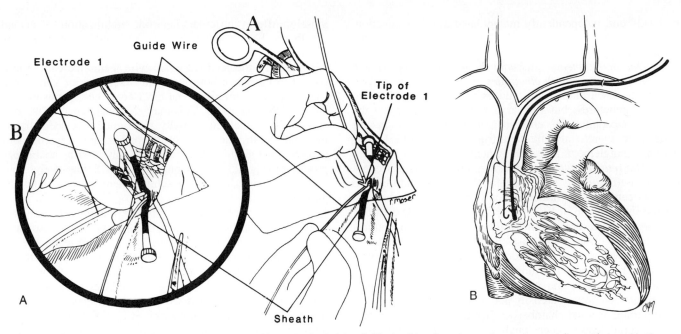

Figure 25–40. *A,* The guide wire with dilator removed remains in the sheath. The lead has been inserted and advanced *(inset B)* alongside the guide wire. *B,* Both the guide wire and the lead are advanced to the vicinity of the middle right atrium. Additional introducers can be advanced over this retained guide wire to place additional leads. (*A* from Belott PH: Retained guide wire introducer technique, for unlimited access to the central circulation. Clin Prog Pacing Electrophysiol 1:59, 1983.)

the unpeeled sheath can be used to pin the lead to the drapes during threshold testing, preventing inadvertent dislodgment of the lead onto the floor. With the sheath withdrawn completely from the circulation, hemostasis is achieved by applying tension to the pursestring or figure-of-eight suture or by applying skin compression over the entry site.

A variation of the introducer technique involves retaining the guide wire. Instead of removing the guide wire together with the dilator, it is left in place, so that the lead is passed through the sheath alongside the guide wire. The sheath is subsequently removed and peeled away (Fig. 25–40). Occasionally, the size of the electrode and the sheath precludes the passage of the lead alongside the guide wire. In this case, the guide wire is removed, the lead is passed down the sheath, and the guide wire is reinserted behind the electrode. The reason this can work is that, in most cases, it is the electrode that will not pass alongside the guide wire, whereas the lead body is thinner and leaves enough room to accommodate both guide wire and lead body. Certain leads (especially those with bipolar electrodes) and sheath combinations are too tight to allow passage of both the electrode and guide wire. In this case, a larger-sized sheath can be used. When reintroducing the guide wire, the tip occluder is not used because it can wind up in the central circulation fairly easily. It works well to reuse the dilator as a tip occluder when reinserting the guide wire. The retained guide wire may provide unlimited venous access and the ability to exchange or introduce additional electrodes by simply applying another sheath set to the guide wire. The retained guide wire should be held to the drape by a clamp to avoid inadvertent dislodgment. The retained guide wire can serve as a ground for unipolar threshold analysis instead of a grounding plate. It can also be used as an intracardiac lead

for recording of the atrial electrogram (to confirm atrial capture) or as an electrode for emergency pacing. It is our routine practice to retain an intravascular guide wire in both single-chamber and dual-chamber procedures until a satisfactory lead position is obtained.

The percutaneous approach is particularly useful in dual-chamber pacing and has eliminated the earlier dilemma of having to introduce two leads into a vein exposed by cutdown that may barely accommodate a single lead and the resultant need for a second venous access site. The options for dual-chamber venous access are shown in Table 25–12. For dual-chamber pacing, there are now at least four methods that involve the percutaneous approach. These techniques, except for the fourth, can be used with any of the previously described percutaneous approaches.

1. *Two separate percutaneous sticks and the use of two sheath sets.*[75] Two separate punctures increase the risk for complications related to the venipuncture process, and there is also the possibility of not finding the vessel the second time. The advantage of this method (which one of us preferentially uses) is that even relatively large bipolar leads can

Table 25–12. Venous Access for Single- and Dual-Chamber Pacing

Venous cutdown: Isolate one or two veins
Percutaneous: Two separate sticks and sheath applications
Percutaneous: Two electrodes down one large sheath
Percutaneous: Retained guide wire (Belott technique)
Percutaneous access to the extrathoracic portion of the subclavian vein (Byrd technique)
Cutdown with cephalic vein guide wire (Ong-Barold technique)

be easily and independently manipulated after introduction, with little risk of unwanted and frustrating movement of the other lead.

2. *One percutaneous stick and the use of a large sheath with the passage of both electrodes.*[76, 77] The passage of two electrodes down one sheath reduces the risk of making two separate punctures, but the large sheath may increase the risk for substantial air embolism and blood loss. In our experience, there is also frequent frustration from lead interaction, entanglement, and dislodgment.

3. *The retained guide wire technique.*[78, 79] This procedure can be used alone as a method for the introduction of two leads or can be incorporated into any of the other techniques for the introduction of two leads. One of us (PHB) uses this technique alone, preferentially for dual-lead introductions, and the other of us (DWR) uses it as backup in combination with the two separate puncture techniques described previously. This approach is most desirable because it provides unlimited access to the central circulation. The implanter using this technique can easily add and exchange leads. This is important in dual-chamber pacing in which the initially chosen atrial lead is occasionally unacceptable for a given anatomic situation. Less commonly, it is also helpful to be able to exchange ventricular leads. When using the retained guide wire technique for dual-chamber implantation, the ventricular electrode is usually positioned first. This is practical and safe. The ventricular electrode can be more easily stabilized and is less susceptible to dislodgment from positioning of the second electrode. The ventricular electrode can then be stabilized by leaving the stylet pulled back in the lead in the vicinity of the lower right atrium (Fig. 25–41). A stitch should be placed proximally around the lead and suture sleeve and secured about 1 to 2 cm from the puncture site in the subcutaneous tissue on the surface of the pectoral muscle. After ventricular electrode stabilization, a second sheath can be advanced over the retained guide wire. The atrial electrode is introduced, positioned, tested, and secured. Alternatively, the retained guide wire technique can be employed to introduce both leads into the superior vena cava, right atrium, or inferior vena cava areas before positioning either of the electrodes. This may eliminate some of the risk of dislodgment of the initially positioned electrode that is incurred by introduction of the second sheath. Regardless of variation, the guide wire is removed only after a satisfactory procedure (Fig. 25–42). A pursestring or figure-of-eight suture can be tied loosely to achieve hemostasis around the puncture site.

4. *The sheath set technique in conjunction with the cutdown approach.*[80, 81] Ong and Barold and their associates described a modified cephalic vein guide wire technique for the introduction of one or more electrodes. The Ong-Barold technique appears to be a safe and reasonable alternative to the percutaneous subclavian vein introducer technique. It is particularly recommended for the inexperienced implanter. It is also recommended in patients at high risk for complications from the percutaneous approach and in situations in which one can anticipate the percutaneous approach to be difficult if not impossible. This requires an initial cutdown to the cephalic vein as previously described. For a single-lead introduction, the size of the vein is irrelevant. All that is necessary is the introduction of the guide wire, which is accomplished using needle puncture under direct visualization. The cephalic vein is sacrificed because it seems to invaginate into the subclavian vein with advancement of the sheath set over the guide wire (Fig. 25–43). Hemostasis is achieved by pressure or the application of a figure-of-eight stitch. Despite sacrificing the cephalic vein, there have been no reported venous complications. When two leads are required, the retained guide wire technique and sheath set technique can be used in this approach.

Complications of Venous Access and Blind Subclavian Puncture

There is ongoing debate with respect to the safety and efficacy of the blind subclavian puncture. Although the blind subclavian puncture technique has proved very useful, it has generated considerable controversy with respect to the incidence of serious complications and even mortality (Table 25–13). Parsonnet and Bernstein reported a 0.4% incidence of serious complications in a survey of 11 implanting physicians in a review of 2500 cases.[82] Furman[83] has demonstrated the remarkable efficiency of the cutdown approach for single-chamber and dual-chamber pacing, particularly with unipolar leads. The cutdown technique, however, was less useful for the introduction of bipolar leads by a single cephalic vein. Furman[84] reported no vascular or pleural complications in a large series of 3500 cases using the cutdown approach for single-chamber and dual-chamber pacemaker implantations. Parsonnet[85] analyzed the pacemaker implantation complication rates with respect to contributing factors. He reviewed 632 consecutive implantations over a 5-year period performed by 29 implanting physicians at a single institution. There were 37 perioperative complications. Complications were analyzed with respect to experience of the implanting physician. Percutaneous venous access was associated with the highest complication rate and contributed significantly to

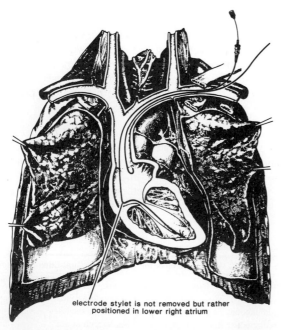

electrode stylet is not removed but rather positioned in lower right atrium

Figure 25–41. The ventricular lead has been placed first. The guide wire has been retained, and the lead stylet is positioned in the lower right atrium for stability.

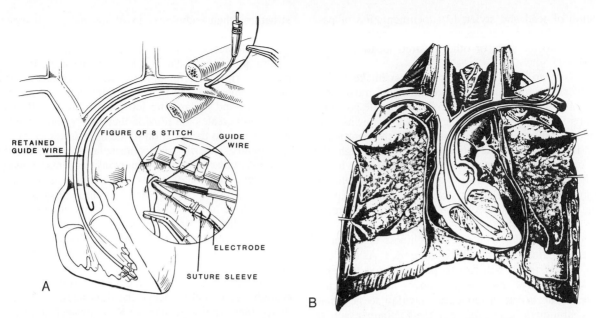

Figure 25–42. *A*, The ventricular electrode and retained guide wire are demonstrated in the main drawing. The *inset* demonstrates the ventricular lead anchored by suture around its suture sleeve and the second sheath advancing over the retained guide wire. A hemostat on the figure-of-eight suture maintains hemostasis. *B*, The atrial and ventricular electrodes have been positioned, yet the guide wire is still retained. (*A* from Barold SS, Mugica J: New Perspectives in Cardiac Pacing 2. Mt Kisco, NY, Futura, 1991, p 110.)

a 5.7% overall complication rate. When the complications related to the percutaneous approach were excluded, the complication rate dropped to a more acceptable 3.5%. The highest complication rate was among physicians implanting fewer than 12 pacemakers a year with the least pacing experience.

Sutton and Bourgeos,[86] in reviewing complications of pacemaker insertion, noted an overall 1% incidence of sub-clavian vein puncture leading to pneumothorax. Arterial puncture occurred more commonly, at a rate of about 3%, but generally was not associated with any morbidity. Similarly, in their analysis of thrombotic complications, axillary vein thrombosis was rare, occurring in 0.5% to 1% of cases. Interestingly, partial venous obstruction in the great veins was almost the rule and occurred to some degree in up to 100% of cases. Clinical pulmonary embolism, however, was extremely rare. As a rule, partial or silent inconsequential thrombosis is considered extremely common but generally of no clinical significance.[87]

Ventricular Electrode Placement

There are many techniques for placing the ventricular electrode described throughout the published pacing literature,[87] essentially reflecting the approach with which any particular author has facility. There is no one correct technique. Ventricular electrode placement is largely independent of the route of venous access. The implanting physician must draw on experience to deal with the variety of situations that will be encountered in any given patient. In time, one develops one's own technique. There are some fundamental principles and maneuvers that are common to all: (1) simultaneous

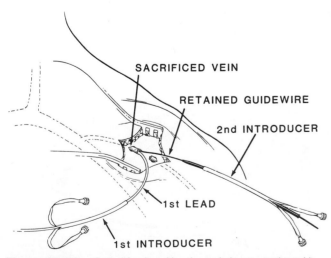

Figure 25–43. Cephalic vein guide wire technique uses the guide wire as access to the vein for one or more electrodes. The distal connection of the cephalic vein is sacrificed (Ong-Barold technique). (From Barold SS, Mugica J: New Perspectives in Cardiac Pacing 2. Mt Kisco, NY, Futura, 1991, p 112.)

Table 25–13. Percutaneous Complications

1. Pneumothorax	6. Nerve injury
2. Hemothorax	7. Thoracic duct injury
3. Hemopneumothorax	8. Chylothorax
4. Laceration, subclavian artery	9. Lymphatic fistula
5. Arteriovenous fistula	

manipulation of lead and stylet, (2) documentation of passage into the right side of the heart, and (3) manipulation of the electrode into the apex or other desired location of the right ventricle.

It is necessary to grasp the concept that pacemaker placement involves a "symphony" of lead and stylet movement. Without the two working together, proper electrode positioning is impossible. The lead without stylet is somewhat like a limp piece of spaghetti. When positioning the ventricular electrode, the lead must negotiate a course through the chambers of the right side of the heart and ultimately to the apex of the right ventricle. This is typically accomplished by preforming the lead stylet. This enables easier manipulation of the lead and is probably the best way to position a pacemaker electrode effectively. A curve is applied to the distal aspect of the stylet. The size or tightness of the curve and how it is created are a personal preference. As a rule, a curve that is too gentle will fail to negotiate the tricuspid valve, making passage into the pulmonary artery difficult. Conversely, a curve that is too tight may fail to negotiate the venous structures in the superior mediastinum, such as the innominate vein and superior vena cava. At times, however, unusual circumstances will call for extremes of wire curvature to position the electrode effectively. In every case, the ideal curve will be slightly different. There are several ways to form the curve on the stylet. Some implanters choose to use a blunt instrument, such as the tip of a clamp or scissors. The stylet is pulled between the thumb and the blunt instrument with a rotary motion of the wrist forming the curve. Another method is to form the curve by pulling the guide wire between the thumb and index finger, gently shaping the curve. Whatever method is used, the curve should be a bend that is not sharp because a sharp bend in a stylet will generally preclude its passage through the lead. In making the curve, the aim is that the curved stylet will direct the electrode to the appropriate position.

Unlike diagnostic catheters, the pacemaker lead cannot be steered or torqued into position. Positioning of a pacemaker electrode is solely dependent, therefore, on the manipulation of lead and stylet together. The basic technique of lead positioning involves advancing the electrode, with curved stylet in place, through the chambers of the right side of the heart. A more sophisticated variation of this technique involves simultaneously advancing the electrode while retracting and readvancing the stylet. The retraction of the stylet renders the lead tip floppy. Using a slightly retracted although curved stylet and pointing the electrode body in the proper direction, the lead, with 1 to 2 cm of its floppy tip, in most instances, can make for more precise and expeditious electrode placement. An alternative, related technique, and one that can expedite ventricular lead implantation, although it is clearly more difficult to master, involves the use of a straight stylet. The stylet is retracted to allow the floppy lead tip to "catch" on a structure in the right atrium, with subsequent advancement of the lead. The lead body then prolapses through the tricuspid valve into the right ventricle. The stylet can then be cautiously advanced to stiffen the lead body and, generally, free the tip from the catch. It is possible, even likely, that these techniques involving prolapse of the leads across the tricuspid valve present less likelihood of damaging the valve or entangling subvalvular

structures than techniques involving direct advancement of stiff-tipped leads.

The fluoroscope should be used for the entire lead positioning process and can be used initially in the PA projection or in the right anterior oblique (RAO) projection. The latter helps delineate the apex of the right ventricle to the left of the spine and toward the left lateral chest wall. The RAO projection creates the illusion that our "mind's eye" expects with respect to the location of the apex of the right ventricle, specifically, that the right ventricular apex is near the apex of the cardiac silhouette. In many patients, however, the right ventricular apex tends to be more anterior than leftward. Much time can be wasted trying to position a ventricular electrode to the left of the spine toward the apex of the cardiac silhouette (in the PA projection) when, in reality, the right ventricular apex is directly anterior to the spine. This anterior position results in an electrode position that is over the spine or nearly so and appears in the PA projection to be erroneously placed in the right atrium or in the less desirable proximal aspect of the right ventricle. Rotating the image intensifier unit into the RAO projection in this situation superimposes the right ventricular apex over the apex of the cardiac silhouette in the left side of the chest, confirming the appropriate position (Fig. 25–44). Whether or not the initial choice of projection is the RAO, it should be used freely to facilitate ventricular lead placement.

We recommend that the electrode be passed initially across the tricuspid valve and then out into the pulmonary artery (Fig. 25–45A to C). This maneuver confirms passage into the right side of the heart and precludes erroneous placement in the coronary sinus. The RAO projection is also helpful in making certain the lead is not in the coronary sinus. If the lead is appropriately in the apex of the right ventricle, there will be no posterior component of the course of the lead in the RAO projection. If the lead is in the coronary sinus, it will have a posterior course in this projection. If it courses down the middle cardiac vein, it will have a posterior course as it traverses the coronary sinus and then an anterior course as it traverses this branch.

There are several techniques for the actual placement of the electrode into the right ventricular apex. They involve the combined manipulation of the lead stylet and electrode body. If one chooses to pass the electrode to the pulmonary

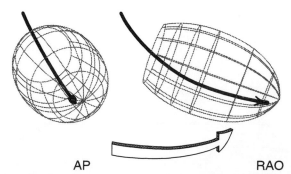

Figure 25–44. Wire frame demonstrating the orientation of the lead in the right ventricular apex in the anteroposterior (AP) and right anterior oblique (RAO) projections. Note that in the AP projection, the electrode appears to be vertical, whereas in the RAO, the lead is horizontal from right to left.

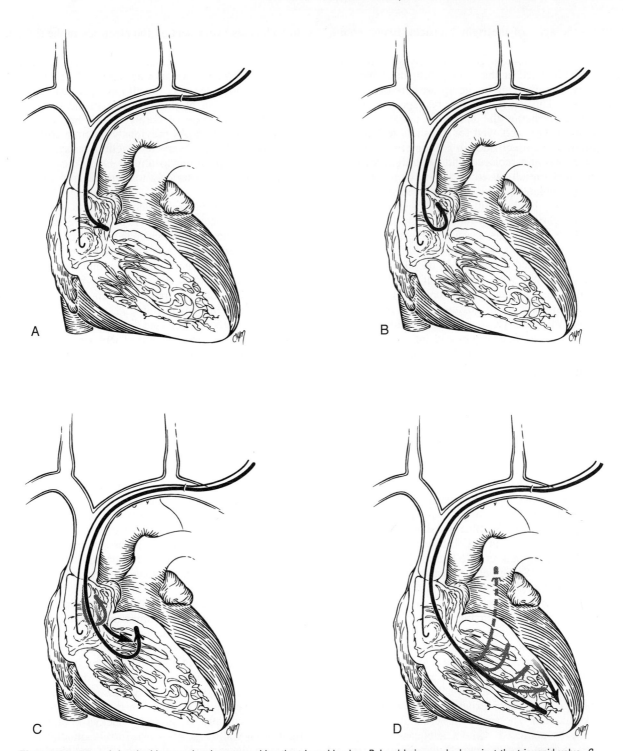

Figure 25–45. *A*, Lead with curved stylet approaching the tricuspid valve. *B*, Lead being pushed against the tricuspid valve. *C*, Lead snapping across the tricuspid valve into the right ventricle. *D*, Lead passed to the pulmonary artery, then withdrawn to the right ventricular apex.

artery as an indicator of being across the tricuspid valve, the next maneuver is to advance the stylet to the tip of the electrode. With the stylet advanced to the electrode tip and the electrode tip in the pulmonary artery, the electrode is slowly withdrawn from the pulmonary artery, dragging the tip down along the interventricular septum. This may result in premature ventricular contractions or runs of nonsustained ventricular tachycardia. When the electrode tip has reached the lower third of the septum, the stylet may be retracted about 2 to 3 cm, making the tip floppy. This can be done with a curved or straight stylet (see Fig. 25–45D). The lead tip can be observed to move up and down with the flow of blood, the motion of the tricuspid valve, and the contractions of the right ventricle. As it does so, it will intermittently point toward the apex of the right ventricle. If one coordinates the advancing of the lead body (with or without the stylet fully inserted, although generally only straight stylets should be fully inserted at this point) with the appropriate lead trajectory, the tip can be gently seated in the right ventricular apex. This maneuver can be repeated by withdrawing and readvancing the electrode until the desired fluoroscopic location is achieved for threshold testing.

After satisfactory electrode tip placement, the curved stylet is withdrawn and replaced with a straight stylet if a curved stylet was initially used and if it was not already replaced (some implanters replace the curved stylet with a straight one while the lead tip is still in the pulmonary artery). The straight stylet is advanced to the electrode tip, and the electrode with stylet in place is gently advanced toward the right ventricular apex until it is fully inserted and resistance is encountered. Care should be taken not to dislodge the electrode tip with the straight stylet. This is a common occurrence, especially in patients with an enlarged right atrium. In the process of advancing the straight stylet to the electrode tip, the stylet can force the electrode body inferiorly to the lower right atrium and inferior vena cava, consequently dragging the tip of the electrode out of the right ventricular apex back into the right atrium. This phenomenon can obviously be extremely frustrating. Ways to avoid this problem include using a more flexible stylet that will be guided more easily by the electrode coil than will the stiff stylet. Also, before advancing the stylet, the lead body is straightened as it crosses the tricuspid valve by gently pulling back on the lead. This usually avoids the looping of the lead in the lower right atrium.

Right ventricular lead fixation can be validated by gently pulling on the electrode until resistance, both tactile and visual, is encountered. This is a good method for ensuring reliable fixation if a tined or other passive-fixation lead is being used. In the case of an active-fixation lead, the best method for determining that reliable fixation is accomplished is a subject of debate. Some believe that threshold measurements, and not retraction of the lead tip to the point of resistance, is a better way of validating fixation. It is argued that the strength of fixation in the tissue with a screw-in electrode is impossible to gauge by the sensation of resistance on retraction and that, all too often, the bond is disrupted by pulling back on the screw-in electrode to the point of resistance. Conversely, others argue that the same gentle lead retraction, coupled with achievement of acceptable thresholds, is more appropriate validation for achievement of active fixation. The argument here is that acceptable thresholds may be achieved without adequate fixation and that adequate fixation easily prevents the disruption of an acceptable bond by gentle retraction.

If the initial stylet choice was straight, or after the electrode with the curved stylet has been passed to the pulmonary artery and is replaced with a stiff, straight stylet, the tip of the straight stylet can be positioned just across the tricuspid valve. It will usually point to the right ventricular apex. Simultaneous advancement of the stylet and retraction of the electrode drags the electrode tip down the interventricular septum to the end of the stylet, which is tracking toward the right ventricular apex. Once the electrode tip has snapped into a straight position, now in line with the trajectory of the stylet, both are advanced to the right ventricular apex.

In both cases, when seating the electrode in the right ventricular apex, perforations can be more easily avoided by simultaneously advancing the electrode body while retracting the stylet. Thus, the stylet is not acting as a battering ram but is merely pointing the way. In all cases, if there is any doubt about the location of the electrode in the right ventricular apex, the fluoroscope is merely rotated into the steep RAO or lateral projection. As previously noted, a correctly placed electrode will be observed to curve anteriorly, with the electrode tip appearing to almost touch the sternum. If the electrode curves posteriorly toward the spine, it is likely in the coronary sinus.

Although the means of venous access has little bearing on electrode placement, there is some difference when comparing left and right sides. Placement of the ventricular electrode after venous access has been achieved from the left side generally appears to be more expeditious. The ventricular lead with a curved stylet in place will track in a gentle curve from the point of venous entry through to the superior vena cava, right atrium, right ventricle, and pulmonary outflow tract (see Fig. 25–16A). Typically, little or no difficulty is encountered. There are generally no acute bends or angles. The only occasional impediment is the tricuspid valve, which can be negotiated using one of several techniques. One may be able to advance the tip across the valve without hang-up. If the lead tends to hang up on the valve, retracting the stylet and using the floppy tip technique already described will frequently avoid this impasse. There is also the possibility of using a technique in which the curved tip of the electrode is pushed across the valve by building a loop. Whatever technique is used, because of the anatomic configuration, passage from the left typically presents little difficulty. One exception is the elderly patient with an extremely tortuous left subclavian innominate venous system. In this case, the venous structure may have one or more sharp angles or bends in the superior mediastinum before entry into the right atrium. It would be a truly extreme case for such tortuosity to preclude passage of the electrode from the left.

Passage and placement of the ventricular electrode after right venous access may be much more challenging. Intrinsic to this approach is one acute angle or bend in the venous system (see Fig. 25–16B). This bend occurs at the junction of the right subclavian vein and internal jugular vein, where the innominate vein is formed. More important is the fact that this bend is clockwise. Because of this, when a lead with a curved stylet is placed in the vein from the right, the electrode typically is directed clockwise or to the lateral right atrial wall (Fig. 25–46A). In this situation, routing the tip across the tricuspid valve, which is in the other direction, may call on all of one's skill, ingenuity, and luck. One method involves building a loop in the right atrium in an attempt to prolapse the lead and to back the electrode across the valve, with the tip ultimately flipping into the right ventricle (see Fig. 25–46B). If the lead has tines, they may get caught on the tricuspid valve and prevent transit to the right ventricle. Another method of crossing the tricuspid valve that is somewhat more successful is the floppy-tip technique. If the curved stylet is withdrawn to the high right atrium, with the lead tip in the lower right atrium, the lead will no longer point to the lateral atrial wall. Its trajectory may now be medial toward the tricuspid valve. Advancing

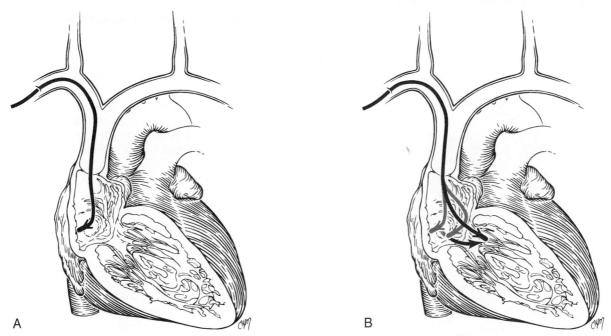

Figure 25–46. *A,* Acute bends encountered with right venous access orient the lead to the lateral wall of the right atrium when a stylet with a modest curve is inserted into the electrode. *B,* The lead must be backed into the right ventricle, across the tricuspid valve when approaching from the right. Rotating or partial withdrawal of the stylet is sometimes helpful in getting the electrode across the valve.

the body of the lead, even though the tip is floppy, allows the lead tip to cross the tricuspid valve into the right ventricle. With this approach, it is important to avoid extreme stylet curves, which serve to increase the tendency for the lead tip to move toward the lateral right atrial wall. It is hoped that future lead designs will incorporate some steering mechanism in either the stylet or the lead.

A benefit of modern lead design is the various fixation mechanisms that have resulted in a near 0% dislodgment rate. One should become familiar with the lead handling characteristics of the various active-fixation and passive-fixation designs. It is important to become familiar with the passive-fixation mechanism of tines. Learning to recognize when tines are stuck on an endocardial structure and to not be intimidated by the resistance encountered when traction is applied is a must. There has yet to be a reported case of endocardial trauma from a tined electrode, even though one may occasionally get the impression that the tines have permanently attached themselves to an endocardial structure during attempts at lead placement. It is this same feeling of resistance that ensures us that the electrode will not dislodge once an ideal location is found. When the tip of a tined lead becomes caught on a structure in an undesirable position, it is usually impossible to advance the lead. The lead must be pulled free and usually withdrawn to the right atrium, no matter what force must be applied. Sometimes, it may take multiple electrode advances and withdrawals with the tines hanging up and preventing placement in the right ventricular apex. Subtle adjustments in the stylet manipulation, as well as persistence, will ultimately overcome this problem.

The active-fixation leads offer a new set of problems. There are some unique problems in placement directly related to design. There are basically two types of active-fixation leads in use, both involving a helix or "screw" as the fixation mechanism. First, there is the fixation tip design with an exposed or fixed screw. Because the screw is continually exposed, its tip may catch onto any endocardial structure. As one would expect, this type of helix has a high propensity for getting caught, particularly on the chordae of the tricuspid valve. Unlike tines, the screw, when caught, cannot be pulled free without some fear of damaging endocardial structures. It can usually be freed easily by counterclockwise rotation of the lead body, which results in unscrewing the tip (the available screws are made with a clockwise helix). Some manufacturers have attempted to resolve this problem by coating the exposed screw with a sugar compound that ultimately dissolves, exposing the screw. This can work well provided that one is consistently able to place the lead in an optimal position quickly. This requires significant skill and experience, among other things, including luck. Once the coating has dissolved, the screw can hook endocardial structures if there is a difficult positioning or a need to reposition or withdraw to the right atrium. The exposed screw does, however, offer a reliable fixation mechanism. The second type of active-fixation lead employs an extendible-retractable screw that is mechanically extended from its "resting" retracted position. This lead is generally easier to work with because the problem of helix hang-up is avoided. In fact, the extendible-retractable screw-in type of leads may be the easiest of all leads to position. Placement of both types of fixation mechanisms use the stylet techniques previously described.

When the implanting physician is satisfied with electrode placement, the stylet may be withdrawn to the vicinity of the lower right atrium (Fig. 25–47)[88] or, alternatively, completely removed. Threshold testing is then carried out. If thresholds

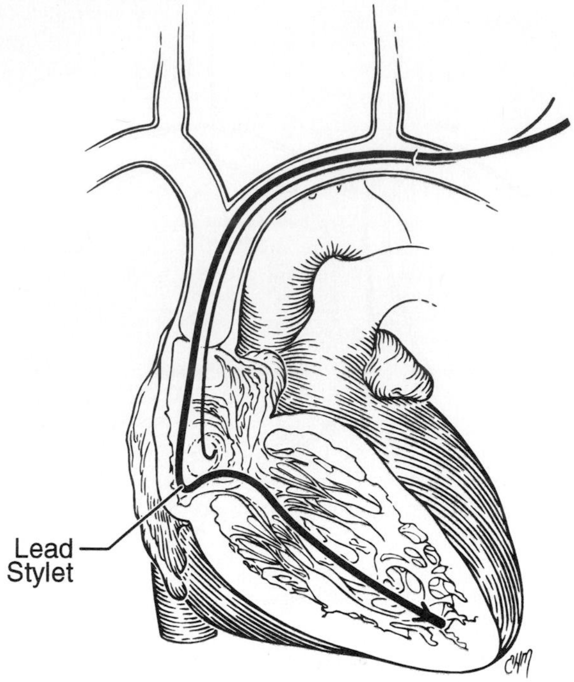

Figure 25–47. The stylet of the ventricular electrode is left in the lead but is withdrawn to the lower right atrium to permit threshold testing and assessment of the appropriate amount of lead redundancy.

are acceptable, the ventricular electrode may be secured. Some implanters leave the stylet in the lead with the tip in the lower right atrium and secure the lead with the anchoring sleeve. This reduces the risk for ventricular lead dislodgment during placement and positioning of the atrial lead. Other implanters remove the stylet completely for testing and securing the lead but not for atrial lead placement and positioning because there is general agreement that the stylet helps stabilize the ventricular lead during atrial lead manipulation, which can frequently dislodge the ventricular lead otherwise.

The suture sleeve is advanced down the shaft of the lead body to the vicinity of venous entry. One to three ligatures are applied around the suture sleeve and lead, incorporating a generous amount of pectoral muscle (Fig. 25–48). It has been our experience that multiple ligatures that are not excessively tight make lead slippage as well as lead damage less likely compared with a single, tightly applied ligature. Securing the ventricular electrode immediately after satisfactory positioning is important. Early securing helps prevent inadvertent dislodgment whether or not an atrial electrode is to be placed. The ventricular electrode should be oriented somewhat horizontally in a plane roughly parallel to the clavicle. This avoids excessive bending of the lead at the point where it exits the vein.

Atrial Electrode Placement

Atrial electrode placement can be extremely easy but has been the nemesis of many implanting physicians. It has even been responsible for many resisting the dual-chamber approach to cardiac pacing. This, we believe, is largely because the clinician has not been exposed to proper place-

ment technique. Once again, it must be appreciated that the proper placement of any pacemaker electrode is a symphony of lead and stylet. The lead, by itself, cannot be steered or twisted into place. There are two fundamental techniques that relate directly to lead design. The first is placement of an electrode with a preformed curve or atrial J electrode.[89] This electrode can have either active-fixation or passive-fixation mechanisms. More commonly, a lead with passive-fixation tines is used. After insertion into the venous system, the lead tip is positioned with a straight stylet fully inserted in the middle to lower right atrium. The preformed J has been straightened with the straight stylet. Fluoroscopy can be in either the PA or the RAO projection. Under fluoroscopic observation, the straight stylet is withdrawn several centimeters. The atrial lead tip can be observed to begin assuming its J configuration with the tip beginning to point upward. The lead body is then slowly advanced at the venous entry site (Fig. 25–49). On fluoroscopy, the lead tip is observed to continue its upward motion, eventually seating in the atrial appendage. If the lead tip is too low in the right atrium, it may catch on or cross the tricuspid valve as the stylet is withdrawn. In this case, the lead is simply withdrawn a bit and the maneuver repeated slightly higher in the right atrium. If the lead tip is too high in the right atrium or is in the superior vena cava, the tip will not move upward adequately. In this case, the electrode is repositioned more inferiorly. As one gains comfort with this maneuver, it can be repeated over and over. With experience, the act of retracting the stylet slightly can be performed briskly. This "snaps" the lead tip into the atrial appendage, at times resulting in better electrode–endocardial contact. Frustration and failure may occur if atrial placement is attempted by briskly removing the entire stylet and expecting the electrode to jump into the atrial appendage. This maneuver usually results in the electrode's coiling on itself in the superior vena cava or right atrium. Further attempts at positioning are impossible until the stylet has been reinserted and the process begun again.

Good atrial positioning consists of a generous J loop, with the tip moving medial to lateral in a to-and-fro fashion

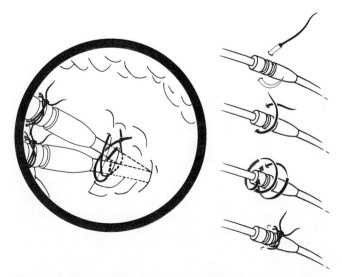

Figure 25–48. Securing the ventricular electrode to the pectoral muscle using the suture sleeve.

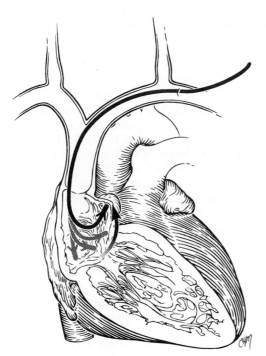

Figure 25–49. Positioning a preformed atrial J electrode by partial withdrawal of the lead stylet.

in the PA radiographic projection (Fig. 25–50).[90, 91] In the lateral projection, the tip should be anterior and observed to "bob" up and down. With the firmly seated tip in the atrial appendage, the lead body should be twisted or torqued to

the left and right to establish a position of neutral torque. Sometimes, in the process of positioning, torque can build up. If it is not released, electrode dislodgment could result. This same maneuver of twisting can also result in better electrode–myocardium contact. With experience, one gets a sense of the proper J or loop size. This can be a source of frustration. Too much or too little loop can result in dislodgment. This may vary somewhat with the lead model. Another frustrating event can occur in relation to conformational changes in the vasculature with postural movement. With the patient supine, just the right loop appears to have been created, but as soon as the patient becomes upright, the conformational change occurs, and it appears as though the mediastinal vasculature shifts inferiorly, pulling up on the lead, and obliterating the loop. Unfortunately, this situation may not be discovered until the postimplantation chest radiograph is seen. Attempts at gauging the loop size by having the patient take deep inspirations is frequently unrewarding. As a general rule, it is better to create a more generous loop.

Positioning the preformed J lead with an active-fixation screw-in mechanism uses the same basic technique described earlier. After positioning in the atrial appendage, however, the active-fixation mechanism must be activated. This usually involves the extension of a screw or helix. The exposed or fixed screw described previously is not available in a preformed atrial J configuration.

The second technique of placing an atrial electrode involves the use of a straight or nonpreformed lead. This lead is positioned in the atrium by use of a stylet that is preformed into a J shape and can be modified into other configurations. The stylets typically come with the lead already preformed into the J shape or, if desired, a straight stylet can be shaped into the J or other configurations using the same technique described for curving the ventricular lead stylet. It can then be positioned in the atrium, frequently in the atrial appendage, although it has become increasingly evident that other locations in the atrium, especially the anterior and lateral free walls, can be easily and safely targeted.[92] Manipulation of the stylet is required to gain access to the various atrial locations. Not uncommonly, modification of the preformed stylet shape is required. At the University of Oklahoma, we have found that modification of the J stylet into a shape similar to that of an Amplatz coronary artery catheter (several varieties) is most helpful in gaining access to a number of positions in the right atrium. The principal advantage of the nonpreformed leads (using various shapes of stylets) with active-fixation mechanisms is that one is not restricted to the atrial appendage. This is discussed in more detail later. With a straight or nonpreformed active-fixation lead, either a fixed screw or an extendible-retractable screw can be used.

Reports have been made of successful placement of a straight, tined lead in the atrial appendage without dislodgment, but because of the risk for dislodgment and the high success rate of both the active-fixation and preformed atrial J leads, this is not recommended, especially early in one's experience. The use of an active-fixation lead in the atrium is ideal in patients who have undergone open heart surgery during which the atrial appendage was amputated.

There are several other advantages to using an active-fixation lead in the atrium. The first, as already noted, is the ability to choose the placement site or to map the atrium for

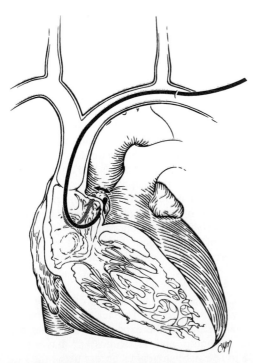

Figure 25–50. The to-and-fro, medial to lateral motion of a well-placed atrial lead in the atrial appendage when viewed in the posteroanterior projection.

optimal electric threshold, or both. By extending and retracting an extendible-retractable screw or attaching and detaching a fixed screw, multiple positions can be analyzed. The straight active-fixation lead can be placed essentially anywhere in the atrium. On the other hand, the preformed atrial J lead can typically and easily be placed only in the atrial appendage. The second advantage of the active-fixation lead is its ease of retrievability. The ability to remove a chronically implanted lead, if it becomes necessary in the future, is probably more easily accomplished with this lead.

Proper or adequate placement of active-fixation leads is reflected by good electric threshold measurements. As discussed in the section on ventricular electrode placement, there are differences of opinion about whether, in addition to achieving optimal electric parameters, a gentle tug on the lead after fixation is helpful in determining whether good mechanical fixation is achieved. Although some implanters use a floppy-tip technique for unusual or precise lead placement, or for both, some types of active-fixation leads (especially of the extendible-retractable variety) require full insertion of the stylet to activate the screw-in mechanism. The floppy-tip approach is not effective in this situation. The fixed screw and some of the extendible-retractable screws do not have this problem.

Occasionally, difficulty is encountered while attempting placement of leads in the atrial appendage with the preformed atrial J stylet. In certain situations, the lead with J stylet in place does not assume an adequate J shape to enter the atrial appendage or make contact with atrial muscle. This may be because the stylet is too limp or does not have enough curve or because the atrium is large. In this situation, one may have to use a stiffer stylet and preform it with an exaggerated curve or J. Problems can be encountered trying to maneuver stiffer stylets down through the electrode as well as during negotiation of the venous system in the superior mediastinum. Trial and error with multiple stylet configurations is almost always ultimately rewarded by success.

The side of venous access has little effect on trial electrode placement. Whether placement is from the right or left, the preformed J electrode or straight electrode with preformed J stylet can generally provide easy access to the atrial appendage. Venous access may affect placement of the electrode in unusual atrial positions. Precise placement by use of stylet and electrode manipulation may be more difficult from the right side. As discussed with ventricular lead placement, the electrode, depending on the shape of the stylet curve, may seek a right lateral orientation.

Securing the atrial lead is similar to securing the ventricular lead. When securing the atrial lead after percutaneous venous access and placement, like the ventricular lead, it should be oriented in a generally horizontal plane, roughly parallel to the clavicle. If the pocket has not already been made, the infraclavicular space is opened by means of dissection with Metzenbaum scissors. Dissection is carried to the surface of the greater pectoral muscle near its attachment point under the clavicle. The fibers of the platysma muscles are severed. A 1–0 silk suture is placed in a generous "bite" of the pectoral muscle under the anticipated site of attachment. The suture sleeve is advanced down the lead to the vicinity of the suture. Care should be taken not to dislodge or change the atrial lead position in the process.

Occasionally, the suture sleeve will bind to the electrode, making it difficult to position. This is best managed by lubricating the lead with sterile saline or other fluid and using smooth forceps to then slide the sleeve into position. Once in position, the suture is secured around the suture sleeve. Many implanters first put a knot in the suture on the surface of the muscle. The two ends of the suture are then wrapped around the suture sleeve and tied. This second tie is directly around the lead and is designed to prevent lead slippage. Some implanters use multiple sutures rather than a single one, as discussed in the section Ventricular Electrode Placement. Care must be taken to make the tie snug and yet avoid injury to the lead. It is important to orient the electrode horizontally. As with ventricular leads, this orients the lead in a plane similar to that of the axillary vein, reduces the bend of the lead, and may decrease the likelihood of the crush phenomenon or other stress-related lead damage.

If venous access and electrode placement have been achieved by venous cutdown, there is essentially no risk of the classic crush injury. Generally, the suture sleeve and lead are anchored to the pectoral muscle parallel to the vein. Similar precautions concerning lead injury should be observed. The securing process is the same, and one should avoid acute angulation of the lead and the creation of points of lead stress.

Upgrading Techniques

An upgrading procedure is necessary in patients with the pacemaker syndrome. With the increasing acceptance of dual-chamber pacing, all patients with initial VVI systems who have intact atrial function are now being considered for a pacemaker system upgrade with the addition of an atrial lead. Generally, this is deferred until the time of pulse generator power depletion, but increased awareness of the pacemaker syndrome has resulted in earlier pacemaker system upgrades. The upgrade procedure requires new venous access for the introduction of an atrial lead. It may also involve the introduction of a new ventricular lead because of problems with the chronic lead. Most pacemaker system upgrades require the replacement of the pulse generator, although occasionally, the chronic pulse generator used in the ventricle can be used for atrial pacing. Most of the time, upgrade procedures involve a conventional approach using one of the previously described percutaneous techniques or a venous cutdown. If the patient has had an initial ventricular lead placed through the cephalic vein, the percutaneous approach is almost mandatory for the upgrade. Conversely, patients with an initial percutaneous subclavian approach can have the atrial lead introduced either by cutdown of the cephalic vein or percutaneous venous access. In the case of an initial percutaneous approach, the ventricular electrode can serve as a map. Using fluoroscopy, the trajectory of the percutaneous needle is guided by the chronic ventricular electrode. Care should be taken not to touch or damage the first lead with the needle. The lead should be used as a reference landmark for the expected location of the subclavian vein. Bognolo and associates[93, 94] have described a technique to re-establish venous access using the old ventricular lead. The patency of the venous structures can be assessed as previously described with the injection of radiographic contrast material.[72]

If access to the subclavian vein cannot be obtained using the axioms of the safe introducer technique previously described by Byrd,[58] an extrathoracic puncture of the axillary vein can be carried out. The puncture of the vein can be expedited by a simple technique. A guide wire or catheter is passed to the vicinity of the subclavian vein through a vein in the arm. The guide wire or catheter can be palpated or viewed fluoroscopically, or both, thus serving as a reference for venous access. In the case of a cutdown on a previously unused cephalic vein, the Ong-Barold percutaneous sheath set technique can be used.[80]

Lead compatibility is important when considering a pacemaker system upgrade. To avoid embarrassment, one must be aware of the new pulse generator's compatibility with the chronic lead system.

Occasionally, ipsilateral venous access is impossible. Either the vessel is thrombosed or there is some form of obstruction that precludes the addition of a second (atrial) lead from the same side. In this case, contralateral venous access can be achieved and the lead tunneled back to the original pocket (Fig. 25–51). Early injection of radiographic contrast material may expedite the decision to use this approach. The use of the contralateral subclavian (rather than cephalic) vein is recommended for this approach.[95] The distance to the original pocket is less, and the new lead is not as susceptible to dislodgment. The same percutaneous techniques and precautions are used as previously described for the percutaneous approach. The only difference is the size of the skin incision, which is limited to about 1 to 1.5 cm. The incision need only be large enough to allow anchoring of the lead and securing of the suture sleeve. Similar to

an initial implantation, the incision should be carried down to the pectoral fascia. Once the lead has been positioned and secured, it can be tunneled to the original pocket.

The maneuver of passing an electrode or catheter through tissue from one location to another is referred to as *tunneling*. It always involves the passage of a catheter from one wound through tissue to a second wound remote from the first. An example is the placement of a pacemaker lead through the internal jugular vein. The lead is passed from the jugular incision through the tissue over (or under) the clavicle to the pacemaker pocket in the pectoral area. Recently, with the development of nonthoracotomy-implantable defibrillator lead and patch systems, tunneling has become popular and necessary.

A number of techniques are available for tunneling. They differ in the degree of trauma to the tissue and lead. As a rule, the least traumatic technique is desirable. A popular technique is to place the proximal end of the lead or leads to be tunneled in a 14-inch Penrose drain (Fig. 25–52A). A gentle, nonconstricting tie is applied around the drain just distal to the lead connector (see Fig. 25–52B). The tract of the tunnel is infiltrated with local anesthesia using an 18-gauge spinal needle from the satellite wound to the pocket. The free end of the Penrose drain is then brought to the receiving wound from the satellite wound in the subcutaneous tissue. This can be accomplished by several techniques. The first technique involves the use of a Kelly clamp or uterine packing forceps. The tip of the clamp is pushed bluntly in the subcutaneous tissue from the receiving wound directly to the satellite wound. Care is taken to keep the tunnel as deep as possible, usually on the surface of the

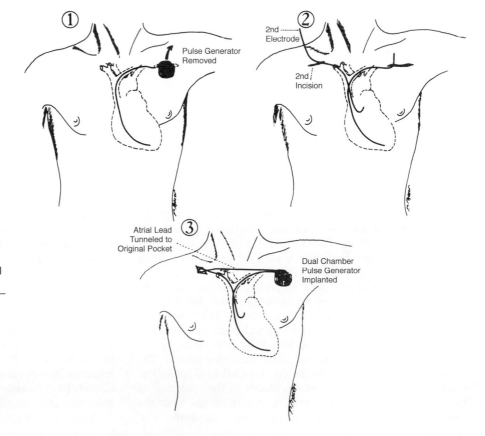

Figure 25–51. Pacemaker upgrade using the contralateral subclavian vein: (1) the pacemaker pocket is opened, and the old pulse generator and lead are dissected free, externalized, and disconnected; (2) the second lead is inserted by means of the contralateral subclavian vein; and (3) the second lead is tunneled back to the initial pocket. (From Belott PH: Use of the contralateral subclavian vein for placement of atrial electrodes in chronically VVI paced patients. PACE 6:781, 1983.)

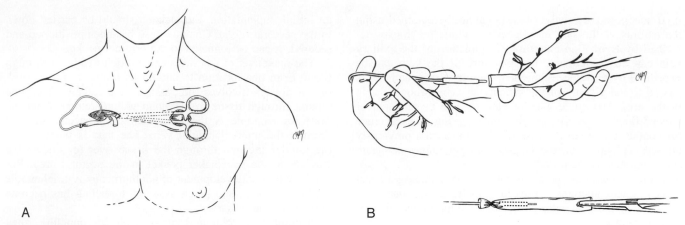

Figure 25–52. *A,* Penrose drain and lead grabbed by clamp that has been passed from the recipient wound to the donor site. The Penrose drain and lead(s) are pulled back to the recipient wound. *B,* Tunneling from one wound to another by placing the electrode(s) in a Penrose drain. The lead(s) are placed in a 14-inch Penrose drain and tied. The Penrose drain is then grabbed with a long clamp.

muscle. The free end of the Penrose drain is grasped and pulled back from the satellite wound to the receiving wound. The remainder of the Penrose drain containing the electrode connector pin is pulled through the tract to the receiving wound. The tie is released, and the Penrose drain is removed.

A second technique delivers the Penrose drain to the receiving wound by use of a "passer," usually a knitting needle or dilator. In this technique, the free end of the Penrose drain is fixed to the back end of the passer by use of a tie. The pointed tip of the passer is inserted into the satellite wound and pushed to the receiving wound. The tip of the passer is grasped and pulled into the receiving wound with the Penrose drain attached. The remainder of the Penrose drain with the lead is pulled into the receiving wound.

A variation of this technique uses the percutaneous technique to establish the tunnel. After infiltrating the tract of the tunnel with an 18-gauge spinal needle, the needle is passed from the wound of origin to the receiving wound. A guide wire is passed through the needle into the receiving wound. A standard peel-away introducer is then passed over the guide wire from the satellite incision to the receiving wound, and the sheath can then be used to pass the lead, with the sheath eventually being removed and peeled.

Another variation uses the dilator of the sheath set to tunnel and the guide wire to pull the Penrose drain from wound to wound. After tunneling from one wound to the other with the dilator, the guide wire is passed through the dilator. The dilator is removed and the guide wire attached to the loose end of the Penrose drain. The Penrose drain is then brought to the receiving wound by pulling the guide wire.

A technique that is similar in principle to the use of the Penrose drain, but that may be more traumatic, involves the use of a small chest tube and Pean clamp. The size of the chest tube is determined by the size and number of leads to be tunneled at one time. The length is determined by the distance from the initial wound to the receiving wound. The tube may be cut to size and the end beveled to a point. The leads at the wound of origin are placed in the back end of the chest tube. The Pean clamp is bluntly passed from the receiving wound to the wound containing the leads. The

pointed end of the chest tube is grasped by the Pean clamp and is pulled into and through the receiving wound. Although more traumatic to tissue, the technique is protective of the electrodes.

Another related technique involving the use of a chest tube requires blunt passage of the chest tube, with trocar in place, through the subcutaneous tissue from the site of origin to the receiving wound with the lead or leads placed in the "back end" of the tube after removal of the trocar. The tube can then be pulled through into the receiving wound.

Finally, new tunneling tools have been developed for use with implantable defibrillators. These tools may be used for pacemaker lead tunneling also.

The preceding techniques and principles are used whenever tunneling is required. Tunneling with a clamp and directly grasping the lead should always be avoided because of the risk of damage to the lead.

Epicardial Electrode Placement

Epicardial pacemaker implantation was the earliest, and once the most common, implantation technique, but it has limited use and utility today. This is largely due to the unparalleled success of transvenous implantation. Today, epicardial implantation is reserved mainly for patients undergoing cardiac surgery. in fact, in many centers, even patients undergoing cardiac surgery who also need permanent pacing have temporary epicardial electrodes applied with subsequent permanent transvenous pacing systems implanted. Modern transvenous leads have largely eliminated the problems of exit block and dislodgment. These leads have proved more reliable than epicardial leads. In addition, the abdominal pacemaker location of epicardial systems may cause more discomfort than a prepectoral one. Today, only unusual circumstances dictate an epicardial implantation. These circumstances include (1) patients undergoing cardiac surgery for another indication (with the preceding caveat), (2) patients with recurrent dislodgments of transvenous systems, and (3) patients with prosthetic tricuspid valves or congenital anomalies, such as tricuspid atresia.

Although this chapter has dealt extensively with transvenous electrode placement, epicardial placement is treated more superficially.

There are several epicardial surgical approaches. The most common is probably the median sternotomy performed as a secondary procedure at the time of other related cardiac surgery. In this case, both atria and ventricles are mapped for optimal pacing thresholds and other electrophysiologic parameters. The electrodes are attached directly to the epicardium. The electrode is tunneled by the chest tube technique to a subcutaneous pocket in the upper abdomen.

As a primary procedure, there are three distinct approaches: the subxiphoid, left subcostal, and left anterolateral thoracotomy. The first two avoid a "formal" thoracotomy. The pericardium is entered through an abdominal incision that is supradiaphragmatic. The subxiphoid approach exposes the diaphragmatic surface of the heart and mainly the right ventricle. The right ventricle can be thin, and care should be taken to avoid laceration that can require urgent thoracotomy and possibly cardiopulmonary bypass. The left subcostal approach exposes more of the left ventricle. The left lateral thoracotomy favors left ventricular electrode placement. With this approach, an incision is made in the fifth intercostal space. The incision extends from the left parasternal border to the left anterior axillary line. Care must be taken to avoid the phrenic nerve.

All of the epicardial pacemaker implantation techniques require general anesthesia. The median sternotomy and left lateral implantation procedures generally require chest tube placement. The epicardial procedures are performed in an operating room by a thoracic surgeon trained specifically in epicardial pacemaker implantation.

Securing Leads, Creating Pockets, and Closure

When all electrodes are in position, it is time to establish permanent venous stasis and secure the leads. These maneuvers pertain to the transvenous approach only. In the epicardial procedures, the electrodes have already been secured directly to the heart, and no vascular structure has been entered that requires comparable attainment of venous stasis. In the case of the transvenous approach, one or more leads must be secured and the venous port of entry must be permanently sealed. If the cutdown approach has been used, the proximal and distal ligatures must be tied. Care should be taken not to injure or cut the lead when securing the ligature around the vein containing the lead. The venous ties are merely to effect hemostasis, not to secure the lead. These ties should be gentle and as nonconstricting as possible. The securing process using the anchoring sleeves has already been described. It is reiterated that the leads should be secured and oriented in a plane that is roughly parallel to the subclavian or axillary vein to reduce the risk for subclavian crush injury. As with the ligatures around the leads, the suture sleeves should be secured snugly but not overtightened (Fig. 25–53).

If the figure-of-eight or pursestring suture has been used in conjunction with the percutaneous approach, it can be tied after all leads are in position and no further venous entry is desired. Also at this time, the retained guide wire can be removed, although it is not essential to do so. The retained guide wire can be removed later, just before wound closure.

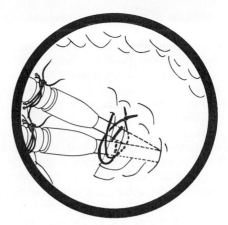

Figure 25–53. Secured atrial and ventricular electrodes using the suture sleeves. Hemostasis is effected at the puncture site, when necessary, with a loose nonconstricting tie.

In this case, if the figure-of-eight or pursestring suture has been tied properly, there will be no back-bleeding. The guide wire should, in any case, be retained until the last moment when no further venous access is required. It should be removed only after the implanter is completely satisfied with electrode placement and there is no need for replacement or exchange. Like the venous ligatures used in the cutdown technique, the figure-of-eight or pursestring suture requires only enough tension to collapse the vein or the tissue surrounding the leads near the point of entry of the leads into the vein. It is not intended to anchor the leads. If tied too tightly, it may injure the lead or leads. It is not essential that the retained guide wire be removed before tying the figure-of-eight stitch. The retained guide wire can be removed much later, just before wound closure. In this case, if the figure-of-eight stitch has been tied properly, there will be no back-bleeding.

Once the leads have been secured, it is time to create the pacemaker pocket if this has not already been accomplished. Traditionally, this is performed at the end of the procedure. The actual timing of the pocket creation, however, is at the discretion of the implanting physician. Some implanters prefer to create the pocket early in the procedure, even as the initial step in a pacemaker implantation. In this case, a rudimentary pocket is created and packed with gauze, allowing time for natural hemostasis. Toward the end of the procedure, the packing is removed, and the pocket is reinspected for hemostasis and surgically modified as necessary. The alternative approach involves creation of the pacemaker pocket after the lead or leads have been secured. There are arguments for both approaches. Proponents of the early pocket approach argue that bleeding is more easily controlled, and the risk for damage to leads is lower. Proponents of the late pocket approach argue that to make the pocket early is "putting the cart before the horse" and that the highest priority is to establish pacing early to protect the patient. Creation of the pacemaker pocket is of lower priority. In addition, early creation of the pocket may result in embarrassment if the pocket is not used because of unsuccessful venous access.

A reasonable modification of the early pocket approach

exists that avoids the risk of embarrassment should the vein on that side not be used for access. It involves percutaneous venous access with placement and maintenance of an intravenous guide wire before pocket creation, which, in turn, precedes placement of the leads using the guide wire. This approach ensures venous access before formation of the pocket and achieves the advantages of early pocket formation noted previously.

Before creation of the pacemaker pocket, the area is generously infiltrated with a local anesthetic agent, assuming local anesthesia is used. If an earlier incision has already been made to facilitate lead placement and securing of the lead, anesthesia is best achieved by infiltrating along the edge of the incision directly into the subcutaneous tissue. The incision is carried down to the anterior surface of the pectoral fascia. The pacemaker pocket is best formed predominantly inferior and medial to the incision, although many implanters also form a small portion of the pocket superior and lateral to an incision directed from the venipuncture site in an inferolateral vector. The advantage of this approach is that the pulse generator, with leads coiled deep, can then be placed directly under the incision, making subsequent pacing procedures, such as pulse generator replacement, both easy and safe with an incision at the same site.

A plane of dissection is created at the junction of the subcutaneous tissue and pectoral fascia. This is best achieved by putting the subcutaneous tissue under slight tension with some form of retraction. This maneuver better defines the plane of dissection. Initially, the Senn retractor can be used and then replaced by the Goulet retractor. The plane of dissection can be started by using the Metzenbaum scissors or the cutting function of electrocautery. After a plane of dissection has been established, the remainder of the pocket can be created by blunt dissection. Some argue that blunt dissection is less traumatic to the tissues. The problems with blunt dissection are the lack of adequate visualization and the lack of control with respect to tissue depth. Optimally, the pacemaker pocket should be as deep as possible, right on top of the fascia of the pectoral muscle. This offers the optimal subcutaneous tissue thickness necessary to avoid erosion. Unfortunately, with blunt dissection, this ideal plane can be lost, creating inconsistent pocket thickness with its increased risk of erosion. Today's pacemaker is small, limiting the amount of dissection required and the pocket size needed. The pocket can easily be created by direct visualization instead of blindly. As previously noted, the subcutaneous tissue is held under gentle tension, defining the plane of dissection. Sharp dissection with Metzenbaum scissors or the cutting function of electrocautery, or both, is then used to form the pocket. This technique is less traumatic than blunt dissection. The pocket created by precise dissection over the pectoral muscle provides optimal tissue thickness. Thus, the pocket is created by visual inspection, and the plane of dissection is well controlled. The head lamp as a light source can be helpful here. There is less risk for hematoma because all bleeding is directly visualized and managed with electrocautery.

Occasionally, the patient has little or no subcutaneous tissue. In this situation, a subpectoral muscle implantation should be considered. Fortunately, with the dramatically reduced size of today's pacemakers and the availability of the Parsonnet pouch (see Fig. 25–5), this approach is rarely

necessary.[96] If required, the placement of the pacemaker under the pectoral muscle represents only a slight departure from the techniques already described. The one major concern with using this approach is the increased bleeding that is typically encountered, resulting in increased risk for hematoma formation. In subpectoral implantation, the incision has already been carried down to the surface of the pectoral muscle and the leads secured. An incision is made through the muscle parallel to the muscle fibers. The muscle is separated, and a plane of dissection is established on the chest wall. This pocket is best created by blunt dissection. As already described, considerable bleeding can be encountered with subpectoral implants. This bleeding is best controlled with electrocautery. Careful visual inspection using a Goulet retractor and good lighting is important. All bleeding sources should be identified and either sutured or coagulated. Pocket drainage is frequently required.

Use of electrocautery has been a traditional taboo in cardiac pacing. It can cause fibrillation or burns at the myocardium–electrode interface and can reprogram or even irreparably damage the pulse generator. However, electrocautery can be extremely useful in a pacemaker procedure in both coagulation and cutting modes. It is the surest and most expeditious way to control bleeding and create the pacemaker pocket. It can be used safely provided that one is aware of the dangers and takes a few precautions. Today's electrocautery systems are extremely safe from an electric hazard point of view. Built-in mechanisms protect against improper grounding. A few simple rules should be followed that are specific to the use of electrocautery systems in pacemaker implantation procedures. First, the use of electrocautery should be avoided when the pulse generator is in the surgical field. Second, the cautery must never touch the exposed pin of the pacemaker lead. Finally, the cautery must never touch the retained guide wire if it is in the heart.

Wound drainage is required in patients who manifest excessive bleeding. The term *wet pocket* has been used to describe this condition. This situation is being encountered more frequently with the increasing use of anticoagulants. Patients taking aspirin, warfarin, or heparin frequently manifest a wet pocket, and medical indications often preclude cessation of such drugs. If a patient is taking warfarin, a prothrombin time 1 to 1.5 times the control level is less likely to cause a problem than if it is greater than 1.5 times the control level. In the latter situation, the procedure should be postponed until the prothrombin time reaches a more reasonable level. Heparin and platelet antagonists appear to cause the greatest problem. Despite diligent efforts to establish hemostasis, the pockets may continue to ooze diffusely. In this circumstance, some implanters have resorted to the topical application of thrombin.

Patients taking anticoagulants and those receiving a subpectoral implantation should be considered for some form of drainage. As a general rule, if reasonable hemostasis cannot be achieved, the pacemaker pocket should be drained (although drainage should not be considered an alternative to adequate attempts to attain hemostasis). This is accomplished by placing a Jackson-Pratt drain or Hemovac system. A trocar connected to the drainage tubing is passed from the inferior aspect of the pacemaker pocket to a satellite exit wound remote from the pacemaker pocket. The distal end of the tubing in the pacemaker pocket is specially designed of soft rubber with multiple drainage ports. This end can be cut to desired size to avoid excessive tubing in the pocket. After the pacemaker pocket is closed, the proximal end of the drainage tubing is connected to a closed suction system. The Jackson-Pratt system is preferred because it has a one-way valve that allows emptying yet prevents inadvertent flushing of old drained fluids back into the pocket. It is small and of little encumbrance to the patient. To avoid infection, the drainage system is removed within 24 hours. If drainage is copious, a longer period may be required. In the case of persistent bloody drainage, the wound should be re-explored and the culprit bleeder ligated or cauterized.

Wound irrigation is largely a personal preference, with no clearly established mandate by investigations to do so. There is a spectrum from simple saline lavage to concentrated solutions of multiple antibiotics. It is likely that such antibiotic solutions are unnecessary, especially if systemic antibiotics are used. This issue has been previously addressed. In addition to irrigation of the wound, some implanters place antibiotic-soaked gauze pads in the pocket early to achieve not only antibiosis but also hemostasis by compression with the pads.

Closure of the pacemaker pocket consists of initial approximation of the subcutaneous tissue and subsequent skin closure. The subcutaneous tissue can be approximated by single or multiple layers of interrupted or running sutures. The number of layers is a function of the thickness of the subcutaneous tissue. The suture material used by most implanters for subcutaneous closure is an absorbable semisynthetic product that is fairly strong, usually 2–0 or 3–0. There are several techniques of skin closure. The choice of technique relates to the desired cosmetic effect and time spent. An ideal cosmetic effect can be achieved by use of the subcuticular suture. This is best accomplished using 4–0 semisynthetic absorbable suture material, which does not require removal. The use of interrupted sutures has the least pleasing cosmetic result, and the sutures require removal. The resulting scar may have visible crosshatches. Many skin closures are performed with surgical staples or clips. This closure is cosmetically appealing and extremely fast. The only drawback to the use of staples is that they require removal in 7 to 10 days. After closure of the skin, the wound is coated with an antiseptic ointment, and a dry sterile dressing is applied. Because a pocket has been created that can fill with blood, some form of pressure dressing may be used, although maintaining the pressure is frequently not easily accomplished in an ambulatory or otherwise active patient.

Immediate Postoperative Care

There is considerable center-to-center variability in the intensity of monitoring after implantation. There is general agreement that intensive care monitoring postoperatively is not usually required. Patients who were in the intensive care unit before implantation may be transferred to a bed on a nursing unit for continuous cardiac rhythm monitoring postoperatively unless, of course, there is another reason for the patient to be in an intensive care setting. Other patients electively admitted to the hospital specifically for pacemaker implantation are also returned to a cardiac monitoring area. Basic rhythm monitoring would appear to be all that is

necessary. The activity level allowed the patient in the immediate postoperative period is subject to personal preference and philosophy. In the early days of pacing, the patient was kept on strict bed rest with restricted activity for many days. Today's lead systems with both active-fixation and passive-fixation mechanisms offer a new dimension of security. The historical dislodgment rates of nearly 20% have been dramatically reduced. In most centers, the current philosophy is to have the patient active immediately or shortly after arrival at the monitoring area. The intention is early detection of patients with potential pacemaker system malfunctions. The patient with a precariously placed electrode who is kept on strict bed rest may not demonstrate malfunction, giving a false sense of security at the time of discharge. The active patient will give a better indication that reliable pacemaker sensing and capture are occurring. This approach is important in the patient being managed on an ambulatory basis. If the patient is to stay in the hospital postoperatively, noninvasive pacemaker evaluation and programming may be carried out. This might include re-evaluation of sensing and pacing thresholds as well as initial activation and setup of the rate-adaptive system. If the patient is to be managed as an outpatient, these functions can be carried out at the time of the initial postoperative visit to the pacemaker clinic.

The documentation of the pacemaker procedure is crucial from both a clinical and a medicolegal point of view. An operative report that identifies indications; pacemaker and lead manufacturer, make, and model; details of the implantation procedure; and pacemaker-programmed settings is essential. A clear description of the procedure, including problems encountered as well as electric testing data, is important. Copies of the operative report should be sent to the pacemaker clinic as well as to the referring and follow-up physicians. Further documentation includes the manufacturer's registration form and, in the United States, the hospital registry or log required by the Food and Drug Administration. Copies of the manufacturer's registration form should also be forwarded to the pacemaker clinic and any physician following the patient. It is extremely important to have multiple resources for retrieving pacemaker implantation information. Many manufacturers supply convenient stickers containing pulse generator and lead data for the patient's chart.

A postoperative chest radiograph is extremely important for documentation of the lead position immediately after surgery. It can be used for comparison if subsequent dislodgment is suspected. In the case of a percutaneous procedure, it is essential to rule out a pneumothorax. Generally, it is useful to obtain both PA and lateral films for documentation of lead position. We ask that the postoperative radiograph be overpenetrated and that the patient's arms not be raised above shoulder level.

Similarly, a 12-lead ECG with and without magnet application is essential to document initial appropriate pacemaker sensing and capture. The chest radiograph and ECG also have medicolegal value should a question arise subsequently.

The timing of discharge is controversial, with considerable variability among institutions. Today, there is a trend toward a more abbreviated hospital stay. For example, at the University of Oklahoma, patients are now discharged routinely the day after implantation unless there is a specific reason for prolonging the hospital stay. During the short hospital stay, the patient ambulates within 2 hours of completion of the procedure, a chest radiographic study and ECG are performed, and preliminary interrogation, threshold testing, and programming are accomplished. Even markedly pacemaker-dependent patients are approached this way. We have experienced no complications or morbidity following discharge that would have been averted by longer hospitalization. Some centers use the first and second postoperative days for more extensive testing of the pacemaker system and the patient–pacemaker system interface. Such testing might include Holter monitoring, extensive reprogramming with particular attention to pacing and sensing thresholds, and exercise testing to adjust rate-adaptive parameters. In some centers, the pacemaker-dependent patient may be hospitalized longer.

At the other end of the spectrum is a completely ambulatory approach. Patients are discharged on the same day immediately after the pacemaker procedure regardless of whether or not they are pacemaker dependent. This has been the approach at the El Cajon Pacemaker Center. This experience in the United States, in addition to a large series of ambulatory procedures in Europe, has been very encouraging. The El Cajon experience is now longer than 10 years and includes 658 ambulatory pacemaker procedures. There have been no postoperative pacemaker deaths or pacemaker emergencies. The El Cajon experience suggests that between 70% and 75% of pacemaker procedures can be safely conducted on an ambulatory basis. It is likely that patients referred for a pacemaker on an ambulatory basis are at no greater risk from the bradyarrhythmia than they were before they entered the hospital in the unlikely event the entire system were to fail postoperatively. If there are specific concerns about the pacemaker-dependent patient, the hospital stay can always be extended. As previously noted, it is important to have ambulatory-based patients active during the monitored postoperative period so that potential problems can be detected. This philosophy also applies to any patient who is considered to be at higher risk for a problem or complication.

The timing of initial follow-up varies depending on the timing of discharge and which physician is going to perform follow-up of the pacing system. If the implanting physician is to discharge the patient and perform the follow-up, there should be excellent continuity of care. Parenthetically, we have a strong bias that implanting physicians must be involved substantially in both acute and chronic follow-up of pacemaker patients to understand and appreciate many important aspects of the process as they relate to implantation.

Even if the discharging physician did not perform the procedure but is responsible for the follow-up, there may again be good continuity of care. Of concern is the situation in which the implanting physician discharges the patient to someone else for follow-up. In this case, there is the possibility that ideal pacemaker follow-up will not take place. This is common when a patient is discharged to a nursing home. In this case, it is imperative that the implanting or discharging physician arrange some form of reliable follow-up. It is important that patients whose procedure has been performed on an ambulatory basis be seen the following day for an initial follow-up visit. At the other extreme are patients who have been hospitalized and evaluated intensively for days

postoperatively with Holter monitoring and extensive reprogramming. These patients may not need to be seen for a week or even a month.

Special Considerations and Situations

If initial venous access is unsuccessful, jugular venous access may be considered.[77] This is less desirable than subclavian, axillary, or cephalic vein placement because of the increased risk for lead fracture and the potential for erosion. An acute bend must be created in the lead after it exits the venous structure and is brought down to the pacemaker pocket under or over the clavicle. In addition, some form of tunneling is required to bring the lead to the pacemaker pocket. If one tunnels under the clavicle, there is increased risk of vascular injury. If the lead is tunneled over the clavicle, the tissue is typically thin, and there is a greater chance of erosion.

Both the internal and external jugular veins have been used. Generally, the right jugular approach is preferred (Fig. 25–54). For a jugular venous approach, two separate incisions are required, above and below the clavicle. Many detailed descriptions have been published of anatomic dissection including both the internal and external jugular veins. In these, there is particular attention paid to precise anatomic landmarks. An alternative percutaneous technique is proposed that is simple, requiring little attention to anatomic landmarks or dissection. Additionally, an initial supraclavicular incision is not required. This approach involves the percutaneous access of the right internal jugular vein.

Once the decision is made to place the electrodes through the jugular vein, the neck must be prepared and draped in a sterile fashion accordingly. To save time, this may be performed in the initial preparation. If done in such a manner, the sterile field can be moved directly to the right supraclavicular area. If not, an effective sterile barrier can be created by use of an iodoform-impregnated see-through plastic drape. Access to the internal jugular vein is best obtained with the patient in the normal anatomic position, with the head facing anteriorly. Turning the head to the left should

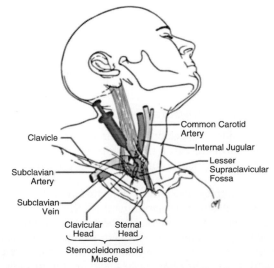

Figure 25–54. Venous anatomy of right internal jugular approach.

be avoided because this may distort the anatomy. The carotid artery is palpated in the lower third of the neck. The internal jugular vein is lateral to the common carotid artery. The two structures are parallel and lie side by side. Standing on the right side of the patient (for a right jugular vein approach), the implanting surgeon places the left middle finger along the course of the common carotid artery. The course of the internal jugular vein will be under the index finger. In fact, the index and middle fingers are, side by side, generally analogous in size and orientation on the surface of the skin to the internal jugular vein and common carotid artery as they run side by side underneath the skin. A puncture anywhere along this course should enter the internal jugular vein. The higher the puncture is in the neck, the less is the risk of pneumothorax. Some prefer to make the needle puncture roughly perpendicular to the plane of the neck rather than angled. This also helps to avoid a pneumothorax.

Once the vein is entered, the needle and syringe can be gently angled inferiorly for passage of the guide wire. If the carotid artery is inadvertently punctured, the needle is removed, pressure over the puncture site is maintained briefly, and a reattempt at venipuncture is made a little lateral to the initial stick. The remainder of the lead placement technique is essentially identical to the previously described percutaneous technique. A small incision is carried laterally down the shaft of the needle to the surface of the muscle (sternocleidomastoid). If more tissue depth is required, the muscle can be split and the incision carried down to the vein. A small Weitlander retractor is used for retraction. A figure-of-eight or pursestring suture can be applied for hemostasis. Two leads for dual-chamber pacing can be placed by the retained guide wire technique. After the leads have been placed, the hemostasis suture is tied and the leads anchored to the muscle using the anchoring sleeve. A second incision for pocket formation is made infraclavicularly. A pacemaker pocket is created with conventional techniques. The leads are then tunneled to the pocket by the techniques previously described.

The tunneling technique described by Roelke and colleagues[97] for submammary pacemaker implantation may also be used for transclavicular tunneling. A long 18-gauge spinal needle can be passed from the infraclavicular incision to the supraclavicular incision. The guide wire is passed, and the sheath set is applied and tunneled to the supraclavicular incision. The rubber dilator is removed. The lead to be used is inserted in the distal end of the sheath and tied. Once secured, the lead and sheath are pulled through the infraclavicular incision (Fig. 25–55). The external jugular vein is less frequently used for venous access because it is more inferiorly located and there is a high risk of pneumothorax and vascular complication. Its location, as previously stated, is less precise, and successful cannulation may be frustrating. If the electrodes are tunneled under the clavicle, care must be taken to avoid vascular trauma. Conversely, when tunneling over the clavicle, every effort should be made to ensure optimal tissue thickness.

Ellestad and French[98, 99] reported a 90-patient experience using the iliac vein as an alternative source of venous access for both single-chamber and dual-chamber pacemaker implantation (Fig. 25–56). It can be used for transvenous lead placement when an abdominal pocket is desired, such as when patients have little pectoral tissue, in bilateral radical

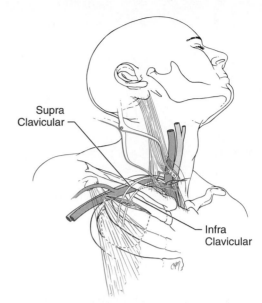

Figure 25–55. Lead(s) tunneled over and under the clavicle to the infraclavicular pocket. (From Belott PH: Pacemaker implantation: The old and new. *In* Singer L, Barold S, Camm AJ: Nonpharmaceutical Therapy of Arrhythmias for the 21st Century. Armonk, NY, Futura, 1998, p 726.)

mastectomy patients after surgery, in patients with extensive pectoral radiation damage, and for a variety of cosmetic reasons. A small incision is made just above the inguinal ligament over the vein (just medial to the palpable artery) and carried down to the fascia above the vein. The vein is punctured by the sheath set technique with the guide wire retained for dual-chamber implants. A figure-of-eight or pursestring suture is placed for hemostasis through the fascia around the lead as it enters the vein. Long (85-cm) leads are positioned in a conventional manner and secured to the fascia by use of a tie around the suture sleeve and lead. A second horizontal incision is made lateral to the umbilicus and is carried to the surface of the rectus sheath. A pacemaker pocket is created by blunt dissection. Preparations are made to tunnel the leads from the initial incision to the pacemaker pocket by use of one of the previously described techniques.

Active-fixation leads are recommended for both atrial and ventricular lead placement. Lead dislodgment is the major weakness of this approach, with 9 of 42 (21%) of the atrial and 5 of 67 (7%) of the ventricular leads in the Ellestad and French experience requiring repositioning.[98] Lead fracture and venous thrombosis do not appear to be problems, although the published experience with this approach is relatively small and the latter especially could be difficult to discern. The complication of pneumothorax essentially does not exist. Extraction of these leads can be challenging because many of the conventional tools used for extraction of leads placed in the axillary subclavian and cephalic veins are not long enough to handle these significantly longer systems.

If the patient is greatly concerned about the negative cosmetic effects of standard pacemaker pocket location, at least two alternative techniques exist.[100] Both can be performed with local anesthesia, but they may best be performed with general or modified general anesthesia for pa-

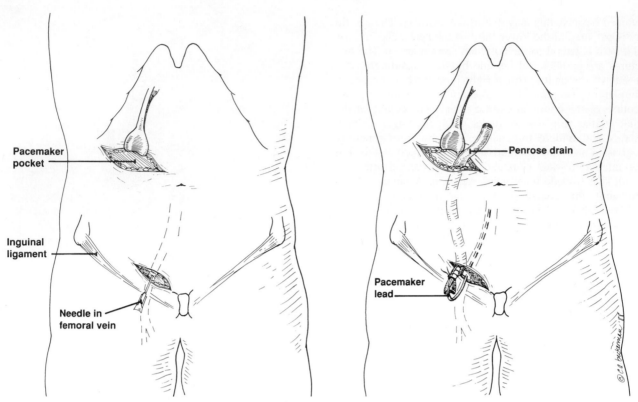

Figure 25–56. Use of the right iliac vein for placement of pacemaker lead(s). Percutaneous capture of the iliac vein is performed, and the lead is tunneled up to an upper-quadrant pacemaker pocket with the use of a Penrose drain. (From Ellestad MH, French J: Iliac vein approach to permanent pacemaker implantation. PACE 12:1030, 1989.)

tient comfort because they involve more extensive surgery. Both of these procedures lend themselves well to the percutaneous approach for both single-chamber and dual-chamber pacing. In both procedures, after the subclavian vein is accessed, a limited (1.5-cm) initial skin incision is made. The incision is carried to the surface of the pectoral muscle, allowing only enough room to secure the lead or leads. A second incision is then made. For one of the alternative pocket locations, an incision is made under the breast along the breast fold or reflection. A standard pacemaker pocket is created under the breast with care taken to stay on the pectoral fascia (Fig. 25–57). The pocket is carefully inspected for hemostasis. Similarly, as another alternative pocket location, a second incision can be made in the axilla with the arm abducted 60 degrees. This incision can be carried to a depth that exposes the muscle fascia, where a pocket can be formed with appropriate attention to hemostasis. With either of these approaches, tunneling of leads can be carried out using the previously described techniques.

As previously noted, Roelke and colleagues[101] have described a submammary pacemaker implantation technique that uses unique tunneling. In this technique, a 1-cm horizontal incision is made over the deltopectoral groove 1 cm inferior to the clavicle. A direct subclavian-axillary puncture or cephalic cutdown for venous access is carried out. The electrodes are positioned and anchored. A 2–3 cm horizontal incision is made in the medial third of the inframammary crease. The incision is carried down to the level of the pectoralis fascia, and blunt dissection is used to create a pocket superficial to the pectoralis fascia behind the breast.

A 20-cm, 18-gauge pericardiocentesis needle is directed from the inframammary pocket to the infraclavicular incision. A 145-cm J wire is then passed from the submammary pocket through the needle and to the infraclavicular incision.

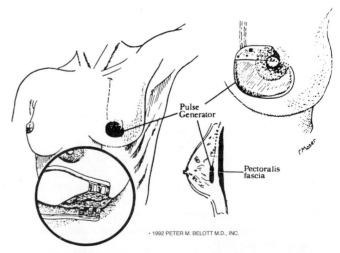

• 1992 PETER M. BELOTT M.D., INC.

Figure 25–57. Inframammary placement of pulse generator after percutaneous lead placement for optimal cosmetic effect. A small incision is made near the clavicle, and the pocket incision is made in the hidden fold under the breast. The lead is tunneled deep to the breast, between the incisions. (From Belott PH, Bucko D: Inframammary pulse generator placement for maximizing optimal cosmetic effect. PACE 6:1241, 1983.)

The needle is removed and, using the retained guide wire technique, two appropriate-sized introducer dilators are passed consecutively over the guide wire. The free ends of the atrial and ventricular electrodes from the infraclavicular incision are placed in the sheaths and secured with a suture (Fig. 25–58). The sheath sets are then withdrawn to the infraclavicular pocket. This innovative tunneling technique has been extremely successful and well tolerated.

Shefer and associates[102] have described a retropectoral transaxillary percutaneous technique for optimal cosmetic effect. This technique is performed under local anesthesia and conscious sedation. Venography is used to confirm the relationship of the axillary vein to the surface anatomy. A marker is then placed in the axillary vein through the antecubital fossa (Fig. 25–59). This usually consists of a temporary transvenous pacing wire or an 0.03 guide wire. The patient is then prepped and draped in the ipsilateral axilla. Under local anesthesia and fluoroscopic control, a 16-gauge thin-walled needle is inserted and guided medially in a cranial and anterior direction to meet and cross the temporary pacing wire marker in the axillary vein (Fig. 25–60). The axillary vein is punctured when the tip of the needle touches and moves the marker wire. Venipuncture is confirmed by aspiration of venous blood. A 0.038 guide wire is then introduced and the needle discarded. A longitudinal incision is made along the posterior border of the pectoralis muscle in the axilla (Fig. 25–61). The pectoralis fascia is then exposed by blunt dissection and the retropectoral space opened. One or two pacing electrodes can then be placed by conventional techniques. The electrodes are secured by their suture sleeve to the pectoralis fascia. The leads are then connected to the pacemaker and inserted in the retropectoral pocket. At the

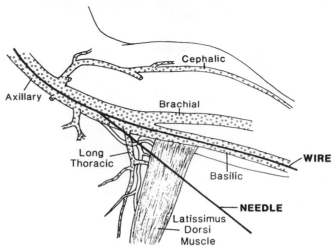

Figure 25–59. Stylized illustration of axillary venipuncture using the guide wire as a landmark.

completion of the operation, the temporary pacing lead and guide wire marker are removed. This technique offers excellent cosmetic results, and there has been no restriction in physical activity or movement of the shoulder joint (Fig. 25–62).

With any of these techniques, the pulse generator and leads are connected and the incisions closed. A polyester (Dacron) or Parsonnet pouch (C. R. Bard, Inc., Billerica, MA; see Fig. 25–5), can be used to avoid rotation of the pulse generator and leads in the tissue. To avoid the problems of diaphragmatic stimulation, a bipolar system should be used, especially with the inframammary pocket.

Historically, the predominance of epicardial pacing has persisted substantially longer in children than it has in adolescents and adults. Explanations for this are manifold. Much

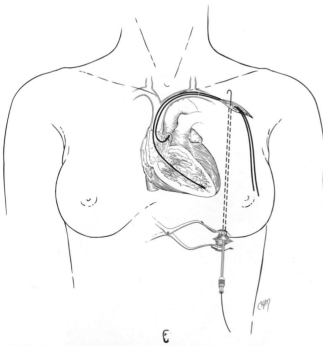

Figure 25–58. Subcutaneous tunneling with guide wire and sheath. (Redrawn from Roelke M, Jackson G, Hawthorne JW: Submammary pacemaker implantation: A unique tunneling technique. PACE 17:1793, 1994.)

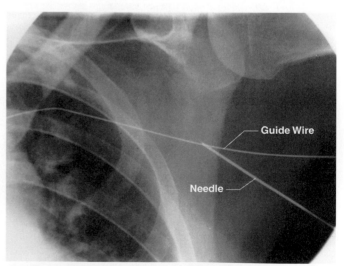

Figure 25–60. Radiograph of needle accessing the axillary vein using guide wire as a landmark. (From Shefer A, Lewis SB, Gang ES: The rectopectoral transaxillary permanent pacemaker: Description of a technique for percutaneous implantation of an invisible device. PACE 16:1646, 1996.)

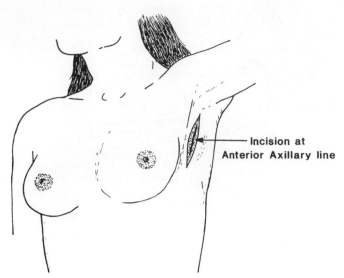

Figure 25–61. Incision in the anterior axillary line for optimal cosmetics. (From Shefer A, Lewis SB, Gang ES: The rectopectoral transaxillary permanent pacemaker: Description of a technique for percutaneous implantation of an invisible device. PACE 16:1646, 1996.)

of the need for pacemaker implantation during infancy and childhood has occurred as a comorbidity of cardiac surgery for congenital heart disease.[103] In this context, epicardial implantation at the time of surgery has been typical. Additionally, certain forms of congenital heart disease (e.g., tricuspid atresia) make transvenous pacing difficult if not impossible. Expertise in transvenous pacing in children has also been difficult to acquire because of the relatively smaller number of patients in this age group who require pacemaker therapy.[104] Also, there has been a perception that the relatively rapid growth in body size that occurs in childhood

makes transvenous pacing problematic with respect to the intravascular length of leads. There has also been a reluctance by parents and physicians to place pacemakers in the traditional prepectoral area in children with, instead, a preference for abdominal pulse generator implantation. Finally, the lead diameters for transvenous pacemaker system implantation and pulse generator sizes have been thought to be excessive for conventional techniques of transvenous implantation. Conversely, as problems with epicardial pacemaker implantation have been more clearly elucidated, especially the problems of epicardial lead fracture and epicardial exit block, transvenous approaches have been appropriately reconsidered.[105] Encouraging in this reconsideration is the evolution of transvenous pacemaker implantation expertise by pediatric cardiologists or in concert between pacemaker implantation experts and pediatric cardiologists. More sophisticated lead placement techniques, coupled with smaller-diameter leads and pulse generators, have also encouraged this relatively recent trend toward transvenous implantation in this age group.[106] New technologies in electrodes that help prevent the exit block problem have also been a motivator for the trend toward transvenous systems. Finally, the clear capacity to implant transvenous pacing systems successfully in patients in a variety of pediatric age groups with a variety of congenital cardiac problems has been a crucial factor. With all of these considerations, especially with anticipated future developments in pacing technology, there is little question that transvenous pacing will become progressively dominant in children as it has in adolescents and adults.

As noted previously, the relative infrequency of pediatric pacemaker implantation, compared with the frequency in the adult population, makes acquisition of expertise in implantation difficult. It is, perhaps, ideal when individuals specifically expert in pediatric implantation can be used, although the degree of regionalization necessary to accomplish this might be unrealistic. A team approach is a reasonable alter-

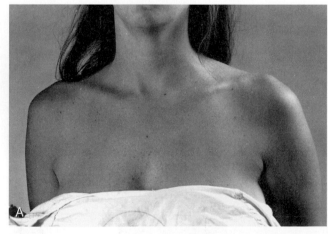

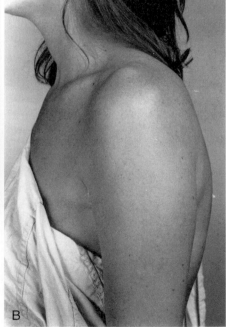

Figure 25–62. Frontal (A) and lateral (B) views of patient after transaxillary retropectoral pacemaker implantation. There are no visible scars. (From Shefer A, Lewis SB, Gang ES: The rectopectoral transaxillary permanent pacemaker: Description of a technique for percutaneous implantation of an invisible device. PACE 16:1646, 1996.)

native, pairing an expert in pacemaker implantation (adult cardiologist or cardiac surgeon) with an invasive pediatric cardiologist or pediatric electrophysiologist. Although this type of redundancy in physician services is generally inefficient and not often well compensated, it may be the most attractive of a variety of options.

Pediatric pacemaker implantation can be carried out with local anesthesia and relatively substantial intravenous sedation and pain control without the services of an anesthesiologist. Conversely, although uncommon in children, excessive sedation must be monitored closely by someone experienced in doing so. It is appropriate to consider general anesthesia for pediatric pacemaker implantation, and in many cases, general anesthesia is the safest approach to use.[107]

For transvenous pacemaker implantation in children, the techniques of venous access are precisely those described for adults. Smaller venipuncture needles and guide wires are available although typically are not necessary except, perhaps, in infants. An important consideration in children is blood loss. Generally speaking, the younger and smaller the patient, the more crucial is blood loss. Special attention to this is warranted in young patients in comparison to their older counterparts.

The choice of pacemaker leads for pediatric implantation is also worthy of brief discussion. The five most important considerations in this regard involve the choice of bipolar or unipolar leads, the lead diameters, the fixation mechanisms (active versus passive), the higher incidence of exit block in children, and lead length. Although bipolar leads and the resulting bipolar (and optional unipolar) pacing systems have distinct advantages, in small infants or in certain situations in which maximal lead flexibility is necessary, unipolar leads and pacing systems may be appropriately chosen. Most small children beyond infancy tolerate not only the thicker bipolar systems but also dual-chamber bipolar systems. As lead (and pulse generator) technology moves toward smaller diameters, bipolar dual-chamber systems may be more comfortably used in even smaller patients. The fixation mechanism is another important consideration. The advantages of the types of fixation are not categorically different from those previously discussed. The flexibility for placement of leads in a variety of locations using active-fixation leads is attractive. It is also an unproven hypothesis that active-fixation leads may be less likely to become dislodged than their passive counterparts in a population of patients not able to understand the importance of temporary immobilization of the shoulder and arm after implantation. In contrast, electrode technologies such as that of steroid elution have proved useful in reducing the problem of exit block, which occurs in substantially greater frequency in children. This steroid elution technology has been married more effectively with passive-fixation leads. Finally, and possibly most importantly, lead length is a crucial issue in children. Excessive lead that must be coiled in the pacemaker pocket beneath the pulse generator creates formidable bulk in these small patients. Leads of variable lengths should be available and the choices for a specific patient carefully made. In this regard, it should be remembered that these patients will grow significantly and an adequate extra length of lead to accommodate this growth is desirable. One of the advantages in unipolar lead technology is that leads can be shortened or lengthened by splicing techniques, although this is certainly an imperfect solution to this vexing problem.

Once the leads have been positioned, the implanter may secure them (if such a procedure is desired) in the manner previously described using the anchoring sleeve. Alternatively, one may use an absorbable suture material for securing the leads using the anchoring sleeve. This approach has the advantage of good security of the lead during the time when the electrode–myocardium interface is unstable and dislodgment is most likely; it also provides for eventual elimination of the fixation to the pectoral fascia and muscle by dissolution of the suture material, facilitating movement of the lead through the anchoring sleeve and into the vein as growth occurs. Another alternative is to use active fixation leads and avoid the anchoring sleeve completely.

The formation of the pacemaker pocket follows the same guidelines outlined previously. There has been greater enthusiasm for subpectoral muscle implantation in children, although as pulse generators decrease in size, this trend may wane.

There are certain unusual situations, especially those that relate to congenital anomalies and their surgical correction, that mitigate creativity. One example involves the need to pace the left ventricle or atrium, or both, in patients who have undergone a Mustard-type baffle procedure for transposition of the great arteries. Another example is successful transvenous pacing in patients with tricuspid atresia. This can be accomplished by passage of a transvenous lead through the right atrium into the coronary sinus and, respectively, into one of the posterior ventricular veins, such as the middle cardiac vein. A caveat here relates to the higher risk for diaphragmatic pacing, especially if a unipolar system is employed. In children with congenital heart disease, intracardiac shunting creates the need for special concern about the risks of systemic embolization related to placement of endocardial pacing systems. Normally, placement of endocardial systems should not be the procedure of choice in these patients before surgical correction of the shunts.

Although a question often arises about the minimum age or size that would be considered acceptable for transvenous pacing, the answer is not easily provided. At the University of Oklahoma (and in many other medical centers), transvenous implantation is considered appropriate for infants weighing 10 pounds or more, although it is likely that as lead and pulse generator technologies are progressively downsized, this minimum size will also decrease.

The use of radiography may be problematic in certain situations, such as during pregnancy. The prospect of implanting a pacemaker in such patients becomes particularly challenging. Guldal and colleagues have described an implantation technique for single-chamber (ventricular) pacemakers using two-dimensional echocardiography and intracardiac electrocardiography.[107] The technique involves subcostal visualization of the structures of the right side of the heart and the lead by two-dimensional echocardiography. The electrode position is verified by recording an intracardiac electrogram, and adequate capture is ensured by intermittent pacing. More recently, Lau and Wong[108] used ultrasound to position an electrode in a patient with severe pulmonary tuberculosis. In this patient, collapse of the right side of the chest caused deviation of the heart to the right, making fluroscopic visualization impossible. A passive-fixation lead was introduced by means of a left cephalic cutdown and was passed with fluoroscopic visualization to an ill-defined cardiopulmonary shadow in the right side of the chest. The lead could then apparently no longer be visualized adequately by fluoroscopy. Two-dimensional echocardiography identified the lead in relation to the anatomy and assisted in final placement. Lead placement was verified by the intracardiac electrogram.

Repositioning of a malpositioned or dislodged permanent pacemaker electrode traditionally requires a surgical procedure. The pacemaker pocket must be surgically reopened. The pacemaker and leads are freed of adhesions and disconnected. A nonsurgical approach has been described by Morris and associates.[109] The technique uses principles similar to those of lead extraction through the femoral vein. The malpositioned lead is hooked and pulled into the inferior vena cava using a 3-mm J-shaped deflecting wire passed through a catheter placed in the femoral vein. This is accomplished by forming a closed loop in the deflecting wire and "capturing" the lead tip with the loop. The lead tip in the inferior vena cava is snared by a loop formed with a 300-cm 0.021 exchange wire. The loop is passed through an 8F catheter with a 2-cm radius curve steamed at its tip. The snared lead tip is then repositioned in the apex of the right ventricle. Iatrogenic repeated dislodgment is avoided by releasing the snare, which is accomplished by advancing one end of the 0.021 guide wire, forming a large loop, while retracting the other end of the wire from the catheter.

Transvenous endocardial lead placement is occasionally contraindicated, impractical, or impossible. Westerman and Van Devanter[110] described a transthoracic technique requiring general anesthesia and a limited thoracotomy for electrode placement. The electrodes are passed and positioned transatrially through the sixth intercostal space (Fig. 25–63). The right atrium is identified, and the electrode is passed transatrially through an incision or by using a sheath set. Hemosta-

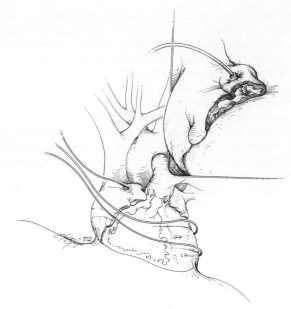

Figure 25–64. Transatrial endocardial atrial pacing in congenital heart disease. The ventricular leads were epicardial because the patient required a prosthetic tricuspid valve. (From Hayes, DL, Vliestra RE, Puga FJ, et al: A novel approach to atrial endocardial pacing. PACE 12:125, 1989.)

sis is effected by a pursestring suture around the entry site. Fluoroscopy can be used for the ventricular placement of a tined or screw-in electrode. All of the electrodes are secured to the endocardial surface. A tined electrode can be directly secured to the atrial endocardium. Double-ended sutures are tied around the leads under the tines of the electrode. Before introduction of the lead, the needles are driven through the atriotomy into the atrial cavity and then out of the atrial muscle at the point of desired endocardial atrial fixation. The electrode is then pulled through the incision into the atrium and "snugged" to the endocardium by retracting and tying the double-ended suture. In many situations, this approach may have more merit than the epicardial approach because better chronic electric thresholds are typically achieved. This technique may be useful for some pediatric implantations.

Hayes and colleagues[111] described a similar technique of endocardial atrial electrode placement at the time of corrective cardiac surgery (Fig. 25–64), avoiding atrial epicardial pacing because of poor pacing and sensing thresholds. In this description, a dual-chamber pacemaker patient with severe tricuspid regurgitation and chronic endocardial electrodes required removal of all four previously implanted endocardial leads and placement of a prosthetic tricuspid valve. New epicardial electrodes were placed on the ventricle. Stable atrial pacing and sensing were achieved by a transatrial endocardial placement in the right atrial appendage. In this case, the lead was secured by pursestring ligatures around the incision.

Byrd and Schwartz[112] described another epicardial approach based on experience in five patients. The technique also allows conventional transvenous leads to be implanted in patients requiring an epicardial approach, including those with superior vena cava syndrome or anomalous venous

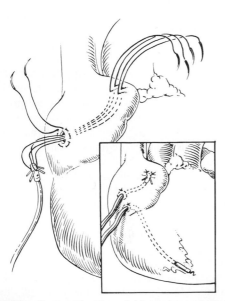

Figure 25–63. Transatrial endocardial lead placement during thoracotomy allows low-threshold transvenous leads to be implanted at the time of thoracic surgery. (From Barold SS, Mugica J: New Perspectives in Cardiac Pacing. Mt Kisco, NY, Futura, 1988, p 271.)

drainage and young patients with one innominate vein occluded by thrombosis. The technique uses a limited surgical approach with general anesthesia. The right atrial appendage is exposed through a 4- to 5-cm incision. The third and fourth costal cartilages are excised. A sheath set is placed inside an atrial pursestring suture and secured in a vertical position. The atrial and ventricular leads are passed down the sheath into the atrium (Fig. 25–65). Using standard techniques, including fluoroscopy, the electrodes are positioned. Once the electrodes are positioned, the sheath is removed, and the pursestring suture around the atriotomy is secured. The pacemaker is placed in a pocket created at the incision on the anterior chest wall. The advantage of this technique for patients in whom conventional transvenous systems are contraindicated or impossible is that it provides for implantation of a more conventional transvenous pacing system with minimal morbidity compared with a standard epicardial implantation. The chest is not entered (except for the atrium), and the time required is similar to that required for transvenous implantation. The disadvantages (although not necessarily in relation to other nonstandard transvenous techniques) include the requirement of general anesthesia, violation of the pericardia and epicardia, and the necessity of a right-sided approach (this may not be possible because of prior infection, mastectomy, and so on).

Occasionally, one encounters an anomalous venous structure, such as a persistent left superior vena cava. Embryologically, the normal left superior vena cava becomes atretic. There is, however, a 0.5% incidence of structural persistence of patency connected with the coronary sinus. Persistence of the left superior vena cava usually represents failure in the development of the left innominate vein. This vein normally forms by communication of the right and left anterior

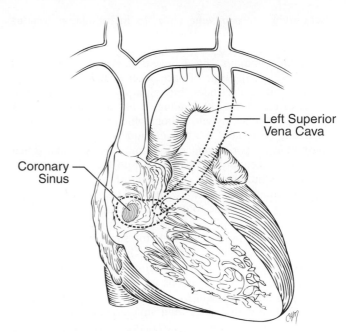

Figure 25–66. Persistent left superior vena cava.

cardinal veins. In this situation, the left anterior cardinal vein persists and continues to drain to the brachiocephalic veins and sinus venosus. This ultimately develops into a left superior vena cava, which empties directly into the coronary sinus (Fig. 25–66). Normally, the left innominate vein develops as an anastomosis between the left and right anterior cardinal veins. Occasionally, with persistent left superior vena cava, there is an associated atresia and incomplete absence of the right superior vena caval system (Fig. 25–67). In 10% to 15% of patients, one will encounter a totally

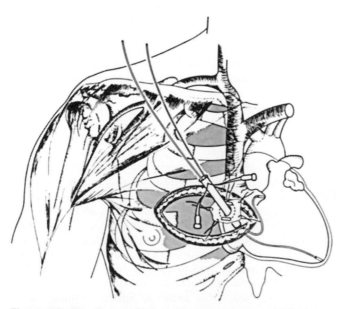

Figure 25–65. Endocardial lead placement by means of limited thoracotomy with removal of only the third and fourth costal cartilages. Standard fluoroscopy and peel-away introducer techniques are used with transatrial access. (From Byrd CL, Schwartz SJ, Siviona M, et al: Technique for the surgical extraction of permanent pacing leads and electrodes. J Thorac Cardiovasc Surg 89[1]:142, 1985.)

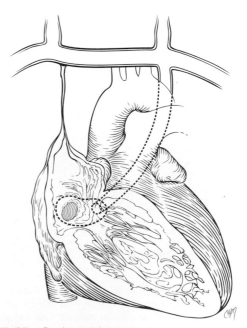

Figure 25–67. Persistent left superior vena cava with absent right superior vena cava.

absent right superior vena cava. In this situation, venous access for pacing from the right is virtually impossible. Despite the fact that there are reported classical physical and radiographic findings, the diagnosis is typically discovered unexpectedly at the time of pacemaker or ICD implantation.

Placement of electrodes through a persistent left superior vena cava can prove challenging, if not impossible.[113–118] A knowledge of anatomy and radiographic orientation is essential. If one proceeds from the left and is confronted with a persistent left superior vena cava, it must be appreciated that lead or leads actually are advanced into the coronary sinus and out its ostium into the right atrium. For right ventricular apical positions to be achieved, the lead must then be manipulated at an acute angle to cross the tricuspid valve. This is best accomplished by having the lead form a loop on itself, using the lateral right atrial wall for support (Fig. 25–68). This maneuver can prove extremely challenging. Depending on anatomy, occasionally, such efforts prove unsuccessful, and changing the site of venous access must be considered. At this point, it is prudent to assess the patency of the right venous system with contrast and angiographic techniques.[119] This can be carried out by advancing a standard end-hole catheter from the left superior vena cava to the vicinity of the right superior vena cava. Occasionally, such communication does not exist. If a right superior vena cava is absent, the iliac vein approach, as previously described by Ellestad,[98] or one of the epicardial approaches is recommended.

In the case of persistent left superior vena cava in which an atrial electrode is required, a positive-fixation screw-in electrode is recommended.[120, 121] The use of a preformed atrial J wire will prove difficult if not impossible. Dislodgment of the preformed J is also a concern. When using a positive-fixation electrode, care should be taken to avoid

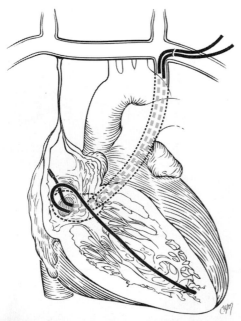

Figure 25–68. Placement of atrial and ventricular electrodes through persistent left superior vena cava and absent right superior vena cava. (From Belott PH: Unusual access sites for permanent cardiac pacing. *In* Barold S, Mugica J: Recent Advances in Cardiac Pacing for the 21st Century. Armonk, NY, Futura, 1998.)

pacing of the right phrenic nerve. This can be accomplished by high-output pacing after fixation. As a rule, the anterior right atrial position is preferred.

An absent right superior vena cava from a right-sided approach may also require changing approach sites. In this case, if an attempt is to be made from the right, the expected venous tortuosity of the persistent left superior vena cava should alert one to request longer electrodes. At times, an 85-cm lead will be required. Again, it is advisable to use positive-fixation leads in anticipation of dislodgment problems.

Permanent pacemakers have also been implanted through the inferior vena cava using a retroperitoneal approach. West and associates[122] reported the case of a 48-year-old man with congenital heart disease. The patient had undergone multiple procedures to correct transposition of the great vessels with a functional single ventricle and subvalvular pulmonic stenosis. The patient had multiple surgical procedures, including a palliative Blalock shunt and Glenn procedures. At 47 years of age, the patient developed a complete AV block. Given the complex congenital anomalies and subsequent corrective procedures, venous access to the right atrium and ventricle was complicated by loss of continuity between the right atrium and superior vena cava. This precluded a standard transvenous access. An epicardial approach was also less desirable, given the patient's multiple surgical procedures. It was elected to perform a retroperitoneal approach through a transvenous right flank incision. The inferior vena cava was infiltrated and cannulated retroperitoneally (Fig. 25–69). Bipolar active-fixation screw-in electrodes were used in both the atrium and the ventricle. The venous insertion site was secured and hemostasis effected by pursestring sutures. The pulse generator was implanted in a subcutaneous pocket formed in the anterior abdominal wall.

In similar fashion, pacemaker leads have been placed through transhepatic cannulation. Fischberger and colleagues[123] have reported percutaneous transhepatic cannulation using fluoroscopic guidance (Fig. 25–70). Once venous access has been achieved percutaneously with the guide wire transhepatically, a sheath set is applied, affording the subsequent introduction of a permanent pacemaker electrode. This procedure has been reserved for complex congenital anomalies that preclude venous access through a superior vein and avoid an unnecessary thoracotomy.

The coronary sinus has been used for pacing both by design and by accident (Fig. 25–71). The coronary sinus, per se, is unreliable for ventricular pacing and should generally be avoided, although posterolateral coronary veins and the middle cardiac vein are used more commonly now to achieve left ventricular pacing. It can be an acceptable location for atrial pacing.[124, 125] The problem with coronary sinus atrial pacing has been access and lead stability. Before the development of reliable atrial electrodes, the coronary sinus was a popular site of lead placement for atrial pacing. The best place for atrial pacing is the proximal coronary sinus. It is also the least stable location. Special coronary sinus leads have been developed to enhance position stability. These leads have a flexible, elongated tip that reaches deep into the coronary sinus, wedging in the great cardiac vein for stability. Gaining access to the coronary sinus requires experience (unless one is trying to avoid it, in which case it seems to be routinely entered). With the growing number of

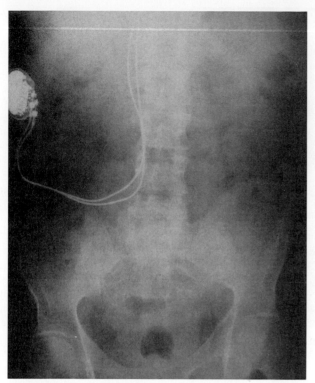

Figure 25–69. Posteroanterior abdominal radiograph showing the position of the pacemaker and generator lead inserted into the inferior vena cava. (From West JNW, Shearmann CP, Gammange MD: Permanent pacemaker positioning via the inferior vena cava in a case of single ventricle with loss of right atrial to vena cava continuity. PACE 16:1753, 1993.)

the mislocation of the lead on the left side of the heart (see Fig. 25–72D). If the mislocation is promptly detected, repositioning within 24 hours is the reasonable course of action. If the detection delay is longer, long-term anticoagulation without repositioning the lead is advisable.

■ IMPLANTABLE CARDIOVERTER-DEFIBRILLATOR IMPLANTATION

A variety of ICD implantation techniques have been developed and essentially involve an epicardial or transvenous approach. Initially, all ICD systems were placed using an epicardial approach for placement of rate sensing and pacing leads as well as defibrillation patch electrodes. The mere size of the ICD pulse generator required an abdominal pocket. With the development of the transvenous pacing and defibrillating electrodes and active can systems, there has been a shift to a nonthoracotomy approach. The radical reduction in ICD device size has allowed pectoral pocket placement. Today, the overwhelming majority of ICD systems are placed by a nonthoracotomy approach.[127–130] The epicardial approach is reserved for unique and extenuating circumstances. Many more ICD procedures are now performed in the electrophysiology or catheterization laboratory under conscious sedation.[131, 132] The various ICD epicardial and nonthoracotomy implantation techniques are reviewed next. The required equipment, personnel, and preparation for safe and expeditious ICD implantation are also reviewed.

implanting electrophysiologists who use the coronary sinus routinely for diagnostic studies, this experience becomes a moot point. In addition, as more implantations are performed in the catheterization laboratory, which is equipped with sophisticated radiographic equipment, including biplane fluoroscopy, the required beneficial fluoroscopic projections for placement are easily achieved.[126]

Placement of a coronary sinus lead is easier from the left side. A generous curve is required on the lead stylet. Coronary sinus placement is confirmed by a posterior lead position on lateral fluoroscopy. In addition, lead placement will not be associated with ventricular ectopy.

Although it was once a popular approach to atrial pacing, the coronary sinus is used infrequently today. This is largely the result of extremely reliable atrial leads equipped with fixation devices and tips that preclude dislodgment and ensure effective capture.

A final cautionary note on lead placement involves the risk of inadvertently placing a permanent ventricular pacing lead in the left rather than right ventricle (Fig. 25–72A). This can occur if the lead is passed from the right atrium through a patent foramen ovale into the left atrium and then advanced into the left ventricle across the mitral valve. The radiographic appearance can be deceptive in an anteroposterior projection. A lateral radiographic projection (see Fig. 25–72B) and an ECG showing an RBBB QRS pattern during ventricular pacing (see Fig. 25–72C) can usually clarify this occurrence. Computed tomography scans can also identify

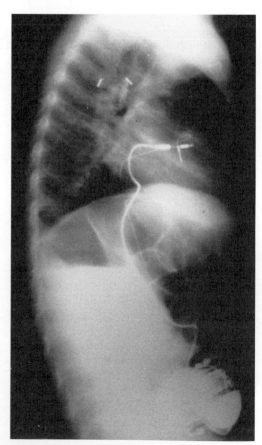

Figure 25–70. Lateral view demonstrating transhepatic lead implantation.

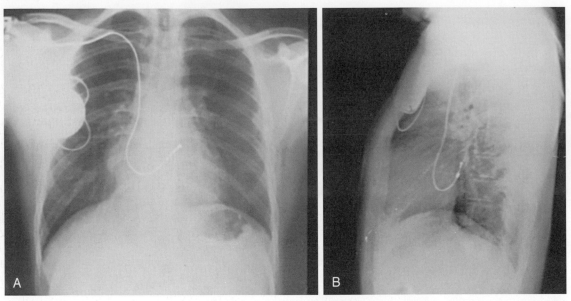

Figure 25–71. *A,* Posteroanterior radiograph of a patient with a coronary sinus permanent pacemaker electrode. The lead tip is superior and to the left side across the midline. *B,* Lateral film showing that the coronary sinus and the lead curve posteriorly and superiorly, precluding right ventricular placement.

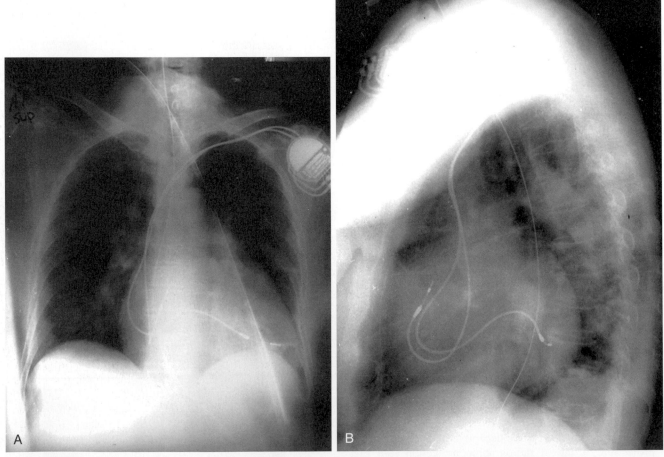

Figure 25–72. *A,* Anteroposterior chest radiograph with the ventricular electrode placed in the lateral wall of the left ventricle. This view can be very deceiving. At first glance, the electrode appears to be appropriately placed in the apex of the right ventricle. The high takeoff across the tricuspid valve gives one a clue that the lead is in reality crossing a patent foramen ovale. *B,* Lateral radiographic projection of the same patient clearly demonstrates the posterior placement of the ventricular electrode.

Illustration continued on opposite page

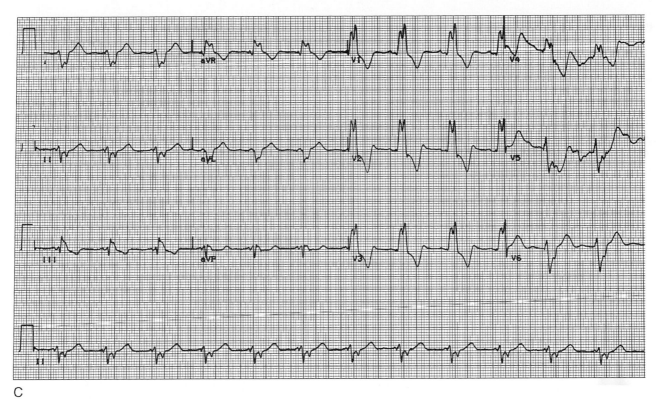

Figure 25–72 *Continued.* *C,* Twelve-lead electrocardiogram of the same patient with a left lateral ventricular pacing electrode placement. Note the prominent right bundle-branch block pattern in the precordial leads.

Personnel and Equipment

The personnel required for insertion of an ICD are similar to those needed for pacemaker implantation. The primary surgeon may be an electrophysiolgist, cardiologist, or a

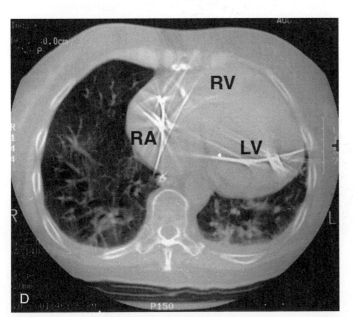

Figure 25–72 *Continued.* *D,* Computed tomography (CT) scan of the same patient with the ventricular pacing electrodes placed in the lateral wall of the left ventricle.

cardiothoracic surgeon. Of course, if an epicardial approach is instituted, the cardiothoracic surgeon is mandatory. In addition, an electrophysiologist should also be available.[133, 134] Although controversial, the ICD manufacturer's representative can be an important member of the implantation team and can prove to be invaluable for providing leads, defibrillators, and support equipment. The earlier ICD implantations that were limited to epicardial placement required a minimum of two trained physicians: an electrophysiologist and a cardiothoracic surgeon. With the transition to the nonthoracotomy approach, a device specialist (electrophysiologist, cardiologist, or cardiothoracic surgeon) working with the ICD manufacturer's representative may be all that is required. If general anesthesia is to be used, a nurse anesthetist or anesthesiologist is also required.[135] The ideal constitution of an ICD implantation team is listed in Table 25–14.[136]

Each member of the ICD implantation team should be completely familiar with the unique requirements of an ICD

Table 25–14. **Personnel Required for ICD Implantation and Testing**

Implanting physician (cardiothoracic surgeon, electrophysiologist)
Anesthesiologist
Electrophysiologist
Technical support personnel
  Engineer
  Technician
  EP nurse
  Manufacturer's representative

implantation. This includes a protocol for patient rescue should this be required. The circulating nurse should be responsible for operating the external defibrillator for rescue as directed by an electrophysiologist or implanting physician. Similarly, the manufacturer's representative should be responsible not only for equipment and supplies but also for threshold testing, programming, arrhythmia induction, and even rescue. This is all under the guidance of the implanting physician or electrophysiologist.

As the ICD implantation procedure becomes less electrophysiologically complex, there is a growing desire on the part of nonelectrophysiologist to implant ICDs. The ICD implantation technique has become very similar to that of a permanent pacemaker. There are no formal published guidelines with respect to obtaining privileges for the insertion of an ICD. It must be remembered that there are two parts to ICD implantation. First, the implantation of a lead and device, and second, the intraoperative electrophysiologic measurements that include not only pace and sense threshold determinations but also arrhythmia induction, defibrillation threshold determination, patient rescue, and finally, defibrillator programming. The second part of an ICD implantation can best be performed by a trained electrophysiologist; in any case, one should be immediately available. It is anticipated that in the future, organizations such as NASPE, the American College of Cardiology, and the American Heart Association will establish formal guidelines with respect to ICD implantation and credentialing.

Although the initial ICD implantations took place solely in the operating room under general anesthesia, ICD implantation now may take place either in the cardiac catheterization laboratory or the operating room. The choice of the implantation facility is subject to operator bias, hospital policy, and economics. The safety and efficacy of ICD implantation in the cardiac catheterization laboratory has been well established.[137-141] In many institutions, the ICD implantation may take place in either venue under conscious sedation. The concerns about infection appear to be unfounded even with complex tunneling and abdominal ICD placement. As previously stated, it is well accepted that the operating room offers a strict sterile environment and unlimited surgical supplies as well as ease of emergency thoracotomy, but these do not preclude the procedure being performed in the cardiac catheterization laboratory, where there is optimal imaging and support equipment. It would also appear that the catheterization laboratory offers a less expensive procedure with lower hospital charges.[142, 143] The basic required equipment for nonthoracotomy ICD insertion is identical to that for permanent pacemaker insertion. Additional considerations include arterial blood pressure monitoring as well as the equipment and supplies unique to the ICD, such as high-voltage cables, programmable stimulator, external defibrillator with sterile external and internal paddles, AC fibrillator, sterile programming wand for ICD communication, an external programmer, and the tunneling tools unique to ICD implantation (Table 25–15).[144, 145]

Similar to the pacemaker implantation procedure, one cannot have too many supplies and spare parts.

ICD Implantation: General Considerations

By and large, the general considerations are identical to those of a permanent pacemaker implantation. There are

Table 25–15. Recommended ICD Supplies

AC fibrillator box
Lead adapter sleeves and caps
External defibrillator
Large Parsonnet Dacron pouches (1.5″ × 6″)
Guide wires
Imaging contrast material
Introducers (long and short lengths, 9, 10, 11, 12, and 14F)
Jackson-Pratt drainage system
Multiple stylets
Multiple torque wrenches
Tunneling tool with multiple lead adapters
Transvenous rate sensing lead
Subcutaneous patches
Y-Adapters
Subcutaneous array
Extra transvenous rate sensing leads
Lead extensions
Lead repair kit

some subtle additional differences. Although not mandatory, many centers require intra-arterial blood pressure monitoring for ICD insertion. In addition, appropriate device selection and choice of anesthesia must be determined. Because of the drastically reduced ICD size and required surgery, as well as protocols for more expeditious device testing, the procedures are now even performed on an outpatient basis.

The choice of anesthesia is related to operator preference or, in some cases, hospital protocol.[146-148] As previously mentioned, the procedure may be performed under general anesthesia or with conscious sedation. In a patient who requires multiple defibrillation threshold determinations as well as subpectoral dissection, general anesthesia might be a better selection.[149] General anesthesia offers optimal patient comfort and airway control. At many centers where subcutaneous prepectoral muscle ICD implantation is performed, conscious sedation with local anesthesia for periods of ventricular fibrillation arrhythmia induction is used and the patient receives brief periods of deeper sedation with short-acting medications such as midazolam, methohexital, propofol, or fentanyl.[150-152]

Epicardial Approach

The identical epicardial approaches that were used for cardiac pacing have been employed for ICD implantation. In addition to those approaches previously mentioned, the median sternotomy[143-155] has become the approach of choice for combination of open heart surgery and ICD implantation.[156, 157] The common approaches for epicardial ICD implantation include the subxiphoid, subcostal, left lateral thoracotomy, and sternotomy. The goal of the epicardial approach is to configure the fibrillation patches around the heart for optimal defibrillation thresholds. Historically, the first clinical implants used an epicardial cup electrode on the ventricular apex in conjunction with a helical spring electrode in the superior vena cava (Fig. 25–73).[158] High defibrillation thresholds from this system ultimately led to the preference of two epicardial patch electrodes.[159] The epicardial patches may even be placed extrapericardially. This modification reduces epicardial adhesions. The epicardial patches come

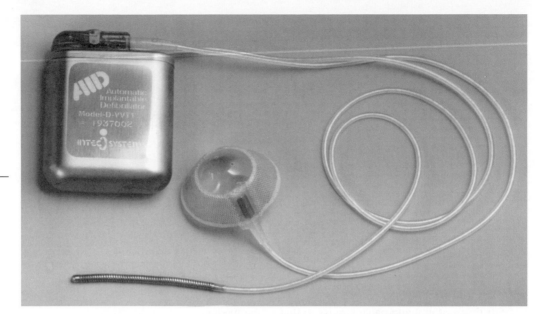

Figure 25–73. Epicardial cup and helical spring electrodes.

in a variety of sizes and shapes and vary among manufacturers (Fig. 25–74). The basic principle is for each patch to cover as large a surface of myocardium as possible. The patches must not touch each other because this would result in short-circuiting. In addition to the patches, rate-sensing leads must also be applied. Usually, this involves the placement of two sutureless screw-in electrodes side by side (Fig. 25–75). These electrodes serve both pacing and sensing functions. Because epicardial pacing and sensing electrodes have less optimal long-term performance characteristics, the rate-sensing and pacing electrodes may be placed transvenously using standard techniques. These leads are then tunneled to the device pocket using the standard tunneling technique previously outlined. Epicardial lead and patch

placement has historically involved an abdominal pocket because of the larger sizes of the devices. Abdominal pockets could be achieved by creation of either a subcutaneous pocket or, if optimal comfort and cosmetics are desired, subrectus muscle placement.

Median Sternotomy Approach

The median sternotomy is preferred by most cardiothoracic surgeons because it provides optimal exposure and access to the entire heart. It is generally used in patients undergoing an open heart procedure who also require ICD implantation. A median sternotomy incision is not necessary for satisfactory placement of defibrillator leads. This approach is usually well tolerated and associated with much less patient discomfort. The median sternotomy usually allows for the place-

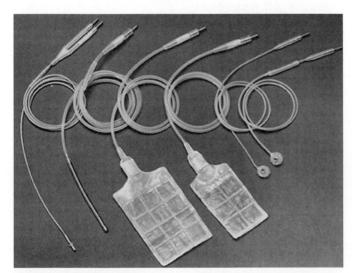

Figure 25–74. Assortment of electrodes available for automatic implantable cardioverter-defibrillator. From left to right: Endocardial bipolar rate-sensing lead, superior vena cava shocking coil, large epicardial patch lead, small epicardial patch lead, and epicardial screw-in rate-sensing electrodes. (Courtesy of Guidant, Inc., St. Paul, MN.)

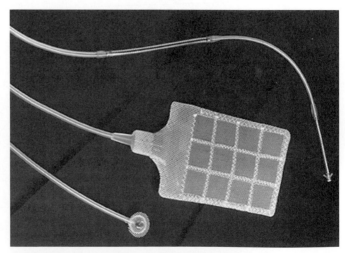

Figure 25–75. Implantable cardioverter-defibrillator (ICD) leads and electrodes. *Left,* Epicardial screw-in, rate-sensing electrode. *Center,* Rectangular epicardial patch electrode. *Right,* Transvenous rate-sensing electrode. (Courtesy of Guidant, Inc., St. Paul, MN.)

ment of two large patches extrapericardially (Fig. 25–76). Because this approach is usually performed while under cardiopulmonary bypass, the lungs can be deflated and excellent exposure achieved. The phrenic nerves and coronary artery bypass graft should be identified to avoid their injury. The rate-sensing electrodes are directly screwed into the surface of the heart. These can be placed on either the right or left ventricle. One patch is typically placed on the surface of the right ventricle. Because of the smaller right ventricular surface area, smaller patch sizes are frequently required. The patches are then sutured to the pericardium (or, in the case of an intrapericardial implant, on the surface of the ventricles directly). The median sternotomy approach for ICD placement is the procedure of choice for most cardiothoracic surgeons. This is true even in a setting of an isolated ICD implantation because the median sternotomy results in less pain and optimal exposure.[160]

Left Anterolateral Thoracotomy Approach

The left thoracotomy approach, similar to that of the median sternotomy, is attractive because it allows for excellent exposure of the heart and, more specifically, the left ventricle. The heart is exposed through an incision created in the fifth intercostal space (Fig. 25–77). The skin incision is made along the inframammary fold. This approach is ideal for the extrapericardial placement of a large patch electrode over the posterior surface of the left ventricle as well as a smaller patch anteriorly between the sternum and pericardium. Occasionally, a small right minithoracotomy is required for additional exposure and placement of a patch electrode on the right side of the heart.

The anterior thoracotomy is associated with considerable

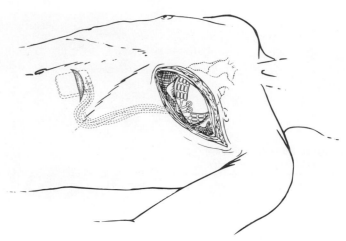

Figure 25–77. Left lateral thoracotomy with epicardial rate-sensing and patch electrodes tunneled to subcutaneous pocket in the left upper quadrant.

postoperative pain, and this is its major detraction. This pain can also result in atelectasis and transient pleural effusions. Postoperative wound pain can be reduced by working through a more lateral incision. An additional disadvantage of the left thoracotomy is seen in patients who have had prior cardiac surgery. The common postoperative adhesions usually preclude the anterior placement of an extrapericardial patch and also raise the hazard of damaging coronary bypass grafts. A more lateral approach has been adapted that eliminates pain associated with division of the latissimus dorsi. The more lateral incision offers an excellent exposure of the left ventricle and avoids injury to the costal cartilages and division of thoracic musculature. The leads are tunneled to the abdominal pocket by the use of a small chest tube and hemostat.

Subxiphoid Approach

The subxiphoid approach was developed for patients undergoing an isolated ICD implantation. This approach offers decreased morbidity and discomfort when compared with the median sternotomy and thoracotomy.[161] Although this approach is associated with a slight increase in defibrillation thresholds, it offers less postoperative wound discomfort and morbidity.[162] This approach requires the least surgical dissection.

A midline incision is made just above the xiphosternal junction and is carried inferiorly for about 6 cm. The xiphoid process is usually excised. Using traction, the sternum is elevated and the pericardium identified. The pericardium is incised with an anterior or transverse incision. Patches are placed over the right anterior and diaphragmatic surfaces of the heart (Fig. 25–78). The pocket is created by merely extending the subxiphoid incision and creating a subcutaneous or subfascial pocket. It can also be created by using a separate incision in the left upper quadrant with the leads tunneled to the pocket. The major disadvantage of this approach is limited surgical exposure and the requirement for intrapericardially placed patches. Occasionally, because of unacceptable defibrillation thresholds, an additional transve-

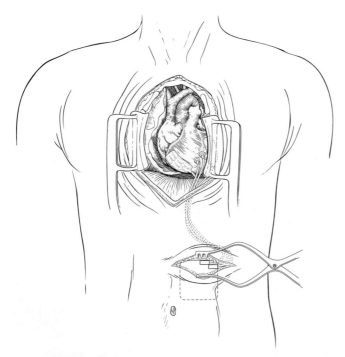

Figure 25–76. Median sternotomy with epicardial rate-sensing and patch electrodes tunneled to implantable cardioverter-defibrillator pocket in the left upper quadrant.

nous coil must be placed. This requires substantial subcutaneous tunneling from the subclavian vein to the abdominal pocket. Also, because of limited exposure, this approach is generally not used in patients having undergone prior cardiac surgery.[163]

Left Subcostal Approach

The left subcostal approach was originally developed for placement of epicardial pacing and sensing electrodes.[164] A technique has been developed expanding this approach for the placement of ICD patches. Like the subxiphoid approach, this approach is associated with minimal morbidity.[165, 166] Surgical exposure is somewhat better than with the subxiphoid approach. The left subcostal approach is carried out with an incision in the left subcostal area (Fig. 25–79). This incision is carried down to the rectus muscle. The rectus muscle is divided. The posterior rectus sheath is identified. Using blunt dissection under the costal margin, the pericardium is exposed. Retraction of the costal margin enhances exposure. With proper dissection, patches may be placed extrapericardially. This approach can be used in patients who have had prior cardiac surgery.[167, 168] Because the posterior rectus sheath has been left intact, a subrectus pocket may be created for pulse generator placement.

The advantages of the subrectus approach are similar to those of the subxiphoid approach. Because the left subcostal approach is extrathoracic, it avoids the complications of a thoracotomy. As previously mentioned, the exposure of the subcostal approach is somewhat better than that of the subxi-

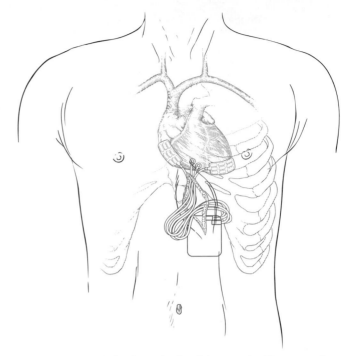

Figure 25–79. Left subcostal epicardial approach with rate-sensing and patch electrodes tunneled to subcutaneous pocket in the left infracostal space.

phoid technique. Because the subcostal approach requires division of the left rectus muscle, there is greater postoperative discomfort. In essence, the subcostal approach improves exposure over the subxiphoid approach while at the same time minimizing pulmonary complications and problems. This approach also affords the ability of inserting the defibrillator through the same incision. A transdiaphragmatic approach has been described that offers the same advantages and disadvantages of the subcostal approach.[169, 170] This approach uses a longitudinal epigastric extraperitoneal incision for access to the heart. An initial skin incision is carried to the surface of the peritoneum. The diaphragm is identified, and an incision is made through its central tendon. Possibly because of potential violation the abdominal cavity, this approach has not gained popularity.

Thoracoscopic Approach

ICD patches can be placed using a thoracoscope.[171, 172] A small incision is made on the left anterior chest, and the defibrillator patches are introduced into the left pleural space (Fig. 25–80). The thoracoscope is then used to grab the patches, guide them, and subsequently attach them to the surface of the pericardium. This is a relative new approach, and its safety and efficacy have not been fully defined. Because this approach avoids thoracotomy and sternotomy, it carries the lowest morbidity of all the epicardial approaches.[173]

Endocardial Approach

The endocardial, or nonthoracotomy, approach was initially introduced in 1987 when the Endo-Tak (CPI, St. Paul, MN)

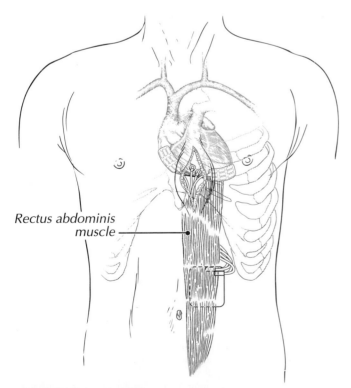

Rectus abdominis muscle

Figure 25–78. Subxiphoid epicardial approach with rate-sensing and patch electrodes tunneled to a subrectus pocket in the left upper quadrant.

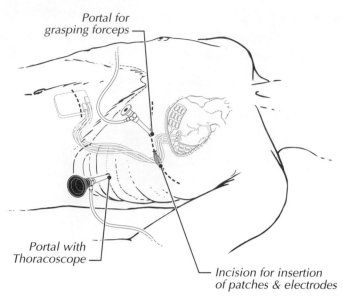

Portal for grasping forceps

Portal with Thoracoscope

Incision for insertion of patches & electrodes

Figure 25–80. Thoracoscopic epicardial rate-sensing and patch electrode placement. Electrodes tunneled subcutaneously to implantable cardioverter-defibrillator pocket in the left upper quadrant.

was introduced (Fig. 25–81). Unfortunately, the early experience was associated with a high incidence of lead fractures and slowed its initial acceptance.[174] Today, most manufacturers offer an endocardial pacing and shocking electrode, and the endocardial approach has become the technique of choice. Initially, the endocardial and transvenous electrode system required a subcutaneous patch to achieve effective acceptable defibrillation thresholds.[175, 176] With the development of new electrical defibrillation wave forms, lead configurations, electrically active can systems, and efficient energy delivery systems, the transvenous approach is now the main technique for ICD implantation.[177, 178] The transvenous lead systems vary in configuration from manufacturer to manufacturer, but venous access is identical and lead positioning nearly identical to those previously described for the ventricular pacing electrode. Because of concerns about the

subclavian crush syndrome, cephalic cutdown or percutaneous access of the axillary vein are recommended.[179, 180] If more than one electrode is to be inserted, a simple venous puncture with the retained guidewire technique or two separate punctures can be used. Left-sided venous access is preferred. Similar to pacemaker systems, the left-sided venous access offers a more direct and facile approach to the right ventricular apex. If a two-coil system is used, the proximal coil is more easily and effectively positioned against the lateral right atrial wall or in the left innominate or subclavian veins from the left subclavian venous approach. Finally, defibrillation thresholds appear to be higher if using an active "hot" can when approached from the right side.[181–183]

The techniques for endocardial defibrillator electrode placement are identical to those for pacing. A right ventricular apical position is desired. Once again, this can frequently be facilitated with a right anterior oblique fluoroscopic projection. Once positioned, the leads are secured to the pectoralis muscle using the suture sleeve. Because the leads are frequently tunneled and there is a risk of dislodgment, a strain-release S can be fashioned with the lead just proximal to the venous entry site. This provides slack to prevent dislodgment from manipulation of the pulse generator. One should avoid a complete loop because this tends to form pressure points that may lead to erosion. The need for a strain-release S has been lessened by the use of pectoral pockets and smaller generators.

Pocket Creation

Initially, ICD pockets were created almost exclusively in the left upper quadrant of the abdomen. This was because of the predominant epicardial approach and the rather generous size of the device. With the advent of the nonthoracotomy approach, the ICD pocket is almost exclusively placed in the left pectoral area. Most abdominal pockets are subcutaneous, but if excellent cosmetics and comfort are desired, an intrarectus sheath or even a submuscular approach can be used. In the pectoral area, because of device size, many centers initially used a submuscular approach. With the radical reduction in device size, the subcutaneous pocket is becoming much more common. The concern associated with a subcutaneous pocket, whether abdominal or pectoral, is the increased risk for erosion (Table 25–16).

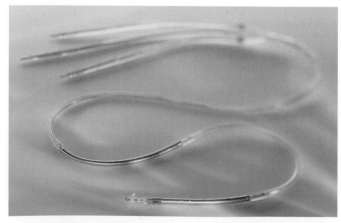

Figure 25–81. Endo-Tak transvenous endocardial pace and shock electrode.

Table 25–16. Subcutaneous v. Submuscular ICD Pocket

Site	Advantages	Disadvantages
Subcutaneous	Limited surgery	Less cosmetic
	Better control of bleeding	Increased risk of erosion
	Better analgesia	Increased risk of dislodgement from twiddler's syndrome
	Easier pulse generator change	
Submuscular	Optimal cosmetics	Increased problems with hemostasis
	Less risk of dislodgement from twiddling	Greater postoperative pain
	Greater patient acceptance	Potential migration laterally to the axilla

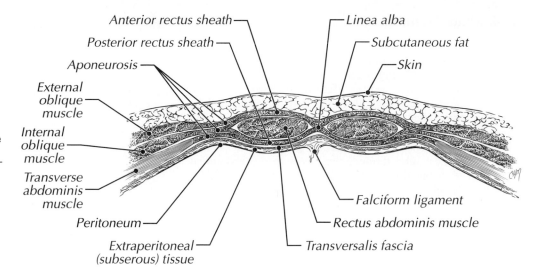

Figure 25–82. Cross-sectional anatomy of the rectus sheath above the arcuate line.

Anterior rectus sheath
Posterior rectus sheath
Aponeurosis
External oblique muscle
Internal oblique muscle
Transverse abdominis muscle
Peritoneum
Extraperitoneal (subserous) tissue
Linea alba
Subcutaneous fat
Skin
Falciform ligament
Rectus abdominis muscle
Transversalis fascia

Abdominal Pocket

If an abdominal pocket is to be created, the implanting surgeon must be completely familiar with the anatomy of the anterior abdominal wall. This includes the multiple muscular and fascial layers (Fig. 25–82). One must be able to identify the anterior rectus sheath, rectus muscle, posterior rectus sheath, linea alba, and peritoneum. Failure to understand the anatomy of the abdominal wall may result in inadvertent access of the peritoneal cavity. An abdominal pocket is created with an initial 3- to 4-inch transverse incision high in the left upper quadrant. This incision is carried through the subcutaneous tissue and fat to the surface of the anterior rectus sheath. The incision can be held apart by use of one or two Weitlaner retractors. A Goelet or Richardson retractor may then be applied to retract the subcutaneous tissue, and using the electrocautery unit cutting function, an inferior pocket is created just on top of the anterior rectus sheath. A plane is created directly on top of the anterior rectus sheath, and an attempt is made not to violate this structure. The subcutaneous tissue is separated from the anterior rectus sheath, creating a pocket large enough to accommodate the particular pulse generator. The pocket is carefully inspected for hemostasis and lavaged with antibacterial solution. The pocket should be low enough to avoid the costal margin and yet above the belt line. The pocket receives the leads, using standard tunneling techniques (see later). When epicardial approaches are used, most leads are tunneled using a small chest tube and Kelly clamp for guidance. In the case of tunneling transvenous leads to an abdominal pocket, a special tunneling tool may be used (Fig. 25–83). Whether using a tunneling tool or elongated clamps, care should be taken to achieve optimal depth of the tunneling tract so as to avoid future lead erosion.

A modification of the subcutaneous approach calls for the creation of a submuscular abdominal pocket. This pocket allows placement of the ICD device in a space created between the posterior rectus sheath and rectus muscle. This space may be approached by a vertical incision through the anterior rectus sheath at either its medial or lateral margin. The muscle can then be easily retracted off of the posterior rectus sheath. Occasionally, vascular pedicles will be encountered; these should be clipped with vascular staples. Once this submuscular compartment has been carefully inspected for hemostasis, the device may be inserted. A redundant lead can be placed in a separate subcutaneous space. The aponeuroses and subcutaneous tissue are then reapproximated using standard closure techniques. Once again, the deeper submuscular approach is associated with potential violation of the peritoneal cavity as well as postoperative erosion into the peritoneal cavity (Fig. 25–84). As a general rule, the abdominal pocket should not be located or placed over previous abdominal surgery. This includes previous abdominal incisions or drain sites. Such scar tissue increases the risk of direct communication between the ICD pocket and the peritoneal cavity. Similarly, one should avoid placement of an abdominal pocket in the vicinity of abdominal hernias, which have the propensity of extending into an ICD pocket. Finally, if one is aware of potential future abdominal surgical requirements, an alternate abdominal location or pectoral approach should be considered.

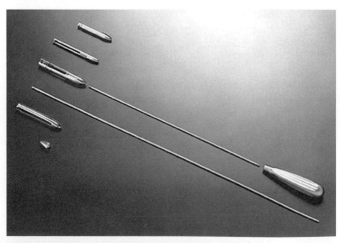

Figure 25–83. Subcutaneous tunneling tool with interchangeable handle, tunneling rod, and tunneling bullet. (Courtesy of Guidant, Inc., St. Paul, MN.)

Tunneling Techniques

The initial epicardial ICD systems required tunneling of leads from the epicardium to an abdominal pocket. This was usually carried out using a large chest tube. The proximal ends of the electrodes were stuffed into the back end of a chest tube for protection, and the chest tube was guided by a large clamp subcutaneously to the abdominal pocket. The tip of the chest tube was grasped with a large, curved Kelly clamp, and using an index finger for palpation, the clamp guided the chest tube through the tissue to the abdominal pocket. The distance from the epicardium to the abdominal pocket was relatively short, and this tunneling technique proved simple and expeditious.

This is not the case when tunneling from a transvenous insertion site in the upper chest to an abdominal pocket. To assist in long stretches of tunneling, CPI developed a tunneling tool to resolve this problem. The tunneling tool had multiple components and basically consisted of a rod with a handle at one end and a distal bullet that could be replaced with a lead adapter (see Fig. 25–83). Tunneling should never be carried out until acceptable lead position and defibrillation thresholds have been achieved. Even with the tunneling tool, tunneling over large areas can prove to be extremely challenging. It is important to maintain optimal depth of the tunneled tract. Care should be taken to avoid intrathoracic entry as well as superficial cutaneous exit. The tunneling device may be introduced either through the abdominal pocket or a venous access incision. Care should be taken to avoid an intramuscular tract to prevent hematoma formation (Fig. 25–84). Once the tunneling tract has been established, the bullet is exchanged for the lead adapter. With the leads placed in the adapter, a suture is sometimes required to secure them in place. After the leads are secured to the adapter, the tunneling tool is retracted back to the abdominal pocket, and the leads are released from the adapter. If the tunneling tool was initially passed from the venous entry incision, the handle and bullet locations must be exchanged. The tunneling tool comes with two rod sizes: the shorter size, 12 inches in length, is used for tunneling over short distances, and the longer 20-inch length is used for pectoral to abdominal communication. The short rod is reserved for tunneling subcutaneous array, for pocket-to-pocket communication, or for venous entry site to pectoral pocket communication. After tunneling, pacing and defibrillation parameters should be reconfirmed.

Subcutaneous Patch and Array

Occasionally, the endocardial lead system alone fails to provide an adequate defibrillation threshold. In this case, a small electrode patch may be added through a small left anterior chest incision (Fig. 25–85).[184] This incision is usually placed along the left inframammary skin fold. A subcutaneous pocket is developed in the vicinity of the anterior axillary line. The patch is sutured to the chest wall and the proximal lead tunneled to the ICD pocket. A variation on this system is the subcutaneous array developed by CPI (Fig. 25–86).[185] The array consists of three flexible defibrillator leads that are joined at a common connector. The leads are designed to be placed subcutaneously along the contour of the left chest wall. The leads fuse as a common electrode

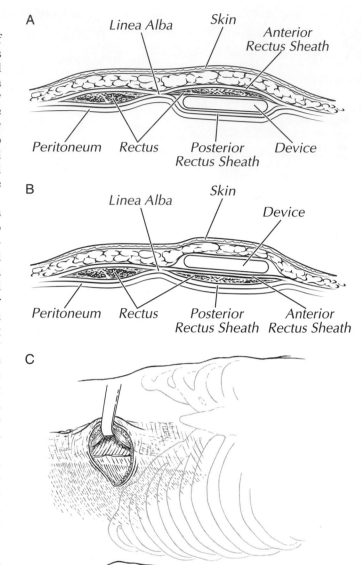

Figure 25–84. Cross-sectional anatomy of the rectus sheath above the arcuate line with implantable cardioverter-defibrillator placement. *A,* Implantable cardioverter-defibrillator (ICD) placed on top of the posterior rectus sheath beneath the rectus muscle. *B,* ICD placed anterior to the anterior rectus sheath in a subcutaneous pocket above the rectus muscle. *C,* Smooth retractor exposing the posterior rectus sheath by gentle retraction of the rectus muscle positioned anterior.

that connects to the ICD. The array is placed by creating a small incision to the left lateral inframammary skin fold. The incision is created down to the muscular fascia. Three subcutaneous tracts are created using a blunt-tipped malleable stylet. The stylet is then loaded with a sheath, which is advanced down each of the tracts. The stylet is removed, and the limbs of the array are passed down each sheath. The sheaths are split and retracted, leaving the array limb in position (Figs. 25–87 and 25–88). The proximal end of the array lead is connected to the ICD, and additional ICD defibrillation thresholds are carried out. The hub of the array is fixed to the chest wall to prevent dislodgment. Once

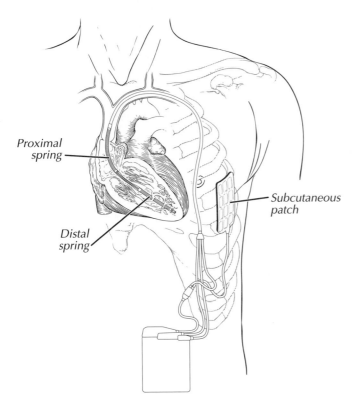

Proximal
spring

Distal
spring

Subcutaneous
patch

Figure 25–85. Endocardial pacing and shocking electrode positioned in the apex of the right ventricle. The electrode has been tunneled to the implantable cardioverter-defibrillator (ICD) in the right upper quadrant; subcutaneous patch has been placed and similarly tunneled to the ICD.

acceptable defibrillation thresholds have been achieved, the proximal end of the lead is tunneled to the device pocket.

Pectoral Pocket

The creation of a pectoral pocket is generally reserved for ICDs inserted by the endocardial approach. The success and acceptance of the pectoral pocket is largely due to the considerable downsizing of the ICD pulse generator. The ICD has now reached the size of the permanent transvenous pacemakers that were routinely placed in pectoral pockets in the early 1970s. Occasionally, because of the downsized ICD pulse generator, epicardial leads have been tunneled to a pectoral pocket. With the ICDs of 40 to 50 cm³ and a thickness of 1.5 cm, pectoral pockets can easily be achieved. The pocket can be created in either the right or left pectoral area, but the left pectoral area is preferred. This is because of lower achievable defibrillation thresholds with an active can device.[186] The pocket created can be either subcutaneous or submuscular. If the subcutaneous approach is used, it is identical to that described for a permanent transvenous pacemaker. The benefit of a subcutaneous pocket is its simplicity and avoidance of deep dissection. The pocket is created identical to that described for the permanent transvenous pacemaker. It cannot be overemphasized that maximum subcutaneous depth should be achieved with the pocket created directly on top of the pectoralis muscle. This is required to avoid potential erosion. The disadvantage of the subcutaneous approach is the concern of erosion. If the

pocket is not created deep enough, the corners of the ICD can create pressure points and potential erosion. If the pocket is not made large enough and the pocket is under tension, once again there is a great risk for erosion. The final disadvantage of the subcutaneous pocket with the ICD at its current size is one of cosmetics. The subcutaneous approach results in a visible bulge that does not occur with a deeper submuscular approach. The less attractive cosmetic result from a subcutaneous placement of an ICD has been a concern of some patients.

If there is any concern with respect to the twiddler syndrome, the Parsonnet pouch can be used.[187] This is a Dacron pouch that is specifically designed for the ICD. The Parsonnet pouch is also of benefit in the asthenic patient with little subcutaneous tissue, hopefully precluding potential erosion. When creating a subcutaneous pocket, some attention should be directed toward appropriate incision length as well as pocket size to avoid skin tension along the suture line that can result in erosion. The management of pocket hematomas in the setting of an ICD pocket is the same as that for a permanent pacemaker. When recognized, the hematoma should be evacuated early and a Jackson-Pratt drain placed. This drain is removed within 24 hours. Antibiotic lavage of the pocket is also identical to that of a permanent pacemaker. One cannot excessively underscore the necessity for strict adherence to antiseptic technique.

Submuscular Pectoral Pocket

The submuscular pectoral pocket remains a popular ICD approach. This is because of its optimal cosmetics and virtual freedom from erosion. Vital to the submuscular pectoral approach is a complete understanding of the regional anatomy.[188] The superficial landmarks of the clavicle, deltoid muscle, pectoralis muscle, and deltopectoral groove should be clearly identified (Fig. 25–89). The pectoralis major muscle is superior to the pectoralis minor. The pectoralis major muscle has two major subdivisions. There is a clavicular head that attaches to the clavicle and a sternal head that attaches to the lateral border of the sternum. Both heads

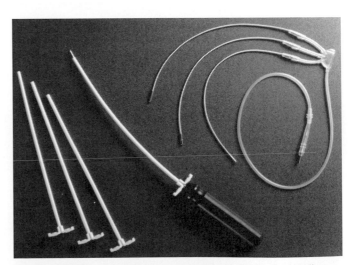

Figure 25–86. Subcutaneous array system. *Left*, sheaths; middle, tunneling tool loaded with sheath; *right*, subcutaneous array. (Courtesy of Guidant, Inc., St. Paul, MN.)

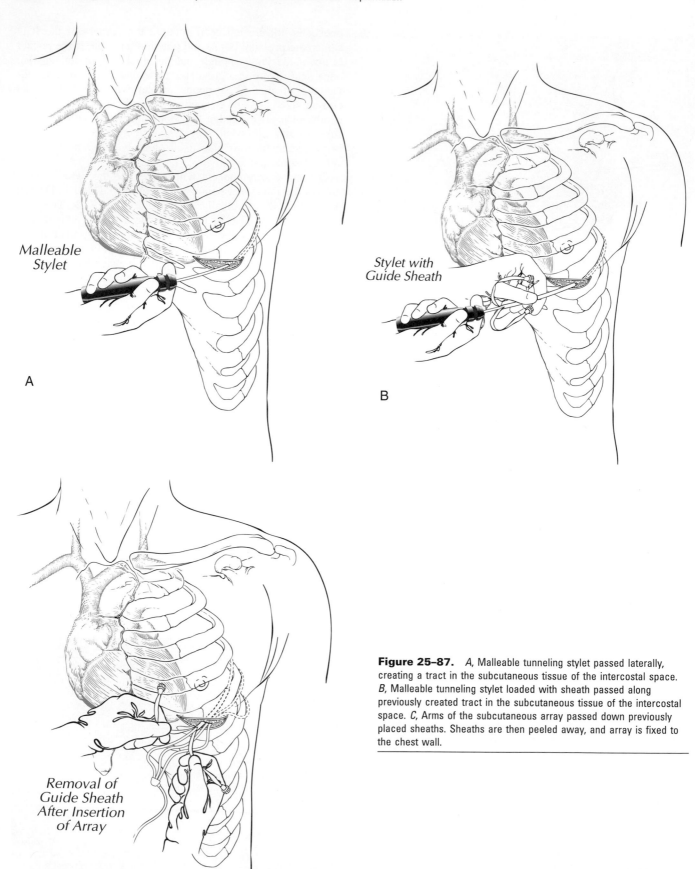

Malleable Stylet

A

Stylet with Guide Sheath

B

Removal of Guide Sheath After Insertion of Array

C

Figure 25–87. *A*, Malleable tunneling stylet passed laterally, creating a tract in the subcutaneous tissue of the intercostal space. *B*, Malleable tunneling stylet loaded with sheath passed along previously created tract in the subcutaneous tissue of the intercostal space. *C*, Arms of the subcutaneous array passed down previously placed sheaths. Sheaths are then peeled away, and array is fixed to the chest wall.

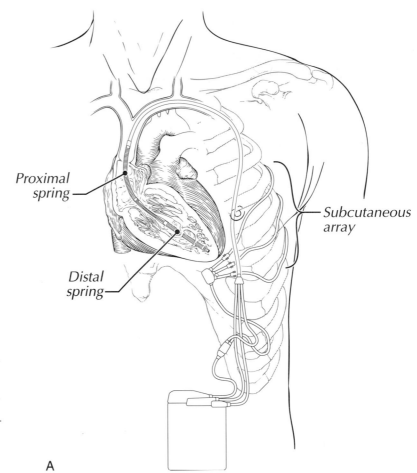

Proximal spring

Subcutaneous array

Distal spring

A

Figure 25–88. *A,* Endocardial pacing and shocking electrode tunneled to the pocket in the left upper quadrant. Subcutaneous array similarly positioned and fixed to the left anterior chest wall and tunneled to the device. *B,* Anteroposterior and lateral radiographic views of the Endo-Tak subcutaneous array system.

ENDOTAK® SQ Array

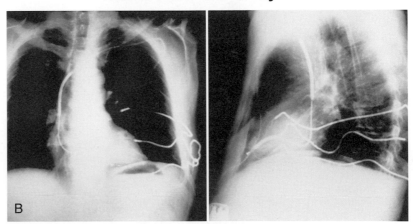

B

Anterior-Posterior View   Lateral View

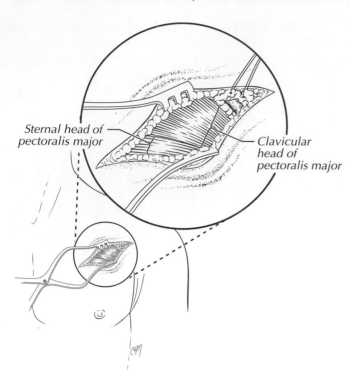

Figure 25–89. Initial incision for subpectoralis implantable cardioverter-defibrillator placement. Insert demonstrates the deltopectoral groove and the clavicular and sternal heads of the pectoralis major muscle.

ultimately fuse and attach to the humerus. The fascial plane that separates these two heads represents an attractive plane of dissection for access to the subpectoral space for creation of a pocket. The much smaller pectoralis minor has two connections. Its superior head is attached to the coracoid process. The muscle then fans out inferiorly, attaching to the anterior ribs. The thoracoacromial neurovascular bundle can be easily identified on the outer surface of the pectoralis minor muscle (Fig. 25–90). With this technique, this bundle should always be identified and avoided because it is a

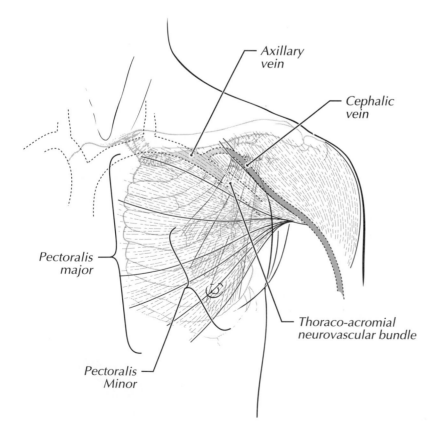

Figure 25–90. Superficial and deep anatomy of the deltopectoral area demonstrating the relationship of the superficial pectoralis major, deep pectoralis minor, axillary and cephalic veins, and thoracoacromial neurovascular bundle.

potential source of complication. Tearing the artery or vein may result in pocket hematoma, and interruption of the nerve may result in pectoral muscle dysfunction. The deltopectoral groove is defined by the lateral border of the clavicular head of the pectoralis major. The anterior axillary fold is defined by the inferolateral border of the sternal pectoralis major muscle head. Today, with the active can and in combination with the dual-coil lead system, the submuscular pectoral approach may be performed from both the right and left pectoral areas. The left pectoral approach, however, results in lower defibrillation thresholds.[189] Occasionally, if the right submuscular pectoral approach is used, a patch or array system may be required.

There are three distinct submuscular pectoral approaches. The first is the anterior subpectoral approach created between the clavicular and sternal heads of the pectoralis major (Fig. 25–91). The second submuscular pectoral approach is by a lateral reflection of the clavicular head of the pectoralis major (Fig. 25–92) and the third is by a lateral submuscular pectoral approach or anterior axillary approach through the inferolateral border of the pectoralis major muscle (Fig. 25–93). Each approach has its benefits and potential complications. The anterior approach is similar to that of a subcutaneous pacemaker pocket creation. It requires the creation of a dissection plane between the sternal and clavicular portions of the pectoralis muscle. The resultant pocket is anterior and does not interfere with the axilla. The lateral approach requires dissection of the pectoralis major along the deltopectoral groove. Because this approach is more lateral, there is a tendency for the ICD to drift into the axilla. Similarly, the axillary approach requires dissection and establishment of a plane at the anterior axillary fold. Once again, there is a tendency for the device to drift into the axilla and cause discomfort, although surgical techniques to help prevent this from occurring have been described. Both the lateral and axillary approaches also run the risk of interrupting the long thoracic nerve, which can result in "wing" scapula.

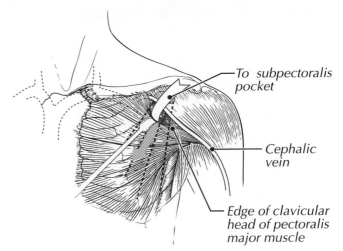

Figure 25–92. Deltopectoral groove, subpectoral approach. The lateral border of the pectoralis major clavicular head is gently retracted, and a plane of dissection is established medially, behind the pectoralis muscle.

The skin incision for the anterior approach is similar to that for a permanent pacemaker. One palpates the coracoid process and notes the angle of the deltopectoral groove. The incision is initiated just medial to the coracoid process and carried from the level of the coracoid process inferomedially perpendicular to the deltopectoral groove for about 3 inches. Using a Weitlaner retractor for retraction and electrocautery, the incision is carried down to the surface of the pectoralis fascia. With this approach, one may access the cephalic vein, the axillary vein, or the subclavian vein. After venous access is achieved and the leads positioned, the leads are anchored to the pectoralis muscle by use of the suture sleeve. The submuscular pectoral pocket is created by identifying the

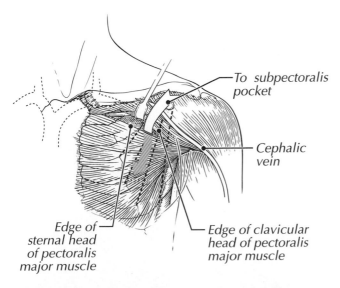

Figure 25–91. Anterior subpectoralis muscle approach. The clavicular and sternal heads of the pectoralis major are gently retracted, and a plane of dissection is established postpectorally.

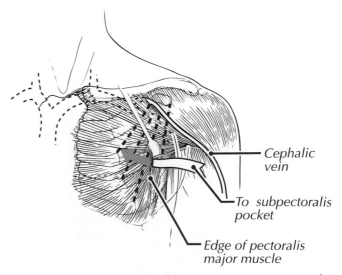

Figure 25–93. Anterior axillary fold, subpectoralis muscle approach. The lateral border of the pectoralis major sternal head at the anterior axillary fold is gently retracted, and a plane of dissection is established retropectorally.

border between the clavicular and sternal heads of the pectoralis muscle. Usually, this is identified by a line of fat. Using the smooth end of two Senn retractors, a plane of dissection is established between the two heads of muscle, which are gently peeled back until the surface of the chest wall is visualized as a clear plane of fatty tissue (Fig. 25–94). One can then insert a finger and continue the dissection bluntly. Underneath the pectoralis major muscle, one can palpate superiorly the leads entering the axillary vein and identify the fibers of the pectoralis minor as well as the thoracoacromial neurovascular bundle. Occasionally, this bundle may be torn, and electrocautery or vascular clamps may be applied to effect hemostasis. Care should be taken to avoid interrupting the nerve. Once the subpectoral pocket has been

established, a Goulet clamp may be inserted and the pocket visually inspected for any unusual bleeding. The leads are connected to the ICD, which is inserted into the submuscular pectoral pocket. It is recommended that longer lead lengths be used for this anterior pocket. Particularly in an AV ICD system, the atrial electrodes should be a minimum of 52 cm long. After successful, thorough device testing, the device may be rendered inactive and removed from the pocket. The pocket is carefully inspected for hemostasis as well as lavaged with antiseptic solution. The device is then reinserted into the pocket, and a multilayer closure is effected. This usually involves the placement of several interrupted sutures to approximate the clavicular and sternal portions of pectoralis muscle and then standard subcutaneous and skin closure.

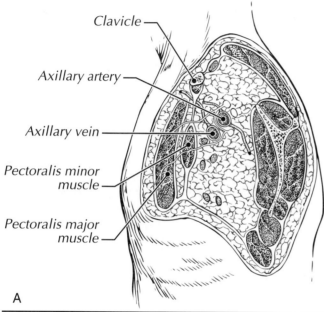

A

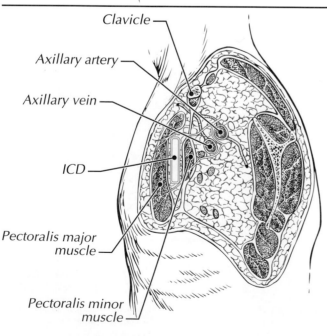

B

Figure 25–94. *A,* Sagittal section of the shoulder girdle demonstrating the superficial and deep anatomy. *B,* Sagittal section of the shoulder girdle demonstrating superficial and deep anatomy with automatic implantable cardioverter defibrillator placement under the pectoralis major muscle.

If the lateral submuscular approach through reflection of the lateral clavicular head is to be used, an initial vertical incision along the deltopectoral groove is recommended. Dissection is carried down to the surface of the pectoralis fascia. After achieving venous access and lead placement through the cephalic, axillary, or subclavian vein, the lateral border of the clavicular head of the pectoralis major is retracted medially once again using a retractor, and a plane of dissection on top of the pectoralis is established. Care should be taken to extend the pocket sufficiently medially to avoid interference with the abductor motion of the lateral humeral head. After through device testing and careful pocket inspection for hemostasis, again a multilayer closure is effected.

The lateral anterior axillary submuscular pectoral approach calls for creation of a dissection plane in the anterior axillary fold.[190] If this approach is to be used, careful sterile skin preparation of the entire axilla should be carried out. Some operators prefer this approach because it is less traumatic. A dissection plane is easily established as the pectoralis major is separated at the planes created between the pectoralis major and minor muscles. This approach is usually carried out with the left arm in abduction. A skin incision is created inferiorly along the anterolateral axillary fold. The incision is carried down to the surface of the pectoralis major muscle, the pectoralis major and minor muscles are identified and separated, and a plane of dissection is created between them. This approach usually requires a separate incision for venous access and tunneling to the axillary fold incision. Once again, one has the option of cephalic, axillary, or subclavian venous access. Some operators also create a small subcutaneous pocket for placement of the strain-relief loop and excess lead. The inferolateral margin of the pectoralis major muscle is easily separated from the adjacent subcutaneous tissue for establishing a large plane of dissection. The plane of blunt dissection is created on top of the pectoralis minor muscle. After pocket creation, the electrodes and ICD are united, and thorough device testing is carried out. The ICD should be placed as medially as possible with the leads lateral to the generator to avoid the risk of can abrasion. With the ICD in the pocket, a multilayer closure is used. The lateral margin of the anterior axillary soft tissue and pectoralis major muscle are approximated. Care should be taken to avoid suturing the pectoralis major and minor muscles together because this will limit motion of the upper extremity. The leads are anchored to the pectoralis muscle through the separate incision for venous access. As mentioned previously, with this approach as well as the lateral approach, care should be taken to avoid the long thoracic nerve.

All three approaches call for a multilayer closure. The submuscular layer is closed by gentle approximation of the muscular heads. Care is taken to avoid tight ties that may damage the muscular tissue. The subcutaneous tissue and skin are approximated as previously discussed.

REFERENCES

1. Schecter DC: Modern era of artificial cardiac pacemakers. *In* Schecter DC: Electrical Cardiac Stimulation. Minneapolis, Medtronic, 1983, pp 110–134.
2. Senning A: Discussion of a paper by Stephenson SE Jr, Edwards WH, Jolly PC, Scott HW: Physiologic P-wave stimulator. J Thorac Cardiovasc Surg 38:639, 1959.
3. Furman S, Schwedel JB: An intracardiac pacemaker for Stokes-Adams seizures. N Engl J Med 261:948, 1959.
4. Littleford PO, Spector SD: Device for the rapid insertion of permanent endocardial pacing electrode through the subclavian vein: Preliminary report. Ann Thorac Surg 27:265, 1979.
5. Mirowski M, Reid PR, Mower MM, et al: Termination of malignant ventricular arrhythmias with an implantable automatic defibrillator in human beings. N Engl J Med 303:322–324, 1980.
6. Parsonnet V, Furman S, Smyth NP, Bilitch M: Optimal resources for implantable cardiac pacemakers. Pacemaker Study Group. Circulation 68(1):226A, 1983.
7. Parsonnet V, Bernstein AD, Lindsay B: Pacemaker implantation complication rates: An analysis of some contributing factors. J Am Coll Cardiol 13:917, 1989.
8. Harthorne JW, Parsonnet V: Seventeenth Bethesda Conference: Adult cardiac training. Task Force VI: Training in cardiac pacing. J Am Coll Cardiol 7:1213, 1986.
9. Parsonnet V, Bernstein AD: Pacing in perspective: Concepts and controversies. Circulation 73:1087, 1986.
10. Parsonnet V, Bernstein AD, Galasso D: Cardiac pacing practices in the United States in 1985. Am J Cardiol 62:71, 1988.
11. Hayes DL, Naccarelli GV, Furman S, et al: Training requirements for permanent pacemaker selection, implantation, and follow-up. PACE 17:6, 1994.
12. Bernstein AD, Parsonnet V: Survey of cardiac pacing in the United States in 1989. Am J Cardiol 69:331, 1992.
13. Stamato NJ, O'Toole MF, Enger EL: Permanent pacemaker implantation in the cardiac catheterization laboratory versus the operating room: An analysis of hospital charges and complications. PACE 15:2236, 1992.
14. Hess DS, Gertz EW, Morady F, et al: Permanent pacemaker implantation in the cardiac catheterization laboratory: The subclavian approach. Cathet Cardiovasc Diagn 8:453, 1982.
15. Andersen FH, Crossland S, Alexander MB: Use of a three-channel electrocardiographic recorder for limited intracardiac electrocardiography during single- and double-chamber pacemaker implantation. Ann Thorac Surg 39:485, 1985.
16. Sutton R, Bourgeois I: Techniques of implantation. *In* Sutton R, Bourgeois I (eds): The Foundations of Cardiac Pacing: An Illustrated Practical Guide to Basic Pacing, vol I, pt 1. Mt Kisco, NY, Futura, 1991.
17. Levine PA, Balady GJ, Lazar HL, et al: Electrocautery and pacemakers: Management of the paced patient subject to electrocautery. Ann Thorac Surg 41:313, 1986.
18. Belott PH, Sands S, Warren J: Resetting of DDD pacemakers due to EMI. PACE 7:169, 1984.
19. Chauvin M, Crenner F, Brechenmacher C: Interaction between permanent cardiac pacing and electrocautery: The significance of electrode position. PACE 15:2028, 1992.
20. Hauser RG, Edwards LM, Guiffe VW: Limitation of pacemaker system analyzers for evaluation of implantable pulse generators. PACE 4:650, 1981.
21. Dreifus LS, Fisch C, Griffin JC, et al (eds): Guidelines for implantation of cardiac pacemakers and antiarrhythmic devices: A report of the ACC/AHA task force on assessment of diagnostic and therapeutic cardiovascular procedures. Circulation 84:455, 1991.
22. Zegelman M, Kreyzer J, Wagner R: Ambulatory pacemaker surgery: Medical and economical advantages. PACE 9:1299, 1986.
23. Belott PH: Outpatient pacemaker procedures. Int J Cardiol 17:169, 1987.
24. Dalvi B: Insertion of permanent pacemakers as a day case procedure. Br Med J 300(6717):119, 1990.
25. Hayes DL, Vliestra RE, Trusty JM, et al: Can pacemaker implantation be done as an outpatient? J Am Coll Cardiol 7:199, 1986.
26. Hayes DL, Vliestra RE, Trusty JM, et al: A shorter hospital stay after cardiac pacemaker implantation. Mayo Clin Proc 63:236, 1988.
27. Haywood GA, Jones SM, Camm AJ, et al: Day case permanent pacing. PACE 14:773, 1991.
28. Belott PH: Ambulatory pacemaker procedures: a 13-year experience. PACE 19:69, 1996.
29. Belott PH: Ambulatory pacemaker procedures. Mayo Clin Proc 63:301, 1988.
30. Goldstein DJ, Losquadro W, Spotnitz HM: Outpatient pacemaker procedures in orally anticoagulated patients. PACE 21:1730, 1998.
31. Philip BK, Corvino BG: Local and regional anesthesia. *In* Wetchler

BV (ed): Anesthesia for Ambulatory Surgery, 2nd ed. Philadelphia, JB Lippincott, 1991, pp 309–334.

32. Bubien RS, Fisher JD, Gentzel JA, et al: NASPE expert consensus document: Use of IV (conscious) sedation/analgesia by nonanesthesia personnel in patients undergoing arrhythmia-specific diagnostic, therapeutic, and surgical procedures. PACE 21:375, 1998.

33. Page CP, Bohen JMA, Fletcher R, et al: Antimicrobial prophylaxis for surgical wounds: Guidelines for clinical care. Arch Surg 128:79, 1993.

34. Muers MF, Arnold AG, Sleight P: Prophylactic antibiotics for cardiac pacemaker implantation: A prospective trial. Br Heart J 46:539, 1981.

35. Ramsdale DR, Charles RG, Rowlands DB: Antibiotic prophylaxis for pacemaker implantation: A prospective randomized trial. PACE 7:844, 1984.

36. Bluhm G, Jacobson B, Ransjo U: Antibiotic prophylaxis in pacemaker surgery: A prospective trial with local and systemic administration of antibiotics at pulse generator replacement. PACE 8:661, 1985.

37. Antimicrobial prophylaxis in surgery. Med Lett Druggs Ther 34(862):5–8, 1992.

38. Golightly LK, Branigan T: Surgical antibiotic irrigations. Hosp Pharm 24:116, 1989.

39. Smyth NPD: Techniques of implantation: Atrial and ventricular, thoracotomy and transvenous. Prog Cardiovasc Dis 23:435, 1981.

40. Smyth NPD: Pacemaker implantation: Surgical techniques. Cardiovasc Clin 14:31, 1983.

41. Netter FH: Atlas of Human Anatomy, fifth printing. West Caldwell, NJ, Ciba Geigy Medical Education, 1992, pp 174–176, 186, 200, and 201.

42. Gray H, Pick TP, Howden RE: Anatomy, Descriptive and Surgical, 1901 edition. Philadelphia, Running Press 1974, p 60.

43. Byrd C: Current clinical applications of dual-chamber pacing. In Zipes DP (ed): Proceedings of a Symposium. Minneapolis, Medtronics, 1981, p 71.

44. Netter FH: The Ciba Collection of Medical Illustrations, vol 5. Heart. Summit, NJ, Ciba Medical Education Division, 1981, pp 22–26.

45. Furman S: Venous cutdown for pacemaker implantation. Ann Thorac Surg 41:438, 1986.

46. Feiesen A, Kelin GJ, Kostuck WJ, et al: Percutaneous insertion of a permanent transvenous pacemaker electrode through the subclavian vein. Can J Surg 10:131, 1977.

47. Littleford PO, Spector SD: Device for the rapid insertion of permanent endocardial pacing electrodes through the subclavian vein: Preliminary report. Ann Thorac Surg 27:265, 1979.

48. Littleford PO, Parsonnet V, Spector SD: method for rapid and atraumatic insertion of permanent endocardial electrodes through the subclavian vein. Am J Cardiol 43:980, 1979.

49. Miller FA Jr, Homes DR Jr, Gersh BJ, Maloney JD: Permanent transvenous pacemaker implantation via the subclavian vein. Mayo Clinic Proc 55:309, 1980.

50. Belott PH, Byrd CL: Recent developments in pacemaker implantation and lead retrieval. In Barold SS, Mugica J (eds): New Perspectives in Cardiac Pacing. 2 Mt Kisco, NY, Futura, 1991, pp 105–131.

51. Stokes K, Staffeson D, Lessar J, et al: A possible new complication of the subclavian stick: Conductor fracture. PACE 10:748, 1987.

52. Fyke FE III: Simultaneous insulation deterioration associated with side by side subclavian placement of two polyurethane leads. PACE 11:1571, 1988.

53. Fyke FE III: Infraclavicular lead failure: Tarnish on a golden route. PACE 16:445, 1993.

54. Jacobs DM, Fink AS, Miller RP, et al: Anatomical and morphological evaluation of pacemaker lead compression. PACE 16:373, 1993.

55. Magey JE, Flynn DM, Parsons JA, et al: Anatomical mechanisms explaining damage to pacemaker leads, defibrillator leads, and failure of central venous catheters adjacent to the sternoclavicular joint. PACE 16:445, 1993.

56. Subclavian venipuncture reconsidered as a means of implanting endocardial pacing leads. Angleton, TX, Issues Intermedics, December 1987, pp 1–2.

57. Subclavian puncture may result in lead conductor fracture. Medtronic News, 16:27, 1986–1987.

58. Byrd CL: Safe introducer technique for pacemaker lead implantation. PACE 15:262, 1992.

59. Nichalls RWD: A new percutaneous infraclavicular approach to the axillary vein. Anesthesia 42:151, 1987.

60. Taylor BL, Yellowlees I: Central venous cannulation using the infraclavicular axillary vein. Anesthesiology 72:55, 1990.

61. Byrd CL: Clinical experience with the extrathoracic introducer insertion technique. PACE 16:1781, 1993.

62. Magney JE, Staplin DH, Flynn DM, et al: A new approach to percutaneous subclavian needle puncture to avoid lead fracture or central venous catheter occlusion. PACE 16:2133, 1993.

63. Belott PH: Blind percutaneous axillary venous access. PACE 21:873.

64. Varnagy G, Velasquez R, Navarro D: New technique for cephalic vein approach in pacemaker implants. PACE 18:1807a, 1995.

65. Spencer W III, Kirkpatrick C, Zhu DWX: The value of venogram-guided percutaneous extrathoracic subclavian venipuncture for lead implantation. PACE 19:700, 1996.

66. Spencer W III, Zhu DWX, Kirkpatrick C, et al: Subclavian venogram as a guide to lead implantation. PACE 21:499, 1998.

67. Ramza BM, Rosenthal L, Hui R, et al: Safety and effectiveness of placement of pacemaker and defibrillator leads in the axillar vein guided by contrast venography. Am J Cardiol 80:892, 1997.

68. Fyke FE III: Doppler-guided extrathoracic introducer insertion. PACE 18:1017, 1995.

69. Gayle DD, Bailery JR, Haistey WK, et al: A novel ultrasound-guided approach to the puncture of the extrathoracic subclavian vein for surgical lead placement. PACE 19:700, 1996.

70. Nash A, Burrell CJ, Ring NJ, Marshall AJ: Evaluation of an ultrasonically guided venipuncture technique for the placement of permanent pacing electrodes. PACE 21:452, 1998.

71. Lamas GA, Fish DR, Braunwald NS: Fluoroscopic technique of subclavian venous puncture for permanent pacing: A safer and easier approach. PACE 11:1398, 1987.

72. Higano ST, Hayes DL, Spittell PC: Facilitation of the subclavian-introducer technique with contrast venography. PACE 15:731, 1992.

73. Belott PH: Implantation techniques: New developments. In Barold SS, Mugica J (eds): New Perspectives in Cardiac Pacing. Mt Kisco, NY, Futura, 1988, pp 258–259.

74. Bognolo DA: Recent advances in permanent pacemaker implantation techniques. In Barold SS (ed): Modern Cardiac Pacing. Mt Kisco, NY, Futura, 1985, pp 206–207.

75. Parsonnet V, Werres R, Atherly T, et al: Transvenous insertion of double sets of permanent electrodes. JAMA 243:62, 1980.

76. Bognolo PA, Vijayanagar RR, Eckstein PR, et al: Two leads in one introducer technique for A-V sequential implantation. PACE 5:217, 1982.

77. VanderSalm TJ, Haffajee CI, Okike ON: Transvenous insertion of double sets of permanent electrodes through a single introducer: Clinical application. Ann Thorac Surg 32:307, 1981.

78. Belott PH: A variation on the introducer technique for unlimited access to the subclavian vein. PACE 4:43, 1981.

79. Gessman LJ, Gallagher JD, MacMillan RM, et al: Emergency guide wire pacing: New methods for rapid conversion of a cardiac catheter into a pacemaker. PACE 7:917, 1984.

80. Ong LS, Barold S, Lederman M, et al: Cephalic vein guide wire technique for implantation of permanent pacemakers. Am Heart J 114:753, 1987.

81. August DA, Elefteriades JA: Technique to facilitate open placement of permanent pacing leads through the cephalic vein. Ann Thorac Surg 42:112, 1986.

82. Parsonnet V, Bernstein AD: Cardiac pacing in the 1980's: Treatment and techniques in transition. J Am Coll Cardiol 1:399, 1983.

83. Furman S: Venous cutdown for pacemaker implantation. Ann Thorac Surg 41:438, 1986.

84. Furman S: Subclavian puncture for pacemaker lead placement. PACE 9:467 1986.

85. Parsonnet V, Bernstein AD, Lindsay B: Pacemaker–implantation complication rates: an analysis of some contributing factors. J Am Coll Cardiol 13:917, 1989.

86. Sutton R, Bourgeois I: The foundations of cardiac pacing. I. An illustrated practical guide to basic pacing. Mt Kisco, NY, Futura, 1991, pp 235–243.

87. Barrold SS, Mugica J: Recent advances in cardiac pacing: Goals for the 21st century, vol 19. Mt Kisco, NY, Futura, 1998, pp 213–231.

88. Belott PH: Retained guide wire introducer technique, for unlimited access to the central circulation: A review. Clin Prog Electrophysiol Pacing 1:59, 1991.

89. Bognolo DA, Vijayanagar R, Ekstein PF, et al: Anatomical suitability of the right atrial appendage for atrial J lead electrodes. In Proceedings of the Second European Pacing Symposium, Florence, Italy. Cardiac Pacing. Padova, Italy, Piccin Medical Book, 1982, p 639.

90. Bognolo DA, Vigayanagar R, Ekstein PF, et al: Implantation of permanent atrial J lead using lateral fluoroscopy. Ann Thorac Surg 316:574, 1981.

91. Thurer RJ: Technique of insertion of transvenous atrial pacing leads: The value of lateral fluoroscopy. PACE 4:525, 1981.

92. Jamidar H, Goli V, Reynolds DW: The right atrial free wall: An alternative pacing site. PACE 16:959, 1993.

93. Bognolo DA, Vijaranagar RR, Eckstein PF, Janss B: Method for reintroduction of permanent endocardial pacing electrodes. PACE 5:546, 1982.

94. Bognolo DA, Vijay R, Eckstein P, Jeffrey D: Technical aspects of pacemaker system upgrading procedures. Clin Prog Pacing Electrophysiol 1:269, 1983.

95. Belott PH: Use of the contralateral subclavian vein for placement of atrial electrodes in chronically VVI paced patients. PACE 6:781, 1983.

96. Parsonnet V: A stretch fabric pouch for implanted pacemakers. Arch Surg 105:654, 1972.

97. Roelke M, Jackson G, Hawthoren JW: Submammary pacemaker implantation: A unique tunneling technique. PACE 17:1793, 1994.

98. Ellestad MH, French J: Iliac vein approach to permanent pacemaker implantation. PACE 12:1030, 1989.

99. Antonelli D, Freedberg NA, Rosenfeld T: Transiliac vein approach to a rate-responsive permanent pacemaker implantation. PACE 16:1637, 1993.

100. Belott PH, Bucko D: Inframammary pulse generator placement for maximizing optimal cosmetic effect. PACE 6:1241, 1983.

101. Roelke M, Jackson G, Hawthorne JW: Submammary pacemaker implantation: A unique tunneling technique. PACE 17:1793, 1994.

102. Shefer A, Lewis SB, Gang ES: The retrospectoral transaxillary permanent pacemaker: Description of a technique for percutaneous implantation of an invisible device. PACE 16:1646, 1996.

103. Young D: Permanent pacemaker implantation in children: Current status and future considerations. PACE 4:61, 1981.

104. Smith RT Jr: Pacemakers for children. In Gillette PC, Garson A Jr (eds): Pediatric Arrhythmias: Electrophysiology and Pacing. New York, Grune & Stratton, 1990, pp 532–558.

105. Smith RT Jr, Armstrong K, Moak JP, et al: Actuarial analysis of pacing system survival in young patients. Circulation 74(Suppl II):120, 1986.

106. Gillette PC, Zeigler VL, Winslow AT, Kratz JM: Cardiac pacing in neonates, infants, and preschool children. PACE 15(11 pt 2):2046, 1992.

107. Guldal M, Kervancioglu C, Oral D, et al: Permanent pacemaker implantation in a pregnant woman with guidance of ECG and two-dimensional echocardiography. PACE 10:543, 1987.

108. Lau CP, Wong CK, Leung WH, et al: Ultrasonic assisted permanent pacing in a patient with severe pulmonary tuberculosis. PACE 12:1131, 1989.

109. Morris DC, Scott IR, Jamesson WR: Pacemaker electrode repositioning using the loop snare technique. PACE 12:996, 1989.

110. Westerman GR, Van Devanter SH: Transthoracic transatrial endocardial lead placement for permanent pacing. Ann Thorac Surg 43:445, 1987.

111. Hayes DL, Vliestra RE, Puga FJ, et al: A novel approach to atrial endocardial pacing. PACE 12:125, 1989.

112. Byrd CL, Schwartz SJ: Transatrial implantation of transvenous pacing leads as an alternative to implantation of epicardial leads. PACE 13:1856, 1990.

113. Dosios T, Gorgogiannis D, Sakorafas G, et al: Persistent left superior vena cava: A problem in transvenous pacing of the heart. PACE 14:389, 1991.

114. Hussaine SA, Chalcravarty S, Chaikhouni A: Congenital absence of superior vena cava: Unusual anomaly of superior systemic veins complicating pacemaker placement. PACE 4:328, 1981.

115. Ronnevik PK, Abrahamsen AM, Tollefsen J: Transvenous pacemaker implantation via a unilateral left superior vena cava. PACE 5:808, 1982.

116. Cha EM, Khoury GH: Persistent left superior vena cava. Radiology 103:375, 1972.

117. Colman AL: Diagnosis of left superior vena cava by clinical inspection: A new physical sign. Am Heart J 73:115, 1967.

118. Dirix LY, Kersscochot IE, Fiernen SH, et al: Implantation of a dual-chambered pacemaker in a patient with persistent left superior vena cava. PACE 11:343, 1988.

119. Giovanni QV, Piepoli N, Pietro Q, et al. Cardiac pacing in unilateral left superior vena cava: Evaluation by digital angiography. PACE 14:1567, 1991.

120. Robbens EJ, Ruiter JH: Atrial pacing by unilateral persistent left superior vena cava. PACE 9:594, 1986.

121. Hellestrand KJ, Ward DE, Bexton RS, et al: The use of active fixation electrodes for permanent endocardial pacing via a persistent left superior vena cava. PACE 5:180, 1982.

122. West JNW, Shearmann CP, Gammange MD: Permanent pacemaker positioning via the inferior vena cava in a case of single ventricle with loss of right atrial to vena caval continuity. PACE 16:1753, 1993.

123. Fishberger SB, Cammanas J, Rodriguez-Fernandez H, et al: Permanent pacemaker lead implantation via the transhepatic route. PACE 19:1124, 1996.

124. Moss AJ, Rivers RJ Jr: Atrial pacing from the coronary vein: Ten-year experience in 50 patients with implanted pervenous pacemakers. Circulation 57:103, 1978.

125. Greenberg P, Castellanet M, Messenger J, Ellestad MH: Coronary sinus pacing. Circulation 57:98, 1978.

126. Hewitt MJ, Chen JTT, Ravin CE, Gallagher JJ: Coronary sinus atrial pacing: Radiographic considerations. Am J Radiol 136:323, 1981.

127. Trappe H, Pfitzner P, Heintze J, et al: Cardioverter-defibrillator implantation in the catheterization laboratory: Initial experiences in 46 patients. Am Heart J 129:259–264, 1995.

128. Koukal C, Hemmer W, Oertel F, et al: Endotak lead alone configuration, a new standard when using biphasic shocks? [Abstract] PACE 18(Pt II):1189, 1995.

129. Bardy GH, Johnson G, Poole JE, et al. A simplified, single-lead unipolar transvenous cardioversion-defibrillation system. Circulation 88:543–547, 1993.

130. Raitt MH, Bardy GH: Advances in implantable cardioverter-defibrillator therapy. Curr Opin Cardiol 9:23–29, 1994.

131. Parsonnet V, Bernstein AD, Lindsay B: Pacemaker-implantation complication rates: An analysis of some contributing factors. J Am Coll Cardiol 13:917, 1989.

132. Bernstein AD, Parsonnet V: Survey of cardiac pacing in the United States in 1989. Am J Cardiol 69:331, 1992.

133. Flowers NC, Abildskov JA, Armstrong WF, et al: ACC Policy Statement. Recommended guidelines for training in adult clinical cardiac electrophysiology. J Am Coll Cardiol 18:637, 1991.

134. Scheinman M, Akhtar M, Brugada P, et al: Teaching objectives for fellowship programs in clinical electrophysiology. Report for the Ad Hoc Committee of the North American Society of Pacing and Electrophysiology. J Am Coll Cardiol 12:255, 1988.

135. Natale A, Kearney MM, Brandon MJ, et al: Safety of nurse-administered deep sedation for defibrillator implantation in the electrophysiology laboratory. J Cardiovasc Electrophysiol 7:301–306, 1996.

136. Lehmann MH, Saksena S: Implantable cardioverter defibrillators in cardiovascular practice: Report of the Policy Conference of the North American Society of Pacing and Electrophysiology. PACE 14:969, 1991.

137. Fitzpatrick AP, Lesh MD, Epstein LM, et al: Electrophysiological laboratory, electrophysiologist-implanted, nonthoracotomy-implantable cardioverter defibrillators. Circulation 89(6):2503–2508, 1994.

138. Strickberger SA, Hummel JD, Daoud E, et al: Implantation by electrophysiologist of 100 consecutive cardioverter-defibrillators with nonthoracotomy lead systems. Circulation 90(2):868–872, 1994.

139. Strickberger SA, Niebauer M, Ching Man K, et al: Comparison of implantation of nonthoracotomy defibrillators in the operating room versus the electrophysiology laboratory. Am Heart J 75:255–257, 1995.

140. Bardy GH, Hofer B, Johnson G, et al: Implantable cardioverter-defibrillators. Circulation 87:1152–1168, 1993.

141. Brooks R, Garan H, Torchiana D, et al: Determinants of successful nonthoracotomy cardioverter-defibrillator implantation: Experience in 101 patients using two different lead systems. J Am Coll Cardiol 22:1835–1842, 1993.

142. Luceri RM, Zilo P, Habal SM, David IB: Cost and length of hospital stay: Comparisons between nonthoracotomy and epicardial techniques in patients receiving implantable cardioverter defibrillators. PACE 18(1 Pt 2):168–171, 1995.

143. Stanton MS, Hayes DL, Munger TM, et al: Consistent subcutaneous prepectoral implantation of a new implantable cardioverter defibrillator. Mayo Clin Proc 69(4):309–314, 1994.

144. Mower M, Mirowski M, Pitt, et al: Ventricular defibrillation with a single intravascular catheter system having distal electrode in left pulmonary artery and proximal electrode in right ventricle or right atrium [Abstract]. Clin Res 20:389, 1972.

145. Schuder JC, Stoeckle H, West JA, et al: Ventricular defibrillation with catheter having distal electrode in right ventricle and proximal electrode in superior vena cava [Abstract]. Circulation 43–44:99, 1971.

146. Tung RT, Bajaj AK: Safety of implantation of a cardioverter-defibrillator without general anesthesia in an electrophysiology laboratory. Am J Cardiol 75:908–912, 1995.

147. Lipscomb KJ, Linker NJ, Fitzpatrick AP: Subpectoral implantation of a cardioverter defibrillator under local anesthesia. Heart 79:253–255, 1998.

148. Pacifico A, Cedillo-Salazar FR, Nasir N Jr, et al: Conscious sedation with combined hypnotic agents for implantation of implantable cardioverter-defibrillators. J Am Coll Cardiol 30:679–773, 1997.

149. Moerman A, Herregods L, Foubert L, et al: Awareness during anaesthesia for implantable cardioverter defibrillator implantation: Recall of defibrillation shocks. Anaesthesia 50:733–735, 1995.

150. Hunt GB, Ross DL: Comparison of effects of three anesthetic agents on induction of ventricular tachycardia in a canine model of myocardial infarction. Circulation 78:221, 1988.

151. Natale A, Jones DL, Kim Y-H, et al: Effects of lidocaine on defibrillation threshold in the pig: Evidence of anesthesia related increase. PACE 14:1239, 1991.

152. Gill RM, Sweeney RJ, Reid PR: The defibrillation threshold: A comparison of anesthetics and measurements methods. PACE 16:708, 1993.

153. Shepard RB, Goldin MD, Lawrie GM, et al: Automatic implantable cardioverter defibrillator: surgical approaches for implantation. J Card Surg 7(3):208–224, 1992.

154. Watkins L Jr, Taylor E Jr: The surgical aspects of automatic implantable cardioverter-defibrillator implantation. PACE 14(5 Pt 2):953–960, 1991.

155. Watkins L Jr, Guarnieri T, Griffith LS, et al: Implantation of the automatic implantable cardioverter defibrillator. J Card Surg 3(1):1–7, 1998.

156. Daoud EG, Strickberger SA, Man KC, et al: Comparison of early and late complications in patients undergoing coronary artery bypass graft surgery with and without concomitant placement of an implantable cardioverter defibrillator. Am Heart J 130:780–785, 1995.

157. Trappe HJ, Klein H, Wahlers T, et al: Risk and benefit of additional aortocoronary bypass grafting in patients undergoing cardioverter-defibrillator implantation. Am Heart J 127:75–82, 1994.

158. Watkins L Jr, Mirowski M, Mower MM, et al: Automatic defibrillation in man: The initial surgical experience. J Thorac Cardiovasc Surg 82:492, 1981.

159. Troup PJ, Chapman PD, Olinger GN, et al: The implanated defibrillator: Relation of defibrillating lead configuration and clinical variable to defibrillation threshold. J Am Coll Cardiol 6:1315, 1985.

160. Shepard RB, Goldin MD, Lawrie GM, et al: Automatic implantable cardioverter defibrillator: Surgical approaches for implantation. J Cardiac Surg 7:208, 1992.

161. Watkins L Jr, Mirowski M, Mower MM, et al: Implantation of the automatic defibrillator: The subxiphoid approach. Ann Thorac Surg 35:515, 1982.

162. Flaker G, Boley T, Walls J, et al: Comparison of subxiphoid and traditional approaches for ICD implantation. PACE 15:1531, 1992.

163. Beckman DJ, Crevey BJ, Foster PR, et al: Subxiphoid approach for implantable cardioverter defibrillator in patients with previous coronary bypass surgery. PACE 15:1637, 1992.

164. Lawrie GM, Griffin JC, Wyndham CRC: Epicardial implantation of the automatic implantable defibrillator by the left subcostal thoracotomy. PACE 7:1370, 1984.

165. Shahian DM, Williamson WA, Streitz JM Jr, Venditti FJ: Subfascial implantation of implantable cardioverter defibrillator generator. Ann Thorac Surg 54(1):173–174, 1992.

166. O'Neill PG, Lawrie GM, Kaushik RR, et al: Late results of the left subcostal approach for automatic implantable cardioverter. Am J Cardiol 67(5):387–390, 1991.

167. Lawrie GM, Kaushik RR, Pacifico A: Right mini-thoracotomy: An adjunct to left subcostal automatic implantable cardioverter defibrillator implantation. Ann Thorac Surg 47(5):780–781, 1989.

168. Damiano RJ Jr, Foster AH, Ellenbogen KA, et al: Implantation of

169. Obadia JF, Claudel JP, Rescigno G, et al: Subdiaphragmatic implantation of implantable cardioverter defibrillator generator. Ann Thorac Surg 59:239–242, 1995.

170. Shapira N, Cohen AI, Wish M, et al: Transdiaphragmatic implantation of the automatic implantable cardioverter defibrillator. Ann Thorac Surg 48:371, 1989.

171. Frumin H, Goodman GR, Pleatman M: ICD implantation via thoracoscopy without the need for sternotomy or thoracotomy. PACE 16(2):257–260, 1993.

172. Krasna MJ, Buser GA, Flowers JL, et al: Thoracoscopic versus laparoscopic placement of defibrillator patches. Surg Laparosc Endosc 6(2):91–97, 1996.

173. Tobin M, Ching E, Firstenberg M, et al: Thoracoscopy ICD implantation compaired to a subxyphoid approach [Abstract]. Eur J Cardiac Pacing Electrophysiol 4:118, 1994.

174. Saksena S, Parsonnet V: Implantation of a cardioverter/defibrillator without thoracotomy using a triple electrode system. JAMA 259:69, 1988.

175. McCowan R, Maloney J, Wilkoff B, et al: Automatic implantable cardioverter-defibrillator implantation without thoracotomy using an endocardial and submuscular patch system. J Am Coll Cardiol 17:415–421, 1991.

176. Trappe H, Klein H, Fieguth H, et al: Initial experience with a new transvenous defibrillation system. PACE 16:134, 1993.

177. Bhandari AK, Isber N, Estioko M, et al: Efficacy of low-energy T wave shocks for induction of ventricular fibrillation in patients with implantable cardioverter defibrillators. J Electrocardiol 31:31–37, 1998.

178. Saksena S, Tullo NG, Krol RB, Mauro AM: Initial clinical experience with endocardial defibrillation using an implantable cardioverter/defibrillator with a triple-electrode system. Arch Intern Med 149:2333–2339, 1989.

179. Roelke M, O'Nunain SS, Osswald S, et al: Subclavian crush syndrome complicating transvenous cardioverter defibrillator systems. PACE 18(10):1968–1970, 1995.

180. Lawton JS, Wood MA, Gilligan DM, et al: Implantable transvenous cardioverter-defibrillator leads: The dark side. Pacing Clin Electrophysiol 19:1273–1278, 1996.

181. Kirchhoffer JB, Cook JR, Kabell GG, et al, for the Jewel Investigators: Right-sided implantation of defibrillators using nonthoracotomy lead system is feasible. PACE 18(II):874, 1995.

182. Epstein AE, Kay GN, Plumb VJ, et al, for the Endotak Investigators: Elevated defibrillation threshold when right-sided venous access is used for nonthoracotomy implantable defibrillator lead implantation. J Cardiovasc Electrophysiol 6:979–986, 1995.

183. Bardy GH, Yee R, Jung W, for the Active Can Investigators: Multicenter experience with a pectoral unipolar transvenous cardioversion-defibrillation. J Am Coll Cardiol 28:400–410, 1996.

184. Saksena S, DeGroot P, Krol RB, et al: Low-energy endocardial defibrillation using an axillary or a pectoral thoracic electrode location. Circulation 88:2655, 1993.

185. Jordaens L, Vertongen P, van Belleghem Y: A subcutaneous lead array for implantable cardioverter defibrillators. PACE 16:1429, 1993.

186. Bardy GH, Yee R, Jung W, for the Active Can Investigators: Multicenter experience with a pectoral unipolar implantable cardioverter-defibrillator. J Am Coll Cardiol 28:400–410, 1996.

187. Crossley GH, Gayle DD, Bailey JR, et al: Defibrillator twiddler's syndrome causing device failure in a subpectoral transvenous system. Pacing Clin Electrophysiol 19:376–377, 1996.

188. Eastman DP, Selle JG, Reames MK Sr: Technique for subpectoral implantation of cardioverter defibrillators. J Am Coll Surg 181:475–476, 1995.

189. Bardy GH, Yee R, for the International Active Can Investigators: World wide experience with the Jewel 7219C unipolar, single lead active can implantable pacer-cardioverter/defibrillator. PACE 18(II):806, 1995.

190. Foster AH: Technique for implantation of cardioverter defibrillators in the subpectoral position. Ann Thorac Surg 59:764–767, 1995.

cardioverter fibrillators in the post-sternotomy patient. Ann Thorac Surg 53(6):978–983, 1992.

Chapter 26

Approach to Generator Change

Steven P. Kutalek, Bharat K. Kantharia, and J. March Maquilan

At some time in the life of any pacemaker or defibrillator patient, replacement of the pulse generator may be required. Although this is most often the result of the finite life-span of the battery, replacement of the device may be precipitated by such diverse causes as infection,[1–9] erosion,[10] trauma,[11–13] device malfunction or migration,[14–20] and the need for system upgrade (Table 26–1).[21, 22] Lead replacement or revision may also result secondarily in generator change.[23–28] Although device or lead replacement includes surgery, the success of the surgery depends on an accurate preoperative evaluation as well as on good surgical technique. Therefore, this chapter addresses the preoperative evaluation of the patient and pacing or defibrillation system and the surgical process of device replacement and revision.

Because of the variety of indications for pacemaker or defibrillator generator replacement, considerations regarding the approach to be used for generator change or lead revision begin at the initial implantation of the system. Meticulous technique in the positioning of endocardial leads to minimize pacing thresholds and maximize sensing capabilities allows optimal programming of the pacing function of the pulse generator to reduce chronic battery drain, thereby prolonging the life of the generator.[29] Careful lead positioning also reduces the likelihood of lead dislodgment that would require reoperation.[26, 27, 30, 31] Cautious venous entry, lead fixation, lead–generator connection, pocket location, and handling of components enhances long-term pacing and sensing function. Ensuring that coiled leads in the generator pocket are placed posterior to the pulse generator improves the likelihood of expeditious pulse generator replacement without damage to the lead. Bulkier defibrillator leads or lead headers may be placed in the same surgical plane next to the device. Thus, the primary implanting physician prepares the stage for successful reoperation (Table 26–2).

■ SPECIAL CONSIDERATIONS FOR IMPLANTABLE CARDIOVERTER DEFIBRILLATORS

Since the first surgical placement of an implantable cardioverter defibrillator (ICD) in 1980,[32] the role of ICDs in the management of patients with life-threatening ventricular tachyarrhythmias has become well established. Advances in engineering technology and implantation methods—particularly the nonthoracotomy approach—have enabled widespread use of ICDs in clinical practice. Furthermore, the indications for ICD implantation have been expanding. Many patients outlive the life span of their first ICD generator. Like pacemakers, ICDs are also prone to complications such as infection and malfunction, necessitating replacement or revision of generator or leads. Although the approach to ICD generator change and lead evaluation and reoperation can be extrapolated from the approach to pacemaker revision, certain aspects of ICD generator change and revision deserve special consideration. These include indications for replacement or revision, the need to upgrade to more complex algorithms or pacing modes, lead malfunction, inadequate defibrillation thresholds, change of implantation site, and interchangeability of devices from various manufacturers. Each of these issues is addressed in the chapter in relation to special considerations for ICD devices.

■ PATIENT EVALUATION

Noninvasive Evaluation

Before performing a surgical procedure for pacemaker or defibrillator revision or generator replacement, the need for intervention must be documented. Specific indications are approached with a well-defined plan of evaluation.

Table 26–1. Indications for Pacemaker or ICD Generator Replacement

Primary
Generator end of service
    Elective replacement indicators
    Loss of output
    Sensing malfunction
Generator upgrade
    Unipolar to bipolar (pacemaker)
    Single to dual chamber
    Addition of rate modulation
    Need for high-energy ICD
Pocket twitch (especially unipolar)
    Due to generator insulation break
    Due to lead insulation break
    Due to unipolarity of system
Unanticipated generator failure
Device recall

Secondary*
Pocket relocation or generator migration
Pronounced pocket effusion or hematoma
Erosion
Infection of pacing system
Need for lead revision
    High thresholds (pacing or sensing)
    High defibrillation threshold
    Lead conductor fracture
    Lead insulation break
    Trauma
    Loose lead–generator connection
    Myopotential sensing
    Diaphragmatic pacing
    Diaphragmatic sensing
    Change bifurcated bipolar to unipolar pacemaker due to malfunction of one conductor
    Twiddler's syndrome

*These are due to factors other than the pulse generator itself. They require reoperation but may or may not require generator replacement.

Table 26–2. Technical Factors at Initial Device Implantation That May Reduce Need for Reoperation

Tissues
Hemostasis
Secure closure
Pocket large enough for generator and leads

Generator
Integrity of generator insulation
Active surface toward skin (pacemakers)
Set screws secure
Intruding on neither clavicle nor axilla

Leads
Meticulous care in positioning for
    Thresholds: pacing and sensing
    Threshold: defibrillation
    Fixation
Lead selection appropriate for patient
Integrity of lead insulation
Gentle handling of stylets
Secured by anchoring sleeve
Nonabsorbable suture tie
Placement posterior to, or beside, pulse generator
Appropriate connections: (A, V) to generator
Appropriate connections: proximal and distal high-energy coils, array, patch leads fully advanced into generator head
Adapters secure and not kinked
Set screw sealed

Documentation of Pacemaker Pulse Generator Battery Depletion

Most bradycardia pacemaker pulse generators provide direct or indirect indicators of various degrees of battery depletion, documenting the need for enhanced follow-up, elective generator replacement, or incipient battery failure. Additionally, certain nonspecific indicators may alert the physician to early signs of battery wear (Table 26–3). Because most pacemaker patients are followed by means of a transtelephonic monitoring system more frequently than by full evaluation in the physician's office, it is not surprising that battery depletion for permanent pacemaker patients is most often detected through transtelephonic recording.[33–37] Methods for transtelephonic evaluation of defibrillator systems are also being developed to allow interrogation after arrhythmic events and to assess battery capacity.

A change in the magnet-activated paced rate remains the most common indicator of reduced battery output voltage for pacemakers (Table 26–4). Some pacemaker pulse generator models respond to declining voltages through a gradual reduction in magnet-activated pacing rate; reduced rates indicate the need for enhanced follow-up, with still slower rates suggesting elective or obligatory replacement. Other models

demonstrate an abrupt shift in the magnet-activated paced rate at the enhanced follow-up period or at the time of elective replacement. A demand mode switch from DDD to VVI (DOO to VOO in magnet mode) may occur at the elective replacement time or as an obligate replacement indicator for dual-chamber systems before complete battery failure (Table 26–5). Inability to reprogram the device may also occur as the generator approaches obligate replacement time.

In the office, other secondary parameters suggest gradual battery depletion. The usual battery impedance in a new pulse generator is less than 1000 Ω. As lithium iodide batteries are depleted, internal battery impedance increases, providing a secondary indicator (Fig. 26–1). With high internal battery impedance, some devices compensate for reduced

Table 26–3. Pacemaker Battery Depletion Indicators

Primary
Abrupt decrease in magnet-paced rate
Gradual decrease in magnet-paced rate
Mode switch (especially DDD to VVI or DOO to VOO magnet mode)
Abrupt loss of pacing or sensing capability
Interrogated marker of battery depletion

Secondary
Rise in internal battery impedance
Fall in battery voltage
Pulse width stretch
Battery depletion curve

Table 26–4. General Magnet Responses of Pulse Generators

Pacemaker
Battery depletion indicator
  Mode switch (DOO to VOO)
  Rate change
    Gradual
    Abrupt
Mode
  AOO, VOO
    Usual asynchronous operation in single-chamber system
    May represent mode switch of battery depletion
    Noise reversion mode
  DOO
    Usual asynchronous operation in dual-chamber system
  AAT, VVT
    P, R synchronous
  OOO
    Inhibited, especially useful with antitachycardia system to avoid initiation of tachyarrhythmia with magnet application
    Common magnet mode for ICDs
Rate
  Fixed
  Variable
  First few complexes faster
  Last few complexes faster
Output
  Fixed
  Variable
    Voltage or pulse width decremented in first or last few complexes for threshold margin test, or pulse width reduced after magnet withdrawal
Duration
  Continuous as long as magnet applied
  Fixed number of paced complexes

ICD
Inhibition
  Of tachyarrhythmia sensing
  Of pacing output
Reset of tachyarrhythmia sensing
Activation/Inactivation of device

current output by increasing the pulse width to maintain adequate energy delivery to the lead tip. The degree of pulse width stretching is measurable and may be precipitated by high-output pacing; it serves as another secondary indicator of battery depletion. Replacement is not required, however, until more definitive indicators appear, such as a change in magnet-activated pacing rate or a mode switch.

Telemetered battery depletion curves (Fig. 26–2) or internal calculations of anticipated device longevity at current programmed settings, as well as a general knowledge of the expected performance of various generators, assists in anticipating and documenting pacemaker generator end of service. Ultimately, loss of sensing and pacing capabilities occurs with battery exhaustion.

Implantable Cardioverter-Defibrillator Generator Replacement Indicators

Because the rate of defibrillator generator depletion depends on both the frequency of bradycardia pacing and the delivery of high-energy shocks to terminate tachyarrhythmias, the precise longevity of ICD battery systems is more difficult to predict on a clinical basis. Nevertheless, documentation of ICD battery drain remains crucial to the safe function of the defibrillator system. Accordingly, various manufacturers have developed relatively straightforward methods of documenting impending battery depletion for ICDs. These fall into three major categories, namely (1) a measurable reduction in battery voltage that can be acquired through telemetry, (2) an increase in measured charge times to levels that indicate elective replacement time, and (3) various device-specific markers that are indicative of a particular degree of generator depletion (Table 26–6).

Measurement of charge time to a maximal voltage on the device capacitors is the oldest method for estimating the remaining longevity of an ICD. Most early-generation systems included such markers. This method of determining elective replacement time, however, requires fully charging the capacitors and usually necessitates an office visit. Charge times can also be obtained if the device spontaneously charges and delivers therapy at maximum output, but this does not always occur opportunely between office visits.

Recording a reduced battery voltage provides a more readily useful method of determining generator depletion; the value can be obtained telemetrically. This method is now the most common for marking elective replacement time and end of service for ICDs. Specifically, telemetered voltage can be obtained on initial interrogation of the device and may be retrievable transtelephonically.

Some specific ICD models use battery voltage to produce labels that indicate the beginning, middle, or end of service for pulse generators. These labels can be obtained directly through interrogation of the device in the office. End of service is clearly indicated (see Table 26–6).

Regardless of the method used by the device to document an approach to the end of its service, the clinician has the responsibility to increase the frequency of follow-up as the unit nears elective replacement time to ensure continued safe function of the system and protection from tachyarrhythmias. In the event that the patient receives frequent shocks just before the need for device replacement, one must keep in mind that the elective replacement time may occur earlier than was originally anticipated.

Pacing rate		60	ppm
Pacing interval		1003	ms
Cell voltage		2.61	volts
Cell impedance		6.75	KOhms
Cell current		20.9	UA
	ATRIAL (Uni)	VENTRICULAR (UNI)	
Sensitivity	1.6	1.5	mV
Lead impedance	613	504	ohms
Pulse amplitude	2.49	4.97	volts
Pulse width	0.50	0.50	ms
Output current	3.8	9.3	mA
Energy delivered	4.4	20.8	UJ
Charge delivered	1.94	4.66	UC

Figure 26–1. Acquired telemetry data from an Intermedics (Angleton, TX) Cosmos II 284-05 dual-chamber (DDD) pacemaker programmed to the unipolar mode. Cell impedance has increased to 6750 Ω, a secondary indicator of battery depletion. Pulse amplitude and pulse width are maintained. Lead impedance in both chambers is acceptable.

Table 26–5. **Examples of Specific Magnet Responses**

		Mode			Rate (ppm)				
Manufacturer	**Model**	**BOL**	**ERI**	**EOL**	**BOL**	**ERI**	**EOL**	**Output (<ERI)**	**Duration of Magnet Response**
Biotronik	178	DOO	VDD	VOO	PR	PR − 11% (AD)	PR − 11%	PO	Cx
Cardiac Control Systems	505	DOO	DOO	VOO	80[a]	80–70 (AD) (alternate cycles)	50	PO	Cx
Cook	500	VOO	VOO	[d]	100	90 (AD)	[d]	PO	Cx
Cordis	233GL	DOO	DOO	Voo	70	62.5 (AD)	52.5[b]	PO	Cx
CPI	1230	DOO	DOO	DOO	100	90 (AD)	85	PO	Cx
ELA	6034	DOO	DOO	DOO	96	80 (GD)	69.8	PO[c]	Cx
Intermedics	294-09	DOO	VOO	VOO	5C @ 90, then PR	4C @ 90, then 80	80	PW 50% on 5th C	64 C (+ 5C @ 90)
Medtronic	7960	DOO	VOO	[d]	3C @ 100, then 85	65 (AD)	[d]	PW 25% on 3rd C	Cx
Pacesetter	2028L	DOO	DOO	[d]		PR PRI + 100 ms (AD)[d]		PO	Cx
Telectronics	1256	DOO	DOO	DOO	100	82.5 (GD)	80 (GD)[e]	PO	Cx

[a]80 ppm × 16 C, then PR for 16 C, then 80 ppm.

[b]62.5 ppm for serial numbers ≥4000.

[c]Output is increased to 5.0 V and 0.49 ms (if programmed for less than these values) during magnet application, then is reduced to PO for 6 complexes at the magnet rate after magnet removal with shortening of the AV interval.

[d]No specific additional EOL indicator before battery failure.

[e]At EOL, rate response suspends and the device goes to VVI at 63 ppm, nonprogrammable.

AD, abrupt decrease; BOL, beginning of life; C, complexes; Cx, continuous; EOL, end of life; ERI, elective replacement indication; Fx, fixed; GD, gradual decrease—indicated rate defines ERI or EOL; PO, programmed output; ppm, pulses per minute; PR, programmed rate; PRI, programmed rate interval; PW, pulse width.

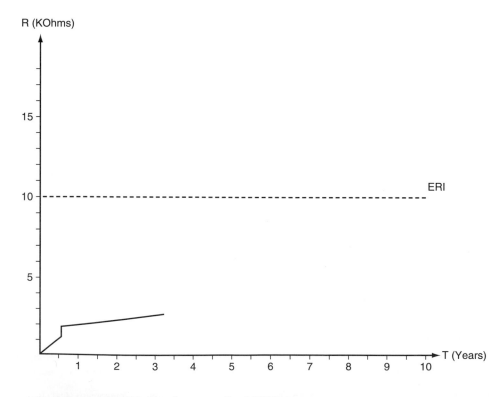

Figure 26–2. Example of a battery depletion curve from an ELA Chorus RM 7034 dual-sensor DDDR pacemaker. The curve graphically presents the true increase in internal battery impedance (R) over time, with an indication of the anticipated impedance at elective replacement time (ERI). Changes in programming that affect battery current drain alter the slope of the battery depletion curve. In this example, the battery impedance has reached about 2.5 KOhms after 3.5 years of use.

Last measured battery impedance was R = 2.5 KOhms
T = time elapsed since initialization.

Table 26–6. Elective Replacement Indicators of Commonly Used ICDs

Manufacturer	Model	Elective Replacement Indicator
Guidant CPI	Ventak 1500, 1510, 1520	CT = 1.2× CT at 8 months*
	Ventak 1550, 1555, 1600	CT = 1.33× BOL CT†
	Ventak 1625, 1630, 1635	Indicated by programmer
	Ventak PRx; 1700, 1715, 1720, 1721, 1725	Indicated by programmer
	Ventak Mini, Mini+ 1740, 1745, 1746	Indicated by programmer
	Ventak Mini II, 1742, 1753, 1762, 1763	Indicated by programmer
	Ventak AV, 1810, 1815	Indicated by programmer
Medtronic	CD, 7201B, 7201D	BV ≤ 4.97V, or second CT ≥ 11 seconds
	JewelCD; 7202C, 7202D, 720E	BV ≤ 4.97V, or second CT ≥ 14.5 seconds
	PCD; 7217B, 7217D	BV ≤ 4.97V, or second CT ≥ 11 seconds
	Jewel PCD; 7218C, 7219C, 7219D, 7219E	BV ≤ 4.91V, or second CT ≥ 14.5 seconds
	Jewel Plus; 2770B, 7220C, 7220D, 7220E	BV ≤ 4.91V, or second CT ≥ 14.5 seconds
	MicroJewel, 7221B, 7221Cx, 722E, 7223Cx	BV ≤ 4.91V, or second CT ≥ 60 seconds
Ventritex	Cadence, V-100, V-110 and V-112 (B, C, D)	BV, 5.1 Volts
	Cadet LT, V-105AC, C, D	BV, 2.55 Volts
	Cadet V-115, AC, B, C, D	BV, 2.55 Volts
	Contour, V-135AC, D, V-145AC, D	BV, 2.55 Volts
Intermedics	Res Q, 101-01, 101-01R	CT = 30 seconds†
	Res-Q Micron, 101-05, 101-09	BV ≤ 4.75 V
Telectronics	Guardian, 4202, 4203	Second CT ≥ 23.5 seconds
	Guardian ATP, 4210	Remaining battery life ≤ 5%
	Guardian ATPII, ATPIII, 4211, 4215	Remaining cell capacity ≤ 20%

BOL, beginning of life; BV, battery voltage; CT, charge time; * both performed during second magnet test, † after capacitor reform.

Documentation of Lead Malfunction

A variety of causes of lead malfunction require reoperation,[29, 38] owing to primary lead dysfunction or secondarily to premature battery depletion as a result of excessive current drain (see Table 26–1). Primary lead malfunction may be due to outer insulation break,[39–45] inner insulation break in a bipolar lead,[46, 47] lead conductor fracture,[11, 13, 48] or lead dislodgment.[26, 27, 30, 31, 49] Current drain may be increased by high pacing thresholds[23, 25, 50] through a need to increase output voltage, by failure to optimize generator output for chronic pacing after lead maturation (about 3 months after implantation), or by inner insulation break with a resultant low pacing impedance; all of these scenarios can result in premature battery depletion. Before reoperation for lead malfunction is performed, consideration should be given to upgrading or replacing the pulse generator, especially if the battery is old.

Lead malfunction can usually be documented by noninvasive telemetric evaluation.[21, 51] A measured bipolar pacing lead impedance below 200 Ω suggests an inner insulation break. An outer insulation break may be the result of lead wear or may have been inadvertently produced during surgery; an inner insulation break between the two coils of a bipolar system occurs most commonly at the subclavian insertion site as the result of crush injury to the lead, especially with leads inserted into the subclavian vein and tied securely in a far medial position in patients with a tight clavicle–first rib space. Telemetry for lead diagnostics may demonstrate markedly low impedance in bipolar pacing in patients with an inner insulation break. The impedance may vary with manipulation of the pacemaker, which causes intermittent shorting of the two lead conductors (Fig. 26–3).

High pacing lead impedance (more than 1200 Ω) may be the result of lead conductor fracture or an incomplete circuit caused by a loose lead–pulse generator connection. The introduction of high-impedance leads makes it essential to compare the impedance at implantation with follow-up impedance measurements. Depending on the point of discontinuity, lead impedance may vary with manipulation of the pulse generator or with respiration. Lead conductor fractures may be evident on chest radiographs or fluoroscopy; however, absence of visual evidence does not exclude lead fracture. A break in the connection of the lead to the generator, or within the lead itself, can produce intermittent loss of energy delivery to the heart. This results in absence of

Pacing rate	68	ppm
Pacing interval	876	ms
Average cell voltage	2.63	volts
Cell impedance	<1.00	KOhms
Sensitivity	8	mV
Lead impedance	41	ohms
Pulse amplitude	7.42	volts
Pulse width	0.45	ms
Output current	96.5	mA
Energy delivered	173.2	UJ
Charge delivered	42.85	UC
Tachycardia detected	No	

Figure 26–3. Acquired telemetry data from an Intermedics Intertach 262-14 VVICP antitachycardia pacemaker connected through a bipolar coaxial lead to the right ventricular apex. Battery voltage and cell impedance are normal. Measured lead impedance of 41 Ω is, however, extremely low. In this patient, measured lead impedance was normal in the supine position but decreased with sitting or when the device was pulled inferiorly. This indicates a break in the inner insulator between the coaxial conductor strands in the area of the clavicle. With movement, the conductors contact one another, resulting in low impedance and preventing delivery of electric current to the heart. Because output voltage is fixed, the low lead impedance results in a high delivered current (96.5 mA) and energy.

pacemaker spikes. Undersensing, or oversensing due to chatter, may also occur with lead conductor fracture.

Lead dislodgment produces intermittent noncapture or failure to sense that may be related to respiration. Pacing thresholds needed to achieve consistent capture may increase significantly. Lead impedance increases or remains unchanged. Fluoroscopy may demonstrate a loose or displaced lead tip but is not always diagnostic.

Special Issues Regarding Implantable Cardioverter-Defibrillator Leads

Evaluation of the ICD generator and its lead system poses a special problem in patients who remain free of arrhythmic events and ICD therapy. The ICD lead remains the weak link in the ICD system for the patient. Oversensing due to diaphragmatic impulses or extraneous signals may lead to inhibition of pacing therapy or to inappropriate "documentation and treatment" of ventricular tachyarrhythmias due to noise sensing (Figs. 26–4 and 26–5).[52] Further, although fracture and degradation of transvenous leads are not as commonly seen as with epicardial ICD lead systems, they can occur with some frequency, necessitating reprogramming or reoperation.[53]

Although depleted battery status is evident on routine ICD follow-up (as described previously and in Table 26–6), and integrity of the ICD lead *pacing* and *sensing* thresholds can be readily evaluated, determining the integrity of the shocking conductors is not as straightforward in current devices. Shocking electrode integrity may be documented by demonstrating a normal shocking lead impedance. Very high shocking electrode impedance measurements may indicate lead discontinuity due to conductor fracture or a lead–generator interface problem. Less severe elevations of high-energy electrode impedance can occur at implantation with inadequate positioning of the high-energy electrodes, leading to reduced current delivery to the heart to terminate arrhythmias.

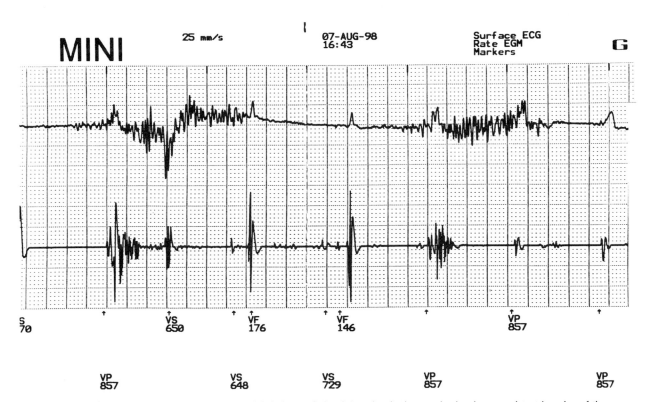

Figure 26–4. Sensing of diaphragmatic myopotential during periods of deep inspiration can lead to inappropriate triggering of the antitachycardia functions of an implantable cardioverter-defibrillator (ICD) (Endotak, CPI, St. Paul, MN). These electrograms are recorded from an ICD placed with a passive-fixation endocardial lead that incorporates integrated bipolar sensing and high-energy shocking coils in the right ventricular apex and the superior vena cava. Surface electrocardiogram, rate-sensing electrograms, and marker channels all record spurious signals that represent inappropriate sensing of extracardiac electrical potentials. The frequency of these signals is high, and they occur after paced events as well as after sensed events. Pacing increases the gain of the device to avoid undersensing low-amplitude signals of ventricular fibrillation.

An underlying paced rhythm exists at a cycle length of 857 msec, but even this is altered by oversensing. The first paced complex (VP 857) is followed by two inappropriately sensed events (VS-650 and VS-648) that inhibit ventricular pacing output. Because the next native QRS complex occurs close to an inappropriately sensed signal, it is interpreted by the device to represent sensing in the ventricular fibrillation zone (VF 176). Following that, another myopotential is inappropriately sensed (VS-729), and the native QRS is again sensed in the VF zone (VF 146). Finally, three sequential paced events occur at intervals of 857 msec, despite the presence of spurious electrical signals, which are not of sufficient amplitude to trigger sensing.

Repetitive events such as these could lead to inappropriate antitachycardia therapies or prolonged periods of inhibition of pacing. This lead was extracted and replaced with an active-fixation endocardial defibrillation lead positioned distally on the lower region of the interventricular septum. (Photography by Todd Forkin, Hahnemann University Hospital, Philadelphia, PA.)

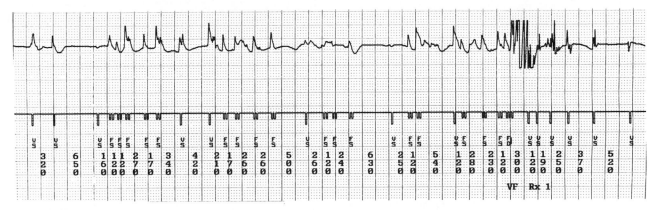

Figure 26–5. Conductor fracture with intermittent contact of the broken ends of the lead wire may result in inappropriate sensing of noise chatter, as demonstrated in this example. Underlying native QRS complexes are difficult to discern. Noise sense intervals vary from 120 to 650 msec. The high degree of variability of sensed intervals, as well as frequent nonphysiologic intervals shorter than 200 msec, lead to the diagnosis of noise sensing. In this example, the number of sensed intervals in the ventricular fibrillation zone is great enough to trigger the VF detection algorithm of the device; this is recorded by the marker channel (FD). Ventricular fibrillation therapy was inappropriately delivered (VF Rx 1). Lead replacement, or placement of a new rate sensing lead, is indicated. The top tracing is a ventricular electrogram, and the bottom tracing is an interpretation channel with interval measurements. (Photography by Todd Forkin, Hahnemann University Hospital, Philadelphia.)

Measuring high-energy electrode impedance has traditionally required delivery of a shock, either for a clinical tachyarrhythmia event or as part of a testing protocol that can be performed noninvasively. In the absence of consensus or strict guidelines for performing noninvasive programmed stimulation routinely during follow-up (when shock electrode integrity may be documented),[54] it is not uncommon for a patient with infrequent shocks to have first documentation of high-energy conductor fracture at the time of presentation for generator replacement. About 10% of patients undergoing ICD generator replacement due to battery depletion may be found to have a previously undetected sensing or defibrillation system failure.[55] The operator hence should test the lead system carefully during the replacement procedure and be prepared to deal with malfunctioning leads at the time of generator change. Newer systems provide the opportunity to measure high-energy lead impedance at device interrogation by the delivery of low-energy pulses through the shocking electrodes; the device then measures impedance in a manner similar to that used for standard pacing and sensing electrodes. The lower-energy impulse delivered by these devices may be more sensitive to the detection of microfractures because higher energies delivered during a shock might readily jump over a microfracture gap, with the device indicating a relatively normal lead impedance.

Determination of Pulse Generator–Lead Interface Malfunction

Pulse generator–lead interface problems can be grouped into three categories, as follows: (1) loose, incomplete, or uninsulated connections; (2) reversal of atrial and ventricular leads in the pulse generator connector block (for ICDs, reversal of shocking electrode polarity may also occur), and (3) improper pulse generator–to-lead match.

A loose pace and sense lead connection should become apparent by noninvasive testing. The device may fail to deliver pacing spikes when appropriate, it may intermittently fail to sense, it may oversense as a result of chatter caused by intermittent contact with the set-screw, or all of these can occur. Atrial and ventricular pace and sense lead problems are similar, although oversensing by an atrial lead can result in inappropriately high tracking rates rather than inhibition of ventricular output. Capture or sensing problems may be exacerbated by manipulation of the device. An uninsulated connection most commonly produces current leakage (an electrical short circuit in the system) that inhibits pacing or sensing. This can occur if a set-screw is not properly insulated or tightened or if sealing rings on the lead header do not prevent body fluid from oozing into the pulse generator connector block around a loosely fitting lead. Leakage around lead header sealing rings may result from a loose lead connection or lead–pulse generator mismatch. Some ICD devices have also used sealing rings around caps placed over set-screws that prevent body fluids from entering to cause a short circuit at the set-screws.

Lead impedance in pulse generator–lead interface problems varies, depending on the specific situation. A loose, unconnected lead that remains in the pulse generator connector block, so that lead header sealing rings prevent fluid from entering, causes a break in the electric circuit and thus a very high impedance. If fluid enters the pulse generator connector block around a loose lead or at the level of a set-screw and maintains contact with body fluids, however, the resultant electric short circuit can produce a very low measured impedance. As with lead fractures, impedance can vary with manipulation of the device.

Reversed lead connections (i.e., atrial lead in the ventricular port, and vice versa) should be readily evident before leaving the implantation laboratory, allowing immediate correction. Some atrial and ventricular leads are marked to allow easy identification; however, it is not uncommon to place "generic" leads into both chambers, especially straight screw-in leads, which may not be so marked. Likewise, atrial and ventricular lead headers for insertion into ICD ports are both of the IS-1 standard, so that the implanter must exercise care in placing these leads properly into the appropriate locations in the ICD generator connector block.

It is also possible, in patients in whom a pacemaker or ICD remains inhibited because of native electrical activity, to see no pacing spikes initially after implantation. To be certain that the pulse generator–lead system functions appropriately immediately after implantation, the device should be programmed to an atrioventricular (AV) delay shorter than the intrinsic PR interval, or (for a pacemaker) a magnet should be placed over the device after the leads are attached, to document appropriate function before the pocket is closed. Caution exercised at implantation should avoid reversed leads; for example, we always connect the ventricular lead first to ensure pacing in the proper chamber.

Beyond ensuring the presence of adequate and appropriate lead connections to the pulse generator, the battery connector block and leads must be compatible[56–58] (see later section). Incompatibility can result in fluid leakage or loose connections, with resultant loss of pace and sense or shocking capabilities, requiring reoperation.

Detection of Need for Reoperation for Other Reasons

Other indications for pacemaker or ICD generator replacement or lead revision (see Table 26–1) are generally apparent through careful patient evaluation. Abrupt pulse generator failure with no antecedent sign of battery depletion is rare but can occur, producing symptoms in pacemaker-dependent patients. In others, abnormal pacing output or rate, lack of pacing output, or inappropriate sensing due to generator malfunction may be detected transtelephonically or in the office.[17] Of particular importance to ICD patients are the possibilities of no output when required to terminate tachyarrhythmias, inappropriate shocks due to oversensing of diaphragmatic or lead chatter artifact (see Figs. 26–4 and 26–5), and oversensing of extraneous electromagnetic signals, such as surveillance systems and cellular phones, that can be sensed as ventricular fibrillation or inhibit ventricular pacing output.[59, 60]

Development of pacemaker syndrome in patients with implanted ventricular demand (VVI), ventricular rate-responsive (VVIR), or atrial rate-responsive (AAIR)[22] pacemakers should be apparent through the history and physical examination, although confirmatory blood pressure or cardiac output measurements may be required. Documentation of hemodynamic improvement with dual-chamber synchronization may require placement of a temporary atrial lead before reoperation for upgrading to a dual-chamber system. Pacemaker syndrome occurring with an implanted functioning dual-chamber pacemaker must be managed by reprogramming.[61, 62]

Interchangeability of Products From Different Manufacturers

Until the present time, unlike leads available in pacemaker systems, most ICD leads from different manufacturers had been 100% compatible only with ICD pulse generators from the same manufacturer. The operator, therefore, has had limited ability to choose different components of the ICD system to meet patient needs. More recently, manufacturers have adhered to more standard header designs for ICDs, including IS-1 ports for the pace and sense lead heads from both atrial and ventricular leads. Defibrillation ports now also follow a standard for defibrillation lead headers, namely DF-1, which involves a 6.5-mm unipolar lead head with

sealing rings. For procedures involving old, nonstandard ICD connector blocks, however, the operator must be familiar with the existing system of leads and generator in the patient before surgery, and technical support from the manufacturer at the time of the operation may be required. A full range of adapters, or various header designs, to mate a replacement generator to the existing leads must be available. Attention to tight and proper connections between the generator and the lead, and any adapters and lead extenders, avoid malfunction and current leak. Although older adapters used an uncured medical adhesive to seal set-screws in the connector block of the device, newer adapters use set-screw seals similar to those found in pacemaker pulse generators.

Special Indications for Implantable Cardioverter-Defibrillator Generator Replacement

In addition to the indications outlined in Table 26–1, the ICD generator may need to be replaced for the following reasons:

Malfunction of the Generator With or Without Lead Malfunction. Hardware or software errors in the ICD generator—or, more commonly, defective ICD leads—may result in malfunction of the ICD system. The overall incidence of lead-related complications has been reported in a range of 2% to 28%.[63, 64] These complications may manifest as being due to inappropriate shocks resulting from oversensing of noise (see Fig. 26–5) or to ineffective shocks from the shunting of defibrillation energy as a result of an inner insulator breach.

Upgrading the Device to Incorporate Tiered Therapy and Multiple Zones of Therapy. Older devices incorporated monophasic shock energy for defibrillation, which was more likely to achieve an inadequate defibrillation threshold (DFT) compared with biphasic lead systems. The success of current ICD generators is attributed primarily to the use of biphasic shocking waveforms.[65–68] Furthermore, certain older ICD systems were designed to deliver only shock therapy. These generators may require replacement by newer ICDs, which offer more sophisticated therapies, including tiered therapies for different arrhythmia zones, antitachycardia pacing, and pacing for bradyarrhythmia.

Upgrading to a Higher-Energy Device, or by Addition of Hardware, for an Inadequate Defibrillation Threshold. Occasionally, through invasive or noninvasive testing, the physician determines that the best function of the device may be achieved through a change in its hardware configuration. This may involve reoperation to place a generator capable of delivering higher defibrillation energy to respond to an elevated DFT, repositioning of the right ventricular apical (RVA) lead, or the addition of various other lead systems, including superior vena cava coils or subcutaneous arrays or patches. Clearly, location of the RVA lead as close to the cardiac apex as possible affords the lowest DFT. Similarly, addition of various other leads to better distribute current around the heart can also reduce the DFT,[69, 70] often concomitantly reducing shocking electrode impedance. Finally, if these invasive adjustments fail to reduce the DFT, waveform adjustments[65] or replacement of the pulse generator with a higher-energy system may be warranted.

Many patients with ICDs continue to require treatment

with antiarrhythmic medications, which can have an effect on the appropriate functioning of ICDs. The most common antiarrhythmia–ICD interaction observed is that of elevation of the DFT. This is particularly evident with potent sodium channel–blocking drugs and with amiodarone.[71, 72] In this regard, reoperation may be required for antiarrhythmic drug changes that lead to substantial alterations in the DFT, although elimination of the offending medication provides a more straightforward solution. When that is not possible, the physician may consider use of a device that delivers high energy for defibrillation. "Active can" technology, in which the ICD pulse generator can acts as an active electrode in the system, also improves defibrillation ability.

Upgrading to Incorporate Dual-Chamber Pacing Capability. With an established role for β-blockers in the treatment of congestive heart failure and coronary artery disease, as well as a baseline frequency of developing sinus node dysfunction or AV conduction disorders, substantial numbers of patients with implanted defibrillators require dual-chamber bradycardia pacing backup. This problem is easily resolved in the new implant but can require considerable deliberation when substantial hardware is already in place. Several scenarios may be encountered, each with unique potential solutions. Some of these situations, with possible approaches, are as follows:

The patient may have a previously implanted abdominal single-chamber ICD with a fully functional epicardial lead system. In this situation, the operator has three primary options, namely (1) place an endocardial atrial pacing lead through the subclavian system and tunnel the lead subcutaneously to the abdominal pocket, while upgrading the device to a dual-chamber ICD; (2) abandon the abdominal ICD and place an entirely new AV sequential ICD system in the pectoral area; or (3) place a totally separate dual-chamber permanent pacemaker system with atrial and ventricular leads and perform device interaction testing to ensure that neither of the two devices inhibits the other.

There are various advantages and disadvantages of each of these techniques: (1) The advantage of long-term stability of thresholds for endocardial pace and sense leads speaks for the approach of adding an endocardial atrial lead and tunneling it to the abdomen, but it also requires that the lead be long enough to tunnel to the abdominal site. This makes manipulation and positioning of the lead in the atrium more challenging. Alternatively, a lead extender may be attached to a shorter lead, but this adds another weak link in the system in the form of an adapter. Finally, this approach requires opening both the abdominal pocket and the subclavian site simultaneously; this could increase the risk for cross-infection of the abdominal site. Accordingly, we prefer not to have two pockets open at the same time, especially when one involves an epicardial lead system, where infection could be disastrous. (2) Abandoning the abdominal site altogether may be the preferred technique because it avoids the need to open two pockets simultaneously; it also eliminates the need to depend on *any* epicardial leads, which have a higher failure rate than endocardial leads. The new pulse generator and lead system are placed in the standard manner in the pectoral area, and DFT testing is performed at implantation; the previous abdominal pocket remains closed at

this operative setting, eliminating the possibility of cross-infection between sites. Electrical shielding afforded by the epicardial patches may affect the endocardial DFT. This problem may well be offset, however, by the improved long-term reliability of the endocardial lead system. The abdominal generator may be turned off and left in place, or it can be removed at a separate operative setting. This approach is particularly useful in patients in whom a new high-energy ventricular coil is needed, which can be placed endocardially. (3) Placement of a totally endocardial dual-chamber pacemaker system with atrial and ventricular bradycardia pacing leads also avoids the need to open both pockets simultaneously; it affords the advantages of prolonging ICD battery life (through a separate pacemaker battery) and provides consistent and separate bradycardia pacing backup through a device designed primarily for bradycardia support. Implantation of a separate pacemaker and an ICD may, however, lead to various device–device interactions, including undersensing of ventricular fibrillation.[72] The availability of combined dual-chamber pacemaker and ICD systems should reduce the physician's concern about device interaction.

Change of Implantation Site. Older ICD generators, because of their bulky nature, were routinely implanted in the abdominal wall. With the availability of active can electrodes and ICD generators of smaller size, consideration should be given to changing the implantation site to the pectoral area when leads need to be revised. This was addressed previously with respect to placement of atrial leads; it should also be considered when ventricular lead malfunction necessitates reoperation. One example of this situation includes malfunction of epicardial ventricular sensing electrodes, especially due to conductor fracture, high pacing threshold, or oversensing. Options here include placing a single ventricular endocardial sensing electrode, tunneling it to the abdominal pocket, or abandoning the abdominal pocket to place an entirely new and complete endocardial ICD system in a pectoral location. We prefer the latter approach, again because it avoids the need to open both pockets simultaneously in a patient with epicardial leads and patches, in whom infection could be devastating.

Implantation site may also need to be changed in the event of incipient erosion, or outright infection, of the ICD site. Clearly, a staged approach here is most useful. Unless the site is infected with a malignant organism such as *Staphylococcus aureus*, one should consider revision of the pocket or removal of the pulse generator, under appropriate antibiotic coverage, followed at a separate surgical procedure by implantation of a pectoral ICD system. Again, both pockets should not be opened at the same operation. Most commonly, removal of the entire system is required for cure of the infection.

Tunneling a lead from an abdominal location to one in the pectoral area can damage the tunneled lead, especially the header. There is no definitive way to avoid this risk, although gentleness with respect to lead manipulation and use of a standard dilator or tunneling tool during this occasionally difficult procedure reduces the tendency to damage. Usually, the lead needs first to be positioned in the ventricle by manipulating it at the shoulder because a long lead would be difficult to maneuver from an abdominal location through

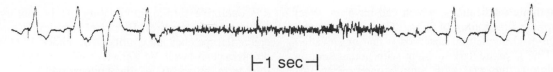

├─1 sec─┤

Figure 26–6. Myopotential inhibition in a unipolar dual-chamber pacing system induced by pectoral muscle contraction in a patient who noted recurrent lightheadedness with activity. Atrial sensitivity is programmed to 0.5 mV and ventricular sensitivity to 2.5 mV. Two atrially tracked complexes are followed by a ventricular premature depolarization. The fourth QRS complex occurs early as a result of atrial myopotential tracking. Thereafter, ventricular pacing output is inhibited by myopotentials for nearly 6 seconds, after which normal DDD function resumes. Intrinsic QRS complexes occurring during the period of inhibition may be obscured by myopotential activity. Programming the ventricular sensitivity to 5 mV avoided myopotential inhibition and the need for lead revision. Although atrial sensitivity could not be adjusted owing to the low intrinsic P-wave amplitude, atrial myopotential tracking remained asymptomatic.

a tunnel. Only after it is carefully positioned can it be tunneled; this means, therefore, that the connector head of the lead will be tunneled from the shoulder to the abdominal pocket. This can place significant stress on the lead connector, which could damage it. When pre-existing tunneled leads need to be replaced, the tract can be dilated using extraction sheaths, although this procedure is time-consuming and complex. Whenever possible, adapters should be avoided because they merely add another weak link in the chain of possibilities for lead malfunction.

Complications Requiring Pacemaker or Implantable Cardioverter-Defibrillator Reoperation

Reoperation may be required for complications resulting from the initial implantation procedure.[10, 15, 16, 73–80] Decisions about surgery in patients with large unresolving pocket hematomas or effusions, cardiac chamber perforation by a lead, or a need to reposition the pulse generator must be made on an individual basis. Most small to moderate hematomas resolve; the risk of secondarily introducing infection through reoperation or aspiration can thus be avoided. Large hematomas or effusions that do not resolve and that compromise the blood supply through pressure on the overlying skin of the pacemaker or ICD pocket may require evacuation; however, primary closure should be attempted because the pocket cannot be left open with a device in place. Bolus dosing of heparin and large loading doses of warfarin should be avoided to reduce hematoma risk.

Pocket twitch (due to lead insulation break, loose lead–generator connection, exposed set-screw, battery insulation break, inverted unipolar pacemaker pulse generator, or the need for high-output pacing in a unipolar system), diaphragmatic pacing, or myopotential pacing or inhibition[81] (Fig. 26–6) may require repeat surgical intervention if such problems cannot be solved by reprogramming.

Identification of Pulse Generator Make and Model

The most straightforward means of identifying a pulse generator showing signs of malfunction or operating in a mode suggesting end of service is to obtain information directly from the patient (Table 26–7). An identification card is provided by the manufacturer for each pacemaker and ICD patient, specifying the type of device, the model and serial number, implantation date, the implanting or following physician, and often the lead model and serial numbers. This information may also be obtained from records kept by the

implanting physician, the following physician, the transtelephonic service that follows the patient, or the institution at which the device was placed. If none of these sources of information is helpful, alternative methods must be used to identify the pulse generator. Identification of the make and model of the existing pulse generator is crucial to determine its true functional status and to have the necessary information to select a replacement or upgraded device or compatible lead system. In the rare situation in which a pulse generator cannot be identified before surgery, the implanting physician must have available a full array of leads, generators, and adapters at the time of reoperation.

Magnet Response. The response of a bradycardia pacemaker pulse generator to placement of a magnet adjacent to the device can assist in the identification of its manufacturer

Table 26–7. Identification of the Pulse Generator

Implant Data
ID card
Transtelephonic monitoring records
Manufacturer's implant records
Following physician's records

Noninvasive Testing
Size, shape, thickness
Magnet response (pacemakers)
Interrogation (if manufacturer identified)

Fluoroscopy
Size, shape
Connector block
    Unipolar or bipolar (pacing)
    Single or dual chamber
    Number of ICD lead ports
Identifying markings/codes

Lead
    Unipolar or bipolar (pacing)
    Active or passive fixation
    Number of high-energy coils

Invasive
Direct identification of pulse generator
Lead
    Manufacturer code and serial number code
    Type of connector
    Size of lead header

(Fig. 26–7; see Table 26–5). Most pacemaker pulse generators respond to magnet application by entering a fixed-rate single-chamber or dual-chamber pacing mode corresponding to the type of generator and the programmed mode. Magnet rates vary among manufacturers and may provide a clue to the origin of the device. To undergo a magnet-activated test, the patient must be connected to an electrocardiographic recorder *before* the magnet is applied and remain connected until after the magnet is removed. The first few paced complexes after magnet application may occur at a rate or an output other than that seen later in the recording, providing identification data as well as information regarding the integrity of the pulse generator and lead system (e.g., the delivered pulse width may be reduced during the first few paced complexes to ensure that capture still occurs with an adequate safety margin). Furthermore, with constant magnet application over the pacemaker, some devices continue to pace at a fixed rate, whereas pacing ceases after a programmed number of intervals in others. Devices temporarily reprogrammed to a backup mode by electrical interference (e.g., electrocautery during surgery) may exhibit magnet responses that vary from the standard for devices that are not in a backup mode.

Radiographic or Fluoroscopic Identification of the Pulse Generator. Most pulse generators—both pacemakers and ICDs—can be identified by their appearance under radiography. The shape and size of the generator may characterize a particular manufacturer (e.g., square, oval, elongated ellipse, round). Pulse generator shape can vary significantly from one device model to another, however, even when produced by the same manufacturer. Considering that the life span of some pacemaker devices may exceed 10 or 12 years, various shapes and sizes may be encountered.

More specific to identification of the pulse generator are radiopaque markings placed near the connector block that code for manufacturer and device model. These markings appear under fluoroscopic or radiographic examination when the device is positioned perpendicular to the x-ray beam (Fig. 26–8).

The shape and orientation of internal components, which can often be identified radiographically, provide further clues to the device type, manufacturer, and model. Comparison of these radiographic features (size and shape, identification markings, internal components) with compiled x-ray photographs available from manufacturers facilitates identification of the pulse generator.

Radiographic or Fluoroscopic Identification of Leads. Radiographic examination of leads serves two purposes.[82] First, it allows the physician to ascertain the presence of unipolar versus bipolar distal electrodes and, frequently, the fixation mechanism. Distal active-fixation screws may be evident by their radiographic appearance, whereas passive-fixation leads often demonstrate a bulbous tip. Second, radiographic examination identifies evident lead conductor fractures where the conductor has clearly separated, leaving a gap; this may require magnified views. Lead information of this sort is important for programming (bipolar versus unipolar), for selecting an appropriately compatible generator, and for identifying leads for extraction. Fluoroscopy also gives some indication of the degree of fibrosis evident through the course of the lead, information that could be useful if extraction is required.

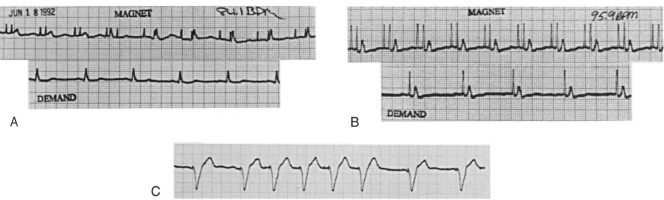

Figure 26–7. Examples of normal pacemaker generator magnet response. Tracings A and B were recorded transtelephonically during routine follow-up. Upper tracings in both A and B show magnet response (DOO), and lower tracings show demand mode with the magnet off. Tracing C was recorded by real-time surface electrocardiography at follow-up in the office. *A,* Representative tracings from Medtronic dual-chamber pacing systems, here from a model 7070 Synergyst II device programmed DDD. The first three atrioventricular (AV) sequentially paced complexes are delivered at a rate 10% higher than the magnet rate; the AV interval is shortened to ensure both atrial and ventricular capture. The first two AV complexes are delivered at programmed atrial and ventricular outputs, whereas the delivered pulse width of the third complex is reduced by 25% ("threshold margin test"). Thereafter, the device delivers AV sequentially paced complexes at a fixed rate of approximately 85 bpm at programmed output. The device in this example remains entirely inhibited in the demand mode. *B,* Representative tracings from ELA dual-chamber pacing systems, here from a model 6034 Chorus device programmed DDD. Magnet application results in fixed-rate DOO pacing at a rate of 96 bpm at the programmed AV interval. The AV interval in this example is short owing to activation of the rate-adaptive AV delay. Output during magnet application may be increased but reverts to programmed levels for six complexes after magnet withdrawal (see Table 26–5). The pacemaker appropriately tracks in the demand mode. *C,* Representative electrocardiographic recording from Intermedics dual-chamber pacing systems, here from a model 294-03 Relay device programmed DDD. The first four complexes are delivered at 90 bpm with a shortened AV delay. Programmed pulse width for the fourth complex is reduced by 50%. Thereafter, the device delivers AV sequential paced complexes in a fixed mode (DOO) at the programmed rate while the magnet remains in place for a total of 60 AV complexes in the DOO mode.

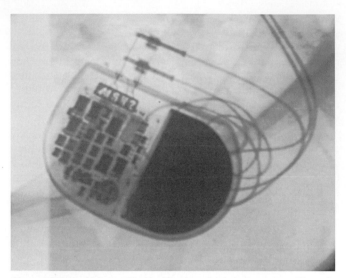

Figure 26–8. Radiographic identification of a pulse generator. The unit is clearly connected to two leads, and each lead has only a single electrically active pole (i.e., unipolar). Although the shape and arrangement of electronic components assist in identification, the specific radiopaque code block inside the pulse generator provides the primary means of identifying the device. Here, a Medtronic logo, followed by S W 2, indicates that the pulse generator is a Synergyst II model 7071 DDDR unit with a connector block that will accept two (atrial and ventricular) 5-mm or 6-mm unipolar leads.

Radiography of leads must involve an examination of the insertion site (e.g., subclavian, cephalic, jugular, or epicardial for some ICD systems) for acute bends or fractures in the lead, the location of lead coils beneath the pulse generator in the event that they need to be freed for lead repositioning or extraction, the position of the pulse generator connector block, and a general preview of the character of the connector block–lead interface (see Fig. 26–8). Fluoroscopically, the lead should be examined throughout its course for kinking, fracture, or excessive tension as well as for fixation at the distal tip. A thorough radiographic examination of lead integrity and pulse generator–lead interface before reoperation in pacemaker and ICD patients saves much distress when the pocket is opened.

Invasive Evaluation

After as much information as possible has been gathered noninvasively regarding the hardware of the pacing system and functional status of all its components, further invasive evaluation may proceed at the time of reoperation. Invasive evaluation does not supplant noninvasive analysis but adds to it. Invasive evaluation involves (1) measuring the functional capacity of implanted leads, (2) examining the structural integrity of leads and the lead–generator interface, and (3) venography.

Measuring the Functional Capacity of Implanted Leads

By far one of the most crucial parts of invasive analysis during reoperation involves measurement of pacing, sensing, and DFTs in existing chronic leads. Vigorous noninvasive evaluation should provide the operator with a significant amount of information regarding lead viability and func-

tional status as well as a determination of pulse generator end of life.[28, 29, 35, 43, 51] Verification of lead integrity and precise DFT determination must, however, be performed at reoperation. If surgery is undertaken for pulse generator replacement, demonstrating viability of existing leads is vital to the appropriate long-term performance of the new battery. Surgery for lead repair or revision itself involves extensive testing of chronic leads to confirm the lead as the source of malfunction, ensure normal operation of other leads, and evaluate new leads for optimal positioning inside the heart.

After the pacemaker or ICD pocket is opened, the pulse generator is disconnected from the leads to enable testing of lead sensing and pacing functional capacity.[83] Disconnecting the lead from the pulse generator must be done cautiously in pacemaker-dependent patients; to avoid prolonged ventricular asystole, the operator must be prepared to connect the lead immediately to a cable attached to a functioning external pacing system. The external device should be activated and should be delivering pacing impulses before the ventricular lead is disconnected from the pulse generator in a pacemaker-dependent patient. Alternatively, although it is not usually necessary, a temporary pacing wire may be placed before disconnecting the lead in a pacemaker-dependent patient; such additional instrumentation, however, may increase the risk of infection. Of course, the operator must exercise care in the removal of the pulse generator and dissection of the lead to maintain lead integrity.

Invasive Testing of the Sensing and Pacing Capabilities of Chronically Implanted Leads

One of the most important aspects of invasive testing involves measurement of pacing and sensing thresholds in chronically implanted pacemaker and ICD leads. Chronic pace and sense lead thresholds rarely remain as low as those at initial lead implantation. Most leads show some deterioration in pacing and sensing thresholds during the first 4 to 8 weeks after implantation, then reach a relatively stable level for the long term.[23, 50] It is possible, however, for chronic thresholds to continue to increase over time, a change that may not be recognized by transtelephonic monitoring alone. The change in chronic threshold from baseline appears greatest with active-fixation, non–steroid-eluting leads; threshold increases are reduced with passive-fixation and steroid-eluting leads, even if the steroid is applied to active-fixation systems. Noninvasive testing should give the operator some clues to the usefulness of chronic leads, but invasive testing confirms their functional utility.

Both atrial and ventricular leads must be tested. If bipolar, they should be evaluated in both unipolar and bipolar configurations. The external pacing analyzer is connected to the lead; pacing and sensing thresholds and lead impedance are determined. The voltage pacing threshold at a fixed pulse width is recorded as that which produces reliable capture. Delivered current can then be measured. Pacing lead impedance is best determined at an increased output voltage (e.g., 5 V) to ensure accuracy.

Low-voltage pacing thresholds are desirable for chronic leads. This allows programming of the pulse generator output to a reduced level, enhancing battery longevity. For leads that have been in place for several years, the operator may decide to accept a pacing threshold (at 0.5-msec pulse width) of up to 2.5 V because this provides a two-times pacing safety margin for most pulse generators and because chronic leads generally show little additional increase in threshold over time. However, a pacing threshold of 2.5 V that occurs early after implantation (e.g., within 6 months) may not be acceptable. This situation suggests excessive early fibrosis around the lead tip and the possibility of developing exit block and noncapture in the future if the pacing threshold continues to increase. Care at initial implantation helps ensure lower chronic pacing thresholds and improved sensing capabilities.

Thresholds for sensing likewise tend to increase after lead implantation. Acceptable measurable intracardiac electrogram amplitudes depend on the maximum programmable sensitivity of the new pulse generator. For most systems, P-wave amplitude of 1 mV or more and R-wave amplitude of 3 mV or more constitute minimally acceptable chronic values. Such low amplitudes, however, leave little room for further deterioration in lead function. Values of 1.5 mV or more and of 4 mV or more for P and R sensing, respectively, provide an additional safety margin. If atrial or ventricular ectopy is present, the operator should determine electrogram amplitude of ectopic complexes to ensure that they will be sensed by the pacemaker. In patients with paroxysmal atrial fibrillation, excellent atrial sensing may be required to detect atrial fibrillation reliably when it occurs, without signal dropout. Higher-amplitude electrograms are required for unipolar (versus bipolar) leads to allow programming of lower sensitivities to avoid myopotential sensing interference.

Inadequate sensing or pacing thresholds at the time of generator replacement are indications for placement of a new lead in the affected chamber. This may entail capping an old lead while leaving it in place or removing it. The new lead can usually be placed through the same subclavian vein, although it is preferable to avoid having too many leads (especially more than three) pass through the same vessel, to reduce the chance of venous occlusion and thrombosis. A single new lead may also be placed through the internal jugular vein, external jugular vein, or contralateral subclavian vein. The proximal tip can be tunneled to the original pocket to meet a second, functional chronic lead for a dual-chamber pacemaker system if required. Alternatively, an entirely new generator or lead system may be placed on the contralateral side.[84]

Invasive Testing of the Defibrillation Capability of Chronically Implanted High-Energy Leads

ICD lead DFT testing can be performed after evaluation of the pace and sense functions of the multifunctional lead and proceeds according to standard DFT testing techniques. Stability of the intracardiac electrogram recording should be ensured, and visual inspection should demonstrate no significant abnormalities in lead appearance, consistent with lead structural integrity.

Examining the Structural Integrity of Leads and the Lead–Generator Interface

Visual inspection provides clues to lead integrity. Fluid inside the lead body suggests an insulation break. Undue tension on the lead near the fixation site may cause kinking, conductor uncoiling, conductor fracture, or thinning of the electric insulator. A hazy appearance of the insulator surrounding an area of tension or repeated stress is common in older leads. This represents surface erosion of the lead insulator and does not itself imply lead malfunction. It should, however, alert the operator to the possibility of lead damage in areas of stress to the insulation. An examination of the suture location ensures that the ligature remains around the suture sleeve, and gentle tension on the lead body ensures its fixation at the venous entry site. Visual inspection of the specific course of a coiled lead in the pocket may be hampered by a significant thickness of overlying capsule scar; fluoroscopy can assist in this regard.[39–42]

Direct examination of the lead connector can assist in the identification of the lead model if not previously known.[56–58] This is particularly important for lead models that have been found to have excessive premature failure rates; such leads in the ventricular position should be replaced in pacemaker-dependent patients.

Venography

Venography is not commonly required as part of the device replacement procedure. It does, however, play an important role when insertion of replacement leads into the subclavian vein is rendered difficult because it can ensure patency of the subclavian and superior vena cava systems, demonstrate the point of venous occlusion, or show the course of the axillary venous system for direct access.

Venography is indicated when the subclavian or cephalic veins cannot be accessed (to demonstrate their locations) and when the veins are accessed but a guide wire cannot be passed into the superior vena cava. Inability to access the subclavian vein that carries a chronically implanted lead suggests either an incorrect needle insertion angle or an occluded subclavian or innominate venous system.[85–89] Finding an appropriate location to insert the access needle can be facilitated by advancing the needle fluoroscopically in the direction of the chronic electrode site under the clavicle, taking care not to damage the chronic lead. The vein should be approached with the bevel of the needle facing the chronic lead. If access is not possible, venography may provide better definition of the course of the subclavian vein. In this situation, radiopaque dye must be injected distal to the subclavian vein, that is, into the basilic or median cubital vein.

Occasionally, access to the subclavian vein is possible, but the guide wire will not pass freely to the superior vena cava. Assuming adequate needle placement in the vessel, this suggests proximal venous occlusion.[90–94] Venography demonstrates whether occlusion is indeed present and the site of occlusion. Chronic venous occlusion may occur asymptomatically concomitant with the development of collateral venous circulation around the shoulder. Delineation of the location and length of occlusion indicates to the operator an appropriate needle insertion site for placement of a new lead. It also ensures patency of the superior vena cava. Dye is injected directly into the subclavian vein. Occlusion of the subclavian system proximal to the junction of the internal jugular vein excludes the ipsilateral jugular system as an alternative site for a new lead. Alternatively, if the subclavian vein is occluded and the internal jugular vein remains patent, a new lead may still be placed using the jugular approach. Occlusion of the superior vena cava precludes the use of any new endocardial lead placed from a superior site unless dilated after lead extraction.[95]

Table 26–8. **Common Endocardial Lead Connector Configurations**

Designation	Unipolar/ Bipolar	Linear/ Bifurcated (Bipolar)	Pin: Long/ Short	Connector Diameter (mm)	Sealing Rings	Fixation Active/ Passive	Atrial J Available
IS-1	U or B	L	S	3.2	Yes	A or P	Yes
VS-1	U or B	L	S or L*	3.2	Yes	A or P	Yes
3.2-mm low profile	U or B	L	L	3.2	Yes or No	A or P	Yes
5-mm	U	—	L	5	Yes	A or P	Yes
5-mm	B	B	L	5	Yes	A or P	Yes
6-mm	U or B	L or B	S or L	6	Yes	A or P	Yes
DF-1	U	—	S	3.2	Yes	N/A	No

IS-1, International Standard for pacemaker lead connectors; DF-1, Standard for high energy defibrillator lead connectors; VS-1, Voluntary Standard for pacemaker lead connectors.

Anomalies of the left superior vena cava (which may enter the coronary sinus) make placement of right ventricular endocardial leads difficult or impossible.[96, 97] Venography defines the anatomy of the venous system in such a situation, which may be suggested by an unusual intravascular guide wire course. Finally, leakage of venography dye into perivascular tissues or into the pericardial space suggests vessel or cardiac chamber perforation, respectively.

The technique is performed by injecting 10 to 20 mL of radiopaque dye (a 50% dilution generally suffices) into a vein distal to the occlusion site. The dye may be injected directly into the subclavian vein if accessed, or into the antecubital or brachial vein if subclavian access is not possible. Fluoroscopy and permanent storage of images is necessary to evaluate flow.

■ GENERATOR LEAD ADAPTABILITY

Lead Connectors

Replacing a pulse generator onto one or more chronic leads requires that the pulse generator connector block be compatible with the proximal lead tip.[56–58] Through years of development by multiple manufacturers, pacemaker leads have evolved to an International Standard (IS-1) proximal lead connector configuration, which involves the following: (1) a

3.2-mm lead connector with a short pin that is electrically connected to the distal electrode tip, (2) a lead connector ring wired to the proximal pacing pole (the ring is electrically active in a bipolar lead), and (3) sealing rings. The proximal lead connector configuration is the same for unipolar or bipolar leads, except that the ring is inactive in unipolar leads. Modern pulse generators have connector block specifications that conform to IS-1 leads and that also fit the prior Voluntary Standard (VS-1) lead type. Thus, generator replacement onto implanted leads of either of these two types poses no difficulty because of the wide array of compatible pulse generators from multiple manufacturers.

In like manner, ICD leads have evolved to incorporate IS-1 pace and sense connectors with concomitant IS-1 atrial and ventricular ports in the generator connector block to attach these leads. Early-generation ICDs, however, used a wide variety of lead port sizes and configurations, requiring the operator to have available generators with various header port sizes, adapters, and upsizing sleeves for reoperation of old ICD generators implanted before the adoption of a uniform standard.

High-energy defibrillation lead headers have also evolved into a standard configuration, DF-1, including the following: (1) a lead pin that is electrically connected to the corresponding high-energy coil or patch, (2) sealing rings, and (3) a single lead head for each coil of an endocardial lead to allow

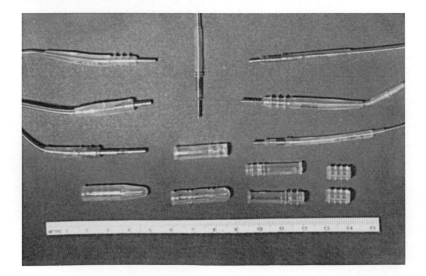

Figure 26–9. A variety of pacemaker lead connectors *(top)*, nonconducting adapters *(bottom right, five)*, and lead caps *(bottom left, two)*. Lead connectors shown are *(clockwise from bottom left)*: Intermedics 6-mm linear bipolar, Intermedics 6-mm unipolar, Medtronic 5-mm unipolar, Cordis 3.2-mm linear bipolar, Pacesetter IS-1, Medtronic atrial 5-mm unipolar, Medtronic IS-1. Lead caps include 5-mm cap *(bottom left)* and 3.2-mm low-profile or IS-1/VS-1 *(bottom left, center)*. Upsizing sleeves include 5- to 6-mm *(top left, center)*, 3.2- to 5-mm *(top right, center)*, 3.2- to 6-mm *(bottom right, center)*. Unipolarizing sleeves for 6-mm bipolar leads are shown on bottom right. (Photography by Andrew C. Floyd, Hahnemann University Hospital, Philadelphia.)

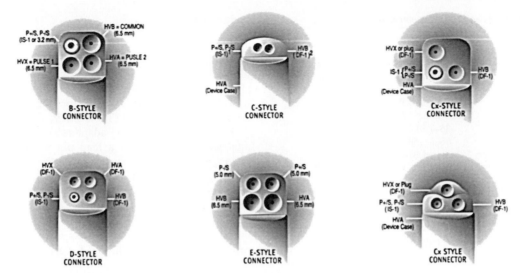

Figure 26–10. Examples of a variety of implantable cardioverter-defibrillator header connector block configurations. These various styles of header configurations are designed to connect directly to different types of implanted rate-sensing and pacing leads (pace and sense, P/S) and to high-voltage lead connectors (HVA, HVB, HVX). All rate/sense lead ports are of the IS-1 configuration. This means that any rate/sense leads that are of different connector configurations must be adapted to fit into these ports. Likewise, high-energy lead ports are of the DF-1 or 3.2-mm configuration. Adapters may be required here as well to provide a direct connection into the implantable cardioverter-defibrillator header. Many forms of adapters are available for pace and sense leads (see Fig. 26–11). A variety of adapters for high-energy leads are also available (see Fig. 26–12). (From ICD Replacement Guide. Minneapolis, Medtronic, Inc., 1997.)

various hardwire configurations. A single DF-1 connector attaches to all three coils of a subcutaneous array or to a single patch. Before the adoption of the DF-1 standard, like pace and sense leads, defibrillator lead heads had a variety of different end configurations, resulting in increased complexity at the time of generator or lead replacement.

Because a variety of other lead connector configurations had previously been developed (Table 26–8; Fig. 26–9) and because implanted leads may remain useful for many years, a number of these older lead connector configurations remain implanted. If sensing and pacing thresholds are adequate, old leads with such configurations may be used, but a pacemaker or ICD pulse generator with a compatible connector block should be selected. Like pacemakers, ICD generator connector blocks from some manufacturers are available in a variety of configurations and port sizes to attach directly to existing implanted leads (Fig. 26–10). An alternative (but less desirable) approach involves using an adapter to fit odd-sized lead connectors into available ports on an ICD header block. Most old pacemaker leads are unipolar; upgrading to a bipolar system should be considered but is not always necessary.

Before the availability of IS-1 and VS-1 lead connector configurations,[56, 57] the most commonly used pacemaker leads included 3.2-mm low-profile leads (unipolar or linear bipolar), 5-mm or 6-mm unipolar or linear bipolar leads, and bifurcated bipolar systems. Pacemaker pulse generators available from some manufacturers remain compatible with each of these lead models, especially 3.2-mm and 5- to 6-mm linear bipolar or unipolar leads. Precise compatibility, however, is essential to ensuring that no fluid leaks into the pulse generator connector block and that electric continuity to proximal and distal poles remains intact. The physician

must be particularly cautious to ensure that sealing rings are located either on the lead connector or in the pulse generator connector block because not all older lead models had sealing rings placed on the lead connector itself.

Review of manufacturers' specifications of devices should provide the necessary details regarding lead and pulse generator compatibility. Because the lead model may not always be known before reoperation and because it may not be determined even with visual inspection, careful evaluation of the lead connector configuration may be required in the laboratory after the old pulse generator has been removed. Although the lead and pulse generator should have been compatible at the initial implantation, the physician cannot make this assumption without visual inspection of the type of lead connector at reoperation. Lead–generator incompatibility may be the cause of presumed lead malfunction or premature generator depletion.

Bifurcated bipolar leads were implanted primarily with ventricular demand pacing systems with 5- to 6-mm lead connectors that plugged side by side into the pulse generator connector block. Some of these leads continue to function. Replacement of the pulse generator entails selection of a new battery with a compatible connector block to maintain bipolar capability, use of an adapter to convert the bifurcated bipolar lead to a linear bipolar system, or conversion to unipolar by using only one pole of the bifurcated lead, capping the other. The last option is particularly useful in the event that only one pole of a bifurcated bipolar lead functions well. This also allows conversion to a unipolar dual-chamber pacing system, if desired, by placing a new atrial unipolar lead with a 5- to 6-mm connector, or by placing an IS-1 atrial lead (unipolar or bipolar) and adapting the functional pole of the old lead in a unipolar configuration

Table 26–9. *Common Pacemaker Adapter Configurations*

From (Lead)	To (Generator)
Conducting adapters	
6-mm UNI	5-mm UNI
6-mm BIF	3.2-mm LP BI
6-mm BI	3.2-mm LP BI
5-mm BIF	3.2-mm LP BI
5-mm BIF	IS-1 BI
5-mm UNI	IS-1 UNI
3.2-mm LP BI	5-mm BIF
3.2-mm LP	IS-1 BI
Nonconducting upsizing sleeve adapters	
3.2-mm LP BI	5-mm or 6-mm UNI (± pin extender)
IS-1 UNI or BI	5-mm or 6-mm UNI
5-mm UNI	6-mm UNI

BI, linear bipolar; BIF, bifurcated bipolar; LP, low profile; UNI, unipolar.

to an IS-1 connector. If the bifurcated bipolar lead is adapted to linear bipolar, placing a linear bipolar atrial lead can convert the system to bipolar DDD.

Other lead types may be used only with particular pulse generators that have specific rate-responsive sensors, including the following: (1) temperature sensors having a thermistor within the lead body, (2) oxygen saturation sensor systems that measure by photometry, (3) respiratory (minute ventilation) sensors that require a particular (bipolar) lead configuration (although some newer systems can function using unipolar leads), and (4) intracavitary pressure–recording leads. Each of these sensor systems can require specific lead types that may be compatible with pulse generators available only from a particular manufacturer. Most such leads require additional connections into the pulse generator. This information must be available preoperatively.

Adapters

Two general categories of adapters are available: electrically conducting units that change the size or configuration of lead connectors to fit specific pulse generators, and upsizing sleeves that allow IS-1 or 3.2-mm low-profile leads to fit into 5- to 6-mm pulse generator connector blocks while maintaining a fluid seal (Table 26–9; Fig. 26–11).

Electrically conducting adapters necessarily contain wires attached on one end to a lead pin to enter the new pulse generator and a socket on the other to accept the old lead as well as a mechanism to connect the old lead, generally a set-screw. Produced by most manufacturers, an array of adapter types exists (see Table 26–9). The most common pacemaker adapters downsize 5- to 6-mm leads to IS-1 unipolar or bipolar configurations or adapt 3.2-mm low-profile connectors to the IS-1 variety. Adapters are also available to convert bifurcated bipolar leads to the linear IS-1 bipolar configuration. This may be particularly useful for a patient who requires upgrading from VVI to DDD pacing when maintenance of bipolar pacing is important, as occurs when a permanent pacemaker is placed in conjunction with an implanted defibrillator, or to avoid myopotential sensing.

Adapters for ICD leads may be used for either the rate sensing (pace and sense) leads or for the high-energy leads, patches, or arrays (Fig. 26–12). These small units are most helpful when adapting epicardial lead connectors found in an abdominal pocket to newer-generation ICD batteries, that is, attaching nonstandard lead connectors to IS-1 pacing and DF-1 shocking ports in an ICD header block. The adapters may also be used when older transvenous leads must be attached to newer, standard-connect ICD pulse generators. One additional special use for ICD lead adapters involves connecting high-energy leads in parallel to enable them to function as a single unit with the same polarity. For example, a subcutaneous patch or array may need to be added to a

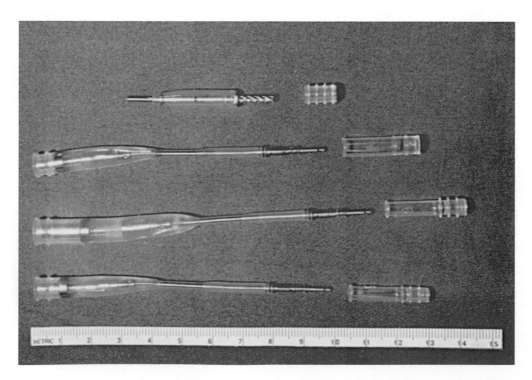

Figure 26–11. Eight pacing lead adapters: four conducting *(left)*, and four nonconducting *(right)*. Conducting adapters shown include *(top to bottom):* 6-mm lead pin replacement, 3.2-mm low-profile linear bipolar (to accept a lead connector without sealing rings) to VS-1 linear bipolar, 6-mm linear bipolar to 3.2-mm linear bipolar, and 3.2-mm low-profile linear bipolar to VS-1 linear bipolar. Nonconducting adapters shown are *(top to bottom):* unipolarizing sleeve for 6-mm bipolar lead, upsizing from 5- to 6-mm, upsizing unipolarizing sleeve from 3.2 to 6 mm, upsizing unipolarizing sleeve from 3.2 to 5 mm. (Photography by Andrew C. Floyd, Hahnemann University Hospital, Philadelphia.)

AICD Lead Adapters

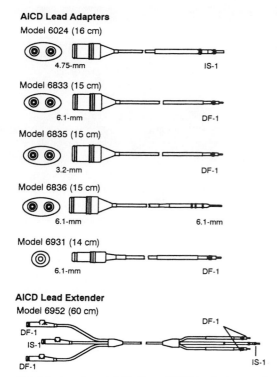

Model 6024 (16 cm)

4.75-mm   IS-1

Model 6833 (15 cm)

6.1-mm   DF-1

Model 6835 (15 cm)

3.2-mm   DF-1

Model 6836 (15 cm)

6.1-mm   6.1-mm

Model 6931 (14 cm)

6.1-mm   DF-1

AICD Lead Extender

Model 6952 (60 cm)

DF-1
DF-1
IS-1
DF-1   IS-1

Figure 26–12. A variety of defibrillator (AICD) lead adapters. As indicated, several different sizes of lead connectors can be inserted side by side to be adapted to the appropriate size to fit directly into the implantable cardioverter-defibrillator (ICD) header port. Additionally, linear adapters used merely to change the size of a lead connector may also be required, as indicated. Lead extenders are used to attach rate sensing and high-energy leads placed through the subclavian system to an ICD pulse generator inserted in the abdomen. As the size and weight of ICDs has been reduced, however, the need to place the ICD pulse generator in the anterior abdominal wall has diminished markedly. (From Multiple Options for Customized Therapy. Guidant Corporation, Cardiac Pacemakers (CPI), St. Paul, MN, 1996.)

system because of a high DFT. This additional hardware can be connected in parallel with a proximal high-energy coil located in the superior vena cava. Lead connectors from both the subcutaneous lead and the proximal coil are inserted side by side into the adapter, which then attaches to a *single* port in the ICD header. This lead system thereby functions as a single electrically connected unit with the same polarity.

Despite the available variety of electrically conducting adapters, these units prove bulky in the pacemaker or ICD pocket. Furthermore, they provide another weak link, that is, one additional set of connections in the pacing circuit for delivery of current to the patient and for sensing, increasing the chance of malfunction, as compared with direct attachment of a lead into a pulse generator connector block. Some adapter set-screws need to be sealed with medical adhesive after being fastened to the lead; a poor seal can result in a short circuit in the system. Because of internal connections, not all adapters have the reliability inherent in most pacemaker or ICD leads.

Tools

Several specially designed tools assist the operator in replacing pacemaker and ICD pulse generators and repairing leads

(Table 26–10; Fig. 26–13). Most important are wrenches to loosen set-screws in the pulse generator connector block to allow the old lead to be withdrawn. If the old generator manufacturer and model are known, a specific wrench may be obtained. If these are not known, it is best to have available an array of small Allen wrenches to remove the hexagonal set-screw. Some pulse generators must be removed from the lead by using a small flat screwdriver. The new battery can often be attached using wrenches available in the sterile packet housing the new device. Some pulse generators are connected to the lead without set-screws by pressing an attachment unit into place; to loosen this unit requires that a small probe be inserted into the side of the connector block to push open the locking mechanism. It is unusual to lose set-screws because they are generally held in place by a seal. It is advisable, however, to have additional set-screws available in a busy pacing laboratory.

Occasionally, repair can salvage an old lead, as long as the conductor fracture or insulation break is accessible at least several centimeters from the point at which the lead enters the vascular system. Lead insulation breaks can be repaired by gluing over a Silastic sleeve with medical adhesive. Conductor fracture can be repaired by severing the lead; placing the two cut conductor ends into an electrically conducting sleeve, which is crimped down onto both ends of the lead conductor; and gluing a Silastic sleeve over the insulator with medical adhesive. This procedure is recommended only for a lead on which the patient is not entirely dependent because recurrent conductor fracture may occur. It is also not recommended for repair of high-energy defibrillation lead conductors. Repair of polyurethane leads can prove functionally inadequate because adhesive may not bond properly with the lead insulator. A more viable ap-

Table 26–10. Commonly Used Tools for Generator or Lead Replacement or Revision or for Lead Repair

Allen wrenches*
   0.035 inch (No. 2)
   0.050 inch (No. 4)
   0.062 inch (No. 6)
   0.093 inch (No. 10)
Screwdrivers
   0.100 inch
   0.200 inch
Set screws
Probes (to unlock lead connector block in some devices)
Anchoring sleeves
Lead repair kit
   Conductor with crimp ends
   Crimping tool
   Insulating sleeve
Medical adhesive
Lead end caps
   6.5 mm
   5 mm
   3.2 mm LP
   IS-1

*Specific torque wrenches may be available from some manufacturers; these are especially important for tightening set screws with appropriate force. Wrench numbers are standardized for ease in identification.

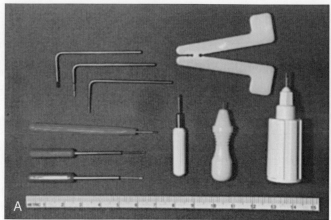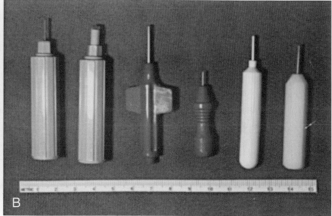

Figure 26–13. Tools commonly required for reoperation. *A,* Three nondeformable Allen wrenches *(top left)* of various sizes; a pinch-on tool (Medtronic) *(top right)* to extend and retract the distal screw of an active-fixation lead; three wrenches *(bottom left)*, two torque wrenches (Medtronic and CPI) *(bottom right)* on either side of a probe (Intermedics) used to unlock a pacemaker connector block. Some wrenches are deformable to avoid placing excess torque on the set screw, whereas others are not; caution is required in using the various systems (see text). *B, left to right,* Intermedics ratchet torque wrench; Intermedics flat-bladed ratchet torque screwdriver; Cordis No. 6 Allen wrench; unlocking probe; two Allen wrenches with handles (not deformable). (Photography by Andrew C. Floyd, Hahnemann University Hospital, Philadelphia.)

proach may be to extract or cap the culprit lead and replace it entirely.

■ SURGICAL CONSIDERATIONS

Device replacement or revision in a tertiary care institution with an active electrophysiology service and long-term follow-up may constitute more than a quarter of all pacemaker or ICD procedures (Table 26–11). The timing of intervention depends on the specific indication. Most patients require reoperation for elective battery replacement or battery or lead revision, whereas 1% to 6% of patients return to the laboratory for other problems, such as pocket hematoma, pocket twitch, diaphragmatic pacing, and pocket relocation (Table 26–12).

Chronic or Elective Intervention

Most reimplantation procedures fall into this category. Preoperative blood work is performed, aspirin is stopped for at least 5 days, and other anticoagulants are discontinued. The patient fasts from midnight and receives preoperative antibiotics, most commonly being admitted on the day of the procedure. Elevated coagulation times may be corrected with fresh-frozen plasma if necessary. Procedures are routinely performed with local or regional anesthesia, supplemented by intravenous conscious sedation. For ICDs, the patient is

placed under general anesthesia for ventricular fibrillation induction and testing of shock therapies. Most institutions use a combination of a short-acting, amnestic benzodiazepine with an intravenous narcotic. Continuous electrocardiographic monitoring, pulse oximetry, and sterile preparation and draping are standard procedure. Preoperative antibiotics are administered intravenously.

General Guidelines and Techniques

There is no substitute for careful surgical planning in approaching the chronic pacemaker pocket and gentle handling

Table 26–11. Pacemaker Pulse Generator Implants and Revisions or Replacements

DDD implants	51%
VVI implants	23%
Revisions or replacement	26%

The frequency of dual-chamber (DDD) and single-chamber (VVI) pulse generator implantations and battery or lead revisions or replacements over 5½-year period at Hahnemann University Hospital, Philadelphia.

Table 26–12. Pacemaker Reoperations: Frequency of Various Indications

Generator Indications	
Battery end of service	53%
DVI to DDD conversion	2.2%
Battery insulation break	1.1%
DDD to VVIR conversion	1.1%
Lead Indications	
Lead revision	17%
Exit block	
Lead injury	
Diaphragmatic pacing	2.2%
Lead fracture	1.1%
Lead insulation break	1.1%
Battery or Lead Indications	
Battery end of service and lead replacement	6.8%
VVI to DDD conversion	4.4%
Unipolar DDD to bipolar DDD	1.1%
Pocket twitch	1.1%
Surgical	
Pocket relocation	5.6%
Pocket effusion	2.2%

The frequency of indications for pacemaker reoperation over a 5½-year period at Hahnemann University Hospital, Philadelphia.

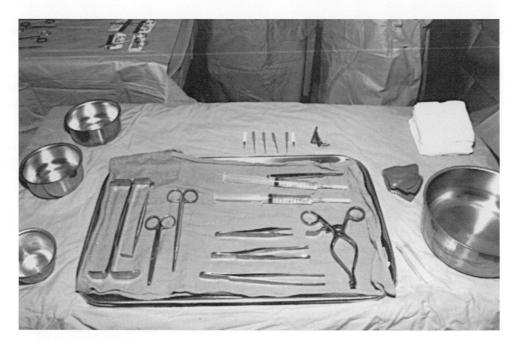

Figure 26–14. Preparation for surgery. A typical array of instruments required for reoperation. *Foreground*, Retractors, scissors, forceps, scalpel, syringes filled with lidocaine anesthetic, sterile saline solution, sponges, and a variety of wrenches. *Background*, Hemostats and absorbable and nonabsorbable sutures. (Photography by Andrew C. Floyd, Hahnemann University Hospital, Philadelphia.)

of the tissues. Perfect hemostasis, avoidance of a tight-fitting pacemaker or ICD pocket, and multilayered incision closure are the basic principles that help prevent future difficulties. These principles are similar to those required at initial implantation (see Table 26–2). Electrocautery must not be used directly over an implanted pulse generator to avoid induction of ventricular fibrillation, development of fibrosis at the lead tip, and damage to the generator itself. Electrocautery must also not be used during battery changes with the generator disconnected when pacemaker leads are grounded to the patient for testing because current may be shunted directly to the heart. Hemostasis at reoperation can usually be secured by direct ligature. Use of surgical absorbable cellulose or topical thrombin assists in treating persistently oozy pockets. Clinical judgment should be used in the application of various technical approaches (Fig. 26–14).

Specific Techniques

Local anesthesia is administered most commonly as 1% lidocaine (Xylocaine) infiltrated into the scar line from the previous procedure; additional lidocaine may be given under direct vision once the capsule of the pocket has been defined.

The surgical incision is placed directly over the previous incision. The skin and subcutaneous tissues are opened with sharp dissection, which is required to penetrate the tough scar tissue and dermal layer. Deeper dissection with Metzenbaum scissors is carried out to delineate the pacemaker capsule. Once the pocket is reached, the fibrous capsule is sharply incised with a blade to make a small opening, which is then extended with scissors under direct visualization of the implanted pulse generator and leads Fig. 26–15). The capsule must be opened far enough to allow extraction of the pulse generator and lead connector assembly without undue force. The posterior capsule may need to be carefully dissected away from the leads to allow mobility. Access to leads and generator may be facilitated through the use of self-retaining retractors. Extreme care is required throughout the procedure to preserve the integrity of the leads and

lead connectors; they must not be punctured with anesthetic needles or cut with blades or scissors.

Once the generator is delivered (out of the pocket, the leads are disconnected and analyzed, as described earlier. Leads from pacemaker-dependent patients need to be expeditiously reconnected to an external pacemaker (Fig. 26–16). Unipolar pacemaker leads require direct grounding to subcutaneous tissue; the active part of the unipolar generator must remain in contact with the patient before the lead is disconnected. Grounding can best be accomplished through a large surface area ground electrode placed directly into the open pocket. Making contact with this electrode onto the active surface of a unipolar pulse generator allows the generator to be removed safely from the pocket before the lead is disconnected, even in a pacemaker-dependent patient.

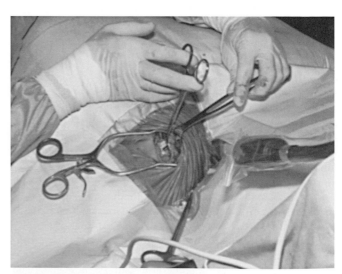

Figure 26–15. Opening the capsule of the chronic generator pocket to expose the pulse generator. (Photography by Andrew C. Floyd, Hahnemann University Hospital, Philadelphia.)

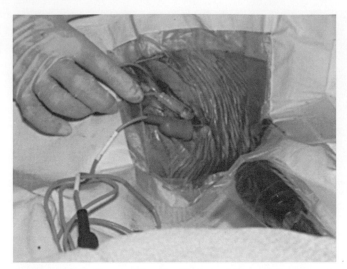

Figure 26–16. Disconnecting the chronic lead. The active surface of the unipolar pacemaker pulse generator remains in contact with the open pocket to maintain pacing output until the lead is withdrawn from the connector block. The surgeon has adequately mobilized the proximal portion of the 5-mm lead to allow rapid connection to an external pacing cable, one end of which has already been securely grounded to the patient. A ligature previously placed around the lead connector block entry post has been removed. After the external pacemaker has been activated, the surgeon will loosen the set-screw (here covered by a seal on the top right side of the connector block) and withdraw the lead from the pulse generator, immediately connecting it to the negative pole of the external pacing cable. (Photography by Andrew C. Floyd, Hahnemann University Hospital, Philadelphia.)

After being secured to temporary pacing cables, leads can be completely freed from adhesions up to their entry point into the subclavian vein, if necessary, to examine lead integrity or for extraction. We use low-energy electrocautery sparingly to dissect the leads free from adhesions because the scar tissue could be especially tough and adherent to lead structures. If lead replacement or repair is not necessary, and if chronic lead function is adequate, dissection of the complete course of each lead may not be necessary. The physician, however, must ascertain whether the lead connector mobility is sufficient to attach it to a new pulse generator without tension.

Inadequate chronic lead pacing or sensing thresholds may require placement of one or two new leads. Upgrading from a single-chamber to a DDD pacemaker system may require placement of one additional lead. If a chronic lead is extracted through a dilating sheath, the new lead or a guide wire can usually be inserted into the vascular system through the extraction sheath. In other cases, repeated subclavian puncture, brachiocephalic cutdown, or an internal jugular approach provides an alternative means of inserting a new lead. If new leads are placed through the same subclavian system by direct puncture, the operator must be cautious to avoid lead damage.

After the old pulse generator has been detached from leads and the lead integrity and functional status have been ascertained, a new pulse generator can be attached. The principles of generator–lead adaptability must be maintained (Fig. 26–17). Redundant lead coils are placed posterior to the pulse generator, and the pocket is closed with three

layers of absorbable suture—two subcutaneous and one subcuticular. ICD leads also require defibrillation testing before, or concomitant with, final pocket closure.

In generator replacement the chronic pacemaker or ICD pocket location is used most commonly, usually opposite the patient's dominant side. Because most pacemakers and most ICDs are placed inferior to the clavicle in a subcutaneous location anterior to the pectoralis fascia, the location of replacement devices is similar. Various modifications suit individual patient needs. In very thin patients, subpectoral

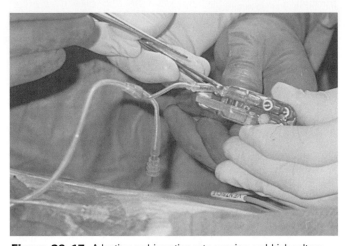

Figure 26–17. Adapting and inserting rate-sensing and high-voltage defibrillator leads into the implantable cardioverter-defibrillator (ICD) connector block. The incision is made in the left upper quadrant of the abdomen over the scar line from the previous device implant. The old ICD generator has been removed, and the leads have been freed up by gentle electrocautery to allow them to be easily manipulated and to be placed into the header of the new pulse generator without undue tension or bending. Basic pacing and sensing thresholds have been tested; this also includes delivery of low-energy (5-V) pacing impulses through the high-energy leads to measure lead impedance and thus ensure structural integrity of the high-voltage conductors. The new ICD device to be implanted has been placed on the surgical field, and connection to the lead system has begun. First, a plug is inserted into the upper right port because it will not be used. The set-screw has already been tightened onto this plug and a required cap has been placed over the set-screw. The surgeon is inserting a unipolar lead connector from the rate-sensing portion of the defibrillator lead into the ICD connector block. This lead head is connected to the distal tip of a right ventricular endocardial integrated lead system (497-05 lead, Intermedics); it is inserted into the appropriate sensing port of the ICD. Sealing O-rings are evident on the ICD header and are used in this device to prevent fluid leakage around a cap placed over the set-screw. Also evident just within the forceps is a thickened area of the lead that represents a sleeve glued in place with medical adhesive to cover a minor break in the outer insulator of the lead (i.e., an insulator repair). A plug has been inserted into an unused port of the ICD connector block; the sealing cap has already been placed over the set-screw for this plug.
The dangling high-voltage lead connector has been inserted through an upsizing sleeve before placing it in the ICD connector block. The original lead connector is a 4-mm configuration; the sleeve passes over the insulator on the head to increase its diameter to fit into a 6-mm high-voltage port in the ICD connector block. The remaining lead connector evident on the patient attaches to a subcutaneous high-voltage patch used in the defibrillation circuit. The tip of this lead is also upsized using a similar sleeve to fit a 6-mm port. (Photography courtesy of Todd Forkin, Hahnemann University Hospital, Philadelphia, PA.)

or axillary locations may be required. The subpectoral plane can be accessed by locating the junction between the sternal and clavicular heads of the pectoralis major and entering at that point, taking care to avoid damage to penetrating neurovascular bundles. Alternatively, the muscle fibers of the pectoralis major can be teased apart longitudinally to enter the subpectoral plane. Axillary placement of pacing devices is generally avoided because of the possibility of lateral migration of the device, which can be uncomfortable for the patient and can, especially with larger ICDs, lead to erosion. When required, however, the axillary location can be entered by direct extension from a subclavian pocket or through a separate axillary incision. The device may be placed in a subpectoral location at that site. The abdominal wall, subcostal, and intrathoracic positions represent other alternatives for a replacement pulse generator. Nevertheless, a subcutaneous approach is appropriate in most patients for both pacemaker and ICD implantation.

For replacement of an abdominal ICD, dissection can be difficult if the device is located behind the rectus abdominis muscle. We usually begin over the area where the device is most easily palpated, carefully spreading the muscle apart in the area of prior scarring. The scar tissue is carefully divided to expose the pulse generator, which is then handled in the usual manner. The physician must be cautious not to exert undue force to remove the generator in order to avoid rupture into the peritoneal cavity. Electrocautery is avoided over the muscle if the patient is not under general anesthesia.

Approach to the Eroding Device

Although relatively uncommon, chronic erosion through the skin of the pulse generator or lead can occur.[1, 10, 77] Incipient erosion manifests as localized erythema in an area of thinned skin that is adherent to the underlying device. The area gradually becomes necrotic and may drain serosanguineous fluid. Outright erosion and drainage necessarily imply that the pacemaker pocket is no longer sterile[1,98]; in such instances, the system (generator and leads) should be removed if possible.[5, 8] Occasionally, the pocket heals with removal of the pulse generator alone, but only when skin integrity has not been breached. After removal of the pulse generator and leads, eroded pockets are packed for secondary closure. Administration of intravenous antibiotics proceeds for 1 to 6 weeks (the longer duration if bacteremia has occurred). A new device should be implanted on the contralateral side only after all signs of infection have resolved at the old pacemaker site, if the patient has not developed recurrent fever, and if there is no elevation of white blood cell count. Five to 7 days of intravenous antibiotic administration appears sufficient before device replacement so long as bacteremia is absent and there are no large intracardiac vegetations. Replacement of the pulse generator on the original side is not recommended but may be possible if complete erosion did not occur, the pocket could be closed after primary generator removal, and there are no signs of active infection after antibiotics have been discontinued. Alternative approaches are discussed in Chapter 28.

Antibiotic Prophylaxis

Compared with pacemaker generator change, the overall procedure time for ICD generator change may be lengthier because of the added time required for DFT testing during the procedure. The surgical wound may, therefore, be open for a longer time, although closure may be started before all testing is complete. Furthermore, the generator change may involve a larger incision in an abdominal site. We recommend routine use of broad-spectrum antibiotics for antimicrobial prophylaxis during all procedures involving generator or lead revision, especially because these procedures use combinations of previously implanted hardware with new equipment. Whether and how long to use postoperative antibiotic prophylaxis has been debated.[98]

Acute Intervention

Indications for acute intervention include primary complications of pacemaker or ICD implantation (e.g., pocket hematoma, infection,[1-3] or cardiac perforation[73-77]) as well as other, less crucial indications, such as iatrogenic lead damage and lead dislodgment.

Pocket hematomas occur most frequently in patients receiving anticoagulants, including aspirin, and in patients with platelet dysfunction, which is common in those undergoing chronic hemodialysis. The range in hematoma size varies from a contained, small amount of fluctuance and ecchymosis to a large hematoma that may drain through the skin. A minor hematoma requires only observation, whereas a breach of skin integrity after operation may require complete removal of the generator and lead system. If the patient remains pacemaker dependent, a temporary wire must be placed when the original system is removed; after an appropriate course of intravenous antibiotic therapy, the old pocket can be closed and a new pacemaker placed on the contralateral side. Prolonged antibiotic therapy may be required in some cases. Antibiotic therapy alone and conservative surgical approaches other than complete removal of the eroded or infected generator and leads prove unsatisfactory.[5-8]

Acute reoperation may also be required for cardiac perforation.[73-77, 79] Perforation is suggested by curvature of the lead beyond the confines of the right ventricular apex, an abrupt rise in pacing threshold or deterioration of sensing, precordial discomfort, hypotension, or hemodynamic collapse. Although most perforations close spontaneously, development of a large pericardial bleed or tamponade requires immediate intervention.[79] Pericardiocentesis usually suffices, but occasionally a subxiphoid approach to pericardial drainage is necessary. Proper lead selection to match the patient's anatomy and gentle technique are vital to avoiding acute perforation. Subcostal placement of epicardial screw-in leads has been associated with a high incidence of serious or fatal ventricular perforations; chronic perforation of endocardial leads is distinctly rare.[24]

Early surgical exploration is indicated to confirm the diagnosis of iatrogenic lead insulation damage. This is an uncommon complication and manifests early in the form of pocket twitch,[81] failure to capture, or failure to sense, with associated low measured lead pacing impedance.[51] Chronic implantation lead damage has been associated with excessively tight anchoring sutures, especially if they are placed around the lead and not the anchoring sleeve. The damaged lead, whether a passive-fixation or an active-fixation device, should be removed and replaced, if possible; alternatively, it may be repaired, although this is difficult if damage has occurred near the venous insertion site.

Lead dislodgment occurs most commonly during the first 24 to 48 hours after system implantation.[26, 27] It can, however, occur later, the result of a loose anchoring sleeve, incomplete fixation of the distal lead tip, excessive diaphragmatic motion, or patient manipulation of the device (i.e., twiddler's syndrome).[49] Before the development of leads with active fixation or a fin-like mechanism at the distal tip, the incidence of lead dislodgment remained as high as 5% to 18%. With careful technique and selection among a variety of active-fixation and passive-fixation leads, the incidence should range no higher than 1% to 2%.[30, 31, 99] Most spontaneous dislodgments occur with atrial passive-fixation leads. The diagnosis may be facilitated by chest radiography or fluoroscopy; pacing analysis reveals an increased pacing threshold with, usually, normal lead impedance. The operator has the option of repositioning or lead replacement. If a distinct cause cannot be identified, placement of an active-fixation lead may avoid a second dislodgment. To prevent recurrent lead dislodgment in twiddler's syndrome, leads must be sutured to prepectoral fascia or firm pacemaker pocket fibrous tissue using nonabsorbable suture around anchoring sleeves at more than two points; the pacemaker connector block may also be anchored to the pectoralis fascia. The use of a polyester (Dacron) pouch can improve device stability in this syndrome and in patients with very loose subcutaneous tissue.[100]

Interval or Unscheduled Intervention

In the course of pacemaker or ICD follow-up and before the patient requires elective replacement, interval intervention may be required to correct other complications. These include pulse generator migration,[15] lead dislodgment,[16, 23, 26, 27, 31, 49] high pacing thresholds,[23, 50] pocket twitch or diaphragmatic pacing,[24, 81] lead insulation break or lead fracture,[11, 13, 26] and premature generator failure (which could be due to intrinsic component failure or the result of externally induced failure, such as that caused by electrocautery, radiation, or cardioversion).[19, 20] The pacemaker clinic may prove particularly useful in recognizing early surgical or functional problems.[37] Evaluation and technique are approached using the principles described earlier.

SUMMARY

Successful pacemaker or ICD replacement is the result of accurate preoperative evaluation and careful surgical intervention. The preoperative status of the pulse generator battery and lead pacing and sensing function and the appropriateness of both to future pacing or defibrillating systems need to be determined to plan the surgery. There should be no surgical surprises, and all the tools, adapters, leads, and generators should be ready for the intervention. The goal should be to avoid reoperation for as long as possible with careful initial implantation and programming. When properly planned, however, surgery is likely to proceed smoothly.

REFERENCES

1. Bonchek LI: New methods in the management of extruded and infected cardiac pacemakers. Ann Surg 176(5):686, 1972.
2. Corman LC, Levison ME: Sustained bacteremia and transvenous cardiac pacemakers. JAMA 233(3):264, 1975.
3. Morgan G, Ginks W, Siddons H, Leatham A: Septicemia in patients with an endocardial pacemaker. Am J Cardiol 44(2):221, 1979.
4. Wohl B, Peters RW, Carliner N, et al: Late unheralded pacemaker pocket infection due to *Staphylococcus epidermidis*: A new clinical entity. PACE 5(2):190, 1982.
5. Prager PI, Kay RH, Somberg E, et al: Pacemaker remnants—another source of infections. PACE 7(4):763, 1984.
6. Mansour KA, Kauten JR, Hatcher CR Jr: Management of the infected pacemaker: Explantation, sterilization, and reimplantation. Ann Thorac Surg 40(6):617, 1985.
7. Buch J, Mortensen SA: Late infections of pacemaker units due to silicone rubber insulation boots. PACE 8(4):494, 1985.
8. Ruiter JH, Degener JE, Van Mechelen R, Bos R: Late purulent pacemaker pocket infection caused by *Staphylococcus epidermidis*: Serious complications of in situ management. PACE 8(6):903, 1985.
9. Vilacosta I, Zamorano J, Camino A, et al: Infected transvenous permanent pacemakers: Role of transesophageal echocardiography. Am Heart J 125(3):904, 1993.
10. Garcia-Rinaldi R, Revuelta JM, Bonnington L, Soltero-Harrington L: The exposed cardiac pacemaker: Treatment by subfacial pocket relocation. J Thorac Cardiovasc Surg 89(1):136, 1985.
11. Kronzon I, Mehta SS: Broken pacemaker wire in multiple trauma: A case report. J Trauma 14(1):82, 1974.
12. Tegtmeyer CJ, Bezirdjian DR, Irani FA, Landis JD: Cardiac pacemaker failure: A complication of trauma. South Med J 74(3):378, 1981.
13. Grieco JG, Scanlon PJ, Pifarre R: Pacing lead fracture after a deceleration injury. Ann Thorac Surg 47(3):453, 1989.
14. Wallace WA, Abelmann WH, Norman JC: Runaway demand pacemaker: Report, in vitro reproduction, and review. Ann Thorac Surg 9(3):209, 1970.
15. Bello A, Yepez CG, Barcelo JE: Retroperitoneal migration of a pacemaker generator: An unusual complication. J Cardiovasc Surg 15(2):256, 1974.
16. Kim GE, Haveson S, Imparato AM: Late displacement of cardiac pacemaker electrode due to heavyweight pulse generator. JAMA 228(1):74, 1974.
17. Austin SM, Kim CS, Solis A: Electrical alternans of pacemaker spike amplitude: An unusual manifestation of permanent pacemaker generator malfunction. PACE 4(3):313, 1981.
18. Campo A, Nowak R, Magilligan D, Tomlanovich M: Runaway pacemaker. Ann Emerg Med 12(1):32, 1983.
19. Venselaar JL, Van Kerkeorle HL, Vet AJ: Radiation damage to pacemakers from radiotherapy. PACE 19(3 Pt 1):538, 1987.
20. Lewinn AA, Serago CF, Schwade JG, et al: Radiation-induced failures of complementary metal oxide semiconductor containing pacemakers: A potentially lethal complication. Int J Radiol Oncol Biol Phys 19(10):1967, 1984.
21. Halperin JL, Camunas JL, Stern EH, et al: Myopotential interference with DDD pacemakers: Endocardial electrographic telemetry in the diagnosis of pacemaker-related arrhythmias. Am J Cardiol 54(1):97, 1984.
22. den Dulk K, Lindemans FW, Brugada P, et al: Pacemaker syndrome with AAI rate-variable pacing: Importance of atrioventricular conduction properties, medication, and pacemaker programmability. PACE 11(8):1226, 1988.
23. Aris A, Shebairo RA, Lepley D Jr: Increasing myocardial thresholds to pacing after cardiac surgery. Surg Forum 24:167, 1973.
24. Gaidula JJ, Barold SS: Elimination of diaphragmatic contractions from chronic pacing catheter perforation of the heart by conversion to a unipolar system. Chest 66(1):86, 1974.
25. Contini C, Papi L, Pesola A, et al: Tissue reaction to intracavitary electrodes: Effect on duration and efficiency of unipolar pacing in patients with A-V block. J Cardiovasc Surg 14(3):282, 1973.
26. Holmes DR Jr, Nissen RG, Maloney JD, et al: Transvenous tined electrode systems: An approach to acute dislodgement. May Clin Proc 54(4):219, 1979.
27. Snow N: Elimination of lead dislodgment by the use of tined transvenous electrodes. PACE 5(4):571, 1982.
28. Alt E, Volker R, Blomer H: Lead fracture in pacemaker patients. Thorac Cardiovasc Surg 35(2):101, 1987.
29. Woscoboinik JR, Maloney JD, Helguera ME, et al: Pacing lead survival: Performance of different models. PACE 15(11,pt2):1991, 1992.
30. Morse D, Yankaskas M, Johnson B, et al: Transvenous pacemaker insertion with a zero dislodgment rate. PACE 6(2 Pt 1):283, 1983.

31. Hakki AH, Horowitz LN, Reiser J, Mundth ED: Improved pacemaker fixation and performance using a modified finned porous surfaced tip lead. Int Surg 69(4):291, 1984.

32. Mirowski M, Reid PR, Mower MM, et al: Termination of malignant ventricular arrhythmias with an implanted automatic defibrillator in human beings. N Engl J Med 303:322–324, 1980.

33. Mond H, Twentyman R, Smith D, Sloman G: The pacemaker clinic. Cardiology 57(5):262, 1972.

34. Starr A, Dobbs J, Dabolt J, Pierie W: Ventricular tracking pacemaker and teletransmitter follow-up system. Am J Cardiol 32(7):956, 1973.

35. Janosik DL, Redd RM, Buckingham TA, et al: Utility of ambulatory electrocardiography in detecting pacemaker dysfunction in the early postimplantation period. Am J Cardiol 60(13):1030, 1987.

36. Mugica J, Henry L, Rollet M, et al: The clinical utility of pacemaker follow-up visits. PACE 9(6 Pt 2):1249, 1986.

37. Byrd CL, Schwartz SJ, Gonzales M, et al: Pacemaker clinic evaluations: Key to early identification of surgical problems. PACE 9(6 Pt 2):1259, 1986.

38. Kertes P, Mond H, Sloman G, et al: Comparison of lead complications with polyurethane tined, silicone rubber tined, and wedge tip leads: Clinical experience with 822 ventricular endocardial leads. PACE 6(5 Pt 1):957, 1983.

39. van Gelder LM, El Gamal MI: False inhibition of an atrial demand pacemaker caused by an insulation defect in a polyurethane lead. PACE 6(5 Pt 1):834, 1983.

40. Sanford CF: Self-inhibition of an AV sequential demand (DVI) pulse generator due to polyurethane lead insulation disruption. PACE 6(5 Pt 1):840, 1983.

41. Timmis GC, Westveer DC, Martin R, Gordon S: The significance of surface changes on explanted polyurethane pacemaker leads. PACE 6(5 Pt 1):845, 1983.

42. Chawla AS, Blais P, Hinberg I, Johnson D: Degradation of explanted polyurethane cardiac pacing leads and of polyurethane. Biomater Artif Cells Artif Organs 16(4):785, 1988.

43. Van Beek GJ, den Dulk K, Lindemans FW, Wellens HJ: Detection of insulation failure by gradual reduction in noninvasively measured electrogram amplitudes. PACE 9(5):772, 1986.

44. Stokes KB, Church T: Ten-year experience with implanted polyurethane lead insulation. PACE 9(6 Pt 2):1160, 1986.

45. Phillips R, Frey M, Martin RO: Long-term performance of polyurethane pacing leads: Mechanisms of design-related failures. PACE 9(6 Pt 2):1166, 1986.

46. Barold SS, Gaidula JJ: Demand pacemaker arrhythmias from intermittent internal short circuit in bipolar electrode. Chest 63(2):165, 1973.

47. Adler SC, Foster AJ, Sanders RS, Wuu E: Thin bipolar leads: A solution to problems with coaxial bipolar designs. PACE 15(11 Pt 2):1986, 1992.

48. Barold SS, Scovil J, Ong LS, Heinle RA: Periodic pacemaker spike attenuation with preservation of capture: An unusual electrocardiographic manifestation of partial pacing electrode fracture. PACE 1(3):375, 1978.

49. Bayliss, CE, Beanlands DS, Baird RJ: The pacemaker-twiddler's syndrome: A new complication of implantable transvenous pacemakers. Can Med Assoc J 99(8):371, 1968.

50. Starr DS, Lawrie GM, Morris GC Jr: Acute and chronic stimulation thresholds of intramyocardial screw-in pacemaker electrodes. Ann Thorac Surg 31(4):334, 1981.

51. Ferek B, Pasini M, Pustisek S, et al: Noninvasive detection of insulation break. PACE 7(6 Pt 1):1063, 1984.

52. Sandler MJ, Kutalek SP: Inappropriate discharge by an implantable cardioverter defibrillator: Recognition of myopotential sensing using telemetered intracardiac electrograms. PACE 17:665–671, 1994.

53. Korte T, Jung W, Spehl S, et al: Incidence of ICD lead related complications during long-term follow-up: Comparison of epicardial and endocardial electrode systems. PACE 18(11):2053–2061, 1995.

54. Schwartzman D, Callans DJ, Gottlieb CD, et al: Early postoperative rise in defibrillation threshold in patients with nonthoracotodefibrillation lead systems: Attenuation with biphasic shock waveforms. J Cardiovasc Electrophysiol 7(6):483–493, 1996.

55. Goyal R, Harvey M, Horwood L, et al: Incidence of lead system malfunction detected during implantable defibrillator generator replacement. PACE 19:1143–1146, 1996.

56. Calfee RV, Saulson SH: A voluntary standard for 3.2-mm unipolar and bipolar pacemaker leads and connectors. PACE 9(6 Pt 2):1181, 1986.

57. Doring J, Flink R: The impact of pending technologies on a universal connector standard. PACE 9(6 Pt 2):1186, 1986.

58. Tyers GF, Sanders R, Mills P, Clark J: Analysis of setscrew and sidelock connector reliability. PACE 15(11 Pt 2):2000, 1992.

59. Hayes DL, Wang PJ, Reynolds DW, et al: Interference with cardiac pacemakers by cellular telephones. N Engl J Med 336(21):1473–1479, 1997.

60. Fetter JG, Ivans V, Benditt DG, Collins J: Digital cellular telephone interaction with implantable cardioverter-defibrillators. J Am Coll Cardiol 31(3):623–628, 1998.

61. Torresani J, Ebagosti A, Allard-Latour G: Pacemaker syndrome with DDD pacing. PACE 7(6 Pt 2):1183, 1984.

62. Cunningham TM: Pacemaker syndrome due to retrograde conduction in DDI pacemaker. Am Heart J 115(2):478, 1988.

63. Schwartzman D, Nallamothu N, Callans DJ, et al: Postoperative lead-related complications in patients with nonthoracotomy defibrillation lead system. J Am Coll Cardiol 26:776–786, 1995.

64. Lawton JS, Wood MA, Gilligan DM, et al: Implantable cardioverter defibrillator leads: The dark side. PACE 19:1273–1277, 1996.

65. Swartz JF, Fletcher RD, Karasik PE: Optimization of biphasic waveforms for human nonthoracotomy defibrillation. Circulation 88:2646–2654, 1993.

66. Neuzner J, Pitschner HF, Huth C, et al: Effect of biphasic waveform pulse on endocardial defibrillation efficacy in humans. PACE 17:207–212, 1994.

67. Natale S, Sra J, Axtell K, et al: Preliminary experience with a hybrid nonthoracotomy defibrillating system that includes a biphasic device: Comparison with a standard monophasic device using the same lead system. J Am Coll Cardiol 24:406–412, 1994.

68. Block M, Hammel D, Bocker D, et al: A prospective randomized cross-over comparison of mono- and biphasic defibrillation using nonthoracotomy lead configuration in humans. J Cardiovasc Electrophysiol 5:581–590, 1994.

69. Gold MR, Foster AH, Shorofsky SR: Lead system optimization for transvenous defibrillation. Am J Cardiol 80(9):1163–1167, 1997.

70. Bardy GH, Dolack GL, Kudenchuck PJ, et al: Prospective comparison in humans of a unipolar defibrillation system with that using an additional superior vena cava electrode. Circulation 89:1090–1093, 1994.

71. Almassi GH, Olinger GN, Wetherbee JN, et al: Long-term complications of implantable cardioverter defibrillator lead system. Ann Thorac Surg 55:888–892, 1993.

72. Brode SE, Schwartzman D, Callans DJ, et al: ICD-antiarrhythmic drug and ICD-pacemaker interactions. J Cardiovasc Electrophysiol 8:830–842, 1997.

73. Peters RW, Scheinman MM, Raskin S, Thomas AN: Unusual complications of epicardial pacemaker: Recurrent pericarditis, cardiac tamponade and pericardial constriction. Am J Cardiol 45(5):1088, 1980.

74. Foster CJ: Constrictive pericarditis complicating an endocardial pacemaker. Br Heart J 47(5):497, 1982.

75. Phibbs B, Marriott HJ: Complications of permanent transvenous pacing. N Engl J Med 312(22):1428, 1985.

76. Villaneuva FS, Heinsiner JA, Burkman MH, et al: Echocardiographic detection of perforation of the cardiac ventricular septum by a permanent pacemaker lead. Am J Cardiol 59(4):370, 1987.

77. Hill PE: Complications of permanent transvenous cardiac pacing: A 14-year review of all transvenous pacemakers inserted at one community hospital. PACE 10(3 Pt 1):564, 1987.

78. Pizzarelli G, Dernevik L: Inadvertent transarterial pacemaker insertion: An unusual complication. PACE 10(4 Pt 1):951, 1987.

79. Sandler MA, Wertheimer JH, Kotler MN: Pericardial tamponade associated with pacemaker catheter manipulation. PACE 12(7 Pt 1):1085, 1989.

80. Mueller X, Sadeghi H, Kappenberger L: Complications after single- versus dual-chamber pacemaker implantation. PACE 13(6):711, 1990.

81. Ekbom K, Nilsson BY, Edhag O, Olin C: Rhythmic shoulder girdle muscle contractions as a complication in pacemaker treatment. Chest 66(5):599, 1974.

82. Chun PK: Characteristics of commonly utilized permanent endocardial and epicardial pacemaker electrode systems: Method of radiologic identification. Am Heart J 102(3 Pt 1):404, 1981.

83. Angello DA: Principles of electrical testing for analysis of ventricular endocardial pacing leads. Prog Cardiovasc Dis 27(1):57, 1984.

84. Kemler RL: A simple method for exposing the external jugular vein for placement of a permanent transvenous pacing catheter electrode. Ann Thorac Surg 26(3):266, 1978.

85. Sethi GK, Bhayana JN, Scott SM: Innominate venous thrombosis: A

rare complication of transvenous pacemaker electrodes. Am Heart J 87(6):770, 1974.

86. Fritz T, Richeson JF, Fitzpatrick P, Wilson G: Venous obstruction: A potential complication of transvenous pacemaker electrodes. Chest 83(3):534, 1983.

87. Sharma S, Kaul U, Rajani M: Digital subtraction venography for assessment of deep venous thrombosis in the arms following pacemaker implantation. Int J Cardiol 23(1):135, 1989.

88. Antonelli D, Turgeman Y, Kaveh Z, et al: Short-term thrombosis after transvenous permanent pacemaker insertion. PACE 12(2):280, 1989.

89. Spittell PC, Vlietstra RE, Hayes DL, Higano ST: Venous obstruction due to permanent transvenous pacemaker electrodes: Treatment with percutaneous transluminal balloon venoplasty. PACE 13(3):271, 1990.

90. Wertheimer M, Hughes RK, Castle CH: Superior vena cava syndrome: Complication of permanent transvenous endocardial cardiac pacing. JAMA 224(8):1172, 1973.

91. Toumbouras M, Spanos P, Konstantaras C, Lazarides DP: Inferior vena cava thrombosis due to migration of retained functionless pacemaker electrode. Chest 82(6):785, 1982.

92. Blackburn T, Dunn M: Pacemaker-induced superior vena cava syndrome: Consideration of management. Am Heart J 116(3):893, 1988.

93. Goudevenos JA, Reid PG, Adams PC, et al: Pacemaker-induced supe-rior vena cava syndrome: Report of four cases and review of the literature. PACE 12(12):1890, 1989.

94. Mazzetti H, Dussaut A, Tentori C, et al: Superior vena cava occlusion and/or syndrome related to pacemaker leads. Am Heart J 125(3):831, 1993.

95. Pace JN, Maquilan M, Hessen SE, et al: Extraction and replacement of permanent pacemaker leads through occluded vessels: Use of extraction sheaths as conduits—balloon venoplasty as an adjunct. J Interven Cardiol Electrophysiol 1(4):271–279, 1997.

96. Chaithiraphan S, Goldberg E, Wolff W, et al: Massive thrombosis of the coronary sinus as an unusual complication of transvenous pacemaker insertion in a patient with persistent left, and no right superior vena cava. J Am Geriatr Soc 22(2):79, 1974.

97. Kennelly BM: Permanent pacemaker implantation in the absence of a right superior vena cava: A case report. S Afr Med J 55(25):1043, 1979.

98. Wade JS, Cobbs CG: Infections in cardiac pacemakers. Curr Clin Topics Infect Dis 9:44, 1988.

99. Boake WC, Kroncke GM: Pacemaker Complications: Cardiac Pacing. Philadelphia, Lea & Febiger, 1979.

100. Parsonnet V: A stretch fabric pouch for implanted pacemakers. Arch Surg 105:654, 1972.

Chapter 27

Management of Implant Complications

Charles L. Byrd

Management of an implanted device complication has become a subspecialty of cardiology and cardiovascular surgery. Special training is required to acquire those cardiovascular surgical and invasive cardiology skills needed to achieve a successful result.

Implantable electrophysiologic devices for controlling bradyarrhythmias, tachyarrhythmias, or a combination of both have components implanted on the chest and abdominal wall, transvenously in the right side of the heart, in the coronary sinus, in the cardiac veins, or in the pericardial tissues. Complications result from device failure, tissue injury inflicted by the implanter, and the interaction of the device with the tissue. Understanding the causes of device failure and tissue injury, including the associated inflammatory reaction, is important in the prevention and management of these complications.

Management of complications ranges from abandonment of a failed lead and reimplantation of a new lead to removal of all inflammatory tissue, removal of all implanted devices, and reimplantation of new devices. The more extensive treatments comprise techniques for managing both the soft tissue and intravascular portions of the device, including removal of all foreign material.

In the early 1980s, before the development of successful low-morbidity techniques for extracting leads, every attempt was made to salvage the chronic pacemaker site or, at least, to leave the leads in place if the site had to be abandoned. Removing all foreign material, including chronically implanted leads, and abandoning of the site was considered only when the risk of a recurrent complication (e.g., septicemia) exceeded the risk of lead extraction.

During the past decade, effective, low-morbidity techniques have evolved for transvenous extraction of leads. As successful experiences with lead extraction grow, fewer leads are abandoned, and implant sites are readily abandoned when clinically indicated.

■ TISSUE INJURY AND INFLAMMATORY REACTION

Extravascular Tissue Injury

A pacemaker or an implantable defibrillator and its leads are routinely placed into a subcutaneous or submuscular tissue pocket. Tissue injury caused by placing of the incision and dissection of the pocket (tissue disruption) initiates an inflammatory reaction.[1] Tissue injury caused by the device-related mechanical stresses, such as pressure exacerbated by motion, continues the inflammatory reaction. Normally, the incision heals by wound healing, and tissue around the device heals by encapsulation. Ideally, this encapsulated fibrous tissue sheath protects the surrounding tissue from further injury. The goal is to maintain this accord between the encapsulated device and surrounding tissue indefinitely.

Poor tissue nutrition, tissue reaction to the implanted materials, excessive pressures, infection, and recursive reactions cause further tissue injury and a device-related complication (Fig. 27–1). Tissue nutrition associated with device implants is directly related to the blood supply. Poor nutrition is caused by tissue ischemia; the resultant injury ranges from dissolution of fatty tissue to cellular necrosis (gangrene). Except for extremely rare immunologic reactions, a reaction to implanted materials is associated only with conditions such as the thrombogenic properties of lead insulation (e.g., surface texture, silicone rubber versus polyurethane).[2] Excessive pressures are seen with implantation of large pulse generators and large, stiff leads. Both the reactions to materials and excessive pressures are device performance issues.

Infection is a complication not related to a specific device but rather to tissue contamination by bacteria. The susceptibility of the tissues to infection, however, is probably related to the device–tissue reaction. The term *recursive* was originally a mathematical term referring to the mathematical expression describing an equation that has the solution as

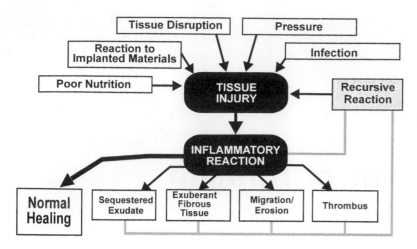

Figure 27-1. Causes of tissue injury. Tissue is injured by a variety of causes. Once tissue is injured, an inflammatory reaction ensues. Depending on the magnitude of the injury and its duration, the tissue will heal "naturally" or "unnaturally," developing one of the recursive reactions. A recursive reaction is defined as a part of the inflammatory reaction, which further injures the tissue and perpetuates the inflammatory reaction.

part of the equation (e.g., $y_{n+1} = y_n + 1$). Some of the products of an inflammatory reaction may cause more tissue injury; this process may be called a *recursive reaction*. For example, sequestered exudate, exuberant fibrous tissue, migration or erosion, and thrombus formation—all products of an inflammatory reaction—may cause further injury to the surrounding tissue and perpetuate the inflammatory reaction. These factors acting individually or together may alter the accord between the encapsulated device and the surrounding tissue, resulting in a complication.

Properties of an Inflammatory Reaction

An inflammatory reaction is a localized protective response elicited by injury or destruction of tissues.[3] It is an integral part of the body's biologic defense system and serves to destroy (bacteria), dilute (toxins), or wall off the injurious agent (such as foreign bodies). Inflammatory reactions cover a broad spectrum but are usually separated into acute and chronic. In acute reactions, vascular and exudative processes predominate. Acute reactions often mature into chronic reactions, in which the formation of stable fibrous tissue predominates. Figure 27–2 summarizes the inflammatory reaction processes.

Exudative Response (Natural or Unnatural)

The exudative process is secondary to the vascular effects and results in a collection of blood plasma, cells, and cellular debris. Depending on the magnitude of the injury and the cellular response, the exudate ranges from an inflammatory edema to pus. Based on the exudative response, I further subdivide inflammatory reactions into natural and unnatural reactions. A natural reaction matures without the formation of a sequestered exudative effusion. The exudate is reabsorbed or organized in a timely fashion. In an unnatural reaction, the exudative process predominates, causing sequestration of the exudative effusion. For a given tissue type, the difference between a natural and an unnatural reaction is a matter of the magnitude and duration of the inflammatory reaction and the presence of "dead space" around the device.

Unnatural reactions are caused by excessive production, poor reabsorption, or retarded organization. For example, the exudative effusion formed by tissue injured by virulent bacteria or collections of necrotic tissue may progress to an abscess or discharge spontaneously. Pathogenic organisms cause varying degrees of tissue injury. Mechanisms include a direct destructive interaction with the tissue, such as intracellular replication, poisoning by toxins, damage by the immunologic defense response, or starvation by passive means, such as competitive metabolism.

The accumulation of exuberant inflammatory tissues (fibrous and granulation tissue) caused by smoldering infections or mechanical stresses occurring over an extended period of time may form a sequestered exudative effusion. These chronic effusions usually contain less cellular debris. Retarded organization also includes cases in which a space large enough to prevent organization of the exudate is created by the device. For example, leads coiled in some configurations may create a space. The unnatural reaction encapsulates this space and causes a cyst, usually filled with edema fluid.

Organization

Organization refers to the replacement of the exudate, necrotic material, and thrombus—first with granulation tissue and then fibrous tissue. Granulation is the beginning of the healing phase of an inflammatory reaction. It is the reddish, granular, collagenous tissue formed by elongated fibroblasts and buds of endothelial cells forming fibrous tissue and capillaries. The amount of granulation tissue present is dependent on the magnitude and duration of the tissue injury. In a natural inflammatory reaction associated with an uncomplicated device implantation, the granulation tissue is rapidly replaced by fibrous tissue. The incision and pacemaker pocket may appear pink for a few weeks after implantation, but exuberant granulation tissue should not be present.

A foreign body reaction occurs when any durable foreign body (too large for phagocytosis) injures tissue. A foreign body reaction is characterized by macrophages adhering to the surface, differentiating into foreign body giant cells, and attempting to surround the foreign body. For example, a foreign body reaction occurs when the pulse generator and leads are placed within disrupted pocket tissue and when an electrode is implanted in the heart. The chronic pacemaker pocket is the encapsulation of the pacemaker and leads by fibrous tissue and foreign body giant cells, resulting from the organization process and foreign body reaction.

Exuberant Fibrous Tissue

A gradual build-up of exuberant fibrous tissue is caused by a continuing, low-grade chronic inflammatory reaction. Two examples of this type of reaction are a smoldering (occult) infection and a continuous mechanical stress. Over time, the scar tissue increases both in mass and in tensile strength; it may even calcify after 8 to 10 years in adults or after 3 to 4 years in children.[4, 5] Although the role of fibrous tissue is to form a protective barrier or increase the tissue's tensile strength, aging exuberant fibrous tissue may cause further injury to the normal tissue and may predispose the tissue to another complication, such as infection or erosion (recursive reaction).

Anti-inflammatory agents such as glucocorticosteroids suppress the inflammatory reaction. In general, inflammatory reactions are protective and should not be suppressed. However, in some situations, local application of a glucocorticoid to suppress a low-grade natural reaction is beneficial. For example, steroid-eluting electrodes in most cases eliminate the clinically apparent reaction at the electrode–myocardial interface without causing any adverse consequences.

Mechanical Stress

Compliant tissues may be compressed and stretched by mechanical stress (positive or negative pressures), directly injuring the tissue. Compliant tissues are compressed at the positive pressure point and stretched some distance away. Negative pressure from pulling on a device stretches and then compresses the tissue. The stretching and compression continue until the forces balance. Excessive pressures may compromise the tissue's blood supply and thereby cause additional tissue injury.

The physical properties of the implanted device (size, weight, configuration, and surface texture) determine the pressure applied to the tissue. Weight is a force, and combined with size and configuration, it determines the resultant applied pressure (force/area). Large, heavy, blunt objects and small, light, sharp objects can both cause the same pressures. Motion and other external forces accentuate the force applied to the tissue. Surface texture can also influence pressure. Current devices are smooth, but, if placed within a Dacron mesh pouch, tissue growth within the interstices of the mesh more uniformly distribute the forces and help negate size, weight, and configuration problems.

Creation of a pocket of sufficient size minimizes the pressure applied to the surrounding tissues by an implanted device. Forcing a device in too small a pocket stretches the tissue, and the resultant tension (force/length) may injure the tissue. In contrast, too large a pocket leaves disrupted tissue, not occupied by the device, that will be filled with an exudate, increasing the amount of granulation tissue.

Wound Healing

Healing of reapproximated disrupted tissue occurs through an inflammatory reaction called *wound healing*. The magnitude of this reaction is related to the severity of tissue injury.

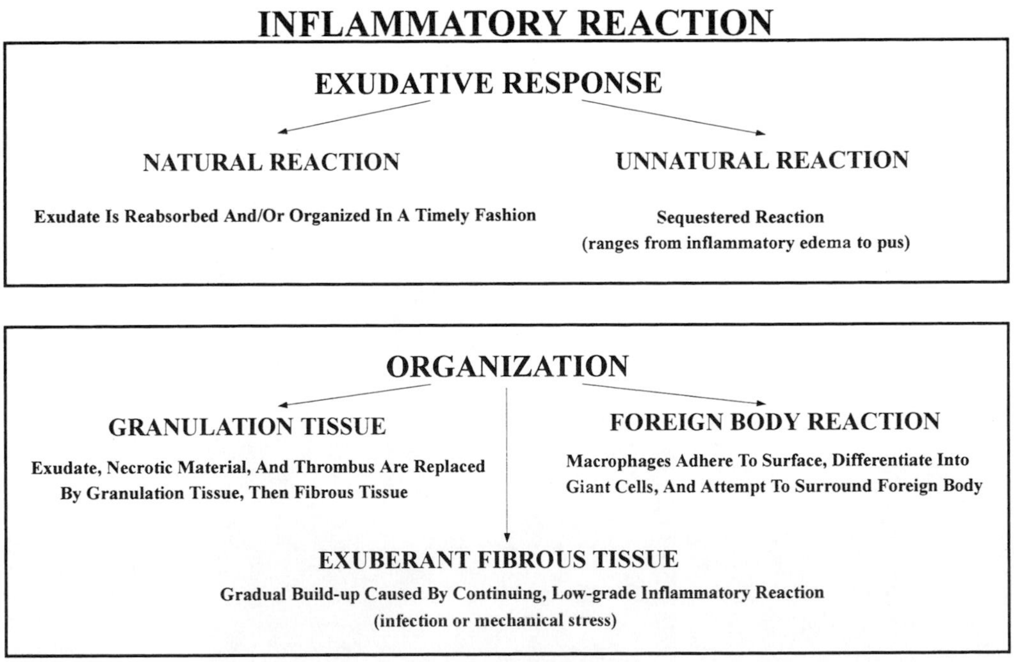

Figure 27–2. Tissue response to injury. The initial response to tissue injury is the exudative response. If the exudate is absorbed or organized in a timely fashion, it is classified as natural. If the exudate is sequestered, it is classified as unnatural. All unnatural reactions represent a complication of wound healing.
Organization of the exudate and inflammatory debris begins with the formation of granulation tissue. In natural reactions, the granulation tissue matures into fibrous tissue. In most unnatural reactions, some granulation tissue persists. The foreign-body reaction begins in the initial stages of the inflammatory reaction with macrophages adhering to the surface of the foreign body. During the maturation of the organization process, giant cells are formed in an attempt to surround the foreign body. If the inflammatory reaction is chronic (e.g., infection, mechanical), exuberant fibrous tissue is formed.

Sharp dissection using a scalpel, electrosurgery, or a laser causes minimal damage; the tissue heals by a predictable natural reaction called *first intention*. Tissue disruption from blunt trauma that causes significant tissue injury, including tissue necrosis, may heal poorly. A large sequestered exudate (unnatural reaction) frequently develops in injuries of this magnitude. Spontaneous drainage of these collections effectively exteriorizes the wound, resulting in an open granulating wound that heals by *second intention*. Healing by second intention is not compatible with a successful device implant, and the device must be removed. Large wounds with skin loss healing by second intention may not heal, leaving only granulation tissue as the protective barrier. This by definition is a *perpetual inflammatory reaction*. These wounds must be covered by a skin graft.

Intravascular Tissue Injury

Permanent transvenous leads are an example of a device causing both extrathoracic and intravascular injury by disruption and mechanical stress. The intravascular interaction injures tissue by endothelial contact and, in some cases, disruption.

Encapsulation With Fibrous Tissue

Depending on the insulation material, 30% to 80% of the intravascular portions of leads may be encapsulated with fibrous tissue initiated by thrombus formation.[6, 7] Fibrous tissue encapsulation ranges from a thin collagenous sheath to thick circumferential bands that bind the lead to the vein or heart wall and to other leads (Fig. 27–3). Leads injure the intima of the veins and cardiac wall by mechanical stress, activating the coagulation mechanism and causing thrombus

formation. The slightest touch is sufficient to start the process. Slowing (stasis) or eddying of the blood flow around the lead also has the potential to cause thrombus. In addition, lead materials, such as silicone rubber (Silastic), tend to be more thrombogenic than polyurethane (Fig. 27–4). The inflammatory reaction associated with organization of thrombus is responsible for encapsulation with fibrous tissue.

Tissue injury from an implanted lead starts at the entry site (tissue disruption) and occurs at each point where the lead body touches the vein and cardiac wall (mechanical stress). At points where the lead does not remain in contact with the wall, the thrombus lyses. At points where the vein remains in contact with the wall, a chronic microthrombus and organization process continues with encapsulation of the lead at that point. As the vein curves, the lead body contacts the wall. The greater the curvature, the greater the area of contact and potential for tissue injury.

With time, the encapsulating fibrous tissue increases its tensile strength through maturation of the collagen. Some of the thicker tissue differentiates from dense collagen into cartilage and finally into bone. Mineralized tissues (usually crystallized calcium deposits) are seen in adult humans in 6 to 8 years and in young children in 3 to 4 years.[4, 5] These findings are routinely observed in animal models, and human observations are similar.[6–9]

Properties of the Electrode–Myocardium Interface

The electrode is placed against the myocardial tissue, forming the electrode–myocardium interface. The electrode exerts mechanical stress against the myocardial tissue, causing injury. Electrodes implanted in the ventricular chamber are

Lead Encapsulation

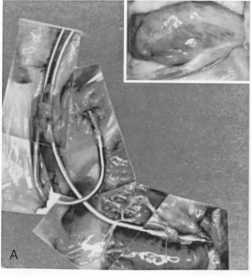

Acute

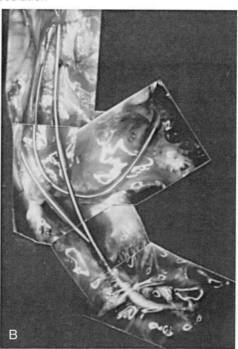

B

Chronic

Figure 27–3. Thrombus formation. *A,* Acute thrombus formation 1 week after implantation in a dog. Thrombus forms at each site where the lead touches the wall and in some regions where there was stasis or eddying of blood flow. Most of this early thrombus lyses. It persists and organizes at sites of continued pressure on the wall and in areas with stagnant blood flow. *B,* Organized fibrous tissue encapsulating the lead forms chronically at sites of pressure, motion, and stasis of blood flow. This material progresses with time from fibrous tissue, to cartilaginous tissue, and finally to bone.

Encapsulation at 12 Weeks

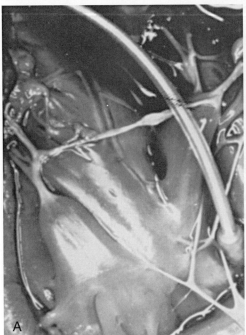 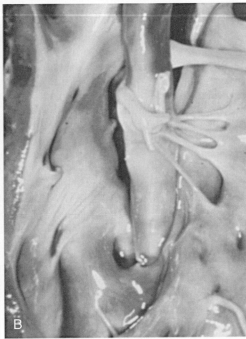

Figure 27–4. Reaction to polyurethane and silicone rubber. Polyurethane and silicone rubber leads implanted for 12 weeks. *A,* The polyurethane lead has minimal encapsulation, and the silicone rubber lead is completely encapsulated. *B,* This is a surface thrombogenicity phenomenon and not related to the mechanical properties of the lead. The magnitude of the surface encapsulation is probably related to silicone leads being more difficult to extract than polyurethane in the first 2 to 3 years after implantation.

Polyurethane   Silicone

subjected to more mechanical stress than are those in the atrium during contraction. The magnitude and duration of the inflammatory reaction, also known as *electrode maturation,* varies. If the inflammatory response is not excessive, steroid-eluting electrodes will suppress the maturation reaction.

Passive-Fixation Devices

Passive-fixation devices, such as tines or fins, hold the electrode in position by entrapment of the fixation device within the trabeculated musculature along the heart wall. The injury caused by the fixation mechanism results in an inflammatory reaction and thrombus formation. Stasis of blood in the trabeculated musculature along the lead body and around the tines also causes thrombus formation. In the ventricle, the passive-fixation devices alone acutely secure the electrode. In most cases in the atrium, the tension on a J configuration is usually needed to ensure stability (straight flexible leads can be successfully implanted in trabeculated atrial tissue in some cases). Chronically, the encapsulating fibrous tissue formed by the inflammatory reaction and organization of thrombus secures the electrode.

Passive-fixation devices are separated from the electrode–myocardium interface. The tissue reaction and organization of clot does not appear to influence the maturation reaction at the electrode–myocardium interface. In some cases, the tines or fins absorb some of the mechanical stresses, reducing the pressures at the electrode–myocardium interface.

Active-Fixation Devices

Current active-fixation devices are wire helices screwed into the myocardium. The inflammatory reaction is initiated by tissue disruption, when the helix is screwed into the myocardium, and is continued by mechanical stress. With active-fixation devices, the wire helix may also serve as the elec-

trode or as part of the electrode, or it may be contiguous with but isolated from the electrode. The injury caused by the active fixation device adds in varying degrees to the electrode maturation reaction. Steroid-eluting electrodes are not always successful in eliminating maturation phenomena of this magnitude. All of the acute stability and most of the chronic stability is dependent on the helix. Chronically, fibrous tissue is supportive, but it may not be sufficient to stabilize the electrode if the helix is not screwed into the tissue.

■ COMPLICATIONS ASSOCIATED WITH THE SUBCUTANEOUS TISSUE AND SUBMUSCULAR POCKETS

The term *pocket* is used to describe the placement site for the pulse generator classically within the subcutaneous or submuscular tissues. Usually, the pocket is placed on the anterior chest wall for transvenous implants or abdominal wall for epicardial implants. However, transvenous leads can be tunneled to an abdominal pocket and epicardial leads tunneled to a chest wall pocket. Pulse generators can also be placed in more exotic locations, such as inside the thorax or abdomen, in the axilla, or on the back. Fortunately, exotic implantations are rare. Complications associated with submuscular pockets are technically more difficult to deal with than those associated with subcutaneous tissue pockets. New pockets include both the pulse generator and all portions of the leads placed within the same tissue plane. Chronic (old) pockets include the pulse generator and only the contiguous leads.

Implant pockets usually heal uneventfully and mature, reaching an accord with the surrounding tissue. Healing starts with wound healing and encapsulation of the implant devices. The tissue is subjected to mechanical stresses during both the healing and maturation of the pocket. The maturation process lasts the duration of the implant. It is a dynamic process with the device–tissue interaction determining the lysis, deposition, and composition of the encapsulating tissue. Normal capsules are made up primarily of fibrous tissue; however, with aging some become lined with calcified plaques.

Pocket complications are summarized in Table 27–1 and include pocket hematoma, wound dehiscence, migration, erosion, pain, and infection. Hematoma formation and wound dehiscences are acute events and are usually related to implantation technique. A pocket hematoma may form late in anticoagulated patients if the pocket is subjected to trauma. Migration, erosion, and pain are related to device–tissue interaction. Infection is caused by contamination of the pocket and is associated with implantation technique and tissue made susceptible by an abnormal device–tissue interaction.

Pocket Hematoma

A hematoma developing immediately after implantation is one of the most common complications associated with a device implant. Although this is a technique-related complication, experienced implanters occasionally have difficulty obtaining hemostasis. Three conditions predispose to hematoma formation: a tear outside the fascial plane, arterial bleeding, and extrusion of venous blood back along the leads into the pocket. Electrosurgery is useful for tissue dissection and for the coagulation of small venous bleeders. It is not recommended for other bleeding conditions. Suture ligation is the only sure way to prevent a recurrence of bleeding.

Fascial Plane Between the Subcutaneous Tissue and Pectoralis Major or Abdominal Muscle

The fascial plane between the subcutaneous tissue and muscle is relatively avascular, but occasionally there are perforating vessels crossing the fascial plane. A dissection or tear out of the fascial plane into either the subcutaneous or muscular tissue can, therefore, cause bleeding. In addition, the pectoralis muscle is easily separated in the direction of its muscle fibers, especially in older patients. This leaves the intramural portion of the muscle exposed and frequently causes bleeding. Hemostasis is best obtained by reapproximation of the muscle and fascial tissue using an absorbable running suture.

Plane Beneath the Pectoralis Major or Rectus Abdominis Muscle

The plane beneath the pectoralis major muscle superficial to the pectoralis minor muscle is also avascular. Care must be taken to open the pectoralis major muscle medial and inferior to the second costal cartilage. At this point, the origins of the pectoralis minor muscle are superior and lateral, thus ensuring entering the correct plane. The dissection can then be extended laterally over the pectoralis minor. Staying under the major and on top of the minor not only is relatively avascular but also prevents projection of the pulse generator into the axilla when the arm is lifted.

Beneath the superior portion of the rectus abdominis muscle is a large plane. This plane has large perforating neurovascular bundles passing from the abdomen to the muscle. Bundles in close proximity to the pocket location must be safely secured by suture ligation. The posterior rectus sheath should not be opened. A cut or tear in this sheath could result in herniation of bowel into the pocket.

Table 27–1. Pocket Complications

Complication	Predisposing Factors or Causes	Treatment

Pocket hematoma	Tearing outside of fascial plane
	Arterial bleeding
	Extrusion of venous blood along leads
		If it is large enough to be palpated:
		  Remove clot and debris
		  Obtain hemostasis
		  Reduce pocket size if necessary
		  Use closed drainage system if hemostasis is difficult to achieve
		Avoid repeated needle aspirations

Wound dehiscence	Excessive stress on suture line by hematoma, hemorrhagic effusion, or trauma
	Error in surgical technique
		Immediate:
		  Attempt to salvage site
		Delayed:
		  Treat as infected pocket

Migration	Unknown	No treatment unless another complication exists

Erosion	Device implanted outside correct plane
	Sustained an insult, forcing device out of correct plane (compromised blood supply, trauma, sequestered effusion)
		Before pocket sticks to skin:
		  Débride and relocate pocket
		After pocket sticks to skin or skin is broken:
		  Treat as infected (abandon site)

Pain	??	Relocate pocket if necessary

Infection	Perioperative contamination
	Chronic site may have poorer defenses against infection
	Metastatic (seeding from remote infection or procedure, such as teeth cleaning)
	Chronic occult infection becomes acute
	Note: pocket infection may present as respiratory distress if infection decompresses into venous system
		Most infections:
		  Antibiotic treatment and abandon site (removing device and leads)
		If no septicemia, no inflammatory build-up around leads near insertion site, and >2.5 cm from pocket to suture sleeve:
		  Antibiotic treatment and abandonment of pocket may be sufficient

Arterial Bleeding

Arterial bleeding within the pocket causes the most dramatic hematoma. The hematoma develops rapidly; if it is not corrected immediately, the pressurized pocket enlarges by dissection into the tissue planes or decompresses by rupturing through the incision. In the pectoral region, a small artery running in the direction of the pectoralis muscle fibers, on or just beneath the surface, is commonly involved. Also, if the cephalic vein is used, bleeding from a small artery running parallel to the vein in the deltopectoral groove must be controlled.

Extrusion of Blood

A pocket hematoma can develop from blood forced retrograde out of the implant vein along the leads into the pocket. Although the pocket may be dry, an elevated venous pressure from heart failure, Valsalva maneuver, or coughing can extrude blood along the leads, filling the pocket with venous blood. With an introducer approach, extrusion of blood is prevented by placing a suture around the leads at the muscle entry site. The suture also prevents debris collected within the pocket from being forced back into the venous circulations. If the cephalic vein is used, a suture around the vein and leads at the entry site will suffice.

Organization of Clot

Once clot forms in the pocket, it is subjected to both lysis and organization. Lysis creates particulate debris, increasing the osmotic and oncotic pressures by pulling fluid into the pocket, thereby creating a hemorrhagic effusion. As the hemorrhagic effusion increases, the resultant tension on the pocket wall may continue to enlarge the pocket by dissection into the tissue planes or may rupture the incision. Both these complications require surgical intervention for correction.

Organization of a large clot in a pocket may result in excessive granulation tissue and, eventually, exuberant fibrous tissue. Granulation tissue may be seen years after the organization of a large hematoma. These pockets are not healthy and behave similarly to pockets with exuberant fibrous tissue.

Treatment

A pocket hematoma large enough to be palpated should be treated. The most successful treatment is immediate pocket exploration. All clot and tissue debris must be removed and hemostasis obtained. If the pocket has been enlarged, the dissected region should be excluded, leaving an appropriate-sized pocket. If adequate hemostasis is difficult to achieve, a closed drainage system (e.g., Jackson-Pratt) is placed in the excluded pocket to prevent the hematoma from recurring. The immediate surgical correction of a hematoma and, if necessary, the proper placement of a closed drainage system do not adversely affect the healing of the pocket.

Prolonged observation and procrastination must be avoided. This is especially true when the pocket wall is tense. Needle aspiration decompresses the pocket but does not remove the clot. Repeated needle aspirations increase the risk for infection. Other complications of an untreated hematoma include wound dehiscence, migration and erosion, and infection.

Wound Dehiscence

Wound dehiscence is a rare event. It occurs within the first few days or weeks after implantation. During the acute wound healing phase, suture material is required to reapproximate and reinforce the tissue. Most cases of wound dehiscence are caused by excessive stress placed on the suture line by a hematoma, hemorrhagic effusion, or trauma. Traumatic disruption is rare. Dehiscence without a predisposing cause is due to an error in surgical technique.

Treatment is to attempt to salvage the site by intervening immediately after dehiscence. This is similar to treating a hematoma and is usually successful. A delayed intervention allows gross contamination, and an infection is likely to develop. When intervention is delayed (Fig. 27–5), it is treated as an infected pocket with abandonment and reimplantation on the opposite side, if possible. This is discussed later in the section on the treatment of infected pockets.

Migration

Migration is the movement of a device through the surrounding tissue. In the past, migration was more common, owing to the large size and pointed shape of some devices, even when contained in a Dacron pouch. Most migrations are slow (occurring over a period of years), move in an inferolateral direction, and do not cause complications. The exact mechanism for migration is unclear. One possibility is the weight of the device interacting with the motion of the musculoskeletal system, creating directed forces that compress or stretch the fibrous capsule and surrounding tissues. A cycle of fibrous tissue lysis and formation associated with a low-grade inflammatory reaction might move the foreign body through the tissue. A migrated device is not usually treated unless a complication exists.

Wound Dehiscence

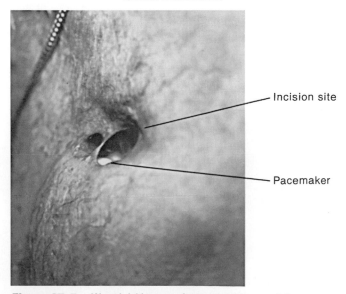

Incision site

Pacemaker

Figure 27–5. Wound dehiscence. A wound dehiscence left unattended for more than a week. The pacemaker pocket developed a hematoma, which evacuated spontaneously, rupturing the incision. The incision was not débrided and re-closed. It became secondarily infected.

Erosion

Erosion is the exteriorization of the device after the loss of integrity of the skin wall. The pacemaker pocket sticks to the skin before erosion (pre-erosion). Before the skin sticks, it can be moved freely over the pocket. At this point, if infection is not present, débridement and relocation of the pocket are usually successful. After the skin sticks, an inflammatory reaction ensues, and bacteria cross the skin, contaminating the pocket. Pockets treated after the skin sticks or after frank erosion occurs are treated as infected pockets.

To erode, the device must migrate outside the normally enclosing tissue plane. For this to occur, it would have to be implanted outside the correct plane or sustain an insult forcing it out of the plane, such as compromise of the blood supply, trauma, or a sequestered effusion.

Implants Outside of Tissue Planes

Flat devices, such as pulse generators, do well when implanted in a natural tissue plane (fascial plane) between two tissue types (subcutaneous tissue and pectoralis muscle or pectoralis muscle and chest wall). Minimal pressures are exerted by the flat surfaces against the two tissue types. The larger pressures are applied by the device's curved surfaces. The forces applied to the curved surfaces tend to keep the device within this tissue plane. It may migrate, but not erode.

Poorly positioned implants with a portion of their curved surface extending out of the fascial plane tend to migrate, and many erode. Erosions occurring within the first few months after an initial implantation are not uncommon in these situations. A trend is to make the pocket within the subcutaneous tissue, especially in obese patients. This pocket has to be perfect and without applied stress, or it is free to migrate in any direction. Most of the eroding pockets that I have seen were placed in the subcutaneous fatty tissue.

Pacemaker pulse generators placed under the pectoralis major muscle sometimes protrude into the axilla when the muscle is flexed. This is because the device was placed under both the pectoralis major and minor. The result may be migration into the axilla, pain, or erosion. This complica-

tion is avoided by placing the device more medially under the pectoralis major and over the pectoralis minor.

Compromised Blood Supply

Compromise of the blood supply causes tissue loss. Blood supply is compromised by mechanical factors and by exuberant fibrous tissue causing pressure. When the blood supply to a region of subcutaneous tissue and skin is compromised, the resultant dissolution of the subcutaneous tissue (pre-erosion) is caused by lack of nutrition. If severe enough, tissue necrosis occurs, leaving only ischemic or gangrenous skin (Fig. 27–6).

Trauma and Sequestered Effusion

Trauma and sequestered effusion may rupture the fibrous capsule barrier around the device. A traumatic rupture is intuitively obvious, resulting in device migration through the rupture site. A sequestered effusion in an infected pocket or a hematoma, however, can generate sufficient pressure to erode through the subcutaneous tissue and skin, draining to the outside. Other contributing mechanisms include tissue ischemia and an intense inflammatory reaction.

Pain

Occasionally, patients complain of pain in or near the pocket, which can be severe. A worst-case scenario for a normal healing process occurs in the patient who is involved in strenuous physical activity. This type of patient should be given more time for postimplantation pain to subside. If the pain is caused by the physical activities, it will subside when the body adjusts to the applied stresses. Patients seem to get through the period of pain just as fast when they are encouraged to continue their activities.

Chronic pain is not normal, and patients complaining of pain should be taken seriously. An implanted device is like a watch: the patient should be aware of its existence only when something draws attention to it. Pain on the chest wall can cause other symptoms. For example, chronic chest wall pain can cause muscle spasm. Spasm of the neck muscles can cause a thoracic outlet syndrome. Spasm of the pectoralis

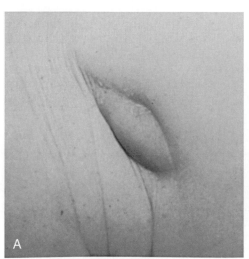

Pre-erosion

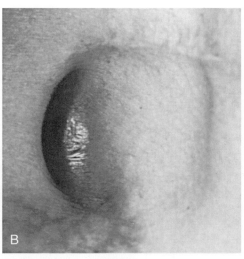

Gangrene

Figure 27–6. Compromised blood supply. Compromise of the blood supply to the subcutaneous tissue and skin causes a decrease in the supply of nutrients to these cells. *A,* In the early stages (pre-erosion), the fatty tissue begins to lose mass. During the latter pre-erosion stages, the tissue becomes ischemic with skin changes. The last stage before erosion is adhesion of the skin to the fibrous tissue pocket. *B,* Complete loss of blood supply to the skin results in gangrene of the skin before erosion.

muscles causes discomfort on moving the arm and tenderness at its insertion site on the humerus.

There is no quantitative diagnostic test for the cause of the pain; history and physical examination make the diagnosis. The cause of pain may be nerve entrapment, inflammation of the scar tissue, migration, or injury to the musculoskeletal system. Pain associated with no physical signs may be related to nerve entrapment. Because nerves cannot be seen, a diagnostic exploration of the pocket is not an option. The best chance for a successful treatment is to remove the generator and leads, abandon the side, and reimplant the device on the opposite side.

Inflammation of the scar tissue is usually obvious. The scar is exuberant, red, and painful to the touch. Injection with steroid reduces the inflammation and eventually alleviates the symptoms.

Pain associated with injury to the musculoskeletal system can be related to the initial placement of the pocket or to migration. Placement of the pocket near the deltopectoral groove is common. The pulse generator injures the structures contiguous with the deltopectoral groove. These areas are tender to touch, and the symptoms can be elicited by moving the arm medially. Pain is usually caused, not by the migration per se, but rather by some traumatic event associated with the new anatomic position. For example, trauma to a rib or at the costochondral junctions is the most common pain complaint. Pocket relocation to another subcutaneous area or to a site beneath the pectoralis major muscle may be effective.

Another cause is injury to the pectoralis major muscle from sutures, tears, or erosions into the muscle. In most cases, the pain is typical of muscle spasm, and the insertion site on the humerus is tender. Spasm of the neck muscle is not uncommon in this situation. This pain usually subsides when the muscle injury heals.

Infected Pocket

Infections involving implanted devices are challenging, not only because of the severity and duration of the inflammatory reaction but also because of the sequelae. The incidence of reported cardiac pacing system infection ranges from 0% to 19%.[10-15] Patients presenting with a device infection are classified in one group encompassing a spectrum that ranges from contaminated tissue to cellulitis with marked tissue loss. In this classification, dry pocket erosion with a positive culture is placed in the same group as acute pocket infection with *Staphylococcus aureus*, cellulitis, a marked purulent effusion, and septicemia. The management of these two "infections" is entirely different. The former is not a tissue infection. This pocket probably had ischemic erosion with some bacterial contamination but no cellulitis; that is, the tissue was not invaded by bacteria or their toxins. These examples demonstrate the two extremes in managing infected pacing systems.

Classification of Infections

Infections associated with implanted devices may be extravascular, intravascular, or both. To avoid ambiguities in discussing infections, I have classified them as class I through class IV (Table 27–2). This classification was designed to reflect the potential morbidity and mortality associated with the type of infection. It does not necessarily relate to the magnitude of the infection for a given tissue type, its acute or chronic nature, nor how extensive the treatment required to eradicate the infection.

Table 27–2. Classes of Device-Related Infections

Class		Definition
I		Endocarditis
	Ia	Infected cardiac tissue
	Ib	Infected vegetation
	Ic	Broken lead fragment in heart
II		Septicemia without endocarditis
III		Extravascular tissue infection
IV		Chronic contamination of extravascular tissue

For example, a class II extravascular infection in a subcutaneous tissue pocket (subcutaneous tissue abscess) with marked cellulitis, a massive suppurative effusion, and septicemia causes significant local morbidity and may cause a lethal systemic condition through metastatic spread. An identical extravascular infection in a subcutaneous tissue pocket without septicemia is a class III infection. The same infection may evolve into class IV by spontaneously draining and forming a chronic draining sinus without cellulitis. A class IV pocket is lined with granulation tissue and contaminated with bacteria. The pocket is not infected, however, in the sense that bacteria or their toxins invade the tissue, causing cellulitis.

The initial treatment is essentially the same for all classes. The only differences are the intensity of the antibiotic therapy before and after the surgical procedures and the potential for incision and drainage of an abscess in classes I through III to ensure resolution of the cellulitis. Curative therapy for all classes includes removal of all inflammatory and foreign material, both extravascular and intravascular. This includes intracardiac vegetation.

Infection of an Initial Implantation Site

Acute infections after an initial implantation in normal tissue are rare and usually result from some breach of technique, contaminating the pocket with a virulent bacterium (Fig. 27–7). *Acute* is a clinically descriptive term meaning of rapid onset, severe, and of short duration. For example, inadvertent contamination of the pocket or devices with *S. aureus* will probably cause an acute infection. Most surgical sites are contaminated by mainly nonvirulent bacteria, such as *Staphylococcus epidermidis*, and do not become infected. The body's defenses can eradicate a small inoculum of these bacteria. However, a large inoculation or the presence of a culture medium such as devitalized tissue or hematoma can negate the body's defenses, and an infection will ensue.

An acute infection involving an implanted pulse generator and leads in a subcutaneous tissue pocket causes the most severe tissue reactions. They are characterized by cellulitis, a suppurative effusion within the pocket (abscess), and, in some cases, decompression into the blood, causing septicemia or discharge through the skin and thus a draining sinus. If septicemia is present, the infection is life-threatening and demands immediate treatment. The magnitude of the cellulitis reflects the tissue reaction to the bacteria and their toxins.

Pocket Infections

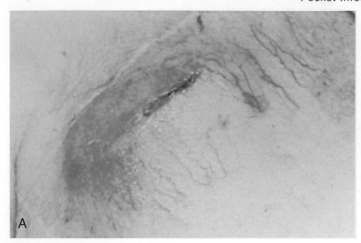

Acute infection

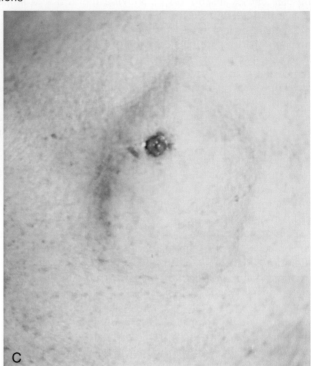

Chronic draining sinus

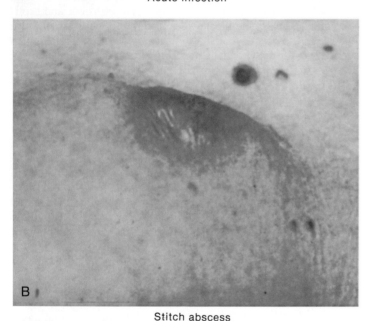

Stitch abscess

Figure 27–7. Infected pocket. *A,* An acute pocket infection caused by a virulent organism immediately after a device implantation or reimplantation is rare and is a result of some form of pocket contamination (breach of sterile technique or metastatic). These infections are equivalent to an abscess with cellulitis and a sequestered purulent exudate. Treatment includes antibiotics and I & D, if the exudate is large, applying pressure to the surrounding tissue, or both.

B, A local abscess around suture or other isolated implanted object decompresses and forms a chronic draining sinus. In these cases, the implanted devices may not be infected. It is impossible to be sure, however, and these local infections are treated as if the device is involved.

C, Chronic draining sinus is a continuously draining infection. In most cases, some part of the implanted device (pulse generator or leads) is infected. While draining, an accord is reached, and the infection is controlled. If drainage stops, the infection is uncontrolled, and an abscess develops.

Infection of a Chronic (Old) Implantation Site

An acute infection involving a chronic pocket is more common. Chronic infection is a clinical condition implying persistent, of less severity, and of long duration. Acute infections can evolve into chronic infections, and chronic infections can change into acute infections. Most infections begin after an invasive reintervention procedure, usually after replacement of a new device (pulse generator or lead) back into the old pocket. Again, during a surgical procedure, tissue is normally exposed to some degree of contamination, such as skin bacteria. Some chronic pacemaker pockets cannot tolerate minimal levels of contamination without developing an infection. For example, pockets with exuberant fibrous tissue exposed to bacteria such as *S. epidermidis* frequently become infected.

Metastatic Infections

Another cause of pocket infection is seeding of the pocket by bacteria from a remote infection or from a procedure such as teeth cleaning.[16] The question of covering patients with prophylactic antibiotics in these situations is still unanswered in the literature.[17–20] I believe that prophylactic antibiotics should be used. The antibiotic therapy used should be similar to the protocols published for patients with diseased or prosthetic heart valves.

The same logic used for prophylactic therapy for chronic implants also applies to acute implants and chronic reimplants. The same probability for metastatic spread exists for both these procedures. In addition, phlebitis and lymphadenitis caused by an infected intravenous fluid administration site have the potential to infect a new device implant pocket and probably a chronic pocket. Therefore, intravenous fluids probably should not be administered on the same side as the implant.

Chronic Occult Infection

Smoldering or occult infections, causing no signs or symptoms, are defined as chronic infections within the pocket. In these low-grade infections some sort of balance is usually reached between the bacteria and the body's defenses. Such chronic infections are usually caused by *S. epidermidis*. On pocket exploration, exuberant fibrous tissue with or without an exudative effusion is present. Granulation tissue may also be present. Bacteria are difficult to culture from small exudates within these pockets. Once the infection has reached a stage where it cannot be suppressed by the body's defenses, it becomes symptomatic. Chronic infections are reclassified as acute when signs and symptoms are present (cellulitis and suppuration).

Chronic Draining Sinus

A chronic draining sinus stabilizes a chronic infection (see Fig. 27–7). An acute infection of a pacemaker pocket behaves like an abscess with a suppurative effusion and cellulitis. The walled-off cavity contains the pulse generator and leads. If the effusion drains through the skin, the abscess cavity is decompressed, the concentration of bacteria and their toxins is decreased, and the cellulitis resolves (usually with the help of antibiotics). With time, a draining sinus develops. The pacemaker pocket is lined with fibrous and granulation tissue. The tissue surrounding the pocket is protected as long as the exudative debris is drained. A balance is achieved, and the infection is tolerated. If the sinus stops draining, the abscess cycle is repeated. Patients with chronic draining sinuses must have lifelong medical management and, in many cases, continuing antibiotic treatment.

In some cases, the entire pocket may not be infected. For example, an infected silk suture (stitch abscess) at the suture sleeve causes a localized abscess, which subsequently forms a draining sinus. In these cases, although the lead and pocket may not be directly involved, there is no way to be absolutely sure, and it should probably be treated the same as an infected lead or pocket.

Respiratory Distress

Pocket infections, which decompress episodically into the venous system, cause fever and pulmonary symptoms. The pulmonary symptoms are from an interstitial reaction caused by the filtering of bacteria and debris in the pulmonary capillary bed. An interstitial reaction is apparent on chest radiographs. Some patients develop significant respiratory distress, especially when the problem persists for a long period of time. Diagnosis is difficult. Patients presenting initially with fever and a persistent cough are sometimes treated for a flulike illness. With antibiotics and time the symptoms improve but then recur after the next episode of bacteremia.

Management of a Device-Related Infection (Author's Experience)

Treatment of class I infected intravenous pacing and defibrillator pockets has been straightforward. The treatment consists of antibiotic therapy, removal of implanted devices, débridement of all inflammatory tissue, abandonment of the pocket, and reimplantation using epicardial leads.[21] Treatment of an infection localized to a soft tissue pocket with or without septicemia (class II and IV) is difficult because of the risk associated with lead removal and the confusing plethora of anecdotal information found in the literature. Treatment with antibiotics, local surgeries, and combinations has been reported to be successful in selected patients.

My experiences were confined to antibiotic therapy combined with procedures designed to either salvage or abandon the implantation site. Antibiotic therapy was never used as the sole modality of therapy. From this experience, a protocol evolved that included preparation of the patient with antibiotic therapy, abandonment of the site, interim antibiotic therapy, reimplantation of a device in a remote site, and predischarge and postdischarge antibiotic therapy. This treatment protocol was used successfully for all class infections (class I through IV). Anything less resulted in a significant failure rate.

Evolution of a Treatment Protocol Using Antibiotics Alone

Antibiotic therapy should not be tried alone as a curative approach. The negative historical experience of others, as well as my own, was the rationale for combining antibiotics with invasive procedures. Antibiotics may cause a remission of the clinical signs and symptoms. However, the remission with virulent bacteria, such as *S. aureus*, may be incomplete, and the clinical manifestations of the infection return as soon as the antibiotic therapy is stopped. The remission with less virulent bacteria, such as *S. epidermidis*, may last for months. The length of the remission is usually related to the condition of the pocket. For example, smoldering infections with a thick layer of encapsulating fibrous tissue usually recur within 1 or 2 weeks after the antibiotics are stopped. These infections in more normal pockets have longer remissions because of the ability of the body's biologic defense systems to engage the bacteria.

Another compelling reason for avoiding treatments with antibiotics alone is the development of resistance to the antibiotics. A high percentage of patients treated for long periods of time with antibiotics are resistant to most of the commonly used antibiotics. It is not uncommon for *S. epidermidis* treated for months to be susceptible to vancomycin and only one or two orally administered antibiotics, such as tetracycline or trimethoprim-sulfamethoxazole (Bactrim). Mutation of bacterium to strains resistant to conventional antibiotics is a nonabstract, real-world reason to avoid this type therapy.

Antibiotic Therapy Protocol

The antibiotic protocol is given in Figure 27–8. The protocol is specific for the abandonment of the implantation site

Antibiotic Protocol

Treatment Segments

Preparation	Abandonment procedure	Interim	Re-implantation procedure	Pre-discharge	Post-discharge

Preparation

Intravenous Antibiotics
Continue pre-admission IV antibiotics or start vancomycin

Procedures

Intravenous Antibiotics
Vancomycin
Gentamicin (Satisfactory renal function)
Cipro or equivalent (Unsatisfactory renal function)

Figure 27–8. Antibiotic protocol. The antibiotic protocol is divided into clinical treatment segments for a device infection. Each segment corresponds to a clinical treatment, which must be completed before starting the next. The rationale for administering a specific antibiotic is given in the text.

Interim and Pre-discharge

Intravenous antibiotics
  Vancomycin
  Add gram-negative coverage if indicated (e.g., culture results, GU instrumentation)
Oral Antibiotics
  Interim   None
  Pre-discharge None if on intravenous gram-negative coverage
                     Cipro or culture specific if resistant or allergic to Cipro

Post-discharge

Class I	Up to 8 weeks appropriate intravenous antibiotics
Class II	5 to 10 days oral Cipro or culture-specific antibiotic
Class III-IV	5 days oral Cipro or culture-specific antibiotic

procedure. All infections are treated with intravenous antibiotics before the invasive procedures. Because the infecting bacterium and its susceptibilities are usually not known when therapy is instituted, antibiotics having the highest probability of being effective should be chosen. Vancomycin is used in all patients unless medically contraindicated. Most staphylococci are susceptible to vancomycin. For gram-negative coverage, gentamicin is administered in addition to vancomycin. The choice of gentamicin was arbitrary and not based on the need to cover any specific organism.

There is a growing national effort being made to limit the use of vancomycin. On rare occasions during chronic

SALVAGING THE IMPLANTATION SITE

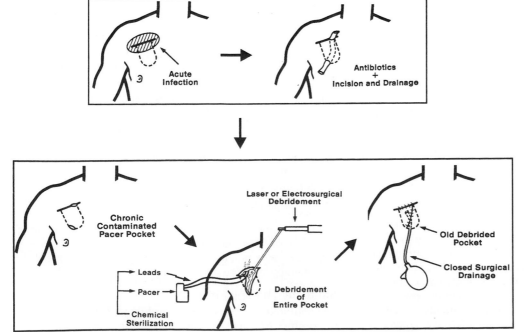

Figure 27–9. Salvaging the site. Acute infections must first be converted into chronic, smoldering infections with a minimal amount of sequestered exudate. In some cases, an incision and drainage (I & D) is performed and the drain left in place.

Chronic smoldering pockets are débrided of all inflammatory tissue using a CO$_2$ laser. The pulse generator is decontaminated using Cidex, and the leads are cleaned using Betadine. The pulse generator is reimplanted in the débrided pocket, and the old portion of the débrided pocket is excluded. A closed drainage system (Jackson-Pratt) is used in all cases.

use of this antibiotic, enterococci and staphylococci have become resistant to it. I still recommend its continued use in treating device-related infections. Patient morbidity, potential mortality, and economic considerations demand that these types of infections be given the same maximal therapeutic regimens as other serious systemic infections.

The offending organism is unknown when the patient first presents for treatment, and in the hospital environment, it is imperative that an antibiotic with the highest probability of success be used. Vancomycin has been effective as the primary antibiotic against most staphylococcal species. Also, as mentioned previously, a high percentage of the staphylococcal species subjected to long-term antibiotic therapies are resistant to most other antibiotics.

Ciprofloxacin was chosen as the preferred oral antibiotic for treatment before and after discharge from the hospital. This was an arbitrary choice based on its broad-spectrum effectiveness against most offending organisms as well as patient acceptance. Many other antibiotics are effective but not well tolerated by patients and, consequently, not taken. When organisms are resistant to ciprofloxacin, an effective antibiotic is chosen from the culture susceptibility data.

The duration of antibiotic therapy before the procedure was determined by the magnitude of the infection. For example, patients with an acute *S. aureus* cellulitis, marked suppuration, and septicemia may require a week of antibiotic therapy, with or without an incision and drainage of the pocket, to resolve the cellulitis and render the patient afebrile. In contrast, a patient with dry gangrenous erosion without cellulitis would need only the few hours required to reach an appropriate blood level of antibiotic. Regardless of the type of infection, two clinical conditions must be met before a surgical procedure: first, the cellulitis must be almost completely resolved to allow a primary intention closure; and second, the patient's temperature must be at most low grade.

Historical Experiences With Salvaging the Implantation Site

Salvaging an implantation site is no longer a viable option: the failure rate is too high, the potential morbidity and mortality are too risky, and economic considerations are prohibitive. Formerly, salvage procedures were designed to correct a pocket infection surgically, leaving the device at the site. A salvage procedure, at a minimum, includes débridement of all inflammatory tissue and debris, leaving only normal viable tissue (Fig. 27–9). A decontaminated old device or a new device is reimplanted in the débrided pocket, and the pocket is closed with or without a closed drainage system.

Débridement of Inflammatory Tissue

All encapsulating and inflammatory tissue must be removed, including the fibrous sheaths tracking the leads into the muscle to near the lead's vein entry site (Fig. 27–10). Successful débridement of encapsulating and inflammatory tissue includes leaving a viable bed of normal tissue and obtaining meticulous hemostasis. Although all tissue dissections are now performed using an electrosurgical unit, my first successful attempts involved the use of CO_2 laser. The surgical principles that must be followed regardless of the dissecting instrument are to minimize the injury to the nor-

Salvage and Abandonment

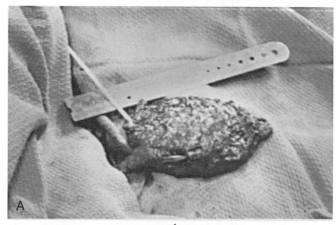

Surgical débridement

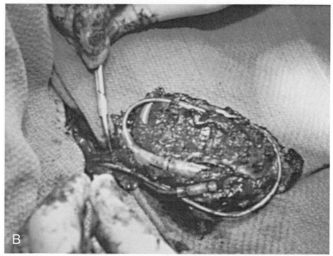

Inflammatory tissue

Figure 27–10. Salvaging the site. *A,* Surgical débridement. To attempt to salvage the site, all inflammatory tissue must be removed, including the tissue around the leads near the vein entry site. *B,* Inflammatory tissue. In this case, the inflammatory tissue extended down near the vein entry site, and the pocket was abandoned. To abandon the site, the pulse generator, leads, and any other retained debris (e.g., suture material, suture sleeves, insulation boot) must be removed in addition to the débridement.

mal tissue and to suture-ligate visible veins and all arteries. Care must be taken to reapproximate separated muscle tissue by direct surgical suturing techniques. Reconstitution of this tissue is necessary to achieve hemostasis.

Decontamination of Devices

In my earlier experience, the pulse generator was decontaminated using glutaral (Cidex), and the leads were wiped clean with povidone-iodine (Betadine) and saline. Although Cidex had the potential to sterilize the pacemaker, it was applied for only a short time and sterility was not assured. The efficacy of lead decontamination by cleaning the surface was dependent on the integrity of the insulation. Insulation with a rough surface or cracks, such as degraded polyurethane, could not be cleaned.

Decontamination and reuse of a pulse generator are no longer done. The warranty provided by the company is usually void if an attempt is made to resterilize the pulse generator. Chemical resterilization may affect the polymers used to insulate the case, the header, and the grommets used to seal the set-screws. Sterilization using ethylene oxide voids the warranty because of the potential for heat-related damage. Therefore, if a device is to be reused after ethylene oxide resterilization, the patient must be made aware of the changes in the warranty and the potential for damaging the device.

Reimplantation Using the Same Site

The pacemaker was reimplanted in the pocket. Most pockets were enlarged after the extensive tissue débridement. If necessary, a portion of the débrided pocket was excluded using interrupted sutures, and the pacemaker was replaced in an appropriately sized space. A closed drainage system (e.g., a flat Jackson-Pratt drain) was routinely used to prevent fluid collection before the adherence of tissue flaps. An exudative or hemorrhagic effusion jeopardizes the success of the procedure by separating the tissues and acting as a culture medium. The closed drainage system was left in place until the drainage stopped and tissue flaps were stuck together (2 to 3 days). All incisions were closed primarily.

Experience With Attempts to Salvage the Implantation Site

The early salvage procedures involved pacemaker erosions or pocket infections with chronic draining sinuses. All were classified as class III and IV infections. Although a few were successfully treated, most failed with immediate recurrence of the infection. In addition, many early successes suffered a recurrence of the infection 6 months to a year after the procedure. A success was then defined as no recurrence of a complication for at least 1 year following the salvage procedure.

Patients must be carefully selected to salvage an infected pocket successfully (Fig. 27–11). Preselection criteria for exclusion were based on experience and included septicemia

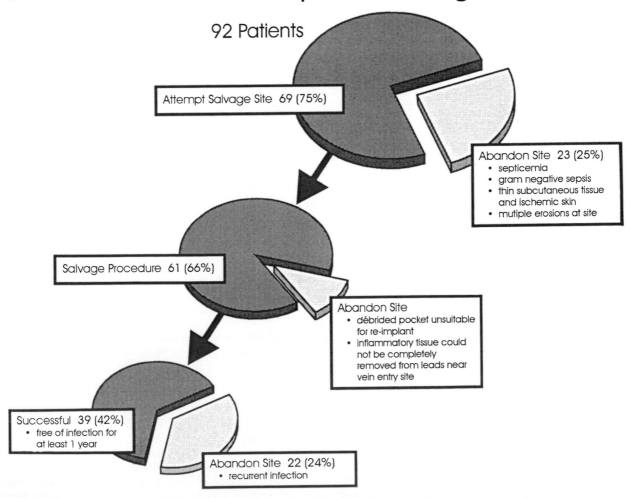

Figure 27–11. This series contains 92 patients presenting with a pocket infection. Only 42% of these patients were successfully treated by the salvage procedure. Of the 69 preselected patients, 57% had a successful result. The salvage procedure was performed on 61 patients, and 39 (64%) were successful.

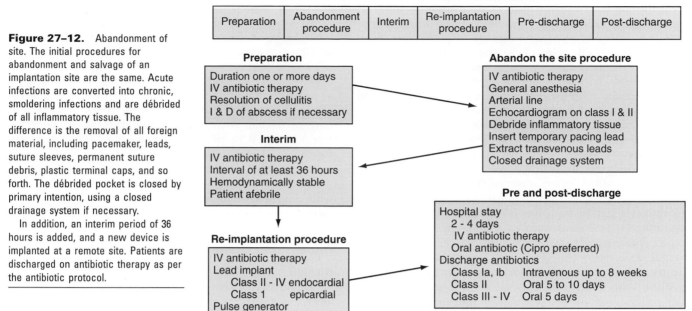

Figure 27–12. Abandonment of site. The initial procedures for abandonment and salvage of an implantation site are the same. Acute infections are converted into chronic, smoldering infections and are débrided of all inflammatory tissue. The difference is the removal of all foreign material, including pacemaker, leads, suture sleeves, permanent suture debris, plastic terminal caps, and so forth. The débrided pocket is closed by primary intention, using a closed drainage system if necessary.

In addition, an interim period of 36 hours is added, and a new device is implanted at a remote site. Patients are discharged on antibiotic therapy as per the antibiotic protocol.

(class I and II), gram-negative sepsis, thin subcutaneous tissue and ischemic skin, and a history of previous erosion at the site. These preselection criteria excluded 25% of the patients.

Further selection occurred during the attempted salvage procedure, excluding another 9%. In these cases, the débrided pocket was judged not suitable for a pacemaker reimplantation, or the inflammatory tissue could not be completely removed from the leads near the vein entry site. The exclusion of these patients required a judgment decision based on experience and the ability to recognize inflammatory changes.

The success rate was 45% for all presenting infections. After excluding 33% of the patients, the success rate for the remaining 67%, those judged suitable for the salvage procedure, was 64%. Excluded patients were treated by an abandonment procedure, which included removal of all foreign material, abandonment of the site, and reimplantation of a new device at a remote site.

During the early and middle 1980s, 45% salvage was an impressive cure rate. Unfortunately, accurately predicting those patients who would have a successful result is not possible. Patients with dry erosions had the highest yield, and those with acute infections had the lowest. Today, the success rate for lead extraction procedures makes salvage procedures, with their 55% failure rate, an unacceptable alternative for the routine management of pocket infections.

Experience With Abandonment of the Site and Remote Reimplantation of a New Device

This modality of management of device-related infections evolved into a protocol, which has been followed for more than 10 years and more than 500 patients (Fig. 27–12). This protocol is divided into treatment segments, each of which must be satisfactorily completed before starting the next.

The antibiotic protocol is a part of this general management protocol. Every attempt was made to maintain consistency in the use of antibiotics. A cephalosporin was used before the availability of ciprofloxacin as the oral antibiotic of choice. To date, this management protocol has been successful in all patients in whom the leads were removed intact. About 10% of the leads broke during removal, leaving broken lead fragments in the heart. Three (<10%) of these retained foreign bodies were subsequently found to be infected. Two were removed by ventriculotomy and one at open heart surgery, combined with a tricuspid valvuloplasty, in another institution.

Abandonment of the Implantation Site

In conjunction with antibiotic therapy, abandonment of the implantation site includes débridement of all inflammatory tissue and primary closure of the site using the procedure performed in salvaging a site. In addition, the pulse generator and leads must be removed and reimplanted at a remote site (usually on the other side). Removal of a device such as a pulse generator or defibrillator from an implant pocket is a minor procedure. Débridement of all inflammatory tissue may occasionally evolve into an extensive surgical procedure.

In the past, the limitation of abandoning the site was the removal of chronically implanted transvenous leads. Today, with the evolution of lead extraction techniques, this is no longer a limitation. In my experience, 95% of leads are successfully extracted using percutaneous transvenous techniques, whereas only 5% require more extensive surgery, such as a transatrial or a ventriculotomy procedure. Open heart procedures, using cardiopulmonary bypass, have not been needed.

Initially, leads were removed by mechanical ablation procedures. Although enough of the lead could be removed to treat the infection in more than 99% of patients, many of these procedures were long, and the level of difficulty limited the number of physicians capable of performing them. Today, the use of an excimer laser (laser ablation) has greatly simplified the procedure. An experienced physician can remove greater than 95% of the leads intact through the vein entry site. Calcification of encapsulating tissue, lead breakage, potential damage to the superior veins, and the presence of intravascular vegetation of the leads are examples of situations in which an alternate procedure is used (about 5% of patients). Currently, the mortality rate for lead removal using mechanical and laser ablation techniques is 0.2% nation wide.[22] In our series of 500 patients, there were no deaths related to the lead removal procedure. Five patients (1%) had a tear of the superior vena cava or right atrium requiring an emergency median sternotomy and a surgical repair. These patients had uneventful recoveries.

All incisions are closed primarily, using a closed drainage system when necessary. Historically, infected abandoned pockets were rarely débrided and were treated by leaving the pocket open to heal by second intention. Healing by second intention was slow, caused some morbidity, and required continued antibiotic therapy and medical attention. Also, a transient bacteremia caused by manipulating the wound could infect a remote implantation site (metastatic infection). Unfortunately, this archaic technique still persists today.

Abandonment of the Pocket Without Removing Leads

Closure of the Pocket and Cure of the Infection

In one specific situation, the pocket can be abandoned removing the proximal portion of the leads and leaving the distal portion intact.[6] The infected chronic pocket must be remote (greater than 2.5 cm from the lead insertion site) and free of any visible inflammatory response. Through a separate incision at the lead insertion site the leads are inspected and, if found free of inflammatory tissue, are cut, clipped, and abandoned. Leads should not be allowed to retract into the superior veins. Leads not anchored in the superior veins may migrate, causing another complication. This incision is closed. The pocket is then opened, the proximal portion of the leads removed, and all inflammatory tissue débrided; and the pocket is closed primarily.

Closure of the Pocket Creating a Permanent Pocket Infection With a Chronic Draining Sinus

Some patients with class III and IV infections are not candidates for one of the previously described procedures. An alternative for these patients is to create a stable class IV infection. A class IV infection becomes class III when the draining sinus closes. The goal is to create a chronic draining sinus, which stays open and drains. This is accomplished by removal of the pulse generator; débridement of the pocket, cutting the leads long; and closure of the pocket around the lead, creating a chronic draining sinus. The leads should be anchored to the skin. As long as the leads protrude from the sinus tract, the chronic draining sinus will persist. The only care is chronic dressing changes. Antibiotic therapy is instituted only for the 7 to 10 days required for the incision to heal. Although this procedure is palliative, it is effective in controlling class III and IV infections.

These patients usually meet one of two criteria. The first criterion is a concomitant disease process, precluding general anesthesia. General anesthesia may not be required for an uneventful lead removal procedure, but it is required in a cardiovascular emergency. For example, a tear of the great veins or heart causing a hemothorax or pericardial tamponade must be corrected immediately by means of a thoracotomy or median sternotomy. Although these accidents are rare (less than 0.5% of cases), the patient must be a candidate for such a procedure to ensure survival. A second criterion is having only a short life expectancy, for example, patients with a terminal illness or patients confined to a nursing home with dementia. In these two examples, it is hard to justify subjecting patients to a curative procedure.

Pacemaker Reimplantation

Reimplantation of the pacemaker system at a distant site is an integral part of abandoning the site. Pacemakers and leads are reimplanted on the opposite side when possible. If the leads cannot be implanted transvenously on the opposite side, they are implanted using a transatrial, epicardial, or transfemoral approach. The pacemaker is then implanted on the chest wall or in the abdomen. I do not use the transfemoral approach. Although some promote this approach, it is potentially dangerous. Those transvenous lead implant complications occurring in the superior veins can occur in the inferior veins. Thrombus formation and venous occlusion occurring in the inferior vena cava, iliac, and femoral veins have life-threatening sequelae.

If there is no infection, a new device is implanted as part of the abandonment procedure. With infection, it is essential that the new system be implanted without risking a subsequent infection. In these patients antibiotic therapy is continued, and reimplantation is delayed for an interval of about 36 hours. Before reimplantation, two clinical conditions must be met: the patient must be hemodynamically stable and have a near-normal temperature. The 36-hour time period was initially an arbitrary choice, and it has been successful. Those patients spiking a temperature after removal of the infected material must have their temperature return to near normal (judgment decision) before a new device can be inserted.

Pre-discharge and Post-discharge Care

Hospital stay for a typical patient presenting with an infection (class II through IV) was 5 days. On the first postimplantation day, the intravenous antibiotic was stopped and the oral antibiotic continued. The patient was then discharged on oral antibiotics for a maximum of 10 days. If the lead could not be extracted using transvenous techniques, a cardiac surgical approach added an average of 2 days to the postimplantation hospital convalescence. Some class II patients were continued on intravenous antibiotics for an additional 2 to 3 days, and some patients with a concomitant disease process required a longer stay to treat this disease. Class I patients required a longer stay to recover from the epicardial lead implantation through a left anterior thoracotomy and to receive intravenous antibiotics.

In my opinion, continued antibiotics are not required for class II through IV infection. The treatment outlined in the protocol described previously was sufficient for pacemaker and implantable cardioverter-defibrillator (ICD) infections. The only subset of patients at risk of a recurrent infection are those whose lead broke, leaving a lead fragment in the heart, and those who have an undetected true class Ia bacterial endocarditis. Less than 10% (three patients) of the retained lead fragments were infected. These infections are not evident at discharge and cannot be cured with antibiotics. The infected lead fragment (class Ic), when detected, must be removed to eradicate the infection. I have had only one patient (not in this series) who had a fungal infection that involved the tricuspid valve (class Ia). If Class Ia endocarditis or some other remote infection does exist, symptoms recur when the antibiotics are stopped, and that infection can be identified and treated. These types of infections also usually require more than just antibiotic therapy to eradicate them.

Septic emboli to the lung after débridement and lead extraction are another potential complication increasing hospital stay. A febrile response increases the duration of intravenous antibiotic therapy. Two patients with septic emboli superimposed on chronic lung disease developed respiratory insufficiency and required a ventilator postoperatively.

■ COMPLICATIONS OF PERMANENT TRANSVENOUS LEADS

The integrity of the electrophysiologic device is dependent on the proper implantation and performance of permanent transvenous leads. Lead-related complications are associated both with implantation and performance. Proper lead implantation includes obtaining an uneventful, stable lead position and satisfactory electrical parameters. After proper implantation, lead performance includes issues such as lead–tissue interaction and device failures (insulation, conductor coil, adaptor, and electrode). Complications related to device failure are not discussed in this chapter.

Primary implantation-related complications include problems such as dislodgments, perforations, and poor electrical parameters. Primary performance-related complications (excluding device failures) are primarily associated with lead–tissue interaction. Most chronic complications are performance related; however, it is sometimes difficult to separate implantation from performance complications. For example, a very stiff lead may be associated with both high implantation and performance complication rates. Currently, the only method of differentiating between the two is statistics along with the opinions of experts. Unfortunately, statistics on human implantations were not available early in the design process.

Complications are grossly divided into device failures, lead infections, vein thrombosis, and problems related to the electrode–myocardium interface (Table 27–3). Although a new lead must be implanted in many cases, the rationale for abandoning or extracting failed leads is based only on those tissue-related complications described subsequently.

Device Failures

Historically, lead failures were breaches in the insulation or a fracture of the conductor coil. The mechanisms for insulation

Table 27–3. Treatment of Lead-Related Complications

Infection
  Remove lead
  Implant new system on opposite side
Vein thrombosis
  Acute venous occlusion
    Anticoagulate (IV heparin, converting to Coumadin)
    Remove lead if abandoned or if clinical events occur (e.g., pulmonary emboli or progressive swelling of the arm)
    May elect to remove lead after fibrous organization occurs
  SVC syndrome
    Administer thrombolytic agents and systemic heparin
    If necessary, perform surgical correction
  Chronic venous occlusion
    Remove abandoned leads
Complications at the electrode–myocardial interface
  Acute dislodgment
    Reposition lead
  Lead migration
    Remove lead
  Acute penetration
    Reposition lead
  Acute perforation
    Immediate pericardiocentesis if there is gradual onset of tamponade
    Immediate cardiac surgery if acute tamponade with low cardiac output occurs

failure (environmental stress cracking [ESC], metal-ion induced oxidation [MIO], compression erosion or abrasion, cold flow, and tears) or conductor coil fracture (crush injury, binding, or traction) are not discussed here. These defects compromise the electrical integrity of the lead, causing a malfunction of the pacing or sensing function of the lead. To correct this type of problem, a new lead has to be implanted. The defective lead becomes a superfluous lead and can be abandoned or removed as discussed later.

Recently, a new and potentially dangerous type of lead failure occurred. Several Telectronics lead models (Table 27–4), most prominently models 330-801 and 330-854, have a component called a *retention wire* designed to hold a J configuration in the atrium. This wire had the potential of breaking (fractures) and eroding through the insulation without a loss of its electrical integrity. Its pacing and sensing characteristics were unchanged. If the retention wire eroded through the insulation, it could penetrate the superior veins, atrium, or aorta, causing a cardiovascular emergency. This type of failure was the first example of a destructive lead. It had the potential to be destructive (penetrating or tearing tissue locally or remotely after migration) but did not cause a problem with the electrical performance of the lead.

Infected Leads

The sequelae of an infected permanent pacing lead range from subcutaneous tissue erosion resulting in a draining sinus (class IV) to a life-threatening systemic infection (class Ib and II) (see Table 27–2). The mortality rate of persistent infection when infected leads are not removed can be as high as 66%.[21] Because of this statistic, it has been recommended that infected leads be removed, even in the elderly high-risk patient, using open heart surgery if necessary.[23, 24]

An infected pacing system is considered either a manda-

Table 27–4. Telectronics Lead Models With Retention J Wire

Model Name	Model Number	Lead Type	Fixation	Distribution
Accufix	033–802	Bipolar	Retractable screw	Non-US
Accufix DEC	033–812	Bipolar	Retractable screw	Non-US
Accufix	329–701	Bipolar	Retractable screw	US and worldwide
Accufix	330–801	Bipolar	Retractable screw	US and worldwide
Encor DEC	033–856	Bipolar	Tines	Non-US
Encor	327–747	Bipolar	Tines	US and worldwide
Encor	327–754	Bipolar	Tines	US and worldwide
Encor	329–749	Bipolar	Tines	US and worldwide
Encor	329–754	Bipolar	Tines	US and worldwide
Encor	330–848	Bipolar	Tines	Non-US
Encor	330–854	Bipolar	Tines	US and worldwide
Encor DEC	033–757	Unipolar	Tines	Non-US
Encor	327–745	Unipolar	Tines	US and worldwide
Encor	327–745P	Unipolar	Tines	US and worldwide
Encor	327–752	Unipolar	Tines	US and worldwide
Encor	327–752P	Unipolar	Tines	US and worldwide
Encor	328–752	Unipolar	Tines	US and worldwide
Encor	328–752P	Unipolar	Tines	US and worldwide
Encor	329–748	Unipolar	Tines	US and worldwide
Encor	329–748A	Unipolar	Tines	US and worldwide
Encor	329–748P	Unipolar	Tines	US and worldwide
Encor	329–755A	Unipolar	Tines	US and worldwide
Encor	330–748	Unipolar	Tines	US and worldwide
Encor	330–755	Unipolar	Tines	US and worldwide
EnGuard/Atrial DF	040–022	ICD	Tines	US investigation, non-US
EnGuard/Atrial DF	040–069	ICD	Tines	Non-US
EnGuard/Atrial DF	040–112	ICD	Tines	US investigation, non-US

tory or necessary condition for lead extraction, depending on the clinical manifestation of the infection.[21, 25–28] An infection involving only the extravascular portion of leads with no systemic symptoms may be treated as described previously for a device pocket infection. However, septicemia may result from a pocket infection with infected tissue along the intravascular portion of the lead or drainage into the bloodstream. Drainage into the bloodstream may occur along the lead, through breaks in the insulation connected by the lead lumen, and by indirect lymphatic or venous drainage. Lead-related septicemia is a mandatory condition for lead extraction. Pockets with negative cultures in the presence of potentially infected leads have only a slightly lower complication rate than those with positive cultures.[29]

An acute infection involving the leads within the vascular space is rare but, if present, causes septicemia. Leads can be infected by vegetation attached to the lead or by actual bacterial growth within the interstices of a degraded insulation polymer or within the lumen if a breach in the insulation is present.[30] If the insulation has failed and bacteria growth is in the lumen, it can extend the entire length of the lead. Treatment is to remove the lead (mandatory condition).

A fresh thrombus may become secondarily infected after lead implantation, causing a suppurative phlebitis or an infected vegetation. These are dangerous infections that can cause septicemia, septic pulmonary emboli, and endocarditis. Controlling the infection with systemic antibiotic therapy and then removing the lead is the best way to treat this problem. If the infection cannot be controlled, lead removal is mandatory. One of the risks of removing a lead with a fresh infected thrombus is to deposit the infected thrombus at the vein entry site, causing a suppurative phlebitis. Although this infection can be successfully treated, the associated morbidity is great.

Infected vegetation may be attached to a chronic lead with or without an insulation fault. This vegetation is seen most commonly in patients with poor cardiac function and a large right atrium. It may be massive, measuring several centimeters in length and diameter. The vegetation is connected to the heart wall or to tissue near the tricuspid valve; it is rarely attached to the leaflets of the valve. In my experience, the vegetation may involve one or more leads (or other chronically implanted catheter) but is not primarily attached to a lead. Most of these vegetations are found in patients with a history of septicemia. Some have had small pulmonary emboli.

Lead removal (mandatory condition) is the treatment of choice but is complicated by the vegetation. A small vegetation can be snared and removed; large vegetations should be removed using the transatrial approach (although this technique is investigational) or open heart surgery. The consequences of a vegetation embolus to the lung should be considered. If this would not be a significant insult to the patient, a snare can be used. Otherwise, a more invasive procedure is necessary.

Vein Thrombosis

Transvenous leads may cause vein thrombosis. The incidence of clinically undetected vein thrombosis has been reported to be as high as 44%.[31]

Acute Vein Thrombosis

Acute reactions of the vein wall at or near the lead entry site can cause thrombosis of the subclavian and brachiocephalic veins. These thrombosed veins usually heal without sequelae. If axillary and brachial vein thrombosis occurs, collateral drainage paths are usually not sufficient, and residual swelling of the arm is a frequent complication.

Treatment of an acute vein thrombosis consists of anticoagulating the patient by administering intravenous heparin, converting to warfarin sodium (Coumadin). The warfarin is continued for at least 3 months. Clinical statistics supporting either leaving or removing the lead are not available, although leaving the lead in place does not appear to alter the course. Immediate removal of the lead may extend the clot both proximally and distally. If thrombus on the distal portion of the lead is pulled back toward the subclavian vein, the thrombosis is extended proximally. Pulling the electrode back through a recently thrombosed subclavian vein may push thrombus distally into the axillary or brachial veins. Lead removal once in the fibrous tissue stage of organization is probably safer.

Leads in thrombosed veins should not be removed unless there are clinical events (acute or chronic), such as pulmonary emboli or progressive swelling of the arm while on anticoagulant therapy. As mentioned previously, removal may worsen the thrombosis. In addition, a new pacing system will have to be implanted on the opposite side, and although unlikely, the new system may have the same problem. Therefore, if clinical events occur or if the leads are abandoned, they should be removed (necessary condition).

In my experience, acute thrombosis of the superior vena cava (SVC) does not occur without a pre-existing condition damaging the vein. For example, the presence of a chronic pacing lead in the vein or the recent extraction of a lead with thrombus formation along the vein wall predisposes the vein to an acute thrombosis.[32] Treatment of SVC syndrome involves thrombolytic agents, anticoagulation, and a major surgical procedure. The initial treatment is to administer a thrombolytic agent in an attempt to reopen the lumen. If successful, the syndrome resolves. In either case, the patient is placed on systemic heparin and prepared for a surgical correction. In my experience, débridement of all thrombotic material from the SVC and brachiocephalic veins and a vein patch angioplasty, using the saphenous vein, have been successful.[33] Construction of a vein conduit (Doty procedure) is an alternative procedure, if the remaining surface area of the vein is inadequate.[34]

Chronic Venous Occlusion

Exuberant fibrous tissue forms when transvenous leads cause an exaggerated inflammatory reaction with thrombus formation at sites of contact with the vein or cardiac wall. Mechanical stress is probably the initial cause of this reaction. It is exacerbated by stasis and eddying of blood flow. The consequences of exuberant intravenous fibrous tissue include gradual obliteration of the lumen and acute vein thrombosis with the possibility of pulmonary emboli. Obliteration of the subclavian and brachiocephalic veins is common. Occlusion of the SVC is uncommon (Fig. 27–13), but when it occurs, if the lumen is narrowed slowly, development of collateral venous flow prevents SVC syndrome.

Exuberant fibrous tissue formation along the heart wall does not cause a problem in situ, but it increases the risk and difficulty of removal. Chronic lead extractions from this exuberant fibrous tissue have a high incidence of thrombus formation, and some sites progress to vein thrombosis.

Multiple leads in one vein increase the incidence of venous occlusion.[35] There are additional sites of vein wall contact, and leads bound together apply even greater mechanical stress to the tissue. This is also exacerbated by stasis and eddying of blood flow. In my experience, the incidence is related to the size and stiffness of the leads and the duration of their implantation. The left brachiocephalic vein is found to be occluded more frequently than the right, and small supple leads cause less fibrous tissue reaction than large stiff leads. Abandoned leads should be removed.

Complications at the Electrode–Myocardium Interface

All complications involving the electrode–myocardium interface present clinically with changes in pacing or inappropriate stimulation of another muscle. These failures are usually due to the electrode causing excessive tissue injury or to dislodgment of the electrode from its implantation site. Stimulation of other muscles may represent a serious problem, such as penetration of the electrode, or it may result from the electrode placed in close proximity to a nerve.

Dislodgment and Migration

Electrode dislodgment is probably the most common complication. Electrode instability is usually a complication of implantation and not a lead–tissue problem (inflammatory reaction). Implantation includes lead performance issues, such as stiffness and fixation devices. Most lead dislodgments that alter the leads' electrical performance are detected and corrected immediately by lead repositioning.

Migration of a dislodged lead out of the heart may go undetected for months in poorly managed patients with an intermittent dysrhythmia. Migrations into the pulmonary artery, a cerebral vein, or an iliac vein cause complications such as pulmonary emboli and thrombosis of the vein.[36] Once discovered, these leads should (necessary condition) be removed and new leads implanted.

Leads break, and abandoned leads are sometimes cut and left unsecured. Although the incidence of migration is probably low, migration of severed or broken transvenous leads does occur and is potentially dangerous. Fatality secondary to lead migration has been reported, but I have not seen it.[21] For example, if the proximal lead tip is bouncing in the right ventricle, causing a ventricular arrhythmia, it is life-threatening. Migrating severed leads have perforated the heart, causing hemorrhage or hemopericardium, and have formed vegetation, causing emboli to the lungs.[37–40] These are mandatory conditions for lead extraction. A severed lead coiled in the right ventricle may not cause acute symptoms, but the scar tissue that develops between the leads or between the lead and the heart wall will compromise ventricular function over time. In symptom-free patients, the potential exists for one of these complications to occur, making lead extraction a necessary condition.

Penetration and Perforation

Exaggerated inflammatory reactions, especially those not controlled by steroid-eluting electrodes, represent significant

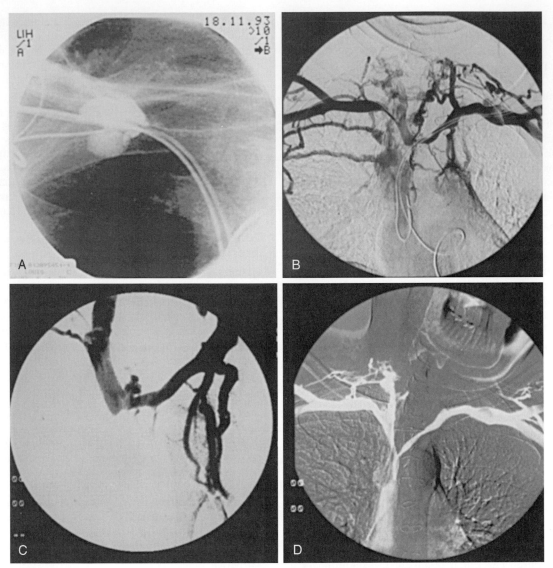

Figure 27–13. Occlusion of the superior veins. *A,* The subclavian vein is the most commonly occluded superior vein. A chronic thrombosis and occlusion of the subclavian vein at the lead entry site is shown in this figure.

B, Chronic thrombosis and occlusion of the superior vena cava (SVC) is unusual. This occlusion is 8 years old and the collateral venous return is complete. The collateral drainage was inadequate when this young patient exercised, causing swelling of the upper extremities, neck, and head.

C, The leads were extracted using countertraction through the femoral vein. The post-extraction venogram shows the SVC occlusion more clearly.

D, The brachiocephalic vein and SVC are shown to be patent 6 months after surgical correction. The veins were repaired by débridement of the organized intravenous inflammatory tissue and a vein patch angioplasty. The patient is symptom free and has a marked reduction of the collateral venous drainage.

tissue injury. For example, stiff or unstable bouncing leads implanted within the ventricle may apply excessive pressure directly to the electrode–myocardium interface. Tissue injury of this magnitude heals with scarring and poor, if any, electrode performance. Clinically, exaggerated reactions result in loss of capture (exit block), loss of sensing, or both.

Penetration

The most severe reactions occur when the electrode penetrates the tissue. In these cases, the pressure at the electrode–myocardium interface is great enough to force the electrode into the cardiac muscle. As the electrode works its way

through the muscle fibers, the resultant tissue injury causes an intense inflammatory reaction. The intensity of the reaction is sufficient to cause exit block (threshold exceeds the output of the pulse generator). As the electrode nears the epicardial surface, it frequently stimulates the diaphragm. Patients usually present with threshold elevation and diaphragmatic stimulation. Penetrations rarely progress to perforation of the electrode into the pericardial space. The preferred treatment for acute penetration is to reposition the electrode or to replace the lead with a more supple model.

Chronic problems with penetration are not common. Usually, the clinical manifestations of the acute presentation are so severe that the problem must be corrected. In addition, the penetration is slow, and the tissue reaction causes a localized pericarditis that obliterates the pericardial space and prevents perforation. Removal of these leads may be dangerous, and the patient should be prepared for an immediate cardiac procedure before the extraction. If the penetration is to the epicardium and the pericardial reaction is not extensive, extraction by traction or countertraction could avulse the remaining cardiac wall, causing hemorrhage and tamponade.

Limited penetration, however, does occur. For example, an electrode with tines recessed 2 to 3 mm may penetrate to the level of the tines. Although the lead is usable, the resultant chronic reaction causes significant fibrosis and a poor chronic stimulation threshold.

Perforation

A perforation is usually an inadvertent misadventure caused by the electrode being pushed through the heart wall. At routine pacemaker implantation, patient monitoring is not adequate to diagnose a perforation unless it is seen on fluoroscopy. It may not be detected until the onset of cardiac tamponade. Unrecognized perforations present chronically with pericarditis or a hemorrhagic effusion with or without tamponade. Chronic perforation of a pacemaker lead is rare.

Gradual onset of cardiac tamponade is treated differently from a marked hemorrhage with tamponade. The treatment is immediate pericardiocentesis, leaving a catheter in the pericardial space and monitoring the blood loss. Preparations for cardiac surgery should be made, although surgery is usually not required. The lead is pulled back into the heart and the blood loss monitored. Treatment of an acute cardiac tamponade with a low cardiac output is more radical. Hemorrhage of this magnitude requires immediate cardiac surgery to ensure a successful result.

Intracardiac Fibrous Tissue Reactions

Reaction to the leads inside the heart is the same as that in the veins. The differences are related only to the size of the chambers. For example, a major exuberant reaction inside the heart will not be occlusive and impede blood flow. There is one exception—stenosis of the tricuspid valve. Multiple leads crossing the tricuspid valve have been demonstrated to cause valvular stenosis. The mechanism for this event is fibrous tissue binding the leads to the valvular or perivalvular tissue, and binding of one lead to the other. With time and contraction of the scar tissue, the valvular orifice is narrowed, creating a gradient. Removal of the leads eliminates the gradient.

Tricuspid valve regurgitation may be seen with ventricular lead implantation. Usually, there are multiple leads crossing the valve. Although the abandoned leads are usually removed, changes in the magnitude of the valvular regurgitation are not seen acutely. The current chronic information is anecdotal (not statistically valid) and does not show an improvement with time. Consequently, the leads should be removed, but a clinical change in the tricuspid valvular insufficiency should not be expected. When a patent foramen ovale is present, a right to left shunt across the septum is frequently evident.

▪ RATIONALE FOR REMOVING CHRONICALLY IMPLANTED LEADS

Regardless of the rationale used for removing leads, there has been a marked expansion of indications in recent years. Some of the reasons for this expansion are given in Table 27–5. A decrease in the risk and morbidity of the procedure, increased experience of the extractor, and availability of more sophisticated equipment are all related. The increase in the number of leads extracted provides more experience, allowing procedures to be done in a safer and more expeditious manner. As the number of procedures increases, more extractors will be trained, and the procedure will hopefully become more economic.

The word *rationale* is used instead of indications. *Indication* is a broad term used in a clinical setting to mean those circumstances considered acceptable for removing a lead. The indications for lead extraction are based on the rationale or reason for removing the lead. Indications are in a state of flux and confusion because their rationales are changing. A logical paradigm accepted by everyone has not evolved. Confusion about the rationale for removing leads is directly related to the fear of doing harm and the intuitive logic that the lead should be removed (even superfluous leads). Initial indications were based on a need *to justify removing a lead*. This philosophy is slowly being replaced by a need *to justify not removing a lead*. Although the latter is a clinical reality, it is based on intuitive logic and not on strong clinical data.[41]

For example, today the treatment of an actual lead-related complication as well as of the potential for a lead-related complication is to remove the lead. In the past, only life-threatening complications, such as infections causing septicemia, were considered indications for lead removal because the justification was clinically supported by clear mortality and morbidity data. Now, in contrast, some leads are extracted and replaced for poor performance, to avoid having too many leads passing through the same vein or valve, and even just because a lead has been abandoned. Lead removal in these situations is based on the potential for a lead-related complication. Clear mortality and morbidity data do not exist to support this rationale. Large gray areas exist between these two extremes in logic.

In hopes of resolving this dilemma, I am presenting the evolution of my rationale for removing leads. It began with the need to justify removing leads and has evolved into the need to justify not removing a lead. The latter arguments are based primarily on clinical experience. In my practice, a paradigm has evolved.

Rationale Based on Justifying Removing Leads

To justify lead removal, the rationale must contain the necessary risk-benefit issues and time constraint information es-

Table 27–5. Reasons for Expansion of Lead Extraction Indications

Extraction equipment is more efficient and easier to use.
Number of leads under recall is increasing.
Number of reimplantation-related infections is increasing.
Extractors are more experienced.
Indications are expanding (superfluous leads removed).
Risk and morbidity of procedure when performed by experienced physicians are low.

sential to making those kinds of clinical decisions. To provide the qualifying statements for risk-benefit comparisons, lead-related complications were grouped empirically into defined clinical conditions (mandatory, necessary, and discretionary). Defined categories for time constraints were already in existence (emergency, urgent, elective).

The need to justify removing leads is based on two false assumptions. The first is the perception that leads are well tolerated by the body, and the second is that the risk associated with removing leads is high. The concept was that implanted leads were designed to last for the patient's lifetime and, consequently, should do no harm. Lifetime performance by a lead implied by manufacturers is a misconception. The lack of data on the natural history of long-duration lead implantation and the lack of an acceptable method of removing leads perpetuated it. Unfortunately, leads were shown to have a limited life expectancy because of materials failure, biophysical interface complications, and incompatibility with evolving pulse generator technology. The risk of removing some leads was high using the conventional techniques available during the early 1980s, especially when inexperienced physicians performed the extractions. Today, the new extraction procedures and increased experience have greatly reduced the risk. In addition, national databases allow a means of separating real from perceived risk.

Classifying the indications into those graded clinical conditions considered mandatory, necessary, and discretionary was the first attempt at justifying the need to remove a lead.[26, 27, 42] This was an attempt to weigh the risk and morbidity of extracting the leads against the medical risk and morbidity of leaving the leads in place. Using this abstract group of clinical conditions, all lead indications can be placed empirically in one of three groups:

- *Mandatory* indications mean that leads *must* be removed. Mandatory conditions are those in which leaving the leads in place would be life-threatening or disabling.
- *Necessary* indications mean the leads *should* be removed. Necessary conditions are those in which the lead removal would correct a problem or prevent a life-threatening situation from developing, but the existing problem is not considered life-threatening.
- *Discretionary* indications mean the leads *could* be removed. Discretionary conditions are those in which it is preferable to remove the leads but in which it would rarely be considered a medical necessity.

In general, the indications for lead extraction for an individual are directly related to the risk and morbidity of the extraction procedure. When cardiopulmonary bypass was necessary to extract the leads, only those patients having mandatory conditions had their leads extracted. After proficiency was gained with the transvenous extraction techniques, patients with most necessary and some discretionary conditions had their leads extracted. Experts are now extracting most abandoned leads (superfluous leads). Those not routinely extracted include discretionary and noninfected necessary conditions associated with leads implanted for longer than 8 to 10 years. Table 27–6 lists the indications and conditions for lead extraction in both the Byrd and Cook Databases. Table 27–7 lists clinical examples of mandatory, necessary, and discretionary conditions.

Table 27–6. Indications and Conditions for Lead Extraction

Indications	Byrd 264 Patients (%)	National 856 Patients (%)	Conditions M	N	D
Lead replacement	25.8	38.7		X	X
Infection	24.6	34.7		X	X
Septicemia/ endocarditis	21.6	10.5	X		
Erosion	7.6	5.0		X	
Pain	5.7	1.9			X
Pre-erosion	4.5	2.2		X	
Chronic draining sinus	4.5	2.0		X	
Free-floating or migrating lead	2.6	1.4	X	X	
Thrombosis	0.8	0.5		X	X
Tricuspid regurgitation	0.0	0.5		X	X
Other*	2.3	2.6		X	X

*Includes isolated presenting conditions such as cancer and trauma and those unknown conditions that could not be classified.

This table combines the Byrd and Cook databases for indications and conditions for lead extraction. Indications are listed as the presenting condition. M, N, and D refer to the mandatory, necessary, and discretionary conditions for lead extraction (see text). In some cases, the indication group depends on the magnitude of the condition and may be listed in more than one group.

Rationale Based on Justifying Not Removing Leads

During the past several years, the philosophy to justify not removing leads has evolved. Based on this supposition, all leads causing some biologic interface complication and all abandoned leads should be removed. This is a reversal of the previous argument. For this supposition to have clinical relevance, the only contraindication to lead removal should be related to the patient's physical condition and ability to undergo a lead extraction procedure safely. The hypothesis is that the biophysical interface reaction is detrimental.

Table 27–7. Indications for Lead Extraction

Mandatory (life-threatening)
  Septicemia
  Endocarditis
  Lead migration (e.g., perforating, causing arrhythmia, causing emboli)
  Device interference (e.g., abandoned implantable defibrillator lead)
  Obliteration of all usable veins
Necessary (significant morbidity)
  Pocket infection
  Chronic draining sinus
  Erosion
  Vein thrombosis
  Lead migration (not presently causing life-threatening problem)
  Potential device interference
  Lead replacement (e.g., supernumerary, extract and implant thrombosed vein)
Discretionary (optional)
  Pain
  Malignancy
  Lead replacement (e.g., abandoned lead for less than 3 to 4 years)

Therefore, for each patient it must be shown that the morbidity and mortality (risk) associated with the lead removal is a valid issue. I believe the clinical data support the statement that the risk associated with lead extraction is predictable.

The mandatory, necessary, and discretionary conditional statements are useful in qualifying the patient's indication but do not relate to the risk factors and magnitude of the procedures involved in lead removal. A rationale was devised relating indication, patient's physical status, lead condition, and social constraints. Table 27–8 is a summary of my current indications for lead extraction based on justifying not removing the lead. It reflects the probability of the worst-case scenario of having a complication and of surviving a surgical corrective procedure. If a patient can survive this worst-case scenario, a routine lead extraction should be uneventful. It also reflects issues relating to the magnitude of the procedure. For example, assume a procedure is performed under general endotracheal anesthesia and a median sternotomy is required to correct a complication. To justify removing a superfluous lead, the probability of an operative complication must be extremely low (near zero), and if a complication does occur, the patient must be able to tolerate the corrective procedure without cardiac, pulmonary, or renal sequelae. In addition, if an extensive surgical procedure is required to remove the lead, the magnitude of the procedure becomes a factor. This philosophical approach must be used with each patient to ensure a successful outcome.

The patient's physical status is the primary indicator for a successful result: the patient's ability to tolerate general anesthesia and not the lead extraction and associated surgical experiences constitutes the major risk factor. For example, if a patient can tolerate general anesthesia, adding a lead extraction, a transatrial approach, and a median sternotomy does not measurably increase the risk factor. One method of grading a patient's physical condition is to use the physical status class I through V as proposed by the American Society of Anesthesiologists (ASA) (Table 27–9).[43] It essentially shows that the only patients who are not candidates for general anesthesia are class V moribund. This would, therefore, be the only absolute contraindication to lead extraction. Class IV patients are at risk of exacerbation of their life-threatening underlying disease process and would not be

Table 27–9. American Society of Anesthesiologists Physical Status Classification

Class	System Disease	Activity Restrictions
I	None	None
II	Mild	None on therapy
III	Moderate	Moderate on therapy
IV	Severe	Maximal on therapy
V	Moribund	Total (patient is terminal)

candidates for lead removal unless the indication or required long-term medical treatment was also life-threatening. Consequently, patients in class I through IV would be candidates for all mandatory and most necessary procedures.

The risk associated with anesthesia for class I through III should be negligible, as should the risk for a procedure-associated mortality. In my experience removing leads from more than 1000 patients, 5 patients developed a procedural complication requiring an emergency median sternotomy with surgical correction. None of these patients died. For class IV patients with end-stage cardiac, pulmonary, or renal disease, the risk is finite but not prohibitive. Two class IV patients had an exacerbation of their underlying condition resulting in death. Although the exact statistics are not known, the gross statistics support the contention that the risk is negligible for class I through III. It also supports the need for a mandatory or necessary condition to justify removing leads from patients with class IV infection.

Lead-related conditions are relative contraindications and not well defined. They include lead properties, such as size, fragility, and integrity. Lead conditions affect the magnitude of the procedure. They influence the technical aspects of the lead extraction and not the risk.

The lead interaction with the biophysical interface influences both the magnitude and risk of the procedure. A lead entrapped in calcified encapsulating tissue is another type of problem. Leads encapsulated with calcified tissue are difficult to remove. The lead may not be removable using a vein-entry procedure. The addition of a femoral approach or a transatrial procedure adds time and morbidity, but the risk factors associated with the procedure are not changed.

Final considerations are the social constraints on the patient, such as decreased life expectancy, dementia, and economics. The aggressiveness of the approach taken with these patients is based on the standard of care in the community and judgment issues. It does not reflect the risk or magnitude of the procedure and is presented here only to include all the variables used in decision making.

Indications Based on the Rationale, the Biophysical Interface, and the Lead Status

Current indications are based on the condition of the lead's biophysical interface and the lead's status (functional utility) (Fig. 27–14). There are only three events related to the biophysical interface (infection, migration, and destruction) and one event associated with the lead's status (superfluous). It is obvious that a compatible intact essential lead with a nonhazardous or safe biophysical interface will not have an indication for removal.

These conditions can be presented by combining the

Table 27–8. Protocol to Justify Not Removing Leads

Biophysical Interface		Physical Status					Social Constraints
Event	Modifier	I	II	III	IV	V	
Infection	Intravascular	+	+	+	+	−	+
Infection	Extravascular	+	+	+	?	−	−
Migration	Actual	+	+	+	+	−	+
Migration	Potential	+	+	+	−	−	−
Destruction	Actual	+	+	+	+	−	+
Destruction	Potential	+	+	+	?	−	−
Leads Status							
Superfluous	Noncalcified	+	+	+	?	−	−
Superfluous	Calcified	?	?	?	−	−	−

The table summarizes the author's current indications and rationale for removing leads. Both the physical status and social conditions must be met for the lead to be removed, i.e., both must be (+).

(+), the leads are removed; (−), the leads are not removed; (?), the leads would be removed only in extenuating circumstances.

INDICATIONS

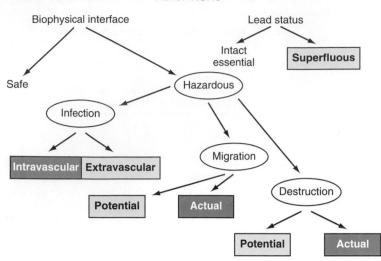

Figure 27–14. Biophysical interface. Indications are based on the lead's interaction at the biophysical interface and the lead's status.

Hazardous conditions at the biophysical interface are infection, migration, and destruction. Lead status conditions are device failure or integrity issues causing the lead to be abandoned, making it superfluous. Lead removal indications are based on these four conditions.

events occurring at the biophysical interface and the lead status with the two clinically descriptive modifiers, as shown in Table 27–7. The modifiers are self-explanatory. The biophysical interface modifiers relate to the grading conditions (mandatory, necessary, and discretionary). The lead status modifiers relate to the magnitude of the procedure. Calcification is the only common lead status condition and is listed as a modifier. Iatrogenic lead destruction, which leaves the lead mangled or lead fragments embedded in scar tissue, is rare and is not included as a modifier. The table also adds the rationale for needing a justification for not removing a lead, that is, ASA physical status and social constraints. The hypothesis is that all leads should be removed; therefore, only those factors influencing the risk and magnitude of the procedure are required.

The major advantage of this approach is the stratification of risk factors in an organized manner. It is apparent that lead conditions considered mandatory are removed from all patients but those with ASA class V infection (only class I through IV infections have clinical applicability). Leads with necessary conditions are removed in patients with ASA class I through III infection and, in some cases, from those with class IV infection, if there are no social constraints. Unique to this rationale, noncalcified superfluous leads are similar to leads with necessary conditions. Also, a calcified superfluous lead is the only category similar to the discretionary condition. This approach is new and a departure from previous indications using the initial grading conditions.

The pathophysiology at the biophysical interface of the lead includes infection, vein thrombosis, vegetation associated with leads, effects from lead migration, tissue destruction, and calcification of the encapsulating tissue. Acute complications, such as penetration and perforation of the heart or vascular wall, are also included as tissue destruction. Applying these examples to the protocol is useful in assessing the validity of this approach.

Infections are probably the most common hazardous condition at the biophysical interface. The modifiers separate infections into intravascular and extravascular. Intravascular infections, defined as causing life-threatening septicemia (class I and II), are a mandatory condition for lead removal.

Because only ASA class I through IV infections are clinically applicable, there are no contraindications to removing these leads. Extravascular infections (class III and IV) causing significant morbidity are a necessary condition for lead removal. Only in patients with ASA class IV infection is lead removal conditional. In all patients with social constraints and in those rare patients with an excessively high anesthetic risk, creating a chronic draining sinus is probably preferable.

Chronically implanted "destructive leads" are a new group. The only examples seen thus far are the Telectronics Accufix (Accufix Research Institute, Englewood, CO) and Encor leads (see Table 27–4). They have a J-shape retention wire that may fracture and protrude from the lead. A protruding retention wire has the potential to puncture or tear the wall of the heart or great vessels or to migrate. Indications for removal of destructive leads and migrating leads are subdivided by whether the event has actually occurred or has the potential to occur. Actual events are mandatory conditions, whereas potential events are necessary conditions.

Vein thrombosis is a lead-related destructive complication at the biophysical interface. All leads have the potential for being destructive by causing vein thrombosis. Except for unilateral thromboses of the subclavian vein (which is common), the actual modifier is usually applied and the lead removed. This is especially true for distal propagation of the thrombus into the brachial vein or involvement of the SVC. It is a situation that must be taken seriously in young patients because of the potential damage to the superior veins due to the long duration of lead implantation. Superfluous leads have the potential for destruction, and the potential modifier is used.

Vegetation is another destructive process associated with leads in the heart and is related to those factors causing clot formation. The actual modifier is used for vegetation. Vegetation is a mandatory indication with or without the presence of infection because of its natural history of increasing in size and embolization. Also, large vegetations, such as those forming on a coiled lead in the ventricle or between multiple leads in the ventricle, may decrease the chamber's volume or the compliance of the wall after maturation of the clot into contracted scar tissue.

Migration of leads is assigned an actual or potential modifier. Migrating leads cause complications by mechanically stimulating the heart or migrating to a region such as the pulmonary artery, where thrombosis of the vessel or embolization would be a serious complication. For example, an actual modifier (mandatory condition) is assigned to a migrating lead bouncing in the heart causing a malignant ventricular tachyarrhythmia. A potential modifier (necessary indication) would be assigned to a migrating lead with the potential of causing this complication. Another example is a lead or lead fragment migrating into the cerebral veins. This is a mandatory indication and should be assigned an actual modifier.

Calcification of the encapsulating tissue represents a different type of problem. Complications associated with its presence have been related to the difficulty of removing leads. Calcified tissue cannot be dilated or torn free. The only way to remove this tissue is to pass a sheath over the calcified region, peel it from the vein or heart wall, and include it with the extracted lead body. The risk associated with this approach is the risk of tearing vascular tissue or creating a false passage after a misadventure while applying excessive force.

Primary complications from calcified encapsulating tissue have not been reported in the literature, probably because tissue calcification is a progression of the natural encapsulation process from a supple to a rigid structure, occurring over a long period of time. This allows surrounding tissues time to compensate. However, multiple rigid leads in the right ventricle could compromise the compliance of the right heart wall and reduce the contractile motion (diastolic and systolic dysfunction). Although a theoretical possibility, this condition has not been documented to my knowledge. If it existed, calcification would become a modifier related to the grading conditions.

The status of an implanted lead is based on its condition and function. A lead must be both intact and essential to the electrical performance of the pulse generator to maintain a satisfactory lead status. Leads that are not intact, structurally or functionally, are either abandoned or removed. All abandoned leads are superfluous. Superfluous leads have the same risk as any other implanted lead of developing a time-dependent biologic interface complication. In addition, these leads may interfere with the electrical performance of essential leads. For example, a retained ICD lead may electrically interfere with the function of an essential lead.

Removal of superfluous leads, in the absence of a biologic interface complication, is controversial.[25] Some physicians prefer to set qualifying conditions for removal of superfluous leads. These include setting a limit on implantation duration or on the maximum number of leads considered safe to abandon in the superior veins, to pass through the tricuspid valve, or to reside in the right ventricle. These qualifying conditions are intuitive. Data concerning these qualifying conditions do not exist and would be extremely difficult to collect.

A positive argument for removing superfluous leads is to relate the dangers of lead extraction to the duration of implantation, to the number of chronic leads implanted, and to the experience of the extractor. For example, it is less dangerous to remove leads implanted for less than 4 to 6 years than to remove leads implanted for greater than 8 to 10 years. It is more dangerous to remove multiple leads implanted for varying lengths of time. The implication of this argument is to remove leads when it is safer. The risk and morbidity are related to physician experience and are low for most experienced extractors. Calcification is the only common modifier, and it relates only to the magnitude of the procedure.

Summary

Implantable electrophysiologic devices consisting of a pulse generator and leads are designed to be *biocompatible*. This general term implies that an accord is reached with the implanted tissue for an extended period of time (permanent implantation). Unfortunately, these devices are not completely biocompatible. Tissue is injured acutely during the implantation procedure and chronically by the device–tissue interactions. When these reactions are excessive, complications may develop. Although some complications continue to remain biocompatible (e.g., excessive inflammatory tissue and migration), others require surgical intervention (e.g., lead dislodgment, pocket hematoma, and wound dehiscence). Many complications are not biocompatible, and the device must be removed and a new device implanted at a remote site.

Managing electrophysiologic device-related complications covers a spectrum of techniques, encompassing both invasive cardiology and cardiac surgery. Techniques involving the implantation site include both salvaging and abandoning the site. Techniques involving leads include repositioning leads (of short implantation duration) and extraction of leads (regardless of the implantation duration). Some of these procedures have the potential for tearing the heart or veins, precipitating a life-threatening complication. To minimize the incidence of these complications and to ensure a satisfactory resolution, prior training in these procedures and the availability of the appropriate surgical support, should a problem arise, is essential. The goal of managing complications is to understand the mechanical, biologic, and technical factors responsible for their occurrence in order to design biocompatible devices and develop complication-free implantation techniques.

REFERENCES

1. Anderson JM: Inflammatory response to implants. ASAIO 11(1): 101–107, 1988.
2. Hecker JR, Scandrett LA: Roughness and thrombogenicity of the outer surfaces of intravascular catheters. J Biomed Mater Res 19:381–395, 1985.
3. Gallin JI, Goldstein IM, Snyderman R (Eds): Inflammation: Basic Principles and Clinical Correlates. New York, Raven Press, 1988.
4. Saab SB, Jung JY, Almond CH: Retention of pacemaker electrode complicated by serratia marcescens septicemia: Removal with total cardiopulmonary bypass. J Thorac Cardiovasc Surg 73:404–407, 1977.
5. Schoen FJ, Harasaki H, Kim KM, et al: Biomaterial-associated calcification: Pathology, mechanisms, and strategies for prevention. J Biomed Mater Res 22(A1): 11–36, 1988.
6. Robboy SJ, Harthorne JW, Leinbach RC, et al: Autopsy findings with permanent pervenous pacemakers. Circulation 39: 495–501, 1969.
7. Huang TY, Baba N: Cardiac pathology of transvenous pacemakers. Am Heart J 83:469–474, 1972.
8. Becker AE, Becker MJ, Caludon DG, et al: Surface thrombosis and fibrous encapsulation of intravenous pacemaker catheter electrode. Circulation 46:409–412, 1972.

9. Fishbein MC, Tan KS, Beazell JW, et al: Cardiac pathology of transvenous pacemakers in dogs. Am Heart J 93:73–81, 1977.

10. Jara FM, Toledo-Pereyra L, Lewis JW, et al: The infected pacemaker pocket. J Thorac Cardiovasc Surg 78:298–300, 1979.

11. Goldman BS, Macgregor DC: Management of infected pacemaker systems. Clin Prog Pacing Electrophysiol 2:220–235, 1984.

12. Cohen TJ, Pons VG, Schwartz J, et al: *Candida albicans* pacemaker site infection. PACE 14:146–148, 1991.

13. Hartstein AI, Jackson J, Gilbert DN: Prophylactic antibiotics and the insertion of permanent transvenous cardiac pacemakers. J Thorac Cardiovasc Surg 75:219–223, 1978.

14. Kennelly BM, Piller LW: Management of infected transvenous permanent pacemakers. Br Heart J 36:1133–1140, 1974.

15. Morgan G, Ginks W, Siddons H, et al: Septicemia in patients with an endocardial pacemaker. Am J Cardiol 44:221–224, 1979.

16. Firor WB, Lopez JF, Nanson EM, et al: Clinical management of the infected pacemaker. Ann Thorac Surg 6:431–436, 1968.

17. Muers MF, Arnold AG, Sleight P: Prophylactic antibiotics for cardiac pacemaker implantation: A prospective trial. Br Heart J 46:539–544, 1981.

18. Ramsdale DR, Charles RG, Rowlands DB, et al: Antibiotic prophylaxis for pacemaker implantation: A prospective randomized trial. PACE 7:844–849, 1984.

19. Bluhm GL: Pacemaker infections: A 2-year follow-up of antibiotic prophylaxis. Scand J Thorac Cadiovasc Surg 19:231–235, 1985.

20. de Lalla F, Bonini W, Broffoni T, et al: Prophylactic mezlocillin-netilmicin combination in permanent transvenous cardiac pacemaker implantation: A single-center, prospective, randomized study. J Chemother 2:252–256, 1990.

21. Rettig G, Doenecke P, Sen S, et al: Complications with retained transvenous pacemaker electrodes. Am Heart J 98:587–594, 1979.

22. Personal communication with Joanne Fee. Detailed information on Telectronics Atrial 'J' Leads. Accufix Research Institute, PAC meeting, May 5, 1998.

23. Choo MH, Holmes DR, Gersh BJ, et al: Permanent pacemaker infections: Characterization and management. Am J Cardiol 48:559–564, 1981.

24. Brodman R, Frame R, Andrews C, et al: Removal of infected transvenous leads requiring cardiopulmonary bypass or inflow occlusion. J Thorac Cardiovasc Surg 103:649–654, 1992.

25. Furman S, Behrens M, Andrews C, et al: Retained pacemaker leads. J Thorac Cardiovasc Surg 94:770–772, 1987.

26. Byrd CL, Schwartz SJ, Hedin N: Lead extraction: Indications and techniques. Cardiol Clin 10:735–748, 1992.

27. Byrd CL, Schwartz SJ, Hedin NB: Lead extraction: Techniques and indications. *In* Barold SS, Mugica J (eds): New Perspectives in Cardiac Pacing. Mount Kisco, NY, Futura, 1993, pp 29–55.

28. Myers MR, Parsonnet V, Bernstein AD: Extraction of implanted transvenous pacing leads: A review of a persistent clinical problem. Am Heart J 121:881–888, 1991.

29. Parry G, Goudevenos J, Jameson S, et al: Complications associated with retained pacemaker leads. PACE 14:1251–1257, 1991.

30. Marrie TJ, Nelligan J, Costerton JW: A scanning and transmission electron microscopic study of an infected endocardial pacemaker lead. Circulation 66:1339–1341, 1982.

31. Lee ME, Chaux A: Unusual complications of endocardial pacing. J Thorac Cardiovasc Surg 80:934–940, 1980.

32. Mazzetti H, Dussaut A, Tentori C, et al: Superior vena cava occlusion and/or syndrome related to pacemaker leads. Am Heart J 125:831–837, 1993.

33. Yakirevich V, Alagem D, Papo J, et al: Fibrotic stenosis of the superior vena cava with widespread thrombotic occlusion of its major tributaries: An unusual complication of transvenous cardiac pacing. J Thorac Cardiovasc Surg 85:632–634, 1983.

34. Doty DB, Doty JR, Jones KW: Bypass of superior vena cava: Fifteen years' experience with spiral vein graft for obstruction of superior vena cava caused by benign disease. J Thorac Cardiovasc Surg 99:889–895, 1990.

35. Pauletti M, Di Ricco G, Solfanelli S, et al: Venous obstruction in permanent pacemaker patients: An isotopic study. PACE 4:36–42, 1981.

36. Toumbouras M, Spanos P, Konstantaras C, et al: Inferior vena cava thrombosis due to migration of retained functionless pacemaker electrode. Chest 82:785–786, 1982.

37. Dalal JJ, Robinson CJ, Henderson AH: An unusual complication of the unremoved unwanted pacing wire. PACE 4:14–16, 1981.

38. Dalvi BV, Rajani RM, Lokhandwala YY, et al: Unusual case of pacemaker lead migration. Cathet Cardiovasc Diagn 21:95–96, 1990.

39. Lassers BW, Pickering D: Removal of an iatrogenic foreign body from the aorta by means of a ureteric stone catcher. Am Heart J 73:375–378, 1967.

40. Wolfram T, Wirtzfeld A: Pulmonary embolization of retained transvenous pacemaker electrode. Br Heart J 38:326–329, 1976.

41. Byrd CL: Is there an optimal method of lead extraction? Rosenqvist M (ed): Cardiac Pacing: New Advances. Philadelphia, WB Saunders, 1997, pp 293–317.

42. Byrd CL, Schwartz SJ, Hedin N: Intravascular techniques for extraction of permanent pacemaker leads. J Thorac Cardiovasc Surg 101:989–997, 1991.

43. Prause G, Ratzenhofer-Comenda B, Pierer G, et al: Can ASA grade or Goldman's cardiac risk index predict peri-operative mortality? A study of 16,227 patients. Anaesthesia 52:203–206, 1997.

Chapter 28

Techniques and Devices for Extraction of Pacemaker and Implantable Cardioverter-Defibrillator Leads

Charles L. Byrd and Bruce L. Wilkoff

The extraction of chronic pacemaker and defibrillator leads has become a challenging endeavor. The goal is to ensure the safe extraction of all transvenous leads. Extraction techniques range from a simple procedure requiring only a few minutes under local anesthesia, to a complicated procedure lasting hours under general anesthesia. For example, a simple procedure would be unscrewing an active fixation lead implanted for a few months, applying minimal traction. A complicated procedure would be extracting multiple leads implanted for 10 years or longer. Some lead extractions may require one or more extraction techniques or approaches, including in some cases a more involved surgical procedure to ensure a safe and successful extraction.

Lead extraction is potentially dangerous. Complications include failure to extract an infected lead, low cardiac output, lead breakage and migration, avulsion of veins and myocardial tissue (e.g., muscle, tricuspid valve), and tears of the veins and heart wall with resultant hemothorax, tamponade, and death. The goal of modern extraction techniques is to present an approach that is successful in extracting all leads and minimizes or eliminates these complications.

▪ ABLATION TECHNIQUES AND EQUIPMENT

To remove (extract) a chronically implanted intravascular device, the device must be separated (extirpated) from the encapsulating inflammatory tissue. This process of extirpating the lead from the encapsulating tissue is a form of ablation. Three ablation techniques are currently used: mechanical, laser, and electrosurgical.

Mechanical Ablation

Mechanical ablation includes traction to pull the lead free of the encapsulating tissue. To focus the traction force to a specific binding site, countertraction and counterpressure techniques and devices were developed.

Traction

All current lead extraction procedures use some form of traction, a pulling force. Pulling on leads was a successful method of extracting leads during the early years of pacing, when leads lacked efficient fixation devices and were implanted for short periods of time. Traction proved unsafe and had a high incidence of failure when applied to leads with efficient fixation devices and leads implanted for longer periods of time.[1, 2] The required amount of traction increases, becoming more dangerous as the duration of time since implantation becomes longer and the tensile strength of the fibrous tissue increases. Leads with efficient passive-fixation devices may be difficult to remove 4 to 6 months after implantation. Failure to extract a lead frequently damages the lead, making future extraction attempts more difficult.

Traction must be applied judiciously to minimize the risk to the patient. The pulling force applied to the proximal portion of the lead is distributed to sites where fibrous tissue binds the lead, where the lead or electrode makes contact with the vein or heart wall. Multiple leads may be bound to the vein or heart wall and to each other. Because the pulling force is not focused, the distribution of force to the binding sites is unknown. It is possible to inadvertently tear a vein or the heart wall.

Accidents are not predictable and frequently happen without warning, in part because it is impossible to judge the force applied to the lead. The applied force varies with lead size, the method of grasping the lead, and, most important, the catecholamine level (stress level) of the physician. Consequently, the use of procedures such as pulling until you feel the heart contraction or applying "just a little tug" to see if the lead will come out may not be safe.

Direct Traction on the Proximal Portion of the Lead

Traction can be applied directly to the proximal lead segment, directly to a locking stylet, or indirectly by means of intravascular snares. Direct traction is applied by pulling on the proximal exposed portion of the lead (Fig. 28–1). Special instrumentation is not required for this type of direct traction. Traction may be applied for minutes manually to days using various weights or elastic bands.[3–5]

Most direct traction techniques try to apply sufficient force to feel the rhythmic tugging of the heart without producing arrhythmias, hypotension, or chest pain. The force applied is limited by the tensile strength of both the lead and the tissue. Exceeding this force results in a broken lead, a tear of a vein, or an avulsion or tear of the heart wall.

Another danger is the inability to relax the tension placed on a ventricular lead after traction is removed. If the lead is withdrawn some distance but the electrode is not freed from the myocardium, the lead may become bound so that it cannot return to its original position. If the ventricular wall is pulled toward the tricuspid valve during traction, it causes a decrease in blood flowing into the ventricle and a low cardiac output. If the lead is bound in its withdrawn position, the reduced blood flow causes a cardiovascular emergency.

A successful removal of the lead from the heart wall may terminate with the lead wedged in fibrous tissue within the atrium or a superior vein. An infected lead must be completely removed. If a part of the lead protrudes distally, it can be snared and removed. For example, a Dotter basket snare or a loop inserted through the femoral vein is frequently successful. If the snare fails, cardiovascular surgery is the only option.

Applying excessive traction to dislodge a lead wedged in a vein may tear the vein or break the lead. Parts of a broken lead may become dislodged and float freely in the bloodstream. The density of the material influences its be-

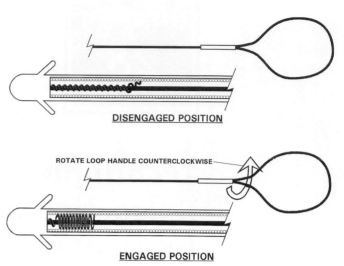

DISENGAGED POSITION

ROTATE LOOP HANDLE COUNTERCLOCKWISE

ENGAGED POSITION

Figure 28–2. The locking stylet is passed ideally to the electrode and secured. The locking mechanism is a wire secured to the tip and wrapped around the stylet. When the stylet is turned counterclockwise, the wire bundles together, binding the stylet to the conductor coil. The locking stylet acts primarily as a lead extender for applying traction and secondarily to keep the lead intact during the extraction. When the stylet is positioned at the electrode, the lead has its best chance of remaining intact. When the stylet is positioned near the proximal end, the fragile leads are pulled apart when traction is applied.

havior. Segments of lead body are usually moved by the blood flow and tend to migrate into the pulmonary artery. Pieces of metal such as the electrodes tend to fall under the influence of gravity, migrating into a dependent position.

Direct Traction With Locking Stylets

The development of locking stylets has greatly simplified the methods of applying traction. The locking stylet also functions as a lead extender and as a handle for applying traction, greatly reducing the extraction time and in most cases eliminating the need to improvise.

Before these stylets were available, traction was applied by grasping the lead and pulling. The tensile strength of the leads was usually not sufficient, and they would break when subjected to extraction forces. Broken leads were removed in pieces, complicating the extraction procedure and frequently resulting in an incomplete extraction. Applying traction to a stylet locked within the lumen of the lead near the electrode resulted in more leads being extracted intact.

The Cook locking stylets (Cook Vascular Inc., Leechburg, PA) are successful because of the simplicity and strength of the locking mechanism (Fig. 28–2). The locking mechanism is a small wire attached to the tip of the stylet and wrapped clockwise. To lock the stylet, it is turned counterclockwise, causing the small wire to bundle together, binding the stylet to the conductor coil. The locking does not weaken the conductor coil or reduce the tensile strength of the lead. It is possible to reverse this lock by forcing a clockwise rotation of the stylet, although forced removal of the stylet may damage the conductor coil and prevent insertion of another stylet.

To insert the stylet, the lead is cut and the insulation trimmed back to expose the conductor coil. For bipolar leads

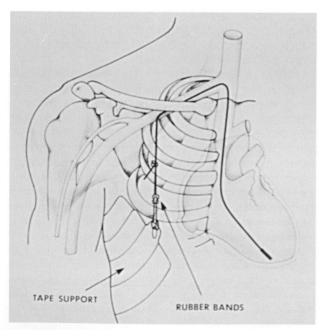

TAPE SUPPORT

RUBBER BANDS

Figure 28–1. Direct traction is being applied by pulling on the proximal portion of the lead. Rubber bands are used in this case. Variations include using free weights and applying weights using an orthopedic traction apparatus. If a locking stylet is inserted, the traction point is moved distal to the locking site, usually near the electrode.

with coaxial conductors, the inner coil is isolated. The lumen of the conductor coil is measured with the measuring pins provided in the kit. The appropriately sized locking stylet is then advanced down the lumen. While the stylet is being advanced, if a damaged conductor coil binds it, clockwise rotation will sometimes screw the stylet through the area. If the locking wire is uncoiled and stretched, it may not bundle or lock when rotated counterclockwise. To prevent this, the stylet should be advanced a few centimeters then pulled back to bundle the wire partially, forming a loose reversible lock. This maneuver is repeated until the electrode is reached.

Failure to lock the stylet is usually caused by improperly measuring the lumen size and inserting too small a stylet. The success in passing the locking stylet is dependent on the condition of the conductor coil. If it is damaged, the stylet may only pass to the damage site. Although it is ideal to pass the stylet to the electrode, passage any distance down the lumen provides a lead extender and traction handle superior to a suture attached to the outside of the lead.

A second mechanism for locking onto the tip of the conductor coil has been manufactured as the Wilkoff locking stylet (Cook Vascular Inc., Leechburg, PA). These stylets have a small flange at the tip, which is designed to stay flat against the stylet until the preloaded thin cylinder is advanced and deflects the flange to lock into the conductor coil (Fig. 28–3).

Several distinctions can be made between the Cook and Wilkoff locking stylets. Sizing, advancement down the conductor, and locking the stylet are simplified, and thus reliability of the locking is improved with the Wilkoff stylets.

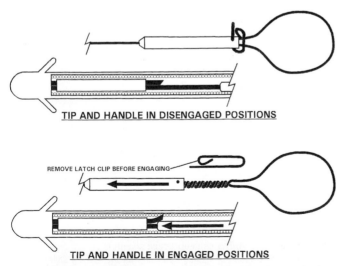

TIP AND HANDLE IN DISENGAGED POSITIONS

REMOVE LATCH CLIP BEFORE ENGAGING

TIP AND HANDLE IN ENGAGED POSITIONS

Figure 28–3. The Wilkoff Locking Stylet employs another mechanism for applying traction to the lead conductor at the tip of the lead. It also functions as a lead extender to lengthen the lead so that the sheaths can be advanced to the endocardial surface. The locking mechanism does not require the precision of measurement of the internal diameter of the conductor coil and bridges three sizes of the original locking stylet for each size of the Wilkoff stylet. The mechanism is activated by advancement of the thin cylinder, which nudges the hook to the side, engaging it between the coils of the conductor. This mechanism can be reversed and relocked but does not tolerate rotation. The response to rotation can be an advantage if the stylet needs to be removed.

These stylets are also more easily removed by retracting the cylinder mechanism or by simply rotating the stylet, which breaks off the flange without damaging the coil lumen. The Wilkoff locking stylets cannot be used for conductor coils that size to 0.016 inches or less in diameter. In addition, the ability to rotate the conductor coil is particularly useful for active-fixation leads. Thus, the Wilkoff locking stylets are best used for passive-fixation leads, retractable screw-in leads, and leads with conductor coils 0.017 inches in diameter and larger.

Traction on a stylet locked at the electrode allows the applied force to be delivered to the electrode. Applying the force at the electrode has helped to maintain the integrity of the lead but does not by itself eliminate those complications associated with traction. Although more leads are removed intact, the risk of the proximal binding sites absorbing the force or binding a withdrawn lead is still present. Electrodes successfully freed from the heart wall may still become impacted in the fibrous tissue within the atrium or a superior vein, and the tensile strength of the heart wall and lead still limit the amount of force applied.

Another stylet that comes in only one size, made by VascoMed (Weil am Rhein, Germany), is being used in Europe.[6] The stylet is reported to have sufficient tensile strength to support lead extractions. We have no experience with this device. The mechanism for locking consists of two flanges that are forced open and become entrapped within the conductor coil. This locking mechanism is also reported to be removable using a motorized tool.

The original traction tool, the suture, still has an important role when tied onto the lead insulation. This is particularly true of Silastic insulation, which has a greater tendency to bunch up or "snowplow" as the extraction sheaths are advanced. Ideally, the suture is tied onto the insulation and also to the extended loop end of the locking stylet. The locking stylet does not always work, and the suture still is an important traction tool.

Indirect Traction

Indirect traction is traction applied by an instrument such as a snare passed into the heart, usually through a femoral vein. The lead is entrapped in the snare, and traction is applied by pulling or pushing.[7–13] The safety of this technique is enhanced by the ability to avoid those problems associated with the binding sites in the superior veins and right atrium. Also, it is more successful than direct traction. The difficulty is in grasping the lead in a manner that allows sufficient traction to be applied. Only a few snares, such as the Dotter basket snare, have sufficient strength to support extraction forces. Techniques for safely applying chronic indirect traction have not evolved.

The lead must be freed from the superior veins and the heart. One technique is to pull the lead out of the superior veins into the atrium or inferior vena cava. The lead is then regrasped and traction applied to the heart. The techniques for applying indirect traction are the same techniques required for grasping and manipulating the leads for the countertraction approach and are described in the countertraction discussion.

Indirect traction has the same potential as direct traction for breaking the lead or tearing the heart wall, if their tensile strength is exceeded. However, the risks eliminated by this approach are tearing of superior veins, wedging the lead in the atrium or in a superior vein, and creating a low cardiac output that is caused by a failure of the lead to return to its original position after traction. Commonly, the lead stretches and breaks and multiple regrasping attempts are required before the lead is completely removed.

Intravascular Counterpressure and Countertraction Techniques

Countertraction is a method of safely extracting an electrode entrapped in fibrous tissue at the electrode–myocardial interface (Fig. 28–4). It is defined as the countering of the traction on the lead by a sheath. A sheath of slightly larger diameter is passed over the lead to a point about 1 cm from the heart wall. Traction is applied on the lead, pulling the myocardial wall to the edge of the sheath, which counters the traction. The edge of the sheath must be blunt; a sharp edge could inadvertently cut myocardial tissue or cut the lead and cause it to break.

Countertraction applied to the heart wall at the electrode–myocardium interface focuses the force perpendicular to the heart wall. Because only scar tissue is present between the sheath and the heart wall, cardiac tissue is not in jeopardy. The amount of traction applied to the lead is limited only by the tensile strength of the lead. When the operator counters the traction, the remainder of the heart wall is not subject to this force. Once sufficient traction is applied, the electrode is torn out of the scar tissue at the electrode–myocardium interface and pulled up into the lumen of the sheath. When

the electrode breaks free, the stationary countertraction sheath remains in the ventricular or atrial cavity and is no longer in contact with the heart wall. We do not believe that it is possible to tear or perforate the heart wall if countertraction is applied at the myocardium perpendicular to the wall.

Byrd Dilator Sheaths

Passage of the sheaths over the lead and down to the electrode is a prerequisite to applying countertraction. To reach a point near the electrode, the sheaths must pass through the fibrous tissue–binding sites along the vein and heart wall. To pass the sheaths safely and prevent problems similar to those associated with direct traction, proper sheaths and techniques must be used. The same sheaths are used for applying counterpressure at the binding sites along the lead and for applying countertraction at the electrode–myocardial interface.

Counterpressure at the Binding Sites

Counterpressure is the pressure applied by the sheath to the tissue at a binding site countered by the tissue resistance (Fig. 28–5). The force applied to the fibrous tissue–binding sites at the vein entry point and along the veins and heart wall fundamentally differs from countertraction, as applied at the electrode–myocardial interface, because the sheath is not stationary. Rather, it is pushed into the vein against the fibrous tissue at the binding site, creating pressure. The tissue resistance countering this pressure is some combination of

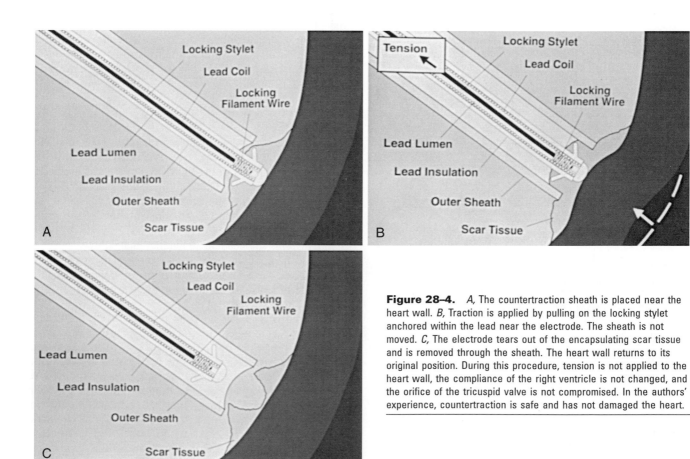

Figure 28–4. *A,* The countertraction sheath is placed near the heart wall. *B,* Traction is applied by pulling on the locking stylet anchored within the lead near the electrode. The sheath is not moved. *C,* The electrode tears out of the encapsulating scar tissue and is removed through the sheath. The heart wall returns to its original position. During this procedure, tension is not applied to the heart wall, the compliance of the right ventricle is not changed, and the orifice of the tricuspid valve is not compromised. In the authors' experience, countertraction is safe and has not damaged the heart.

Counterpressure

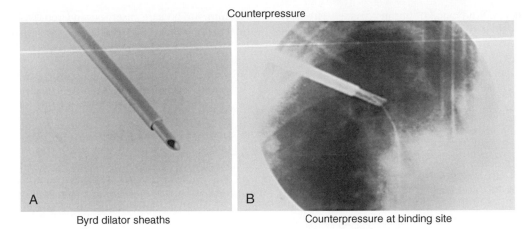

A	B
Byrd dilator sheaths	Counterpressure at binding site

Figure 28–5. *Counterpressure* is defined as the pressure applied (pushing) by the telescoping sheaths countered by tissue. Counterpressure is the opposite of countertraction; the sheath is pushed and the lead is used for support only. *A,* The Byrd dilator telescoping sheaths are used to apply counterpressure. These sheaths are made of metal (stainless steel) and plastic (Teflon and polypropylene). The metal sheaths are used to pass through the soft tissue and the vein entry site. Once inside, they are replaced by the plastic sheaths. *B,* A radiograph of the sheaths being passed to the right brachiocephalic vein. The telescoping sheaths apply counterpressure at a binding site. The sheaths are being manipulated and pushed against the binding site. When the applied pressure exceeds the tensile strength of the binding site, the binding site dilates, tears, or peels (shears) off the wall.

the tensile strength of the fibrous tissue binding the lead and the strength of the vein or heart wall.

Counterpressure is applied tangentially as a shearing force. Properly applied, it dilates and tears the fibrous tissue or shears it off the wall. Shearing forces are not as safe as a force applied perpendicular to an electrode at the heart wall. If an excessive shearing force is applied, a misdirected tear might create a false passage, tearing the vein or heart wall. Good judgment and experience are required for safety.

To focus the pressure, the sheaths must be properly guided and supported. Direct traction on the lead is used to guide the sheath along the lead, focusing the pushing force to the fibrous tissue binding the lead and not to the vein or heart wall. Direct traction should be limited to the amount needed to supply this support. If too much traction is applied to the lead, the traction has the same attendant risk as that associated with direct traction. If excessive traction is required, this approach should be abandoned. Good judgment and experience are required to avoid applying excessive force.

In some situations, countertraction may be used in the veins and along the heart wall. If the lead is firmly bound by fibrous tissue that prevents its being pulled through the binding site, countertraction is applied. Traction is applied to the lead and countered by the sheaths at the bound site. This is a common occurrence when leads pass through chronically occluded veins. It is extremely difficult to pass the sheaths through these areas. If excessive force must be used, this approach should be abandoned. Rotation of the sheaths with the pin vise greatly increases the efficacy of counterpressure and countertraction in the venous structures.

Using the Counterpressure-Countertraction Sheaths

Sheaths passed over the lead and down to the heart must be strong enough to be forced through the scar tissue and supple

enough to make sharp turns. Use of telescoping sheaths allows one sheath to work against the other. Various sizes of plastic sheaths are available; an 11-French (F) inner sheath and a 16-F outer sheath are adequate for most leads. The inner sheath is supple and the outer sheath more rigid. To break through the scar tissue at the vein entry site, a telescoping set of rigid stainless steel sheaths is used. Once inside the vein, the stainless steel sheaths are changed to the flexible plastic sheaths.

Stainless Steel Sheaths: Telescoping stainless steel sheaths are passed over the lead in the subcutaneous tissue and used to break through the tissue at the vein entry site. The material at the vein entry site ranges from fibrous tissue capsule, of varying tensile strength, to bone. These sheaths were designed to allow a sufficient longitudinal force to be applied to just break into the vein. Both countertraction and counterpressure techniques are applied. A single stainless steel sheath was tried for a period of time but was difficult to use and not as successful as the telescoping sheaths.

Fluoroscopic visualization is essential to follow the lead path and avoid creating a false passage. A false passage does not allow entry into the vein and may damage the lead. Once in the vein, these sheaths are exchanged for the more flexible plastic sheaths. Failure to change to the more flexible sheaths can be dangerous.

Plastic Sheaths: The flexible telescoping sheaths are for maneuvering around curves and forcing through the circumferential bands of fibrous tissue. Sufficient traction is applied to support the smaller supple sheath for maneuvering around curves in the vein. The smaller sheath then acts as a guide, supporting the advancement of the larger, more rigid outer sheath. Fluoroscopic visualization is again essential to avoid creating a false passage, tearing the vein or heart wall.

As the sheaths are advanced, fibrous tissue with low tensile strength is dilated. As the tensile strength increases, the fibrous tissue is torn. After the circumferential bands of fibrous tissue begin to calcify, the sheaths cannot tear through the calcified tissue around the lead, but a larger diameter sheath can be advanced over it (inclusion). It peels the calcified bands off the vein or heart wall.

As discussed, counterpressure subjects the tissue to a shearing force. The shearing force must be judiciously applied. The flexible Teflon sheaths, which are easier to maneuver around curves, limit the applied shearing force. If the counterpressure force is more than can be easily applied with these sheaths, this approach is often abandoned. Stiffer sheaths can be used only if care is taken to have the sheaths follow the course of the lead instead of allowing the sheath to alter the course of the lead.

Passage of sheaths along the circuitous route down the lead to the heart is successful for most leads that have been implanted for 6 to 8 years or less. Leads implanted for a greater length of time have an increasing incidence of failure to extract because of the tensile strength of the scar tissue. Old, large-diameter leads allow only one large-diameter sheath to be passed over them. The advantages of using telescoping sheaths are lost, and the incidence of failure to extract increases.

Byrd Femoral Workstation: The transvenous approach through the femoral vein requires a special sheath set that functions as an introducer, as a workstation for manipulation of snares, and as countertraction sheaths. The Byrd Femoral Workstation set consists of an introducer needle, guide wire, 16-F workstation, 11-F tapered dilator, 11-F telescoping sheath, a Cook deflection snare, and a Dotter basket snare.

The workstation serves many functions. Initially, it acts as a protective sheath, preventing the insertion, withdrawal, and manipulation of the other sheath and snares from damaging the veins or heart. To prevent clot formation, the workstation has a "check-flo" valve to irrigate the sheath continuously. The workstation and snares form a reversible loop to pull the proximal portion of the lead out of the superior veins; it also acts as the outer telescoping countertraction sheath.

Insertion: The safe insertion and removal of the workstation is a prerequisite to extraction through a femoral vein. The workstation is 16 F in size and must be inserted with care. Fluoroscopic monitoring is mandatory. Once the guide wire is passed into the heart, the workstation with its tapered dilator must be maneuvered through the iliac vein and inferior vena cava (IVC) and into the right atrium. The route can be circuitous, especially from the left side. In rare cases, the curvature may too sharp for the stiff dilator to follow the guide wire. Forcing the dilator in this situation is unsafe, and the approach should be abandoned. A torn retroperitoneal iliac vein or IVC is a serious complication. Once the workstation is inserted, irrigation fluids are run continuously through the check-flo valve to prevent clotting.

Dotter and Deflection Snare

Reversible Loop: A reversible loop is created around the lead body to pull the proximal end of the lead out of the superior veins into the IVC, without placing traction on the electrode–myocardium interface (Fig. 28–6). A loop must be created and bound to the lead body. It is mandatory that the binding and the loop itself are reversible. Irreversible binding of the lead or the inability to remove the loop from around the lead may result in dangerous traction maneuvers performed in desperation while the operator tries to extract the lead and snare. Failure to extract the lead subjects the patient to more invasive procedures to remove both the lead and snare.

Creating a reversible loop using two snares is a complicated maneuver, requiring practice to perfect. One technique is to use a Cook deflecting wire guide and a Dotter basket snare. The Cook deflecting wire guide is wrapped more than 360 degrees around the lead body. Next, the tip of the deflection catheter is passed into the Dotter basket snare. When the basket snare is pulled into the workstation, the basket closes, grasping the deflection catheter and completing the loop. The loop is pulled into the workstation, tightly binding the lead body to the workstation, and traction is applied. If needed, the loop is relaxed and repositioned on the lead body. This sequence is repeated until the lead is pulled out of the superior veins, through the right atrium,

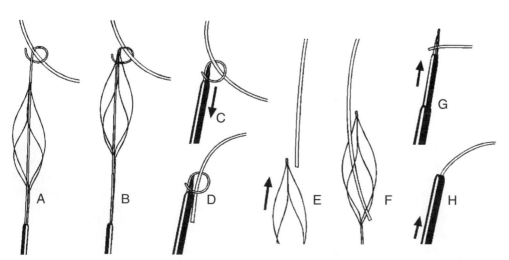

Figure 28–6. *A*, The Cook deflection catheter encircles the lead. *B*, The Dotter snare grasps the tip of the deflection catheter, forming a loop. *C*, The loop is pulled into the workstation. *D*, The lead is bound and pulled out of the superior vein into the heart or inferior vena cava. *E*, The loop is reversed by pushing it out of the workstation and separating the catheter and snare. *F*, The catheter is removed and the proximal portion of the lead grasped by the snare. *G*, The lead is pulled back into the workstation. *H*, The 11-F catheter and workstation are advanced into the heart to apply countertraction, extracting the lead.

and into the IVC. The reversible loop is then released and the deflection catheter removed.

Pulling the Lead Down and Out of the Superior Veins: The maneuver of pulling leads down and out of the superior veins has been remarkably successful. Many leads freed from the heart cannot be pulled up through these same veins. Lead binding by the circumferential bands of fibrous tissue is the same in both directions. The hypothesis for this difference is the free upward mobility of the mediastinal structures. The mediastinum is easily pulled upward, compressing the veins, but is limited in its downward motion. Compression of the fibrous tissue bands around the lead as they bunch together is postulated to increase the binding strength.

Failures to extract the proximal lead from the superior veins using this technique are rare and are usually caused by other complicating factors. Examples of complicating factors are thrombosis of the superior veins and excessive fibrosis around the lead caused by a previous extraction attempt that left the conductor coil exposed or pulled the lead taut against the heart and vein wall. These leads are removed using approaches such as transatrial, reserved for more complicated extractions.

Countertraction

To apply countertraction through the workstation, the proximal end of the lead must be entangled in the basket snare. This is accomplished by placing the basket snare in close proximity to the lead and rotating it slowly. The lead flips into the basket. The basket closes by advancing the 11-F sheath over the snare. For most leads, the snare and lead are pulled into the 11-F sheath. The workstation and 11-F sheath are then worked in a telescoping fashion to a point near the electrode. At this point, countertraction is applied to extract the electrode as previously described.

Removal

Removal of the workstation must be carefully performed. Once the lead is extracted, clot and debris may be attached to the end of the tubing. If this material dislodges in the femoral vein entry site, it can act as a nidus, forming a thrombus or initiating thrombophlebitis and its sequelae. To prevent this complication, blood is aspirated during the withdrawal of the workstation. If the entry site does not bleed freely after withdrawal of the workstation, a surgical exploration of the vein is recommended. Bleeding is controlled by applying slight pressure over the vein entry site. A suture is required to close the skin.

The risk for thrombophlebitis and pulmonary embolus after an IVC approach was the stimulus for using the workstation. The standard precautions are taken. Patients are given antiembolism stockings (pneumatic, if possible) and are placed on subcutaneous heparin, 5000 U twice daily.

Precision

The technique of grasping the lead in a reversible loop using a Cook deflection catheter and a Dotter snare is a more complicated maneuver. Once mastered, however, it is an effective method of performing a precision extraction. For example, a patient may have six leads in the heart. Two new leads are connected to a pacemaker and are to be saved.

Four leads are abandoned and are to be extracted. The abandoned atrial and ventricular leads can be extracted, leaving the newly implanted leads intact. The IVC approach allows this level of precision.

Needle's Eye Snare

The Needle's Eye Snare (Cook Vascular Inc., Leechburg, PA) is another apparatus that can be inserted through the Byrd Femoral Workstation. Like the tip-deflecting guide wire and Dotter basket, this tool is intended to grasp the lead within the cardiac structures and pull the lead down from the superior venous structures and then from the heart with countertraction. Both the preloaded countertraction sheaths (tip-deflecting guide wire and Dotter basket) and the Needle's Eye Snare can be used with a straight or curved sheath. The Needle's Eye Snare makes it easier to grasp the lead with a reversible loop, as described previously. The hook is draped over the lead, the "needle" is advanced through the hook, and the inner sheath is advanced, trapping the lead body between the hook and the needle. This is easily reversed but requires maintaining some distance from the endocardium to work the mechanism (Fig. 28–7).

Laser Ablation

The Spectranetics excimer laser (Spectranetics Corp., Colorado Springs, CO) is effective in separating the lead from the fibrous tissue–binding sites. The laser delivers a 308-nm laser beam through a fiberoptic sheath. The circumferential zone of optic fibers at the end of the sheath delivers a 308-nm laser beam that is effective for about 1 mm. This frequency laser light beam primarily vaporizes water molecules, disrupting the encapsulating fibrous tissue. Some photochemical disruption of the protein bonds takes place, but this is not the primary mechanism for disrupting the tissue. These sheaths are available in three sizes, 12 F, 14 F, and 16 F. These sizes are sufficient to remove the leads currently in use.

In an ideal situation, the sheath is passed over the lead, vaporizing each binding site until the sheath reaches a point about a few millimeters from the heart wall. The lead is then removed from the heart wall using countertraction.

Most leads cannot be removed using the laser sheath as depicted in this idealized situation. Instead, the laser sheath must be combined with an outer plastic sheath. The outer sheath acts as a workstation for maneuvering the laser sheath and for applying countertraction at the myocardial-endocardial surface. Counterpressure is occasionally used by working one sheath against the other, combining the techniques of laser and mechanical ablation. It is especially effective at calcified binding sites, where the encapsulating tissue is peeled off the wall and included within the sheath.

Laser ablation can be used with both the superior vena cava approach through the vein entry site and the transatrial approach. The sheath is not long enough to use with the femoral approach. For cut or broken intravascular leads, the laser sheaths can be used in combination with snares. The snare entraps the lead and becomes a traction device over which the laser sheath is passed.

Electrosurgical Ablation

The electrosurgical sheaths are used to ablate the encapsulating fibrous tissue in a manner similar to the laser sheaths

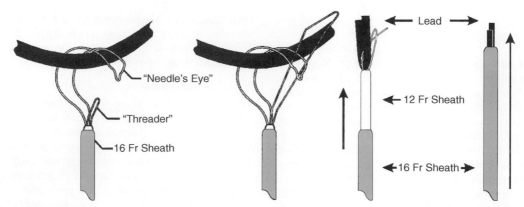

Figure 28–7. The Needle's Eye Snare is looped over the lead body, and the threader is advanced, closing the open segment of the circle. The 12-F sheath is then advanced, closing the snare and trapping the lead body in the snare. The proximal segment of the lead is pulled down from the subclavian system. Sometimes, the lead needs to be released and snared on a more proximal segment to complete the removal from the superior veins. The 16-F sheath is then advanced over the lead body to the endocardial surface to provide countertraction.

method. The differences are in the method of ablation and the configuration of the ablation device at the tip of the sheath. The electrosurgical sheath works as a bipolar electrosurgical cutting instrument, similar to the conventional devices used for hemostasis and cutting. The electrical arc placed at the tip of the beveled end at the tip of the sheath cuts the fibrous tissue. An outer sheath is used as a workstation and for counterpressure and countertraction.

This device is new and does not have a proven track record. Its utility and advantages over the laser sheath will have to be demonstrated. For example, it is postulated that this device will be less expensive and more supple and will allow for precision cutting of the fibrous tissue (Fig. 28–8).

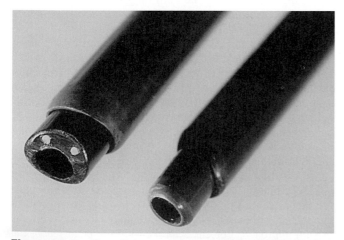

Figure 28–8. The radiofrequency energy causes a spark at the tip of the inner electrosurgical sheath. The energy is conducted to two small tungsten wires at the tip of the inner sheath. The outer sheath provides strength and limits the tendency for kinking, as it does for all telescoping sheath sets. The current delivery at the tip is controlled with a sophisticated transformer, which adjusts the output in relation to the tissue impedance.

■ EXTRACTION PROCEDURES

Intravascular Extraction Procedures

To apply the new, successful countertraction extraction procedures safely, it is important to understand the problems associated with direct and indirect traction techniques (Fig. 28–9). Countertraction is applied by means of the implant vein through the superior vena cava (SVC) approach, and indirectly, by means of the femoral vein through the IVC approach. Occasionally, a more invasive transatrial approach is combined with countertraction. The following is a detailed discussion of these techniques.

A series of transvenous and thoracic surgical procedures have evolved using countertraction. Countertraction extraction approaches include the SVC, the IVC, and the transatrial.[14-20] To date, cardiopulmonary bypass has not been necessary. Most leads can be removed using the transvenous SVC and IVC approaches individually or in combination. In some situations, both the SVC and IVC approaches fail, and countertraction is applied through a transatrial approach using a small anterior thoracotomy.[16, 17, 21] Table 28–1 lists the considerations that should be kept in mind to perform lead extraction safely.

Preparation for the Procedure

Patients who undergo lead extractions are prepared for multiple approaches, including an emergency cardiac surgical procedure. Although routine lead extractions do not require surgical intervention, a complication such as tearing of a large vein or the heart wall may precipitate a cardiovascular emergency. These emergencies must be handled in an expeditious manner to ensure a successful resolution.

Some operators prefer general endotracheal anesthesia, although many lead extractions are done with local and intravenous sedation. General endotracheal anesthesia and either peripheral or conventional techniques for cardiopulmonary bypass must be available. The chest and groin areas

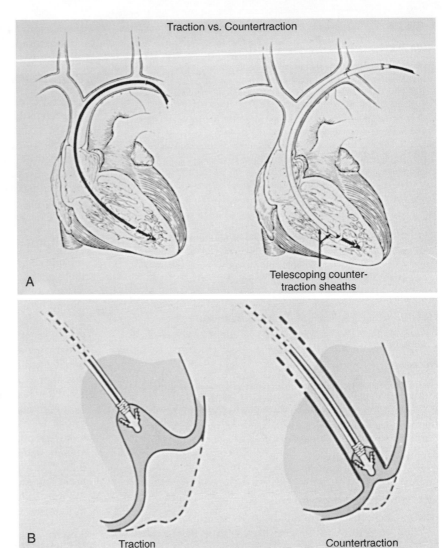

Figure 28–9. *A* and *B,* Traction is a pulling force. The lead is grasped at any point and pulled. As the lead is pulled, the right ventricle is everted, and tension is applied to the heart wall. Eversion decreases compliance and compromises the tricuspid valve, both of which cause a low cardiac output. The tension is relieved by the tissue tearing. If the scar tissue surrounding the electrode tears, the electrode is freed; if the heart wall tears, a cardiovascular emergency ensues. Countertraction is the countering of the traction force by the countertraction sheaths. Countertraction focuses the traction force at the electrode myocardial interface. Countertraction prevents eversion of the right ventricle and allows only the tissue surrounding the electrode to tear, freeing the electrode.

are shaved and prepared. Venous and arterial lines are placed for monitoring and vascular access. The patient is monitored by electrocardiography, oxygen saturation, and often carbon dioxide sensors. Additional tools include a Foley catheter, instruments for pacing and defibrillation, an electrosurgical unit, and a sternal saw for emergencies. Blood is typed and screened but not cross-matched.

Temporary Pacing Lead

A temporary pacing lead is inserted in all patients who need a pacemaker. An exception is made for patients with an implanted permanent pacemaker whose leads are not to be extracted. Because of the maneuvering required to extract some leads, conventional temporary pacing leads are not used. Instead, a permanent unipolar or bipolar active-fixation lead is implanted. If a unipolar lead is used, a temporary epicardial lead, the same as is used in cardiac surgery, is sutured into the skin over the deltoid muscle and used as an indifferent electrode. The newer transvenous bipolar temporary pacing wires with active-fixation screws are less expensive, flexible tools for both atrial and ventricular stimulation.

The active-fixation lead is placed on the same side as the lead to be extracted, even if the pacemaker site is infected, to avoid contaminating the other side. It is inserted into the subclavian or internal jugular vein using standard introducer techniques. If the lead must be placed on the opposite side, the internal jugular vein is used. The lead is secured in a reversible manner for the duration of the procedure. Alternatively, a temporary pacing lead can be placed using femoral venous access; the infected leads are then removed, and a clean transvenous active-fixation lead (permanent or temporary, as described previously) is then placed by way of the internal jugular vein.

Fluoroscopy

Fluoroscopy should be used to visually monitor all transvenous maneuvers. Most complications involving transvenous insertion and extraction can be avoided if the procedures are performed using fluoroscopy. This is especially true for extraction procedures. If the applied forces are misdirected, the heart or vein wall can be torn. Bleeding into the pleural cavity can be seen using fluoroscopy. The lead being extracted may break, with pieces floating in the bloodstream. If the break is seen immediately, the objects can be retrieved

Table 28–1. Precautions to Consider for Lead Removal Procedures

Preparations

Thorough patient history, including the manufacturer, model number, and implantation date of lead to be removed

Radiographic evaluation of lead condition, type, and position; ECG evaluation as appropriate

Patient preparation for vein entry approach, possible femoral approach, and possible thoracic approach

Patient typed and screened for possible emergency transfusion; preparations made for possible emergency surgery

Backup pacing established as necessary

Extensive collection of sheaths, locking stylets, snares, and accessory equipment

Procedure Room

High-quality fluoroscopy, pacing equipment, defibrillator, pericardiocentesis tray, and thoracotomy tray

Rapidly available: ECG, appropriate blood products, emergency cardiovascular surgery

Monitoring

Fluoroscopy during all lead and sheath manipulations

ECG and blood pressure (arterial line preferred) during procedure and recovery

Procedure

Use proper sheath technique and maintain tension on locking stylet

If scar tissue is severe, consider an alternate approach

If lead breaks, evaluate fragment; retrieve as indicated

If hypotension develops, release tension on lead, and rapidly evaluate for possible tamponade or hemothorax; treat as appropriate

ECG, electrocardiography.

while in a large vein or in the right atrium. They may be difficult to remove if lodged in a vein in the head, liver, extremities, or lungs.

Emergency Surgery

Cardiovascular emergencies are caused by tearing a vein or the heart wall, resulting in life-threatening hemorrhage. Bleeding into the pericardium causes tamponade. Marked bleeding with rapid onset of tamponade is treated by an immediate median sternotomy and surgical repair of the torn heart or vein wall. To achieve a successful result, contingency plans must be made to treat these complications in an expeditious manner.

Tearing the vein extrapleurally or in the extrapericardial portion of the mediastinum will probably not cause a problem because of the low venous pressure. Tearing the vein wall and puncturing the pleural cavity is a potential complication of this procedure, caused by pushing the sheaths and creating a false passage. Tearing outside the vein and into the pleura can result in life-threatening hemorrhage into the pleural cavity. Treatment is emergency surgery. These surgical approaches are generally more difficult, and the approach depends on the location of the tear. A tear in the subclavian vein is the most difficult to access. The safest approach is probably a median sternotomy. The brachiocephalic veins can be reached through this incision. The subclavian vein is approached by combining this incision with an anterior

thoracotomy through the second intercostal space, creating an anterosuperior chest wall flap.

Superior Vena Cava Approach

The SVC approach is the initial approach used by most physicians (Fig. 28–10). The SVC approach combines the pocket abandonment procedure with passage of the dilator sheaths to the electrode. In all cases, the leads are exposed, débrided of inflammatory tissue, and freed from restraining sutures as part of the abandonment procedure. A locking stylet is passed to the electrode and locked. Stainless steel telescoping sheaths are passed over the lead entering the vein, then exchanged for the plastic sheaths. These sheaths are used to pass through the tissue-binding sites to the electrode–myocardium interface. The electrode is extracted by applying countertraction, and the lead is removed through the sheaths. In general, if any difficulty is encountered in advancing the countertraction sheaths, the SVC approach should be abandoned.

The rationales for using the SVC approach are greater speed, less fluoroscopic exposure, and a high success rate for undamaged leads implanted less than 6 to 8 years. Almost all undamaged leads implanted 8 to 10 years are extracted using this approach. The tensile strength at the tissue-binding sites for older leads sometimes prohibits passage of the sheaths. In some cases, the amount of scar tissue continues to increase with time and, after 8 to 10 years, starts to calcify. Consequently, the forces needed to advance the sheaths are greater, and the lead needs greater tensile strength to remain intact during the extraction. Leads implanted 10 years or more and leads damaged in previous extraction attempts are the most difficult to remove and have the highest extraction failure rate using this approach.

Inferior Vena Cava Approach

The IVC approach is a more versatile approach (Fig. 28–11). The procedure is performed by inserting a sheath workstation and extracting the leads through the sheath using snares. The IVC approach is the procedure of choice for broken or cut leads floating freely in the veins, heart, or pulmonary artery and for leads passing through occluded veins. A grossly contaminated vein entry site is another indication. Using the SVC approach and pushing sheaths through this contaminated debris is unsafe. It has the potential of causing septicemia and showering pulmonary emboli. The IVC approach is also used in cases in which the SVC approach has failed. Physicians who have had extensive training in transfemoral catheter procedures may feel more comfortable using it as their initial approach.

Transatrial Approach

The transatrial approach is a cardiovascular surgical procedure first described by Byrd 1985.[21] It is a primary approach for noninfected patients who are candidates for a transatrial lead implantation. Younger patients with occlusion of one brachiocephalic vein or with an SVC syndrome have the old leads extracted through a transatrial approach, followed by implantation of new leads. The advantage of the transatrial approach is the ability to remove leads not accessible or

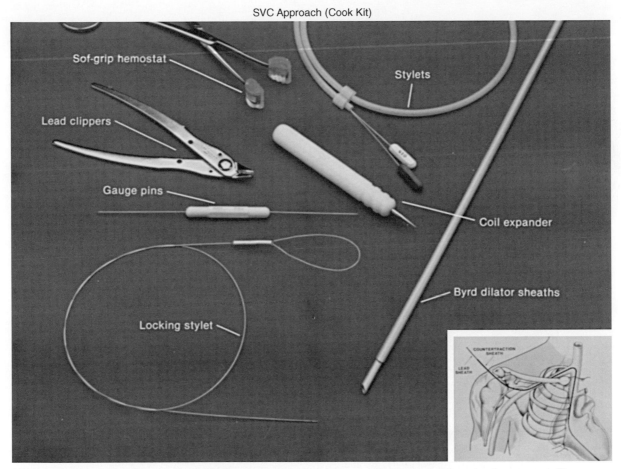

Figure 28–10. The superior vena cava (SVC) approach is the most common initial countertraction extraction approach. The procedure includes insertion of Byrd dilator sheaths over the lead and passage through the implant site to the electrode. The Cook Extraction Kit is used for an SVC approach. Tools provided include a wire cutter, lead holder, conductor coil dilator, conductor coil sizing pins, locking stylet, and counterpressure-countertraction sheaths.

The *inset* shows the proximal portion of the lead exposed down to the vein entry site: the vein for a cephalic or external jugular venotomy approach, the pectoralis muscle for an introducer approach, and the tissue near the vein for an internal jugular approach. The counterpressure-countertraction sheaths are passed over the lead, through the vein entry site, and through the veins and heart to a site near the electrode.

removable by the SVC or IVC approach. Most of the transatrial extractions are failures of the IVC approach. Rarely, in a case in which an SVC approach failed, the operator proceeds directly to a transatrial approach—for example, in situations in which the workstation cannot be passed through the femoral veins into the heart. Infected patients who are candidates for transatrial lead implants have the leads extracted by an SVC or IVC approach, and the transatrial implantation is performed after the infection is properly treated.

Procedure

The transatrial approach is performed as originally described, through a limited surgical approach (Fig. 28–12). The right atrium is exposed by removing the third or fourth right costal cartilage. The pericardium is opened and suspended, and a pledgeted pursestring suture is placed in the right atrium. Using fluoroscopy, a pituitary biopsy instrument is inserted through the pursestring, and the lead body is grasped and pulled out of the atrium. The lead is then cut, extracting

both the proximal and distal segments separately. The proximal portion can usually be pulled out by traction. On rare occasions, the countertraction sheaths are required. The distal segment is extracted by inserting a locking stylet, advancing countertraction sheaths around the lead, and applying countertraction at the electrode–myocardium interface. This procedure is repeated for each lead to be extracted.

Thrombus or Infected Material Attached to Leads

The presence of large masses of vegetation connected to the leads is a limitation of all extraction procedures. Passing sheaths over the lead may shear the vegetation from the lead, causing a pulmonary embolus. This is a dangerous maneuver if the mass is large or contains infection. Most of these large masses are an organizing thrombus formed on or around the lead and attached to the heart wall. Techniques for extraction of these leads along with the vegetation are being evaluated but have not been perfected. The risk for embolism needs to be compared with the risks associated with other techniques.

IVC Approach (Byrd Workstation)

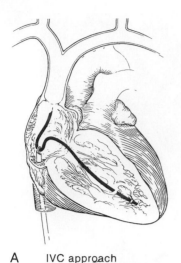

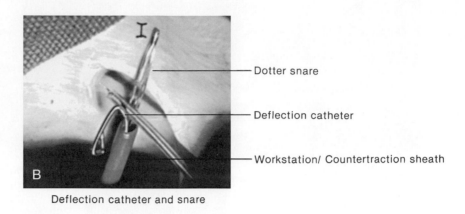

A   IVC approach

Deflection catheter and snare

— Dotter snare

— Deflection catheter

— Workstation/ Countertraction sheath

Byrd workstation

Figure 28–11. *A*, The inferior vena cava (IVC) approach. The workstation is passed through a femoral vein into the heart. The lead is grasped, pulling the proximal end into the heart or IVC. *B* and *C*, The Byrd workstation. The workstation consists of a 16-F Teflon sheath with a check-flow valve and intravenous site. Components are inserted into the workstation as needed. For insertion, a tapered dilator is inserted, and the workstation is passed over the guide wire (standard introducer approach) into the right atrium. The dilator is replaced by an 11-F sheath, through which the Cook deflection catheter and Dotter snare (*B*) are passed. The deflection catheter and snare are used to maneuver the lead, form a reversible loop, and snare the lead for applying countertraction.

Patient Management

After transatrial extraction, patient management is more involved than for the transvenous extraction techniques. The pericardium must be drained in most cases by a closed drainage system, such as a Jackson-Pratt system. The thoracic cavity is occasionally entered, and a chest tube is inserted to drain both the pericardium and pleura. These drainage tubes are removed in 2 to 3 days. Although the morbidity is not great, the hospital stay is increased 1 or 2 days.

Ventriculotomy

A lead extracted by this approach is considered a failure of conventional extraction techniques. A ventriculotomy is a cardiovascular surgical procedure (Fig. 28–13). It is reserved for infected broken leads not reachable by the other approaches, or it is used in conjunction with an emergency

repair of the heart wall. Some leads are fragile, and if they break near the ventricular wall or within a fibrous tissue tunnel along the ventricular wall, they are impossible to grasp using transvenous or transatrial techniques. If the heart wall tears during an extraction attempt, the lead is extracted through a ventriculotomy after the median sternotomy and repair of the tear.

The heart is exposed through a median sternotomy incision. The heart is then elevated on a pad, exposing the right ventricle. The tip of the electrode is localized by fluoroscopy and by using needles for triangulation of the electrode. A pursestring suture is placed around the electrode, and a ventriculotomy incision is made to the electrode. The electrode is grasped with a clamp and pulled out of the heart.[22] Because the lead segment is being pulled in the direction of the tines, the tines slip out of the embedding scar without resistance.

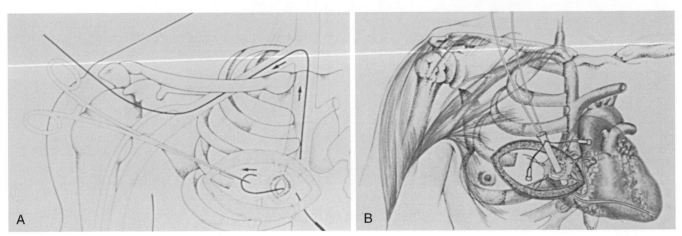

Figure 28–12. *A,* Transatrial extraction. The atrium is exposed through the third or fourth costal cartilage. Through a pursestring suture, the lead is grasped using a pituitary biopsy instrument and pulled out of the atrium. The lead is then cut. The proximal portion is removed using direct traction, and the distal portion is removed using countertraction. *B,* Transatrial implantation. An introducer sheath is placed in the atrium, and the pacing or defibrillator lead is implanted when indicated.

Results of Lead Extraction

U.S. Extraction Database

A database was established in 1988 to track removal of cardiac leads by any intravascular extraction technique. The database is a voluntary registry, funded by Cook Vascular Incorporated. A growing body of experience at multiple centers demonstrates the widespread effectiveness of intravascular extraction techniques. Intravascular extraction procedures were reported for 6420 leads in 4090 patients at more than 400 centers from January 1994 through December 1997. Of the 6420 leads, 93% were completely extracted, 5% were partially extracted, and 2% were not removed.

Success was correlated with shorter duration of implantation, greater physician experience, atrial lead placement, absence of infection, and lower patient age (Table 28–2).

Extraction from the implantation vein was used alone for 94% of the leads implanted for 1 year or less, 86% of the leads implanted for 2 to 4 years, 83% of the leads implanted for 5 to 7 years, and 76% of the leads implanted for 8 to 26 years. Femoral venous access was used as the primary approach for 2% of the leads implanted for 1 year, increasing to 10% for leads implanted for 8 to 26 years. A combination of both approaches was used for 4% of the leads implanted for 1 year and for 14% of leads implanted for 8 to 26 years.

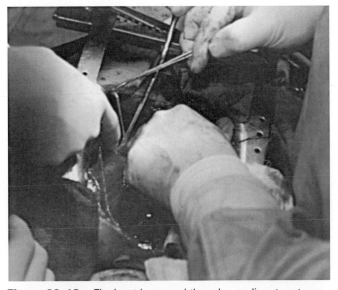

Figure 28–13. The heart is exposed through a median sternotomy incision. The electrode is located by palpation and triangulation using fluoroscopy. A pursestring suture is applied, and the electrode is grasped through a small ventriculotomy incision, removing the electrode and lead. Cardiopulmonary bypass is not required.

Table 28–2. Lead and Patient Characteristics Affecting Lead Extraction Outcome for 6420 Leads

Variable	Extraction Outcome (%)		
	Complete	Partial	Failed
Implant Duration			
1 yr	98.8	0.8	0.4
2–4 yr	95.4	3.0	1.6
5–7 yr	91.2	6.0	2.8
8–26 yr	83.6	12.9	3.5
Experience			
First case	89.9	6.5	3.6
>20 Cases	94.2	4.7	1.1
Placement			
Atrial	95.1	3.4	1.5
Ventricular	91.2	6.5	2.3
Indication			
Infection	93.8	4.7	1.5
Other	92.7	5.1	2.2
Patient Age			
<40 yr	88.4	8.4	3.2
40–59 yr	92.8	4.9	2.3
60–79 yr	94.0	4.4	1.6
80–97 yr	94.5	4.1	1.4

Data from the U.S. Extraction Database, January 1994 through December 1997.

Table 28–3. Extraction Indications for 4090 Patients

Indication	Percentage of Patients
Infection	
Septicemia or endocarditis	5.0
Infection	24.0
Chronic draining sinus	0.3
Erosion	3.3
Total	32.7
Removal of nonfunctional/failed leads	
J-wire related	35.1
Other leads	29.6
Total	64.7
Other indications	
Pre-erosion	0.1
Pain	0.7
Displaced or free floating	0.5
Thrombosis or superior vena cava occlusion	0.4
Tricuspid insufficiency or regurgitation	0.1
Other	0.9
Total	2.6

Data from the U.S. Extraction Database, January 1994 through December 1997.

The transatrial approach was not performed on a national level. The indications for lead extraction are listed in Table 28–3.

Major complications occurred in 1.6% of patients, including a 0.2% mortality rate (Table 28–4). Women with more than two leads appear to be at highest risk for major complications.[23] For women undergoing removal of one or two leads, the incidence of major complications was 2%; the small cohort of women undergoing removal of 3 or more leads (109 patients) had a major complication rate of 7.3%. Major complication rates were lower for men (1% for re-

Table 28–4. Description of Major Complications for 4090 Patients

Description	Percentage of Patients
Death (3 tamponade; 2 hemothorax; 1 AV fistula; 1 pulmonary embolism; 1 acute renal failure; 1 death on day 26 after transfusion on day 10)	0.2
Nonfatal hemopericardium or tamponade	0.6
Nonfatal hemothorax (includes 1 AV fistula)	0.3
Transfusion (without hemothorax or tamponade)	0.2
Other nonfatal major complications (3 pneumothorax treated with chest tube; 3 pulmonary embolism; 2 subclavian AV fistula [includes 1 renal failure]; 1 femoral AV fistula; 1 femoral artery pseudoaneurysm; 1 stroke; 1 respiratory arrest; 1 defibrillator lead entrapped in sheaths)	0.3
Total	1.6

AV, atrioventricular.
Data from U.S. Extraction Database, January 1994 through December 1997. Data include complications associated with reimplantation during the same procedure.

moval of one or two leads, 2% for removal of three or more leads). Further research is needed to determine whether this effect is due to gender or to vessel or patient size.

Implantable Cardioverter-Defibrillator Leads

One special group of patients is worth singling out: those with ICD leads. In the attempted removal of 443 implantable cardioverter-defibrillator (ICD) leads from 373 patients, 96% were completely removed, 2% were partially removed, and 2% were not removed. Although the rate of complete removal was higher than that for pacing leads (93% complete removal), the difference was not significant when the effect of implantation duration was considered in multivariate analysis. The implantation durations for ICD leads were substantially less than those for pacing leads (25 ± 18 months versus 54 ± 46 months).

Despite the substantially shorter implantation durations for ICD leads, the rate of major complications for patients with ICD leads was 2.1%, compared with 1.6% for patients with pacing leads. Further research is needed to determine whether ICD patients are at higher risk of extraction complications.[24]

Excimer Laser Results

The safety and effectiveness of PLEXES (*p*acemaker *l*ead *ex*traction with the *e*xcimer *s*heath) was compared with lead extraction using conventional locking stylet and telescoping sheath tools in a prospective randomized trial.[25] Complete removal was achieved in 94% of laser leads and in 64% of nonlaser leads ($P = .001$) (Table 28–5). The time for complete removal was reduced—10.1 ± 11.5 minutes versus 12.9 ± 19.2 minutes, respectively ($P < .04$). Potentially life-threatening complications occurred in none of the nonlaser and three of the laser patients, including one death (P = value not significant). The potential for complications requires further evaluation; however, excimer laser sheaths improved the effectiveness and reduced the time for pacemaker lead extraction.[25] There was no evidence that the Telectronics J wire (Accufix and Encor Telectronics Inc., Englewood, CO) leads were more difficult or dangerous to remove with the 12-F sheaths. Indeed, because these leads are more fragile than most other leads, the laser sheath was greatly preferred by the investigators for these leads.

Additional trials of the 14-F and 16-F laser sheaths had similar extraction rates of leads too large to fit into the 12-F laser sheath. The complication rates were no different, and

Table 28–5. Laser Extraction Outcomes and Reasons for Failure

	No. of Patients (%)	
	Nonlaser	Laser
No. of leads	221	244
Complete extraction*	142 (64)	230 (94)
Partial extraction	4 (1.8)	6 (2.5)
Failure*	75 (34)	8 (3.3)
Crossover to 12-F laser	72 (33)	—
Crossover to 16-F laser	1 (0.5)	—
Crossover to femoral	2 (0.9)	5 (2.0)
Clinical success of procedure	142 of 148 (95.9)	145 of 153 (94.8)

*$P = .001$.

the extraction times were only 2 to 4 minutes longer per lead. Most unipolar leads are best removed with the 12-F laser, whereas almost all bipolar pacing leads are best removed with the 14-F sheaths. ICD leads, which constitute a large and increasing percentage of lead extraction attempts, almost always require the 16-F sheaths.[26-28]

Summary

The informal development of transvenous extraction techniques continues, with the general availability of formally developed tools since 1988. The techniques have been disseminated to a modestly large number of physicians and have come into common use. The awareness of the need for these tools coincides with the recall of several lead models for insulation failure, the recall of J-wire leads, the appearance of relatively fragile ICD leads, and the ongoing need to treat pacemaker and ICD infections.

As implantable devices prove to be increasingly useful in the treatment of bradyarrhythmias and tachyarrhythmias, the use of these techniques will become widespread. The tools are still developing, but they are adequate for the safe removal of leads. New techniques will be required and are under development for the removal of multisite atrial and ventricular pacing electrodes and coronary sinus defibrillating electrodes.

Despite the excellent tools, great respect for the potential morbidity and mortality of this procedure is required. There is nothing trivial about this procedure, and serious precautions must be used, along with consideration given to actions to be taken if there are complications.

Finally, the patient should be considered as a whole being. Patients who require lead extraction may be best served with medications, different kinds of devices, or devices with specific features. All of the patient's cardiac and particularly arrhythmia diagnoses must be considered before the incision is made. In addition, the time should be taken to ensure that all of the equipment required to complete the procedure is at hand before it is begun.

REFERENCES

1. Madigan NP, Curtis JJ, Sanfelippo JF, et al: Difficulty of extraction of chronically implanted tined ventricular endocardial leads. J Am Coll Cardiol 3:724–731, 1984.
2. Jarvinen A, Harjula A, Verkkala K: Intrathoracic surgery for retained endocardial electrodes. Thorac Cardiovasc Surg 34:94–97, 1986.
3. Bilgutay AM, Jensen MK, Schmidt WR, et al: Incarceration of transvenous pacemaker electrode: Removal by traction. Am Heart J 77:377–379, 1969.
4. Imparato AM, Kim GE: The trapped endocardial electrode. Ann Thorac Surg 14:605–608, 1972.
5. Kaizuka H, Kawamura T, Kasagi Y, et al: An experience of infected catheter removal with continuous traction method and silicon rubber wearing. Kyobu Geka 36:309–311, 1983.
6. Alt E, Theres H, Busch U, et al: Entfernung von drei infizierten Elektroden mit Hilfe eines neuen Extraktionsstiletts: Ein Fallbericht. Herzschr Elektrophys 2:29–34, 1991.
7. Ramo BW, Peter RH, Kong Y, et al: Migration of a severed transvenous pacing catheter and its successful removal. Am J Cardiol 22:880–884, 1968.
8. Rossi P: "Hook catheter": Technique for transfemoral removal of foreign body from right side of the heart. Am J Radiol 109:101–106, 1970.
9. Taliercio CP, Vlietstra RE, Hayes DL: Pigtail catheter for extraction of pacemaker lead. J Am Coll Cardiol 5:1020, 1985.
10. Foster CJ, Brownlee WC: Percutaneous removal of ventricular pacemaker electrodes using a Dormier basket. Int J Cardiol 21:127–134, 1988.
11. Zehender M, Buchner C, Geibel A, et al: Diagnosis of hidden pacemaker lead sepsis by transesophageal echocardiography and a new technique for lead extraction. Am Heart J 118:1050–1053, 1989.
12. Kratz JM, Leman R, Gillette PC: Forceps extraction of permanent pacing leads. Ann Thorac Surg 49:676–677, 1990.
13. Deutsch LS, Dang H, Brandon JC, et al: Percutaneous removal of transvenous pacing lead perforating the heart, pericardium, and pleura. AJR Am J Roentgenol 156:471–473, 1991.
14. Goode LB, Clarke JM, Fontaine JM, et al: Explantation of chronic transvenous pacemaker leads. PACE 12:677, 1989.
15. Byrd CL, Schwartz SJ, Hedin N: Intravascular techniques for extraction of permanent pacemaker leads. J Thorac Cardiovasc Surg 101:989–997, 1991.
16. Byrd CL, Schwartz SJ, Hedin N: Lead extraction: Indications and techniques. Cardiol Clin 10:735–748, 1992.
17. Byrd CL, Schwartz SJ, Hedin NB: Lead extraction: Techniques and indications. In Barold SS, Mugica J (eds): New Perspectives in Cardiac Pacing. Mount Kisco, NY, Futura Publishing Company, 1993, pp 29–55.
18. Brodell GK, Castle LW, Maloney JD, et al: Chronic transvenous pacemaker lead removal using a unique, sequential transvenous system. Am J Cardiol 66:964–966, 1990.
19. Fearnot NE, Smith HJ, Goode LB, et al: Intravascular lead extraction using locking stylets, sheaths, and other techniques. PACE 13:1864–1870, 1990.
20. Byrd CL, Schwartz SJ, Hedin NB, et al: Intravascular lead extraction using locking stylets and sheaths. PACE 13:1871–1872, 1990.
21. Byrd CL, Schwartz SJ, Sivina M, et al: Technique for the surgical extraction of permanent pacing leads and electrodes. J Thorac Cardiovasc Surg 89:142–144, 1985.
22. Dubernet J, Irarrazaval MJ, Lema G, et al: Surgical removal of entrapped endocardial pacemaker electrodes. Clin Prog Pacing Electrophysiol 4:147–152, 1986.
23. Wilkoff BL, Byrd CL, Love CJ, et al: Risks of intravascular extraction of chronic pacemaker and ICD leads: A multicenter analysis of 1895 patients. PACE 21(4 Pt 2):826, 1998.
24. Niebauer M, Wilkoff B, VanZandt H, et al: Nonthoracotomy defibrillator lead extraction: Comparison with ventricular pacing leads. PACE 20(4 Pt 2):1071, 1997.
25. Wilkoff BL, Byrd CL, Love CJ, et al: Pacemaker lead extraction with the laser sheath: Results of the PLEXES Trial. J Am Coll Cardiol 33:1671–1676, 1999.
26. Niebauer MJ, Al-Khadra A, Chung MK, et al: The Spectranetics laser sheath reduces extraction time for nonthoracotomy defibrillator leads. J Am Coll Cardiol 31(Suppl 2):1047–1073, 1998.
27. Al-Khadra AS, Wilkoff BL, Byrd CL, et al: Extraction of nonthoracotomy defibrillator leads using the spectranetics® laser sheath: The US experience. PACE 21(4 Pt II):889, 1998.
28. Epstein LM, Byrd CL, Wilkoff BL, et al. Initial experience with larger laser sheaths for removal of transvenous pacemaker and defibrillator leads. Circulation (In press).

Chapter 29

Pacemaker and Implantable Cardioverter-Defibrillator Radiography

Margaret A. Lloyd and David L. Hayes

The chest radiograph can provide valuable information regarding the type and integrity of the pacing and implantable cardioverter-defibrillator (ICD) systems as well as patient anatomy. The evaluation of the chest radiograph should be thorough to obtain important information about the system and to avoid missing significant details. The bony structure of the thorax, cardiac silhouette, lung fields, diaphragm, relative position of the trachea and aortic knob, and location of pre-existing hardware should all be noted (Fig. 29–1). Clues to significant prior cardiac or thoracic surgery, such as surgical clips, wires, and prosthetic valves, should be obtained.

It is important that this type of approach be employed even before the system is implanted: the preoperative chest radiograph can provide essential anatomic information for the implanting physician. After implantation of the pacing or ICD system, a chest radiograph should be obtained to ascertain the correct position of the generator and leads.[1] Additionally, complications of implantation, such as ipsilateral pneumothorax (Fig. 29–2), ipsilateral pleural effusion and hemothorax (Fig. 29–3), pericardial effusion, or retained surgical sponge (Fig. 29–4), should be noted.[2] Pneumothorax is best demonstrated on a posteroanterior (PA) view in full expiration. Although it is important to inspect the cardiac silhouette and compare it to the preimplantation chest radiograph for any significant change in size, the chest radiograph should not be relied on for a diagnosis of pericardial effusion. If there is clinical suspicion of a pericardial effusion, an echocardiogram should be obtained.[3]

It is not uncommon for a patient to have a pacing system, an ICD, and a variety of functional and abandoned leads. The type and position of the generators and the type, position, and integrity of all leads should be determined. A thorough examination requires both PA and lateral chest radiographs.

■ PULSE GENERATORS

The initial evaluation includes the location of the pulse generators and the ICD. Most current implants are prepectoral in location, and the pulse generator is located in the upper chest, inferior to the clavicle and medial to the axilla. An excessively large generator pocket may allow for rotation of the generator, either spontaneously or by patient manipulation (twiddler's syndrome), leading to knotting and coiling of the leads (Fig. 29–5).[4] The pacing pulse generator is sometimes placed in the abdomen, either subcutaneously or below the rectus abdominus in children (usually the left upper quadrant); many early ICDs were also implanted in the abdomen. Complete radiographic evaluation in these cases may require an anteroposterior (AP) and lateral radiograph of the abdomen (Fig. 29–6).

The generator manufacturer and type can be identified from the chest radiograph. At one time, each manufacturer had a relatively unique "can" shape that allowed recognition on that basis. Internal circuitry patterns were at one time also helpful for pulse generator recognition. Although these identifiers may still be helpful, all current pulse generators and ICDs have a radiopaque code identifying the manufacturer and model of the device (Fig. 29–7), and this marker is the most reliable radiographic identifier.[5] If the manufacturer can be determined, the technical support division of that manufacturer can help identify the device. (All manufacturers have a toll-free support number that should be answered 24 hours a day.) The manufacturer may be able to provide additional information obtained at the time of implant (e.g., leads used, configurations, and thresholds). Some patients may have both pacing and ICD systems implanted; the devices may come from different manufacturers, and careful inspection of both is important.

The relationship of redundant, coiled leads in the generator pocket relative to the generator should be noted. The

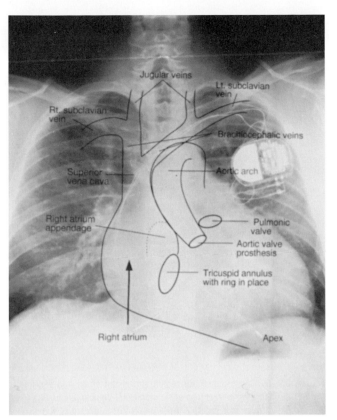

Figure 29–1. Overlay of diagram on a posteroanterior chest radiograph demonstrating the typical location for the formation of the subclavian veins, brachiocephalic veins, the superior vena cava, and the right atrium along with their associated osseous landmarks. Rt, right, Lt, left. (From Castle LW, Cook S: Pacemaker radiography. *In* Ellenbogen KA, Kay GN, Wilkoff BL [eds]: Clinical Cardiac Pacing. Philadelphia, WB Saunders, 1995, p 538.)

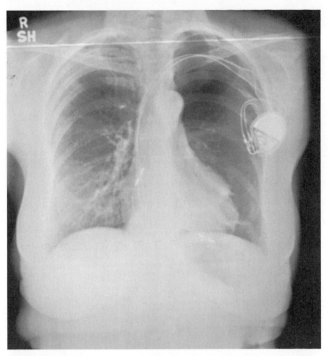

Figure 29–2. Posteroanterior chest radiograph demonstrating a dual-chamber pacing system in place with fixed electrodes in both the right atrial appendage and the right ventricular apex. Note the relative radiolucency over the left chest compared with the right. There is a moderate-sized pneumothorax on the left, with evidence of subsegmental atelectasis in the lingula and in the left lower lobe. Note absence of lung markings superiorly. (From Castle LW, Cook S: Pacemaker radiography. *In* Ellenbogen KA, Kay GN, Wilkoff BL [eds]: Clinical Cardiac Pacing. Philadelphia, WB Saunders, 1995, p 538.)

position of the leads relative to the generator is important when system revision is contemplated and is best appreciated on the lateral chest radiograph. Using external radiographic markers at either edge of the surgical scar helps to define the relationship of leads in the pocket to the incision in the PA view.

Radiographic evaluation of the pulse generator and ICD connector block should also be performed routinely. The connector pin should be advanced beyond the set screws, and the screws should be in contact with the pin. The polarity of pacing pulse generators can be ascertained by the number and type of connector pins (unipolar, coaxial bipolar, bifurcated bipolar).

▪ LEADS

Lead assessment is perhaps the most difficult and the most crucial component of the radiographic evaluation of a pacing or ICD system. Radiographic assessment is useful when evaluating the functional status of the lead in pacing or ICD system failure as well as when planning lead revision or extraction.[6] Standard radiographic techniques may not clearly demonstrate lead components, and higher radiographic penetration may be required. The number, types, location, and radiographic integrity of all leads should be

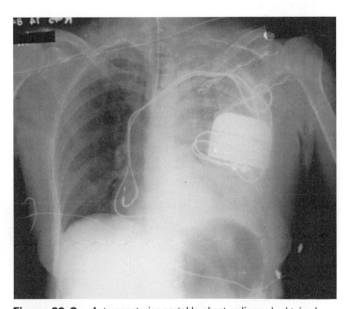

Figure 29–3. Anteroposterior portable chest radiograph obtained immediately after pacemaker insertion demonstrates a large hemothorax on the left secondary to perforation of the left subclavian artery. There is almost complete opacification of the left hemithorax. (From Castle LW, Cook S: Pacemaker radiography. *In* Ellenbogen KA, Kay GN, Wilkoff BL [eds]: Clinical Cardiac Pacing. Philadelphia, WB Saunders, 1995, p 538.)

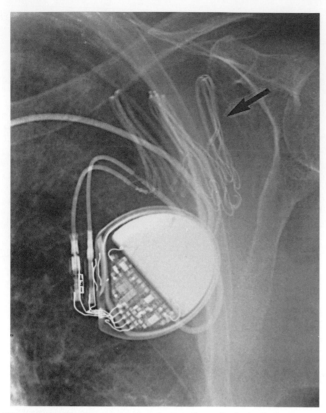

Figure 29–4. Posteroanterior chest radiograph obtained the day after pacemaker implant. Arrow designates imbedded radiopaque material in a surgical sponge retained in the generator pocket.

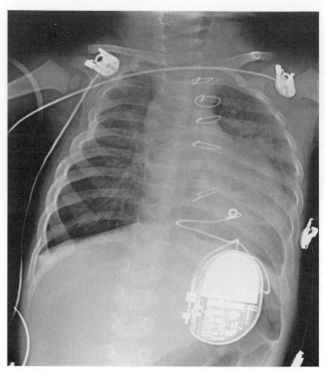

Figure 29–6. Anteroposterior radiograph of the chest and abdomen of a young child after placement of an epicardial ventricular pacing lead, with the pulse generator located in the upper left quadrant of the abdomen. Sternotomy wires are present; the pacing system was implanted as part of a corrective cardiac surgical procedure.

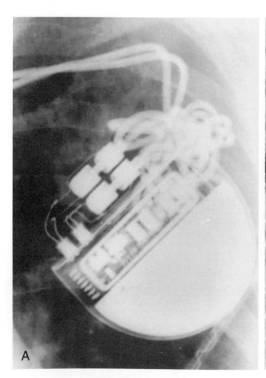

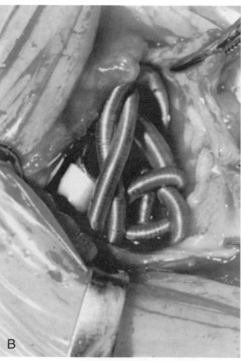

A   B

Figure 29–5. *A,* Magnified view of a radiograph of a patient with "twiddler's syndrome." *B,* During surgical exploration, the pacer had to be twisted 18 revolutions to uncoil the leads. Note the wormlike characteristic of the multiple loops of electrode wires, which are coiled on themselves. (From Castle LW, Cook S: Pacemaker radiography. *In* Ellenbogen KA, Kay GN, Wilkoff BL [eds]: Clinical Cardiac Pacing. Philadelphia, WB Saunders, 1995, p 538.)

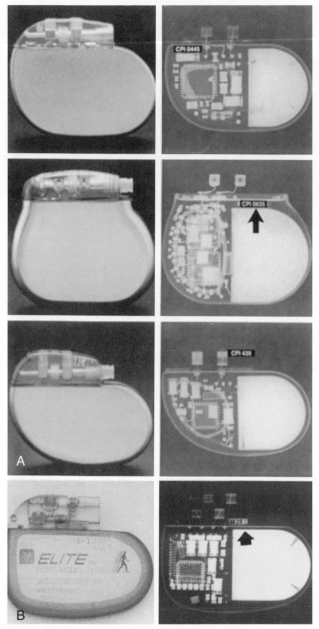

Figure 29–7. Radiographic appearance of various pacing pulse generators. Arrows denote manufacturer's identification symbol and device code number. (From Castle LW, Cook S: Pacemaker radiography. *In* Ellenbogen KA, Kay GN, Wilkoff BL [eds]: Clinical Cardiac Pacing. Philadelphia, WB Saunders, 1995, p 538.)

cephalic vein, and rarely via the internal or external jugular or femoral veins. Clues to the insertion site can sometimes be obtained on the chest radiograph by a change in the directional contour of the lead. A more medial site suggests a subclavian vein insertion, whereas a more lateral site suggests a cephalic vein insertion. If the lead sleeve suture has been placed tightly enough to crimp the lead, it may be visible on the chest radiograph and suggest the insertion site of the lead (Fig. 29–8). The term *pseudofracture* is used by some to describe such crimping of the lead by anchoring sutures.[7] (Pseudofracture has also been used to describe the point at which coils come together in a bifurcated bipolar lead.) Despite the designation as a pseudofracture, a ligature placed too tightly on the lead may result in damage to the lead insulation and true fracture of the coil over time. Insertion into the jugular veins can usually be easily identified by the course of the pacing lead over or under the clavicle and into the neck.

The radiopaque coil should be inspected in its entirety. There should be no discontinuity of the coil, nor should there be any sharp angulation or kinking. Such findings suggest lead fracture or the potential for fracture. Special attention should be paid to the area between the clavicle and first rib because this area is a common site of lead fracture (subclavian crush syndrome) (Fig. 29–9). Unfortunately, it is not possible to visualize the lead insulation radiographically.

Atrial leads should have minimal redundancy present, whereas ventricular leads should have a modest amount of redundancy. Undue tension on leads may result in dislodgment from the endocardial surface or poor pacing thresholds (Fig. 29–10). Generous lead redundancy is usually preferred in children to accommodate subsequent growth and minimize the number of lead revisions usually required during a lifetime of pacing therapy.[8]

The chest radiograph (Fig. 29–11) can often determine the type of transvenous lead fixation. Active-fixation leads have a radiopaque screw that may be fixed (extended) or retractable. Passive-fixation leads have a variety of fins and tines, which cannot be visualized radiographically. Unipolar leads have a single electrode (cathode) at the tip of the lead, whereas bipolar leads have two electrodes separated by an interelectrode space. Extracardiac location of the tip of the pacing lead suggests cardiac perforation with migration of the lead outside of the heart. An extracardiac position cannot always be determined by the chest radiograph and may require other imaging modalities as well as clinical troubleshooting techniques to determine if the lead is indeed extracardiac.[9]

Although most pacing systems use one or two leads, investigational pacing for arrhythmia or hemodynamic optimization may incorporate systems that use novel transvenous lead placement, including dual atrial leads and coronary sinus leads (Fig. 29–12).[10] Therefore, the presence of three or more leads does not necessarily imply that one or more of the leads has been abandoned. In abandoned leads, the proximal portion of the lead is free in the generator pocket and not attached to the generator. Additionally, it should be determined whether the abandoned lead is present in its entirety or a proximal portion of it has been amputated.

Although used less frequently than in the past, epicardial pacing leads are still used in patients with some congenital abnormalities (sometimes as part of a corrective or palliative

determined. Unlike pulse generators, leads do not have characteristic radiopaque markings to aid in their identification; however, much information can be obtained about the type (active versus passive fixation; unipolar, bipolar, tripolar) and functional status of a lead by its radiographic appearance.

Pacemaker Leads

Most current pacing leads are transvenous, with the intravascular insertion usually through the subclavian, axillary, or

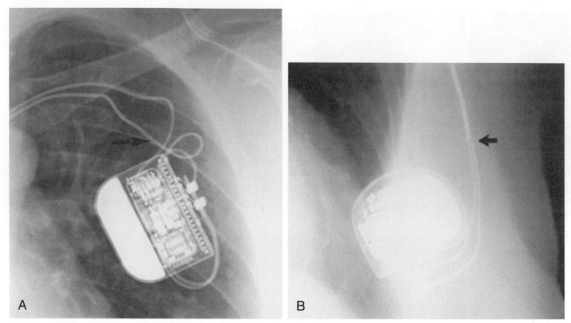

Figure 29–8. *A,* Magnified view of the ventricular lead near the generator showing a localized indentation *(arrow)* superior to the generator. This does not represent disruption of the wire but merely too tight a placement of the ligature. *B,* Example of pseudofracture *(arrow).* This appearance is related to the design and construction of the coaxial system and not to a disruption of the pacing coil. (From Castle LW, Cook S: Pacemaker radiography. *In* Ellenbogen KA, Kay GN, Wilkoff BL [eds]: Clinical Cardiac Pacing. Philadelphia, WB Saunders, 1995, p 538.)

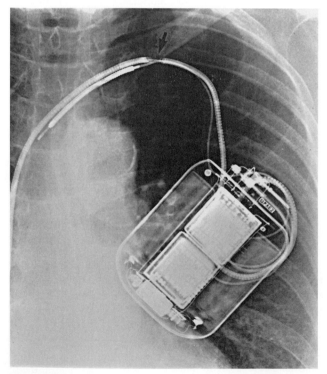

Figure 29–9. Posteroanterior radiograph of a left pectoral implantable cardioverter-defibrillator system (generator, high-voltage lead, and superior vena cava lead). The high-voltage coil is fractured as it passes under the clavicle *(arrow).* The patient presented with inappropriate shocks; interrogation of the device revealed a lead impedance of more than 2000 Ω.

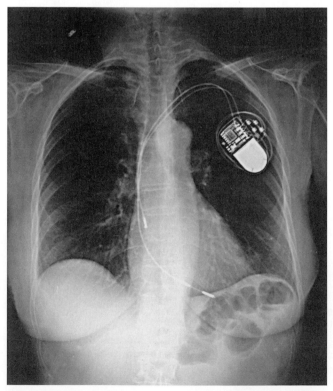

Figure 29–10. Posteroanterior chest radiograph of a dual-chamber pacing system. Both the atrial and ventricular leads have inadequate redundancy, which may result in poor pacing thresholds or lead dislodgment.

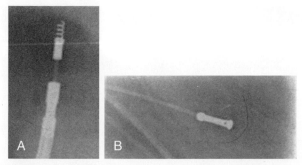

Figure 29–11. Radiographic appearance of transvenous pacing leads. *A,* Active fixation, bipolar lead. *B,* Passive fixation, bipolar lead. (Courtesy of Medtronic, Inc., Minneapolis, MN.)

surgical procedure) and in patients with prosthetic tricuspid valves. Historically, epicardial leads have carried a higher incidence of malfunction than transvenous pacing leads. Epicardial leads are distinctly exterior to the cardiac silhouette; they may be positioned over the atrium or the ventricle (see Fig. 29–6). The leads are then tunneled to the pulse generator either in the pectoral or abdominal area. Evaluation of the lead requires that it be inspected in its entirety, which sometimes necessitates that both chest and abdominal radiographs be obtained.

Transvenous Atrial Leads

Most atrial leads have a J shape and are placed in the right atrial appendage.[11] On the PA chest radiograph, the lead most commonly has a gentle curve to the left, and on the lateral view, it has J-shaped curve anteriorly. A large poste-

rior curve in the atrial lead suggests coronary sinus placement, or placement across a patent foramen ovale or atrial septal defect into the left atrium (Fig. 29–13). In patients who have undergone prior cardiac surgery, the right atrial appendage is often surgically truncated. In these cases, the lead may be placed septally or on the lateral wall, wherever optimal thresholds and mechanical stability can be obtained. Active-fixation leads are most frequently employed in this situation; unlike the appendage, the remainder of the right atrium is not trabeculated, and it is difficult to obtain satisfactory mechanical stability with passive-fixation leads. Investigational pacing for the prevention of atrial fibrillation may employ active-fixation leads placed on the septum or two atrial pacing leads. Regardless of the atrial leads employed, they should follow the gentle contour of the vascular system without excess redundancy.

Special note of the appearance of the atrial lead should be made if it is one of the Telectronics Pacing Systems (Englewood, CO) atrial leads under advisory.[12, 13] The Accufix active-fixation atrial lead and the Encor passive-fixation atrial lead have retention wires in the distal portion of the lead to maintain the J shape; in the Accufix lead, the retention wire is within the insulation, and in the Encor lead, it is inside the coil. The retention wire may fracture, with protrusion and rarely migration of the wire, leading to perforation of cardiac and vascular structures. The shape of the distal portion of the Accufix lead should be noted because data suggests that an open J shape may be more conducive to fracture of the retention wire than a more closed J shape. The retention wire itself is difficult to visualize radiographically, even with significant protrusion or migration of the retention wire. Coned-in views with higher penetration may aid in visualization. Digital fluoroscopy has proved to be a more reliable technique to assess the status of the retention wire (Fig. 29–14).

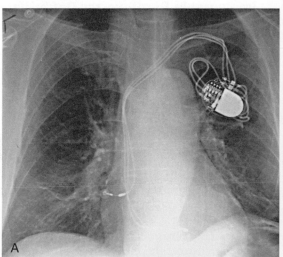
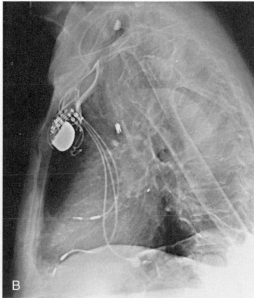

Figure 29–12. *A,* Posteroanterior chest radiograph of patient with a dual-site atrial pacing system for the prevention of atrial fibrillation. *B,* Lateral chest radiograph of the same patient. Leads are present in the lateral right atrium, the coronary sinus, and the right ventricular apex.

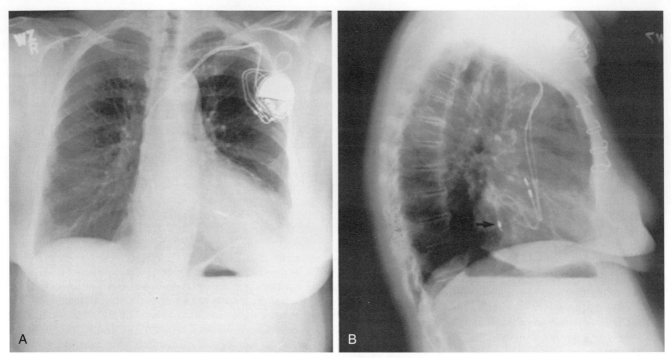

Figure 29–13. Posteroanterior *(A)* and left lateral *(B)* views demonstrating a dual-chamber pacing system. The ventricular wire has an unusual curve on the posteroanterior view, and on the lateral view it is noted to extend in a posterocranial direction, only then to curve back on itself with the tip of the wire in the wall of the left ventricle *(arrow)*. This is an example of improper ventricular lead placement, with the wire traversing the foramen ovale and extending through the body of the left atrium, through the mitral valve, and into the left ventricle. (From Trohman RG, Wilkoff B, Byrne T, Cook S: Successful percutaneous extraction of a chronic left ventricular pacing lead. PACE 14:1448, 1991).

Fracture of the retention wire in the Encor lead is difficult to detect, even using fluoroscopy, because of the position of the wire within the coil; however, fracture has been associated with angulation in the interelectrode space (Fig. 29–15). Fracture and protrusion of the retention wire have also been noted in this area of the lead. Although chest radiographs may demonstrate linear disruption of the interelectrode space, digital fluoroscopy provides optimal imaging. High-magnification and orthogonal views should be used for optimal visualization of the retention wire in these leads.

Transvenous Ventricular Leads

Transvenous ventricular leads are traditionally placed in the right ventricular apex. Radiographically, the lead should have a gentle contour with the tip of the lead pointing downward in the PA view. On the lateral view, the lead should point anteriorly; posterior angulation of the lead suggests positioning in the coronary sinus (Fig. 29–16). Occasionally, it may be desirable to position the lead on the right ventricular septum or in the outflow tract (Fig. 29–17). These alternative positions are commonly used when adequate thresholds cannot be obtained at the apex, or an ICD lead is present and the pacing lead is positioned away from the ICD lead to prevent system interactions.[14] An additional bipolar sensing electrode on the lead in the right atrial area (Fig. 29–18) can identify single lead VDD or DDD systems.[15] Ventricular leads employ previously mentioned fixation techniques; special note should be made of the appearance of active fixation mechanisms.

Positioning of the ventricular pacing lead in alternative sites will undoubtedly become more common in the near future. In addition to outflow tract and septal positions already mentioned, positioning a lead in one of the cardiac veins in an attempt to stimulate the left ventricle directly might become a more common practice.

Implantable Cardioverter-Defibrillator Leads

Most ICD systems use a single transvenous lead placed in the right ventricle and connected to a generator located in the pectoral region.[16] Like ventricular pacing leads, gentle redundancy should be present, and the tip of the lead should be directed toward the right ventricular apex. Transvenous defibrillator leads may have two high-voltage coils (one in the area of the superior vena cava and right atrium and one in the right ventricle) or a single high-voltage coil (in the right ventricle). An additional subclavian lead with or without a subcutaneous patch or array may be used (Fig. 29–19). In one manufacturer's lead, the continuation of the lead immediately after the proximal high-voltage coil may appear fractured; this so-called phantom fracture is a result of this lead design and is normal (Fig. 29–20).

Coronary sinus leads are rarely used in standard ICD systems because of the relative mechanical instability of these leads and a high incidence of lead dislodgment. Because of their larger diameter relative to pacing leads, defibrillation leads may be more susceptible to subclavian crush syndrome, and this area should be scrutinized carefully. All

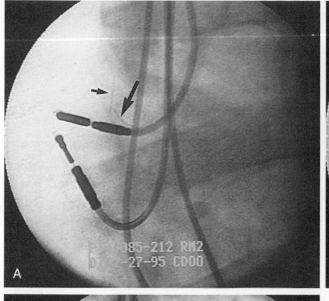

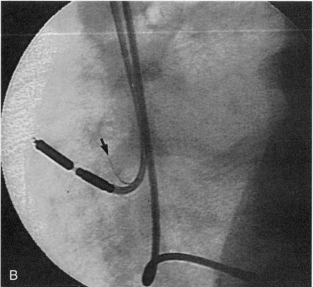

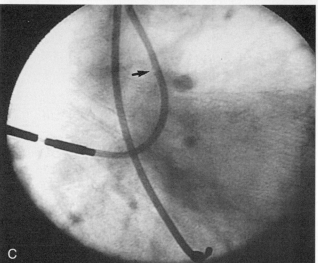

Figure 29–14. *A,* Digital fluoroscopic image of distal Accufix (Accufix Research Institute, Englewood, CO) atrial lead. The J retention wire is fractured; one portion of the wire has migrated out of the lead and is imbedded in the right atrial wall *(small arrow).* A second portion of the wire is protruding from the lead *(large arrow). B,* Digital fluoroscopic image of distal Accufix atrial lead. The retention wire is protruding from the lead *(arrow). C,* Digital fluoroscopic image of distal Accufix atrial lead. There is irregularity of the inner surface of the lead, indicating insulation damage from fractured retention wire *(arrow).*

leads and patches should be inspected for fracture and any unusual bending or kinking of the leads noted. Subcutaneous patches and arrays are usually placed posterior and inferior to the axilla, and customized lateral and oblique views may be necessary to visualize them in their entirety.

The evolution of defibrillation systems from epicardial to transvenous has been rapid; therefore, there are many functional epicardial systems in today's patient population (see Fig. 29–20). Many patients with epicardial systems have the generator placed in the abdomen, and abdominal radiography is needed to visualize the entire lead. Radiopaque markers are incorporated into the perimeter of some epicardial patches for radiographic location; however, they are not part of the defibrillation system, and fractures do not signify lead failure.

New devices incorporate dual-chamber pacing, atrial defibrillation algorithms, and ventricular defibrillation capacity. Radiographically, a coronary sinus lead or an atrial lead or both usually are present in addition to the ventricular defibrillation lead see (Fig. 29–19).

■ MISCELLANEOUS CONSIDERATIONS

Congenital cardiovascular anomalies may require implantation techniques that result in unusual appearances of the pacing or ICD system on the chest radiograph. Knowledge of the native and corrected anatomy is essential when interpreting the chest radiograph in these circumstances.

The most common cardiovascular anomaly encountered de novo by the implanting physician is persistent left superior vena cava (Fig. 29–21), in which the atrial lead is placed through the left vena cava, through the coronary sinus, and into the right atrium. The ventricular lead follows the same course, usually looping in the right atrium to direct the tip into the right ventricle (Fig. 29–22). The diagnosis of persistent left superior vena cava can be suspected by the finding of an enlarged coronary sinus at echocardiography, and confirmed by injecting contrast material into peripheral intravenous lines in the upper extremities. Observed under fluoroscopy, the course of the contrast material into the central circulation outlines the venous anatomy. If the diagnosis is

Text continued on page 723

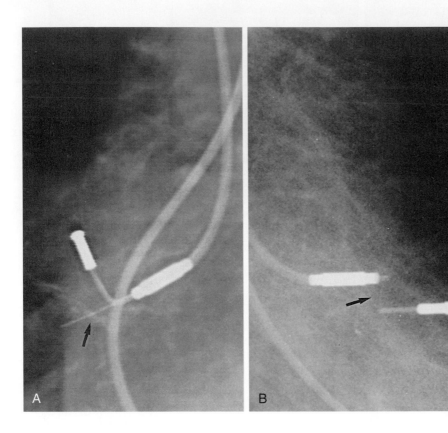

Figure 29–15. *A,* Digital fluoroscopic image of distal Encor lead. The interelectrode area is angled, and the retention wire is protruding *(arrow). B,* Digital fluoroscopic image of distal Encor lead. The lead is transected in the interelectrode space as a result of fracture of the retention wire *(arrow).* (Courtesy of Accufix Research Institute, Englewood, CO).

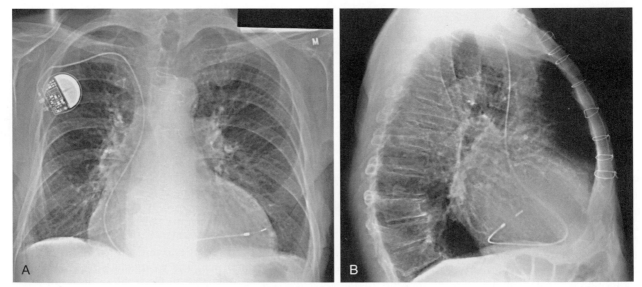

Figure 29–16. *A,* Posteroanterior chest radiograph of a ventricular pacing system. *B,* Lateral chest radiograph of the same patient. The lead courses posteriorly in the coronary sinus and into a cardiac vein.

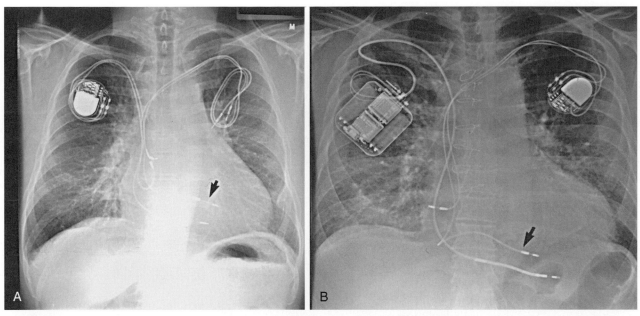

Figure 29–17. *A,* Posteroanterior chest radiograph. The original pacing system on the left has been abandoned. Note that the leads have not been amputated. A second pacing system has been implanted on the right. The second ventricular lead has been implanted high on the right ventricular septum *(arrow)*, owing to poor pacing thresholds at the apex. *B,* Posteroanterior chest radiograph. A dual-chamber pacing system is implanted on the left, and an implantable cardioverter-defibrillator (ICD) system is implanted on the right. The ventricular pacing lead is implanted higher on the septum and away from the high-voltage ICD lead *(arrow)*; this allows the high-voltage ICD lead to be placed in the apex, where better defibrillation thresholds are usually obtained.

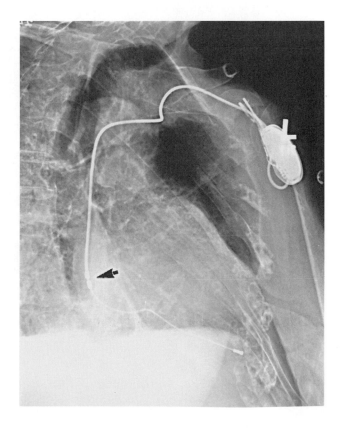

Figure 29–18. Oblique chest radiograph of a single lead VDD pacing system. The system uses a bipolar atrial sensing electrode *(arrow)* and unipolar ventricular pacing.

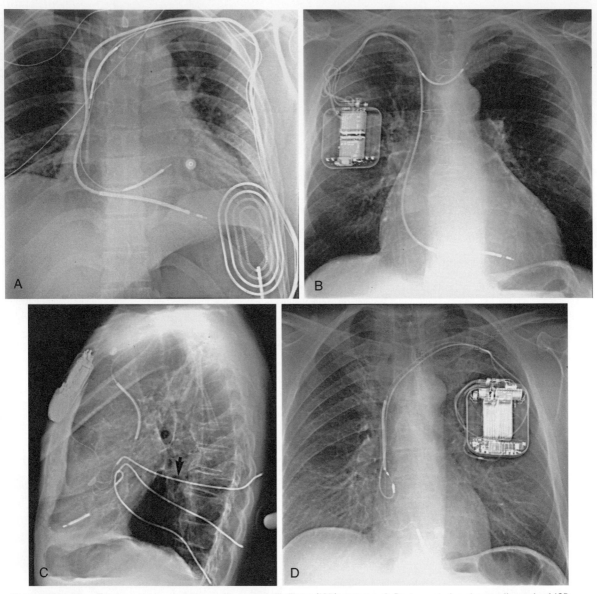

Figure 29–19. Transvenous implantable cardioverter-defibrillator (ICD) systems. *A,* Posteroanterior chest radiograph of ICD system. A ventricular high-voltage lead is present as well as a superior vena cava (SVC) lead, a coronary sinus lead, and a subcutaneous patch. The generator (not shown) is implanted in the abdomen. *B,* ICD system implanted in the right pectoral area. An SVC lead (positioned into the left subclavian vein) and a ventricular lead are present. *C,* Lateral chest radiograph of an ICD system. A single lead incorporating SVC (proximal) and ventricular (distal) shocking coils is present as well as the posteriorly directed three-pronged subcutaneous array (CPI, St. Paul, MN) *(arrow). D,* Combination DDD pacing and ICD device. An atrial lead is present for atrial sensing and pacing. A single ICD lead incorporating proximal and distal shocking coils is present.

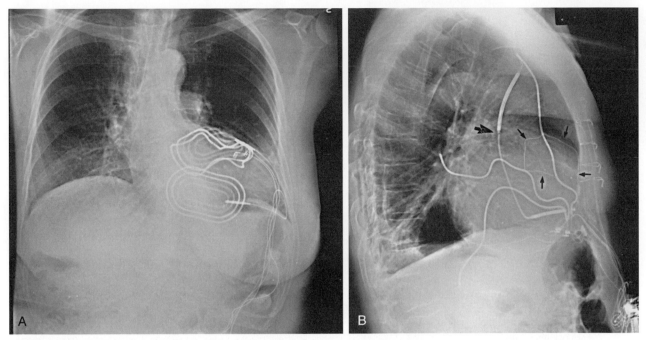

Figure 29–20. Epicardial patches. *A,* Posteroanterior chest radiograph. Epicardial defibrillator patches are present as well as ventricular screw-in pacing leads. The generator is in the abdomen. *B,* Lateral chest radiograph. An epicardial defibrillator patch is seen *(small arrows).* This model of patch is radiolucent; a radiopaque marker is placed around the perimeter of the patch but is not functional; therefore, fractures of this marker are functionally irrelevant. Also noted is "phantom fracture" of the high-voltage transvenous lead just distal to the proximal shocking coil *(large arrow).*

Figure 29–21. Schematic representation of the three different types of persistent left superior vena cava (SVC) with various insertions of the left SVC into the right heart system. IVC, inferior vena cava; PV, pulmonary vein; Rt, right; Lt, left; c.s., coronary sinus; VV, veins. (From Castle LW, Cook S: Pacemaker radiography. *In* Ellenbogen KA, Kay GN, Wilkoff BL [eds]: Clinical Cardiac Pacing. Philadelphia, WB Saunders, 1995, p 538.)

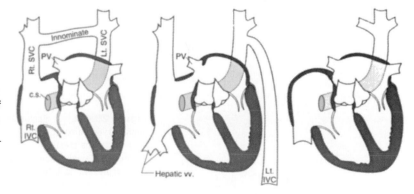

Persistent Left Superior Vena Cava

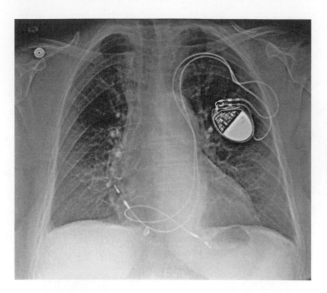

Figure 29–22. Posteroanterior chest radiograph of DDD pacing system in patient with persistent left superior vena cava (SVC). The atrial lead courses through the left SVC, through the coronary sinus, and into the right atrium. The ventricular lead follows the same path but is then looped into the right ventricle. (Courtesy of Dr. Raul E. Espinosa, Mayo Clinic, Rochester, MN.)

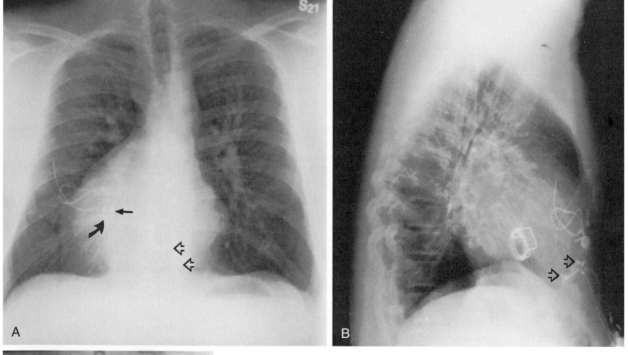

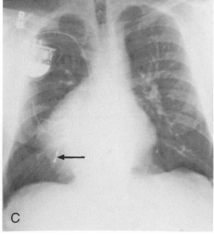

Figure 29–23. *A,* Posteroanterior chest radiograph obtained in August 1985 demonstrating dextrocardia with a prosthetic mitral valve in place. There are remnant stab electrodes identified overlying the right precordium *(small curved* and *straight black arrows).* The single-chamber pacing system has two screw-in epicardial leads *(open arrows)* present. *B,* Lateral view of same patient. *C,* Posteroanterior chest radiograph dated July 1989 demonstrates abandonment of the previously placed epicardial system. A single-chamber bipolar system is now present, with the new transvenous lead near the right ventricular apex *(narrow arrow).* (From Castle LW, Cook S: Pacemaker radiography. *In* Ellenbogen KA, Kay GN, Wilkoff BL [eds]: Clinical Cardiac Pacing. Philadelphia, WB Saunders, 1995, p 538.)

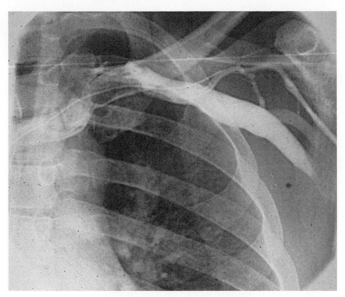

Figure 29–24. Fluoroscopic image of the left axillary and subclavian venous system after injection of contrast material into an ipsilateral upper extremity intravenous line. Although the patient did not have symptoms, the vessel has near obliteration of the lumen around the pacing lead, making it unlikely that a new lead would pass through this area.

suspected preoperatively, other imaging modalities, such as computed tomography, may be useful. Another congenital abnormality that may be encountered is dextrocardia, which should be recognized on the preoperative chest radiograph (Fig. 29–23).

Occasionally, it may be difficult to locate the subclavian vein, or the patency of the cephalic-axillary-subclavian venous system may be in question. Contrast material injected into a peripheral intravenous line in the ipsilateral upper extremity outlines the venous system under fluoroscopy and can guide location of the subclavian vein and determine the status of the subclavian-cephalic venous systems (Fig. 29–24).[17]

Summary

The chest radiograph can provide important information about pacing and ICD systems. Preoperative radiographs can provide important anatomic information to the implanting physician. Lateral and PA chest radiographs should be obtained after implantation to confirm correct lead placement

and to note any potential complications of the implantation procedure. The chest radiograph is an important component of system troubleshooting. During such evaluation, the position and type of generator, the position and type of all functional and abandoned leads, and the radiographic integrity of all components of the system should be determined. Abdominal films may be required if any portion of the pacing or ICD system is in the abdomen. A systematic evaluation of the anatomy and system components is essential.

REFERENCES

1. Grier D, Cook PG, Hartnell GG: Chest radiographs after permanent pacing: Are they really necessary? Clin Radiol 42:244, 1990.
2. Steiner RM, Tegtmeyer CJ, Morse D, et al: The radiology of cardiac pacemakers. Radiographics 6:373, 1986.
3. Iliceto S, Antonelli G, Sorino M, et al: Two dimensional echocardiographic recognition of complications of cardiac invasive procedures. Am J Cardiol 53:846, 1984.
4. Roberts JS, Wagner NK: Pacemaker twiddler's syndrome. Am J Cardiol 63:1013, 1989.
5. Hayes DL: Pacemaker radiography. In Furman S, Hayes DL, Holmes DR Jr (eds): A Practice of Cardiac Pacing. New York, Futura Publishing, p 361.
6. Filice R, Hutton L, Klein G: Cardiac pacemaker leads: A radiographic perspective. Can Assoc Radiol J 35:20, 1984.
7. Heckt S, Berdoff R, Van Tosh A, Goldberg E: Radiographic pseudofracture of bipolar pacemaker wire. Chest 88:302, 1985.
8. Gheissari A, Hordof AJ, Spotnitz HM: Transvenous pacemakers in children: Relation of lead length to anticipated growth. Ann Thorac Surg 52:118, 1991.
9. Sussman SK, Chiles C, Cooper C, Lower JR: CT demonstration of myocardial perforation by a pacemaker lead. J Comput Assist Tomogr 10:670, 1986.
10. Daubert C, Gras D, Leclercq C, et al: Biatrial synchronous pacing: A new approach for prevention of drug refractory atrial flutter. Circulation 92:1-532, 1995.
11. Hertzberg BS, Chiles C, Ravin CE: Right atrial appendage pacing: Radiographic considerations. AJR 145:31, 1985.
12. Lloyd MA, Hayes DL, Holmes DR Jr: Atrial "J" pacing lead retention wire fracture: Radiographic assessment, incidence of fracture, and clinical management. PACE 18:958, 1995.
13. Gross J, Hildner F, Brinker J, et al: Multi-center passive fixation lead study: Fluoroscopic screening and clinical event update. PACE 20:1064, 1997.
14. Epstein, AE, Kay GN, Plumb V, et al: Combined automatic implantable cardioverter-defibrillator and pacemaker systems: implantation techniques and follow-up. J Am Coll Cardiol 13:121, 1989.
15. Graeter TP, Wahlers T, Uthoff K, Trappe HJ: Early clinical results with VDD pacing in patients with atrioventricular block. Thorac Cardiovasc Surg 43:108, 1995.
16. Stanton MS, Hayes DL, Munger TM, et al: Consistent subcutaneous prepectoral implantation of a new implantable cardioverter-defibrillator: Techniques of implantation and results. Mayo Clin Proc 696:309, 1994.
17. Higano ST, Hayes DL, Spittell PC: Facilitation of the subclavian-introducer technique with contrast venography. PACE 13:681–684, 1990.

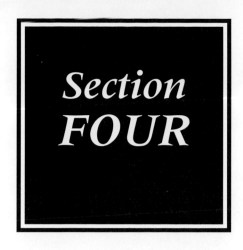

Pacemaker and

Defibrillator

Electrocardiography

Chapter 30

Timing Cycles and Operational Characteristics of Pacemakers

S. Serge Barold

Understanding the timing cycles of pacemakers is important because "all comprehension of pacemaker electrocardiography depends on the interpretation of pacemaker timing cycles," as emphasized by Furman.[1] Characterization of the various timing cycles that control pacemaker function must be clear and unambiguous to reflect the mathematical behavior of the timing circuits.[2–7] The increasing complexity of pacemakers and their timing cycles has led to the pacemaker code[8] that has become the essential language of pacing.

■ PACEMAKER CODE

Pacemakers are categorized according to the site of pacing electrodes and the mode of pacing[8] (Table 30–1). The letters in the identification code are few and easy to remember: V = ventricle, A = atrium, D = double (A and V), I = inhibited, T = triggered, and 0 = none. The first position denotes the chamber or chambers paced. The second position indicates the chamber or chambers sensed. The third position describes the response to sensing, if any, with I response indicating an inhibited response (output suppressed by a sensed signal), T indicating a triggered response (output discharged by a sensed signal, either P or QRS), and D indicating both inhibited and triggered functions. Both I and T responses reset the timing circuit. In the third position, 0 indicates that the pulse generator is not influenced by cardiac events because it does not sense. Therefore, when the third position is 0, the second one must always be 0, and vice versa. Occasionally, the letter S is used in the first and second positions to indicate that a single-chamber unit is suitable for either atrial or ventricular pacing, depending on how its parameters are programmed. For most pacemakers, the first three positions contain all the information of practical importance. The fourth and fifth positions describe additional functions, but the letters are infrequently stated in

practice except for R, which indicates a rate-adaptive, sensor-driven pulse generator. The pacemaker codes are described in detail in Chapter 13.

■ OPERATIONAL CHARACTERISTICS OF SINGLE-CHAMBER PACEMAKERS

Asynchronous AOO and VOO Modes

In the AOO and VOO modes, pacemaker stimuli are generated asynchronously at a "fixed rate" with no relationship to the spontaneous rhythm. During VOO pacing, stimuli capture the ventricle only when they fall outside the ventricular myocardial refractory period that follows spontaneous ventricular beats (Fig. 30–1). The VOO and AOO modes require only one timing interval (automatic interval). Dedicated VOO or other asynchronous pacemakers that cannot sense are now obsolete. However, asynchronous modes are often used temporarily during testing, when a special magnet is applied over the pacemaker, or by programming the asynchronous mode with an external programmer. The asynchronous mode can be used over a wide range of rates (but usually fast) for competitive pacing to terminate reentrant tachycardia. Rarely, a multiprogrammable pacemaker is permanently programmed to the asynchronous mode to prevent undesirable oversensing.

VVI Mode

In the early 1970s, sensing circuits were added to ventricular pacemakers to allow stimulation only when required or on demand whenever the sensing circuit detects no underlying ventricular activity. A VVI, or ventricular demand pacemaker, senses the intracardiac ventricular depolarization or electrogram, that is, the potential difference between the two electrodes (anode and cathode) also used for pacing (Fig.

Table 30–1. The NASPE/BPEG Generic Pacemaker Code

Position Category	I Chamber(s) Paced	II Chamber(s) Sensed	III Response to Sensing	IV Programmability, Rate Modulation	V Antitachyarrhythmia Function(s)
	0 = none	0 = none	0 = none	0 = none	0 = none
	A = atrium	A = atrium	T = triggered	P = simple programmable	P = pacing (antitachyarrhythmias)
	V = ventricle	V = ventricle	I = inhibited	M = multiprogrammable	S = shock
	D = dual (A + V)	D = dual (A + V)	D = dual (T + I)	C = communicating	D = dual (P + S)
				R = rate modulation	
Manufacturer's designation only	S = single (A or V)	S = single (A or V)			

BPEG, British Pacing and Electrophysiology Group; NASPE, North American Society of Pacing and Electrophysiology.

30–2). A VVI pacemaker programmed to a predetermined rate of 70 pulses per minute (ppm) will pace with a cycle length of 857 msec whenever the spontaneous rate falls below 70 ppm or the RR interval lengthens beyond 857 msec. The timing cycle (or internal clock) of a VVI pulse generator begins with either a sensed or paced ventricular event. The initial portion of the cycle consists of a refractory period (usually 200 to 350 msec), during which the pulse generator cannot sense any signals. The refractory period prevents the pulse generator from sensing its own stimulus waveform, the paced or spontaneous QRS complex, T waves, and the decaying residual voltage (polarization or afterpotential) at the electrode–myocardium interface because of an electrochemical process.[9–11] Beyond the pacemaker refractory period, a sensed ventricular event inhibits and resets the pacemaker, so that its timing clock returns to the baseline; a new pacing cycle is initiated, and the output circuit therefore remains inhibited for a period equal to the programmed pacemaker (or lower rate) interval. Any ventricular event within the ventricular pacemaker refractory period cannot reset the timer responsible for the lower rate interval (LRI). If no signal is sensed, the timing cycle ends with the delivery of a ventricular stimulus, and a new cycle is started. The sensing function prevents competition between pacemaker and intrinsic rhythm and conserves battery capacity.

Single-Chamber Pacemakers: Intervals and Rates

There are several basic intervals or rates in single-chamber pacemakers. The *automatic interval* is the period between two consecutive stimuli during continuous pacing and corresponds to the programmed free-running or lower rate. For the sake of simplicity, the *escape interval* is measured in the ECG from the onset of the sensed QRS complex (or other signal) to the succeeding pacemaker stimulus. In the case of a VVI pulse generator, sensing ventricular activity, the exact time when the ventricular electrogram activates the sensing circuit (when the timing clock returns to the baseline as in Fig. 30–2) and initiates a new (electronic) escape interval cannot be determined precisely from the surface ECG.[12] Consequently, in pacemakers with identical automatic and "electronic" escape intervals, the escape interval determined

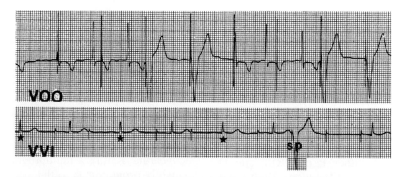

Figure 30–1. *Top*, VOO pacing. The pacemaker competes with the spontaneous rhythm. Pacemaker stimuli capture the ventricle only beyond the myocardial refractory period. *Bottom*, Supernormal phase (sp). The recording shows a ventricular demand (VVI) pacemaker with ineffectual pacemaker stimuli. The high pacing threshold was close to the output of the pulse generator. The third last stimulus captures the ventricle in the supernormal phase when the excitability threshold attains its lowest value. Spontaneous QRS complexes falling within the pacemaker refractory period (350 msec after the stimulus) are not sensed; those beyond the pacemaker refractory period are sensed and recycle the pacemaker. (From Barold SS, Zipes DP: Cardiac pacemakers and antiarrhythmic devices. *In* Braunwald E [ed]: Heart Disease: A Textbook of Cardiovascular Medicine. Philadelphia, WB Saunders, 1992, pp 726–755.)

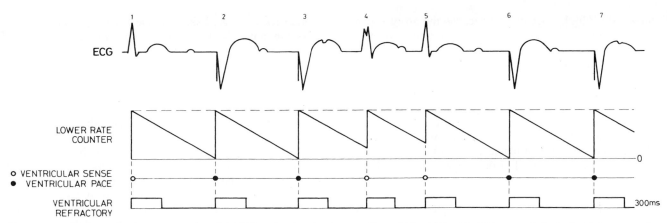

Figure 30–2. Diagrammatic representation of the VVI mode of pacing (rate = 80 ppm). The QRS marked 1 is sensed. Beats 2 and 3 are paced complexes. A ventricular extrasystole (4) and a normal QRS (5) are then sensed. The sixth and seventh beats are paced. The pacemaker ventricular refractory period (300 msec) is shown by a rectangle. Complexes 4 and 5 reset and start the lower rate counter before the zero level has been reached, that is, before completion of the escape or automatic interval. The pacemaker emits its stimulus only from the zero level. (From Lindemans FW: Diagrammatic representation of pacemaker function. *In* Barold SS [ed]: Modern Cardiac Pacing. Mt Kisco, NY, Futura, 1985, pp 323–353.)

from the surface ECG must of necessity be slightly longer than the automatic interval by a value ranging from a few milliseconds to almost the entire duration of the QRS complex, depending on the time of intracardiac sensing according to the temporal relationship of the intracardiac electrogram and the surface ECG. It is evident that a VVI pacemaker requires only two timing intervals: an LRI (automatic interval, usually equal to the electronic escape interval) and the pacemaker refractory period.

Application of a special magnet over a pulse generator closes a magnetic reed switch that inactivates the sensing function with conversion to the asynchronous mode.[13] The *magnet rate* (interval) varies according to the manufacturer and is generally faster (shorter interval) than the programmed rate to override the spontaneous rhythm. The magnet interval is often used for assessment of battery status; it lengthens with impending battery depletion. The *interference rate* is the rate (often equal to the lower rate) at which a pulse generator will revert automatically in the presence of continually sensed extraneous interference.

Rate or Interval?

The pulse generator and the pacemaker physician both "think" in terms of intervals rather than rate.[1, 2] We must do away with "rate" (bpm for intrinsic rate and ppm for pacing rate) in the definition of timing cycles. In this respect, Furman has indicated that "timing cycles must be individu-

ally interpreted. Only collectively do they make up a pacing rate. When considering any timing cycles or analyzing any ECG for pacemaker function, it is necessary to analyze function as a series of intervals between sensed or paced events rather than as a continuous rate. Rate is a relatively simple designation during continuous pacing or continuous inhibition but is of little worth and confusing if pacing and sensing alternate."[1] Yet for ease of programming, manufacturers have expressed parameters in terms of rate rather than interval. The terms lower rate and upper rate should be de-emphasized but not completely discarded because the traditional rate terminology can be useful under certain circumstances. For example, programmed rates may provide useful information when communicating with the patient or the referring physician with little or no knowledge of cardiac pacing who simply wants to know the upper and lower rates (in the case of rate-adaptive single-chamber or dual-chamber devices) without having to understand the complexity and timing cycles of contemporary pacemakers.

AAI Mode

AAI pacing may be used for patients with sick sinus syndrome and intact atrioventricular (AV) conduction. The AAI mode is identical to the VVI mode except that it paces the atrium and senses atrial electric activity (Fig. 30–3). AAI pacemakers differ from VVI pacemakers in two respects:

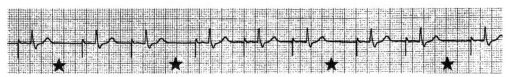

Figure 30–3. AAI pacing. Pacemaker rate = 70 ppm (automatic interval = 857 msec), and refractory period = 250 msec. There is intermittent prolongation of the interstimulus interval because the atrial lead senses the far-field QRS complex just beyond the 250 msec pacemaker refractory period. When the refractory period was programmed to 400 msec, the irregularity disappeared, with restoration of regular atrial pacing at a rate of 70 ppm. (From Barold SS, Zipes DP: Cardiac pacemakers and antiarrhythmic devices. *In* Braunwald E [ed]: Heart Disease: A Textbook of Cardiovascular Medicine. Philadelphia, WB Saunders, 1992, pp 726–755.)

(1) they need a higher sensitivity because the atrial electrogram is considerably smaller than the ventricular one, and (2) the pacemaker refractory period should be longer (400 msec) to prevent sensing of the conducted QRS complex or the "far-field" ventricular electrogram (registered by the atrial lead), which may cause inappropriate inhibition of the pacemaker.[14] Ideally, an AAI pacemaker should not sense ventricular activity. Oversensing of ventricular activity is more common with unipolar systems than with bipolar systems[15] and can often be corrected by lengthening the pacemaker atrial refractory period or decreasing atrial sensitivity.

VVT Mode

In the VVT mode, a sensed ventricular event causes immediate release or triggering of a pacemaker stimulus. The VVT mode therefore requires at least three timing intervals: (1) an LRI, (2) an upper rate interval (URI), and (3) a refractory period. In a simple VVT design, the pacemaker refractory period determines the maximal pacing rate according to the following formula:

$$\text{Upper rate (ppm)} = \frac{60}{\text{refractory period (sec)}}$$

On sensing a QRS complex, a VVT pacemaker discharges its stimulus during the absolute refractory period of the ventricular myocardium (Figs. 30–4 and 30–5). Such ineffectual stimulation wastes battery capacity and distorts the ECG. As in the VVI mode, if no QRS is sensed during the LRI, the pacemaker delivers its impulse at the completion

of the LRI. Dedicated single-mode VVT (AAT) pulse generators are now obsolete, but in the early days of pacing, they constituted important systems because they prevented prolonged inhibition (exhibited by unsophisticated VVI pacing systems) secondary to detection of extraneous or electromagnetic interference (EMI). The triggered VVT mode therefore ensures stimulation (i.e., prevents inhibition) whenever the pulse generator senses signals other than the QRS complex.

The triggered function is generally available in contemporary single- and dual-chamber pacemakers as a programmable mode for either temporary or permanent use. The VVT (AAT) mode of some pulse generators possesses a short inhibitory window beyond the pacemaker refractory period in which sensed signals can inhibit rather than trigger the output circuit.[16] As a rule, this occurs when the URI is longer than the programmed refractory period.[16] In the temporary VVT (AAT) mode, the capability of triggering an implanted pacemaker by the application of chest wall stimuli (generating signals for sensing) from an external pacemaker provides a way of performing noninvasive electrophysiologic studies or terminating reentrant tachycardias by appropriately timed stimuli or burst pacing[17–19] (see Fig. 30–5). The temporary VVT or AAT mode may also delineate the presence and exact time of sensing by "marking" the sensed signals with a stimulus, a function useful in the diagnosis of oversensing spurious signals (invisible on the surface ECG) generated by a fractured or defective lead.[14] Rarely, the VVT (AAT) mode is used to prevent inhibition of a unipolar pulse generator by myopotentials (musculoskeletal electric activity

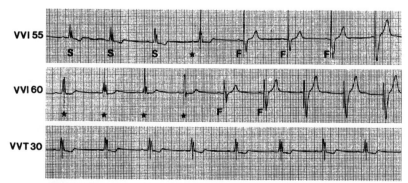

Figure 30–4. *Top,* VVI pacemaker at a rate of 55 ppm. The first three beats are sensed, and the fourth beat (*star*) is a pseudofusion beat (i.e., superimposition of a pacemaker stimulus on the surface QRS complex because the intracardiac ventricular electrogram registered by the pacing lead has not yet developed sufficient amplitude to inhibit the pacemaker output). The fifth, sixth, and seventh complexes are ventricular fusion beats (F). *Middle,* VVI pacemaker at a rate of 60 ppm. The first three beats (*stars*) are pseudofusion beats. The fourth beat (*star*) appears to be a pseudofusion beat because the initial QRS vector occurs just before the stimulus. Note that in beat 4, the T wave is identical to that of the previous beats, suggesting that depolarization was also identical. The fifth and sixth complexes are fusion beats (F), and the last three beats are pure ventricular paced beats. *Bottom,* Same patient. The pacemaker was programmed to the VVT mode, rate = 30 ppm. The pacemaker emits a stimulus immediately on sensing each QRS complex. Thus, a stimulus marks the precise time of sensing in the VVT mode. This may be correlated with the pseudofusion beats in the middle tracing in which the first pseudofusion beat is deformed by a stimulus just before the R wave returns to the baseline, that is, just before sensing would have occurred as determined from the VVT mode in the lower tracing. (From Barold SS, Zipes DP: Cardiac pacemakers and antiarrhythmic devices. *In* Braunwald E [ed]: Heart Disease: A Textbook of Cardiovascular Medicine. Philadelphia, WB Saunders, 1992, pp 726–755.)

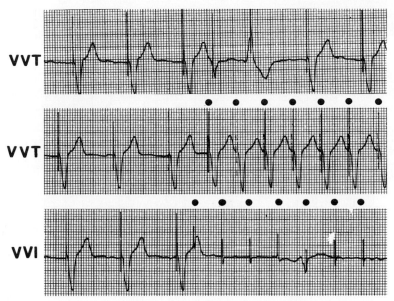

Figure 30–5. VVI pacemaker programmed to the VVT mode, rate = 70 ppm. *Top*, There are two sensed ventricular extrasystoles, both deformed by ventricular stimuli. *Middle*, VVT mode. Chest wall stimulation (*solid black circles*) delivered from an external pacemaker (to electrodes on the chest) provides signals detected by the implanted VVT pacemaker, which thereupon discharges its stimuli in synchrony with the sensed signals. This leads to an increase in the rate of ventricular pacing equal to the rate of chest wall stimulation. *Bottom*, Same patient. The pacemaker was reprogrammed back to the VVI mode, rate = 70 ppm. Chest wall stimulation at the same rate and amplitude as in the *middle tracing* now causes inhibition, with the emergence of a slow spontaneous rhythm. (From Barold SS: Single- and dual-chamber pacemakers: Electrophysiology, pacing modes, and multiprogrammability. *In* Singer I, Kupersmith J [eds]: Clinical Manual of Electrophysiology. Baltimore, Williams & Wilkins, 1993, pp 231–273.)

originating near the anodal electrode on the pacemaker case) when programming of sensitivity in the VVI (AAI) mode cannot correct the problem without compromising QRS (or P) sensing.[16] In the VVT mode, a unipolar pulse generator will increase its pacing rate on sensing myopotentials, which is a better trade-off than ventricular inhibition.

Hysteresis

When the escape interval is significantly longer than the automatic interval, the pacemaker is said to operate in the (positive) hysteresis mode[20] (Fig. 30–6). The original purpose of hysteresis was to maintain sinus rhythm (i.e., AV synchrony) for as long as possible at a spontaneous rate lower (e.g., 50 ppm) than the automatic rate of the pacemaker (e.g., 70 ppm). Thus, when the spontaneous rate drops below 50 bpm, the pacemaker will take over and pace at a rate of 70 ppm. The pacemaker will continue to pace at a rate of 70 ppm until the spontaneous rate exceeds the automatic rate, that is, when the spontaneous QRS complex occurs before the 857-msec automatic interval has timed out. Thus, if the spontaneous rate never exceeds 70 bpm, ventricular pacing will continue indefinitely at a rate of 70 ppm.

In some advanced systems, a device with hysteresis (e.g., 50 ppm/70 ppm) lengthens one or more pacing cycles automatically (to 1200 msec) after a given number of paced cycles at the programmed value (857 msec) to allow the return of a slower spontaneous rhythm (search hysteresis). The length of the extended interval (or "search" interval) corresponds to the programmed hysteresis rate, that is, 50 ppm. If no event is sensed during a search interval (1200 msec), the pulse generator delivers a stimulus at the end of that interval or intervals (depending on the number of search intervals programmed for the search function) and resumes pacing at the programmed rate of 70 ppm. Periodic activation of the search hysteresis function eventually promotes the return of the spontaneous rhythm.

Hysteresis is a frequent source of confusion in ECG interpretation of pacemaker function. Although hysteresis is available as a programmable option in many contemporary pacemakers, it is probably used infrequently because its advantages are more theoretical than real and because it may predispose the patient to undesirable arrhythmias.[21, 22] Indeed, hysteresis appears to have no advantage over simply decreasing the pacing rate in patients with symptoms due to loss of AV synchrony.[23] When pacing is required for carotid sinus syndrome or malignant vasovagal syndrome (neurally mediated syncope), however, a dual-chamber pulse generator with search hysteresis is often recommended to provide rapid pacing only during the episodes.[24, 25]

Fusion and Pseudofusion Beats

Ventricular fusion beats occur when the ventricles are depolarized simultaneously by spontaneous and pacemaker-

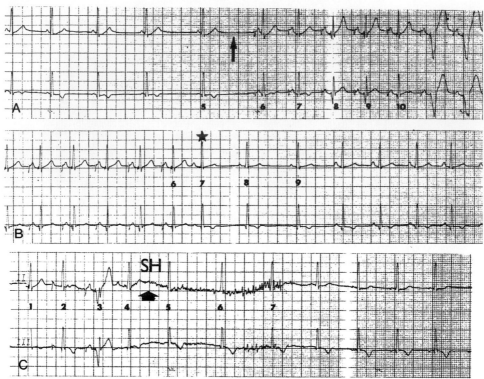

Figure 30–6. Two-lead ECG of a patient with cardioneurogenic syncope who received an Intermedics Relay DDDR pacemaker programmed to the DDD mode with hysteresis (50/85 ppm). The pacemaker is programmed to pace in the (AV sequential) DDD mode at 85 ppm (AV interval = 200 msec) whenever the spontaneous rate falls below 50 ppm (RR interval > 1200 msec) as shown in *A* (*arrow*), where the RR interval initiated by the fifth QRS complex is longer than 1200 msec. With standard 50/85 ppm hysteresis, the pacemaker should continue pacing at 85 ppm indefinitely unless the spontaneous rate exceeds 85 ppm to inhibit the device. In panel *B*, the pacemaker senses a relatively early spontaneous beat (*star*) with an RR interval of 600 msec (6–7), shorter than the 705 msec interval corresponding to the pacing rate of 85 ppm. Consequently, pacing is inhibited, and the device remains inhibited by sensing of a spontaneous rate faster than 50 ppm. In *C*, the search hysteresis function was programmed. After 255 paced beats, the search hysteresis (SH) option is activated, and the pacemaker automatically extends the pacing interval (in this case it was programmed for three intervals). The length of the extended or search intervals corresponds to a programmed hysteresis rate of 50 ppm, that is, 1200 msec. Sensed events in the search intervals inhibit the pacemaker and allow resumption of a spontaneous rhythm of less than 85 ppm. If no event is sensed during a search interval, the pacemaker delivers a stimulus at the end of the interval and resumes pacing at the programmed rate after the last search interval. In *C*, the three intervals (4–5, 5–6, 6–7) during the search intervals are all shorter than 1200 msec. Consequently, the pacemaker is inhibited. Note that when the search option is selected (*C*), the patient's intrinsic rate need not exceed the programmed pacing rate (as in *B*) to inhibit the pulse generator with hysteresis function. In panel *A*, beat 6 shows ventricular inhibition from a conducted QRS complex (see Fig. 30–10). Beat 7 is a ventricular pseudofusion beat. Beats 8, 9, and 10 are ventricular fusion beats, as are all the paced beats in panel *B*. In panel *C*, beat 1 is a ventricular fusion beat, beat 2 is a ventricular pseudofusion beat, and beat 3 is a ventricular fusion beat. Beat 4 may be a ventricular fusion beat.

induced activity. A ventricular fusion beat is often narrower than a pure paced beat and can exhibit various morphologic features depending on the relative contribution of the two foci to ventricular depolarization. Ventricular fusion can mimic lack of capture if it produces an isoelectric complex in a single ECG lead: ventricular depolarization should be obvious in other leads, and the presence of a T wave (repolarization) indicates that preceding depolarization has taken place.

Pseudofusion beats consist of the superimposition of an ineffectual pacemaker stimulus on the surface QRS complex originating from a single focus; they represent a normal

manifestation of VVI pacing.[12, 26] A substantial portion of the *surface* QRS complex can be inscribed before *intracardiac* electric activity or the electrogram monitored by the pacing lead generates the required voltage or signal to inhibit the output circuit of a VVI pacemaker (Fig. 30–7). Therefore, a VVI pacemaker functioning normally according to its programmed timing mechanism can deliver its impulse within a spontaneous surface QRS complex (mimicking undersensing) before the pulse generator has the opportunity to sense the "delayed" *intracardiac* signal or electrogram at the right ventricular apex. In a pseudofusion beat, the pacemaker stimulus falls within the absolute refractory period of the myocardium. In the presence of normal ventricular sensing, striking examples of ventricular pseudofusion beats with pacemaker stimuli released late within the surface QRS complex can occur in right bundle-branch block, left ventricular extrasystoles, and deranged intraventricular conduction (such as hyperkalemia) because of delayed arrival of activation at the sensing electrode or electrodes at the right ventricular apex.[27] Whenever pseudofusion beats are observed, true sensing failure must be excluded with long electrocardiographic recordings. Pacemaker stimuli falling clearly beyond the surface QRS complex indicate undersensing. Fusion and pseudofusion atrial beats can also occur with atrial pacing but are more difficult to recognize in view of the smaller size of the P wave in the ECG.

■ OPERATIONAL CHARACTERISTICS OF A SIMPLE DDD PULSE GENERATOR

The function and timing intervals of the various modes of dual-chamber pacing are best understood by focusing first on the DDD mode, in which pacing and sensing occur in the atrial and ventricular "electric" chambers.

Ventricular Channel (Lower Rate Interval and Ventricular Refractory Period)

As in a standard VVI pacemaker, the ventricular channel of a DDD device requires two basic timing cycles. The first is the LRI that corresponds to the programmed lower rate. In most dual-chamber pacemakers, lower rate timing (LRT) is

ventricular based (V-V timing) in that the LRI is controlled and initiated only by a paced or sensed ventricular event.[28, 29] In this situation, the LRI is the longest interval from a paced or sensed ventricular event to the succeeding ventricular stimulus (without any intervening atrial or ventricular sensing events). The second timing cycle is the period when the pacemaker cannot sense (ventricular refractory period [VRP]), traditionally defined as the time when the pulse generator is insensitive to incoming signals.[11] Yet many contemporary pulse generators can sense during part of the refractory period (as discussed later) and use such signals to initiate or reset certain timing cycles with the exception of the inviolable LRI.

VVI Pacing With an Atrial Channel (Atrioventricular Interval and Upper Rate Interval)

The addition of an atrial channel to a VVI system (the latter supplying the LRI and VRP) creates a simple DDD pulse generator. Two new intervals are required: an AV interval (the electronic analog of the PR interval) and a URI (the speed limit) to control the response of the ventricular channel to sensed atrial activity. The AV interval is initiated either by an atrial-paced or an atrial-sensed event. If the pulse generator does not detect ventricular activity during the AV interval, it emits a ventricular stimulus at the end of the programmed AV delay (Fig. 30–8).

If the URI of a DDD pacemaker is 500 msec (upper rate = 120 ppm), a P wave occurring earlier than 500 msec

Figure 30–7. *A,* Diagrammatic representation of the mechanism of pseudofusion. The surface electrocardiogram (ECG) and ventricular electrogram are recorded simultaneously. The electrogram generates the necessary intracardiac voltage to inhibit the pacemaker (yz, assumed at 4 mV) at a point corresponding to the descending limb of the surface QRS complex in its second half (*at dotted line*). Consequently, it is possible for a pacemaker stimulus to occur at the apex of the R just before the dotted line (or point of sensing) because the ventricular electrogram has not yet generated the voltage required to inhibit the pulse generator. *B,* Diagrammatic representation of the mechanism of pseudopseudofusion. Assume a DVI pulse generator with an AV interval of 155 msec and an atrial escape (pacemaker VA) interval of 678 msec. The atrial channel cannot sense in the DVI mode. The first beat shows atrial and ventricular capture by the atrial and ventricular stimuli. The relatively early occurrence of a spontaneous P wave and the ensuing conducted QRS complex allow the atrial stimulus to fall within the surface QRS complex according to the programmed atrial escape interval (AEI) of 678 msec. The ventricular electrogram generates the necessary voltage for sensing (yz) relatively late in relation to the surface QRS complex (corresponding to the dotted line). Consequently, the pulse generator delivers its atrial stimulus within the surface QRS complex (before the point of sensing at the *dotted line*) according to its programmed VA interval because the electrogram has not yet generated sufficient intracardiac voltage to suppress the pulse generator. In a DVI (or DDD) pulse generator, release of the atrial stimulus initiates a short ventricular refractory period (known as the *blanking period*) to prevent the ventricular channel from sensing the atrial stimulus as crosstalk. If a substantial portion of the ventricular electrogram falls within the ventricular blanking period, the ventricular channel will not sense the QRS complex, leading the pacemaker to deliver its ventricular stimulus on the ascending limb of the T wave at the completion of the programmed AV delay (*asterisk*). The atrial stimulus within the QRS may be called *pseudopseudofusion* because two chambers are involved. The same mechanism can occur during DDD pacing with ventricular extrasystoles or atrial undersensing (see Figs. 30–13 and 30–14). (In ventricular pseudofusion, the ventricular stimulus deforms the QRS complex.) (From Barold SS, Falkoff MD, Ong LS, et al: Electrocardiographic analysis of normal and abnormal pacemaker function. Cardiovasc Clin 14:97, 1983.)

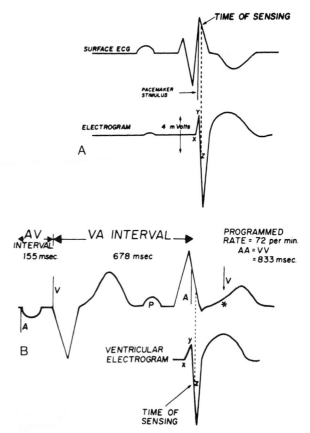

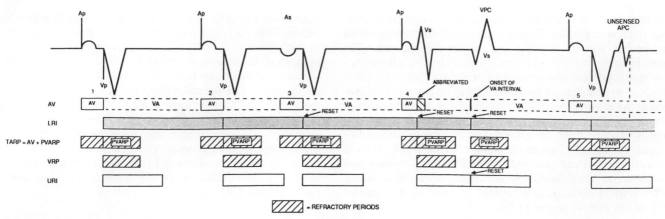

Figure 30–8. Diagram showing the function of a simple DDD pacemaker with only four basic intervals. Lower rate timing is ventricular based and controlled by ventricular events (paced or sensed). Ap, atrial paced beat; As, atrial sensed event; Vp, ventricular paced beat; Vs, ventricular sensed event. The four fundamental intervals are as follows: LRI, lower rate interval; VRP, ventricular refractory period; AV, atrioventricular delay; PVARP, postventricular atrial refractory period. The two derived intervals are atrial escape (pacemaker VA) interval = LRI − AV; total atrial refractory period (TARP) = AV + PVARP. Reset refers to the termination and reinitiation of a timing cycle before it has timed out to its completion according to its programmed duration. Premature termination of the programmed AV delay by Vs is indicated by its abbreviation. The upper rate interval (URI) is equal to TARP. As (third beat) initiates an AV interval terminating with Vp; As also aborts the atrial escape interval initiated by the second Vp. The third Vp resets the LRI and starts the PVARP, VRP, and URI. The fourth beat consists of Ap, which terminates the atrial escape interval (AEI) initiated by the third Vp, followed by a sensed conducted QRS (Vs). The AV interval is therefore abbreviated. Vs initiates the AEI, LRI, PVARP, VRP, and URI. The fifth beat is a ventricular extrasystole (ventricular premature contraction) that initiates AEI, PVARP, and VRP and resets the LRI and URI. The last beat is followed by an unsensed atrial extrasystole because it occurs within the PVARP. (From Barold SS, Zipes DP: Cardiac pacemakers and antiarrhythmic devices. *In* Braunwald E [ed]: Heart Disease: A Textbook of Cardiovascular Medicine. Philadelphia, WB Saunders, 1992, pp 726–755.)

from the previous atrial event will not be followed by a ventricular stimulus. Such an arrangement allows atrial sensing with 1:1 AV synchrony between the LRI and URI. In such a simple DDD pulse generator with only four intervals, the URI is equal to the refractory period of the atrial channel, or total atrial refractory period (TARP), which is initiated by a paced or sensed atrial event. As before, if the TARP is equal to 500 msec, the pacemaker will maintain 1:1 AV synchrony up to an atrial rate of 120 ppm, corresponding to a PP interval of 500 msec. When the atrial rate exceeds 120 ppm, P waves will fall within the TARP, and 1:1 AV synchrony can no longer occur. The TARP actually provides the URI.

The atrial escape (pacemaker ventriculoatrial [VA]) interval is a *derived* timing interval obtained by subtracting the programmed AV delay from the LRI (see Fig. 30–8). In a pacemaker with ventricular-based (V-V) LRT, the atrial escape (pacemaker VA) interval always remains constant and starts with a sensed or paced ventricular event and terminates (in the absence of sensed atrial or ventricular activity) with the release of an atrial stimulus[30–32] (see Fig. 30–8). The behavior of the atrial escape interval (AEI) of pacemakers with atrial-based (A-A) LRT is more complicated and discussed later.

Influence of Events of One Chamber on the Other

The functions of the two channels of a DDD pacemaker are intimately linked, and an event detected by one channel generally influences the other.[30–32] A sensed atrial event alters pacemaker response in two ways: (1) it triggers a ventricular stimulus after the completion of the programmed AV interval, provided that the ventricular channel senses no signal during the AV interval; and (2) it inhibits the release of the atrial stimulus expected at the completion of the AEI (pacemaker VA) because there is no need for atrial stimulation. Thus, the atrial channel functions simultaneously in the triggered mode by delivering ventricular stimulation (it triggers a ventricular output after a sensed P wave) and in the inhibited mode by preventing competitive release of an atrial stimulus when a P wave is sensed; that is, the AEI does not time out in its entirety. When the ventricular channel senses a signal, both atrial and ventricular channels are inhibited simultaneously. A sensed ventricular event inhibits release of the atrial stimulus (the AEI does not time out) and initiates a new AEI and LRI.

If a sensed ventricular event occurs during the AV interval, there is obviously no need for a ventricular stimulus at the completion of the programmed AV interval. The AV interval is therefore terminated (i.e., abbreviated), and the pacemaker initiates a new AEI and LRI. The ventricular channel of a DDD pulse generator functions in the inhibited mode under all circumstances. The code DDTI/I was originally proposed for the DDD mode because the atrial channel functions both in the triggered and inhibited modes, whereas the ventricular channel is restricted to the inhibited mode. This designation, although correct, was considered unwieldy and was eventually replaced by a simpler but less descriptive DDD mode requiring that the last position be labeled D (double) if both T and I responses occur, regardless of other considerations.

Refractory Periods

In a DDD pulse generator, an atrial sensed or atrial paced event initiates the AV interval and atrial refractory period.

The atrial channel of a DDD pulse generator must remain refractory during the entire AV interval to prevent initiation of a new AV interval while one is already in progress. Thus, the first part of the atrial refractory period lasts for the duration of the AV interval in the form of Ap-Vs, Ap-Vp, As-Vp, As-Vs (Ap = atrial paced event, As = atrial sensed event, Vp = ventricular paced event, Vs = ventricular sensed event). The AV interval terminates with a ventricular event (Vp or Vs), which immediately restarts (or continues) the atrial refractory period. The part of the atrial refractory period initiated by a ventricular event is called the postventricular atrial refractory period (PVARP). The PVARP is designed to prevent the atrial channel from sensing a variety of signals, such as retrograde P waves related to retrograde VA conduction, very early atrial extrasystoles, and far-field ventricular signals registered in the atrial electrogram.[33, 34] The TARP is equal to the sum of the AV delay and the PVARP. Thus, programming a long PVARP limits the upper rate of the pacemaker by lengthening the TARP.

In a DDD pulse generator, does a paced or sensed event in one channel initiate a refractory period in both atrial and ventricular channels to ensure that a given paced or sensed event in one (electric) chamber or channel does not interfere with the function of the other? Four possible events may be considered: Ap, As, Vs, and Vp.

1. Vs or Vp initiates the VRP and the PVARP simultaneously.

2. Ap initiates the AV interval and the atrial refractory period and simultaneously initiates a short ventricular blanking period to avoid sensing of the atrial stimulus by the ventricular channel (interference known as *crosstalk*).[30, 35, 36] Thus, the ventricular channel can sense throughout most of the AV interval because the ventricular blanking period is relatively short. This allows intrinsic ventricular activity to inhibit the ventricular output if sensed before the AV interval times out.

3. As is the only one of the four possible events (As, Ap, Vs, Vp) that generates a refractory period only in the atrial channel. No ventricular blanking period is needed after As because ordinarily it cannot be sensed by the ventricular electrode and therefore cannot directly disturb the function of the ventricular channel.

Control of Upper Rate Interval in a Simple DDD Device

In a simple DDD pulse generator (without a separately programmable URI), the URI is equal to the TARP. The TARP (AV delay + PVARP) and URI are interrelated according to the following formula:

$$\text{Upper rate (ppm)} = \frac{60,000}{\text{TARP (msec)}}$$

In the previously discussed example, if TARP is equal to 500 msec (AV delay = 200 msec; PVARP = 300 msec), the pulse generator will sense atrial signals (P waves) 500 msec or longer apart up to a repetition rate of 120 ppm. An atrial signal occurring earlier than 500 msec (the URI) from the previous atrial event will fall in the atrial refractory period and will not be sensed.[30, 31]

Basic and Derived Timing Cycles of DDD Pulse Generators

Although the URI was previously considered a basic timing cycle, it is preferable at this stage to use the PVARP as a fundamental interval and relegate the URI and TARP to derived functions. At this point in the discussion, a simple DDD pulse generator can be built with only four basic intervals: LRI, AV interval, VRP, and PVARP, and with three derived intervals: AEI, TARP (AV delay + PVARP), and URI (equal to the TARP). Theoretically, a DDD pulse generator equipped with these timing cycles should function well provided that the ventricular channel does not sense the atrial stimulus (crosstalk).[35, 36] Prevention of crosstalk is mandatory and requires the addition of a fifth fundamental timing interval in the form of a brief ventricular refractory (blanking) period starting with the release of the atrial stimulus. Indeed, a DDD device with only these five basic intervals was successfully used clinically in early DDD pulse generators manufactured by the Cordis Corporation (Miami, FL) (purchased by Telectronics [Englewood, CO] and then St. Jude Medical [Sylmar, CA]). Further refinements related to crosstalk and the upper rate response created the need for two other basic intervals: the ventricular safety pacing (VSP) period (to complement the ventricular blanking period in dealing with crosstalk) and a URI that is programmable independently of the TARP for an upper rate response smoother than the sudden mechanism provided only by the TARP[30–32, 37, 38] (Fig. 30–9).

Crosstalk Intervals

Crosstalk with self-inhibition refers to the inappropriate detection of the atrial stimulus by the ventricular channel. It occurs more commonly in unipolar than in bipolar dual-chamber pacemakers. In patients without an underlying ventricular rhythm, inhibition of the ventricular channel by crosstalk could be catastrophic by causing ventricular asystole.

Ventricular Blanking Period

The prevention of crosstalk requires a basic timing cycle called the *ventricular blanking period,* which consists of a brief absolute VRP starting coincidentally with the release of the atrial stimulus (Fig. 30–10). The duration of the ventricular blanking period varies from 10 to 60 msec according to the manufacturer and is generally programmable.[33] A QRS occurring soon after Ap within the ventricular blanking period will be unsensed, whereupon the pulse generator will emit a competitive ventricular stimulus. Thus, if the programmed AV interval is relatively long, this particular ventricular stimulus could fall on the T wave of the unsensed ventricular beat (whose QRS falls within the ventricular blanking period). There is no need for ventricular blanking after atrial sensing. Sensing of a ventricular stimulus or QRS complex by the atrial channel (VA crosstalk), which is the reverse of AV crosstalk, is also prevented in conventional devices by appropriate blanking of the atrial channel provided automatically by the PVARP.

Ventricular Safety Pacing

In many dual-chamber pulse generators, the AV interval initiated by an atrial stimulus contains an additional safety

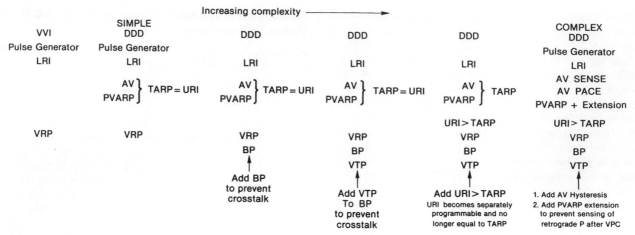

Figure 30–9. The progressive addition of new timing cycles to a simple DDD pacemaker (*left*) creates a more complex device (*right*) (see text for details). Abbreviations as in Figure 30–8: AV pace, AV interval initiated by Ap; AV sense, AV interval initiated by As; BP, blanking period; VTP, ventricular triggering period or ventricular safety pacing period. (From Barold SS, Falkoff MD, Ong LS, et al: Timing cycles of DDD pacemakers. *In* Barold SS, Mugica J [eds]: New Perspectives in Cardiac Pacing. Mt Kisco, NY, Futura, 1988, pp 69–119.)

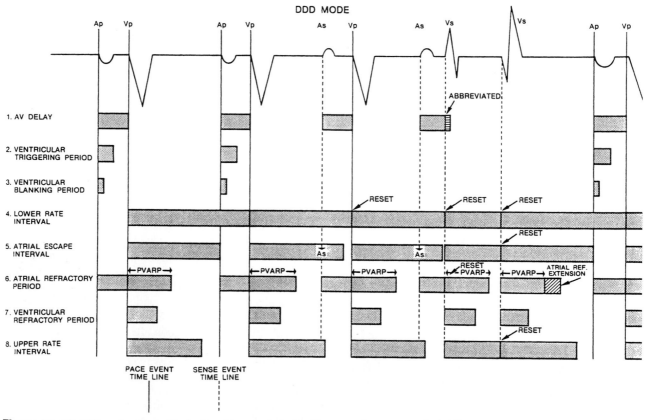

Figure 30–10. DDD mode with ventricular-based lower rate timing. Diagrammatic representation of timing cycles. REF, refractory; ventricular triggering period-ventricular safety period. The second Vs event is a sensed ventricular extrasystole. The fourth AV interval initiated by As is abbreviated because Vs occurs before the AV interval has timed out. The PVARP generated by the ventricular extrasystole is automatically extended by the atrial refractory period extension. This design is based on the concept that most episodes of endless-loop tachycardia (pacemaker macroreentrant tachycardia due to repetitive sensing of retrograde atrial depolarization) are initiated by ventricular extrasystoles with retrograde ventriculoatrial conduction. Whenever possible, the AV interval and atrial escape (pacemaker VA) interval are depicted in their entirety for the sake of clarity. The arrow pointing down within the atrial escape (pacemaker VA) interval indicates that As has taken place; As inhibits the release of the atrial stimulus expected at the completion of the atrial escape interval (AEI). The abbreviations and format used in this illustration are the same as those for Figures 30–19, 30–21, 30–28, 30–33, 30–36, and 30–53. (From Barold SS, Falkoff MD, Ong LS, et al: All dual-chamber pacemakers function in the DDD mode. Am Heart J 115:1353, 1988.)

mechanism to prevent the potentially serious consequences of crosstalk. The AV delay initiated by an atrial stimulus is divided into two parts (see Fig. 30–10). The first part is the VSP period (also known as the *nonphysiologic AV delay, ventricular triggering period,* or *crosstalk sensing window*).[36, 39, 40] Traditionally, the VSP period encompasses the first 100 to 110 msec of the AV interval and is programmable in some devices. During the traditional model of the VSP period, a signal (crosstalk, QRS, and so forth) sensed by the ventricular channel does not inhibit the pulse generator. Rather, the signal initiates or triggers a ventricular stimulus delivered prematurely only at the completion of the VSP period, producing a characteristic abbreviation of the paced AV (Ap-Vp) interval (usually 100 to 110 msec)[39] (Fig. 30–11). In this way, if the ventricular channel detects crosstalk beyond the ventricular blanking period, activation of the VSP mechanism prevents ventricular asystole by delivering an early Vp. Consequently, during continual crosstalk in pacemakers with ventricular (V-V) LRT, because the atrial escape (pacemaker VA) interval remains constant and the AV interval shortens, the AV sequential pacing rate becomes faster than the programmed lower rate[28] (Fig. 30–12; see Fig. 30–11). When a QRS complex is sensed during the VSP period, the early triggered ventricular stimulus is supposed to fall harmlessly during the absolute refractory period of the myocardium because of the abbreviated AV interval (Figs. 30–13 and 30–14).

Although the duration of the VSP is generally described as beginning from the atrial stimulus, obviously, ventricular sensing cannot occur until termination of the initial ventricular blanking period. A sensed ventricular signal beyond the VSP period in the second part of the AV interval inhibits rather than triggers the ventricular output. Pulse generators without a VSP period generally require a relatively long ventricular blanking period to prevent crosstalk. A long ventricular blanking period (being an absolute refractory period) predisposes to undersensing by the ventricular channel (see Fig. 30–13). Consequently, VSP provides a backup mechanism to deal with crosstalk and allows the use of relatively short ventricular blanking periods to optimize ventricular sensing. Figures 30–15 and 30–16 show further refinements of the VSP response of contemporary dual-chamber pacemakers[41] (Fig. 30–16).

In pulse generators (ventricular-based LRT) without a VSP mechanism, crosstalk produces the following distinctive electrocardiographic manifestations[42, 43]:

1. There is unexpected prolongation of the interval between the atrial stimulus and the succeeding conducted (spontaneous) QRS complex to a value greater than the programmed AV interval. If there is no AV conduction, ventricular asystole will occur. Myopotential interference sensed during the AV interval of unipolar DDD pulse generators can superficially resemble crosstalk (Fig. 30–17).

2. The rate of atrial pacing increases compared with the programmed free-running AV sequential (lower) rate. There is no paced QRS complex. The atrial stimulus (sensed by the ventricular channel) initiates a new atrial escape (pace-

COSMOS DDD

LOWER RATE = 80 ppm (750 ms)
AV INTERVAL = 300 ms
ATRIAL ESCAPE INTERVAL = 450 ms
VTP = 100 ms

| VENTRICULAR SENSITIVITY = 2 mV | VENTRICULAR SENSITIVITY = 5 mV |
| CROSSTALK VV = 550 ms (109 ppm) | VV = 750 ms (80 ppm) |

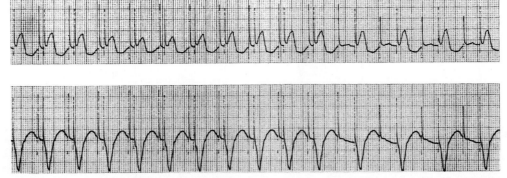

Figure 30–11. The Intermedics Cosmos I unipolar DDD pulse generator (ventricular-based lower rate timing) with ventricular safety pacing mechanism (ventricular triggering period [VTP]) showing on the *left* crosstalk characterized by abbreviation of the AV interval to 100 msec. The lower rate interval (LRI) is controlled by ventricular events. Consequently, the AEI remains constant at 450 msec. The interval between two consecutive ventricular stimuli (Vp-Vp) therefore shortens from 750 to 450 + 100 = 550 msec, increasing the AV sequential pacing rate from 80 to 109 ppm during continual crosstalk. In the *right* panel, crosstalk disappears when the ventricular sensitivity is reduced from 2 to 5 mV (less sensitive setting). Two ECG leads were recorded simultaneously. (From Barold SS: Single- and dual-chamber pacemakers: Electrophysiology, pacing modes, and multi-programmability. *In* Singer I, Kupersmith J [eds]: Clinical Manual of Electrophysiology. Baltimore, Williams & Wilkins, 1993, pp 231–273.)

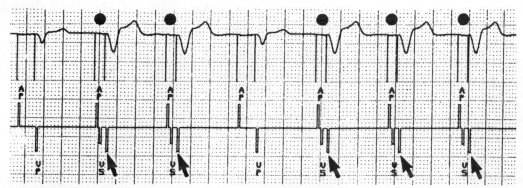

Figure 30–12. Ventricular safety pacing during DDD pacing (ECG leads V1, V2, and V3). *A,* In the absence of crosstalk, the first, fourth, and last AV intervals are equal to the programmed value of 200 msec. Intermittent crosstalk *(solid black circles)* leads to activation of the ventricular safety pacing mechanism so that the AV interval of the second, third, fifth, sixth, and seventh beats *(solid black circles)* is abbreviated to 110 msec. The marker channel below the ECG confirms the presence of crosstalk with ventricular sensing (Vs) of the atrial stimulus (Ap) within the ventricular safety pacing period but beyond the short ventricular blanking period initiated by Ap. The arrows point to Vp triggered at the end of the ventricular safety pacing period (110 msec after the release of Ap). In a DDD pulse generator with ventricular-based lower rate timing, activation of the ventricular safety pacing mechanism due to continual crosstalk leads to an increase in the pacing rate (although the atrial escape interval remains constant). (From Barold SS, Zipes DP: Cardiac pacemakers and antiarrhythmic devices. *In* Braunwald E [ed]: Heart Disease [5th ed]. Philadelphia, WB Saunders, 1997, pp 705–741.)

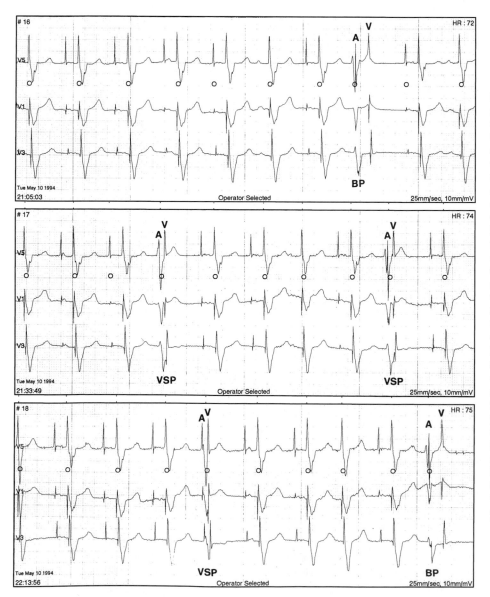

Figure 30–13. Holter recording of DDD pacemaker showing the effect of crosstalk timing cycles during normal pacemaker function. Three ECG leads were recorded simultaneously. The eighth beat is a ventricular premature contraction (VPC) deformed by an atrial stimulus (A). The effective electrogram of the VPC (of adequate amplitude to be sensed) occurs within the ventricular blanking period (BP) initiated by the atrial stimulus. The VPC is therefore unsensed by the ventricular channel of the pacemaker. The last beat in the *bottom panel* (BP) shows the same response. The delivery of the atrial stimulus within the QRS complex (capable of being sensed) is called a *pseudopseudofusion* beat. In the *middle panel*, the ventricular electrogram of the VPCs (fourth and ninth beats) is of sufficient amplitude to be sensed. The VPCs are deformed by an atrial stimulus as in the *top panel*. However, the atrial stimulus occurs earlier than it does in the *top panel*, thereby allowing the pacemaker to sense the effective ventricular electrogram beyond the ventricular blanking period but still within the ventricular safety pacing (VSP) period. The abbreviated Ap-Vp interval provides proof that the VPCs are sensed in the VSP. A similar response occurs with the fifth beat (VSP) in the *bottom panel.* A, atrial stimulus; V, ventricular stimulus.

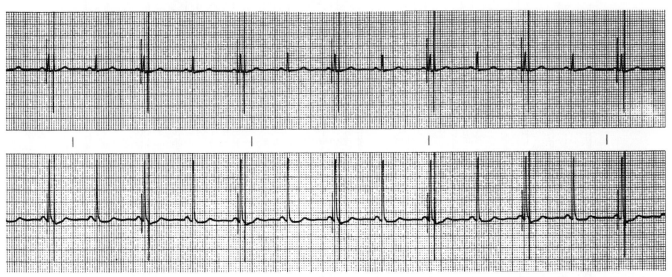

Figure 30–14. Intermittent atrial undersensing during DDD pacing with delivery of atrial stimulus within the terminal portion of every second P wave. The conducted QRS complex following Ap falls within the ventricular safety pacing period of 110 msec The ventricular channel therefore senses the QRS complex and triggers Vp with the expected abbreviated Ap-Vp interval of 110 msec (programmed Ap-Vp = 200 msec).

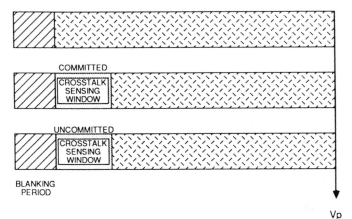

Figure 30–15. Behavior of the ventricular safety pacing (VSP) mechanism of DDD pacemakers. The VSP period actually begins at the completion of the ventricular blanking period, but its total duration is generally expressed as starting from the atrial stimulus with the onset of the ventricular blanking period. Medtronic dual-chamber pulse generators (Medtronic, Inc., Minneapolis, MN) possess a VSP period of 110 msec, while other pulse generators have a VSP period with a nominal value of 100 ms. In the Medtronic and Intermedics Cosmos I pulse generators, a signal sensed at any time during the VSP period (beyond the blanking period) by the ventricular channel of these pulse generators triggers an obligatory (committed) ventricular stimulus at the termination of the VSP period. In the Intermedics Cosmos II and Relay DDDR pulse generators, the VSP period contains an initial crosstalk sensing window. When the ventricular channel senses a signal during the crosstalk window, the pulse generator triggers a committed ventricular stimulus at the termination of the VSP period regardless of any other ventricular events sensed during the VSP period beyond the crosstalk sensing window. In contrast, an isolated ventricular signal sensed in the VSP beyond the crosstalk sensing window inhibits the ventricular output. In the Pacesetter Siemens Paragon DDD and Synchrony DDDR pulse generators, the crosstalk sensing window functions as in the Cosmos II pulse generator. A signal sensed by the ventricular channel during the crosstalk sensing window triggers a ventricular stimulus at the termination of the VSP period. In contrast to the Cosmos II pulse generator, the ventricular output triggered by sensing in the VSP is uncommitted. Thus another ventricular event sensed in the VSP (beyond the crosstalk sensing window) will inhibit the triggered ventricular response initiated by ventricular sensing within the crosstalk sensing window. (From Barold SS: Single- and dual-chamber pacemakers: Electro-physiology, pacing modes, and multi-programmability. *In* Singer I, Kupersmith J [eds]: Clinical Manual of Electrophysiology. Baltimore, Williams & Wilkins, 1993, pp 231–274.)

Patient: Nurse, Vivian   Report No: 94-000

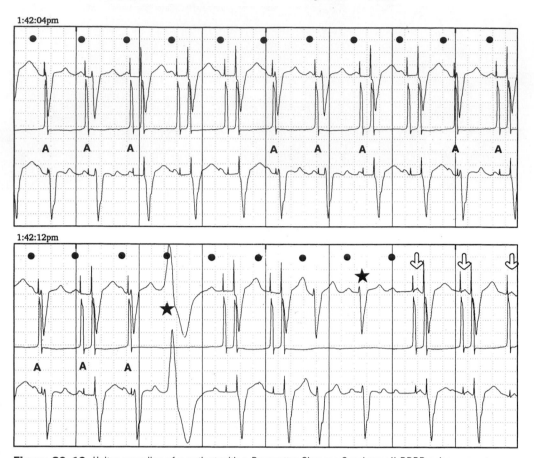

Figure 30–16. Holter recording of a patient with a Pacesetter-Siemens Synchrony II DDDR pulse generator (programmed to the DDD mode) showing intermittent atrial undersensing (lower rate timing is ventricular-based) and unusual behavior during sensing in the ventricular safety pacing interval (lower rate interval [LRI] = 750 msec; AV = 175 msec; A, atrial stimuli). *Solid black circles* indicate sinus P waves. Atrial stimuli are ineffectual when they occur in the atrial myocardial refractory period of a preceding unsensed atrial depolarization. Only the last three atrial stimuli in the *bottom panel* capture the atrium. The first effective atrial stimulus *(first arrow)* close to the previous spontaneous P wave proves the efficacy of atrial capture and rules out the coincidental occurrence of an ineffectual stimulus followed by a spontaneous P wave (i.e., apparent atrial pacing). The pacemaker senses only the second last P wave in the *upper panel* and the third P wave in the *bottom panel.* In the *bottom panel,* the atrial escape interval initiated by the first VPC *(star)* measures 830 msec, substantially longer than the atrial escape interval initiated by the succeeding ventricular paced beat. In this pacemaker, a sensed ventricular premature contraction (VPC, defined as two successive ventricular events without an intervening sensed P wave) initiates a fixed atrial escape of 830 msec (regardless of the programmed value) and automatic prolongation of the postventricular atrial refractory period (PVARP) to 480 msec (+PVARP on VPC). This feature was designed to prevent sensing of a VPC-related retrograde P wave and the initiation of endless-loop tachycardia (discussed later). The longer atrial escape interval after VPC promotes AV synchrony (and prevents competitive atrial pacing) by delaying the atrial stimulus from unsensed atrial activity in the PVARP. A spontaneous QRS complex preceded by a sensed P wave initiates an atrial escape interval equal to the programmed value. *Bottom panel,* The star on the right in the bottom panel refers to a conducted QRS complex preceded by a P wave. The pacemaker interprets this QRS as a VPC because it fails to sense the preceding P wave. Consequently, the QRS initiates an atrial escape interval of 830 msec. In the *bottom panel,* it appears that the pacemaker senses the first P wave and triggers a ventricular stimulus with apparent ventricular capture. However, the first stimulus is atrial, and the QRS is spontaneous and not paced. The pacemaker does not identify the first QRS complex as a VPC because it is preceded by Ap. This pacemaker functions with ventricular-based lower rate timing, so that the atrial escape interval remains constant except after a pacemaker-defined VPC. The first spike-to-spike interval is longer than the atrial escape interval, so that the first stimulus cannot be ventricular because the second one is atrial. The pacemaker actually senses the first QRS complex beyond the 64-msec crosstalk window (measured from the atrial stimulus and including the ventricular blanking period) but before termination of the ventricular safety pacing (VSP) period (120 msec). The VSP feature of this device is uncommitted, so that ventricular sensing in the VSP beyond the first 64 msec inhibits the ventricular channel rather than triggers a ventricular stimulus at the completion of the entire VSP interval as in many other devices. Other Ap-Ap intervals (without an intervening Vp) behave similarly *(top panel).* (From Barold SS: Evaluation of pacemaker function by Holter recordings. *In* Moss AJ, Stern AJ [eds]: Noninvasive Electrocardiology: Clinical Aspects of Holter Monitoring. Philadelphia, WB Saunders, 1996, p 107.)

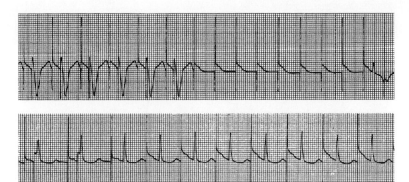

Figure 30–17. Crosstalk during DDD pacing without a ventricular safety pacing (VSP) mechanism (ventricular-based lower rate timing). *Top strip*, The lower rate was increased to test for crosstalk (lower rate interval [LRI] = 580 msec; AV = 170 msec). During crosstalk, the interval between atrial stimuli on the right becomes shorter than the LRI because the ventricular channel initiates a new atrial escape interval (AEI) on sensing the atrial stimulus. Crosstalk, therefore, causes an increase in the atrial pacing rate faster than the free-running AV sequential LRI on the left. Continual crosstalk causes prolonged ventricular asystole. *Bottom strip*, Crosstalk with AV conduction (LRI = 857 msec; AV interval = 200 msec). Crosstalk occurs with the third atrial stimulus and produces characteristic prolongation of the interval between the atrial stimulus and the succeeding conducted QRS complex to a value longer than the programmed AV interval. The rate of atrial pacing increases because the sensed atrial stimulus by the ventricular channel initiates a new AEI just beyond the termination of the ventricular blanking period. Consequently, the interval between two consecutive atrial stimuli becomes equal to the AEI of 657 msec (857 − 200) plus the duration of the ventricular blanking period (50 msec), providing a total of about 700 msec. (From Barold SS, Zipes CP: Cardiac pacemakers and antiarrhythmic devices. *In* Braunwald E [ed]: Heart Disease: A Textbook of Cardiovascular Medicine. Philadelphia, WB Saunders, 1992, pp 726–755.)

maker VA) interval. Consequently, the interval between two consecutive atrial stimuli (AA interval) becomes equal to the AEI (pacemaker VA), ignoring the negligible duration of the blanking period.

Prevention of Crosstalk

Crosstalk is best prevented by using bipolar dual-chamber devices. The presence of crosstalk and effective (ventricular) blanking is tested by reprogramming the atrial output to its maximal value and the ventricular sensitivity to its most sensitive setting.[43] To avoid competition, the lower rate is set above the patient's own spontaneous rate, and the AV delay is shortened to less than the spontaneous PR interval. If crosstalk is observed, the atrial voltage output should be decreased before decreasing the atrial pulse duration and the ventricular sensitivity. If these maneuvers are unsuccessful or undesirable, the blanking ventricular period should be prolonged, provided it is programmable. Some pulse generators automatically adjust the duration of the blanking period according to the programmed atrial output (volts and pulse duration), ventricular sensitivity, and polarity (unipolar versus bipolar).

■ UPPER RATE RESPONSE OF DDD PACEMAKERS

In the DDD mode, the *atrial*-driven URI refers to the shortest Vs-Vp or Vp-Vp, in which the second Vp is triggered by a sensed *atrial* event. The URI always refers to the shortest *ventricular* paced interval. The second Vp can be released only at the completion of the atrial-driven *ventricular* URI initiated by a preceding Vs or Vp. In the DDD mode, URI always refers to the *atrial*-driven (ventricular) URI because there are no sensor-driven intervals (SDIs) in a device without a nonatrial sensor.

No Separately Programmable Upper Rate Interval

In a DDD pacemaker without a separately programmable URI, the TARP is equal to the (ventricular) URI and provides a simple way of controlling the paced ventricular response to a fast atrial rate. This upper rate response is often called *fixed-ratio AV block* (Fig. 30–18). The TARP defines the fastest atrial rate associated with 1:1 pacemaker response or the fastest paced ventricular rate associated with 1:1 AV synchrony.[31, 33, 37] As the atrial rate increases, any P wave falling within the PVARP is unsensed. The degree of block depends on the atrial rate and where the P waves occur in the pacemaker cycle. The AV interval (As-Vp) always remains constant and equal to its programmed value. As the atrial rate increases, more P waves fall within the TARP, and the degree of block increases. If the upper rate is 120 ppm (TARP = 500 msec) and the lower rate is 70 ppm, the rate will not drop by half to 60 ppm (i.e., 2:1) when atrial tachycardia occurs because the paced ventricular rate cannot fall below the lower rate. This

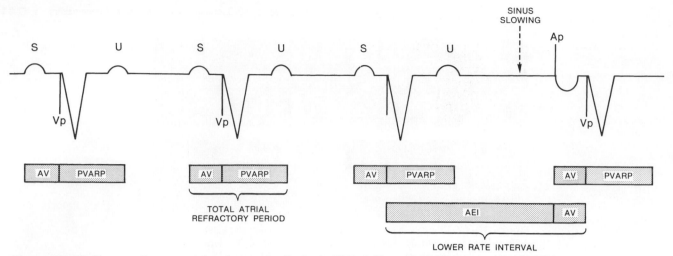

Figure 30–18. Diagrammatic representation of pacemaker fixed-ratio AV block. The total atrial refractory period (TARP) (AV + postventricular atrial refractory period [PVARP]) controls the upper rate interval (URI). Every second P wave is unsensed because it falls within the PVARP (2:1 block). When sinus slowing occurs on the right, the pacemaker functions according to the programmed lower rate interval (LRI), thereby delivering an atrial stimulus that terminates the pause. AEI, atrial escape interval; Ap, atrial paced event; S, sensed P wave; U, unsensed P wave; Vp, ventricular paced event. (From Barold SS, Falkoff MD, Ong LS, et al: Electrocardiography of contemporary DDD pacemakers. A. Basic concepts, upper rate response, retrograde ventriculoatrial conduction, and differential diagnosis of pacemaker tachycardias. *In* Saksena S, Goldschlager N [eds]: Electrical Therapy for Cardiac Arrhythmias: Pacing, Antitachycardia Devices, Catheter Ablation. Philadelphia, WB Saunders, 1990, pp 225–264.)

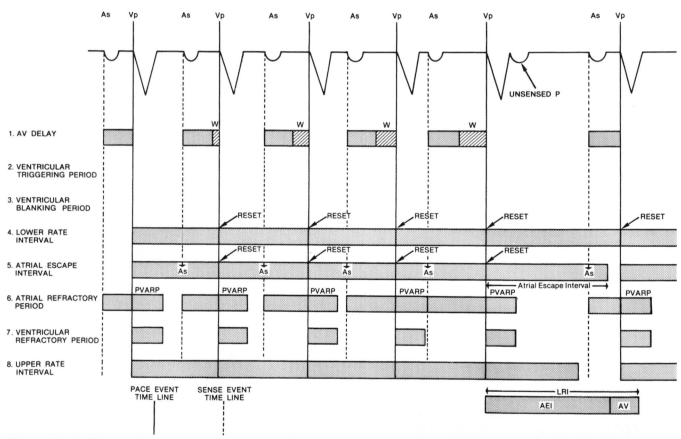

Figure 30–19. DDD mode (ventricular-based lower rate timing). Upper rate response with pacemaker Wenckebach AV block. AEI, atrial escape interval. The upper rate interval (URI) is longer than the programmed total atrial refractory period (TARP). The PP interval (As-As) is shorter than the URI but longer than the programmed TARP. The As-Vp interval lengthens by a varying period (w) to conform to the URI. During the Wenckebach response, the pacemaker synchronizes Vp to As, and because the pacemaker cannot violate its (ventricular) URI, Vp can be released only at the completion of the URI. The AV delay (As-Vp) becomes progressively longer as the ventricular channel waits to deliver its Vp until the URI has timed out. The maximum prolongation of the AV interval represents the difference between the URI and the TARP (see Fig. 31–20). The As-Vp interval lengthens as long as the As-As interval (PP) is longer than the TARP. The sixth P wave falls within the postventricular atrial refractory period (PVARP) and is unsensed and not followed by Vp. A pause occurs, and the cycle restarts. In the first four pacing cycles, the intervals between ventricular stimuli (Vp-Vp) are constant and equal to the URI. When the PP interval becomes shorter than the programmed TARP, Wenckebach pacemaker AV block cannot occur, and fixed-ratio pacemaker AV block (e.g., 2:1) supervenes. Same format as Figure 30–10. (From Barold SS, Falkoff MD, Ong LS, et al: All dual-chamber pacemakers function in the DDD mode. Am Heart J 115:1353, 1988.)

response is often called *2:1 block,* although it is really a misnomer. Actually, the paced ventricular rate will be exactly half the atrial rate or equal to the lower rate of the pacemaker, whichever is higher. When half the atrial rate is slower than the programmed lower rate, the pulse generator must pace AV sequentially according to the LRI; that is, an atrial stimulus rather than a sensed P wave initiates the AV interval. An upper rate response using fixed-ratio AV block can be inappropriate in young or physically active patients because the sudden reduction of the ventricular rate with activity may be poorly tolerated.

Wenckebach Upper Rate Response

Only DDD pulse generators with an independently programmable upper rate (interval) produce a Wenckebach (or pseudo-Wenckebach) response to faster atrial rates. For a Wenckebach response to occur with *prolongation* of the AV interval (As-Vp), the URI must be *longer* than the TARP[31-33, 37, 38, 40, 44-47] (Fig. 30–19). The maximal prolongation of the AV interval during a Wenckebach sequence represents the difference between these two intervals (Fig. 30–20). If As-Vp as programmed is less than Ap-Vp as programmed, the maximum extension of the basic As-Vp interval can be calculated as follows:

$$[(Ap\text{-}Vp) - (As\text{-}Vp)] + [URI - TARP]$$

where TARP = PVARP + Ap-Vp as programmed; that is, maximal AV extension = URI − (PVARP + As-Vp).

When the separately programmable URI becomes equal to the TARP, a Wenckebach response cannot occur, and the URI becomes a function of the programmed TARP, thereby creating fixed-ratio AV block. With a progressive increase in the atrial rate, the Wenckebach response of a pacemaker with a URI longer than the TARP eventually switches to (2:1) fixed-ratio AV block when the PP interval becomes shorter than the TARP (Fig. 30–21).

During the Wenckebach response, the pacemaker synchronizes its ventricular stimulus to sensed atrial activity. The ventricular stimulus can be released only at the completion of the URI because the pacemaker cannot violate its (ventricular) URI. The AV delay (initiated by a sensed P wave) becomes progressively longer as the ventricular channel waits to deliver its stimulus until the URI has timed out (see Fig. 30–19). The atrial channel remains refractory and therefore insensitive to incoming signals through the entire duration of the AV interval, regardless of its duration. Eventually, a P wave falling within the PVARP is not followed by a ventricular output, and a pause occurs. In other words, Wenckebach behavior limits the paced ventricular rate by extending the AV interval. The Wenckebach upper rate re-

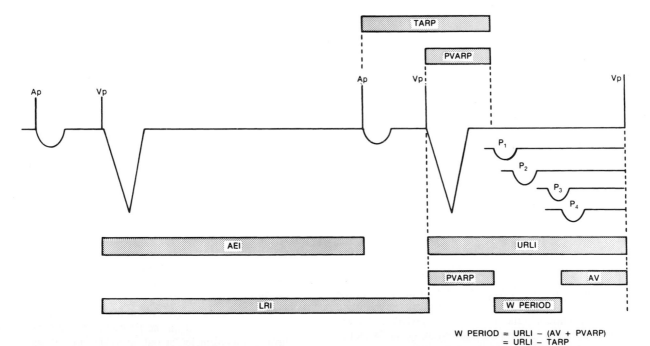

W PERIOD = URLI − (AV + PVARP)
= URLI − TARP

Figure 30–20. Diagrammatic representation of the mechanism of AV interval prolongation in a pulse generator with a separately programmable total atrial refractory period (TARP) and upper rate interval (URI). Lower rate timing is ventricular based. The maximum AV extension, or waiting period (W), = URI − (AV + postventricular atrial refractory period [PVARP]) = URI − TARP. A P wave (P₁) occurring immediately after the termination of the PVARP exhibits the longest AV interval, that is, AV + W. A P wave just beyond the W period (P₄) initiates an AV interval equal to the programmed value. P waves occurring during the W period (P₂ and P₃) exhibit varying degrees of AV prolongation to conform to the URI depicted as the shortest interval between two consecutive ventricular-paced beats. If the pacemaker is programmed with As-Vp shorter than Ap-Vp, W becomes URI − (As-Vp) − PVARP; that is, AV extension becomes longer if basic As-Vp is shorter than Ap-Vp. However, the maximum As-Vp duration is URI − PVARP, regardless of programmed AV interval. AEI, atrial escape interval; LRI, lower rate interval; Ap, atrial-paced beat; Vp, ventricular pacing beat. (From Barold SS, Falkoff MD, Ong LS, et al: Electrocardiography of contemporary DDD pacemakers. A. Basic concepts, upper rate response, retrograde ventriculoatrial conduction, and differential diagnosis of pacemaker tachycardias. *In* Saksena S, Goldschlager N [eds]: Electrical Therapy for Cardiac Arrhythmias: Pacing, Antitachycardia Devices, Catheter Ablation. Philadelphia, WB Saunders, 1990, pp 225–264.)

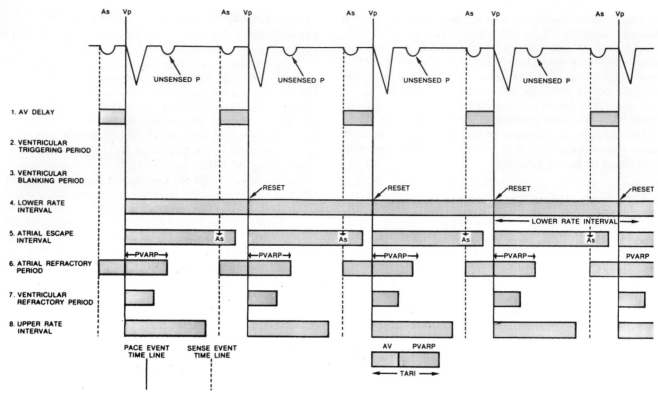

Figure 30–21. DDD mode with ventricular-based lower rate timing. *Top,* Upper rate response with fixed-ratio pacemaker AV block. The upper rate interval (URI) is longer than the total atrial refractory period (TARP) (AV + postventricular atrial refractory period [PVARP]), and the PP interval (As-As) is shorter than the TARP. Thus, a Wenckebach upper rate response cannot occur. Every second P wave falls within the PVARP and is unsensed. The AV interval remains constant. Same format as Figure 30–10. (From Barold SS: Management of patients with dual-chamber pulse generators: Central role of pacemaker atrial refractory period. Learning Center *Highlights* (Heart House, American College of Cardiology) 5:10, 1990.)

sponse provides a smoother transition rather than a sudden decrease in the ventricular rate as the pacemaker shifts from a 1:1 ventricular response to fixed-ratio AV block. The Wenckebach upper rate response also allows some degree of AV synchrony.

The pacemaker Wenckebach upper rate response exhibits variability of the AV (As-Vp) interval, a sustained fast-paced ventricular rate (the programmed upper rate), and an occasional abrupt change in the ventricular beat-to-beat interval. Basically, a pacemaker Wenckebach sequence contains only two ventricular intervals: (1) Vp-Vp pacing at the URI and (2) Vp-Vp longer than the URI following the undetected P wave in the PVARP. The actual duration of the pause can be calculated with a formula published by Higano and Hayes[48] by knowing the PP interval, TARP, and URI. The *maximal* duration of the pause terminating the Wenckebach cycle measured between two consecutive ventricular stimuli (after a blocked or unsensed P wave) is equal to the sum of the PVARP, PP interval, and programmed AV interval, provided that the pulse generator senses the P wave that follows the unsensed one in the PVARP at the end of the Wenckebach sequence.[49] Should a P wave not occur before the end of the atrial escape (pacemaker VA) interval, the pause will be equal to the LRI, and the pacemaker will release Ap.

Artificial Versus Natural Wenckebach Phenomenon

There are important differences between the artificial and the natural Wenckebach phenomena:

1. Although a spontaneous, atypical AV nodal Wenckebach phenomenon may occasionally cause some regularization of the RR intervals, it is never associated with absolutely constant RR intervals, as seen with the pacemaker response to a rapid atrial rate. The intervals between the pacemaker stimuli are constant because they are locked at the URI.

2. There appears to be AV dissociation during the pacemaker Wenckebach period because the P waves march through the ventricular cycle. In contrast to spontaneous AV dissociation, in which atrial and ventricular events are unrelated, in pacemaker Wenckebach periods, there is a definite link between each P wave and its triggered ventricular stimulus.

3. The blocked P wave is not really blocked but is unsensed when it falls within the PVARP. The pacemaker then synchronizes its ventricular output to the next P wave.

Disadvantages of the Wenckebach Upper Rate Response

1. In patients with retrograde VA conduction, progressive lengthening of the AV delay to conform to the URI during the Wenckebach response may result in the atria being "ready" to accept a retrograde impulse generated by the ventricular-paced beat. Critical prolongation of the AV interval during a pacemaker Wenckebach sequence may therefore initiate endless-loop tachycardia (discussed later). Rarely, the same mechanism may also initiate endless-loop tachycardia during exercise in predisposed patients.[50, 51]

2. The hemodynamic benefit of AV synchrony is attenu-

ated or even lost because of the wide variability of the As-Vp intervals.

3. The pause at the end of a Wenckebach sequence may not be tolerated during exercise in some active patients. (The pause can be reduced or eliminated by sensor-driven rate smoothing during DDDR pacing, as discussed later.)

Mathematics of the Wenckebach Upper Rate Response

If w is equal to the increment of the AV interval per cycle during the Wenckebach upper rate response, w = URI − (PP interval). If W is equal to the maximal increment of the AV (As-Vp) interval, W = URI − TARP. Thus, the AV interval will vary from the basic value of As-Vp (as programmed) to a value equal to (As-Vp) + (URI − TARP). For example, if the URI = 600 msec, the AV interval = 200 msec, the PVARP = 200 msec, and the PP interval = 550 msec, the increment per cycle w = URI − (PP interval) = 50 msec. The maximal increment of the AV interval, W = URI − TARP = 600 − 400 = 200 msec. Thus, the As-Vp interval will vary from 200 to 400 msec. The Wenckebach ratio can be calculated according to the formula of Higano and Hayes[48] as follows: n = W/w = 4. If N is the next integer above n, N = 5, Wenckebach ratio = N + 1/N = 6/5. Thus, with the preceding parameters, a DDD pulse generator will exhibit 6:5 Wenckebach pacemaker AV block. The pacemaker will respond to an atrial rate faster than 100 ppm and less than 150 ppm with a Wenckebach upper rate response. When the atrial rate reaches 150 ppm, the Wenckebach upper rate response gives way to fixed-ratio AV block.

In contrast, if a DDD pulse generator were programmed with an AV interval equal to 200 msec, a PVARP equal to 250 msec, and an upper rate equal to 125 ppm (URI = 480 msec), it would be difficult to produce an actual pacemaker Wenckebach effect. Maximal prolongation of the AV interval during Wenckebach behavior (W interval) would be only 30 msec (480 − 450). The maximal duration of the AV interval would therefore be 230 msec. In the preceding situation in which the TARP is equal to 450 msec (corresponding to a rate of 133 ppm), the pulse generator will respond with a Wenckebach response to an atrial rate higher than 125 ppm but less than 133 ppm. When the atrial rate exceeds 133 ppm, fixed-ratio AV block will occur without a Wenckebach response. A short W period means that the pulse generator will respond basically with fixed-ratio AV block.

Relationship of Upper Rate Interval and Total Atrial Refractory Period: An Overview

Upper Rate Interval Shorter Than the Total Atrial Refractory Period

When the URI is programmed to a shorter value than the TARP (despite the fact that the programmer and the pulse generators may seem to have accepted the command), the pacemaker obviously cannot exhibit Wenckebach pacemaker AV block. The URI will be the longer of the two intervals; that is, equal to the TARP. The programmer should alert the operator that such values are not acceptable in the DDD mode. However, this paradoxical relationship (TARP > URI) may actually be programmable and clinically useful in some DDDR pacemakers, as discussed later.

Upper Rate Interval Equal to the Total Atrial Refractory Period

If a separately programmable URI is equal to the TARP, a Wenckebach upper rate response cannot occur, and the pulse generator will respond to fast atrial rates with only a fixed-ratio pacemaker AV block.

Upper Rate Interval Longer Than the Total Atrial Refractory Period

When the URI is longer than the TARP, the upper rate response of a DDD pulse generator depends on the duration of three variables: TARP, URI, and PP interval (corresponding to the atrial rate) and three situations can occur:

1. PP interval is longer than the URI. The pulse generator maintains 1:1 AV synchrony because the atrial rate is slower than the programmed upper rate.
2. PP interval is shorter than the URI. When the PP interval becomes shorter than the URI but remains longer than the TARP (i.e., the URI is longer than the PP interval, which is longer than the TARP), the pulse generator responds with a Wenckebach pacemaker AV block.
3. PP interval is shorter than the TARP. When the PP interval is shorter than the TARP (and therefore also shorter than the URI), a Wenckebach upper rate response cannot occur, and the upper rate response consists of only a fixed-ratio pacemaker AV block regardless of the duration of the separately programmable URI (Fig. 30–21). Therefore, when the URI is longer than the TARP, a progressive increase in the atrial rate (shortening of the PP interval) causes first a pacemaker Wenckebach upper rate response (when PP < URI); when the PP interval becomes equal to or shorter than the TARP, the upper rate response switches from pacemaker Wenckebach AV block to fixed-ratio pacemaker AV block.

Upper Rate and Duration of the Atrioventricular Interval

The AV interval initiated by atrial sensing As (i.e., As-Vp), and not the one initiated by Ap (i.e., Ap-Vp) (either equal to or longer than the As-Vp interval), determines the point at which fixed-ratio pacemaker AV block occurs, that is, when the PP interval becomes equal to or shorter than the TARP, where TARP = (As-Vp) + PVARP. In many pacemakers, As-Vp can be programmed to a value shorter than the Ap-Vp interval, thereby shortening the TARP during atrial sensing. In some pulse generators, the TARP can shorten further on exercise by one of three mechanisms: (1) the As-Vp decreases with an increase in the sensed atrial rate, sensor activity, or both (adaptive AV interval); (2) the PVARP shortens on exercise (adaptive PVARP); or (3) both the As-Vp interval and PVARP shorten on exercise. In terms of the upper rate response, abbreviation of the TARP, especially in relation to the AV interval initiated by atrial sensing (As-Vp < Ap-Vp), provides important advantages.

1. There is a shorter TARP duration (As-Vp + PVARP) compared with the situation in which As-Vp is equal to Ap-Vp. The shorter TARP induces fixed-ratio pacemaker AV block only at faster sensed atrial rates whenever the PP interval becomes equal to or shorter than the TARP.

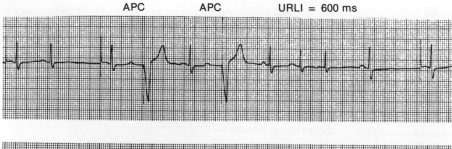

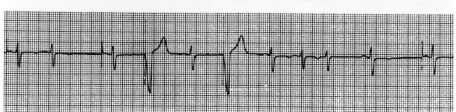

Figure 30–22. Two-lead electrocardiogram showing DDD pacing (ventricular-based lower rate timing) with sensed atrial premature contractions (APC) (lower rate interval [LRI] = 1000 msec; AV = 200 msec; upper rate interval [URI] = 600 msec; postventricular atrial refractory period [PVARP] = 155 msec). Note the extended AV interval generated by the APCs to conform to the URI. This response with single beats should not be called a Wenckebach upper rate response; rather, it is best called an AV extension upper rate response.

2. With a constant separately programmable URI, a shorter TARP widens the range of atrial rates associated with pacemaker Wenckebach AV block, that is, the Wenckebach upper rate response begins at the same atrial rate (determined by URI), but fixed-ratio pacemaker AV block begins at a faster atrial rate (determined by TARP).

3. A shorter TARP allows programming of a shorter (separately programmable) URI (keeping URI > TARP), with preservation of the Wenckebach pacemaker AV block response at faster atrial rates.

So-Called Wenckebach Upper Rate Response in Single Cycles

The response of a DDD pacemaker (with URI > TARP) to a sensed atrial extrasystole may at first appear complicated (Fig. 30–22). The AV interval engendered by a sensed premature atrial depolarization depends on its timing within the pacing cycle, bearing in mind that the release of a triggered ventricular stimulus must wait until the URI has timed out. Thus, an atrial extrasystole prolongs the As-Vp for a single

Table 30–2. Types of Wenckebach Upper Rate Responses

	ADURI Times Out to Completion	Partial or Complete AV Extension*	Event Terminating AV Interval	AV Intervals	P Wave in PVARP†	Variability of Vp-Vp or Vs-Vs Intervals	Pause at End of Wenckebach Sequence‡
Traditional Wenckebach Upper Rate Response							
DDD	Yes	Complete	Vp	Variable	Yes	Yes	Yes (≤LRI)
DDDR	Yes	Complete	Vp	Variable	Yes	Yes	Yes (<LRI)
LRI > SDI > ADURI							
DDDR	Yes	Complete	Vp	Variable	Yes	No	No
SDI = ADURI							
Repetitive Pre-empted Wenckebach Upper Rate Response							
1. Ventricular sensed form	No	Partial	Vs	Relatively constant	No	No	NA
2. Ventricular paced form (DDDR)							
ADURI > SDURI							
PP < SDI < ADURI	No	Partial	Vp	Variable	Yes	No	No
PP = SDI < ADURI	No	Partial	Vp	Relatively constant	No	No	NA

ADURI, atrial-driven upper rate interval; LRI, lower rate interval; NA, not applicable; PP, interval between two consecutive P waves; PVARP, postventricular atrial refractory period; SDI, sensor-driven interval; SDURI, sensor-driven upper rate interval.

Ventricular-based lower rate timing. Pacemakers with atrial-based lower rate timing in the DDDR mode allowing As-Vp > Ap-Vp are not available.

*Partial AV extension: AV interval terminates before ADURI has timed out to its entirety. Complete AV extension occurs when the AV interval terminates coincidentally with completion of the ADURI. An upper rate response with extension of the AV interval can occur only when TARP < PP < ADURI.

†P wave in the last cycle of Wenckebach sequence.

‡End of Wenckebach sequence is defined as the cycle containing the unsensed P wave in the PVARP. No pauses occur when P waves do not fall periodically within the PVARP.

From Barold SS: Wenckebach upper rate response of dual chamber pacemakers: A reappraisal and proposed new terminology. PACE 18:244, 1995.

cycle to conform to the URI. The URI can be identified on the ECG by moving calipers from a premature ventricular stimulus back to the previous ventricular event. If this interval corresponds to the URI, it provides presumptive proof that an atrial-sensed event occurred between the two ventricular events bracketing the URI.

Some workers have called this response a manifestation of Wenckebach upper rate behavior, creating potential confusion because a Wenckebach sequence does not actually occur. Rather, a single-cycle response is best described as an "AV extension" upper rate response (to conform to the relationship URI > TARP).

Repetitive Pre-Empted Wenckebach Upper Rate Response

In a traditional Wenckebach upper rate response, the As-Vp intervals (except for the one terminating a pause) lengthen progressively beyond the basic programmed duration and terminate coincidentally with completion of the atrial-driven URI (the shortest Vs-Vp or Vp-Vp interval when the last Vp is triggered by an As; the pacemaker releases the terminal Vp only at the completion of the atrial-driven URI initiated by the preceding Vs or Vp) (Table 30–2). In contrast, a repetitive pre-empted Wenckebach upper rate response consists of an attempted Wenckebach upper rate response characterized by the continual partial or incomplete extension of the programmed AV interval (see Table 30–2). The term *pre-empted* is preferable to "aborted," previously used to describe this type of pacemaker behavior. In a pre-empted response, the AV intervals terminate before completion of the atrial-driven URI (Fig. 30–23). In other words, the extended AV intervals never acquire the full extension dictated by the atrial-driven URI (partial extension, in which the AV interval is extended but an early Vp or Vs event terminates the AV interval before the atrial-driven URI has timed out; this is the hallmark of a repetitive pre-empted Wenckebach upper rate response). In a pre-empted response, an early sensed or early paced ventricular event (Vs or Vp) continually usurps delivery of the ventricular output, so that the atrial-driven URI is continually reset before timing out in its entirety.[52, 53] Thus, all other factors remaining constant, the elimination of the early Vs or Vp event would allow full extension of the As-Vp interval and transform a repetitive pre-empted Wenckebach upper rate response into a typical Wenckebach upper rate response with emission of Vp at the completion of the atrial-driven URI (except during the pause). Repetitive pre-empted Wenckebach upper rate sequences can be classified as either ventricular sensed or ventricular paced according to the events that end the partially extended AV intervals.

Ventricular-Sensed Repetitive Pre-Empted Wenckebach Upper Rate Response

In patients with complete AV block (or substantial prolongation of AV conduction), a classic Wenckebach upper rate response occurs during DDD or DDDR pacing only when TARP < PP < atrial-driven URI. However, in patients with preserved AV conduction when TARP < PP < atrial-driven URI, a DDD pacemaker can continually sense the conducted QRS complex (Vs) before the atrial-driven URI times out in its entirety (or in the case of a DDDR, provided that the

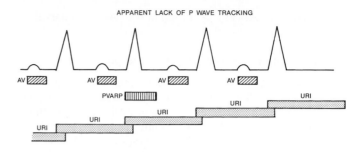

APPARENT LACK OF P WAVE TRACKING

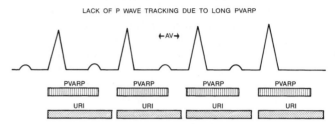

LACK OF P WAVE TRACKING DUE TO LONG PVARP

Figure 30–23. *Top panel,* Diagrammatic representation of a ventricular-sensed repetitive pre-empted Wenckebach upper rate response by a DDD pacemaker. The spontaneous RR interval is shorter than the upper rate interval (URI). A relatively early P wave initiates an extended AV interval to conform to the relationship URI > total atrial refractory period (TARP). However, the next QRS complex (Vs) occurs before the URI has timed out, so that the partially extended AV interval cannot attain the full duration dictated by the URI. Vs, therefore, usurps control of the ventricular channel from the URI, and the pacemaker cannot deliver Vp. The process perpetuates itself as long as the RR interval remains shorter than the URI (spontaneous rate faster than the programmed upper rate). The sequence simulates P-wave undersensing due to a long postventricular atrial refractory period (PVARP; *lower diagram*) or low-amplitude atrial electrogram outside the PVARP. (From Barold SS, Falkoff MD, Ong LS, et al: Electrocardiography of DDD pacemakers. B. Multiprogrammability, follow-up and troubleshooting. *In* Saksena S, Goldschlager N [eds]: Electrical Therapy for Cardiac Arrhythmias: Pacing, Antitachycardia Devices, Catheter Ablation. Philadelphia, WB Saunders, 1990: 265–301.)

SDI is longer than the atrial-driven URI, as discussed later). In this situation, it is the sensed conducted QRS complex that prevents the development of a typical Wenckebach upper rate response that would otherwise occur if AV conduction were sufficiently impaired. Continual sensing of the conducted QRS complex before completion of the atrial-driven URI creates a repetitive pre-empted Wenckebach upper rate response because it leads to continual partial extension of the AV interval.[53] Figure 30–23 shows the mechanism of this form of Wenckebach upper rate response. An early Vs resets the atrial-driven URI, then initiates a self-perpetuating mechanism, with Vs continually pre-empting the expected Vp dictated by the atrial-driven URI. This sequence represents a ventricular-sensed form of repetitive pre-empted Wenckebach upper rate response simply because ventricular-sensed events terminate the partially extended AV intervals.

A ventricular-sensed repetitive pre-empted Wenckebach upper rate response thus has the following characteristics:

- RR or Vs-Vs interval < atrial-driven URI (spontaneous ventricular rate faster than pacemaker atrial-driven upper rate)

- PR interval (As-Vs) > programmed As-Vp interval (a feature simulating atrial undersensing)
- No unsensed or "dropped" P waves (in the PVARP), as in a typical Wenckebach upper rate response

The process continues until the sinus rate slows to a critical value. When the Vs-Vs interval lengthens beyond the atrial-driven URI, the pacemaker will emit Vp after a nonextended As-Vp interval. Leung and colleagues[54] recently described the same phenomenon in two patients with DDDR pacemakers and called it a modified upper rate behavior with pseudoextension of the AV interval. These investigators argued that this phenomenon was due to a sensor-based algorithm against supraventricular tachyarrhythmias. In fact, their observations can be simply explained in terms of a relatively long atrial-driven URI without invoking sensor activity (other than the possible indirect effect of lengthening the atrial-driven URI as in the conditional ventricular tracking limit of the Relay DDDR device (Intermedics, Inc., Freeport, TX) or the DDDR mode).

The ventricular-sensed form of repetitive pre-empted Wenckebach upper rate response is more likely to emerge during exercise testing (or other forms of activity), especially in patients with relatively normal AV conduction. It is an extremely important observation in patients treated with dual-chamber pacemakers for obstructive hypertrophic cardiomyopathy (Figs. 30–24 and 30–25). In this respect, Leung and colleagues[54] emphasized that this form of upper rate response, which occurs in patients with relatively normal AV conduction, is favored by a relatively long atrial-driven URI (slow atrial-driven upper rate), a short programmed AV interval, and an increased sinus rate faster than the atrial-driven upper rate at rest or with slight exercise.

Ventricular Paced Repetitive Pre-empted Wenckebach Upper Rate Response

This form of Wenckebach upper rate response can only occur in the DDDR mode under certain circumstances when delivery of Vp occurs before termination of the atrial-driven URI[52, 53] (discussed later). In this context, shortening or obliteration of the pause at the end of a Wenckebach sequence during DDDR pacing (discussed later) is best called an "aborted Wenckebach pause" rather than an "aborted Wenckebach upper rate response."

Wenckebach Upper Rate Response and Tachycardia Termination Algorithm

When the sinus rate produces a PP interval essentially equal to the URI but longer than the TARP (URI > TARP), the pacemaker continues to function with an extended As-Vp interval (longer than the programmed As-Vp) to conform to the URI. In this situation, Wenckebach "progression" can occur for a long time without discernible prolongation of the AV (As-Vp) delay. In the absence of the characteristic pause at the end of the pacemaker Wenckebach block upper rate response, this type of upper rate behavior can resemble a ventricular paced repetitive pre-empted Wenckebach upper rate response (discussed later) but differs from the latter

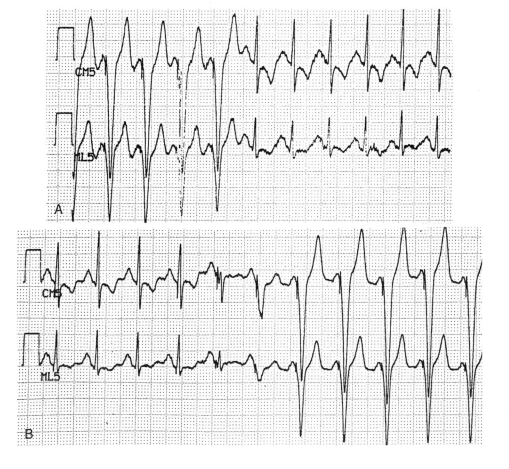

Figure 30–24. *A,* Apparent loss of atrial tracking related to upper rate limitation shown in ECGs from a patient with an Intermedics Cosmos II DDD pacemaker implanted for obstructive hypertrophic cardiomyopathy. Lower rate interval (LRI) = 1000 msec; upper rate interval (URI) = 500 msec; AV = 75 msec. The ECG was recorded during a treadmill stress test. The P waves on the right were sensed (documented later by markers during repeated exercise, not shown), but the pacemaker does not emit Vp because a QRS complex occurs before the termination of the 75-msec AV interval, thereby producing a sensed repetitive pre-empted Wenckebach upper rate response. *B,* Same patient as panel A. During recovery of the stress test, as the sinus rate slows, the AV interval gradually shortens in a few cycles until it reaches 75 msec. This produces a "reverse Wenckebach" response with gradually more ventricular capture (fusion beats) until full ventricular capture is re-established, preceded by As-Vp of 75 msec. (*A* and *B* from Douard H, Barold SS, Broustet JP: Too much protection may be a nuisance. Stimucoeur 25:183–187, 1997.)

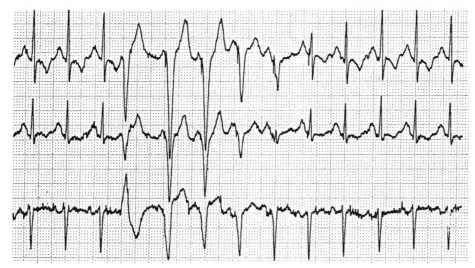

Figure 30–25. Same patient as in Figure 30–24. At the end of exercise during a sensed repetitive pre-empted Wenckebach upper rate response on the left, a ventricular premature contraction (VPC; fourth beat) disrupts the regularity of the rhythm. The sinus rhythm is not disturbed, but the fourth P wave falls in the postventricular atrial refractory period (PVARP) generated by the VPC. Therefore, the P wave following the VPC triggers Vp because the post VPC-pause permitted the upper rate interval (URI) to time out. Because the sinus rate is still faster than the URI, a typical Wenckebach upper rate response then occurs, with gradual increase in the AV interval. The Wenckebach upper rate response does not progress to its completion because the longer AV interval allows the emergence of spontaneous ventricular activation. The Vs-Vs interval remains shorter than the URI, and the sensed repetitive pre-empted Wenckebach upper rate response returns. (From Douard H, Barold S, Broustet JP: Too much protection may be a nuisance. Stimucoeur 25:183–187, 1997.)

because the As-Vp interval and the URI both time out in their entirety.

Some pulse generators possess a tachycardia-terminating algorithm to abolish endless-loop tachycardia automatically (discussed later). In one device, after 15 paced ventricular beats (triggered by sensed P waves) at the URI, the 16th paced ventricular beat is blocked by inhibiting the delivery of the 16th ventricular stimulus.[17] This pause terminates endless-loop tachycardia by re-establishing AV synchrony with the next pacing cycle. This algorithm is based on the concept that endless-loop tachycardia occurs at the programmed upper rate. Although this is frequently the case, it is not always true. An algorithm linked to the URI does not come into play when the cycle length of the endless-loop tachycardia is longer than the URI; that is, the sum of the retrograde VA conduction time and the programmed AV interval is longer than the URI. Occasionally, the tachycardia termination algorithm comes into play during sinus tachycardia, particularly when the programmed upper rate is relatively slow. Sinus tachycardia with a PP interval slightly shorter than the URI can cause a Wenckebach progression without discernible prolongation of the AV delay, especially if the programmed AV interval is relatively long and the P wave is concealed within the T wave of the previous beat. This Wenckebach sequence does not terminate in the usual fashion with a P wave ultimately falling within the PVARP (Fig. 30–26). Rather, after 15 cycles at the URI, the pulse generator activates the tachycardia termination algorithm and omits the 16th ventricular stimulus. The P wave never falls in the PVARP, but a pause occurs, although its mechanism differs from that seen in the classic pacemaker Wenckebach block upper rate response (see Fig. 30–26).

Such premature termination of a Wenckebach sequence could be called an aborted Wenckebach upper rate response. The same terminology would apply in other circumstances, e.g., when Wenckebach-like block is terminated by a ventricular extrasystole.

Wenckebach-Related Timing Cycles

The plethora of terms used to describe Wenckebach-related timing cycles, at times contradictory, is bound to generate confusion. For the sake of clarity, the maximum AV interval increment during Wenckebach-like block (URI − TARP) could simply be labeled W, whereas any AV interval increment < W could be labeled w.[53] Because the last cycle in a Wenckebach sequence (associated with the unsensed P wave) can now become close to, equal to, or even shorter than (discussed under rate-adopting pacing) the prevailing Vp-Vp interval, one can no longer describe it in terms of a *Wenckebach pause*. The term *last interval* also loses its meaning when all the intervals in a Wenckebach sequence remain constant. The terms *Wenckebach interval, Wenckebach cycle, Wenckebach escape interval,* and *Wenckebach escape rate* are also inappropriate to characterize the interval containing the unsensed P wave, and these terms should be removed from the pacemaker lexicon. In a Wenckebach sequence with varying AV intervals, the last cycle is the only one that contains the unsensed P wave. Consequently, this last interval could be called the *atrial unsensed interval* or *cycle*, a more precise term applicable to all forms of Wenckebach sequences during DDD or DDDR pacing regardless of the type of LRT.

```
LOWER RATE  =  70 ppm (857 ms)
UPPER RATE  =  94 ppm (638 ms)
AV INTERVAL =  200 ms
PVARP       =  270 ms
```

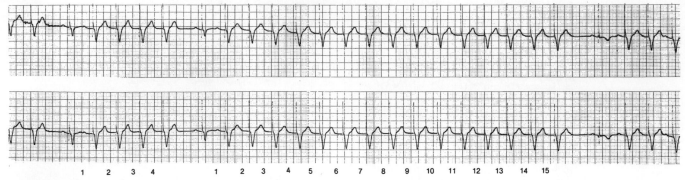

Figure 30–26. Operation of the tachycardia termination algorithm of the Intermedics Cosmos I DDD pulse generator during sinus rhythm (atrial escape interval [AEI] = 657 msec). The sinus rate is close to the programmed upper rate of 94 ppm. On the *left,* there is a pacemaker Wenckebach sequence with four cycles (indicated by the numbers 1–4). The P wave following cycle 4 falls in the PVARP and is unsensed. The subsequent AEI is equal to 657 plus the VA extension (300 msec for this particular pulse generator after a preceding cycle at the upper rate interval [URI]). This is equal to 957 msec. The extended AEI or VA interval terminates prematurely because of P-wave sensing. The next sequence is another pacemaker Wenckebach response with very small increments of the AV (As-Vp) interval, so that all the cycles occur at the URI and no P waves fall in the postventricular atrial refractory period (PVARP). The pulse generator activates the tachycardia-terminating algorithm after detecting 15 cycles at the URI. The pause at the end of the tachycardia-terminating algorithm is equal to the URI (638) + AEI (657) = 1295 msec. This interval is aborted by sensing of a P wave about 1000 msec after the previous ventricular stimulus. Note that the pause (Vp-As) after the tachycardia termination algorithm is longer than the maximum extended AEI or VA interval; that is, 1000 msec is longer than 957 msec, the maximum duration of the extended AEI from the previous 6:5 Wenckebach sequence. Note that the sinus P wave that follows the 15th ventricular-paced beat does not fall in the PVARP. (From Barold SS, Falkoff MD, Ong LS, et al: Upper rate response of DDD pacemakers. *In* Barold SS, Mugica J [eds]: New Perspectives in Cardiac Pacing. Mt Kisco, NY, Futura, 1988, pp 121–172.)

■ RATE-ADAPTIVE PACEMAKERS

Single-Chamber Pacemakers: Lower Rate Interval

In the VVIR (AAIR) mode, the LRI is variable and changes according to the activity of the sensor (which monitors activity in terms of body vibration, minute ventilation volume, temperature, and so forth) designed to increase the pacing rate with effort. At any given time, the duration of the LRI can be either its basic programmed value or the constantly changing sensor-controlled LRI, whichever is shorter (Fig. 30–27). The shortest sensor-driven LRI is equal to the programmed sensor-driven URI.

Dual-Chamber Pacemakers: Lower Rate Interval

In the DDDR mode (as in the VVIR mode), the LRI varies as the sensor-driven rate varies. At any given time, the duration of the LRI can be either the programmed LRI or the constantly changing sensor-driven LRI, whichever is shorter (see Fig. 30–27). The shortest sensor-driven LRI is equal to the programmed sensor-driven URI.

DDDR Pacemakers: Upper Rate Response

Control of the upper rate involves (1) only two intervals (TARP and PP intervals) with a simple DDD pacemaker; (2) three intervals (TARP, PP interval, and URI) with a more complex DDD pacemaker with a separately programmable URI that is longer than the TARP; and (3) four intervals

(TARP, PP interval, atrial-driven URI, and sensor-driven URI) in DDDR devices.[6, 52]

A DDDR device may function with either a common ventricular URI or two separate ventricular URIs, as follows: (1) atrial-driven URI (sometimes known as the maximum tracking rate) and (2) sensor-driven URI. The *atrial-driven* URI refers to the shortest Vs-Vp or Vp-Vp interval in which the last Vp is triggered by an atrial-sensed event (As). The pacemaker releases the terminal Vp output only at the completion of the atrial-driven URI initiated by the preceding Vs or Vp. The *sensor-driven* URI refers to the shortest Vs-Vp or Vp-Vp interval in which the last Vp is controlled by *sensor* activity. The pacemaker releases the last Vp output only at the completion of the sensor-driven URI initiated by the preceding Vs or Vp. Note that both the sensor-driven URI and the atrial-driven URI begin with either Vs or Vp and are therefore ventricular intervals.

The relationship between the sensor-driven URI and atrial-driven URI can take one of three forms[52, 53]: (1) a sensor-driven URI that is longer than the atrial-driven URI, that is, a sensor-driven upper rate that is slower than the atrial-driven upper rate; (2) a sensor-driven URI that is equal to the atrial-driven URI (common upper rates); or (3) a sensor-driven URI that is shorter than the atrial-driven URI, that is, a sensor-driven upper rate that is faster than the atrial-driven upper rate. The upper rate behavior of DDDR pacemakers is described in detail later in the text.

■ TYPES OF DUAL-CHAMBER PACEMAKERS

Simpler pacing modes can be derived by the removal of "building blocks" from the DDD mode and equalizing cer-

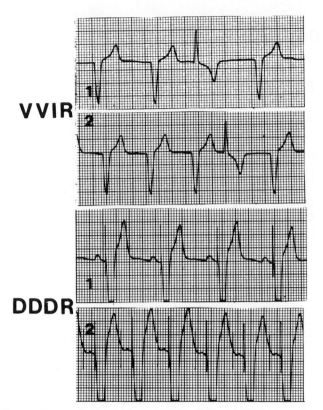

VVIR

DDDR

Figure 30–27. Response of rate-adaptive VVIR and DDDR pacemakers to exercise. *Top,* VVIR. The tiny bipolar stimuli cannot be discerned. *Panel 1* shows pacing at the programmed lower rate interval (LRI)—857 msec (corresponding to a rate of 70 ppm). The third beat is a ventricular extrasystole sensed by the pacemaker. The escape interval is essentially equal to the automatic interval. *Panel 2* shows the response on exercise when the ventricular rate increases to about 88 ppm (sensor-driven interval = 680 msec), so that the sensed ventricular extrasystole now recycles the pacemaker with an escape interval of about 680 msec. *Bottom,* DDDR. *Panel 1* shows DDD pacing with sensing of P waves (LRI = 1000 msec). In *panel 2,* during exercise, the AV sequential pacing rate increases to 107 ppm (cycle length, 560 msec). (From Barold SS, Falkoff MD, Ong LS, et al: Cardiac pacing in the nineties: Technologic, hemodynamic, and electrophysiologic considerations in the selection of the optimal mode of pacing. *In* Rackley CE [ed]: Challenges in Cardiology I. Mt Kisco, NY, Futura, 1992, pp 39–83.)

tain timing intervals.[44] A DDD pacemaker may have to be downgraded to a simpler mode for the treatment of certain complications. In contrast, a DDDR pacemaker consists of a DDD system upgraded with the addition of a non–P-wave sensor to provide an increase in the pacing rate in patients with abnormal atrial chronotropic function on exercise.

DVI Mode

Dedicated permanent DVI pacemakers (but not the DVI mode as a programmable option) are now obsolete. The DVI mode may be considered as the DDD mode with the PVARP extending through the entire AEI[44] (Fig. 30–28). Thus, in the DVI mode, the TARP in effect lasts through the entire LRI because during the AV interval, the atrial channel of a DDD pacemaker always remains refractory. The URI cannot exist because a DVI pacemaker cannot sense atrial activity.

In the DVI mode, therefore, the LRI, TARP, and URI are equal. Asynchronous atrial pacing may precipitate atrial fibrillation.

In the uncommitted DVI mode,[55] the ventricular channel can sense through the entire duration of the AV interval (no ventricular blanking period), whereas in the partially committed DVI mode, the ventricular channel can sense only during part of the AV interval beyond the initial ventricular blanking period[56] (see Fig. 30–28). In contrast, a committed DVI pacemaker may be regarded as having a ventricular blanking period that encompasses the entire AV interval, rendering crosstalk impossible.[57] These modes are mostly of historical interest and are rarely used nowadays.

DDI Mode

The DDI mode, which conforms to the original three-letter identification code drafted long before this pacing mode was considered, was first mentioned by Levine and Seltzer[58] in 1983. A year later, Floro and colleagues[59] described the DDI mode in detail, characterizing it as "less complex, and easier to understand than the DDD mode." This statement is not really true because the functional characteristics, limitations, and adverse effects of and indications for the DDI and DDIR modes are still not fully appreciated. The reason for this lack of understanding stems in part from the widely divergent descriptions of the DDI mode in the literature[60, 61] (Table 30–3).

Unlike the ventricular response of the traditional DDD and VDD modes, the *paced* ventricular rate must always remain constant regardless of the atrial rate and it cannot exceed the programmed lower rate during normal function. In the DDIR mode it is always equal to the sensor-driven rate.

In the DDI mode when the pacemaker senses spontaneous atrial activity beyond the PVARP, it inhibits release of the atrial stimulus at the completion of the AEI. The subsequent Vp can *only* occur at the completion of the LRI. In this way, it prevents competitive atrial pacing characteristics of the

Table 30–3. Characterizations of DDI Mode in the Literature

AAI mode with ventricular backup
AAI and VVI modes
DVI mode without the potential for atrial competition by virtue of atrial sensing
Improved or upgraded DVI with atrial sensing
Upgrade of DVI noncommitted pacing
Intermediate pacemaker between DVI and DDD modes
Hybrid of DVI and DDD modes
DDD mode without P-wave tracking capability
Non–P-synchronous DDD pacing
Dual-chamber pacing and sensing, nontracking
AV sequential, non–P-synchronous pacing with dual-chamber pacing
Dual-sequential, atrial-, and ventricular-inhibited pacing
Atrial- and ventricular-inhibited dual-chamber pacing
Demand atrial and ventricular pacing with disabling of atrial triggering of ventricular stimulation
DDD mode (ventricular-based lower rate timing) with identical upper rate (interval) and lower rate (interval)

From Barold SS: Optimal pacing in the brady-tachy syndrome. Cardiol Rev 5:63, 1997.

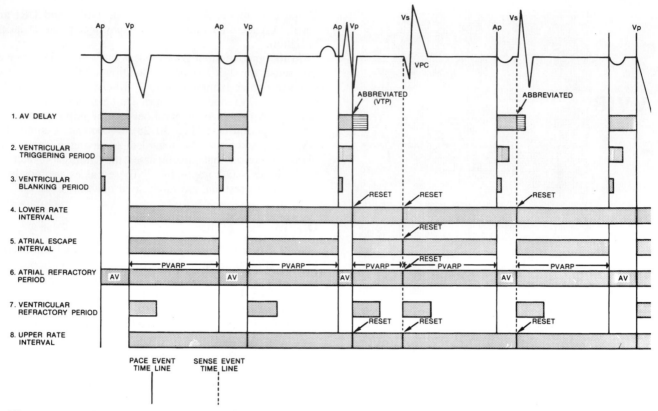

Figure 30–28. DVI mode (partially committed). The total atrial refractory period (TARP), lower rate interval (LRI), and upper rate interval (URI) are equal. Atrial pacing is asynchronous. The AV interval is longer than the ventricular safety pacing (VSP; triggering) period, and the latter is in turn longer than the ventricular blanking period. The third P wave is unsensed because the atrial channel functions asynchronously. The first spontaneous QRS complex (between the third Ap and the third Vp) is sensed within the VSP period (ventricular triggering period [VTP]), so that the ventricular channel delivers Vp at the completion of the VSP period. Therefore, the third AV interval (Ap-Vp) is abbreviated by premature delivery of Vp. The fourth Ap initiates an AV interval that is terminated prematurely because Vs occurs before the AV interval has timed out; premature emission of Vp does not occur because Vs is sensed beyond the VSP period. The fourth beat is a ventricular extrasystole (ventricular premature contraction [VPC]) sensed by the ventricular channel. In an uncommitted DVI device, the ventricular blanking period and VTP are absent. In a committed DVI device, the ventricular blanking period is equal to the AV interval. Same format as Figure 30–10. (From Barold SS, Falkoff MD, Ong LS, et al: All dual-chamber pacemakers function in the DDD mode. Am Heart J 115:1353, 1988.)

DVI mode in which atrial sensing does not occur. A DDI pacemaker senses atrial signals but does not track them (Fig. 30–29). In other words, the pacemaker does not use a sensed atrial signal to generate a *physiologic* AV interval according to its programmed value. Therefore, in the DDIR mode, only the AV delay starting with an atrial stimulus can be programmed. Because atrial sensing in effect does not trigger ventricular pacing in the traditional sense, a shorter AV interval after atrial sensing than atrial pacing cannot occur.

Timing Cycles

Constancy of the paced ventricular rate in the DDI mode is best achieved with ventricular-based LRT after a paced or sensed ventricular event; that is, LRI starts with Vp or Vs, and the AEI always remains constant.

With ventricular-based LRT, the DDI mode can be considered the same as the DDD mode with identical URI and LRI.[62] Like the DDD mode, the DDI mode requires an LRI, AV delay, PVARP, VRP, and crosstalk intervals (ventricular blanking and safety pacing), but no URI, because LRI equals URI. A sensor-driven URI is obviously required for the DDIR mode (i.e., the shortest rate-adaptive LRI). An atrial-

sensed event may be considered to initiate an AV interval that terminates (as in the DDD mode) only at completion of the URI (identical to the LRI) with the release of the ventricular stimulus—hence the long As-Vp intervals with sensing of early sinus P waves or atrial extrasystoles. The pacemaker cannot increase its ventricular pacing rate in response to an atrial rate faster than the programmed lower rate because the URI and LRI are identical. Similarly, a DDIR pacemaker cannot increase its ventricular pacing rate in response to an atrial rate faster than the prevailing sensor-driven (lower) rate.

The above statements do not really contradict the traditional concept that atrial tracking does not occur in the DDI mode because in both conceptual models of the DDI mode, tracking with a *physiologic* AV interval does not exist. Levine[41] has indicated that the designation of the DDI mode as an equivalent to the DDD mode with equal URI and LRI is erroneous. Yet the circuit designer creates the DDI mode from the DDD mode by simply equalizing the URI and LRI electronically on the pacemaker chip. Similarly, in a DDI pacemaker without a specifically programmable DDI mode, the latter can be obtained clinically by programming identi-

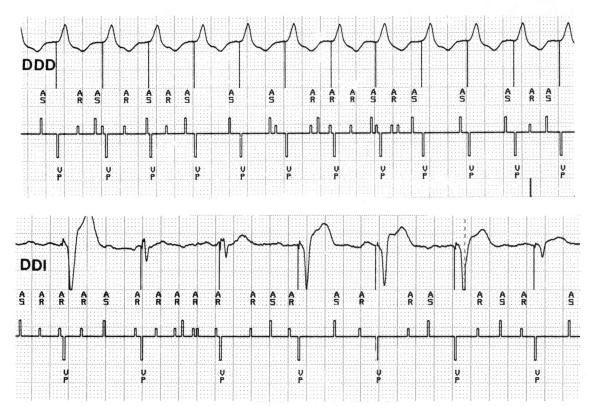

Figure 30–29. *Top,* DDD pacing in a patient with paroxysmal atrial flutter-fibrillation. The pacemaker tracks atrial activity, resulting in a fast-paced ventricular rate. The rate-adaptive AV delay shortens the As-Vp interval according to the sensed atrial rate (third As-Vp interval). The As-Vp intervals are variable because Vp-Vp intervals cannot violate the upper rate interval (URI). URI = 500 msec, programmed As-Vp interval = 200 msec. *Bottom,* DDI pacing in a different patient with paroxysmal atrial flutter-fibrillation. The ventricular paced rate remains constant at 70 ppm. Most of the paced beats exhibit fusion with supraventricular QRS complexes. Note that the DDI mode is indistinguishable from the VVI mode (ignoring event markers). Lower rate interval (LRI) = 857 msec (rate = 70 ppm); postventricular atrial refractory period (PVARP) = 380 msec. (From Barold SS: DDI and DDIR modes of pacing: An overview. Med Intell Cardiac Pacing Electrophysiol 14(4):2, 1996.)

cal upper and lower rates, provided that the LRT is ventricular-based.

Behavior of the DDI Mode

Atrial and Ventricular Stimuli. The DDI mode provides AV synchrony when the programmed rate exceeds the spontaneous atrial rate and AV conduction is slower than the programmed AV delay, so that both channels pace sequentially, a situation that provides no advantage over DDD pacing.

No Stimuli With Relatively Normal Atrioventricular Conduction. If the spontaneous atrial rate exceeds the programmed lower rate (PP interval < LRI), the P waves and conducted QRS complexes inhibit the pulse generator, a situation that provides no advantage over DDD pacing.

Normal Atrial Chronotropic Function With Atrioventricular Block. When the sinus rate exceeds the programmed lower rate in patients with AV block and normal atrial chronotropic function, AV synchrony (at the programmed AV interval) does not occur in the DDI mode. P waves sensed by the atrial channel gradually march through the pacing cycles, moving closer and closer to the preceding paced ventricular beat, a situation that produces constantly

changing AV intervals, mostly unphysiologic in duration regardless of the programmed AV interval (Fig. 30–30). More obvious AV dissociation occurs with faster atrial rates. The pacemaker therefore functions like the VVI mode (with AV dissociation), except when the P wave falls in the PVARP (and is unsensed), whereupon the pulse generator delivers an atrial stimulus at the termination of the AEI (ventricular stimuli with occasional atrial stimuli).

The relatively long periods of AV dissociation favored by a relatively short PVARP (because release of atrial stimuli is inhibited by the sensed P waves) may not be tolerated in some patients because they create a pacemaker syndrome at rest (even in the absence of retrograde VA conduction). In this respect, in patients with implanted pacemakers, Sulke and associates[63] demonstrated that "mode switching" from the DDI mode (with AV sequential pacing) to the functional VVI mode with mild exertion associated with an increase in atrial rate (faster than the paced ventricular rate) was not acceptable to most patients. The perceived general sense of well-being was similar when the DDI mode was compared with the VVI mode. A comparable situation associated with the pacemaker syndrome can occur in the DDIR mode on exercise in patients with complete AV block when the sinus rate exceeds the sensor-driven rate and the pacemaker functions essentially as if in the VVIR mode.

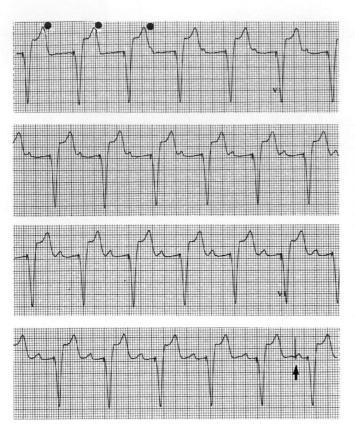

Figure 30–30. DDI pacing in a patient with complete AV and VA block. (The four ECG strips are continuous.) In this patient the PP interval was shorter than the LRI before the ECG was recorded. However, this ECG was registered when the sinus rate was only slightly slower than the programmed lower rate. The pacemaker senses all the P waves that gradually move away from the preceding QRS complexes until the last beat, when an atrial stimulus probably causes an atrial fusion beat. Note that the movement of the P waves is opposite to that in Figure 31; however, in both cases, DDI pacing causes AV dissociation. Barring the last beat, the ECG resembles VVI pacing with AV dissociation. The solid black circles correspond to sensed sinus P waves just beyond the PVARP. LRI = 857 msec (rate = 70 ppm); AV = 200 msec, PVARP = 300 msec. (From Barold SS: DDI and DDIR modes of pacing: An overview. Med Intell Cardiac Pacing Electrophysiol 14(4):2, 1996.)

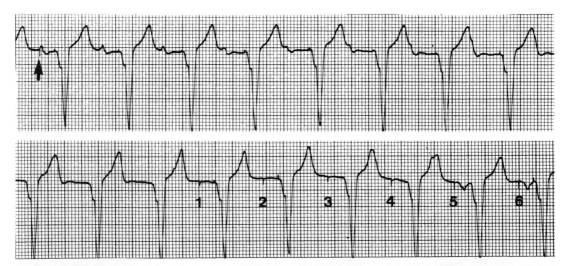

Figure 30–31. DDI pacing in a patient with complete AV and VA block. (The *top* and *bottom* ECG strips are continuous.) The first ventricular-paced beat is preceded by Ap *(arrow)*. The P waves then march through the pacing cycles, gradually getting closer and closer to the preceding QRS complexes. The atrial channel senses the P waves and inhibits atrial output until a P wave falls within the postventricular atrial refractory period (PVARP) and is therefore unsensed. At that point, the pacemaker releases an atrial stimulus (1) at the termination of the atrial escape interval. The first (1) and next three (2 to 4) atrial stimuli are ineffectual because they occur in the atrial myocardial refractory period generated by unsensed atrial depolarization (sinus P waves) within the long PVARP. The fifth and sixth atrial stimuli (5 and 6) are effectual because the sinus P waves within the PVARP are now sufficiently removed from the succeeding atrial stimuli. This form of competitive atrial pacing can be prevented with a rate-adaptive PVARP that shortens with an increasing pacing rate. Lower rate interval (LRI) = 750 msec (rate = 80 ppm); AV = 180 msec, PVARP = 400 msec, PP < LRI. (From Barold SS: DDI and DDIR modes of pacing: An overview. Med Intell Cardiac Pacing Electrophysiol 14(4):2, 1996.)

Ventricular Stimuli Only: Paroxysmal Supraventricular Tachycardia. When supraventricular tachycardia (SVT) is not particularly fast, the response of the pacemaker will be basically similar to that in sinus rhythm with occasional atrial stimulation. The latter does not occur when the pacemaker senses a rapid atrial rate. During rapid SVT, an unsensed P or f wave is quickly followed by another that is sensed beyond the PVARP but before termination of the AEI. In this way, rapid SVT continually inhibits the atrial output of the pacemaker, which therefore emits no atrial stimuli[60, 61] (see Fig. 30–29). Then, a DDIR pacemaker merely paces at the programmed lower ventricular rate or at the sensor-driven ventricular rate. For example, during atrial fibrillation, when the pacemaker continually senses atrial activity, the DDI mode looks exactly like VVI pacing without any atrial stimuli whatsoever (ventricular stimuli only).

Duration of Atrioventricular Intervals. An AV interval that is shorter after atrial sensing than after atrial pacing—an important feature of DDD (DDDR) systems—is incompatible with the DDI mode. With atrial sensing, the As-Vp interval becomes variable, but it is never equal to or shorter than the programmed Ap-Vp interval. Thus, the As-Vp interval (with no tracking) is always longer than the programmed Ap-Vp interval. During DDIR pacing, when the Ap-Vp interval shortens according to sensor input, the As-Vp interval at any given time will also be longer than the abbreviated rate-adaptive Ap-Vp interval.

Atrial Competition. No atrial competition occurs except with a substantial increase in the ventricular pacing rate in the DDI or DDIR mode when the pacemaker can discharge its atrial stimulus relatively close to a preceding P wave unsensed in a relatively long PVARP. Atrial stimulation may then fall in the atrial vulnerable period or may be ineffectual if delivered in the myocardial atrial refractory period generated by the preceding atrial depolarization (Fig. 30–31). During DDIR pacing, competitive atrial pacing may be reduced or eliminated by incorporating an adaptive PVARP that shortens as the pacing rate increases.[64]

Ventriculoatrial Synchrony. In the DDI mode, sensing of retrograde P waves due to VA conduction (beyond the PVARP) produces a pacemaker endless-loop arrangement

(obviously at the programmed lower rate) similar to its counterpart (endless-loop tachycardia) in the DDD mode, an arrangement capable of causing the pacemaker syndrome, as in the VVI mode with retrograde VA conduction[65, 66] (Figs. 30–32 and 30–33).

Atrial Stimuli Only (Ventricular Inhibition). In the DDI mode, as in the DDD mode with ventricular-based LRT, when Ap-Vs is shorter than Ap-Vp, the sequence Ap-Vs-Ap-Vs causes an increase in the atrial pacing rate and an increase in the ventricular rate (the Vs-Vs interval shortens), but the ventricular-paced rate cannot increase by definition[28, 29] (Fig. 30–34).

Increase in Paced Ventricular Rate. In the DDIR mode, the pacemaker increases the paced ventricular rate only in response to sensor input. In the DDI mode (with ventricular-based LRT) during VSP, the paced AV interval shortens, usually to 100 to 110 msec, and the AEI remains constant. Therefore, continual safety pacing causes an increase in the paced ventricular rate, so that the intervals between two consecutive paced ventricular beats (Vp-Vp) shorten by the difference between the programmed Ap-Vp interval and the shorter AV interval during safety pacing.

Ventricular Undersensing. In the first generation of pulse generators offering the DDI mode (Pacesetter AFP [283] and Genisis [285], Pacesetter Inc., Sylmar, CA), a ventricular blanking period is generated upon completion of the AEI even when release of Ap is inhibited by a sensed P wave (Fig. 30–35). This design eccentricity may cause ventricular undersensing but can often be corrected by programming the blanking period to its shortest value of 13 msec.[67, 68] Many of the pacemakers that exhibit this phenomenon are still in operation.

Despite their limitations, the DDI mode and its rate-adaptive counterpart, the DDIR mode, achieved some degree of success in the treatment of patients with alternating bradycardia and tachycardia, as in the sick sinus syndrome.[69–72] In the latter, the DDI mode provides atrial pacing and AV synchrony (in the absence of atrial tachyarrhythmias), with the potential of preventing atrial tachyarrhythmias by overdrive suppression. During episodes of atrial tachyarrhythmias, a DDI (DDIR) pacemaker simply paces at the constant

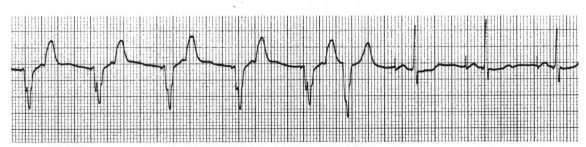

Figure 30–32. DDI pacing with endless loop. Ventricular pacing causes retrograde VA conduction. The pacemaker senses the retrograde P wave beyond the postventricular atrial refractory period (PVARP). Atrial sensing inhibits the atrial output, and the process repeats itself until a ventricular extrasystole *(arrow)* causes retrograde VA conduction block because of its prematurity. This allows release of Ap with successful atrial capture followed by ventricular fusion. On the *left*, the electrocardiogram resembles VVI pacing with retrograde VA conduction. Lower rate interval (LRI) = 857 msec (rate = 70 ppm); AV = 150 msec, PVARP = 200 msec. (From Barold SS: DDI and DDIR modes of pacing: An overview. Med Intell Cardiac Pacing Electrophysiol 14(4):2, 1996.)

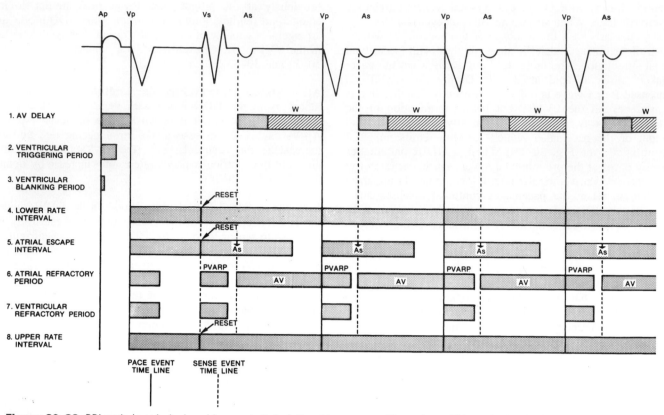

Figure 30–33. DDI mode (ventricular-based lower rate timing). Repetitive reentrant VA synchrony. This mechanism is identical to that of endless-loop tachycardia (see Fig. 30–53), but no tachycardia occurs in the DDI mode because the upper rate interval (URI) equals the lower rate interval (LRI). A sensed ventricular extrasystole (Vs) generates retrograde VA conduction (As). The pacemaker senses As and initiates an extended AV interval lengthened by W to conform to the URI (Vp-Vp), also equal to the LRI. Same format as Figure 30–10. (From Barold SS, Falkoff MD, Ong LS, et al: All dual-chamber pacemakers function in the DDD mode. Am Heart J 115:1353, 1988.)

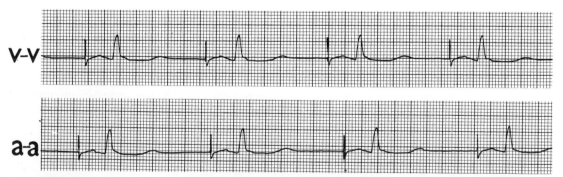

Figure 30–34. *Top*, DDI mode with ventricular-based lower rate timing (V-V). The sensed QRS terminates the AV interval and initiates an atrial escape interval of 557 msec, which always remains constant. In this Ap-Vs-Ap-Vs sequence, the Ap-Ap or the Vs-Vs intervals are shorter than the lower rate interval (LRI). In the DDI mode, the Vs-Vs interval, but not the Vp-Vp interval, can be shorter than the LRI. LRI = 857 msec, AV = 300 msec. *Bottom*, DDI mode with hybrid lower rate timing (atrial-based lower rate timing after Ap-Vs, with Ap initiating the LRI). The sensed QRS terminates the AV interval and initiates an atrial escape interval longer than its basic duration of 557 msec, so that the Ap-Ap interval remains equal to LRI. The Ap-Ap and Vs-Vs intervals are both equal to the LRI (857 msec). Remember that in the DDI mode, AV intervals longer than the programmed Ap-Vp must be associated with ventricular-based lower rate timing to provide a constant paced ventricular rate. (From Barold SS: DDI and DDIR modes of pacing: An overview. Med Intell Cardiac Pacing Electrophysiol 14(4):2, 1996.)

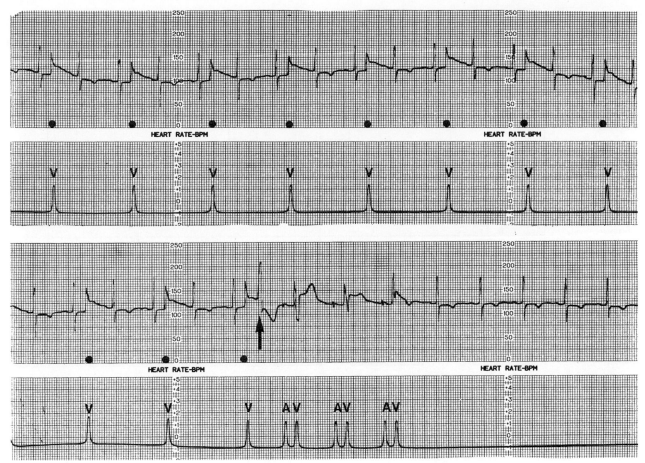

Figure 30–35. Undersensing during DDI pacing of a Pacesetter-Genisis DDD pacemaker due to blanking period eccentricity. Each *solid black circle* depicts a ventricular stimulus that completes the lower rate interval (LRI) initiated by a sensed QRS that precedes it by 857 msec. The QRS complexes immediately preceding the ventricular stimuli (and *black circles*) that fall within the ventricular blanking period generated at the time an atrial stimulus would have fired in the absence of sinus P waves. The pacemaker actually sensed the P waves and inhibited the atrial output, yet the timing cycles behaved as if Ap had been released. The pacemaker, therefore, creates a ventricular blanking period starting at the implied Ap. The QRS complexes just before the ventricular stimuli fall within the ventricular blanking period and are therefore unsensed. In this case, programming the blanking period to its shortest value (13 msec) reduced but did not eliminate this eccentricity, which appeared to be of no clinical importance. Such eccentricity does not occur with subsequent generations of Pacesetter dual-chamber pacemakers. LRI = 857 msec (rate = 70 ppm), AV = 200 msec. (From Barold SS: DDI and DDIR modes of pacing: An overview. Med Intell Cardiac Pacing Electrophysiol 14(4):2, 1996.)

programmed (lower) ventricular rate (or sensor-driven rate). In patients with paroxysmal supraventricular tachyarrhythmias with a normal sinus mechanism and AV block, AV dissociation can be prevented by implanting a DDD or DDDR unit (that maintains AV synchrony) with the capability of recognizing pathologic SVT and designed with automatic mode switching (AMS). This mechanism controls the paced ventricular rate by virtue of temporary self-programming to a new pacing mode without atrial tracking capability, with or without rate-adaptive response (e.g., VVI, VVIR, DDI, DDIR modes, discussed later).

The advent of AMS has rendered the DDIR mode virtually obsolete as a primary pacing mode for sick sinus syndrome. It is still useful in patients with carotid sinus syndrome and malignant vasovagal syncope when used with hysteresis.[73–75] However, contemporary pacemakers with AMS should be programmed to the DDI or DDIR mode to provide a backup function in case problems arise with the AMS algorithm.

VDD Mode

The VDD mode functions like the DDD mode except that the atrial output is turned off[44] (Fig. 30–36). The VDD mode is a programmable option in many dual-chamber pacemakers. If not, it can be obtained by programming the atrial output to zero. If the design does not allow the latter, the lowest pulse duration and atrial voltage usually do not capture the atrium, and the pulse generator then functions essentially in the VDD mode. In the case of bipolar atrial pacing, the stimuli often become invisible, and the VDD mode is mimicked. In the VDD mode, failure to deliver an atrial stimulus precludes initiation of crosstalk intervals (ventricular blanking and safety pacing periods). The required timing cycles of the VDD mode include LRI, URI, AV interval, VRP, and PVARP.[44] As far as the timing cycles are concerned, the omitted atrial stimulus begins an implied AV interval during which, according to design, the atrial channel is refractory, as in the DDD mode. This behavior explains

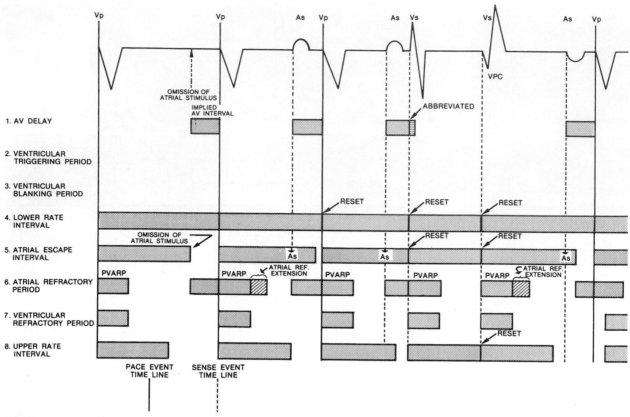

Figure 30–36. VDD mode. In the DDD mode, an atrial stimulus is released at the completion of the atrial escape interval (AEI) whenever no As occurs within the atrial escape interval. In the VDD mode (equivalent to the DDD mode without an atrial output), the atrial stimulus is omitted. Nevertheless, the pulse generator initiates an implied AV interval with the same characteristics as in the DDD mode. Most pacemakers do not sense (or track) a P wave falling in the implied AV interval. In the first Vp-Vp cycle, the pacemaker extends its PVARP automatically, as after a sensed ventricular extrasystole (see Fig. 31–10), because Vp terminating the implied AV interval is not preceded by Ap or As. No ventricular blanking and ventricular safety pacing (VSP; triggering) periods are needed because there are no atrial stimuli in the VDD mode. With the omission of Ap at the end of the implied AV interval and the absence of As, the pulse generator effectively paces in the VVI mode at the programmed DDD lower rate interval (first cycle). Same format as in Figure 30–10. (From Barold SS, Falkoff MD, Ong LS, et al: All dual-chamber pacemakers function in the DDD mode. Am Heart J 115:1353, 1988.)

why in many contemporary VDD designs, a P wave occurring during the implied AV interval (after an aborted atrial stimulus) cannot initiate a new AV interval. In some DDD pulse generators programmed to the VDD mode, however, a P wave during the implied AV interval can be sensed and can actually reinitiate an entirely new AV interval, so that the Vs-Vp or Vp-Vp interval becomes longer (maximum extension equal to As-Vp interval) than the programmed (ventricular-based) LRI, producing a form of hysteresis.[1, 41]

In the absence of sensed atrial activity, the VDD mode will continue to pace effectively in the VVI mode (at the LRI of the DDD mode) because the VDD mode preserves all the other timing cycles of the DDD mode despite the missing atrial output. Dedicated VDD devices became obsolete with the introduction of DDD pacemakers. However, single-lead AV systems with floating atrial electrodes on the intra-atrial portion of the ventricular lead can provide reliable VDD pacing and have led to a renaissance of dedicated VDD devices.[76]

■ TYPES OF LOWER RATE TIMING

Traditional dual-chamber pacemakers are designed with ventricular-based LRT, or simply *V-V timing*, a term often used interchangeably with *VA timing* to emphasize constancy of the AEI. With ventricular-based LRT, a ventricular-paced (Vp) or ventricular-sensed (Vs) event initiates the LRI, which is, therefore, the longest Vp-Vp or Vs-Vp interval without intervening atrial- and ventricular-sensed events. Although basically correct, Furman's definition of LRI as "the longest interval between sensed ventricular events without a ventricular pacemaker stimulus"[1] is somewhat awkward and less satisfactory than the previously given definition.

The AEI (Vp-Ap or Vs-Ap; where Ap = atrial-paced event) always remains constant, provided that there are no intervening atrial-sensed or ventricular-sensed events (As or Vs). A ventricular-sensed event either in the AV interval or during the AEI resets both the LRI and the AEI. Despite the well-established performance of dual-chamber pacemakers with ventricular-based LRT, a number of manufacturers have

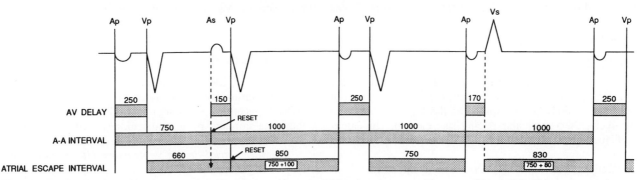

Figure 30–37. Diagrammatic representation of the timing cycles of a DDD pulse generator with pure atrial-based (A-A) lower rate timing showing the effect of differential AV delays (lower rate interval [LRI] = 1000 msec; basic atrial escape interval [AEI] = 750 msec during free-running AV sequential pacing; As-Vp = 150 msec; and Ap-Vp = 250 msec). The second Vp terminates the As-Vp interval that is equal to 150 msec and initiates an AEI of 750 + (250 − 150) = 850 msec to maintain constancy of the A-A or Ap-Ap interval. On the *right*, the third Ap initiates an Ap-Vs interval equal to 170 msec. The corresponding AEI becomes 750 + (250 − 170) = 830 msec to maintain constancy of the A-A or Ap-Ap interval. The last interventricular interval (Vs-Vp) = 830 + 250 = 1080 msec and is longer than the atrial-based LRI (1000 msec). (From Barold SS, Falkoff MD, Ong LS, et al: A-A and V-V lower rate timing of DDD and DDDR pulse generators. *In* Barold SS, Mugica J [eds]: New Perspectives in Cardiac Pacing 2. Mt Kisco, NY, Futura, 1991, pp 203–247.)

introduced dual-chamber pulse generators with atrial-based LRT (A-A timing)[2–5, 28, 29] designed to avoid or minimize perturbations in the pacing rate or cycle-to-cycle fluctuations primarily related to ventricular inhibition during the programmed AV delay[29] (Fig. 30–37) and differential AV delays (As-Vp < Ap-Vp) when the faster sinus rate approaches the lower rate (Table 30–4).

With atrial-based LRT, the LRI is initiated and therefore controlled by atrial (As or Ap) rather than ventricular events, so that the LRI is the longest Ap-Ap or As-Ap interval (without an intervening As or ventricular extrasystole). Other forms of lower rate control include a variety of hybrids with either atrial or ventricular LRT according to circumstances. These new designs have introduced new complexities in the understanding of timing cycles related to lower rate function of dual-chamber pacemakers.

Lower Rate Timing in Single Cycles

For descriptive purposes, the behavior of a single pacemaker cycle initiated by any combination of atrial and ventricular

Table 30–4. Rationale for Atrial-Based Lower Rate Timing

	Ventricular-Based Lower Rate Timing	Atrial-Based Lower Rate Timing
1. Ventricular Inhibition (Ap-Vs-Ap-Vs sequence) Atrial Pacing Rate	Faster than lower rate (atrial cycle length < LRI). The discrepancy widens during DDDR pacing without a rate-adaptive AV interval when the sensor-controlled atrial pacing rate can exceed the sensor-driven upper rate by a substantial value.	Equal to the lower rate (atrial cycle length = LRI). During DDDR pacing, the sensor-controlled atrial pacing rate never exceeds the sensor-driven upper rate.
2. Differential AV Delays (As-Vp < Ap-Vp) (As-Vp-As-Vp sequence)	In the DDD mode, oscillations in ventricular cycle length can occur when the faster sinus rate approaches the programmed lower rate. When LRI > PP > (As-Vp) + (Vp-Ap), Ap occurs before the expected P wave. In this situation, smooth 1 : 1 AV synchrony associated with P-wave sensing is prevented before the atrial rate reaches the programmed lower rate. This behavior becomes more pronounced with a faster programmed lower rate and a larger difference in the programmed As-Vp and Ap-Vp intervals.	Stabilizes the heart rate. When LRI > PP, the pacemaker maintains 1 : 1 AV synchrony with As until the lower rate is attained because As-Ap interval = LRI.

Ap, atrial-paced event; As, atrial-sensed event; Vp, ventricular-paced event; Vs, ventricular-sensed event; LRI, lower rate interval; PP, interval between two consecutive P waves in sinus rhythm.
From Barold SS: Ventricular- versus atrial-based lower rate timing in dual chamber pacemakers: Does it really matter? PACE 18:83, 1995.

events (As-Vs, As-Vp, Ap-Vs, Ap-Vp, or isolated Vs) can be considered in terms of two basic LRT mechanisms. Tables 30–4 and 30–5 outline the differences between the two LRT mechanisms.

Pacemaker Rate

As already discussed, description of pacemaker behavior for only one cycle in terms of rate should be discouraged, but the practice is likely to continue. On the basis of only one pacing cycle, the ventricular pacing rate can only be calculated if the cycle consists of Vp-Vp or Vs-Vp with V-V timing.

Calculation of ventricular *pacing* rate is impossible from a single-cycle Vs-Vs or Vp-Vs that terminates with Vs. Yet the misconception that the paced ventricular rate can be derived from a single cycle terminating with a ventricular-sensed event has slipped into the literature.[4, 77] During atrial-based LRT, a sequence of Ap-Vp-Ap-Vs causes the Vp-Vs interval to become shorter than the atrial LRI; that is, the interventricular interval shortens. In this situation, a statement that ventricular pacing rate increases on the basis of a Vp-Vs cycle would be illogical. Yet, Stroobrandt and coauthors[77] specified wrongly that during atrial-based LRT in an Ap-Vp-Ap-Vs sequence, the resulting ventricular paced rate will accelerate by a small amount.

Escape Intervals

With dual-chamber pulse generators, the escape interval should always be qualified as either atrial or ventricular. Regardless of the type of LRT, the definition of the AEI as the interval from Vp or Vs to the succeeding Ap remains identical for all LRT mechanisms. Some workers have used AEI to describe the LRI or the Ap-Ap interval of devices with atrial-based LRT.[78] This potentially misleading terminology must be abandoned. The term *lower rate VA interval* to depict the longest AEI during activity rate-adaptive pacing is also inappropriate.[79]

With regard to DDD pacing, Sinnaeve[80] defined the escape interval of DDD pacemakers as "the longest period of time between a sensed spontaneous atrial depolarization and the subsequent paced atrial event," that is, As-Ap interval, without specifying whether it applies to ventricular-based or

atrial-based LRT. This statement is correct only if As is not followed by Vs and As-Vp = Ap-Vp, but incorrect with As-Vp < Ap-Vp.

Lower Rate Timing Versus Upper Rate Timing

Control of the LRI by either an A-A or V-V response should not be confused with behavior of the URI. All DDD and DDDR pacemakers possess a URI that is controlled and therefore initiated by a ventricular (paced or sensed) event regardless of the LRT mechanism.

The term *atrial-driven ventricular URI* is not contradictory because, as already emphasized, it refers to the shortest Vs-Vp or Vp-Vp whereupon an *atrial-sensed* event (As) triggers or drives the terminal Vp output. The pacemaker can release the last Vp output only at the completion of the *ventricular* URI initiated by the preceding Vs or Vp. An atrial-based LRT does not mean that the URI is also atrial based because no DDD or DDDR pacemakers can function with a URI solely controlled by atrial events. (Some DDD pacemakers function with separate but linked atrial and ventricular URIs, which may become evident only under exceptional circumstances.)

Ventricular-Based LRT (V-V Response)

Vp or Vs determines the duration of the succeeding pacing cycle; that is, Vp or Vs initiates a constant AEI (Vs-Ap or Vp-Ap). If Ap terminating the AEI is followed by Vp, the Vs-Ap-Vp or Vp-Ap-Vp intervals are constant and equal to the programmed (ventricular-based) LRI. An isolated Vs, that is, a ventricular premature contraction (VPC) not preceded by an atrial event, initiates a constant AEI and therefore a ventricular-based LRT response.

Analysis of Pacemaker Function on a Cycle-to-Cycle Basis

The behavior of a DDD pulse generator can be analyzed on a cycle-to-cycle basis (Fig. 30–38). In any given cycle, a DDD pulse generator with ventricular-based LRT can be considered to function in one of the following modes: AAI,

Table 30–5. Characteristics of Lower Rate Timing

	Ventricular Based	Atrial Based
1. Ap-Vs-Ap-Vs, As-Vp-Ap-Vp, and As-Vs-Ap-Vp sequences*		
Ap-Ap and As-Ap intervals	<LRI	Equal to LRI
Vp-Vp and Vs-Vp intervals	Constant and equal to LRI	>LRI
Vs-Vs intervals	<LRI	Equal to LRI
2. Continuous ventricular safety pacing (Ap-Vp < programmed Ap-Vp)		
Pacing rate	Faster than programmed lower rate	Equal to programmed lower rate
3. 2 : 1 AV block during atrial pacing (alternating Ap-Vp and Ap-Vs intervals)*		
Interventricular intervals (Vs-Vp and Vp-Vs)	Alternates between value equal to LRI and value < LRI	Alternates between value > LRI and value < LRI

Ap, atrial-paced event; As, atrial-sensed event; Vp, ventricular-paced event; Vs, ventricular-sensed event; LRI, lower rate interval.
* Ap-Vs < Ap-Vp, As-Vp < Ap-Vp, As-Vs < Ap-Vp as programmed.
From Barold SS: Ventricular- versus atrial-based lower rate timing in dual chamber pacemakers: Does it really matter? PACE 18:83, 1995.

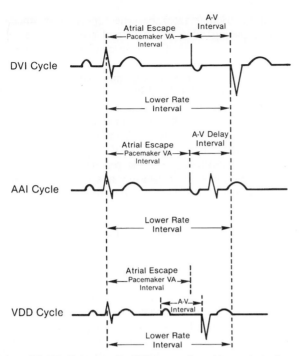

Figure 30–38. Behavior of a DDD pacemaker with ventricular-based (V-V) lower rate timing based on examination of a single cycle at a time in a continuous electrocardiogram. The DDD mode incorporates the essentials of three simpler modes: DVI, AAI, and VDD. In any one pacemaker cycle, starting with either a sensed or a paced ventricular event (Vs or Vp), one of these three modes may be seen. The descriptive mode for a single pacemaker cycle is determined only by the way the cycle terminates: (a) DVI mode if there are two stimuli. The DVI mode occurs with a slow atrial rate and abnormal AV conduction. (In this context, the DVI mode refers to a partially committed system.) (b) AAI mode. If there is only an atrial stimulus, the pacemaker functions in the AAI mode. The AAI mode occurs if the atrial rate is slow, with intact AV conduction. (c) VDD mode. If there is only a ventricular stimulus, the pacemaker functions in the VDD mode. The VDD mode occurs with a normal atrial rate but abnormal AV conduction. If there are no stimuli, the pacemaker is fully inhibited, and the mode for a given cycle cannot be determined. Thus, if there are no stimuli, the pacemaker could be operating in any one of its three modes for any given cycle (AAI, VDD, or DVI). In this situation, the RR interval (Vs-Vs) is shorter than the lower rate interval (LRI), and the PR interval is shorter than the programmed AV interval. However, inhibition does not always mean that the pulse generator senses both ventricular and atrial signals. Thus, during total inhibition, a DDD pulse generator may actually be working continuously in the DVI mode with atrial undersensing (if the atrial signal is too small to be sensed), if the RR interval is shorter than the AEI. (From Barold SS, Falkoff MD, Ong LS, et al: Electrocardiography of contemporary DDD pacemakers. A. Basic concepts, upper rate response, retrograde ventriculoatrial conduction, and differential diagnosis of pacemaker tachycardias. *In* Saksena S, Goldschlager N [eds]: Electrical Therapy for Cardiac Arrhythmias: Pacing, Antitachycardia Devices, Catheter Ablation. Philadelphia, WB Saunders, 1990, pp 225–264.)

DVI, VVI, or inhibited mode. Under exceptional circumstances, a DDD pulse generator can also function in the VVI, VOO, DOO, or DDT mode.

No Pacemaker Stimuli

If there are no stimuli, the pacemaker could be operating in any one of its three modes for any given cycle (AAI, VDD,

or DVI) or in all of them together. In this situation, the RR interval is shorter than the LRI, and the PR interval is shorter than the AV interval. However, pacemaker inhibition does not always mean that the device senses both ventricular and atrial signals. Thus, during total inhibition, a DDD pulse generator may actually be working continuously in the DVI mode; that is, if the atrial signal is too small to be sensed and if the RR interval is shorter than the AEI, atrial undersensing can be masked.[43]

One Pacemaker Stimulus

If there is only one stimulus, the pacemaker could be operating in any one of three modes:

AAI Mode. If there is only one atrial stimulus, the pacemaker functions in the AAI mode. This occurs if the atrial rate is slow, with intact AV conduction. The conducted QRS causes ventricular inhibition.

VDD (VAT) Mode. If there is only a ventricular stimulus, the pacemaker functions in the VDD (VAT) mode. This occurs with a normal atrial rate but abnormal AV conduction.

VVI (VOO) Mode. If there is a single ventricular stimulus, the pacemaker may also be functioning in the VVI or VOO mode rather than the VDD mode. Automatic conversion of a DDD or DDDR pulse generator to the VVI (or VOO) mode (pacemaker reset) can occur as a result of sensing extraneous interference or battery depletion.[81] In the latter situation, the reset mode (VVI or VOO) functions as the elective replacement indicator. The VVI (VOO) mode can usually be ignored in the routine electrocardiographic analysis of pacemaker function because it occurs only under unusual circumstances. Some DDD pulse generators convert to the VOO mode on application of the magnet.

Two Pacemaker Stimuli

If there are two pacemaker stimuli, three possibilities exist:

DVI Mode. This is the most likely mode, and it occurs with a slow atrial rate and abnormal AV conduction. In this context, the DVI mode refers to a partially committed system; that is, the pulse generator is capable of sensing ventricular activity during part of the AV interval (after termination of the ventricular blanking period to prevent detection of the atrial stimulus or crosstalk).

DOO Mode. This may occur in the presence of excessive noise or interference or on application of the test magnet.

DDT (Triggered) Mode. Under certain circumstances, a DDD pulse generator may be considered to be working in the DDT mode, a code suggested by Garson and colleagues[82] to denote VSP.

The duration of a DVI cycle (initiated by Vs or Vp and terminating with Ap-Vp) is equal to the (ventricular) LRI and always remains constant. AAI and VDD cycles are variable and produce interventricular intervals shorter than the LRI. In the case of VDD cycles, shortening of the ventricular cycles is due to early P wave sensing (i.e., Vp-As-Vp or Vs-As-Vp), and with AAI cycles, it is due to early sensing of the conducted QRS by the ventricular lead (Vp-

Ap-Vs or Vs-Ap-Vs). In dual-chamber devices, the AAI cycles are shorter than the LRI, in contrast to single-chamber AAI pacing, in which the pacing cycles remain constant (Ap-Ap is equal to the LRI) because the far-field QRS should be unsensed (by the atrial lead) with appropriate programming of the refractory period, sensitivity, and the use of a bipolar lead.

Rate Fluctuation Due to Ventricular Inhibition During Programmed Atrioventricular Delay

During traditional DDD, DVI, and DDI pacing with ventricular-based LRT, when AV conduction is relatively normal, atrial capture (Ap) may give rise to a normally conducted QRS complex that may, in turn, inhibit the ventricular channel (Vs). In this situation, the QRS complex must occur before the completion of the programmed AV interval (Ap-Vp). Because the sensed QRS complex also starts a new LRI and AEI, this situation causes a faster atrial pacing rate (i.e., faster than the constant programmed lower rate for ventricular pacing) either on a beat-to-beat basis or continually when atrial pacing is followed by ventricular inhibition (Ap-Vs-Ap-Vs, etc.).[28, 29, 83–86] Ventricular intervals, such as Vp-Ap-Vs or Vs-Ap-Vs, become shorter than the programmed lower rate for ventricular pacing (Vs-Ap-Vp or Vp-Ap-Vp). With atrial-based LRT, the atrial pacing rate remains constant and independent of ventricular inhibition (discussed later).

In pulse generators with a ventricular-based LRT, an increase in the paced atrial rate (and therefore the conducted ventricular rate) due to ventricular inhibition is slight when pacing occurs according to the LRI interval (Fig. 30–39). An increase in the atrial pacing rate (and therefore the

conducted ventricular rate) becomes more pronounced at faster basic pacing rates, an important consideration in the design of rate-adaptive DDDR pulse generators with ventricular-based LRTs. Figure 30–39 shows how a programmed DDDR pulse generator with a common upper rate of 120 ppm (equal sensor- and atrial-driven upper rates) can actually result in a faster atrial pacing rate of 150 ppm with exercise because of ventricular inhibition (in the absence of Ap-Vp adaptation on exercise). Rate-adaptive shortening of the Ap-Vp and As-Vp intervals during DDDR pacing on exercise diminishes or eliminates this discrepancy and allows the maximum ventricular rate (during a sequence of Ap-Vs-Ap-Vs) to remain close to the programmed upper rate for ventricular pacing[84] (Fig. 30–40).

Modified Ventricular-Based Lower Rate Timing

The Vigor DDDR pacemaker (Cardiac Pacemakers, Inc., St. Paul, MN) was designed with modified ventricular-based LRT. This modification eliminates the potential for the atrial pacing rate to exceed the programmed sensor-driven upper rate in the presence of intact AV conduction at high rates. The AEI is automatically extended by the difference between the programmed AV delay and the Ap-Vs interval.[85] This results in sensor-driven pacing that cannot exceed the maximum sensor-driven rate regardless of AV conduction (Fig. 30–41).

Rate Fluctuation Due to Ventricular Safety Pacing

In ventricular-based LRT pulse generators with a VSP mechanism, activation of VSP (by ventricular sensing of signals such as crosstalk) also causes an increase in the pacing rate,

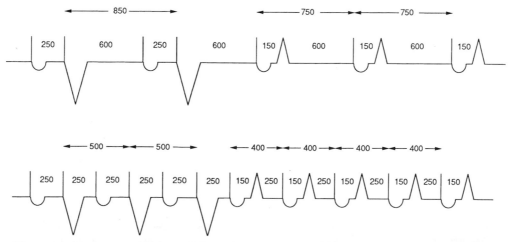

Figure 30–39. Diagrammatic representation of the function of a DDDR pacemaker with ventricular-based (V-V) lower rate timing showing the effect of ventricular inhibition. *A,* DDD mode: lower rate interval (LRI) = 850 msec; AV = 250 msec; atrial escape interval (AEI) = 600 msec. On the *right,* when Ap is followed by a conducted QRS complex, the PR (Ap-Vs) interval shortens to 150 msec, but the AEI remains constant at 600 msec. Therefore, the Ap-Ap interval decreases to 750 msec; that is, the atrial pacing rate increases from 70 to 80 ppm. *B,* DDDR mode: the programmed maximum sensor-driven rate is 120 ppm (500 msec). The AV interval remains at 250 msec, so the AEI shortens to 250 msec. On the *right,* when Ap is followed by a conducted QRS complex, the PR (Ap-Vs) interval shortens to 150 msec, but the AEI remains constant at 250 msec. Therefore, the Ap-Ap interval decreases to 400 msec; that is, the atrial pacing rate increases from 120 to 150 ppm. (From Barold SS, Falkoff MD, Ong LS, et al: A-A and V-V lower rate timing of DDD and DDDR pulse generators. *In* Barold SS, Mugica J [eds]: New Perspectives in Cardiac Pacing 2. Mt Kisco, NY, Futura, 1991, pp 203–247.)

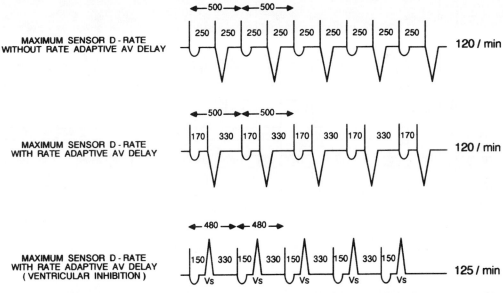

MAXIMUM SENSOR D - RATE
WITHOUT RATE ADAPTIVE AV DELAY
120 / min

MAXIMUM SENSOR D - RATE
WITH RATE ADAPTIVE AV DELAY
120 / min

MAXIMUM SENSOR D - RATE
WITH RATE ADAPTIVE AV DELAY
(VENTRICULAR INHIBITION)
125 / min

Figure 30–40. Diagrammatic representation of the function of a DDDR pacemaker with ventricular-based (V-V) lower rate timing showing the effect of a rate-adaptive AV delay that shortens on exercise. The maximum sensor-driven rate is 120 ppm (500 msec). The basic AV interval is 250 msec. *Top,* Maximum sensor-driven rate without rate-adaptive AV delay. *Middle,* Maximum sensor-driven rate with rate-adaptive AV delay. Note that the AV delay has shortened from 250 to 170 msec, and the sensor-driven atrial escape interval (AEI) has lengthened from 250 msec (top) to 330 msec. *Bottom,* The maximum sensor-driven rate is 120 ppm (500 msec). The AV interval shortens to 150 msec because a conducted QRS complex (Vs) is sensed before termination of the rate-adaptive AV interval. As in the *middle example,* the sensor-driven AEI remains at 330 msec, so that the atrial pacing rate increases to only 125 ppm (compare with the atrial pacing rate of 150 ppm in Fig. 30–39). (From Barold SS: Single- and dual-chamber pacemakers: Electrophysiology, pacing modes, and multiprogrammability. *In* Singer I, Kupersmith J [eds]: Clinical Manual of Electrophysiology. Baltimore, Williams & Wilkins, 1993, pp 231–273.)

due to abbreviation of the Ap-Vp interval, with the AEI (Vp-Ap) remaining constant (see Fig. 30–11).

■ A-A LOWER RATE TIMING (A-A RESPONSE)

When the LRI of a DDD pacemaker with atrial-based LRT is equal to the LRI of a DDD pacemaker with ventricular-based LRT, the basic AEI of both types of devices is identical during the free-running state with continuous atrial and ventricular pacing, that is, DVI cycles terminate with an atrial stimulus (Ap) when there is no spontaneous ventricular activity or Ap-Vp-Ap-Vp sequences.

Ap or As determines the duration of the succeeding pacing cycle; that is, As or Ap initiates a constant LRI

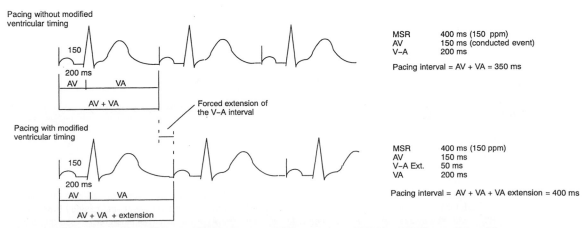

Pacing without modified
ventricular timing

150

200 ms
AV | VA

AV + VA

Forced extension of
the V–A interval

Pacing with modified
ventricular timing

150

200 ms
AV | VA

AV + VA + extension

MSR	400 ms (150 ppm)
AV	150 ms (conducted event)
V–A	200 ms

Pacing interval = AV + VA = 350 ms

MSR	400 ms (150 ppm)
AV	150 ms
V–A Ext.	50 ms
VA	200 ms

Pacing interval = AV + VA + VA extension = 400 ms

Figure 30–41. Mechanism of extension of atrial escape (VA) interval in the CPI Vigor DDDR pacemaker. When 1:1 AV conduction occurs at the maximum sensor rate, the pulse generator maintains the paced rate at the maximum sensor rate by extending the VA interval. This prevents the atrial pacing rate from exceeding the maximum sensor rate. This is often referred to as *modified ventricular-based timing.* (Courtesy of Guidant Corporation, St. Paul, MN.)

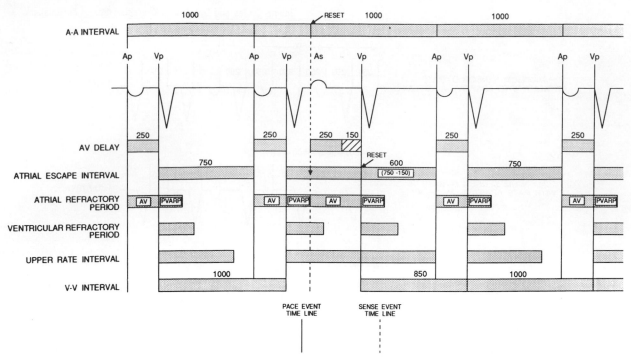

Figure 30–42. Diagrammatic representation of timing cycles of a DDD pulse generator with pure atrial-based (A-A) lower rate timing (lower rate interval [LRI] = 1000 msec; basic atrial escape interval [AEI] = 750 msec during free-running AV sequential pacing). An atrial extrasystole (As) initiates an AV interval of 400 msec (As-Vp) to conform to the ventricular upper rate interval [URI]. Therefore, the pulse generator emits Vp at the completion of the URI. Vp initiates an AEI of 750 + (250 − 400) = 750 − 150 = 600 msec. The A-A interval (As-Ap) remains constant at 1000 msec and equal to the LRI. However, the Vp-Vp interval from the third Vp to the fourth Vp is equal to 850 msec, a value shorter than the programmed LRI. The postventricular refractory period (PVARP; 200 msec) was deliberately shortened to demonstrate the effect of AV extension upper rate response (URI > total atrial refractory period [TARP]) on the timing of Vp. (From Barold SS, Falkoff MD, Ong LS, et al: A-A and V-V lower rate timing of DDD and DDDR pulse generators. *In* Barold SS, Mugica J [eds]: New Perspectives in Cardiac Pacing 2. Mt Kisco, NY, Futura, 1991, pp 203–247.)

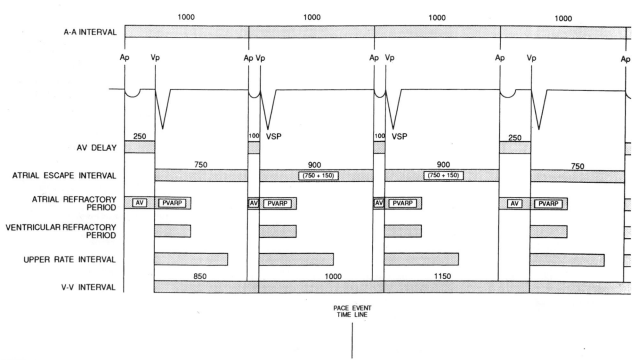

Figure 30–43. Diagrammatic representation of timing cycles of a DDD pulse generator with pure atrial-based (A-A) lower rate timing (LRT). (Lower rate interval [LRI] = 1000 msec; atrial escape interval [AEI] = 750 msec during free-running AV sequential pacing.) Crosstalk induces ventricular safety pacing (VSP) with abbreviation of the Ap-Vp interval to 100 msec. The Ap-Ap interval remains constant, so that the AEI lengthens to 750 + (250 − 100) = 900 msec. During VSP, the pacing rate of a pulse generator with A-A LRT remains constant, in contrast to an increase in the pacing rate in a DDD pulse generator with V-V LRT (see Fig. 30–17). At the termination of crosstalk, the Vp-Vp interval lengthens to 1150 msec, longer than the atrial LRI. (From Barold SS, Falkoff MD, Ong LS, et al: A-A and V-V lower rate timing of DDD and DDDR pulse generators. *In* Barold SS, Mugica J [eds]: New Perspectives in Cardiac Pacing 2. Mt Kisco, NY, Futura, 1991, pp 203–247.)

(As-Ap or Ap-Ap) disregarding any Vs or Vp that immediately follows the atrial event (As or Ap) opening the pacing cycle (Figs. 30–42 to 30–44; see Fig. 30–37). The Vs related to intrinsic AV conduction does not reset the LRI timer. Consequently, the AEI must adapt its duration (longer, shorter, or unchanged) to maintain a constant Ap-Ap or As-Ap interval equal to the atrial-based LRI (see Figs. 30–37 and 30–44). The actual AEI of a given pacing cycle becomes equal to the sum of the basic AEI (as defined previously) plus an extension equal to the difference of the programmed AV delay (Ap-Vp) and the actual PR interval (As-Vs, As-Vp, Ap-Vs, or Ap-Vp) that immediately precedes the AEI in question. Alternatively, the duration of the AEI can be calculated as the LRI minus the AV interval immediately preceding the AEI in question.

The atrial-based LRI or AA interval (As-Ap) remains constant under all circumstances, even when the sensed AV interval (As-Vp) and the paced AV interval (Ap-Vp) are different. During AA timing in pacing sequences consisting of As-Vs-Ap-Vp or Ap-Vs-Ap-Vp, the interventricular (or V-V) interval (Vs-Vp or Vp-Vp) can be longer than the programmed atrial-based LRI (see Figs. 30–37 and 30–43). When a pulse generator with atrial-based LRT senses a late VPC preceded by a (nonconducted) P wave, it actually detects a short AV interval (i.e., Ap-Vs or As-Vs). In this situation, constancy of the atrial-based LRI mandates delay of the subsequent Ap. The AEI initiated by the VPC therefore lengthens and produces a form of hysteresis with regard to the interval between the VPC and the subsequent Vp output. Such slowing of the ventricular rate predisposes to ventricular bigeminy and may be undesirable in some patients.

Analysis of Pacemaker Function on a Cycle-to-Cycle Basis

During atrial-based LRT, in the pacing sequence Ap-Vs-Ap-Vs, the atrial pacing rate remains constant at the programmed lower rate and independent of ventricular inhibition, in contrast to ventricular-based LRT in which the atrial pacing rate increases. Any given cycle may be considered to start with an atrial-paced or atrial-sensed event and terminate either with As or Ap (see Figs. 30–37, 30–42, and 30–43). A DVI cycle begins with Ap-Vp, a VDD cycle begins with As-Vp (even if As-Vp is shorter than Ap-Vp), and an AAI cycle begins with Ap-Vs. To qualify as AAI, DVI, or VDD cycles, the cycle must terminate with Ap. In cases terminating with As, the cycle is considered to be an inhibited or aborted AAI, DVI, or VDD cycle. All three cycles (AAI, DVI, and VDD) terminating with Ap exhibit constant AA intervals

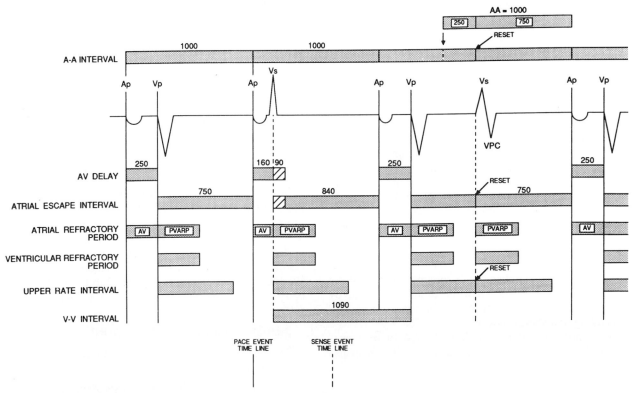

Figure 30–44. Diagrammatic representation of timing cycles of a DDD pulse generator with pure atrial-based (A-A) lower rate timing (LRT). Lower rate interval (LRI) = 1000 msec; AV = 250 msec (As-Vp = Ap-Vp); basic atrial escape interval (AEI) = 750 msec (during free-running pacing). The second Ap is followed by a conducted QRS complex Vs, and Ap-Vs = 160 msec. Ap initiates an A-A (Ap-Ap) interval of 1000 msec. Consequently, the AEI is equal to 750 + (250 − 160) = 840 msec. Note that the Vs-Vp interval is equal to 1090 msec and is longer than the atrial LRI. A ventricular extrasystole (ventricular premature contraction; VPC) beyond the AV interval initiates an AEI of 750 msec, equal to the basic value. The VPC response is similar to that seen in devices with a ventricular-based (V-V) LRT. (From Barold SS, Falkoff MD, Ong LS, et al: A-A and V-V lower rate timing of DDD and DDDR pulse generators. *In* Barold SS, Mugica J [eds]: New Perspectives in Cardiac Pacing 2. Mt Kisco, NY, Futura Publishing Co., 1991, pp 203–247.)

equal to the atrial LRI regardless of As-Vp being programmed to be shorter than Ap-Vp. In this respect, the timing behavior of an AAI cycle resembles that of a single-chamber AAI system that ignores the far-field QRS complex. In circumstances already described, DDD pacemakers with an atrial-based LRI, like those with a ventricular-based LRI, can function in the VVI, VOO, DOO, or DDT mode.

Ventricular Premature Beats and Atrial-Based Lower Rate Timing

In defining atrial-based LRT, Hayes and colleagues[3-5] and other workers[84, 87] stated categorically that "when a ventricular premature beat (defined as Vs without a preceding As) is sensed during the VA or AEI interval, the timers are also reset but now it is the AA interval rather than the VA interval that is reset." This statement actually violates the concept that AA timing is based on atrial rather than ventricular events. The definition of Hayes and coworkers[3-5] is probably based on the behavior of the original and now defunct Siemens 674 and 740 DDD pulse generators (Siemens-Elema, Solna, Sweden) designed with an atrial-based LRT.[28, 78] The now defunct Cyberlith committed DVI pulse generator (Intermedics, Inc., Angleton, TX) also exhibited AA timing only in response to a sensed ventricular event, initiating an AEI equal to the sum of the basic (as programmed) AEI (Ap-Ap) and the AV (Ap-Vp) interval.[57] These original designs created the erroneous notion that in a contemporary pure atrial-based LRT system, the AEI initiated by a VPC should be equal to the LRI.

In an atrial-based LRT system, a VPC-initiated AEI equal to the LRI constitutes a form of obligatory hysteresis. Yet the atrial-based LRT of contemporary pacemakers was designed primarily to avoid rate fluctuation, especially during ventricular inhibition, and sensing of a VPC constitutes ventricular inhibition. Furthermore, many contemporary pulse generators with pure atrial-based LRT or a hybrid LRT system (atrial- or ventricular-based according to circumstances) exhibit mostly V-V or VA timing in response to a VPC (see Fig. 30–44). For these reasons, the definition of pure atrial-based LRT should not require that a VPC-initiated AEI be equal to the LRI. Devices with atrial-based or hybrid LRT systems can therefore be classified into two groups in terms of their VPC response:

1. Common type with VPC-induced V-V or VA response. In this case, the VPC response can be assumed and need not be specified. The term *modified* atrial-based LRT used by some workers[3, 84] to describe this behavior appears awkward and misleading and should not be used.

2. Uncommon type with VPC-induced AA or hysteresis response (AEI = LRI), in which case the VPC response should be specified.

Disadvantages of Pure Atrial Lower Rate Timing

Pure atrial-based LRT maintains constant As-Ap or Ap-Ap intervals (equal to LRI) whenever As or Ap initiates an AV interval shorter or longer than the programmed Ap-Vp interval (see Fig. 30–42). Although devices with pure atrial LRT are no longer manufactured, the following discussion

provides a historical and theoretical basis for understanding atrial LRT (Table 30–5).

Pure atrial-based LRT is compatible with normal pacemaker function in the DVI and VDD modes but incompatible with normal function in the DDIR or even the DDDR(R) mode.

DDI Mode

A conventional DDI pulse generator is really a DDD pulse generator with ventricular-based LRT, in which the ventricular URI and LRI (rates) are identical. The ventricular pacing rate cannot exceed the programmed LRI. The DDI mode with atrial-based LRT (controlling the LRI) creates a paradoxical situation in which the LRI is an atrial interval controlled by atrial events, whereas the URI (which should be equal to the LRI) is a ventricular interval. A DDI pacemaker with atrial-based LRT must, however, retain constancy of the atrial LRI (As-Ap or Ap-Ap) (Fig. 30–45).

Preservation of the atrial LRI takes hierarchical precedence over any other intervals, including the ventricular URI (equal to the atrial LRI), a situation that can produce violation of the URI (whenever Ap-Vp never exceeds its programmed value). For this reason, a dual-chamber pulse generator functioning in the DDI or DDIR mode requires ventricular-based LRT in most circumstances. Actually, the DDI (DDIR) mode can function with a hybrid LRT in which short AV intervals (shorter than programmed Ap-Vp) initiate A-A cycles, whereas AV intervals longer than the programmed Ap-Vp or VPC initiate V-V cycles. With this arrangement in the DDI mode, Ap-Vs-Ap-Vs sequences (ventricular inhibition) will show an atrial pacing rate equal to the programmed lower rate, in contrast to the DDI mode with ventricular-based LRT, in which Ap-Vs-Ap-Vs sequences will show an atrial pacing rate faster than the programmed lower ventricular pacing rate.

As with the DDI and DDIR modes, pure atrial-based LRT does not lend itself to smooth functioning of DDD or DDDR pulse generators.[28, 29, 86]

DDD Mode

In the DDD mode with pure atrial-based LRT, the greater the separation of LRI and URI, the less the likelihood of violation of the atrial-driven URI as seen in the DDI mode. The closer the LRI and URI, the greater the likelihood of violation of the atrial-driven URI. Violation of the URI can occur only with AV interval extension as a response to Wenckebach upper rate limitation (Table 30–6). Mathematically, violation of the atrial-driven URI will occur in the following circumstance:

2 atrial-driven URI > LRI − TARP.

The largest degree of violation Δ msec = (URI − LRI) + W, where

W = URI − TARP as previously defined.[88]

For example, in the case of a DDD pulse generator with pure atrial-based LRT and the following indices, violation of the URI can be calculated mathematically (Fig. 30–46): LRI = 750 msec (80 ppm), URI = 600 msec (100 ppm), AV delay = 200 msec, PVARP = 200 msec

2 URI > LRI + TARP
1200 > 1150

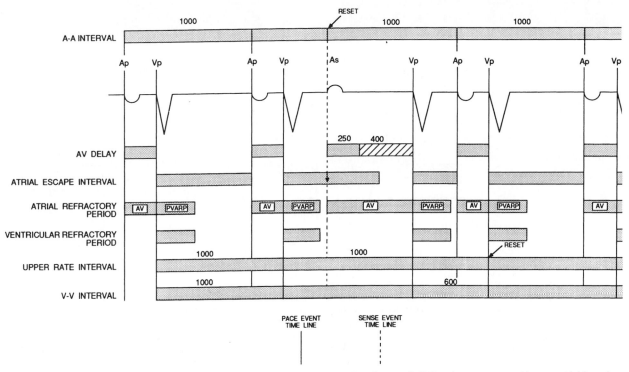

Figure 30–45. Diagrammatic representation of the DDI mode in the Intermedics Cosmos II DDD pulse generator with pure atrial-based (A-A) lower rate timing (LRT). For this generator, the lowest programmable upper rate is 80 ppm, and the closest programmable lower rate is 78 ppm. For the sake of discussion, it was assumed that both the upper rate and the lower rate were programmable to 60 ppm, in an attempt to obtain the DDI mode (lower rate interval [LRI] = 1000 msec; AV = 250 msec). In the DDI mode, the ventricular upper rate interval (URI) should be equal to the LRI, which in this case is atrial based (as opposed to ventricular based in Figs. 30–32 through 30–34). An early As initiates a long As-Vp interval of 650 msec, as in any DDD pulse generator (regardless of LRT), simply to conform to the ventricular URI (1000 msec and equal to LRI). With A-A LRT, because Vp terminates the As-Vp interval, Vp initiates an atrial escape interval (AEI) equal to 750 + (250 − 650) = 350 msec, as shown. The As-Ap interval, however, is maintained at 1000 msec. The Vp-Ap-Vp = 350 + 250 = 600 msec, in violation of the ventricular URI. This illustration demonstrates the incompatibility of A-A LRT with the DDI mode of pacing. (From Barold SS, Falkoff MD, Ong LS, et al: A-A and V-V lower rate timing of DDD and DDDR pulse generators. *In* Barold SS, Mugica J [eds]: New Perspectives in Cardiac Pacing 2. Mt Kisco, NY, Futura, 1991, pp 203–247.)

Therefore, a 50-msec violation of the atrial-driven URI can occur.

$$\Delta = (URI - LRI) + W$$
$$= (600 - 750) + 200 = +50 \text{ msec}$$

If $\Delta = 0$ or negative value, no violation of the atrial-driven URI can occur.

Table 30–6. Disadvantages of Pure Atrial-Based Lower Rate Timing (AV Interval > Programmed Ap-Vp Interval)

	Ventricular-Based Lower Rate Timing	Atrial-Based Lower Rate Timing
URI Violation (early sensed APC or Wenckebach upper rate response)	No	Yes, when 2 URI > LRI + TARP
DDI Mode	Compatible	Incompatible

APC, atrial premature contraction; LRI, lower rate interval; TARP, total atrial refractory period; URI, upper rate interval.

From Barold SS: Ventricular- versus atrial-based lower rate timing in dual chamber pacemakers: Does it really matter? PACE 18:83, 1995.

DDDR Mode

The same argument applies to DDDR pulse generators with pure atrial-based LRI. In the DDDR mode, the LRI obviously gets closer and closer to the URI with increasing sensor activity, and violation of the atrial-driven URI can occur as in the DDD mode. If sensor-driven URI = atrial-driven URI = 500 msec, SDI = 600 msec, AV interval = 150 msec, PVARP = 200 msec, and violation of the common URI will occur if 2 × atrial-driven URI > LRI + TARP, and 1000 > 600 + 350, + 50 msec. This represents a violation of 50 msec. Alternatively, $\Delta = (URI - LRI) + W$, = (500 − 600) + 150 = msec. This represents the maximum violation of the common URI.

In some DDDR pulse generators, the situation is more complex when the atrial-driven URI > sensor-driven URI. When the atrial-driven URI > sensor-driven URI > SDI − W, violation of both the atrial-driven URI and the sensor-driven URI will occur (Fig. 30–47). In this situation, the sensor-driven URI is only slightly shorter than the atrial-driven URI. When the sensor-driven URI becomes substantially shorter than the atrial-driven URI, only the atrial-driven URI can be violated. If the sensor-driven URI < SDI − W, violation of the sensor-driven URI cannot occur.

DDD MODE
PURE ATRIAL-BASED LOWER RATE TIMING. WENCKEBACH UPPER RATE RESPONSE

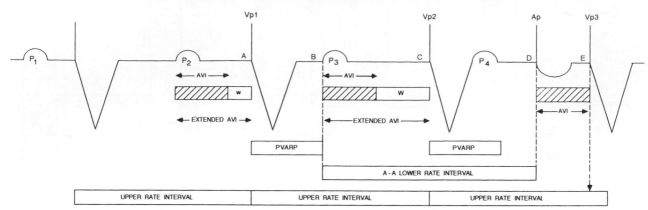

Figure 30–46. Wenckebach upper rate response of a DDD pulse generator with pure atrial-based lower rate timing. Vp, ventricular-paced event; Ap, atrial-paced event; Ap-Vp = programmed As-Vp; AVI, AV interval; W, maximum extension of AVI; w, AV extension shorter than W. (W = upper rate interval [URI] − total atrial refractory period [TARP].) The pacemaker senses the third P wave (P_3) just beyond the postventricular refractory period (PVARP), so that P_3 initiates a maximally extended AVI, i.e., Ap-Vp + W. P_4 falls in the PVARP and is unsensed. The pacemaker initiates an atrial-based lower rate interval (LRI) at P_3. The LRI terminates at D with the release of Ap. Upon completion of the Ap-Vp interval, the pulse generator delivers Vp3, which violates the URI. URI violation occurs because (LRI − URI) < W. (From Barold SS, Fredman CS: Pure atrial-based lower rate timing of dual chamber pacemakers: Implications for upper rate limitation. PACE 18:391, 1995.)

DDDR MODE
ATRIAL-DRIVEN URI LONGER THAN SENSOR-DRIVEN URI
PURE ATRIAL-BASED LOWER RATE TIMING. WENCKEBACH UPPER RATE RESPONSE

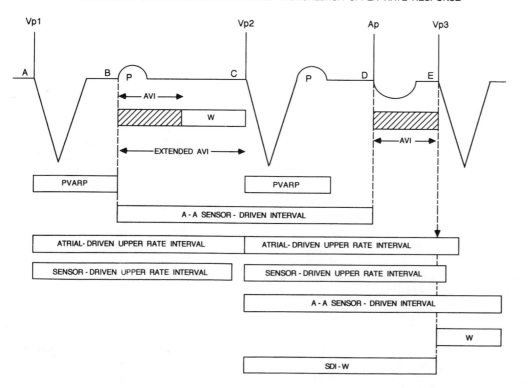

Figure 30–47. End of a Wenckebach upper rate response during DDDR pacing with pure atrial-based lower rate timing. The atrial-driven upper rate interval (URI) is longer than the sensor-driven URI. The pacemaker violates the atrial-driven URI, and Vp3 also violates the sensor-driven URI because the sensor-driven interval (SDI) − W < sensor-driven URI. W = maximal extension of the AV interval (atrial-driven URI minus total atrial refractory period); Ap, atrial-paced event; Vp, ventricular-paced event; AVI, AV interval; PVARP, postventricular atrial refractory period. (From Barold SS, Fredman CS: Pure atrial-based lower rate timing of dual chamber pacemakers: Implications for upper rate limitation. PACE 18:391, 1995.)

Lower Rate Timing: Concept of Committed Atrioventricular Interval

All types of LRT mechanisms can be considered as being ventricular based with or without a committed AV interval (in terms of timing cycles) under specific circumstances. Ventricular-based LRT functions with an uncommitted AV interval and atrial-based LRT functions like a ventricular-based system but with committed AV interval.[29]

Atrial-Based Lower Rate Timing

By definition, the Ap-Vp interval must time out in its entirety because it is committed (Fig. 30–48). For example, when Ap-Vs (< Ap-Vp) initiates a pacing cycle, Vs inhibits the release of Vp. Nevertheless, the Ap-Vp interval times out in its entirety, so that Vp becomes implied (Vpi) (see Fig. 30–48). Medtronic has called Vpi an "impending or scheduled V-pace" event.[28, 29, 89, 90] Vpi controls initiation of the timing cycles that pertain to LRT (AEI, LRI, sensor-driven AEI, and SDI; the last two in the DDDR mode) precisely as if Vp had actually been released. The preceding Vs event

initiates the PVARP, VRP, and URI (Fig. 30–49). Such pacemaker behavior is characteristic of ventricular-based LRT because the implied Vp (Vpi) initiates the timing cycles related to the lower rate. When VSP causes premature delivery of Vp, abbreviation of the Ap-Vp interval occurs. Yet in an atrial-based LRT system with a committed AV interval, the lower rate intervals (LRI, AEI, SDI, and sensor-driven AEI) do not begin with the release of the premature Vp. Consequently, with VSP, as with Vs occurring before the completion of the programmed Ap-Vp interval, the pacemaker waits until the entire programmed Ap-Vp interval has timed out to initiate LRIs coincidentally with Vpi. Nevertheless, with VSP, the early Vp event initiates the PVARP, VRP, and URI. Furthermore, when As-Vs > Ap-Vp or As-Vp > Ap-Vp in an AV extension or Wenckebach upper rate response (TARP < PP interval < URI), the concept of a committed AV interval also applies (see Fig. 30–48). Thus, Vpi at the end of the committed AV interval initiates the AEI and LRI (or sensor-driven AEI and SDI during DDDR pacing), and the delayed Vp or Vs event (consequent to AV extension) initiates PVARP, VRP, and URI.

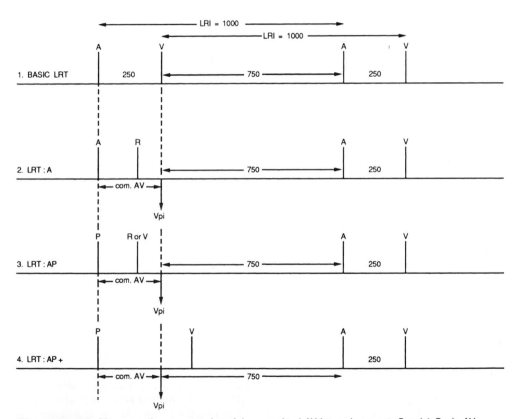

Figure 30–48. Diagrammatic representation of the committed AV interval concept. *Panel 1,* Basic AV sequential pacing with programmed Ap-Vp interval. *Panel 2,* Ap-Vp < programmed Ap-Vp (ventricular safety pacing) or Ap-Vs < programmed Ap-Vp. The atrial escape interval (AEI) and lower rate interval (LRI) begin at Vpi (implied but not released ventricular pacing event at the termination of the programmed committed Ap-Vp interval). *Panel 3,* As-Vp < programmed Ap-Vp or As-Vs < programmed Ap-Vp. As in panel 2, the AEI and LRI begin at Vpi. *Panel 4,* As-Vp > programmed Ap-Vp or As-Vs> programmed Ap-Vp as in a Wenckebach upper rate response. As in panels 2 and 3, the AEI and LRI begin at Vpi. In all the depicted situations, a pacemaker with atrial-based lower rate timing in appropriate circumstances can be conceptualized as functioning with ventricular-based lower rate timing and a committed AV interval. Ap, atrial-paced event; As, atrial-sensed event; Vp, ventricular-paced event; Vs, ventricular-sensed event; com, committed. All values are given in msec. (From Barold SS: Ventricular- versus atrial-based lower rate timing in dual chamber pacemakers: Does it really matter? PACE 18:83, 1995.)

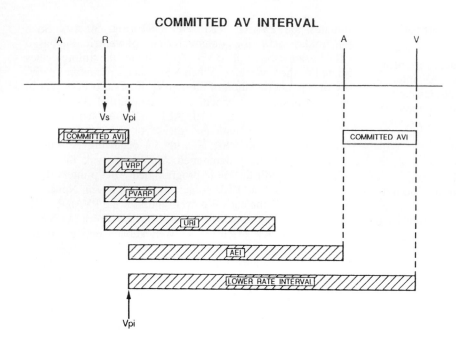

Figure 30–49. Initiation of timing cycles during DDD pacing with atrial-based lower rate timing. The device is considered as functioning with ventricular-based lower rate timing and a committed AV interval (AVI). Ap-Vs < programmed Ap-Vp. The atrial escape interval and the lower rate interval begin with Vpi, the implied but not released ventricular-paced event at the termination of the programmed committed Ap-Vp AVI. Vs initiates the ventricular refractory period (VRP), the postventricular atrial refractory period (PVARP), and the upper rate interval (URI). Ap, atrial-paced event; As, atrial-sensed event; Vp, ventricular-paced event; Vs, ventricular-sensed event. (From Barold SS: Ventricular- versus atrial-based lower rate timing in dual chamber pacemakers: Does it really matter? PACE 18:83, 1995.)

Atrioventricular Combinations for Lower Rate Timing Initiation

Each of the pacing cycles initiated by one of the nine possible A-V combinations shown in Table 30–7 can be translated into a V-V cycle with or without a committed AV interval. In this way, A-A cycles automatically become V-V cycles with a committed AV interval, whereas V-V cycles without a committed AV interval remain V-V cycles.[29] With better understanding of LRT, much of the terminology that includes pseudo A-A timing and modified atrial lower timing becomes of little value because all cycles in hybrid systems can be characterized only in terms of A-A or V-V cycles. Thus, for the understanding of lower rate behavior, one only needs to know what combinations of atrial and ventricular events initiate A-A cycles. Similarly, if one accepts that all pacemakers have ventricular-based LRT, one only needs to know what cycles are associated with a committed AV interval.

As previously emphasized, pure atrial-based LRT that maintains constant As-Ap or Ap-Ap intervals (equal to LRI) whenever As or Ap initiates an AV interval *longer* than the programmed Ap-Vp interval no longer exists in contemporary pacemakers. Atrial-based LRT operative in pacemakers maintains constancy of the As-Ap or Ap-Ap interval initiated by AV intervals (As-Vs, As-Vp, Ap-Vs, and Ap-Vp) *shorter*

Table 30–7. Atrioventricular Combinations Determining Lower Rate Interval Initiation

1. Ap-Vp
2. Ap-Vs
3. Abbreviated Ap-Vp (ventricular safety pacing)
4. As-Vp < programmed Ap-Vp
5. As-Vp > programmed Ap-Vp (as in Wenckebach upper rate response)
6. As-Vs < programmed Ap-Vp
7. As-Vs > programmed Ap-Vp (as in Wenckebach upper rate response)
8. As-Vs = 0
9. Ventricular safety pacing not preceded by As

than the value of the programmed Ap-Vp interval. When atrial-based LRT involves only intervals initiated by Ap or atrial pacing (whenever Ap-Vs and Ap-Vp are shorter than the programmed Ap-Vp), the response could be called the partial type of atrial-based LRT. Exceptions to the rules could be stated in parenthesis. This simple classification makes the various forms of atrial-based LRT easy to remember. Finally, the presence of a hysteresis response to a VPC (AEI = atrial-based LRI) should be specifically stated.

Importance of Atrial-Based LRT

Atrial-based LRT involving long AV intervals (As-Vp or As-Vs > programmed Ap-Vp) serves no useful purpose. Barring the above, the disadvantages of A-A timing are unclear, but they are likely to be minimal. The advantages of atrial-based LRT in devices with differential AV delays is probably marginal. In rate-adaptive devices with a nonadaptive AV interval (no shortening on exercise), the advantage of atrial-based LRT, especially during activity, is easy to understand in the case of Ap-Vs-Ap-Vs sequences (see Fig. 30–39, Table 30–4). However, pacemakers with nonadaptive AV intervals are being replaced by systems with adaptive AV intervals. The performance of devices with ventricular-based LRT and appropriately designed and programmed adaptive AV interval rivals that of systems with atrial-based LRT. In other words, during ventricular-based LRT, an adaptive AV interval reduces the discrepancy between the atrial pacing rate and the sensor-driven upper rate in Ap-Vs-Ap-Vs sequences[91] (see Fig. 30–40). In this respect, a suitably designed DDDR pacemaker with ventricular-based LRT and an adaptive AV interval can maintain the maximum atrial pacing rate in Ap-Vs-Ap-Vs sequences equal to the programmed sensor-driven upper rate by automatic prolongation of the sensor-driven AEI[4] for perfect or nearly perfect compensation. When all is said and done, the real importance of atrial-based LRT lies in knowing its characteristics for the proper electrocardiographic interpretation of pacemaker function because it may occasionally generate complex electrocardiographic recordings (Figs. 30–50 and 30–51).

■ ENDLESS-LOOP TACHYCARDIA

Endless-loop tachycardia (sometimes called *pacemaker-mediated tachycardia*) is a well-known complication of DDD (DDDR, VDD) pacing and represents a form of VA synchrony, or the reverse of AV synchrony.[31, 32, 38, 46, 50, 92–94] Any circumstances causing AV dissociation with separation of the P wave away from the paced or spontaneous QRS complex, coupled with the capability of retrograde VA conduction, can initiate endless-loop tachycardia (Fig. 30–52 and Table 30–8). The most common initiating mechanism is a ventricular extrasystole with retrograde VA conduction (Figs. 30–53 and 30-54). Other initiating mechanisms are outlined in Table 30–8 (Fig. 30–55). The atrial channel of a dual-chamber pacemaker can sense retrograde atrial activation only when it falls beyond the PVARP. Therefore, a short PVARP and a long AV interval predispose to endless-loop tachycardia. A relatively long AV interval allows recovery of the AV conduction system to permit retrograde VA conduction (Fig. 30–56). The following terminology best describes the mechanism of endless-loop tachycardia: repetitive pacemaker reentrant VA synchrony, pacemaker VA reentrant tachycardia,[95] or antidromic reentrant dual-chamber pacemaker tachycardia (the pacemaker acting as an electronic accessory pathway).

Endless-loop tachycardia may terminate spontaneously because of VA conduction block either from a fatigue phenomenon in the conduction system or the occurrence of a ventricular extrasystole sufficiently premature to cause retrograde VA conduction block.

1. Elimination of atrial sensing terminates endless-loop tachycardia by affecting the anterograde limb of the reentrant process in a variety of circumstances:
   a. Magnet application when the pulse generator converts to the DOO or VOO mode. Rarely, the tachycardia recurs on magnet removal.
   b. PVARP prolongation
   c. Decrease of atrial sensitivity
   e. Programming to a nonatrial tracking mode, such as the DVI or VVI mode
2. Disruption of the retrograde limb of the reentrant process can also terminate endless-loop tachycardia by one of two mechanisms:
   a. Direct effect on VA conduction with carotid sinus massage (rarely successful unless VA conduction is already quite prolonged)[96] or the administration of drugs such as adenosine, verapamil, or beta-blockers[97, 98]
   b. Uncoupling of VA synchrony by the following means:
      i. Any ventricular-sensed event unaccompanied by retrograde VA conduction block, such as a sufficiently premature ventricular extrasystole with retrograde VA conduction block, myopotentials (in unipolar pulse generators), or chest wall stimulation[99]
      ii. Omission of a single ventricular stimulus, as in the automatic tachycardia-terminating algorithm of some DDD pacemakers after the detection of a

given number of pacing cycles at the programmed upper rate or other predetermined rate[100]

Uncoupling of VA synchrony allows restoration of AV synchrony by promoting either a paced or sensed atrial event (other than retrograde P waves).

About 80% of patients with sick sinus syndrome and 35% of patients with AV block exhibit retrograde VA conduction.[101, 102] Consequently, more than 50% of patients receiving dual-chamber pacemakers are susceptible to endless-loop tachycardia. The VA conduction time ranges from 100 to 400 msec, rarely longer. All patients should be considered capable of retrograde VA conduction until proved otherwise, with particular emphasis on its unpredictable behavior. Retrograde VA conduction is influenced by various circumstances, including the resting heart rate, level of activity, and changes in autonomic tone, pacing rate, catecholamines, and concurrent drug therapy.[94, 97, 103–105] In some patients, measurements made at the time of pacemaker implantation may have little bearing on future VA conduction patterns because improvement in VA conduction may occur with ambulation and may indeed return when it was absent at the time of implantation. However, only a minority of patients (5% to 10%) with no VA conduction at the time of implantation will subsequently acquire VA conduction.[106]

With appropriate programming of sophisticated contemporary pulse generators, endless-loop tachycardia can now be prevented in most cases.[107–109] Even with appropriate programming, endless-loop tachycardia may still occur because of unpredictable variation of VA conduction that is either spontaneous or secondary to the administration of cardiac drugs.

Evaluation of Retrograde Ventriculoatrial Conduction and Propensity for Endless-Loop Tachycardia

Although the presence and duration of retrograde VA conduction can be determined in the VVI mode (with or without telemetry of the atrial channel), or even automatically by telemetry connected to the programmer of advanced pacemakers, the propensity for endless-loop tachycardia is best tested by programming the parameters of the pulse generator as follows: (1) DDD mode, (2) lower rate faster than the spontaneous rate, (3) highest atrial sensitivity, (4) shortest PVARP, (5) lowest possible atrial output (pulse duration and voltage) to produce subthreshold atrial stimulation.[32, 50, 110] An ineffectual atrial stimulus preceding a paced ventricular beat favors retrograde VA conduction by separating the spontaneous P wave from the paced QRS complex. Endless-loop tachycardia occurs when retrograde VA conduction is sustained and the retrograde P wave falls beyond the PVARP (Figs. 30–57 and 30–58). As an alternative, a pulse generator may be programmed to the VDD mode with the preceding parameters, the VDD mode being equivalent to the DDD mode with zero atrial output. However, the VDD mode is not universally available as a programmable option. Furthermore, in the presence of a relatively fast sinus rate, programming to the VDD mode with a lower rate faster than the sinus rate makes evaluation difficult. Occasionally, in the DDD mode, the threshold for atrial pacing is so low that subthreshold stimulation cannot be achieved by programming

Text continued on page 778

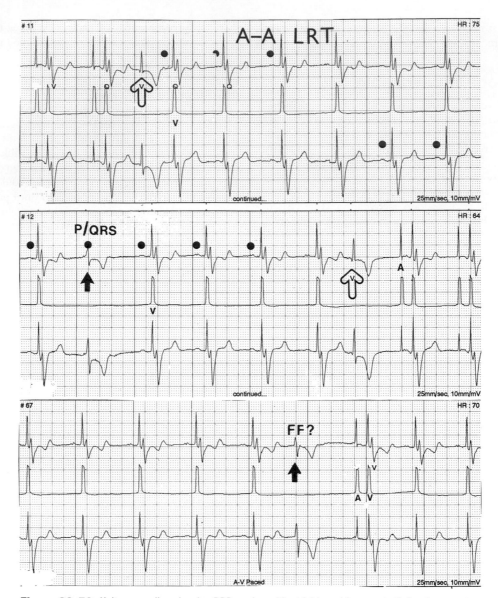

Figure 30–50. Holter recording showing DDD pacing with atrial-based lower rate timing. Lower rate interval (LRI) = 1000 msec, AV = 200 msec. *Solid black circles* depict sinus P waves. *Top,* The open arrow points to a sensed QRS complex followed by a sensed P wave that triggers the third Vp. The early P wave *(first black circle)* aborts the atrial escape interval. *Middle,* The second QRS complex is a spontaneous beat that initiates a Vs-Vp interval longer than the LRI of 1000 msec. According to the sinus rate, it appears that a P wave occurs coincidentally with the second QRS complex *(black arrow).* The pacemaker senses the concealed P wave before the QRS complex. Because of atrial-based lower rate timing, the pacemaker initiates the LRI from the sensed P wave. Thus, the atrial escape interval from the sensed ventricular event lengthens beyond the basic value of 800 msec to maintain constancy of the atrial-based LRI. The *open arrow* points to a QRS complex (without a preceding sensed P wave) that initiates an atrial escape interval corresponding to the basic value of 800 msec. *Bottom,* The QRS at the arrow (far-field sensing [FF?]) appears to initiate an atrial escape interval of 920–940 msec that cannot be explained in terms of late sensing of a narrow QRS complex. The prolonged atrial escape interval represents a manifestation of atrial-based lower rate timing due either to a P wave that is sensed by the pacemaker before it senses the QRS complex or, more likely, to a far-field phenomenon whereby the atrial channel, by sensing the QRS deflection in the atrial electrogram (before the ventricular channel senses it as a near-field signal), initiates the LRI. These normal manifestations of atrial-based lower rate timing should not be misinterpreted as T wave or other forms of oversensing, programmed hysteresis, or malfunction. (From Barold SS: Evaluation of pacemaker function by Holter recordings. *In* Moss A, Stern S [eds]: Noninvasive Cardiology: Clinical Aspects of Holter Monitoring. Philadelphia, WB Saunders, 1996, p 107.)

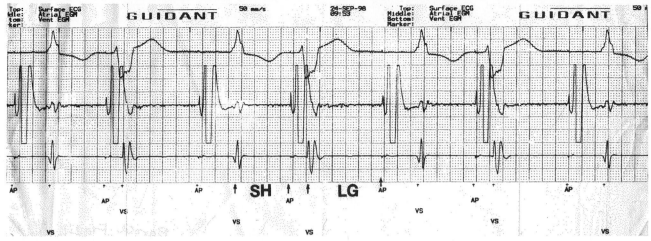

Figure 30–51. Simultaneous recording (50 mm/sec) of surface ECG *(top)*, atrial electrogram *(middle)*, and ventricular electrogram *(bottom)* in a patient with a Guidant Discovery DDDR pacemaker with atrial-based lower rate timing. AV = 300 msec, lower rate interval (LRI) = 700 msec. Paced and spontaneous P waves were invisible on the surface ECG. The Ap-Ap interval remains constant at 700 msec, which is the LRI. The Ap-Vs intervals vary because ventricular premature beats (VPC) occur within the AV delay. Short Ap-Vs intervals are associated with longer atrial escape (Vs-Ap) intervals, creating a form of hysteresis. The question arises as to whether the long ventricular cycles are responsible for the perpetuation of ventricular bigeminy. In this case, programmability from atrial-based to ventricular-based LRT (not yet available in devices) might have been useful.

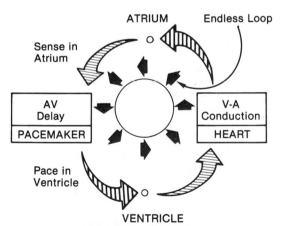

Figure 30–52. Diagrammatic representation of the mechanism of endless-loop tachycardia. When the atrial channel senses a retrograde P wave, a ventricular pacing stimulus is issued at the completion of the programmed AV interval. The pulse generator itself provides the anterograde limb of the macroreentrant loop because it functions as an artificial AV junction. Retrograde VA conduction following ventricular pacing provides the retrograde limb of the reentrant loop. The pulse generator again senses the retrograde P wave, and the process perpetuates itself. Termination of endless-loop tachycardia can be accomplished by disrupting either the anterograde limb (by eliminating atrial sensing) or the retrograde limb (by eliminating retrograde VA conduction). (From Barold SS, Falkoff MD, Ong LS, et al: Pacemaker endless loop tachycardia: Termination by simple techniques other than magnet application. Am J Med 85:817, 1988.)

Table 30–8. Initiating Mechanisms of Endless-Loop Tachycardia

1. Ventricular extrasystoles
2. Subthreshold atrial stimulation
3. Chest wall stimulation selectively sensed by the atrial channel
4. Atrial extrasystole with prolongation of the AV interval (to conform to the programmed upper rate interval > total atrial refractory period)
5. Decrease in atrial sensitivity; undersensing of anterograde P waves with preserved sensing of retrograde P waves
6. Application and withdrawal of the magnet
7. a. Myopotential oversensing by the atrial channel only
   b. Myopotential inhibition of ventricular channel can also initiate endless-loop tachycardia by allowing ventricular escape beats without preceding atrial depolarization, thereby favoring retrograde VA conduction
8. Programmer-generated electromagnetic interference sensed by the atrial channel only
9. Excessively long programmed AV interval
10. Paradoxical induction with excessively long PVARP, also with automatic PVARP extension
11. Programming to the VDD mode when the sinus rate is slower than the programmed lower rate
12. Exercise treadmill stress testing with development of pacemaker Wenckebach upper rate response with lengthening of the AV interval initiated by a sensed P wave
13. Sensing of a far-field QRS signal by the atrial lead, i.e., far-field endless-loop tachycardia without atrial participation (only with inappropriate abbreviation of the PVARP)

PVARP, postventricular atrial refractory period.
Modified from Barold SS: Repetitive reentrant and nonreentrant ventriculoatrial synchrony in dual chamber pacing. Clin Cardiol 14:754, 1991.

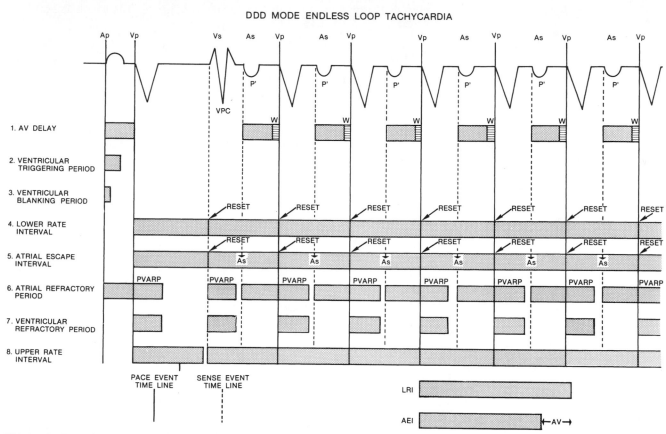

Figure 30–53. DDD mode with ventricular-based lower rate timing. Endless-loop tachycardia initiated by a ventricular extrasystole (VPC, second beat) with retrograde VA conduction (As). The atrial channel senses the retrograde P wave (P′), and a ventricular pacing stimulus (Vp) is issued after extension of the AV interval to conform to the upper rate interval (URI). Vp generates another retrograde P wave, again sensed by the pulse generator, and the process perpetuates itself. The pulse generator itself provides the anterograde limb of the macroreentrant loop because it functions as an artificial AV junction. Retrograde VA conduction following ventricular pacing provides the retrograde limb of the reentrant loop. The cycle length of the endless-loop tachycardia may occasionally be longer than the URI if retrograde VA conduction is prolonged (see Figs. 30–54 and 30–57). Same format as in Figure 30–10. (From Barold SS, Falkoff MD, Ong LS, et al: All dual-chamber pacemakers function in the DDD mode. Am Heart J 115:1353, 1988.)

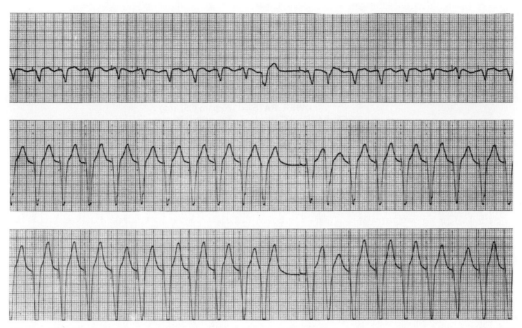

Figure 30–54. Endless-loop tachycardia terminated and reinitiated by a ventricular extrasystole. The three ECG leads were recorded simultaneously. Upper rate interval (URI) = 500 msec (120 ppm); lower rate interval (LRI) = 857 msec (70 ppm); AV delay = 150 msec. The cycle length of the tachycardia is longer than the URI. (From Barold SS, Falkoff MD, Ong LS, et al: Electrocardiography of contemporary DDD pacemakers. A. Basic concepts, upper rate response, retrograde ventriculoatrial conduction, and differential diagnosis of pacemaker tachycardias. *In* Saksena S, Goldschlager N [eds]: Electrical Therapy for Cardiac Arrhythmias: Pacing, Antitachycardia Devices, Catheter Ablation. Philadelphia, WB Saunders, 1990, pp 225–264.)

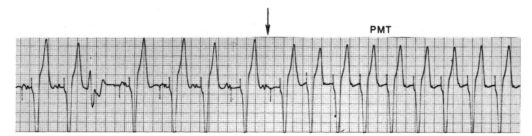

Figure 30–55. Initiation of endless-loop tachycardia or pacemaker-mediated tachycardia (PMT) due to undersensing of sinus P waves and normal sensing of retrograde P waves. The *arrow* points to the unsensed P wave responsible for initiation of endless-loop tachycardia. (From Barold SS, Falkoff MD, Ong LS, et al: Electrocardiography of contemporary DDD pacemakers. A. Basic concepts, upper rate response, retrograde ventriculoatrial conduction, and differential diagnosis of pacemaker tachycardias. *In* Saksena S, Goldschlager N [eds]: Electrical Therapy for Cardiac Arrhythmias: Pacing, Antitachycardia Devices, Catheter Ablation. Philadelphia, WB Saunders, 1990, pp 225–264.)

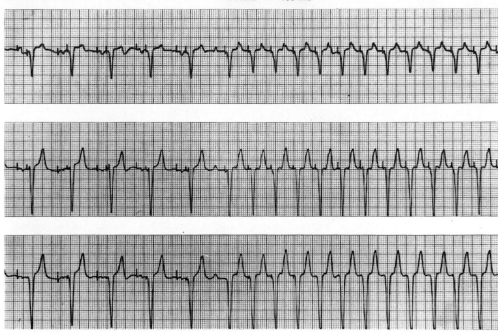

SYMBIOS 7006 DDD
LOWER RATE = 70 ppm (857 ms)
UPPER RATE INTERVAL = 125 ppm (480 ms)
AV INTERVAL = 200 ms
PVARP = 155 ms

Figure 30–56. "Spontaneous" endless-loop tachycardia in a patient with a Symbios 7006 DDD pulse generator. The programmed parameters are shown above the 3-lead ECG. The paced AV (Ap-Vp) interval is not associated with retrograde VA conduction. When the AV interval is initiated by a sensed sinus P wave (As-Vp), retrograde VA conduction occurs and initiates an endless-loop tachycardia. This initiating mechanism was repeatedly documented in long ECG recordings. Endless-loop tachycardia was prevented (on a short-term basis) by programming the AV interval to 150 msec without changing the postventricular atrial refractory period (PVARP). No atrial extrasystoles were observed. The sequence of events suggests that a sinus impulse reaches the AV junction earlier than a paced atrial depolarization. Earlier recovery of the AV junction permits retrograde VA conduction only after a sinus P wave. The relatively late recovery of the AV junction after a paced atrial depolarization prevents retrograde VA conduction. (From Barold SS, Falkoff MD, Ong LS, et al: Electrocardiography of contemporary DDD pacemakers. A. Basic concepts, upper rate response, retrograde ventriculoatrial conduction, and differential diagnosis of pacemaker tachycardias. *In* Saksena S, Goldschlager N [eds]: Electrical Therapy for Cardiac Arrhythmias: Pacing, Antitachycardia Devices, Catheter Ablation. Philadelphia, WB Saunders, 1990, pp 225–264.)

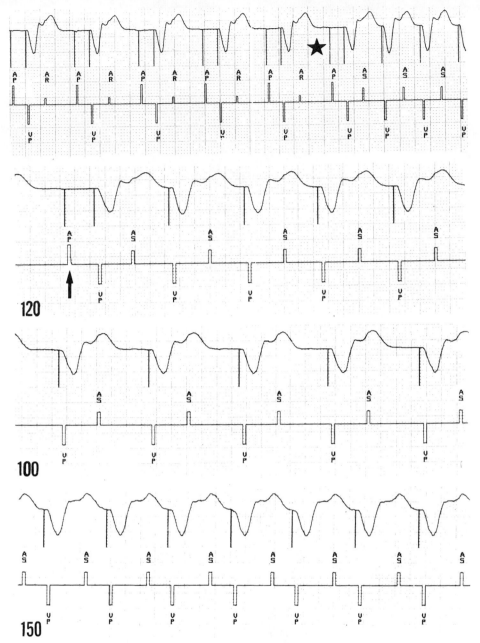

Figure 30–57. DDD pacing with endless-loop tachycardia. Lower rate interval (LRI) = 857 msec; AV = 200 msec after atrial pacing and 150 msec after atrial sensing; postventricular atrial refractory period (PVARP) = 300 msec, upper rate interval (URI) = 500 msec (120 ppm). *Top panel,* Subthreshold atrial stimulation (AP). Ventricular pacing causes retrograde VA conduction. On the *left,* the retrograde P waves fall within the PVARP and are unsensed (A_R). The PVARP is shortened to 200 msec at the *star.* The pacemaker then senses the retrograde P waves (A_S) and initiates endless-loop tachycardia. *Second panel,* Recording at 50 mm/sec also shows the initiation of endless-loop tachycardia by subthreshold atrial stimulation. The markers indicate that the retrograde VA time measures about 240 msec. The As-Vp interval is prolonged to conform to the URI, so that the Vp-Vp interval = URI = 500 msec (120 ppm). *Third panel* (50 mm/sec), The URI is programmed to 600 msec (100 ppm). The retrograde VA conduction time during endless-loop tachycardia remains constant at 240 msec, but the As-Vp interval lengthens further to conform to the URI, so that the Vp-Vp interval = 600 msec. *Bottom panel* (50 mm/sec), The upper rate is programmed to 150 bpm (URI = 400 msec). The retrograde VA conduction time is now slightly longer at about 260 msec. The programmed As-Vp remains at 150 msec and is not extended. The tachycardia interval represents the sum of the VA conduction time and the programmed As-Vp, and it is slightly longer (410–420 msec) than the URI. Endless-loop tachycardia was no longer induced by subthreshold atrial stimulation when the PVARP was again programmed to 300 msec, as in the *top panel* on the *left.* (From Barold SS, Zipes DP: Cardiac pacemakers and antiarrhythmic devices. *In* Braunwald E [ed]: Heart Disease [5th ed]. Philadelphia: WB Saunders, 1997, pp 705–741.)

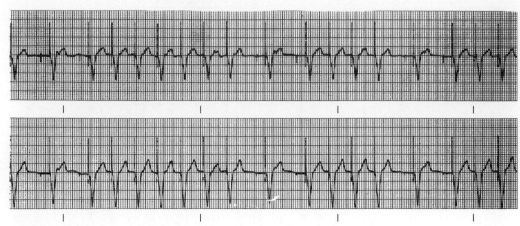

Figure 30–58. Subthreshold atrial stimulation in the DDD mode leading to unsustained endless-loop tachycardia in a patient with a Cosmos (Intermedics) DDD pulse generator (two-lead ECG). The programmed parameters were as follows: lower rate interval = 880 msec; upper rate interval = 480 msec; postventricular atrial refractory period = 200 msec; AV interval = 180 msec. The retrograde VA conduction time is just over 200 msec, so that the retrograde P wave is sensed by the atrial channel, thereby initiating runs of unsustained endless-loop tachycardia. Two ECG leads were recorded simultaneously. (From Barold SS, Falkoff MD, Ong LS, et al: Function and electrocardiography of DDD pacemakers. *In* Barold SS [ed]: Modern Cardiac Pacing. Mt Kisco, NY, Futura, 1985, pp 645–675.)

the lowest atrial output. In this situation, chest wall stimulation (with an external pacemaker providing signals sensed selectively by the atrial channel) can easily precipitate endless-loop tachycardia in susceptible patients by separating the P wave from the paced QRS complex[19, 99, 111, 112] (Fig. 30–59). Other techniques, such as application and withdrawal of the magnet, isometric muscle exercise (unipolar devices), maximum prolongation of the AV interval, tread-

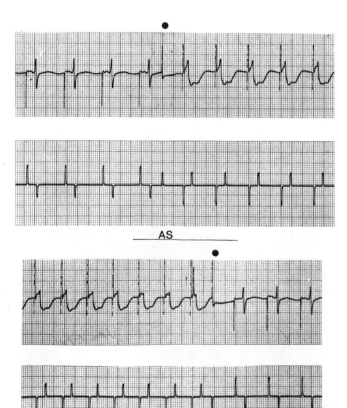

Figure 30–59. Effect of chest wall stimulation (CWS) on unipolar DDD pulse generator. Real-time event markers are shown below the electrocardiogram, with atrial events on top and ventricular events at the bottom. The markers depicting sensed events are smaller than those related to paced events. *Top,* CWS (*solid black circle*) sensed only by the atrial channel initiates endless-loop tachycardia. *Bottom,* Endless-loop tachycardia terminated by the second CWS (*solid black circle*) sensed by the ventricular channel. The first CWS falls within the refractory period of the ventricular channel. As, atrial-sensed event; Vs, ventricular-sensed event. (From Barold SS, Falkoff MD, Ong LS, et al: Electrocardiography of contemporary DDD pacemakers. A. Basic concepts, upper rate response, retrograde ventriculoatrial conduction, and differential diagnosis of pacemaker tachycardias. *In* Saksena S, Goldschlager N [eds]: Electrical Therapy for Cardiac Arrhythmias: Pacing, Antitachycardia Devices, Catheter Ablation. Philadelphia, WB Saunders, 1990, pp 225–264.)

mill exercise, and chest thumping 3(to produce ventricular extrasystoles), are inconsistently effective and are not recommended.[32]

Prevention of Endless-Loop Tachycardia

Maneuvers to initiate endless-loop tachycardia are repeated until appropriate programming of the pacemaker prevents induction of tachycardia (Table 30–9). The rate of the tachycardia is often equal to the programmed upper rate. When the rate of endless-loop tachycardia is slower than the programmed upper rate, the retrograde VA conduction time is equal to the difference between the tachycardia cycle length and the AV interval, which in this case is equal to the programmed value.[113] Telemetry by means of event markers with automatic measurements of intervals and transmission

Table 30–9. Programmability for the Prevention of Endless-Loop Tachycardia

Parameter	Advantages	Disadvantages
1. Programmable PVARP	Applicable to all patients unless VACT is excessively long	Limits programmable upper rate. Long TARP precludes pacemaker Wenckebach upper rate response and may cause sudden undesirable 2 : 1 pacemaker AV block at relatively low levels of exercise
2. Automatic PVARP extension for one cycle after a ventricular premature event, i.e., ventricular extrasystole*	Standard PVARP remains unchanged. Upper rate not compromised. Useful with long VACT or if short PVARP is required	(a) Not operative with ventricular paced beat (b) Cannot be programmed "off" in some units† (c) Long PVARP may cause atrial undersensing with perpetuation of PVARP extension if the pacemaker senses only ventricular events (d) Long PVARP may paradoxically induce ELT (e) Delivery of atrial stimulus close to the preceding unsensed P wave may theoretically induce supraventricular arrhythmias
3. DDX mode after a ventricular premature event (DVI cycle)	As above	As above except for (b). The DVI mode is not necessarily restricted to one cycle. The pacemaker will remain in the DVI mode until emission of an atrial stimulus.
4. Synchronous atrial pacing upon sensing a ventricular premature event	As above Preempts atrial depolarization so that retrograde impulse encounters refractory atrium	(a) Not operative after a ventricular paced beat (b) May cause pacemaker orthodromic tachycardia
5. Programmable atrial sensitivity	Upper rate not compromised. Allows shorter PVARP. 60%–75% of anterograde P waves are at least 0.5 mV larger than retrograde P waves.	Requires device with extensive selection of atrial sensitivity to allow fine tuning. This approach never became popular, probably for technical reasons.
6. Shortening of AV interval	Allows a faster programmable upper rate by shortening TARP. If the atrial sensed ventricular paced AV interval is shorter than the atrial paced ventricular paced AV interval and further decreases on exercise, a faster upper rate can be programmed.	Limited value
7. Faster upper rate to induce VA conduction block at faster ventricular rates	ELT either unsustainable or of shorter duration and better tolerated	Limited application. Sustained rapid ELT may occur with improvement of VA conduction
8. Adaptive TARP (AV, PVARP, or both can shorten on exercise)	Longer TARP at rest limits upper rate often with fixed-ratio block if TARP = URI. Shortening of PVARP on exercise allows a high programmed upper rate. ELT much less likely on exercise	More complex pacemaker behavior. Rarely, prolonged VA conduction may be absent at rest or may occur only on exercise.
9. Elimination of effective atrial tracking by programming to another mode, e.g., VVI (VVIR), DVI (DVIR), DDI (DDIR)	Ventricular pacing rate always remains at the programmed lower rate	(a) VVI (VVIR) and DVI (DVIR) are unphysiologic paced modes. (b) DDI (DDIR) mode may not prevent repetitive reentrant VA synchrony at lower rate (ELT without tachycardia)

TARP, total atrial refractory period; PVARP, postventricular atrial refractory period; VACT, ventricular atrial conduction time; ELT, endless-loop tachycardia

* Interpreted by a pacemaker as two ventricular events without an intervening sensed atrial event.

† Automatic PVARP extension may also come into effect with magnet removal, VVD mode without a preceding atrial event, inhibition of atrial output in the DDI mode, and noise sensed by atrial channel.

In some pulse generators, automatic PVARP extension is accompanied by a longer atrial escape interval to favor AV synchrony and prevent ELT.

Modified from Barold SS: Repetitive reentrant and nonreentrant ventriculoatrial synchrony in dual chamber pacing. Clin Cardiol 14:754, 1991.

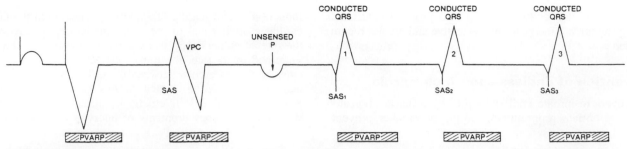

Figure 30–60. Diagram illustrating the mechanism of orthodromic pacemaker tachycardia during DDD pacing with a synchronous atrial stimulation (SAS) algorithm to prevent endless-loop tachycardia. SAS delivers an atrial stimulus on detection of a ventricular premature contraction (VPC). In this way, retrograde VA conduction engendered by a VPC cannot cause atrial depolarization because it is pre-empted by SAS that renders the atrium refractory. A ventricular extrasystole (VPC) is sensed by the ventricular electrode, thereby triggering SAS. This is followed by an unsensed P wave outside the PVARP. The unsensed P wave is conducted and gives rise to the first conducted QRS complex that is sensed beyond the ventricular refractory period of the pacemaker. The pulse generator interprets this conducted QRS complex as a VPC and delivers SAS. This again leads to a conducted QRS complex (2) with a very long PR interval. The second QRS complex causes SAS 2, and SAS 2 causes QRS 3, and so forth, and the process perpetuates itself. The reentrant loop is composed of an anterograde limb in the heart (AV junction), and the retrograde limb occurs in the pacemaker (sensing by the ventricular channel). Such an orthodromic pacemaker tachycardia could also be initiated by a sensed VPC (without retrograde conduction) or any other signal sensed by the ventricular channel and interpreted as a VPC (e.g., myopotentials in a unipolar system), provided SAS causes prolonged but successful AV conduction. A related pacemaker tachycardia can occur during single-chamber AAT pacing. In this particular case, the far-field QRS complex is sensed in the atrium, and the pacemaker delivers an atrial stimulus synchronously with sensing of the QRS complex. (From Barold SS: Repetitive reentrant and nonreentrant ventriculoatrial synchrony in dual-chamber pacing. Clin Cardiol 14:754, 1991. Copyrighted and reprinted with the permission of Clinical Cardiology Publishing Company, Inc., P.O. Box 832, Mahwah, NJ 07430.)

of the atrial electrogram permit determination of the retrograde VA conduction time. Programmability of the PVARP constitutes the most effective way of preventing endless-loop tachycardia at present. In general, the PVARP should be programmed at 50 to 75 msec beyond the duration of the retrograde VA conduction time determined noninvasively. A PVARP of 300 msec offers protection against endless-loop tachycardia in most patients with retrograde VA conduction. If possible, patients without demonstrable retrograde VA conduction at the time of the implantation should have a PVARP programmed to 300 msec, provided that there is no compromise of the upper rate. A long PVARP limits the upper rate of the pacemaker. This is true at rest, but upper rate limitation may be partially circumvented with automatic shortening of the As-Vp interval as the sinus rate increases (rate-adaptive AV delay) and shortening of an adaptive PVARP during exercise, both of which abbreviate the TARP. As discussed later, a long PVARP can also cause atrial undersensing and the induction of repetitive nonreentrant VA synchrony and induce competitive atrial stimulation during DDDR pacing.

Other measures to prevent endless-loop tachycardia (see Table 30–9) include (1) a shorter AV interval, (2) differential discrimination of the larger anterograde P wave from the smaller retrograde atrial depolarization,[114, 115] or a programmable change in the bandpass filter for sensing,[116] and (3) response to ventricular extrasystoles. A sensed ventricular event (outside the AV delay) that the pacemaker interprets as a ventricular extrasystole activates a special mechanism consisting of either automatic extension of the PVARP for one cycle to ensure containment of retrograde atrial depolarization[30, 32, 40, 117] (discussed later in the section on the atrial refractory period) or delivery of synchronous atrial stimulation (to pre-empt retrograde atrial depolarization).[117, 118]

The measures listed in Table 30–9 can be useful in min-

imizing or eliminating endless-loop tachycardia, but they may also create new problems, as shown in Figure 30–60. A contemporary DDD pacemaker should rarely if ever be downgraded to a simpler mode (e.g., DVI or VVI) to prevent endless-loop tachycardia. Rarely, refractory endless-loop tachycardia can be treated by catheter ablation of the AV junction.[119]

Automatic Termination and Prevention of Endless-Loop Tachycardia

Algorithms for the detection and termination of endless tachycardia should not be based solely on the detection of the programmed upper rate because some tachycardias are slower than the upper rate in the presence of relatively prolonged VA conduction. Furthermore, the pulse generator should recognize the nature of tachycardia because pacing at the upper rate obviously does not discriminate endless-loop tachycardia from tracking of a normal sinus tachycardia.

In a basic algorithm, on detection of the upper rate or a programmed slower rate for a given number of cycles (6 to 16), the pacemaker uncouples VA synchrony by withholding a single ventricular output or extending the PVARP for one cycle. Termination of endless-loop tachycardia in the DDD mode, therefore, produces a pause, which has been minimized in a recent algorithm.[120]

Another algorithm uses stability of the Vp-As interval shorter than a given value as a diagnostic parameter of ELT regardless of the rate. In one algorithm (ELA Chorus), the pacemaker automatically shortens one As-Vp interval (As = retrograde P wave in case of endless-loop tachycardia). Such AV interval modulation, regardless of the rate,[121–123] with automatic shortening of a single AV interval by advancing ventricular activation may occasionally terminate tachycardia by causing retrograde VA conduction block. The pacemaker identifies endless-loop tachycardia if the same Vp gives rise to a Vp-As interval that remains constant; that is, retrograde VA conduction remains constant after shortening of the AV interval. In an SVT, the Vp-As lengthens by the amount the As-Vp interval is shortened by the pacemaker algorithm. The Trilogy DR + (St. Jude Medical, Sylmar, CA) uses the same principle but lengthens the As-Vp interval for its diagnostic function.[120] After diagnosis by AV modulation, the pacemaker omits a single ventricular stimulus for tachycardia termination.

Smart Pacemakers

A smart pacemaker should know when the automatic tachycardia-terminating algorithm is being activated too frequently, whereupon it could automatically increase the PVARP permanently, a change that would be telemetered at the time of the next follow-up interrogation of the device.

A smart DDDR pacemaker can differentiate physiologic from nonphysiologic rate variations.[124, 125] This discrimination can be achieved in the passive sensor mode, with the pulse generator itself not necessarily functioning in the rate-adaptive mode. During endless-loop tachycardia, the atrial channel senses a rapid rate, but the input to the nonatrial sensor indicates physical inactivity and therefore no need to increase the pacing rate. The pulse generator can use this information to increase its PVARP for one cycle to terminate endless-loop tachycardia immediately. If tachycardia persists, the pulse generator would then identify it as an SVT other than endless-loop tachycardia, whereupon it might switch its pacing mode automatically to avoid rapid ventricular pacing. A smart pacemaker will also analyze the relationship between atrial and ventricular events. The smart pacemaker will then automatically lengthen the PVARP or omit the Vp related to an atrial-sensed event in situations favoring retrograde VA conduction, for example, lack of atrial capture (detected by evoked response recognition) or detection of early atrial events, such as retrograde P waves,[126] with prolongation of AV conduction. A smart pacemaker may eventually be capable of differentiating anterograde from retrograde P waves in all cases, and it should also detect atrial signals other than the P wave by improved electronics for better signal discrimination. Further refinements of these designs may eliminate the need to compromise the upper rate of the pacemaker by programming a long PVARP to contain relatively slow retrograde VA conduction.

Repetitive Nonreentrant Ventriculoatrial Synchrony

VA synchrony can occur without endless-loop tachycardia when a paced ventricular beat engenders an unsensed retrograde P wave falling within the PVARP of a DDD (DDDR, DDI, DDIR) pacemaker. Under certain circumstances, this form of VA synchrony may become self-perpetuating because the pacemaker continually delivers an ineffectual atrial stimulus during the atrial myocardial refractory period generated by the preceding retrograde atrial depolarization[95, 127–131] (Fig. 30–61). By definition, the amplitude of the atrial stimulus must exceed the atrial pacing threshold tested during atrial pacing with a normal relationship of atrial and ventricular events. This form of VA synchrony has been called *AV desynchronization arrhythmia*,[129] *repetitive nonreentrant VA synchrony,* or *VA synchrony nonreentrant arrhythmia.*[95] Schüller and Brandt have called this situation *pseudoatrial exit block.*[132]

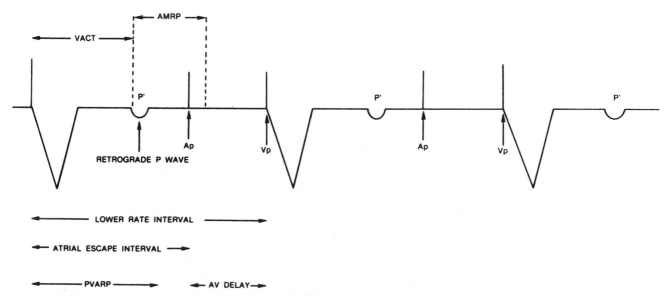

Figure 30–61. Diagrammatic representation of nonreentrant VA synchrony or AV desynchronization arrhythmia. There is relatively slow retrograde VA conduction. The first ventricular-paced beat causes retrograde VA conduction. The retrograde P wave (P) is unsensed either because it falls within the postventricular atrial refractory period (PVARP) or because the magnet causes asynchronous DOO pacing. At the completion of the AEI, the pacemaker delivers an atrial stimulus (Ap), falling too close to the preceding P wave and therefore still within the atrial myocardial refractory period (AMRP) engendered by the preceding retrograde atrial depolarization. Ap is therefore ineffectual. Barring any perturbations, this process becomes self-perpetuating. VACT, retrograde VA conduction time; Vp, ventricular stimulus. (From Barold SS, Falkoff MD, Ong LS, et al: Magnet unresponsive pacemaker endless loop tachycardia. Am Heart J 116:726, 1988.)

LOWER RATE INTERVAL = 750 ms

AV DELAY = 250 ms

PVARP = 400 ms

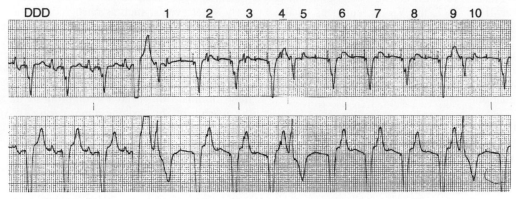

Figure 30–62. Initiation of nonreentrant VA synchrony by ventricular extrasystole (ventricular premature contraction, VPC) during DDD pacing (parameters shown above the ECG). The numbers indicate retrograde P waves. The fourth and fifth complexes are VPCs. The second VPC initiates retrograde VA conduction (1). The succeeding atrial stimulus is ineffectual because it falls within the myocardial atrial refractory period related to retrograde P wave 1. The accompanying ventricular paced beat perpetuates retrograde VA conduction (2), thereby starting repetitive nonreentrant VA synchrony. VPCs with retrograde VA conduction (5 and 10) during nonreentrant VA synchrony do not disturb the basic mechanism. Two electrocardiographic leads were recorded simultaneously. (From Barold SS: Repetitive reentrant and nonreentrant ventriculoatrial synchrony in dual-chamber pacing. Clin Cardiol 14:754, 1991. Copyrighted and reprinted with the permission of Clinical Cardiology Publishing Company, Inc., P.O. Box 832, Mahwah, NJ 07430.)

During repetitive nonreentrant VA synchrony, the pacemaker provides an anterograde pathway (atrial stimulus followed by ventricular stimulus), whereas the conduction system provides a retrograde pathway back to the atrium (Fig. 30–62). In contrast to endless-loop tachycardia, the potential reentrant circuit does not close because the pacemaker does not sense the retrograde P wave. The process repeats itself with each cardiac cycle, and release of the ventricular stimulus does not depend on the timing of the retrograde P wave.

A long AV interval, a relatively fast lower rate (or sensor-driven rate with DDDR pacing), or both favor the development of repetitive nonreentrant VA synchrony, usually in the setting of relatively long retrograde VA conduction with retrograde P waves in the PVARP. A retrograde P wave

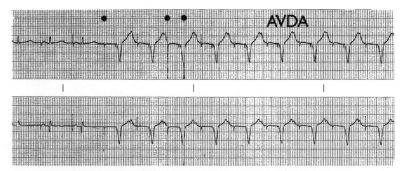

Figure 30–63. Initiation of repetitive nonreentrant VA synchrony or AV desynchronization arrhythmia (AVDA) by chest wall stimulation adjusted to be sensed selectively by the atrial channel. Chest wall stimuli are depicted by *solid black circles*. The first chest wall stimulus sensed by the atrial channel triggers a ventricular paced beat followed by retrograde VA conduction. The retrograde P wave falls within the long postventricular atrial refractory period (PVARP; 400 msec) and deforms the apex of the T wave. The succeeding atrial stimulus falls within the atrial myocardial refractory period. The second and third chest wall stimuli fall within the pacemaker atrial refractory period and are unsensed by the atrial channel. Two ECG leads were recorded simultaneously. (From Barold SS: Nonreentrant ventriculoatrial synchrony in dual-chamber pacing. *In* Santini M, Pistolese M, Alliegro A [eds]: Progress in Clinical Pacing 1990. Amsterdam, Excerpta Medica, 1990, pp 451–471.)

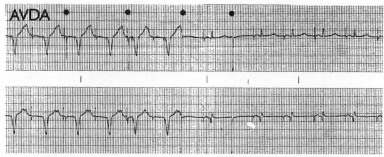

Figure 30–64. Termination of repetitive nonreentrant VA synchrony or AV desynchronization arrhythmia (AVDA) by chest wall stimulation. Same patient and parameters as in Figure 30–63. Chest wall stimuli are depicted by *solid black circles.* The first chest wall stimulus is unsensed. The amplitude of chest wall stimulation was increased, so the second chest wall stimulus is sensed by the ventricular channel activating the ventricular safety pacing mechanism, with resultant abbreviation of the AV interval. The ventricular channel of the DDD pulse generator senses the third chest wall stimulus, and nonreentrant VA synchrony terminates immediately. Two ECG leads were recorded simultaneously. (From Barold SS: Repetitive nonreentrant ventriculoatrial synchrony in dual-chamber pacing. *In* Santini M, Pistolese M, Alliegro A [eds]: Progress in Clinical Pacing 1990. Amsterdam, Excerpta Medica, 1990, pp 451–471.)

beyond the PVARP, but unsensed because of low amplitude or low sensitivity of the atrial channel, can also initiate the same form of VA synchrony. Rarely, AV synchrony (with atrial capture) and VA synchrony (retrograde P waves) coexist in the same cardiac cycle whenever a relatively long AV interval (e.g., 250 msec) favors retrograde VA conduction. Endless-loop tachycardia and repetitive nonreentrant VA synchrony depend on retrograde VA conduction and are physiologically similar (Figs. 30–63 to 30–65). Both share

similar initiating and terminating mechanisms, and under certain circumstances, one arrhythmia may convert spontaneously to the other.[95] Termination of repetitive nonreentrant VA synchrony rarely occurs spontaneously, secondary to VA conduction block or improved VA conduction (situations that displace the atrial stimulus away from the atrial myocardial refractory period generated by the preceding retrograde conduction).

Once initiated, two scenarios are possible during repeti-

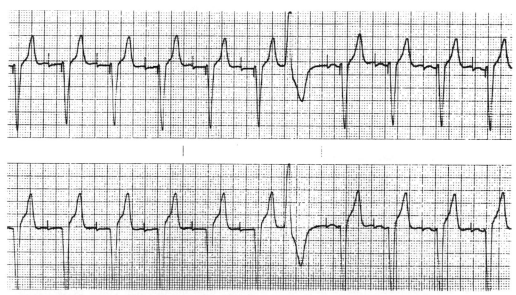

Figure 30–65. Two-lead ECG showing termination of repetitive nonreentrant VA synchrony or AV desynchronization arrhythmia at 80 ppm by ventricular extrasystole (ventricular premature contraction, VPC). On the left, the atrial stimuli are ineffectual because they fall in the atrial myocardial refractory period generated by the preceding retrograde atrial depolarization. The VPC restores AV synchrony (on the right). It is impossible to determine from the ECG whether the VPC is associated with retrograde VA conduction block (because of prematurity) or retrograde conduction that is sufficiently removed from the subsequent atrial stimulus to allow it to capture the atrium.

tive nonreentrant VA synchrony: (1) The atrial stimulus continually falls in the absolute atrial myocardial refractory period and is always ineffectual even if the atrial output of the pacemaker is increased to its maximal value. (2) The atrial stimulus falls within the relative refractory period of the atrial myocardium, so that the threshold for atrial pacing is increased. After the induction of repetitive nonreentrant VA synchrony, the higher atrial pacing threshold appears to decrease gradually and then stabilize (all other parameters remaining unchanged) over a period of less than 1 minute to a value greater than the one tested during atrial pacing with a normal relationship of atrial and ventricular events. The mechanism of such threshold behavior is unknown. One of two situations can then occur: (1) spontaneous return of atrial capture without altering any of the pacemaker parameters when the diminishing atrial pacing threshold attains a value equal to the atrial output of the pacemaker (indeed, repetitive nonreentrant VA synchrony is often unsustained for this reason), or (2) repetitive nonreentrant VA synchrony persists until a deliberate increase in the atrial output of the pacemaker promotes atrial capture with all other parameters remaining constant.

When sustained, repetitive nonreentrant VA synchrony can cause unfavorable hemodynamics similar to the pacemaker syndrome during normal function of a DDD/DDI (DDDR/DDIR) pulse generator.[133, 134] Because the duration of the AEI (pacemaker VA) and AV interval can be easily controlled, repetitive nonreentrant VA synchrony should not be an important problem with conventional DDD or DDI pulse generators. However, DDDR or DDIR pulse generators could induce repetitive nonreentrant VA synchrony on exercise when the sensor-driven increase in pacing rate shortens the atrial escape (pacemaker VA) interval. Conceivably, during exercise, a ventricular extrasystole could precipitate repetitive nonreentrant VA synchrony with perpetuation of retrograde VA conduction, thereby negating the beneficial effect of AV synchrony by producing a VVIR-like pacemaker syndrome.

Prevention and termination of repetitive nonreentrant VA synchrony can be achieved by a number of algorithms discussed later in the section on the atrial refractory period.

Magnet-Unresponsive Endless-Loop Tachycardia

When magnet application causes relatively fast DOO pacing, endless-loop tachycardia may convert to a slower repetitive nonreentrant VA synchrony without disturbing VA conduction. On withdrawal of the magnet and restoration of atrial sensing, repetitive nonreentrant VA synchrony is immediately converted to an endless-loop tachycardia that cannot be terminated by magnet application[130] (Fig. 30–66A and B). Other causes of magnet-unresponsive endless-loop tachycardia include inadvertent programming of the "magnet off" operation and insufficient magnetic field when a magnet is applied over the pulse generator of an obese patient. In the absence of an appropriate programmer, magnet-unresponsive endless-loop tachycardia can be terminated in a variety of ways. Carotid sinus massage may occasionally be successful by causing block of retrograde VA conduction.[96] Pharmacologic therapy to block retrograde VA conduction is not recommended, but adenosine may work accurately.[97] Uncoup-

ling of VA synchrony with immediate termination of endless-loop tachycardia can be accomplished easily by chest wall stimulation sensed by the ventricular channel.[99] Without special equipment, chest wall stimulation can be easily and reliably delivered by transcutaneous external pacing (pulse width, 20 to 40 msec), with the large pad electrodes separated by 10 to 15 cm and an output invariably less than 20 mA (well below the external pacing threshold).[99]

Coexistence of Repetitive Reentrant and Nonreentrant Ventriculoatrial Synchrony

Manipulation, such as application or removal of the magnet, may convert an endless-loop tachycardia to nonreentrant VA synchrony and vice versa. Occasionally, conversion of nonreentrant VA synchrony to endless-loop tachycardia and back to nonreentrant VA synchrony can occur spontaneously. The predisposing factors for spontaneous conversion include (1) PVARP close to the retrograde VA conduction time. Minor variations of P-wave timing may cause periods of P-wave sensing alternating with undersensing; (2) progressive prolongation of the retrograde VA conduction time with eventual stabilization (repetitive nonreentrant VA synchrony converts to sustained endless-loop tachycardia when the retrograde P wave falls beyond the PVARP); and (3) borderline voltage for atrial sensing provided by the retrograde P wave. Endless-loop tachycardia occurs with P wave sensing, but when the P wave is unsensed, the subsequent atrial stimulus falls within the refractory period of the atrial myocardium and creates a situation akin to repetitive nonreentrant VA synchrony. A situation like repetitive nonreentrant VA synchrony will continue until the pulse generator resumes sensing the P wave.

■ UPPER RATE RESPONSE OF DDDR PULSE GENERATOR

In DDDR pulse generators, the sensor-driven URI can be longer or shorter than or equal to the atrial-driven URI.[52, 135, 136] There appears to be no clinical use for a sensor-driven upper rate slower than the atrial-driven upper rate except perhaps to attenuate the effect of sudden deceleration of the sinus rate after effort. As a rule, a sensor-driven URI greater than atrial-driven URI should not be programmed, and this combination will not be discussed further.

Sensor-Driven Upper Rate Equal to Atrial-Driven Upper Rate

When the sensor-driven URI is equal to the atrial-driven URI, three responses can occur: (1) Wenckebach pacemaker AV block if TARP < PP interval < atrial-driven URI < SDI, (2) fixed-ratio pacemaker AV block if the PP interval < TARP < SDI; (3) AV sequential pacing if the SDI < PP interval, with the AV sequential (Ap-Vp-Ap-Vp) pacing rate faster than the one that could be provided by atrial sensing with 1:1 AV synchrony (Table 30–10). The maximal AV sequential pacing rate is equal to both the sensor-driven URI and the atrial-driven URI.

Pacemaker Wenckebach Atrioventricular Block

A Wenckebach pacemaker upper rate response occurs only when TARP < PP interval < atrial-driven URI < SDI.

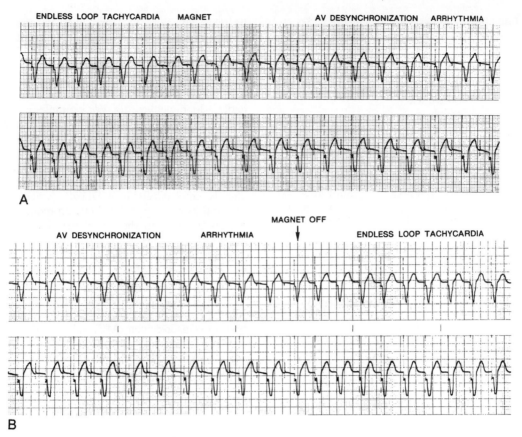

Figure 30–66. *A,* Inability to terminate endless-loop tachycardia (ELT) by magnet application in a patient with a Medtronic 7000 DDD pulse generator. Application of the magnet converts ELT to repetitive nonreentrant VA synchrony or AV desynchronization arrhythmia. Two ECG leads were recorded simultaneously. The pulse generator was programmed to the following settings: lower rate interval (LRI) = 750 msec (rate, 80 ppm); upper rate interval (URI) = 480 msec (rate, 125 ppm); AV interval = 250 msec; postventricular atrial refractory period (PVARP) = 155 msec (nonprogrammable); atrial output = 5.0 V at 0.3 msec (threshold for atrial pacing was less than 5.0 V at 0.05 msec). The rate of the ELT is about 107 ppm (cycle length = 560 msec). Retrograde P waves are not discernible, but the retrograde VA conduction time (VACT) can be calculated because the ELT is slower than the programmed upper rate. Therefore, the cycle length of the ELT (560 msec) must be equal to the sum of the VACT and the AV interval. Consequently, the VA conduction time is about 560 − 250 = 310 msec. *Top,* Application of the magnet converts the DDD pulse generator to the DOO mode for three cycles at a rate 10% above 85 ppm (93.5), with an AV interval of 100 msec. Then, DOO pacing continues at a rate of 85 ppm (faster than the programmed rate) at the programmed AV interval (250 msec). During magnet application, all atrial stimuli appear ineffectual. Retrograde VA conduction continues because the atrial stimuli fall within the atrial myocardial refractory period initiated by the preceding retrograde atrial depolarization. This results in repetitive nonreentrant VA synchrony (AV desynchronization arrhythmia). *B,* ELT recurs on magnet removal in same patient as in panel *A.* Nonreentrant VA synchrony or AV desynchronization arrhythmia continues as long as the magnet remains in place. Magnet removal (*arrow*) causes immediate return of ELT. Identical responses were observed with repeated application and removal of the magnet. Two ECG leads were recorded simultaneously. (From Barold SS, Falkoff MD, Ong LS, et al: Magnet-unresponsive pacemaker endless loop tachycardia. Am Heart J 116:726, 1988.)

During the Wenckebach block upper rate response in the DDD mode, the atrial-driven URI times out with each constant Vp-Vp cycle (equal to URI) until a pause occurs, that is, Vp-Vp lengthens only when a P wave falls in the PVARP. Thus, the atrial-driven URI controls Vp release except in the pause terminating the Wenckebach sequence. In contrast to the DDD mode, DDDR pacing shortens the pause, terminating the Wenckebach sequence to a value equal to the SDI (Fig. 30–67). Higano and colleagues[137] have called this effect "sensor-driven rate smoothing." Unlike true rate smoothing, sensor-driven rate smoothing occurs only at atrial rates faster than the atrial-driven upper rate (PP < atrial-driven

URI).[137, 138] In the DDDR mode, the duration of the pause terminating the Wenckebach cycle depends on sensor activity, and it becomes progressively shorter as the SDI shortens or as the sensor-driven rate increases.

A DDDR pulse generator working with a shorter sensor-driven AEI delivers Ap earlier in relation to the preceding ventricular event (Vs or Vp) than in the conventional DDD mode. The consequences of sensor-controlled earlier release of the atrial stimuli (when the preceding P wave falls in the PVARP) is discussed later. The pause at the end of the Wenckebach cycle disappears when the SDI eventually becomes equal to the sensor-driven URI. At that point, the

Table 30–10. DDDR Upper Rate Response: Atrial-Driven = Sensor-Driven Upper Rate Interval

Parameters	Response	Comments
1. PP < TARP = atrial-driven URI < SDI	Fixed-ratio (2 : 1) AV block with sensor-induced rate smoothing	
2. PP < TARP < atrial-driven URI < SDI	As above	
3. PP < TARP ≥ SDI	Atrial sensing cannot occur	Functions in DVIR mode
4. TARP < PP < atrial-driven URI = sensor-driven URI < SDI	Wenckebach block upper rate response with sensor-driven rate smoothing and shorter pause at end of sequence	Atrial-driven URI times out. The pause at the end of Wenckebach sequence is equal to SDI
5. TARP < PP < atrial-driven URI = sensor-driven URI = SDI	Wenckebach block upper rate response *without* a pause at the end of sequence; Vp-Vp remains constant	Identical to DDIR mode and therefore functionally equivalent to VVIR mode: atrial-driven URI times out

TARP, total atrial refractory period; URI, upper rate interval; SDI, sensor-driven interval; PP, interval between two consecutive P waves; Vp-Vp, interval between two consecutive ventricular paced beats

Modified from Barold SS: Electrocardiography of rate-adaptive dual chamber (DDDR) pacemakers: Upper rate behavior. *In* Alt E, Barold SS, Stangl K (eds): Rate-Adaptive Cardiac Pacing. Heidelberg, Berlin, Springer-Verlag, 1993, pp 195–221.

pulse generator continues to pace the ventricle regularly with constant Vp-Vp intervals at the sensor-driven URI (equal to the atrial-driven URI) and functions as if it were in the DDIR mode (with a constant ventricular pacing rate and P waves marching through the cardiac cycle) (Fig. 30–68). In the DDD mode, some otherwise healthy young patients do not tolerate the beat-to-beat variations in cycle length due to the pause at the end of a Wenckebach block upper rate response. In these patients without atrial chronotropic incompetence, an appropriately programmed DDDR pacemaker will shorten the pause, with its minimum value being equal to the sensor-driven URI. At that point, the pacemaker functions basically in the DDIR mode (see Fig. 30–68).

Pacemaker Fixed-Ratio Atrioventricular Block

When the PP interval < TARP < SDI, fixed-ratio pacemaker AV block occurs. During DDD pacing, rapid acceleration of sinus rate may cause shortening of the PP interval to a value less than the TARP, whereupon sudden fixed-ratio pacemaker AV block will occur. The abrupt fall in the paced ventricular rate seen in the DDD mode is attenuated in a DDDR system in the same way as the SDI abbreviates the pause at the end of Wenckebach cycles during DDDR pacing[139] (Fig. 30–69).

Sensor-Controlled Rate Smoothing and Atrial Competition

During DDDR pacing, the shorter SDI and sensor-driven AEI generate an Ap earlier than in the DDD mode (Ap can

be relatively close to a preceding unsensed P wave in the PVARP). Ap occurs earlier in abbreviated pauses related to (1) fixed-ratio pacemaker AV block and (2) the cycle terminating Wenckebach pacemaker AV block.

Sensor-controlled rate smoothing[137] can be useful in active patients who require a long PVARP for the prevention of endless-loop tachycardia. For example, in the DDD mode in a pulse generator with the following parameters (lower rate = 70 ppm, PVARP = 350 msec), if As-Vp shortens to 100 msec at the programmed (common) upper rate, a TARP of 450 msec will produce fixed-ratio pacemaker AV block when the atrial rate exceeds 140 bpm. In this circumstance, as already emphasized, in a DDDR device, the sensor-driven rate and its corresponding SDI can reduce or even eliminate the abrupt drop in the paced ventricular rate produced by fixed-ratio pacemaker AV block in the DDD mode.

On the basis of the preceding considerations, in the DDDR mode, fixed-ratio and Wenckebach pacemaker AV block can create complex electrocardiographic patterns with various combinations of (1) ineffectual Ap (no capture) when an early sensor-controlled Ap (delivered at the completion of sensor-driven AEI) falls in the atrial myocardial refractory period generated by the preceding unsensed P wave in the PVARP, and (2) effectual Ap with atrial capture but close to the previous P wave, that is, atrial competition. Stimulation in the atrial vulnerable period (with the risk of inducing an atrial arrhythmia) is more a theoretical concern than a practical problem.[140] Thus, at any one time in the DDDR mode, Vp can be preceded by one of the following: (1) ineffectual Ap, (2) effectual Ap sometimes close to the previous P wave, (3) sensed P wave (As) triggering Vp, or (4) sensed P wave (As) with Vp controlled by the SDI and not triggered by atrial activity (discussed later). Furthermore, a DDDR pulse generator can release Ap either in the PVARP or beyond the PVARP (discussed later). Atrial competition during Wenckebach or fixed-ratio pacemaker AV block can be reduced or minimized with correct selection of the pacing mode (is the DDDR mode really indicated?) and programmable settings.

Total Atrial Refractory Period Longer Than the Upper Rate Limit

Patients with atrial chronotropic incompetence and paroxysmal supraventricular tachyarrhythmias may benefit from a DDDR pulse generator programmed with (1) a relatively slow atrial-driven upper rate to avoid tracking of fast unphysiologic atrial rates at rest, and (2) a faster sensor-driven upper rate to provide an increase in the pacing rate on exercise. However, in some DDDR pulse generators with equal atrial-driven and sensor-driven upper rates, the two upper rates (intervals) cannot be dissociated.

In the DDD mode, a TARP > atrial-driven URI cannot exist because the atrial-driven URI becomes equal to the TARP. Consequently, one could easily conclude that the two upper rates (atrial-driven and sensor-driven) in a DDDR device with a common upper rate are inextricably linked and cannot be uncoupled. Indeed, as in the conventional DDD mode, some DDDR pulse generators with a common URI permit programming of the TARP to a value equal to or shorter than, but not longer than, the atrial-driven URI (equal to the sensor-driven URI). In other DDDR pulse generators, the TARP can actually be programmed to a value longer

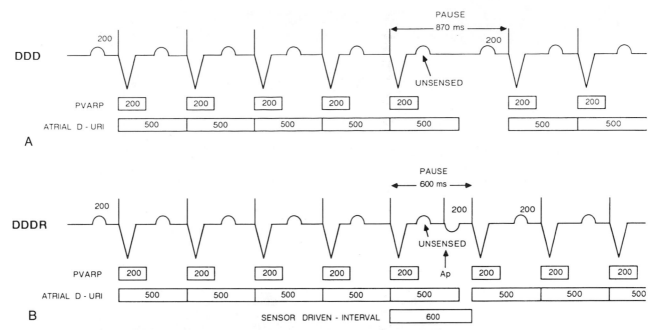

Figure 30–67. DDD (a) and DDDR (b) pacing with pacemaker Wenckebach block upper rate response. Lower rate interval (LRI) = 1000 msec; atrial-driven upper rate interval (URI) = 500 msec; postventricular atrial refractory period (PVARP) = 200 msec; AV interval = 200 msec. (As-Vp = Ap-Vp in both the DDD and the DDDR modes.) A Wenckebach upper rate response occurs because the atrial-driven URI is longer than the total atrial refractory period (TARP). *A,* DDD pacing with typical Wenckebach upper rate response. The pulse generator does not sense the sixth P wave in the PVARP but senses the succeeding P wave, so that the pause at the end of the Wenckebach cycle measures about 870 msec. *B,* In the DDDR mode with the same basic parameters as in the DDD mode in panel *A,* the sensor-driven interval (SDI) is equal to 600 msec and is longer than the atrial-driven URI. The pulse generator does not sense the sixth P wave in the PVARP. The pause at the end of the Wenckebach sequence is shorter than that in the DDD mode because the SDI = 600 msec and the sensor-driven atrial escape interval (AEI) = 400 ms. Thus, Ap occurs earlier (and closer to the preceding P wave in the PVARP) because its release is sensor controlled. The pause at the end of the Wenckebach sequence therefore shortens to the 600 msec (SDI). (From Barold SS: Electrocardiography of rate-adaptive [DDDR] pacemakers. 2. Upper rate behavior. *In* Alt E, Barold SS, Stangl K [eds]: Rate-Adaptive Cardiac Pacing. Berlin, Springer-Verlag, 1993, pp 195–221.)

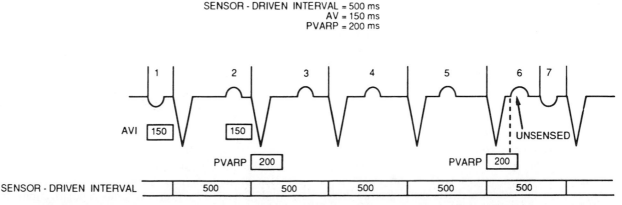

Figure 30–68. DDIR mode. The sinus rate is faster than the sensor-driven rate; that is, the PP interval is shorter than the sensor-driven interval (SDI; 500 msec). In the DDI or DDIR mode, the ventricular-paced rate (or the Vp-Vp interval) always remains constant and equal to the programmed lower rate interval (LRI) or (lower rate) SDI. The first atrial stimulus captures the atrium. The pulse generator senses the subsequent P waves (2 to 5). The P waves march through the pacing cycle with progressive prolongation of the AV interval. The sixth P wave falls in the 200-msec postventricular atrial refractory period (PVARP) and is therefore unsensed. The pacemaker delivers its next atrial stimulus (which captures the atrium and generates the seventh P wave) at the end of the sensor-driven atrial escape interval (AEI; 500 − 150 = 350 msec). Because the ventricular pacing rate (or Vp-Vp interval) remains constant, the DDIR mode is functionally equivalent to the VVIR mode (with AV dissociation), with the occasional occurrence of atrial extrasystoles (premature beats) when the pulse generator delivers Ap relatively close to the preceding (unsensed) P wave in the PVARP. (From Barold SS: Electrocardiography of rate-adaptive (DDDR) pacemakers. 2. Upper rate behavior. *In* Alt E, Barold SS, Stangl K [eds]: Rate-Adaptive Cardiac Pacing. Berlin, Springer-Verlag, 1993, pp 195–221.)

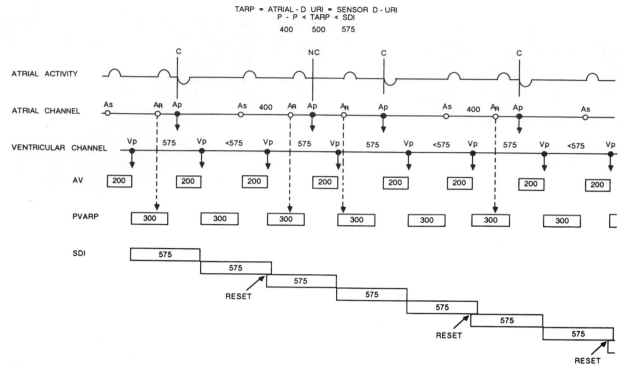

Figure 30–69. Pacing by a DDDR pulse generator showing an upper rate response with fixed-ratio AV block. Atrial-driven upper rate interval (URI) = sensor-driven URI = total atrial refractory period (TARP). Fixed-ratio pacemaker AV block occurs because the PP interval (400 msec) is shorter than the TARP (500 msec). The Vp-Vp remains constant and equal to the sensor-driven interval (SDI; 575 msec). The second P (A$_R$) falls in the postventricular atrial refractory period (PVARP) and is therefore unsensed. The succeeding Ap is delivered at the end of the sensor-driven atrial escape interval (AEI) and captures the atrium (C) very near the preceding spontaneous P (A$_R$). The fourth (As) P wave falls beyond the PVARP and initiates an AV interval of 200 msec. The Vp-Vp interval between the second Vp and the third Vp is shorter than 575-msec Vp-Vp SDI because the third Vp is controlled by As and not the sensor. The fifth P wave (A$_R$) falls in the PVARP. The pulse generator fires Ap at the end of the sensor-driven AEI, but Ap falls too close to the previous P wave (in the PVARP). Ap delivery within the atrial myocardial refractory period produces no capture (NC). Note that the SDI is reset whenever Vp occurs prematurely (earlier than the SDI of 575 msec) when triggered by As. Competitive atrial pacing produces complex electrocardiographic patterns. (From Barold SS: Electrocardiography of rate-adaptive (DDDR) pacemakers. 2. Upper rate behavior. *In* Alt E, Barold SS, Stangl K [eds]: Rate-Adaptive Cardiac Pacing. Berlin, Springer-Verlag, 1993, pp 195–221.)

than the common URI. Obviously, if the TARP is ≥ common URI, no Wenckebach upper rate response can occur. When the TARP > common URI, the TARP actually becomes equal to the atrial-driven URI. This manipulation allows programming of a sensor-driven upper rate faster than the atrial-driven upper rate in pacemakers without a separately programmable atrial-driven URI and sensor-driven URI. The atrial-driven URI becomes equal to the TARP and corresponds to the rate at which fixed-ratio pacemaker AV block supervenes. Thus, the atrial-driven URI can be *functionally* separated from the sensor-driven URI by programming a TARP longer than the common URI, that is, atrial-driven URI = TARP > sensor-driven URI. In this way, fixed-ratio pacemaker AV block will occur at atrial rates slower than the programmed sensor-driven upper rate. This approach may be useful in limiting the atrial-driven upper rate in patients with paroxysmal supraventricular tachyarrhythmias in devices without automatic mode switching (AMS) (Table 30–11).

Atrial Pacing in the PVARP

During DDD pacing, the delivery of Ap cannot occur in the PVARP because Ap can be released only at the completion

of the AEI, that is, after the completion of the PVARP. In the DDDR mode, atrial pacing can occur in the PVARP only when the sensor-driven URI < TARP, allowing an SDI < TARP (Figs. 30–70 and 30–71). When the PP interval shortens to a value less than the TARP, P waves fall in the terminal portion of the PVARP and are therefore unsensed. The DDDR pulse generator then takes over control of the atrial rhythm. Sensor-driven release of Ap may occur either in the PVARP or beyond it, according to the SDI at any given time. As previously stated, an earlier Ap may result in lack of capture (i.e., Ap in atrial myocardial refractory period generated by previous atrial depolarization) or atrial capture with competition. Note that it is possible for Ap to fall in the *myocardial* atrial refractory period generated by a preceding unsensed P wave and also within the *pacemaker* atrial refractory period (or PVARP). Techniques to avoid competitive atrial pacing are discussed later in the section on noncompetitive atrial pacing (NCAP).

Sensor-Driven Upper Rate Faster Than Atrial-Driven Upper Rate

In pacemakers that allow programming of separate atrial-driven URI and sensor-driven URI, when sensor-driven URI

Table 30–11. DDDR Upper Rate Response: Atrial-Driven URI = Sensor-Driven Upper Rate Interval

Relationship of Total Atrial Refractory Period and Sensor-Driven Intervals

Parameters	Response	Comments
PP < sensor-driven URI < TARP < SDI	Fixed-ratio AV block with sensor-driven rate smoothing	Ap beyond PVARP
PP* < sensor-driven URI < SDI < TARP†	DVIR pacing	Ap in PVARP
PP* < TARP = SDI	DVIR pacing	Ap at end of PVARP
PP* > TARP = SDI	As above	As above

TARP, total atrial refractory period; PVARP, postventricular atrial refractory period; URI, upper rate interval; PP, interval between two consecutive P waves; SDI, sensor-driven interval.

* Duration of PP interval is immaterial because pacer functions in DVIR mode; atrial sensing cannot occur because SDI is ≤ TARP.

† Capability of programming TARP ≥ common URI is required. In this way, sensor-driven URI < TARP, i.e., sensor-driven URI < SDI < TARP is possible in devices that allow programming of TARP > common URI.

Modified from Barold SS: Electrocardiography of rate-adaptive dual chamber (DDDR) pacemakers: Upper rate behavior. *In* Alt E, Barold SS, Stangl K (eds): Rate-Adaptive Cardiac Pacing. Heidelberg, Berlin, Springer-Verlag, 1993, pp 195–221.

< atrial-driven URI, the upper rate response of a DDDR pulse generator depends on the interplay of four variables: PP interval, TARP, atrial-driven URI, and sensor-driven URI.[84, 141–143] (Table 30–12). A sensor-driven upper rate faster than an atrial-driven upper rate can be useful in patients with paroxysmal supraventricular tachyarrhythmias in devices without AMS and in patients requiring a very long PVARP to prevent endless-loop tachycardia.[143] When the TARP < atrial-driven URI, a Wenckebach block upper rate response can occur (with extension of the As-Vp interval) only when the TARP < PP interval. When the SDI ≤ atrial-driven URI, no pause occurs at the end of a Wenckebach block upper rate sequence. This contrasts with the occurrence of pauses during DDDR pacing when the atrial-driven URI = the sensor-driven URI and the SDI > atrial-driven URI.

Atrial-Driven Upper Rate Limit Longer Than the Total Atrial Refractory Period

1. PP interval longer than SDI. When the PP interval is longer than the SDI, the pulse generator paces AV sequentially. Complexity occurs when the PP interval is equal to or shorter than the SDI and sensor-driven URI.

2. PP interval shorter than SDI. When the atrial rate exceeds the sensor-driven rate (PP interval < SDI), the SDI may also become shorter than the atrial-driven URI (i.e., PP interval < SDI < atrial-driven URI). Such a relationship cannot occur when the sensor-driven URI and atrial-driven URI are common and cannot be uncoupled.

Sensor-Driven Interval Shorter Than the Atrial-Driven Upper Rate Interval

In the absence of atrial activity, when SDI < atrial-driven URI, a pulse generator delivers an atrial stimulus (Ap) at the completion of the sensor-driven AEI and an accompanying Vp at the completion of the Ap-Vp interval. Vp occurs

URI = 400 ms
TARP = 550 ms
SDI = 450 ms

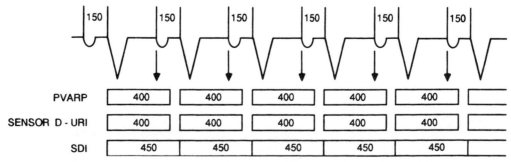

Figure 30–70. Pacing by a DDDR pacemaker with a total atrial refractory period (TARP) longer than the common upper rate interval (URI). (Ap-Vp = 150 msec.) The atrial-driven URI and sensor-driven URI should be equal (400 msec) according to pacemaker specifications when a 400-msec URI is programmed. However, TARP (AV + postventricular refractory period [PVARP]) = 550 msec. (TARP > URI is allowed only in certain DDDR pulse generators.) A 550 msec TARP actually represents an atrial-driven URI of the same duration, and a Wenckebach upper rate response cannot occur. At that particular level of activity with an SDI of 450 msec, the sensor-driven atrial escape interval (AEI; 300 msec) is shorter than the 400 msec PVARP. Therefore, the atrial stimulus is continually delivered with the PVARP. (From Barold SS: Electrocardiography of rate-adaptive [DDDR] pacemakers. 2. Upper rate behavior. *In* Alt E, Barold SS, Stangl K [eds]: Rate-Adaptive Cardiac Pacing. Berlin, Springer-Verlag, 1993, pp 195–221.)

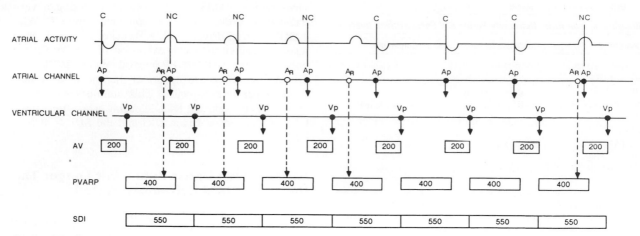

Figure 30–71. Pacing in the DDDR mode with a common upper rate interval (URI) of 450 msec, an AV of 200 msec, a postventricular atrial refractory period (PVARP) of 400 msec, a total atrial refractory period (TARP) of 600 msec, and a sensor-driven interval (SDI) of 550 msec. Provided that the pulse generator allows programming a TARP > common URI, these parameters indicate that the atrial-driven URI (600 msec = TARP) > sensor-driven URI (450 msec = programmed common URI). There is an atrial sensing window beyond the PVARP, but it closes when SDI ≤ TARP. In this example, because the SDI < TARP, the pulse generator cannot sense spontaneous atrial activity (A_R). Atrial pacing is asynchronous, and Ap competes with A_R, producing a response functionally equivalent to the DVIR mode. Therefore, both Ap-Ap and Vp-Vp intervals remain constant. C, capture; NC, no capture (when Ap in atrial myocardial refractory period). (From Barold SS: Electrocardiography of rate-adaptive [DDDR] pacemakers. 2. Upper rate behavior. *In* Alt E, Barold SS, Stangl K [eds]: Rate-Adaptive Cardiac Pacing. Berlin, Springer-Verlag, 1993, pp 195–221.)

Table 30–12. DDDR Upper Rate Response: Sensor-Driven Upper Rate Interval Is Shorter Than Atrial-Driven Upper Rate Interval and Total Atrial Refractory Period Is Shorter Than Atrial-Driven Upper Rate Interval

Parameters	Atrial-Driven URI Times Out	Pause at End of Wenckebach Sequence	Ventricular-Paced Repetitive Preempted Wenckebach Upper Rate Response	Vp-Vp Interval Solely Controlled by Sensor or SDI	Comments
1. PP < SDI < atrial-driven URI. Sensor-driven URI < TARP* < PP < SDI < atrial-driven URI.	No	No	Yes	Yes	Functionally equivalent to DDIR
TARP* < sensor-driven URI < PP < SDI < atrial-driven URI	As above	As above	As above	As above	As above
2. PP < SDI = atrial-driven URI. Sensor-driven URI < TARP* < PP < SDI = atrial-driven URI	Yes	No	No	No because Vp-Vp = atrial-driven URI = SDI	Functionally equivalent to DDIR
TARP* < sensor-driven URI < PP < SDI = atrial-driven URI	As above	As above	As above	As above	As above
3. PP = SDI < atrial-driven URI. Sensor-driven URI < TARP* < PP = SDI < atrial-driven URI	No	No	Yes	Yes; Vp-Vp controlled by SDI < atrial-driven URI	Apparent P-wave tracking above atrial-driven upper rate, i.e., at the sensor-indicated rate; extended As-Vp interval
TARP* < sensor-driven URI < PP = SDI < atrial-driven URI	As above	As above	As above	As above	

URI, upper rate interval; TARP, total atrial refractory period; PP, interval between two consecutive P waves; SDI, sensor-driven interval; Vp-Vp, interval between two consecutive ventricular paced beats.
* TARP < atrial-driven URI permits Wenckebach block upper rate response with extension of As-Vp longer than programmed value.
Modified from Barold SS: Electrocardiography of rate-adaptive dual chamber (DDDR) pacemakers: Upper rate behavior. *In* Alt E, Barold SS, Stangl K [eds]: Rate-Adaptive Cardiac Pacing. Heidelberg, Berlin, Springer-Verlag, 1993, pp 195–221.

at the end of the SDI initiated by the preceding ventricular event, but before completion of the atrial-driven URI, also initiated by the same preceding ventricular event (Fig. 30–72).

Ventricular-Paced Repetitive Pre-Empted Wenckebach Upper Rate Response

In this form of repetitive pre-empted Wenckebach upper rate response, it is an early sensor-controlled ventricular-paced beat (Vp), rather than Vs, that prevents the development of a classic Wenckebach upper rate response. Therefore, such a pre-empted response can occur with DDDR pacing only when sensor-driven URI < atrial-driven URI.[53] The ventricular-paced pre-empted responses can be classified according to behavior of the AV intervals (see Table 30–11).

Variable Atrioventricular Intervals

When SDI < atrial-driven URI, a DDDR pacemaker delivers Vp at the completion of the SDI but before the atrial-driven URI has timed out in its entirety (see Fig. 30–72). When PP < SDI < atrial-driven URI, sensed P waves (As) inhibit release of sensor-controlled Ap. Consequently, the As-Vp

interval extends beyond its programmed value, a response analogous to the classic Wenckebach block upper rate behavior (possible only if atrial-driven URI > TARP). In this response, when the PP interval < SDI < atrial-driven URI, P waves march through the pacing cycles and initiate As-Vp intervals of progressively longer duration until a P wave falls in the PVARP and is unsensed, a behavior resembling the typical pacemaker Wenckebach block upper rate response. However, the partially extended As-Vp intervals never attain the full duration dictated by the atrial-driven URI. This response occurs only because the SDI or sensor-driven URI usurps control of the paced ventricular rate. Such a sequence produces a "ventricular-paced" repetitive pre-empted Wenckebach upper rate response (with varying AV intervals) in which paced ventricular beats (issued at the completion of the SDI) continually terminate the partially extended AV intervals before completion of the atrial-driven URI. (Compare this response with the previously described ventricular-sensed repetitive pre-empted Wenckebach upper rate behavior.) P waves march through the pacing cycles and initiate partially extended As-Vp intervals of progressively longer duration until a P wave falls in the PVARP. At that point, no pause occurs because the pacemaker releases the subsequent Ap and Vp events according to the sensor-driven

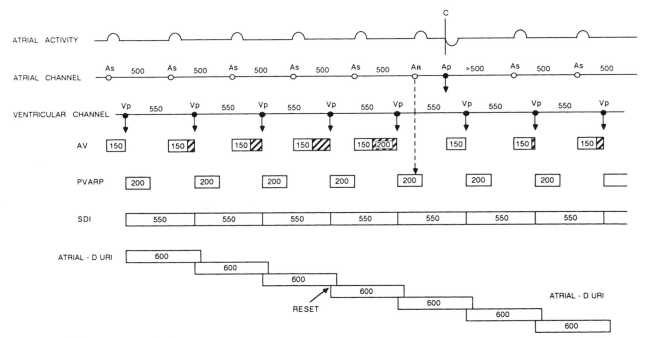

Figure 30–72. Pacing by a DDDR pulse generator with the sensor-driven upper rate interval (URI; 400 msec) shorter than the atrial-driven URI (600 msec). Sensor-driven URI (400 msec) is shorter than the PP interval (500 msec), which is shorter than the sensor-driven interval (SDI; 550 msec), which is in turn shorter than the atrial-driven URI (600 msec). As-Vp = Ap-Vp = 150 msec; postventricular atrial refractory period (PVARP) = 200 msec; total atrial refractory period (TARP) = 350 msec. The TARP is shorter than the PP, which is shorter than the atrial-driven URI. The maximal increment of the AV interval during the Wenckebach upper rate response is 600 − 350 = 250 msec. The first P wave initiates an AV interval of 150 msec. The second P wave initiates an AV interval extended beyond 150 msec to conform to the atrial-driven URI, which does not time out because the SDI is shorter than the atrial-driven URI. Thus, the delivery of Vp is sensor controlled, and the Vp-Vp interval is controlled by the sensor or the SDI. The AV interval cannot fully extend to the completion of the atrial-driven URI because an earlier Vp (sensor controlled) terminates the AV interval. This response may be called a *ventricular-paced repetitive pre-empted Wenckebach upper rate response.* The sixth P wave falls in the PVARP and is therefore unsensed (A$_R$). The next Ap released at the end of the sensor-driven escape interval (550 − 150 = 400 msec) occurs 400 msec from the previous Vp, close to the sixth P wave, but capable of atrial capture. There is no pause at the end of the Wenckebach sequence because the Vp-Vp interval is reset by the earlier Vp. On the *right,* the process repeats itself. (From Barold SS: Electrocardiography of rate-adaptive [DDDR] pacemakers. 2. Upper rate behavior. *In* Alt E, Barold SS, Stangl K [eds]: Rate-Adaptive Cardiac Pacing. Berlin, Springer-Verlag, 1993, pp 195–221.)

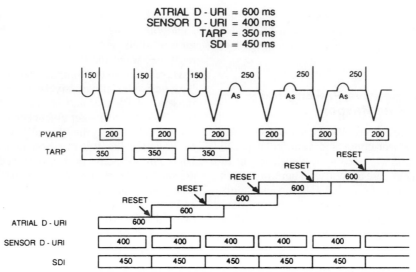

Figure 30–73. Pacing with a DDDR pulse generator showing apparent P-wave tracking. Atrial-driven upper rate interval (URI) is longer than sensor-driven URI. As-Vp = Ap-Vp = 150 msec. The sinus rate is equal to the sensor-driven rate (PP interval = sensor-driven interval [SDI] = 450 msec). The pulse generator senses the last three spontaneous P waves (As). A sensed P wave initiates an AV interval of 150 msec, but at the completion of the 150-msec AV interval, the atrial-driven URI (600 msec) has not yet timed out. Consequently, the pacemaker extends the AV interval to conform to the atrial-driven URI (600 msec). The latter does not time out because the pulse generator emits Vp at the termination of the 450 msec SDI initiated by the preceding ventricular event. The As-Vp interval is stretched to 250 msec. (In the absence of sensor activity or SDI, the As-Vp interval would have stretched to 400 msec to conform to the atrial-driven URI.) Delivery of the last three ventricular stimuli is sensor controlled. The atrial-driven URI is repeatedly reset by the early delivery of sensor-controlled Vp, producing apparent P-wave tracking at a rate faster than the programmed atrial-driven upper rate. (From Barold SS: Electrocardiography of rate-adaptive [DDDR] pacemakers. 2. Upper rate behavior. *In* Alt E, Barold SS, Stangl K [eds]: Rate-Adaptive Cardiac Pacing. Berlin, Springer-Verlag, 1993, pp 195–221.)

AEI and SDI. Thus, all Vp-Vp intervals (including the one containing the unsensed P wave in the PVARP) remain constant and equal to the prevailing SDI (which, according to circumstances, can be either longer than the sensor-driven URI or equal to it) but shorter than the atrial-driven URI. The pacemaker, therefore, effectively functions in the DDIR mode[53] (Fig. 30–72). Calling this behavior a *DDIR-like Wenckebach upper rate response*, although technically correct, would be too confusing because the functional DDIR mode also occurs when atrial-driven URI = SDI = sensor-driven URI, a situation in which the atrial-driven URI does time out in its entirety.

Sensor-Driven Interval Equal to the Atrial-Driven Upper Rate Interval: Variable Atrioventricular Intervals

When PP < atrial-driven URI = SDI, a Wenckebach upper rate response will also occur, with no pause at the end of the sequence in the cycle containing the unsensed P wave within the PVARP (see Table 30–11). The Vp-Vp interval remains equal to the SDI and to the atrial-driven URI. Therefore, both the SDI and the atrial-driven URI time out, but the sensor-driven URI does not. The effect is therefore identical to the situation in which atrial-driven URI = sen-

sor-driven URI = SDI, which also creates a classic Wenckebach upper rate response without a pause at the end of the sequence, provided that TARP < PP < SDI. In the latter situation, all three intervals (atrial-driven URI, sensor-driven URI, and SDI) time out at the end of every Vp-Vp cycle.

PP Interval Equal to the Sensor-Driven Interval
Constant Atrioventricular Intervals

When PP = SDI and continual atrial sensing inhibits the emission of Ap, P waves followed by Vp give the appearance of P-wave tracking at a rate faster than the programmed atrial-driven upper rate (a situation called "apparent tracking" by Higano and Hayes[137]). Apparent P-wave tracking occurs with partially extended but constant As-Vp intervals that never attain the full duration dictated by the atrial-driven URI because SDI < atrial-driven URI[53] (Fig. 30–73). The Vp-Vp interval is shorter than the atrial-driven URI. No P waves fall in the PVARP as long as PP = SDI. Therefore, the Vp-Vp intervals remain constant. During this form of ventricular-paced repetitive pre-empted Wenckebach upper rate response (with constant AV intervals), the pacemaker also effectively functions in the DDIR mode. When the sinus rate increases (PP < SDI), the sequence is transformed into a ventricular-paced repetitive pre-empted

Wenckebach upper rate response with variable AV intervals as already described (Fig. 30–74).

Other Considerations and Overview

During DDD or DDDR pacing (atrial-driven URI > TARP and SDI > atrial-driven URI), when the PP interval is equal to the atrial-driven URI (but longer than the TARP), the pacemaker continually functions with an extended As-Vp interval to conform to the atrial-driven URI. Such upper rate behavior, without discernible progressive prolongation of the AV (As-Vp) interval, can superficially resemble a ventricular-paced repetitive pre-empted Wenckebach upper rate response with constant AV intervals.[53] However, the mechanism is different because the As-Vp intervals are fully extended and the atrial-driven URI times out in its entirety. Similarly, during DDDR pacing, if atrial-driven URI = sensor-driven URI, a ventricular-paced repetitive pre-empted Wenckebach upper rate response cannot occur because the atrial-driven URI is always permitted to time out completely under the appropriate circumstances. In contrast, the DDIR mode is electrocardiographically and mechanistically identical to both types of ventricular-paced repetitive pre-empted Wenckebach upper rate responses (with either constant or inconstant AV intervals) because in the DDI mode (with ventricular-based LRT), LRI = atrial-driven URI, and in the DDIR mode other than at rest, SDI < atrial-driven URI, which in turn is equal to the LRI.

When sensor-driven URI < atrial-driven URI, the response of a DDDR pacemaker depends on the relationship of the PP interval to SDI, and there are five situations, provided that PP > TARP, that make AV extension possible:

1. PP > SDI: AV sequential pacing
2. PP < SDI < atrial-driven URI: modified Wenckebach upper rate response with P waves marching through the pacing cycle and no pauses. (Ventricular-paced repetitive pre-empted Wenckebach upper rate response.) The P waves start an AV interval, but unlike the Wenckebach response in the DDD mode, the pulse generator never completes the expected AV interval (although it is extended to some extent) because the pulse generator emits Vp at the completion of the SDI. This causes continual reset of the atrial-driven URI by the sensor-controlled Vp. The Vp-Vp interval is sensor-driven, and the atrial-driven URI does not time out.
3. PP < SDI = atrial-driven URI. The response is as in number 2, except that the atrial-driven URI times out and is similar to the situation where atrial-driven URI = SDI = sensor-driven URI.
4. PP = SDI < atrial-driven URI: sustained apparent P wave tracking with a fixed but extended As-Vp interval
5. Fluctuation of PP interval to a value equal to, longer, or shorter than the SDI leads to irregular patterns with intermittent inhibition of Ap creating complex ECGs. In numbers 4 and 5, apparent P-wave tracking should not be misinterpreted as pacemaker malfunction.

■ DDDR PACING: FUNCTIONAL MODE VERSUS PROGRAMMED MODE

During DDDR pacing, a particular programmed pacing mode may effectively function in another mode according to circumstances. A DDDR pacemaker can switch its functional pacing mode in the following situations.

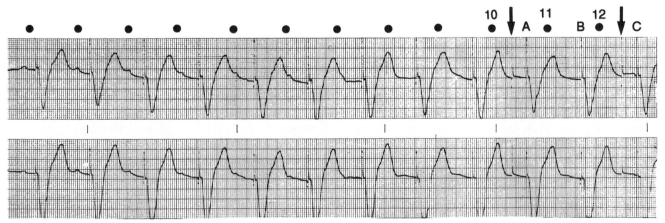

DDDR SYNCHRONY

LOWER RATE INTERVAL = 857 ms
ATRIAL D - URI = 600 ms
SENSOR D - URI = 400 ms
PVARP = 225 ms

Figure 30–74. Repetitive ventricular-sensed pre-empted Wenckebach upper rate response during pacing with a Pacesetter Synchrony DDDR pacemaker. *Solid black circles* represent P waves. PP interval < sensor-driven interval of 540-550 msec (Vp-Vp) < atrial-driven upper rate interval (URI). The device senses P waves 1–9 and generates progressively longer As-Vp intervals. The As-Vp intervals are partially extended because sensor-controlled Vp occurs before the atrial-driven URI (600 msec) has timed out. P wave 10 falls in the postventricular atrial refractory period (PVARP) and is unsensed. Therefore, the sensor-controlled atrial escape interval terminates with the release of Ap. There is no pause at the end of this type of Wenckebach sequence because the sensor forces the release of Vp (A) after Ap and the Vp-Vp interval remains constant. P wave 11 is sensed and inhibits Vp, whereas P wave 12 is unsensed in the PVARP and permits the emission of Ap. The Vp-Vp intervals (A-B, B-C) remain unchanged and equal to the sensor-driven interval.

DDDR to DVIR Mode

When the SDI ≤ TARP, the atrial channel paces asynchronously, and the DDDR mode functions as a DVIR mode. For example, if AV is equal to 200 msec, the PVARP is equal to 400 msec, and the TARP is equal to 600 msec; when the SDI reaches 600 msec or less, the pacemaker functions in the DVIR mode because these parameters obliterate the atrial-sensing window.

DDIR to DVIR Mode

In the DDIR mode with an AV equal to 150 msec, PVARP equal to 350 msec, and LRI equal to 1000 msec, the atrial-sensing window is equal to the LRI minus the TARP, which equals 500 msec. As the sensor-driven LRI shortens with exercise, the atrial-sensing window also shortens. Eventually, when the SDI reaches 500 msec (corresponding to a rate of 120 ppm), the programmed indices obliterate the atrial-sensing window, and the pacemaker then functions in the DVIR mode.

DDDR to DDIR Mode

1. Any Wenckebach upper rate response without a pause at the termination of the cycle (when the P wave falls within the PVARP) is functionally equivalent to the DDIR mode. In a pulse generator with equal atrial-driven URI and sensor-driven URI, shortening of the SDI (i.e., sensor-driven LRI) on exercise brings it closer to the atrial-driven or common URI. The pacing mode begins to resemble the DDIR mode. When the difference between the URI and the SDI diminishes, the pause at the end of a Wenckebach cycle becomes inconspicuous, so that the pacing mode looks like the DDIR mode (constant rate of ventricular pacing) with an occasional, hardly discernible, slight prolongation of the Vp-Vp interval at the end of the Wenckebach sequence. When the SDI is equal to the atrial-driven URI, which is equal to the sensor-driven URI, no pauses occur at the end of the Wenckebach cycle, and the pacing mode becomes effectively DDIR. In this situation, the Vp-Vp interval becomes equal to the common URI.

2. A Wenckebach upper rate response without pauses (functionally equivalent to the DDIR mode) can also occur when PP < SDI < atrial-driven URI, provided that the TARP < atrial-driven URI. The SDI becomes the Vp-Vp interval when the SDI < atrial-driven URI. The atrial-driven URI times out only when the SDI is equal to the atrial-driven URI, the Vp-Vp interval being equal to the SDI.

■ AUTOMATIC MODE CONVERSION

Conventional or specially designed pacemakers can convert automatically to another pacing mode in a variety of circumstances.[144-154] Automatic conversion of the pacing mode of single- and dual-chamber devices may be classified as follows:

Apparent. A VDD pulse generator effectively paces in the VVI mode in the presence of sinus bradycardia slower than the programmed lower rate, whereas a DDI pacemaker appears to function in the VVI mode in the presence of an atrial tachyarrhythmia when the atrial channel consistently senses P or f waves beyond the PVARP.

Temporary. When the mechanism causing the automatic change of pacing mode no longer exists, the pulse generator reverts immediately to its original pacing mode. In this way, a VVI pacemaker can revert to the VOO mode and a DDD pacemaker to the VOO or DOO mode as a temporary response to sensed EMI or other extraneous signals (interference mode). Additionally, a pacemaker in the VDD, DDD, or DDDR mode may respond to an atrial rate faster than the programmed upper rate by automatic conversion to a nontracking mode (such as VVI), with a gradual or sudden reduction of the pacing rate to a predetermined level; reversion to the DDD mode subsequently occurs when the atrial rate drops below the tachycardia detection. In patients with sick sinus syndrome, AV interval hysteresis allows conversion from the DDD(R) to the functional AAI mode by automatic prolongation of the AV delay if relatively normal AV conduction is detected by the pacemaker (discussed later). Tachycardia-terminating pacemakers also belong to this group.

Permanent until reprogrammed (pacemaker reset). The DDD mode can be converted to the VVI or VOO mode, and the VVIR mode to the VVI mode, as a permanent (unless reprogrammed) response to the sensed EMI or as an indicator of the elective replacement time (ERT).[81]

Permanent and unresponsive to reprogramming. Conversion to the reset mode with inability to reprogram the pulse generator to its original mode may occur with advanced battery depletion (end of life) or component malfunction (including damage from defibrillation, therapeutic radiation, and electrocautery).

■ AUTOMATIC MODE SWITCHING

Fallback algorithms were introduced more than a decade ago in certain dual-chamber pacemakers to provide protection against rapidly paced ventricular rates during SVT. Such systems were rarely used because, at the time, paroxysmal SVT was considered a contraindication to dual-chamber pacing. According to the original concept of fallback when the atrial rate exceeds either the programmed upper rate or tachycardia detection rate for a given duration, the pulse generator activates a mechanism that produces a slower paced ventricular rate. The latter occurs either in the same pacing mode or by conversion to the nontracking VVI mode.[37] Now that dual-chamber pacemakers are widely recommended for all forms of bradycardia-tachycardia syndrome, many devices come equipped with a more refined "atrial tachy response," popularly known as *automatic mode switching* (AMS), with algorithms specific to each manufacturer.[152]

AMS in response to SVT controls the paced ventricular rate by virtue of temporary self-programming to a new pacing mode without atrial tracking capability, and it functions with or without a rate-adaptive response (e.g., VVI, VVIR, DDI, DDIR modes) (Fig. 30–75). During AMS, the DDI or DDIR modes do not provide hemodynamic benefit from AV synchrony. When the sensed atrial rate drops below the tachycardia detection rate, the pulse generator automatically returns to its previous dual-chamber mode with 1:1 AV synchrony.

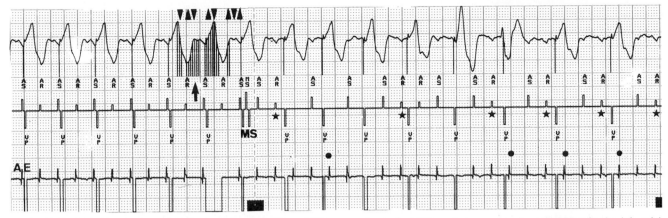

Figure 30–75. Automatic mode switching of a Medtronic Thera DDDR pacemaker to the DDIR mode in response to atrial flutter. On the *left*, atrial flutter (cycle length = 260 msec) causes rapid ventricular pacing. Note that the AV interval initiated by an atrial-sensed event is only 30 msec, a rate-adaptive response related to sensing a fast atrial rate. Every second atrial event (A_R) falling in the postventricular atrial refractory period is counted as an atrial signal. Automatic mode switching was externally programmed at the arrow. The pacemaker immediately detects a fast atrial rate and begins its automatic mode-switching function with gradual slowing of the ventricular rate to 70 ppm in the DDI(R) mode on the right. Had activation of automatic mode switching started from sinus rhythm followed by the abrupt onset of supraventricular tachycardia (SVT), the diagnosis of SVT by the tachycardia counter would have required a few more seconds. Note that the atrial flutter signals falling in the postventricular atrial blanking period of 150 msec are not detected and therefore do not generate event markers. A_R signals are detected during the AV interval only beyond a short initial blanking period *(stars)*. (From Barold SS: Optimal pacing in the brady-tachy syndrome. Cardiol Rev 5:63, 1997.)

Pacemaker Diagnosis of Supraventricular Tachycardia

Most contemporary dual-chamber pacemakers use only the atrial sensor for the detection of unphysiologic atrial rates.

In DDDR devices, the relative contributions from the nonatrial sensor and atrial inputs can also be used for the diagnosis of pathologic SVT (Table 30–13), but relatively simple algorithms based on this concept are still being developed. In conventional devices with AMS, the sensing window of the atrial channel is extended to include part of the pacemaker atrial refractory period (relative refractory period) and, in some cases, part of the AV interval during which the pacemaker is able to detect atrial signals solely for SVT diagnosis.[60, 150]

The criteria used for SVT diagnosis vary considerably in design and complexity from manufacturer to manufacturer.[155–159] Some devices make the diagnosis of SVT when the sensed atrial cycles are equal or shorter than a given number of programmed SVT detection intervals. In some algorithms, the number of detected short cycles need not be consecutive. The required number of short cycles to activate

AMS is usually programmable. However, some devices use complex nonprogrammable algorithms for the detection of the programmed SVT rate rather than a specific number of SVT intervals. In some devices, the algorithm compensates for the occasional prolongation of the atrial cycle length longer than the tachycardia detection interval to ensure sensing of irregular signals with varying amplitude, especially during atrial fibrillation (so-called short–long sequences).[156, 157]

Timing Cycle Related to Automatic Mode Switching

A ventricular-paced or ventricular-sensed event initiates the PVARP and a blanking interval called the *postventricular atrial blanking period,* which usually lasts 150 msec or less from the onset of the PVARP. The postventricular atrial blanking period is designed to ignore the far-field QRS registered by the atrial electrogram to avoid false counting of nonatrial events. In some designs, the duration of the blanking periods or "blind spots" prevents the pacemaker from detecting SVT, if the SVT cycle does not match the

Table 30–13. Interactions of Atrial and Sensor Activity During DDDR Pacing

Atrial Rate	Slow	Slow	Fast	Fast
Sensor 1 response	Slow	Fast	Slow	Fast
Sensor 2 response	Fast	Fast	Slow	Fast
Pacemaker interpretation	Sinus bradycardia, patient at rest	Sinus bradycardia, patient active	Pathologic atrial tachycardia	Sinus tachycardia
Pacemaker response	Pace or sense according to lower rate timing or blunted sensor response	Pace in accord with sensor response	Place cap on maximum tracking rate, mode switch to nontracking mode	Rate controlled by either sinus or sensor depending on programmed parameters

From Levine PA, Barold SS: Pacemaker automaticity, enabled by a multiplicity of new algorithms. *In* Singer I, Barold SS, Camm AJ (eds): Nonpharmacological Therapy of Arrhythmias for the 21st Century: The State of the Art. Armonk, NY, Futura, 1998, pp 845–880.

sensing window of the pacemaker. In other words, the duration of the postventricular atrial blanking period imposes mathematical limits on the detection of SVT for AMS (Fig. 30–76). If AV delay + postventricular AB period > atrial cycle length, the pacemaker will exhibit 2:1 atrial sensing of SVT. For example, if AV delay = 160 msec and postventricular atrial blanking period = 150 msec, the pacemaker cannot sense atrial flutter at a rate of 280/bpm (cycle length = 214 msec) on a 1:1 basis because 160 + 150 > 214 msec. Sensing will therefore occur, with alternate atrial beats.[160] Restoration of 1:1 atrial sensing requires programming of the AV interval to 60 msec (if postventricular atrial blanking period is nonprogrammable). Now, the sum of the AV delay and the postventricular atrial blanking period, or 60 + 150, is shorter than the atrial flutter cycle length of 214 msec. The pacemaker will now sense atrial flutter on a 1:1 basis and activate AMS. Restoration of AMS function by shortening of the AV delay to circumvent a long postventricular atrial blanking period produces unfavorable hemodynamics for long-term pacing if the AV delay remains permanently short. For this reason, a design that allows substantial shortening of the AV delay (atrial sensed and ventricular paced), only with increasing sensed atrial rates, optimizes sensing of SVT and yet preserves a physiologic AV interval at rest and low levels of exercise. During SVT when AV delay + postventricular atrial blanking period = 30 + 150 = 180 msec, this combination allows sensing of atrial flutter with a cycle length of up to 180 msec (rate = 333/bpm).

Programmability of Automatic Mode Switching

Programming and troubleshooting of AMS requires a wide range of atrial sensitivities and detailed knowledge of pacemaker specifications, especially the duration of the atrial blanking periods and related timing cycles. Incorrect reprogramming of AMS parameters (or suboptimal design) may create a number of problems. These include loss of specific-

ity, such as sensing sinus tachycardia on exercise as pathologic tachycardia, with obvious hemodynamic consequences, or withholding AMS because of inappropriate selection of atrial sensitivity or atrial blanking (absolute refractory) periods—the "blind spots" during which the pacemaker cannot sense SVT.

The effective atrial electrogram during SVT can have a lower amplitude than that in sinus rhythm.[161–163] Indeed, in atrial fibrillation, effective AMS often requires more sensitive settings than in sinus rhythm to ensure consistent atrial sensing.[164, 165] Therefore, pacing with AMS requires a higher atrial sensitivity and bipolar atrial leads to minimize atrial oversensing of myopotentials or the far-field QRS complex.[166–168] Despite seemingly appropriate programming, a pacemaker can still sense sufficient atrial activity during SVT to produce an unphysiologic ventricular pacing rate yet fail to activate its AMS function because the criteria for tachycardia detection are not met. Intermittent AMS, especially during atrial fibrillation, can cause marked oscillations in the pacing rate.[160, 164]

Specificity of Automatic Mode Switching

Specificity remains a problem and depends a great deal on the design of the AMS algorithm. Unipolar atrial-sensing systems can induce AMS from myopotential oversensing and should not be used. Barring myopotential oversensing, far-field sensing of the tail end of the QRS complex by the atrial channel is the most common cause of a false-positive AMS response (Fig. 30–77). Such far-field sensing of the QRS complex (almost always from a paced beat) causes VA crosstalk in the opposite direction to the well-known form of AV crosstalk.[169] VA crosstalk occurs only when the postventricular atrial blanking period is too short or the QRS too long. Any circumstance that prolongs the QRS complex (administration of flecainide or amiodarone; hyperkalemia) favors VA crosstalk.

Less commonly, oversensing of atrial signals can occur within the AV delay. In such cases, the atrial blanking period connected to the AV interval must terminate before the AV interval has timed out. Thus, double sensing of the P wave (near-field) or sensing of the early part of the QRS complex can occur within the AV delay. Far-field sensing of the spontaneous QRS complex during the AV delay is far less common than sensing the terminal part of the QRS complex beyond the postventricular atrial blanking period. During the AV delay, the atrial channel can sense the early part of the spontaneous QRS only if it is detected before the ventricular channel senses it as a near-field signal (Fig. 30–78). In some devices, AMS can occur after a series of short–long cycles, in which the short cycles occur within the AV delay (As-A_R or A_R-As) despite the fact that the long cycles exceed the duration of the tachycardia detection interval. Problems related to sensing within the AV delay could be eliminated by extending the blanking period to encompass the entire AV delay either as a factory-set feature or a programmable option. Signal detection during the AV delay was originally designed to optimize the detection of atrial fibrillation. Improved AMS algorithms should make sensing within the AV interval unnecessary and obviate atrial oversensing during the AV delay.

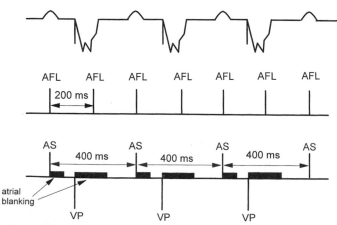

Figure 30–76. 2:1 sensing of atrial flutter by a Medtronic Thera pacemaker. The atrial flutter cycle length is shorter than the sum of the AV interval plus the postventricular atrial blanking period. The blanking periods are depicted in black. Every alternate f wave falls in the postventricular atrial blanking period. (Courtesy of Medtronic, Inc., Minneapolis, MN.)

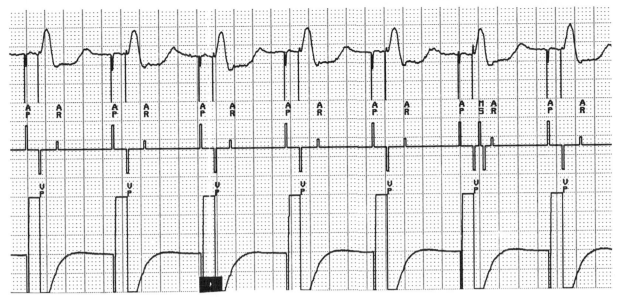

Figure 30–77. VA crosstalk. Far-field atrial sensing of the tail end of the paced QRS complex beyond the 150 msec postventricular atrial blanking period. During the period of far-field R-wave sensing, the matching atrial interval (MAI) is decreasing on the short intervals ($As-A_R$) by 24 msec and increasing on the long intervals (A_R-As) by 8 msec. The net change is a 16-msec decrease per cycle. This continues until the MAI shortens beyond the tachycardia detection interval and automatic mode switching occurs. Far-field sensing can be eliminated by programming a longer postventricular atrial blanking period in devices capable of such programming.

Testing for Ventriculoatrial Crosstalk

After pacemaker implantation, the propensity for VA cross-talk should be tested during ventricular pacing. The AV delay is shortened to provide continual paced ventricular depolarization. The pacemaker is then programmed to the highest atrial sensitivity and the largest ventricular output (voltage and pulse duration). These settings should be evaluated at several pacing rates to at least 110 to 120 ppm because faster ventricular pacing rates impair dissipation of the afterpotential. Such parameters enhance the afterpotential and therefore provide a voltage superimposed on the tail end of the paced QRS complex. The combined voltage from these two sources may be sensed as a far-field signal by the atrial channel. In devices with a programmable postventricular atrial blanking period, this procedure is positive for VA crosstalk and can be performed at various durations of the postventricular atrial blanking period until VA crosstalk is eliminated.

Does Undersensing of Supraventricular Tachycardia Eliminate the Need for Automatic Mode Switching?

Undersensing of SVT protects the patient against rapidly paced ventricular rates automatically. However, this situation should not be considered an acceptable substitute for AMS because it robs the system of diagnostic data stored in the pacemaker memory in terms of the duration, nature, and device treatment of SVT, especially when atrial fibrillation is asymptomatic.[170–173] Some contemporary pacemakers can already store in their RAM memory a brief sequence of atrial electrograms and marker chain to characterize the SVT or the abnormal processes that initiate AMS.

DDI and DDIR Modes Versus Automatic Mode Switching

With present AMS systems, SVT management can occasionally be difficult despite extensive trials of programmability and concomitant administration of antiarrhythmic drugs.

Patients with paroxysmal common atrial flutter, especially if atrial flutter is unresponsive to AMS, should be considered for curative ablation. The few patients refractory to AMS require permanent pacing in the DDI or DDIR mode.

AMS has made primary pacing with the DDI and DDIR modes virtually obsolete in the management of the bradycardia-tachycardia syndrome. However, AMS algorithms require further refining for greater specificity and sensitivity. Algorithms will become more complex to ensure consistent sensing of atrial fibrillation that generates signals irregular in timing and amplitude. More extensive programmability of atrial blanking periods, adaptive AV delays, and a very wide range of high atrial sensitivity and complex electronic averaging algorithms will be required.

The first widely available commercial device for AMS, the Meta DDDR 1250, 1254, and 1256 devices (Telectronics),[160, 174–176] used an algorithm with a counter to keep track of the number of atrial signals at a rate above the tachycardia detection rate. The first model was too sensitive, and AMS could occur after only one cycle.[150] In subsequent models, when the number of beats was programmed to n (e.g., 4), the counter would increment by 1 whenever an atrial cycle was shorter than the tachycardia detection interval. A sensed atrial interval longer than the tachycardia detection interval would decrease the counter by 1. AMS occurred when the counter registered the programmed number of tachycardia detection intervals (e.g., 4) (Fig. 30–79).

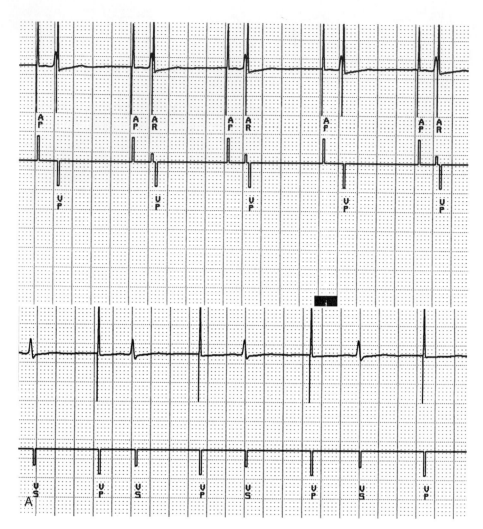

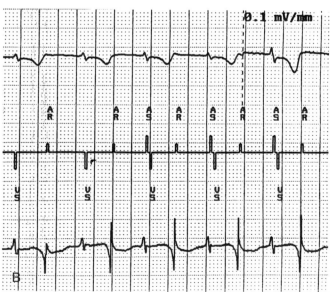

Figure 30–78. *A,* Early far-field atrial sensing of the QRS complex before sensing of the QRS complex within the AV interval as a near-field signal by the ventricular channel. This produces an atrial signal (A_R) that can be counted by the tachycardia detection mechanism of a pacemaker. *Top,* Medtronic Elite unipolar DDDR pacemaker showing atrial pacing followed by Vp, producing a pseudofusion beat. The atrial channel senses the early part of the spontaneous QRS complex. *Bottom,* Same patient. The device was programmed to the subthreshold VVI mode on the right with the same ventricular sensitivity as in panel *A.* There is normal ventricular sensing. *B,* AV junctional rhythm showing early far-field atrial sensing of the QRS complex before ventricular sensing occurs, almost immediately afterward. The lower tracing shows the atrial electrogram, which confirms the absence of atrial activity coincidentally with the QRS complex. Postventricular atrial refractory period (PVARP) = 310 msec.

Figure 30–79. Diagrammatic representation of the Telectronics automatic mode-switching algorithm with failure during atrial fibrillation. The pacemaker counts a tachycardia cycle only when the interval between successive sensed f (P) waves becomes shorter than the programmed tachycardia interval to activate automatic mode switching. One short cycle increments the counter by 1. When a sensed atrial cycle > tachycardia interval for automatic mode switching, the counter is decreased by 1. Irregular atrial sensing prevents the tachycardia counter from registering five short intervals, the programmed value to activate automatic mode switching for this particular algorithm. (From Ellenbogen KA, Mond HG, Wood MA, et al: Failure of automatic mode switching: Recognition and management. PACE 20:268, 1997.)

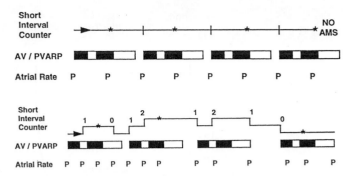

Illustrative Algorithms

A description of all available algorithms from a variety of manufacturers is beyond the scope of this discussion. Two recent reviews outline the specifications of the AMS function of current pacemakers.[157, 158] This discussion focuses mainly on the algorithms developed by Medtronic, Inc. (Minneapolis, MN), the largest manufacturer in the world, to illustrate their complexity and evaluation.

Medtronic AMS Function

The manufacturer indicates that the pacemaker uses the mean atrial rate to activate AMS in the Thera and Kappa 400 family of pacemakers. Actually, the *mean atrial rate* is a misnomer because the device measures a changing artificial atrial interval that bears a constantly changing relationship to the true atrial rate. This artificial atrial interval must eventually match the tachycardia detection interval for AMS to occur. Consequently, the so-called mean atrial rate is best described in terms of a *matching atrial interval* (MAI). When AMS is programmed on, the pacemaker continuously monitors the interval between two atrial-sensed beats. It translates this into the mean atrial rate, or the MAI. With each cycle the MAI is compared with the spontaneous atrial cycle. If the MAI is longer than the atrial cycle, the MAI shortens by 24 msec. If the MAI is shorter than the atrial cycle, the MAI increases by 8 msec (Fig. 30–80). The process continues until the duration of the MAI has short-

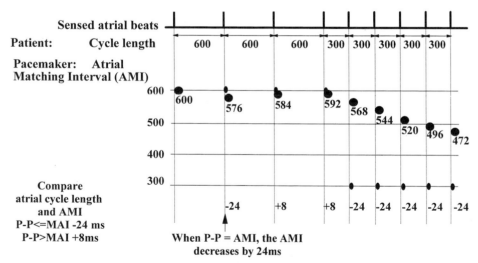

Figure 30–80. *A,* Diagrammatic representation of the matching atrial rate (MAR) of Medtronic Thera pacemaker during supraventricular tachycardia. The *large solid circles* represent the value of the matching atrial intervals (MAI). The *smaller oval circles* represent the instantaneous atrial interval. On each interval, the MAI is compared with the instantaneous interval, resulting in a change. *First beat:* The MAI is the same as the atrial interval, resulting in a decrease of 24 msec in the MAI. *Second beat:* The MAI is shorter (corresponding rate faster) than the atrial interval, resulting in an increase of 8 msec in the MAI. *Third beat:* The MAI is again shorter than the atrial interval, resulting in an increase of 8 msec in the MAI. *Fourth beat:* The 300 msec atrial interval is shorter (corresponding rate faster) than the MAI, resulting in a decrease of 24 msec in the MAI. *Fifth to eighth beats:* the same. The MAI decreases by 24 msec with each cycle. *B,* Should the postventricular atrial blanking period cause failure to sense an occasional atrial signal, the sensed atrial interval would double to 600 msec. In that case, an 8-msec addition to the MAI would occur, but the 24-msec subtractions on shorter 300-msec atrial intervals guarantee that the MAI continues to shorten to meet the spontaneous tachycardia interval. Mode switching occurs when the MAI reaches the tachycardia detection interval. (Courtesy of Medtronic, Inc., Minneapolis, MN.)

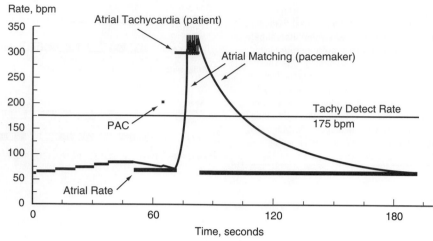

Figure 30–81. Matched atrial interval (MAI) of the Medtronic Thera pacemaker is limited in the speed at which it can track the detected atrial rate. Isolated events, such as premature atrial contractions (PACs), leave the MAI essentially unaffected. The precipitous onset of atrial tachycardia results in a rapid increase in the MAI. Automatic mode switching occurs when it reaches the tachycardia detection rate. (Courtesy of Medtronic, Inc., Minneapolis, MN.)

ened to the value of the tachycardia detection interval (Fig. 30–81). At this point, AMS occurs. Actually, MAI variation or dithering occurs around the rate of the tachycardia, not the tachycardia detection rate. If the atrial rate (sinus or SVT) is stable, the dither is always a 3:1 ratio (Fig. 30–82). The algorithm is designed to weather intermittent sensing. Several long intervals due to oversensing can be compensated for with just one fast interval. In other words, the MAI is resistant to sudden changes in atrial rate. When MAI is equal to the PP interval, the MAI shortens by 24 msec (Fig. 30–83). The subsequent three MAI values are shorter than the PP intervals, and each increments by 8 msec (8 × 3 = 24). The third 8-msec increment causes the MAI to equal

the PP interval, which triggers a 24-msec subtraction in the MAI, and the process repeats.

The time to AMS depends on the following parameters: (1) starting atrial rate—a faster rate requires less ground to cover to reach the tachycardia detection rate; (2) tachycardia detection rate (interval); (3) rate of atrial tachycardia. The biased nature of the algorithm was designed to promote intermittent sensing because several long intervals due to undersensing can be compensated for with just one fast interval. Exit from AMS at the termination of tachycardia depends on the reverse process, with the MAI gradually lengthening with each cycle until resynchronization occurs (Table 30–14).

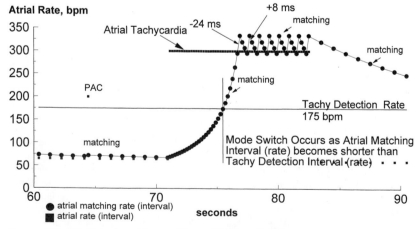

Figure 30–82. Behavior of the matching atrial interval of Medtronic Thera pacemakers during supraventricular tachycardia. The MAI variation (dithering) actually occurs at the rate of the atrial tachycardia, not at the tachycardia detection rate. The dither (if the atrial rate is constant) is always a 3:1 ratio. The 24-msec decrease causes the MAI to be shorter than the atrial interval; three subsequent 8-msec additions then occur. The third 8-msec addition causes the MAI to lengthen beyond the atrial tachycardia interval, triggering another 24-msec subtraction. (Courtesy of Medtronic, Inc., Minneapolis, MN.)

Modeswitching Medtronic Thera*i*

Patient		Pacemaker	Increment for Next AM
P-P		AMI	
600	=	600	− 24
600	>	576	+ 8
600	>	584	+ 8
600	>	592	+ 8
600	=	600	− 24
600	>	576	+ 8
600	>	584	+ 8
600	>	592	+ 8
600	=	600	− 24

Figure 30–83. Behavior of the mode-switching algorithm of the Medtronic Thera pacemakers. When MAI = P-P cycle, the matched atrial interval (MAI) decreases by 24 msec. There is one MAI decrement, followed by three MAI increments, the last of which causes the MAI to equal the initial value. Because the PP interval = MAI, the MAI restarts the same cycle. The MAI returns to 600 msec every fourth beat.

When AMS of the Thera device is programmed, the obligatory rate-adaptive AV algorithm shortens the AV delay according to the sensed atrial rate to a minimum of 30 msec to enhance atrial sensing, especially the detection of atrial flutter. AV delay abbreviation is controlled by the same algorithm as the MAI. Thus, with an AV interval of 30 msec and postventricular atrial blanking period of 150 msec (150 + 30 = 180 msec), the pacemaker can sense atrial flutter up to a cycle length of 180 msec or rate of 333/bpm.

Blanking of the AV Interval

In the Medtronic Thera and Kappa 400 devices, blanking following Ap or As varies from 50 to 100 msec and is a function of the size of the sensed signal (see Table 30–14). The purpose of sensing in the AV interval was to provide an opportunity to detect additional A_R events for updating the MAI. However, such a window may cause double sensing of P waves, sensing of far-field R waves preceding ventricular-sensed R waves, and possible detection of polarization after atrial pacing.[177] The AV interval of the Kappa 700 is now essentially blanked in the DDD and DDDR modes. The marker channel will show A_R for events in the AV interval, but unlike A_R events in the PVARP, they are completely ignored by the device for the purpose of counting. The pacemaker believes that in the DDIR mode, atrial sensing inhibits Ap, and there is no "real" AV interval. Therefore, counting takes place in the As-Vp interval.

Long–Short Sequences

A long–short sequence is characterized by an atrial interval < tachycardia detection interval alternating with an atrial interval > tachycardia detection interval (Fig. 30–84). The algorithm of the Thera and Kappa 400 devices, therefore, adds 24 msec to the MAI, alternating with an 8-msec subtraction to the MAI. This process eventually allows the MAI (because the system is biased toward tachycardia) to reach

Table 30–14. Automatic Mode-Switching Algorithms of Medtronic Pacemakers

Feature	Thera, Thera*i*	Kappa 400	Kappa 700
Programmable AV delays	Rate-adaptive* AV—ON Maximum SAV—170 msec	Rate-adaptive* AV—On/Off Maximum SAV—350 msec	Rate Adaptive* AV—On/Off Maximum SAV—250 msec
Programmable PVAB	Fixed	Programmable	Programmable 120–220 msec
AV blanking	First 50–100 msec (function of the size of the sensed signal)	First 50–100 msec (function of the size of the sensed signal)	Mostly blanked in DDD, DDDR modes, but not in the DDIR mode.
PVARP outside AMS	Fixed 270–310 msec depending on tachycardia detection rate	Programmable nominally 270–310 msec according to tachycardia detection rate	Adaptive—varies according to sensed *atrial* rate Programmable (nominal value is adaptive)
Detection algorithm	MAR faster than tachycardia detection rate	MAR faster than tachycardia detection rate	4 of the last 7 atrial intervals faster than tachycardia detection rate or using blanked flutter search
Detection time	7–10 sec (depends on starting point and rate of tachycardia)	7–10 sec (depends on starting point and rate of tachycardia)	3 sec in most cases
Tachycardia detection rate	120–190	120–190	120–200
Resynchronization after AMS	MAR < upper rate or 5 consecutive atrial-paced events	MAR < upper rate or 5 consecutive atrial-paced events	7 consecutive atrial beats < upper rate or 5 consecutive atrial paced events

AMS, automatic mode switching; MAR, matched atrial rate.

* All switch to DDIR (when permanent programmed mode is DDD or DDDR) or VVIR (if permanent mode is VDD). Based on atrial rate–matched atrial rate algorithm. The rate-adaptive paced AV interval is based on the sensor rate.

Note: Programmability of AV interval in the Kappa 400 device was introduced in response to physician request about the Thera interlocks. The maximum sensed AV of 170 msec in the Thera series may cause pseudofusion with a conducted QRS complex. Programmability of the AV interval in the Kappa 400 may interfere with AMS function under certain circumstances. Warnings are displayed on the programmer when parameters are selected that may have deleterious effects on AMS. The Kappa 700 device is immune to these problems by virtue of the "blanked flutter search" feature because it anticipates that 2 : 1 sensing can occur and adapts. Thus, the Kappa 700 pacemakers require few or no interlocks. Rate-adaptive AV intervals are not as essential for AMS in the Kappa 700 as in the 400. The Thera programmer restricts selection of parameters that may compromise AMS behavior.

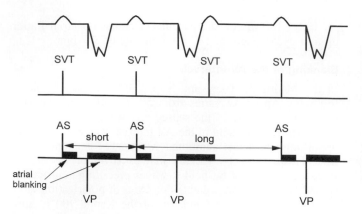

Figure 30–84. Long-short-long-short sequences can cause automatic mode switching in Medtronic Thera and Kappa 400 devices even when long cycles exceed the tachycardia detection interval. A 3:2 Wenckebach upper rate response may result in pacemaker detection of alternating long and short intervals. The third atrial supraventricular tachycardia (SVT) signal is not detected because it falls in the postventricular atrial blanking period. The matched atrial interval decreases by 24 msec, then increases by 8 msec, then decreases by 24 msec, then increases by 8 msec, until it reaches the tachycardia detection interval. (Courtesy of Medtronic, Inc., Minneapolis, MN.)

the tachycardia detection rate and AMS to be established. Although this algorithm is helpful in detecting an irregular tachycardia with detection gaps (some atrial beats undetected in the blanking period or one associated with intermittent undersensing), it may also induce AMS in circumstances without tachycardia.

The new Medtronic Kappa 700 DDDR pacemaker features a different AMS algorithm that is characterized by the following features[177] (Tables 30–14 and 30–15):

Statistical detection method. Four of the last seven intrinsic atrial intervals must be shorter than the tachycardia detection interval (corresponding to the mode switch rate). The pacemaker continually reviews the most recent seven atrial-sensed intervals. Intervals that begin with an atrial-sensed event (As or A_R) and end with Ap are not counted as part of the seven intervals.

Automatic PVARP controlled by sensed atrial rate (not the sensor rate). The pacemaker determines the sensed atrial rate using the "mean atrial rate" or atrial matching rate (AMR) designed in the Thera and Kappa 400 devices. The pacemaker calculates a desired 2:1 AV block point (30 beats faster than the atrial matching rate), but never less than 100 ppm and never more than 35 ppm above the upper tracking rate (subject to Wenckebach operation above upper rate). The PVARP is adjusted so that the

TARP provides the desired 2:1 block point. If the sensed AV interval is too long and PVARP would need to be very short, PVARP is shortened to a programmed minimum value, and then the sensed AV interval is shortened to maintain the desired 2:1 block response.

Every 4 beats, a new TARP is calculated equal to the atrial matching rate + 30 bpm.

There is a minimum value to which PVARP can be reduced to achieve this new TARP. For example:

AMR = 80 bpm; SAV = 200 msec; minimum PVARP = 220 msec.
The desired TARP for 80 bpm would be equivalent to 110 bpm (80 + 30), or 550 msec: 550 msec − SAV = 350 msec. Thus, PVARP would be set equal to 350 msec. Later, AMR = 100 bpm; SAV = 200 msec; minimum PVARP = 220 msec.
The desired TARP for 100 bpm would be equivalent to 130 bpm (100 + 30), or 460 msec: 460 msec − SAV = 260 msec. Thus, PVARP would be set equal to 260 msec. Now, under a different scenario: MAR = 110 bpm; SAV = 200 bpm; minimum PVARP = 250 msec.
The desired TARP for 110 bpm would be equivalent to 140 bpm (110 + 30), or 430 msec: 430 msec − SAV = 230 msec, which is lower than the minimum PVARP of 250 msec.

Table 30–15. Characteristics of the Postventricular Atrial Refractory Periods of Medtronic Pacemakers

PVARP Status	Thera	Kappa 400	Kappa 700
AMS not programmed	Programmable or *sensor* rate adaptive	Programmable or *sensor* rate adaptive	Programmable or *sensor* rate adaptive (DDIR) or *atrial* rate adaptive (DDD/R)
AMS programmed			
1. During sinus rhythm	PVARP fixed 270–310 msec according to tachycardia detection rate	PVARP programmable, nominally 270–310 msec according to tachycardia detection rate	PVARP programmable or *atrial* rate adaptive
2. During SVT before AMS has converted pacer to DDIR mode	PVARP fixed 270–310 msec according to tachycardia detection rate	PVARP programmable, nominally 270–310 msec according to tachycardia detection rate	PVARP programmable or *atrial* rate adaptive
3. During AMS (DDIR)	VA interval: 300 msec; VA interval is sensor controlled	VA interval: 300 msec; VA interval is sensor controlled	VA interval: 300 msec; VA interval is sensor controlled

AMS, automatic mode switching; SVT, supraventricular tachycardia; VA interval, atrial escape interval; PVARP, postventricular atrial refractory period.

MODE SWITCHING - TACHY DETECTION

- Blanked Flutter Search:
   Technique to assess true atrial rate

- High Atrial Rate "Suspected" when atrial interval is less than 2 * (SAV + PVAB)

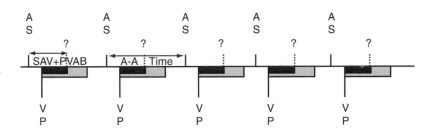

Figure 30–85. Diagrammatic representation of blanked flutter search of Medtronic Kappa 700 pacemaker. A high atrial interval is suspected when the atrial interval is less than 2 × (sensed AV interval + postventricular atrial blanking interval). Then, the pacemaker extends the postventricular atrial refractory period (PVARP), as shown in Fig. 30–86. The postventricular atrial blanking period is depicted in black. (Courtesy of Medtronic, Inc., Minneapolis, MN.)

In this case, PVARP = 250 msec, and SAV is reduced 20 msec to 180, so the resultant TARP is equal to 430 msec.

A long PVARP enhances sensing of SVT by diminishing the total blanking periods (in AV delay and PVARP) per cycle. A long PVARP at rest provides control of the ventricular response at the onset of an arrhythmia.

Blanked Flutter Search

This algorithm is based on modification of synchronization for one cycle to bring out atrial signals (F waves) masked by blanking of the pacemaker. The pacemaker continuously reviews atrial intervals in comparison to the AV interval and postventricular atrial blanking period (Figs. 30–85 to 30–87). When PP interval < than 2 × (AV + postventricular atrial BP) or 2 × total atrial blanking period (AV interval is totally blanked), it is possible that an atrial rate is being sensed on a 2:1 basis. If this condition persists for 8 beats, PVARP is extended to interrupt the rhythm and detect the true PP interval (Fig. 30–88, see Table 30–14).

Other Automatic Mode-Switching Algorithms

The Trilogy DR+ (Pacesetter) uses the same principle as the MAI technique of Medtronic devices.[178–179] Pacesetter calls the MAI the *filtered atrial rate interval* (FARI). If the PP < FARI, FARI is decreased by 38 msec, and if PP > FARI, FARI is increased by up to 25 msec. As the atrial rate reaches the maximum tracking rate, the PVARP "opens up"

to enhance sensing beyond the postventricular atrial blanking period. This function may lead to 2:1 sensing of atrial flutter. Several other systems use a programmable tachycardia detection rate and number of beats (Figs. 30–89 to 30–92). The Intermedics algorithm allows rapid detection of SVT and AMS within as little as one ventricular cycle. However, atrial undersensing during atrial fibrillation may cause mode-switching oscillations because a rapidly switching device may become repeatedly unswitched and switched.[157, 158] The combined use of the SmarTracking feature can be helpful to provide smooth transition in the pacing rates at the onset and termination of mode switching. Patients appear to prefer an AMS algorithm that results in mode switching in 4 to 7 beats.[180] Devices that use an averaging technique, such as the MAI, usually provide a stable and smooth decrease in pacing rate during atrial fibrillation.[157, 181] Such devices take longer to achieve AMS and to exit from it.[181]

Pacemaker Diagnosis of Atrial Arrhythmias Using a Nonatrial Sensor

Table 30–13 shows how a rate-adaptive device can determine whether a high atrial rate is physiologic. Pacemakers using a nonatrial sensor would be more specific but more complex and would probably increase the time to mode switching.[157]

The Intermedics Marathon DDDR pacemaker incorporates a new SmarTracking algorithm in which sensor activity

Extend PVARP to prevent tracking of next beat this will reveal true atrial interval

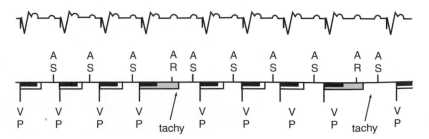

Figure 30–86. Diagrammatic representation of blanked flutter search of Medtronic Kappa 700 pacemaker. Following the events in Fig. 30–85, the pacemaker extends the postventricular atrial refractory period (PVARP) for one cycle. An atrial signal (which previously generated As) is now sensed in the PVARP as A$_R$ and the succeeding one beyond the PVARP as As, thereby revealing the A$_R$-As atrial flutter or tachycardia cycle. The postventricular atrial blanking period is depicted in black. (Courtesy of Medtronic, Inc., Minneapolis, MN.)

If No Tachy is present, atrial pace escapes near expected atrial event

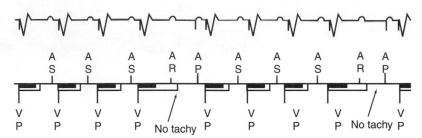

Figure 30–87. Diagrammatic representation of blanked flutter search of Medtronic Kappa 700 pacemaker after events in Fig. 30–86 in a patient without atrial tachycardia or flutter. A_R is followed by Ap after the postventricular atrial refractory period (PVARP) extension for one cycle. The postventricular atrial blanking period is depicted in black. (Courtesy of Medtronic, Inc., Minneapolis, MN.)

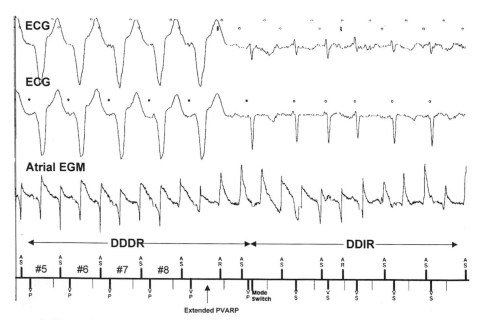

Figure 30–88. Automatic mode switching of a Medtronic Kappa 700 pacemaker secondary to a blanked atrial flutter search. Whenever eight atrial intervals are less than twice the total atrial blanking interval (AV + postventricular atrial blanking period), the pacemaker extends the PVARP. This uncovers A_R in the extended postventricular atrial refractory period (PVARP) followed by As at an A_R-As interval half the previous As-As intervals. The device makes the diagnosis of atrial flutter on the basis of the true atrial interval and activates mode switching to the DDIR mode. The end of the PVARP is shown on the Marker Channel as an unlabeled negative tick. Atrial depolarization not marked on the Marker Channel falls within the postventricular atrial blanking period. EGM, electrogram. (Courtesy of Medtronic, Inc., Minneapolis, MN.)

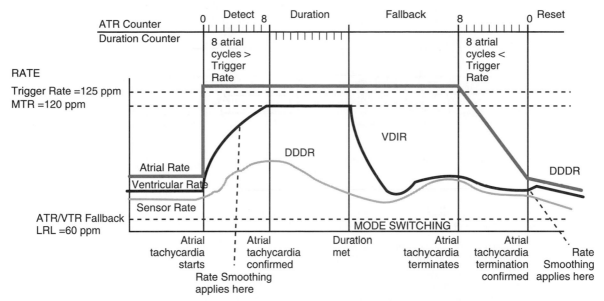

Figure 30–89. Diagrammatic representation of the atrial tachycardia automatic mode switching (AMS) response of the CPI (Guidant) Vigor, Discovery, and Meridian pacemakers. The pacemaker requires detection of eight cycles at a rate exceeding the programmed upper rate (there is no separate tachycardia detection rate) to diagnose tachycardia. Pacing then continues for a programmable duration of 10 to 2000 ventricular cycles. During this period, the pacemaker continues to function at the programmed upper rate (Wenckebach or fixed-ratio block) and then switches to the VVI(R) mode during a fallback period of 1–5 minutes, with a progressive slowing of the pacing rate. AMS terminates when eight cycles are longer than the programmed upper rate. Rate smoothing can also be used to provide smooth transitions before AMS and when returning to the synchronized DDDR mode. (Courtesy of Guidant Corporation.)

Figure 30–90. Diagrammatic representation of the Intermedics Marathon automatic mode-switching (AMS) algorithm. The device truly uses *consecutive* intervals. The postventricular atrial blanking period is 100 msec. The T2 interval starts from each atrial-sensed event and is only interrupted by another atrial event (paced or sensed). If the atrial event is a sensed signal, the counter is incremented, and another T2 interval is started, provided that the As-As interval is shorter than the tachycardia detection T2 interval. If the atrial event is paced, the counter is returned to 0, and T2 is terminated. A low number of detection cycles allows the diagnosis of supraventricular tachycardia (SVT) when the atrial rate is fairly low. The number of cycles is programmable from 1 to 7. AMS occurs at the sensor-indicated rate. An adaptive AV delay enhances sensing of SVT. (Courtesy of Intermedics, Inc.)

Programmable Parameters:

Non-physiolgic Atrial Rates $\geq$ *nnn* bpm
Number of consecutive cycles = *x*

In the DDD(R) or VDD(R) modes, the device will switch ( ) to VVI(R) mode pacing when:

The sensed atrial interval is less than $\dfrac{60,000}{nnn}$ msec for x consecutive cycles

[These atrial sense events must occur outside the absolute atrial refractory period (aarp)]

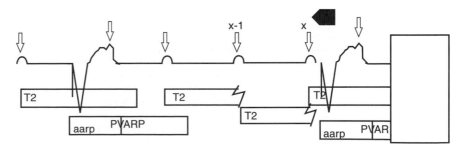

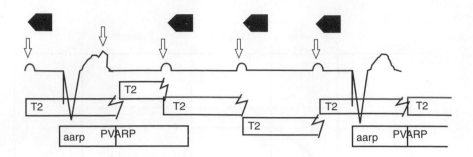

To remain in the VVI(R) 'switched' mode:

An atrial sense event must be sensed during the T2 interval;

If switched (◀), and a ventricular event occurs, a T2 interval
is started at the end of aarp to stay in VVI(R) despite 'blind spot'

Figure 30–91. Diagrammatic representation of the Intermedics Marathon automatic mode-switching (AMS) algorithm. During AMS, it was assumed that an atrial event would fall in the atrial blanking or absolute atrial refractory period (AARP) and that missing an atrial event would cause a "dropout" from AMS. Therefore, the T2 interval starts at the end of the 100-msec AARP when mode switching is active. T2 ignores ventricular events. AMS ends when the T2 interval ends without an atrial-sensed event or when an atrial-paced event occurs. If there is no sensed atrial event within T2, the next atrial-sensed event will be tracked in the usual DDD(R) pacing mode. (Courtesy of Intermedics, Inc., Angleton, TX.)

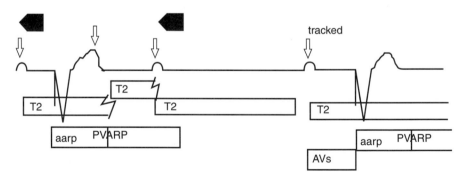

Mode switching ends when:

A *T2* interval ends without a sensed atrial event;

or

An atrial pace occurs

Figure 30–92. Schematic diagram of Intermedics Marathon SmarTrackingJ algorithm. The SmarTracking algorithm results in a continuously changing ventricular tracking limit based on sensor input. For example, if an atrial tachyarrhythmia occurs at a rate of 110 bpm (below the programmed automatic mode-switching rate), the SmarTracking algorithm will limit the ventricular tracking rate to a rate that the sensor determines is appropriate for that level of activity. If SmarTracking determines that the rate of 110 is "inappropriate" for that level of activity, it will not track the atrial rate. This algorithm limits ventricular tracking of atrial rates not due to exercise, particularly those below the upper rate limit. The SmarTracking algorithm has a programmable lower rate, response curve, and decay curve. (From Ellenbogen KA, Wood MA, Mond HG, et al: Clinical applications of mode switching for dual-chamber pacemakers. *In* Singer I, Barold SS, Camm AJ [eds]: Nonpharmacological Therapy of Arrhythmias for the 21st Century: The State of the Art. Armonk, NY, Futura, 1998, p 819.)

determines the upper atrial tracking rate.[157, 158] The difference between the upper atrial tracking rate and the sensor-indicated rate is programmable. The slope of the curve relating the sensor-indicated rate to the upper tracking rate is programmable from a value of one (least responsive) to four (most responsive). Thus, the upper tracking rate is continuously adjusted according to the sensor-indicated rate. If there is no sensor activity, the upper tracking rate is relatively low.

SmarTracking prevents tracking of unphysiologic rapid atrial rates unless the sensor detects that the patient is active. This feature complements the associated AMS algorithm and may cause less variation and oscillation of the ventricular rate owing to intermittent atrial undersensing during atrial fibrillation.[154, 182]

Indications for Pacemakers With Automatic Mode Switching

Overall experience with AMS has been satisfactory so far.[160, 183–194] Barring economic considerations, all pacemakers should possess an AMS function as one of the many programmable options. These devices are indicated in all patients with the bradycardia-tachycardia syndrome. They should also be considered in patients with sick sinus syndrome without paroxysmal SVT, obstructive hypertrophic cardiomyopathy, or any condition that predisposes patients to paroxysmal SVT.[194] Indeed, like the rate-adaptive function (R), it could be argued that all patients should receive a device with AMS capability because one cannot predict which patients will eventually develop SVT (or atrial chronotropic incompetence in the case of the rate-adaptive function).

Rate Smoothing

Rate smoothing is a programmable option that is not specifically an upper rate response because it is designed to eliminate pronounced variations in cycle length and therefore functions over all rate ranges. At the upper rate, rate smoothing prevents marked change in cycle length.[195] This mode of operation is complex, and its clinical advantages and disadvantages are not fully known, especially in the DDDR mode. Rate smoothing can provide an effective ventricular response to pathologic atrial rates (Fig. 30–93). Rate smoothing is an attempt to replace abrupt changes in rate with gradual transition by limiting the maximal change in the pacing rate from cycle to cycle to some percentage of the previous RR interval (smoothing factor). Rate smoothing

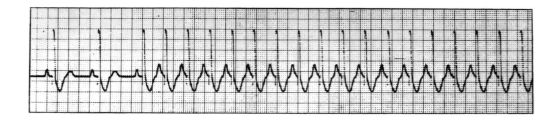

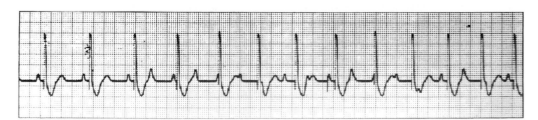

Figure 30–93. Rate smoothing with the CPI Delta 925 DDD pulse generator (Cardiac Pacemakers, Inc., St. Paul, MN). The programmed parameters were as follows: lower rate = 65 ppm; upper rate = 150 ppm; AV interval = 150 msec, and postventricular atrial refractory period (PVARP) = 250 msec. The top tracing shows 1:1 P-wave tracking during supraventricular tachycardia without rate-smoothing operation. The bottom strip shows the same supraventricular tachycardia with rate-smoothing operation (smoothing factor of 6%). The pulse generator stores in its memory the most recent RR interval, either paced or sensed. It then calculates "rate control windows" for the next cycle based on the RR interval and the programmed rate-smoothing value (6% in this example). Separate windows are calculated for the atrium and the ventricle. Atrial synchronization window = (previous RR interval ± rate-smoothing value) − AV delay. Ventricular synchronization window = previous RR interval ± rate-smoothing value. The timing for both windows is initiated at the end of a ventricular event. For example, if the previous RR interval is 800 msec, with a 6% rate-smoothing factor, the ventricular window would be 800 ± 6% = 800 ± 48 msec. The window would therefore extend from 752 to 848 msec. Paced activity (atrial or ventricular), if it is to occur, must occur during these rate control windows. When an atrial event occurs before the atrial synchronization window, the ventricle is paced after an interval that equals the previous RR interval less the rate-smoothing value. When an atrial event occurs within the synchronization window, the programmed AV delay is initiated, and the ventricle is paced at the end of the AV delay period. When no atrial event occurs during the synchronization window, the interval becomes equal to (previous RR interval + rate-smoothing value) − AV delay, so that the atrium is paced at the end of this interval, followed by ventricular pacing at the end of the programmed AV delay. (Courtesy of Cardiac Pacemakers, Inc., St. Paul, MN.)

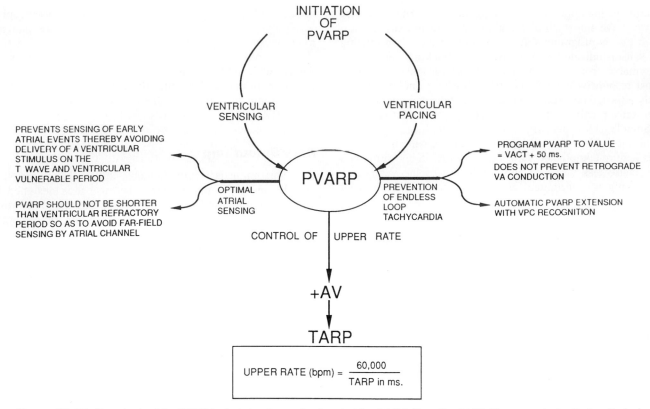

Figure 30–94. Central role of the PVARP in dual-chamber pacing (see text for details). (From Barold SS: Management of patients with dual-chamber pulse generators: Central role of pacemaker atrial refractory period. Learning Center *Highlights* [Heart House, American College of Cardiology] 5[4]:8, 1990.)

controls the response of a pulse generator because of increases and decreases in the intrinsic rate. Rate smoothing may be useful in patients who cannot tolerate marked fluctuations of paced rate with fixed-ratio or Wenckebach block response during the upper rate response of a DDD pulse generator or at the onset of tachycardia before AMS.[138, 196, 197] Rate smoothing may prevent the sudden deceleration of the ventricular rate during exercise, as with the development of 2:1 or 3:1 fixed-ratio block. During rate smoothing, the pulse generator loses effective AV synchrony and thus sacrifices optimal AV relationships to maintain pacing rates. For increasing atrial rates, rate smoothing will look similar to a Wenckebach response, with prolonged AV delays and occasional unsensed P waves falling in the PVARP.

Rate smoothing modifies the onset of endless-loop tachycardia by preventing abrupt variations in the paced rhythm. Actually, rate smoothing may itself precipitate endless-loop tachycardia because of its propensity to induce AV dissociation.

■ ATRIAL REFRACTORY PERIOD

The total refractory period (AV interval + PVARP) is the most important timing cycle of dual-chamber pacemakers, and many factors influence its duration[30, 33, 34, 40] (Fig. 30–94). The various factors determining the duration of the AV

interval are discussed later in the section on AV interval, and those determining PVARP duration are described in the discussion herein.

The shortest possible TARP (AV + PVARP) occurs when the AV interval is 0 (i.e., TARP = PVARP). In a DDD pacemaker when URI > TARP, the longest possible TARP (excluding PVARP extension) is equal to the separately programmable URI. The PVARP was originally designed as an absolute refractory period during which the pulse generator cannot sense. However, a number of contemporary designs permit atrial sensing during the PVARP to fulfill a number of functions (by definition, a sensed atrial event within the PVARP cannot be tracked and thus cannot initiate an AV interval). The first part of the PVARP (sometimes programmable) now becomes the postventricular atrial blanking period or an absolute refractory period, as described in the section on AMS. Published pacemaker specifications by manufacturers are somewhat confusing because some refer to the atrial refractory period as the TARP, whereas others refer only to the PVARP.

Upper Rate Limitation

As previously discussed, the TARP defines the longest PP interval (corresponding to the slowest atrial rate) that will produce an upper rate response characterized by pacemaker fixed-ratio AV block (e.g., 2:1) whether or not the pacemaker can respond to a longer PP interval with Wenckebach block upper rate behavior.

Postventricular Atrial Refractory Period

Automatic Extension

Many DDD pulse generators incorporate an automatic extension of the PVARP (for one cycle only) after a sensed ventricular event (outside the AV delay) that the pacemaker interprets as a VPC (two ventricular events without an intervening P wave). In some pulse generators, PVARP extension after a VPC is programmable ("off," "on," and to a variety of durations), and in others, it is automatic and nonprogrammable. PVARP extension is based on the concept that most episodes of endless-loop tachycardia are initiated by VPCs with retrograde VA conduction. Another design related to PVARP extension, the so-called DDX mode, consists of conversion to the DVI mode (i.e., asynchronous atrial channel)[30] (Fig. 30–95). The DDX mode in effect functions like an automatic PVARP extension after a VPC, with the atrial channel remaining refractory for a complete cycle (corresponding to the programmed lower rate). The pacemaker may continue to function in the DVI mode indefinitely as long as the RR interval between two consecutive sensed ventricular events remains shorter than the pacemaker AEI (Vs-Ap or Vp-Ap).[198] Termination of the DVI mode requires delivery of an atrial stimulus either spontaneously or by application and removal of the magnet (Fig. 30–95).

Advantages: Automatic PVARP extension or the DDX mode may play a role in the prevention of endless-loop

tachycardia. Automatic PVARP extension does not sacrifice the atrial tracking capability (upper rate) because the standard PVARP remains unchanged.

Limitations: PVARP extension does not provide protection when the first retrograde P wave is engendered by a ventricular-paced event. Although atrial sensing does not occur during the lengthened PVARP, the algorithm may postpone an endless-loop tachycardia for one cycle if the subsequent atrial stimulus falls in the atrial myocardial refractory period generated by retrograde atrial depolarization contained in the extended PVARP. Retrograde VA conduction then becomes possible with emission of the ventricular stimulus.

Disadvantages: Under certain circumstances, both the DDX and excessive extension of the PVARP may paradoxically increase susceptibility to endless-loop tachycardia[199] (Fig. 30–96). Automatic PVARP extension can also cause atrial undersensing despite a large intracardiac signal[200] (Fig. 30–97) (discussed later).

Apparent or Functional Undersensing

The differential diagnosis of atrial undersensing, not an uncommon problem in dual-chamber pacing, requires knowledge of atrial refractory period behavior under a variety of circumstances to avoid unnecessary surgical intervention to correct an apparent problem when the amplitude of the atrial signal is actually sufficiently large for sensing by the atrial channel. Apparent or functional atrial undersensing (or lack of P-wave tracking in the presence of an adequate atrial signal) originates from two main sources: (1) atrial signal in the PVARP, and (2) upper rate limitation (Table 30–16; see Fig. 30–23).

DDX MODE, LOWER RATE = 45 ppm, AV = 165 ms, UPPER RATE = 145 ppm

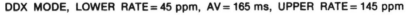

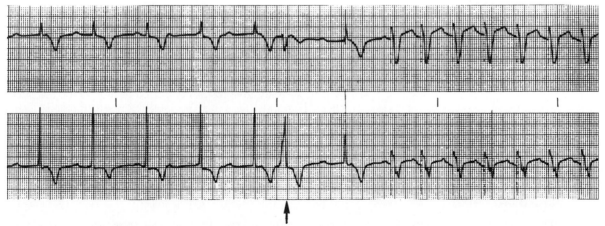

Figure 30–95. DDX mode of operation of the 283 AFP Pacesetter DDD pulse generator (Siemens-Pacesetter, Inc.). The programmed parameters are shown above the electrocardiogram, with two leads recorded simultaneously. The DDX mode of operation initiated the DVI mode after sensing of a ventricular extrasystole. The DVI mode can terminate only with the emission of an atrial stimulus. This stimulus does not occur because the RR interval of the AV junctional escape rhythm (about 1000 msec) is shorter than the atrial escape interval (AEI; 1333 − 165 = 1168 msec). A ventricular extrasystole *(arrow)* induces a longer pause, thereby allowing the release of an atrial stimulus at the termination of the AEI. The atrial stimulus produces a pseudopseudofusion beat. This atrial stimulus terminates the DVI mode, with the return of P-wave tracking in the DDX (or DDD) mode. (From Barold SS, Falkoff MD, Ong LS, et al: Electrocardiography of contemporary DDD pacemakers. A. Basic concepts, upper rate response, retrograde ventriculoatrial conduction, and differential diagnosis of pacemaker tachycardias. *In* Saksena S, Goldschlager N [eds]: Electrical Therapy for Cardiac Arrhythmias: Pacing, Antitachycardia Devices, Catheter Ablation. Philadelphia, WB Saunders, 1990, pp 225–264.)

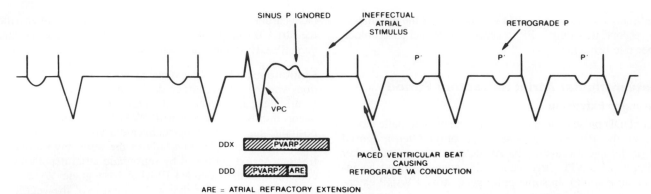

Figure 30–96. Diagrammatic representation of the mechanism of paradoxical induction of endless-loop tachycardia by excessive prolongation of the postventricular atrial refractory period (PVARP) with either atrial refractory period extension (ARE) or the DDX mode, in which the PVARP extends for the entire duration of the pacemaker cycle. The unsensed sinus P wave renders the succeeding atrial stimulus ineffectual because the stimulus falls within the atrial myocardial refractory period. This ineffectiveness of the atrial stimulus causes AV dissociation followed by retrograde VA conduction and initiation of endless-loop tachycardia. (From Barold SS, Falkoff MD, Ong LS, et al: Electrocardiography of contemporary DDD pacemakers. A. Basic concepts, upper rate response, retrograde ventriculoatrial conduction and differential diagnosis of pacemaker tachycardias. *In* Saksena S, Goldschlager N [eds]: Electrical Therapy for Cardiac Arrhythmias: Pacing, Antitachycardia Devices, Catheter Ablation. Philadelphia, WB Saunders, 1990, pp 225–264.)

Atrial Undersensing Related to the Refractory Period: P-wave undersensing can occur in the presence of an adequate atrial electrogram if the PVARP is excessively prolonged, especially when the atrial rate is relatively fast because it pushes the P wave toward the preceding PVARP. This form of undersensing is more likely with prolongation of spontaneous AV conduction (long PR interval), bringing the P wave closer to the prior PVARP (Fig. 30–98). Occasionally, P-wave undersensing can occur when the programmed basic PVARP is short (e.g., 155 msec). This paradox is explained by the onset of P-wave undersensing within

an automatically extended PVARP (e.g., 400 msec) initiated by a VPC or any other signal (e.g., sinus conducted QRS complex, false signal), not preceded by a detected P wave and interpreted as a VPC by the pacemaker. The unsensed P wave in the PVARP gives rise to a spontaneous conducted QRS complex that is then interpreted by the pacemaker as a VPC (no preceding sensed P wave), thereby generating another automatically extended PVARP (Figs. 30–99 and 30–100). This excessively long PVARP is perpetuated from cycle to cycle (the pacemaker continually interprets the spontaneous conducted QRS as a VPC), especially if the atrial

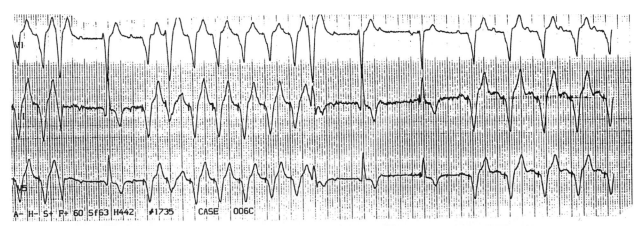

Figure 30–97. Effect of automatic postventricular atrial refractory period (PVARP) extension on exercise. Three-lead ECG recorded during exercise in a patient with a Pacesetter Synchrony DDDR pacemaker programmed to the DDD mode. Lower rate interval (LRI) = 1000 msec; upper rate interval (URI) = 387 msec; AV = 150 msec; PVARP = 250 msec, + PVARP on ventricular premature contraction (VPC) measures (480 msec); Beat 3 is a VPC that activates a PVARP extension of 480 msec, whereupon the succeeding P wave is unsensed because it falls in the automatically extended PVARP. QRS complex 4 is a ventricular escape beat not preceded by a sensed P wave, so that the PVARP is again extended. However, the succeeding P wave is sensed because it occurs just beyond the 480-msec PVARP. The 12th beat is again a VPC, and the extended PVARP prevents sensing of the next P wave. The 13th beat is a ventricular escape beat without a preceding sensed P wave, and the PVARP is extended again with loss of the following P within the PVARP. This is followed by Ap and Vp (with fusion), and the sinus rate slows down, but AV synchrony returns (As-Vp). The atrial escape interval (AEI) depicted by the arrow measures about 850 msec and is equal to the constant 850 msec AEI after automatic PVARP extension, but this is not seen because the basic AEI is 850 msec. A shorter LRI would have demonstrated the extended AEI.

Table 30–16. Postventricular Atrial Refractory Period and Atrial Undersensing

Normal PVARP Duration

Relatively fast sinus rate with long PR interval (P wave falls close to the preceding QRS, i.e., within PVARP).

Long PVARP

As programmed, or DDX mode.

Automatic PVARP Extension

(Secondary to two ventricular events without an intervening P wave, interpreted by pacemaker as a ventricular extrasystole.) P-wave undersensing may be perpetuated from cycle to cycle if the pulse generator continually interprets the spontaneous supraventricular QRS complex (i.e., preceded by a P wave) as a ventricular extrasystole or premature ventricular event and P waves occur consistently within the extended PVARP and remain undetected.

Some contemporary devices allow atrial sensing in the PVARP. If a pacemaker thus detects a P wave in the PVARP, it prevents VPC status for any subsequent intrinsic ventricular event, i.e., PVARP does not lengthen automatically.

PVARP Reinitiation by Inapparent Ventricular Signals

Oversensing by ventricular channel, e.g., T wave, myopotentials, etc. With relatively low-voltage signals, decrease in ventricular sensitivity may restore atrial sensing.

Retriggerable Atrial Refractory Period

Atrial sensing occurs in the PVARP during the noise-sampling period. This mechanism creates overlapping atrial refractory periods and asynchronous atrial pacing when PP interval is shorter than the TARP.

Oversensing of far-field QRS complex initiates a new TARP that can cause atrial undersensing. A decrease in atrial sensitivity often eliminates atrial sensing of far-field QRS complex with correction of atrial undersensing.

PVARP, postventricular atrial refractory period; VPC, ventricular premature contraction; TARP, total atrial refractory period.

---

rate remains relatively fast and AV conduction is delayed, so that P waves consistently occur within the extended PVARP. The relatively long PR interval suggests lack of atrial tracking.[200–203]

The implantation of a pacemaker with an appropriate AV interval in patients with markedly prolonged PR interval can therefore cause the pacemaker syndrome, with the pacemaker itself as a bystander (Fig. 30–101). In other words, the pacemaker can initiate a pacemaker syndrome, but the device is not necessary for its perpetuation. A long PVARP can thus recreate the original hemodynamic disturbance for which the pacemaker was implanted. This self-perpetuating mechanism can be unlocked by slowing of the atrial rate, improvement of AV conduction, or VPC (without retrograde VA conduction), circumstances that create a new and premature PVARP. The PVARP, by starting earlier, finishes earlier, thereby giving the succeeding P wave an opening for being sensed outside the PVARP, whereupon AV synchrony is immediately restored.

A similar situation can occur on exercise following the last unsensed P wave (in the PVARP) of a Wenckebach block upper rate response (see Fig. 30–99). If the unsensed P wave is conducted to the ventricle, the pacemaker can interpret the QRS as a VPC because it ignores the preceding P wave. Such a situation leads to automatic PVARP extension, perpetuated by each succeeding QRS complex as the P wave continually falls within the extended PVARP. The ECG, therefore, suggests lack of atrial tracking. After exercise, as the sinus rate decreases, P-wave sensing is restored only when the PP interval ≥ PR interval + PVARP as programmed + PVARP extension.

Ventricular oversensing (e.g., T wave, P wave, myopoten-

LOWER RATE = 70 ppm (857 ms)
UPPER RATE INTERVAL = 135 ppm
AV INTERVAL = 150 ms
PVARP = 400 ms
VRP = 250 ms

Figure 30–98. Lack of P-wave tracking due to long PVARP (PVARP = 400 msec). The sinus rate is about 85 ppm, and there is first-degree AV block. The P waves fall within the PVARP initiated by the preceding sensed QRS complex. Shortening the PVARP to 375 msec *(bottom)* restores 1:1 atrial tracking with the programmed AV interval (150 msec). VRP, ventricular refractory period. (From Barold SS, Falkoff MD, Ong LS, et al: Timing cycles of DDD pacemakers. *In* Barold SS, Mugica J [eds]: New Perspectives in Cardiac Pacing. Mt Kisco, NY, Futura, 1988, pp 69–119.)

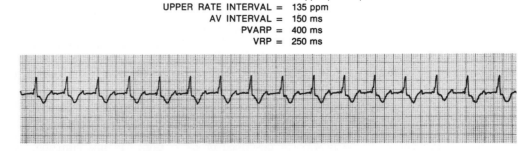

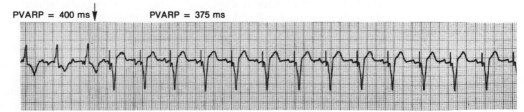

PVARP = 400 ms   PVARP = 375 ms

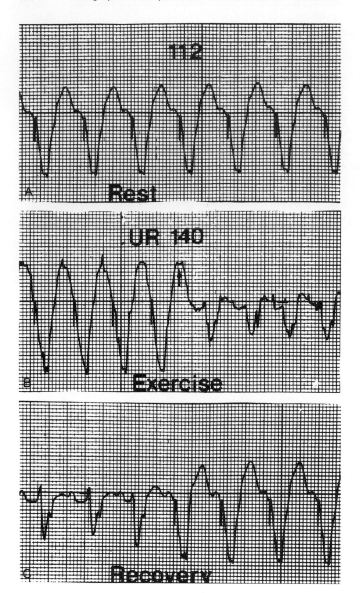

Figure 30–99. Apparent P-wave undersensing in an Intermedics Cosmos II DDD pacemaker on exercise in a patient with intermittent AV block. Lower rate = 60 ppm; upper rate = 140 ppm; AV delay after P-wave sensing = 135 msec (adaptive AV delay with minimum AV delay of 75 msec); postventricular atrial refractory period (PVARP) = 320 msec; automatic PVARP extension = 100 msec. A, At rest, the atrial rate is 112 bpm, causing atrial sensing and ventricular pacing with AV interval of about 100 msec. B, After 1 minute of exercise, Wenckebach block upper rate response occurs, and the pacemaker does not sense a P wave *(arrow)* in the PVARP. The P wave in the PVARP allows spontaneous AV conduction with a PR interval of about 260 msec. The pacemaker interprets the spontaneous QRS as a ventricular premature contraction (VPC) and therefore automatically lengthens the PVARP to 320 + 100 = 420 msec. Subsequent events all are spontaneous, that is, P-wave and conducted QRS complex with PR interval longer than the programmed As-Vp interval at that particular atrial rate (apparent lack of atrial tracking). The spontaneous QRS complex continually activates the PVARP extension as the P waves continually fall within the extended PVARP. C, In the recovery phase, the electrocardiogram shows sinus rhythm (PR = 200 msec) and conversion to an atrial synchronous ventricular-paced rhythm with an AV interval of 100 msec. The PR interval preceding ventricular pacing shows an abrupt shortening of about 40 msec without a change in the PP interval. This results in earlier detection of the conducted QRS complex and subsequently the next P wave falls outside the extended PVARP of 420 msec. (From VanGelder BM, VanMechelen R, DenDulk K, et al: Apparent P wave undersensing in a DDD pacemaker after exercise. PACE 15:1651, 1992.)

tials, false signals) causes reinitiation of the PVARP, as occurs with any ventricular-sensed event. The new PVARP can in turn cause atrial undersensing. This diagnosis is confirmed when a decrease in ventricular sensitivity restores atrial sensing.[30]

Optimal Pacing in Patients With Symptomatic First-Degree Atrioventricular Block: This subject has become important because the 1998 American College of Cardiology/American Heart Association guidelines for implantation of pacemakers classify first-degree AV block as a class IIA indication.[204] Prevention of the previously described problems in patients with a long PR interval requires the following measures[205]: (1) A relatively short PVARP if clinically advisable because most patients with marked prolongation of the PR interval have disease of the AV node and impaired retrograde VA conduction; (2) capability of programming "off" the automatic postventricular extrasystole PVARP extension; (3) elimination of the post-VPC PVARP extension whenever a P wave is detected within the extended PVARP immediately before the next ventricular-sensed event; (4)

prolongation of AEI after a pacemaker-defined PVC to permit atrial capture followed by ventricular capture, which eliminates PVC-induced PVARP extension; (5) noncompetitive pacing (discussed later); and (6) ablation of the AV junction. Kuniyashi and colleagues[206] used such an innovative approach with a resultant complete AV block, a procedure conceptually similar to AV nodal ablation for the prevention of endless-loop tachycardia in which a P wave also occurs close to the preceding QRS complex.[133]

Apparent Atrial Undersensing and Upper Rate Limitation: In this situation, as previously discussed, P waves are sensed outside the PVARP, but the pacemaker does not emit its ventricular stimulus at the end of the programmed AV interval (ventricular-sensed repetitive pre-empted Wenckebach upper rate response) (see Figs. 30–23 to 30–25). Apparent atrial undersensing occurs during continual AV conduction when the PP and RR intervals are shorter than the URI.[52, 53] P waves are actually sensed beyond the PVARP and give rise to a conducted QRS complex, but the PR interval is longer than the programmed value of the AV

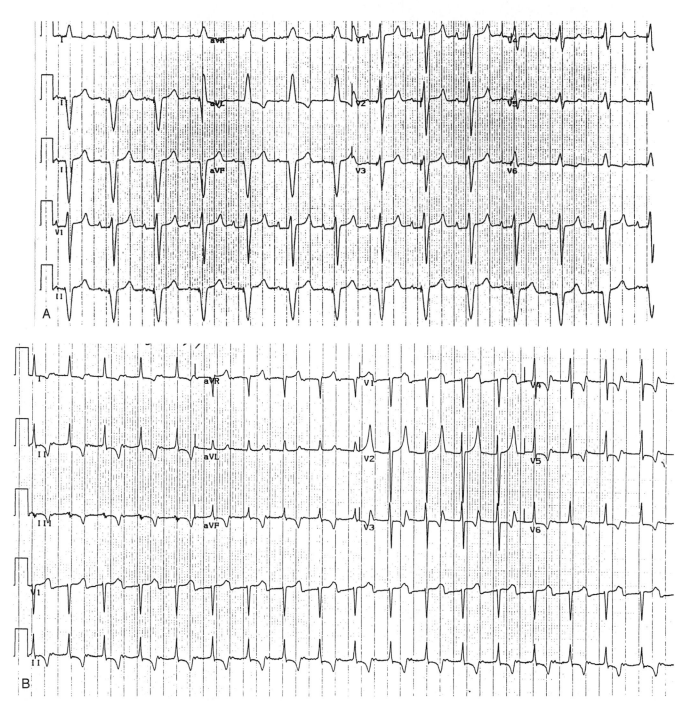

Figure 30–100. *A,* Twelve-lead ECG showing normal DDD pacing with atrial sensing followed by ventricular sensing. Lower rate interval = 1000 msec; AV = 150 msec; postventricular atrial refractoryperiod (PVARP) = 200 msec; post VPC PVARP extension = 400 msec. *B,* Same patient as in panel *A* presenting with dyspnea. There is a sinus tachycardia and marked first degree AV block. The P waves are unsensed because they fall within an extended 400-msec PVARP, probably initiated by a series of ventricular premature complexes (VPCs). The pacemaker interprets each conducted QRS complex as a VPC because it detects no atrial activity between two consecutive sensed ventricular events. A pacemaker capable of detecting the P wave within the PVARP could automatically terminate this situation by canceling the PVARP extension. Alternatively, this locked rhythm can be disrupted by the delivery of a noncompetitive atrial stimulus, as discussed in the text. In this case, the PVARP extension was programmed "off" because it was not needed in the presence of VA conduction block. The sinus tachycardia was probably secondary to the hemodynamic derangement related to inappropriate AV synchrony. (From Levine PA, Barold SS: Pacemaker automaticity, enabled by a multiplicity of new algorithms. *In* Singer I, Barold SS, Camm AJ [eds]: Nonpharmacological Therapy of Arrhythmias for the 21st Century: The State of the Art. Armonk, NY, Futura, 1998, pp 845–880.)

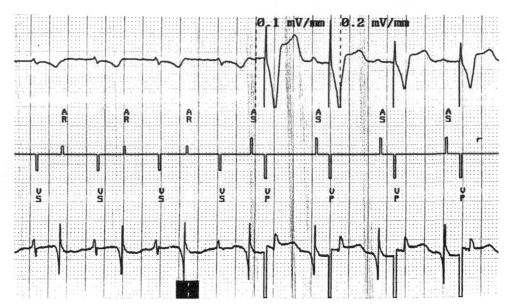

Figure 30–101. ECG of a patient with sinus rhythm and marked first-degree AV block who developed pacemaker syndrome with a DDDR pacemaker as a bystander. AV = 150 msec; postventricular atrial refractory period (PVARP) = 310 msec. Automatic PVARP extension after a ventricular premature contraction (VPC) was programmed "off." The sinus P wave (not discernible on the surface ECG) falls within the PVARP (A_R) and cannot initiate an AV interval. Slight slowing of the sinus rate in the middle of the tracing moves the sinus P wave out of the PVARP, and resynchronization returns. When sequences of VS-A_R occur, the hemodynamic derangement often causes a reflex sinus tachycardia, which compounds the problem by pushing the P wave even closer to the preceding QRS complex because the PR interval does not shorten and may even lengthen.

interval. The pulse generator cannot emit a ventricular stimulus at the end of the programmed AV interval (As-Vp) because it cannot violate the URI. This relationship represents another cause of lack of P-wave tracking or sensing.[53]

Prevention of Undesirable Atrial Sensing

Early Sensing

If the PVARP is too short, very premature atrial extrasystoles can be sensed and cause triggering of a ventricular pacing beat very close to the apex of the T wave linked to the previous beat; a short URI and long AV interval favor ventricular capture beyond the myocardial VRP. Such a situation could lead to repetitive ventricular responses and potentially serious unsustained or sustained ventricular tachyarrhythmias.[33, 207, 208]

Far-Field Sensing

A ventricular event (Vs or Vp) may generate a substantial QRS deflection in the atrial electrogram registered by the atrial lead. When the ventricular channel senses the tail end of the near-field QRS complex before the atrial channel can sense its far-field counterpart, the pulse generator responds only to Vs because the far-field QRS signal (delivered to the atrial electrode) then falls in the PVARP initiated by ventricular sensing (Vs). If sufficiently large, the far-field QRS complex (paced or spontaneous) picked up by the atrial electrogram can be sensed by the atrial channel under certain circumstances,[209–211] including the following: (1) relatively short PVARP or, more specifically, the postventricular atrial blanking period; (2) low ventricular sensitivity preventing or

delaying ventricular sensing, and (3) atrial channel sensing the far-field QRS signal before the ventricular channel senses the near-field QRS signal. Atrial sensing of the far-field QRS complex is far more common in unipolar than in bipolar sensing systems. With far-field atrial sensing, the signal delivered to the atrial channel beyond the atrial refractory period initiates an AV interval. At the completion of the programmed AV delay, the pulse generator releases a ventricular stimulus that falls within the ST segment or the T wave (Fig. 30–102). A long programmed AV delay favors early ventricular capture. Repetitive atrial sensing of the far-field tail end of the QRS complex may also cause a sustained endless-loop tachycardia in the absence of regular retrograde VA conduction (Figs. 30–103 and 30–104). During normal DDD pacing (in the absence of lead displacement), far-field sensing of the QRS complex generally occurs only when the PVARP is relatively short and the VRP is subsequently longer than the PVARP, a situation favoring selective atrial sensing of the far-field events. Thus, the PVARP should not be less than 200 msec and should always be equal to or longer than the VRP to avoid far-field sensing by the atrial channel. These recommendations do not apply to the AMS algorithm, in which the postventricular atrial blanking period can be shorter than the total VRP.

Optimal Duration of Atrial and Ventricular Refractory Periods

As mentioned previously, the duration of the VRP should not exceed the value of the PVARP to avoid far-field sensing by the atrial channel. A relatively long VRP $\geq$ 300 msec predisposes to undersensing of early ventricular events. A

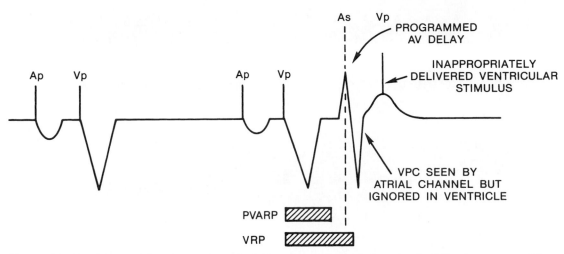

Figure 30–102. Diagrammatic representation of far-field sensing by the atrial electrode of a DDD pulse generator. When the ventricular refractory period is substantially longer than the postventricular atrial refractory period (PVARP), it creates a window within which a ventricular signal can be sensed by the atrial channel and ignored by the ventricular channel. On sensing the ventricular premature contraction (VPC), the atrial channel initiates an AV interval, with the ultimate delivery of the ventricular stimulus on the T wave of the VPC. The likelihood of delivering a ventricular stimulus at the apex of the T wave is increased by programming a relatively long AV interval. Ap, atrial-paced event; As, atrial-sensed event; Vp, ventricular-paced event. (From Barold SS, Falkoff MD, Ong LS, et al: Electrocardiography of DDD pacemakers. B. Multiprogrammability, follow-up, and troubleshooting. *In* Saksena S, Goldschlager N [eds]: Electrical Therapy for Cardiac Arrhythmias: Pacing, Antitachycardia Devices, Catheter Ablation. Philadelphia, WB Saunders, 1990, pp 265–301.)

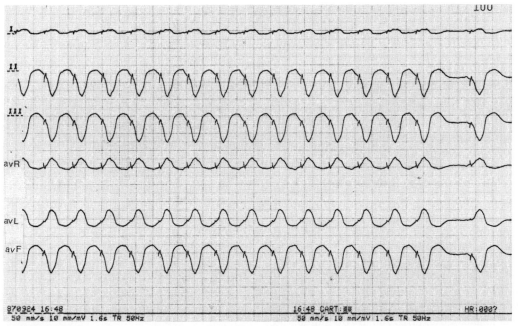

Figure 30–103. Six-lead ECG showing far-field endless-loop tachycardia with a 925 Delta DDD pulse generator (Cardiac Pacemakers, Inc.). Lower rate interval (LRI) = 857 msec; upper rate interval (URI) = 330 msec; AV = 130 msec; postventricular atrial refractory period (PVARP) = 125 msec. The atrial channel senses far-field ventricular depolarization and not retrograde P waves. This diagnosis cannot be made from the surface ECG because there was no clear-cut evidence of AV dissociation during the tachycardia. (From Barold SS, Falkoff MD, Ong LS, et al: Electrocardiography of contemporary DDD pacemakers. A. Basic concepts, upper rate response, retrograde ventriculoatrial conduction, and differential diagnosis of pacemaker tachycardias. *In* Saksena S, Goldschlager N [eds]: Electrical Therapy for Cardiac Arrhythmias; Pacing, Antitachycardia Devices, Catheter Ablation. Philadelphia, WB Saunders, 1990, pp 225–264.)

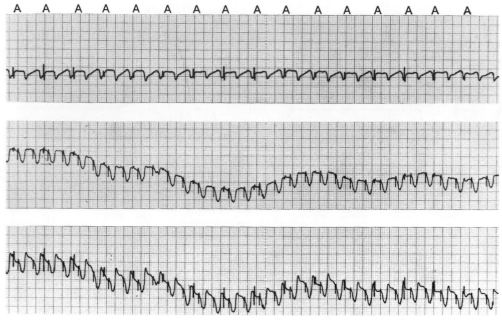

Figure 30–104. Same patient as in Figure 30–103. Three-lead ECG with bipolar esophageal recording in the upper strip and compound leads below. A, Atrial depolarization. AV dissociation excludes the usual type of near-field endless-loop tachycardia related to sensing of retrograde P waves. The tachycardia was terminated and prevented by lengthening the postventricular atrial refractory period (PVARP). (From Barold SS, Falkoff MD, Ong LS, et al: Electrocardiography of contemporary DDD pacemakers. A. Basic concepts, upper rate response, retrograde ventriculoatrial conduction, and differential diagnosis of pacemaker tachycardias. *In* Saksena S, Goldschlager N [eds]: Electrical Therapy for Cardiac Arrhythmias: Pacing, Antitachycardia Devices, Catheter Ablation. Philadelphia, WB Saunders, 1990, pp 225–264.)

VPC may be unsensed when it falls within a relatively long VRP. However, if the VPC engenders retrograde VA conduction, the atrial channel can sense the retrograde P wave if it falls beyond the PVARP. In this situation, the retrograde P wave can trigger an undesirable ventricular stimulus falling within the T wave of the unsensed VPC.

Adaptive Postventricular Atrial Refractory Period

Automatic Refractory Period Abbreviation With Exercise

Wittkampf and Boute[212] suggested that a DDD pulse generator could be designed with shortening of the PVARP on exercise whenever the atrial channel interprets atrial activity as being physiologic according to the actual rate and rate of change of atrial-sensed events. PVARP abbreviation during exercise, coupled with adaptive shortening of the AV interval (As-Vp) on exercise, would therefore produce substantial shortening of the TARP. A long PVARP and TARP at rest provide protection against atrial arrhythmias (by limiting the upper ventricular-paced rate) in patients with bradycardia-tachycardia syndrome. A shorter PVARP on exercise allows programming of a faster upper rate.

Mathematically, the timing of pacemaker and spontaneous events makes initiation of endless-loop tachycardia by retrograde VA conduction (from a VPC) highly unlikely at atrial-driven fast ventricular pacing rates because the retrograde P wave cannot arrive at the atrium before the occurrence of the next spontaneous P wave. There is, therefore, no need in most cases for the PVARP on exercise to equal the required

duration at rest to prevent endless-loop tachycardia. Thus, under normal circumstances at rest, the URI could be equal to the TARP because there is no need for a Wenckebach upper rate response at rest. With this arrangement at rest, an early atrial extrasystole would not prolong the AV interval (As-Vp) and would minimize the potential of inducing endless-loop tachycardia present when the URI > TARP. With a constant URI, TARP shortening on exercise would establish a Wenckebach upper rate response only on exercise.

Automatic PVARP Prolongation With Atrial Tachyarrhythmias

Some DDD pulse generators are designed with an automatic PVARP extension (and therefore longer TARP if the AV interval does not shorten) upon sensing a nonphysiologic atrial rate with consequent reduction in the maximum ventricular pacing rate.[37] This response avoids an unnecessarily fast ventricular-paced response to unphysiologic atrial tachyarrhythmias and represents a form of fallback.

Retriggerable Atrial Refractory Period

In some DDD pulse generators, the first part of the PVARP consists of the absolute refractory period during which atrial sensing cannot occur. However, atrial sensing may take place in the second and terminal portion of the PVARP, sometimes known as the *noise sampling period*. A sensed P wave within the noise sampling period does not initiate a new AV interval as ordinarily occurs in all DDD pulse generators by a P wave outside the TARP. Rather, a sensed P wave in the

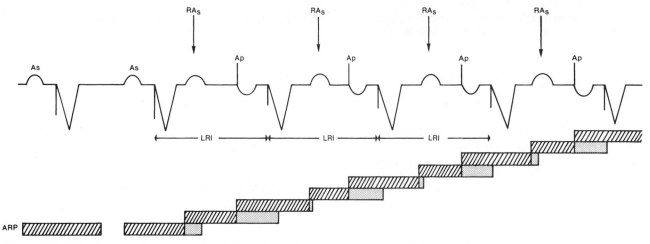

Figure 30–105. Diagrammatic representation of the retriggerable atrial refractory period (ARP) of the Siemens 674 DDD pulse generator (Siemens-Pacesetter, Inc.). As, atrial-sensed event outside ARP; RA$_s$, atrial-sensed event within ARP; Ap, atrial-paced event. The first 125 msec of the PVARP represents the absolute refractory period during which signals cannot be sensed. The second part of the PVARP (and AV interval) consists of the noise sampling period. P waves falling within the noise sampling period may be sensed, and although they do not initiate a new AV interval, they retrigger a full ARP. Continual retriggering of the ARP causes the DDD pulse generator to operate in the atrial asynchronous mode at the lower rate, that is, DVI mode when the PP interval is shorter than the ARP. (From Barold SS, Falkoff MD, Ong LS, et al: Upper rate response of DDD pacemakers. *In* Barold SS, Mugica J [eds]: New Perspectives in Cardiac Pacing. Mt Kisco, NY, Futura, 1988, pp 121–172.)

noise sampling period retriggers a complete TARP (i.e., AV + PVARP) (Fig. 30–105). In a pulse generator with a retriggerable TARP of 500 msec, when the PP interval becomes slightly shorter than 500 msec, every alternate P wave will fall within the noise sampling period generated by the preceding P wave. Sensing of the P wave within the noise sampling period restarts another full TARP of 500 msec (not just the AV interval). As long as the PP interval remains shorter than the 500-msec TARP, the atrial refractory periods overlap. In effect, the pulse generator reverts to the DVI mode (asynchronous atrial pacing) and provides an effective way of avoiding a faster paced ventricular rate in response to atrial tachyarrhythmias by automatic mode conversion to the DVI mode.[213] When the PP interval becomes shorter than the TARP, a pulse generator with a retriggerable atrial refractory period cannot exhibit a fixed-ratio AV block upper rate response because the P waves never occur beyond the TARP. Conceptually, this design is similar to that of automatic tachycardia-terminating dual-demand pacemakers with overlapping refractory periods and activation of the pulse generator to pace at the same lower rate automatically in response to both bradycardia and tachycardia.[214]

In pulse generators with a retriggerable atrial refractory period, atrial sensing of a far-field QRS signal may cause reinitiation of the TARP and loss of atrial sensing. In this situation, decreasing atrial sensitivity may paradoxically restore atrial sensing, whereas decreasing ventricular sensitivity produces no effect. Decrease of atrial sensitivity abolishes atrial sensing of the far-field QRS complex, so that the additional TARP initiated by the previously sensed far-field QRS complex cannot occur. This response is in sharp contrast to loss of atrial sensing secondary to PVARP (not TARP) reinitiation by ventricular oversensing. The diagnosis of PVARP reinitiation is certain if a decrease in the ventricular sensitivity restores atrial tracking, as previously described, whereas reduction of atrial sensitivity alone produces no effect.

Advantages of Atrial Sensing During the Postventricular Atrial Refractory Period

1. To make the diagnosis of physiologic or pathologic atrial rates to provide an appropriate pacemaker response as with AMS.

2. To achieve noncompetitive atrial pacing (NCAP) during DDDR pacing. An unsensed P wave in the PVARP can be followed by an atrial stimulus either in the PVARP (according to design) or beyond it according to the SDI. The sensor-driven atrial output may thus occur within the vulnerable period of atrial depolarization and carries the potential of inducing atrial arrhythmias (Fig. 30–106).

In the Medtronic Thera and Kappa DDDR pacemakers,

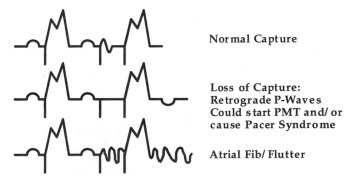

Normal Capture

Loss of Capture: Retrograde P-Waves Could start PMT and/ or cause Pacer Syndrome

Atrial Fib/ Flutter

Figure 30–106. Competitive atrial pacing. *Middle panel,* Lack of capture (LOC) by an atrial stimulus falling in the atrial myocardial refractory period generated by a preceding atrial depolarization may cause retrograde VA conduction with pacemaker-mediated tachycardia (PMT, or endless-loop tachycardia) or repetitive nonreentrant VA synchrony that may cause pacemaker syndrome. *Bottom panel,* An atrial stimulus falling in the vulnerable period of the atrium may precipitate atrial fibrillation or flutter. The vulnerable zone is < 300 msec. (Courtesy of Medtronic, Inc., Minneapolis, MN.)

NCAP is a programmable feature to prevent atrial pacing from being closely coupled to atrial activity within the PVARP (see Fig. 30–106). NCAP is available only in the DDDR mode. Even if it is not programmed, NCAP is automatically enabled for 1 beat after endless-loop tachycardia termination or a PVC response, both of which use an extended PVARP of 400 msec. A refractory sensed atrial event falling in the PVARP starts a 300-msec NCAP period, during which no atrial pacing may occur (Fig. 30–107). If an atrial stimulus is scheduled to occur during the NCAP period, the AEI is extended until the NCAP period expires. If no pacing stimulus is scheduled to occur during the NCAP period, timing of the AEI is unaffected. When an atrial stimulus is delayed by NCAP, the pacemaker attempts to maintain a stable ventricular rate by shortening the paced AV interval (to no less than 30 msec in the Kappa device). When a relatively short LRI and long PVARP are programmed, NCAP operation may cause ventricular pacing with an interval slightly longer than the LRI.

A similar concept was incorporated in the Telectronics Meta 1254 pacemaker, which minimizes the possibility of competitive atrial pacing by ensuring that the TARP will never be more than 70% of the sensor-controlled interval.

3. To prevent inappropriate automatic PVARP extension by a conducted atrial extrasystole or sinus beat (P wave unsensed in the PVARP followed by a sensed conducted QRS falling beyond the VRP) when the pulse generator interprets the ventricular signal as a ventricular extrasystole. Sensing of a preceding P wave in the PVARP would eliminate the PVARP extension applied to the succeeding conducted and sensed QRS complex (a feature incorporated in some contemporary pacemakers). This arrangement would therefore avoid atrial undersensing perpetuated by P waves continually falling within an automatically extended (and long) PVARP (e.g., as in relatively fast sinus rhythm associated with first-degree AV block).

4. Extension of the AEI. This promotes sensing of spontaneous atrial activity or atrial pacing beyond the atrial myocardial refractory period engendered by the preceding atrial depolarization contained in the PVARP. Pacesetter devices in the DDD and DDDR modes provide some protection

in the form of +PVARP on PVC, a feature designed to prevent endless-loop tachycardia related to sensing retrograde P waves after a PVC. Atrial sensing occurs beyond the PVARP, but a similar response secondary to atrial sensing in the PVARP is theoretically possible. Upon detecting a PVC, the Pacesetter pacemaker lengthens the PVARP cycle regardless of the programmed rate, thereby providing an 830 − 480 = 350 msec window for the detection of native atrial activity or effective (delayed) atrial capture (see Fig. 30–97). This protection is limited to a pacemaker defined PVC.

In the first-generation Telectronics Meta DDDR (1250) pacemaker, a single retrograde P wave sensed in the PVARP inhibited the release of the succeeding stimulus. The device was designed to increase the duration of the AEI by 240 msec after detecting eight consecutive P waves not necessarily retrograde in the PVARP, whereupon Ap was delivered beyond the atrial myocardial refractory period generated by the preceding atrial depolarization.

5. Detection and treatment of repetitive nonreentrant VA synchrony by initiating responses 2, 3, or 4

6. Initiation of a new URI. By design, the upper rate circuit governs only the rate of atrial triggered ventricular pacing.

When a ventricular signal is detected during the noise sampling period, it retriggers another complete VRP. With continual retriggering, the pulse generator will eventually time out at the LRI and appear to be pacing asynchronously. Such VRP design is particularly effective in preventing inhibition of the pacing output by electromagnetic or skeletal muscle interference.[16]

■ ATRIOVENTRICULAR INTERVAL

Recent Refinements
Positive Atrioventricular Interval Hysteresis

Positive AV interval hysteresis allows a long AV interval to be the dominant interval when AV conduction is relatively intact and a shorter AV interval when there is AV block.

New algorithms provide a long AV delay when AV nodal conduction is intact and a shorter, more physiologic AV delay when AV block and ventricular pacing are required.[215–219] The result is functional single-chamber atrial pacing when conduction is intact (with the aim of improving hemodynamics) and appropriate dual-chamber pacing in the presence of delayed AV conduction. With these new algorithms, after the first cycle of AV pacing (Ap-Vp or As-Vp) at the long AV interval, the next AV interval is delivered at a shorter and more physiologic duration (Figs. 30–108 and 30–109). Because the paced or sensed AV delay may be shorter than the intrinsic conduction, it locks the device into pacing at the shorter AV delay until the device automatically determines whether intrinsic AV conduction has returned by a search mechanism. After either a set number of cycles or a programmable period of time, the system automatically extends the AV interval to the longer base interval. If a native R wave occurs within this extended interval, the longer base AV interval is again engaged, thus inhibiting the ventricular output and re-establishing functional single-chamber atrial pacing with more physiologically appropriate backup ventricular support.

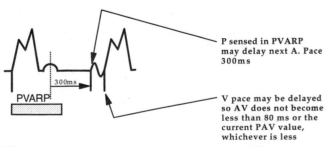

P sensed in PVARP may delay next A. Pace 300ms

V pace may be delayed so AV does not become less than 80 ms or the current PAV value, whichever is less

Figure 30–107. Operation of the Medtronic noncompetitive atrial pacing (NCAP) feature. This algorithm becomes operative when the device senses a P wave in the postventricular atrial refractory period (PVARP). The atrial pacing stimulus is delayed if necessary, and the AV interval is compressed to compensate for the delayed atrial stimulus. In the Thera series, the paced AV (PAV) interval is maintained at 80 msec (or the programmed value if less), and in the Kappa 400 device, the paced AV interval does not shorten to less than 30 msec. (Courtesy of Medtronic, Inc., Minneapolis, MN.)

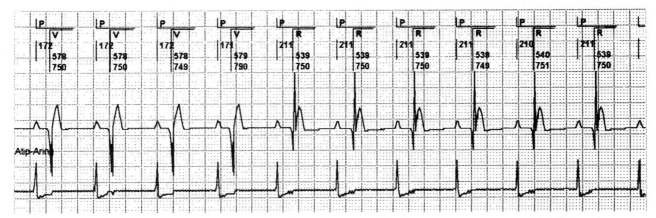

Figure 30–108. Positive AV/PV or ApVp — AsVp hysteresis in the Pacesetter Affinity DR pacemaker. After a period of pacing, a search mechanism is initiated where the system automatically extends the paced or sensed AV delay. If a native R wave occurs within the extended AV delay, the longer AV delay is maintained restoring intact AV conduction and allowing for a normal ventricular activation sequence. Although the PR interval is longer than the PV interval, there is intact AV conduction. When the AV delay is extended on the 256th cycle, a sensed R wave is seen by the pacemaker, thus inhibiting the ventricular output and re-establishing the longer AV/PV delay engendered by adding the positive hysteresis interval to the programmed intervals. This results in functional AAI pacing or *inhibited pacing*, except in the presence of AV block. Although this could be accomplished with a fixed long AV or PV delay, when and if AV block develops, the pacing system will be functioning in a hemodynamically deleterious long AV/PV delay until intact conduction resumes. P = As; R = Vs; V = Vp. (Courtesy of St. Jude Cardiac Rhythm Management Division, Sylmar, CA.)

Two such algorithms have been introduced.[120, 220, 221] The ELA Chorum system functions in the AAI(R) mode, but learns the Ap-Vs interval. If the Ap-Vs interval + 31 msec expires without a sensed R wave, AV pacing is initiated with a search performed every 100 cycles if spontaneous AV nodal conduction is not previously identified. In St. Jude Medical's Trilogy DR + in the DDD(R) modes, the basic paced or sensed AV delay is programmed, and an additional hysteresis interval is then added to this to promote functional single-chamber atrial pacing. If AV block develops, one cycle occurs with Ap-Vp or As-Vp pacing at the long interval followed by pacing at the shorter Ap-Vp/As-Vp interval until either intact conduction spontaneously resumes or after

255 cycles when a search is performed in which the Ap-Vp/As-Vp interval is lengthened looking for resumption of conduction.

Negative Atrioventricular Interval Hysteresis

Negative AV interval hysteresis is a capability unique to the St. Jude Medical Trilogy DR + pacemaker. The intent is to maintain full ventricular capture for patients paced for hypertrophic obstructive cardiomyopathy.[120, 221] A short AV delay usurps control of ventricular activation from the normal conduction system. However, during physiologic stress, one cannot predict the degree of shortening of AV nodal conduction to ensure complete ventricular capture by the

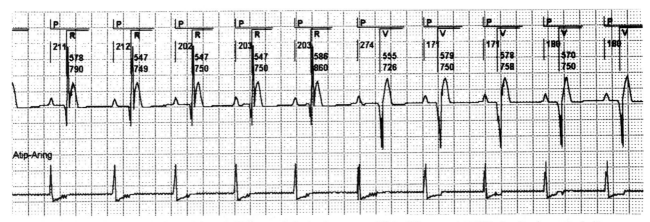

Figure 30–109. Positive AV/PV or ApVp — AsVp hysteresis in the Pacesetter Affinity DR pacemaker. With the development of either overt AV block or even first-degree AV block (to the extent defined by the extended AV or PV delay), the first cycle of AV or PV pacing at the longer interval results in a shortening of the paced or sensed AV delay to the programmed value. This will continue for 255 cycles unless a spontaneous R wave occurs within the shortened AV delay. On the *left*, the pacemaker is inhibited by the intrinsic rhythm. In the middle of the tracing, there is a single cycle of PV pacing at a long AV delay (274 msec), presumably owing to the transient development of AV block. This is followed by atrial-sensed ventricular pacing at a PV delay of 171 msec, which is shorter than the PR interval identified by the pacemaker of 200–210 msec. P = As; R = Vs; V = Vp. (Courtesy of St. Jude Cardiac Rhythm Management Division, Sylmar, CA.)

pacemaker. In negative AV delay hysteresis, one programs a hysteresis interval by which the pacemaker will shorten the paced or sensed AV delay if an R wave, presumably a conducted R wave, is sensed within the AV interval (Fig. 30–110). The system measures this interval and, on the next cycle, automatically shortens the AV delay by a programmable interval, such that it is shorter than the measured As-Vs interval. After a set number of cycles, the system automatically searches for the intrinsic AV interval. If there is Ap-Vs or As-Vs pacing at the longer interval, the pacemaker restores the original programmed AV timing.

Variability of the Atrioventricular Interval

Variability of the AV interval is common during DDD and DDDR pacing, and its interpretation requires a thorough understanding of pacemaker timing cycles. Evaluation of the AV interval can be complex. One must consider the following events that constitute the AV interval: As, Ap, Vs, Vp, as already defined, as well as P wave and QRS complex not necessarily sensed at the correct time.

Differential Diagnosis of Variable Atrioventricular Intervals During Dual Chamber Pacing

Obviously, during normal function As-Vs < As-Vp and Ap-Vs < Ap-Vp, according to the status of AV conduction. Application of the magnet produces changes in the AV interval specific to a particular device.

1. Spontaneous activity
   a. Normal stimulation: As-Vs < As-Vp
   b. Ventricular-sensed repetitive pre-empted Wenckebach sequence. The P wave is sensed. URI has not timed out when Vs occurs: As-Vs > As-Vp as programmed. As-Vs > AP-Vp as programmed.
   c. The P wave falls in the PVARP and is therefore unsensed despite an adequate atrial electrogram: P-Vs > Ap-Vp (P = P wave)
   d. Ventricular oversensing during the AV interval. R is unsensed in the VRP generated by the sensed signal: As-R (R = QRS complex)

2. Atrial stimulation followed by spontaneous ventricular activity
   a. Normal situation: Ap-Vs < Ap-Vp (Ap-Vp is constant)
   b. Positive AV interval hysteresis: Ap-Vs < Ap-Vp (Ap-Vp changes because of hysteresis)
   c. Negative AV interval hysteresis: Ap-Vs > Ap-Vp (Ap-Vp changes because of hysteresis)
   d. Oversensing during AV interval including crosstalk: Ap-R > Ap-Vs or Ap-Vp as programmed

3. Paced AV interval
   a. VSP and rate-adaptive (sensor controlled) shortening: Ap-Vp < Ap-Vp as programmed
   b. Noncompetitive atrial pacing: Ap-Vp < Ap-Vp as programmed
   c. Positive and negative AV hysteresis: Ap-Vp can be shorter or longer than base Ap-Vp
   d. During DDD pacing in devices with pure atrial-based LRT, some pacemakers deliver Ap on time, but delay Vp to avoid violation of the URI[222]: Ap-Vp > Ap-Vp as programmed

4. Spontaneous atrial activity followed by ventricular stimulation
   a. Wenckebach block upper rate limitation. AV extension can occur with a single APC: As-Vp > As-Vp as programmed. As-Vp > Ap-Vp as programmed.
   b. A rate-adaptive AV delay mimics the physiologic shortening of the PR interval during physiologic increase in the atrial rate. The pacemaker AV interval can shorten progressively secondary to an increase in the atrial rate (duration of previous cycle) and/or increase in the sensor-controlled rate related to increase in sensor activity: As-Vp < As-Vp as programmed.
   c. This occurs during VDD pacing when the P wave is late and falls in the implied AV interval that has already started. The pacemaker therefore does not sense the P wave. The pacemaker releases Vp at the end of the LRI. The P wave does not trigger Vp: P-Vp < As-Vp as programmed.
   d. Atrial oversensing before the P wave initiates the AV

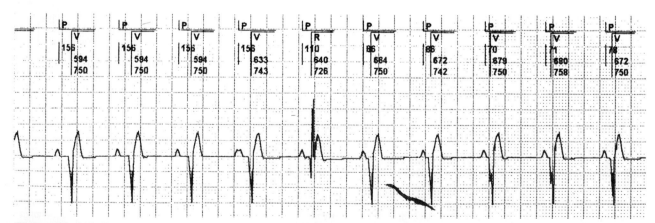

Figure 30–110. Negative AV/PV hysteresis in the Pacesetter Affinity DR pacemaker. Stable PV pacing is interrupted by one PR cycle (110 msec) at a shorter As-Vs interval than the PV interval (150 msec). This causes shortening of the As-Vp (PV) interval by the programmed value restoring PV pacing with full ventricular capture. After a period of pacing, the system extends the AV/PV interval to determine whether intact conduction is still present or will allow the longer interval to remain in effect. P = As; R = Vs; V = Vp. (Courtesy of St. Jude Cardiac Rhythm Management Division, Sylmar, CA.)

interval. The P wave is unsensed because it falls in the already initiated and refractory AV interval: P-Vp < As-Vp (P = P wave).

■ VENTRICULAR REFRACTORY PERIOD

With the advent of sophisticated pulse generators, the definition of the VRP has changed and is now known as the period during which the lower rate timer cannot be reset or restarted. Therefore, a pulse generator can actually recognize ventricular signals during the second part of the VRP (also known as the relative refractory period or noise sampling period) beyond the first part or the absolute refractory period. The detected signals can only reset timing intervals other than the inviolable LRI.[223] In most cases, the duration of the VRP initiated by a ventricular stimulus is equal to the VRP initiated by a ventricular sensing (with or without a preceding P wave).

The noise sampling (or noise interrogation) period may be considered as a relative refractory period (usually in the terminal portion of the VRP), with design function and duration varying from manufacturer to manufacturer. Single- and dual-chamber pacemakers (sometimes both the atrial and ventricular channels) can be designed with a noise sampling period. There are at least three types of responses when a signal is sensed within the noise sampling period[223]: (1) the sensed signal may reset the entire refractory period (retriggerable refractory period); (2) the sensed signal resets only the noise sampling period, rather than the entire refractory period. Repetitive retriggering of the noise sampling eventually leads to asynchronous pacing; (3) the sensed signal may cause reversion to asynchronous pacing for one full cycle, that is, the refractory period is extended for the duration of one pacing cycle only.

The VRP of Medtronic's dual-chamber pulse generators provides good examples of a retriggerable design.[213] The VRP is composed of an initial nonprogrammable 50- to 100-msec absolute refractory period (also called the *ventricular blanking period* by Medtronic), followed by the noise sampling period, a programmable interval that occupies the second part of the VRP. Sensing cannot occur during the ventricular blanking period. Such terminology is potentially misleading because this particular blanking period could be confused with the brief ventricular blanking period occurring coincidentally with the atrial stimulus and designed to prevent crosstalk. When Medtronic DDD pulse generators sense a VPC in the noise sampling period (VPC defined as two successive ventricular events without any sensed intervening atrial activity), an entirely new VRP is reinitiated. A signal sensed during the noise sampling period is represented by a telemetered marker pulse indicating a refractory ventricular sense event (V_R event). Such a signal does not reset the lower rate timer but resets (restarts) basic intervals, as follows:

- Initiation of a complete VRP with the blanking period occupying the first part as defined previously
- A new PVARP, together with (programmable) automatic extension to 400 msec, because the pacemaker interprets the sensed signal (in the refractory period) as a VPC unless there is a preceding As or A_R event

REFERENCES

1. Furman S: Comprehension of pacemaker timing cycles. *In* Furman S, Hayes DL, Holmes DR Jr (eds): A Practice of Cardiac Pacing (3rd ed). Mt. Kisco, NY, Futura, 1993, pp 135–194.
2. Barold SS: Lower rate and related timing cycles of dual chamber pacemakers: The need for precise definitions and language. Eur J Cardiac Pacing Electrophysiol 3:278, 1993.
3. Hayes DL: Timing cycles of permanent pacemakers. Cardiol Clin 10:593, 1992.
4. Hayes DL, Ketelson A, Levine P, et al: Understanding timing systems of current DDDR pacemakers Eur J Cardiac Pacing Electrophysiol 3:70, 1993.
5. Hayes DL, Levine PA: Pacemaker timing cycles. *In* Ellenbogen KA (ed): Cardiac Pacing (2nd ed). Cambridge, MA, Blackwell Scientific, 1996, pp 278–332.
6. Lau CP: DDDR pacing: Lower and upper rate behaviors. *In* Lau CP (ed): Rate-Adaptive Cardiac Pacing: Single and Dual Chamber. Mt. Kisco, NY, Futura, 1993, pp 271–290.
7. Barold SS, Zipes DP: Cardiac pacemakers and antiarrhythmic devices. *In* Braunwald E (ed): Heart Disease: A Textbook of Cardiovascular Medicine (5th ed). Philadelphia, WB Saunders, 1997, pp 705–741.
8. Bernstein AD, Camm AJ, Fletcher R, et al: The NASPE/BPEG generic pacemaker code for antibradyarrhythmia and adaptive-rate pacing and antitachy-arrhythmia devices. PACE 10:794, 1987.
9. Barold SS, Carol M: "Double reset" of demand pacemakers. Am Heart J 84:276, 1972.
10. Barold SS, Falkoff MD, Ong LS, et al: Oversensing by single-chamber pacemakers: Mechanisms, diagnosis and treatment. Cardiol Clin 3:565, 1985.
11. Barold SS: Clinical significance of pacemaker refractory periods. Am J Cardiol 28:237, 1971.
12. Barold SS, Gaidula JJ: Evaluation of normal and abnormal sensing functions of demand pacemakers. Am J Cardiol 28:201, 1971.
13. Driller J, Barold SS, Parsonnet V: Normal and abnormal function of the pacemaker magnetic switch. J Electrocardiol 6:1, 1973.
14. Barold S, Mugica J, Falkoff MD, et al: Multiprogrammability in cardiac pacing. *In* Barold SS (ed): Modern Cardiac Pacing. Mt. Kisco, NY, Futura, 1985, pp 377–409.
15. Brandt J, Fahraeus T, Schüller H: Far-field QRS complex sensing in the atrial pacemaker lead. II. Prevalence, clinical significance and possibility of intraoperative prediction in DDD pacing. PACE 11:1540, 1988.
16. Barold SS, Falkoff MD, Ong LS, et al: Interference in cardiac pacemakers: Endogenous sources. *In* El-Sherif N, Samet P (eds): Cardiac Pacing and Electrophysiology (3rd ed). Philadelphia, WB Saunders, 1991, pp 634–651.
17. Barold SS, Falkoff MD, Ong LS, et al: Cardiac pacing for the treatment of tachycardia. *In* Barold SS (ed): Modern Cardiac Pacing. Mt. Kisco, NY, Futura, 1985, pp 693–725.
18. Barold SS, Falkoff MD, Ong LS, et al: Termination of ventricular tachycardia by chest wall stimulation during DDD pacing. Am J Med 84:549, 1988.
19. Barold SS: Clinical uses of chest wall stimulation in patients with DDD pulse generators. Intelligence Reports in Cardiac Pacing and Electrophysiology 7:2, 1988.
20. Friedberg HD, Barold SS: On hysteresis in pacing. J Electrocardiol 6:1, 1973.
21. Rosenqvist M, Vallin HO, Edhag KO: Rate hysteresis pacing: How valuable is it? A comparison of the stimulation of 70 and 50 beats per minute and rate hysteresis in patients with sinus node disease. PACE 7:332, 1984.
22. Thompson ME, Shaver JA: Undesirable cardiac arrhythmias associated with rate hysteresis pacemakers. Am J Cardiol 38:685, 1976.
23. Hollins WJ, Leman RB, Kratz JM, et al: Limitations of the long-term clinical application of rate hysteresis. PACE 10:302, 1987.
24. Barold SS: Cardiac pacing in special and complex situations: Indications and modes of stimulation. Cardiol Clin 10:573, 1992.
25. Katritsis D, Ward DE, Camm AJ: Can we treat carotid sinus syndrome? PACE 14:1367, 1991.
26. Spritzer RC, Donoso E, Gadboys HI, et al: Arrhythmias induced by pacemaking on demand. Am Heart J 77:619, 1969.
27. Vera Z, Mason DT, Awan NA, et al: Lack of sensing by demand pacemakers due to intraventricular conduction defects. Circulation 51:815, 1975.
28. Barold SS, Falkoff MD, Ong LS, et al: A-A and V-V lower rate

timing of DDD and DDDR pulse generators. *In* Barold SS, Mugica J (eds): New Perspectives in Cardiac Pacing. Mt. Kisco, NY, Futura, 1991, pp 203–247.

29. Barold SS: Ventricular- versus atrial-based lower rate timing in dual chamber pacemakers: Does it really matter? PACE 18:83, 1995.
30. Barold SS, Falkoff MD, Ong LS, et al: Timing cycles of DDD pacemakers. *In* Barold SS, Mugica J (eds): New Perspectives in Cardiac Pacing. Mt. Kisco, NY, Futura, 1988, pp 69–119.
31. Barold SS, Falkoff MD, Ong LS, et al: Function and electrocardiography of DDD pacemakers. *In* Barold SS (ed): Modern Cardiac Pacing. Mt. Kisco, NY, Futura, 1985, pp 645–676.
32. Barold SS, Falkoff MD, Ong LS, et al: Electrocardiography of contemporary DDD pacemakers. A. Basic concepts, upper rate response, retrograde ventriculoatrial conduction and differential diagnosis of pacemaker tachycardias. *In* Saksena S, Goldschlager N (eds): Electric Therapy for Cardiac Arrhythmias, Pacing, Antitachycardia Devices, Catheter Ablation. Philadelphia, WB Saunders, 1990, pp. 225–264.
33. Barold SS: Management of patients with dual chamber pacemakers: Central role of the pacemaker atrial refractory period. Learning Center Highlights (Heart House). Am Coll Cardiol 5:8, 1990.
34. Levine PA: Postventricular atrial refractory periods and pacemaker mediated tachycardias. Clin Prog Pacing Electrophysiol 1:394, 1983.
35. Furman S, Reicher-Reiss H, Escher DJW: Atrio-ventricular sequential pacing and pacemakers. Chest 63:783, 1973.
36. Barold SS, Ong LS, Falkoff MD, et al. Crosstalk or self-inhibition in dual-chamber pacemakers. *In* Barold SS (ed): Modern Cardiac Pacing. Mt. Kisco, NY, Futura, 1985, pp 615–623.
37. Barold SS, Falkoff MD, Ong LS, et al: Upper rate response of DDD pacemakers. *In* Barold SS, Mugica J (eds): New Perspectives in Cardiac Pacing. Mt. Kisco, NY, Futura, 1988, pp 121–172.
38. Furman S, Gross J: Dual chamber pacing and pacemakers. Curr Prob Cardiol 15:119, 1990.
39. Barold SS, Belott PH: Behavior of the ventricular triggering period of DDD pacemakers. PACE 10:1237, 1987.
40. Levine PA: Normal and abnormal rhythm associated with dual-chamber pacemakers. Cardiol Clin 3:595, 1985.
41. Levine PA: Base rate behavior of dual chamber pacing systems. *In* Barold SS, Mugica J (eds): New Perspectives in Cardiac Pacing: 3. Mt. Kisco, NY, Futura, 1993, pp 215–232.
42. Barold SS, Falkoff MD, Ong LS, et al: Arrhythmias caused by dual chambered pacing. *In* Steinbach K (ed): Proceedings of the 7th World Symposium on Cardiac Pacing. Darmstadt, Steinkkopff Verlag, 1983, pp 505–510.
43. Barold SS, Falkoff MD, Ong LS, et al: Electrocardiography of DDD pacemakers. B. Multiprogrammability, follow-up and troubleshooting. *In* Saksena S, Goldschlager N (eds): Electrical Therapy for Cardiac Arrhythmias: Pacing, Antitachycardia Devices, Catheter Ablation. Philadelphia, WB Saunders, 1990, pp 265–301.
44. Barold SS, Falkoff MD, Ong LS, et al: All dual-chamber pacemakers function in the DDD mode. Am Heart J 115:1353, 1988.
45. Furman S: Dual-chamber pacemakers: Upper rate behavior. PACE 8:197, 1985.
46. Luceri RM, Castellanos A, Zaman L, et al: The arrhythmias of dual chamber cardiac pacemakers and their management. Ann Intern Med 99:354, 1983.
47. Stroobandt R, Willems R, Holvoet G, et al: Prediction of Wenckebach behavior and block response to DDD pacemakers. PACE 9:1040, 1986.
48. Higano ST, Hayes DL: Quantitative analysis of Wenckebach behavior in DDD pacemakers. PACE 13:1456, 1990.
49. Fearnot NE, Smith HJ, Geddes LA: A review of pacemakers that physiologically increase rate: The DDD and rate-responsiveness pacemakers. Prog Cardiovasc Dis 29:145, 1986.
50. DenDulk K, Lindemans FW, Wellens HJJ: Noninvasive evaluation of pacemaker circus movement tachycardia. Am J Cardiol 53:537, 1984.
51. Warren J, Falkenberg E: Wenckebach type upper rate behavior: A mixed blessing [Abstract]. PACE 8:A-37, 1985.
52. Barold SS: Electrocardiography of rate-adaptive dual-chamber (DDDR) pacemakers: Upper rate behavior. *In* Alt E, Barold SS, Stangl K (eds): Rate-Adaptive Pacing. Heidelberg, Berlin, Springer-Verlag, 1993, pp 195–221.
53. Barold SS: Wenckebach upper rate response of dual chamber pacemakers: a reappraisal and proposed new terminology. PACE 18:244, 1995.
54. Leung SK, Lau CP, Leung WH, et al: Apparent extension of the atrio-

55. Barold SS, Falkoff MD Ong LS, et al: Characterization of pacemaker arrhythmias due to normally functioning AV demand (DVI) pulse generators. PACE 3:712, 1980.
56. Barold SS, Falkoff MD, Ong LS, et al: Function and electrocardiography of DVI pacing systems. *In* Barold SS (eds): Modern Cardiac Pacing. Mt. Kisco, NY, Futura, 1985, pp 625–644.
57. Barold SS, Falkoff MD, Ong LS, et al: Interpretation of electrocardiograms produced by a new unipolar multiprogrammable "committed" AV sequential (DVI) pulse generator. PACE 4:692, 1981.
58. Levine PA, Seltzer JP: AV universal (DDD) pacing and atrial fibrillation. Clin Prog Pacing Electrophysiol 1:275, 1983.
59. Floro J, Castellanet M, Florio J, et al: DDI: A new mode for cardiac pacing. Clin Prog Pacing Electrophysiol 2:255, 1984.
60. Barold SS: Optimal pacing in the brady-tachy syndrome. Cardiol Rev 5:63, 1997.
61. Barold SS: DDI and DDIR modes of pacing: An overview. Med Intell Cardiac Pacing Electrophysiol 14(4):2, 1996.
62. Barold SS: The DDI mode of cardiac pacing. PACE 9:480, 1987.
63. Sulke N., Dritsas A, Bostock J, et al: Subclinical pacemaker syndrome: A randomized study of symptom free patients with ventricular demand (VVI) pacemakers upgraded to dual-chamber devices. Br Heart J 67:57, 1992.
64. Sutton R, Markowitz TM: Toward physiologic stimulation in sinus node disease. Eur J Cardiac Pacing Electrophysiol 4:126, 1994.
65. Ellenbogen KA, Gilligan DM, Wood MA, et al: The pacemaker syndrome: A matter of definition. Am J Cardiol 79:1226, 1997.
66. Cunningham TM: Pacemaker syndrome due to retrograde conduction in a DDI pacemaker. Am Heart J 115:478, 1988.
67. Erlbacher JA, Stelzer P: Inappropriate ventricular blanking in a DDI pacemaker. PACE 9:519, 1986.
68. Irwin M, Harris L, Cameron D, et al: DDI pacing: Indications, expectations and follow-up. PACE 17:274, 1994.
69. Vanerio G, Maloney JD, Pinski SL, et al: DDIR versus VVIR pacing in patients with paroxysmal atrial tachyarrhythmias. PACE 14:1630, 1991.
70. Sutton R, Ingram A, Kenny RA, et al: Clinical experience of DDI pacing. *In* Belhassen B, Feldman S, Cooperman Y (eds): Cardiac Pacing and Electrophysiology. Proceedings of the VII World Symposium on Cardiac Pacing and Electrophysiology. Jerusalem, Keterpress Enterprises, 1987, pp 161–163.
71. Dodinot B, BarrosCosta A: Interets et limites du mode DDI. Stimucoeur 20:205, 1992.
72. Bana G, Locatelli V, Piatti L, et al: DDI pacing in bradycardia-tachycardia syndrome. PACE 13:264, 1990.
73. Clarke M, Sutton R, Ward D, et al: Recommendations for pacemaker prescription for symptomatic bradycardia. Br Heart J 66:185, 1991.
74. Petersen M, Chamberlain-Weber R, Fitzpatrick AP, et al: Permanent pacing for cardioinhibitory malignant vasovagal syncope. Br Heart J 71:274, 1994.
75. Benditt DG, Petersen M, Lurie KG, et al: Cardiac pacing for prevention of recurrent vasovagal syncope. Ann Intern Med 122:204, 1995.
76. Antonioli GE: Single lead atrial synchronous ventricular pacing: A dream come true. PACE 17:1531, 1994.
77. Stroobandt R, Willems R, Vandenbulcke, et al: DDDR pacemakers: A framework for the understanding of atrial and ventricular based device timing. Eur J Cardiac Pacing Electrophysiol 2:151, 1992.
78. Siemens 674 DDD Pulse generator, Technical Manual. Solna, Sweden, 1984.
79. Technical Manual, Elite II 7084/85/86. Activity response dual chamber pacemaker with telemetry. Minneapolis, Medtronic Inc., 1992.
80. Sinnaeve A: From VVI to DDD pacemakers: Glossary of terms and normal functions. *In* Andries E, Brugada P, Stroobandt R (eds): How to face "The Faces" of Cardiac Pacing. Dordrecht, The Netherlands, Kluwer, 1992, pp 41–81.
81. Sanders R, Barold SS: Understanding elective replacement indicators and automatic parameter conversion mechanisms in DDD pacemakers. *In* Barold SS, Mugica J (eds): New Perspectives in Cardiac Pacing. Mt. Kisco, NY, Futura, 1991, pp 203–227.
82. Garson A Jr, Coyner T, Shannon CE, et al: A systematic approach to the fully automatic (DDD) pacemaker electrocardiogram. *In* Gillette PC, Griffin JC (eds): Practical Cardiac Pacing. Baltimore, Williams & Wilkins, 1986, pp 181–270.
83. Markowitz T, Prest-Berg K, Betzold R, et al: Clinical implications of

dual chamber responsive rate pacing. *In* Belhassen B, Feldman S, Cooperman Y (eds): Cardiac Pacing and Electrophysiology. Proceedings of the VII World Symposium on Cardiac Pacing and Electrophysiology. Jerusalem, Keterpress, 1987, pp 165–170.

84. Levine PA, Hayes DL, Wilkoff BL, et al: Electrocardiography of rate-modulated pacemaker rhythms. Sylmar, CA, Siemens-Pacemaker, Inc., 1990, pp 1–90.

85. Merillat JC: Understanding and assessing DDDR pacing systems in adaptive rate pacing: Perspectives in cardiac rhythm management, St. Paul, MN, Cardiac Pacemakers, Inc., 1993, pp 53–85.

86. Barold SS: Electrocardiography of rate-adaptive dual chamber (DDDR) pacemakers. 1. Lower rate behavior. *In* Alt E, Barold SS, Stangl K (eds): Rate Adaptive Pacing. Heidelberg, Berlin, Springer-Verlag, 1993, pp 173–194.

87. Goldschlager NF, Hayes DL, Ellenbogen KA: Cardiac Pacing Electrophysiology Self-Assessment Program. American College of Cardiology and North American Society of Cardiac Pacing and Electrophysiology, 1996, pp 6.4–6.66.

88. Barold SS, Fredman CS: Pure atrial-based lower rate timing of dual chamber pacemakers: Implications for upper rate limitation. PACE 18:391, 1995.

89. Technical manual: Synergyst II 7070/7071 activity responsive dual chamber pacer with telemetry. Minneapolis, Medtronic Inc., 1989.

90. Synergystics: Synergyst II guidelines to operations and patient management. Minneapolis, MN, Medtronic Inc., 1989.

91. Barold SS: Single- and dual-chamber pacemakers: Electrophysiology pacing modes, and multiprogrammability. *In* Singer I, Kupersmith J (eds): Clinical Manual of Electrophysiology. Baltimore, Williams & Wilkins, 1993, pp 231–273.

92. Tolentino AO, Javier RP, Byrd C, et al: Paced-induced tachycardia associated with an atrial synchronous ventricular inhibited (ASVIP) pulse generator. PACE 5:251, 1982.

93. Furman S, Fisher JD: Endless loop tachycardia in an AV universal (DDD) pacemaker. PACE 5:476, 1982.

94. Akhtar M, Gilbert C, Mahmud R, et al: Pacemaker-mediated tachycardia: Underlying mechanism, relationship to ventriculoatrial conduction, characteristics and management. Clin Prog Pacing Electrophysiol 3:90, 1985.

95. Barold SS: Repetitive reentrant and nonreentrant ventriculoatrial synchrony in dual chamber pacing. Clin Cardiol 14:754, 1991.

96. Friart A: Termination of magnet-unresponsive pacemaker endless loop tachycardia by carotid sinus message. Am J Med 87:1, 1989.

97. Conti JB, Curtis AB, Hill JA, et al: Termination of pacemaker-mediated tachycardia by adenosine. Clin Cardiol 17:47, 1994.

98. Perrins EJ, Morley CA, Dixy J, et al: The pharmacologic blockade of retrograde atrioventricular conduction in paced patients [Abstract]. PACE 6:A-112, 1983.

99. Barold SS, Falkoff MD, Ong LS, et al: Pacemaker endless loop tachycardia: Termination by simple techniques other than magnet application. Am J Med 85:817, 1988.

100. Fontaine JW, Maloney JD, Castle LW, et al: Noninvasive assessment of ventriculoatrial conduction and early experience with the tachycardia termination algorithm in pacemaker-mediated tachycardia. PACE 9:212, 1986.

101. Hayes DL, Furman S: Atrioventricular and ventriculoatrial conduction times in patients undergoing pacemaker implant. PACE 6:38, 1983.

102. Westveer DC, Stewart JR, Goodfleish R, et al: Prevalence and significance of ventriculoatrial conduction. PACE 7:784, 1984.

103. Altamura G, Boccadamo R, Toscano S, et al: Incidence of and drug effect on ventriculoatrial conduction in patients with bradyarrhythmias. *In* Pérez Gómez F (ed): Cardiac Pacing: Electrophysiology: Tachyarrhythmias. Mt Kisco, NY, Futura Media Services, 1985, pp 735–742.

104. Harriman RJ, Pasquariello JL, Gomes JAC, et al: Autonomic dependence of ventriculoatrial conduction. Am J Cardiol 56:285, 1985.

105. Cazeau S, Daubert C, Mabo P, et al: Dynamic electrophysiology of ventriculoatrial conduction: Implications for DDD and DDDR pacing. PACE 13:1649, 1990.

106. VanMechelen RV, Ruiter J, Vanderkerckhove Y, et al: Prevalence of retrograde conduction in heart block after DDD pacemaker implantation. Am J Cardiol 57:797, 1986.

107. Hayes DL, Holmes DR, Vliestra RE, et al: Changing experience with dual-chamber (DDD) pacemakers. J Am Coll Cardiol 4:556, 1984.

108. Calfee RV: Pacemaker-mediated tachycardia: Engineering solutions. *In* Barold SS, Mugica J (eds): New Perspectives in Cardiac Pacing. Mt Kisco, NY, Futura, 1988, pp 357–373.

109. Hayes DL: Endless loop tachycardia: The problem has been solved? *In* Barold SS, Mugica J (eds): New Perspectives in Cardiac Pacing. Mt Kisco, NY, Futura, 1988, pp 375–386.

110. Barold SS, Falkoff MD, Ong LS, et al: Programmability in DDD pacing. PACE 7:1159, 1984.

111. Littleford P, Curry RC Jr, Schwartz KM, et al: Pacemaker-mediated tachycardia: A rapid bedside technique for induction and observation. Am J Cardiol 52:287, 1983.

112. Greenspon AJ, Greenberg RM: Noninvasive evaluation of retrograde conduction times to avoid pacemaker tachycardia. J Am Coll Cardiol 5:1403, 1985.

113. Gabry MD, Klementowicz P, Furman S: Balanced endless loop tachycardia. PACE 9:294, 1986.

114. Klementowicz PT, Furman S: Selective atrial sensing in dual-chamber pacemakers eliminates endless loop tachycardia. J Am Coll Cardiol 7:590, 1986.

115. Bernheim C, Markewitz A, Kemkes BM: Can reprogramming of atrial sensitivity avoid an endless loop tachycardia? [Abstract] PACE 9:293, 1986.

116. Rognoni G, Occhetta E, Perucca A, et al: A new approach to the prevention of endless loop tachycardia in DDD and VDD pacing. PACE 14:1828, 1991.

117. DenDulk K, Lindemans FW, Wellens HJJ: Merits of various antipacemaker circus movement tachycardia features. PACE 9:1055, 1986.

118. DenHeijer P, Grinjns HJGM, VanBinsbergen EJ, et al: Orthodromic pacemaker circus movement tachycardia. PACE 10:955, 1987.

119. Timmermans C, Rodriguez LM, DenDulk K, et al: Cure of incessant pacemaker circus movement tachycardia by radiofrequency catheter ablation. J Cardiovasc Electrophysiol 7:862, 1996.

120. Levine PA, Barold SS: Pacemaker automaticity, enabled by a multiplicity of new algorithms. *In* Singer I, Barold SS, Camm AJ (eds): Nonpharmacological Therapy of Arrhythmias for the 21st Century: The State of the Art. Armonk, NY, Futura, 1998, pp 845–880.

121. Goldschlager N: Advances in avoidance and termination of pacemaker-mediated tachycardia. *In* Barold SS, Mugica J (eds): New Perspectives in Cardiac Pacing. Mt Kisco, NY, Futura, 1991, pp 459–471.

122. Bonnet JL, Limousin M: A new algorithm to solve endless loop tachycardia (ELT): A multicenter study of 1816 ELTs. PACE 13:555, 1990.

123. Nitzsché R, Gueunoun M, Lamaison D, et al: Endless loop tachycardia: Description and first clinical results of a new fully automatic protection algorithm. PACE 13:1711, 1990.

124. Mugica J, Barold SS, Ripart A: The smart pacemaker. *In* Barold SS, Mugica J (eds): New Perspectives in Cardiac Pacing. 2. Mt Kisco, NY, Futura, 1991, pp 545–577.

125. Goy J, Vogt P, Kappenberger L: Activity sensing for prevention of pacemaker-mediated tachycardia in DDD pacing. PACE 11:531, 1988.

126. Nitzsché R, Girodo S, Limousin M, et al: Use of a new fallback function to prevent endless loop tachycardia: First clinical results. The Investigators of the Multicenter Study. PACE 15:1851, 1992.

127. VanGelder LM, El Gamal MIH: Ventriculoatrial conduction: A cause of atrial malpacing in AV universal pacemakers. A report of two cases. PACE 8:140, 1985.

128. Sudduth B, Goldschlager N: Retrograde ventriculoatrial conduction in atrial refractoriness: Cause of apparent failure of atrial capture. Pacing 4:56, 1986.

129. Barold SS, Falkoff MD, Ong LS, et al: AV desynchronization arrhythmia during DDD pacing. *In* Belhassen S, Feldman S, Cooperman Y (eds): Cardiac Pacing and Electrophysiology. Jerusalem, Keterpress Enterprises, 1987, pp 177–184.

130. Barold SS, Falkoff MD, Ong LS, et al: Magnet-unresponsive pacemaker endless loop tachycardia. Am Heart J 116:726, 1988.

131. Barold SS: Repetitive non-reentrant ventriculoatrial synchrony in dual-chamber pacing. *In* Santini M, Pistolese M, Alliegro A (eds): Progress in Clinical Pacing 1990. Amsterdam, Excerpta Medica, 1990, pp 451–471.

132. Schüller H, Brandt J: The pacemaker syndrome: Old and new causes. Clin Cardiol 14:336, 1991.

133. Chien WW, Foster E, Phillips B, et al: Pacemaker syndrome in a patient with DDD pacemaker for long QT interval. PACE 14:1209, 1991.

134. Barold SS: Pacemaker induced repetitive nonreentrant ventriculoatrial synchrony: Initiation and termination by ventricular extrasystole. PACE 20:989, 1997.

135. Hayes DL: DDDR timing cycles: Upper rate behavior. In Barold SS, Mugica J (eds): New Perspectives in Cardiac Pacing: 3. Mt. Kisco, NY, Futura, 1993, pp 233–257.

136. Hayes DL: Pacemaker electrocardiography. In Furman S, Hayes DL, Holmes DR (eds): A Practice of Cardiac Pacing (3rd ed). Mt Kisco, NY, Futura, 1993, pp 309–359.

137. Higano ST, Hayes DL, Eisinger G: Sensor-driven rate smoothing in a DDDR pacemaker. PACE 12:922, 1989.

138. VanMechelen R, Ruiter J, DeBoer H, et al: Pacemaker electrocardiography of rate smoothing during DDD pacing. PACE 8:684, 1985.

139. Hanich RF, Midei MG, McElroy BP, et al: Circumvention of maximum tracking limitations with a rate-modulated dual-chamber pacemaker. PACE 12:392, 1989.

140. Feuer JM, Shandling AH, Ellstad MH: Sensor-modulated dual-chamber cardiac pacing: Too much of a good thing too fast? PACE 13:816, 1990.

141. Higano ST, Hayes DL: P-wave tracking above the maximum tracking rate in a DDDR pacemaker. PACE 12:1044, 1989.

142. Hayes DL, Higano ST, Eisinger G: Electrocardiographic manifestations of a dual-chamber rate-modulated (DDDR) pacemaker. PACE 12:555, 1989.

143. Higano ST, Hayes DL, Eisinger G: Advantages of discrepant upper rate limits in a DDDR pacemaker. Mayo Clin Proc 64:932, 1989.

144. Lescault G, Frank G, Girodo S, et al: Tachycardie atriales et stimulation double chambre: Utilité potentielle de l'algorithme de repli. Stimucoeur 18:8, 1990.

145. Van Wyhe G, Sra J, Rovang K, et al: Maintenance of atrioventricular sequence after His bundle ablation for paroxysmal supraventricular rhythm disorders: A unique use of the fallback mode in dual-chamber pacemakers. PACE 14:410, 1991.

146. Barold SS: Automatic switching of pacing mode. Cardiostimolazione 9:121, 1991.

147. Mayumi H, Uchida T, Shinozaki K, et al: Use of a dual chamber pacemaker with a novel fallback algorithm as an effective treatment for sick sinus syndrome associated with a transient supraventricular tachyarrhythmia. PACE 16:992, 1993.

148. Barold SS: Automatic mode switching during antibradycardia pacing in patients without supraventricular tachycardia. In Barold SS, Mugica J (eds): New Perspectives in Cardiac Pacing: 3. Mt. Kisco, NY, Futura, 1993, pp 455–481.

149. Barold SS, Mond HG: Optimal antibradycardia pacing in patients with paroxysmal supraventricular tachyarrhythmias: Role of fallback and automatic mode switching mechanisms. In Barold SS, Mugica J (eds): New Perspectives in Cardiac Pacing: 3. Mt. Kisco, NY, Futura, 1993, pp 483–518.

150. Mond HG, Barold SS: Dual chamber rate-adaptive pacing in patients with paroxysmal supraventricular tachyarrhythmias: Protective measures for rate control. PACE 16:2168, 1993.

151. Barold SS, Mond HG: Fallback responses of dual chamber (DDD and DDDR) pacemakers: A proposed classification. PACE 17:1160, 1994.

152. Furman S: Automatic mode change. PACE 16:2079, 1993.

153. Sutton R: Mode switching in DDDR pacing. In Aubert AE, Ector H, Stroobrandt R (eds): Cardiac Pacing and Electrophysiology. Dordrecht, The Netherlands, Kluwer Academic Publishers, 1994, pp 363–370.

154. Fahraeus T, Bruls A: A new dual protection mechanism against high rate ventricular pacing during atrial tachyarrhythmias [Abstract]. PACE 20:1534A, 1997.

155. Deharo JC, Macaluso G, Djiane P: Les systemes de protection des stimulateurs double chambre contre les arythmies atriales. Arch Mal Coeur Vaiss 89:465, 1996.

156. Bonnet J-L, Brusseau E, Limousin M, et al: Mode switch despite undersensing of atrial fibrillation in DDD pacing. PACE 19:1724, 1996.

157. Ellenbogen KA, Wood MA, Mond HG, et al: Clinical applications of mode-switching for dual-chamber pacemakers. In Singer I, Barold SS, Camm AJ (eds): Nonpharmacological Therapy of Arrhythmias for the 21st Century: The State of the Art. Armonk, NY, Futura, 1998, pp 819–844.

158. Kay GN, Bubien RS: Algorithms for management of atrial fibrillation in patients with dual-chamber pacing systems. In Rosenqvist M (ed): Cardiac Pacing: New Advances. Philadelphia, WB Saunders, 1997, pp 61–82.

159. DenDulk K: Automatic mode switching in DDDR pacemakers. In Oto A (ed): Practice and Progress in Cardiac Pacing and Electrophysiology. Dordrecht, Kluwer, 1996, pp 151–160.

160. Ellenbogen KA, Mond HG, Wood MA, et al: Failure of automatic mode switching: Recognition and management. PACE 20:268, 1997.

161. Walfridsson H, Aunes M, Edvardsson N, et al: Sensed atrial amplitude during atrial fibrillation by a dual chamber pacemaker with mode-shift capabilities [Abstract]. PACE 18:1807, 1995.

162. Palma EC, Kedarnath V, VanKawalla V, et al: Effect of varying atrial sensitivity, AV interval, and detection algorithm on automatic mode switching. PACE 19:1734, 1996.

163. Wood MA, Moskovljevic P, Stambler BS, et al: Comparison of bipolar atrial electrogram amplitude in sinus rhythm, atrial fibrillation, and atrial flutter. PACE 19:150, 1996.

164. Ricci R, Puglisi A, Azzolini P, et al: How should atrial sensitivity be programmed in automated mode switching pacemakers? PACE 20:1063, 1997.

165. Leung SK, Lau CP, Lam C, et al: How should atrial sensitivity be programmed for optimal automatic mode switching? [Abstract] J Am Coll Cardiol 29:149A, 1997.

166. Fröhlig G, Kindermann M, Heisel A, et al: Mode switch without atrial tachyarrhythmia. PACE 19:592, 1996.

167. Baerman JM, Ropella KM, Sahakian AAV, et al: Effect of bipole configuration on atrial electrograms during atrial fibrillation. PACE 13:78, 1990.

168. Lewalter T, Schimpf R, Jung W, et al: Prospective evaluation of mode switch behavior in patients with dual chamber pacing and unipolar atrial leads: Relevance of atrial fibrillation/flutter potentials and myopotential triggering [Abstract]. PACE 19:642A, 1996.

169. Dijkman B, DenDulk K, Wellens HJJ: Importance of farfield QRS sensing evaluation for the functioning of automatic mode switching algorithms [Abstract]. PACE 18:829, 1995.

170. Kamalvand K, Tan K, Willems R: Use of pacemaker diagnostic functions for recognition and management of cardiac arrhythmias. PACE 19:514, 1996.

171. Waktare JE, Malik M: Holter loop recorder and event counter capabilities of implanted devices. PACE 20:2658, 1997.

172. Barold SS, Bornzin G, Levine P: Development of a true pacemaker Holter. In Vardas PE (ed): Cardiac Arrhythmias: Pacing and Electrophysiology. Dordrecht, Kluwer, 1998, pp 421–426.

173. Mabo P, Daubert C, Limousin M, et al: Atrial electrogram storage: A new tool for atrial arrhythmia diagnosis in pacemaker patients [Abstract]. PACE 19:721A, 1996.

174. Meta DDDR Model 1254 multiprogrammable minute ventilation volume rate responsive pulse generator with telemetry. Physician's Manual. Englewood, CO, Telectronics, 1994.

175. Pitney MR, May CD, David MJ: Undesirable mode switching with a dual chamber rate response pacemaker. PACE 16:729, 1993.

176. Lau CP, Tai YT, Fong PC, et al: Atrial arrhythmia management with sensor controlled atrial refractory period and automatic mode switching in patients with minute ventilation sensing dual-chamber rate-adaptive pacemakers. PACE 15:1504, 1992.

177. Hess M: Personal communication. Minneapolis, Medtronic Inc., 1996, 1997, 1998.

178. Levine PA, Bornzin GA, Barlow J, et al: A new automode switch algorithm for supraventricular tachycardias. PACE 17:1895, 1994.

179. Levine PA, Florio J, Bornzin GA: Automatic mode switching in the Pacesetter Trilogy DRT and DC+ pulse generators. In Sethi KK (ed): VI Asian-Pacific Symposium on cardiac pacing and electrophysiology. Bologna, Monduzzi Editore, 1997, pp 167–173.

180. Kay GN, Hess M, Marshall H, et al: Effect of mode switching algorithm in patient symptoms [Abstract]. PACE 20:1064A, 1997.

181. Leung S-K, Lam T-F, Tse H-F, et al: Different responses to atrial fibrillation in three automatic mode switching algorithms [Abstract]. PACE 20:1497A, 1997.

182. Kamalvand K, Kotsakis A, Tan K, et al: Evaluation of a new pacing algorithm to prevent rapid tracking of atrial tachyarrhythmias. PACE 19:1714, 1996.

183. Brignole M, Gianfranchi L, Menozzi C, et al: A new pacemaker for paroxysmal atrial fibrillation treated with radiofrequency ablation of the AV junction. PACE 17:1889, 1994.

184. DenDulk K, Lindemans FW, Wellens HJJ: Initial experience with mode switching in a dual sensor, dual chamber pacemaker in patients with paroxysmal atrial tachyarrhythmias. PACE 17:1900, 1994.

185. Ovsyshcher IE, Katz A, Bondy C: Initial experience with a new algorithm for automatic mode switching from DDDR to DDIR mode. PACE 18:1908, 1994.

186. Delay M, Brüls A, Mounier C, et al: Evaluation of a new sensor-based algorithm to protect against atrial arrhythmias. PACE 19:1704, 1996.

187. Ricci R, Puglisi A, Azzolini P, et al: Reliability of a new algorithm for automatic mode switching from DDDR to DDIR pacing mode in sinus mode disease patients with chronotropic incompetence and recurrent paroxysmal atrial fibrillation. PACE 19:1716, 1996.

188. Provenier F, Jordaens L, Verstraeten T, et al: The "automatic mode switch" function in successive generations of minute ventilation sensing dual chamber rate responsive pacemakers. PACE 17:1913, 1994.

189. Gencel L, Geroux L, Clementy J, et al: Ventricular protection against atrial arrhythmias in DDD pacing based on a statistical approach: Clinical results. PACE 19:1729, 1996.

190. Brignole M, Gianfranchi L, Menozzi C, et al: Assessment of atrioventricular function ablation and DDDR mode-switching pacemaker versus pharmacological treatment in patients with severely symptomatic paroxysmal atrial fibrillation: A randomized study. Circulation 96:2617, 1997.

191. Kamalvand K, Tam K, Kotsakis K, et al: Is mode switching beneficial? A randomized study in patients with paroxysmal atrial tachyarrhythmias. J Am Coll Cardiol 30:496, 1997.

192. Schuchert A, vanLangen H, Michels K, et al: DDD(R) pacing with automatic mode switch in patients with paroxysmal atrial fibrillation following AV nodal ablation. Cardiology 88:323, 1997.

193. Marshall HJ, Harris ZI, Gammage MD: The increasing use of mode-switching. PACE 20:3012, 1997.

194. Love CJ, Wilkoff BL, Kevin S, et al: Incidence of mode switch in a general pacemaker population [Abstract]. PACE 20:1131, 1997.

195. Azara D, Girardi C, Ruffa H, et al: Assessment of rate smoothing in dual chamber pacemakers. Am J Cardiol 70:548, 1992.

196. Papp MA, Mason T, Gallastegni J: Use of rate smoothing to treat pacemaker mediated tachycardias and symptoms due to upper rate response of a DDD pacemaker. Clin Prog Pacing Electrophysiol 2:547, 1984.

197. Giudici MC, Orias DW: Mode switching anomalies: A patient who remained symptomatic during paroxysmal atrial tachyarrhythmias despite a mode switching pacemaker. PACE 20:1883, 1997.

198. Satler LF, Rackley CE, Pearle DL, et al: Inhibition of a physiologic pacing system due to its antipacemaker-mediated tachycardia mode. PACE 8:806, 1985.

199. DenDulk K, Wellens HJ: Failure of the postventricular premature beat DVI mode in preventing pacemaker circus movement tachycardia. Am J Cardiol 54:1371, 1984.

200. Greenspon AJ, Volasin KJ: "Pseudo" loss of atrial sensing by a DDD pacemaker. PACE 10:943, 1987.

201. Wilson JH, Lattner S: Undersensing of P waves in the presence of adequate P wave due to automatic postventricular atrial refractory period extension. PACE 12:1729, 1989.

202. VanGelder BM, VanMechelen R, DenDulk K, et al: Apparent P wave undersensing in a DDD pacemaker post exercise. PACE 15:1651, 1992.

203. Dodinot B, Beurrier D, Simon JP, et al: "Functional" loss of atrial sensing causing sustained first to high-degree AV block in patients treated with dual-chamber pacemakers [Abstract]. PACE 16:1189, 1993.

204. Gregoratos G, Cheitlin MD, Freedman RA, et al: ACC/AHA guidelines for implantation of cardiac pacemakers and antiarrhythmia devices. A report of the American College of Cardiology/American Heart Association Task Force on Practice Guidelines (Committee on Pacemaker Implantation). J Am Coll Cardiol 31:1175, 1998.

205. Barold SS: Indications for permanent cardiac pacing in first-degree AV block. Class I, II or III? PACE 19:747, 1996.

206. Kuniyashi R, Sosa E, Scanavacca M, et al: Pseudo-sindrome de marcapasso. Arch Bras Cardiol 62:111, 1994.

207. Freedman RA, Rothman MT, Jason JW: Recurrent ventricular tachycardia induced by an atrial synchronous ventricular inhibited pacemaker. PACE 5:490, 1982.

208. Furman S, Fisher JD: Repetitive ventricular firing caused by AV universal (DDD) pacing. Chest 83:586, 1983.

209. Dodinot BP, Medeiros P, Galv̄ao SS, et al: Endless loop dual-chamber pacemaker tachycardias related to R-wave sensing by the atrial circuit. PACE 8:301, 1985.

210. Dodinot B, Medeiros P, Galv̄ao S, et al: Dual-chamber pacemaker sustained tachycardias related to "cross ventricular sensing." Stimucoeur Med 14:15, 1986.

211. Pimenta J, Soldá R, Britto Pereiva C: Tachycardia mediated by an AV universal (DDD) pacemaker triggered by a ventricular depolarization. PACE 9:105, 1986.

212. Wittkampf FHM, Boute W: Return to Wenckebach: Improved timing cycles for dual-chamber pacemakers. *In* Barold SS, Mugica J (eds): New Perspectives in Cardiac Pacing. Mt Kisco, NY, Futura, 1988, pp 173–186.

213. Ahmed R, Worzewski W, Ingram A, et al: A new pacemaker algorithm preventing atrial tracking during atrial flutter/fibrillation in DDD pacing [Abstract]. Eur Heart J 12:414, 1991.

214. Curry PVL, Rowland E, Krikler DM: Dual demand pacing for refractory atrioventricular reentry tachycardias. PACE 2:137, 1979.

215. Leclerq C, Gras D, LeHelloco A, et al: Hemodynamic importance of preserving the normal sequence of ventricular activation in permanent cardiac pacing. Am Heart J 129:1133, 1995.

216. Rosenqvist M, Isaaz K, Botvinick EH, et al: Relative importance of activation sequence compared to atrioventricular synchrony in left ventricular function. Am J Cardiol 67:148, 1991.

217. Rosenqvist M, Bergfeldt L, Haga Y, et al: The effect of ventricular activation sequence on cardiac performance during pacing. PACE 19:1279, 1996.

218. Jutzy RV, Feenstra L, Pai R, et al: Comparison of intrinsic versus paced ventricular function. PACE 15:1919, 1992.

219. Vardas PE, Simantirakis EN, Parthenakis FI, et al: AAIR versus DDDR pacing in patients with impaired sinus mode chronotropy: An echocardiographic and cardiopulmonary study. PACE 20:1762, 1997.

220. Mayumi H, Kohno H, Yasui H, et al: Use of automatic mode change between DDD and AAI to facilitate native atrioventricular conduction in patients with sick sinus syndrome or transient atrioventricular block. PACE 19:1740, 1996.

221. Linde C: The clinical utility of positive and negative AV/PV hysteresis. *In* Santini M (ed): Progress in Clinical Pacing 1996. Armonk, NY, Futura Media Services, 1997, pp 339–345.

222. Fredman CS, Bjerregaard P, Janosik DL, et al: Unusual Wenckebach upper rate response of an atrial-based DDD pacemaker. PACE 15:975, 1992.

223. Barold SS, Falkoff MD, Ong LS, et al: Interference in cardiac pacemakers: Exogenous sources. *In* El-Sherif N, Samet P (eds): Cardiac Pacing and Electrophysiology (3rd ed). Philadelphia, WB Saunders, 1991, pp 608–633.

Chapter 31

Pacemaker Diagnostics and Evaluation of Pacing System Malfunction

Paul A. Levine and Charles J. Love

Pacemakers have advanced from nonprogrammable single-chamber asynchronous devices (VOO) to dual-chamber systems with extensive programmability. They now include the ability to adjust automatically the pacing rate on the basis of signals that are independent of the intrinsic heart rhythm (DDDR). The analysis of a pacing system was comparatively easy during the early days of pacing, whereas the challenge in evaluating the modern pacemaker has increased to a degree that is concordant with the sophistication of the current devices.

To facilitate these evaluations, manufacturers have incorporated a multitude of diagnostic tools in the pacemaker. The various capabilities commonly complement one another, either eliminating the need for ancillary testing or providing the direction for additional testing. Occasionally, a given feature provides absolutely unique information that is not readily available by any other technique. These tools, which are integral to the implanted device, can be accessed by the programmer and are the subject of the first part of this chapter. To take advantage of these diagnostic features and to determine the appropriate function of a pacing system, the clinician must have an in-depth knowledge of the system components, including not only the pulse generator but also the leads, programmed parameters, sensors, connectors, and other implanted devices, as well as the patient's physiology. It is crucial that the clinician understand the importance of evaluating the entire system rather than focusing on isolated individual components. The evaluation of malfunctioning pacemaker systems is the subject of the second part of this chapter.

■ BIDIRECTIONAL TELEMETRY

Telemetry is the ability to transmit information or data from one device to another, a capability that was essential to the introduction of programmability. This is the ability to noninvasively change the functional parameters of the pacing system by coded commands transmitted to the pacemaker from a programmer.[1-4] The first generation of programmable pacemakers used unidirectional telemetry from the programmer to the pacemaker but was not able to transmit data from the pacemaker to the programmer. This limited the confirmation of a programming change, such as the sensitivity or refractory period that was electrocardiographically silent, when a parameter was programmed. To serve as a marker that the programming command was both received and acted on, another standard recommendation was to program a parameter, such as rate, that could be easily measured using the electrocardiogram (ECG). The introduction of bidirectional telemetry also allowed the pacemaker to communicate with the programmer. The successful programming of sensitivity, refractory periods, sensor parameters, and other parameters that could not be easily identified on a standard ECG recording can now be programmed with confidence that the command will be appropriately received and acted on by the implanted pacemaker.

Bidirectional telemetry is communication in two directions. With respect to pacing systems, this means that the pacemaker and programmer can communicate with each other, an essential capability for the development of the multiple diagnostic capabilities that are the subject of this chapter.[5, 6] First implemented in rechargeable pacemakers, bidirectional telemetry was developed to confirm the proper alignment of the recharging head with the implanted pacemaker. When the recharging wand was not aligned properly with the pacemaker, there was an audible beep from the charging unit to notify the patient and whoever was in attendance of this condition. When the two devices were properly aligned, the system was silent.

This capability was next applied to confirmation of programming. This was particularly valuable for those parameters that did not result in an overt change in pacing system

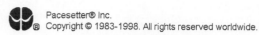

Page 5a
Affinity™ DR Model: 5330 Serial: 11300
3500 Serial: 3500 (APS® III 3303 - 0.15)

Basic Parameters

	Initial	Present	
Mode	DDDR	DDDR	
Base Rate	60	60	ppm
Hysteresis Rate	Off	Off	ppm
Rest Rate	45	45	ppm
Max Track Rate	140 =>	170	ppm
2 :1 Block Rate	175	175	ppm
AV Delay	170	170	ms
PV Delay	150	150	ms
Rate Resp. AV/PV Delay	Medium	Medium	
Shortest AV/ PV Delay	70	70	ms
Ventricular Refractory	250	250	ms
Atrial Refractory	275	275	ms
Ventricular:			
V. AutoCapture	Off	Off	
V. Pulse Amplitude	2.00	2.00	V
V. Pulse Width	0.6	0.6	ms
V. Sensitivity	2.0	2.0	mV
V. Pulse Configuration	Bipolar	Bipolar	
V. Sense Configuration	Bipolar	Bipolar	
Atrial:			
A. Pulse Amplitude	2.00	2.00	V
A. Pulse Width	0.6	0.6	ms
A. Sensitivity	0.2	0.2	mV
A. Pulse Configuration	Bipolar	Bipolar	
A. Sense Configuration	Bipolar	Bipolar	
Magnet Response	Snapshots+Batt.	Snapshots+Batt.	

Extended Parameters

	Initial	Present	
AutoIntrinsic Conduction Search™	Off	Off	ms
Negative AV/PV Hysteresis / Search	Off	Off	ms
Auto Mode Switch	DDIR	DDIR	
Atrial Tachycardia Detection Rate	225	225	ppm
Post Vent. Atrial Blanking (PVAB)	100 =>	60	ms
Vent. Safety Standby	On =>	Off	
Vent. Blanking	12	12	ms
PVC Options	Off	Off	
PMT Options	Off =>	Auto Detect	
PMT Detection Rate	* =>	110	bpm

Sensor Parameters

	Initial	Present	
Sensor	On	On	
Max Sensor Rate	140 =>	160	ppm
Threshold	Auto (+0.0)	Auto (+0.0)	
Meas. Average Sensor	2.5	2.5	
Slope	8 =>	Auto (+0)	
Measured Auto Slope	* =>	8	
Reaction Time	Fast =>	Slow	
Recovery Time	Medium =>	Fast	

*	Not Applicable	
=>	Initial value differs from Present value	
T=>	Temporary programmed value	
---	Unknown/Invalid values	

Patient Data

Vent. Lead Type	Unipolar/Bipolar
Atrial Lead Type	Unipolar/Bipolar
Implant Date:	14 Jul 1998 12:06

Patient Information

    JOHN Q. PUBLIC ID# 123-45-6789
    DOI: 14 JULY,1998 AT SW MED CNTR
    A LEAD: SJM 1388T-46 AB223345
    V LEAD: SJM 1388T-52 BC199887
    DX:COMPLETE HEART BLOCK, S/P AV
       NODE ABLATION, PMKR DEPENDENT
       SEVERE PMKR SYNDROME WITH VVI
    DR.PAUL A LEVINE 818-493-2900

Measured Data

Date Last Programmed	18 Sep 1998 07:35	
Magnet Rate	98.5	ppm
Ventricular:		
Pulse Amplitude	1.9	V
Pulse Current	3.6	mA
Pulse Energy	3.3	μJ
Pulse Charge	2	μC
Lead Impedance	538	Ω
Atrial:		
Pulse Amplitude	2.0	V
Pulse Current	3.6	mA
Pulse Energy	3.5	μJ
Pulse Charge	2	μC
Lead Impedance	542	Ω
Battery Data	(W.G. 9438 - nom. 0.95 Ah)	
Voltage	2.76	V
Current	12	μA
Impedance	<1	kΩ

Test Results

Atrial Capture Threshold	<0.25	V
Atrial Capture Test Pulse Width	0.6	ms
Atrial Capture Test Polarity	Bipolar	
Atrial Capture Safety Margin	>8.0 : 1 @ 2.00V	
Vent. Capture Threshold	0.50	V
Vent. Capture Test Pulse Width	0.6	ms
Vent. Capture Test Polarity	Bipolar	
Vent. Capture Safety Margin	4.0 : 1 @ 2.00V	
P-Wave Amplitude	2.5	mV
Atrial Sense Test Polarity	Bipolar	
Atrial Sense Safety Margin	12.5 : 1 @ 0.20mV	
R-Wave Amplitude	>12.5	mV
Vent. Sense Test Polarity	Bipolar	
Vent. Sense Safety Margin	>6.3 : 1 @ 2.00mV	

Figure 31–1. Final interrogation of a Pacesetter Affinity DR model 5330 (St. Jude Medical CRMD, Sylmar, CA) with the programmed parameters and the changes identified from the initial evaluation, measured data telemetry, model, serial number, date, and time, patient information entered by the medical staff, and summary of capture and sensing threshold results performed during the evaluation.

performance and that could not be independently identified on an ECG recording. This ability is essential for the DDDR pacemaker and modern implantable cardioverter-defibrillators (ICDs) because these devices may have 20 to 30 or more independently programmable parameters, most of which are not readily identifiable on the ECG (Fig. 31–1). Bidirectional telemetry allows the unit to be interrogated about its programmed parameters when the patient is seen during follow-up or is evaluated for a suspected pacing system malfunction. Without this feature, there would be no way to determine the current settings of a device for features other than rate and pulse width. It also makes the retrieval of detailed data collected by the pacemaker in its various event counters feasible.

Measured Data

Complementing the interrogation of programmed data is the provision of measured data, including data obtained from the pacemaker detailing information concerning lead and battery function at the time of evaluation. Information regarding demand and asynchronous rates may also be measured (Fig. 31–2). Telemetry allows this information to be transferred from the pacemaker to the programmer for evaluation by the clinician.

Battery Status

Although not all systems provide the same information, data concerning battery function often include a measure of battery voltage, impedance, and current drain.[7–11] All three parameters are interrelated. The battery current drain is a measure of the average current being drawn from the battery assuming 100% pacing at the programmed rate and output settings. Inhibition or pacing at higher rates, as might occur with sensor drive, directly affects the functional battery current drain, as do changes in the lead or stimulation imped-

ance. The reported current drain is only an estimate of the actual battery current drain.

The measured current drain of the battery at a known set of parameters can be used to qualitatively assess the effect of programming changes on the longevity of the system. After the rate or output or both are changed, the measured data can be reassessed and the effect of the programming change on longevity estimated. A simple calculation may be used to obtain an estimate of the pacemaker battery longevity when the pacemaker is relatively new. Most manufacturers provide the usable battery capacity reported in ampere-hours (Ah). For this calculation, the battery's capacity is converted to microampere-hours (μAh). This number is divided by the measured battery current drain. The result is the anticipated number of hours of normal function at the programmed rate and output. This number, divided by 8760 (the number of hours in 1 year), yields an estimate of the longevity of the system in years. This calculation is best performed with a new system before there has been significant battery depletion.

Virtually every pacemaker incorporates a change in either the magnet or demand rates (and sometimes mode or other functions) to signal a level of battery depletion that warrants pulse generator replacement. Most of these changes occur when the battery's voltage reaches a predefined level, which is specific for each manufacturer and even for each model of pacemaker. These changes are termed elective replacement time (ERT), recommended replacement time (RRT), and elective replacement indicator (ERI), with further changes in rate or function associated with continued battery depletion being labeled either end of life (EOL) or end of service (EOS). Although these changes may occur abruptly, there is commonly a 3- to 6-month period between activation of the ERT indicator and erratic behavior or device nonfunction caused by continued battery depletion. A marker to determine when to increase the frequency of pacing system surveillance, either transtelephonically or in the office, is included in some systems and is commonly an intermediate rate between a fully functional battery and the ERT indicator. This is termed an *intensified follow-up indicator* and provides an indication of changing battery status even before the ERT is reached.

Given the degree of programmability of most current pacemakers, a dual-chamber pacemaker programmed to a rapid base rate with a maximal output on each channel may last only 2 years. The identical model programmed to a low base rate with outputs of 2.5 V or lower on each channel that are inhibited a significant portion of the time may be anticipated to function properly for 15 years or longer. It would be inappropriate to follow the second unit on a monthly basis beginning 1 year after implantation, whereas it would be equally inappropriate to plan only annual checks on a pacing system programmed with high outputs and rapid rates. By following some measure of the status of the battery, either directly or indirectly, the clinician can achieve a qualitative assessment about when to increase the frequency of pacing system follow-up.[12]

There are two primary indicators of battery status. One is the battery voltage, which progressively decreases over time (see Chapter 6). A lithium-iodine power cell is now used in virtually all pulse generators, whereas the power source in an ICD is vanadium pentoxide. The nominal unloaded output

294-03-001024		APR 13 '93	11:46 AM	*
RELAY	TELEMETRY DATA			I
PACING RATE			70 PPM	N
PACING INTERVAL	860 MSec			T
CELL VOLTAGE			2.48 VOLTS	E
CELL IMPEDANCE			< 2.5 KOHMS	R
CELL CURRENT			40.1 UA	M
	ATRIAL (Bi)		VENTRICULAR (Bi)	E
SENSITIVITY	1.3		3.0 MV	D
LEAD IMPEDANCE	501		Low OHMS	I
PULSE AMPLITUDE	3.43		3.13 VOLTS	C
PULSE WIDTH	0.45		0.45 MSEC	S
OUTPUT CURRENT	6.5		HIGH MA	
ENERGY DELIVERED	9.1		HIGH UJ	I
CHARGE DELIVERED	2.94		HIGH UC	N
				C

| RETURN | *

Figure 31–2. Measured data telemetry from a Relay model 294-03 rate-modulated dual-chamber pacemaker (Sulzer Intermedics, Angleton, TX) reporting a low impedance on the ventricular lead as a result of an insulation failure. This also results in an increase in the battery or cell current caused by a higher output current, charge, and energy being delivered by the pacemaker, whether or not it reaches the heart. This system reports extreme values as high or low, whereas as other systems report specific numbers.

voltage of the lithium-iodine cell is 2.8 V, with each manufacturer triggering the RRT indicator at a specified battery voltage based on circuit design considerations. The battery voltage and programmed output voltage are not identical. The programmed output voltage is achieved by modifying the 2.8-V battery output with either voltage multipliers or charge pumps to provide a higher voltage. The battery voltage can also be divided to deliver a voltage lower than 2.8 V. As energy is consumed, the battery voltage progressively decreases. Most manufacturers have included circuitry to maintain the stability of the delivered programmed voltage to the patient, whereas the ability to track the progressive decrease in battery voltage provides an effective guide to the physician regarding the frequency with which the pacing system should be routinely checked for signs of battery depletion. This, in part, is affected by the battery current drain. The higher the current drain, the lower the battery voltage.

Inversely related to battery voltage is battery impedance. In the lithium-iodine power cell, the release of electrons is generated by the combination of the lithium ion with two iodine atoms. The result of this chemical reaction is the release of two electrons (negatively charged particles) and the formation of lithium iodide. As the lithium iodide accumulates, it forms a resistive barrier between the anode and the cathode. With progressive cell depletion, the increasing amount of lithium iodide results in a rise in the internal impedance of the battery, which some pacemakers can measure and report in the telemetry data. The higher the battery impedance, the lower the cell voltage.

Either or both of these parameters—battery voltage and impedance—may be tracked. If these measurements are provided to the manufacturer's technical service engineers, along with the programmed parameters and an estimate of the percentage of pacing versus inhibition, the remaining longevity of that pacing system can be estimated with reasonable accuracy, assuming that the various parameters remain stable. These calculations have also been incorporated into some programmers to provide an on-line estimate of longevity. In present systems, this is based on the assumption of 100% pacing. Systems are being developed that use the historic percentage of pacing as acquired from the event counter diagnostics to provide a more accurate longevity estimate based on the actual device use. This prediction is dependent on the tolerances and accuracy of the measurements of battery status. Even with this enhanced capability, the longevity estimate remains as an approximation because projections of a battery's function are determined from accelerated testing and not long-term monitoring under normal conditions.

Lead Status

Although many systems provide data concerning lead function, including pulse voltage, current, charge, and energy, the measurement that is used most frequently is that of lead or stimulation resistance (impedance). Changes in lead impedance affect the other measures of lead function. The terms *resistance* and *impedance*, although technically different, are often used interchangeably by the clinical community. Impedance is a complex concept reflecting a changing environment involving a variety of factors. This results in fluctuations in the moment-to-moment resistance. The resistance to electron flow in a pacing system progressively rises during the delivery of the stimulation pulse as a result of polarization at the electrode–myocardial interface and, as a continuously changing variable, is appropriately termed impedance. Many pulse generators and pacing system analyzers make this measurement at a specific point within the pacing stimulus; this is a resistance. Other devices report the resistance as an average of the impedance throughout the pulse. The actual resistance to current flow imparted by the conductor coil is fixed and represents a small portion of the total stimulation resistance. The polarization at the electrode–myocardium interface, which is due in part to the surface area and geometry of the electrode, and the impedance associated with conduction of the pulse through the body's tissues play a larger role in the overall resistance of the system. All this is incorporated in the single measurement termed either *lead impedance,* or more accurately, *stimulation impedance.*

Stimulation impedance is affected by many factors, not the least of which are electrode size, configuration, and materials. Manufacturers have designed electrodes with high impedance values. For any given output, a high impedance system reduces the overall current drain of the battery and effectively increases the unit's longevity. Other leads have been designed with low polarization to allow for detection of capture with each pace stimulus. Polarization and impedance are not the same phenomenon, although one affects the other. For any given lead model, there is a range of normal impedance values that may be broad, whereas for a specific lead within that model series, the impedance should fall within a relatively narrow range.

The clinician can use knowledge of the lead impedance to follow and identify a developing mechanical problem with the lead. This requires baseline or historical data to recognize subtle changes that may reflect a conductor fracture or a breach of the insulation. It is essential to know what device is being used to make these measurements. As noted previously, different devices may obtain these data at different points of the pacing stimulus. Because of these differences, the impedance measurement obtained with a pacing system analyzer at the time of implantation may be significantly different from that obtained by telemetry from the implanted pacemaker moments, if not years, later. This difference does not necessarily imply a problem. Furthermore, impedance may evolve over time, with a fall in impedance occurring in the days to weeks after implantation, followed by a gradual rise toward the initial measurements on a chronic basis.

Multiple factors may affect impedance, particularly in a unipolar system. For example, measurements obtained during deep inspiration may significantly differ from those obtained during maximal exhalation. In the same patient, impedance measurements obtained that are based on a single-output pulse may vary by 100 Ω or even more during the same follow-up evaluation while remaining consistent with normal function. If a marked change in lead impedance from previous measurements (e.g., more than 300 Ω) is encountered during a routine follow-up evaluation, further evaluation of the pacing system is advisable, although even these changes may be normal.[13, 14] If the patient has no clinical symptoms and has stable capture and sensing thresholds, operative intervention would be premature, although a more frequent follow-up schedule would be prudent. A dramatic change in telemetered lead impedance in the presence of a clinical problem, however, directs the physician toward the likely source of the difficulty (see Fig. 31–2).

A dramatic fall in impedance usually reflects a break in the insulation.[15–17] This effectively increases the surface area of the electrode, resulting in lower impedance. In a unipolar system, an insulation problem provides an alternative pathway for current flow, starting closer to the pulse generator and resulting in less energy reaching the heart, possibly causing a loss of capture. The amplitude of the stimulus artifact as recorded by the ECG is determined by the distance the current travels in the tissues from the cathode (tip electrode) to anode (ring electrode or housing of the pulse generator). Hence, a bipolar pacing system in which both active electrodes are inside the heart, separated only 1 to 2 cm, results in a small stimulus artifact, whereas the pacing spike recorded in a unipolar system in which the current travels from the tip electrode to the housing of the pulse generator is large despite equivalent output settings. It is also affected by the recording system: some of the newer digital designs result in a marked signal-to-signal variation in amplitude or in the generation of a uniform amplitude artifact, with any high-frequency electrical transient precluding differentiation of a bipolar and a unipolar pacing system based on the analysis of the ECG recording.

In a previously stable system, a mechanical problem developing with the lead—either a breach in the insulation or a conductor fracture—results in a change in the stimulation impedance, which may be reflected by a change in the ECG recorded stimulus artifact (Fig. 31–3). In a bipolar pacing system, an insulation defect between the proximal conductor and the tissues of the body is not likely to affect capture thresholds, but it results in a larger stimulus artifact, making it appear unipolar. Depending on the actual location of the insulation failure in either the bipolar or unipolar lead, stimulation of the extracardiac muscle contiguous to the insulation defect may occur. Insulation failures may also attenuate the electrical signal reaching the pacemaker, possibly resulting in sensing failure.

In a bipolar lead, an insulation defect developing between the proximal and distal conductors can present as a variety of clinical manifestations. Intermittent contact between the two conductors generates a voltage transient, which the pacemaker can sense, resulting in inhibition or triggering, depending on the programmed sensing mode and the channel on which the problem has occurred. This signal is not seen on the surface ECG and is appropriately termed *oversensing*. If the two conductors remain in contact, current flowing down the distal conductor is short-circuited to the proximal conductor and never reaches the electrodes. This may result in a loss of capture and a further reduction in the amplitude of the normally diminutive bipolar stimulus artifact. In addition, loss of appropriate sensing may also occur.

Programming the output configuration to unipolar (in

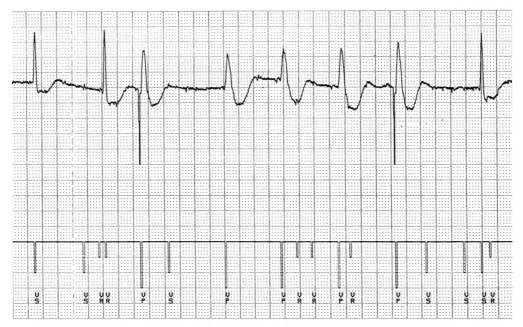

Figure 31–3. Simultaneous electrocardiogram (ECG) and event markers from a Medtronic Activitrax model 8400 single-chamber bipolar rate-modulated pacemaker (Medtronic, Minneapolis, MN) with an internal insulation failure of the lead. There is both oversensing (VS and VR) and functional undersensing when the true native complex coincides with the refractory period initiated by the oversensing. During the intervention for lead replacement, the measured lead impedance was 125 Ω. The event markers are both labeled (VP, ventricular pacing; VS, ventricular sensing; VR, sensed event occurring during the refractory period) and identified by different amplitudes of the marker artifacts. The surface ECG should also be examined. This recording system generates a large-amplitude "artifact" to simulate the paced output with any high-frequency transient that is detected independent of the output configuration of the pulse. If no stimulus is detected, no artifact is generated. There are paced QRS complexes identified by the event markers that have no "pacing stimulus" on the ECG, whereas others have a large "unipolar" pacing stimulus visible. The identification of the pacing system malfunction was facilitated by the simultaneous event markers.

those systems that have this capability) may prevent the loss of capture and possibly undersensing from an internal short circuit. This does not prevent the oversensing behavior associated with make-break electrical transients generated by intermittent contact between the two conductors, which is allowed to occur because of a failed inner insulation. Typically, a bipolar lead with failed internal insulation exhibits a higher impedance when pacing is programmed to the unipolar rather than the bipolar output configuration.[18, 19] This is opposite to the expected higher impedance of a bipolar system. Although programming to unipolar may result in an apparent resolution of a malfunction, it is not a cure and should only be considered a temporary measure, allowing the observed problem to be managed on an elective rather than emergent basis. The malfunctioning lead should be replaced expeditiously.

An increase in lead impedance may be the result of a conductor fracture or a connector problem.[20] When this occurs, the lead impedance often rises to high levels. It is inappropriate, however, to assume that a normal lead impedance is 500 Ω. New leads are being introduced that are designed to be high impedance with values ranging from 1500 to 2500 Ω. Other leads, at implantation, have a relative impedance level in the range of 300 Ω and even 200 Ω. Thus, it is essential to look for a trend in serial lead impedance measurements in conjunction with the stability or changes in capture and sensing thresholds. A mechanical problem with the lead—either a conductor fracture resulting in a high impedance or an insulation failure resulting in a low impedance—eventuates in an overt clinical problem that can be identified by telemetric measurement of the stimulation impedance. When the impedance is sufficiently high, there is no current flow and no effective output, although the telemetered event markers indicate an output and therefore loss of capture. The reduced current flow also results in a fall in the measured current drain of the battery. Any problem, however, may be intermittent. This typically occurs when the two broken ends make contact at times but are separated at other times, or in the case of an insulation failure, when lead movement either opens the compromised area or pushes the edges of the break together, resulting in normal function.

Before the availability of telemetry for lead impedance measurements, physicians could obtain similar information by oscilloscopic analysis of the pacemaker stimulus. In the 1970s, some manufacturers included a photograph of the pulse wave contour at a variety of different impedance values with the technical manual accompanying each pacemaker. Some more recent computer-based ECG systems are able to record and display the pacemaker pulse at an expanded scale, so that its waveform can be recorded and tracked as a routine part of the periodic pacing system evaluation. Although available, this is not routinely used, given the ready access to lead impedance measurements provided by the implanted pacing system.

Lead impedance measurements have an indeterminate incidence of false-negative results when the lead problem is only intermittently manifested. The measurement system forces the pacemaker to function asynchronously in an effort to obtain the measurements. The measurements, however, are made over a few cycles. If there is a true lead problem, but it is intermittent and was not present when the measurements were being made, the telemetered lead impedance may be normal. Thus, if a problem is suspected, repeated measurements are required. In addition, using provocative maneuvers, such as placing manual pressure along the subcutaneous course of the lead or having the patient raise or in other ways manipulate the ipsilateral arm, may be required to unmask a problem. It is often awkward to obtain measurements during these maneuvers.

Some older pacemakers were able to report lead impedance measurements on a beat-by-beat basis, allowing the physician to observe the digital read-out of lead impedance on the programmer screen over a protracted number of cycles. This capability is being incorporated in future devices, allowing the physician to look for an intermittent unexpected fluctuation at the time of routine follow-up. Like the oscilloscopic monitoring of the pulse wave morphology, this technique will reduce but not eliminate the incidence of false-negative results. A further enhancement is the automatic periodic monitoring of lead impedance, resulting in a graphic display reporting the history of lead impedance performance and potentially automatically programming the pacemaker from the bipolar output configuration to unipolar in the presence of either a marked rise in impedance reflecting a conductor fracture[21] or a marked drop in impedance consistent with an insulation failure. Some newer systems may be set to monitor only lead impedance on a periodic basis or to monitor and revert to the unipolar output and sensing configuration if out-of-bounds measurements are obtained. This increases the frequency with which measurements can be obtained, increasing the likelihood of diagnosing an intermittent lead problem and possibly intervening on an automatic basis (Fig. 31–4).

Event Marker Telemetry

The challenges associated with interpreting the paced ECG have markedly increased with the expanded use of dual-chamber multisensor rate-modulated systems. Even with the simplest pacing systems, multiple assumptions had to be made. Most clinicians are comfortable evaluating a surface ECG composed of P waves representing native atrial depolarizations and QRS complexes (or R waves) representing native ventricular depolarizations. The pacemaker does not respond to the P or R wave but to the intrinsic deflection of the electrical potential inside the heart that occurs as the wave of depolarization passes by the pacing electrode (see Chapter 3). Although the events inside the heart frequently correspond to events recorded by the ECG, there may be events inside the heart that are not visible on the ECG. In addition, the pacemaker senses and responds to events occurring outside the heart if detected by the sense amplifier. Standard ECG recordings may not depict these internal and external electrical events, yet these events affect the behavior of the pacing system. Similarly, standard ECG recordings do not detect the usual sensor signals that may also drive the pacemaker to a variety of different rates and timing settings.

The introduction of dual-chamber pacing significantly increased the level of complexity of the paced rhythm. The interaction between the two channels of the pacing system with the spontaneous rhythms occurring in either the atria or ventricles added to the potential for confusion. The addition of rate-modulated pacing (i.e., allowing the pacemaker

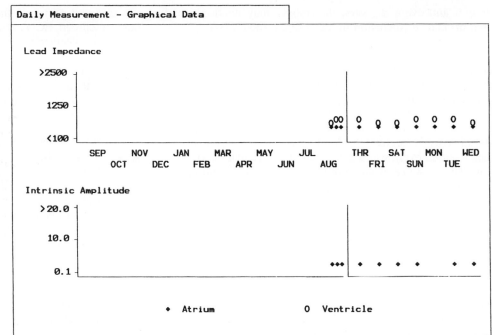

Figure 31-4. Graphic display and tabular summary of serial automatic atrial and ventricular lead impedance measurements as well as intrinsic signal amplitude from an implanted Guidant Discovery DDDR model 1273 pacemaker (CPI Guidant, St. Paul, MN). This event counter reports measurements made on a daily basis for the past 7 days and the mean weekly measurements before that time, with the potential for extending back a full year. This was retrieved at a follow-up evaluation.

Guidant				DISCOVERY
				03-SEP-98 14:21
Institution	JER^{DY} L. PETTIS V.A. MEDICAL CENTER			
Patient			CPI Programmer	001580
Model	1273 Serial	303566	2890 Software	1.20

Daily Measurement - Data Table

Date	Atrium Amplitude (mV)	Atrium Impedance (Ω)	Ventricle Amplitude (mV)	Ventricle Impedance (Ω)
02-SEP-98	>3.5	480	PACED	680
01-SEP-98	>3.5	500	PACED	710
31-AUG-98	PACED	500	PACED	710
30-AUG-98	>3.5	480	PACED	710
29-AUG-98	>3.5	500	PACED	680
28-AUG-98	>3.5	470	PACED	670
27-AUG-98	>3.5	470	PACED	710
21-AUG-98	>3.5	480	PACED	710
14-AUG-98	>3.5	480	PACED	720
07-AUG-98	>3.5	480	PACED	680

to respond also to one or more sensor signals that are invisible on the ECG) further contributes to the challenge of interpreting the paced ECG because these sensor signals are invisible on the ECG.

In the modern pacemaker, interpretation of the paced rhythm requires knowledge of the basic timing intervals. A variety of refractory periods, including postventricular atrial refractory period (PVARP), postventricular atrial blanking period, ventricular refractory period, ventricular blanking period, and paced and sensed atrioventricular (AV) intervals, must also be considered. Some intervals may change depending on the rate, such as the AV interval, atrial escape interval (when under sensor drive or with special features), and PVARP. The clinician also needs to be aware of a number of device-specific responses to protect the system from a variety of anticipated but undesirable behaviors or clinical events. These include crosstalk, a premature ventricular beat initiating a pacemaker-mediated tachycardia (PMT), mode switching, and multiblock upper rate behavior.

To facilitate interpretation of the paced rhythm, increasing numbers of pacing systems incorporate the ability to transmit information regarding real-time pacing system behavior to the programmer on a virtually continual basis and to display this information on a screen or other recording system. Both paced and sensed events are communicated to the programmer. Displayed as a series of positive or negative marks, with or without alphanumeric annotation, these are generically termed *event markers*. These have the greatest diagnostic value when superimposed above or below a simultaneously recorded surface ECG (see Fig. 31-4). Some systems also display the duration of the atrial and ventricular refractory periods and interval measurements. Others show events that are sensed during the refractory period but do not play a role in altering the system timing (sensed but not used). These may be displayed in either in a real-time manner or after the tracing has been frozen on the programmer screen by using cursors to identify the interval of interest. If the real-time monitor screen method is used to show the rhythm and event markers, the tracing may be frozen and then printed for inclusion in the medical record (Fig. 31–5).

Event markers (also called *marker channels*, *annotated event markers*, and *main timing events*) are most effectively used when displayed with a simultaneously recorded ECG rhythm.[22-25] Without the ECG, the event marker simply reports the behavior of the pacemaker. This information is valuable in showing that an output has been released or that sensing has occurred. What it does not confirm is that the stimulus was effective–that is, that it resulted in capture or that a sensed event was a true atrial or ventricular depolarization. The presence of an output marker does not confirm that the stimulus even reached the heart because it is transmitted directly from the pacemaker to the programmer by way of the telemetry module. An open circuit (e.g., a fractured conductor coil) may preclude the output pulse from reaching the heart, yet the pacemaker would indicate that an output pulse was released. Similarly, there may have been a native depolarization that was not sensed, allowing the pacing stimulus to be released at a time when the myocardium was physiologically refractory. If the markers reported that an event was sensed on the atrial channel followed by a ventricular output pulse after a preset delay (known as *P-wave synchronous ventricular pacing* or *tracking*), the clinician would know that the pacemaker was capable of sensing in the atria and pacing in the ventricles. Without a simultaneously recorded ECG, however, it would be impossible to determine whether the pacemaker was responding to inappropriate signals on the atrial channel, whether the ventricular stimulus was effective, or whether a native QRS was present but not sensed. Hence, telemetered event markers are most effective when displayed with a simultaneously recorded ECG.

Event Marker Displays

A variety of different displays have been used over the years. Although not intended for this purpose, the simplest event marker for sensed events was achieved with triggered mode pacing, particularly if the output configuration was unipolar. A sensed event would be marked by the simultaneous release of a pacing stimulus coincident with sensing. This was easily recorded on an ECG because the stimulus artifact distorted the morphology of the native sensed complex. The next evolutionary step in this technology involved the pacemaker emitting a series of varying-amplitude subthreshold stimuli to represent the release of an output pulse, a sensed event, and the end of the refractory period. Both of these systems, the triggered mode and the series of markers, were limited by the fact that the signals required an intact lead system, allowing the pulse to be delivered to the heart

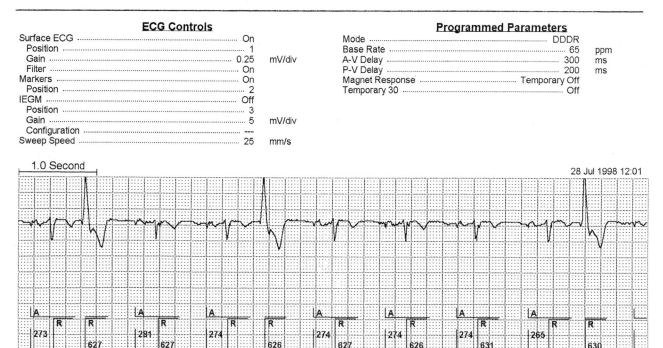

ECG Controls

Surface ECG	On
Position	1
Gain	0.25 mV/div
Filter	On
Markers	On
Position	2
IEGM	Off
Position	3
Gain	5 mV/div
Configuration	---
Sweep Speed	25 mm/s

Programmed Parameters

Mode	DDDR
Base Rate	65 ppm
A-V Delay	300 ms
P-V Delay	200 ms
Magnet Response	Temporary Off
Temporary 30	Off

Figure 31–5. Surface electrocardiogram and simultaneous event marker telemetry from a Pacesetter Trilogy DR+ model 2360 (St. Jude Medical CRMD, Sylmar, CA) showing an atrial-paced rhythm with intact atrioventricular nodal conduction and isolated ventricular ectopic beats. Key programmed parameters are shown at the upper right and recording parameters at the upper left. The numbers refer to the millisecond intervals automatically measured and displayed by the programmer. The horizontal lines following the alphabetic label (A, atrial-paced output; R, sensed ventricular event) represent the length of the programmed or functional refractory period.

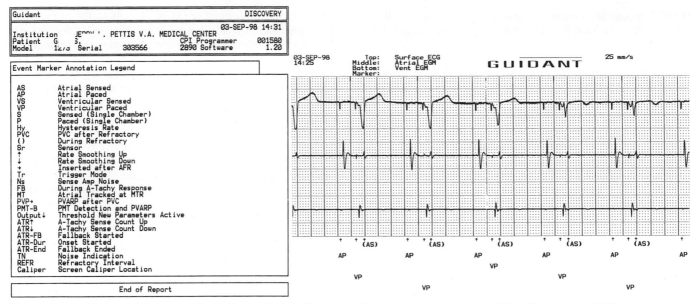

Figure 31–6. Event marker annotation legend from a Guidant Discovery DDDR model 1273 pacing system (CPI Guidant, St. Paul, MN) are shown on the left. These labels are placed under the simultaneously recorded electrocardiogram (ECG) to identify the specific event reflecting the behavior of the pacemaker as shown on the right. Also displayed are simultaneously recorded atrial and ventricular electrograms. AP, atrial-paced event; VP, ventricular-paced event; (AS), atrial-sensed event occurring during atrial refractory period—in this case, it is a far-field R wave that is also visible on the atrial electrogram channel (middle channel on ECG recording).

through the lead and thus recorded for display by the ECG. If the output pulse was bipolar, the diminutive signal might not be readily visible, particularly in the triggered mode, because it would be obscured by the larger native complexes. In addition, if there were an open circuit (most commonly a conductor fracture) or an internal insulation failure involving a coaxial bipolar lead, no marker would be visible.

The next improvement was to transmit coded signals representing paced and sensed events from the pacemaker to the programmer. The programmer reconstituted these signals into a series of varying-amplitude pulses or alphanumeric labels representing paced or sensed events. These could be either displayed on a monitor screen or recorded using a printer integral to the programming system, which allowed for the simultaneous recording of a surface ECG acquired by way of a separate set of cables. The simultaneous ECG and markers allow the clinician to correlate the behavior of the pacemaker directly with the patient's rhythm to determine whether the system is functioning properly. A calibration signal composed of a series of different amplitude pulses or a legend of the cryptic labels allows the clinician to interpret the various markers. In an early series of markers, the largest pulse represented a pacing output, the intermediate one indicated a sensed event, and the smallest represented either the end of the refractory period or a sensed complex that occurred during the refractory period. With the advent of dual-chamber pacing systems, a marker pulse extending above the baseline identified atrial events, and ventricular events were labeled with a pulse extending below the baseline.

A further refinement to this system was the addition of alphanumeric annotations. Two common sets of notations have been used and are summarized later. These are not the only possibilities because some manufacturers use a unique set of symbols to identify paced and sensed events, with the location of the symbol on the recording identifying whether it represents atrial or ventricular events. Others have expanded on the set of labels and, on command, provide a detailed explanation.

Many of the single-chamber pacing systems with event marker telemetry used the letter P to reflect a paced event and S to represent a sensed event. This has the potential for causing confusion with other dual-chamber systems in which the letter P reflects a sensed atrial event indicative of a native P wave (with which most medical personnel are familiar, based on their knowledge of the standard ECG). The interpretation of the alphanumeric event markers is often product specific, and the clinic personnel who evaluate the pacing system must take this into account (Fig. 31–6).

In the case of dual-chamber pacing or when the pacemaker knows that it is providing atrial pacing and sensing, a native atrial depolarization may be identified as either the letter P or the combination AS. P is taken from the standard ECG identifier for an atrial depolarization. AS is one abbreviation for an atrial-sensed event. An atrial stimulus may be identified by either the letter A or the combination AP for atrial-paced event.

Analogous lettering is used on the ventricular channel. Again, single-chamber pacing in some systems might still use the letters P to represent a paced event and S to refer to a sensed event. Other systems use R to refer to a native ventricular depolarization, which is generically called an R wave on the standard ECG. This may also be identified by the letter combination VS for a ventricular-sensed event. The letter V in one system might be used to represent a ventricular pacing stimulus, whereas the identical event may be labeled VP for ventricular pacing in other systems.

Other symbols may be used for a paced or sensed event;

these symbols are commonly displayed with an identifying key on the resultant printout. Each paced or sensed event may also be identified by a vertical line, going up in the case of atrial events and down for ventricular events. In some cases, a difference in the amplitude of these lines has been retained in conjunction with the alphanumeric lettering. Indeed, as the complexity of the devices increases, the variety of symbols and letters identifying specific events and behaviors is also increasing (see Fig. 31–6).

In many systems, interval measurements between the various events either are calculated automatically and displayed or are measured after cursors are aligned with specific events. There may be a time delay between the actual sensed or paced event and the release of the event marker. This is due to a finite period that is required for the pacemaker to recognize the event and then transmit the appropriate information to the programmer through the telemetry channel. In most cases, priority is given to the normal function of the pacemaker, with the diagnostic marker feature being delayed. Differences of up to 40 msec between the actual event and the resultant marker have been noted.

Laddergramming

Laddergramming is a standard adjunct to the interpretation of clinical arrhythmias. It is now being incorporated in some programming systems by using the known programmed parameters of the pacemaker combined with the event marker information telemetered from the implanted pacemaker (Fig. 31–7).[23–26] For all the elegance of these graphic interpretations of the pacemaker's behavior, they still require the simultaneously recorded ECG rhythms. Although the pacemaker may be functioning normally, in that it is behaving properly with respect to its programmed parameters, failure to capture or properly sense would not be diagnosed from the various diagrams and markers without the simultaneously recorded surface ECG.[27]

Event Marker Limitations

A number of limitations are associated with event marker telemetry. The first is that by itself, markers report the behavior of the pacemaker but do not allow the clinician to determine whether this behavior is appropriate for the patient.[27] In this regard, it is analogous to the small hand-held digital counters that report pacing rates and intervals. The counters only detect and report the pacing stimuli, not whether these output pulses are effective in causing a cardiac depolarization or that native events are properly and consistently sensed. There is no information about whether a long interval between consecutive pacing stimuli reflects normal function because the pacemaker responded appropriately to a native complex, or whether it represents a system malfunction with oversensing or no output (e.g., from an intermittent lead fracture). Neither event marker telemetry nor the digital counters should be used independently of a simultaneously monitored ECG rhythm.

The second limitation is that the report of a stimulus output does not mean that there is appropriate capture. Confirmation of capture requires an ECG or concomitant hemodynamic pulse monitoring. In addition, the markers may report that the pacemaker is sensing a signal, but if this signal is not visible on the surface ECG, there is cause for concern. Is it an appropriate signal that the pacemaker should sense because some intrinsic atrial rhythms may not be visible on the specific lead that is being monitored, or is the system responding to an inappropriate or nonphysiologic signal, such as the make-break potentials associated with a breach of the internal insulation in a coaxial bipolar lead?

Most pacemaker event marker telemetry is limited to real-time recordings. The markers must be telemetered from the pacemaker to the programmer or another display system while the rhythm is being actively monitored. Neither the pacemaker nor the programmer can retrospectively provide markers for a previously recorded rhythm. If the pacemaker is responding to events that are not visible on the surface ECG, the event marker simply confirms this fact but does not identify the specific signal. An evaluation of sensed but otherwise invisible events requires electrogram (EGM) telemetry or an invasive procedure to record the signal from the implanted lead. More recently, pacemakers have been introduced that have the capability of storing event markers

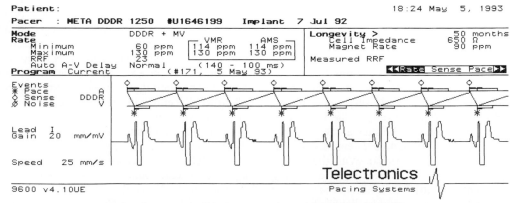

Figure 31–7. Laddergram from a META DDDR model 1250 rate-modulated dual-chamber pacing system (Telectronics Pacing Systems, now Pacesetter, St. Jude Medical CRMD, Sylmar, CA) displayed with a model 9600 programmer. The event markers are identified by a variety of symbols displayed in a key to the left of the tracing. In addition, battery (cell) impedance and projected longevity are reported in the upper right portion of the tracing; selected programmed parameters are shown in the upper left quadrant. AV, atrioventricular; RRF, rate response factor.

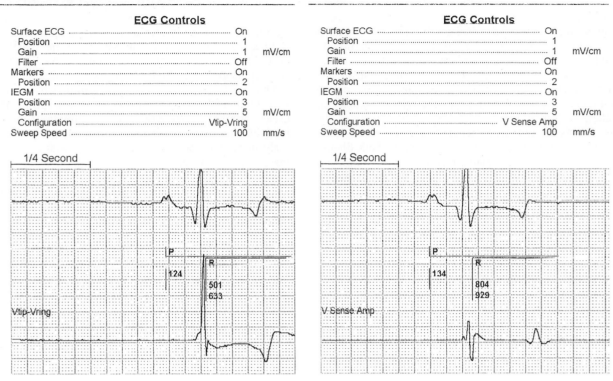

Figure 31–8. Side-by-side display of telemetered bipolar ventricular electrograms before being processed by the sense amplifier (Vtip-Vring) on the left or after being processed by the sense amplifier (V Sense Amp). The simultaneously recorded surface electrocardiogram and telemetered event markers are also shown (P, native atrial depolarization; R, native ventricular depolarization) with the horizontal lines representing the atrial *(top)* and ventricular *(bottom)* refractory periods. The circuitry of the sense amplifier has a narrow band-pass filter that modifies the raw signal, which can also be telemetered. These signals were telemetered from a Pacesetter Affinity DR pacemaker, model 5330 (St. Jude Medical CRMD, Sylmar, CA).

with or without EGMs. These may be stored by the use of a patient trigger such as magnet application,[28] use of a simple battery-operated radio-frequency transmitter, or on spontaneous activation of specific predefined algorithms or sequence of sensed or paced events.

Electrogram Telemetry

The clinician evaluates a pacing system based on an analysis of the ECG, but the pacemaker does not respond to P waves or QRS complexes. The latter are surface manifestations of the atrial and ventricular depolarization. The recorded signal that enters the pacemaker's sense amplifier by way of the electrode located within or on the heart is termed an *EGM* or *intracardiac EGM*. The EGM is composed of a number of elements. The portion that is sensed by the pacemaker is termed the *intrinsic deflection* and reflects the rapid deflection that occurs when the wave of cardiac depolarization passes by the electrode. The intrinsic deflection can be characterized by both the amplitude and slew rate. The change in voltage amplitude divided by the time duration of this portion of the signal is the known as the *slew rate*. The unit of measurement for slew rate is volts per second or millivolts per millisecond. Most implanted pacemakers require a slew rate of more than 0.5 V/sec for proper sensing.

The other portions of the cardiac depolarization, as reflected by the EGM, are termed the *extrinsic deflection*. Although the extrinsic deflection may have an adequate amplitude, the slew rate is usually too low, precluding this portion of the cardiac signal from being sensed by the pacemaker (see Chapter 3).

At the time of implantation, the amplitude of the EGM is commonly measured with a pacing system analyzer that reports a millivoltage amplitude. The pacing system analyzer uses its own unique set of filters, which may not be identical to those in the pacemaker's sense amplifier. Thus, the analyzer's reported signal, at best, provides an approximation of what the pacemaker effectively sees. Likewise, the morphology of the EGM observed on a high-fidelity monitor is not identical to the signal as seen by the pacemaker because filters in the pacemaker's sense amplifier usually have a narrower bandpass and therefore block out some of the frequencies (Fig. 31–8). Examining the EGM recorded with a physiologic recorder or telemetry with a wide bandpass can provide valuable information on the slew rate, splintering of the intrinsic deflection, and other morphologic abnormalities.

Measuring the peak-to-peak amplitude of the EGM, as recorded at the time of implantation or as telemetered from the already implanted pacemaker, is commonly used to determine the sensing threshold. This may be inappropriate when the frequency content of the signal is outside the constraints of the bandpass filter of the sense amplifier. If the clinician wants to determine the sensing threshold for a given patient, the sensitivity of the system should be progressively reduced until the system no longer consistently senses the native signal. The highest number of the sensitivity settings (usually identified by a millivolt amplitude) at which there is consistent sensing is the sensing threshold. The precision of this measurement is limited by the number and range of the programmable sensitivity options in the specific model of pacemaker.[29–31]

Other EGMs are obtained after the signal is processed by the pacemaker's sense amplifier. In some cases, both filtered and unfiltered EGMs are available (see Fig. 31–8). Although the telemetered EGM should not be used to determine the sensing threshold, it has many other roles.[32, 33] A primary value is identifying signals that are being sensed but are not visible on the surface ECG. Another is to facilitate an analysis of the timing of the pacing system because the sensed intrinsic deflection resets one or more timers. The intrinsic deflection at which sensing occurs can be best identified from the EGM and only indirectly measured from the surface ECG. Under unique circumstances, the telemetered EGM has been used to confirm capture (particularly atrial) when the evoked complex is not visible in any lead of the surface ECG.[34, 35] This requires a unique output pulse configuration either to cancel the residual polarization artifact or to record the signal through electrodes that are not directly involved with the output pulse. The output pulse has a tendency to overload the telemetry or sense amplifier, driving the signal off scale. This is then followed by a refractory period within the telemetry amplifier before anything can again be recognized.

The telemetered EGM has been effectively used to diagnose native arrhythmias in which the pacemaker is simply an innocent bystander or to identify retrograde P waves not visible on the surface ECG. The latter may facilitate programming of the PVARP to prevent PMTs.[35–43] The telemetered EGM provides clues to why episodes of undersensing may be occurring. Reasons include splintering of the EGM and low slew rates that may place the signal outside the tight constraints of the pacemaker's sense amplifier despite an adequate peak-to-peak amplitude (Fig. 31–9).[44]

The telemetered EGM can also be followed on a periodic basis to monitor the progression of the patient's intrinsic disease process. A decrease in the amplitude of the telemetered EGM was reported to identify early rejection effectively in cardiac transplant recipients. A return to the baseline amplitude correlated with a resolution of the rejection process.[45] Preliminary work on the signal-averaged EGM, either atrial or ventricular, suggests that this may be helpful in identifying disease in the respective chamber that may be beyond the resolution of signal-averaging of the surface ECG.[46]

Limitations of Electrogram Telemetry

That the telemetered EGM appears to be of adequate amplitude for sensing does not mean that the pacemaker will sense it. The telemetry amplifier may use filters different from those in the sensing circuit, providing qualitative rather than quantitative data concerning the EGM (see Fig. 31–9). In most pacing systems, telemetered EGMs also suffer from limitations that are similar to those of event markers. They are real-time recordings and cannot be retrospectively provided by the programmer to facilitate the interpretation of an earlier ECG.

Real-time telemetry allows the physician to analyze the behavior of the pacing system when the patient is in the physician's office or clinic while these diagnostics are being accessed with the programmer. This is impractical over a

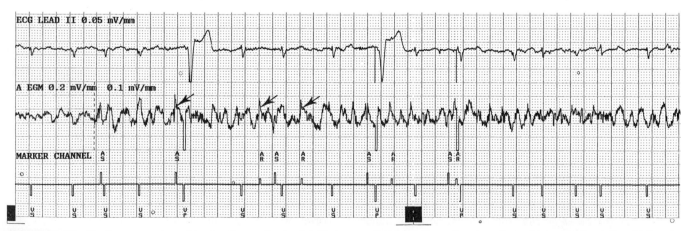

Figure 31–9. Simultaneous surface electrocardiogram *(top)*, atrial electrogram *(middle)*, and event markers *(bottom)* from a patient with a Medtronic Prodigy DR model 7860 pulse generator (Medtronic Inc., Minneapolis, MN). Although the Automatic Mode Switch algorithm was enabled, this system did not mode switch despite the persistence of atrial fibrillation; the reason is clearly identified from the atrial electrograms. These electrograms are telemetered before being processed by the sense amplifier. The atrial fibrillatory signal is a predominantly low-frequency signal identified by the slow rise deflections, even though the peak-to-peak amplitude should have been adequate to sense as this was well above the programmed sensitivity. These low-frequency signals are filtered out by the sense amplifier as demonstrated by the event markers—very few of the fibrillatory signals are sensed (AS or AR), and hence, the rhythm never fulfills the rate criteria necessary to initiate mode switching. Note that the signals with a discrete rapid deflection (arrows) are properly sensed, whereas those that are not sensed have a relatively slow deflection.

long period. In addition, it does not allow the patient to move around much while these recordings are being obtained. Long-term monitoring of pacing system behavior requires either a Holter monitor, which is expensive and cumbersome, or event counter telemetry, depending on the degree of precision that is desired. Pacemakers with microprocessors and significant random access memory (RAM) can now store selected EGMs[47, 48] as well as event markers when triggered by the patient or by a predefined set of circumstances. This may markedly reduce the need for Holter or other monitoring techniques to evaluate intermittent symptoms in the paced patient.

Event Counter Telemetry

Simplistically put, the pacemaker "knows" when it has released an output pulse or responded to a sensed event. The availability of high-density, low-power RAM and read only memory (ROM) integral to microprocessors that can be incorporated in the pacemaker have given pacemakers the ability to store information about system performance for retrieval at a later date. The objective of the event counters is to facilitate the clinician's ability to analyze and manage the patient's pacing therapy more effectively. Although this may add to the time required for the evaluation, namely to retrieve and interpret these data, the additional time is usually minimal. This technology can provide the clinician with information that is crucial to understanding the performance of the system over time to direct the programming of the system and to achieve optimal performance. Other techniques, such as standard Holter monitor recordings or repeated exercise tolerance tests, although valuable, are impractical, arduous, and relatively expensive to acquire on a routine as well as repeated basis.

The first use of stored diagnostic data in cardiac pacemakers was associated with the introduction of multiparameter programmability. Simple data using codes to identify implant indications and medications were able to be downloaded into the pacemaker for retrieval at subsequent follow-up evaluations. This ability has been expanded, allowing entry of free text (the date of implantation, lead model numbers, pharmacologic regimens, and even acute implant measurements, including capture and sensing thresholds and lead impedances) (see Fig. 31–1). This information is printed with the programmed parameters each time the pacemaker is interrogated.

Event counters have been expanded since these early efforts. There are now a variety of different diagnostic counters. Some provide information concerning the overall performance of the system, whereas others focus on a specific algorithm or subsystem. Still others provide detailed information on the basis of the time course of events. The number of individual event counters that are currently available from a multiplicity of different devices is too numerous to detail in this chapter. Thus, selected examples are used to illustrate these capabilities.

Total System Performance Counters

Some systems keep track of the number of times a pacing stimulus is released or a native complex is sensed. This allows for an assessment of the degree to which the pacemaker was used. A refinement of this ability allows the

pacemaker to diagnose bradycardia and, in the dual-chamber modes, to tell whether the bradycardia was the result of sinus node dysfunction or AV block. Event counters with this ability have also been termed *diagnostic data, implanted Holter systems*, and *data logging*.[49–55]

With the introduction of dual-chamber pacing (specifically the DDD mode), the potential interactions between the pacemaker and the patient increased from two (pacing or sensing in one chamber) to five (pacing or sensing in the atria or ventricles and sensing ventricular activity without pre-existing atrial activity). Knowledge of how the pacing system has behaved over time, combined with the clinician's knowledge of the patient, provides invaluable information toward assessing the overall performance of the implanted system.

The various annotations described in the event marker section were combined to provide a cryptic description of the different operational states of the DDD mode. These include an atrial-sensed event followed by a ventricular-sensed event (AS-VS or PR) indicating that the pacemaker is inhibited on both channels. Atrial sensing followed by a ventricular-paced event (AS-VP or PV) refers to P-wave synchronous ventricular pacing. Atrial pacing with intact AV nodal conduction or functional single-chamber atrial pacing would be indicated by AP-VS or AR. Base-rate pacing in both chambers would be represented by AP-VP or AV. A ventricular-sensed event not preceded by atrial activity, either paced or sensed, is a premature ventricular event (PVE), identified by the letter R or combination VS. Some systems label these premature ventricular contractions (PVCs).

This information may be collected in conjunction with events occurring in specific rate bins, allowing for a detailed report of heart rate distributions. Additional data that have been collected include the percentage of pacing in the atrium and ventricle, the amount of time at the maximum tracking rate, and the number of episodes in which the pacing system reached the programmed upper rate limit, in which mode switching has occurred, or in which the PMT termination algorithm was used, or the number of times any one of a number of other special features was been activated. The counters are able to continue to accumulate data until one of the pacing state bins is full and cannot accept one additional bit of information; at this point, one or more of the counters are frozen (Fig. 31–10). The volume of data that can be stored depends on the memory capacity of the pacemaker that is dedicated to these features.

The following example provides a general idea about the amount of data that can be stored or the quantity of memory. All data are stored in a binary code, represented by a series of 1s and 0s. A binary unit of memory is called a *bit*. Eight bits are a *byte* and result in 256 combinations of 1s and 0s. If each series of combinations represents a single item of data, a total of 256 pieces of information can be stored in a system with eight bits of memory. As the number of bits increases, the amount of data that can be stored increases geometrically. If each pacing state is represented by a single combination of bits, and there are 24 bits in the RAM devoted to these counters, upward of 17 million events can be counted and stored in memory for retrieval at the time of routine pacing system follow-up. Reading the counters requires access to the memory banks in the pacemaker by using specific coded commands from the programmer. One

Page 2a
Synchrony® II Model: 2022 Serial: 54440
3500 Serial: 2024 (APS™ III 3302 - 1.02)

Mode	DDD	
Sensor	Passive	
Base Rate	50	ppm
Max Track Rate	145	ppm
Max Sensor Rate	135	ppm
A-V Delay	250	ms
Rate Resp. A-V Delay	Enable	

Note: The above values were obtained
when the histogram was interrogated.

Date Read:	10 Aug 1998 14:57
Total Time Sampled:	388d 19h 4m 22s
Sampling Rate	Every Event
Percent of counts paced in atrium	7%
Percent of counts paced in ventricle	19%
Total Time at Max Track Rate	0d 0h 0m 0s

Event Histogram

Event Histogram, Percent of Total Time

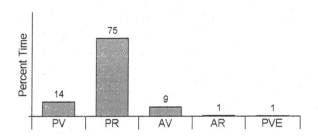

Heart Rate Histogram

Heart Rate Histogram, Percent of Total Time

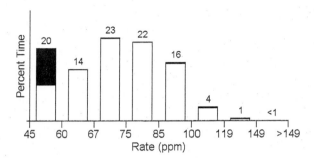

Event Counts

Rate (ppm)	PV	PR	AV	AR	PVE
45 - 60	997,091	1,888,457	2,621,941	237,669	0
61 - 67	1,791,645	3,252,366	60	44	553
68 - 75	1,821,846	7,182,349	0	0	7,330
76 - 85	410,361	9,349,618	0	0	14,901
86 - 100	56,251	8,170,791	0	0	87,023
101 - 119	8,477	2,213,554	0	0	157,939
120 - 149	214	468,215	0	0	55,365
> 149	0	10,675	0	0	1,758
Total:	5,085,885	32,536,025	2,622,001	237,713	324,869

Total Event Count: 40,806,493

Heart Rate Histogram, Percent Of Time Per Rate Bin

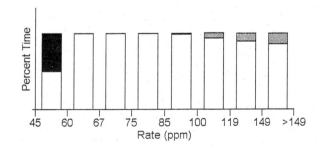

Sensed (PV/PR)
Paced (AV/AR)
PVE

Figure 31–10. Event and Heart Rate Histogram retrieved from a patient with a Pacesetter Synchrony II model 2022 (St. Jude Medical CRMD, Sylmar, CA) programmed to the DDD mode. The key programmed parameters are shown in the upper left, whereas other information is shown at the upper right. These data represent the performance of the pacing system over the preceding 388 days with monitoring of every event. The Event Histogram is a graphic display of the relative percentage of events within each of the five basic pacing states, whereas the Heart Rate Histogram is a graphic display of the rate distribution based on atrial-sensed or atrial-paced events. This bimodal distribution reflects normal chronotropic function of the sinus node in this patient, whose pacemaker was placed for intermittent atrioventricular block. The precise number of events in each rate bin and pacing state is shown in the Event Count table, whereas the Percent of Time per Rate Bin represents a normalized display of the relative percentage of atrial-paced or atrial-sensed events and premature ventricular-sensed events in each rate bin during this period of time.

DDD system introduced in the mid-1980s had this ability, with sufficient memory to provide a summary of the pacing system behavior for about a 6-month period. As their memory capacity increases, these systems are able to store much more data for longer periods (see Fig. 31–10).

Storing a simple marker of the pacing state and rate requires relatively little memory compared with that required to store waveform data representing the rhythm, as depicted by a consecutive series of EGMs. A theoretical 100-Hz bandwidth with 200 samples per cardiac cycle at eight bits of resolution per sample, recording the entire rhythm during a 24-hour period, would require 140,000,000 bits/day and, then, only if the heart rate was a steady 60 bpm.[47] Most implantable defibrillator systems now store a series of EGMs preceding and following the delivery of antitachycardia therapy. An older method used to save memory was to provide "snapshots" of representative complexes; the trigger to store these data was the delivery of antitachycardia therapy. Extensive storage of cardiac rhythm data within pacemakers becomes possible with increasingly sophisticated data compression algorithms and more memory than was previously available. Higher-bandwidth data transmission channels are required for this volume of data storage, particularly long series of rhythms, so that transmission can be accomplished efficiently and as quickly as possible.

An implanted Holter monitor complete with stored rhythms is now available as a stand-alone device, in ICDs, and in high-end pacemakers. Most pacemakers, however, continue to store only data reflecting the total number of times a pacing state was encountered and, in some systems, the distribution of rates or intervals, rate ranges, or mean rates within these pacing states. This information provides the physician with an overview of the function of the system in the patient. Predominant base-rate pacing is expected in patients with marked sinus node dysfunction or in patients receiving anti-ischemia medications. On the other hand, predominant base-rate pacing, AP-VP, in patients whose primary indication for pacing was complete heart block, suggests either the development of sinus node dysfunction or primary atrial undersensing. In these same patients with high-grade AV block, frequent counts of AS-VS and PVEs, particularly in the absence of known ventricular ectopy, suggests episodes of ventricular oversensing or the resolution of the AV block. Large numbers of counts regarding PMTs warrant a reassessment of retrograde conduction and possible adjustment of the programmed PVARP or PMT prevention and termination algorithm programming. A large number of counts at the maximum tracking rate suggests that the upper rate limit should be reassessed. Event counter telemetry can provide an insight into the overall function of the pacing system; a variation from the clinician's knowledge of the patient may suggest the need for a further evaluation.

When the additional ability to monitor a series of rates and pacing states is added, chronotropic function can be assessed by the distribution of atrial-sensed rates (AS-VS or PR and AS-VP or PV; see Fig. 31–10). Furthermore, atrial pacing at rates above the programmed base rate reflect sensor drive in the DDDR pacing systems providing an overview of the sensor behavior. When there is the ability to report both rates and pacing states, the clinician can obtain a better insight into the cause of PVEs as well as overall pacing system function. True premature ventricular contractions tend to occur at short coupling intervals, which is equivalent to a rapid rate. Large numbers of PVEs might suggest recurrent ventricular arrhythmias.[58, 59] If there are large numbers of PVE counts at relatively low rates, the clinician should consider episodes of atrial undersensing or accelerated junctional rhythms, which would also fulfill the pacemaker's criteria for a PVE (i.e., a sensed R wave not preceded by an atrial event).

Subsystem Performance Counters

An increasing number of specific algorithms and capabilities are used either intermittently or potentially independently of the functional performance of the pacing system. An early counter representative of this capability is the sensor indicated rate histogram, reporting the distribution of pacing rates that would have occurred had the sensor been totally controlling the pacing rates.[56, 57] This counter reports the sensor-defined rates, even if the pacemaker was inhibited by a faster native rhythm or the actual functional rate was being controlled by the sensed atrial activity.

Other subsystem performance counters include automatic mode switch histograms, reports of the cumulative duration that the system functioned at the maximum tracking rate, the number of times the PMT algorithm was enabled, high atrial or ventricular rate episodes (Fig. 31–11), and sudden rate-drop episodes to identify some of these. These diagnostic counters provide detailed information about the use of a specific algorithm or system behavior that may not be activated on a daily basis or not visible on the ECG, making identification difficult using standard recording techniques such as a Holter monitor.

The principal limitation associated with the two types of counters described to this point is that counts are placed in a bin, either the pacing state alone or the pacing state and rate, which provides a one-dimensional view of the system's behavior. If the period of monitoring is short, as during a casual or brisk walk, the clinician can reasonably assess the behavior of the pacing system. Longer periods of monitoring accumulate and overlap the results of many activities, precluding an assessment of the pacing system's behavior during a specific activity or the identification of a symptomatic episode occurring at an earlier time. The ability of the system to store pacing state and rate data with respect to time (identified as time-based event counters) has been variably termed *event record* or *pacemaker Holter systems*.[60–62] Technically, this is not yet a true Holter monitor because continuous rhythm recordings are not retained in memory, even though rate data may be available.

Time-based System Performance Counters

Time-based event counters require an extensive amount of memory. Not only are the pacing state and rate stored, these data must be stored with respect to the preceding and subsequent events. The data cannot be simply dumped into a rate or pacing state bin. Each piece of data (i.e., every cardiac event) must have a time reference, which takes significantly more memory than simple histogram-type counters.

Two techniques are available for storing real-time data. One is to continue to accumulate the data until the memory is full and then to freeze the recorded events. Freezing all of the counters at the same time maintains the ratios between

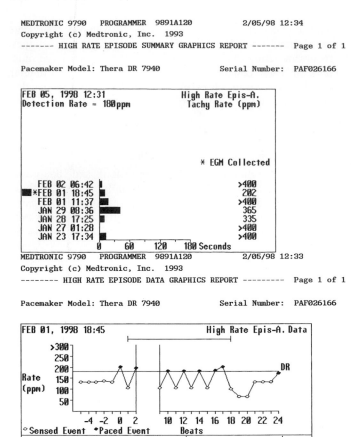

Pacemaker Model: Thera DR 7940   Serial Number: PAF026166

Pacemaker Model: Thera DR 7940   Serial Number: PAF026166

Figure 31–11. High-rate episode summary *(top)* and high-rate episode graphic with stored atrial electrogram *(bottom)* from a Medtronic Thera DR model 7940 (Medtronic Inc, Minneapolis, MN). This facilitates the clinician's ability to assess the behavior of the pacing system between office visits. In this case, the specific episode associated with the atrial electrogram reports atrial-paced events occurring above the trigger level for this event counter, which is also above the maximum sensor rate. The electrogram demonstrates atrial pacing with a large far-field R-paced ventricular event, and presumably, the labeled high-rate episode is due to far-field sensing. This knowledge may be helpful in further programming the pacemaker.

the events. A clearing function is usually provided to reset the counters. In some devices, reprogramming of any parameter or specific parameters (e.g., rate or pacing mode) can result in the automatic clearing of these data. This "initial" or "frozen" recording technique is especially useful for short-term monitoring, as in office-based exercise evaluations. It also allows the system's response to exercise to be evaluated, often without the need for simultaneous ECG monitoring.

The other option is to collect the data continuously. As the counters fill, new data are added at the expense of the oldest data (Fig. 31–12). This has been called a *rolling trend* or *continuous data storage* and is based on the "first in, first out" (FIFO) principle. When the patient is seen in follow-up, the data acquired over the time immediately preceding

the interrogation of the system are available for review. The patient can often recall symptoms and activities during this period. These can be correlated with the behavior of the pacing system at the time of the symptoms. In this manner, the clinical staff caring for the patient may further assess chronotropic function, the behavior of the pacemaker during a variety of special or usual activities, and whether the sensor is behaving appropriately. The clinician may gain insight into the cause of palpitations and other symptoms that may have occurred during this time by correlation of the recorded data and the patient's complaints or activities.[51, 58–62]

Combining sensor-input data with the actual rates that have been achieved has been used to facilitate reprogramming of the sensor parameters. Once acquired, the data from an exercise session are retained in the memory of the programmer, uploaded to the programmer, then displayed on a screen. The system's performance is based on a given set of sensor parameters that were in effect at that time. Because the pacemaker has the actual sensor-signal data, it can calculate how the unit would perform in response to a different set of sensor parameters. If a new set of sensor parameters is entered into the programmer, the curves that are based on the original input data are redrawn to display the system's behavior in response to the new set of parameters. The clinical staff can then determine which are the best set of sensor parameters for the individual patient without having the patient perform repeated activities (Fig. 31–13). This feature has been termed *redraw*,[63] *exercise test,* or *prediction model.*[64]

Limitations of Event Counter Telemetry

The major value of event counters is that they provide a review of system performance over time. This is not available from the real-time diagnostic features of measured data and event counter and EGM telemetry. The data, however, are only interpretable after a detailed assessment of the capture and sensing thresholds in a manner analogous to event marker telemetry. The pacemaker can only store information that it knows about, namely output and sensed events, sensor data, and activation of unique algorithms. If there is a problem with undersensing, the pacemaker releases a pacing pulse, and the counters report a paced rhythm. Similarly, a large number of sensed events may cause the pacemaker to be inhibited on the respective channel. The counter simply reports a large percentage of sensed events, but this may be clinically inappropriate if the cause is oversensing.

With respect to pacing, if the rhythm is predominantly composed of AV- or PV-paced complexes, this does not necessarily indicate complete heart block. It might result from a programmed AV delay that was not sufficiently long to allow for full conduction through the AV node. Although the ventricular complex could have been fully paced, it could also have been a fusion or pseudofusion beat. The counters cannot differentiate between these complexes because the native complex had not yet been sensed, the timer had been completed, and an output was delivered. Another situation would be a total loss of ventricular capture with intact AV nodal conduction (Fig. 31–14). The conducted R wave would not have been sensed because it occurred during the refractory period that followed the ventricular output pulse.

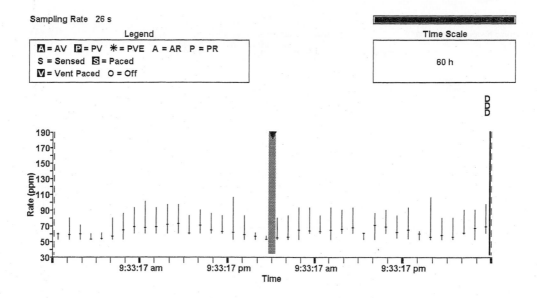

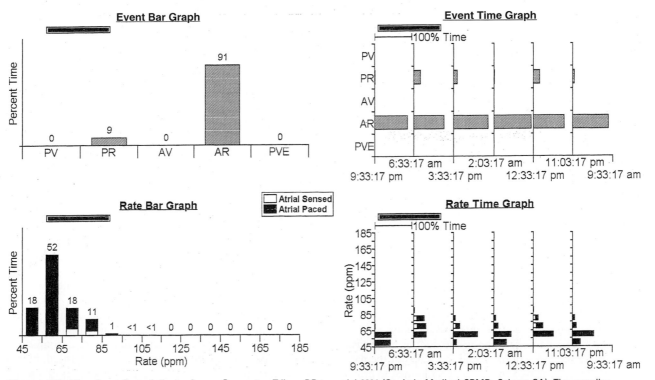

Figure 31–12. Event Record display from a Pacesetter Trilogy DR + model 2364 (St. Jude Medical CRMD, Sylmar, CA). The sampling interval was 26 seconds, which provides a detailed overview of the behavior of the pacing system for the preceding 60 hours. The top display is an overview of the moment-to-moment behavior of the pacing system, with the vertical lines representing the maximum and minimum rates during each time period (the total displayed interval is divided into 40 equal time segments) and with the cross-bar representing the mean heart rate. The vertical line is displayed if there are two or more complexes in the specific time bin. The display scale can be expanded to display individual events, in which case a specific alphanumeric label is shown consistent with the legend in the upper left. The same data may be displayed as an Event Bar Graph equivalent to the Event Histogram, a Rate Bar Graph which is equivalent to the Heart Rate Histogram. The solid bars represent atrial-paced events; hence, atrial rates above the programmed base rate represent sensor drive. Atrial rates below the programmed base rate represent "sleep mode" behavior that had also been programmed. The Time Graphs automatically divide the overall monitoring period into six equal segments.

Pacemaker Model: Medtronic.Kappa KDR401/403
Serial Number: PER101148

Exercise Test Report   Page 1

Exercise Test   Collected: 06/11/98 9:22:20 AM

	During Exercise	CurrentValues *
Mode	DDDR	DDDR
Lower Rate	60 ppm	60 ppm
ADL Rate	90 ppm	90 ppm
Upper Sensor Rate	115 ppm	125 ppm
Upper Tracking Rate	130 ppm	130 ppm
Optimization	On	On
RR Sensor	Integrated	Integrated
ADL Rate Setpoint	11	11
Upper Sensor Rate Setpoint	15	15

* Note: Current values depicted by Exercise Test Graph

Additional Data

Maximum Achieved Rate	108 bpm
Maximum MV Counts	14
Maximum Activity Counts	5

Figure 31–13. Exercise test report from a patient with a Medtronic Kappa KDR model 401 (Medtronic Inc., Minneapolis, MN). The circles represent the actual behavior of the pacing system, with open circles representing atrial-sensed events, solid circles representing atrial-paced events, and shaded circles representing a combination of both sensed and paced events. The thin line represents the behavior of the pacemaker under sensor drive at the current sensor values that had been modeled.

Pacemaker Model: Medtronic.Kappa KDR401/403
Serial Number: PER101148

Exercise Test Report   Page 2

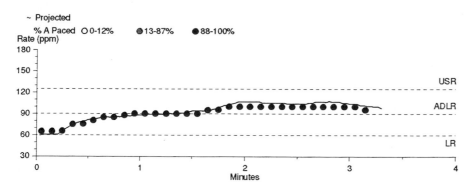

An identical result in the counters would occur with intact AV nodal conduction but with ventricular undersensing.

The event counters simply report the system's performance without making any statement or judgment about the appropriateness of this behavior. The information provided by the event counters can be interpreted only after the programmed parameters are known, the pacing and sensing thresholds have been determined, and the status of the native rhythm is known. If the pacemaker is programmed to provide a good margin of safety for both pacing and sensing, the event counters are likely to be an accurate reflection of the patient's clinical rhythms. This also provides insight into the degree to which the patient requires pacing support at the current programmed parameters, the chronotropic function of the sinus node, and responsiveness of the sensor. Evidence of oversensing or lead dysfunction renders the event counter data suspect with regard to these findings, although a marked

change in the event counter data can provide the clinician with a clue to a developing problem.

The event counter data cannot be adequately interpreted without knowledge of how these data are collected, the clinical status of the patient, and any unique behavioral performance of the implanted pacemaker. This is illustrated by Figure 31–11, which is an atrial high-rate graphic from a Medtronic Thera DR pacemaker. The reported high rates were more than 200 bpm, yet the graphic suggests that these were atrial-paced events at this high rate and that the device is not capable of being programmed to rates this high. It is essential to know how the manufacturer calculates rates. In this case, the device measures the interval between atrial events; if the event preceding the atrial output were an event occurring during the refractory period (labeled AR by the markers), the reported atrial-paced rate would be based on the AR–AP interval. With this knowledge, the graphic report

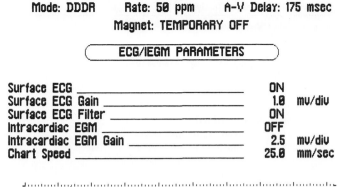

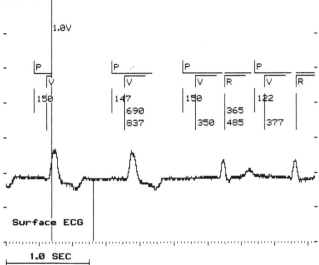

Figure 31–14. Although obtained during a ventricular capture threshold test in a Pacesetter Synchrony II model 2022 dual-chamber pacing system (St. Jude Medical CRMD, Sylmar, CA), this printout demonstrates the limitations of some of the telemetry data in the absence of a simultaneously recorded electrocardiogram (ECG). The last two ventricular output pulses were subthreshold, resulting in a loss of capture. The endogenous P wave conducted, but with a marked first-degree atrioventricular (AV) block, placing the R wave outside the ventricular refractory period that was initiated by the subthreshold ventricular output, thus allowing it to be sensed. Based on event marker and event counter data, this patient would be interpreted as having frequent premature ventricular events (PVEs) interspersed in a stable atrial-sensed ventricular-paced rhythm; however, in actuality, there was a loss of ventricular capture and intact AV nodal conduction. Key programmed and recording parameters are also included with each printout to facilitate its interpretation. EGM, electrogram.

can be understood. If this were not known, it would suggest a pacing system malfunction.

■ PACING SYSTEM MALFUNCTION

Interrogating the pacemaker about programmed parameters, measured data, and retrieval of any and all event count data and the use of the event markers and EGM telemetry capabilities is essential in a routine office-based follow-up evaluation. It is equally important when evaluating a suspected pacing system malfunction. Knowledge of the present programmed settings, combined with the baseline data against which the current results can be compared, is ex-

tremely important. Many devices have special programming features and idiosyncrasies that may appear to be malfunctions to clinicians not completely familiar with the particular system under scrutiny. It is not unusual to hear about devices being explanted and returned to the manufacturer for failure to pace at the programmed rate, only to find that hysteresis had been enabled. The latter is but one of many examples of pseudomalfunctions, which are discussed in greater detail later.[65–69] The remainder of this chapter focuses on a discussion of pacing system malfunction.

Historical Clues

The first step in the evaluation of the patient with a suspected pacing system problem is to gather as much information about the patient as is possible (Table 31–1). This includes the indications for the pacemaker, the operative record of the implantation, the model and possibly serial numbers of all portions of the implanted pacing system, the current programmed parameters, and any and all measured data. The programmed parameters and measured data are absolutely crucial to the correct evaluation of the device.

Even in the current high-technology environment of cardiac pacing, the history and physical examination continue to be important. The patient should be asked about symptoms relating to potential device malfunction. These include presyncope, syncope, palpitations, slow or fast pulse rates, pain or erythema around the implanted devices, fevers, chills, night sweats, and extracardiac stimulation. It is also important to obtain any history of trauma to the area where the device is located, exposure to intense electromagnetic signals or therapeutic radiation, use of electrocautery or defibrillation (internal or external), programming changes by other medical personnel, or exposure to environmental extremes.

Information related to the actual implantation procedure can be important with respect to making clinical decisions. If the implanting physician was unable to obtain an adequate

Table 31–1. Evaluation of the Patient With a Potential Pacing System Malfunction

Know the Patient
    Cardiac and noncardiac diagnoses
    Exposure to environmental extremes
    Exposure to sources of electromagnetic interference
    Programming changes performed by others
Know the Pacemaker
    Manufacturer
    Model and serial number
    Alerts or recalls
    Current programmed settings
    Device idiosyncrasies
    Mode and algorithm indiosyncrasies
Know the Leads
    Manufacturer
    Model and serial number
    Alerts or recalls
    Connector type
    Polarity
    Insulation material
    Fixation mechanism
    Radiographic appearance

EGM in the atrium for sensing, then atrial undersensing of P waves by the device would be expected. Knowledge of such a situation might prevent a second futile operation for the patient. Another common situation occurs with unusual radiographic findings. What may appear to be a lead dislodgment might actually be the intentional site of placement because of poor sensing or capture thresholds in the "standard" location. In addition, ventricular leads are being implanted with increasing frequency in areas other than the right ventricular (RV) apex. These areas include the RV outflow tract, RV septum, and coronary sinus. Thus, an otherwise stable and normal system might be interpreted as a potential problem resulting in an inappropriate intervention in the absence of this crucial historical information.

The full analysis of a suspected pacing system malfunction is facilitated by access to telemetry and programming information, allowing a detailed noninvasive evaluation. Despite this, an invasive evaluation may sometimes be required (Tables 31–2 and 31–3). The model numbers of the pulse generator and leads should be determined before proceeding with an invasive evaluation of the system because there may be unique device eccentricities that are known to the manufacturer and reflect normal function, or unique tools or replacement devices may be required. Hence, before an operative intervention for an unexpected behavior in an otherwise clinically stable patient, the manufacturer's technical service group should be contacted.

With respect to a noninvasive system evaluation followed by subsequent programming, serious errors may occur in the absence of full knowledge of the programmed parameters, measured data, and clinical information. Although most patients carry an identification card that identifies the pulse generator and lead models and serial numbers, this does not provide the current programmed settings. If the patient has had more than one device implanted, it is important to determine whether the identification card is the most recent one. Many patients like to keep their old and invalid identi-

Table 31–3. Invasive Analysis

Visual Inspection
  Connector
  Set-screws
  Grommets
  Insulation
  Conductor
  Suturing sleeve
Measurements
  Capture threshold
    Strength–duration curve
    Evoked-response amplitude
    Polarization amplitude
  Sensing threshold
    Pacing system analyzer measurement
      Peak-to-peak amplitude
      Slew rate
    Electrogram recording
  Stimulation impedance

fication cards as mementos of their previous pacemakers. If chronic leads had been reused, the data relating to the leads may or may not be on the new card for the pulse generator, yet a large percentage of pacemaker problems are the result of lead malfunction. Certain leads are less reliable than others, and there have been multiple recalls and alerts regarding leads, making such information vital.

In that the observed system problem may be due to a lead malfunction, an electrode–tissue interface problem, or the manner in which the pacemaker was programmed for the individual patient, it is prudent to think about this as a system. Rather than labeling an observed abnormal behavior as a pacemaker malfunction, it should be termed a *pacing system malfunction,* which expands the focus of the evaluation from the pulse generator to all components of the system.

In the absence of an identification card, model and serial number information may be obtained from the operative report or from adhesive labels (provided with each pulse generator and lead) if they had been included in the medical record at the time of implantation. Finally, if none of these is available, a radiograph of the patient, including the area of the pulse generator, allows the clinician to match the identification label inside the pulse generator to those in a reference source (Fig. 31–15).[70–72] Although not all pulse generators have these labels, many have a distinct radiographic "skeleton" or radiopaque alphanumeric labels from which the clinician can determine the name of the manufacturer if not the model. All manufacturers provide toll-free numbers that the clinician may call to obtain further information regarding the pulse generator and the leads that are implanted.

Increasing numbers of manufacturers' programmers and devices are capable of automatically identifying the model and serial number of the pacemaker. Certain pulse generators are also capable of storing data concerning the patient, implantation date, and lead model (see Fig. 31–1). These data need to be downloaded into the pacemaker by the clinician or support staff. If the pacemaker and programmer have this capability, the programmer provides much of the data necessary for finding additional patient data. It may be

Table 31–2. Noninvasive Testing

Office Evaluation
  Multichannel rhythm strips or 12-lead electrocardiogram
  Pulse generator interrogation
    Programmed parameters
    Measured data—lead and battery function
    Event counters
    Rhythm monitoring with telemetered electrograms
    Event markers
  Pacing system evaluation
    Capture threshold assessment
    Sensing threshold assessment
    Sensor evaluation
    Special algorithm evaluation
    Provocative maneuvers
Ancillary Testing
  Posteroanterior and lateral chest radiographs
    Fluoroscopy
  Continuous rhythm monitoring
    Telemetry
    Holter monitoring
    Event or transient arrhythmia monitoring
Transtelephonic monitoring

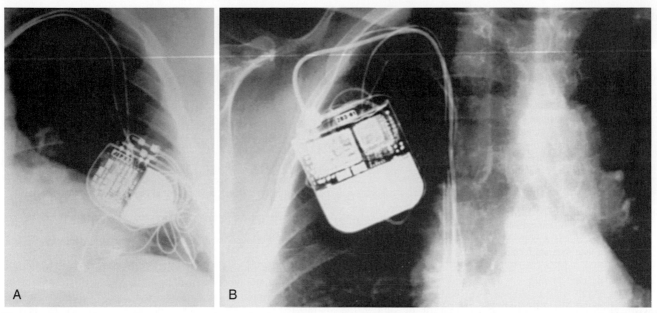

Figure 31–15. *A* and *B*, Roentgenograms of two pulse generators showing radiopaque identification tags. Some units may not have this helpful feature, but they can still be identified by the appearance of their unique radiographic "skeletons." Also note that the leads exit the connector block of the pulse generator in a clockwise direction, indicating that the pulse generator is properly situated with the anode facing the subcutaneous tissue. On panel *A*, also note that the terminal pins of the leads extend through the set-screw connector block, indicating that they are properly and fully inserted into the pulse generator connector. One cannot determine, however, if the set-screw is fully secured based on the radiograph. *A*, Medtronic (Minneapolis, MN); *B*, Sulzer Intermedics (Angleton, TX).

possible to obtain further information from the manufacturer's patient tracking database. Finally, pulse generators often have a characteristic magnet response signature that can be recorded on an ECG strip, which may provide clues to the manufacturer or model. The clinician should never "blindly" interrogate a device without knowing at least the name of the manufacturer. Unexpected and possibly disastrous reprogramming results have been reported when one manufacturer's programmer was used on another manufacturer's pacemaker.

Knowing the specifics about the implanted pacing system's components is a crucial first step. It is also important to know what, if any, special considerations apply to the device. These might include recalls, alerts, known idiosyncrasies, and the functions of specialized programmable features and rate-modulation sensors.[73–79] Any of these items may affect the observed behavior and guide the further evaluation of the system as well as any decisions regarding parameter adjustment. For example, a pulse generator that is exhibiting its elective replacement parameters would typically be replaced using the same lead system if the latter had a good capture threshold, a good sensing threshold, and a normal stimulation impedance. If it is known that the lead is under a safety alert or recall, however, the clinician should follow recommended guidelines and, when appropriate, replace the vulnerable lead system at the time of generator replacement. There have been patients who required a second operation to revise another element of the pacing system simply because the implanting physician was unaware of previously reported potential product deficiencies.

Virtually every device may exhibit idiosyncratic behavior that may be mistaken for malfunctions. In addition, functional undersensing as a result of a variety of normal refractory and blanking periods, pauses due to normal hysteresis, a change in the spontaneous functional behavior of the pacemaker as with automatic mode switching, rate-drop response, and endless-loop tachycardia (ELT) prevention and termination algorithms are but a few examples of features that may cause confusion if the clinician is not aware of these capabilities.

Physical Examination and Telemetry

After the history has been obtained and the pacemaker system's specifics are known, the patient should be examined. The implantation site is examined for proper healing; erosion of suture material, leads, or the generator; erythema; hematoma; seroma; excessive pain on palpation; evidence of trauma; pocket stimulation; device mobility; and generator displacement.

The precordium is inspected for chest wall or diaphragmatic stimulation. The presence of the latter may indicate a number of possible problems (Table 31–4). If the system is unipolar, the pacemaker may have the anode facing the skeletal muscle or be considered to be upside down in the pocket. The malpositioning of a pacemaker sitting upside down in the pocket may have occurred inadvertently at implantation, may have developed spontaneously (most commonly in conjunction with lax subcutaneous tissues), or may have resulted from the patient manipulating the pacemaker within the pocket, a condition known as *twiddler's syndrome*.[80–84] Alternatively, the unidirectional insulated coating on the pulse generator or the grommets protecting the set-screws may have been damaged or may have degraded over time. In some situations, pocket stimulation may occur even with the generator in the correct position and the insulation

Table 31–4. **Causes of Extracardiac Stimulation**

Improper Lead Position
Gastric vein
Cardiac vein
Diaphragmatic Stimulation
Lead in cardiac vein
Thin right ventricular wall combined with high output
Myocardial perforation
Lead position near phrenic nerve
Active fixation lead—right atrium
Lead withdrawal to innominate vein and superior vena cava
Pacemaker Pocket Stimulation
Delamination of insulating coating
Device movement (twiddler's syndrome)
Device inserted in pocket upside down
Unipolar output configuration at high output
Irritable skeletal muscles—low stimulation threshold
Breach of lead external insulation

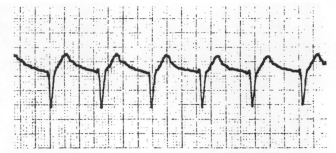

Figure 31–16. An electrocardiographic rhythm strip of a patient with 100% ventricular pacing. The pace artifact is not readily identified as a result of the small electrical potential generated by the bipolar pacing polarity.

intact.[85] High-output settings, placement in or below the pectoral musculature, or high-current delivery as a result of low lead impedance may be at fault. Outer lead insulation failure may also allow problematic current leakage and local extracardiac muscle stimulation.

The neck veins should be evaluated for distention or the presence of cannon A waves. The latter might indicate an atrial lead problem, inappropriate programming in a dual-chamber system with too long or short an AV delay assuming otherwise normal electrical function, or the pacemaker syndrome in a single-chamber system. Auscultation of the heart for variable intensity heart sounds, rubs, or gallops may also give clues to the physiology related to the patient–device interaction.[86, 87]

Physical maneuvers may be useful to unmask an intermittent symptom or malfunction during an examination. Carotid sinus massage and other vagal maneuvers may slow the intrinsic rhythm so that device function or malfunction becomes evident. Positional changes (sitting or standing up) or having the patient perform in-place exercise or isometric maneuvers may accelerate the heart rate to allow observation for sensing (proper tracking and inhibition). Manipulation of the device and lead may disclose an intermittent lead fracture, loose connection, or insulation failure that was not evident while the patient was lying quietly on the examination table. Other helpful maneuvers include movement of the patient's ipsilateral arm (reaching overhead or reaching behind the back), isometric exercise (pressing hands together in front of the chest or reaching around the chest to scratch the opposite side), and doing sit-ups in the case of an abdominal implant are helpful in identifying an intermittent problem.[88, 89] If the patient develops symptoms during the induced abnormal behavior, and these symptoms reproduce those that occurred spontaneously, there is a high likelihood that the cause of the symptoms has been identified.

A 12-lead ECG is required to document the pacemaker-evoked morphology of the atrial and ventricular depolarizations at baseline. It may then be helpful to repeat a 12-lead or at least multiple-lead ECG, instead of a single-lead rhythm strip, when evaluating a suspected malfunction. A myocardial infarction or progressive cardiomyopathy may have occurred, resulting in a change of capture or sensing thresholds.

A change in the paced QRS axis may be a clue to lead dislodgment, whereas a change in the intrinsic axis (a new bundle-branch block) may be associated with sensing problems. Multiple leads are frequently necessary to recognize the relatively low-amplitude atrial depolarization. In addition, the pacing artifact may not be visible in any given lead, especially if the pacing system is bipolar[90] (Figs. 31–16 and 31–17). Care should be taken in the interpretation of the ECG tracing with regard to the type of recording system used. The older-style analog systems provide a consistent reproduction of the pacing stimulus, varying the relative amplitude of the stimulus with the delivered energy of the system. An unstable paced artifact on an analog ECG is a sign of potential problems. The same cannot be said for digital recording systems, which have generally replaced the older-generation analog systems. Although these allow computer interpretation of the ECG, they can introduce a multiplicity of artifacts and have several idiosyncrasies that have been misinterpreted as a device malfunction when it was actually a recording system artifact (Fig. 31–18).[90–96]

After the baseline ECG rhythm strip is obtained, it should be closely inspected for any abnormalities of rate, sensing, loss of capture, or change in paced axis. A tracing with the magnet applied to the pulse generator should also be performed. This provides information about the status of the battery and, if the device were otherwise inhibited, allows for a quick assessment of capture and whether the output was being delivered to the appropriate chamber. If no output

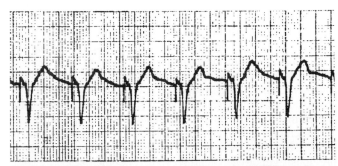

Figure 31–17. Electrocardiographic rhythm strip of a patient with 100% ventricular pacing. The pace artifact is easily identified because of the large electrical potential generated by the unipolar pacing polarity.

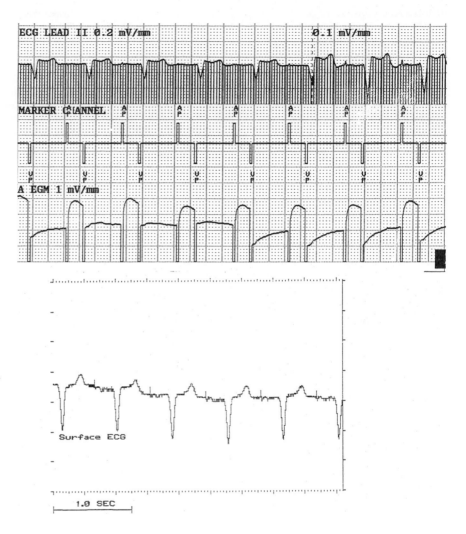

Prodigy DR 7860/61/62   8/06/98   9:08
CHART SPEED 25.0 mm/s

Figure 31–18. Recording of the same rhythm with two different systems. The cause of the high-frequency artifact was never identified but was amplified by the design of the Medtronic 9790 programmer when evaluating a patient with a Prodigy DR 7860 pacemaker (Medtronic Inc., Minneapolis, MN). The simultaneous event markers identify atrial pacing followed by ventricular pacing. The paced output saturates the telemetry amplifier for the atrial electrogram. The electrocardiogram (ECG) cable was disconnected from the electrodes, and the Pacesetter APS II model 3003 programmer (St. Jude Medical CRMD, Sylmar, CA) was connected to these same electrodes and used as a monitor for the pacing system evaluation. The ECG display in the APS II programmer uses analog recording technology without any artificial amplification of high-frequency transients. Hence, the bipolar outputs are small on the atrial channel and even smaller, such that they are not visualized, on the ventricular channel in this specific lead that was being monitored.

is seen during application of the magnet, several possibilities should be considered: the battery may be depleted, the device may be nonfunctional, or an open circuit (such as a lead fracture) may be present. In some models, the magnet response is programmable to be turned on or off. If the magnet function is disabled, placement of a magnet over it does not result in an overt change in its demand behavior. Alternatively, the magnet may not have been positioned properly, the reed switch may be stuck open, or an inappropriate magnet may have been used.

The magnet function of each device is unique with regard to the rate and mode of response. This may differ by manufacturer, model, and programmed mode of the pacemaker. The magnet response may also be programmable not only to whether a response will occur but also to the type of response. The clinician should not assume that a DDD device will exhibit a DOO response to application of the magnet. Some earlier generations of Cordis DDD devices responded with asynchronous behavior during the atrial escape interval such that an atrial output would always be delivered but

with restoration of sensing during the effective AV delay, whereas other devices would revert to the VOO mode at rates that may be significantly different from the programmed base rate. If there are questions about the appropriate response to magnet application, the physician's manual that is supplied with the pacemaker, other reference sources, or the manufacturer should be consulted to determine the expected response.

In pacemakers capable of telemetry or communication, programmed settings should be both retrieved and printed.[97, 98] The latter is important because it documents the initial settings and serves as a reference in case the clinician wishes to restore the device to the same settings when the evaluation is complete. If measured telemetry is available, these data should be requested and printed. The same recommendation holds for models that have extensive histograms, trend data, or other diagnostic counters. If the settings are routinely retrieved at the beginning of the evaluation, the various programming changes that may be required during the evaluation and that may cause the clearing of these counters do not result in the loss of these critical data. Indeed, on completion of this task, the counters should be cleared so that they reflect the subsequent behavior of the implanted pacing system in response to any changes made by the end of the evaluation.

When reviewing the results of the interrogation, an evaluation of the programmed setting data should be the first step. What are the mode and base rate? Are any special algorithms enabled? Many suspected device malfunctions have been eliminated once the programmed parameters are known. These may have been changed by another medical professional since the last evaluation, accounting for the concern. This has been referred to as *phantom reprogramming*, which most often is caused by another physician who did not notify the physician responsible for following the patient of the changes made to the pacemaker. Depletion of the battery may also cause a change in the mode, rate, or other parameters. Other causes of mode changes are listed in Table 31–5. Some dual-chamber devices change to a single-chamber mode to conserve power when the battery's voltage drops below a manufacturer-defined value. In other devices, the sensor, data storage, and telemetry may be disabled to slow the rate of battery depletion in an effort to protect the patient from a no-output state.

In cold climates and high altitudes, new devices that are shipped or transported may cool sufficiently to allow the

Table 31–5. Causes of Apparent Mode and Parameter Changes

Programming
Special Algorithms
  Upper rate behavior
    Wenckebach
    Fixed block
    Fallback
    Rate smoothing
  Base-rate behavior
    Sensor drive
    Hysteresis
    Sudden rate-drop response
    Sleep or rest mode
    Postventricular atrial refractory period extension post–premature
      ventricular contraction algorithms
  Automatic mode switch algorithms
  Functional AAI[R] pacing
    Autointrinsic conduction search
    DDD/AMC
  Pacemaker-mediated tachycardia prevention and termination algorithms
  Lead surveillance and configuration change
Battery Depletion
  Recommended replacement time indicator
  End-of-life indicator
Stuck Reed Switch (DOO, VOO, AOO)
Electromagnetic Interference
  Electrocautery
  Cardioversion and defibrillation
    External
    Internal
  Airport security systems
  Electronic article surveillance
  Cellular telephone
  Magnetic resonance imaging
Cold

Table 31–6. Causes of Rate Change

Programming
  DDD mode with atrial-paced ventricular-sensed complex pacing in
    ventricular-based timing system
  Sensor drive
  P-wave tracking modes (DDD, VDD)
    Sinus
    Atrial tachyarrhythmias
  Triggered modes
  Special algorithms
    Rate hysteresis
    Overdrive algorithms
  Rate smoothing
Circuit Failures
  Runaway
Recording Artifacts
  Paper or tape speed errors
  Pulse enhancement artifact
Rate Slowing
  Sensed premature (ectopic) beats
  Hysteresis
  Oversensing
  Open circuit
  Battery depletion
Rate Acceleration—Malfunction
  Crosstalk—ventricular based timing
  Inappropriate sensor drive
    Pressure on piezocrystal sensor
    Hyperventilation—minute ventilation sensor
  Runaway malfunction

battery's voltage to drop, triggering elective replacement behavior even though the device is new. Normal function either spontaneously returns or can be reset using the programmer once the device has warmed up to at least room temperature. Attempting to accelerate the warming of the pulse generator by placement in an oven may damage the pacemaker. Electrocautery and defibrillation can cause mode and polarity changes to occur on some models and may also trigger the elective replacement indicator of the pacemaker. Pacing rate changes may also occur for many other reasons (Table 31–6). Thus, any assumption about the expected operating characteristics of a device cannot be made without the knowledge of the mode and rate.

After the mode and rate have been verified, an evaluation of the remaining programmed parameters is appropriate. The identified output, pulse width, sensitivity, and refractory periods should be reviewed for each channel and correlated with the ECG. The presence and status of any special programmable features should be checked. The latter includes rate-modulation behavior, ELT prevention and termination algorithms, hysteresis, search hysteresis, time-of-day–dependent or circadian sensor–based rate changes, rate-adaptive AV delay, differential paced and sensed AV delay, rate smoothing, and others. An evaluation of the device's function in relation to all programmed data is performed by comparing the programmed data with ECG and event counter data. In many cases, the event counter diagnostics may minimize if not eliminate the requirement for routine screening Holter monitor studies.

The measured data are reviewed.[5, 44, 99] Lead or stimulation impedance is one of the most important elements of the measured data. Proper interpretation of lead impedance, however, is dependent on the manufacturer and model of the lead used, the method of measurement, and the historical values of an individual lead's impedance. The other parameters of the lead's performance, including pulse voltage, pulse charge, pulse energy, and current, should also be correlated with the measured impedance and internal consistency assessed. A marked discrepancy between observed and expected values may identify a telemetry error or measurement error within the pacemaker rather than a primary problem with the lead. It is prudent to repeat the measurements several times if a conflict is noted.[15]

Another important data set that may be available measures the battery's status. This can include a measured magnet rate; measured base-rate pacing; projected longevity; elective replacement indicator or status message; and the voltage, impedance, and mean current drain of the battery. The latter measurement may be useful to corroborate the measured data from the lead. If the mean current drain remains unchanged, despite a major change in the lead's impedance or current, then a telemetry or measurement error should be suspected. Normal mean current drains vary greatly among generator models, the lead system implanted, and the programmed settings. Once again, tracking these data over time provides the greatest clinical benefit.

After the telemetry and measured data are obtained and reviewed, a meticulous assessment of the pacing and sensing thresholds is warranted. A complete threshold evaluation should be performed for each lead present. Marked changes in capture or sensing thresholds may imply a malfunction of a lead or of the lead–tissue interface when lead impedance values are stable. Other causes of both permanent and transient increases in threshold are discussed subsequently.

If a pacing system problem is suspected, posteroanterior and lateral chest radiographs should be obtained. It is usually best to request a slightly overpenetrated exposure to visualize the intracardiac segment of the pacing leads for position and integrity. Requesting a thoracic spine exposure technique provides optimal penetration for visualization of the pacing leads. The film should be inspected for evidence of conductor disruption, insulation failure as inferred from a deformity in the conductor coil because the insulation is radiolucent (Fig. 31–19), proper lead placement in the generator connector block, adequate slack in the lead system, electrode perforation, dislodgment or malposition of a lead, generator movement, and proper orientation of the coated side of the can positioned against the muscle (i.e., leads exiting in a clockwise direction, except in devices specifically designed for implantation on the left side of the chest; see Fig. 31–15).[100] The latter is especially important when evaluating pocket stimulation in unipolar systems. The fact that some new pacemakers and most implantable cardioverter defibrillators are constructed such that the leads exit in a counterclockwise manner may confuse this issue. Knowledge of the construction of the specific device in question is essential to establishing the proper diagnosis. Close attention should be paid to the infraclavicular area, where pressure from the clavicle and first rib may cause lead failure (see Chapter 4).[101–115]

On occasion, a fluoroscopic evaluation of the patient may be useful. This shows many of the mechanical or positional problems and defects listed earlier. It also provides a dynamic view of the lead system, facilitating identification of

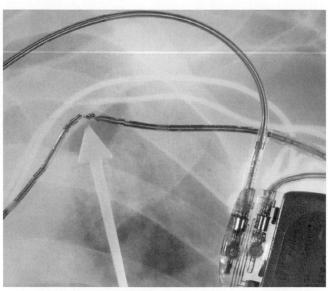

Figure 31–19. Focused view of a posteroanterior chest radiograph showing attenuation of the ventricular lead where it crosses between the clavicle and the first rib. Superimposed on this radiograph is the explanted pulse generator and both atrial and ventricular leads. The attenuation of the conductor coil visualized on the radiograph is associated with a marked disruption of the insulation and conductor coil of the explanted lead at this position, although the extraction process itself may have contributed to some of the disruption of the lead, exacerbating the abnormality seen on the radiograph. In some cases, overlapping leads or leads overlying other structures may make it difficult to visualize a deformity of the conductor coil. If a problem is suspected, multiple views, including oblique and lordotic views, using either standard radiograph techniques or fluoroscopy may be required.

excessive electrode movement consistent with an unstable lead, or there may be insufficient slack with respiratory movement placing traction on the lead and tension at the electrode–tissue interface. Either of these would provide an explanation for an intermittent capture or sensing problem.

Differential Diagnosis of Pacing System Malfunction

Although many pacing system malfunctions are common to single-chamber and dual-chamber devices, the latter present a greater challenge. The section that follows deals with problems seen in both single-chamber and dual-chamber devices. The subsequent section deals with problems unique to dual-chamber devices.

Failure of Output (No Artifact Present)

In the pacemaker-dependent patient, failure to pace represents a potentially catastrophic and lethal situation. The ECG appearance in a single-chamber system is that of no pacing artifact, with an intrinsic rate below the lower rate limit of the device. This may be intermittent or continuous. In a dual-chamber device, the clinician may see an atrial pace alone, ventricular pace alone, or no pacing artifacts at all. The latter may be entirely normal, depending on the patient's sinus rate, AV nodal conduction, AV interval settings, enabling of hysteresis or one of its analogs such as sleep mode

Table 31-7. **Failure to Pace (No Output or Rate Slowing)**

Normal System Function	**Open Circuit**
Hysteresis	Conductor (lead) fracture
Sleep or rest mode	Failure to tighten set-screw
Postventricular atrial refractory period extension after	Failure to insert lead fully in connector block
premature ventricular contraction	Component malfunction
Oversensing	Incompatible lead and pulse generator
Electromagnetic interference (see Table 31–8)	Air in pocket—unipolar pulse generator
Inappropriate physiologic signals	Pacemaker not in pocket—unipolar pulse generator
Myopotentials	**Battery Depletion**
T waves	**Recording Artifact**
Afterpotentials	Isoelectric ectopic beats—properly sensed
Far-field signals	Isoelectric paced beats
Make-break signals	Rapid recording speed—longer interval between complexes
Internal insulation failure	
Lead chatter	
Partial conductor fracture	
Crosstalk—in the presence of atrioventricular block	
Safety pacing either not available or disabled	

or rate drop response, and sensor settings. The causes of a no-output condition are listed in Table 31–7. In evaluating this situation, the clinician must be certain that a malfunction truly exists before taking any corrective action. Remember that the ECG (especially as visualized in a single-surface lead) may not display the pacing artifact because of technical factors (Fig. 31–20). This is particularly common in bipolar systems and systems programmed to a lower-than-nominal

voltage output. It is important to recognize that the problem may be failure to capture rather than failure to output. Access to telemetered event markers and measured data facilitates the evaluation. Event markers identify the release of an output pulse or recycling resulting from a sensed event, even if not visualized on the ECG. If lead impedance is normal (with the previously noted caveat that the problem may be intermittent and multiple measurements should be obtained),

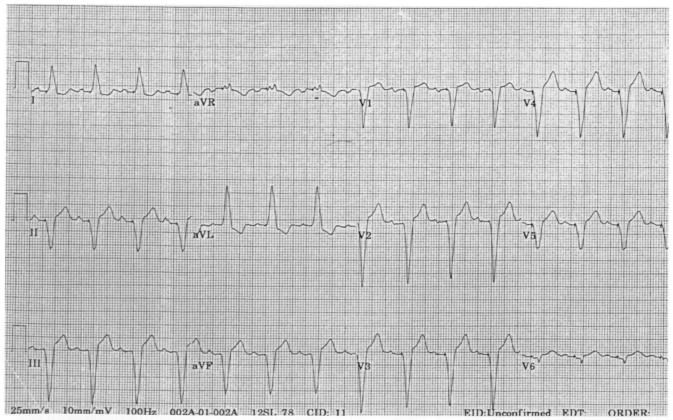

Figure 31-20. A 12-lead electrocardiogram of a patient with a normally functioning bipolar pacing system. Note that a small pace artifact is seen in lead V4, whereas other leads do not show it at all.

this probably reflects a capture problem if there is an output or an oversensing problem if there is a sensed event. If the impedance is high, it favors an open circuit, whereas a low impedance suggests an insulation failure, both probable mechanical problems with the lead, particularly if the lead is coaxial bipolar.

If the markers fail to demonstrate either an ineffective output or an inappropriate sensed event, consider normal function such as hysteresis. At this point, double check the programmed parameters to determine whether hysteresis or one of its analogs had been programmed. Pacemakers have been returned to their manufacturers as defective when hysteresis was enabled. In these cases, the physician was either not aware of the programming or did not understand this feature.[112–114] Other causes of intermittent prolongation of the pacing interval are listed in Table 31–7.

Another source of evaluation error is failure to recognize intrinsic complexes that are present and are properly sensed, causing an appropriate device inhibition. This problem is not uncommon in the hospital's telemetry unit, in which only a single lead is monitored. Premature beats may be present, with the ectopic complexes appearing nearly isoelectric (Fig. 31–21). Although the observer may not recognize the PVC or premature atrial contraction (PAC) on casual observation, the pacemaker senses these events and is appropriately inhibited. The use of multiple leads or a 12-lead ECG recording virtually eliminates this cause of pseudomalfunction.

The lack of an output pulse, most commonly in unipolar systems, is frequently caused by oversensing. The pacemaker, for all of its complexity, operates from a relatively simple set of rules. Any event that generates an electrical signal of adequate strength and frequency content and occurs during the alert period is sensed and resets the timing cycle. Oversensing is the sensing of a physiologically inappropriate or nonphysiologic signal. A cause of intracardiac oversensing in AAI systems is the sensing of the far-field QRS complex[116] (Fig. 31–22). This is most common in unipolar systems when the lead is placed in close proximity to the tricuspid valve, with high sensitivity settings, and with short atrial refractory periods. In systems that can deliver antitachycardia pacing therapy, oversensing may result in an inappropriate diagnosis of a tachycardia and therapy delivery.[117] Far-field sensing is uncommon in VVI systems because of the diminutive size of the P wave, as seen electrically from the ventricle, although this too has been reported,

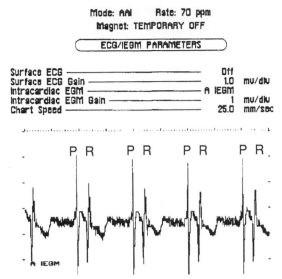

Figure 31–22. An intracardiac electrogram (IEGM) recorded from a unipolar atrial lead. Note the large size of the far-field ventricular electrogram (EGM) (R). If the near-field atrial EGM (P) was not as large, the device could undersense the atrium, sensing the ventricular EGM in error. ECG, electrocardiogram.

usually associated with other problems such as an insulation abrasion on the atrial portion of the ventricular lead.[15] Sensing of the intracardiac T wave may occur in VVI systems with similar results (Fig. 31–23), although this was a more common problem in the early days of pacing, as was the polarization artifact generated by the output pulse. Chapters 1 and 3 provide a description of polarization and the evoked response. Oversensing of this event occurred with short refractory periods combined with high outputs on certain lead systems and has also been reported in ICD systems that require short refractory periods and broad bandpass filters in the sense amplifier.

The most common source of a physiologic extracardiac signal that causes oversensing is myopotential inhibition. The pacemaker is capable of sensing muscle depolarizations of not only the heart but also noncardiac structures, such as the pectoralis, rectus abdominis, and diaphragmatic muscles. Myopotential inhibition of pacemaker output can be seen during arm movements (prepectoral implantation) or when the patient sits up (abdominal implantation; Fig. 31–24).

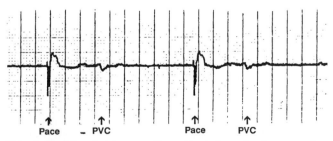

Figure 31–21. An electrocardiographic rhythm strip of a pacemaker programmed to VVI with a demand rate of 50 bpm. This appears to show an inappropriate bradycardia. Note the low-amplitude waves that map out to the escape interval. These are premature ventricular contractions (PVCs) that appeared almost isoelectric in this lead.

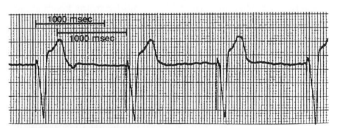

Figure 31–23. Electrocardiographic rhythm strip of a device programmed VVI at 60 bpm. T-wave oversensing is present. The last sensed event can always be determined by mapping back by the escape interval.

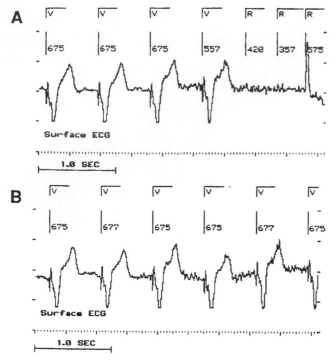

Figure 31–24. *A*, An electrocardiogram (ECG) rhythm strip showing inappropriate inhibition caused by myopotential oversensing. *B*, An ECG rhythm strip of the same pacing system with a magnet placed over the pulse generator. If a loss of output was still evident with the magnet on, then the problem is not likely to be oversensing.

This primarily occurs in unipolar systems because the anode is the pacemaker's case, which remains in close proximity to these muscular structures.[88, 89, 118–124] Nonphysiologic electrical signals may also cause oversensing. Formerly, electromagnetic interference (EMI) from microwave ovens was a significant problem when pacemakers were encased in plastic or epoxy, with the net relatively large antenna created by the discrete components. Newer devices are shielded from EMI by their metal cases and filters and smaller antenna due to integrated circuits, although strong EMI sources can still cause oversensing. A summary of EMI sources and their potential effects is presented in Table 31–8.[125–142]

It has been well documented that intermittent metal-to-metal contact can create electrical signals. These make-break signals may be of sufficient amplitude to be detected by pacing systems. Signals exceeding 25 mV have been recorded in some cases (Fig. 31–25). The latter presents a major problem because this false signal cannot be managed by programming a lower sensitivity, the nonphysiologic signal being far greater than the physiologic atrial or ventricular depolarization. The sources of these electrical signals include a loose set-screw, fracture of the conductor coil, failed insulation between the anodal and cathodal conductors in a bipolar system, interaction between an active and abandoned pacing electrodes, and a loose retractable fixation screw.[142–150] There are studies under way at this time to investigate the origin of these signals because there may be other mechanisms operating in addition to the make-break phenomenon.

Oversensing need not result in pacing system inhibition. In the dual-chamber mode, if oversensing occurs on the atrial channel, it can result in ventricular pacing in response to this false P wave, which, in the patient who is susceptible to retrograde conduction, can precipitate an ELT. If the pacemaker were programmed to the triggered mode (which is one way to manage an oversensing problem that cannot be safely eliminated by reducing the programmed sensitivity), there would be periods of irregular pacing at a rate exceeding the programmed base rate in the presence of oversensing.

Oversensing can be confirmed by use of the magnet or by reprogramming to an asynchronous mode. If the cause of the pauses or slow rate is oversensing, regular pacing resumes during asynchronous pacing. If a lead failure, open circuit, or other cause of no output exists, then this maneuver does not result in asynchronous pacing. The use of intracardiac EGMs and event marker telemetry can quickly identify the cause of the pause, whether it is an output pulse that failed to reach the heart or the presence of oversensing. In the case of oversensing, the telemetered EGM may provide a clue to the source of the extraneous signal. This is useful for differentiating the causes of oversensing and thus deciding on the proper remedy (see Fig. 31–24). The normal refractory period timing cycle initiated by the oversensing may give the overt appearance of undersensing because the native complex that coincides with the electrocardiographically invisible refractory period is not sensed (normal behavior), allowing for time-out of the pacing escape interval and delivery of an output pulse; this is termed *functional undersensing* (see Fig. 31–3). The output pulse, if delivered during a period of physiologic refractoriness initiated by the native cardiac depolarization, may not capture, a phenomenon appropriately termed *functional noncapture*. The true cause of the observed behavior is readily appreciated with telemetered event markers but may be otherwise difficult to decipher from the free-standing ECG or rhythm strip.

Primary component failure of the pulse generator circuit is the least common of all the causes of pacing system failure, but it too can result in failure to output (Table 31–9). Patients who had been lost to follow-up may present with complete exhaustion of the power source (battery) and a virtually dead system. As the power source begins to fail, slowing of the pacing rate and erratic behavior may occur (Fig. 31–26). The latter may also be associated with mode and rate changes with or without sensing problems.

Several problems may be mistaken for pulse generator failure, resulting in a no-output situation. These are generally related to problems at the time of implantation. If the lead is not positioned properly in the connector block of the pacemaker, or if an improper lead is used, the electrical connection may not be complete. This is still an open circuit, but in the presence of a technically normal pulse generator and normal lead, the two are simply not connected appropriately, which is a physician error at the time of implantation. A transient situation has been reported in unipolar systems after wound closure. It is possible for air to be present in the pocket, especially when a large generator is replaced by a smaller one. Air is an effective insulator and prevents contact of the anterior anodal surface of the pacemaker's case with the body's tissues. This results in an incomplete circuit until the air is absorbed. Subcutaneous emphysema has also been reported to be responsible for loss of anodal contact.[151, 152] A similar pseudofailure occurs when a unipolar

Table 31–8. **Causes of Potential Electromagnetic Interference**

Source	Pacer Damage	Total Inhibition	One-Beat Inhibition	Asynchrony Noise	Rate Increase	Unipolar/Bipolar
Ablation	Y	Y	N	N	Y	U/B
Antitheft device	N	N	Y	N	N	U
Arc welder	N	Y	Y	Y	N	U/B
Cardiokymography	N	Y	Y	N	Y	U/B
Cardioversion	Y	N	N	N	N	U/B
Citizen's band radio	N	N	Y	N	N	U
Defibrillation	Y	N	N	N	N	U/B
Dental scaler	N	N	Y*	Y*	Y§	U
Diathermy	Y	Y	Y	Y	Y	U/B
Electroconvulsive therapy	N	Y	Y	Y	Y§	U
Electric blanket	N	N	N	Y†	N	U
Electric power tools	N	N	N	Y§	N	U
Electric shaver	N	N	Y§	N	N	U
Electric switch	N	N	Y*	N	N	U
Electric toothbrush	N	N	Y	N	N	U
Electrocautery	N	N	Y*	N	N	U
Electrolysis	Y	Y	Y	Y	Y§	U/B
Electronic Article Surveillance	N	Y	Y	Y	Y	U/B
Electrotome	N	N	Y	Y	N	U
Ham radio	N	N	Y*	N	N	U
Heating pad	N	N	Y	N	N	U
Lithotripsy	Y§	Y*	Y*	Y*	Y‡	U/B
Magnetic resonance imaging scanner	Y	N	Y	Y	Y‡	U/B
Positron emission tomographic scanner	Y	N	N	N	N	U/B
Powerline (high voltage)	N	N	N	Y	N	U/B
Pulp tester	N	Y*	Y*	Y	N	U
Radar	N	N	Y*	N	N	U
Radiation (therapeutic)	Y	N	N	N	Y	U/B
Radiotransmission (AM)	N	N	Y*	N	N	U
Radiotransmission (FM)	N	N	Y*	Y*	N	U
Stun gun	N	N	Y	N	N	U/B
Telephone						
Cellular	N	Y	Y	Y	Y‡	U/B
Cordless	N	Y	Y	Y	Y‡	U/B
Transcutaneous electrical nerve stimulation	N	Y	N	Y	Y‡	U
Television transmitter	N	Y*	Y*	Y*	N	U
Ultrasound (therapeutic)	Y§	N	Y*	N	N	U
Weapon detector	N	N	Y*	N	N	U

*Remote potential for interference.
†Impedance-based sensors.
‡DDD mode only.
§Piezocrystal-based sensors.
Data updated from Telectronics, now Pacesetter Inc., St. Jude Medical, Sylmar CA, technical note.

pulse generator is out of the pocket. If one were able to measure the stimulation impedance in each of these settings, it would be extremely high and well above the standard measurement for the particular lead being used. Event markers would report the release of an output pulse even though the circuit was open, precluding effective pacing.

It is important to keep in mind that although a pulse generator is bipolar, it may be programmed to function in the unipolar mode. Failure to output may also be seen with bipolar pacemakers that are connected to a unipolar pacing lead. This is more likely with the VS-1 or IS-1 leads because the bipolar and unipolar connectors are similar. Some unipolar leads now have a protective metal band where the anodal screw of the pacemaker connector block is located to prevent an inadvertent tightening of this screw from damaging the lead. This gives the appearance of a bipolar lead, even

though no anodal conductor is present, and is potentially misleading. Some configuration programmable pulse generators allow the user to designate the output configuration as unipolar in a separate field of the programming system. Then, when the standard programmed parameter page is accessed, the bipolar lead option is locked out, minimizing the chance that the device will be accidentally programmed to the bipolar configuration because the pulse generator, with the appropriate lead, can otherwise support bipolar pacing.

In dual-chamber systems, sensing an event on one channel triggers refractory periods on both channels. Oversensing on the ventricular channel initiates both a ventricular refractory period and a PVARP. Depending on its precise timing, the PVARP initiated by the oversensed ventricular event may result in failure to sense a native P wave, yet another example of functional undersensing. A similar phenomenon may

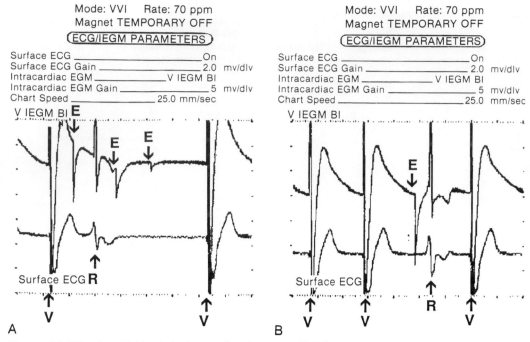

Figure 31–25. *A and B,* Ventricular intracardiac electrogram (IEGM) as telemetered by a pulse generator, recorded simultaneously with a surface electrocardiogram (ECG). Note the large artifacts (E) on the intracardiac channel seen without ventricular activity (R, native QRS; V, pace output). These were caused by failing inner insulation in a bipolar coaxial lead system. EGM, electrogram.

be seen in single-chamber systems in the presence of relatively rapid intrinsic rhythms. Oversensing starts a refractory period that may coincide with a native complex. Although this same complex is otherwise perfectly capable of being sensed, the pacemaker's refractory period precludes its being sensed, with the result being apparent undersensing when the true cause of the problem is oversensing. This is most readily identified if the phenomenon is occurring while the rhythm can be monitored with the simultaneous display of event markers.

Failure to Capture (Artifact Is Present)

With the advent of the newer ECG recording systems and the use of pulse artifact enhancement, the clinician must first be certain that the pace artifact seen is truly from the pacing system. The newer recording and monitoring systems have unique pacemaker pulse detectors that generate a discrete pacemaker pulse in response to any high-frequency transient. There are many extraneous signals that can cause the enhanced ECG, telemetry system, or Holter recorder to place an erroneous pace artifact on the ECG. EMI (including

programmer telemetry), loose ECG electrode connections, and subthreshold pulses, as are seen with the minute ventilation sensors associated with normal pacemaker function, are examples of situations associated with spurious ECG artifacts (see Fig. 31–18). The use of event marker telemetry and intracardiac EGMs can assist in differentiating the true pacemaker output from a recording system artifact, whereas retrospective analysis of a previously recorded rhythm may prove challenging.

A common cause of functional noncapture is undersensing, with a resultant delivery of the pacemaker impulse during the physiologic refractory period of the myocardium. Although the output does not elicit a depolarization, the problem in this case is related to sensing, not output, and should be evaluated as such (Fig. 31–27). This is best identified as undersensing, but if one insists on commenting on capture, it is functional noncapture. No matter how high the energy content of the output pulse, the myocardium is physiologically refractory and incapable of being depolarized.

When true noncapture is documented, the patient's safety

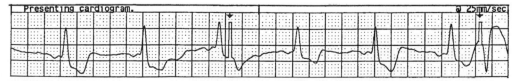

Figure 31–26. Rhythm strip from a patient whose pulse generator is beyond the elective replacement interval. Not only is the pacing rate below the programmed rate of 70 bpm, the device is not sensing properly. The leads were found to function normally when the device was replaced.

Table 31–9. **Causes of Pulse Generator Failure**

Battery depletion
Component malfunction
Direct trauma
Loss of hermeticity
Therapeutic radiation
Electrocautery
Defibrillation and cardioversion
Lithotripsy

Table 31–10. **Causes of Loss of Capture***

Lead Dislodgement or Malposition
Microinstability
Macrodislodgment
Perforation
Elevated Capture Thresholds
Lead maturation
Chronic
Progressive cardiac disease
Myocardial infarction
Cardiomyopathy
Metabolic abnormality
Electrolyte abnormality
Drugs
Local Damage at Electrode–Myocardial Interface
Electrocautery
Defibrillation and cardioversion
Battery Depletion
Circuit Failure
Inappropriate Programming
Too low a safety margin
Pseudomalfunction
Recording artifacts mimicking a pacing stimulus
Isoelectric evoked potential with visible pacing stimulus
Functional noncapture—delivery of output during physiologic refractory period
Functional Noncapture
True undersensing
Functional undersensing

*Pulse artifact present but no evoked potential.

must be ensured. If the patient is pacemaker dependent or is intolerant of the subsequent bradycardia associated with complete or intermittent loss of capture, the device should be programmed to its highest output. This can often be rapidly achieved by activating emergency VVI mode through the programmer. In most systems, even with a dual-chamber device, this programs the pacemaker to the highest available output in a unipolar output configuration. If consistent capture is still not secured, placement of a temporary pacemaker may be required. Increasing numbers of bipolar devices allow programming to the unipolar mode. This may acutely correct the situation, particularly in the presence of an internal insulation failure, with a resultant short circuit or an open circuit associated with a fracture of the proximal conductor. Although this eliminates the need for an emergency operative intervention, it is a temporizing measure only, and a lead with a mechanical failure should be replaced.

The causes of noncapture are listed in Table 31–10. The onset of noncapture relative to the implantation of the device and lead system can provide valuable clues to identification of the cause of the loss of capture. If this occurs within 24 to 48 hours of implantation, dislodgment, malposition, or perforation of the heart by the lead should be high on the list of possible problems. Elevated thresholds occurring during the first several weeks after implantation were more common in the early days of pacing, and although the incidence of this problem has markedly decreased with the introduction of steroid-eluting electrodes and other electrode materials and designs, a significant rise in capture threshold may still occur (see Chapter 4). The capture threshold rise is attributed to the inflammatory reaction resulting from two factors: the pressure and hence trauma applied by the elec-

trode to the endocardium, and a standard foreign-body reaction. The peak of the early threshold rise usually occurs between 2 and 6 weeks after implantation. Using a higher output during this acute period minimizes the likelihood of noncapture until the threshold improves to its chronic level. A rise in threshold occurring after 6 weeks is usually considered to be in the chronic phase of the lead maturation process. The threshold may rise steadily over time until noncapture occurs or until the threshold exceeds the pacemaker's maximum output. This is commonly referred to as *exit block.*[153–159] Older lead models and some epicardial leads are more likely to develop elevated capture threshold levels.[160–163] Some patients demonstrate repeated episodes of this phenomenon and have required multiple lead revisions or replacements. Children with epicardial implants are especially prone to this condition.[153, 164] Steroid-eluting leads are useful in minimizing the development of exit block.[166–173] There have been some anecdotal reports proposing the use of high-dose systemic steroids to lower high thresholds, continued for months and then slowly tapered, but there have been no formal prospective randomized trials to evaluate this pharmacologic intervention.[174–176]

There are many causes of threshold rise in both the acute and chronic phases. Any severe metabolic or electrolyte derangement can lead to acute threshold changes (Table 31–11).[177–188] These are not uncommon in critically ill patients or during and immediately after cardiac arrest. Thus, noncapture may be secondary to the hypoxemia, acidemia, or hyperkalemia rather than the primary event leading to the arrest. In addition, some medications may affect capture

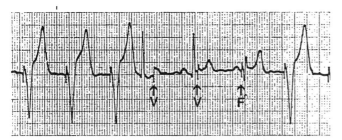

Figure 31–27. Electrocardiogram rhythm strip showing functional noncapture. The problem in this case is the pacing system's failure to sense the QRS. A pace output (V) then occurs during the myocardial refractory period and should not be expected to capture. The second to last QRS represents fusion (F) between the pace artifact and the native QRS.

Table 31–11. Metabolic Factors That May Increase Capture Thresholds

Major Changes	Minor Changes
Acidosis	Sleep
Alkalosis	Viral infections
Hypercarbia	Eating
Hyperkalemia	
Severe hyperglycemia	
Hypoxemia	
Myxedema	

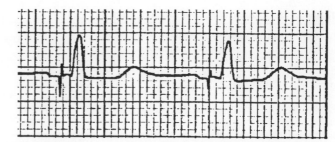

Figure 31–28. Electrocardiogram rhythm strip showing latency. Note the prolonged period from the pace artifact until the evoked QRS. This patient had a serum potassium concentration of 7.1 mEq because of renal failure.

thresholds, resulting in significant changes from the patient's baseline (Table 31–12).[189–194] The recent availability of beat-by-beat AutoCapture, an algorithm that allows the implanted pacemaker to monitor and track the capture threshold, has been reported to identify patients with transient late rises in capture threshold, such as those with decompensated congestive heart failure that would have resulted in loss of capture had the implanted pacemaker been programmed to a standard 2:1 safety margin.[195] As experience continues using systems with these capabilities, our understanding of factors that may affect the chronic capture threshold will increase.

Although the clinician might expect a fracture of a lead to present as the absence of any visible pacing artifact, this is frequently not the case. The ECG may display failure to capture, especially in unipolar systems. This occurs because of the current passes across the gap in the conductor coil through the fluid in the lead; however, the resistance is high, and the delivered output is likely to be subthreshold. Unipolar systems virtually always have the anode intact (the pulse generator surface), which provides enough of an electrical transient to trigger the artificial pace artifact circuitry of many monitoring systems. One can also see stimulus artifacts in the setting of a total disruption of both the conductor and the insulating sheath, which allows the output to be delivered to some local tissue, resulting in a stimulus on the ECG even though there is noncapture.[145] In the setting in which the entire lead is severed, the impedance may be in a normal range because conductor material is exposed, allowing a flow of current.

Although modern pulse generators attempt to maintain the programmed voltage output until the battery is exhausted, a reduction in the delivered voltage may occur before the elective replacement indicator is activated. At advanced stages of depletion of the battery, this may result in an ineffective pacing stimulus. This is now independent of the programmed output setting.

Latency is a finding that may be mistaken for failure to capture. This is defined as the delay between the delivery of the pacing impulse and the onset of the evoked potential or electrical systole.[196] Some antiarrhythmic agents or severe electrolyte disturbances, such as hyperkalemia, may cause latency (Fig. 31–28). A Wenckebach type of prolongation, leading to a noncapture and a repeat of the cycle, has also been reported.

Failure to Sense

To comprehend undersensing, it is necessary to understand how the sense amplifier works, where in the cardiac cycle the

Table 31–13. Causes of Undersensing

Poor Intrinsic Signal From Implant
  Signal amplitude
  Slew rate
Deterioration of Intrinsic Signal Over Time
  Lead maturation
  Progression of disease
    Cardiomyopathy
    New bundle-branch block
    Myocardial infarction
  Respiratory or motion variation
  Ectopic complexes not present at implantation
Transient Decrease in Signal Amplitude
  Postcardioversion or defibrillation
  Metabolic derangement, i.e., hyperkalemia
Component Malfunction
  Sensing circuit abnormality
  Stuck reed switch
Battery Depletion
Mechanical Lead Dysfunction
  Insulation failure
  Partial open circuit
Pseudomalfunction
  Recording artifact
Normal Device Function—Misinterpreted
  Triggered mode
  Fusion and pseudofusion beats
  Functional undersensing
    Long refractory periods
    Blanking period
    Safety pacing
    Oversensing
    DVI mode (particularly committed DVI)
Oversensing Initiated Functional Undersensing

Table 31–12. Effect of Specific Drugs on Pacing Thresholds

Increase Threshold	Possibly Increase Threshold	Decrease Threshold
Bretylium		Atropine
Encainide	β-Blockers	Epinephrine
Flecainide	Bretylium	Isoproterenol
Moricizine	Lidocaine	Glucocorticoids
Propafenone	Procainamide	
Sotalol	Quinidine	
Mineralocorticoids		

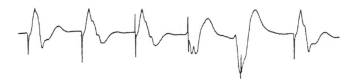

Figure 31–29. Electrocardiogram rhythm strip showing pseudofusion beats. The premature ventricular contractions have a right bundle-branch block morphology; thus, right ventricular depolarization occurs late within the overall cardiac activation sequence. The QRS complexes cannot be sensed by the pacemaker until late into the surface QRS, resulting in pseudofusion complexes when the escape interval "times-out" before the intrinsic deflection has occurred. Hence, even though the ventricle has started to depolarize, the pacemaker was not yet capable of sensing it.

sensing can occur, and where it cannot occur (see Chapter 3). Prerequisite for proper sensing is the EGM; the signal must possess both an adequate amplitude and frequency content (slew rate) to be sensed properly. A signal of apparently adequate peak-to-peak amplitude may be markedly attenuated by the sense amplifier because of its poor slew rate. The resultant "filtered" signal may be of insufficient size to be recognized as a valid event.[197–202] Table 31–13 lists the causes of sensing failure.

It is often assumed that the pacemaker senses a cardiac event at the beginning of the P wave or QRS complex, as seen on the surface ECG. This is not the case. The surface P wave or QRS is a summation of all electrical events occurring at the cellular level over a period of time (80 to 120 msec or longer). If the clinician looks at the intracardiac EGM as recorded from a pacing electrode, it appears as a large amplitude relatively rapid deflection (see Fig. 31–8). If one did not know that the recording was an EGM, an atrial signal could be easily mistaken for a QRS complex presumed to have been recorded with a standard surface ECG. It is thus helpful to record both the atrial and ventricular EGMs simultaneously, the EGM with the simultaneous surface ECG, or telemetered event markers. This event, the intrinsic deflection of the QRS or P wave, is generated as the wave of depolarization passes by the electrode. This is the complex that is sensed even if it occurs well after the onset of the native depolarization. An excellent example of this delayed sensing is in the patient who has right bundle-branch block and a pacing electrode in the right ventricle. The native depolarization occurs late in the right ventricle

because of the conduction delay, and thus, the pacemaker does not sense this event until that event reaches the pacing lead, which is late in the timing of the QRS complex. By assuming that sensing occurred earlier, this has been incorrectly labeled *late sensing*. Measurements made from the onset of the QRS complex misinterpret the timing cycle by more than 100 msec. Thus, an ECG with a pacing artifact in the QRS (pseudofusion and fusion) can occur in the presence of absolutely normal sensing (Fig. 31–29).[203, 204]

The refractory period is integral to understanding sensing and whether a native complex is even potentially capable of being sensed. Long programmed refractory periods may cause undersensing of events coinciding with the refractory period, a timing interval during which the pacemaker, for technical reasons is not capable of sensing (Fig. 31–30). This might occur in the case of a closely coupled PVC or PAC or very rapid intrinsic rhythms. Although there may be resultant competition, this is not a lead or pulse generator malfunction in that both devices are functioning properly and in accord with their design. This is clinically undesirable and reflects inappropriate programmed settings in the pacemaker, a behavior amenable to correction by programming. This should also be termed *functional undersensing* because the pacemaker is not capable of sensing at the time the native signal occurred. On the other hand, the failure to sense the native complex allows the timing period to complete, with the resultant release of an output pulse that may prove to be ineffective because it was delivered at a time of physiologic refractoriness. Functional undersensing commonly results in functional noncapture. A classic example of this phenomenon was the committed DVI pacing system, an early-generation AV sequential pacing system that was not capable of sensing on the atrial channel but, with release of an atrial output, was committed to release a ventricular output even in the presence of a native R wave.[203, 222]

As in noncapture, the onset of undersensing relative to the implantation of the pacemaker and lead system may direct the clinician to the correct diagnosis of the malfunction. The undersensing that occurs close in time to the implantation should lead the physician to suspect dislodgment, malposition, or perforation of the electrode. Problems occurring in chronic systems are frequently caused by mechanical problems with the lead or, if the lead is normal, programming errors, or they are attributable to a change in the morphology of the intrinsic cardiac signal associated with disease progression. Inappropriate programmed settings are not uncommon, particularly when sensitivity threshold

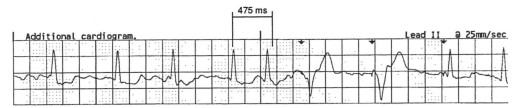

Figure 31–30. Electrocardiogram rhythm strip showing undersensing of the QRS complexes in a patient with atrial fibrillation. The device is programmed to VVI with a demand rate of 70 bpm and a refractory period of 475 msec. Because of a long programmed ventricular refractory period, this does not represent a pacemaker malfunction. The pacemaker will not respond to intrinsic events during the refractory period, a phenomenon termed *functional undersensing*.

testing has been performed during follow-up. The clinician may forget to return the sensitivity to the appropriate setting and leave it at or above the threshold setting. Occasionally, the sensing threshold may show a slow decline in the amplitude of the native signal as the lead–tissue interface changes over time.[205–212]

The vector of depolarization can affect the amplitude and the slew rate of the intracardiac EGM. Any change in the vector may result in significant changes in the sensing threshold. If a patient with a ventricular pacemaker has a myocardial infarction, develops a bundle-branch block, or has PVCs, the intracardiac signal may be insufficient to allow sensing at the previous appropriate setting (Fig. 31–31).[206–208] The same may be seen with atrial implants and PACs. Another cause of vector change is movement of the lead's position associated with respiration. Marked changes in the intracardiac signal can be documented in some patients as the angle of the lead relative to the heart changes with body position or diaphragmatic motion (Fig. 31–32).[209–212] Evaluating the quality of the intracardiac signal associated with the sensing failure is greatly facilitated by access to the telemetered intracardiac EGM.

As the pacemaker's battery begins to deplete, erratic behavior may occur, including persistent or intermittent undersensing. Failure of a circuit component may also cause sensing failure. Rarely, the reed switch that activates the

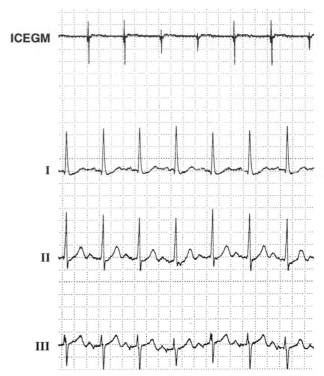

Figure 31–32. Intra-atrial electrogram and surface electrocardiogram. Note the profound variation of the intracardiac signal without apparent change of the surface P-wave morphology. This was synchronous with respiratory movements. This may be seen in either the atrium or the ventricle. ICEGM, intracardiac electrogram.

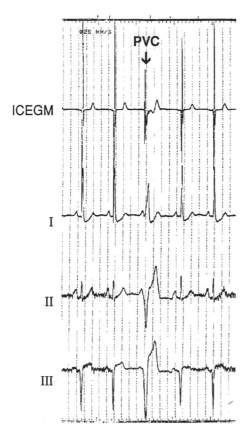

Figure 31–31. The intracardiac electrogram (ICEGM) and surface electrocardiogram (I, II, III) of intrinsic beats and a premature ventricular contraction (PVC). In this example, the PVC electrogram has a peak-to-peak amplitude that is a significantly lower amplitude than the normal beats and may lead to undersensing.

magnet mode may stick in the closed position, causing (in most cases) asynchronous pacing. For the same reason, when reviewing a rhythm strip, the clinician must know whether the magnet was over the device when the recording was made. Asynchronous pacing may also be seen during the interference or noise mode function of the device. The latter obligates pacing when the presence of electrical noise is sensed by the pulse generator. Typically, this is defined as multiple sensed events occurring within the terminal portion of the ventricular refractory period. The device then paces asynchronously to protect the pacemaker-dependent patient against inappropriate device inhibition.[142, 213]

One frequently misinterpreted reason for failure to sense involves pacemakers that use impedance plethysmography as a rate-modulation sensor. This applies primarily to minute ventilation sensors. Because the system uses the pacemaker's case as the anode for the impedance sensing impulses, when the case is out of the pocket, a great deal of electrical noise is generated because the system is not grounded. This results in asynchronous pacing until the device is placed into the pocket. If the clinician is not aware of this idiosyncrasy, a malfunction of the pulse generator might be inappropriately diagnosed.

Finally, the use of either external or internal defibrillation may cause temporary or permanent loss of the sensing function. This may be caused by transient saturation of the sensing amplifier pacemaker, circuit damage, and lead–myocardium interface damage. This phenomenon is caused when the large electrical current delivered by the defibrillator is diverted from the pacemaker's circuitry to the pacing lead by way of zener diodes, which are included in the pacemaker circuitry to protect the pulse generator from large voltage surges. The result may cauterize the myocardium and thus reduce or eliminate the local EGM. It may also cause a marked elevation in the capture threshold or result in exit block. Capacitive coupling is another mechanism that may allow a current to be induced into the pacing lead by either a shock or nearby electrocautery use.[214–216]

Dual-Chamber Pacemaker Issues

Crosstalk Inhibition

Crosstalk is a potentially catastrophic form of ventricular oversensing that can occur in any dual-chamber mode in which the atrium is paced and the ventricle is sensed and paced. Consider the fact that the common output voltages for the atrial channel range from 2.5 to 5 V. This is the same as 2500 to 5000 mV. The ventricular lead is just several centimeters away from this atrial lead and is "looking" for an electrical event of about 2 mV, which would represent a ventricular depolarization. If the ventricular channel senses the pacing impulse delivered to the atrium, it interprets the event as a R wave. The ventricular output is inhibited, and

the patient is left without pacing support if crosstalk occurs in a patient with complete AV block; ventricular asystole could result in the absence of an escape rhythm with only paced P waves visible.[217–220] Conversely, crosstalk is more difficult to detect when AV nodal conduction is intact, but in the system that uses ventricular based timing, it may result in an acceleration of the paced atrial rate with ventricular output inhibition even in the presence of a first-degree AV block that exceeds the programmed AV delay.[220]

As demonstrated in Figure 31–33, crosstalk can be recognized by an acceleration of the atrial-paced rate in a non–sensor-driven dual-chamber system using ventricular-based timing. Note that ventricular sensing occurs virtually simultaneously with atrial output. The AV delay is immediately terminated with ventricular sensing, and the atrial escape interval is started. Thus, the pacing interval with this type of timing is equal to the atrial escape interval (programmed pacing interval minus the AV delay) plus the ventricular blanking period. Rate-modulated pacing systems that use ventricular-based timing have a rate acceleration that is seen at the base pacing rate. Crosstalk may not be readily diagnosed in patients with rate-modulated pacing systems and intact AV nodal conduction because the increased atrial pacing rate may be thought to be caused by the sensor.

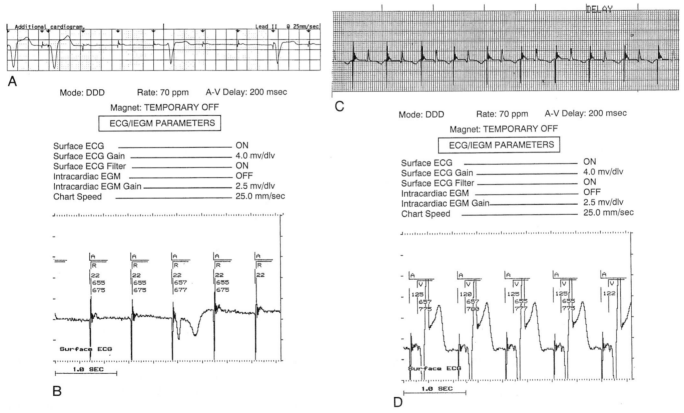

Figure 31–33. *A,* Electrocardiogram (ECG) rhythm strip showing crosstalk in a patient with complete atrioventricular (AV) block, with a ventricular-based pacing system. Note the presence of an atrial output without a ventricular output. A comparison of the interval from the first atrial pulse until the second with the second until the third demonstrates that the pacing interval is shortened by the AV interval minus the blanking period (120 msec). *B,* ECG strip with event markers during crosstalk. Note that the ventricular sensing (R) occurs immediately after the atrial output pulse (A). Safety pacing was turned off. *C,* ECG rhythm strip showing crosstalk in a patient with intact AV conduction. Because this pacemaker operates with ventricular-based timing, the atrial escape interval resets with each atrial output, elevating the frequency of atrial stimulation. *D,* ECG rhythm strip and event markers during crosstalk and ventricular safety pacing. Note that despite the AV interval being set to 200 msec, the event markers demonstrate the ventricular stimulus at 125 msec after the atrial output pulses. EGM, electrogram; IEGM, intracardiac electrogram.

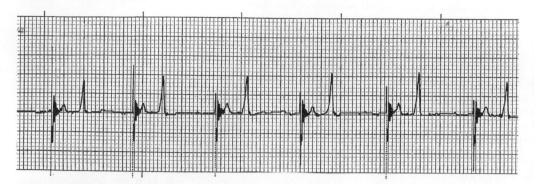

Figure 31–34.
Electrocardiogram rhythm strip showing crosstalk with a pacemaker operating with atrial-based timing. Note that the atrial pacing rate remains at the programmed rate of 70 bpm. The atrioventricular interval was programmed to 175 msec.

Pacing systems that use atrial-based timing do not exhibit this rate increase. Although ventricular sensing of the atrial output inhibits the ventricular output, the portion of the AV interval not used is added to the atrial escape interval, maintaining atrial pacing at the programmed interval (Fig. 31–34). Without access to event marker telemetry, ventricular output inhibition due to crosstalk cannot be differentiated from failure to output, as with an open circuit.

Several factors increase the likelihood of crosstalk (Table 31–14). Programmed settings that increase either the ventricular sensitivity or the atrial energy output predispose to this problem. Insulation failure on the atrial lead also increases the chances of crosstalk by increasing the pulse charge and energy. The clinician must be aware that certain pacemaker models are more prone to this phenomenon than are others. This is related to differences in circuit designs and the degree of isolation between the two channels within the pulse generator.[217] Crosstalk may occur within the circuitry of the pulse generator rather than between the pacing leads. Unipolar systems are also significantly more prone to crosstalk because of the larger electrical signal, as sensed by the ventricular channel.[218, 221–223]

There are two approaches to the problem of crosstalk: (1) prevention of crosstalk, and (2) prevention of the consequences of crosstalk.

Prevention of Crosstalk. Prevention of crosstalk is approached by proper programming of the device and proper lead placement. Atrial amplitude and pulse width settings that provide an appropriate safety margin without being excessive and ventricular sensitivity settings that are not unnecessarily sensitive are helpful. Newer circuit designs are much more resistant to this problem. Even under ideal circumstances, however, crosstalk may still occur.

The use of an additional ventricular refractory period, known as the *blanking period*, is fundamental to prevention.[221] The blanking period begins with the atrial output and usually lasts from 12 to 51 msec. In many devices, this is a

Table 31–14. Factors Promoting Crosstalk

High atrial output settings
  Pulse amplitude
  Pulse width
  Pulse current as with low impedance
High ventricular sensitivity setting
Short ventricular blanking period

programmable parameter. During this time, nothing (including the atrial output) can be sensed on the ventricular channel. Short blanking periods help to prevent the undersensing of intrinsic ventricular activity but may allow crosstalk to occur. Long blanking periods virtually ensure the prevention of crosstalk but may cause intrinsic events to not be sensed, a potential problem if the native beat is a late-cycle PVC and the AV interval is programmed to a long length. Functional failure to sense PVC (because the intrinsic deflection of the PVC coincided with the ventricular blanking period) may be followed by a ventricular output beyond the myocardial refractory period and on the vulnerable zone of the T wave. This might result in the induction of a ventricular arrhythmia, which may also occur with atrial undersensing when a normally conducted QRS falls into the blanking period. The latter event would not be detected, and an unnecessary stimulus would be delivered (Fig. 31–35).

Prevention of Crosstalk Sequelae. The earliest approach to the prevention of ventricular output loss as a result of crosstalk was the introduction of the DVI-committed mode (DVI-C). In this version of DVI, ventricular sensing is completely disabled during the AV interval that follows an atrial output pulse. After the termination of the AV interval, a ventricular output pulse is committed whether or not an intrinsic ventricular event has occurred. Thus, with DVI-C, there can never be an inhibition of the ventricular output by an atrial output. Although this approach worked, it resulted in confusing ECGs and wasted energy because of the delivery of unnecessary pacing impulses.[203, 222] It is also not practical for DDD devices for similar reasons. With the development of the DDD mode, however, manufacturers were able to provide brief refractory periods (blanking periods) starting with the atrial output. Even blanking periods, however, are not a guaranteed prevention for ventricular output inhibition associated with crosstalk.

To ensure patient safety, a unique circuit was integrated to the ventricular channel. The most common approach is the use of a safety output pulse. This is referred to by multiple names, depending on the manufacturer of the device (safety pacing, nonphysiologic AV delay, or ventricular safety standby). This method uses a brief sensing period (crosstalk sensing window) after the blanking period. Any electrical event sensed during this crosstalk sensing period is assumed to be crosstalk. A ventricular output is then triggered to be delivered after a shortened AV delay[223, 224] (Fig. 31–36). Other events may cause a safety output pulse to occur. These include premature ventricular beats, premature

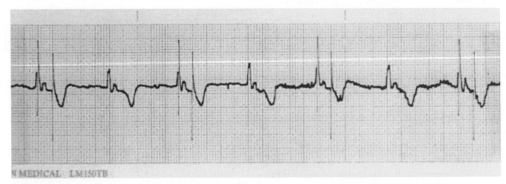

Figure 31–35. Electrocardiogram rhythm strip showing undersensing of native QRS. The device was programmed to the DVI mode; thus, there is no atrial sensing. When the atrial escape interval expires, the atrial output coincides with the onset of the native QRS. The ventricular blanking period is triggered by the release of the atrial output; this precludes ventricular sensing for 38 msec after the atrial output. If the intrinsic deflection of the native QRS coincides with the ventricular blanking period, it will not be sensed, and a ventricular output will be delivered at the end of the programmed atrioventricular interval.

junctional beats, and normally conducted ventricular events that may occur after undersensed intrinsic atrial beats (see Fig. 31–35). After one of the latter events, if the safety output pulse were delivered using a long AV interval, there would be a potential for delivering a tightly coupled and potentially arrhythmogenic stimulus to the ventricle. Therefore, a shortened AV interval is used (typically, between 100 and 120 msec) to deliver the stimulus harmlessly into the depolarizing ventricle while maintaining the ability to rescue the patient in the presence of actual crosstalk. In the presence of a long programmed AV delay and intact AV nodal conduction, crosstalk is signaled by AV pacing at the abbreviated AV delay. Reducing the atrial output or ventricular sensitivity or lengthening the ventricular blanking periods should reduce, if not totally eliminate, episodes of crosstalk.

As in crosstalk, the delivery of the safety output pulse causes a shortening of the base pacing interval because of the shortening of the AV interval. If the baseline AV interval is programmed to the same duration as that of the safety output pulse, or if a rate-modulated or differential AV interval is present, the presence of safety pacing (thus, crosstalk) may be difficult, if not impossible, to discern on the standard ECG. The use of event marker telemetry documents the presence of crosstalk or safety output pulses in these situations (see Fig. 31–36).

Finally, delivery of a safety output pulse does not prevent crosstalk. It is designed to prevent the sequelae of crosstalk

by preventing ventricular asystole. It is unwise to allow a patient to use this backup mechanism continually. If crosstalk is suspected or documented, the clinician should pursue the potential causes and make the necessary adjustments to terminate this condition. In some situations, such as failure of the lead's insulation, programming changes may not be adequate, and surgical intervention may be required.

Pacemaker-Mediated Tachycardia

Any undesired rapid pacing rate caused by the pulse generator or by an interaction of the pacing system with the patient may be considered PMT. This has classically been associated with the ELT seen in dual-chamber devices. PMT, however, should be assumed to be a more general term. The following are several conditions that are well-documented causes of PMT.

Runaway Pacemaker. The runaway pacemaker is a pacemaker malfunction that may occur in single-chamber or dual-chamber pacing systems. It is usually the result of a minimum of at least two separate component failures within the pulse generator. The result is the rapid delivery of pacing stimuli to the heart, with the potential for inducing lethal arrhythmias, such as ventricular tachycardia or fibrillation. Newer devices incorporate a runaway protect circuit that prevents stimulation above a preset rate, typically between 180 and 200 bpm. Although extremely rare with modern

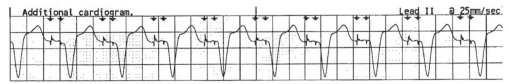

Figure 31–36. Electrocardiogram rhythm strip showing safety pacing. Sensing is occurring on the ventricular channel during the crosstalk sensing window. This causes a ventricular output to be delivered at a shortened atrioventricular (AV) interval. In a ventricular-based timing system, the pacing interval is shortened by the difference between the programmed AV interval and the safety-paced AV interval because the atrial escape interval is reset by any sensed or paced ventricular event. This results in an AV-paced rate of 93 bpm, even though the device is programmed DDD at 75 bpm and not capable of rate modulation.

pacing devices, this represents a medical emergency. Emergent surgical intervention to replace the device or, if all else fails, cut the lead, must be performed. Obviously, a patient who is pacemaker dependent presents a new challenge as soon as the defective pacing system is disabled.[225, 226]

Sensor-Driven Tachycardia. Sensor-driven tachycardia is a rapid heart rate occurring in rate-modulated pacemakers. This can occur with any type of sensor-driven pacing system (Table 31–15). Interaction between the patient and external stimuli may cause the rate-modulation system to over-react and pace at high rates. The most common cause of this PMT type is inappropriate programming of the sensor parameters. In piezoelectric devices, a threshold setting that is too low or a slope setting that is too high results in high pacing rates for low levels of activity. It also exposes the patient to increased pacing rates for nonphysiologic events, such as riding in a car, exposure to loud noise or music, and sleeping on the ipsilateral side to the device implant.[227–237]

One unpublished incident concerns a patient with a bipolar piezoelectric VVIR device. The emergency medical squad had been summoned to treat an unconscious patient. They arrived to find the patient with tonic seizure activity. On viewing the ECG, they found the patient's condition to be wide complex tachycardia at 150 bpm. The patient received repeated direct current cardioversion for this tachycardia without reversion to sinus rhythm. In this case, the seizures were caused by epilepsy, and the vibration-based sensor responded to the seizure by pacing at its upper rate. No spikes had been noted on the ECG because the output configuration was bipolar, which resulted in a diminutive artifact on the monitor (Fig. 31–37).

Patients with pacing systems responsive to central venous temperature changes may respond to a fever spike with upper rate pacing. This requires a nulling feature to restore a more appropriate pacing rate after a specified time at the upper rate has occurred. Similarly, devices that respond to changes in the evoked QT interval use this nulling feature, although for different reasons. As the QT interval shortens because of catecholamine increases and changes in the autonomic nervous system, the pacing rate is increased by the device; however, this may cause further shortening of the QT interval by a rate-dependent mechanism. The latter further increases the pacing rate, which may then spiral to the upper rate limit.

Table 31–15. Causes of Sensor-Driven Pacemaker Tachycardia

Vibration Sensor—Piezocrystal
Pressure on device
  Patient lying on device as during sleep
  Tapping on device
Submuscular implantation
Loud, low-frequency music
Bumpy ride as in tractor, lawn mower, helicopter
Use of vibration generating tools
Impedance-Based Sensors—Minute Ventilation
Hyperventilation
Electrocautery
Environmental 50- to 60-Hz electrical interference
Evoked QT Interval
Rate-dependent QT shortening spiral

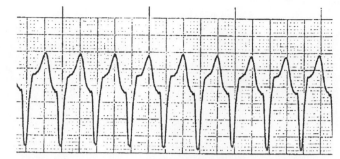

Figure 31–37. Electrocardiogram rhythm strip of pseudoventricular tachycardia caused by rapid ventricular pacing using a bipolar device. Note that the pace artifact is not well seen, leading to this potential misdiagnosis.

Devices that use thoracic impedance plethysmography to determine changes in minute ventilation may pace at the upper rate during marked hyperventilation, use of electrocautery, hyperventilation during anesthesia induction, and when in close proximity to an electrical power supply. Thus, it is strongly recommended that any patient have the rate-modulation feature disabled before undergoing virtually any surgical procedure (even if electrocautery is not used because there is a multiplicity of electrical equipment in most operating room suites), treatment with a mechanical ventilator, or treatment in a critical care unit.[236]

Magnetic Resonance Imaging. Exposure to magnetic resonance imaging (MRI) scanners has been reported to cause inappropriately high pacing rates when tested in animals. Some pacemakers have been noted to pace at the pulse rate of the scanner. This situation resolves immediately with the cessation of the radiofrequency output by the scanner.[238–243] MRI may also result in the inhibition of the pacing output during the scanning process. Because of these issues, such scanning has been cautioned against by all manufacturers of pacemakers. This is true even though some patients have inadvertently or intentionally undergone MRI without sequelae. Some physicians have programmed nonpacemaker-dependent patients to the OOO mode or to a subthreshold voltage output or pulse width, effectively disabling the pacemaker, whereas pacemaker-dependent patients have had the device programmed to an asynchronous mode. Although this may help, the induced current from having a wire in a moving magnetic field can theoretically stimulate the heart without being connected to the generator. A recent study, which looked at this very issue, reported that the induced current was subthreshold,[244] even though the potential exists (see Chapter 35).

Myopotential Tracking. Myopotential tracking is caused by oversensing of muscle potentials by the atrial channel in a dual-chamber pacing system capable of P-wave tracking. This has become far less common with the use of bipolar sensing, which is preferred by many implanting physicians. It is a greater problem with unipolar dual-chamber systems, but a new sensing modality (Combipolar sensing, which is sensing between the atrial and ventricular electrodes for a form of wide dipole bipolar sensing with the entire system

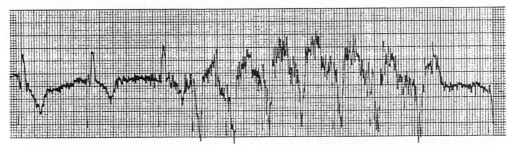

Figure 31–38. Electrocardiogram rhythm strip of myopotential tracking. The electrical activity of the muscle adjacent to the pacemaker case in a unipolar system is sensed by the atrial channel. This causes repeated initiation of the atrioventricular interval up to the maximum tracking rate. Higher-amplitude myopotentials may also cause the inhibition of the ventricular channel.

restricted to the heart) has reduced the incidence of atrial myopotential oversensing.[245] Myopotential tracking occurs when the atrial channel senses the electrical activity of the muscle underlying the pulse generator. Those same signals, if sensed on the ventricular channel, would result in myopotential inhibition. Because the atrial sensitivity setting is usually higher (more sensitive) than that in the ventricular channel, atrial sensing is more likely in the unipolar configuration; and although the atrial output is inhibited, this pseudo–P wave repeatedly triggers the ventricular output. Ventricular pacing may occur up to the programmed maximum P-wave tracking rate (Fig. 31–38). If the myopotential inhibitions are of sufficient amplitude, they may be sensed on the ventricular channel, in which pacing system inhibition may also occur.[88, 89, 120]

Atrial Arrhythmias. A common cause of rapid pacing in a dual-chamber pacemaker capable of tracking the atrium is atrial fibrillation. Any rapid atrial rhythm, such as flutter or ectopic atrial tachycardia, may also cause a similar situation. The pacemaker attempts to track the atrium to the upper rate limit if one of these arrhythmias occur. This is not a pacemaker malfunction, although it may manifest as rapid ventricular pacing and be clinically undesirable. Suppression of the arrhythmia with medication or cardioversion may be necessary. Urgently placing a magnet over the pacemaker stops the high-rate tracking. After a programmer is obtained, a nontracking mode my be programmed, or features such as automatic mode switching may be enabled. The latter is most useful in patients with AV block and intermittent atrial arrhythmias. In other cases, modes such as DDI or VVI have proved to be effective.

Endless-loop Tachycardia. The classic form of PMT is ELT, which can occur in dual-chamber pacemakers that are capable of atrial tracking modes, most commonly DDD or VDD. Only patients who are capable of retrograde ventriculoatrial conduction through the AV node or an AV accessory pathway are capable of sustaining this rhythm. The mechanism is identical to any macroreentrant tachycardia seen in the heart in which two electrical pathways exist between the atria and ventricles. Pacemaker ELT is classically initiated by a PVC. The depolarization is then conducted in a retrograde manner to the atria. If the PVARP has ended and the retrograde complex is of sufficient amplitude to be sensed, the atrial channel senses the event and initiates an AV interval. At the end of the AV interval, the pacemaker then delivers a stimulus to the ventricle, and the loop is reinitiated (Fig. 31–39). Although PVC is the classic cause of PMT initiation, any situation that results in AV dissociation, allowing a ventricular depolarization to occur without a normally coupled atrial-paced or atrial-sensed event, may begin the loop (Table 31–16). The latter includes atrial noncapture, oversensing, and undersensing. In addition, if the programmed AV interval is long (some units allow programming of up to a 350-msec interval), it may be possible for the AV node to recover in time to conduct the subsequent ventricular-paced event in a retrograde direction, thus initiating another ELT (Fig. 31–40). The absence of anterograde AV nodal conduction does not rule out retrograde conduction over the AV node or a concealed AV accessory pathway. Patients may also exhibit intermittent retrograde conduction or have variations in the retrograde conduction time relative to their sympathetic tone and catecholamine status.[246–255]

The rate of ELT depends on the conduction velocity and refractory period of the retrograde AV pathway. If the

Table 31–16. Endless-Loop Tachycardia Summary

Initiation
Premature ventricular ectopic beat
Atrial undersensing
Atrial oversensing
Atrial noncapture
Long programmed AV delay with echo beats

Prevention
PVARP
PVARP extension after ventricular ectopic beat detection
Differential atrial sensing
Rate-responsive AV delay allowing longer PVARP
Adaptive PVARP
High maximum tracking rate—retrograde fatigue

Detection
P tracking at upper rate limit
P tracking at intermediate rate
AV interval modulation
Discrepancy between sensed atrial rate and sensor-indicated rate

Termination
PVARP extension
Withhold of ventricular output
Withhold of ventricular output with early A pace

PVARP, postventricular atrial refractory period.

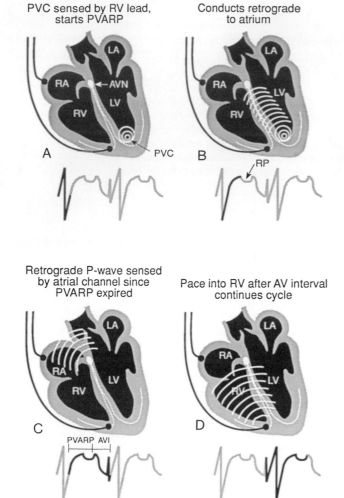

PVC sensed by RV lead, starts PVARP

Conducts retrograde to atrium

Retrograde P-wave sensed by atrial channel since PVARP expired

Pace into RV after AV interval continues cycle

Figure 31–39. Diagram showing the classic initiation of endless-loop tachycardia by a premature ventricular contraction (PVC) in a patient with retrograde atrioventricular (AV) conduction. *A,* A PVC occurs. *B,* The event is conducted in a retrograde fashion to the atrium, as seen by the inverted (retrograde) P wave. *C,* The retrograde event is sensed by the atrial channel, which causes an AV interval to be started. *D,* At the end of the AV interval, a stimulus is delivered to the ventricle if or when the maximum rate limit is not violated, resulting in retrograde conduction and the perpetuation of this cycle. RV, right ventricle; RA, right atrium; LA, left atrium; LV, left ventricle; AVN, atrioventricular node; PVARP, postventricular atrial refractory period; AVI, atrioventricular interval.

retrograde AV conduction is the same as or shorter than the upper rate interval (but not shorter than the PVARP), the tachycardia rate is at the programmed upper rate. If the retrograde AV conduction time is slower than the upper rate interval, the tachycardia rate is below the upper programmed rate (Fig. 31–41). Thus, although the rate of the ELT can never exceed the programmed upper rate of the pacemaker, it may be lower.[254–256] When the rate is lower than the maximum tracking rate, the rhythm has been termed a *balanced* ELT.

As with crosstalk, there are two approaches to ELT management: (1) prevention of ELT initiation, and (2) termination of ELT once it occurs.

Prevention of Endless-loop Tachycardia. The main defense against ELT is the use of an appropriate PVARP

interval. During the PVARP, the atrial channel cannot sense the retrograde depolarization that would, in a different set of circumstances, initiate the ELT. This is independent of the source of that atrial event. If retrograde conduction is present during implantation or follow-up, it is a simple matter to measure the ventriculoatrial time and program PVARP to an interval that is longer.[250] Many patients, however, exhibit only intermittent ventriculoatrial conduction, making an accurate assessment difficult. The major limitation of using a long PVARP is that it limits the upper tracking rate of the device (2:1 blocking rate). Some patients in our clinics have ventriculoatrial times in excess of 430 msec. Thus, using a PVARP of 450 msec and an AV interval of 150 msec, the total atrial refractory period is 600 msec. This causes 2:1 blocking at an atrial rate of 100 bpm, which is far too low for an active patient but which may be appropriate for a sedentary patient.

One solution to this problem is the use of ELT prevention algorithms.[257, 258] The most common algorithm is PVARP extension on PVE detection. A PVE is defined as a ventricular-sensed event that is not preceded by an atrial-paced or atrial-sensed event. When a PVE is detected, the device prolongs PVARP by a fixed or programmable value for the following cycle. It allows a shorter baseline PVARP to be used, with associated higher 2:1 blocking rates. A variation on this technique is to proceed with one DVI cycle after the PVE. This is the ultimate PVARP extension because the atrial channel remains refractory to sensing throughout the entire atrial escape interval. A problem with most of the

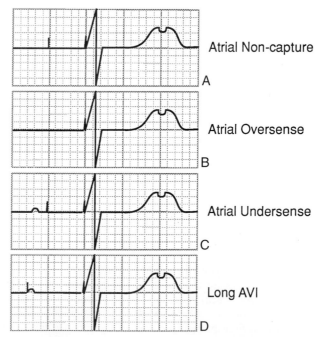

Atrial Non-capture

Atrial Oversense

Atrial Undersense

Long AVI

Figure 31–40. Diagram of different initiating events leading to retrograde P-wave conduction and the potential for endless-loop tachycardia. *A,* Atrial noncapture causes ventricular stimulation without the atrioventricular (AV) node being blocked by an anterograde event. *B,* Atrial oversensing inhibits atrial output and provides just a ventricular output with the same results as in *A. C,* Atrial undersensing allows a long AV interval, allowing the AV node time to recover and conduct retrograde. *D,* A long programmed AV interval may also allow the AV node to recover.

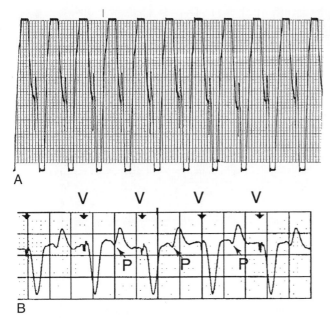

Figure 31–41. *A,* Electrocardiogram rhythm strip of endless-loop tachycardia (ELT) with fast ventriculoatrial (VA) conduction, resulting in a rapid ELT at the upper programmed rate of 155 bpm. Lower rate, 60 ppm; sensed atrioventricular (AV) interval, 150 msec; postventricular atrial refractory period (PVARP), 275 msec; VA time, 300 msec. *B,* Electrocardiogram rhythm strip of ELT with slow VA conduction, resulting in ELT below the programmed upper rate. As a result of the slow retrograde conduction, the ELT rate is significantly slower than the programmed upper rates. Retrograde P wave (P); ventricular output (V); lower rate, 60; upper rate, 145; AV interval, 165 msec; PVARP, 250 msec.

or PACs) and sinus tachycardia with exertion.[259–261] Even in the absence of rate modulation, rate-responsive AV delay algorithms allow a shorter total atrial refractory period and thus a higher maximum tracking rate, even with a fixed long PVARP.

A comparison of P-wave morphology can allow discrimination between sinus and retrograde atrial depolarizations in some cases; this is referred to as *differential atrial sensing*.[262–266] Mapping of the atrium may allow positioning of the lead at a site that has a large P wave when generated by the sinus node, although the retrograde P waves appear small in comparison. The pacemaker may be programmed to be sensitive enough to allow sensing of the anterograde P wave but be sufficiently insensitive so as to not sense the retrograde P wave. Thus, ELT cannot be initiated or sustained because the loop cannot be completed. Although the retrograde P wave is usually of lower amplitude than the anterograde P wave, this is not always the case and needs to be evaluated before attempting to use atrial sensitivity as a discriminating factor. In addition, it has been noted that the atrial EGM may decrease in amplitude as the sinus rate increases under physiologic stress. Programming a reduced atrial sensitivity to facilitate discrimination between anterograde and retrograde P waves may compromise sensing of rapid intrinsic atrial rhythms.[246]

Another preventive mechanism has been to program a high maximum tracking rate in the hope of inducing retrograde fatigue and spontaneous termination of an ELT if this is allowed to start. Careful assessment of the patient's ability to conduct retrograde should be performed, however, because some patients may have superior retrograde conduction as compared with anterograde conduction and be able to sustain extremely rapid ELTs.[246]

Termination of Endless-loop Tachycardia. The most difficult aspect of applying an ELT termination protocol is having the device determine whether ELT is present rather than a native atrial tachycardia that is being appropriately tracked. This has been approached by several different criteria by different manufacturers. Some of these are simple; others are more complex. The following are some of the most common techniques for identifying the presence of ELT.

The first is sustained P-wave tracking at the upper rate. This is the most common method of ELT detection. If the pacemaker tracks the P waves at the upper rate for a specific number of intervals, either the PVARP is prolonged for one cycle, DVI is used for one cycle, or the ventricular output is withheld. The number of events at the upper rate that trigger an ELT termination attempt depend on the particular pulse generator. Some algorithms use a fixed number of beats, whereas this is a programmable option in other systems. The method of ELT termination may also be programmable (PVARP extension or DVI cycle).[267, 268]

The second method to identify ELT is sustained P-wave tracking at a specific rate that is lower than the upper rate. As previously noted, not all ELTs occur at the upper programmed tracking rate. An ELT rate is always limited by the slowest point in the loop. If the patient has a ventriculoatrial conduction time that is longer than the upper tracking interval, the resulting ELT is slower than the upper tracking rate that is programmed. This presentation of ELT is not

PVARP extension algorithms is that functional atrial noncapture may occur. Because there was an atrial output, the system returns to the shorter PVARP, thus allowing for retrograde conduction to be sensed after the AV-paced cycle, simply postponing the ELT for one cycle. In the latter case, the pacemaker does not maintain the long PVARP because it has delivered an atrial stimulus (although ineffective) before a ventricular event. The subsequent ventricular-paced event then leads to ELT (Fig. 31–42). A refinement to the standard PVARP extension algorithm is to add an alert period to the end of the extended PVARP.[246] On release of the atrial output at the end of the alert period, the atrial myocardium will have recovered, allowing for capture precluding retrograde conduction on the next ventricular cycle.

Newer approaches have been made possible by the advent of sensor-driven pacing systems. With a DDDR system, even though the maximum tracking rate may be limited by a long PVARP, faster AV sequentially paced rates may be possible through the sensor. Even though atrial sensing does not occur during the PVARP, sensor-driven atrial pacing may occur. Another alternative in some DDDR pulse generators is to use an adaptive PVARP that is long when the sensor determines that the patient is at rest. When the patient's sensor-indicated rate increases along with the need for higher heart rates, the PVARP is shortened proportionately, allowing higher rates before a 2:1 block upper rate behavior occurs. This approach allows the device to discriminate between early atrial depolarizations at rest (possibly retrograde beats

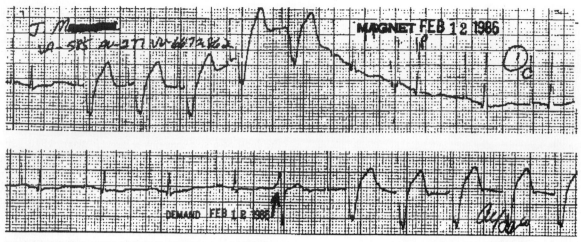

TRANSTELEPHONIC EVALUATION   J.M. 283-01-03155

Figure 31–42.   Dual-chamber Cosmos (model 283-01) (Sulzer Intermedics, Angelton, TX) pulse generator programmed with postventricular atrial refractory period (PVARP) extension on premature ventricular event (PVE) detection. Top tracing shows behavior of pacemaker with magnet application. AV delay is programmed to a long value to allow functional single chamber atrial pacing. Bottom tracing shows demand mode. A ventricular premature contraction occurs *(arrow)* causing PVARP extension. The retrograde P wave coincides with the extended PVARP and, appropriately, is not sensed and not tracked. When the atrial output was delivered at the end of the atrial escape interval, it was ineffective (functional noncapture) because the native atrial depolarization had rendered the atrial myocardium physiologically refractory. The delivery of the atrial output caused the pacemaker to shorten the PVARP with the next ventricular paced event by which time atrial refractoriness had resolved; retrograde conduction followed the paced ventricular complex and initiated an ELT at this time. Thus, the PVARP extension simply postponed the initiation of the ELT rather than preventing it. (From Levine PA, Selznick L: Prospective Management of the Patient With Retrograde Ventriculoatrial Conduction: Prevention and Management of Pacemaker Mediated Endless Loop Tachycardias. Sylmar, CA, Pacesetter Systems, 1990.)

identified by the sustained upper rate method. Some devices allow an initiation of the ELT termination algorithm at a P-wave tracking rate that is lower than the upper tracking rate. This lower rate is typically a programmable option to provide for the termination of ELT in this subset of patients.

The third is a modulation of the AV interval during sustained P-wave tracking at or above a specific rate. The technique used is based on the observation that the ventriculoatrial conduction time in an individual patient is relatively constant. When the device is P-wave tracking at a high rate, the system first assesses the stability of the retrograde interval. The AVI is then either shortened or lengthened, and the effect on the subsequent retrograde interval is assessed. If an ELT is present and the V-pace to P-sense interval remains constant (the atrial cycle length is shortened by the shortening of the AV interval), the device confirms ELT and initiates a termination algorithm (Fig. 31–43) composed of either withholding the ventricular output or delivering an atrial output after a period of time sufficient to allow for atrial recovery.[260, 261] If the V-pace to A-sense interval changes by more than a preset amount (the atrial cycle length being unaffected by the AV interval shortening), however, the ELT is not confirmed, and the device continues to track the atrium normally (see Fig. 31–43).

Cross-Stimulation

Cross-stimulation can be defined as stimulation of one cardiac chamber when stimulation of the other is expected (Fig. 31–44). An embarrassing cause of this phenomenon is the inadvertent placement of the ventricular lead into the atrial connector and the atrial lead into the ventricular connector of the pulse generator. Dislodgment of either lead into the other chamber may also be a cause. These are both true system malfunctions. Coronary sinus placement of either lead, either intentionally or accidentally, may cause continued or intermittent cross-stimulation. For all of these situations, surgical revision of the pacing system is the only option for correction. Several reports of cross-stimulation have been reported that are not related to these situations.[269–272] Internal crossover within the pulse generator circuitry may be the cause. This can be seen in dual unipolar systems with the leads connected but before placement in the pocket as the current crosses from one electrode to the other and then back to the pulse generator through the other lead. In this case, because the atrial output is first, atrial capture is obscured by ventricular capture. Because the impedance in this system is high, it requires a high output with a very low capture threshold. After the pulse generator is implanted, this phenomenon ceases. There is also a system that has internal energy crossover when a magnet is applied to the pacemaker. Here too, the amount of energy crossover is minimal, and capture can only be demonstrated when the capture threshold is very low. In all cases, this resolved after several weeks, and lead maturation resulted in a rise in the capture threshold.

Repetitive Nonreentrant Ventriculoatrial Synchronous Rhythm

The repetitive nonreentrant ventriculoatrial synchronous rhythm is becoming increasingly common with the growth

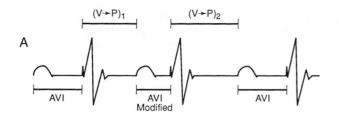

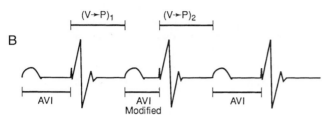

Figure 31–43. Diagram of ELA (Paris, France) endless-loop tachycardia (ELT) detection scheme. *A,* Rapid tracking of sinus tachycardia. The device causes the atrioventricular (AV) interval to be varied. When the atrioventricular interval is shortened (AVI modified), there is a prolongation of the V-P interval (V-P2 is longer than V-P1) because the sinus node rate is not affected. *B,* ELT caused by tracking of retrograde P waves. The device again causes the AV interval to be varied. In this case, shortening of the AV interval has no effect on the next retrograde event (V-P2 is the same as V-P1). This is defined by the device as ELT, and a termination algorithm is activated.

of the DDDR mode. It represents a classic example of an adverse interaction between a normally functioning DDDR pacemaker and the patient. A prerequisite for this rhythm is intact retrograde conduction. Further, the pacemaker is programmed with a sufficiently long PVARP such that retrograde conduction does not induce ELT. The second prerequisite is a sufficiently high base rate such that there will be a relatively short atrial escape interval and an even shorter interval from the native but retrograde atrial depolarization that renders the atrial tissue physiologically refractory. The

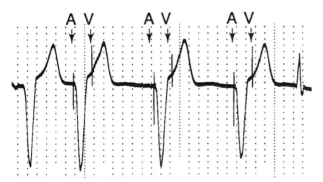

Figure 31–44. Electrocardiogram rhythm strip showing cross-stimulation as a result of lead reversal due to a misconnection at the time of implantation. Although the leads were properly situated in the heart, the atrial lead was placed into the ventricular connector, and the ventricular lead was placed into the atrial connector. Note that the first output delivered stimulated the ventricle, and the second falls into the ST segment when it is delivered into the atrium at the end of the atrioventricular interval because it is delivered through the atrial lead.

retrograde P wave is not sensed because it coincides with the PVARP. This represents functional undersensing. Because of the relatively high rate and the failure to reset the atrial timing cycle because the retrograde P wave is not sensed, an atrial output is delivered when the atrial myocardium is physiologically refractory. This results in functional atrial noncapture. The retrograde P wave occurs so early that it finds the AV node physiologically refractory, and it is not conducted. Hence, after the ineffective atrial output, the AV interval times out, and a ventricular-paced event occurs, by which time the AV node and atrial myocardium have fully recovered, allowing retrograde conduction to occur. The result is an AV-paced rhythm with repeated functional atrial noncapture and functional atrial undersensing, all due to a coincidence of various key timing intervals. This rhythm is called either *repetitive nonreentrant ventriculoatrial synchrony* or *AV desynchronization arrhythmia.*[273–275] The effect on the patient is the same as that of high-rate ventricular pacing with retrograde conduction but in a DDDR pacing system. This can lead to symptoms of palpitations, dyspnea, and even syncope. Effectively, the resultant rhythm is a classic rhythm associated with pacemaker syndrome, but unless one recognizes the problem, either normal pacemaker function is diagnosed and the symptoms are unexplained or the disorder is labeled *atrial noncapture,* and efforts are directed toward correcting this "malfunction."

Management requires allowing sufficient time for the atrial tissue to recover. This means either a short AV delay at the higher rates or limiting of the specific rates. When AV nodal conduction is intact, the clinician may consider single-chamber AAIR pacing, which would totally avoid this rhythm. If the rhythm is repeatedly triggered by a VPC with retrograde conduction, use of a PVARP extension algorithm that also slows the escape rate, allowing time for the atrium to physiologically recover, would be indicated.

It is absolutely essential that the clinician fully understand the interaction between the timing circuits in the pacemaker and those in the heart. One of the authors recently saw a patient in consultation who had been taken back to the operating room for an atrial lead repositioning on two additional occasions after the initial implantation because of this rhythm and the failure by the implanting physician to understand the adverse interaction between the various programmed parameters and the patient's intrinsic rhythms. This was not a lead dislodgment or malposition, although the latter was the working diagnosis. As such, it could not be solved by repositioning the lead, yet that was the diagnosis by the referring physicians because of repeated failure to capture on the atrial channel at the highest outputs that the pacemaker would allow. At the first consultation, this rhythm was suspected because the referring physician described losing atrial capture at 0.5 V and then not being able to regain it at 7.5 V when the base rate was 90 ppm but having absolutely no problems with capture when the base rate was 60 ppm. The referring physician sought advice about where the lead could be positioned (on a fourth operative procedure) to prevent repeated loss of atrial capture. Rather than reoperate, it was advised to leave the rate low and disable the rate modulation. The patient was then sent for a detailed evaluation, at which time it was easy to induce and demonstrate this phenomenon with the aid of the telemetered atrial EGM and event markers (Fig. 31–45). Management was

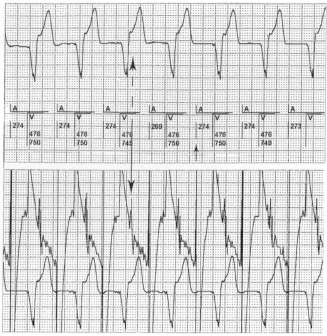

Figure 31–45. Induced during an atrial capture threshold test, functional atrial noncapture persisted when the output was returned to the previously effective programmed level. This is an example of repetitive nonreentrant ventriculoatrial synchronous rhythm. The retrograde P wave seen as a negative deflection in the ST segment of the paced QRS complex, as seen on the surface electrocardiogram *(top)* and the rapid deflection on the atrial electrogram *(bottom) (arrow)* coincides with the atrial refractory period as identified by the event markers. This is consistent with the programmed settings of the pacemaker. Hence, the failure to sense this P wave is normal allowing delivery of an atrial output pulse (functional undersensing). The atrial output pulse occurs at a time when the atrial myocardium is still physiologically refractory from the native atrial depolarization; hence, there is failure to capture, but on a functional basis, not as a sign of a malfunction. By the time the ventricular output is delivered, the atrium has recovered, allowing retrograde conduction to again occur. This rhythm persists until the base rate slows or is reduced, allowing the atrium to physiologically recover so that the atrial output effectively captures the atrium.

more of a challenge in that the maximum sensor rate had to be limited to preclude atrial pacing at a high rate, which meant that there would be a relatively short atrial escape interval. This patient's adverse rhythm was triggered by early atrial premature beats.

▪ Summary

Pacing system malfunction, although seemingly difficult to assess, can be categorized in relation to the dysfunction of the leads or the generator and apparent dysfunction related to the idiosyncratic characteristics of the pacemaker's timing algorithms. In contrast to the relative frequency of lead failure, either as a result of implantation error or deterioration of the lead materials, primary malfunction of the pulse generator is rare. Patient-specific problems or inappropriate program settings are relatively common as well. Consequently, the key to understanding the unexpected pacemaker behavior is related to meticulous evaluation of the integrity

of the leads, assessment of capture and sensing thresholds, and an understanding of the timing cycles of the specific pacemaker, which is facilitated by access to event marker telemetry.

Clues to the problem and its cause are found in the patient's history, physical examination, and the various diagnostic tests integral to the pacemaker and retrieved through bidirectional telemetry. With respect to the hardware, the answer is usually lead dysfunction or is a behavioral eccentricity detailed in the pacemaker's technical manual. One must always keep the patient's physiology and pathophysiology in mind because this also affects the function of the pacing system. Furthermore, all components of the system may be normal, with the pacemaker programmed to a set of parameters that are no longer optimal for the patient.

When the clinician is presented with a suspected pacing system malfunction, it is essential to proceed in a meticulous and orderly manner, carefully assessing each component of the system. This includes the pulse generator, the programmed settings, any unique algorithms, the leads, and the patient. If a complete assessment of capture and sensing thresholds, lead impedance, sensor response, and the behavior of any unique algorithms is performed on a periodic basis as part of the routine surveillance of the patient's pacing system, the baseline data will be available for comparison with the results of the evaluation when and if a problem is suspected.

REFERENCES

1. Furman S: Pacemaker programmability. PACE 1:161, 1978.
2. Furman S, Escher DJW, Fisher JD: Seven-year experience with programmable pulse generators. *In* Meere C (ed): Cardiac Pacing. Montreal, Pacesymp Publications, 1979, Chap 19-1.
3. Levine PA: Why Programmability? Indications for and Clinical Utility of Multiparameter Programmability. Sylmar, CA, Pacesetter Systems, 1981.
4. Gold RD, Saulson SH, MacGregor DC: Programmable pacing systems: The medium and the message. PACE 5:777, 1982.
5. Sholder J, Levine PA, Mann BM, Mace RC: Bidirectional telemetry and interrogation in cardiac pacing. *In* Barold SS, Mugica J (eds): The Third Decade of Cardiac Pacing: Advances in Technology and Clinical Applications. Mt Kisco, NY, Futura Publishing, 1982, pp 145–166.
6. Levine PA (ed): Proceedings of the Policy Conference of the North American Society of Pacing and Electrophysiology on Programmability and Pacemaker Follow-up Programs. Clin Prog Pacing Electrophysiol 2:145, 1984.
7. Del Marco CJ, Tyers GFO, Brownlee RR: Lithium pacers with self-contained multiparameter telemetry: First year followup. *In* Meere C (ed): Cardiac Pacing. Montreal, Pacesymp Publications, 1979, Chap 28-1.
8. Tanaka S, Nanba T, Harada A, et al: Clinical experience with telemetry pacing systems and long-term followup: Clinical aspects of lead impedance and battery life. PACE 6:A30, 1983.
9. Castellanet MJ, Garza J, Shaner SP, Messenger JC: Telemetry of programmed and measured data in pacing system evaluation and followup. J Electrophysiol 1:360, 1987.
10. Marco D: Pacemaker output settings for lowest current drain and maximum longevity. Reblampa 8:159–162, 1995.
11. Crossley GH, Gayle D, Simmons TW, et al: Reprogramming pacemakers enhances longevity and is cost-effective. Circulation 1996, 94(Suppl II):II-245–II-247.
12. Freedman RA, Marks ML, Chapman P, King C: Telemetered pacemaker battery voltage preceding generator elective replacement time: Use to guide utilization of magnet checks [Abstract]. PACE 18:863, 1995.
13. Ben-Zur UM, Platt SB, Gross JN, et al: Direct and telemetered lead impedance. PACE 17:2004–2007, 1994.

14. Danilovic D, Ohm OJ: Pacing impedance variability in tined steroid eluting leads. PACE 21:1356–1363, 1998.
15. Levine PA: Clinical manifestations of lead insulation defects. J Electrophysiol 1:144, 1987.
16. Clarke M, Allen A: Early detection of lead insulation breakdown. PACE 8:775, 1985.
17. Winoker P, Falkenberg E, Gerard G: Lead resistance telemetry: Insulation failure prognosticator. PACE 8:A85, 1985.
18. Phlippin F, O'Hara GE, Gilbert M: Lead impedance measured bipolar vs unipolar: A method to identify lead insulation failure [Abstract]. PACE 18:817, 1995.
19. Pickell D, Siegler K, Brewer L, et al: Suspect polyurethane insulated bipolar pacing leads: Clinical management [Abstract]. PACE 18:866, 1995.
20. Schmidinger H, Mayer H, Kaliman J, et al: Early detection of lead complications by telemetric measurement of lead impedance. PACE 8:A23, 1985.
21. Mauser JF, Huang SKS, Risser T, et al: A unique pulse generator safety feature for bipolar lead fracture. PACE 16:1368–1372, 1993.
22. Kruse I, Markowitz T, Ryden L: Timing markers showing pacemaker behavior to aid in the follow-up of a physiologic pacemaker. PACE 6:801, 1983.
23. Olson W, McConnell M, Sah R, et al: Pacemaker diagnostic diagrams. PACE 8:691, 1985.
24. Levine PA, Schuller H, Lindgren A: Pacemaker ECG: Utilization of pulse generator telemetry. Solna, Sweden, Siemens Elema AB, 1988.
25. Furman S: The ECG interpretation channel [Editorial]. PACE 13:225, 1990.
26. Olson WH, Goldreyer BA, Goldreyer BN: Computer-generated diagnostic diagrams for pacemaker rhythm analysis and pacing system evaluation. J Electrocardiol 1:376, 1987.
27. Levine PA: Pacemaker diagnostic diagrams [Letter]. PACE 9:250, 1986.
28. Machado C, Johnson D, Thacker JR, Duncan JL: Pacemaker patient-triggered event recordings: Accuracy, utility and cost for the pacemaker follow-up clinic. PACE 19:1813–1818, 1996.
29. Furman S, Hurzeler P, DeCaprio V: Cardiac pacing and pacemakers. III. Sensing the cardiac electrogram. Am Heart J 93:794, 1977.
30. Levine PA, Klein MD: Discrepant electrocardiographic and pulse analyzer endocardial potentials: A possible source of pacemaker sensing failure. In Meere C (ed): Cardiac Pacing. Montreal, Pacesymp Publications 1979, Chap 18-1.
31. Levine PA, Podrid PJ, Klein MD, et al: Pacemaker sensing: Comparison of signal amplitudes determined by electrogram telemetry and noninvasively measured sensing thresholds [Abstract]. PACE 12:1294, 1989.
32. Levine PA, Sholder J, Duncan JL: Clinical benefits of telemetered electrograms in the assessment of DDD function. PACE 7:1170, 1984.
33. Clarke M, Allen A: Use of telemetered electrograms in the assessment of normal pacemaker function. J Electrophysiol 1:388, 1987.
34. Edery T: Clinical applications of pacemaker-telemetered intracardiac electrograms: Technical concept paper. Minneapolis, MN, Medtronic Inc, 1991.
35. Hughes HC, Furman S, Brownlee RR, Del Marco C: Simultaneous atrial and ventricular electrogram transmission via a specialized single-lead system. PACE 7:1195, 1984.
36. Feuer J, Florio J, Shandling AH: Alternate methods for the determination of atrial capture thresholds utilizing the telemetered intracardiac electrogram. PACE 13:1254, 1990.
37. Sarmiento JJ: Clinical utility of telemetered intracardiac electrograms in diagnosing a design dependent lead malfunction. PACE 13:188, 1990.
38. Marco DD, Gallagher D: Noninvasive measurements of retrograde conduction times in pacemaker patients. J Electrophysiol 1:388, 1987.
39. Nalos PC, Nyitray W: Benefits of intracardiac electrograms and programmable sensing polarity in preventing pacemaker inhibition due to spurious screw-in lead signals. PACE 13:1101, 1990.
40. Halperin JL, Camunas JL, Stern EH, et al: Myopotential interference with DDD pacemakers: Endocardial electrographic telemetry in the diagnosis of pacemaker-related arrhythmias. Am J Cardiol 54:97, 1984.
41. Gladstone PJ, Duxbury GB, Berman ND: Arrhythmia diagnosis by electrogram telemetry: Involvement of dual-chamber pacemaker. Chest 91:115, 1987.
42. Hassett JA, Elrod PA, Arciniegas JG, et al: Noninvasive diagnosis and treatment of atrial flutter utilizing previously implanted dual-chamber pacemaker. PACE 11:1662, 1988.
43. Luceri RM, Castellanos A, Thurer RJ: Telemetry of intracardiac electrograms: Applications in spontaneous and induced arrhythmias. J Electrophysiol 1:417, 1987.
44. Levine PA: The complementary role of electrogram, event marker, and measured data telemetry in the assessment of pacing system function. J Electrophysiol 1:404, 1987.
45. Pirolo JS, Tweddel JS, Brunt EM, et al: Influence of activation origin, lead number, and lead configuration on the noninvasive electrophysiologic detection of cardiac allograft rejection. Circulation 84(Suppl III):344, 1991.
46. Berbari EJ, Lander P, Geselowitz DB, et al: Correlating late potentials from the body surface with epicardial electrograms. Eur J Cardiac Pacing Electrophysiol 2:A156, 1992.
47. Barold SS, Bornzin G, Levine P: Development of a true pacemaker Holter. In Vardas PE (ed): Cardiac Arrhythmias, Pacing and Electrophysiology: The Expert View. Dordrecht, The Netherlands, Kluwer Academic Publishers, 1998, pp 421–426.
48. Sermasi S, Marconi M: Temporary RAM programming of pacemaker capabilities. In Santini M (ed): Progress in Clinical Pacing 1996. Armonk, NY, Futura Publishing, 1997, pp 85–91.
49. Sanders R, Martin R, Frumin H, et al: Data storage and retrieval by implantable pacemakers for diagnostic purposes. PACE 7:1228, 1984.
50. Levine PA, Lindenberg BS: Diagnostic data: An aid to the follow-up and assessment of the pacing system. J Electrocardiol 1:396, 1987.
51. Levine PA: Utility and clinical benefits of extensive event counter telemetry in the follow-up and management of the rate-modulated pacemaker patient. Sylmar, CA, Siemens-Pacesetter, January 1992.
52. Newman D, Dorian P, Downar E, et al: Use of telemetry functions in the assessment of implanted antitachycardia device efficiency. Am J Cardiol 70:616, 1992.
53. Wang PJ, Manolis A, Clyne C, et al: Accuracy of classification using a data log system in implantable cardioverter defibrillators. PACE 14:1911, 1991.
54. Luceri RM, Puchferran RL, Brownstein SL, et al: Improved patient surveillance and data acquisition with a third-generation implantable cardioverter defibrillator. PACE 14:1870, 1991.
55. Stangl K, Sichart U, Wirtsfeld A, et al: Holter functions for the enhancement of the diagnostic and therapeutic capabilities of implantable pacemakers, Vitatext. Dieren, The Netherlands, Vitatron Medical, 1987, pp 1–6.
56. Hayes DL, Higano ST, Eisinger G: Utility of rate histograms in programming and follow-up of a DDDR pacemaker. Mayo Clin Proc 64:495, 1989.
57. Levine PA, Sholder JA, Florio J: Obtaining maximal benefit from a DDDR pacing system: A reliable yet simple method for programming the sensor parameters of Synchrony. Sylmar, CA, Siemens-Pacesetter, 1990.
58. Lascault GR, Frank R, Fontaine G, et al: Ventricular tachycardia using the Holter function of a dual-chamber pacemaker [Abstract]. PACE 16:918, 1993.
59. Lascault GR, Frank R, Barnay C, et al: Clinical usefulness of a "diagnostic" dual-chamber pacemaker [Abstract]. PACE 16:918, 1993.
60. Levine PA: Holter and pacemaker diagnostics. In Aubert AE, Ector H, Stroobandt R (eds): Cardiac Pacing and Electrophysiology: A Bridge to the 21st Century. Dordrecht, The Netherlands, 1994, pp 309–324.
61. Novak M, Smola M, Kejrova E: Pacemaker built-in Holter counters match up to ambulatory Holter recordings. In Sethi KK (ed): Proceedings of the Sixth Asian-Pacific Symposium on Cardiac Pacing and Electrophysiology. Bologna, Italy, Monduzzi Editore S.P.A., 1997, pp 61–64.
62. Limousin M, Geroux L, Nitzsche R, et al: Value of automatic processing and reliability of stored data in an implanted pacemaker: Initial results in 59 patients. PACE 1997, 20:2893–2898.
63. Intermedics Technical Manual: Relay DDDR Pacing System. Angleton, TX, Intermedics, 1992.
64. Trilogy DR+ 2364L Pulse Generator Technical Manual. Sylmar, CA, Pacesetter Inc, 1996.
65. Garson A Jr: Stepwise approach to the unknown pacemaker ECG. Am Heart J 119:924, 1990.
66. Furman S: Cardiac pacing and pacemakers. VI. Analysis of pacemaker malfunction. Am Heart J 94:378, 1977.

67. Mond HG: The Cardiac Pacemaker: Function and Malfunction. New York, Grune & Stratton, 1983.

68. Barold SS: Modern Cardiac Pacing. Mt Kisco, NY, Futura Publishing, 1983.

69. Levine PA: Pacing system malfunction. *In* Ellenbogen KA (ed): Cardiac Pacing. Boston, Blackwell Scientific, 1992, pp 309–382.

70. Morse DP, Steiner RM, Parsonnet V: A Guide to Cardiac Pacemakers. Philadelphia, FA Davis, 1983.

71. Morse DP, Steiner RM, Parsonnet V: A Guide to Cardiac Pacemakers: Supplement 1986–1987. Philadelphia, FA Davis, 1986.

72. Morse DP, Parsonnet V, Gessment LJ, et al: A Guide to Cardiac Pacemaker, Defibrillator and Related Products. Durham, NC, Droege Computing Services, 1991.

73. Van Gelder LM, El Gamal MIH: Myopotential interference inducing pacemaker tachycardia in a DVI programmed pacemaker. PACE 7:970, 1984.

74. Lindenberg BS, Hagan CA, Levine PA: Design dependent loss of telemetry: Uplink telemetry hold. PACE 12:823, 1989.

75. Levine PA, Lindenberg BS: Upper rate limit circuit-induced rate slowing. PACE 10:310, 1987.

76. Levine PA, Lindenberg BS, Mace RC: Analysis of AV universal (DDD) pacemaker rhythms. Clin Prog Pacing Electrophysiol 2:54, 1984.

77. Bertuso J, Kapoor A, Schafer J: A case of ventricular undersensing in the DDI mode: Cause and correction. PACE 9:685, 1986.

78. Erlbacher JA, Stelzer P: Inappropriate ventricular blanking in a DDI pacemaker. PACE 9:519, 1986.

79. Ajiki K, Sagara K, Namiki T, et al: A case of a pseudomalfunction of a DDD pacemaker. PACE 14:1456, 1991.

80. Meyer JA, Fruehan CT, Delmonico JE: The pacemaker twiddler's syndrome: A further note. J Thorac Cardiovasc Surg 67:903, 1974.

81. Veltri EP, Mower MM, Reid PR: Twiddler's syndrome: A new twist. PACE 7:1004, 1984.

82. Lal RB, Avery RD: Aggressive pacemaker twiddler's syndrome: Dislodgment of an active fixation ventricular pacing electrode. Chest 97:756, 1990.

83. Roberts JS, Wenger NK: Pacemaker twiddler's syndrome. Am J Cardiol 63:1013, 1989.

84. Ellis GL: Pacemaker twiddler's syndrome: A case report. Am J Emerg Med 8:48, 1990.

85. Ekbom K, Nilsson BY, Edhag O: Rhythmic shoulder girdle muscle contractions as a complication in pacemaker treatment. Chest 66:599, 1974.

86. Gelleri D: Retrograde (ventriculoatrial) conduction, premature beats, pseudotricuspid regurgitation, systolic atrial sounds, and pacemaker sounds observed together in two patients with ventricular pacing. Acta Med Hung 48:157, 1991.

87. Flickinger AL, Peller PA, Deran BP, et al: Pacemaker-induced friction rub and apical thrill. Chest 102:323, 1992.

88. Jalin P, Kaul U, Wasir HS: Myopotential inhibition of unipolar demand pacemakers: Utility of provocative maneuvers in assessment and management. Int J Cardiol 34:33, 1992.

89. Levine PA, Caplan CH, Klein MD, et al: Myopotential inhibition of unipolar lithium pacemakers. Chest 82:461–465, 1982.

90. Levine PA: Electrocardiography of bipolar single- and dual-chamber pacing systems. Herzschrittmacher 8:86–90, 1988.

91. Cherry R, Sactuary C, Kennedy HL: The question of frequency response. Ambulatory Electrocardiol 1:13, 1977.

92. Sheffield LT, Berson AL, Bragg Remschel D, et al: AHA special report: Recommendation for standards of instrumentation and practice in the use of ambulatory electrocardiography. Circulation 71:626A, 1985.

93. Lesh MD, Langberg JJ, Griffin JC, et al: Pacemaker generator pseudomalfunction: An artifact of Holter monitoring. PACE 14:854–857, 1991.

94. Van Gelder LM, Bracke FALE, El Gamal MIH: Fusion or confusion on Holter recordings. PACE 14:760–763, 1991.

95. Engler RL, Goldberger AL, Bhargava V, Kapelusznik D: Pacemaker spike alternans: An artifact of digital signal processing. PACE 5:748–750, 1982.

96. Slack JP: Identification of recording artefact in a dual chamber (DDD) paced rhythm: Clues from the electrocardiogram. Clin Prog Pacing and Electrophysiol 2:384–387, 1984.

97. Schüller H, Fåhraeus T: Pacemaker EKG: A clinical approach. Solna, Sweden, Siemens Elema, 1980.

98. Levine PA, Schüller H, Lindgren A: Pacemaker ECG: An introduction and approach to interpretation. Solna, Sweden, Siemens-Pacesetter, 1986.

99. Wilkoff BL, Firstenberg MS, Moore S, Ching B: Lead impedance velocity as a predictor of pacing lead instability. PACE 16:930, 1993.

100. Karis JP, Ravin CE: Counterclockwise exit of cardiac pacemaker leads: Sign of pulse-generator flip. Radiology 174:711, 1990.

101. Suzuki Y, Fujimori S, Sakai M, et al: A case of pacemaker lead fracture associated with thoracic outlet syndrome. PACE 11:326, 1988.

102. Stokes K, Staffenson D, Lessar J, et al: A possible new complication of subclavian stick: Conductor fracture. PACE 10:748, 1987.

103. Anonymous: Subclavian puncture procedure may result in lead conductor fracture. Medtronic News Winter 16(2):27, 1986/87.

104. Magney JE, Flynn DM, Parsons JA, et al: Anatomical mechanisms explaining damage to pacemaker leads, defibrillator leads, and failure of central venous catheters adjacent to the sternoclavicular joint. PACE 16:445, 1993.

105. Jacobs DM, Fink AS, Miller RP, et al: Anatomical and morphological evaluation of pacemaker lead compression. PACE 16:434, 1993.

106. Arakawa M, Kambara K, Ito HA, et al: Intermittent oversensing due to internal insulation damage of temperature sensing rate-responsive pacemaker lead in subclavian venipuncture method. PACE 12:1312, 1989.

107. Antonelli D, Rosenfeld T, Freedberg NA, et al: Insulation lead failure: Is it a matter of insulation coating, venous approach or both? PACE 21:418–421, 1998.

108. Fyke FE: Simultaneous insulation deterioration associated with side-by-side subclavian placement of two polyurethane leads. PACE 11:1571, 1988.

109. Kranz J, Crystal DK, Wagner CL, et al: Thoracic outlet compression syndrome: The first rib. Northwest Med 68:646, 1969.

110. Witte A: Pseudofracture of pacemaker lead due to securing suture: A case report. PACE 4:716, 1981.

111. Deering JA, Pederson DN: A case of pacemaker lead fracture associated with weightlifting. PACE 15:1354, 1992.

112. Schuger CD, Mittleman R, Habbal B, et al: Ventricular lead transection and atrial lead damage in a young softball player shortly after the insertion of a permanent pacemaker. PACE 15:1236, 1992.

113. Papa LA, Abkar KB, Chung EK: Pacemaker hysteresis. Heart Lung 3:982–984, 1974.

114. Bornzin GA, Arambula ER, Florio J, et al: Adjusting heart rate during sleep using activity variance. PACE 17:1933–1938, 1994.

115. Gammage MD, Hess M, Markowitz T: Initial experience with a rate drop algorithm in malignant vasovagal syndrome. Eur J Cardiac Pacing Electrophysiol 5:45–48, 1995.

116. Brandt J, Fåhraeus T, Schüller H: Far-field QRS complex sensing via the atrial pacemaker lead. I. Mechanism, consequences, differential diagnosis and countermeasures in AAI and VDD/DDD pacing. PACE 11:1432–1438, 1988.

117. Wolpert C, Jung W, Scholl C, et al: Electrical proarrhythmia: Induction of inappropriate atrial therapies due to far-field R wave oversensing in a new dual chamber defibrillator. J Cardiovasc Electrophysiol 9:859–863, 1998.

118. Halperin JL, Camunas JL, Stern EH, et al: Myopotential interference with DDD pacemakers: Endocardial electrographic telemetry in the diagnosis of pacemaker-related arrhythmias. Am J Cardiol 54:97, 1984.

119. Williams DO, Thomas DJ: Muscle potentials simulating pacemaker malfunction. Br Heart J 38:1096, 1976.

120. Ohm OJ, Morkrid L, Hammer E: Amplitude-frequency characteristics of myopotentials and endocardial potentials as seen by a pacemaker system. Scand J Thorac Cardiovasc Surg 22(Suppl):41–46, 1978.

121. Ohm OJ, Bruland H, Pedersen OM, et al: Interference effect of myopotentials on function of unipolar demand pacemakers. Br Heart J 35:77, 1974.

122. Gabry MD, Behrens M, Andrews C, et al: Comparison of myopotential interference in unipolar-bipolar programmable DDD pacemakers. PACE 10:1322, 1987.

123. Gross JN, Platt S, Ritacco R, et al: The clinical relevance of electromyopotential oversensing in current unipolar devices. PACE 15:2023, 1992.

124. Volosin KJ, Rudderow R, Waxman HL: VOOR: Nondemand rate-modulated pacing necessitated by myopotential inhibition. PACE 12:421, 1989.

125. Dodinot B, Godenir JP, Costa AB: Electronic article surveillance: A possible danger for pacemaker patients. PACE 16:46, 1993.

126. Inbar S, Larson J, Burt T, et al: Case report: Nuclear magnetic resonance imaging in a patient with a pacemaker. Am J Med Sci 305:174, 1993.
127. Marco D, Eisinger G, Hayes DL: Testing of work environments for electromagnetic interference. PACE 15:2016, 1992.
128. Toivonen L, Valjus J, Hongisto M, et al: The influence of elevated 50 Hz electric and magnetic fields on implanted pacemakers: The role of the lead configuration and programming of the sensitivity. PACE 14:2114, 1991.
129. Mellenberg DE Jr: A policy for radiotherapy in patients with implanted pacemakers. Med Dosim 16:221, 1991.
130. Mangar D, Atlas GM, Kane PB: Electrocautery-induced pacemaker malfunction during surgery. Can J Anaesth 38:616, 1991.
131. Teskey RJ, Whelan I, Akyurekli Y, et al: Therapeutic irradiation over a permanent pacemaker. PACE 14:143, 1991.
132. Salmi J, Eskola HJ, Pitkanen MA, et al: The influence of electromagnetic interference and ionizing radiation on cardiac pacemakers. Strahlenther Onkol 166:153, 1990.
133. Chin MC, Rosenqvist M, Lee MA, et al: The effect of radiofrequency catheter ablation on permanent pacemakers: An experimental study. PACE 13:23, 1990.
134. McDeller AG, Toff WD, Hobbs RA, et al: The development of a system for the evaluation of electromagnetic interference with pacemaker function: Hazards in the aircraft environment. J Med Eng Technol 13:161, 1989.
135. Godin JF, Petitot JC: STIMAREC report: Pacemaker failures due to electrocautery and external electric shock. PACE 12:1011, 1989.
136. Belott P, Sands S, Warren J, et al: Resetting of DDD pacemakers due to EMI. PACE 7:169, 1984.
137. Erdman S, Levinsky L, Strasberg B, et al: Use of the new Shaw scalpel in pacemaker operations. J Thorac Cardiovasc Surg 89:304, 1985.
138. Gascho JA, Newton MC: Electromagnetic interference in dynamic electrocardiography caused by an electric blanket. Am Heart J 95:408, 1978.
139. Irnich W: Interference in pacemakers. PACE 7:1021, 1984.
140. Kuan P, Kozlowski J, Castellanet MJ, et al: Interference with pacemaker function by cardiographic testing. Am J Cardiol 58:362, 1986.
141. Leeds CJ, Akhtar M, Damato AN, et al: Fluoroscope-generated electromagnetic interference in an external demand pacemaker. Circulation 55:548, 1977.
142. Warnowicz-Papp M: The pacemaker patient and the electromagnetic environment. Clin Prog Pacing Electrophysiol 1:166, 1983.
143. Van Gelder LM, El Gamal MIH: False inhibition of an atrial demand pacemaker caused by insulation defect in a polyurethane lead. PACE 6:834, 1983.
144. Sanford CF: Self-inhibition of an AV sequential demand pulse generator due to polyurethane lead insulation disruption. PACE 6:840, 1983.
145. Salem DN, Bornstein A, Levine PA, et al: Fracture of pacing electrode mimicking failure of pulse generator. Chest 74:673, 1978.
146. Coumel P, Mujica J, Barold SS: Demand pacemaker arrhythmias caused by intermittent incomplete electrode fracture. Am J Cardiol 36:105, 1975.
147. Barold SS, Scovil J, Ong LS, et al: Periodic pacemaker spike attenuation with preservation of capture: An unusual electrocardiographic manifestation of partial pacing electrode fracture. PACE 1:375, 1978.
148. Sarmiento JJ: Clinical utility of telemetered intracardiac electrograms in diagnosing a design dependent lead malfunction. PACE 13:188, 1990.
149. Nalos PC, Nyitray W: Benefits of intracardiac electrograms and programmable sensing polarity in preventing pacemaker inhibition due to spurious screw-in lead signals. PACE 13:1101, 1990.
150. Chew PH, Brinker JA: Oversensing from electrode "chatter" in a bipolar pacing lead: A case report. PACE 13:808, 1990.
151. Santomauro M, Ferraro S, Maddalena G, et al: Pacemaker malfunction due to subcutaneous emphysema: A case report. Angiology 43:873, 1992.
152. Giroud D, Goy JJ: Pacemaker malfunction due to subcutaneous emphysema. Int J Cardiol 26:234, 1990.
153. Shepard RB, Kim J, Colvin HC, et al: Pacing threshold spikes months and years after implant. PACE 14:1835, 1991.
154. Trautwein W: Electrophysiological aspects of cardiac stimulation. In Schaldach M, Furman S (eds): Advances in Pacemaker Technology. New York, Springer-Verlag, 1975, pp 11–23.
155. Siddons H, Sowton E: Threshold for stimulation. In Cardiac Pacemakers. Springfield, IL, Charles C Thomas, 1967, pp 145–174.
156. Ohm OJ, Breivik K, Anderssen KS: Strength-duration curves in cardiac pacing. In Meere C (ed): Proceedings of the Sixth World Symposium on Cardiac Pacing. Montreal, January 1979, Chap 20.
157. Irnich W: The chronaxy time and its practical importance. PACE 3:292, 1980.
158. Davies JG, Sowton E: Electrical threshold of the human heart. Br Heart J 28:231, 1966.
159. Furman S, Hurzeler P, Mehra R: Cardiac pacing and pacemakers. IV. Threshold of cardiac stimulation. Am Heart J 94:115, 1977.
160. Helguera ME, Maloney JD, Woscoboinik JR, et al: Long-term performance of epimyocardial pacing leads in adults: Comparison with endocardial leads. PACE 16:412, 1993.
161. Esperper HD, Mahmoud PO, von der Emde J: Is epicardial dual-chamber pacing a realistic alternative to endocardial DDD pacing? Initial results of a prospective study. PACE 15:155, 1992.
162. Bianconi L, Boccadamo R, Toscano S, et al: Effects of oral propafenone therapy on chronic myocardial pacing threshold. PACE 15:148, 1992.
163. Szabo Z, Solti F: The significance of the tissue reaction around the electrode on the late myocardial threshold. In Schaldach M, Furman S (eds): Advances in Pacemaker Technology. New York, Springer-Verlag, 1975, pp 273–287.
164. DeLeon SY, Ilbawi MN, Backer CL, et al: Exit block in pediatric cardiac pacing: Comparison of the suture-type and fishhook epicardial electrodes. J Thorac Cardiovasc Surg 99:905, 1990.
165. Stojanov P, Djordjevic M, Velimirovic D, et al: Assessment of long-term stability of chronic ventricular pacing thresholds in steroid-eluting electrodes. PACE 15:1417, 1992.
166. Karpawich PP, Hakimi M, Arciniegas E, et al: Improved epicardial pacing in children: Steroid contribution to porous platinized electrodes. PACE 15:1551, 1992.
167. Johns JA, Fish FA, Burger JD, et al: Steroid-eluting epicardial pacing leads in pediatric patients encouraging early results. J Am Coll Cardiol 20:395, 1992.
168. Stamato NJ, O'Tolle MF, Petter JG, et al: The safety and efficacy of chronic ventricular pacing at 1.6 volts using a steroid-eluting lead. PACE 15:248, 1992.
169. Hamilton R, Gow R, Bahoric B, et al: Steroid-eluting epicardial leads in pediatrics: Improved epicardial threshold in the first year. PACE 14:2066, 1991.
170. Anderson N, Mathivanar R, Skalsky M, et al: Active fixation leads: Long-term threshold reduction using a drug-infused ceramic collar. PACE 14:1767, 1991.
171. Kruse IM, Terpstra B: Acute and long-term atrial and ventricular stimulation thresholds with a steroid-eluting electrode. PACE 8:45, 1985.
172. Mond H, Stokes K, Helland J, et al: The porous titanium steroid-eluting electrode: A double-blind study assessing the stimulation threshold effects of steroid. PACE 11:214, 1988.
173. Klein HH, Steinberger J, Knake W: Stimulation characteristics of a steroid-eluting electrode compared with three conventional electrodes. PACE 13:134, 1990.
174. Beanlands DS, Akyurekli Y, Keon WJ: Prednisone in the management of exit block. In Meere C (ed): Proceedings of the Sixth World Symposium on Cardiac Pacing. Montreal, January 1979, Chap 18.
175. Nagatomo Y, Ogawa T, Kumagae H, et al: Pacing failure due to markedly increased stimulation threshold two years after implantation: Successful management with oral prednisolone, a case report. PACE 12:1034, 1989.
176. Preston TA, Judge RD, Lucchesi BR, et al: Myocardial threshold in patients with artificial pacemakers. Am J Cardiol 18:83, 1966.
177. Schlesinger Z, Rosenberg T, Stryjer D, et al: Exit block in myxedema, treated effectively with thyroid hormone therapy. PACE 3:737, 1980.
178. Lee D, Greenspan K, Edmands RE, Fisch C: The effect of electrolyte alteration on stimulus requirement of cardiac pacemakers. Circulation 38:VI124, 1968.
179. Gettes LS, Shabetai R, Downs TA, et al: Effect of changes in potassium and calcium concentrations on diastolic threshold and strength-interval relationships of the human heart. Ann N Y Acad Sci 167:693, 1969.
180. O'Reilly MV, Murnaghan DP, Williams MB: Transvenous pacemaker failure induced by hyperkalemia. JAMA 228:336, 1974.
181. Dohrmann ML, Godschlager N: Metabolic and pharmacologic effects on myocardial stimulation threshold in patients with cardiac pacemakers. In Barold SS (ed): Modern Cardiac Pacing. Mt Kisco, NY, Futura Publishing, 1985, pp 161–170.

182. Sowton E, Barr I: Physiologic changes in threshold. Ann N Y Acad Sci 167:679, 1969.

183. Finfer SR: Pacemaker failure on induction of anaesthesia. Br J Anaesth 66:509, 1991.

184. Hughes JC Jr, Tyers GFO, Torman HA: Effects of acid-base imbalance on myocardial pacing thresholds. J Thorac Cardiovasc Surg 69:743, 1975.

185. Preston TA, Judge RD: Alteration of pacemaker threshold by drug and physiologic factors. Ann N Y Acad Sci 167:686, 1969.

186. Preston TA, Fletcher RD, Lucchesi BR, et al: Changes in myocardial threshold: Physiologic and pharmacologic factors in patients with implanted pacemakers. Am Heart J 74:235, 1967.

187. Emilsson K, Oddsson II, Allared M, Brorson L: An unusual cause of high threshold values at pacemaker implantation. PACE 20:366–367, 1977.

188. Perry GY, Parsonnet V, Werres R, Flowers NC: Transient loss of sensing and capture during coronary angiography in two patients with permanent pacemakers. PACE 18:108–112, 1995.

189. Hellestrand KJ, Burnett PJ, Milne JR, et al: Effect of the antiarrhythmic agent flecainide acetate on acute and chronic pacing thresholds. PACE 6:892, 1983.

190. Levick CE, Mizgala HF, Kerr CR: Failure to pace following high-dose antiarrhythmic therapy: Reversal with isoproterenol. PACE 7:252, 1984.

191. Nielsen AP, Griffin JC, Herre JM, et al: Effect of amiodarone on acute and chronic pacing thresholds. PACE 7:462, 1984.

192. Montefoschi N, Boccadamo R: Propafenone-induced acute variation of chronic atrial pacing threshold: A case report. PACE 13:480, 1990.

193. Salel AF, Seagren SC, Pool PE: Effects of encainide on the function of implanted pacemakers. PACE 12:1439, 1989.

194. Guarnieri T, Datorre SD, Bondke H, et al: Increased pacing threshold after an automatic defibrillatory shock in dogs: Effects of class I and class II antiarrhythmic drugs. PACE 11:1324, 1988.

195. Clarke M, Liu B, Schüller H, et al: Automatic adjustment of pacemaker stimulation output correlated with continuously monitored capture thresholds: A multicenter study. PACE 21:1567–1575, 1998.

196. Grant SC, Bennett DH: Atrial latency in a dual-chambered pacing system causing inappropriate sequence of cardiac chamber activation. PACE 15:116, 1992.

197. Furman S, Hurzeler P, DeCaprio V: Cardiac pacing and pacemakers III: Sensing the cardiac electrogram. Am Heart J 93:794, 1977.

198. Ohm OJ: The interdependence between electrogram, total electrode impedance, and pacemaker input impedance necessary to obtain adequate functioning demand pacemakers. PACE 2:465, 1979.

199. Kleinert M, Elmqvist H, Strandberg H: Spectral properties of atrial and ventricular endocardial signals. PACE 2:11, 1979.

200. Myers GH, Kresh YM, Parsonnet V: Characteristics of intracardiac electrograms. PACE 1:90, 1978.

201. Evans GL, Glasser SP: Intracardiac electrocardiography as a guide to pacemaker positioning. JAMA 216:483, 1971.

202. Levine PA, Klein MD: Discrepant electrocardiographic and pulse analyzer endocardial potentials: A possible source of pacemaker sensing failure. *In* Meere C (ed): Proceedings of the Sixth World Symposium on Cardiac Pacing. Montreal, January 1979, Chap 34.

203. Levine PA, Seltzer JP: Fusion, pseudofusion, pseudo-pseudofusion and confusion: Normal rhythms associated with atrioventricular sequential "DVI" pacing. Clin Prog Pacing Electrophysiol 1:70, 1983.

204. Barold SS, Falkoff MD, Ong LS, et al: Characterization of pacemaker arrhythmias due to normally functioning AV demand (DVI) pulse generators. PACE 3:712, 1980.

205. Breivik K, Ohm OJ, Engedal H: Long-term comparison of unipolar and bipolar pacing and sensing, using a new multiprogrammable pacemaker system. PACE 6:592, 1983.

206. Ohm OJ: Demand failures occurring during permanent pacing in patients with serious heart disease. PACE 3:44, 1980.

207. Griffin JC, Finke WL: Analysis of the endocardial electrogram morphology of isolated ventricular beats. PACE 6:315, 1983.

208. Barold SS, Gaidula JJ: Failure of demand pacemaker from low-voltage bipolar ventricular electrograms. JAMA 215:923, 1971.

209. Van Mechelen R, Hart CT, De Boer H: Failure to sense P waves during DDD pacing. PACE 9:498, 1986.

210. Bricker JT, Ward KA, Zinner A, Gillette PC: Decrease in canine endocardial and epicardial electrogram voltage with exercise: Implications for pacemaker sensing. PACE 11:460, 1988.

211. Frohlig G, Schwerdt H, Schieffer H, et al: Atrial signal variations and pacemaker malsensing during exercise: A study in the time and frequency domain. J Am Coll Cardiol 11:806, 1988.

212. van Gelder BM, van Mechelen R, den Dulk, et al: Apparent P-wave undersensing in a DDD pacemaker post exercise. PACE 15:1651, 1992.

213. Sager DP: Current facts on pacemaker electromagnetic interference and their application to clinical care. Heart Lung 16:211, 1987.

214. Lau FYK, Bilitch M, Wintroub HJ: Protection of implanted pacemakers from excessive electrical energy of D.C. shock. Am J Cardiol 23:244, 1969.

215. Levine PA, Barold SS, Fletcher RD, Talbot P: Adverse acute and chronic effects of electrical defibrillation and cardioversion on implanted unipolar cardiac pacing systems. J Am Coll Cardiol 1:14130–1422, 1993.

216. Van Lake P, Levine PA, Mouchawar GA: Effect of implantable non-thoracotomy defibrillation system on permanent pacemakers: An in-vitro analysis with clinical implications. PACE 18:182–187, 1995.

217. De Keyser F, Vanhaecke J, Janssens L, et al: Crosstalk with external bipolar DVI pacing: A case report. PACE 14:1320, 1991.

218. Sweesy MW, Batey RL, Forney RC: Crosstalk during bipolar pacing. PACE 11:1512, 1988.

219. Coombs WJ, Reynolds DW, Sharma AJ, Bennett TD: Crosstalk in bipolar pacemakers. PACE 12:1613–1621, 1989.

220. Levine PA, Venditti FJ, Podrid PJ, Klein MD: Therapeutic and diagnostic benefits of intentional crosstalk mediated ventricular output inhibition. PACE 11:1194–1201, 1988.

221. Batey FL, Calabria DA, Sweesy MW, et al: Crosstalk and blanking periods in a dual-chamber pacemaker. Clin Prog Pacing Electrophysiol 3:314, 1985.

222. Barold SS, Falkoff MD, Ong LS, et al: Interpretation of electrocardiograms produced by a new unipolar multiprogrammable "committed" AV sequential demand (DVI) pacemaker. PACE 4:692, 1981.

223. Levine PA: Normal and abnormal rhythms associated with dual-chamber pacemakers. Cardiol Clin 3:595–616, 1985.

224. Barold SS, Belott PH: Behavior of the ventricular triggering period of DDD pacemakers. PACE 10:1237–1252, 1987.

225. Heller LI: Surgical electrocautery and the runaway pacemaker syndrome. PACE 13:1084, 1990.

226. Mickley H, Andersen C, Nielsen LH: Runaway pacemaker: A still existing complication and therapeutic guidelines. Clin Cardiol 12:412, 1989.

227. Snoeck J, Beerkhof M, Claeys M, et al: External vibration interference of activity based rate-responsive pacemakers. PACE 15:1841, 1992.

228. Lamb LS Jr, Judson EB: Maximal rate response in a permanent pacemaker during chest physiotherapy. Heart Lung 21:390, 1992.

229. Lau CP, Tai YT, Fong PC, et al: Pacemaker-mediated tachycardias in single-chamber rate-responsive pacing. PACE 13:1575, 1990.

230. Madsen GM, Andersen C: Pacemaker-induced tachycardia during general anaesthesia: A case report. Br J Anaesth 63:360, 1989.

231. Fetter J, Patterson D, Aram G, et al: Effects of extracorporeal shock wave lithotripsy on single-chamber rate-response and dual-chamber pacemakers. PACE 12:1494, 1989.

232. Lau CP, Linker NJ, Butrous GS, et al: Myopotential interference in unipolar rate-responsive pacemakers. PACE 12:1324, 1989.

233. French RS, Tillman JG: Pacemaker function during helicopter transport. Ann Emerg Med 18:305, 1989.

234. Volosin KJ, O'Connor WH, Fabiszewski R, et al: Pacemaker-mediated tachycardia from a single-chamber temperature-sensitive pacemaker. PACE 12:1596, 1989.

235. Fearnot NE, Kitoh O, Fujita T, et al: Case studies on the effect of exercise and hot water submersion on intracardiac temperature and the performance of a pacemaker which varies pacing rate based on temperature. Jpn Heart J 30:353, 1989.

236. Seeger W, Kleinert M: An unexpected rate response of a minute ventilation dependent pacemaker [Letter]. PACE 12:1707, 1989.

237. Hayes DL: Rate adaptive cardiac pacing: Implications of environmental noise during craniotomy. Anesthesiology 87:1243–1245, 1997.

238. Holmes DR, Hayes DL, Gray JE, Merideth J: The effects of magnetic resonance imaging on implantable pulse generators. PACE 9:360, 1986.

239. Hayes DL, Holmes DR, Gray JE: Effect of 1.5 Telsa nuclear magnetic resonance imaging scanner on implanted permanent pacemakers. J Am Coll Cardiol 10:782, 1987.

240. Erlebacher JA, Cahill PT, Pannizzo F, Knowles RJR: Effect of magnetic resonance imaging on DDD pacemakers. Am J Cardiol 57:347, 1986.

241. Gimbel JR, Johnson D, Levine PA, Wilkoff BL: Safe performance of magnetic resonance imaging on five patients with permanent cardiac pacemakers. PACE 19:913–919, 1996.

242. Achenbach S, Moshage W, Diem B, et al: Effects of magnetic resonance imaging on cardiac pacemakers and electrodes. Am Heart J 134:467–473, 1997.

243. Shellack F, Kanal E: Politics, guidelines and recommendations for MR imaging safety and patient management. J Magn Reson Imaging 11:97–104, 1991.

244. Lauck G, von Smekal A, Wolke S, et al: Effects of nuclear magnetic resonance imaging on cardiac pacemakers. PACE 18:1549–1555, 1995.

245. Schüller H, Binner L, Linde C, et al: Combipolar™ sensing in DDD pacemakers: Do we still need bipolar atrial leads? In Sethi KK (ed): Proceedings of the Sixth Asian Pacific Symposium on Cardiac Pacing and Electrophysiology. Bologna, Italy, Monduzzi Editore S.P.A., 1997, pp 75–79.

246. Levine PA, Selznick L: Prospective Management of the Patient With Retrograde Ventriculoatrial Conduction: Prevention and Management of Pacemaker Mediated Endless Loop Tachycardias. Sylmar, CA, Pacesetter Systems, 1990.

247. Limousin M, Bonnet JL: A multicentric study of 1816 endless loop tachycardia (ELT) responses. PACE 13:555, 1990.

248. Oseran D, Ausubel K, Klementowicz PT, et al: Spontaneous endless loop tachycardia. PACE 9:379, 1986.

249. Rubin JW, Frank MJ, Boineau JP, et al: Current physiologic pacemakers: A serious problem with a new device. Am J Cardiol 52:88, 1983.

250. Levine PA: Postventricular atrial refractory periods and pacemaker-mediated tachycardias. Clin Prog Pacing Electrophysiol 1:394, 1983.

251. Furman S, Fisher JD: Endless loop tachycardia in an AV universal (DDD) pacemaker. PACE 5:486, 1982.

252. Den Dulk K, Lindemans FW, Bar FW, et al: Pacemaker-related tachycardias. PACE 5:476, 1982.

253. Luceri RM, Castellanos A, Zaman L, et al: The arrhythmias of dual-chamber cardiac pacemakers and their management. Ann Intern Med 99:354, 1983.

254. Ausubel K, Gabry MD, Klementowicz PT, et al: Pacemaker-mediated endless loop tachycardia at rates below the upper rate limit. Am J Cardiol 61:465, 1988.

255. Denes P, Wu D, Dhingra R, et al: The effects of cycle length on cardiac refractory periods in man. Circulation 49:32, 1974.

256. Amikam S, Furman S: Programmed upper rate limit dependent endless loop tachycardia. Chest 85:286, 1984.

257. Haffejee C, Murphy J, Gold R, et al: Automatic extension vs. programmability of the atrial refractory period in the prevention of pacemaker-mediated tachycardia. PACE 8:A56, 1985.

258. Den Dulk K, Hamersa M, Wellens HJJ: Role of an adaptable atrial refractory period for DDD pacemakers. PACE 10:425, 1987.

259. Rognoni G, Occhetta E, Perucca A, et al: A new approach to the prevention of endless loop tachycardia in DDD and VDD pacing. PACE 14:1828, 1991.

260. Nitzsche R, Gueunoun M, Lamaison D, et al: Endless-loop tachycardias: Description and first clinical results of a new fully automatic protection algorithm. PACE 13:1711, 1990.

261. Cameron DA, Gentzler RD, Love CJ, et al: Initial clinical experience with a new automatic PMT detection and termination algorithm to discriminate between pacemaker mediated tachycardia due to ventriculo-atrial conduction and normal sinus tachycardia. HeartWeb 2(1), article 96110035, 1996; http://www.webaxis.com/heartweb/1196/pacing0018.htm.

262. Klementowicz PT, Furman S: Selective atrial sensing in dual-chamber pacemakers eliminates endless loop tachycardias. J Am Coll Cardiol 7:590, 1986.

263. Pannizzo F, Amikam S, Bagwell P, et al: Discrimination of antegrade and retrograde atrial depolarization by electrogram analysis. Am Heart J 112:780, 1986.

264. McAlister HF, Klementowicz PT, Calderon EM, et al: Atrial electrogram analysis: Antegrade versus retrograde. PACE 11:1703, 1988.

265. Bernheim C, Markewitz A, Kemkes BM: Can reprogramming of atrial sensitivity avoid endless loop tachycardia? PACE 9:293, 1986.

266. Throne RD, Jenkins JM, Winston SA, et al: Discrimination of retrograde from anterograde atrial activation using intracardiac electrogram waveform analysis. PACE 12:1622, 1989.

267. Van Gelder LM, El Gamal MIH, Sanders RS: Tachycardia-termination algorithm: A valuable feature for interruption of pacemaker-mediated tachycardia. PACE 7:283, 1984.

268. Duncan JL, Clark MF: Prevention and termination of pacemaker-mediated tachycardia in a new DDD pacing system (Siemens-Pacesetter model 2010T). PACE 11:1679, 1988.

269. Puglisi A, Ricci R, Azzolini P, et al: Ventricular cross stimulation in a dual-chamber pacing system: Phenomenon analysis. PACE 13:993, 1990.

270. Goldschlager N, Francoz R: Ventricular cross stimulation using a pacing system analyzer. PACE 13:986, 1990.

271. Doi Y, Takada K, Nakagaki O, et al: A case of cross stimulation. PACE 12:569, 1989.

272. Levine PA, Rihanek BD, Sanders R, et al: Cross-stimulation: The unexpected stimulation of the unpaced chamber. PACE 8:600, 1985.

273. Van Gelder LM, El Gamal MIH: Ventriculoatrial conduction: A cause of atrial malpacing in AV universal pacemakers. A report of two cases. PACE 8:140–143, 1985.

274. Barold SS: Repetitive non-reentrant ventriculoatrial synchrony in dual chamber pacing. In Santini M, Pistolese M, Alliegro A (eds): Progress in Clinical Pacing 1990. Amsterdam: Exerpta Medica, 1990, p 451.

275. Levine PA: Pacing system malfunction: Evaluation and management. In Podrid PJ, Kowey P (eds): Cardiac Arrhythmia, Mechanisms, Diagnosis and Management. Baltimore, Williams & Wilkins, 1995, pp 582–610.

Chapter 32

Evaluation of Implantable Cardioverter-Defibrillator Malfunction, Diagnostics, and Programmers

Igor Singer

Since its introduction to the clinical practice in the early 1980s, the implantable cardioverter-defibrillator (ICD) has undergone significant evolution from a therapeutic modality of last resort to the therapeutic tool of choice for treatment of aborted sudden cardiac death and sustained ventricular arrhythmias. The original device (AID, Intec, Pittsburgh, PA) lacked any programmability and had virtually no diagnostic capabilities. With the emergence of sophisticated therapies, including bradycardia and antitachycardia pacing, the need for diagnostic capabilities and features has grown exponentially with the therapeutic sophistication of the ICD. The need to recognize and define the initiating and resulting arrhythmias after ICD intervention is but one of the reasons that sophisticated telemetric features were developed; the other reasons were the need to diagnose ICD malfunction noninvasively and to evaluate the performance of the ICD components, including battery and lead integrity.

The purpose of this chapter is to review the available methods to diagnose ICD malfunction using the programmer and noninvasive techniques.

■ DIAGNOSTIC TOOLS

Clinical History

As in all other areas of medicine, clinical history provides the cornerstone of rational diagnosis. Historical clues suggesting ICD malfunction, although by themselves nondiagnostic, provide the basis for the presumptive diagnosis and suggest further avenues of inquiry. For example, repeated shocks in asymptomatic patients suggest false signal detection. Certain body positions associated with ICD shocks suggest the possibility of lead fracture or lead instability. ICD model, manufacturer, date of implantation, lead type and location, antiarrhythmic drug history, presence or absence of symptoms of heart failure or angina preceding

therapy, and other historical clues are important to elicit because any or all of these factors may have relevance and can be causally related to inappropriate ICD therapy. The presence of an implanted pacemaker with an ICD raises the specter of device–device interactions.

Physical Examination

The physical examination is rarely helpful in pinpointing the exact cause of ICD malfunction; however, certain aspects of the examination may be helpful. For example, in a patient who reports that certain body positions or movements may elicit ICD shock, it is helpful—indeed sometimes even crucial—to put the patient through the precise maneuvers known to elicit ICD shocks while simultaneously telemetering the device to reproduce the exact circumstances causing the shock occurrence. Occasionally, patients are reluctant to allow the examiner to do this because the prospect of an ICD shock is psychologically threatening and almost universally painful. In such circumstances, it is best to perform the specific maneuvers in the electrophysiology laboratory while the patient is under sedation and where full resuscitative measures are available.

Manipulation of the device pocket or the lead entry point to the subclavian vein may elicit false detection signals, indicating lead conductor fracture (Fig. 32–1). Occasionally, similar symptoms may occur with a loose connection of the set-screw to lead terminal pin in the ICD pulse generator header. Other diagnostic clues may be elicited by the physical examination, such as detection of an irregular pulse suggestive of atrial fibrillation, which may be readily confirmed by electrocardiographic (ECG) recording. Congestive heart failure (CHF) is often associated with exacerbation of ventricular arrhythmias. Therefore, eliciting symptoms and signs of left ventricular (LV) decompensation suggests a possible cause for worsening arrhythmias.

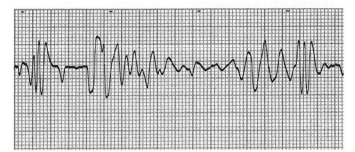

Figure 32–1. Stored electrogram (Ventritex V-100, Sunnyvale, CA) from a patient who presented with multiple implantable cardioverter-defibrillator shocks while moving the left arm. Spurious signals were recorded from conductor fracture of the right ventricular lead. (From Singer I: Complications of ICD surgery, postoperative care and follow-up. *In* Singer I [ed]: Interventional Electrophysiology. Baltimore, Williams & Wilkins, 1997, p 777.)

It is beyond the scope of this chapter to list all possible permutations of physical signs that could suggest reasons for ICD malfunction. It is, however, important to point out that, like a detective, the physician should not overlook all available clues.

Electrocardiographic Recording

Documentary evidence of the arrhythmia and subsequent ICD therapy, or an arrhythmia with absence of the expected ICD response, can be extremely helpful and is usually diagnostic (Fig. 32–2). Unfortunately, such evidence is rarely available unless the patient is hospitalized and monitored at the time of the event. Availability of stored ICD telemetry in modern ICDs has overcome many of the problems resulting from frequently missing corroborative ECG evidence, but on occasion, even retrieved ICD telemetry may be inconclusive or confusing. Nevertheless, whenever such recordings are available, they should be reviewed carefully along with all other available clinical evidence.

Device Telemetry

The advent of device telemetry has revolutionized and greatly simplified analysis of arrhythmias and events suspected of representing ICD malfunction. The early devices (e.g., Ventak, CPI, St. Paul, MN) were able to emit sounds, or beeps synchronous with ventricular electrogram detection, enabling identification of oversensing (Fig. 32–3) or undersensing. Although helpful, these crude attempts at telemetry were quickly supplanted by advances that enabled detailed information, such as RR intervals and ventricular electrograms, to be telemetered out (Fig. 32–4). The complexity and sophistication of these diagnostic tools is increasing with the new generation of ICDs. The addition of the atrial channel has greatly simplified analysis of arrhythmia events (Fig. 32–5).

Other diagnostic information is now routinely available in all ICDs, including battery voltage, lead impedance, charge times, capacitor reformation times, high-voltage lead impedance, and frequency and timing of ventricular events. It is likely that the complexity and the scope of the available information will increase in the future as the technologic advances in ICDs, microcircuitry, and available device memory provide further avenues for storage and retrieval of information.

Radiographic Evidence

Radiographic evidence is helpful when lead malposition or displacement is suspected (Fig. 32–6). It is recommended, whenever possible, that chest radiographs taken after ICD implantation be compared with the current radiographs. Such comparisons may reveal lead malposition and displacement when none are suspected. Radiographs can also be helpful in confirming a loose pin in the device header or rarely in demonstrating conductor fracture. Examining the radiographic "signature" of the device can help identify the device type when the patient is unaware of the ICD model or type.

Figure 32–2. An episode of asymptomatic ventricular tachycardia (VT) recorded during hospitalization in a patient with an implantable cardioverter-defibrillator (ICD). Despite the short cycle length of this tachycardia, the patient, who was sitting in bed watching television, was unaware of the VT until he received the shock from his ICD. This demonstrates the now well-known fact that the absence of symptoms does not preclude rapid VT and ventricular fibrillation in patients receiving asymptomatic shocks. (From Tchou P, Kadri N, Anderson J, et al: Automatic implantable defibrillators and survival of patients with left ventricular dysfunction and malignant ventricular arrhythmias. Ann Intern Med 109:529, 1988.)

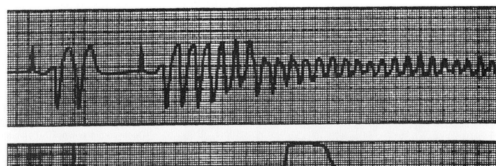
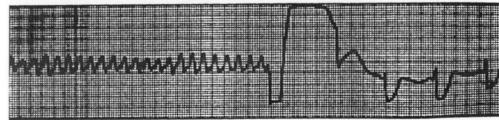

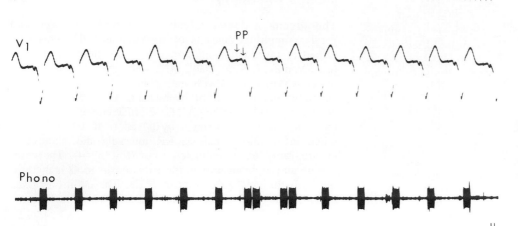

V₁

PP

Phono

T

Figure 32–3. Double sensing occurs with the Ventak (CPI, St. Paul, MN) device as a result of the sensing of the pacemaker artifact and the ventricular depolarization. Top tracing lead V₁; bottom tracing, phonocardiogram. Note the intermittent double counting. (From Singer I: Interactions with antiarrhythmic drugs and pacemakers. *In* Singer I [ed]: Implantable Cardioverter Defibrillator. Armonk, NY, Futura, 1994, p 386.)

■ SUSPECTED MALFUNCTION

ICD malfunction is uncommon. The reasons for inappropriate therapy or the absence of expected therapy usually relates to one of the following: (1) inappropriate programming; (2) lead-related complications; (3) drug–device interactions; (4) device–device interactions; (5) imperfect diagnostic specificity, particularly with single-chamber ICDs; and rarely, (6) true device component malfunction.

Inappropriate Programming

Programming of ICDs is a complex subject; discussion in this chapter is necessarily superficial. Several general comments need to be emphasized at this point. As ICD technology has evolved and has become more complex, the panoply of available therapies has also grown exponentially, providing both choice and challenge to electrophysiologists. Programming of ICDs requires a thorough understanding of the

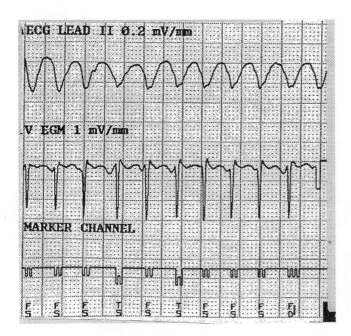

Figure 32–4. Appropriate sensing during ventricular tachycardia in a patient with an implanted PCD Jewel 7219C device (Medtronic, Minneapolis, MN). Top channel, surface lead II; middle channel, ventricular electrogram (V EGM); bottom channel, marker channel; FS, fibrillation sense; TS, tachycardia sense; FD, fibrillation detected. (From Singer I: Complications of ICD surgery, postoperative care and follow-up. *In* Singer I [ed]: Interventional Electrophysiology. Baltimore, Williams & Wilkins, 1997, p 789.)

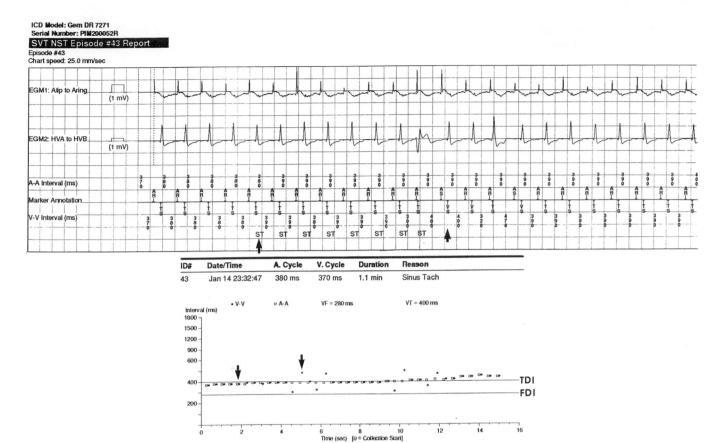

Figure 32–5. A stored supraventricular tachycardia episode from the Gem DR (Medtronic, Minneapolis, MN) implantable cardioverter-defibrillator is shown for sinus tachycardia (ST) that was not detected as ventricular tachycardia (VT) because of the ST dual-chamber detection algorithm. The strip shows the bipolar atrial electrogram (EGM), the right ventricular coil-to-can ventricular EGM, and the marker annotations, including the rhythm annotations. "VT," which begins at the left arrow, shows when dual-chamber detection is withholding therapy. The VT annotations end at the right arrow because the compensatory pause of 480 msec after the premature ventricular contraction resets the VT counter to zero, and detection cannot occur again until the VT counter reaches the number of intervals for detection (NID = 16). The interval versus time graph shows the PP and RR intervals with a 1:1 rhythm close to the tachycardia detection interval, which is equal to 400 msec. Arrows on the strip and plot correspond to the beginning and end of this ST episode that was not detected or treated. (From Olson WH: Dual chamber sensing and detection of ICDs. *In* Singer I, Barold SS, Camm AJ [eds]: Nonpharmacological Therapy of Arrhythmias for the 21st Century. The State of the Art. Armonk, NY, Futura 1998, p 394.)

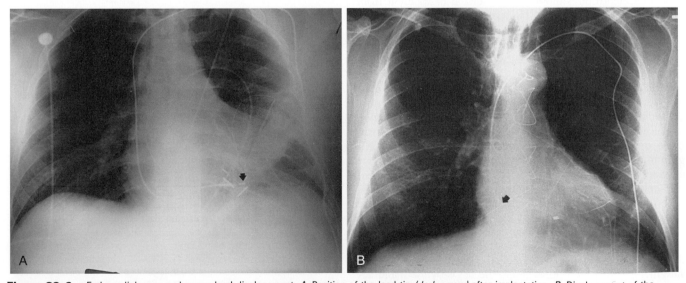

Figure 32–6. Endocardial pace and sense lead displacement. *A,* Position of the lead tip *(dark arrow)* after implantation. *B,* Displacement of the endocardial lead to the atrioventricular junction. (From Singer I: Complications of cardioverter-defibrillator surgery. *In* Singer I [ed]: Implantable Cardioverter Defibrillator. Armonk, NY, Futura, 1994, p 423.)

specific device, the arrhythmic substrate, and the potential for drug–device interactions, device–device interactions, and other clinical variables. Further, the effect of ventricular tachycardia (VT) on hemodynamics and the influence of therapies on cerebral perfusion need to be understood because the most effective and least harmful therapies for VT and ventricular fibrillation (VF) should be programmed.[1] In addition, most ICDs implanted to date have no atrial rhythm discrimination. Consequently, arrhythmia recognition is based on ventricular rate discrimination; in certain circumstances, detection enhancements, such as *rate, stability, suddenness of onset* of arrhythmia, and *arrhythmia duration*, are also used. Although these enhancements increase specificity of VT detection over and above the *rate* criteria, they do so at the expense of decreasing sensitivity and delaying ICD therapy. Therefore, it should be anticipated that whereas near 100% sensitivity is possible for detection of VF,[2] the specificity estimates for detection of VT, using the rate-only criteria, have variously been estimated at 59% to 80%.[3]

Although it is possible that arrhythmia detection specificity will improve with the addition of atrial sensing and complex algorithms for arrhythmia detection based on both the ventricular and the atrial electrogram detection and classification, this is by no means a foregone conclusion. Because atrial sensing introduces additional variables and diagnostic complexities, it could theoretically multiply further possible interpretation errors based on sensing to false signals, complex refractory periods, blanking periods, and other issues. Dual-chamber ICDs, however, hold a promise for further enhancement of arrhythmia detection specificity.

The ability to program ICDs effectively depends on several factors: (1) understanding the specific arrhythmia substrate, such as VT cycle length and hemodynamic consequences of VT (syncopal or hemodynamically well tolerated); (2) presence of supraventricular arrhythmias, such as atrial fibrillation or atrioventricular (AV) node re-entry tachycardia; (3) range of intrinsic heart rates and maximal sinus rate response during exercise; (4) status of LV function; (5) frequency of nonsustained episodes of VT; and (6) need for antiarrhythmic drugs and their effect on VT cycle length and other electrophysiologic parameters. It is apparent from this list of variables that the potential for inappropriate programming is huge and that being "too clever" in programming can potentially lead to either delay in therapy or VT nondetection, with potentially serious or even disastrous consequences.

It is not uncommon for an electrophysiologist to be confronted with the issue of ICD malfunction when a patient is diagnosed clinically to have VT but when the ICD has failed to deliver therapy. On interrogation of the device, however, more often than not it is discovered that the specific programming of the device has precluded VT detection because of inappropriate choice of rate cutoff or because the detection enhancements were programmed in such a way that the criteria for VT detection could not be met under certain conditions. Programming of ICDs by inexperienced personnel holds a real danger to the patient. The ICD may be inadvertently crippled by poor programming decisions, so that the detection of VT is precluded. Fortunately, many fail-safe mechanisms incorporated into the ICDs by the manufacturers prevent the most egregious programming combinations. This by no means precludes all possible programming errors. Therefore, appropriate training and experience are

mandatory for anyone attempting to program or follow patients with implanted ICDs. This is a compelling argument against allowing general cardiologists without specific electrophysiology training and experience to implant ICDs or to follow ICD patients.

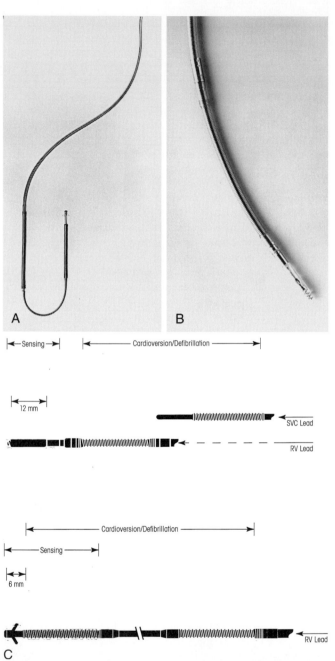

Figure 32–7. Comparison of *(A)* the Endotak-C (Guidant Corp., St. Paul, MN) endocardial electrode, which uses a single-pass endocardial lead with integrated bipolar sensing; and *(B)* the Transvene (Medtronic, Minneapolis, MN) endocardial electrode, which uses true bipolar sensing between the distal screw and the proximal ring electrode. *C,* True bipolar sensing is accomplished between the active screw and the proximal ring electrode with the Transvene lead *(top),* whereas modified bipolar sensing is obtained from the electrogram that is derived from the distal electrode to defibrillation electrode *(bottom).* (From Singer I: Defibrillation threshold testing and intraoperative ICD evaluation. *In* Singer I [ed]: Interventional Electrophysiology. Baltimore, Williams & Wilkins, 1997, p 745.)

Lead-Related Complications

ICD leads serve dual functions. In the conventional sense, the pacing bipolar pair of electrodes is used to sense and pace. Unique to the ICD, however, the same lead also incorporates defibrillation electrodes, which, when coupled to other defibrillation leads or an electrically active ICD can, are used to deliver high-voltage current for defibrillation. A less intense current may be delivered to cardiovert VT. The construction of the ICD leads is therefore more complex than that of the pacemaker leads. Two types of sensing leads have been developed: (1) a true bipolar sensing lead, with an independent defibrillation coil on the same electrode (Fig. 32–7A); and (2) an integrated bipolar lead (see Fig. 32–7B), in which the distal electrode and the more proximal coil to the distal electrode are used as the sensing electrode pair. The additional wire conductors requiring independent insulation mandate electrodes of greater diameter and complexity and, by inference, provide a greater potential for complications. These electrodes are more prone to crush fracture or insulation material failures. Because of the greater diameter and bulk, these electrodes are stiffer and more difficult to maneuver in the intravascular compartment.

Defibrillation occurs when current is delivered between the positively and negatively charged electrodes. The sensing electrode, with defibrillation coil proximal to it, is positioned within the right ventricular (RV) cavity; the other is positioned within the superior vena cava (SVC) or the innominate vein. Alternatively, the subcutaneous or subpectoral electrode is employed, either as a separate electrode, or more commonly as an electrically active titanium ICD shell ("hot can"; Fig. 32–8). Many electrode combinations have been tried, but the simplest configuration is a single RV electrode coupled to an active ICD can shell of opposite polarity.[4]

To test the integrity of the RV electrode, the operator needs to interrogate the sensing and pacing as well as the defibrillation conductors. Sensing and pacing function is tested by using the external programmer. Sensing in sinus rhythm and during VT and VF is analyzed to assess sensing integrity (Fig. 32–9). Oversensing in sinus rhythm may occur as a result of a very small ventricular signal, large T waves, far-field sensing of P waves (Fig. 32–10), interference due to a fractured conductor, or "noise" from a loose terminal pin set-screw. Occasionally, postpacing beats may be undersensed as a result of insufficient autogain amplifier adaptability, that is, ramping up or down of the automatic gain control (AGC). The integrity of the high-voltage electrodes can be verified on the basis of the analysis of impedance values and delivered energies during an ICD shock. It is also possible to administer a low-energy shock in sinus rhythm to obtain the high-voltage lead impedance. Such testing is discouraged in an outpatient setting because of the discomfort that even a low-energy shock is likely to cause to the patient. Less invasive means of testing the high-voltage lead integrity are under clinical investigation.

Conductor Fracture

Conductor fractures may be associated with oversensing and increases in lead impedance and pacing threshold. All or some of these features may be present. When oversensing is recorded in sinus rhythm, and there is also an increase in impedance (more than 1500 Ω), conductor fracture should

be suspected. Intermittent oversensing of high-frequency signals, particularly when the patient assumes certain postures (e.g., sitting, arm abduction, pressure over the lead or ICD), should prompt the physician to suspect lead fracture. The patient may present with ICD shocks in sinus rhythm, usually at rest or on mild physical effort. Radiographs of the ICD leads are usually unhelpful, although they occasionally may demonstrate lead conductor interruption.

Fracture of a high-voltage lead is more difficult to diagnose, although it may have disastrous consequences, resulting in failure of ICD shock to defibrillate (Fig. 32–11). A clue to this problem is an increase in the high-voltage lead impedance after the shock. With high-voltage conductor fracture, the postshock impedance is generally high (more than 150 Ω), and the delivered shock energy is much less than that programmed, because of current shunting. Clues indicating high-voltage conductor fracture may be provided by the data logs, revealing failure to defibrillate at energies previously demonstrated to provide safety margins above the defibrillation threshold (DFT). This situation should be distinguished from other causes of ineffective defibrillation, such as lead displacement or increased DFTs caused by antiarrhythmic drug effect (see later). In this situation, the high-voltage lead impedance that follows defibrillation is unchanged and normal, usually less than 100Ω.

Insulation Breakdown

Lead insulation breakdown is a more subtle diagnosis. Insulation breakdown has a predilection for certain anatomic locations: (1) at the site of the lead entry into the subclavian

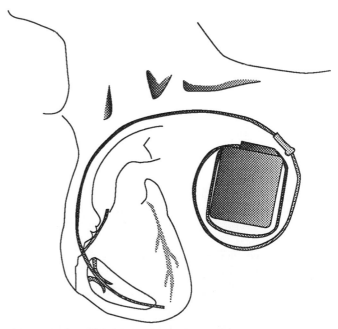

Figure 32–8. PCD Jewel 7219C (Medtronic, Minneapolis, MN) active can device. The external surface of the implantable cardioverter-defibrillator pulse generator acts as the active electrode in conjunction with the implanted right ventricular electrode. (From Singer I: Defibrillation threshold testing and intraoperative ICD evaluation. *In* Singer I [ed]: Interventional Electrophysiology. Baltimore, Williams & Wilkins, 1997, p 761.)

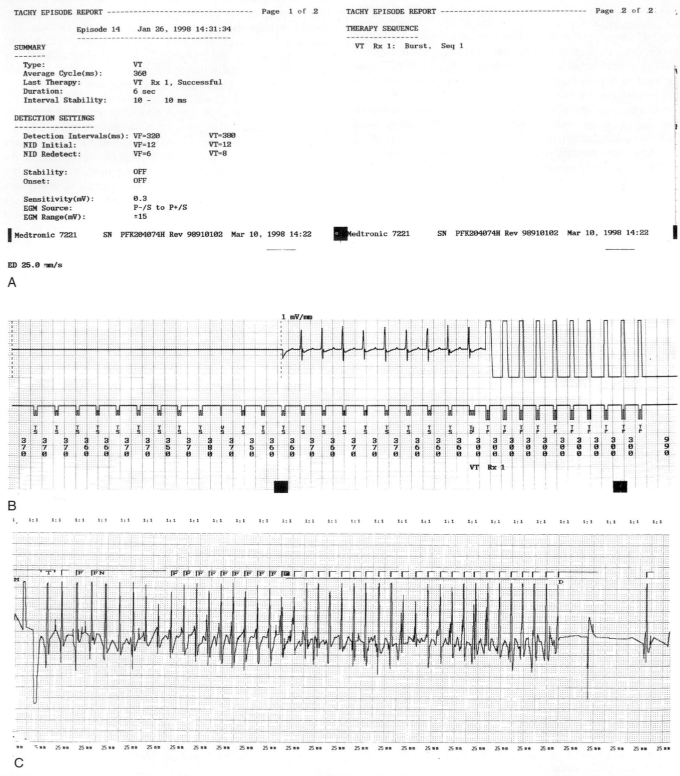

TACHY EPISODE REPORT -------------------------------- Page 1 of 2

        Episode 14   Jan 26, 1998 14:31:34

SUMMARY

  Type: VT
  Average Cycle(ms):   360
  Last Therapy: VT Rx 1, Successful
  Duration: 6 sec
  Interval Stability: 10 -   10 ms

DETECTION SETTINGS

  Detection Intervals(ms): VF=320   VT=380
  NID Initial: VF=12   VT=12
  NID Redetect: VF=6   VT=8

  Stability: OFF
  Onset: OFF

  Sensitivity(mV):   0.3
  EGM Source: P-/S to P+/S
  EGM Range(mV):   ±15

Medtronic 7221   SN PFK204074H Rev 98910102 Mar 10, 1998 14:22

ED 25.0 mm/s

A

TACHY EPISODE REPORT -------------------------------- Page 2 of 2

THERAPY SEQUENCE

  VT Rx 1: Burst, Seq 1

Medtronic 7221   SN PFK204074H Rev 98910102 Mar 10, 1998 14:22

1 mV/mm

VT Rx 1

B

C

Figure 32–9. Examples of typical stored event information during ventricular tachycardia VT (*A* and *B*) and during ventricular fibrillation (VF) *(C)*. *A*, Summary of the logged event. *B*, VT episode is followed by ATP therapy (Medtronic ICD 7221, Minneapolis, MN). *C*, Bipolar electrogram during VF resulting in the defibrillation shock and resumption of sinus rhythm (Micron, Intermedics, Angleton, TX).

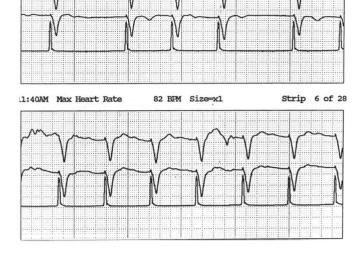

Figure 32–10. Intermittent P-wave oversensing documented on a routine 24-hour Holter monitor in a patient with an implanted Res-Q ICD (Intermedics, Angleton, TX). (From Singer I: Defibrillation threshold testing and intraoperative ICD evaluation. *In* Singer I [ed]: Interventional Electrophysiology. Baltimore, Williams & Wilkins, 1997, p 768.)

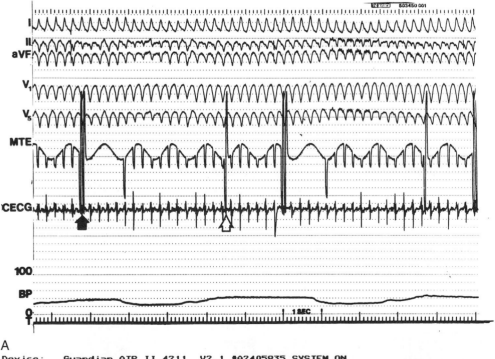

Figure 32–11. *A,* Failure of multiple shocks to terminate ventricular fibrillation due to endocardial defibrillation lead fracture (AccufixDF lead, Telectronics, Englewood, CO). From top to bottom: surface leads I, II, avF, V₁, V₅, main timing events (MTE), intracardiac electrogram (iCECG), blood pressure (BP), and time lines (T); *dark arrow,* an unsuccessful shock; *open arrow,* charging of the capacitors. *B,* Telemetry of the recorded event. Note appropriate detection, followed by the implantable cardioverter-defibrillator shock delivery of 36.1 J (three times) with an actual shock strength of 1.0, 0.5, and 0.5 J, with a lead impedance of >500 Ω, indicative of a high-voltage conductor fracture and current shunting. (From Singer I: Complications of cardioverter-defibrillator surgery. *In* Singer I [ed]: Implantable Cardioverter Defibrillator. Armonk, NY, Futura, 1994, p 429.)

vein; (2) below the ICD pulse generator, where the redundant leads are usually coiled; or (3) along the subcutaneous course, for an ICD located in the abdominal pocket. Insulation break is characterized by a decrease in pacing lead impedance, usually of less than 300 Ω for pace and sense programmed leads, and a decrease in impedance of less than 20 Ω when high-voltage leads are affected. In the case of pacing leads, effective capture may be maintained at the expense of current shunting, resulting in premature battery depletion. The consequence of high-voltage lead insulation failure is potentially more serious. It may result in current shunting and ineffective defibrillation. Therefore, whenever ineffective defibrillation on the first shock is documented clinically a careful scrutiny of data logs is mandatory. When low impedance is recorded during the shock, the clinician should suspect that insulator failure may be the cause. If the insulation failure is confirmed, the definitive treatment is lead extraction and implantation of new leads.

Lead Displacement

Lead dislodgment most commonly occurs immediately after implantation and frequently results from poor lead positioning or ineffective lead anchoring. It may be diagnosed on chest radiograph, or it may manifest as failure to sense, pace, or both (RV lead displacement) or as oversensing with spurious arrhythmia detections (when the lead is displaced to the atrium or to the tricuspid valve level, resulting in intermittent atrial and ventricular sensing) (Fig. 32–12). Displacement of the SVC lead is usually clinically silent and not readily recognized, except when demonstrated radiographically. It may also present as an inability to defibrillate effectively, which is a cause of an increased DFT of "uncertain" etiology. When lead displacement is obvious, particularly when the RV lead is displaced, reoperation is required, with lead repositioning. Stable SVC lead displacement with no adverse consequences on the DFTs may be ignored, provided that the lead position remains stable.

Lead displacement may manifest late, as sensing, pacing, or a combination of sensing and pacing problems. Double sensing may occur when the lead is pulled back to the atrium and is intermittently sensing atrial and ventricular electrograms (Fig. 32–13). Intermittent failure to sense may occur when the ventricular electrogram is too small and deteriorates further during VF. Pacing failure may also result from lead microdisplacement or from subclinical lead perforation. Resultant increases in pacing thresholds may not be crucial in a patient who does not require bradycardia pacing support but may be of great importance in a pacemaker-dependent patient. Microdisplacement may be subtle and is often difficult to diagnose. It is usually characterized by an increase in pacing thresholds, undersensing, or a combination of both problems in the absence of significant changes in the pacing lead impedance or anatomically detectable lead displacement. Noninvasive telemetry is crucial to an accurate diagnosis.

Drug–Device Interactions

The use of antiarrhythmic drugs in conjunction with ICD therapy is common in clinical practice. Antiarrhythmic drugs are used for the following reasons: (1) to suppress frequent episodes of sustained VT, which can result in frequent therapies and possibly frequent ICD shocks; (2) to suppress frequent episodes of nonsustained VT, which can aggravate

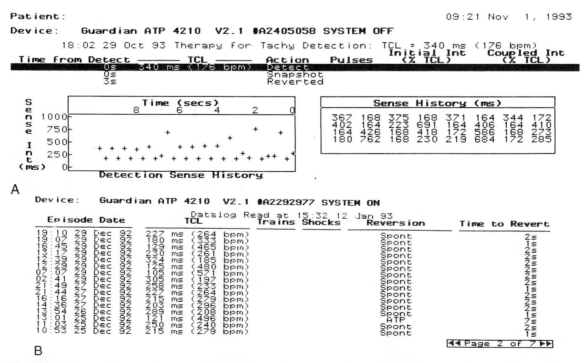

Figure 32–12. *A,* Sensing of both atrial and ventricular electrograms due to the lead displacement. *B,* The result is multiple spurious rhythm detections (Telectronics Guardian ATP 4210, Englewood, CO). (From Singer I: Complications of cardioverter-defibrillator surgery. *In* Singer I [ed]: Implantable Cardioverter Defibrillator. Armonk, NY, Futura, 1994, p 423.)

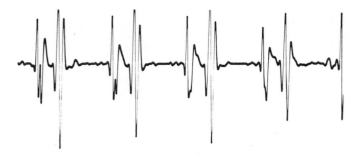

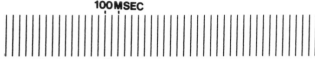

Figure 32–13. Real-time electrograms demonstrate atrial and ventricular sensing by the displaced endocardial lead. Atrial and ventricular electrograms of similar amplitudes suggest proximal displacement of the endocardial lead to the tricuspid area. This was later confirmed by fluoroscopy (Cadence, Ventritex, Sunnyvale, CA). (From Singer I: Complications of cardioverter-defibrillator surgery. *In* Singer I [ed]: Implantable Cardioverter Defibrillator. Armonk, NY, Futura, 1994, p 267).

Table 32–2. Possible Interactions Between Antiarrhythmic Drugs and Implantable Cardioverter-Defibrillators

Alteration in defibrillation threshold
Increase in latency, PR interval, or conduction, leading to double counting
Change in QRS morphology, resulting in satisfaction of PDF criteria for VT
Increase or decrease in VT cycle length
Change from sustained to nonsustained VT, yielding shocks after nonsustained VT (committed devices only)
Alteration in postshock excitability
Increase in pacing thresholds

PDF, probability density function.
Adapted from Singer I, Guarnieri T, Kupersmith J: Implanted automatic defibrillators: Effects of drugs and pacemakers. PACE 11:2250, 1989.

morphology; alter postshock excitability; and increase pacing thresholds (Table 32–2). Detailed discussion of antiarrhythmic drug–device interactions is beyond the scope of this chapter and may be found elsewhere.[5] These potential interactions should be considered when diagnosis of ICD malfunction is suspected.

Device–Device Interactions

Device–device interactions will become largely of historical interest. In the early days of ICDs, pacemakers were often implanted with ICDs to provide bradycardia and antitachycardia pacing capabilities. This is no longer commonly true, except for the addition of dual-chamber and rate-response features, because all modern ICDs incorporate VVI pacing functionality. A substantial number of patients who received ICDs before the advent of these technologic advances are still being followed with implanted single-chamber, dual-chamber, or ATP pacemakers. Therefore, working knowledge of potential device–device interactions is still required for the practicing electrophysiologist. Possible pacemaker and ICD interactions are summarized in Table 32–3. Sensing of pacemaker artifacts can lead to double or triple counting and inappropriate ICD shocks (Fig. 32–14). Similarly, an ATP device can trigger an ICD by simulating VT. Pacemaker reprogramming may occur as a result of an ICD shock. Postshock undersensing and capture failure may also result.

Unipolar pacing should be avoided in patients with ICDs because the ICD can "lock on" to the pacing signal during

CHF and trigger "aborted" ICD shocks, leading to premature battery depletion; (3) to suppress atrial fibrillation, thus preventing inappropriate ICD therapies; (4) to increase VT cycle length, and convert fast VT to hemodynamically better tolerated VT, amenable to antitachycardia (ATP) pacing termination; and (5) to blunt AV node response during atrial fibrillation. Although intended effects are often achieved, other undesirable effects of antiarrhythmic therapy abound. One unintended consequence is the potential for antiarrhythmic drugs to interfere indirectly with ICD function.[5]

Antiarrhythmic drugs may affect defibrillation threshold[6] (Table 32–1); alter VT cycle length, slowing the VT to the point at which the VT may fall below the programmed rate cutoff of the ICD, precluding VT detection; change QRS

Table 32–1. Effects of Antiarrhythmic Drugs on Defibrillation Thresholds

Increase	No change	Decrease
Encainide	MODE	Amiodarone (acute)
ODE	Quinidine	Clofilium
Flecaininde	Procainamide	Isoproterenol
Lidocaine	Bretylium	N-acetyl procainamide
Amiodarone (chronic)	D-Sotalol	
Propafenone		
Phenytoin		
Recainam		

Adapted from Singer I, Guarnieri T, Kupersmith J: Implanted automatic defibrillators: Effects of drugs and pacemakers. PACE 11:2250, 1989.

Table 32–3. Potential Pacemaker and Implantable Cardioverter-Defibrillator (ICD) Interactions

Pacemaker–ICD Interactions
VF nondetection because of pacemaker stimuli.
    Especially true for unipolar pacemakers
    Double, triple, and multiple counting, resulting in false-positive shocks
ICD–Pacemaker Interactions
Pacemaker reprogramming because of ICD discharge
Sensing and capture failure after defibrillation
ICD–Antitachycardia Pacemaker Interactions
Antitachycardia pacing triggering ICD discharge

Adapted from Singer I, Guarnieri T, Kupersmith J: Implanted automatic defibrillators: Effects of drugs and pacemakers. PACE 11:2250, 1989.

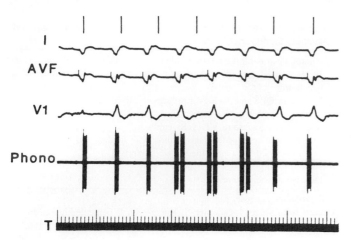

Figure 32–14. Intermittent sensing of pacing stimuli and their evoked QRS responses demonstrated using a phonocardiogram during VVI pacing. Double counting is seen in complexes 4–6. Paper speed is 25 mm/sec; intervals between the elevated lines on time (T) scale are 1 sec. (From Chapman P, Troup P: The automatic implantable defibrillator: Evaluating suspected inappropriate shocks. J Am Coll Cardiol 7:1075, 1986.)

VF and fail to detect the low-amplitude VF signals, resulting in a failure to detect and defibrillate. Another important caveat is that whenever a pacemaker and ICD are contemplated in combination, the physician must not only consider the possibility but also test for possible interactions during the device implantation and testing. The testing should include verification that the pacemaker artifacts are not sensed during either sinus rhythm or VF, with the pacemaker programmed to pace VOO or DOO at maximum output. Assuming that an ICD shock could induce a "power on reset" (POR) condition, usually producing a unipolar VVI mode at modestly high outputs, normal ICD sensing should be verified with the pacemaker programmed to the same settings. Sensing of ventricular pacing artifacts during sinus rhythm may be checked by noninvasive telemetry. ICD sensing of pacing artifacts can usually be eliminated by repositioning the pacemaker leads to a more distant site from the sensing ICD ventricular lead (e.g., the RV outflow tract with the ICD sensing lead located at the right RV apex). Detailed consideration of this subject matter is beyond the scope of this chapter.

Diagnostic Specificity of the ICD

Primary algorithms for VT and VF recognition are based on rate detection in most clinically available ICDs. Less frequently, morphology characteristics of the ventricular electrogram are used. Rate measurement requires that the ventricular electrograms be accurately detected. When the electrograms are classified within a range, for a given number of intervals (specified by programming), the rhythm is identified as VT or VF depending on the specifics of programming. An example of this is shown in Figure 32–15. Although few arrhythmias (other than VF) have ventricular rates faster than 220 bpm in the absence of an atrioventricular (AV) bypass tract, this is clearly not the case with VT, in which ventricular rates may vary significantly, usually between 100 and 200 bpm. Clearly, many arrhythmias may fall within this rate range, including atrial fibrillation, atrial flutter, AV node re-entry tachycardia, and sinus tachycardia. Therefore, rate alone is insufficient to separate VT from supraventricular arrhythmias.

To improve the specificity, certain detection enhancements have been developed, for example, sudden onset,

rate stability, and arrhythmia duration. These concepts are illustrated in Figure 32–16. These detection enhancements may help to screen out sinus tachycardia and atrial fibrillation. Unfortunately, they are not foolproof. For this and other reasons, dual-chamber ICD discrimination has been developed. It is hoped that algorithms using simultaneous information from the atrial and ventricular channels will improve specificity significantly, without sacrificing the sensitivity, a crucial issue for ICDs. An example of dual-chamber ICD sensing is shown in Figure 32–17.

Imperfect specificity has led to inappropriate ICD therapy during atrial fibrillation, sinus tachycardia, or other supraventricular tachycardias. When inappropriate therapies are suspected, it is often helpful to examine the telemetered logs of the ICD. During atrial fibrillation, irregular RR intervals are recorded, and ATP therapies are almost always unsuccessful (Fig. 32–18). Thus, a large number of tachycardia "events" followed by a large number of unsuccessful ATP therapies is the rule in a patient with paroxysmal or chronic atrial fibrillation. Diagnosis of atrial flutter or re-entrant arrhythmias is a more subtle diagnosis. When these arrhythmias are clinically suspected, it is often helpful to use a Holter monitor or an event recorder to aid in the diagnosis.

Dual-Chamber ICDs

Dual-chamber ICDs have been developed to provide DDDR pacing and to provide sensing information from the atrium, with the hope of improving diagnostic specificity for supraventricular arrhythmias, without sacrificing sensitivity for VT and VF detection. Inappropriate detection for supraventricular rhythms has been estimated to occur in 20% to 41% of cases.[1] Atrial electrodes have possible therapeutic potential for ICDs, such as atrial defibrillation and addition of ATP for therapy of re-entrant atrial tachycardias. The benefits of atrial sensing for diagnosis of tachycardias can be seen in Figure 32–19. The price of increased sensitivity, however, is a much greater complexity of ICD timing cycles and possibly an increase in complication rates as a result of the requirement for two ICD leads rather than one. Atrial electrogram amplitude was the most important criterion for DDD pacemaker lead placement; however, in dual-chambered ICDs, atrial electrograms with small far-field R waves can falsely induce a mode-switch condition. Complex refractory period timings and blanking periods in dual-chamber ICDs can occasionally be confusing even to an expert.

ICD Programmers

ICD programmers have undergone an evolution paralleling that of the ICD. Most programmers are software driven and based on the PC platform incorporating the Intel Pentium (Santa Clara, CA) chip technology. The interface is a liquid crystal screen, which is either touch sensitive (Ventritex, St. Jude Medical, Sunnyvale, CA) or a "pen"-activated screen (Medtronic, DISD, Minneapolis, MN) (Fig. 32–20). Other programmers are driven with trackball or a "mouse"-activated cursor (Guidant, St. Paul, MN) (Fig. 32–21). Programmers provide the means to communicate noninvasively with the ICD to retrieve stored information and program the device. Regardless of the specific ICD model, however, these features are common to all programmers: communication wand, surface electrode connection, printer, and pass-through connection available for external slaved pacing or recording.

Data storage to a floppy disk is also available in most programmers.

Interrogation yields the following routine information: (1) programmed parameters; (2) telemetered lead measurements (Fig. 32–22); (3) noninvasive real-time electrograms (Fig. 32–23); (4) data log retrieval and specific information, such as battery status, lead impedance, most recent charge times and capacitor formation times, high-voltage lead impedance after the shock, and individual electrogram replay of stored arrhythmia events (Fig. 32–24); (5) noninvasive tests of leads, including sensing and pacing thresholds, pacing lead impedance values, and tests of battery integrity; (6) noninvasive programmed stimulation facilities for VT and VF induction in the electrophysiology laboratory or in the operating room setting. Although each individual programmer has some specific features peculiar to the programmer, the

Text continued on page 892

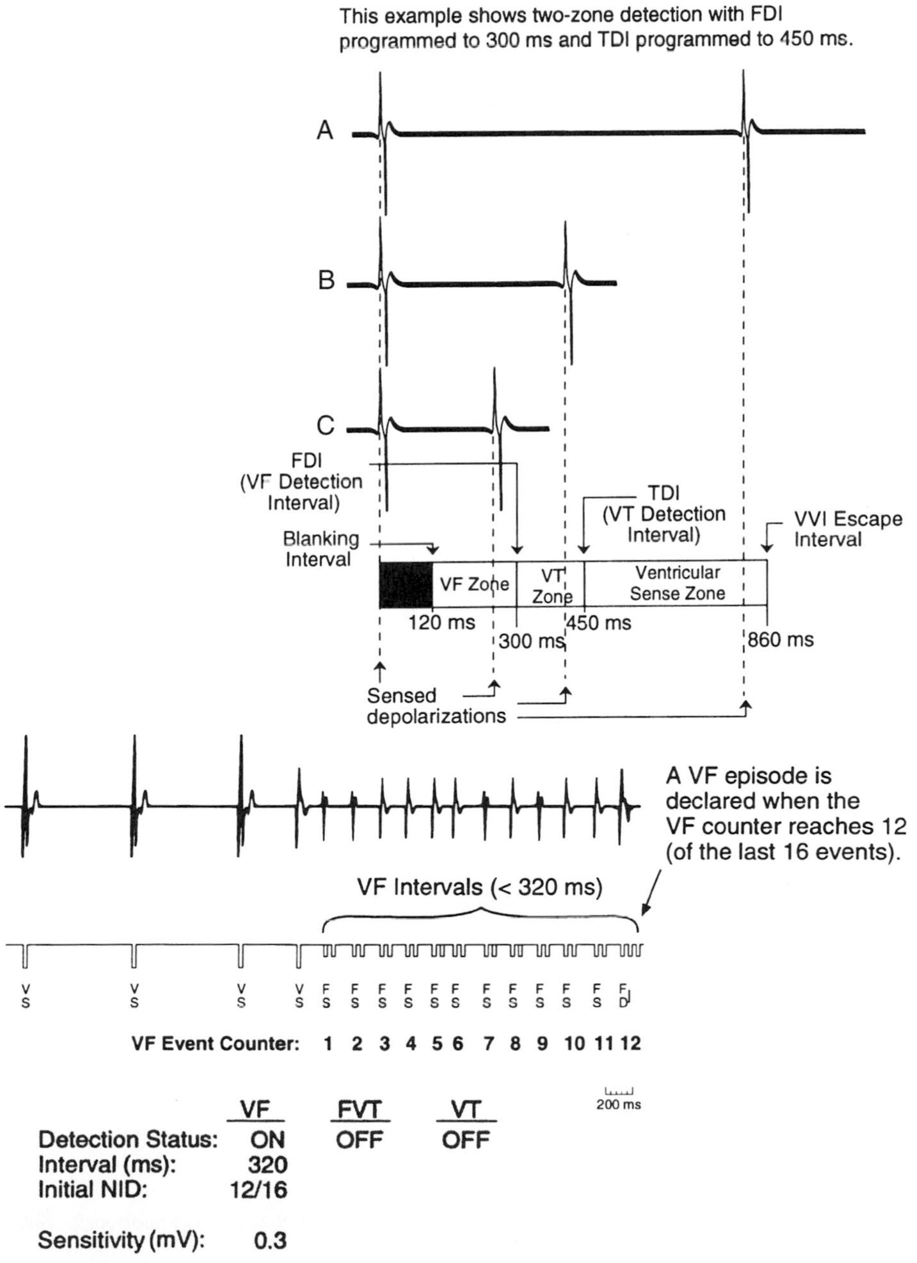

Figure 32–15. *Upper panel,* Jewel PCD (Medtronic, Minneapolis, MN) sensing and electrogram classification. Whether a sensed event is classified as ventricular tachycardia (VT) *(B)*, ventricular fibrillation (VF) *(C)*, or sinus beat *(A)* depends on the interval from the initial sensed ventricular event. *Lower panel,* VF sensing is based on the VF criterion being fulfilled. When 12/16 intervals are detected in the VF range (<320 msec), VF detection is fulfilled and declared. (From Jewel PCD Technical Manual. Minneapolis, Medtronic, 1994.)

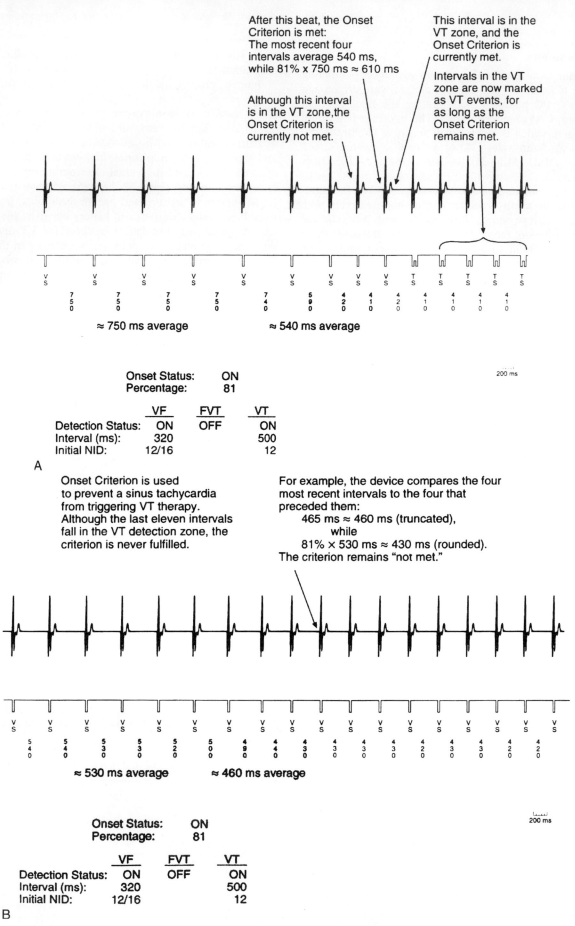

After this beat, the Onset Criterion is met:
The most recent four intervals average 540 ms, while 81% x 750 ms ≈ 610 ms

This interval is in the VT zone, and the Onset Criterion is currently met.

Intervals in the VT zone are now marked as VT events, for as long as the Onset Criterion remains met.

Although this interval is in the VT zone, the Onset Criterion is currently not met.

≈ 750 ms average ≈ 540 ms average

200 ms

Onset Status: ON
Percentage: 81

	VF	FVT	VT
Detection Status:	ON	OFF	ON
Interval (ms):	320		500
Initial NID:	12/16		12

A

Onset Criterion is used to prevent a sinus tachycardia from triggering VT therapy. Although the last eleven intervals fall in the VT detection zone, the criterion is never fulfilled.

For example, the device compares the four most recent intervals to the four that preceded them:
465 ms ≈ 460 ms (truncated),
    while
81% × 530 ms ≈ 430 ms (rounded).
The criterion remains "not met."

≈ 530 ms average   ≈ 460 ms average

200 ms

Onset Status: ON
Percentage: 81

	VF	FVT	VT
Detection Status:	ON	OFF	ON
Interval (ms):	320		500
Initial NID:	12/16		12

B

Figure 32–16. *See legend on opposite page*

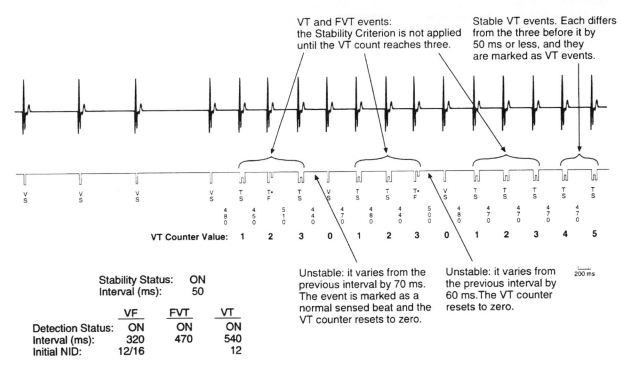

Figure 32–16. *A,* An example, of how *sudden onset* is determined using the PCD Jewel (Medtronic, Minneapolis, MN). *B,* The *sudden onset* is used to prevent sinus tachycardia from triggering ventricular tachycardia therapy. *C, Interval stability* criterion used to prevent the device from being triggered during atrial fibrillation. (From Jewel PCD Technical Manual. Medtronic, Minneapolis, 1994.)

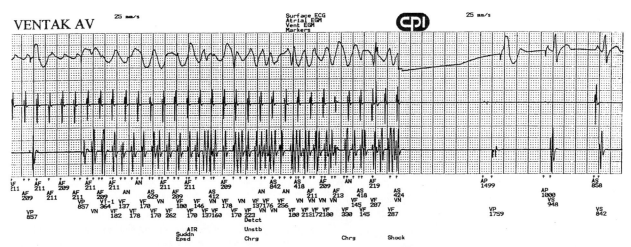

Figure 32–17. This real-time strip from the Ventak AV shows ongoing atrial flutter, initiation of spontaneous ventricular fibrillation (VF) that was detected and shocked. The channels are surface electrocardiogram, atrial electrogram, ventricular electrogram, sense and pace arrows, atrial markers with PP intervals, ventricular markers with RR intervals, and episode annotations. Atrial markers are atrial pace (AP), atrial sense (AS), atrial fibrillation (AF), and atrial noise (AN). Ventricular markers are ventricular pace (VP), ventricular sense (VS), VT-1 zone sense (VT-1), VT zone sense (VT), VF zone sense (VF), ventricular noise (VN), and noise-telemetry (TN). Episode annotation markers are start /end of episode (Epsd), onset-sudden (Suddn), onset-gradual (Gradl), atrial-tachy response mode switch (ATR), duration expired (Dur), stable (Stb), unstable (Unstb), atrial fibrillation met (AFib), V rate faster than A rate (V>A), detection met (Detct), Sustained rate duration expired (SRD), start/end of charge (Chrg), Shock delivered (Shock), Therapy diverted (Dvrt). (From Olson WH: Dual chamber sensing and detection of ICDs. In Singer I, Barold SS, Camm AJ [eds]: Nonpharmacological Therapy of Arrhythmias for the 21st Century: The State of the Art. Armonk, NY, Futura, 1998, p 411.)

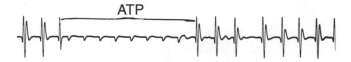

Figure 32–18. Failure of antitachycardia pacing (ATP) to terminate an episode of ventricular tachycardia, as captured on the stored electrograms of a Cadence device. The irregularity of ventricular electrograms is typical of atrial fibrillation, explaining the reason that ATP delivered in the right ventricle is unsuccessful in terminating the tachycardia. (From Nisam S, Fogoros R: Troubleshooting of patients with implantable cardioverter defibrillators. *In* Singer I [ed]: Implantable Cardioverter Defibrillator. Armonk, NY, Futura, 1994, p 453.)

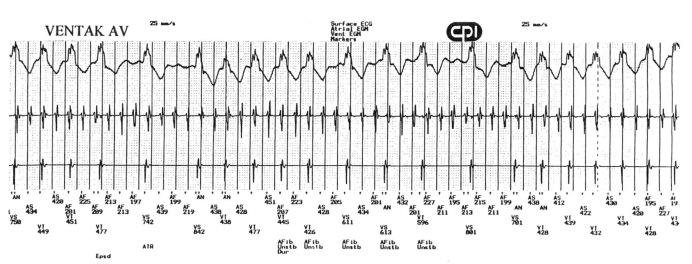

Figure 32–19. Double tachycardia is almost inappropriately detected for atrial fibrillation that transiently conducts rapidly to the ventricle. Enough beats of ventricular tachycardia (VT) (8 of 10) are sensed to initiate an episode (Epsd) of VT that, despite two long RR intervals, satisfied duration (Dur). The atrial fibrillation (AFib) is recognized by the unstable ventricular intervals, and enough atrial intervals are less than the AFib rate interval threshold. After 5 beats of AFib detection, the episode ends because there are less than 6 of the last 10 ventricular events in the VT zone. (From Olson WH: Dual chamber sensing and detection of ICDs. *In* Singer I, Barold SS, Camm AJ [eds]: Nonpharmacological Therapy of Arrhythmias for the 21st Century: The State of the Art. Armonk, NY, Futura, 1998, p 414.)

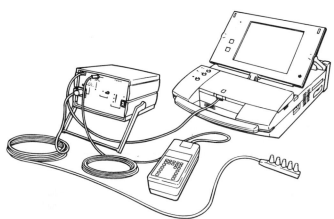

Figure 32–20. Defibrillation implantation support device (DISD) with programmer and pacing system analyzer (PSA). (From 5358 Technical Manual. Medtronic, Minneapolis, MN.)

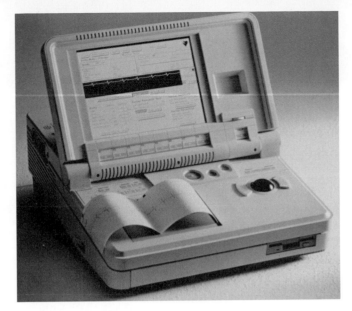

Figure 32–21. Model 2950 Programmer Recorder Monitor (PRM) can be used for device-based testing or outpatient implantable cardioverter-defibrillator interrogation and programming. (Courtesy of Guidant Corporation, St. Paul, MN.)

Date Interrogated: Sep 11, 1995 14:21:36

BATTERY VOLTAGE:
Sep 11, 1995 13:55:24
Last Measured (V): 6.34

MOST RECENT CHARGE:
Sep 11, 1995 14:21:20
Energy (J): 3.2–23.9
Charge Time (sec): 3.82

MIN. BATTERY VOLTAGE
DURING CHARGE:
May 06, 1994 07:20:58
Minimum Measured (V): 4.43

LAST CAPACITOR
FORMATION:
Jul 27, 1995 09:26:27
Energy (J): 0.0–32.7
Charge Time (sec): 9.18

MOST RECENT PACING LEAD
IMPEDANCE:
Sep 11, 1995 13:55:24
Impedance (ohms): 868

MOST RECENT H.V. LEAD
IMPEDANCE:
Sep 11, 1995 14:21:21
Waveform: BIPH
Pathway: AX>B
Delivered Energy (J):   22.7
Impedance (ohms):   83

Figure 32–22. Typical information that may be obtained from stored parameters on routine implantable cardioverter-defibrillator interrogation, including battery status, pacing lead impedance, most recent charge and capacitor reformation times, and most recent high-voltage (H.V.) impedance. (From Singer I: Complications of ICD surgery, postoperative care and follow-up. *In* Singer I [ed]: Interventional Electrophysiology. Baltimore, Williams & Wilkins, 1997, p 784.)

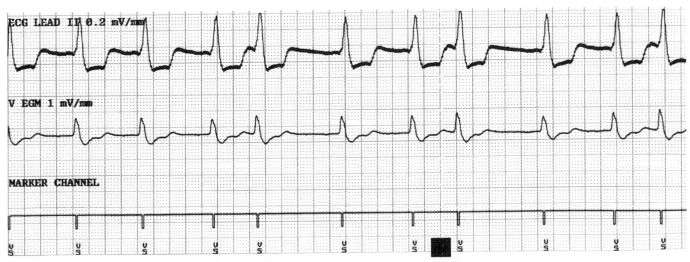

7223   2/18/98 16:27
CHART SPEED 25.0 mm/s

EGM Range(mV): +-15

Figure 32–23. Noninvasive telemetry of Medtronic Jewel PCD 7223 device. Atrial fibrillation with IVCD is noted on the surface electrocardiogram lead II *(top)*. Intracardiac electrogram is displayed *(middle)* with sense markers *(bottom)*.

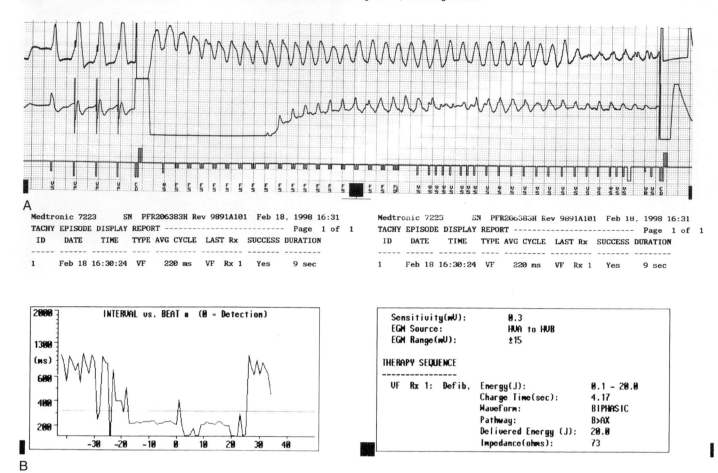

Figure 32–24. *A,* Ventricular fibrillation (VF) induction by shock-T induction method with surface electrocardiogram, intracardiac electrogram recording, and sense markers. *B,* A typical graphic display of the events is shown, demonstrating VF detection and termination *(left)* and details of the energy delivery, shock pathway, and high-voltage (H.V.) lead impedance stored in the device. (Medtronic model 7223, Minneapolis, MN.)

principles evoked are shared by all programmers. Familiarity with the specific programmer can be gained with some experience and by repeated use. The ease of use is directly proportional to an operator's experience.

■ DEVICE-BASED TESTING

With the advent of small pectoral ICDs and the availability of biphasic waveforms, successful primary implantation can be achieved in more than 95% of patients with transvenous leads.[6] When additional leads are used, such as a subcutaneous patch or a subcutaneous array with hot can ICDs, the success rate approaches 100%. Given the high success rates of the primary ICD implant, most manufacturers and implanters feel confident that an ICD implant will be successful. Therefore, to shorten the procedure time and to simplify the implantation procedure, device-based testing is now used routinely. I routinely use this technique because it eliminates the need for connecting cables and the external device simulators and simplifies significantly the implantation procedure. The potential risk of abandoning the device implant because of inadequate DFT safety margins is rarely encountered. Given the simplification of the logistics, the manufacturers

are prepared to absorb the cost of an occasional "wasted" device (an ICD pulse generator opened but not implanted). I have yet to encounter this situation.

Device-based testing has much to recommend it. It is simple to implement and trouble free. It requires only the external programmer and a sterilized communication wand or a plastic sleeve for ICD testing. This technique not only is practical but also, in the long run, is probably more cost-effective than the more elaborate testing techniques that use cables and external simulators, saving operating laboratory room time, sterilization requirements (for cables), and overall, minimizing costs.

■ TROUBLESHOOTING PRINCIPLES

Troubleshooting in a patient with suspected ICD malfunction follows logically from analysis of the index clinical event. Using the "tools" discussed previously, the clinician can usually arrive at the correct diagnosis. Steps for logical analysis have been summarized by Nisam and Fogoros[7] and are shown in Tables 32–4 and 32–5. Proper analysis involves two steps: identification of the problem and analysis of possible causes of the problem. There are four distinct types

Table 32–4. Troubleshooting Suspected Inappropriate Therapy (Shocks or ATP) in Absence of Electrocardiographic Documentation

Possible Causes	Means of Identifying the Source of the Problem
1. Asymptomatic, but appropriate, i.e., sustained VT > R	1.1 Check circumstances leading to Tx. 1.2 Analyze device's therapy history, especially RR intervals, versus settings. 1.3 If cause 1 is eliminated, investigate causes 2–10.
2. Sinus tachycardia	2.1 Can patient under exercise and/or stress exceed R? 2.2 If yes, do 1.2; if no, consider causes 3–10.
3. SVT (atrial fibrillation, atrial flutter, SVT), with rapid ventricular conduction	3.1 Is patient susceptible to SVT? 3.2 If yes, is resulting ventricular rate > R. 3.3 If both 3.1 and 3.2 are yes, check steps 1.1 and 1.2. 3.4 If still unclear, do rapid atrial pacing using "beep-o-grams" and/or marker channels to check ICD detection. 3.5 If either 3.1 or 3.2 are no, consider causes 4–10.
4. NSVT	4.1 Is there evidence (past history or via ECG monitoring) of NSVT? 4.2 If yes, is ICD a "committed" device (or programmed to commit)? 4.3 If 4.1 and 4.2, yes, do 1.2; check in particular whether programmed detection delay exceeds length of NSVT episode 4.4 If cause 4 (and 1–3) can be ruled out, consider causes 5–10.
5. T-wave or P-wave oversensing	5.1 Check "beep-o-gram" and/or marker channels. 5.2 Do 1.2. 5.3 Check for position or dislodgment of ICD sensing leads. 5.4 In devices without AGC, check if sensitivity is the cause.
6. Pacemaker "spikes" or evoked potentials	6.1 Same as 5.1. If necessary, repeat with increased pacer output. 6.2 Same as 1.2.
7. Lead fracture, insulation break, loose set-screws, dislodgment, etc.	7.1 Same as 5.1. Do if necessary, during upper body exercise and/or manipulation near ICD connector. 7.2 Do 1.2. 7.3 Check lead impedance values (also, during body exercise). 7.4 Check radiographs for lead or insulation breaks, dislodgments, etc.
8. Outside sources (EMI, MRI, electrocautery)	8.1 Same as 1.1. 8.2 Do 5.1.
9. Device proarrythmia	9.1 Same as 1.1. 9.2 Same as 1.2.
10. Faulty detection algorithm	10.1 Same as 1.1. 10.2 Same as 1.2. 10.3 Same as 5.1. 10.4 Analyze whether detection algorithm may have been set too sensitive.

Tx, therapy (shocks or ATP); ICD, implantable cardioverter-defibrillation; R, ICD programmed "cutoff rate"; SVT = supraventricular tachycardia; NSVT, nonsustained VT defined arbitrarily as runs of 5+ consecutive ventricular extrasystoles, at rates > R, self-terminating within 30 seconds; AGC, automatic gain control (automatic sensitivity); EMI, electromagnetic interference; MRI, magnetic resonance imaging.
From Nisam S, Fogoros R: Troubleshooting of patients with implantable cardioverter defibrillators. *In* Singer I (ed): Implantable Cardioverter Defibrillator. Armonk, NY, Futura, 1994, pp 433–456.

of ICD-related problems: suspected inappropriate therapy, failure of the ICD to deliver therapy, ineffective ICD therapy, and a deactivated ICD. Using the algorithm outlined in Tables 32–4 and 32–5, the clinician can usually arrive at the correct diagnosis. The only modification to the suggested algorithm is that analysis of atrial electrograms for dual-chamber ICDs and the use of sensed electrograms and markers diagnosed by noninvasive telemetry has for all practical purposes replaced "beep-o-grams" as the means to arrive at a correct diagnosis. With these caveats, however, one can add precious little to the algorithm put forward by these two authors. In many respects, the approach is identical to the time-honored approach for diagnosis, including a complete and thorough analysis of facts based on the clinical history, the physical examination, the ECG and the device telemetry, the radiographic evidence when necessary, and occasionally the data derived from intraoperative ICD lead recordings.

With the improvements in the ICD memory capacity and data retrieval, this process is likely to become easier and even more explicit. Thorough knowledge of the device sensing and therapy algorithms, as well as extensive experience with programming, is required to diagnose ICD malfunction correctly.

Summary

Troubleshooting ICDs is an exercise in systematic analysis of evidence based on history, physical examination, and analysis of retrieved ICD information. The analysis must take into account the specifics of the ICD as well as the sensing and therapy algorithms used to arrive at an accurate diagnosis. Atrial channel analysis is likely to enhance this process further and enhance the specificity for arrhythmia detection by the future dual-chamber ICDs.

Table 32–5. Troubleshooting Therapy Problems in Absence of Electrocardiographic Documentation

Problem	Possible Causes	Means of Identifying the Source of the Problem
A. Failure to deliver Tx (in case Tx delivered but ineffective, see B)	1. Sensitivity problems	1.1 Same as 5 in Table 32–4.
		1.2 In devices without AGC, check whether programmed sensitivity may be responsible for undersensing of R waves (see text for explanation).
		1.3 Do 1.2 from Table 32–4, with VT-induced tachycardia.
	2. Lead problems	2.1 Same as 7 in Table 32–4.
	3. Postshock signal attenuation and undersensing	3.1 Same as 5.1–5.3 in Table 32–4.
		3.2 Verify whether amplitude of R waves is sufficient for good sensing before and after shock (within 5–10 sec).
	4. Separate pacemaker*	4.1 Same as 5.1–5.2 in Table 32–4.
	5. Faulty sensing algorithm or programming	5.1 Same as 1.1–1.2, 5.3 in Table 32–4.
		5.2 Analyze whether detection algorithm set too sensitive; i.e., determine whether detection enhancements† might be inhibiting Tx.
	6. Antiarrhythmic drugs	6.1 Determine effect of change in antiarrhythmic drugs on patient's rate and morphology regarding R and the detection enhancements.
	7. Outside interference	7.1 Same as 8 in Table 32–4.
B. Ineffective Tx (shocks and/or ATP ineffective)	1. Inadequate shock output or programming	1.1 Retest DFT (problem not simply due to probabilistic nature of defibrillation?).
		1.2 Verify that the energy levels set for VF/polymorphic VT are at maximum.
	2. Rise in DFT due to impedance changes	2.1 Check (from device telemetry) impedance of the shocking leads.
		2.2 If increased, check whether device's *delivered* energy is still ample.
		2.3 Check for causes of impedance rise (see 7 in Table 32–4).
	3. Influence of drugs on DFT	3.1 Retest DFTs, following changes in antiarrhythmic drug administration, especially amiodarone.
	4. Lead problems (include "patch crumpling")	4.1 Same troubleshooting techniques as used in 7 from Table 32–4 (but concentrate on both shocking and pacing leads).
	5. Exacerbated CHF or degradation of LVF	5.1 Retest DFTs, and if marginal, revise the shocking lead system.
	6. Failed ATP modes	6.1 Same as 1.1–1.2 in Table 32–4.
		6.2 Retest ATP modes. Have substrate changes altered previous success?
	7. Inadequate pacing output (exit block)	7.1 Retest pacing thresholds, including postshock.
		7.2 Same as 7.3–7.4 in Table 32–4.
C. Device deactivated	1. Inadvertently (via magnet or programmer)	1.1 Check on possibility that hospital staff inadvertently turned off device.
		1.2 Similarly, with patient, family, local physician.
	2. Outside interference (EMI)	2.1 Check patient's environment for EMI (listen for audio tone from the implanted or equivalent device).
	3. Battery depletion	3.1 Test device's battery status.
	4. Circuit failure or shut-down mode	4.1 Interrogate ICD to determine its functional status.

Tx, Therapy (shocks or ATP); DFT, defibrillation threshold; CHF, congestive heart failure; EMI, electromagnetic interference; R, ICD programmed cutoff rate; AGC, automatic gain control (automatic sensitivity).

*Unipolar pacing is generally contraindicated in combination with ICD.

†Sudden onset, stability, "probability density function (PDF) on," "noncommitted," "reconfirmation."

From Nisam S, Fogoros R: Troubleshooting of patients with implantable cardioverter defibrillators. *In* Singer I (ed): Implantable Cardioverter Defibrillator. Armonk, NY, Futura, 1994, pp 433–456.

REFERENCES

1. Singer I, Edmonds H Jr: Changes in cerebral perfusion during third generation ICD testing. Am Heart J 127(4 Part 2): 1052–1057, 1994.
2. Anderson MH, Murgatroyd FD, Hnatkova K, et al: Performance of basic ventricular tachycardia detection algorithms in implantable cardioverter defibrillators. PACE 20(12 Pt I):2957–2983, 1997.
3. Jenkins JM, Caswell SA: Detection algorithms in implantable cardioverter defibrillators. Proc IEEE 84(3):428–445, 1996.
4. Bardy GH, Johnson G, Poole JE, et al: A simplified, single lead unipolar transvenous cardioversion-defibrillation system. Circulation 88:543–547, 1993.
5. Singer I, Guarnieri T, Kupersmith J: Implanted automatic defibrillators: Effects of drugs and pacemakers. PACE 11:2250–2262, 1988.
6. Singer I: Defibrillation threshold testing and intraoperative ICD evaluation. *In* Singer I (ed): Interventional Electrophysiology. Baltimore, Williams & Wilkins, 1997, pp 741–763.
7. Nisam S, Fogoros R: Troubleshooting of patients with implantable cardioverter defibrillators. *In* Singer I (ed): Implantable Cardioverter Defibrillator. Armonk, NY, Futura, 1994, pp 433–456.

Chapter 33

Follow-Up of the Paced Patient

Mark H. Schoenfeld

The fifth decade of permanent transvenous pacemakers is almost upon us. Despite the proliferation of enhanced technologic features, follow-up of the patient with these increasingly complex devices remains woefully inadequate and underappreciated.[1-3] The goals of pacemaker follow-up are, simply put, two-fold: assess the *pacemaker* and assess the *patient*. All too often, the patient is "lost" as attention is focused only on the device. The pacemaker physician needs to elicit symptoms from the patient to determine whether the pacemaker, as originally implanted, is adequately addressing the needs of the patient or, in some cases, whether the pacemaker may actually be causing new symptoms. In addition to documenting an already present pacer-system malfunction, follow-up is designed to *anticipate* future or potential problems *before* they result in patient compromise, allowing for pre-emptive corrective measures to be taken when appropriate. Systematic record keeping plays an indispensable role in this process, both to follow such important parameters as declining generator longevity and to track devices that are under advisory.

A review of the pacemaker literature indicates that little has been written to address the specific concerns encountered in pacemaker follow-up.[4-7] Even less information is available on appropriate training requirements (Table 33–1) and who should be performing pacemaker follow-up.[1, 2, 8] The purposes of this chapter are to explore these and related issues as they apply to both pacemakers and defibrillators and to examine the methodology of follow-up.

■ TRANSTELEPHONIC FOLLOW-UP OF PACEMAKERS AND CLINIC ORGANIZATION

Transtelephonic monitoring (TTM) of the patient's free-running and magnet rates has been increasingly used as a convenient and important method of following pacemaker patients.[9-11] It must be emphasized that this methodology

should not and cannot supplant the role of direct physician–patient contact in the office setting, where certain aspects of physical examination and programming manipulations must be performed (described later). Nonetheless, TTM provides an assessment of free-running sensing and capture capabilities of the device, and through magnet rate evaluation, provides for an assessment of generator viability.[12] TTM thereby

Table 33–1. Core Knowledge Base for Pacemaker Follow-Up (What the Pacing Specialist Must Recognize and Understand)

History: Symptoms that suggest a pacing system complication, e.g., pacemaker syndrome, extracardiac stimulation, and inappropriate rate response.

Physical Examination: Physical signs of pacing system complications. Expected appearance of pacemaker pocket and incision.

Chest Radiography: Assessment of pacing system, i.e., lead and electrode placement, lead integrity, and pulse generator orientation and identification.

Electrocardiography: Thorough understanding of normal, pseudonormal, and abnormal pacemaker function, and of magnet function.

Telemetered Pacemaker Data: Programmed data, measured data, rate histograms, electrograms, and other diagnostic data.

Programming: Sensing threshold, Stimulation threshold, AV conduction assessment, VA conduction assessment, Assessment of chronotropic incompetence, Optimization of physiologic function, Initiation and management of pacemaker-mediated tachycardia, Uses of available programmable pacing modes: rate programming, output programming, sensitivity programming, refractory period programming, rate-adaptive parameters; Complications of programming: rate changes, oversensing, undersensing, crosstalk, noncapture.

Transtelephonic monitoring: Understanding of its role in follow-up.

Troubleshooting: Pulse generator failure (battery depletion), lead failure, rate changes, sensing abnormalities, noncapture, crosstalk.

From Hayes DL, Naccarelli GV, Furman S, et al: Report of the NASPE Policy Conference training requirements for permanent pacemaker selection, implantation, and follow-up. PACE 17:6–12, 1994.

affords a method by which to access information from a patient who may live in a geographically remote area and helps to reduce the frequency of potentially burdensome outpatient visits for patients who are frail or unable to travel. It also allows another means by which to interact with the patient, assessing ongoing symptoms and any new events that may be going on in the patient's life. Increasingly, symptom-initiated TTM has been used to identify potential pacemaker malfunction or arrhythmias that may be responsible for a patient's symptoms—patients are encouraged to call in whenever they have a problem, such as palpitations or dizziness (Figs. 33–1A–C).

As currently undertaken, the transmission entails connecting electrodes (typically placed on wrists, ankles, or fingertips) to a transmitter, over which the telephone mouthpiece is placed. Certain limitations to the technique apply: insufficient voltage depending on the lead used, 60-Hz interference, and noise from telephone or motion artifact, especially in a patient prone to tremors.

Specific Medicare guidelines, although subject to some debate,[13, 14] exist for both pacer clinic follow-up and TTM scheduling. Those for the latter are listed below:

- Guideline I: Applies to most pacers, with either inability to demonstrate or insufficient exposure to demonstrate the following:
  1. A 5-year longevity of greater than 90%, and
  2. Nonabrupt decline of output over 3 or more months of less than a 50% drop in output voltage/less than 20% magnet deviation or a drop by 5 ppm or less

  Single-chamber pacers:
  1st month: every 2 weeks
  2nd to 36th month: every 8 weeks
  Thereafter: every 4 weeks
  Dual-chamber pacers:
  1st month: every 2 weeks
  2nd to 6th month: every 4 weeks
  7th to 36th month: every 8 weeks
  Thereafter: every 4 weeks

- Guideline II: The minority of pacers that do meet the criteria for longevity indicated above.

  Single-chamber pacers:
  1st month: every 2 weeks
  2nd to 48th month: every 12 weeks
  49th to 72nd month: every 8 weeks
  Thereafter: every 4 weeks
  Dual-chamber pacers:
  1st month: every 2 weeks
  2nd to 30th month: every 12 weeks
  31st to 48th month: every 8 weeks
  Thereafter: every 4 weeks.

According to the Medicare Coverage Issues Manual (section 50–1), the frequency of clinic visits is "the decision of the patient's physician, taking into account, among other things, the medical condition of the patient. However, (Medicare carriers) can develop monitoring guidelines that will prove useful in screening claims." Hayes and colleagues[15] from the Mayo Clinic have suggested that less frequent TTM follow-up schedule is adequate for most patients and could result in substantial cost savings. They proposed a follow-up schedule that is weekly for the first month, then every 3

months until the first sign of battery depletion, and then monthly until ERI is reached.

Record keeping is an indispensable aspect of TTM monitoring and outpatient clinic follow-up. Records of these encounters should include such patient demographics as name and address, specifics of the pacer system employed (model and serial numbers), demonstration of free-running and magnet rhythm strips, end-of-life parameters, and programmed settings. These records may often be stored in a computer[16] and retrievable and may also allow for a graphical demonstration of changes in magnet rate (Fig. 33–2).

To accomplish the various goals of follow-up detailed later, the outpatient clinic site should allow history taking and physical examination and be fully equipped to allow demonstration of pacer system function or the lack thereof. This includes facilities for electrocardiographic (ECG) studies, fluoroscopy, and radiography; TTM monitoring; and ambulatory ECG recording. In addition, there should be a physician's manual and programmer available for every pacer model encountered. A routine schedule for pacemaker follow-up should be arranged. This allows for the identification of potential problems with pacer system function well before they become actualized. A separate location for pacemaker records should be established. Important data to register in the outpatient pacemaker record include such patient demographics as name, age, address, and phone number; pacer generator data (model and serial numbers); lead data (model and serial numbers); implantation operative note; notes on history and physical examination; chest radiograms; ECG recordings with and without magnets; generator interrogation printouts; sensing and pacing threshold data; real-time telemetry data and measurements of other interrogated data such as histograms; and printout of final values.

CLINICAL FOLLOW-UP OF THE PACED PATIENT

Follow-up of the paced patient begins with the immediate postimplantation period and extends throughout the life of the patient rather than throughout the life of a particular pacer system per se. The original indications for pacer insertion require periodic re-review and changing technologies, and indications for pacing may dictate the need for a modification of the existing pacemaker system and, rarely, termination of pacemaker therapy.[17] As previously discussed, the physician must evaluate whether those symptoms for which the pacer was originally implanted are being satisfactorily treated and separately determine whether de novo symptoms have been actually created by the pacer system. Most important is the assessment of the continued viability and appropriate functioning of the system.

Immediately after pacer implantation, the patient is generally observed on a cardiac monitor for 1 to 2 days before discharge from the hospital. The length of hospital stay may be dictated by local practices and insurance concerns, and in some cases, more "ambulatory" surgery has been used. Follow-up radiography is undertaken to confirm satisfactory positioning of atrial and ventricular leads and to rule out pneumothorax in the case of subclavian placement. Twelve-lead ECG studies with and without magnet are undertaken to confirm location of the leads (e.g., to rule out a left ventricular location suggested by left bundle-branch block

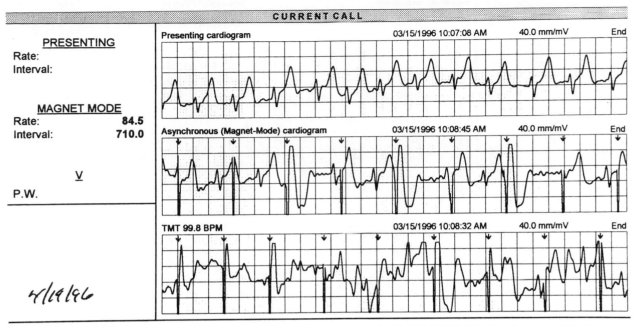

CURRENT CALL

PRESENTING
Rate:
Interval:

MAGNET MODE
Rate: **84.5**
Interval: **710.0**

V

P.W.

Presenting cardiogram 03/15/1996 10:07:08 AM 40.0 mm/mV End

Asynchronous (Magnet-Mode) cardiogram 03/15/1996 10:08:45 AM 40.0 mm/mV End

TMT 99.8 BPM 03/15/1996 10:08:32 AM 40.0 mm/mV End

4/19/96

Patient requested has been lost to PTM f.u. Called reporting "irregular rhythm." Atrial fibrillation (maximum ventricular response 140 BPM). Appropriate magnet response. Report to :
Patient states he "missed some medication doses this week."

A

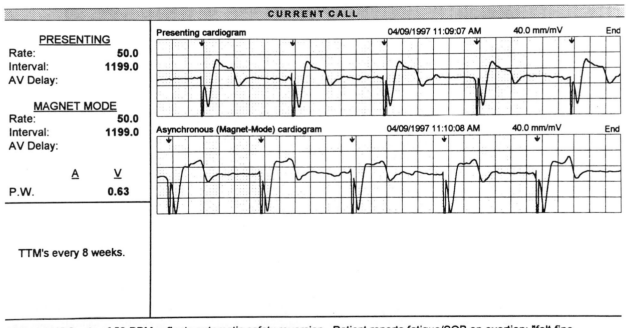

CURRENT CALL

PRESENTING
Rate: **50.0**
Interval: **1199.0**
AV Delay:

MAGNET MODE
Rate: **50.0**
Interval: **1199.0**
AV Delay:

A V

P.W. **0.63**

TTM's every 8 weeks.

Presenting cardiogram 04/09/1997 11:09:07 AM 40.0 mm/mV End

Asynchronous (Magnet-Mode) cardiogram 04/09/1997 11:10:08 AM 40.0 mm/mV End

VVI and VOO rate of 50 BPM reflects automatic safety reversion. Patient reports fatigue/SOB on exertion; "felt fine yesterday." Pacer replacement scheduled for 4/14/97.

B

Figure 33–1. *A,* Transtelephonic transmission for patient symptoms of "irregular rhythm" documenting atrial fibrillation. *B,* Transtelephonic transmission for fatigue actually showing reversion from DDD to VOO pacing, automatic safety reversion, indicating that elective replacement is warranted.

Illustration continued on following page

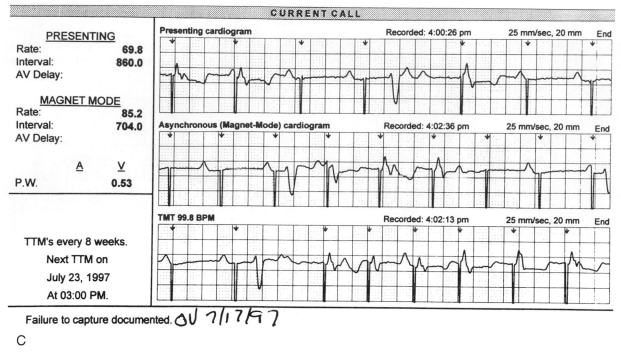

Figure 33–1 *Continued.* *C,* Symptomatic transmission during lightheadedness indicating intermittent failure to capture.

morphology or a right ventricular outflow tract position suggested by right-axis deviation); the magnet tracing is essential to confirm capture in patients whose underlying rhythm normally exceeds the programmed baseline rate.

Most important in the immediate postimplantation setting is the education of the patient. Early on, this includes an emphasis on restricting excessive lifting or abduction ipsilateral to the side of pacer implant for 4 to 6 weeks; close attention to the wound healing with regard to pain, redness, swelling, or drainage at the incision site; and review of symptoms suggestive of possible pacer malfunction. The importance of always carrying a pacemaker identification card (initially a temporary one to be supplanted by a permanent one issued by the manufacturer) is stressed, and identification bracelets are often recommended.

The first outpatient visit, about 2 to 3 weeks after implantation, is primarily directed at the healing wound. This is especially important in patients with diabetes or those taking steroids who may heal more slowly and in patients on anticoagulant therapy, in whom pocket hematomas may pose serious concerns.[18] Follow-up radiography is undertaken to rule out lead dislodgment, which is also a potential issue early after implantation. ECGs are again performed to ensure appropriate pacer function and assess pacer dependence. Rarely, reprogramming may be important if thresholds have risen acutely. At the time of implantation, rate-adaptive features of pacers are often left inactive so as not to result in rate swings at the time of acute pacer generator manipulations; activation of rate-adaptive pacing at the first outpatient visit may be necessary in the patient with chronotropic incompetence.[19] Also at this visit, arrangements for TTM monitoring are made, as are plans for a 3-month checkup. It is at the subsequent visit that chronic thresholds are assessed, allowing for a reprogramming of the device to a lower

output so as to conserve on the longevity of the system. Thereafter, patients are generally seen twice yearly or as otherwise determined by their clinical needs.

Subsequent Outpatient Visits: Interval History

The pacemaker physician must, in essence, function as a detective to elicit symptoms that may go unnoticed by the patient or the patient's other physicians. Perceptions of pain, vigor, or well-being (or the lack thereof) may vary substantially from one patient to another as a function of an individual's threshold for pain or malaise. Patients' expectations following pacemaker implantation may not always be entirely met, and the physician must ascertain whether the pacer system is functioning both *appropriately* and *optimally* and, in some instances, consider whether the patient's original symptoms may have been multifactorial in nature (i.e., not treatable by antibradycardia pacing alone). In some patients, there may be a patient–pacer mismatch, whereby bradycardia is being treated adequately but the system is not addressing some of the patient's needs owing to malprogramming. Thus, for example, upper rate limits may be programmed inappropriately low for younger patients, and rate-adaptive systems may be set to thresholds that are either overly sensitive for some sicker patients or insufficiently sensitive to meet the chronotropic needs of more vigorous patients.

The cardinal symptoms to address include dizziness, presyncope, and syncope, but more subtle concerns include weakness, fatigability, and dyspnea.[20] The symptoms reminiscent of the bradyarrhythmia for which a pacer was inserted may reappear either because of pacer malfunction or, paradoxically, because of appropriate cardiac pacing that is poorly tolerated by the patient. Symptoms of angina may actually be *precipitated* by a pacer system if either the lower or upper rate limits are set too high, thereby limiting time for adequate diastolic coronary perfusion. Conversely, rates may be set too low in certain patients with rate-limited cardiac outputs, resulting in symptoms of congestive heart failure. Optimal atrioventricular (AV) intervals can be determined by right heart catheterization or Doppler assessment in some patients, with reprogramming resulting in optimal cardiac efficiency for patients with either systolic dysfunction or hypertrophic cardiomyopathy to optimize ventricular filling and alleviate outflow obstruction, respectively.

As indicated previously, a pacer system may actually produce symptoms of malaise despite apparent appropriate electrical functioning. This so-called pacemaker syndrome[21-23] typically reflects the loss of optimal atrioventricular synchrony, most often seen in patients with single-chamber ventricular pacing. The resulting pathophysiology observed includes systemic hypotension, AV valvular regurgitation, reduced cardiac output, pulmonary and hepatic congestion, and unpleasant neck pulsations due to atrial contraction against a closed AV valve (cannon A waves). This phenomenon is particularly striking in patients who are critically dependent on ventricular filling because of underlying diastolic heart disease (critical aortic stenosis, hypertrophic cardiomyopathy), whether suffering from heart block or sinus node dysfunction.[24] Even patients with structurally normal hearts, however, may suffer from pacemaker syndrome due to ventricular pacing, particularly if retrograde ventriculoatrial (VA) conduction is present. This is observed in about 80% of patients with sick sinus syndrome and even in a small percentage of patients with antegrade heart block. Less commonly, a type of pacemaker syndrome may arise in single-chamber atrial pacing because of the development of Wenckebach block at relatively slower paced rates in patients with simultaneous sick sinus syndrome and abnormal AV nodal conduction. This may require reprogramming to a slower atrial paced rate or upgrading to a dual-chamber system that will allow for programming of the AV interval.

Nonarrhythmic symptoms related to a pacemaker system may also be encountered. These include diaphragmatic stimulation (due to either direct contact with a perforated ventricular lead, to pacing across a thin ventricular wall, or to

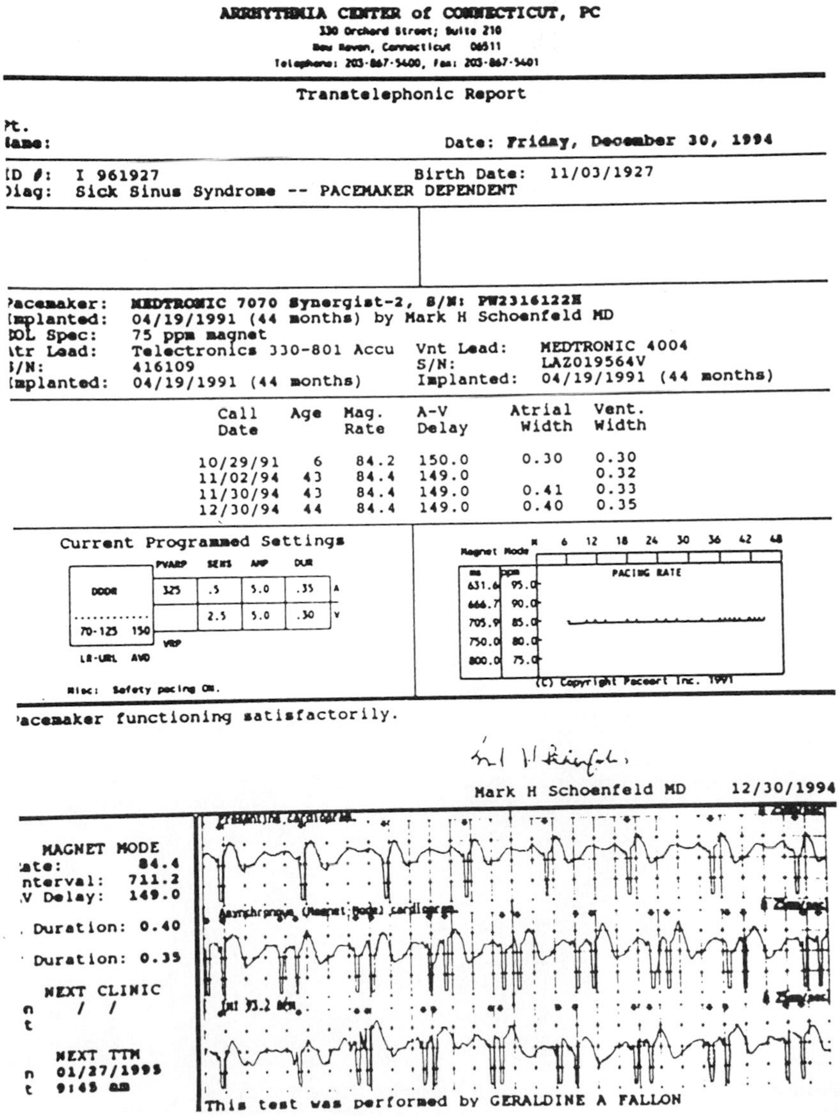

Figure 33–2. Sample computerized transtelephonic monitor report.

phrenic nerve stimulation from an adjacent atrial lead); myopectoral stimulation, especially in patients with unipolar systems; and pocket- or wound-related symptoms, such as pain, swelling, or incipient erosion. Rarely, patients may develop cardiac tamponade late after pacemaker implantation.

Physical Examination

The incision and pacer pocket should be examined for warmth, erythema, tenderness, near-erosion, and hematoma. The viability of the overlying skin and nearby tissue should be examined; adjacent skin infections or cancers or breast malignancies may involve the pacer pocket. Patients may report caudal migration of the generator in the pocket or superficiality to the leads, but these are commonly observed conditions that are rarely of concern. Pocket hematomas are more commonly seen in patients treated with intravenous heparin postoperatively but may also be seen in patients on warfarin sodium (Coumadin) or aspirin therapy. Usually, these pocket hematomas are small; only in exceptional cases (such as expanding hematoma or unrelenting pain) should there be consideration of invasive needling or evacuation because it is usually difficult to aspirate the congealed blood and there is clearly a risk of introducing infection into the pocket. Overt generator or lead erosion (Figs. 33–3A and B) is best managed by complete extraction of the entire system, with replacement by a new system after a period of antibiotic therapy; lesser treatments undertaken to salvage the existing system are invariably associated with a far lower chance of success.

In some patients, myopectoral stimulation may be evident on physical examination. Rarely, this may be due to incorrect placement of a unipolar generator with the uncoated side down, with resulting anodal stimulation of the underlying pectoral muscles; occasionally, patients may "twiddle" their generator upside down,[25] and sometimes there may be an actual lead fracture, allowing for direct conductor stimulation of the adjacent muscle. In most cases in which there is no identifiable problem aside from stimulation of adjacent tissue from the unipolar anodal can, the problem may be managed by reducing the output, particularly the voltage.

Diaphragmatic stimulation may be occasionally evident on physical or fluoroscopic examination or be reported as hiccoughs by the patient. The management approach depends on the cause and may include reducing the ventricular output, reducing or eliminating the atrial output (in cases of phrenic nerve stimulation), or invasive repositioning in the case of displaced or perforated leads.

Physical evaluation should also include an assessment of vital signs (particularly pulse and blood pressure). This is in part to determine (even before the electrocardiogram) whether the patient is paced, what the patient's chronotropic responsiveness may be, and how different conditions are tolerated (e.g., paced versus nonpaced, DDD versus VVI pacing). Signs of pacemaker syndrome or atrial noncapture in a dual-chamber system may include cannon A waves during the neck examination or evidence of congestion in the lung fields, liver, or extremities. On cardiac examination, paradoxical splitting of the second heart sound would be consistent with active right ventricular pacing; the presence of a pericardial rub may suggest perforation of a ventricular (or, less commonly, atrial) lead. It is unusual to produce tricuspid regurgitation murmurs or, for that matter, any hemodynamically significant flow disturbances from endocardial leads. Occasionally, more musical murmurs in systole may reflect movement of a pacing lead within the right ventricular cavity.[26, 27] Carotid sinus massage may occasionally be useful to slow conduction at the level of either the sinus or AV node and thereby elicit and assess adequacy of paced rhythm in a patient whose free-running rhythm is nonpaced. The arm ipsilateral to the generator site should be examined for evidence of central venous thrombosis, which may be initially treated with arm elevation but may ultimately require long-term anticoagulation—it is rare to see pulmonary thromboembolism from cephalic or subclavian vein thrombosis.[28] Rarely, swelling, coupled with inflammation, may represent a gouty attack, which may flare up near the time of pacemaker implantation.

Perhaps the most underappreciated aspect of the physical examination is *direct manipulation* of the system to assess the integrity of the leads and their connection to the generator terminal sites. Traction applied to the can may reveal an

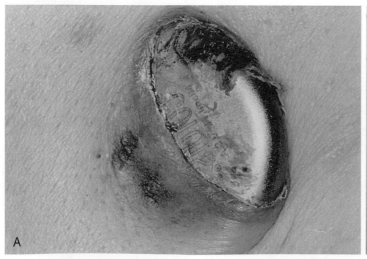
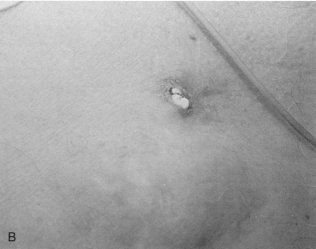

Figure 33–3. *A,* Generator erosion. *B,* Anchoring sleeve erosion.

MEASURED DATA		**MEASURED DATA** with traction on generator	
Pacer Rate...59.7 ppm		Pacer Rate...59.7 ppm	
Ventricular:		Ventricular:	
Pulse Amplitude...3.8 Volts		Pulse Amplitude...3.2 Volts	
Pulse Current...9.8 mAmperes		Pulse Current...40.7 mAmperes	
Pulse Energy..13 μJoules		Pulse Energy..25 μJoules	
Pulse Charge...4 μCoulombs		Pulse Charge...11 μCoulombs	
Lead Impedance..388 Ohms		Lead Impedance..<250 Ohms	
Atrial:		Atrial:	
Pulse Amplitude...3.9 Volts		Pulse Amplitude...3.9 Volts	
Pulse Current...6.0 mAmperes		Pulse Current...6.1 mAmperes	
Pulse Energy...8 μJoules		Pulse Energy...9 μJoules	
Pulse Charge...2 μCoulombs		Pulse Charge...2 μCoulombs	
Lead Impedance..646 Ohms		Lead Impedance..648 Ohms	
Battery Data: (W.G. 8077–NOM. 1.8 AHR)		Battery Data: (W.G. 8077–NOM. 1.8 AHR)	
Voltage..2.80 Volts		Voltage..2.79 Volts	
Current...17 μAmperes		Current...24 μAmperes	
Impedance ....<1 KOhms		Impedance ....<1 KOhms	

Figure 33–4. Problem with insulation defect and consequent low impedance, detectable only with traction on generator.

otherwise unsuspected insulation or conductor fracture or may demonstrate a loose set-screw site, with resulting failure to capture or myopectoral stimulation (Fig. 33–4). Observation of continued pacing should also be undertaken in the upright position and with deep breathing and coughing so as to confirm adequacy of pacing in patients with questionable lead slack or potentially difficult physiognomics and body habitus (e.g., very tall or very short and obese patients). Tapping the generator of a rate-adaptive pacer responsive to activity should translate into an increased pacer rate and serves as yet another "check" on the system. Finally, myopotential inhibition in single-chamber systems or myopotential triggering in dual-chamber systems may be elicited by various pectoral muscle maneuvers, such as pulling, weight lifting, performing abduction, or pressing the hands together (Fig. 33–5). Simultaneous ECG monitoring should be undertaken at the time of such maneuvers. Myopotential inhibition is typically and frequently observed in unipolar systems and may require revision to a bipolar system if inhibition is clinically significant and not reversible by programming; less invasive approaches include reducing sensitivity when possible or programming to either asynchronous or triggered modes in the pacer-dependent patient.

Radiography

The chest radiograph (posteroanterior and lateral positions) remains an indispensable feature of pacer follow-up.[29] During early follow-up, it confirms the stability of lead positioning and confirms, in the case of active-fixation leads, that the screw tip has been advanced appropriately. Anterior positioning of the right ventricular lead is confirmed on the lateral film, to be distinguished from erroneous (posterior) placement into the coronary sinus (or indeed identifying the intentional placement of the lead through the coronary sinus, e.g., in the case of a persistent left superior vena cava, Fig. 33–6). The timing of subsequent films remains subject for debate—certainly they should be performed if there is a specific question of pacer malfunction, but whether preventive or maintenance radiographs should otherwise be taken is less clear.[30] Lead conductor fractures may occasionally be identified radiographically in cases of failure to sense or capture, particularly when an elevated lead impedance is confirmed on telemetry; these occur more commonly at sites of acute lead angulation or at areas of lead compression over (external jugular) or underneath (subclavian) bone or at anchoring sites. Occasionally, real-time fluoroscopy with

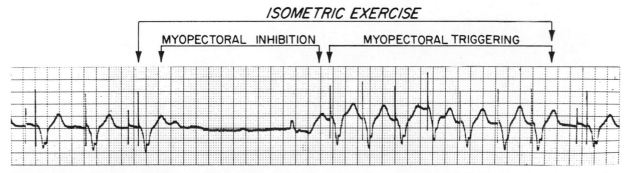

Figure 33–5. Myopectoral inhibition and myopectoral triggering in dual-chamber system elicited by isometric exercise. (Courtesy of Dr. J. Warren Harthorne.)

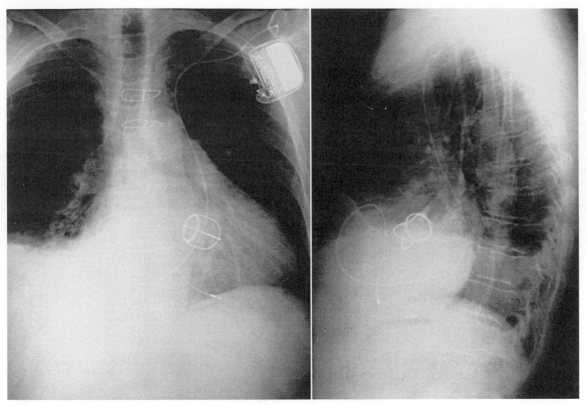

Figure 33–6. Radiograph of active-fixation ventricular lead intentionally placed by way of the coronary sinus through a left persistent superior vena cava, into the right ventricular apex.

traction on the lead may be required to demonstrate the fracture. Fluoroscopy has also been required increasingly to demonstrate fractures of an inner retention wire associated with an advisory in certain active fixation J-shaped atrial leads (Accufix, Telectronics, Englewood, CO; Fig. 33–7). The radiograph also helps to identify the venous insertion site (e.g., external jugular superior to the clavicle versus cephalic or subclavian), which may be useful in cases of subsequent lead revisions, as well as the location of the generator (e.g., occasionally submammary; Fig. 33–8).

Beyond this, the radiograph identifies the number and relative positioning of multiple leads (Figs. 33–9A and B),

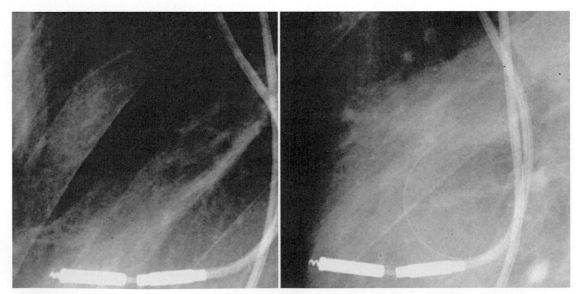

Figure 33–7. Protrusion of inner retention wire in Accufix (Teletronics, Englewood, CO) J-lead *(right),* not apparent on previous film *(left).*

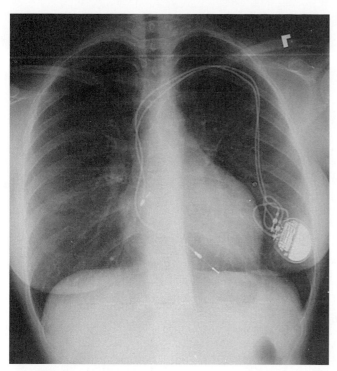

Figure 33–8. Submammary generator implant in young woman with congenital heart block.

the polarity of the leads (although a bipolar system may nonetheless be programmed to unipolar pacing, sensing, or both) and may give a feeling about the security or completeness of lead connection at the set-screw site in the connector block. Importantly, the chest radiograph serves to identify the manufacturer and model of the generator if not otherwise known to the physician—different older models have various characteristic shapes or battery configurations radiographi-

cally, and newer models have identification codes that are manufacturer and model specific.

Electrocardiography and the Use of Magnets

The 12-lead ECG study, both with and without a magnet, is an essential component of pacemaker follow-up.[31, 32] It validates the ability of the system to sense native rhythm and capture as appropriate but also provides important information on the integrity of the leads and positions thereof. For example, right ventricular pacing is typically associated with a left bundle-branch block morphology; right bundle-branch block morphology may suggest a left ventricular location that is associated with epicardial pacing or may reflect inadvertent positioning across a septal defect or by means of perforation (Fig. 33–10). Occasionally, right bundle-branch block paced morphology in the early precordial leads may be consistent with right ventricular pacing, albeit from the apical septum. Ventricular pacing associated with a right axis deviation suggests a position in the right ventricular outflow tract. Analysis of pacemaker spikes may sometimes be helpful as well, such as distinguishing unipolar from bipolar pacing. Evaluation of spike axis, amplitude, and timing may indicate problems with partial electrode conductor fractures (resulting in spike attenuation with prolongation of spike-to-spike intervals exactly by a multiple of the automatic interval) or with defects in insulation (e.g., increased spike amplitude in bipolar systems)[33] (Figs. 33–11A and B).

Magnet application is an extremely important function. It is a typical misconception to medical personnel unfamiliar with pacemakers that magnets "turn off" pacers; clearly, the opposite applies, namely the enabling of asynchronous pacing. Rarely, ventricular ectopy may result from asynchronous ventricular pacing, but this is seldom of clinical significance. Caution should be observed in patients who have, in addition, an implanted cardioverter-defibrillator (ICD) because some ICD models may be inactivated by prolonged magnet

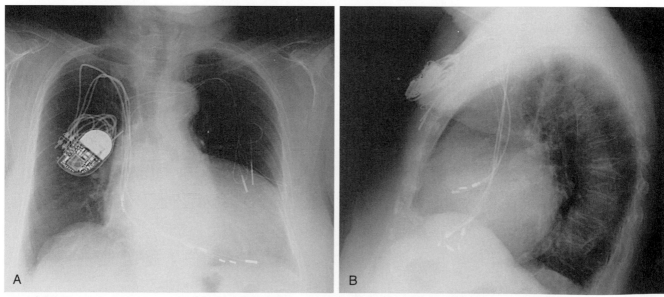

Figure 33–9. Radiograph of patient with five pacer leads (three abandoned), including two atrial and three ventricular. *A,* Posteroanterior view. *B,* Lateral view.

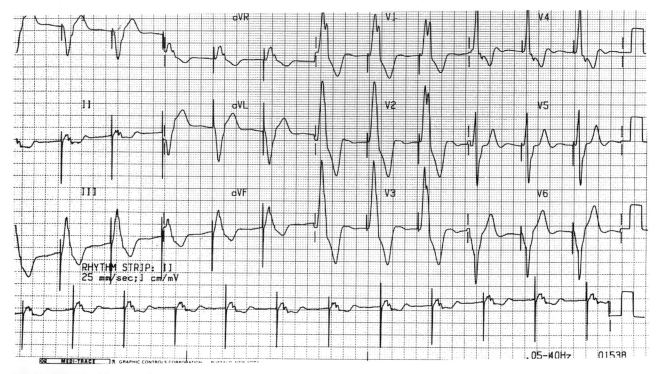

Figure 33–10. Electrocardiogram of epicardial left ventricular pacing.

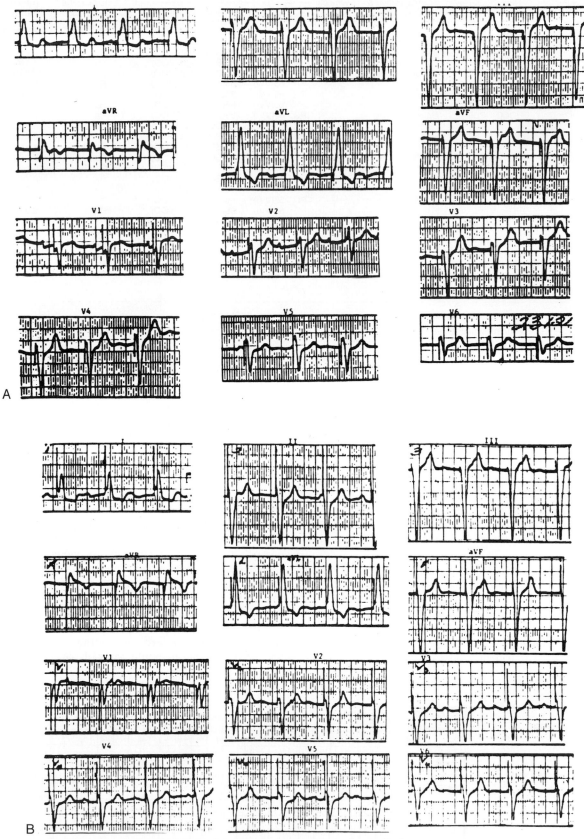

Figure 33–11. *(A)* and after *(B)* insulation defect resulting in increased spike amplitude.

MEDTRONIC   (612) 514-8575 OR FAX: (612) 514-6134

Model Number/ Name	NBG Code	X-Ray* ID	Configuration & Connector	Wrench Size	Rate (ppm)		Magnet Rate (ppm)		ERI/EOL Indicator and Behavior	Theoretical Longevity (Yrs.)
					BOL	ERI/EOL	BOL	ERI/EOL		
7942 Thera DR	DDDRO	PAT	Uni/Bi 3.2 mm LP	2	PR	65(VVI)	85(DOO)	65(VOO)	Ra:	7.4@2.5V
	DDD		IS •1 Compatible		PR	65(VVI)	85(DOO)	65(VOO)	Ra:	5.4@3.5V
	SSIR				PR	65(VVI)	85(SOO)	65(VOO)	Ra:	8.7@2.5V
	SSI				PR	65(VVI)	85(SOO)	65(VOO)	Ra:	7.1@3.5V
7944 Thera D	DDDCO	PBD	Uni/Bi IS • 1	2	PR	65(VVI)	85(DOO)	65(VOO)	Ra:	7.4@2.5V
					PR	65(VVI)	85(DOO)	65(VOO)	Ra:	5.4@3.5V
	SSIR				PR	65(VVI)	85(SOO)	65(VOO)	Ra:	8.7@2.5V
	SSI				PR	65(VVI)	85(SOO)	65(VOO)	Ra:	7.1@3.5V
7945 Thera D	DDDCO	PBE	Unipolar 5 mm	2	PR	65(VVI)	85(DOO)	65(VOO)	Ra:	7.4@2.5V
					PR	65(VVI)	85(DOO)	65(VOO)	Ra:	5.4@3.5V
	SSIR				PR	65(VVI)	85(SOO)	65(VOO)	Ra:	8.7@2.5V
	SSI				PR	65(VVI)	85(SOO)	65(VOO)	Ra:	7.1@3.5V
7946 Thera D	DDDCO	PBF	Uni/Bi 3.2 mm LP	2	PR	65(VVI)	85(DOO)	65(VOO)	Ra:	7.4@2.5V
			IS • 1 Compatible		PR	65(VVI)	85(DOO)	65(VOO)	Ra:	5.4@3.5V
	SSIR				PR	65(VVI)	85(SOO)	65(VOO)	Ra:	8.7@2.5V
	SSI				PR	65(VVI)	85(SOO)	65(VOO)	Ra:	7.1@3.5V
7950 Thera DR	DDDRO	PBR	Uni/Bi IS • 1	2	PR	65(VVI)	85(DOO)	65(VOO)	Ra:	12.0@2.5V
	DDD				PR	65(VVI)	85(DOO)	65(VOO)	Ra:	8.9@3.5V
	SSIR				PR	65(VVI)	85(SOO)	65(VOO)	Ra:	13.9@2.5V
	SSI				PR	65(VVI)	85(SOO)	65(VOO)	Ra:	11.6@3.5V
7951 Thera DR	DDDRO	PBV	Unipolar 5/6 mm	2	PR	65(VVI)	85(DOO)	65(VOO)	Ra:	12.0@2.5V
	DDD				PR	65(VVI)	85(DOO)	65(VOO)	Ra:	8.9@3.5V
	SSIR				PR	65(VVI)	85(SOO)	65(VOO)	Ra:	13.9@2.5V
	SSI				PR	65(VVI)	85(SOO)	65(VOO)	Ra:	11.6@3.5V

77

*Note Medtronic logo precedes and engineering series number follows the radiopaque code (X-Ray ID).

Figure 33–12. Magnet responses and elective replacement indicator (ERI) data for one group of generators of one manufacturer.

exposure. The application of a magnet during ECG monitoring confirms the ability of the system to capture the appropriate cardiac chamber at the programmed output settings. Some systems, in addition, provide for a threshold margin test as the initial phase of magnet application. The exact magnet response (mode and rate) is manufacturer and model specific. Such responses may include asynchronous pacing at the programmed rate, at some other predetermined rate, or at the programmed rate plus a certain percentage. The exact rate (and mode) may also vary depending on whether the device is programmed to single- or dual-chamber pacing (Fig. 33–12).

The magnet response may serve to identify a particular model in patients unfamiliar to the physician, particularly if no other information is available from the patient. Furthermore, the magnet rate is an indicator of end-of-life or elective replacement, again characteristic of each model. In addition, magnets may be helpful both diagnostically and therapeutically. In a patient whose native rhythm inhibits pacer activity, the application of a magnet may serve to identify the programmed mode of the system if the correct programmer is not available for telemetry. In some cases of pacemaker malfunction due to malsensing, asynchronous pacing from magnet application may temporarily correct the problem, confirming the presence of such phenomena as far-field signal sensing, cross-talk inhibition, T-wave sensing, or pacemaker-mediated tachycardias.[34] Magnets can confirm a propensity for pacemaker-mediated tachycardias (see later) by temporarily promoting AV dysynchrony. In pacer-dependent patients, magnet application may ensure pacing during certain situations in which electromagnetic interference may inhibit output, such as from electrocautery during surgery. Finally, magnet application may be used to terminate pacemaker-mediated tachycardias resulting from tracking of retrogradely conducted atrial activity (Fig. 33–13) and may occasionally be helpful in terminating slow ventricular tachycardias by underdrive pacing—in the latter case, backup defibrillation should be available.

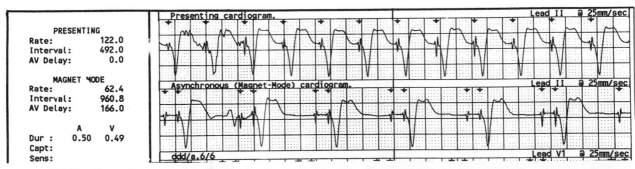

Figure 33–13. Pacemaker-mediated tachycardia *(upper panel)* interrupted with magnet application *(lower panel)*.

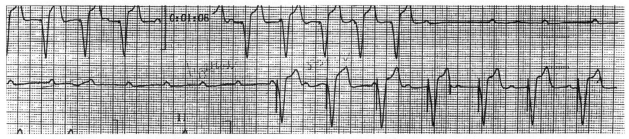

Figure 33–14. Abrupt reduction in output in pacer-dependent patient, resulting in highly symptomatic ventricular asystole.

Determination of Pacemaker Dependency

Strictly speaking, pacemaker dependency is defined as significant bradycardia or ventricular asystole resulting from cessation of pacemaker function. The fact that a patient is 100% ventricular paced at some predetermined rate (e.g., 70 bpm) does not necessarily indicate a condition of being pacemaker dependent—the system must be reprogrammed to assess what native underlying rhythm, if any, is present without pacing. It must be further emphasized that pacemaker dependence may vary over time, reflecting variations in the patient's native sinus or AV nodal conduction or, alternatively, concomitant medications that a patient may be taking that may facilitate or depress conduction. When reprogramming to assess underlying rhythm, *gradual* slowing of the programmed rate is more likely to enable an escape rhythm to emerge than an abrupt termination of pacing. Thus, a sudden programmed reduction in output to subthreshold levels may result in ventricular asystole and define a condition of pacer dependence (Fig. 33–14) when, in fact, an escape rhythm may have otherwise been observed (Fig. 33–15). Associated symptoms should also be observed, even in cases in which an escape rhythm is present; these may be less apparent in the supine compared with upright position. In systems in which the lowest programmable rate (e.g., 45 bpm) is still associated with ventricular pacing

because slower rates (e.g., 30 bpm) are not achievable, an escape rhythm may nonetheless be identified at this point by reducing output to subthreshold values. Alternatively, chest wall stimulation may be applied to skin electrodes overlying the pacer generator by means of alligator clips attached to a temporary pacing box. This may produce enough electromagnetic interference to suppress output from the permanent pacemaker and allow the native rhythm to emerge (Fig. 33–16).

Pacemaker Programmers

Programmability has been defined as a "noninvasive, reversible alteration of the electronic performance of an implanted pacemaker device."[35] The ability to adjust certain parameters to avoid second surgical interventions has received particular emphasis, as in cases of marginal capture or malsensing, as well as achieving other goals, such as optimizing cardiac output or minimizing rate-related angina. Essential now to the capability for programming is the ability to confirm that a programming command has been successfully received by the pulse generator, the so-called concepts of verification and bidirectional telemetry.[36] Although historically, three forms of electromagnetic waves have been used for communication between programmer and pulse generator (magnetic coupling, inductive coupling, and radiofrequency energy),

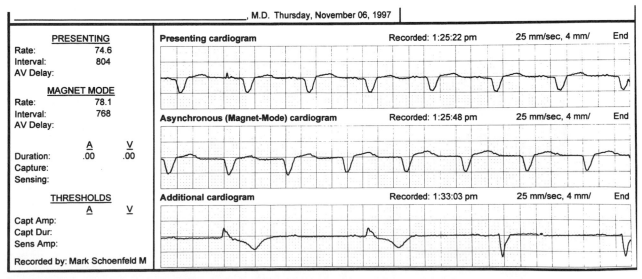

Figure 33–15. More gradual reduction in pacer rate, allowing for emergence of escape rhythm *(lowest panel),* in anticipation of generator replacement without requiring temporary pacer wire placement as backup.

CHEST WALL STIMULATION

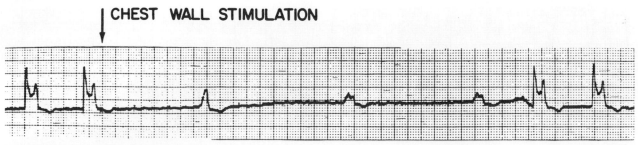

Figure 33–16. Application of chest wall stimulation to suppress pacer activity and reveal underlying rhythm.

radiofrequency waves (ranging from 10 to 175 kHz) have emerged as the dominant carriers because they allow for rapid transmission of large amounts of information.[37] Both the transmitter (in the programmer) and the receiver (in the pulse generator) have antennae for emitting and decoding radiofrequency signals (Fig. 33–17).

The selection of carrier frequencies for use in programmers is variable and manufacturer specific. Certain programming systems employ both a radiofrequency field and a reed switch that must be magnetically dithered to allow detection of the radiofrequency waves by the pulse generator detector antenna coil. In these systems, the requirement for a second electromagnetic field interaction (magnet-actuated reed switch closure) is viewed as a "safety interlock" or an environmental security measure against misprogramming. The receiver circuit in this case does not remain constantly activated because of concern about current drain on the power cell of the pulse generator. A potential limitation of using a reed switch as the receiving element is the requirement for its mechanical motion, a factor that limits its speed. As a result, a relatively long transmission time is required for programming.[38]

Signal attenuation is a potential concern in the interaction of the programmer with the pulse generator. Because the programming signal must pass from the programmer through the air intervening between the transmitter antenna and the skin, the subcutaneous tissues, and the pulse generator can, the signal that is received in the pulse generator may be of lower amplitude than the signal that was transmitted by the programmer. These same barriers may attenuate the signal emitted by the pulse generator during telemetry to the programmer, and the extent to which these signals are attenuated is directly proportional to the distance between programmer and pulse generator. Such attenuation by the pulse generator can be particularly noted at higher radiofrequency carrier frequencies.[39]

The method of encoding information in the carrier input signals by the programmer is a process called *modulation*.[40] Modulation of signal amplitude (turning the carrier on and off between zero amplitude and a predefined value), pulse width, and time between pulses all have been employed in programming systems. When modulation is accomplished by variations in pulse amplitude, encoding is based on the total number of pulses transmitted to the pulse generator. In

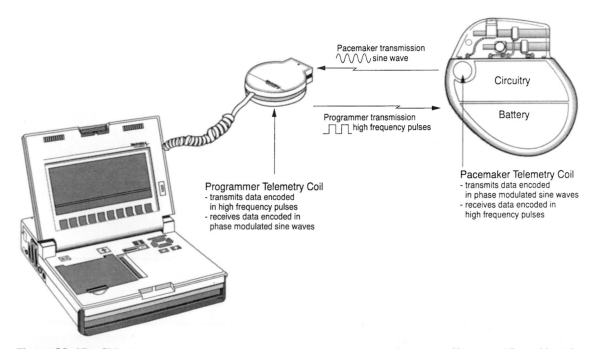

Figure 33–17. Bidirectional telemetry between programmer/programming head and generator. (Courtesy of Trevor Moody.)

such programming schemes, the time required for signal transmission is directly proportional to the number of pulses used for the code; furthermore, a minimum pulse count is required to identify the subsequent pulses as a valid code. Pulse width–modulated programming systems are ideally suited to binary coding, in which narrow and wide pulses may represent bit values of 0 and 1 respectively; the information that can be encoded with x binary digits is 2 to the xth power, allowing more information to be conveyed in a smaller number of pulses.[40]

The programming signal must be designed to be secure, both for proprietary reasons and to protect against misprogramming. Such programming security is of three types: message security, system security, and carrier security.[40] *Carrier* security implies that a pulse generator will respond only to the carrier for which it has been designed to be sensitive—magnetic pulses and low-frequency radiofrequency offer the greatest security from spurious environmental interference, whereas higher-frequency radiofrequency systems may be "confused" by other signal sources, such as radios, televisions, or even garage door openers. One type of *message* security includes the use of the first group of transmitted bits or pulses as an identification or access code. In the case of multiparameter programmability, the linkage of two or more parameters, such as sensitivity and pacing rate, may be used to verify that a change in one programmed value has occurred by verifying a change in another, more easily confirmed pacing parameter (*system* security).

Despite such security measures, spurious programming may nonetheless be observed. This may include *dysprogramming* (from an anomalous source of interference), *misprogramming* (the faulty transmission of programming instructions in which the pulse generator responds to the programmer in unanticipated fashion), *phantom programming* (by another "unknown" physician), and *cross-programming* (reprogramming of pulse generator from one manufacturer by the programmer of another manufacturer).[39, 41–45]

All programming systems, independent of manufacturer, share certain fundamental features (Fig. 33–18). Input is the mechanism by which the user of the programmer sets up or enters the information that is to be conveyed from the programmer to the pulse generator. Typically, the programming instructions are entered by means of a keyboard or a set of pushbuttons accompanied by a video display, such as a light-emitting diode or liquid crystal display. Input of the programmed values may require interaction of the user and the programmer through a light pen or a touch-sensitive computer screen. These programming screens also provide a record of the programming session and are usually sent to an integrated printer. An invariable component of the input feature is a key for emergency programming to high-stimulus output or rapid reprogramming to nominal or standard values.[46]

With telemetry, a coil in the pulse generator serves as the transmitting antenna, and the coil in the telemetry component of the programmer (usually in hand-held format) receives

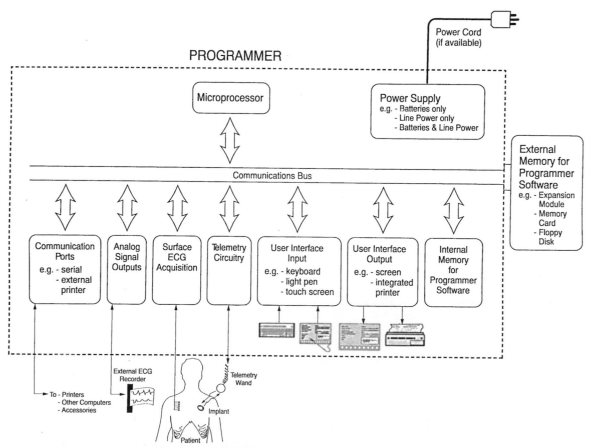

Figure 33–18. Components of a pacemaker programmer system. (Courtesy of Trevor Moody.)

the transmitter signal (see Fig. 33–17).[36] The telemetry circuit may be used to indicate the programmed values in the pulse generator or to confirm that a programming step has been successfully received and executed in the pulse generator. Real-time measurements of battery voltage and impedance, stimulus current, voltage and energy, and lead resistance may be conveyed from the pulse generator to the programmer, as may real-time intracardiac electrograms, marker channels, and stored histograms of paced and sensed events and rate-adaptive sensor data.[4, 47–50]

Although bidirectional telemetry is used in most modern pacing systems to confirm that a programming sequence has been undertaken and completed successfully, it is incumbent on the physician to establish independently that appropriate programming has occurred by inspection of the ECG recording—"what you see (by telemetry) is not always what you get."

Use of the Programmer to Assess Appropriate Functioning of the Pacer System: Sensing and Pacing

Assessing pacing capture thresholds is an important feature of pacer follow-up because longevity of the generator may be considerably enhanced by programming the device to the lowest value that will provide an adequate safety margin for effective pacing. On the other hand, programmability of output will also allow for programming to higher effective outputs in patients with poor chronic thresholds who might previously have required surgical revision to enable safe pacing. Typically, chronic thresholds are reached by 3 months after implantation, and calculation of the strength–duration curve for stimulation requirements allows the physician to determine this lowest safe output value. Some systems have programmable threshold tests, allowing for automatic pulse width or amplitude decrement, whereas other systems require one or the other parameter to be manually programmed to assess capture threshold. Generally, at short pulse durations, small changes in pulse width result in large differences in voltage and current thresholds. Shorter pulse widths result in lower impedance values and increased stimulation efficiency. In the case of devices with fixed-output voltage and programmable pulse width durations, acceptable margins may be achieved by tripling the pulse width threshold if this value is less than 0.4 msec, but four times threshold should be considered for higher pulse width thresholds.

Most modern-day devices allow for programmable voltage, and pulse duration thresholds can be determined at 2.5 V and programmed to that pulse duration at 5 V to provide an adequate safety margin. Another approach is to reduce voltage while extending the pulse width somewhat if the pulse duration is very low (less than 0.1 msec) at a given output voltage. Generally, output voltage of less than 2.5 V does not significantly reduce battery drain but should be considered if diaphragmatic or myopectoral stimulation is present at higher outputs. Conversely, in situations in which the pulse duration threshold is elevated, increasing the output voltage is necessary to allow for safe pacing because the higher pulse widths approaching rheobase are neither effective nor energy efficient. The physician should be aware that certain drugs, most notably the antiarrhythmic agents flecainide and amiodarone, may result in increased pacing thresholds.

Some newer devices allow for frequent automatic self-determination of pacing thresholds with corresponding self-adjustments in pacer output to minimize current drain. In most devices, however, manual determinations of threshold are required.

To assess capture threshold, the paced rate must be programmed, at least temporarily, to exceed the patient's native rate. Atrial capture in atrial-demand systems or dual-chamber systems may sometimes be difficult to confirm because there may be spurious artifact following the atrial spike. It is usually easily made in patients with intact conduction to the ventricle by determining whether the resulting QRS complexes occur at the programmed rate. In patients with AV block, however, programmed rates required to observe atrial capture may result in even higher-degree block with resulting long periods of ventricular asystole, limiting the ability to assess thresholds carefully. In some patients, loss of atrial capture with dual-chamber pacing may be evident because of resulting ventriculoatrial conduction present despite antegrade heart block; this phenomenon may be evident on surface ECG studies or through channel event markers.

Sensing thresholds are determined by programming the inhibited mode to a rate slower than the patient's intrinsic rate and, by decreasing sensitivity, determining at what value pacer output is no longer appropriately inhibited. An alternative approach is to use the triggered mode, in which pacer output is supplied whenever an intrinsic depolarization is sensed; once again, the sensitivity is progressively reduced (i.e., the millivolt values are increased) until a sensed event no longer triggers a pacing spike; in essence, the pacer spike serves as a type of marker channel for sensed activity (Fig. 33–19). Either approach applies to single-chamber or dual-chamber systems. In dual-chamber pacers, furthermore, atrial sensing can be confirmed by programming to a P-wave synchronous ventricular triggered mode, shortening the AV interval so as to ensure ventricular pacing, and then progressively reducing atrial sensitivity until ventricular pacing is no longer triggered. Reprogramming of sensitivity to higher values may on occasion be warranted if oversensing is a clinical problem, as in the case of T-wave sensing or myopotential sensing resulting in inhibition; this is especially the case in the pacer-dependent patient. Rarely, reprogramming of single-chamber systems to the purely triggered mode may be required to prevent undue inhibition of pacer output by oversensing of extraneous signals. More commonly, undersensing is problematic (especially in the atrium where smaller atrial electrograms are typically observed), necessitating a programmed increase in sensitivity.

As previously indicated, the possibility of myopotential inhibition or triggering should be evaluated by isometric deltopectoral muscle maneuvers (see Fig. 33–5). Reprogramming to greater sensitivity may be necessary to demonstrate an otherwise unappreciated potential clinical problem.

Programmability: Changes in Pacing Mode, Polarity, and Atrioventricular Interval

Reprogramming of pacing mode may be required in a variety of clinical scenarios. In patients with oversensing despite programming to the least sensitivity, conversion to the asynchronous or triggered modes may become necessary to ensure pacer output, as already indicated. In patients with atrial undersensing despite maximal settings, dual-chamber pacing may need to be abandoned for ventricular demand pacing. Conversely, where atrial pacing thresholds are unreliable but sensing is adequate, the VDD mode may be selected to

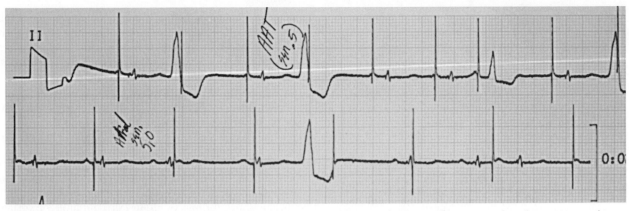

Figure 33–19. Atrial triggered mode with atrial spikes falling on sensed P waves *(upper panel)* but not sensing when programmed to reduced sensitivity *(lower panel).*

preserve AV synchrony. In some dual-chamber systems, the problem of myopotential inhibition may be treated by reprogramming to the DAD mode. In dual-chamber paced patients with rapid atrial fibrillation in whom reprogramming atrial sensitivity and upper tracking rate behavior does not suffice, consideration of the DDI mode may be made.

Programmability of polarity has become increasingly available and may be useful in certain clinical situations (Fig. 33–20). Programming to unipolar pacing allows for larger spikes to be observed electrocardiographically, which may be useful in following patients, but at the same time increases the likelihood of myopectoral stimulation. Programming to bipolar sensing reduces the likelihood of far-field or myopotential inhibition. Programming from bipolar to unipolar modes has been increasingly used in the case of "subclavian crush" syndrome, in which problems with certain polyurethane leads has resulted in insulation defects and an unacceptably low impedance. Programming to unipolar generally increases the impedance to more acceptable values and prevents loss of capture and undersensing; it does not, however, prevent oversensing from make/break electrical transients resulting from contact between the two conductors, and ultimately lead replacement may be required, especially in the pacer-dependent patient.

Reprogramming to a longer AV interval may be temporarily necessary to evaluate atrial capture in the patient with intact AV conduction, as already indicated. Permanent reprogramming to longer intervals may be considered in an effort to minimize ventricular pacing and increase longevity of the device. In general, PR intervals of longer than 240 to 260 msec result in suboptimal hemodynamics, and ventricular pacing should be instituted by reprogramming the AV interval to a shorter value. Reprogramming of the interval to an "optimal" shorter duration may be considered in patients whose cardiac output may be correspondingly enhanced as assessed by Doppler or right heart catheterization techniques, or in the patient with hypertrophic cardiomyopathy.

Other programmable features have become increasingly available as a result of advances in both pacer generators (Fig. 33–21) and their associated programmers. (As stated earlier, it is incumbent on any following physician to have the full complement of programmers available for the many types of pacers being followed in clinic (Fig. 33–22); univer-

sality of programmers has yet to be realized.[37]) The newer programmable features include adjustable AV intervals that allow for physiologic adaptation to shorter AV delays with faster paced heart rates and changing the AV interval as a

294-03		Jan 26 '93 5:12 PM
SN		
001777		
RELAY		TELEMETRY DATA
Pacing Rate		70 ppm
Pacing Interval		857 msec
Cell Voltage		2.72 volts
Cell Impedance		2.67 kohms
Cell Current		17.3 UA
	ATRIAL (Uni)	VENTRICULAR (Bi)
Sensitivity	1.0	5.0 mv
Lead Impedance	635	1815 ohms
Pulse Amplitude	3.99	4.03 volts
Pulse Width	0.35	0.35 msec
Output Current	6.1	2.2 ma
Energy Delivered	8.1	3.0 mj
Charge Delivered	2.15	0.77 mc
294-03 SN 001777		Jan 26 '93 5:14 PM
RELAY		TELEMETRY DATA
Pacing Rate		70 ppm
Pacing Interval		857 msec
Cell Voltage		2.70 volts
Cell Impedance		2.98 kohms
Cell Current		20.3 UA
	ATRIAL (Uni)	VENTRICULAR (Uni)
Sensitivity	1.0	5.0 mv
Lead Impedance	652	508 ohms
Pulse Amplitude	3.97	3.94 volts
Pulse Width	0.35	0.35 msec
Output Current	5.9	7.5 ma
Energy Delivered	7.8	9.6 mj
Charge Delivered	2.09	2.64 mc

RETURN

Figure 33–20. Elevated lead impedance evident on telemetry, temporarily corrected by reprogramming to unipolar mode. More typically, it is an extremely low impedance that may be encountered in lead malfunction ("subclavian crush syndrome" for bipolar leads) with transient correction by changing to unipolar mode.

PARAMETER	Trilogy DR + MODELS 2370, 2371, 2372, 2373, 2374 Range of Parameters	AFP MODEL 283 Range of Parameters
Mode	DDD, DDI, DVI, DOO, AAI, AAT, AOO, VVI, VVT, VOO, OFF	DDD, DDI, VDD, DVI, DOO, AAI, AAT, AOO, VVI, VVT, VOO, OFF
Sensor Modes	DDDR, DDIR, DVIR, DOOR, AAIR, AATR, AOOR, VVIR, VVTR, VOOR, OFF	None
Lower Rate (ppm)	45–130, Temp. 30	45–118, Temp. 30
AV Delay (ms)	31–300	65–240
PV Delay (me)	AV Delay–25 ms	Same as AV Delay
Max Track Rate (ppm)	85–180	90–150
V Pulse Config.	Bipolar/Unipolar	Unipolar–only
V Pulse Width (ms)	0.2–1.6 Auto	0.1–1.6
V Pulse Amp. (V)	0.5–7.5 Auto	1.3–10
V Sense Config.	Flexipolar	Unipolar–only
V Sensitivity (mv)	1.0–10.0	0.5–14.0
V Refractory (ms)	125–325	250–475
A Pulse Config.	Bipolar/Unipolar	Unipolar–only
A Pulse Width (ms)	0.2–1.6	0.1–1.6
A Pulse Amp. (V)	0.5–7.5	1.3–10
A Sense Config.	Flexipolar	Unipolar–only
A Sensitivity (mv)	0.5–5.0	0.5–14.0
A Refractory (ms)	150–500	150–550
V Blanking (ms)	15, 25, 38, 51	13, 25, 83, 50
PVC Options	DDD, + PVARP	DDX
Hysteresis Escape Rate (ppm)	Off, 45–150	35–85, Single Chamber Mode Only
Magnet	On, Off, Temp. Off	On, Off
V Safety Option	Enable	
PMT Options	10 Beats > MTR, Auto Detect, Off	
Programmable RRAVD	1–3 mos/beat > 90	
Minimum AV/PV Delay ms	30–102	
AV/PV Hysteresis w/ Search	80 ms to 100 ms	
V Auto Capture with Auto Threshold	Off, Auto	
Threshold Search Interval	90 min, 9 hrs, 7 days	
Threshold on Magnet Removal	Off, On Single Sequence Only	
Evoked Response Sensitivity	1.0–10 mv	
Threshold Safety Factor	2X, 3X, 4X	
Auto Mode Switch	On (DDI(R) at ATDR) On (VVI(R) at ATDR)	
Atrial Tachycardia Detection Rate	MTR + 20 up to 300 ppm	
Sleep Mode	45 ppm to Base Rate Less 5 ppm	
Activity Threshold	1.0–7.0	
Auto Rate Response Thresh	Auto (0.5 to + 1.5)	
Activity Rate Responsive Slope	1.0–16	
Auto Rate Response Slope	Auto (1.0 to + 3.0)	
Max Sensor Rate (ppm)	80–180	
Reaction Time	9–36 sec	
Recovery Time	2–5 min	

Figure 33–21. Programmable parameters for a newer *(left)* and older *(right)* dual-chamber device from one manufacturer (Pacesetter, St. Jude Medical, Sylmar, CA.)

function of whether the atrial activity is sensed or paced (Fig. 33–23). Circadian functions allow for slowing of the pacer rate at night to minimize nocturnal pacing and conserve energy (Fig. 33–24). Search hysteresis function in certain pacer systems allows the patient's rate to dip down to a low value before pacing at a much faster pacing rate, with automatic scanning for when the endogenous rhythm returns to normal; this feature has been used with great success to treat patients with the severe cardioinhibitory responses associated with vasovagal syncope[51] (Fig. 33–25). Automatic mode switching is a programmable feature incorporated into many of the newer devices that allows for automatic reversion from dual-chamber to single-chamber ventricular pacing when atrial fibrillation is recognized.[52] (Fig. 33–26). These features are beyond the scope of this chapter; needless to say, an awareness of the growing versatility of pacer systems is incumbent on the pacer physician.

Assessing for Crosstalk, Retrograde Ventriculoatrial Conduction, and Pacemaker-Mediated Tachycardia in the Dual-Chamber System

In dual-chamber systems, the propensity for crosstalk[53] (the sensing of electric signals generated in one cardiac chamber by the sense amplifier in the second cardiac chamber) and pacemaker-mediated tachycardias should be explored. To assess for the possibility of crosstalk, the ventricular channel should be programmed to its greatest sensitivity and the atrial output to its highest value. The programmed rate should exceed the native rate, allowing for continuous atrial pacing, and the programmed AV interval should be shorter than the native PR interval to allow for fully AV paced rhythm; if programmable, the ventricular blanking period should be set to the shortest value possible. Typically, crosstalk inhibition is manifested as ventricular sensing of atrial output with corresponding inhibition of ventricular output (Fig. 33–27); the absence of this phenomenon at maximal atrial output and ventricular sensitivity suggests that this is not likely to be a clinical problem for a given patient at usual programmed settings. Caution should be undertaken in evaluating this in the pacer-dependent patient with heart block because transient ventricular asystole may ensue. Conversely, if the phenomenon is demonstrated or was clinically apparent from other (e.g., Holter monitor) data, reprogramming may be necessary; this could include a reduction in atrial output, a reduction in ventricular sensing, a lengthening of the ventricular blanking period, reprogramming from unipolar to bipolar pacing and sensing, or changing to another mode such as VDD. In some patients, an atrial lead insulation defect may result in a low lead impedance and consequent high current output crossing the lead and produce crosstalk in a previously stable pacer system; changing to VDD mode or revision of the atrial lead may be necessary in such cases.

Retrograde ventriculoatrial conduction may be responsible for the aforementioned pacemaker syndrome as well as for pacemaker-mediated tachycardia (PMT). Certain pacer programmers have specific follow-up support programs that evaluate for retrograde VA conduction. If these programs are not available, the propensity for VA conduction should be assessed by programming to either the VVI mode or AV

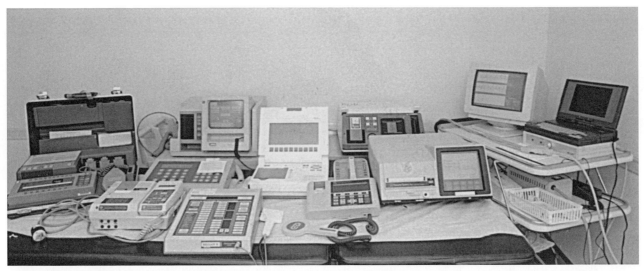

Figure 33–22. Typical array of programmers required for outpatient pacer follow-up.

Short Term A-V Conduction Histogram Report

Pacemaker Model: Medtronic.Kappa KDR401/403   Serial Number: PER211203   Date of Visit: 08/20/97

Patient Name: john smith   **ID: 123456**   **Chart Number: 567890**

Data Collection Period: 08/17/97 12:55 AM - 08/20/97 8:55 AM (Over Last 3 days)

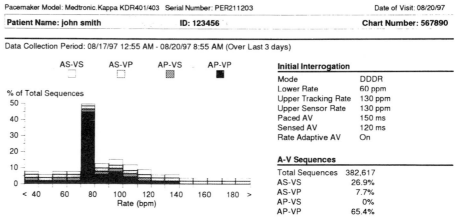

Initial Interrogation

Mode	DDDR
Lower Rate	60 ppm
Upper Tracking Rate	130 ppm
Upper Sensor Rate	130 ppm
Paced AV	150 ms
Sensed AV	120 ms
Rate Adaptive AV	On

A-V Sequences

Total Sequences	382,617
AS-VS	26.9%
AS-VP	7.7%
AP-VS	0%
AP-VP	65.4%

Figure 33–23. Histogram of atrioventricular (AV) conduction in pacer patient with programmable rate adaptive AV delay and programmable paced versus sensed AV intervals.

Rate Range (bpm)	Events	% Total Events	% AS-VS	% AS-VP	% AP-VS	% AP-VP
0 - 39	1,152	0.3	0.3	0	0	0
40 - 49	1,413	0.4	0.3	0	0.0	0
50 - 59	4,460	1.2	1.0	0.2	0	0
60 - 69	8,910	2.3	1.6	0.7	0	0
70 - 79	189,064	49.4	3.3	1.5	0	44.6
80 - 89	37,451	9.8	2.7	1.1	0	6.0
90 - 99	48,010	12.5	3.7	1.1	0	7.7
100 - 109	34,562	9.0	3.6	0.9	0	4.5
110 - 119	21,917	5.7	3.2	0.8	0	1.7
120 - 129	10,918	2.9	1.9	0.4	0.0	0.5
130 - 139	10,607	2.8	2.1	0.4	0.0	0.3
140 - 149	7,213	1.9	1.6	0.2	0.0	0.0
150 - 159	3,752	1.0	0.9	0.1	0.0	0.0
160 - 169	1,605	0.4	0.4	0	0.0	0.0
170 - 179	387	0.1	0.1	0	0.0	0.0
180 - 400	1,196	0.3	0.3	0.1	0.0	0.0

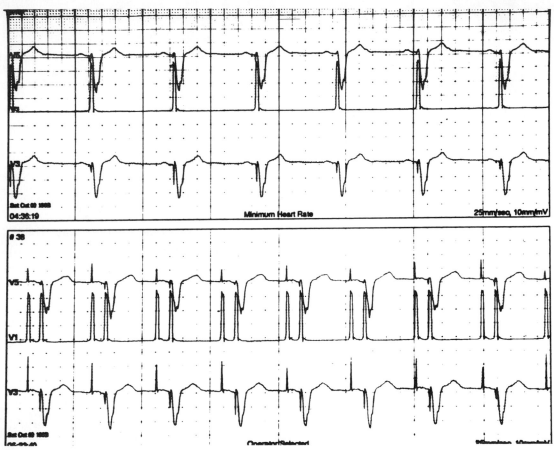

Figure 33–24. Circadian feature demonstrating P-wave synchronous ventricular pacing at slow rates while asleep *(upper panel)* and atrioventricular sequential pacing at faster baseline rates during waking hours *(lower panel)*.

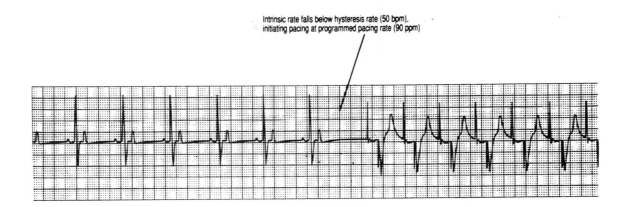

Intrinsic rate falls below hysteresis rate (50 bpm),
initiating pacing at programmed pacing rate (90 ppm)

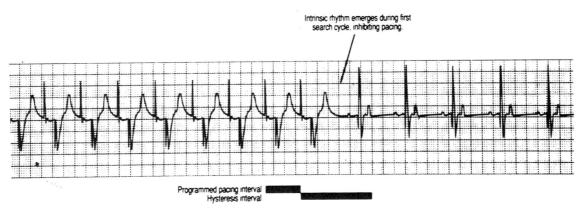

Intrinsic rhythm emerges during first
search cycle, inhibiting pacing.

Programmed pacing interval
Hysteresis interval

Figure 33–25. Search hysteresis. Intrinsic rate falls below hysteresis rate, initiating pacing at fast rate *(upper panel);* eventually, intrinsic rhythm emerges during search cycle, inhibiting pacing *(lower panel).*

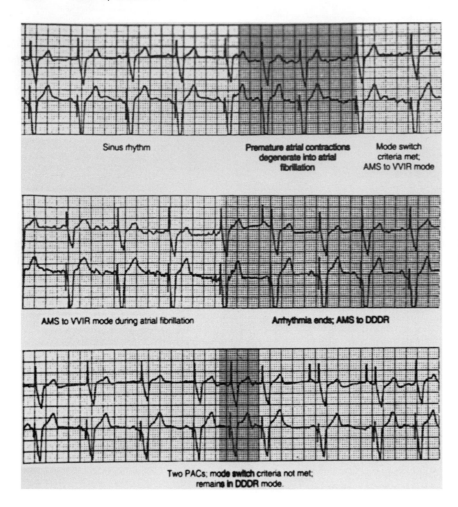

Figure 33–26. Automatic mode switching for one manufacturer (Telectronics).

pacing with the atrial channel output programmed to sub-threshold levels; because this phenomenon may be somewhat dynamic,[54] different pacing rates should be assessed. VA conduction may be apparent either by examining the inferior leads of the 12-lead ECG recording (Fig. 33–28) or by examining the patient for such signs as cannon A waves or AV valvular regurgitation. The use of marker channels in certain pacer systems may facilitate the identification of retrogradely conducted atrial activity, provided the postven-tricular atrial refractory period (PVARP) is programmed suf-ficiently short.

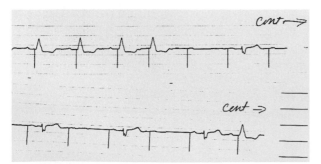

Figure 33–27. Crosstalk inhibition in a unipolar dual-chamber system. Atrial spikes are sensed by the ventricular channel, inhibiting ventricular output and resulting in very slow ventricular escape rhythm.

An extension of this phenomenon is the ability to generate pacemaker-mediated tachycardia (PMT). These require tran-sient AV dysynchrony and the ability thereafter for retro-grade atrial activation to occur. Thus, when programmed to the DDD mode at a sufficiently short PVARP, PMT may be observed if triggered by a spontaneous premature ventricular contraction, if dysynchrony is created by momentary magnet application and removal, or if atrial output is programmed to subthreshold values. In the last case, AV pacing fails to capture the atrium but captures the ventricle, with retrograde conduction resulting in activation of a nonrefractory atrium, which in turn triggers the next ventricular paced beat, setting up PMT. In patients with a propensity for PMT, the ability to terminate with magnet (see Fig. 33–13) or PMT-terminating algorithms should be explored, and the device should be reprogrammed by limiting the upper ventricular tracking rate, extending the PVARP, or changing to a different (i.e., nontriggered) pacing mode such as DDI.

Not infrequently, atrial fibrillation or flutter may be sensed in a dual-chamber system and trigger rapid ventricular paced rhythms that are often irregular or at the upper tracking limit. Measures to address this include reprogramming to a lower upper tracking limit or reprogramming to the VVI mode with plans to re-establish sinus rhythm in the interim either chemically or through direct current cardioversion, thereafter reprogramming back to dual-chamber pacing. Rarely, temporary programming of rapid atrial burst pacing may be attempted by means of the atrial channel in an effort

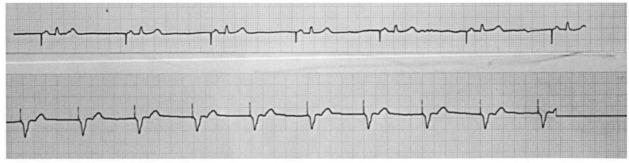

Figure 33–28.   Ventriculoatrial conduction demonstrated by programming from dual-chamber pacing *(upper panel)* to ventricular demand pacing *(lower panel).*

to convert atrial flutter back to sinus mechanism. Activating the automatic mode switch function in devices in which this feature is available is a commonly employed maneuver in patients with frequent paroxysms of atrial fibrillation and flutter.

Telemetry of Programmed Settings, Measured Data, Histograms, Electrograms, and Marker Channels

The device should always be interrogated with regard to *programmed settings* before any reprogramming is undertaken or thresholds evaluated; without documenting the device settings, it may be difficult to appreciate why a device may or may not be "behaving" appropriately. Some older devices with limited telemetry may allow for telemetry of previously programmed settings, but this may not reflect

what the device is actually doing, for example, if end of life has been reached. Again, independent confirmation of telemetered parameters must be made electrocardiographically after all interventions because telemetry will not always reflect true programmed settings. This is particularly true in patients whose systems have come into contact with extreme environmental noise, with subsequent resetting of the device.

The ability to undertake telemetry or programming is device and manufacturer specific and requires the correct programmer and, in some cases, the correct range-of-motion module associated with a given model. If the patient is previously unknown, identification of the device through the patient identification card or radiographic identification becomes indispensable. Some newer programmers allow for automatic model select if at least the manufacturer is known (Fig. 33–29).

In addition to programmed data, previously recorded ini-

Automatic Model Select Screen

With the programming head in position, select this button for automatic model selection.

For manual model selection, select proper button to display model options.

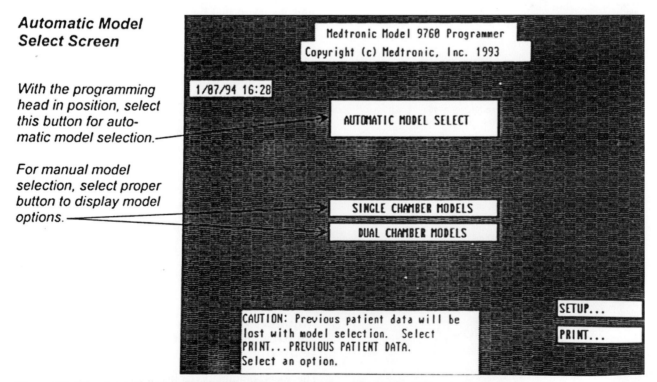

Figure 33–29.   Automatic model select feature available on Medtronics (Minneapolis, MN) programmer.

tial implantation values may be telemetered in certain pacer systems and be available for later recall and comparison. Other "administrative" data features that may also be included are patient demographics, nominal programmed values for certain models, and a screen indicating the full array of programmability inherent in a particular device (Fig. 33–30).

Real-time telemetry of *measured data* is available in most modern pacer systems, including an assessment of battery voltage, current, and impedance as well as lead impedance. These are useful measures in diagnosing or anticipating problems with the pacer system with regard to impending battery depletion or lead integrity.[36, 47, 48] Battery voltage progressively decreases over time, whereas battery impedance is inversely related to battery voltage (Fig. 33–31). Especially problematic in recent years has been the decline in impedance associated with certain bipolar polyurethane leads, particularly those inserted using the subclavian approach; a very low telemetered impedance may suggest a corresponding problem with lead insulation in these cases (Fig. 33–32). Conversely, a very high telemetered lead impedance may indicate conductor fracture or a loose setscrew connection, either one of which may be inapparent

radiographically (see Fig. 33–20). Multiple determinations of impedance should be made when evaluating suspected pacer malfunction because problems with lead impedance may be intermittent. Newly available in some devices is the ability to telemeter trends in lead impedance that have been automatically gathered by the pacemaker (Fig. 33–33).

Telemetry of event counters and histograms may be especially useful in evaluating the percentage of time that a patient spends in a particular rhythm or at a particular rate; this may lead to the conclusion that reprogramming may be necessary to optimize a pacer's clinical performance. Such events may be subdivided into *event histograms/event counts* (which evaluate the frequency of pacing since the last visit—in essence, an assessment of pacer dependence at the programmed settings, see Fig. 33–23); *sensor-indicated rate histograms* (demonstrating how often different rates would occur during rate-adaptive pacing at a particular activity-sensing threshold—allowing for reprogramming to more physiologic rate-responsiveness if required)[55]; and *event records* (allowing for precise determination of when a specific event occurred and at what rate, such as a tachycardia, a search hysteresis episode, or automatic mode switching episodes, Figs. 33–34 and 33–35). The specific pacer systems allowing for retrieval of these data in essence provide the function of a mini-Holter or event recorder (Fig. 33–36).

Real-time intracardiac electrograms are occasionally helpful. The size of the electrogram gives a rough clue to the lead sensing capabilities and may also demonstrate the strength of far-field signals. Intracardiac electrograms may also be used in evaluating retrograde VA conduction and measuring VA conduction intervals, evaluating lead integrity, assisting in rhythm identification (e.g., supraventricular tachycardias, atrial flutter, or AV dissociation in the setting of ventricular tachycardia; Fig. 33–37) and evaluating myopotential or other unusual sensing phenomena. Additional telemetry features include actual measurements of intrinsic signal amplitudes (Fig. 33–38).

From an operational standpoint, *marker channels* are actually more useful than intracardiac electrograms. These channels denote when a particular channel, either atrial or ventricular, is sensing activity or emitting paced output. In so doing, they provide evidence as to what the device is seeing, whether accurate or not, and how it is functioning and reacting, whether appropriately or not. This results in certain limitations; for example, the designation of a paced event on the marker channel does not indicate whether the chamber has actually been successfully depolarized. Marker channels can be very useful, however, in unraveling pacer behaviors and phenomena that may not otherwise be comprehensible to the physician, at least by surface ECG studies. This is particularly true when it delineates sensed events corresponding to extraneous signals (such as polarization voltage) or when signals that seemingly should be sensed are ignored (due to refractory periods; Fig. 33–39).

Adjuncts for Follow-up: Ambulatory Electrocardiographic Recording and Treadmill Testing

The incorporation of Holter monitor–like capabilities into some of the more current devices may preclude the need for

	12:02 Feb 28, 1995	
META		
DDDR		
1254		
META	8 mm 20 cc 48 g vs.1A Uni/Bi X-ray: TBM	
DDDR		
1254		
Lead Config	Sense: unipolar, bipolar Pace: unipolar, bipolar	
Mode	AOO, VOO, DOO, AAI, VVI, VDD, DDD, DDI, VVT, AAIR, VVIR, VDDR, DDDR, DDIR	
Standby Rate	30–50 by 5 ppm; 50–80 by 2.5 ppm	
Minimum Rate	80–165 by 5 ppm	
	50–120 by 5 ppm	
Maximum Rate	80–180 by 5 ppm	
V Max Rate	70–120 by 5 ppm; 120–180 by 10 ppm	
AMS Rate	Off; 150, 175, 200 bpm; for 5 or 11 beats	
Hysteresis	0, 100–500 by 20 ms	
RRF	(Rate response Factor) 1–45	
A–V Delay	0–300 by 20 ms; xDxR modes: Constant or Adaptive	
A Sensitivity	0.3, 0.5, 0.7, 1.0, 1.4, 2.0, 2.8, 4.0 mV	
V Sensitivity	1.0, 1.4, 2.0, 2.8, 4.0, 5.7, 8.0, 11.3 mV	
A Refractory	240–480 by 40 ms	
V Refractory	200–440 by 80 ms	
PVARP	160–600 by 40 ms	
PVARP Base	160–600 by 40 ms	
PEPVARP	OFF, 80, 160, 240, 320 ms, Next A Pace	
Pulse Ampl	2.5, 5.0, 7.5 V	
Pulse Width	0.125–1.000 by 0.125 ms	
Magnet Rates	BOL: > 85 ppm	ER I <=78 ppm
	EOL = 63 ppm	

Telectronics
9600 v4.5 OUE   Pacing Systems

Figure 33–30. Range of programmable features that can be interrogated from Telectronics programmer.

Patient:
Pacer : META   DDD 1230   #U1627876   Implant   23 Apr 91

14:29 Nov 4, 1997

Mode	DDD	
Lead	A Unipolar	V Bipolar
Rate		
Standby	70 ppm	
V Max Rate	120 ppm	
A-V Delay	180 ms	
Measure at	100 ppm	
Sense	**A**	**V**
Configuration	Unipolar	Bipolar
Sensitivity	0.7 mV	2.8 mV
Reset. Refract		280 ms
PVARP	280 ms	
PEPVARP	OFF	
Pace	**A**	**V**
Configuration	Unipolar	Bipolar
Amplitude	5.0 V	5.0 V
Width	0.500 ms	0.500 ms

Program Currrent   (#20, 31 May 96)

MEASUREMENTS

Longevity >		4 months
Cell Impedance		13000 Ω
Magnet Rate		78 ppm

Measured RRF

Counts		521 Day 21.2 Hr
PVC		>65534
	A	**V**
Noise		101
% Paced	73	103

Measured	**A**	**V**
Impedance	730 Ω	660 Ω
Amplitude	4.0 V	3.8 V
Threshold		

9600 v5.5 OUE

Telectronics ⋀
Pacing Systems

Figure 33–31. Elevated battery impedance on telemetry with associated decline in estimated pacer generator longevity.

ambulatory ECG evaluations of pacer function in the future. For the time being, however, such recordings may be particularly useful in disclosing problems with pacer malfunction potentially responsible for a patient's symptoms. Perhaps even more importantly, they may serve to identify potential problems with pacer function that are extant but currently unassociated with symptoms, such as myopotential sensing or atrial undersensing[56, 57] (Figs. 33–40 and 33–41). Assessment of rate adaptiveness with activity in either dual-chamber or rate-adaptive pacer systems may be aided by observation during ambulatory recordings as well as the degree of pacemaker dependence on a random 24-hour period.

Treadmill testing may also be useful in evaluating exercise tolerance in one pacing mode compared with another and as a function of programmed activity sensing thresholds in certain rate-adaptive pacing systems. This may be particularly important to the young patient wishing to be physically active as well as to the more elderly patient in whom an overly sensitive system may result in potentially harmful pacing rates. Upper rate behavior in dual-chamber systems may be better appreciated with exercise testing and may dictate the need for reprogramming, for example, to a higher upper rate limit. Rarely, exercise-provoked arrhythmias may be appreciated.

Elective Replacement Indicators

A pacemaker's end of life indicates gross malfunction or lack of function; this is to be distinguished from the elective

Text continued on page 924

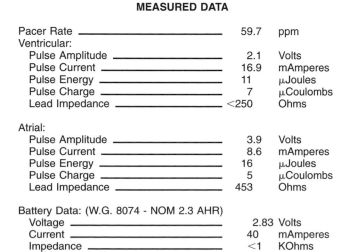

MEASURED DATA

Pacer Rate	59.7	ppm
Ventricular:		
Pulse Amplitude	2.1	Volts
Pulse Current	16.9	mAmperes
Pulse Energy	11	μJoules
Pulse Charge	7	μCoulombs
Lead Impedance	<250	Ohms
Atrial:		
Pulse Amplitude	3.9	Volts
Pulse Current	8.6	mAmperes
Pulse Energy	16	μJoules
Pulse Charge	5	μCoulombs
Lead Impedance	453	Ohms
Battery Data: (W.G. 8074 - NOM 2.3 AHR)		
Voltage	2.83	Volts
Current	40	mAmperes
Impedance	<1	KOhms

Figure 33–32. Interrogated low-lead impedance.

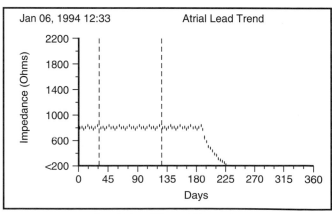

Lead Trend Report Example

The two dashed vertical lines indicate a temporary interruption in data collection caused by application of the programming head (or a magnet) over the pacemaker.

Figure 33–33. Decline in lead impedance demonstrated in a lead trend report from a problematic atrial lead.

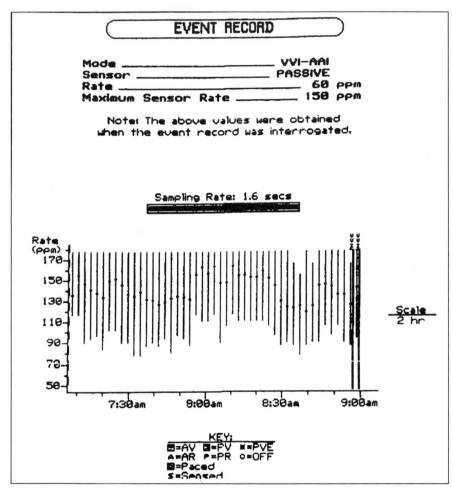

Figure 33-34. Event record demonstrating range in heart rate over time in a paced patient with rapid atrial fibrillation that was symptomatic. (Courtesy of Dr. Paul A. Levine.)

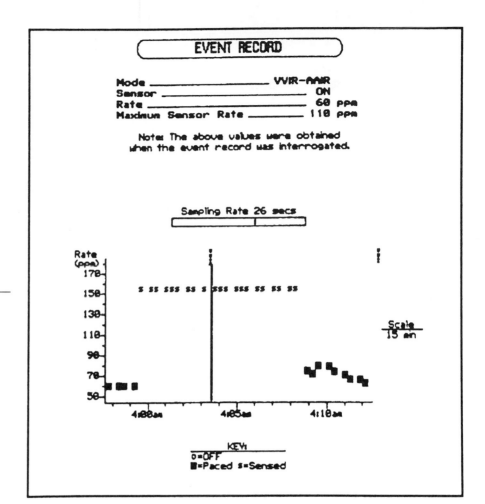

Figure 33–35. Event record demonstrating symptomatic paroxysmal supraventricular tachycardia in a paced patient. (Courtesy of Dr. Paul A. Levine.)

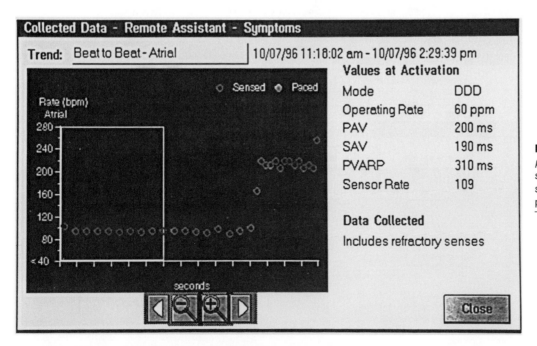

Figure 33–36. Newly available *patient-activated* transmission of symptoms demonstrating supraventricular tachycardia in a paced patient.

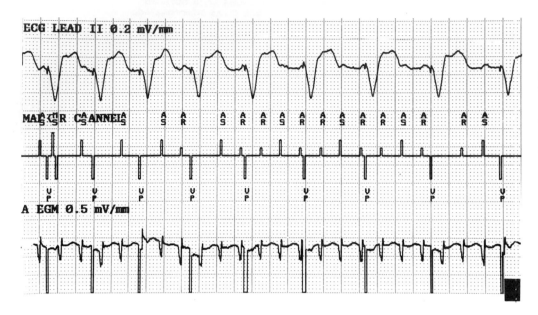

Thera DR 7960i/61i/62i   **10/21/97 12:00**
              CHART SPEED 25.0 mm/s

Figure 33–37. Paced patient with atrial flutter, with atrial intracardiac electrograms *(lowest panel)* and marker channels indicating sensed and refractory atrial events *(middle panel)*.

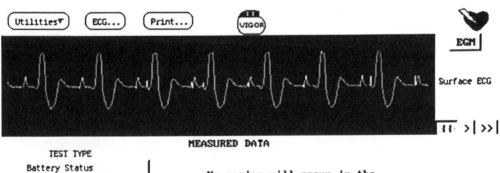

Figure 33–38. Measurement of intrinsic P- and R-wave signals from a CPI system. (Guidant, St. Paul, MN.)

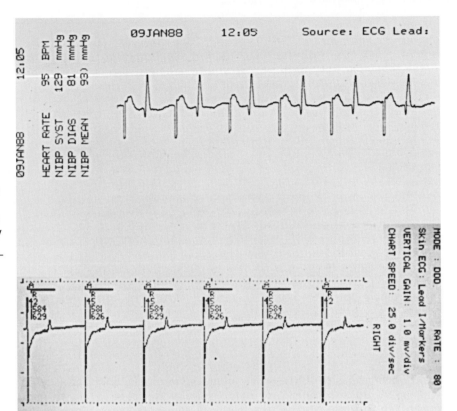

Figure 33–39. Patient programmed to atrioventricular paced rhythm with baseline rate of 80 bpm yet actually pacing at 95 bpm because of crosstalk inhibition, demonstrated by marker channels showing sensing of atrial spike polarization voltage by ventricular channel.

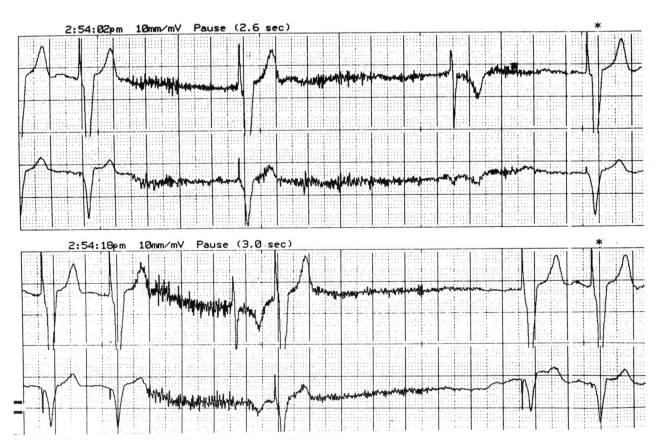

Figure 33–40. Myopotential inhibition demonstrated on Holter recording.

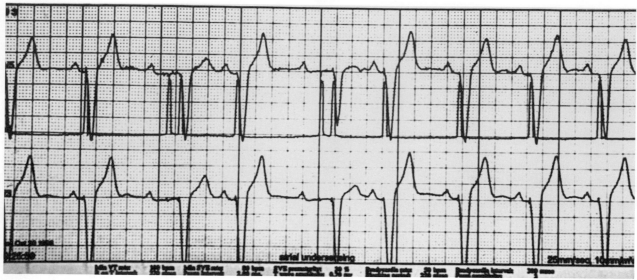

Figure 33–41. Atrial undersensing demonstrated on Holter recording (*middle panel* demonstrates atrial and ventricular spike artifacts, a feature available in certain Holter systems).

replacement indicator (ERI), which provides the physician with an advance "window" of time (typically weeks to months) in which to consider generator replacement before end of life is reached[58, 59] (Fig. 33–42). A variety of indicators have been used in different systems, including gradual or stepwise declines in free-running or magnet-pacing rates, rate drops to a preset value, pulse width stretching, and automatic changes in pacing modes (such as from DDD to VVI or from VVIR to VVI to allow for energy conservation as end of life draws near). These are device and manufacturer specific and may be found by consulting with the manufacturer or physician's manual (see Fig. 33–12). As already indicated, real-time telemetry of battery-measured data may be useful in guiding replacement in that progressive increases in battery impedance are observed.

The mechanism governing ERI may be latched or unlatched.[58] If the battery voltage falls below a minimum trip-point voltage responsible for triggering ERI, a decline in the free-running or magnet rate will be observed. If the mechanism governing this is latched, the newer slower rate is permanent even if the fall in available battery voltage is momentary. In unlatched systems, on the other hand, the

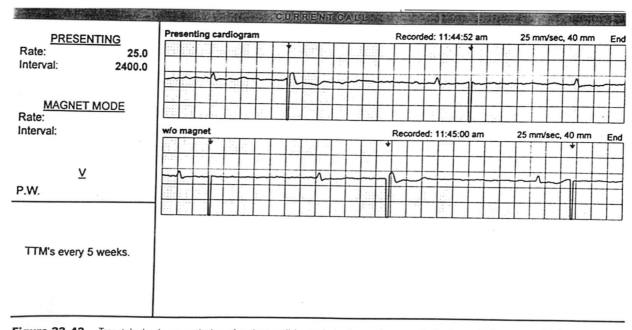

Figure 33–42. Transtelephonic transmission of patient well beyond elective replacement indicators with instances of failure to sense documented.

generator may actually return to the original faster rate if the current drain on the battery diminishes and available battery voltage, even for the moment, increases. Thus, sudden changes in pacing rate may be observed in unlatched systems as a function of changes in available voltage and may be misinterpreted as a pacer malfunction. In addition to appreciating the various types of ERIs, a knowledge of latching versus unlatching behavior, as well as of resetting phenomena, is essential in guiding the physician regarding the need for, and timing of, generator replacement.

Pacer Lead and Generator Advisories and Intracardiac Device Recalls

Advisories, alerts, technical notices, and recalls are inescapable aspects of pacemaker follow-up. The U.S. General Accounting Office issued a report in 1989 citing 1635 medical device recalls between 1983 and 1988, of which intracardiac devices accounted for 226 (14%).[60] Because of manufacturer laxness in reporting such problems and the lack to date of a national device/lead database as originally proposed by the North American Society of Pacing and Electrophysiology (NASPE),[61] it is increasingly incumbent on the pacer physician to keep his own databases, to track pacer system performance, and to be vigilant about potential systematic problems or trends in said performance. If the physician, for example, detects premature and otherwise unsuspected lead failure in a subgroup of paced patients with a given device model, it behooves the physician to scrutinize the systems of other patients with the same model more closely and to consult the appropriate manufacturer.

The responsibilities of the physician in device recalls, as recently codified by a NASPE consensus conference,[62] include confirming all unimplanted versus implanted devices; identifying all followed patients and individual clinical risks (e.g., age, duration of implantation, and sex, as in a recent advisory for patients with potential fracture of the Accufix inner retention wire); notifying centers or physicians to whom patient care may have been transferred; notifying the patient or designate with full disclosure by registered mail and telephone contact; conveying to the patient the problem, natural history, risks of intervention and nonintervention, and plans for investigation and management; ensuring the patient's commitment to clinic appointments and continued follow-up; and providing feedback to recall task forces and manufacturer. In patients who are pacer dependent, as previously defined, closer or more frequent follow-up may be important either in the clinic or transtelephonically. The threshold for (invasively) intervening and revising a potentially affected system is clearly lower in the pacer-dependent patient. Whether and when to intervene must be decided with cognizance of the risks of intervention and considering the statistical likelihood of a *potential* future problem (if not actually thus far identified).

Special Considerations

Electrocautery and cardioversion-defibrillation may adversely affect the function of a pacing system, both temporarily and permanently.[63–66] Resetting of the generator to a backup or noise reversion mode may be observed.[64, 67] The reset mode is device specific and is a feature that the pacer physician must be cognizant of; typically, reprogramming of the generator is sufficient to re-establish normal function, but the unwary physician may misconstrue the situation as a permanent malfunction and unnecessarily commit the patient to a corrective (invasive) intervention. Preoperative and postoperative tracings with and without magnet are essential, lest the physician presume, incorrectly, that the preoperatively programmed settings still apply (Fig. 33–43).

Transient undersensing and changes in pacing threshold, both acute and chronic, may be observed with cautery and defibrillation.[63, 65, 66] (Fig. 33–44). These effects may be due to direct damage to the generator but may also reflect transmission of current down the pacer conductors, resulting in a burn at the local tissue–electrode interface. Transient oversensing, as previously discussed, may also be observed with intraoperative electrocautery. To minimize this phenomenon, cautery should be used sparingly, with the ground plate placed as close as possible to the operating site and remotely from the pacer system, with short bursts at the lower energy possible; *bipolar* cautery is less likely to produce problems. In the pacer-dependent patient, preoperative reprogramming transiently to the asynchronous or triggered modes may be considered to minimize oversensing; if the relevant programmer is not available, continuous magnet application over the generator will ensure asynchronous pacing. Temporary transvenous pacing, although invasive, would offer a suitable alternative if neither programmers nor magnets were available. To minimize damage to the system from cardioversion-defibrillation, anteroposterior application of direct current energy is preferred over two frontal paddles, and the least

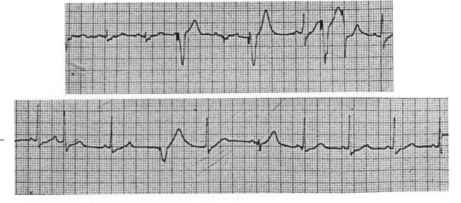

Figure 33–43. Preoperative *(upper panel)* and postoperative *(lower panel)* tracings of patient undergoing coronary artery bypass grafting whose generator was reset by cautery from VVI pacing at 50 bpm to VVI at 76 bpm, the reset mode for this Intermedics (Intermedics, Angleton, TX) device.

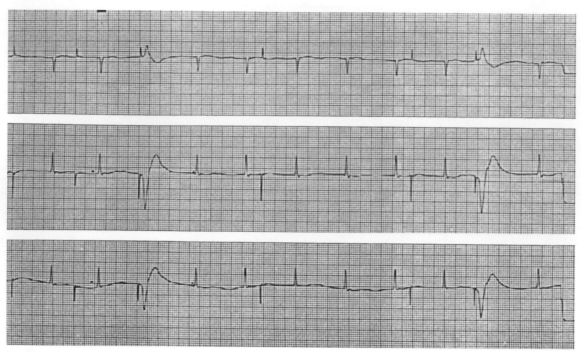

Figure 33–44. Transient ventricular undersensing in paced patient immediately after direct current cardioversion.

amount of energy feasible should be applied; equipment for temporary pacing in the pacer-dependent patient should be nearby.

Radiofrequency current has also been used increasingly in the approach to therapeutic ablation for cardiac arrhythmias. Observed phenomena during such procedures in the paced patient may include pacer inhibition (even when the device has been reprogrammed to the asynchronous mode), device resetting, undersensing, asynchronous pacing, and induction of rapid pacing.[68, 69] In one multicenter trial, no significant changes in pacing nor sensing thresholds were observed, and impedances were unaffected.[69] Again, the ground plate should be placed remotely, a minimum of energy should be applied, and backup temporary pacing should be considered. Reassessment of the pacer system after the procedure is essential.

Ionizing radiation applied to the chest, as in radiation therapy for lung or breast cancer, should be undertaken with appropriate shielding of the generator. In some patients (Fig. 33–45), it may be necessary to reposition the generator if it lies in the radiation field. Damage to the generator is random, unpredictable, and cumulative and may result in sudden loss of output, reprogramming of the device, or pacemaker "runaway" rates.[70–74] Transcutaneous electrical nerve stimulation (TENS) does not apparently interfere with normal pacer function.[75]

Although not typically encountered in the medical environment, cellular telephones constitute a potential source of electromagnetic interference for paced patients. This subject has recently been analyzed in a multicenter study of 980 patients with pacers and five types of telephones.[76] The incidence of any type of EMI was 20% in 5533 tests, with an incidence of symptoms in 7.2%. Interference was more frequent in dual-chamber systems but did not appear to pose

a health risk when placed over the ear contralateral to the pulse generator.

Magnetic resonance imaging (MRI) is an increasingly applied modality; it is generally to be avoided in the paced patient because the associated development of magnetic fields may result in actual physical movement of the internal components of the generator, especially the reed switch.[77–80] Despite this concern, no apparent component damage has been reported in a number of pacer systems tested.[81] The application of MRI will cause most devices to pace asyn-

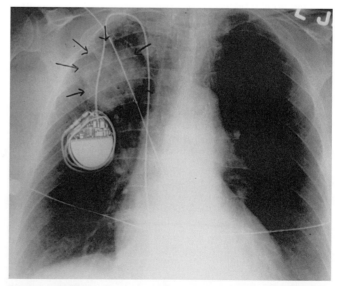

Figure 33–45. Lung cancer patient with pacer generator situated near proposed irradiation site.

chronously[82]; in some patients, radiofrequency pulsing may induce voltage across the pacemaker electrodes and stimulate myocardial tissue at rapid rates approaching the MRI pulsing rate, that is, up to 300 bpm.[79] As with cautery and defibrillation, resetting of generators may be observed.[80] In the rare case in which MRI is unavoidable, certain precautions must be considered. These would include in vitro tests of the generator, which may predict device behavior in vivo; programming the device to "magnet off" if available; and reprogramming of the device to asynchronous mode, especially in the pacer-dependent patient.

Lithotripsy may result in undue inhibition of pacer output or irregular sensing, particularly in the case of rate-adaptive devices employing piezoelectrode crystals.[83, 84] These crystals may oversense extracorporeal shock waves and result in rapid pacing rates; alternatively, they may be susceptible to being shattered by the shock waves. Recommendations for such devices would therefore include avoidance of lithotripsy in patients with abdominal generator implants; reprogramming of generators situated in the chest to inactivate the rate-adaptive mode temporarily; reprogramming of dual-chamber devices to the VVI mode (to avoid triggering of the shock-wave output by the atrial output pulse, which may delay delivery of the shock wave and result in oversensing and inhibition of output on the ventricular channel); distancing of the pacer from the focal point of the lithotripsy and synchronization of the lithotriptor to the QRS or ventricular pacing spike to minimize inhibition or triggering by the discharge spark, which may otherwise occur at other times in the pacer timing cycle (i.e., outside the refractory period of the ventricular channel); continued cardiac monitoring throughout the procedure with backup temporary pacing capabilities available; and re-evaluation of the pacer system subsequent to the lithotripsy procedure.

The physician may be asked to evaluate a paced patient preoperatively. It is important to be familiar with the indications for the pacer and to establish the details of the history and physical examination as outlined previously. A knowledge of the pacemaker model and programmed settings is essential; a chest radiograph may be very helpful. Baseline ECG studies with and without magnet should be analyzed and the patient's underlying rhythm and degree of pacer dependence evaluated. If the patient has no underlying rhythm, then reprogramming to asynchronous or triggered modes may be important, or the application of a magnet over the generator may be made, as indicated previously. Cautery should be minimized and postoperative ECG recordings should be undertaken to ascertain whether device resetting may have occurred and to otherwise confirm appropriate pacer functioning. Occasionally, in the patient with coronary disease, reprogramming may be warranted to examine the native unpaced ECG recording to rule out the interval development of perioperative infarction.

The patient with a pacer may return with new or recurrent episodes of presyncope or syncope. This may reflect pacer malfunction and requires careful assessment of the pacer system as addressed previously, namely an assessment of thresholds and potential inhibition by extraneous signals, such as myopotentials or electromagnetic interference. Pacemaker-*induced* symptoms of presyncope may also arise: PMT should be evaluated for, and not uncommonly, an unappreciated pacemaker syndrome may be extant. Evaluation should include an assessment of VA conduction, hemodynamics during ventricular pacing, and the possibility of PMT, as previously outlined. Reprogramming to reduce pacer dependence, such as to a lower demand rate, may be required, but ultimately an upgrade from single-chamber to dual-chamber pacing may be required. Syncope may clearly be multifactorial and may have nothing to do with the pacer system at all—other arrhythmias may be contributory and other phenomena, such as vasodepressor syncope, may coexist, requiring additional testing, such as Holter monitoring, electrophysiologic study, or tilt-table testing.

Automaticity and the Future of Pacemaker Follow-Up

Automaticity refers to those automatic functions provided by pacemaker systems to modulate function without clinician input. The concept is not new. Indeed, pulse width stretching was one of the first automatic mechanisms incorporated into pacer systems in an effort to maintain constant energy as a battery depleted to maintain an adequate safety margin for pacing. An extension of this concept was mode switching at end of life, particularly important with the advent of dual-chamber pacing, wherein current drains became considerably higher and could be lessened by converting to single-chamber modes automatically near elective replacement time. Reversion to asynchronous pacing upon encountering myopotentials and reversion to reset mode when encountering severe external interference (e.g., electrocautery, as discussed previously) are further historical examples of automaticity. In fact, the very concept of "demand" pacing may be considered an automatic function. More recent examples of automaticity, some discussed previously, have included algorithms for rate-adaptive pacing, rate-adaptive AV intervals, PMT interventions, prevention of atrial competitive pacing, automatic mode switch from dual-chamber to single-chamber pacing when atrial fibrillation is detected, and polarity switch from bipolar to unipolar when a decline in lead impedance is detected (suggesting failure of the bipolar insulation). Automatic determination of both sensing and pacing thresholds is also newly available, coupled with the ability to reduce output so as to maintain pacing safely and yet promote device longevity. To be anticipated is the ability of a pacing system to gather increasing diagnostic information about the patient and pacer system, recognize problems and directly correct them, report such changes to the physician as appropriate, and indicate when the physician must take corrective action.

Simultaneous with enhancements of pacer system automaticity are ongoing advances in programmer technology and automaticity. Already appearing are many elements of the "ideal" programmer: user-friendliness, probability, safety, efficiency. Backward compatibility of programmers with older pulse generator models no longer available and universality of programmers (i.e., manufacturer independent) remain goals for the future. As the number of functions and programmable parameters of pacemakers expands, programmers will be asked to provide programming instructions to the pulse generator, gather and transmit data, analyze the data received from the pulse generator to provide useful information, and transmit this information to other computers for storage in a database. The programmers themselves must be capable of interpreting anomalies in the stored data, such as the implications of increasing or decreasing lead impedance, battery impedance, and the interaction between AV delay and intrinsic AV conduction in any patient. Programmers identify this information to the pacer physician when certain parameter combinations are not feasible ("parameter warnings"). There is ongoing interest in the ability of programmers to update therapies automatically: whenever pacers are programmed, the programmer will update the pacemaker to the latest software and track performance of the pacing system.

As previously stated, the precise timing for optimal pacer follow-up scheduling remains controversial. It is also unclear which of the many specific aspects of follow-up discussed in this chapter should be assessed at each visit. The development of automaticity may free the clinician from "routine" follow-up examinations (avoiding the problem of missed patient appointments) and may potentially correct pacer problems independent of human input or human error (e.g., due to untrained health care providers). It may, however, promote excessive reliance on a technology that to date is not fully proven when compared with the gold standard of direct physician–patient contact. As such, the development of automatic features should be viewed as an exciting and welcome component or enhancement of pacer follow-up, but we must always acknowledge the primacy of the pacer physician's role in the follow-up process.[1, 2]

REFERENCES

1. Schoenfeld MH: Quality assurance in cardiac electrophysiology and pacing: A brief synopsis. PACE 17:267–269, 1994.
2. Schoenfeld MH: Manpower concerns in cardiac electrophysiology and pacing. PACE 18:1977–1979, 1995.
3. Griffin JC, Schuenemeyer TD, Hess KR, et al: Pacemaker follow-up: Its role in the detection and correction of pacemaker system malfunction. PACE 9:387–391, 1986.
4. Schoenfeld MH: Follow-up of the pacemaker patient. In Ellenbogen KA (ed): Cardiac Pacing, 2nd ed. Cambridge, Blackwell Scientific, 1996, pp 456–500.
5. Griffin JC, Schuenenemyer TD: Pacemaker follow-up: An introduction and overview. Clin Prog Pacing Electrophysiol 1:30, 1983.
6. Furman S: Pacemaker follow-up. In Furman S, Hayes DL, Holmes DR (eds): A Practice of Cardiac Pacing, 3rd ed. Mount Kisco, NY, Futura, 1993, pp. 571–603.
7. Levine PA: Proceedings of the policy conference of the North American Society of Pacing and Electrophysiology on programmability and pacemaker follow-up programs. Clin Prog Pacing Electrophysiol 2:145–191, 1984.
8. Hayes DL, Naccarelli GV, Furman S, et al: Report of the NASPE Policy Conference training requirements for permanent pacemaker selection, implantation, and follow-up. PACE 17:6–12, 1994.
9. Strathmore NF, Mond HG: Noninvasive monitoring and testing of pacemaker function. PACE 10:1359–1370, 1987.
10. Zinberg A: Transtelephonic follow-up. Clin Prog Pacing Electrophysiol 2:177, 1984.
11. Dreifus L, Pennock R, Feldman M: Experience with 3835 pacemakers utilizing transtelephonic surveillance. Am J Cardiol 35:133, 1975.
12. Platt S, Furman S, Gross JN, et al: Transtelephone monitoring for pacemaker follow-up 1981–1994. PACE 19:2089–2098, 1996.
13. Medicare Cardiac pacemaker evaluation services. Effective Oct 1, 1984, Coverage Issues Manual HCFA Publication No.6, section 50–1.
14. Vallario L, Leman R, Gillette P, Kratz J: Pacemaker follow-up and adequacy of medical guidelines. Am Heart J 116:11, 1988.
15. Hayes DL, Hyberger LK, Lloyd MA: Should the Medicare transtelephonic pacemaker follow-up schedule be altered? PACE 20:1153, 1997.
16. MacGregor CD, Covvey HD, Noble EJ, et al: Computer-assisted reporting system for the follow-up of patients with cardiac pacemakers PACE 3:568–588, 1980.
17. Iskos D, Lurie KG, Sakaguchi S, Benditt DG: Termination of implantable pacemaker therapy: Experience in five patients. Ann Intern Med 126:787–790, 1997.
18. Byrd CL, Schwartz SJ, Gonzalez M, et al: Pacemaker clinic evaluations: Key to early identification of surgical problems. PACE 9:1259–1264, 1986.
19. Schoenfeld MH: Adaptive-rate patient management: When should the sensor be activated? CPI Pacing Dynamics 1994, First quarter, pp. 6–7.
20. Hoffman A, Jost M, Pfisterer M, et al: Persisting symptoms despite permanent pacing Incidence, causes, and follow-up. Chest 85:207–210, 1984.
21. Ausubel K, Furman S: The pacemaker syndrome. Ann Intern Med 103:420–429, 1985.
22. Kenny RS, Sutton R: Pacemaker syndrome. Br Med J 293:902–903, 1986.
23. Ellenbogen KA, Thames MD, Mohanty PK: New insights into pacemaker syndrome gained from hemodynamic, humoral and vascular responses during ventriculoatrial pacing. Am J Cardiol 65:53–59, 1990.
24. Cohen SI, Frank HA: Preservation of active atrial transport: An important clinical consideration in cardiac pacing. Chest 81:51, 1982.
25. Bayliss CE, Beanlands DA, Baird RJ: The pacemaker-twiddler's syndrome: A new complication of implantable transvenous pacemakers. Can Med Assoc J 99:371, 1968.
26. Misra KP, Korn M, Ghahramani AR, et al: Auscultatory findings in patients with cardiac pacemakers. Ann Intern Med 74:245, 1971.
27. Cheng TO, Ertem G, Vera A: Heart sounds in patients with cardiac pacemakers Chest 62:66, 1972.
28. Mazzetti H, Dussaut A, Tentori C, et al: Superior vena cava occlusion and/or syndrome related to pacemaker leads. Am Heart J 125:831, 1993.
29. Steiner RM, Morse D: The radiology of cardiac pacemakers. JAMA 240:2574–2576, 1978.
30. Grier D, Cook PG, Hartnell GG: Chest radiographs after permanent pacing: Are they really necessary? Clin Radiol 42:224, 1990.
31. Mugica J, Henry L, Rollet M, et al: The clinical utility of pacemaker follow-up visits. PACE 9:1249–1251, 1986.
32. Barold SS, Falkoff MD, Ong LS, Heinle RA: Normal and abnormal patterns of ventricular depolarization during cardiac pacing. In Barold SS (ed): Modern Cardiac Pacing. Mount Kisco, NY, Futura, 1985, pp 545–569.
33. Barold SS, Falkoff MD, Ong LS, Heinle RA: The abnormal pacemaker stimulus. In Barold SS (ed): Modern Cardiac Pacing. Mount Kisco, NY, Futura, 1985, pp 571–586.
34. Van Gelder LM, El Gamal MIH: Magnet application, a cause of persistent arrhythmias in physiological pacemakers: Report of 2 cases. PACE 5:710, 1982.
35. Harthorne JW: Programmable pacemakers: Technical features and clinical applications. In Dreifus L (ed): Pacemaker Therapy, Philadelphia, WB Saunders, 1983, pp 135–147.
36. Sholder J, Levine PA, Mann BM, et al: Bidirectional telemetry and interrogation. In Barold SS, Mugica J (eds): Cardiac Pacing: The Third Decade of Cardiac Pacing. Mount Kisco, NY, Futura, 1982, pp 145–166.
37. Schoenfeld MH: A primer on pacemaker programmers. PACE 16:2044–2052, 1993.
38. Gordon PL, Calfee RV, Baker RG Jr: Multiprogrammable pacemaker technology: A tutorial review and prediction. In Barold SS, Mugica J (eds): The Third Decade of Cardiac Pacing. Mount Kisco, NY, Futura, 1982, pp 127–143.
39. Hardage ML, Barold SS: Pacemaker programming techniques. In Barold SS, Mugica J (eds): The Third Decade of Cardiac Pacing. Mount Kisco, NY, Futura, 1982, pp 1–26.
40. Gold RD, Saulson SH, Macgregor DC: Programmable pacing systems: The medium and the message. PACE 5:776, 1982.
41. Mond H: Programmability. In Mond H (ed): The Cardiac Pacemaker: Function and Malfunction. New York, Grune & Stratton, 1983, pp 169–187.
42. Sinnaeve A, Piret J, Stroobandt R: Potential causes of spurious programming: Report of a case. PACE 3:541, 1980.
43. Fieldman A, Dobrow R: Phantom pacemaker programming. PACE 1:166, 1978.
44. Cameron J, Chisholm A, Froggatt G, et al: Phantom programming. In Meere C (ed): Cardiac Pacing Proceedings of the VI World Symposium on Cardiac Pacing. Montreal, Pacesymp, 1979.
45. Furman S: Spurious pacemaker programming. PACE 3:517, 1980.

46. Sweesy MW, Batey RL, Forney RC: Activation times for "emergency back-up" programs. PACE 13:1224, 1990.

47. Levine PA, Sholder J, Duncan JL: Clinical benefits of telemetered electrocardiograms in assessment of DDD function. PACE 7:1170, 1984.

48. Sanders R, Martin R, Fruman H, et al: Data storage and retrieval by implantable pacemakers for diagnostic purposes. PACE 7:1228, 1984.

49. Duffin EG Jr: The marker channel: A telemetric diagnostic aid. PACE 7:1165, 1984.

50. Levine PA, Vendetti FJ, Podrid PJ, et al: Telemetry of programmed and measured data, electrograms, event markers, and event counters: Luxury or necessity? *In* Barold SS, Mugica J (eds): New Perspectives in Cardiac Pacing. Mount Kisco, NY, Futura, 1988, pp 187–201.

51. Petersen MEV, Chamberlain-Webber R, Fitzpatrick AP, et al: Permanent pacing for cardioinhibitory malignant vasovagal syndrome. Br Heart J 71:274–281, 1994.

52. Lau CP, Tai YT, Fong PC, et al: Atrial arrhythmia management with sensor controlled atrial refractory period and automatic mode switching in patients with minute ventilation sensing dual chamber rate adaptive pacemakers. PACE 15:1504–1514, 1992.

53. Batey FL, Calabria DA, Sweesy MW, et al: Crosstalk and blanking periods in a dual chamber pacemaker Clin Prog Pacing Electrophysiol 3:314–318, 1985.

54. Klementowicz P, Ausubel K, Furman S: The dynamic nature of ventriculoatrial conduction. PACE 9:1050–1054, 1986.

55. Hayes DL, Higano ST, Eisinger G: Utility of rate histograms in programming and follow-up of a DDDR pacemaker. Mayo Clin Proc 64:495, 1989.

56. Famularo MA, Kennedy HL: Ambulatory electrocardiography in the assessment of pacemaker function Am Heart J 104:1086–1094, 1982.

57. Gaita F, Asteggiano R, Bocchiardo M, et al: Holter monitoring and provocative maneuvers in the assessment of unipolar demand pacemaker myopotential inhibition. Am Heart J 107:925, 1984.

58. Barold SS, Schoenfeld MH: Pacemaker elective replacement indicators: Latched or unlatched? PACE 12:990–995, 1989.

59. Barold SS, Schoenfeld MH, Falkoff MD, et al: Elective replacement indicators of simple and complex pacemakers *In* Barold SS, Mugica J (eds): New Perspectives in Cardiac Pacing, 2nd ed. Mount Kisco, NY, Futura, 1991, pp 493–526.

60. General Accounting Office, Report to the Chairman, Subcommittee on Health and the Environment, Committee on Energy and Commerce, US House of Representatives. "Medical Device Recalls," August, 1989.

61. Schoenfeld MH: Recommendations for implementation of a North American multicenter arrhythmia device/lead database. PACE 15:1633–1635, 1992.

62. Goldman BS, Newman D, Fraser J, Irwin M, et al: Management of intracardiac device recalls: A consensus conference. PACE 19:7–17, 1996.

63. Furman S: External defibrillation in implanted cardiac pacemakers. PACE 4:485, 1981.

64. Barold SS, Ong LS, Scovil J, et al: Reprograming of implanted pacemaker following external defibrillation. PACE 1:514, 1978.

65. Levine PA, Barold SS, Fletcher RD, et al: Adverse acute and chronic effects of electrical defibrillation and cardioversion on implanted unipolar cardiac pacing system. J Am Coll Cardiol 1:1413, 1983.

66. Yee R, Jones DL, Klein GJ: Pacing threshold changes after transvenous catheter shock. Am J Cardiol 53:503, 1984.

67. Lamas GA, Antman EM, Gold JP: Pacemaker backup mode reversion and injury during cardiac surgery. Ann Thorac Surg 41:155, 1986.

68. Chin MC, Rosenqvist M, Lee MA, et al: The effect of radiofrequency catheter ablation on permanent pacemakers: An experimental study. PACE 1990:13:23.

69. Ellenbogen KA, Wood MA, Stambler BS, et al: Acute effects of radiofrequency ablation of atrial arrhythmias on implanted permanent pacing systems. PACE 19:1287–1295, 1996.

70. Adamac R, Haefliger JM, Killisch JP, et al: Damaging effect of therapeutic radiation on programmable pacemakers. PACE 5:146, 1982.

71. Calfee RF: Therapeutic radiation in pacemakers. PACE 5:160, 1982.

72. Lee RW, Huang SK, Mechling E, et al: Runaway atrial sequential pacemaker after radiation therapy. Am J Med 81:833, 1986.

73. Shehata WM, Daoud GL, Meyer RL: Radiotherapy for patients with cardiac pacemakers: Possible risks. PACE 9:919, 1986.

74. Venselaar JLM, VanKerkoerle HLMJ, Vet AJTM: Radiation damage to pacemakers from radiotherapy. PACE 10:538, 1987.

75. Rasmussen MJ, Hayes DL, Vlestra RE, et al: Can transcutaneous electrical nerve stimulation be safely used in patients with permanent cardiac pacemakers? Mayo Clin Proc 63:433, 1988.

76. Hayes DL, Wang PJ, Reynolds DW, et al: Interference with cardiac pacemakers by cellular telephones. N Engl J Med 336:1473–1479, 1997.

77. Fetter J, Aram G, Homes DR Jr, et al: The effects of nuclear magnetic resonance imagers on external and implantable pulse generators. PACE 7:720, 1984.

78. Holmes DR, Hayes DL, Gray J, et al: The effects of magnetic resonance imaging on implantable pulse generators. PACE 9:360–370, 1986.

79. Hayes DL, Holmes DR Jr, Gray JE: Effect of 1.5 Tesla nuclear magnetic resonance imaging scanner on implanted permanent pacemakers. J Am Coll Cardiol 10:782, 1987.

80. Erlebacher JA, Cahill PT, Pannizzo F, Knowles JR: Effect of magnetic resonance imaging on DDD Pacemakers. Am J Cardiol 57:437, 1986.

81. Iberer F, Justich E, Stenzl W, et al: Behavior of the Activitrax pacemaker during nuclear magnetic resonance investigation. First International Symposium on Rate-Responsive Pacing, Munich. PACE 10:1215, 1987.

82. Iberer F, Justich E, Tscheliessnigg KH, Wasler A: Nuclear magnetic resonance imaging in pacemaker patients. *In* Atlee JL, Gombotz H, Tschelissnigg KH (eds): Perioperative Management of Pacemaker Patients. Berlin, Springer-Verlag, 1992, pp 86–90.

83. Cooper D, Wilkoff B, Masterson M, et al: Effects of extracorporeal shock-wave lithotripsy on cardiac pacemakers and its safety in patients with implanted cardiac pacemakers. PACE 11:1607–1616, 1988.

84. Langberg J, Arber J, Thuroff JW, Griffin JC: The effects of extracorporeal shock-wave lithotripsy on pacemaker function. PACE 10:1142, 1987.

Chapter 34

Follow-Up of the Patient With a Defibrillator

George H. Crossley, III

When following patients with defibrillators, it is important to concentrate not only on the technologic features of the device and the arrhythmia history but also on the cardiac status and the general health status of the patient. This is even more important in patients with defibrillators than it is in patients with pacemakers because the former virtually always have concomitant cardiac problems, such as congestive heart failure, and often have other medical problems as well.

It is common for the physician following the patient's defibrillator and arrhythmia status to be someone other than the patient's general cardiologist, and it is virtually always the case that these physicians do not provide the patient's primary care. It is, therefore, important for the patient's well-being and peace of mind that clear roles be established for these physicians, ensuring that the patient's medical problems are being addressed as well as the status of the defibrillator. The goals of defibrillator follow-up are listed in Table 34–1.

■ IMMEDIATE POSTIMPLANTATION FOLLOW-UP

In the early follow-up period, attention is focused on the surgical aspects of the defibrillator. Although there are little published data to guide us, our standard practice is to have the patient keep the wound completely dry for 10 days to avoid washing bacteria into the wound. Likewise, we have the patient refrain from reaching above the horizon or reaching back with the affected arm for 10 days. This is to avoid excessive force on the lead. We typically see the patient in the clinic 1 to 2 weeks after implantation to assess the wound. Pulse generator interrogation is usually not done on this visit unless there have been symptoms suggesting arrhythmias. A reasonable amount of time needs to be devoted to this visit for education and patient reassurance.

The other aspects of surgical follow-up depend on the nature of the surgery. If the implantation is abdominal, careful attention must be paid not only to the abdominal pocket but also to the subcutaneous lead tract. These patients (especially men) require education about modification of clothing to avoid tenderness and excessive pressure on the pocket. Men appear to be more comfortable wearing either stretch-waist pants or suspenders, thereby avoiding belts.

Most patients now have their defibrillators implanted in the pectoral region with the pulse generator being placed either submuscularly or subcutaneously. For submuscular implantations, it is important to pay careful attention to the wound because a relatively large hematoma can be hidden. Attention should also be given to the position of the pulse generator. If there are signs of significant movement, the patient should be warned not to "twiddle" the pulse generator.[1] If the implantation was performed by means of thoracotomy, then the usual post-thoracotomy routine is employed.

■ LONG-TERM FOLLOW-UP SCHEDULE

Follow-up of defibrillator patients can be divided into three distinct periods. In the *surgical period*, the follow-up is driven by concerns about the wound, as noted previously. Once the wound is healed, the schedule of the *follow-up period* of a patient with a defibrillator is often driven by other medical concerns, such as the treatment of congestive heart failure. In the past, the follow-up of the pulse generator was linked to the need for manual capacitor reformation and usually occurred at least quarterly and in some cases every 2 months.[2] There remain a few of these implanted devices. Now that most pulse generators perform automatic capacitor reformation, the follow-up is often dependent on patient factors. Although most physician manuals continue to recommend quarterly visits,[3–5] it is our practice to see defibrillator patients, who have other cardiologists, every 6 months

Table 34–1. Goals of Defibrillator Patient Follow-up

Identification and recording of the nature and frequency of the arrhythmias
Identification and recording of device activity
Assessment of pacing and sensing functions
Assessment of the battery status
Enhancement of pulse generator longevity
Optimization of therapeutic parameters based on the device history
Optimization of ancillary parameters, such as diagnostic enhancements
Assessment of general cardiac status

and to increase the frequency of that schedule for patients who need medical care more often and for patients with an active arrhythmia history. One example would be a patient with frequent pacing termination of ventricular tachycardia. As the battery begins to show wear, the patient enters a *late follow-up period*, during which the follow-up schedule is driven by concerns about the battery status. During this period, the follow-up schedule is typically accelerated to a quarterly, bimonthly, and then monthly schedule as the battery approaches its designated elective replacement indicator. Specific recommendations are available from each manufacturer.

■ MAXIMIZING PULSE GENERATOR LONGEVITY

The longevity of a defibrillator pulse generator is dependent on the capacity and efficiency of the power source or sources, the frequency and energy of shocks, the static current drain, the amount of pacing, the efficiency of pacing, and the impact of various ancillary functions, such as electrogram recording. We now know that the longevity of many defibrillators varies considerably[6] and is markedly affected by bradycardia pacing and by some schemes of electrogram recording.[5] The impact of pacing is likely to be amplified as ICDs capable of dual-chamber pacing are implemented. It will become important for physicians to recognize these longevity costs.[7]

■ INTERVAL HISTORY

As with virtually all other areas of internal medicine, the history is the most important part of the evaluation of a patient with a defibrillator.

Symptoms With Shocks

In sorting out whether a shock was appropriate or not, it is important to know about the symptoms before the shock. Patients with ventricular tachycardia may or may not report palpitations before therapy. Although patients with rapid ventricular tachycardia or ventricular fibrillation often have altered sensorium or dizziness before the shock, this is unfortunately far from universal. It is not unusual in patients with ventricular fibrillation to have the shock as their only symptom.

The physician must consider several factors in analyzing symptoms. First, it is important to evaluate patient factors,

such as symptoms with prior known episodes and patient posture and activities at the time of the shock. Second, it is crucial to know how the defibrillator was programmed. Many current generation defibrillators can be programmed to delay the time between the onset of ventricular tachycardia and the initiation of therapy, either by increasing the number of intervals required for detection[5] or by programming a delay between detection and the onset of therapy.[8] In this situation, a patient may have prolonged symptoms before therapy even though the device performed as programmed. In a patient who is programmed in a more traditional manner, however, prolonged symptoms may be an indicator of problems with arrhythmia recognition, such as undersensing or inappropriate detection rates for ventricular tachycardia and ventricular fibrillation. Finally, it is important to know the charge time of a given defibrillator. In some pulse generators, the charge time lengthens considerably when the battery voltage is nearing the elective replacement indicator.

Congestive Heart Failure Symptoms

It is now clear that the most important determinant of the long-term outlook of defibrillator patients is the status of their congestive heart failure. Careful attention must be paid to the traditional symptoms of left-sided congestive heart failure, such as dyspnea and exercise intolerance. It is also crucial to realize that in many patients with severe left ventricular dysfunction, the symptoms of right-sided failure (peripheral edema, hepatic or generalized abdominal distention) may predominate. Likewise, the vegetative symptoms associated with low cardiac output may predominate. These symptoms, which suggest a poor prognosis, are often confused with depression.

The traditional therapies of heart failure, such as diuretics, nitrates, and digoxin, are of obvious importance. Newer therapies, however, are even more crucial to the patient's prognosis. The mortality benefits seen with angiotensin-converting enzyme (ACE) inhibitors in congestive heart failure are almost unmatched in medicine.[9-13] ACE inhibitors have even been demonstrated to decrease the incidence of ventricular tachycardia.[14] The availability of the β-blocker carvedilol adds another modality of therapy that may be even more helpful in patients with ventricular arrhythmias than in the general population of heart failure patients.[15, 16]

Drug History

It is vitally important to obtain a thorough drug history on each patient encounter. There are significant drug–device interactions (see Chapter 23). It is not unusual for a well-intentioned pharmacologic intervention to have detrimental effects on the defibrillator–patient interaction, either by slowing the arrhythmia below the detection window or by increasing the defibrillation threshold.[17]

■ ROLE OF CHEST RADIOGRAPHS

Chest radiography is commonly used in the follow-up of defibrillator patients. It is standard practice to obtain chest radiographs to confirm appropriate lead placement, to look for surgical complications, and to serve as a baseline film for future use. The use of chest radiography in routine follow-up varies widely. In some centers, films are obtained at regular intervals, but in other centers, films are obtained only when problems develop. Although chest radiographs can certainly detect lead fractures and lead dislodgment, late dislodgment is exceedingly rare, and data do not exist concerning the efficacy of chest radiographs for detecting lead problems in the era of modern programmers.[18–22]

■ DETERMINATION OF ADEQUATE FUNCTIONING

Sensing

It is crucial when following a patient with a defibrillator to ensure that there is adequate sensing. In some devices, the gain of the sense amplifier is automatically adjusted to maintain adequate sensing.[3, 8] In others, an automatic algorithm exists, but the maximum sensitivity is programmable.[5] For example, in one device, the sensitivity is decreased to the lesser of 10 times the programmed sensitivity, or 75% of the sensed R wave. It is then rapidly increased to the programmed sensitivity with a time constant of 450 msec. With a paced event, the sensing begins after the postpacing blanking period at the lesser of 4.5 times the programmed value, or at 1.8 mV.[5] Both these schemes have advantages and disadvantages.

A common problem is T-wave oversensing. If this occurs with pacing, as it frequently does, it results in an effectively lower pacing rate than the programmed lower limit. Two possible methods can be used to deal with this. First, the sensitivity can be decreased so that the T wave is not sensed. This has the disadvantage of decreasing the sensitivity for the detection of the low-amplitude signals that are sometimes seen in ventricular fibrillation. It is generally preferable to adjust the postpacing ventricular refractory period modestly.[4] It is important not to overextend the postpacing refractory periods, which can compromise sensing of ventricular fibrillation.[4] T-wave oversensing can also occur in sinus rhythm or with arrhythmias. Figure 34–1 demonstrates T-wave oversensing in ventricular tachycardia. This double counting can lead to inappropriate therapy. If the sensing of the device has changed since the last noninvasive electrophysiologic study, it should be repeated. It is important that sensing during ventricular fibrillation be ensured during an electrophysiologic evaluation of the defibrillator. If significant changes are made in the sensitivity of a defibrillator during follow-up, this mandates a follow-up electrophysiology study.

Stimulation Threshold

As with a cardiac pacemaker, it is important to test the stimulation threshold and to program the device for a sufficient safety margin. In most modern defibrillators, the output settings for postshock pacing, antitachycardia pacing (ATP), and bradycardia pacing are independently programmable. It is not unusual for the pacing threshold to increase somewhat after a shock for ventricular fibrillation. Consequently, the postpacing output is generally programmed to a high-output setting. The bradycardia pacing output settings are typically programmed, as would be a pacemaker.

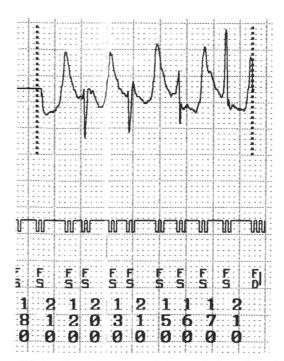

Figure 34–1. T-wave oversensing during ventricular tachycardia. This caused a tachycardia that could have otherwise been terminated by antitachycardia pacing to be treated with a high-energy shock. This was resolved by treating the patient's hyperkalemia.

Episode Review

Much of the focus of a defibrillator follow-up session is dedicated to the analysis of the arrhythmia history. It is important to examine each episode and make a reasonable judgment about the nature of the arrhythmia, the appropriateness of the therapy that was administered, and the efficacy of that therapy. After reviewing the symptoms, it is important to review the hard data supplied by the device. Some older pulse generators provided only counters, and it was virtually impossible to know exactly what happened during a given episode. In most currently implanted devices, either marker channels or electrograms or both are available.[23] These are invaluable in the follow-up of a patient. The electrograms can be analyzed and are often helpful in the discrimination of supraventricular arrhythmias from ventricular arrhythmias (Fig. 34–2). This discrimination, however, is dependent on the wavefront approaching the ventricular sensing lead differently—some ventricular rhythms approach the ventricular lead in a manner similar to sinus rhythm. As illustrated in Figure 34–3, in some cases ventricular tachycardia can appear remarkably similar to sinus rhythm.[24] In others, however, the electrograms can be very helpful (see Fig. 34–2). Now that defibrillators are available with atrial electrograms, the differentiation of supraventricular arrhythmias from ventricular arrhythmias is greatly simplified (Fig. 34–4). Electrograms can also be useful for the evaluation of other problems, as demonstrated in Figure 34–5.

Although electrograms may be beneficial, they may come at a significant longevity cost. There are two important issues concerning longevity and electrograms. First, some pulse generators record the electrogram directly from the sensing

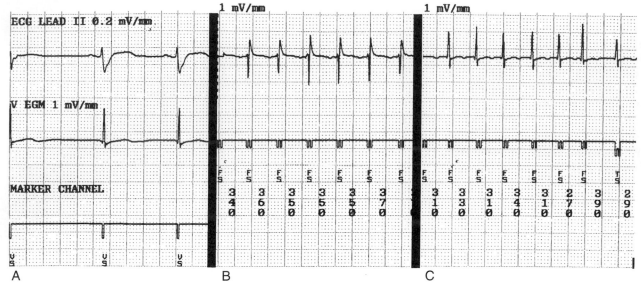

Figure 34–2. Electrograms recorded from a patient with ischemic cardiomyopathy and ventricular tachycardia. *A,* Sinus rhythm, recorded in the clinic. *B,* Ventricular tachycardia. The upper tracing is a ventricular electrogram, and the lower tracing is a marker channel with intervals. The difference in ventricular activation is obvious. *C,* An episode of atrial fibrillation that exceeded the programmed detection criteria. The ventricular electrogram is similar to the previously recorded sinus rhythm electrogram. The irregularity of the rhythm makes the diagnosis obvious.

amplifiers of the pulse generator; others use a separate higher-resolution amplifier that does consume more power but that also supplies a higher-resolution electrogram. Second, some pulse generators have a programmable option that allows the recording of an electrogram before the onset of the arrhythmia. This is similar to a loop recorder and requires that this energy-expensive circuit be continuously powered.[5] It is used mainly in problem solving.

The efficacy of programmed therapy must also be reviewed. If it is found that the programmed parameters are not achieving termination of the arrhythmias, changes must be made. The difficult decision is often whether a noninvasive electrophysiology test is needed. In general, any major change in therapy should be undertaken only after evaluation in the electrophysiology laboratory. Minor changes, such as

using the second ATP train first, after telemetry demonstrates that it has been more efficacious, can be done without further testing. Table 34–2 lists some of the indications for an electrophysiologic test of the implantable cardioverter-defibrillator (ICD).

It is also important to review carefully the episode data for all shocks, making sure that the high-voltage lead impedance is stable. If a significant drop in impedance is detected, there should be concerns about the possibility of insulation breakdown. Conversely, if the impedance increases significantly, conductor problems are suggested.

If patients are found to have frequent episodes of tachycardia that require shocks, it is often necessary to employ adjunctive therapy. The two principal therapies available are the addition of an antiarrhythmic drug and use of catheter

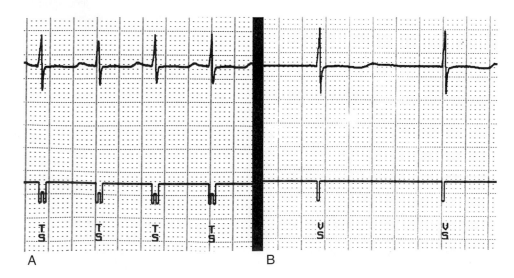

Figure 34–3. Electrograms from a patient in ventricular tachycardia (*A*) and sinus rhythm (*B*). The upper tracing is the ventricular electrogram, and the lower tracing is a marker channel. Notice the similarity of the electrograms. The only significant difference is the amplitude.

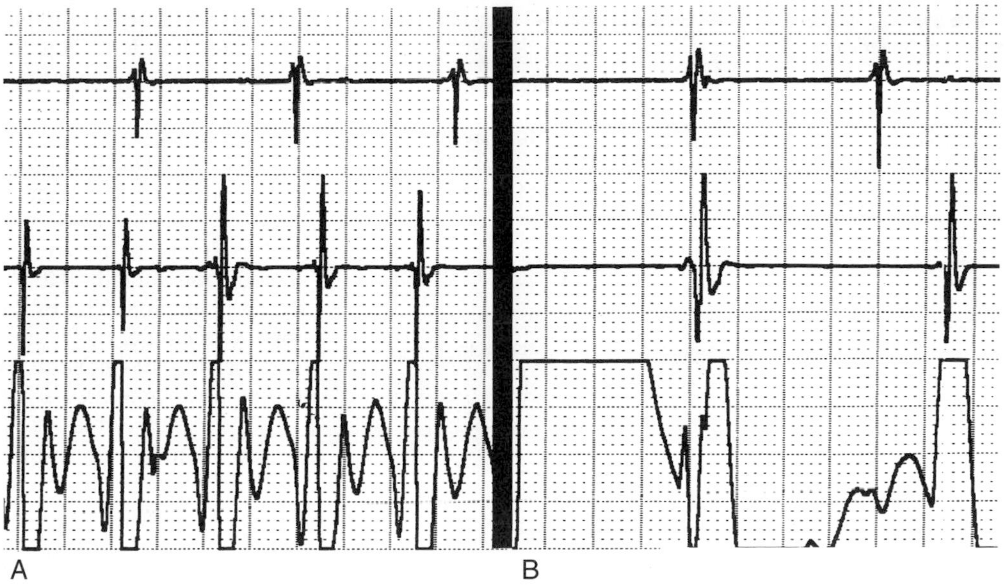

Figure 34–4. Electrograms from a patient with ventricular tachycardia (*A*) and junctional sinus rhythm (*B*). The upper tracing is the atrial electrogram, the middle tracing is the ventricular electrogram, and the lower tracing is a widely spaced electrogram. Note the difference in the ventricular electrogram and the ventriculoatrial dissociation.

A   B

ablation. These may have two beneficial effects. First, the number of episodes of ventricular tachycardia or ventricular fibrillation can be reduced. Second, either of these therapies can slow the cycle length of the ventricular tachycardia so that it can be treated more successfully with ATP rather than shock therapy.

If the frequency or nature of the arrhythmias changes significantly, the clinician may consider investigating the possibilities of a change in the ischemic substrate, the status of the patient's congestive heart failure, or the patient's metabolic status.

Evaluation of Battery Status

An important element of the follow-up of a defibrillator patient is the evaluation of the status of the battery. The silver-vanadium-oxide cells that are used in defibrillators perform differently from the lithium-oxide cells that are commonly used in pacemakers. The decay pattern of a defibrillator battery is illustrated in Figure 34–6. Typically, follow-up is accelerated as the battery begins to reach the plateau. It is common for this plateau to have a significant duration.

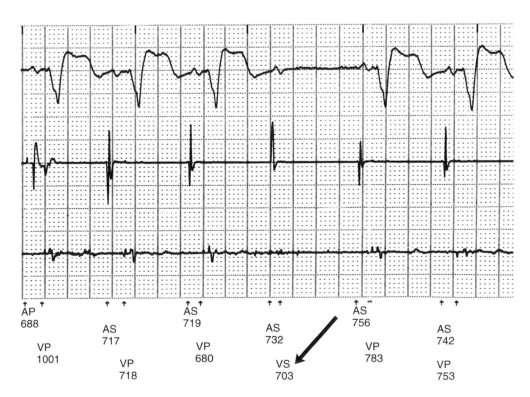

Figure 34–5. Electrograms and markers recorded in clinic from a patient with ventricular tachycardia, a defibrillator that senses both the atrium and ventricle, and a microdislodgment of the ventricular lead. The upper tracing is a surface electrocardiogram, the middle tracing is an atrial electrogram, and the lower tracing is a ventricular electrogram. The marker channel is at the bottom. The ventricular electrogram is small as a result of the microdislodgment; the automatic gain control then allows sensing of diaphragmatic potentials, which causes ventricular oversensing (*arrow*). AS, atrial sense; AP, atrial pace; VS, ventricular sense; VP, ventricular pace.

Table 34–2. Indications for an Electrophysiologic Study of an Implanted Defibrillator

Predischarge testing to prescribe settings, especially for antitachycardia pacing

Any change in primary antiarrhythmic (class I or III) therapy

An episode of ventricular tachycardia or ventricular defibrillation that was not adequately treated by the device and had no reversible cause

After an acute myocardial infarction

Major cardiac surgery, e.g., coronary artery bypass graft, valve surgery

Routine periodic follow-up (possibly controversial)

A need for significant reprogramming, such as a change in sensitivity

Exercise Testing

A difficult problem arises when a patient has ventricular tachycardia with a cycle length that is near the range of sinus rhythm. One useful tool is exercise testing, which can serve two purposes. First, it can help the physician identify the maximum expected sinus rate. Second, it can reassure the patient that exercise is possible. One limitation of exercise testing is the reluctance of the patient and the exercise technician or nurse to allow the patient to reach a near-maximum heart rate, for fear of a shock. It is our practice to have an electrophysiologist or defibrillator follow-up nurse present with the appropriate programmer during all exercise tests.

■ ROLE OF FOLLOW-UP ELECTROPHYSIOLOGIC STUDIES

Noninvasive electrophysiologic studies of patients with implanted defibrillators are indispensable. Table 34–2 lists some of the indications for this. The routine use of these tests was largely driven by investigational protocols in most centers. These protocols almost universally called for defibrillation testing at implantation and testing of defibrillation threshold, cardioversion threshold, and ATP before discharge from the hospital. This testing was repeated at about 3 months, after lead maturity had been achieved. Some centers also employ annual electrophysiologic studies. Few data exist demonstrating the usefulness of this routine testing. It is clear, however, that other events do trigger a need for an electrophysiologic evaluation of the defibrillator and patient; some of these are listed in Table 34–2.

It is crucial to use an electrophysiologic study to establish the efficacy of defibrillation for ventricular fibrillation during the implantation. The evaluation of ATP and cardioversion for the treatment of ventricular tachycardia may be done as part of the implantation procedure or may be performed during a separate predischarge electrophysiologic study.

A prospective study has called into question the necessity of careful follow-up testing of ATP for induced ventricular tachycardia at predischarge testing to predict ATP success during follow-up.[30] In this study, 200 consecutive patients who received ICD implants underwent electrophysiologic testing and randomization to empirically programmed ATP or tested ATP. During follow-up over a 20-month period, 90% of spontaneous ventricular tachycardias were terminated by tested ATP programming in a subgroup of patients. The success for all episodes in individual patients was 90% or higher. Acceleration of ventricular tachycardia by ATP occurred in 2% of the patients with tested ATP and in 5% of the empirically programmed ATP patients. The authors suggest that empiric programming of ATP is safe and effective and does not depend on demonstrated efficacy from follow-up or predischarge electrophysiology testing.

Clinical Situations
Repeated Shocks

One of the most common problems in following a patient with a defibrillator is the evaluation and management of patients with repeated shocks. The differential diagnosis of repeated shocks is as follows:

1. Failure of therapy: the initial shock failed to convert the arrhythmia

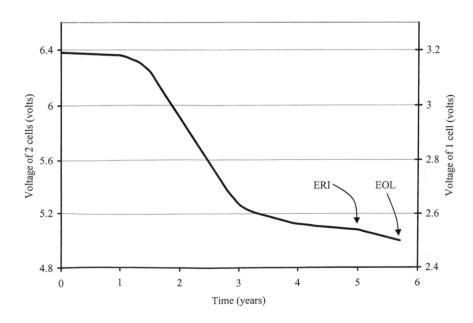

Figure 34–6. The voltage of a typical silver-vanadium-oxide battery is displayed. The battery voltage is displayed over time. On the left is the typical voltage for defibrillators using two cells, and on the right is the typical voltage for a single-cell device. Most defibrillators use two cells and report the voltage of the two in series; others report the voltage of a single cell. Typically, there is a period of slow voltage decline followed by a more rapid decline to a voltage just above the level of the elective replacement indicator. There is typically then a plateau phase that can last for a year or more, during which the voltage decline is gradual. The elective replacement indicator (ERI) is then reached, followed by the end-of-life (EOL) indicator. This is the point at which the reliable operation of the defibrillator may be compromised.

2. Incessant tachycardia: the arrhythmia terminated but quickly reinitiates

3. Device failure, causing the sensing of noise

4. Electromagnetic interference

With first-generation defibrillators, the only data that were available were the counters. Physicians had to rely on the patient's symptoms to determine if the shock was appropriate or inappropriate. With the advent of third-generation defibrillators, markers were available that were of much more help in determining the rhythm that initiated an episode and the result of the therapy. We now have vast quantities of stored electrograms in addition to the counters and markers.

Asymptomatic Shocks

Asymptomatic shocks presented major problems in the past but now present no quandary. With the assistance of stored electrograms and stored markers, this problem can usually be resolved with little work.

Palpitations or Syncope

It is not unusual for patients with defibrillators to present with either sustained palpitations or syncope. The concerns should first focus on the arrhythmia history. If the device memory cannot be used to help, an indispensable tool is the loop recorder. Short-term Holter monitoring is rarely of benefit in this situation, unless the events occur on a daily basis.

Defibrillator Patient Requiring Surgery

Patients with defibrillators often have the need to undergo either cardiac or noncardiac surgery. There are three principle interactions between the defibrillator and surgical cautery. First, the output from the cautery can be sensed as ventricular fibrillation, and the patient may receive an inappropriate shock or, in the case of a pacemaker-dependent patient, the pacing output can be inhibited. Second, the output of the cautery can cause a transient or permanent reprogramming of the defibrillator. Third, the current from the defibrillator can be transmitted down the sense and pace lead and can cause an increase in the stimulation threshold. The first of these is easy to avoid, but the latter two are largely out of the physician's control. Fortunately, the inadvertent reprogramming of a pacemaker or defibrillator with cautery is a very rare event.

The consensus advice for defibrillator patients undergoing surgery is to deactivate the tachyarrhythmia therapies before surgery and reactivate them postoperatively. Our approach is somewhat different. We encourage our anesthesiologists to use a magnet during the surgery, if it is physically feasible, given the nature of the patient's surgery. This has the distinct advantage of allowing the anesthesiologist or surgeon to remove the magnet if the patient develops a tachyarrhythmia intraoperatively. It is important to realize that some defibrillators can be permanently turned off with a magnet.[8] It is always our practice to disable this feature to avoid accidental deactivation.

It is difficult to deal with the intraoperative management of a pacemaker-dependent patient who is pacing with the defibrillator. This has not been a common problem in the past because most pacemaker-dependent patients had a separate pacemaker. With the availability of dual-chamber pacing defibrillators, however, it is becoming more common to allow the patient to pace continuously with the defibrillator. Regardless of the intraoperative management, we always interrogate the defibrillator postoperatively and recheck the stimulation thresholds in 2 to 4 weeks.

Elective Replacement Indicator

As noted previously, it is the usual practice to increase the frequency of follow-up visits as the battery voltage approaches the designated elective replacement indicator. Typically, devices are designed to operate normally for 3 months after the elective replacement indicator has been reached.[3, 5] There is, however, considerable prolongation of the charge time between the elective replacement indicator and the end-of-service indicators. It is therefore important to replace the pulse generator at the first opportunity after the elective replacement indicator is reached. It is also important to see patients who have reached the elective replacement indicator for evaluation with any further shocks.

Educational Aspects

The education of both the defibrillator patient and the family is crucial. The surgical aspects of education are similar to those that are appropriate for a patient with a pacemaker, and these have been reviewed. In addition to the precautions about excessive movements and keeping the wound dry, patients are advised to alert the physician immediately if there are any signs of infection. The hazards of excessive manipulation of the device are also explained. Twiddler's syndrome has even occurred in subpectoral pockets.[1] Patients should be carefully educated about the need to avoid high-power magnetic fields and sources of electromagnetic interference (see Chapter 35).

Psychological Aspects

The psychological aspects of patient care can generally be divided into two parts: the perioperative period and the maintenance period. The reactions of a patient during the perioperative period are related not only to the device and the surgery but also to the event that caused the patient to present for care.[25] When a catastrophic arrest is accompanied by a period of anoxic encephalopathy, the psychological changes are further complicated. Psychological support may be even more important in follow-up. There has been extensive experience with defibrillator patient support groups,[26–28] most of which has been positive. The fear of many electrophysiologists is that a support group will degenerate into a communal session of negative expression. If the group is well coordinated, this can usually be avoided. The principal benefits of a defibrillator patient support group are patient education and the positive feedback of other patients who are doing well.

■ FUTURE DEVELOPMENTS

A number of possibilities exist in the near future for the follow-up of patients with ICDs. Work has already been done on transtelephonic follow-up on several levels of sophistication.[29] One of the most helpful and long-awaited developments will be the ability to assess the impedance and integrity of the defibrillation electrodes without delivering a high-energy shock. This will give physicians much more confidence in the integrity of an ICD and will likely result in an early warning system for defibrillation lead problems. Other advances will involve the automation of follow-up.

REFERENCES

1. Crossley GH, Gayle DD, Bailey JR, et al: Defibrillator twiddler's syndrome causing device failure in a subpectoral transvenous system. PACE 19:376–377, 1996.
2. Cardiac Pacemakers Incorporated: Physician's Manual: Ventak® P AICD™. St. Paul, MN, Cardiac Pacemakers, Inc., 1994.
3. Ventritex Incorporated: Physician's Manual: Cadet™ V-115 Tiered-Therapy Defibrillator System and Cadet™ LT V-105 Cardioverter/Defibrillator System. Sunnyvale, CA, Ventritex, Inc., 1998.
4. Medtronic Incorporated: Principles of Operation: Jewel™ PCD®. Minneapolis, MN, Medtronic Inc., 1998,
5. Medtronic Incorporated: Microjewel™ II Product Information Manual. Minneaplois, MN, Medtronic, Inc., 1998.
6. Karasik P, Steele P, Ellenbogen KA, et al: Longevity variation for implantable defibrillators in the VA database [Abstract]. Circulation 94:I-563, 1996.
7. Crossley GH, Fitzgerald DM: Estimating defibrillator longevity: A need for an objective comparison [Editorial]. PACE 20:1897–1901, 1997.
8. Cardiac Pacemakers Incorporated: Physician's System Manual: Ventak® Mini™ II 1762 and Ventak® Mini™ II+ 1763. St. Paul, MN, Cardiac Pacemakers Inc., 1996.
9. Swedberg K, Kjekshus J: Effects of enalapril on mortality in severe congestive heart failure: Results of the Cooperative North Scandinavian Enalapril Survival Study (CONSENSUS). Am J Cardiol 62:60A–66A, 1988.
10. Anonymous: Effect of enalapril on survival in patients with reduced left ventricular ejection fractions and congestive heart failure. The SOLVD Investigators [see Comments]. N Engl J Med 325:293–302, 1991.
11. Francis GS, Cohn JN, Johnson G, et al: Plasma norepinephrine, plasma renin activity, and congestive heart failure: Relations to survival and the effects of therapy in V-HeFT II. The V-HeFT VA Cooperative Studies Group. Circulation 87:VI40–VI48, 1993.
12. Swedberg K, Held P, Kjekshus J, et al: Effects of the early administration of enalapril on mortality in patients with acute myocardial infarction: Results of the Cooperative New Scandinavian Enalapril Survival Study II (CONSENSUS II). N Engl J Med 327:678–684, 1992.
13. Anonymous: Effect of enalapril on mortality and the development of heart failure in asymptomatic patients with reduced left ventricular ejection fractions. The SOLVD Investigators [Published erratum appears in N Engl J Med 327(24):1768, 1992; see Comments]. N Engl J Med 327:685–691, 1992.
14. Fletcher RD, Cintron GB, Johnson G, et al: Enalapril decreases prevalence of ventricular tachycardia in patients with chronic congestive heart failure: The V-HeFT II VA Cooperative Studies Group. Circulation 87:VI49–VI55, 1993.
15. Taylor SH, Storstein L: Carvedilol: A wide therapeutic potential in cardiovascular syndromes. Introduction. Cardiology 82(Suppl 3):1–2, 1993.
16. Storstein L: Carvedilol: Clinical experience in arrhythmias. Cardiology 82(Suppl 3):29–33, 1993.
17. Greene HL: Interactions between pharmacologic and nonpharmacologic antiarrhythmic therapy. Am J Cardiol 78:61–66, 1996.
18. Eagar G, Gutierrez FR, Gamache MC: Radiologic appearance of implantable cardiac defibrillators. AJR Am J Roentgenol 162:25–29, 1994.
19. Daly BD, Cascade PN, Hummel JD, et al: Transvenous and subcutaneous implantable cardioverter defibrillators: Radiographic assessment. Radiology 191:273–278, 1994.
20. Daly BD, Hummel JD, Langberg J, et al: Nonthoracotomy lead implantable cardioverter defibrillators: Normal radiographic appearance. AJR Am J Roentgenol 161:749–752, 1993.
21. Chmielewski SR, Zegel HG, Gottlieb C, Freiman DB: Cardioverter-defibrillator systems implanted without thoracotomy: Radiographic findings. AJR Am J Roentgenol 161:943–946, 1993.
22. Drucker EA, Brooks R, Garan H, et al: Malfunction of implantable cardioverter defibrillators placed by a nonthoracotomy approach: Frequency of malfunction and value of chest radiography in determining cause. AJR Am J Roentgenol 165:275–279, 1995.
23. Brachmann J, Sterns LD, Hilbel T, et al: Advances in follow-up techniques for implantable defibrillators [Review, 17 refs]. Am Heart J 127:1081–1085, 1994.
24. Rosenthal M, Alderfer T, Marchlinski F: Troubleshooting suspected ICD malfunction. In Kroll MW, Lehmann M (eds): Implantable Cardioverter Defibrillator Therapy: The Engineering–Clinical Interface. Norwell, MA, Kluwer Academic Publishers, 1996, pp 435–476.
25. Aarons D, Veltri EP: Psychological aspects of ICD implantation and ICD support groups. In Naccarelli GV, Veltri EP (eds): Implantable Cardioverter-Defibrillators. Cambridge, MA, Blackwell Scientific Publications, 1993, pp 171–184.
26. Molchany CA, Peterson KA: The psychosocial effects of support group intervention on AICD recipients and their significant others. Prog Cardiovasc Nurs 9:23–29, 1994.
27. Badger JM, Knott JE: Death of a support group member: A practical guide to helping other members cope. J Cardiovasc Nurs 7:63–72, 1993.
28. Sneed NV, Finch NJ, Michel Y: The effect of psychosocial nursing intervention on the mood state of patients with implantable cardioverter defibrillators and their caregivers. Prog Cardiovasc Nurs 12:4–14, 1997.
29. Fetter JG, Stanton MS, Benditt DG, et al: Transtelephonic monitoring and transmission of stored arrhythmia detection and therapy data from an implantable cardioverter defibrillator. PACE 18:1531–1539, 1995.
30. Schaumann A, von zur Muhlen F, Herse B, et al: Empirical versus tested antitachycardia pacing in implantable cardioverter defibrillators. Circulation 97:66–74, 1998.

Electromagnetic Interference With Implantable Devices

David L. Hayes and Neil F. Strathmore

Pacemakers and implantable cardioverter-defibrillators (ICDs) are subject to interference from nonbiologic electromagnetic sources.[1-3] In addition, extremes of temperature or irradiation may cause device malfunction. In general, modern devices are effectively shielded against electromagnetic interference (EMI), and the increasing use of bipolar leads has further reduced the problem. Although there has always been some concern about the EMI that patients may encounter in the nonhospital environment, improvements in pacemaker protection, such as shielding and design changes, have lessened this concern.[1] The principal sources of interference that affect these devices are in the hospital environment.

The portion of the electromagnetic spectrum that may affect implantable devices includes *radiofrequency waves* with frequencies between 0 and 10^9 Hz, such as alternating current electricity supplies (50 or 60 Hz) and electrocautery. The other applicable portion of the electromagnetic spectrum includes *microwaves,* with frequencies between 10^9 and 10^{11} Hz, including ultra high-frequency radio waves and radar, and microwave ovens (2.45×10^9 Hz). Higher-frequency portions of the spectrum, including infrared, visible light, ultraviolet, x-rays, and gamma rays, do not interfere with pacemakers because their wavelengths are much shorter than the pacemaker or lead dimensions. However, high-intensity therapeutic x-rays can damage pacemaker circuitry directly.

EMI enters a pacemaker or ICD by conduction if the patient is in direct contact with the source or by way of radiation if the patient is in an electromagnetic field with the lead acting as an antenna. The devices have been protected from interference by shielding the circuitry, reducing the distance between the electrodes to minimize the antenna, and filtering the incoming signal. If interference does enter the pulse generator, noise protection algorithms in the timing circuit decrease the effect on the patient.

The contemporary pacemaker and ICD is immune from most sources of interference because the circuitry is shielded inside a stainless steel or titanium case. In addition, the body tissues provide some protection by reflection or absorption of external radiation. Therefore, although in vitro studies of pacemaker or ICD interference may at times demonstrate a disturbance of device function, in vivo exposure to the same EMI may not result in any abnormalities.[4]

Bipolar leads sense less conducted and radiated interference because the electrode distance, and thus the antenna, is smaller than that for unipolar leads. Bipolar sensing has effectively eliminated myopotential inhibition and crosstalk as pacemaker problems. In addition, studies have shown that bipolar sensing is associated with considerably less sensing of external electrical fields[5, 6] and less effect from electrocautery during surgery.[7]

Sensed interference is filtered by narrow bandpass filters to exclude noncardiac signals; however, this still leaves signals in the 5- to 100-Hz range, which overlap the cardiac signal range and are not filtered. These signals can give rise to abnormal device behavior if they are interpreted as cardiac signals and inappropriately inhibit or trigger responses.

The possible responses to external interference include the following:

- Inappropriate inhibition of paced output
- Inappropriate triggering of paced output
- Asynchronous pacing
- Reprogramming, usually to a backup mode
- Damage to the device circuitry
- Triggering an ICD discharge

■ DEVICE RESPONSES TO NOISE

Asynchronous Pacing

To protect the patient from inappropriate inhibition of paced output, contemporary devices have the capability of reverting to asynchronous pacing if exposed to sufficient interference. This change is usually activated by signals detected during a noise sampling period (NSP) within the timing cycle (Fig. 35–1). The NSP occurs immediately after the ventricular refractory period (VRP), which follows a ventricular sensed or paced event. The VRP is an "absolute" refractory period, during which the ventricular sensing channel does not detect any signals and in particular does not sense the ventricular pacing pulse afterpotential or the evoked QRS and T waves. The VRP usually lasts between 200 and 400 msec, and events occurring during this period have no effect on pacemaker timing. The NSP or resettable refractory period lasts between 60 and 200 msec. If an event is sensed during this period, it is interpreted as noise, and either the VRP or the NSP is restarted. In addition, in a dual-chamber mode, the postventricular atrial refractory period and the upper rate interval, but not the lower rate interval, are restarted. If a further noise event is detected in the NSP, the VRP or NSP is again restarted, and the pacemaker does not recognize cardiac signals. Repetitive noise events eventually cause the lower rate interval to time out, and a pacing pulse is delivered. Continuous noise thus results in asynchronous pacing at the lower rate limit.

In some pacemakers, rather than timing out the lower rate interval, repetitive detection of noise in the NSP causes temporary switching to a specific "noise reversion mode," which is usually an asynchronous mode (VOO or DOO). In some pacemakers with programmable polarity, the pacing output is unipolar in the noise reversion mode, even if the device is programmed to bipolar pacing.

Whether noise causes inhibition or asynchronous pacing depends on the duration and field strength of the signal.[8] At the lowest field strength, there is no effect. As the field strength increases, there is a greater tendency to inhibition because the noise may be sensed intermittently and may be sensed not in the NSP but in the alert period between the NSP and the next pacing pulse. At higher field strengths, the noise is sensed continuously, including in the NSP, and

asynchronous pacing occurs. There is considerable variation in pacemaker models in their susceptibility to noise.[8, 9]

If the entire VRP is restarted by a sensed event in the NSP, cardiac impulses at a cycle length equal to the VRP could cause asynchronous pacing. In most VVI pacemakers, the VRP is about 250 msec, so that only cardiac rates greater than 240 bpm do this. In some DDD pacemakers, however, the VRP may be prolonged after a ventricular premature beat—that is, as defined by the pacemaker logic, a ventricular event not preceded by an atrial event. In some pacemakers, the VRP is sufficiently prolonged after a ventricular premature beat, allowing faster cardiac rates to be interpreted as noise and to cause asynchronous pacing. For example, if the VRP extension is to 345 msec, cardiac rates greater than 174 bpm could be interpreted as noise. This has been observed clinically during sinus tachycardia, supraventricular tachycardia, atrial fibrillation, and ventricular tachycardia.[10–14]

If the NSP, rather than the VRP, is restarted by noise, only events at this shorter cycle length will cause asynchronous pacing—that is, if the NSP is 200 msec, only rates of 300 bpm cause asynchronous pacing.

Mode Resetting

In addition to the temporary changes already discussed, electrical interference can cause a change to another device mode that persists after the noise stops. This is usually the "backup mode" or "reset mode" and is often the same as the device elective replacement indicator or "battery depletion" mode. Confusion can arise when the backup mode and the settings at battery depletion are the same. A pacemaker that has been affected by interference may be wrongly assumed to have reached battery depletion and be replaced, or an operator believing that the device has been subject to interference may reprogram a pacemaker that has truly reached battery depletion. In both cases, careful attention to the programmer telemetry, when available, can help. If the telemetered cell impedance remains low or the battery voltage is normal, the battery is not exhausted, and interference is the problem. Another test is to stress the pacemaker power supply by reprogramming to the original pacing mode with maximum output and an increased rate. If the battery is truly near depletion, the device quickly reverts to the settings that indicate battery depletion.

The backup or reset mode is usually VVI, and if the pulse generator has programmable polarity, the backup polarity is unipolar. This may be significant in patients with implantable defibrillators and is discussed later. Some pacemakers may reset to VOO mode if subjected to interference, resulting in competition with the intrinsic rhythm.

EMI is not the only inappropriate cause of mode resetting in pacemakers and ICDs. Exposure to low temperatures before implantation causes an increase in the internal battery resistance, with a subsequent decrease in the battery voltage causing the battery depletion indicator or reset mode to be activated.[15] This frequently occurs during shipment in cold climates, so that all devices should be routinely interrogated before implantation and reprogrammed if necessary.

Triggered Mode

A completely different clinical approach to an interference problem is to program one of the triggered modes, VVT or

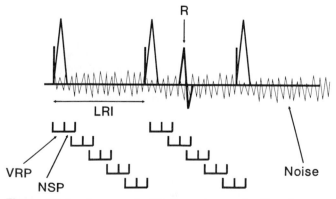

Figure 35–1. Response of a VVI pacemaker to noise. There is no sensing during the ventricular refractory period (VRP). Noise is detected in the noise sampling period (NSP) immediately after the VRP and causes restarting of the VRP. In the next NSP, noise is again detected, and the VRP is again restarted. This continues until the lower rate interval (LRI) times out, and a ventricular pacing pulse is delivered. Because the sensing channel is refractory throughout the LRI, the intrinsic cardiac beat (R) is not sensed, and pacing is asynchronous.

AAT. In these modes, sensed signals trigger, rather than inhibit, a paced pulse. Noise triggers pacing at an upper rate determined by the VRP, which is usually set at about 400 msec to limit the maximum triggered rate to 150 ppm. Although pacemakers are rarely programmed permanently to a triggered mode, the triggered modes may be used to prevent myopotential inhibition in unipolar pacing systems and may be used for patients undergoing surgery to prevent interference by electrocautery.

■ ENVIRONMENTAL ELECTROMAGNETIC INTERFERENCE

Electrical and magnetic signals are emitted by certain industrial and domestic sources with which the pacemaker or ICD patient may have contact. Even though in vitro studies of implantable devices in test rigs may demonstrate susceptibil-

ity to interference from such environmental effects, in vivo studies of the same devices have shown that there are few problems in the domestic area, and problems rarely occur in the industrial area.[16]

Many potential sources of EMI are capable of one-beat inhibition of the pacemaker (Table 35–1). It would be unusual, however, for any of these sources to cause EMI of clinical significance. It would also be unlikely for any of the devices in Table 35–1 to produce sustained effects resulting in clinically significant interference with an ICD; however, anecdotal reports exist.[17–20]

Hospital Environment

The hospital is the most common environment in which sources of potential EMI may cause significant interference with implantable devices (Table 35–2).

Table 35–1. Potential Sources of Electromagnetic Interference

EMI Source	Generator Damage	Complete Inhibition	One-Beat Inhibition	Asynchronous Pacing	Rate Increase
Ablation (RF)	Y	Y	N	N	Y
Acupuncture	N	Y	Y	Y	N
Airport detector	N	N	Y	N	N
Antitheft equipment	?	?	Y	Y	?
Arc welder	N	Y	Y	Y	N
Cardioversion	Y	N	N	Y	Y
Cautery, coagulation	Y	Y	Y	Y	Y*, †
Cellular phone	N	Y	Y	Y	Y
CB radio	N	N	Y	N	N
CT scanner	N	N	N	N	N
Defibrillation	Y	N	N	Y	Y
Diathermy	Y	Y	Y	Y	Y
Drill, electric	N	N	Y‡	N	N
ECT, EST	N	Y	Y	Y	Y†
Electric blanket	N	N	Y‡	N	N
Electric shaver	N	N	Y‡	N	N
Electric switch	N	N	Y‡	N	N
Electrolysis	N	N	Y	Y	N
Electrotome	N	N	Y‡	N	N
Ham radio	N	N	Y	N	N
Heating pad	N	N	N	Y	N
Lithotripsy	Y†	Y‡	Y‡	Y‡	Y§
Metal detector	N	N	Y‡	N	N
Microwave	N	N	N	N	N
MRI	?	N	Y	Y	Y
PET scanner	?	N	N	N	N
Power line	N	N	N	Y	N
Radar	N	N	Y‡	N	N
Radiation, diagnostic	N	N	N	N	Y
Radiation therapy	Y	N	N	N	Y
TENS	N	Y	N	Y	Y
TV remote	N	N	N	N	N
Diagnostic ultrasound	N	N	N	N	N

CB, citizens-band; CT, computed tomography; ECT, electroconvulsive therapy; EMI, electromagnetic interference; EST, electroshock therapy; MRI, magnetic resonance imaging; N, no; PET, positron emission tomography; RF, radiofrequency; Rx, therapeutic; TENS, transcutaneous electrical nerve stimulation; TV, television; Y, yes.
*Impedance-based pulse generators.
†Piezoelectric crystal–based pulse generators.
‡Remote potential for interference.
§DDD mode only.
Modified from Telectronics: Electromagnetic interference and the pacemaker patient. Technical Notes No. 110, 1991.

Table 35–2. Sources of Electromagnetic Interference in the Hospital Environment

- Electrocautery
- Cardioversion, defibrillation
- Magnetic resonance imaging
- Lithotripsy
- Radiofrequency ablation
- Electroshock therapy
- Electroconvulsive therapy
- Diathermy

Electrocautery

Electrocautery continues to be one of the most common potential sources of EMI for patients with implanted devices.[7, 21] Electrocautery involves the use of radiofrequency current to cut or coagulate tissues. It is usually applied in a unipolar configuration between the cauterizing instrument (the cathode) and the indifferent plate (the anode) attached at a distant location on the patient's skin. Bipolar cautery uses a bipolar instrument for coagulation. The frequency is usually between 300 and 500 kHz (at frequencies of less than 200 kHz, muscle and nerve stimulation may occur). Cutting diathermy uses a modulated signal to apply bursts of energy, whereas coagulation diathermy uses an unmodulated signal to heat the tissue. Coagulation diathermy is used in radiofrequency ablation of cardiac tissue for the treatment of arrhythmias.

The current generated by electrocautery is related to the distance and orientation of the cautery electrodes relative to the device and lead.[22] High current is generated if the cautery cathode is close to the pulse generator, and particularly high currents are generated in the circuitry if it lies between the two cautery electrodes.

Electrocautery can result in multiple clinical responses from a permanent pacemaker (Table 35–3). The radiofrequency signal may be interpreted as a cardiac impulse and result in inappropriate inhibition. Prolonged application of cautery causes repetitive stimulation in the NSP and, thus, asynchronous pacing at the lower rate. Pacemaker function returns to normal each time the diathermy is switched off. In addition, ICDs are likely to interpret the electrocautery signal as ventricular fibrillation and induce a shock therapy.

Switching to the backup or reset mode may also occur, and reprogramming is necessary for a return to normal.[23, 24] This switch can cause hemodynamic compromise if the reset mode is VVI and atrioventricular (AV) synchrony is lost or the rate of the reset mode is too slow.[25] If the backup mode is VOO, asynchronous pacing occurs, even after the electrocautery device has been switched off.

Device circuitry can be damaged by electrocautery despite electronic protection, resulting in output failure, pace-maker runaway,[26] or other malfunctions requiring pulse generator replacement.

The electrocautery signal may induce currents in the pacing lead and cause local heating at the electrode, leading to myocardial damage with subsequent elevation of the pacing or sensing threshold (or both). Threshold alteration is often transient. This problem is a cause of concern but appears to be infrequently documented.

To prevent inappropriate inhibition of the pacemaker, a magnet is often applied to the chest over the pacemaker during cautery to convert it to the asynchronous mode. Although this maneuver may be successful, in some models, it may open the pacemaker to reprogramming by the electrocautery signal and is therefore not recommended.

Pacemakers with rate-responsive functions may exhibit unexpected responses during surgery. The electrocautery signal may overwhelm the impedance measuring circuit of a minute ventilation rate-responsive pacemaker and cause pacing at the upper rate limit.[27]

Most reported complications of electrocautery are with unipolar pacemakers. A prospective study of pacemaker patients undergoing surgery suggested that bipolar devices are less susceptible to the effects of electrocautery.[7]

Patients with pacemakers who are to undergo surgery in which electrocautery may be used should be assessed preoperatively (Table 35–4). The crucial step is to identify the pacemaker so that its response to cautery is known and the appropriate programmer is available. In particular, the backup mode should be determined from the manufacturer's literature. If the backup mode might compromise the patient by reducing AV synchrony, pacing asynchronously, or delivering too slow a rate, the programmer must be available in the operating room, the pulse generator must be accessible to the programming head, and someone experienced in programming should be present.

Pacemaker and ICD function should be checked with a programmer preoperatively: the device should be telemetered, programmed settings should be recorded, the underly-

Table 35–3. Effects of Electrocautery

- Reprogramming
- Permanent damage to the pulse generator
- Pacemaker inhibition
- Reversion to a fall-back mode, noise reversion mode, or electrical reset
- Myocardial thermal damage

Table 35–4. Perioperative Management of Pacemakers

Preoperative

- Identify pacemaker and determine "reset" mode
- Check pacemaker program, telemetry, thresholds, battery status
- Deactivate rate response and magnet-induced threshold testing
- Record pacemaker information

Intraoperative

- Position electrocautery indifferent plate away from pacemaker so that pacemaker is not between electrocautery electrodes
- Monitor pulse or oximeter (electrocardiogram will be obscured by artifacts)
- Have programmer readily available
- Use bipolar cautery when possible
- Do not use cautery near pacemaker
- Use cautery in short bursts
- Reprogram if necessary if reset mode is hemodynamically unstable
- Rarely consider use of VVT mode if necessary

Postoperative

- Check pacemaker program, telemetry, thresholds
- Reprogram if necessary

ing rhythm should be determined, and pacing thresholds should be measured. Rate responsiveness and magnet-initiated threshold testing should be turned off. Consideration could be given to programming to an asynchronous mode or triggered mode (VVT), particularly if the patient is pacemaker dependent. The tachycardia response of ICDs should be disabled just before the surgery and restored immediately after surgery.

In the operating room, the indifferent plate of the electrocautery procedure should be placed at a distance from the device, usually on the thigh, and good contact should be ensured. The effect of electrocautery may be difficult to assess because it causes interference on the electrocardiogram (ECG) monitor. Other methods of assessing cardiac rhythm should be used, such as palpation of the pulse, pulse oximetry, or arterial blood pressure monitoring.

Cautery should be used with caution in the vicinity of the device and its leads. The cathode should be kept as far from the pulse generator as possible, the lowest possible amplitude should be used, and the surgeon should deliver only brief bursts.

During electrocautery, pacemaker function and cardiac rhythm should be carefully assessed. The most likely response is transient inhibition or asynchronous pacing during electrocautery, which should not cause a significant hemodynamic problem. If persistent pacemaker inhibition occurs, a magnet can be applied to the device during electrocautery application so long as the pacemaker is not one that might be reprogrammed with the magnet in place.

Postoperatively, the device should be interrogated and, if it is in the reset mode, reprogrammed to the original settings. Ideally, thresholds should be reassessed and compared with preoperative values. If problems are encountered when the pulse generator is interrogated or reprogrammed to its original settings, the manufacturer should be consulted to determine if a malfunction has occurred. In some cases, the device can be reactivated with a special programming sequence or programmer, but if this is not possible, it should be replaced.

Defibrillation

External transthoracic defibrillation produces the largest amount of electrical energy delivered in the vicinity of a device and has the potential to damage both the pulse generator and the cardiac tissue in contact with the lead.[28] Internal defibrillation through epicardial or subcutaneous patches or endocardial defibrillation electrodes delivers smaller amounts of energy but may also interfere with pacemaker function.[29, 30]

Pacemakers are protected from damage from high defibrillation energies by special circuitry incorporating a Zener diode that electronically regulates the voltage entering the circuitry and should prevent high currents from being conducted through the lead to the myocardium. The extremely high energies, however, can overwhelm this protection and damage the pulse generator or the heart. Reports of extensive pacemaker and cardiac damage refer predominantly to older unipolar devices, and it is likely that bipolar pacemakers are more resistant (Fig. 35–2).

Most commonly, the backup or reset mode or the elective replacement or battery depletion indicator is activated. In the backup or reset mode, however, pacemakers with program-

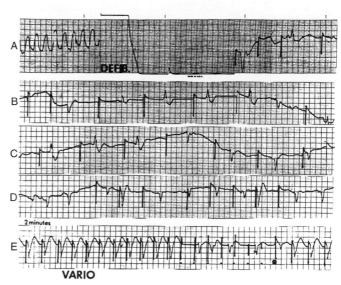

Figure 35–2. Serial electrocardiograms showing transient loss of capture after defibrillation (DEFIB.) in a patient. The loss of capture is followed by intermittent capture, first demonstrated in the supernormal zone of the native beats (*strip D*). Sensing function is normal. The refractory period of the pacemaker was programmed to 437 msec. *Strip E* demonstrates stimulation threshold testing using the Vario function of this pacemaker. This is initiated by placing a test magnet over the implanted pulse generator, which starts a test cycle with two phases repeating themselves as long as the magnet is in place. The first part of testing consists of 16 impulses at the magnet rate of 100 bpm delivered at the full output of the generator. At the end of the first 16 impulses, the Vario mechanism produces pacing at a rate slightly faster than the magnet rate. The output voltage is decreased by a fixed amount successively during the ensuing 16 impulses from the full output to an output of 0 V. The threshold is then calculated by counting the number of ineffective pacing impulses from right to left. At the end of the test cycle, the pacemaker automatically returns to its programmed voltage output. (From Levine PA, Barold SS, Fletcher RD, et al: Adverse acute and chronic effects of electrical defibrillation and cardioversion on implanted unipolar cardiac pacing systems. J Am Coll Cardiol 1:1413, 1983. By permission of the American College of Cardiology.)

mable polarity usually deliver unipolar pacing pulses. Because unipolar pulses are much more likely to be detected by an ICD, it is essential that a pacemaker in a patient with an ICD be paced in a bipolar mode or that the unipolar configuration be thoroughly tested to prevent undersensing and oversensing by the defibrillator. A dedicated bipolar pacemaker without programmable pacing polarity is preferred for such patients. Defibrillation may induce high-energy currents in the pacemaker lead, either by capacitive coupling to the defibrillation shock or by shunting in the pacemaker circuit.[28] This energy may be sufficient to cause trauma to or burning of the myocardium at the myocardium–electrode interface, with subsequent chronic threshold elevation. Transient elevation of capture and sensing thresholds is not uncommon, however, after both external and internal defibrillation. Unipolar pacing systems probably are more prone to this form of damage than are bipolar systems,[28] and there are no reports of extensive cardiac damage with bipolar leads. It has also been suggested that elevation of the pacing threshold after defibrillation is related to the duration of

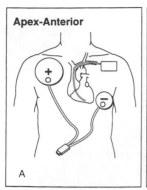
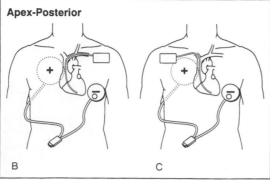

Figure 35–3. Schematic representation of positioning of paddles or R2 pads to minimize damage to the pulse generator and pacemaker lead. *A*, Both paddles are placed anteriorly in positions allowing effective cardioversion while maintaining a safe distance from the implanted device. *B* and *C*, Apex-to-posterior paddle positions are shown with the device in the right prepectoral region (*B*) and the left prepectoral region (*C*).

ventricular fibrillation rather than to the energy of defibrillation.[31]

The degree of damage appears to be related to the distance of the defibrillation paddles from the pulse generator. All device manufacturers recommend that the paddles be placed as far as possible from the generator. When possible, an anteroposterior configuration is preferred (Fig. 35–3). In the anteroanterior configuration, the paddles should be 10 cm away from the pacemaker if possible. After defibrillation, transient loss of capture or sensing should be anticipated. The pulse amplitude may need to be increased, and this increase is automatic in ICDs with backup bradycardia pacing. The pacemaker should be interrogated and the program checked. Transient rises in threshold should be managed by increasing the output energy if necessary. Rarely, prolonged, severe threshold increases occur that necessitate lead replacement. Recommendations for management of patients undergoing cardioversion and defibrillation are summarized in Table 35–5.

Catheter Ablation

Catheter ablation of intracardiac structures to control arrhythmias was first performed with direct current shock. This technique had a higher tendency to affect pacemakers than does external defibrillation. About 50% to 60% of patients in three series experienced problems, including activation of the backup or reset mode, pacemaker circuit failure, and transient rises in pacing and sensing thresholds.[32-34] Direct current catheter ablation should be avoided in patients with permanent pacemakers or ICDs if alternative therapy is available.

Nearly all ablations are now done with radiofrequency current, which is the same as coagulation electrocautery—that is, unmodulated radiofrequency current at a frequency of 400 to 500 kHz. Effects similar to those of surgical electrocautery have been reported, including inappropriate inhibition, asynchronous pacing, and resetting to

Table 35–5. Cardioversion-Defibrillation in the Patient With a Pacemaker or Implantable Cardioverter-Defibrillator

- Ideally, place paddles in the anteroposterior position
- Try to keep paddles at least 4 inches from the pulse generator
- Have the appropriate programmer available
- Interrogate the device after the procedure

backup mode.[35-37] An example of oversensing due to sensing of radiofrequency energy during the NSP is shown in Figure 35–4.

The ablation catheter is usually some distance from the lead, and radiofrequency ablation has been accomplished safely in patients with implanted pacemakers and ICDs and does not appear to result in any significant myocardial damage at the site of the electrode. Some operators actually prefer to place the permanent pacemaker before AV nodal ablation. Performing the procedure in this sequence obviates temporary pacemaker placement.

Before radiofrequency ablation is performed, however, it is essential to interrogate the device, record its programmed settings, and measure thresholds. Rate-modulation sensors should be switched off. A programmer should be available during the procedure. After the procedure, the pulse generator should be checked and reprogrammed if necessary.

Magnetic Resonance Imaging

In magnetic resonance imaging (MRI), a large magnetic field generated by an electromagnet is modulated by a radiofrequency electrical signal of 30 to 3000 Hz. Ferrous metal objects are attracted by the electromagnet and are not allowed near the scanner. Most contemporary devices contain little ferromagnetic material; however, the ferromagnetic content of pacemakers manufactured in the 1980s varied considerably. Patients with pacemakers containing ferromagnetic material could experience torque forces when placed near the strong static magnetic field in the MRI suite.[38]

When a pacemaker is near an MRI scanner with the electromagnet "on," the reed switch closes, and asynchronous pacing occurs, which may compete with the underlying cardiac rhythm. Measuring the effect of the MRI scanner on pacemakers is made difficult because the radiofrequency pulses cause ECG artifacts. Several studies, however, have demonstrated the potential effects by use of pacemakers connected to dogs with special monitoring. In some pacemakers, the only effect was asynchronous pacing.[39] In other pacemakers, however, a signal of about 20 V was induced in the lead,[41] which can cause cardiac pacing at the same frequency or a multiple of the frequency of the radiofrequency current.[39-41] Thus, cardiac pacing may occur at the frequency of the pulsed energy, 60 to 300 bpm. In a dual-chamber pacemaker, this may affect the atrial channel or the ventricular channel or both. The radiofrequency signal is detected by the leads acting as an antenna and is then

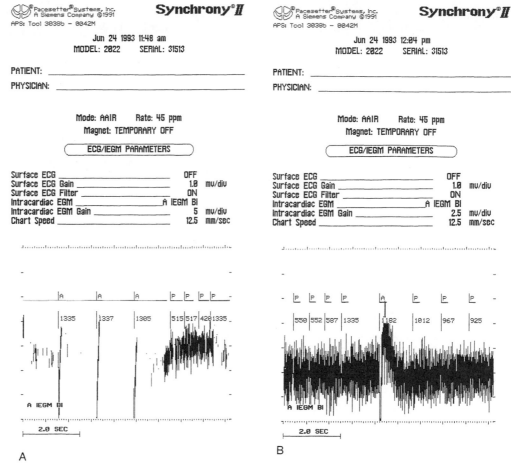

Figure 35–4. Atrial electrograms recorded from a patient with an incessant atrial tachycardia and a Pacesetter Synchrony II generator (model 2022, Sylmar, CA) during radiofrequency ablation. During these recordings, the pacemaker was programmed to the AAI mode at 45 bpm with a sensitivity of 0.5 mV and an atrial refractory period of 225 msec. *A,* In the 11:48 AM recording, asynchronous atrial pacing is due to continuous sensing of noise and extension of the refractory period. These occur intermittently during the delivery of the radiofrequency lesion. *B,* Several minutes later, the patient remains in atrial tachycardia (cycle length, 550 to 587 msec) as radiofrequency energy is applied. There are sensing of noise and extension of the refractory period, which stop several seconds later as the atrial tachycardia is terminated during formation of the radiofrequency lesion. A, atrial pacing; P, atrial sensing; ECG, electrocardiogram; IEGM, intracardiac electrogram.

amplified by the pacemaker circuitry to produce sufficient energy to pace the heart. Because the lead must be attached to a pacemaker for pacing to occur, it is not simply related to the radiofrequency energy in the lead.[40] The lead does not necessarily have to be in use, however, as demonstrated in a canine study in which a dual-chamber pacemaker with both atrial and ventricular leads attached but programmed to the AAI mode produced rapid ventricular pacing in the vicinity of an MRI scanner.[42]

Reported problems of pacemakers in MRI scanners include magnet-activated asynchronous pacing, inhibition by the radiofrequency signal, rapid pacing induced by the radiofrequency signal,[38–43] discomfort at the pacemaker pocket, and death of an unmonitored patient.[44] In the canine model, transient reed switch malfunction has also been seen.[40] There are no published reports of pacemaker reprogramming or of permanent component damage by MRI.

In phantom studies, Achenbach and colleagues[38] demonstrated significant heating of the electrode tip during MRI exposure. The documented temperatures at the electrode tip were as high as 88.8°C, or an increase of 63.1°C from the starting temperature of 25.7°C. They warned that although clinical complications from electrode heating have not been reported, clinicians should be aware of this potentially adverse effect.

External pacemakers are also subject to interference from MRI. If operation is in the inhibited mode, the radiofrequency signal is sufficient to inhibit the pacemaker output.

Pacemaker response to MRI may also vary by manufacturer and by model from an individual manufacturer. Some companies comment on MRI in their technical manuals. Some advocate that MRI be a firm contraindication in the patient, and others suggest that MRI be used with caution. There have been at least five patients with pacemakers who have died during MRI scanning. No precautions were taken to monitor or rescue these patients because the presence of the pacemaker was determined only after the patient had died.[44] On the other hand, many patients have had clinical MRI scans without morbidity or mortality. Many of these patients, who mostly underwent head MRI, were specifically monitored with pulse oximetry and a rescue team with an external defibrillator was available.[45] In general, patients with pacemakers should not routinely undergo MRI scanning until further study results are available. Patients who require head MRI scanning without alternative diagnostic possibilities, however, may be best served in a carefully monitored setting.

Extracorporeal Shock Wave Lithotripsy

Extracorporeal shock wave lithotripsy (ESWL) is a noninvasive treatment for nephrolithiasis and cholelithiasis that delivers multiple, focused hydraulic shocks, generated by an underwater spark gap, to a patient lying in a water bath. The shock is focused on the calculi by an ellipsoid metal reflector. Because the shock wave can produce ventricular extrasystoles, it is synchronized to the R wave. Pacemakers could be subject to electrical interference from the spark gap and mechanical damage from the hydraulic shock wave.

Several investigators[46-48] have studied the effect of ESWL on pacemakers suspended in a water bath and on pacemakers strapped to the bodies of patients undergoing ESWL. Pacemaker output was not inhibited by the synchronous shocks, but asynchronous shocks caused inhibition in both unipolar and bipolar devices.[46, 48] The risk of pulse generator inhibition may be lower with single-chamber devices than with dual-chamber devices. Intermittent reversion to magnet mode and rate during lithotripsy has been reported to occur because of transient closure of the reed switch from the high-energy vibration created by the lithotripsy machine. Other responses noted during in vitro testing were an increase in rate of some pulse generators, failure of output (rare), and malfunction of the reed switch. Activity-sensing pacemakers increased their pacing rate to the upper pacing rate within 1 minute of the shock.[48] When a dual-chamber pacemaker was tested, the shock was synchronized to the atrial pacing pulse but was frequently sensed by the ventricular channel, causing either inhibition of the ventricular output if ventricular safety pacing was not enabled or safety pacing at a shortened AV interval if safety pacing was enabled.[47, 48]

ESWL caused no physical damage to the hermetic seal or the internal components of the pacemakers tested,[47, 48] except that when an activity-sensing pacemaker was placed at the focal point of the ESWL, the piezoelectric crystal was shattered.[47] Patients with piezoelectric crystal activity rate-adaptive pacemakers can probably undergo lithotripsy safely if the device is implanted in the thorax, but lithotripsy should be avoided if the device is located in the abdomen.

Subsequent to these in vitro studies, several reports appeared of patients with implanted cardiac pacemakers undergoing ESWL without any ill effects.[47, 49, 50] In addition, no instances of reprogramming of pulse generators or conversion to reset or backup mode have been reported.

ESWL is safe to use with implanted pacemakers, provided that the shock is given synchronously with the ECG and that dual-chamber pacemakers have safety pacing enabled. An activity-sensing pacemaker may develop an increase in rate after the shock, and if this is considered clinically undesirable, the pacemaker should be programmed to the non–rate-responsive mode. Careful pacemaker follow-up should be continued for the next several months to ensure appropriate function of the reed switch. Physicians should contact the pulse generator's manufacturer to ascertain whether any clinical experience is available with that particular generator in patients undergoing lithotripsy.

Some investigators recommend that if insufficient experience exists with a particular device, in vitro testing may be helpful. In addition, programming of a DDD pulse generator to the VVI, VOO, or DOO mode avoids the rare cases in which irregularities of pacing rate may occur, supraventricular arrhythmias that could be tracked are induced, or triggering of the ventricular output by electromechanical interference occurs.

Implantable defibrillators have also been studied, but to a much lesser extent. It is best to disable the tachycardia detection during lithotripsy and to test the unit thoroughly after the procedure. If the patient is pacemaker dependent, the same precautions taken for the pacemakers is appropriate. Many of the ICDs have piezoelectric crystals to make

sounds instead of the rate response. These devices should not be placed near the focal point of the therapy.[51]

Transcutaneous Electrical Nerve Stimulation

Transcutaneous electrical nerve stimulation (TENS) is now a widely used method for the relief of acute and chronic pain from musculoskeletal and neurologic problems. A TENS unit consists of several electrodes placed on the skin and connected to a pulse generator that applies 20-μsec rectangular pulses of 1 to 200 V and 0 to 60 mA at a frequency of 20 to 110 Hz. To provide maximum relief of pain, the patient can adjust the output and frequency of the unit.

The repetition frequency of the TENS output is similar to the normal range of heart rates, so that it would be expected that TENS pulses might cause pacemaker inhibition. However, a study of 51 patients who were monitored for 2 minutes during TENS stimulation showed no inhibition.[52] Instances of asymptomatic inhibition of pacemaker output by a TENS machine detected by ambulatory monitoring have been reported.[53, 54] These events took place in unipolar pacemakers and were eliminated by increasing the sensing threshold of the pacemaker (in one case to 5 mV). This effect has not been reported in dual-chamber pacemakers.

TENS can probably be used safely in most patients with bipolar pacemakers and ICDs. It is reasonable, however, to take special precautions in ICD and pacemaker-dependent patients and monitor them during initial TENS application. If TENS results in interference in patients with unipolar pacemakers, the testing can be repeated after the sensitivity is reprogrammed to a less sensitive value.

Dental Equipment

Dental ultrasound scalers may cause inhibition or asynchronous pacing in older pacemakers, but a study showed no effect on pacing function.[55] Repetitive activation of other dental equipment may cause inhibition.[56] As would be expected, dental drilling can cause sufficient vibration to increase the pacing rate of an activity-sensing pacemaker.[56]

Radiation

Diagnostic radiation has no effect on pacemakers. Therapeutic radiation did not affect the earliest pacemakers but can cause failure in newer pacemakers that incorporate complementary metal oxide semiconductor–integrated circuit technology.[57-62] Radiation causes leakage currents between insulated parts of the circuit, leading to inappropriate charge accumulation in silicon oxide layers, which eventually leads to circuit failure. ICDs have been shown to fail when exposed to radiation.[59]

Therapeutic radiation involves doses of up to 70 Gy, and pacemakers may fail with as little as 10 Gy. Failure is unpredictable and may involve changes in sensitivity, amplitude, or pulse width; loss of telemetry; failure of output; or runaway rates. If dysfunction occurs, device replacement is required. Although some changes may resolve in hours to days, the long-term reliability of the pulse generator is suspect, and the device should be replaced. Radiation therapy to any part of the body away from the site of the pulse generator should not cause a problem with the pulse generator, but the pulse generator should be shielded to avoid scatter.

Linear accelerators may cause EMI, leading to pacemaker inhibition or reversion to the noise mode in susceptible pacemakers, particularly devices programmed to a unipolar configuration.

Therapeutic radiation centers should have a protocol for patients with pacemakers.[62] Before radiation is delivered, the pacemaker should be identified and evaluated.

The most common clinical situation is development of a malignant lesion in the breast of a patient with a permanent pacemaker on the same side. The pacemaker must be moved out of the field of radiation because shielding the pacemaker would result in suboptimal radiation therapy. The pacemaker can be explanted and a new system implanted on the contralateral side. Alternatively, it is often possible to explant the pacemaker, tunnel the existing permanent pacing lead through the subcutaneous tissues to the contralateral side, form a new pacemaker pocket on the contralateral side, reattach the pacemaker to the tunneled lead, and reimplant the device.

Electroconvulsive Therapy

Electroconvulsive therapy appears safe for ICD and pacemaker function because only a slight amount of electricity reaches the heart owing to the high impedance of body tissues. ECG monitoring and interrogation of the pacemaker appear advisable. In unipolar pacemakers, seizure activity may generate sufficient myopotentials to result in inhibition or ventricular tracking.

Diathermy

Short-wave diathermy consists of therapeutic application of current directly to the skin. Diathermy can be a source of interference and should be avoided near the implantation site because of its high frequency. It has the potential to inhibit the pulse generator or damage the pulse generator circuitry by excessive heating.[1] Short-wave or microwave diathermy may provide signals of high enough frequency to bypass noise protection mechanisms and directly damage the pacemaker's electronic components.

Industrial Environment

Conventional wisdom has been to advise patients to avoid arc welding and close contact with combustion engines. This advice needs to be re-examined as pacemakers become more resistant to external interference. As previously discussed, however, pacemakers of unipolar sensing configuration remain more susceptible to EMI than pacemakers in a bipolar sensing configuration. This basic tenet should always be kept in mind when advising patients about potential EMI from any source. For patients whose livelihood involves equipment with the potential for EMI, a pacemaker with committed bipolar sensing configuration should be implanted.

Industrial environments with significant potential for clinically significant EMI with implantable devices include industrial-strength welding, that is, welding equipment of 500 A or more, degaussing equipment, and induction ovens. If a patient works in one of these environments or potentially some other even more obscure environment that suggests significant potential for EMI, the work environment should be carefully evaluated. If the patient is pacemaker dependent, consideration should be given to assessment of the work environment by an engineer from the pacemaker manufacturer. Most major companies are willing to send someone to the patient's work environment to conduct such testing. If the patient is not pacemaker dependent, assessment may be achieved by ambulatory monitoring during exposure to the environment or by use of patient-triggered event records stored within the pacemaker or ICD (Fig. 35–5).

From a practical standpoint, most patients who claim to do arc welding use low-amperage equipment for hobby welding. If the patient uses welding equipment in the 100- to 150-A range, significant EMI is unlikely to occur.[16] Before giving the patient permission to return to this activity, however, the pacemaker clinician must consider the type of hardware implanted and the dependency status.

Testing methods have been designed to allow exposure of the patient with a pacemaker or an ICD to progressively stronger fields of EMI.[16] Although this testing is not practical for the individual patient, levels of interference have been determined at several programmed sensitivities[16] (Table 35–6). This information could be applied to an individual patient if readings of "milligauss" strengths in the work environment could be obtained.

Nonindustrial and Home Environments

Although few sources are capable of causing clinically significant EMI resulting in pulse generator malfunction, the possibility of interference from cellular phones and electronic article surveillance equipment has been of intense interest because of the potential public health issues. Before these are discussed in detail, several other potential

Table 35–6. Electromagnetic Interference Levels in Work Environments Capable of Pacemaker Interference

| Sensitivity Setting (mV) | Milligauss Units | | | |
| | Atrial | | Ventricular | |
	Unipolar	Bipolar	Unipolar	Bipolar
0.50	4,509	17,984	1,720	14,240
0.75	5,744	20,000	NA	NA
1.00	7,679	20,000	4,705	18,100
1.50	10,143	20,000	NA	NA
2.00	11,790	20,000	7,454	19,630
3.00	15,034	20,000	10,003	20,000

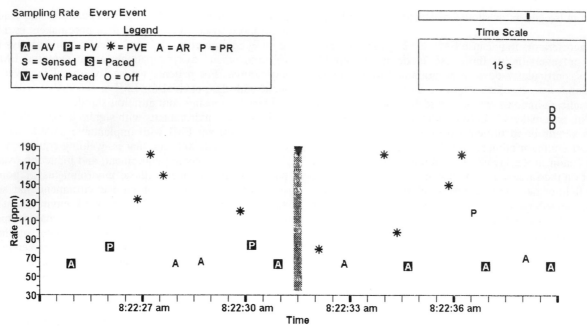

Figure 35-5. Event record obtained from a dual-chamber pacemaker implanted in a pacemaker-dependent patient. Normal pacemaker function was noted before and after electromagnetic interference (EMI) exposure, and the underlying rhythm was P-synchronous pacing at a rate of about 85 ppm. The 15-second event recording displayed was the peak of interference noted during testing. The first event displayed was atrioventricular sequential pacing. This indicated that the atrial sensing circuit was in the noise mode and could not sense intrinsic P waves. The second event was a P-synchronous event at 85 ppm, which was normal for this patient. Events 3, 4, and 5 represented oversensing of the EMI by the ventricular sensing circuit and were interpreted by the pacemaker as premature ventricular events (PVE). Events 6 and 7 were oversensing of EMI in the atrial channel, resulting in operation in the noise mode (in this pacemaker, noise mode operation is asynchronous pacing in the channel in which the oversensing occurs). At the same time, oversensing of the EMI in the ventricular channel resulted in inhibition of ventricular output. The 18th event was oversensing in both channels, inhibiting both atrial and ventricular outputs. Only seven paced events occurred during this 15-second segment, and this resulted in patient symptoms. Because symptoms occurred during exposure to the EMI source, the patient was advised to avoid this source in the future. AV, timing from a paced atrial event to a paced ventricular event; PV, timing from an intrinsic atrial event to a paced ventricular event; AR, timing from a paced atrial event to an intrinsic ventricular event; PR, timing from an intrinsic atrial event to an intrinsic ventricular event.

sources—some of historical importance only—merit discussion.

One of the most common questions still asked by pacemaker recipients today is whether they can use a microwave oven. In many areas, signs are still posted warning the pacemaker patient not to use a microwave oven. The original warnings were put in place because ineffective microwave shielding and less effective shielding of early pacemakers created the potential for pacemaker interference. Microwave ovens are no longer considered a significant source of interference, partly because of effective shielding and interlocking circuitry that prevents them from being switched on while the door is open and partly because of significant advances in shielding of the pacemaker circuitry.

There are no reports of other normally functioning domestic appliances having any significant effect on modern pacemakers.[1] An electric shaver moved over a unipolar pacemaker might cause temporary asynchronous pacing. There are no reports of interference from mobile telephones or portable computers, but as this technology expands, it is possible that interference may be detected.

Metal detectors are frequently mentioned as a potential problem, and warning signs are often seen at airport security stations. However, a study of patients wearing ambulatory ECG monitors while passing through metal detector gates with pacemakers programmed to the most sensitive programmable option showed no effect on pacing.[63] Asynchronous pacing might occur for one or two beats without ill effect to the patient. The major reason to warn patients about metal detectors is that the ICD or pacemaker will likely activate the detector.

In the close vicinity of high-voltage power lines or substations, the electrical field may be strong enough to cause transient inhibition or asynchronous pacing in unipolar pacemakers, but it has no effect on bipolar pacemakers with normal sensitivity settings and only a rare effect at maximum sensitivity.[5] At 40 meters from a 400-kV power line, the field strength is less than 1 kV per meter and has no effect on either a unipolar or a bipolar pacemaker.[5]

Electronic Article Surveillance Equipment

Antitheft devices (electronic article surveillance equipment) in many department stores consist of a tag or marker sensed by an electromagnetic field as the customer walks through or by a "gate." Most systems consist of a "deactivator" that a cashier may use to remove or deactivate the tag after the purchase of an item. This allows the customer to purchase an item and leave the store without activating an alarm. These electronic antitheft devices, through multiple technologic means, generate electromagnetic fields in various ranges. In vitro testing of pulse generators and in vivo studies in patients with permanent pacemakers or ICDs have been done.[64-68] In an earlier study of 32 volunteers with 26 different pacemaker models, 1 of 22 patients with a single-chamber pacemaker experienced inhibition, whereas 7 of 10 patients with dual-chamber generators experienced inhibition of output, with long pauses occurring in most pacemaker-dependent patients.[64] Inhibition occurred when patients were in regions of low- and high-intensity magnetic fields of 10 kHz or at 300 Hz, or in both. Radiofrequency and pulsed electromagnetic fields did not affect pacemaker function. Alterations in pacing thresholds or programmed settings were not noted. The authors concluded that electronic antitheft devices can be dangerous to pacemaker patients, particularly if a unipolar DDD generator is implanted.[64]

In a study of the triggering of pacemakers and ICDs by electronic article surveillance equipment, 35 devices, 18 pacemakers and 17 ICDs, in 33 patients were exposed to six different electronic article surveillance detectors.[67] Of the six detectors, three were radiofrequency, one was magnetoacoustic, and two were magnetic devices. No reprogramming of or damage to the pulse generators was noted. Sixteen of the pacemakers responded with noise reversion, inhibition, or both when they were exposed to a magnetoacoustic system at a close range, that is, less than 18 inches. Reprogramming the sensitivity of the pacemaker could not abolish this effect. In addition, one epicardial, unipolar pacemaker exhibited inhibition or noise reversion in each magnetic device. No EMI effects were found on any of the ICDs. No EMI was detected in any patients during exposure to the radiofrequency system.

Another abstract reported on 53 patients with pacemakers exposed to two security systems, an antitheft device and an electromagnetic access device.[68] The difference between these devices was not described in the abstract. The authors noted pacemaker malfunction in 13% of the monitored patients exposed to the first security system. They then described one patient with a VVIR pacemaker that was reprogrammed to a backup VOO mode. It is not clear whether the one patient accounted for the 13% malfunction rate. With the second security system, a malfunction was detected in 4% of the patients tested. In patients with pacemakers with bipolar sensing configurations, no malfunctions were seen with exposure to any of the equipment. No patients, regardless of pacemaker sensing polarity, had abnormalities with exposure to the antitheft device or the electromagnetic access device. The authors recommended that patients who might be near security systems should preferentially receive pacing systems with bipolar sensing configuration.

Cellular Phones

Since 1994, the potential for wireless phone communication to interfere with pacemakers has been recognized. Beginning with in vitro studies, several investigators demonstrated various forms of interference resulting from handheld wireless phones.[69-71] Several in vivo studies showed that interference could potentially occur with various phones using digital technology, whereas analog phones appeared safe—that is, had no clinically significant EMI.[69, 71-73] At least one case report described injury in a pacemaker-dependent patient who used a digital cellular phone.[74]

In a multicenter study,[75] 980 patients were tested with as many as six telephones for a total of 5533 phone exposures. In this study, a highly variable incidence of interference was observed. The overall incidence, 20%, was high. However, to quote this single percentage out of context would be clinically misleading. Interference at the "normal" ear position used was very low, and none was clinically significant, a finding supporting the safety of normal use. The incidence of interference and, specifically, of clinically significant interference was also highly variable by combination of phone type, pacemaker manufacturer, and pacemaker model. If just one phone, the TDMA-11 (which is not being commercially produced), were eliminated from the analysis, the incidence of interference and clinically significant interference would decrease significantly, to 13.1% and 2.8%, respectively.

Although symptoms were present during 7.2% of the phone exposures, most were due to palpitations. The incidence of presyncope was highest in patients classified as completely dependent. Therefore, the greatest potential risk of presyncope was in patients who were at least intermittently pacemaker dependent. When episodes associated with TDMA-11 phones were eliminated, the incidence of presyncope was lower.

The incidence of interference was highly variable by pacemaker manufacturer. Even for a given manufacturer, the incidence varied by pacemaker model, a reflection of the effect of design on susceptibility to interference.

The highest incidence of interference occurred when the phone was directly over the pacemaker. Although this position might exist if the activated phone were carried in a pocket directly over the pacemaker, it is certainly not a normal position of use and could be consciously avoided. As stated earlier, minimal interference was present at the ear position. This finding was in agreement with findings of other studies examining the effect of distance on interference. Many studies have confirmed that most effects are limited to the space 8 to 10 cm from the pacemaker.[69]

Tracking of phone-induced interference by the atrial sensing circuitry was the most common type of interference (Fig. 35–6). Although tracking resulted in paced rates that were physiologically inappropriate without exertion, the rate of tracking was always limited by the programmed upper rate limit of the pacemaker, which had been set by the patient's physician. Because the atrial channel of a dual-chamber pacemaker is more sensitive, there is a greater opportunity for tracking and noise reversion response to EMI in dual-chamber pacemakers.

Ventricular inhibition was the next most common type of interference (Fig. 35–7). Clinically, ventricular inhibition is potentially one of the most significant forms of interference, and a pause of greater than 3 seconds is frequently considered to be clinically significant. Additionally, the frequency of symptoms, such as presyncope, increased with the duration of ventricular inhibition.

Although it is well known that pacemakers of unipolar

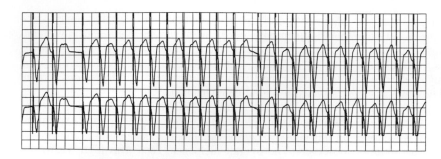

Figure 35–6. Ventricular tracking of noise sensed on the atrial sensing circuit in a patient with a dual-chamber pacemaker exposed to a cellular phone that is not commercially available.

sensing configuration are more susceptible to many forms of electromagnetic energy than pacemakers of bipolar sensing configuration, the multicenter study revealed a similar incidence of interference for pacemakers of unipolar and bipolar sensing configurations. Interference from wireless phones occurs at the header of the pacemaker and does not appear to depend on the distance between the cathode and the anode of the sensing circuit, so that sensing polarity is not a significant factor.

Specific pacemaker design changes, such as feedthrough filters, may limit EMI, as previously reported.[75] Although design changes have significantly reduced rates of interference, new phone technologies could have the potential for pacemaker interference and thus require further testing.

Information on ICD interference from cellular phones remains limited. Recent publications involving relatively small subsets of patients with ICDs or exposure to a limited variety of cellular phone technologies did not demonstrate any significant interference.[76, 77] Larger-scale studies are needed.

■ INTERACTION BETWEEN IMPLANTABLE DEVICES

This chapter has not attempted to consider pacemaker–ICD interactions, although obviously electromagnetic energy generated by a pacemaker could interfere with an ICD implanted in the same patient and vice versa. Recently, reports have appeared of pacemaker or ICD interference by permanently implanted devices for therapeutic purposes other than control of arrhythmia. Specifically, several recent reports considered the interaction of implantable arrhythmia-control devices with devices implanted for neurostimulation.[78, 79] The potential exists for interference from other implantable devices,

and further in vitro and observational in vivo studies are necessary.

Summary

Nearly all patients can be reassured that EMI will not affect their pacemakers during the course of daily life. Patients in specialized industrial environments should be assessed individually. In the course of medical treatment, patients should be carefully assessed and managed if they are to be exposed to electrocautery or have been subject to defibrillation. MRI scanning should continue to be regarded with caution, although some pacemaker manufacturers have reduced their warnings. Lithotripsy and TENS can generally be undertaken without adverse outcomes as long as simple precautions are taken. Regardless of the type of EMI device to which the patient may have been exposed, the pulse generator should always be reinterrogated after the procedure to ensure normal function and expected programming. Therapeutic irradiation in patients with ICDs or pacemakers should be carefully planned to prevent destruction of the circuitry.

Improvements in pacemaker and ICD resistance to EMI should continue to minimize clinical concerns. The potential for EMI should never be taken lightly, however, and appropriate screening and monitoring should be done to avoid adverse clinical outcomes. In addition, despite improvements in pacemaker resistance to EMI, other emerging technologies, such as cellular phones and electronic article surveillance equipment, result in new challenges for the patient with an implanted arrhythmia-control device. Assessment of newer technologies for potential interference to the patient with a pacemaker or ICD must continue.

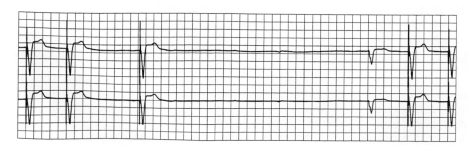

Figure 35–7. Ventricular inhibition in a patient with a single-chamber pacemaker during exposure to a cellular phone that is not commercially available.

REFERENCES

1. Barold SS, Falkoff MD, Ong LS, et al: Interference in cardiac pacemakers: Exogenous sources. *In* El-Sherif N, Samet P (eds): Cardiac Pacing and Electrophysiology, 3rd ed. Philadelphia, WB Saunders, 1991, p 608.
2. Irnich W: Interference in pacemakers. PACE 7:1021, 1984.
3. Grobety M, Perret F, Schlaepfer J, et al: Cardiac pacemaker dysfunction secondary to outside interference: A review [French]. Schweiz Med Wochenschr 126:723, 1996.
4. Toff WD, Edhag OK, Camm AJ: Cardiac pacing and aviation. Eur Heart J 13(Suppl H):162, 1992.
5. Toivonen L, Valjus J, Hongisto M, et al: The influence of elevated 50 Hz electric and magnetic fields on implanted cardiac pacemakers: The role of the lead configuration and programming of the sensitivity. PACE 14:2114, 1991.
6. Astridge PS, Kaye GC, Whitworth S, et al: The response of implanted dual chamber pacemakers to 50 Hz extraneous electrical interference. PACE 16:1966, 1993.
7. Hayes DL, Trusty J, Christiansen J, et al: A prospective study of electrocautery's effect on pacemaker function [Abstract]. PACE 10:686, 1987.
8. Kaye GC, Butrous GS, Allen A, et al: The effect of 50 Hz external electrical interference on implanted cardiac pacemakers. PACE 11:999, 1988.
9. Toff WD, Camm AJ: Implanted devices and aviation. Eur Heart J 9(Suppl G):133, 1988.
10. Falkoff M, Ong LS, Heinle RA, et al: The noise sampling period: A new cause of apparent sensing malfunction of demand pacemakers. PACE 1:250, 1978.
11. Sudduth BK, Morris DL, Gertz EW: Noise mode response at peak exercise in a DDD pacemaker. PACE 8:746, 1985.
12. Frohlig G, Dyckmans J, Doenecke P, et al: Noise reversion of a dual chamber pacemaker without noise. PACE 9:690, 1986.
13. Fontaine JM, Alma-Perri C, el-Sherif N: DDD-pacemaker pseudomalfunction during supraventricular tachycardia. PACE 11:1380, 1988.
14. Glikson M, Trusty JM, Grice SK, et al: Importance of pacemaker noise reversion as a potential mechanism of pacemaker-ICD interactions. PACE 21:1111, 1998.
15. Barold SS, Falkoff MD, Ong LS, et al: Resetting of DDD pulse generators due to cold exposure. PACE 11:736, 1988.
16. Marco D, Eisinger G, Hayes DL: Testing of work environments for electromagnetic interference. PACE 15:2016, 1992.
17. Seifert T, Block M, Borggrefe M, et al: Erroneous discharge of an implantable cardioverter defibrillator caused by an electric razor. PACE 18:1592, 1995.
18. Man KC, Davidson T, Langberg JJ, et al: Interference from a hand held radiofrequency remote control causing discharge of an implantable defibrillator. PACE 16:1756, 1993.
19. Schmitt C, Brachmann J, Waldecker B, et al: Implantable cardioverter defibrillator: Possible hazards of electromagnetic interference. PACE 14:982, 1991.
20. Ferrick KJ, Johnston D, Kim SG, et al: Inadvertent AICD inactivation while playing bingo. Am Heart J 121:206, 1991.
21. Levine PA, Balady GJ, Lazar HL, et al: Electrocautery and pacemakers: Management of the paced patient subject to electrocautery. Ann Thorac Surg 41:313, 1986.
22. Chauvin M, Crenner F, Brechenmacher C: Interaction between permanent cardiac pacing and electrocautery: The significance of electrode position. PACE 15:2028, 1992.
23. Belott PH, Sands S, Warren J: Resetting of DDD pacemakers due to EMI. PACE 7:169, 1984.
24. Lamas GA, Antman EM, Gold JP, et al: Pacemaker backup-mode reversion and injury during cardiac surgery. Ann Thorac Surg 41:155, 1986.
25. Bailey AG, Lacey SR: Intraoperative pacemaker failure in an infant. Can J Anaesth 38:912, 1991.
26. Heller LI: Surgical electrocautery and the runaway pacemaker syndrome. PACE 13:1084, 1990.
27. Van Hemel NM, Hamerlijnck RP, Pronk KJ, et al: Upper limit ventricular stimulation in respiratory rate responsive pacing due to electrocautery. PACE 12:1720, 1989.
28. Levine PA, Barold SS, Fletcher RD, et al: Adverse acute and chronic effects of electrical defibrillation and cardioversion on implanted unipolar cardiac pacing systems. J Am Coll Cardiol 1:1413, 1983.
29. Yee R, Jones DL, Klein GJ: Pacing threshold changes after transvenous catheter countershock. Am J Cardiol 53:503, 1984.
30. Calkins H, Brinker J, Veltri EP, et al: Clinical interactions between pacemakers and automatic implantable cardioverter-defibrillators. J Am Coll Cardiol 16:666, 1990.
31. Reiter MJ, Lindenfeld J, Breckinridge S, et al: Does defibrillation raise the ventricular pacing threshold? [Abstract]. J Am Coll Cardiol 11(Suppl):144A, 1988.
32. Bowes RJ, Bennett DH: Effect of transvenous atrioventricular nodal ablation on the function of implanted pacemakers. PACE 8:811, 1985.
33. Fontaine G, Lemoine B, Frank R, et al: Effects of fulguration on the permanent pacemaker. *In* Fontaine G, Scheinman MM (eds): Ablation in Cardiac Arrhythmias. Mt Kisco, NY, Futura, 1987, p 367.
34. Vanerio G, Maloney J, Rashidi R, et al: The effects of percutaneous catheter ablation on preexisting permanent pacemakers. PACE 13:1637, 1990.
35. Pfeiffer D, Tebbenjohanns J, Schumacher B, et al: Pacemaker function during radiofrequency ablation. PACE 18:1037, 1995.
36. Chin MC, Rosenqvist M, Lee MA, et al: The effect of radiofrequency catheter ablation on permanent pacemakers: An experimental study. PACE 13:23, 1990.
37. Ellenbogen KA, Wood MA, Stambler BS: Acute effects of radiofrequency ablation of atrial arrhythmias on implanted permanent pacing systems. PACE 19:1287, 1996.
38. Achenbach S, Moshage W, Diem B, et al: Effects of magnetic resonance imaging on cardiac pacemakers and electrodes. Am Heart J 134:467, 1997.
39. Gimbel JR, Lorig RJ, Wilkoff BL: Survey of magnetic resonance imaging in pacemaker patients. HeartWeb 1:1, 1996.
40. Holmes DR Jr, Hayes DL, Gray JE, et al: The effects of magnetic resonance imaging on implantable pulse generators. PACE 9:360, 1986.
41. Gimbel JR, Wilkoff BL: Safe performance of magnetic resonance imaging in five patients with permanent cardiac pacemakers. PACE 19:913, 1996.
42. Hayes DL, Holmes DR Jr, Gray JE: Effect of 1.5 Tesla nuclear magnetic resonance imaging scanner on implanted permanent pacemakers. J Am Coll Cardiol 10:782, 1987.
43. Fetter J, Aram G, Holmes DR Jr, et al: The effects of nuclear magnetic resonance imagers on external and implantable pulse generators. PACE 7:720, 1984.
44. Gimbel JR, Lorig RJ, Wilkoff BL: Safe magnetic resonance imaging of pacemaker patients [Abstract]. J Am Coll Cardiol 25(Suppl):11A, 1995.
45. Lauck G, von Smekal A, Wolke S, et al: Effects of nuclear magnetic resonance imaging on cardiac pacemakers. PACE 18:1549, 1995.
46. Langberg J, Abber J, Thuroff JW, et al: The effects of extracorporeal shock wave lithotripsy on pacemaker function. PACE 10:1142, 1987.
47. Cooper D, Wilkoff B, Masterson M, et al: Effects of extracorporeal shock wave lithotripsy on cardiac pacemakers and its safety in patients with implanted cardiac pacemakers. PACE 11:1607, 1988.
48. Fetter J, Patterson D, Aram G, et al: Effects of extracorporeal shock wave lithotripsy on single chamber rate response and dual chamber pacemakers. PACE 12:1494, 1989.
49. Stoller ML, Stackl W, Langberg JJ, et al: Extracorporeal shock wave lithotripsy performed on woman with a cardiac pacemaker. J Urol 140:1510, 1988.
50. Kanazawa T, Kishimoto T, Senju M, et al: A case of stone former with pacemaker treated by extracorporeal shock wave lithotripsy [Japanese]. Acta Urol Jpn 34:1415, 1988.
51. Chung MK, Streem SB, Ching E, et al: Effects of extracorporeal shock wave lithotripsy on tiered therapy implantable cardioverter defibrillators. PACE 22:738, 1998.
52. Rasmussen MJ, Hayes DL, Vlietstra RE, et al: Can transcutaneous electrical nerve stimulation be safely used in patients with permanent cardiac pacemakers? Mayo Clin Proc 63:443, 1988.
53. O'Flaherty D, Wardill M, Adams AP: Inadvertent suppression of a fixed rate ventricular pacemaker using a peripheral nerve stimulator. Anaesthesia 48:687, 1993.
54. Chen D, Philip M, Philip PA, et al: Cardiac pacemaker inhibition by transcutaneous electrical nerve stimulation. Arch Phys Med Rehabil 71:27, 1990.
55. Agarval A, Hewson J, Redding V: Ultrasound dental scalers and demand pacing [Abstract]. PACE 11:853, 1988.
56. Rahn R, Zegelman M: The influence of dental treatment on the Activitrax [Abstract]. PACE 11:852, 1988.
57. Adamec R, Haefliger JM, Killisch JP, et al: Damaging effect of therapeutic radiation on programmable pacemakers. PACE 5:146, 1982.

58. Venselaar JL, Van Kerkoerle HL, Vet AJ: Radiation damage to pacemakers from radiotherapy. PACE 10:538, 1987.

59. Rodriguez F, Filimonov A, Henning A, et al: Radiation-induced effects in multiprogrammable pacemakers and implantable defibrillators. PACE 14:2143, 1991.

60. Last A: Radiotherapy in patients with cardiac pacemakers. Br J Radiol 71:4, 1998.

61. Souliman SK, Christie J: Pacemaker failure induced by radiotherapy. PACE 17:270, 1994.

62. Marbach JR, Sontag MR, Van Dyk J, et al: Management of radiation oncology patients with implanted cardiac pacemakers: Report of AAPM Task Group No. 34. American Association of Physicists in Medicine. Med Phys 21:85, 1994.

63. Copperman Y, Zarfati D, Laniado S: The effect of metal detector gates on implanted permanent pacemakers. PACE 11:1386, 1988.

64. Dodinot B, Godenir JP, Costa AB: Electronic article surveillance: A possible danger for pacemaker patients. PACE 16:46, 1993.

65. Beaugeard D, Kacet S, Bricout M, et al: Interference between cardiac pacemaker and electromagnetic anti-theft devices in stores [French]. Arch Mal Coeur Vaiss 85:1456, 1992.

66. Moraes JC: Effects of electronic autodefense devices on cardiac pacemakers. Artif Organs 19:238, 1995.

67. McIvor M, Johnson D, Reddinger J, et al: Study of pacemaker and implantable cardioverter defibrillator triggering by EAS devices (SPICED TEAS): Part 2 [Abstract]. PACE 20:1109, 1997.

68. Wilke A, Kruse T, Funck R, et al: Security systems: Interferences with pacemakers [Abstract]. Eur Heart J 18(Suppl):482, 1997.

69. Hayes DL, Carrillo RG, Findlay GK, et al: State of the science: Pacemaker and defibrillator interference from wireless communication devices. PACE 19:1419, 1996.

70. Barbaro V, Bartolini P, Donato A, et al: Do European GSM mobile cellular phones pose a potential risk to pacemaker patients? PACE 18:1218, 1995.

71. Irnich W, Batz L, Muller R, et al: Electromagnetic interference of pacemakers by mobile phones. PACE 19:1431, 1996.

72. Wilke A, Grimm W, Funck R, et al: Influence of D-net (European GSM Standard) cellular phones on pacemaker function in 50 patients with permanent pacemakers. PACE 19:1456, 1996.

73. Naegeli B, Osswald S, Deola M, et al: Intermittent pacemaker dysfunction caused by digital mobile telephones. J Am Coll Cardiol 27:1471, 1996.

74. Yesil M, Bayata S, Postaci N, et al: Pacemaker inhibition and asystole in a pacemaker dependent patient. PACE 18:1963, 1995.

75. Hayes DL, Wang PJ, Reynolds DW, et al: Interference with cardiac pacemakers by cellular telephones. N Engl J Med 336:1473, 1997.

76. Sanmartin M, Fernandez Lozano I, Marquez J, et al: The absence of interference between GSM mobile telephones and implantable defibrillators: An in-vivo study. Groupe Systemes Mobiles [Spanish]. Rev Esp Cardiol 50:715, 1997.

77. Fetter JG, Ivans V, Benditt DG, et al: Digital cellular telephone interaction with implantable cardioverter-defibrillators. J Am Coll Cardiol 31:623, 1998.

78. Romano M, Zucco F, Baldini MR, et al: Technical and clinical problems in patients with simultaneous implantation of a cardiac pacemaker and spinal cord stimulator. PACE 16:1639, 1993.

79. Romano M, Brusa S, Grieco A, et al: Efficacy and safety of permanent cardiac DDD pacing with contemporaneous double spinal cord stimulation. PACE 21:465, 1998.

Chapter 36

Pediatric Pacing and Defibrillator Usage

Gerald A. Serwer, Parvin C. Dorostkar, and Sarah S. LeRoy

Permanent cardiac pacemakers have been used in children for more than 30 years.[1] Through advances in pacemaker technology, permitting greater customization of the pacemaker to the patient and a smaller generator size coupled with increased generator longevity, the use of cardiac pacemakers in children has been expanded. Although many aspects of pediatric pacing are similar to their counterparts in adult pacing, major differences exist. Not only are children physically smaller than adults, but also their underlying cardiac diseases are different. Their expected longevity, together with the lives that these children lead, is different. As a consequence of this, differences exist, not only in selection of the optimal pacing system but also in implantation techniques, programming considerations, and follow-up methods.

No pacemakers and only a limited number of electrodes are designed specifically with pediatric patients in mind. As a consequence, the manner in which these devices are used often requires modifications from the standard practice employed in adults. In this chapter, we discuss the unique aspects of pediatric pacing, specifically focusing on pacing indications, electrode and generator selection, implantation techniques, follow-up considerations and methods, and adjustments to the child's lifestyle that are necessitated by pacemaker implantation. Much of the material presented in other chapters is equally applicable to children, and therefore this chapter is intended as a supplement rather than a replacement for chapters dealing with similar material.

We also discuss the expanding use of implantable cardioverter-defibrillators (ICDs) in children. Although the use of ICDs is limited in children compared with adults, these devices are finding increasing utility, especially as their size decreases. Because of differing causes of ventricular tachyarrhythmias, as well as differing patient sizes, there are differences in the manner of ICD use that must be considered in pediatric patients.

■ MIDWEST PEDIATRIC PACEMAKER REGISTRY

Because the number of children requiring pacemakers is small, one difficulty plaguing research into pediatric pacing has been the lack of a large experience in any one center. This has led to conclusions based on limited experience that are susceptible to statistical inaccuracies. To address this problem, the Midwest Pediatric Pacemaker Registry was formed as a voluntary project of the members of the Midwest Pediatric Cardiology Society in 1980. Member institutions of this society submit data on patients requiring pacemaker implantation, consisting of patient demographics, pacing indication, associated structural cardiac disease, type of generator, type of electrode and threshold data at implantation, and device explantation data. No chronic follow-up data are provided. To promote the submission and validity of the data, annual reports are presented to the Midwest Pediatric Cardiology Society at its annual meeting. Concerns about the type of data collected and the method of data acquisition are discussed to ensure uniformity among participating institutions.

To date, the registry contains information on more than 900 patients who have had implantations of more than 1000 pulse generators and more than 1100 electrodes. These data present a representative sample of current pacing practice among pediatric cardiologists and avoid the bias inherent in data obtained from a single institution. The data are obtained at the time of implantation and subsequent invasive electrode evaluation. Figure 36–1 presents a summary of the data collected. Chronic follow-up data are confined to the date and reason that a generator or electrode was removed from service. Noninvasive electrode threshold data and reprogramming information after implantation are not collected. Throughout this chapter, much of the information presented on pacing indications, device selection, and acute thresholds was obtained from this source.

Patient Demographics

- ID number and institution
- Birthdate
- Date of initial implant
- Pacing indication
- Associated structural cardiac disease

Generator Information

- Manufacturer and model
- Implant date
- Programming at implant
- Explant date
- Programming at explant

Electrode Information

- Manufacturer and model
- Implant site and route
- Pacing thresholds (multiple pulse widths)
- Sensing values (RMS amplitude, slew rate)

Figure 36–1. Information collected by the Midwest Pediatric Pacemaker Registry. The data are collected on all new patients entered in the registry; all generators implanted and explanted; and all electrodes implanted, explanted, or invasively tested. ID, identification; RMS, mean spontaneous waveform amplitude.

■ INDICATIONS FOR PERMANENT PACEMAKER IMPLANTATION

Surgically Induced Heart Block

The single largest cause of pacemaker implantation in children remains surgically induced heart block. About 30% to 60% of children undergoing pacemaker implantation do so as a consequence of this.[2–7] Data from the Midwest Pediatric Pacemaker Registry show the indication for initial pacemaker placement to be surgically induced heart block in an average of 32% of patients (Fig. 36–2). The percentage varies from year to year; it reached a low of 20% in 1983 to 1984. There has been no definite downward trend during the past 10 years, although the underlying structural cardiac disease in patients with surgically induced heart block has changed dramatically. Most children acquiring surgical heart block in the last 5 years have complex disease and undergo complex surgical repairs. The surgical procedure resulting in the greatest incidence of heart block is the repair of an atrioventricular (AV) septal defect, which accounted for 17% of patients with surgical heart block since 1988. The other common diagnoses associated with surgical heart block during the past 5 years are listed in Figure 36–3.

Currently, it is unusual for a child with an isolated ventricular septal defect (VSD) to acquire heart block. This was not the case previously. During the past 5 years, VSD closure

accounted for only 14% of children with surgical complete heart block; atrial switch procedures (Mustard or Senning procedure) for the correction of dextro-transposition of the great arteries accounted for 12%. Other common lesions associated with surgical heart block are levo-transposition of the great arteries, repair of tetralogy of Fallot, and aortic valvular replacement, usually associated with the resection of a subaortic obstruction.

Surgical heart block can develop at the time of the initial cardiac repair or at some later point. In addition, the heart block acquired at the time of the repair may be temporary, with return of reliable AV conduction. For this reason, our current practice is to implant only temporary pacing electrodes at the time of the initial surgery and to defer permanent pacemaker implantation for 10 to 14 days in the hope of a return of AV conduction. However, ventricular escape rhythms are unstable, and no child with a permanent surgically acquired complete heart block is discharged without a permanent pacemaker. Even in the hospital, all children are supported with an external pacemaker through temporary pacing wires placed at the time of surgery until consistent AV conduction returns or a permanent pacemaker is inserted. Monitoring should consist of both electrocardiographic (ECG) monitoring and non-ECG monitoring, such as arterial pressure measurements or pulse oximetry. Many ECG monitors detect the pacing artifact and do not recognize the lack of capture with subsequent bradycardia or asystole. This is avoided by the use of a non-ECG method of detecting cardiac ejection.[8]

Congenital Complete Heart Block

The second most common indication for pacemaker implantation is congenital complete heart block. The cause of congenital heart block is variable. In many cases, an autoimmune mechanism can be implicated, with clinical or laboratory evidence of connective tissue disease in the mother.[9] Congenital block is also associated with specific forms of structural disease, particularly those involving abnormalities of the AV junction, such as levo-transposition of the great arteries with AV discordance and atrial situs ambiguous.[10] It is common for fetal heart block to "develop" in utero with intact conduction present in the young fetus and heart block developing at 20 to 30 weeks of gestation.

Data from the Midwest Pediatric Pacemaker Registry indicate that about 25% of patients have congenital heart block as the primary indication for permanent pacing. The age at which the pacing system is implanted varies, ranging from a few hours of age to older than 20 years of age. Most children with associated structural cardiac disease who require pacing before 1 year of age have congestive heart failure requiring an increased heart rate for adequate therapy. The mortality rate in such children is also high, with 43% dying by 2 years of age.[11]

For children with structurally normal hearts and congenital heart block, the incidence of pacemaker implantation is lower for the younger children but increases as the child ages, associated with a gradually decreasing ventricular rate.[12] This is associated with a gradual and steady increase in the need for permanent pacing that continues to increase with advancing age, reaching 75% by age 20 years (Fig. 36–4). The need for permanent pacing is due to the develop-

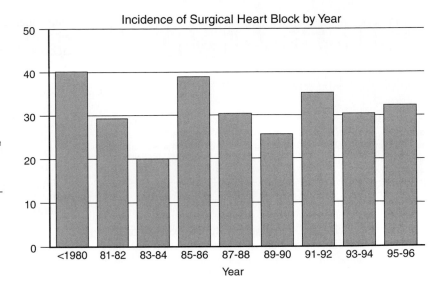

Figure 36–2. The percentage of all children undergoing initial pacemaker implantation in a given period, whose indication was surgically induced complete heart block. There has been no significant change in this percentage during the last 16 years. (Data from the Midwest Pediatric Pacemaker Registry.)

ment of syncope, congestive heart failure, or increasing ventricular ectopy, often associated with prolongation of the corrected QT interval (QTc). Death is rare in children with no structural cardiac disease (only 5% by 20 years of age), but it can occur suddenly.

Current recommendations call for the implantation of a permanent pacemaker system whenever congestive heart failure is present. In addition, implantation is recommended when the average heart rate is less than 50 bpm in the awake young infant, when there is a history of a syncopal or presyncopal event, when significant ventricular ectopy is present, or when there is exercise intolerance.[13, 14] However, symptoms of exercise intolerance can be difficult to elicit. Many children deny such symptoms, as do their parents, when in fact their exercise tolerance would be improved with permanent pacing. Many parents return after pacemaker implantation to relate that the activity level of their child has markedly increased. They are amazed at this change because they did not believe that the child was significantly hindered before pacemaker implantation. Exercise testing is often useful as an indicator of the child's exercise capabilities compared with those of a normal child. The physician should also periodically assess the child for increasing car-

diac size by chest roentgenography and decreasing cardiac function by echocardiography. The presence of either of these should be considered an indication for permanent pacemaker placement.

Finally, some children with congenital complete heart block develop tachydysrhythmias, specifically ventricular tachycardia, which can be controlled only with permanent pacing.[15] The maintenance of a minimal heart rate often suppresses the tendency toward ventricular ectopy, particularly during exercise. The development of tachyarrhythmias with the stress of exercise, even in children with otherwise asymptomatic disease, necessitates pacemaker implantation.

Controversy exists regarding the need for pacing in symp-

Most Prevalent Structural Cardiac Defects Associated with Surgical Complete Heart Block	
• Atrioventricular Septal Defects	17%
• Isolated Ventricular Septal Defect	14%
• D-Transposition of the Great Arteries	12%
• L-Transposition of the Great Arteries	12%
• Tetralogy of Fallot	7%
• Aortic Valve Replacement	3%

Figure 36–3. The most common structural cardiac lesions associated with surgically induced heart block at the time of complete repair for children undergoing initial implantation since 1988. D, dextro; L, levo. (Data from the Midwest Pediatric Pacemaker Registry.)

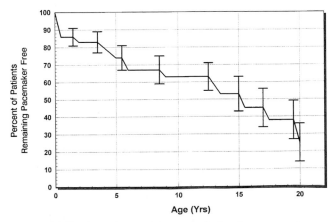

Figure 36–4. Actuarial analysis of months free from pacemaker need for children with congenital complete heart block and structurally normal hearts. By age 20 years, fewer than 30% of patients are pacemaker free. The brackets represent 1 standard error around the mean. (Data from Dorostkar P, Serwer GA, LeRoy S, Dick M II: Long-term course of children and young adults with congenital complete heart block. J Am Coll Cardiol 21:295A, 1993.)

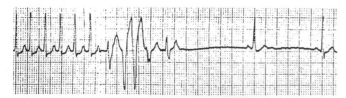

Figure 36–5. Electrocardiogram from a patient with sick sinus syndrome, demonstrating a 1.5-second period of asystole following acute termination of a tachyarrhythmia. Long pauses can result in syncope and are indications for pacemaker implantation. The paper speed is 25 mm/sec.

tom-free older children with bradycardia of less than 50 bpm while asleep. This is not an absolute indication for pacemaker implantation. However, when bradycardias below 50 bpm are present, a detailed history and close follow-up are required to determine the need for pacemaker implantation.

Sick Sinus Syndrome

The next most common indication for cardiac pacing in children is sick sinus syndrome. This indication is listed for about 15% of the patients in the Midwest Pediatric Pacemaker Registry. Most of these patients have undergone cardiac surgery, specifically extensive atrial procedures. The single most common surgical procedure is the atrial switch operation for transposition of the great arteries.[16] The likelihood of needing permanent pacing in this situation increases with the time from surgery.[17] The indications are similar to those for congenital complete heart block. In addition, the presence of tachyarrhythmias, with the subsequent risk for prolonged asystole after acute termination of the tachycardia, is also an indication for pacemaker implantation (Fig. 36–5). In patients with sick sinus syndrome after an atrial switch operation, our practice is to recommend pacemaker implantation in all patients with sleeping heart rates of less than 30 bpm even in the absence of symptoms. The need for medications known to affect AV conduction for the control of tachyarrhythmias in these patients would also necessitate pacemaker placement.[17]

Other Indications

Patients with intermittent complete heart block either secondary to lesions such as cardiac rhabdomyomas associated with tuberous sclerosis (Fig. 36–6) or idiopathic and those with long QT syndrome and uncontrollable ventricular tachycardia may also benefit from pacemaker placement.[18] A chronic increase in heart rate shortens the QT interval and decreases the occurrence of ventricular tachycardia. The combined use of pacing and an ICD may be even more efficacious, particularly with the development of the dual-chamber ICD.

Other indications for pacemaker placement reported in the Midwest Pediatric Pacemaker Registry include the control of atrial tachyarrhythmias unresponsive to pharmacologic therapy, second-degree heart block associated with symptoms, and concern about a sudden loss of AV conduction in patients receiving certain antiarrhythmic therapy known to interfere with AV conduction. Although such indications are rare, the clinician should not restrict pacemaker use to those children with complete heart block. First-degree heart block and trifascicular block with no documented loss of AV conduction are not considered indications for pacemaker implantation.[19]

A relatively new indication for pacemaker placement is symptomatic hypertrophic obstructive cardiomyopathy with significant outflow tract obstruction. Although not effective in all children with this disorder, both hemodynamic and symptomatic improvement have been observed.[20] Decreases in gradient and measures of diastolic performance were observed. Generators used for this indication must allow programming of relatively short AV intervals and rate-adaptive AV intervals to maximize the QRS width and degree of pre-excitation. Younger patients with more rapid heart rates may present insurmountable difficulties.

Categorization of pacing indications is helpful only as a general guide. Each patient must be carefully evaluated to determine the benefits from permanent pacing in light of the risks of implantation and the burden placed on the family and child for the subsequent care needed.

■ SELECTION OF THE APPROPRIATE PACEMAKER SYSTEM

Many factors must be considered in the selection of the most appropriate pacemaker generator and electrode system for an individual child. Unlike that in the adult patient, the 5-year survival rate following pacemaker implantation exceeds 70% in children (Fig. 36–7), and death is usually related to the underlying structural heart defect.[6, 21] Thus, pacing may

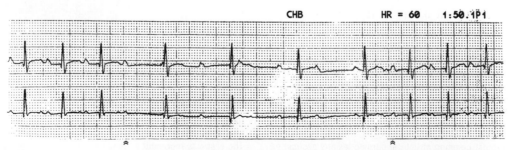

Figure 36–6. Recording from a 24-hour ambulatory electrocardiogram showing a period of complete heart block (CHB) with acute bradycardia (between the *arrowheads*) in a patient with tuberous sclerosis and cardiac rhabdomyomas. The paper speed is 25 mm/sec. HR, heart rate (in beats per minute).

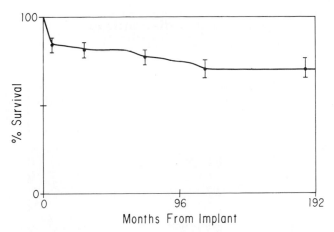

Figure 36–7. Actuarial survival for patients following pacemaker implantation. Excellent patient longevity is demonstrated. The brackets represent 1 standard error around the estimate. (From Serwer GA, Mericle JM: Evaluation of pacemaker pulse generator and patient longevity in patients aged 1 day to 20 years. Am J Cardiol 59:824, 1987.)

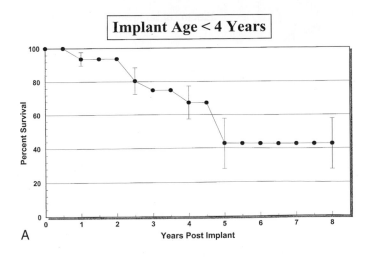

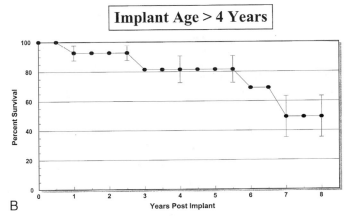

Figure 36–9. DDD generator longevity when using epicardial electrodes as a function of patient age at the time of implantation. Panel *A* provides a life table analysis of longevity when implanted in children younger than 4 years of age. More than half require replacement before 5 years. Panel B provides longevity analysis when implant age is more than 4 years. Half life has risen to 6.5 years, presumably owing to the lower average heart rates in older children.

be needed for more than 50 years in the average child. This affects pacing choices because the number of replacement generators and electrodes may be high. The average longevity of the currently available lithium-powered pulse generators is only 5 years when all children are grouped together (Fig. 36–8). However, when children are divided into those younger than 4 years and older than 4 years at the time of generator implantation, longevity is markedly different (Fig. 36–9). The generator half-life is 5 years in children younger than 4 years of age and increases to 7 years for the older children. This is presumably due to the higher heart rates present in younger patients, when in the dual-chamber mode tracking the atrial rate, or to the higher programmed rates used in younger children.

The average epicardial electrode lasts 7 years.[22] Although the average endocardial electrode's longevity in children is significantly increased, it is still only slightly more than 10 years (Fig. 36–10).[23] In the child undergoing an initial implantation at age 1 year, a minimum of nine electrode changes and 17 generator changes can be expected. The fact that multiple procedures will be needed and the effect of one procedure on subsequent procedures must be considered.

Generator Selection

The major factors to be considered must be the features of the generator that are of significant benefit to the individual child, a battery capacity coupled with a projected generator's longevity, and the size of the generator. Because newer generators are smaller than prior ones, size is becoming less of a factor; yet, all are not the same size. Large generators not only create unsightly protuberances that can have negative psychological consequences but also increase the risk for skin breakdown over the generator because of erosion of

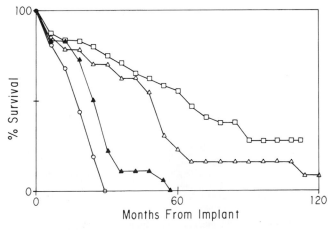

Figure 36–8. Actuarial survival curve for generators using various battery types. Even for lithium-powered generators, only half of generators last 5 years. Current models using lithium batteries; models using mercury-zinc batteries; models using mercury-silver batteries; models using rechargeable batteries. (From Serwer GA, Mericle JM: Evaluation of pacemaker pulse generator and patient longevity in patients aged 1 day to 20 years. Am J Cardiol 59:824, 1987.)

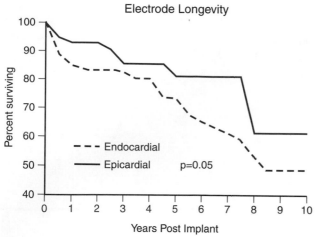

Figure 36–10. Actuarial analysis of endocardial *(solid line)* and epicardial *(dashed line)* electrode survival. Half of epicardial electrodes last about 8 years; for endocardial electrodes, the 50% survival time is greater than 10 years. The curves are significantly different ($P = .05$). (Epicardial electrode data from Serwer GA, Mericle JM, Armstrong BE: Epicardial ventricular pacemaker electrode longevity in children. Am J Cardiol 61:104, 1988; endocardial electrode data from Serwer G, Uzark K, Dick M II: Endocardial pacing and electrode longevity in children. J Am Coll Cardiol 15:212A, 1990.)

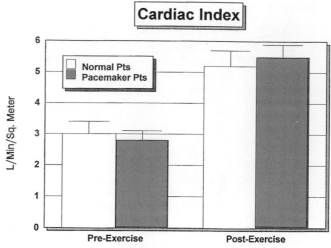

Figure 36–11. Changes in cardiac index as measured by acetylene rebreathing from rest to maximal exercise in normal children and those with fixed-rate ventricular pacing. The cardiac index was identical at rest and maximal exercise. The brackets represent 1 standard error around the mean. Pts, patients. (Data from Serwer G, Dick M II, Eakin B: Cardiac output response to treadmill exercise in children with fixed-rate pacemakers. Circulation 84:II-514, 1991. By permission of the American Heart Association, Inc.)

the generator or trauma to the skin over the generator, especially in the active child, with a subsequent infection leading to pacing system removal.

Generator Mode Selection

The choices concerning the pacing mode to use are related to single-chamber versus dual-chamber pacing and fixed-rate versus rate-variable pacing. In general, it has been our policy to avoid the use of fixed-rate pacemakers, except in situations in which sinus and AV node function are intact for most of the time, with the pacemaker serving only as a backup for those times when such function is not adequate. This is often the situation when sinoatrial (SA) and AV node function is marginal and antiarrhythmic drugs are required. Even in these cases, generators capable of rate-variable operation are preferable because the electrophysiologic state may change, and this allows for a change in mode without replacement of the generator. In addition, should a sudden rate drop occur during exercise, the lower rate of a fixed-rate generator may be inadequate to provide an adequate cardiac output. There is no difference in the size or capacity of the battery between fixed-rate and rate-variable units, and the difference in cost is minimal.

Although cardiac output increases with exercise, even during fixed-rate pacing (Fig. 36–11), this occurs as a result of a large increase in stroke volume (Fig. 36–12), with presumed increased wall stress and potentially increased myocardial work compared with the same change in cardiac output when a heart rate increase is possible.[24] However, enhanced exercise tolerance is achieved when rate-variable pacing is used.[25] This suggests an advantage to rate-variable pacing in the child expected to lead an active life. The rate-responsive mode should always be used unless the patient can demonstrate an adequate intrinsic rate response to exercise by exercise testing or ambulatory ECG.

Single-chamber pacing in either the atrium or the ventricle has been advocated for the treatment of sick sinus syndrome.[13] When atrial pacing is chosen, the presence of normal AV node function must be established by provocative electrophysiologic testing before implantation, especially in the postsurgical patient, because AV nodal disease can ac-

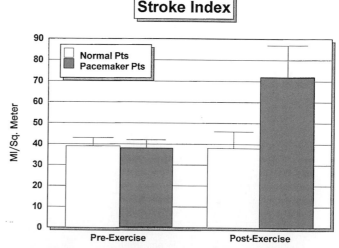

Figure 36–12. Stroke index changes from rest to maximal exercise in normal children and those with fixed-rate ventricular pacemakers. Pre-exercise values were similar; the stroke index increased significantly in the patients with pacemakers to provide an increased output in the face of a fixed heart rate. The brackets represent 1 standard error around the mean. Pts, patients. (Data from Serwer G, Dick M II, Eakin B: Cardiac output response to treadmill exercise in children with fixed-rate pacemakers. Circulation 84:II-514, 1991. By permission of the American Heart Association, Inc.)

company SA nodal disease and may not be apparent in the resting nonprovoked state. AAI(R) pacing has the advantage of preserving the normal ventricular activation sequence with potentially better cardiovascular function. In addition, some evidence in animals points toward the long-term development of myocardial changes when an abnormal pattern of myocardial activation is present.[26] A comparison of cardiac myocyte changes between ventricular free wall pacing and high septal pacing near the bundle of His with a subsequently narrower QRS morphology is striking. However, the clinical implication of these changes is unknown.

Atrial electrodes are less reliable than ventricular electrodes, even when placed endocardially. As such, conditions associated with early atrial electrode failure should serve as a contraindication to AAI pacing. Such conditions include prior extensive atrial surgery in which extensive atrial fibrosis is likely, small atrial size, and prior placement of a large intra-atrial baffle, limiting venous access to viable atrial tissue. After Fontan's procedure (right atrial to pulmonary artery connection), patients also have a low-flow velocity present within the atrium, increasing the risk for venous thrombosis when endocardial electrodes are placed. This is one situation in which long-term anticoagulation may be indicated.

Single-chamber ventricular pacing—VVI(R)—allows the use of more stable electrode systems and, in the rate-responsive mode, still allows rate variability to be maintained. The importance of atrial systole in the maintenance of the cardiac output is debatable and varies from child to child. Because most children have good myocardial function, the atrial contribution is probably minimal. The cardiac output increase with exercise is improved in children with DDD versus VVI pacing. It is unclear, however, whether this increase is the result of atrial synchrony or rate variability. Pacemaker syndrome from VVIR pacing is rare in children and is generally not a concern in choosing between single- and dual-chamber pacing. The major factor to be considered in such a choice is the difficulty in placing an adequate atrial electrode. If prior surgery or underlying structural disease precludes atrial electrode placement, single-chamber pacing is an acceptable alternative. However, dual-chamber pacing should be considered for all patients, with single-chamber pacing used only if contraindications to dual-chamber pacing (as discussed later) exist. Even in patients with sick sinus syndrome, dual-chamber pacing should be considered, particularly if AV nodal function is suspect.

We now consider dual-chamber pacing to be the mode of choice in children and use single-chamber pacing only when a contraindication to dual-chamber pacing exists. The major contraindications to the use of dual-chamber pacing include (1) persistent atrial tachyarrhythmias; (2) changing AV nodal status, making numerous programming changes necessary; and (3) inability to place reliable atrial and ventricular electrodes. Examples of this last contraindication would be (1) the small child in whom endocardial pacing is preferred, but the presence of two electrodes in the superior vena cava might present a high risk for thrombosis, and (2) the child requiring epicardial electrode placement in whom atrial electrode placement would necessitate a greatly enhanced surgical procedure. This is of particular concern in the child who has undergone a median sternotomy with resultant severe mediastinal fibrosis. If the durability of the atrial electrode is a concern, the approach commonly used is to implant a

---

Contraindications to Dual Chamber Pacing

✳ Inability to place both an atrial and ventricular electrode
      Small patient size
      Limited venous access
      Extensive epicardial fibrosis

✳ Persistent atrial tachyarrhythmia
      Uncontrolled atrial flutter
      Arrhythmia easily triggered by atrial pacing
      Pacemaker inability to detect atrial arrhythmia
        and limit ventricular rate

✳ Changing electrophysiologic status of AV conduction

Figure 36–13. Contraindications to dual-chamber pacing in children. AV, atrioventricular.

---

unit with the ability to be programmed to the VVIR mode should the atrial electrode fail. The generator's size and functionality is no longer a consideration because dual- and single-chamber pacemakers are comparable in both regards. Figure 36–13 relates the most common reasons for not implanting a dual-chamber system.

Dual-chamber pacing in children has previously been underused. Midwest Pediatric Pacemaker Registry data show a significant increase in dual-chamber pacing, with 43% of generators implanted in 1991 to 1992 using the DDD or DDDR mode, increasing to a majority (68%) by 1995 to 1996. This is in marked contrast to the years before 1983, when less than 10% of generators were in the DDD mode (Fig. 36–14). Data from 1997 to 1999 showed 66% of implanted generators to be dual-chamber units. This increase in dual-chamber pacing has been the result of improvements in atrial epicardial electrodes, increased experience with endocardial pacing in children, the smaller size of dual-chamber generators, and a better understanding of the benefits of dual-chamber pacing.

Desirable Generator Features

Current pacemakers permit an almost infinite number of possible programming combinations, allowing far more programming possibilities than will ever be used in any given patient. Because of the diversity among pediatric patients, however, such programmability is necessary. There are certain features that are more important for children than for adults. In this section, we discuss those programming features considered to be essential in the pediatric patient, which should influence the choice of the most appropriate pacing generator for a given patient. We begin with a discussion of those features applicable to all generators, both single and dual chamber, and cover features unique to rate-responsive pacemakers and dual-chamber pacemakers.

General Characteristics

The most important consideration is related to the range of energy output available, which includes both the pulse width and the pulse amplitude programmability. Although most

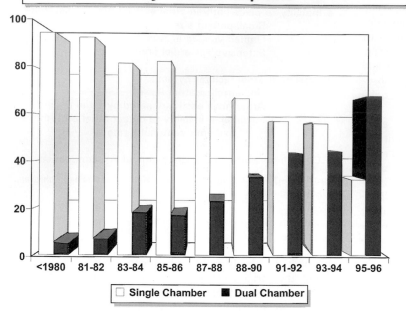

Figure 36–14. Comparison of the percentage of dual-chamber versus single-chamber generators implanted by year. Note the gradual shift from single-chamber to dual-chamber use. (Data from the Midwest Pediatric Pacemaker Registry.)

pacemakers are chronically programmed to have either 2.5 or 5 V of amplitude, the presence of other amplitudes is of key importance. Specifically, when a generator is used with an epicardial electrode, high-output features are mandatory. Although only a minority of children require chronic pacing at outputs greater than 5 V, many children have an initial threshold rise and temporarily require such high outputs. Even with endocardial implants, acute increases in thresholds can occur, and the ability to increase the pacemaker amplitude to 8 V may avert the necessity for emergent electrode replacement. In addition, threshold testing at multiple low-pulse amplitudes allows a more accurate determination of the characteristics of the strength–duration curve. This is mandatory to determine the lowest, but still safe, pulse amplitude and width settings. The strength–duration curve characteristics are not constant and vary not only with time but also in relationship to activity and the time of day.[27] Such changes are discussed more fully in relation to appropriate follow-up. Knowing where the steep part of the strength–duration curve begins is crucial for appropriate programming in which the clinician wants to ensure an adequate safety margin but, at the same time, minimize the energy output to maximize the generator's longevity. The ability to determine thresholds at a multitude of pulse amplitudes is a necessity.

The same argument also applies to the ability to vary duration of the pulse width. Again, although the pacemakers in most children are programmed to a relatively small number of pulse durations, the ability to have a much larger number of such settings available increases the accuracy with which the clinician can characterize the strength–duration curve.

The third universal parameter of key importance to children is the rate. Although the use of fixed-rate pacemakers is becoming less common, the availability of a wide range

of both lower and upper pacing rate limits is important in meeting the varying metabolic demands of the pediatric patient. Programming the upper rate limit of dual-chamber or rate-responsive pacemakers to values less than 150 bpm is inadequate, particularly in the small child. Even older patients can raise their heart rates above this value when exercising maximally in the absence of heart block; therefore, pulse generators must provide an upper rate limit of at least 180 bpm, and preferably higher. The lower rate limit needs are also variable. Immediately after surgery in children, greater lower rate limits are often necessary to maintain an adequate cardiac output. This is especially important after atrial surgery in patients in whom sinus node function may be impaired. In our opinion, lower rates must be programmable from at least 50 to 120 bpm.

Another parameter often overlooked is the refractory period. In single-chamber pacing, this is often fixed to an arbitrary value of 325 msec without much thought being given to whether this is appropriate. For the ventricular channel, this value must be of sufficient duration to prevent inappropriate T-wave sensing and yet not prevent sensing of spontaneous ventricular depolarizations. The measurement of the pace or sensing point to the T-wave interval from the intracardiac electrogram is straightforward (Fig. 36–15). In healthy children, the QT interval decreases with an increasing heart rate. When rate-variable pacing is used, the ventricular refractory period may be appropriate at rest but too long during exercise. Ideally, the ventricular refractory period should vary with the pacing rate. Thus, this value must be long enough to prevent T-wave sensing at the resting heart rate and short enough not to limit the upper pacing rate inappropriately. It is not uncommon for children with complete heart block to have spontaneous ventricular beats during the stress of exercise, which must be appropriately sensed. Appropriate programming is discussed later. Again,

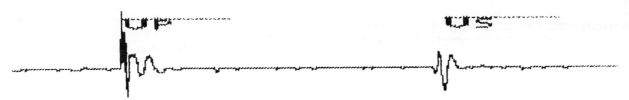

Figure 36–15. Intracardiac electrogram from a patient with VVI pacing showing the duration of the ventricular refractory period (*dashed line*) after either ventricular pacing (VP) or sensing (VS). In this example, the ventricular refractory period extends well beyond the termination of electric activity seen by the electrode to prevent inappropriate T-wave sensing.

the wider the range of available refractory periods that is permitted, the more universally applicable the pacemaker generator is to the entire pediatric population.

For AAI(R) pacing, the refractory period must be long enough to prevent sensing of ventricular events but again not be too limiting in terms of the upper rate. Recording of the intracardiac electrogram shows the extent to which ventricular events are seen by the pacemaker and the minimum value to which the atrial refractory period may be safely programmed (Fig. 36–16). Appropriate programming may be difficult and is a problem with AAI(R) pacing.

Rate-Responsive Pacing

For the single-chamber rate-responsive pacemaker, appropriate settings to mimic the pediatric response to exercise are mandatory. During exercise, the healthy child's heart rate increases in a linear manner with the increasing intensity of exercise (Fig. 36–17).[28] When healthy children are exercised using the Bruce protocol, the heart rate increases an average of 20 bpm with each subsequent increase in exercise stage. This continues throughout the course of the exercise. After an abrupt increase in exercise intensity (i.e., by advancing from stage I to II), the heart rate shows a sudden rapid increase, reaching a plateau value. Thus, the pacemaker increase its rate in an appropriate manner with increasing exercise intensity—and this must occur quickly, reaching a plateau value rapidly for that level of intensity. Therefore, not only must the heart rate increase to an appropriate degree, but also it must increase in an appropriate time frame to mimic the normal physiologic response to exercise in the pediatric patient.

After the termination of exercise, the heart rate decreases in an exponential fashion (Fig. 36–18). Although there is an initial rapid drop, the heart rate does not reach resting levels for at least 10 minutes. Inappropriate rapid declines in the heart rate after exercise termination may not meet the metabolic demands of the body and result in inadequate cardiac output and a syncopal episode.

With these considerations of the normal heart rate response to exercise in children taken into account, the ideal rate-responsive pediatric pacemaker must have the ability to offer a variety of linear increases in heart rate with increasing exercise intensity (rate-response curves). In addition, it should offer a range of acceleration times (the rate of the heart rate increase with increased exercise intensity), with more rapid acceleration times being preferred. Such increases in heart rate should be independent of resting and maximal rates. After the termination of exercise, the heart rate decline should be exponential but slow enough that the lower rate limit is not reached for a minimum of 10 minutes. Finally, the pacemaker must be able to tailor its detection of increasing exercise levels to the individual patient. Different manufacturers have used several approaches to address this problem, and it is unclear which approach is best. However, all manufacturers allow tailoring of exercise detection to the individual patient, realizing that not all patients produce the same characteristics detectable by the pacemaker in response to the same degrees of exercise. Although simplicity in programming is desirable, the clinician must weigh against it the ability to tailor the pacemaker's settings and optimize the pacemaker's performance to a given patient.

Numerous types of sensors have been used, with the most common sensing being either activity (as a function of body vibration), blood temperature, or minute ventilation. Body vibration sensing is the most useful in children because it does not require special electrodes and is not markedly

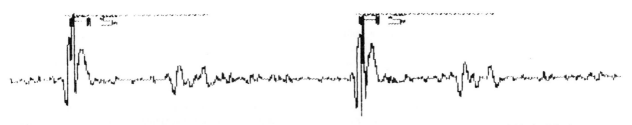

Figure 36–16. Intracardiac atrial electrogram recorded from a patient with AAI pacing. The refractory period (*dashed line*) must be long enough to prevent sensing of ventricular events by the atrial electrode. Note the marked increase in refractory period required compared with VVI pacing. When AAIR pacing is used, the length of this refractory period may significantly restrict the upper rate limit of the pacemaker.

Normal Heart Rate Response to Exercise

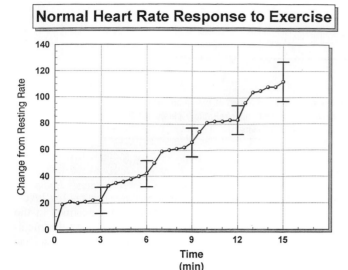

Figure 36–17. Normal heart rate increases from the resting value in normal children exercised using the Bruce treadmill protocol. The brackets represent 1 standard error around the estimate. (Data from Serwer GA, Uzark K, Beckman R, Dick M II: Optimal programming of rate altering parameters in children with rate-responsive pacemakers using graded treadmill exercise testing. PACE 13:542, 1990.)

different in the child than in the adult. Blood temperature and minute-ventilation sensing[29] have been used in children, but to a lesser degree.

Dual-Chamber Pacing

Not only do all the considerations discussed previously apply to dual-chamber pacing, but also additional programmable features must be considered. The first is the ability to program an appropriate AV interval and to decrease it with increasing atrial rate. Such shortening of the AV interval with increasing atrial rate is clearly desirable in children and should occur with changes in the sensed atrial rate and with increases in the paced atrial rate during DDDR pacing. Because this decrease mimics the physiologic response more closely and provides a shorter total atrial refractory period at higher rates, the multiblock rate is higher. This is probably the most important feature of dual-chamber generator selection because children often reach much higher atrial rates than do adults. If the total atrial refractory period is inappropriately long, multiblock occurs during the course of normal exercise, with a subsequent sudden decline in ventricular rate and the potential for syncope. It is common for children to reach atrial rates in excess of 180 bpm during routine exercise. Should the total atrial refractory period, of which the AV delay is a major part, be abnormally long, problems will occur.

In addition, multiple settings for the postventricular atrial refractory period (PVARP) also are considered desirable because of its contribution to the total atrial refractory period (TARP) and, ultimately, the multiblock rate. This parameter must have enough programmability to prevent inappropriate ventricular sensing by the atrial electrode and, at the same time, to allow a multiblock rate of at least 185 bpm (preferably 200 bpm), particularly in younger children.

One closely allied feature that is mandatory is the ability to control the degree of PVARP extension after a spontaneous ventricular depolarization. An automatic extension of the PVARP after the spontaneous ventricular depolarization is often used to prevent sensing of retrograde atrial activation, thus avoiding pacemaker-mediated tachycardia. This is not necessarily desirable in children because the presence of retrograde-only ventriculoatrial conduction is rare and, therefore, the risk for pacemaker-mediated tachycardia is rare. With exercise, spontaneous ventricular depolarizations do occur, and if an inappropriate PVARP extension occurs, normal atrial depolarizations may not be sensed, with a subsequent sudden overall decline in the heart rate. The ability to disable this feature must be present for the generator to be appropriate for use in children. This concern is discussed later when the use of exercise testing in pacemaker follow-up is discussed.

Other features that must be considered include the ability to lower the upper rate limit in the presence of atrial tachycardia. The occurrence of such rhythms, particularly atrial flutter, is not uncommon, particularly in the postoperative patient. Another feature that may find utility in children is the ability to decrease the lower rate limit based on the time of day. Children, who tend to have a much more predictable schedule than adults, can benefit from having their pacemakers programmed to a lower pacing rate during sleep than during the daytime hours, when a higher heart rate may be needed. This is particularly useful for the child with sinus node disease in whom the clinician cannot rely on the intrinsic atrial rate to govern the paced ventricular rate. With an intact sinus node, one can simply set the pacing rate at an appropriately low level for sleep and rest, knowing that it will be at an appropriate rate during waking hours. When sinus node disease is present, however, this may not be the case, and the ability to vary the lower pacing rate with the

Normal Heart Rate Decrease Following Exercise

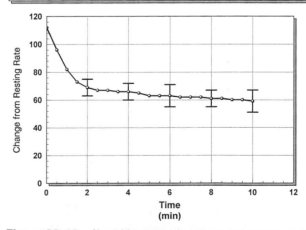

Figure 36–18. Normal heart rate decreases after exercise compared with the pre-exercise value in normal children. Even at 10 minutes after exercise, the heart rate has not reached the resting value. The brackets represent 1 standard error around the estimate. (Data from Serwer GA, Uzark K, Beckman R, Dick M II: Optimal programming of rate altering parameters in children with rate-responsive pacemakers using graded treadmill exercise testing. PACE 13:542, 1990.)

time of day may be helpful because this feature can lower the average daily rate and prolong the generator's life. This feature may also be helpful in the single-chamber rate-responsive pacemaker.

Traditional factors that were once important in pediatric pacing, such as the generator's longevity and size, are now less of a concern in the selection of a generator. All generators are much smaller than previous models, and yet longevity has not been sacrificed. This is a consequence of improved circuit efficiency. The difference in size between single-chamber, dual-chamber, and rate-responsive pacemakers is often undetectable. Pediatric patients generally have long life expectancies, and the ability to have a highly programmable pacemaker implanted to meet changing metabolic demands as a consequence of growth, age, or patient desires is indispensable. The difference in cost between a highly programmable unit and one with fewer features is minimal, particularly when the cost is spread over the lifetime of the pacemaker. Figure 36–19 summarizes the features that must be considered for the appropriate selection of a generator. Thus, the choice of a pacemaker should be based solely on the features it possesses and its ability to meet the demands of the patient.

Pacing Electrode Selection

There are many aspects to the choice of the appropriate electrode system in children. The first obvious choice is between the placement of an endocardial or an epicardial system; yet, other choices are often equally important and overlooked. Such choices include the selection of a unipolar or a bipolar system, the type of electrode fixation to be used, and steroid-eluting versus non–steroid-eluting capabilities.

Endocardial Versus Epicardial Pacing

Initially, almost all electrode systems implanted in children were epicardial. This was a consequence of the large size of the endocardial electrodes and the pacing generators. With

---

```
┌─────────────────────────────────────────────┐
│       Desirable Generator Features in         │
│             Pediatric Pacing                  │
└─────────────────────────────────────────────┘
```

＊ Highly programmable for mode, output, and AV intervals

＊ Rate responsive mode available

＊ Diagnostic rate counters available

＊ Performance indicators provided (battery voltage, battery current drain, electrode impedance)

＊ Intracardiac electrograms provided

＊ Automatic adjustments to changing status such as a change in the upper rate limit with the onset of atrial tachyarrhythmias

＊ Variable AV interval with increasing heart rate - either atrial or sensor driven

Figure 36–19. Generator features desirable in children. AV, atrioventricular.

---

the development of smaller electrodes and generators, this is changing; however, most children still undergo epicardial lead placement as a consequence of small patient size or of other factors that do not permit the placement of an endocardial electrode system. Midwest Pediatric Pacemaker Registry data show a gradual increase in endocardial electrode use, but half of all patients still receive epicardial electrodes (Fig. 36–20). Our basic approach is to assume that all children should undergo the placement of an endocardial system; we then evaluate the child for factors that do not allow endocardial electrode use. The major factors to be considered, in addition to patient size, are (1) venous access to the ventricle, (2) the presence of intracardiac right-to-left shunting, (3) the presence of increased pulmonary vascular resistance, (4) the presence of right-sided prosthetic valves, and (5) the presence of severe right ventricular dysfunction or fibrosis.

Initially, it was believed that children below 15 kg in weight and younger than 4 years of age should not undergo placement of endocardial electrodes.[30] This was based on the concerns that the subclavian vein and superior vena cava are too small, leading to a high risk for thrombosis, and that the large size of the generators made implantation in the subclavicular area impractical. With increased experience and smaller generator and electrode sizes, however, many centers now routinely implant endocardial lead systems in children weighing much less than 15 kg.[7, 31, 32] What the lower range for weight should be is not yet known. From a technical standpoint, children as small as 3 kg in weight can undergo endocardial electrode placement, but the follow-up of such children is too limited to know whether this is in their best interest. The risk for vessel thrombosis appears to be less than what was once thought, at least in the short term.[33] Although superior vena caval thrombosis has been reported,[34, 35] the true incidence is unknown because noninvasive methods of detecting thrombosis are not sensitive and angiography is not routinely done unless thrombosis is suspected clinically (Fig. 36–21). Lead displacement secondary to growth remains a concern, although techniques have been proposed to deal with this problem.[7, 32] The placement of large electrode loops within the atrium was proposed to allow for growth, but they may not be as effective as originally thought because they may fibrose to the cardiac wall and not uncoil with growth.

The major objection to endocardial electrode use in the small child is related to long-term problems. Because young children can be expected to require numerous electrodes over their lifetime, many more than are needed in adult patients, the clinician must consider how many electrodes can be left in place before problems with either vessel obstruction or tricuspid valve dysfunction occur as well as the difficulty with which old electrodes can be extracted. Although lead extraction has become more widely used,[36, 37] it still represents a significant problem in children, with the potential for damage to the cardiac structures, mainly the tricuspid valve. To commit a child to potentially numerous lead extractions is still a worry. In our institution, current guidelines call for the placement of dual-chamber endocardial systems in children weighing 15 kg or more and the placement of single-chamber endocardial systems, when single-chamber pacing is appropriate, in children heavier than 8 kg. These guidelines may change as electrode development

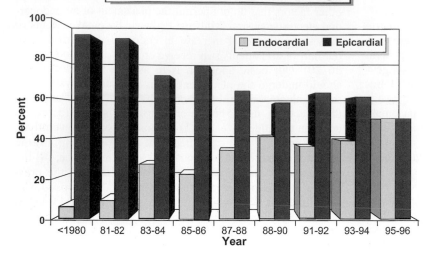

Figure 36–20. Comparison of epicardial and endocardial electrode use during each period in children. Note the gradual increasing use of endocardial electrodes. (Data from the Midwest Pediatric Pacemaker Registry.)

continues and as data on the long-term follow-up of children with endocardially placed electrodes becomes available.

The next factor that must be considered is the presence of intracardiac shunting. Electrodes are potential sources of small particulate matter, with the risk for subsequent embolization until endothelialization occurs.[38] Except in the presence of pulmonary vascular disease, this does not tend to be a problem when such particulate matter goes only to the lungs, where it is filtered out of the circulation and eventually absorbed. In the presence of right-to-left shunting, however, the potential for systemic embolization is great. The general recommendation is to avoid such electrodes in patients with documented right-to-left shunting.[30] This also must be considered in patients with the potential for right-to-left shunting, even if their net intracardiac shunt is left to right. Children with atrial septal defects and VSDs can show right-to-left shunting in the setting of elevated right ventricular pressure, even with a net left-to-right shunt.[39, 40] The specific hemodynamic situation of the individual child must be considered before endocardial electrode implantation is performed.

The same concerns apply to the child with elevated pulmonary vascular resistance in whom pulmonary embolization of small matter may further elevate the pulmonary resistance. Whether or not short-term anticoagulation of such patients until lead endothelialization can occur would prevent such concerns and permit transvenous pacemaker placement has yet to be investigated. In the situation in which epicardial pacing is not possible, this may be an acceptable alternative, but given the current lack of knowledge concerning the benefit of anticoagulation in this setting, it should not be general practice.

The presence of an artificial tricuspid valve prosthesis negates the ability of the clinician to use an endocardial pacing system. There have been isolated reports of endocardial electrode placements at the time of open heart surgery through the perivalvular area.[41] This requires cardiopulmonary bypass and can only be done at the time of valvular placement. This technique cannot be used in the usual transvenous implantation; however, it prevents lead extraction should that become necessary, except during repeat open heart surgery.

Finally, the physician must consider the state of the right ventricle. Severe right ventricular dysfunction and endocardial fibrosis can occur in children with congenital cardiac disease and may prevent adequate pacing of the right ventricle. This tends to be more prevalent in the older child with long-standing disease. In such children, left ventricular pacing and, therefore, epicardial pacing may become necessary. In the setting of severe right ventricular dysfunction and dilation, an appropriate endocardial site that permits both adequate sensing and pacing may not be achievable.

In summary, endocardial pacing is generally preferable

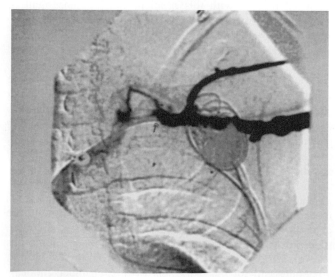

Figure 36–21. Venous angiogram in a patient after endocardial pacemaker implantation through the left subclavian vein. Note the complete obstruction of the subclavian vein at the site of electrode entry *(arrow)*, with collateral flow around the obstruction.

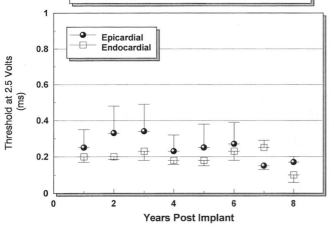

Figure 36–22. Comparison of long-term pulse width thresholds for endocardial versus epicardial electrodes measured at a pulse amplitude of 2.5 V. Thresholds for both groups show no significant rise, and they do not differ significantly from each other. The brackets represent 1 standard error around the mean.

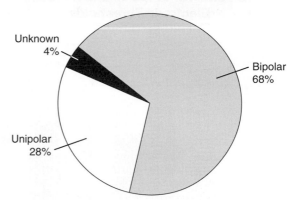

Figure 36–24. Data from the Midwest Pediatric Pacemaker Registry indicating that more than two thirds of endocardial electrode systems use bipolar electrodes.

because of the ease of implantation and the improved longevity of the electrode. Long-term thresholds are as stable as epicardial electrodes and tend to be lower (Fig. 36–22). This permits lower-output programming of the pacing generator, enhancing its longevity. However, there are many situations in which endocardial electrode use is contraindicated (Fig. 36–23). As such, epicardial electrodes still play a significant role in pediatric pacing, which may be reduced in the future but will not be eliminated.

Unipolar Versus Bipolar Pacing

The choice between a unipolar and bipolar electrode configuration only becomes an issue for endocardial implantation. For the epicardial implant, the unipolar configuration is used almost exclusively. To use a bipolar configuration requires that two electrodes be placed on the heart, with an increased

---

Contraindications to Endocardial Pacing

✴ Small patient size (relative)

✴ Presence of intracardiac right-to-left shunting

✴ No venous access

✴ Elevated pulmonary vascular resistance

✴ Prosthetic tricuspid valve

✴ Severe right ventricular dilatation or endocardial fibrosis

✴ Presence of hypercoagulable state

Figure 36–23. Contraindications to endocardial pacing.

---

risk for electrode failure. The data from the Midwest Pediatric Pacemaker Registry document the finding that 95% of all epicardial implants use a unipolar configuration. Were bipolar electrodes to be developed, they might be beneficial.

For endocardial pacing systems, the choice between unipolar and bipolar pacing becomes more controversial. Again, data from the Midwest Pediatric Pacemaker Registry show that most endocardial systems are bipolar (Fig. 36–24). Initially, it was believed that unipolar pacing was preferable because of the smaller size of the unipolar pacing electrode.[42] With recent improvements in electrode design, however, this difference in size has become negligible. Electrode body diameters are the important factor in determining the risk for venous thrombosis, and there is a minimal difference. For example, the model 4057M unipolar screw-in electrode (Medtronic, Minneapolis, MN) has a body diameter of 2.2 mm; the 4058M bipolar version has a body diameter of 2.4 mm. This same minimal difference in body size is also seen in passive-fixation electrodes, such as the 4023 unipolar steroid-eluting electrode (Medtronic), which has a body diameter of 1.2 mm, compared with 1.9 mm for the bipolar version (model 4024). The recently developed ThinLine (Intermedics, Angleton, TX) bipolar electrode has further decreased the lead body diameter and potentially the tendency for interelectrode shorts.[43] In all cases, the diameter of the electrode's head is smaller for a unipolar electrode, which may make insertion easier, but once implanted, the size of the head is of little consequence.

A comparison of acute implantation characteristics between unipolar and bipolar electrodes of similar design from the Midwest Pediatric Pacemaker Registry showed no significant difference for threshold values of voltage, current, or resistance (Fig. 36–25). Long-term thresholds have been thought by some to be improved in unipolar pacing.[42] This has been postulated to be the result of the smaller size of the head and its lower weight, creating less tension on the endocardial surface, particularly when active-fixation electrodes are used, and therefore leading to less tip fibrosis. However, this appears to be unique only to active-fixation leads and has not been reported to be a problem with passive-fixation tined electrodes.

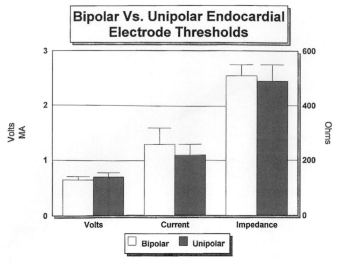

Figure 36–25. Acute implantation thresholds for bipolar versus unipolar endocardial electrodes are not significantly different for voltage, current, or electrode impedance. All were measured at a 0.5-msec pulse width. The brackets represent 1 standard error around the mean. (Data from the Midwest Pediatric Pacemaker Registry.)

It was initially thought that sensing using a bipolar electrode was inferior to unipolar sensing because of the close proximity of the two electrodes; however, data from the Midwest Pediatric Pacemaker Registry show this not to be the case. Acute-implantation R-wave amplitudes and slew rates show no significant difference between the unipolar and bipolar electrodes (Fig. 36–26). Unipolar sensing, however, is more affected by myopotentials and more prone to oversensing and inappropriate pacemaker inhibition. This has been estimated to be a problem in 31% to 93% of patients, as discussed later. Bipolar sensing is rarely affected by such myopotential inhibition from the closer proximity of the electrodes. The degree to which such inappropriate inhibition is seen is dependent on the location of the generator, the provocative tests used, and generator model implanted. All series, however, report a significant incidence of this problem, which can be a particular concern in active children.

Thus, it would appear that, in most active children, bipolar pacing is preferred, particularly with the smaller electrode sizes now available. Sensing does not appear to be a problem, and myopotential inhibition is seen less often. In addition, with bipolar pacing, the risk for extracardiac pacing of the surrounding muscle is minimized, particularly in a child in whom it may be difficult to position the generator in a location where all such stimulation of surrounding muscles is avoided. This is particularly relevant to implantations with the pocket placed in the subclavicular region. In many children, the lack of significant subcutaneous tissue requires the placement of the generator in the subpectoral position, where the risk for extracardiac pacing with a unipolar system increases.

Epicardial Electrode Types

Compared with endocardial electrodes, there are relatively few epicardial electrode types from which to choose. Pre-

viously, all electrodes were intramyocardial in type, with the intramyocardial portion being either a corkscrew coil, a single wire with a barbed end (fishhook), or an intramyocardial wire drawn through the myocardium (suture type).[44–47] Recently, a truly epicardial electrode with steroid-eluting capabilities has been developed.[48–50] This is sutured to the epicardial surface and requires direct contact of the electrode with stimulatable myocardium.

The most widely used electrodes currently, based on data from the Midwest Pediatric Pacemaker Registry, are the screw-in corkscrew type (6917, 471 [Intermedics], or 4312), the barbed fishhook type (4951 or 4951M) and the Medtronic steroid-eluting electrode (4965) (Fig. 36–27). The choice of electrode depends on the chamber to be paced and the preference of the implanting physician.

Atrial epicardial implantation requires an electrode that either sits on the epicardial surface or has only a shallow penetration into the atrial myocardium. Should the electrode extend through the chamber wall into the atrial cavity, a low-resistance circuit is established with an inability to pace reliably. Little data can be found concerning the longevity or thresholds of atrial epicardial electrodes. In part, this is related to their limited use and to the fact that constant change in the electrode design continues, making long-term comparisons difficult. The most widely used atrial electrode is the fishhook or stab-in electrode because it does not penetrate deeply into the myocardium, compared with the screw-in or corkscrew type. The newest version (4951M), which has a platinized coating, has resulted in slightly improved thresholds at acute implantation (Fig. 36–28). The average threshold at implantation is about 1.05 V and 3.3 mA, measured at a pulse width of 0.5 msec. The average acute electrode impedance is 320 Ω. The steroid-eluting electrode is receiving increasing usage as an atrial epicardial electrode and may become the dominant electrode for atrial epicardial pacing.

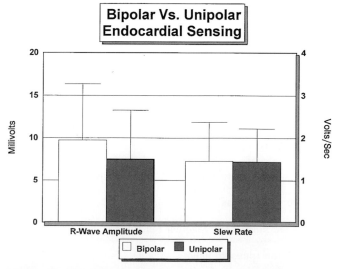

Figure 36–26. Acute implantation electrode sensing for bipolar versus unipolar endocardial electrodes demonstrates no significant difference in either R-wave amplitude (millivolts) or slew rate (volts/sec). The brackets indicate 1 standard error around the mean. (Data from the Midwest Pediatric Pacemaker Registry.)

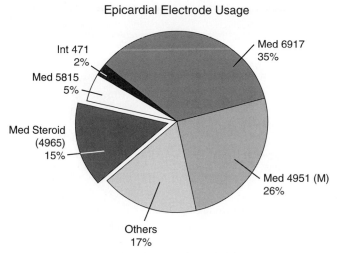

Figure 36–27. Distribution of epicardial electrode types used. The two most common epicardial electrodes are the Medtronic 6917/5069 (screw-in) electrode and the Medtronic 4951(M) (fishhook) electrode. Yet the Medtronic steroid-eluting electrode (exploded slice) is finding increasing use in recent years. Med steroid, epicardial steroid-eluting electrode (4965); Med 5815, myocardial stab-in electrode; Int 471, Intermedics screw-in electrode. (Data from the Midwest Pediatric Pacemaker Registry.)

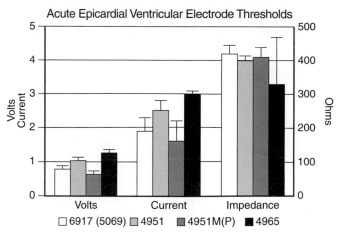

Figure 36–29. Comparison of thresholds for the Medtronic 6917 (now known as 5069) screw-in electrode, the Medtronic 4951 fishhook electrode, the Medtronic 4951M(P) platinized fishhook electrode, and the Medtronic steroid-eluting electrode (4965) when implanted on the ventricle shows no significant difference in voltage threshold, but the impedance is slightly lower for the steroid-eluting electrode, similar to findings for atrial usage. The brackets represent 1 standard error around the mean. (Data from the Midwest Pediatric Pacemaker Registry.)

More diversity exists in the choice of the electrode for ventricular pacing. A comparison of the original nonplatinized fishhook electrode (4951) with the screw-in electrode (6917 or 5069) reveals essentially no difference in acute implantation thresholds. However, implantation thresholds for the currently available platinized fishhook electrode (4951M) are slightly improved (Fig. 36–29). Lead survival appears to be longer for the screw-in electrode than for the fishhook type. Five years after implantation, the lead survival rate of the former was found to be about 84%, whereas that of the fishhook electrode was found to be about 65%.[46] Most failures were found to be exit block. Other studies, however, found little difference in longevity between these two types of electrodes.[45] Some of the discrepancy between the results of these studies was believed to be caused by different surgical modes of implantation for the fishhook electrode. Whether or not the lead was stabilized by being sutured to the myocardium was variable. It has been suggested that a lack of such stabilization leads to more electrode movement within the myocardium and, therefore, greater fibrosis and the risk for exit block.[46] This is discussed further when implantation techniques are considered. Such data for the steroid-eluting electrode have yet to be obtained.

Others authorities have advocated using the suture-type electrode (030-170 [Telectronics, Englewood, CO]).[47] Although implantation thresholds were similar to those of the fishhook electrode, the incidence of exit block was lower. This may also be related to the better electrode stabilization of the suture-type electrode. Because of its increased surface area, however, the electrode's impedance is lower, with a resultant increased current drain from the generator. A recent advance in epicardial pacing is the steroid-eluting electrode.[48–50] This electrode consists of a platinized flat electrode that sits atop the epicardial surface with a silicone plug impregnated with dexamethasone to allow elution of the dexamethasone onto the area of myocardium being stimulated. About 1 mg of dexamethasone is present within the electrode. This electrode is affixed to the epicardial surface by sutures, with the active portion of the electrode not extending into the myocardium as with other epicardial electrodes. This is both advantageous and disadvantageous, de-

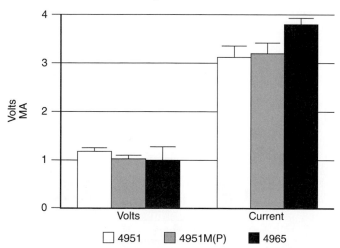

Figure 36–28. Acute implantation voltage and current threshold values measured at a 0.5-msec pulse width for the original fish-hook electrode (Medtronic 4951) compared with the newer platinized version (Medtronic 4951M) and the steroid-eluting electrode (Medtronic 4965) when implanted on the atrium. Acute thresholds are not statistically different. Current at threshold for the steroid electrode is slightly higher, implying a lower impedance. The brackets represent 1 standard error around the mean. (Data from the Midwest Pediatric Pacemaker Registry.)

pending on the patient. For patients whose epicardial surfaces are relatively nonfibrotic, this appears to be an advantage because there is less myocardial injury to provoke subsequent fibrotic formation. However, for patients with markedly fibrotic epicardial surfaces, often present following multiple open heart surgical procedures, these electrodes are difficult to use. In these patients, the surgeon must find an area of myocardium with a limited epicardial fibrotic reaction or attempt to strip away such a fibrotic reaction to expose the myocardium, which simply leads to further subsequent fibrosis.

Initial experience with this electrode is encouraging. Although acute thresholds appear to be comparable to those of other epicardial electrodes (see Fig. 36–29), the threshold rise is less over the first several months after implantation (Fig. 36–30).[49] In selected patients with limited myocardial fibrosis, non-intramyocardial epicardial electrodes appear to be beneficial; however, they are not necessarily ideally suited to all patients, and care must be taken to choose the most appropriate form of ventricular epicardial electrode to fit the individual patient. All three types of ventricular electrodes in current use have advantages and disadvantages, and no one type is ideally suited to all patients.

Endocardial Electrode Types

Similar to the adult population, there are several general types of endocardial electrodes in use in children: passive-fixation non–steroid-eluting, passive-fixation steroid-eluting, and active-fixation electrodes, both non–steroid-eluting and a recently developed steroid-eluting model. Active electrode data presented here are for the non–steroid-eluting model. The most commonly used endocardial electrode type in children continues to be the active-fixation screw-in elec-

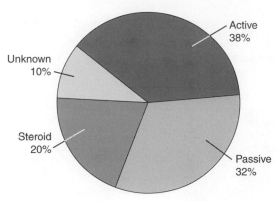

Figure 36–31. Distribution of endocardial electrode type use. Active, active-fixation (screw-in) electrode; passive, passive-fixation (tined) non–steroid-eluting electrode; steroid, passive-fixation steroid-eluting electrode. (Data from the Midwest Pediatric Pacemaker Registry.)

trode (Fig. 36–31). The use of this electrode has been advocated because of its better fixation qualities, given the tremendous range of anatomic variation present in children with congenital heart disease. When implantation is within the morphologic left ventricle in children after an atrial switch repair for transposition of the great arteries or in those with ventricular inversion, the active-fixation electrode is preferable. Also, in children with markedly dilated right ventricles, such that it is difficult to wedge the electrode into the trabecular recesses of the right ventricle, active-fixation electrodes are preferable.

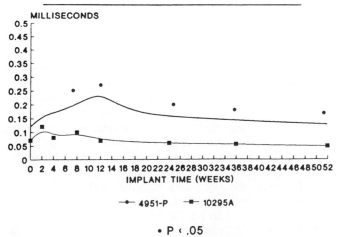

Figure 36–30. Comparative thresholds of the Medtronic 4951P platinized fish-hook electrode versus the epicardial steroid-eluting electrode (10295A, now known as model 4965), showing a lack of significant threshold rise in the first 3 months after implantation for the steroid-eluting epicardial electrode with threshold improvement at 1 year after implantation. (From Karpawich PP, Harkini M, Arciniegas E, Cavitt DL: Improved chronic epicardial pacing in children: Steroid contribution to porous platinized electrodes. PACE 15:1152, 1992.)

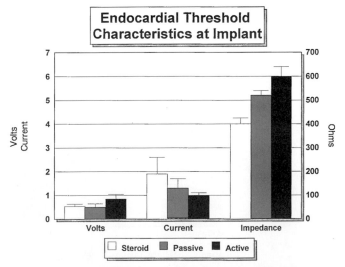

Figure 36–32. Acute thresholds for endocardial electrode types showed a tendency toward lower thresholds in the passive-fixation and steroid-eluting electrodes compared with the active-fixation electrodes. However, the difference in voltage threshold is minimal. The changes become more evident in current and impedance values, with steroid electrodes having the lowest impedance and highest current flow. The brackets represent 1 standard error around the mean. (Data from the Midwest Pediatric Pacemaker Registry.)

This electrode type, however, is not ideal in all children. A comparison of acute threshold data shows that active-fixation electrodes have the highest acute thresholds (Fig. 36–32). Both non–steroid-eluting passive-fixation electrodes and steroid-eluting passive-fixation electrodes have lower acute thresholds. However, they do not differ from each other. The presence of the steroid does not influence the acute implantation thresholds, but with increasing electrode age, this is no longer the case. Follow-up data indicate significantly lower electrode thresholds for the steroid-eluting electrode compared with other types.[51] A comparison of steroid-eluting and non–steroid-eluting electrodes showed no difference in chronic thresholds at 5 V of pulse amplitude but did show significant differences at 2.5 and 1.6 V (Fig. 36–33). Thus, it would appear that the strength–duration curve is significantly shifted leftward for the steroid-eluting electrodes.

Such changes affect generator programming. In one study,[51] only 33% of generators that used non–steroid-eluting electrodes were able to be programmed to 2.5 V of pulse amplitude, compared with 77% of generators that used steroid-eluting electrodes. The remainder required a pulse amplitude of 5 V or greater. Thus, the use of steroid-eluting passive-fixation electrodes allowed chronically lower output settings for the pulse generator, thereby increasing the generator's longevity. The follow-up averaged 3.3 years (median, 3.6 years).

Single-lead VDD systems have been employed in children obviating the need for two electrodes yet maintaining AV synchrony[52]; however, problems exist. The major prob-

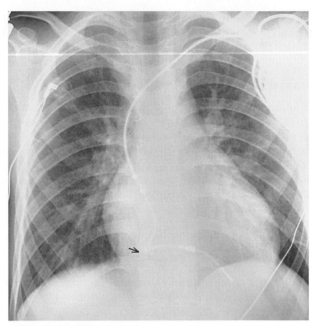

Figure 36–34. Chest radiograph showing placement of a single-pass VDD system. Note the lead buckling in the atrium necessary to place the atrial sensing electrodes *(arrow)* within the atrium.

lem is lack of atrial pacing capabilities when sinus node function is inadequate. Also, the spacing of the atrial electrodes from the electrode tip is often too great for use in small children. This requires that the electrode be buckled such that the atrial dipole is within the ventricle (Fig. 36–34), which may lead to ventricular electrode dislodgment. These problems, together with the increased complexity of the electrode construction with a potential for increased electrode failure, combine to limit the usefulness of this approach in children, especially smaller children.

In summary, we believe that the ideal pacing system in children is a dual-chamber system with the capacity for rate-responsive pacing, using endocardial atrial and ventricular bipolar electrodes with active-fixation electrodes in the atrium and steroid-eluting passive-fixation electrodes in the ventricle. In situations in which the child's size is marginal or it is not thought to be possible to implant an atrial endocardial electrode, we then prefer to use an endocardial single-chamber rate-responsive system. Only in situations in which endocardial pacing is specifically contraindicated do we use epicardial pacing. In these situations, the currently preferred electrode is the steroid-eluting electrode for both the atrium and the ventricle or, in the presence of significant epicardial fibrosis, the platinized version of the fishhook electrode for the atrium and the corkscrew electrode for the ventricle. Long-term data are not yet available to show whether the steroid-eluting epicardial electrode performs better in the long term than the intramyocardial electrode.

■ IMPLANTATION TECHNIQUES

In many ways, implantation techniques in the child are similar to those used in the adult, but differences do exist. This section does not attempt to describe again those tech-

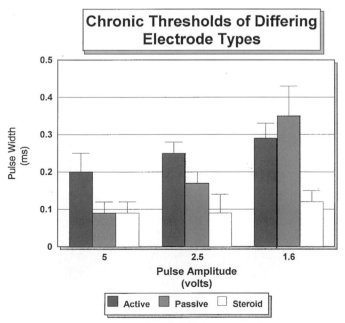

Figure 36–33. Chronic long-term electrode thresholds are significantly higher for active-fixation electrodes than for both passive-fixation and steroid-eluting electrodes. At low pulse amplitudes, steroid-eluting electrodes show significantly lower thresholds than the other types. The brackets represent 1 standard error around the mean. (Data from Serwer GA, Dorostkar PC, LeRoy S, Dick M II: Comparison of chronic thresholds between differing endocardial electrode types in children. Circulation 86:I-43, 1992.)

niques that are similar but instead focuses on describing the differences that are important in the child and must be considered.

Epicardial Implantation Techniques

The approach used for the placement of epicardial electrodes is highly variable, depending on the patient's individual circumstances. Approaches to the epicardial surface that have previously been employed include thoracotomy, sternotomy, and subxiphoid incision. The subxiphoid approach requires the smallest incision, and through the same incision, both the electrode's implantation on the epicardial surface of the heart and the pacemaker's implantation in the abdomen can be accomplished.[53–55] This approach has been used for both ventricular and atrial epicardial electrode implantation. The disadvantage to this approach is that it exposes only a limited ventricular epicardial or atrial surface, and in the patient with extensive epicardial fibrosis as a consequence of prior cardiac surgery, finding a suitable location for implantation of the electrode may be difficult. Such an approach requires a 6- to 7-cm skin incision from the xiphoid tip to a point superior to the umbilicus. The dissection is continued as deep as it is thought to be necessary to provide adequate tissue between the pacemaker and the surface of the skin. Depending on the degree of subcutaneous tissue present, the pacemaker can be implanted above the rectus muscle, below the rectus muscle but above the peritoneum, or in some circumstances, intraperitoneally, housed in a Silastic pouch sutured to the underside of the peritoneum and anchored to the rectus fascia.[53] The depth to which the incision is carried should be governed solely by the tissue

available to cover the pacemaker. When only minimal tissue is present over the pacemaker, not only does an unsightly bulge result, but also the skin is more susceptible to traumatic injury, with a resultant risk for pacemaker erosion and infection.

A left thoracotomy approach is often used in the child who has had prior cardiac surgery in whom the risk for significant epicardial fibrosis is high.[56] This affords an increased myocardial surface from which to choose an appropriate pacing site. Implantation of the generator can either be in the abdomen, in the subclavicular region, or in rare settings, intrathoracically. However, for implantation of a dual-chamber system, this approach affords less exposure of the atrium and requires left atrial pacing. Although this has been accomplished, it introduces complexity into the programming because the postpace AV interval must be prolonged enough to afford adequate time for right ventricular filling caused by the time necessary for left-to-right atrial excitation spread. The postsense AV interval must be short to avoid an excessive AV interval (Fig. 36–35). In this setting, a generator with a rate-adaptive AV delay is mandatory. For this reason, we think that right atrial pacing is preferable but use left atrial pacing if right atrial pacing is not possible. When the thoracotomy approach is used with an abdominal placement of the generator, the electrode must be passed subcostally to a pocket created in the abdomen through a separate incision. The electrode must not be passed over a rib and must be tunneled from the thoracic cavity to the abdomen as medially as possible to minimize the risk for traumatic electrode fracture.

Finally, a median sternotomy approach can be used, but this creates the largest and most obvious scar. However, it

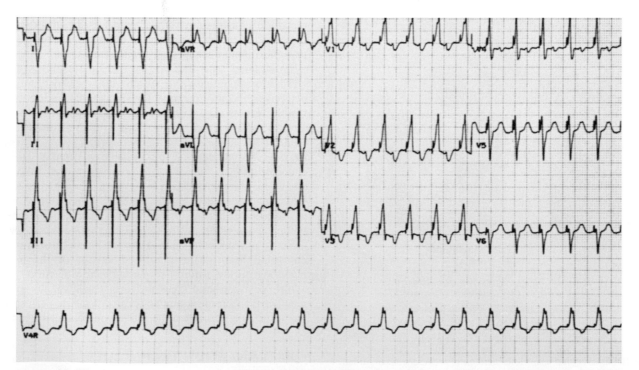

Figure 36–35. Electrocardiogram from a patient with a DDD pacemaker in whom the atrial electrode is on the left atrium. To provide an appropriate time for ventricular filling during both atrial pacing and sensing, either a compromise AV interval must be used or the generator must have the ability to alter the atrioventricular (AV) interval (dynamic AV delay).

affords the best exposure of the epicardial surface of both the ventricle and right atrium. In the patient with significant epicardial scarring and fibrosis, this affords the best likelihood of finding an appropriate pacing site. After implantation of the electrode, it can then be pulled through the subxiphoid region to the abdominal wall, where, through a separate incision or an extension of the medium sternotomy incision, an appropriate pocket can be created.

Regardless of the electrode type chosen, appropriate anchoring of the electrode to the epicardial surface is crucial. Our approach is to insert the electrode into the myocardium and determine the threshold strength–duration curve. If it is acceptable, the electrode is sutured to the epicardial surface, and the thresholds are rechecked. Suturing the electrode to the surface theoretically reduces the movement of the electrode tip within the myocardium, with less formation of fibrotic tissue and better long-term performance of the electrode.[46] When the fishhook electrode is used and there is significant epicardial fibrosis, unbending the barb to permit deeper penetration is often beneficial. There should be several types of myocardial electrodes available during implantation to meet whatever situation is encountered.

When the steroid-eluting electrode is used, a suitable position is found by holding the electrode in contact with the epicardial surface and quickly determining the voltage threshold at a single pulse width. If acceptable, the electrode is sutured to the epicardial surface, and a complete strength–duration curve is determined. Often, several sites must be tested before a suitable one is found.

A gentle loop of the electrode should be left in the thoracic cavity to allow for some growth, but excessive loops should be avoided. Instances of entrapment of vascular structures by pacemaker electrodes have been reported.[57, 58] The extra length of the electrode is easily coiled and placed within the generator's pocket; even this may allow for some growth because the electrode wire slowly uncoils with subsequent growth of the patient.

The exact placement of the abdominal pocket is generally left to the discretion of the surgeon. However, it should be placed away from the belt line and not in the upper right quadrant. Placement in the upper right quadrant interferes with subsequent assessment of hepatic size, which may be important in children with structural cardiac disease. The electrodes should be tunneled from the thorax to the abdomen as near the midline as possible to minimize the risk for electrode fracture.

The placement of unused or redundant electrodes is not recommended. It was once believed that the placement of an unused electrode would provide a "spare" electrode that could be used if the primary electrode failed, thus preventing the need for a second thoracotomy. It was found, however, that if the primary electrode failed, there was a high likelihood that the redundant electrode was also unusable.[13, 59] Thus, the extra electrode that had been placed provided no benefit to the child.

Endocardial Implantation Techniques

Before endocardial implantation, echocardiography should be performed to make certain no contraindications to endocardial implantation exist, specifically tricuspid valve dysfunction, right-to-left shunting, or superior vena caval ob-

struction. Whether the pacemaker is placed under the left or right clavicle is somewhat arbitrary but may be important to some patients, and the location should be discussed with them. Our general policy is to place the pacemaker on the side opposite the patient's handedness (i.e., if the patient is right-handed, the pacemaker is placed on the left side).

The endocardial approach used for implantation in children is similar to that in adults. Before beginning, transcutaneous pacing electrodes are placed to provide emergency pacing ability. A sudden decrease in the intrinsic heart rate caused by the stress of the procedure or the general anesthesia, if administered, is not unusual. Although placement of a temporary transvenous pacing electrode can be done, the stress of this alone may cause bradycardia. In addition, the risk for infection of the permanent system by the temporary electrode must be considered. Transcutaneous pacing electrodes for all sizes of children are now available and function well.

Whether the electrode is introduced into the vascular system by a direct subclavian vein puncture[31, 60, 61] or by a cephalic vein cutdown procedure[7, 32] is guided by the experience of the implanting physician. In our institution, direct subclavian vein puncture is used exclusively. Our approach is to enter the subclavian vein percutaneously and introduce a guide wire. Using the guide wire's entrance through the skin as the proximal point, an incision is made laterally along the deltopectoral groove. The dissection is then carried down to the pectoralis. At this point, the degree of subcutaneous tissue is examined to determine whether there is sufficient tissue to cover the generator. In many children, this tissue is inadequate, and placement of the generator above the pectoralis results in a significant pacemaker bulge as well as an increased risk for pacemaker erosion and traumatic injury to the tissue above the pacemaker.[60] This is also psychologically important because many children are self-conscious about a prominent bulge. When the tissue is believed to be inadequate, the dissection is then carried through the pectoralis, using blunt dissection to separate the muscle fibers, with a pocket created in the subpectoral region. After this pocket is created, a sheath and dilator are introduced into the subclavian vein over the previously positioned guide wire. The electrode is then passed into the right atrium together with a new guide wire. The sheath is then removed. Retention of the guide wire allows for either the introduction of a second electrode, in the case of a dual-chamber implant, or the option to remove the prior electrode and replace it without having to again puncture the subclavian vein. After the electrodes have been positioned and tested, the guide wire can be removed. The electrodes are then connected to the generator, which is placed in the pocket with the uninsulated side placed away from the pectoralis. When the subpectoral approach is used, it may be difficult to avoid extracardiac pacing with a unipolar system, and for this reason, a bipolar system is preferred.

A third implantation approach is a hybrid of both methods. In some patients in whom transvenous implantation would be preferable but in whom there is no venous access, the electrode can be inserted into the atrium through an incision in the atria wall and then advanced into the ventricle across the AV valve.[62] The atrial incision is closed with a pursestring suture after the electrode has been positioned in the ventricle. This provides the advantages of endocardial pacing with improved thresholds when venous access to the ventricle is not available. We have employed this approach in children in whom epicardial electrode thresholds were unacceptable but who had no venous access (Fig. 36–36). This can be especially useful in children after right heart bypass (Fontan's) procedure, even though anticoagulation is necessary because of implantation within the systemic ventricle.[38]

Acute Electrode Evaluation

After placement of the electrode, its electrical characteristics must be determined. For active-fixation or intramyocardial electrodes, 15 minutes should be allowed from the placement of the electrode to threshold testing to permit acute myocardial changes caused by the electrode's entry into the myocardium to subside. All changes do not subside in this amount of time, but this short delay is warranted. Our initial approach is to measure the electrode's impedance and, if possible, intrinsic electrogram amplitudes. The impedance should be between 200 and 600 Ω for the epicardially placed electrode and between 300 and 700 Ω for the endocardially placed electrode. The amplitude of the electrogram should be sufficient to allow appropriate sensing by the generator to be implanted. The minimally acceptable signal amplitude varies, depending on the specific generator. If these measurements are found to be acceptable, threshold testing is performed. It is our general practice to set a given pulse width and then determine the minimum pulse amplitude necessary

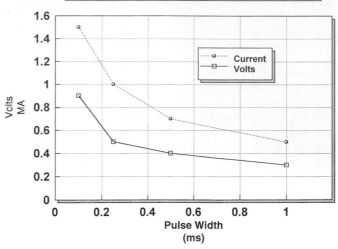

Figure 36–37. Example of a strength–duration curve determined at implantation. From this curve, the minimum voltage needed to pace at any pulse width and the minimum pulse width needed to pace at any voltage can be determined.

to maintain capture. Multiple threshold determinations at differing pulse widths are performed to define the strength–duration curve adequately. We think it is important to determine the shape of the strength–duration curve to be certain that the minimum pulse width necessary to pace at any pulse amplitude and the minimum amplitude necessary to pace at any pulse width are sufficiently removed from the proposed generator settings to allow for some movement in the strength–duration curve without the risk for loss of capture (Fig. 36–37). Data from the Midwest Pediatric Pacemaker Registry suggest that the minimum voltage necessary to pace the ventricle at a 0.5-msec pulse width is below 1 V, and below 1.5 V for the atrium. Such threshold guidelines apply to both endocardial and epicardial electrodes.

Before the pulse generator is connected to the electrodes, it is advisable to pace the ventricle at the maximal output of the pacing system analyzer. In children, because of the close proximity of the diaphragm to the electrode, diaphragmatic pacing can occur. At the maximal pacing system analyzer output, if diaphragmatic pacing should occur, the electrode must be moved. This is particularly relevant to the child with transposition of the great arteries in whom a ventricular electrode is positioned within the left ventricle. Positioning the electrode tip at the left ventricular apex puts it in close proximity to the diaphragm, and there is a high incidence of diaphragmatic pacing. To prevent this, we position the electrode on the midposterior free wall at the approximate level of the papillary muscles (Fig. 36–38). This affords acceptable thresholds with a minimal risk for diaphragmatic pacing. This problem is more often seen in endocardial pacing than in epicardial pacing, but it can occur in either setting.

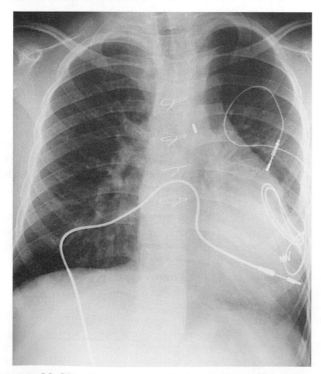

Figure 36–36. Chest radiograph showing placement of an endocardial electrode introduced through the atrial wall, passed through the atrioventricular valve, and secured to the ventricular endocardial surface. The electrode is tunneled to the generator pocket in the abdominal wall.

■ FOLLOW-UP METHODS FOR THE CHILD WITH A PACEMAKER

Proper pacemaker programming and early recognition of inappropriate pacemaker performance require frequent, me-

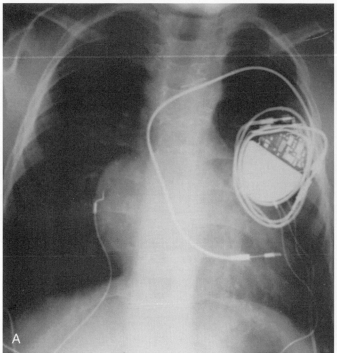

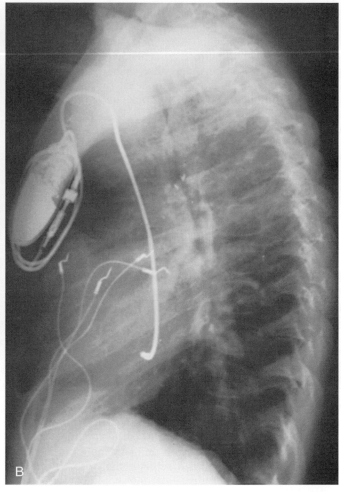

Figure 36–38. Posteroanterior *(A)* and lateral *(B)* chest radiographs from a patient who underwent endocardial electrode implantation after performance of an atrial switch procedure (Senning) for dextro-transposition of the great arteries. Note the electrode position in the left ventricle away from the ventricular apex and the diaphragm to avoid diaphragmatic stimulation.

thodical, and appropriate follow-up. In this section, we discuss the follow-up techniques used and the differences in the follow-up routine with increasing time from implantation.

Pacemaker follow-up can be divided into three periods, based on the length of time from implantation. The two most crucial periods are within the first 2 months after implantation (early follow-up) and when the pacemaker approaches its theoretical life expectancy (late follow-up). Between these two periods, the function of the pacemaker and electrode remain fairly stable, and the generator does not require frequent readjustment. Problems can occur, however, particularly as a result of electrode breakage in the active child. The major components of pacemaker follow-up (i.e., pacemaker clinic visit, 24-hour ambulatory ECG recordings, and treadmill exercise testing) are discussed, followed by a description of the differences between the three follow-up periods.

Pacemaker Clinic Visit

During a pacemaker clinic visit, all patients undergo a complete history and physical examination, pacemaker interrogation, threshold testing, evaluation of electrode sensing, and routine ECG testing. When indicated, other tests, such as chest radiography and echocardiography, are also performed. Specific attention must be paid to obtaining a complete history as it relates to potential pacemaker malfunction.

Symptoms suggesting pacemaker malfunction include sudden exercise intolerance, dizziness, nausea, or loss of consciousness. In particular, parents often note that the child has "less energy" than previously. One of the more common symptoms in patients with intermittent atrial sensing malfunction is a sudden lack of energy or transient dizziness, which is related to a loss of atrial sensing with a resultant acute drop in the rate to the lower rate limit of the pacemaker. This can often be a subtle finding and must be carefully sought, not only in the older child from whom a history can be obtained directly, but also from the parents of the younger child who must be asked whether they have ever noted sudden changes in the child's activity state or temperament, sudden interruptions of play time, interruptions of eating, or sudden staring episodes suggestive of acute decrease in cardiac output.

The physical examination should relate specifically to complications produced by the presence of pacemaker electrodes, such as AV valve incompetence, the acute appearance of pericardial rubs (suggesting lead perforation), irregular heart rates, pocket infections, or in unusual situations, stenotic lesions (suggesting extracardiac compression of vessels by the epicardial implanted pacemaker electrodes).

Pacemaker interrogation must consist of interrogation of programmed settings and pacemaker performance data, consisting of the electrode's impedance, the generator battery's voltage, the generator's measured pulse amplitude, the electrode's current flow, the energy delivered, the pulse width, and the measured magnet rate. Such parameters can often show early signs of electrode dysfunction or an approaching generator end of service. Impedance changes are of particular utility in indicating early exit block (manifested as increasing impedance) and insulation fracture or erosion of the electrode's tip (manifested as a decline in the electrode's impedance).

Following this, interrogation of the pacemaker's diagnostic counters is performed to assess the extent to which the pacemaker is being used and the rate variability the patient is experiencing. Information provided by diagnostic counters is variable, depending on the pacemaker model. The most useful data are those collected over many months to assess the degree to which the pacemaker is providing rate variability and to what extent the patient is dependent on the pacemaker. This information is useful in assessing the appropriateness of the lower rate limit in DDD pacing and sinus node function. A high percentage of atrial pacing with a low programmed lower rate limit suggests significant sinus nodal dysfunction (Fig. 36–39).

Next, intracardiac electrograms are recorded. The utility of such tracings is discussed later. Sensing thresholds are also performed to determine the least sensitive settings that still maintain appropriate sensing.

Finally, threshold determinations from both atrial and ventricular leads are obtained at all pulse amplitudes, producing 100% capture at any pulse width setting. Pulse width thresholds are generally preferred to pulse amplitude thresholds because most pacemakers have many more pulse width settings than pulse amplitude settings; thus, more accurate thresholds can be determined. All threshold determinations are performed in duplicate. Thresholds are reported as the minimum pulse width that maintains 100% capture at each programmable pulse amplitude. From these data, strength–duration curves are constructed and compared with previously obtained curves to detect shifts. From these data, appropriate programming decisions can be made.

Intracardiac Electrogram Determinations

Intracardiac electrograms should be obtained whenever possible. They are obtained both simultaneously with a surface ECG and with telemetered annotation markers that indicate the point during the electrogram at which sensing or pacing occurs and the beginning and length of the refractory periods. Thus, the relationship of programmed refractory periods to the waveform is shown. This is particularly useful for the atrial channel to ascertain the appropriateness of the programmed settings. For example, when the atrial electrode has been implanted in the left atrium, a determination of the appropriate AV interval may be difficult because the spontaneous P wave on the body surface significantly precedes the time at which atrial sensing occurs (Fig. 36–40). This results in a prolonged PR interval, as determined from the surface ECG recording, that could raise concerns about appropriate generator function.

Recording the annotation markers with the intracardiac electrogram also permits minimizing refractory periods as much as possible to maximize the multiblock rate and yet not risk oversensing of ventricular depolarization or repolar-

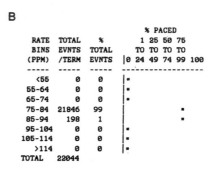

Figure 36–39. Examples of data obtained from generator diagnostic counters showing the number of beats occurring in each rate range. *A,* Data from a patient who had acceptable heart rate variability. *B,* Data from a patient in whom there was minimal heart rate variability and required reprogramming. *C,* Information about the types of atrial and ventricular beats occurring. This patient had predominantly atrial sensing, followed by ventricular pacing, indicating an appropriate lower rate limit.

ization by the atrial channel (crosstalk) (Fig. 36–41). This is of even more concern in young children who experience high atrial rates and are at risk for multiblock, with a subsequent sudden decrease in the ventricular rate and a concomitant decrease in cardiac output. This is demonstrated more fully when the results of exercise testing are discussed.

We also find the intracardiac electrogram to be helpful in determining decreasing atrial amplitudes over time with the potential for loss of atrial sensing. With the electrode's aging and fibrosis of the tip, recorded electrogram amplitudes may decline, and appropriate changes in atrial sensitivity often need to be made. This is particularly relevant to exercise, during which atrial amplitudes may further decline, as discussed later.

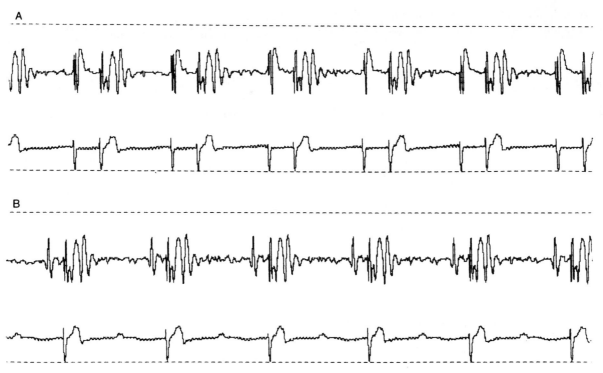

Figure 36–40. Example of an intracardiac electrogram from a patient with left atrial pacing. In both panels, the top trace is the atrial electrogram, and the bottom trace is the body surface electrocardiogram. Panel *A* was recorded during atrial pacing. The atrial electrogram and the surface P wave occur close to each other. Panel *B* was recorded during atrial sensing. The P wave now precedes the atrial electrogram by a considerable time.

Finally, the intracardiac electrogram is also useful in the diagnosis of atrial dysrhythmias. In the active child, the presence of a high-paced rate may not be unusual or suggest an atrial tachycardia. An example of such a situation is in the presence of atrial flutter (Fig. 36–42). In the first example, the rapid atrial rate was apparent on the body surface ECG recording, and the pacemaker is at the upper rate limit. In the second example, the body surface ECG recording showed an apparently regular rhythm at a rate below the upper rate limit; the atrial electrogram showed atrial flutter.

Exercise Testing

Exercise testing should be an integral part of all pacemaker follow-up in children old enough to undergo treadmill test-ing. Such testing often pinpoints inappropriate programming, resulting in inappropriate performance. In one series, 43% of patients had clinically significant inappropriate programming while exercising that was not apparent on routine pacemaker testing.[63] Of these patients, 75% showed an inadequate heart rate increase with the stress of exercising. Although most were paced in the VVIR mode, one patient in the DDD mode was shown to have an inadequate exercise response indicative of chronotropic incompetence. All such patients underwent reprogramming with subsequent appropriate heart rate increases. Other patients were shown to have spontaneous beats at maximal exercise, causing an automatic extension of the PVARP and acute multiblock with an acute decline in the heart rate (Fig. 36–43). The development of multiblock was also seen with an acute decline in the heart

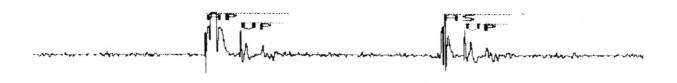

Figure 36–41. Intracardiac electrogram recorded while in the DDD mode together with annotation markers showing the time of onset and termination of the various refractory periods. The dashed line following the denotation of atrial pacing (AP) or atrial sensing (AS) shows the duration of the total atrial refractory period (TARP) and that it is of significant duration to prevent inappropriate sensing by the atrial amplifier of ventricular events. The shorter dashed line following ventricular pacing (VP) shows the duration of the ventricular refractory period but is of little utility in this recording.

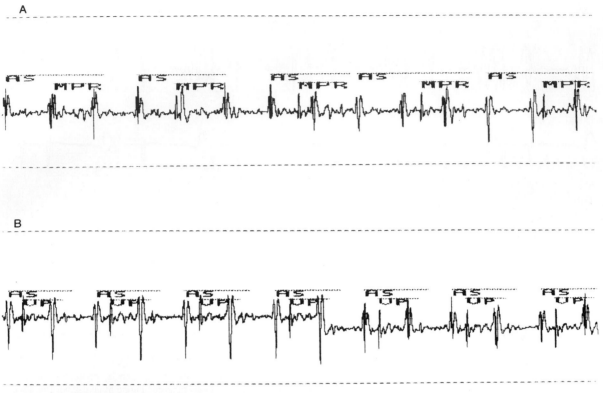

Figure 36–42. Atrial electrograms from two patients while in atrial flutter. *A*, The time of atrial sensing (AS) is variable, as is the atrioventricular (AV) interval, because the pacemaker is at the upper rate limit, or maximal paced rate (MPR). Note the changing total atrial refractory period (TARP) as a result of the Wenckebach behavior imposed by the upper rate limit. *B*, There is a definite 2:1 block, and the pacemaker is not at the upper rate limit. The body surface electrocardiogram was suggestive only of atrial flutter in that the heart rate was completely regular. VP, ventricular pacing.

rate from an inappropriately long total atrial refractory period. The multiblock rate was only slightly above the upper rate limit, causing an abrupt decline in the heart rate (Fig. 36–44). If decreasing the AV interval or the PVARP cannot adequately shorten the TARP, use of the DDDR or VDDR mode may be helpful. When the multiblock rate is reached during the use of either of these pacing modes, the ventricular rate falls to the sensor rate rather than the inappropriately sensed atrial rate, providing a smaller decline in the heart rate. A loss of capture at the maximal heart rate was also observed, even though there had been 100% capture at rest and programming of the pacemaker was believed to be appropriate, based on resting threshold testing (Fig. 36–45).

Changes in pacing thresholds do occur and can either worsen, as the previous example shows, or improve.[26, 64] For fixed-rate pacing, thresholds decline after exercise, and therefore, resting thresholds are not necessarily indicative of those present during the stress of exercise (Fig. 36–46). However, these findings may not be applicable to the patient whose pacemaker is in the rate-responsive mode, as the example in the patient who developed loss of capture at maximal exercise showed. This is a potentially serious problem that would not have been apparent had evaluation only at rest been performed.

Changes in P-wave amplitude were also documented at maximal exercise.[65–67] A decrease in P-wave amplitude can result in a loss of atrial sensing, and in the DDD mode, this can cause an immediate drop to the lower rate limit of the pacemaker. This can result in syncope from a sudden decrease in the cardiac output. Although DDDR pacing can minimize the magnitude of this heart rate drop, the physician should not rely on this mechanism because the sensor rate may not be the same as the atrial rate, especially during activities, such as swimming or cycling. Myopotential sensing by either channel can have similar effects.[68, 69] This is more evident in unipolar systems, but it can occur in bipolar systems.

Ambulatory Electrocardiographic Monitoring

Ambulatory ECG monitoring is also essential in the appropriate follow-up of pediatric patients with pacemakers. This is particularly true in those patients unable to exercise because this may be the only method to evaluate high-rate performance. In many series, 24-hour ambulatory ECG monitoring was the only means by which pacemaker malfunction was detected.[70–72] Such monitoring is particularly valuable in evaluating atrial and ventricular sensing problems and intermittent lack of capture. This is particularly important because myocardial characteristics and, hence, appropriate pacemaker programming may vary, depending on the activity state and time of day.[27] Interactions between the patient's intrinsic rhythm and the pacemaker are also more completely evaluated on ambulatory monitoring, which may result in more optimal programming.

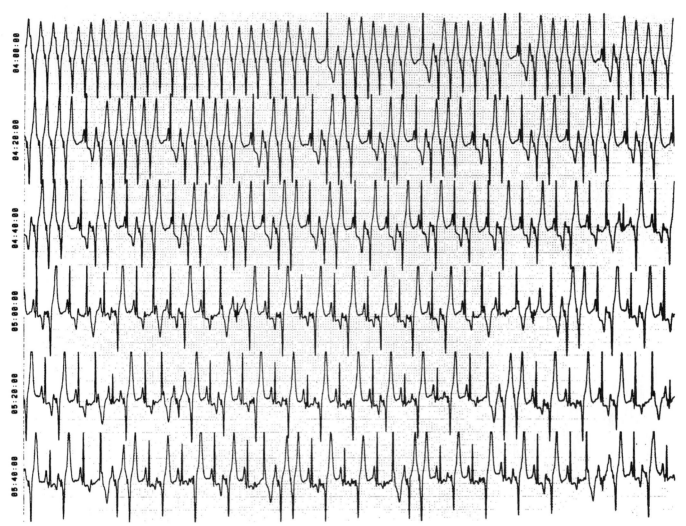

Figure 36–43. Continuous electrocardiographic recording during exercise treadmill testing showing the development of spontaneous beats at maximal exercise. This resulted in automatic extension of the postventricular atrial refractory period, with an overall decline in the heart rate from 167 to 141 bpm. This was associated with sudden fatigue and near syncope and was corrected by the elimination of the automatic postventricular atrial refractory period extension. The paper speed is 12.5 mm/sec, with each row being 20 seconds. The time from the onset of exercise is noted by the numbers in the left margin.

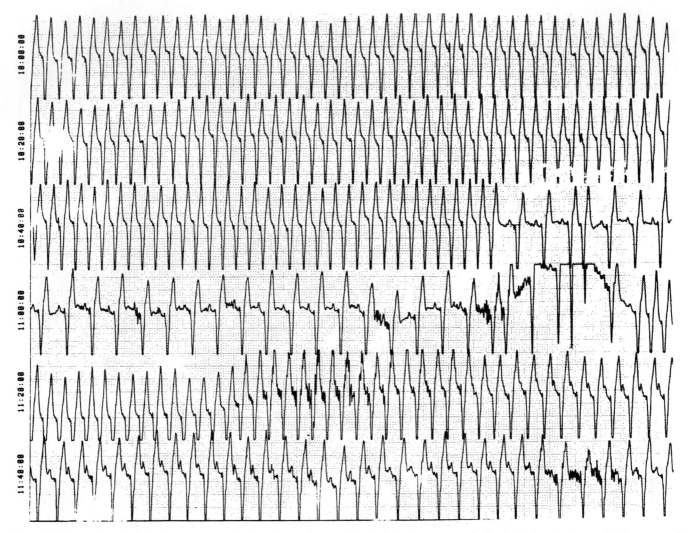

Figure 36–44. Example from an exercise test showing the development of multiblock with an acute decline in the heart rate, resulting in syncope. In this example, the patient's upper rate limit was 180 bpm, with a multiblock rate of 187. This lack of difference between the upper rate limit and the multiblock rate provided no gradual heart rate decline but rather an acute decline in heart rate and cardiac output. The multiblock rate was increased by shortening the postventricular atrial refractory period. The paper speed is 12.5 mm/sec, with each row being 20 seconds. The time from the onset of exercise is noted by the numbers in the left margin.

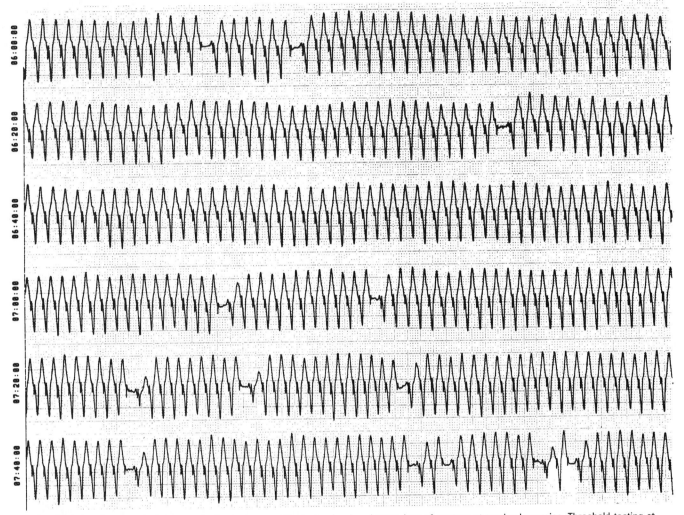

Figure 36–45. An example from an exercise test on a patient who developed acute loss of capture at maximal exercise. Threshold testing at rest revealed excellent thresholds with the minimal pulse width necessary to pace being 0.15 msec at a 5.4-V amplitude. The programmed settings were a pulse width of 0.5 msec at a 5.4-V amplitude. At rest and early exercise, there was 100% capture, with a loss of capture occurring only at maximal exercise. The pulse width was subsequently increased to 1 msec, with no loss of capture on repeat testing. The paper speed is 12.5 mm/sec, with each row being 20 seconds. The time from the onset of exercise is noted by the numbers in the left margin.

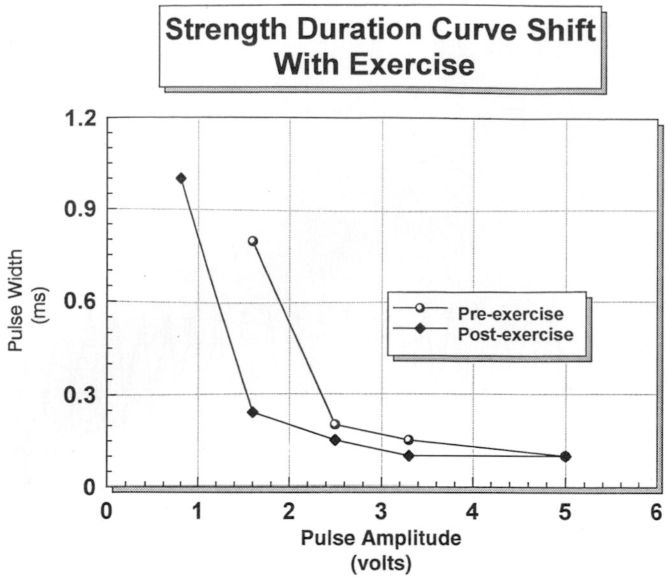

Strength Duration Curve Shift With Exercise

[Graph: Pulse Width (ms) on y-axis from 0 to 1.2; Pulse Amplitude (volts) on x-axis from 0 to 6. Legend shows open circle = Pre-exercise, filled diamond = Post-exercise.]

Figure 36–46. Data from a patient with fixed-rate VVI pacing who demonstrated a decrease in thresholds after termination of exercise compared with pre-exercise values. At higher pulse amplitudes, there was a minimal change, but marked changes were noted at lower pulse amplitudes. This denotes a shift of the strength–duration curve leftward, implying an increased excitability of the heart with exercise. (Data from Serwer GA, Kodali R, Eakin B, et al: Changes in pacemaker threshold with exercise in children and young adults. J Am Coll Cardiol 17:207A, 1991.)

Transstelephonic Electrocardiographic Monitoring

Transtelephonic ECG monitoring also plays an important role in pacemaker follow-up. In most aspects, its use is similar to that in adults. The major differences relate to the difficulty in performing the test because of the uncooperative nature of some children. We find transmitters in which the phone can be placed in a cradle rather than held to be superior. These units consist of a cradle in which the phone is placed and a small electrode plate that is held against the chest (Fig. 36–47). This leaves the parent with a free hand to calm or hold the child. Also, longer rhythm strips must be run to assess the pacemaker's function if a motion artifact is present. Routinely, 60-second strips are run to be sure adequate data are obtained. Both nonmagnet and magnet strips are obtained, as in adult patients. We allow the parents to choose the best time of day to call. They often vary the time they call, based on nap or school schedules. Reminder notes are sent at the beginning of the month in which a recording is due. The follow-up nurse contacts the patient only if a call has not been received within 3 weeks of the notice's mailing. In general, inadequate recordings are seldom obtained because the parents become adept at sending them.

Transtelephonic monitoring decreases cost by decreasing the number of outpatient visits needed and also provides a method to address parent and child concerns about proper pacemaker function. The capability of the child or the parent to detect pacemaker malfunction is very limited.[73] Use of transtelephonic ECG monitoring not only can confirm pacemaker malfunction but also can reassure the parent and child of proper pacemaker function.

Early Follow-Up Period

Follow-up during the crucial early period must be frequent and thorough. This is especially true when a new electrode has been implanted. Our current protocol initially after implantation includes both pacemaker interrogation and noninvasive threshold determination at multiple pulse amplitudes performed at 2 days and 4 and 8 weeks after implantation. During this period, thresholds often vary, and the generator's output may also need to be reprogrammed to maintain reliable pacing. Exit block, in particular, is common during this period, with little to no exit block being noted beyond 3 months after implantation.[72] In other series, there appeared to be a slight increase in threshold noted after 3 months, but this occurred in only 24% of patients.[74] It is important to determine thresholds at multiple pulse amplitudes because the strength–duration curve may move only in a horizontal direction, with thresholds at the higher outputs unchanging and thresholds at lower outputs showing marked increases (Fig. 36–48).

In addition, 24-hour ambulatory ECG monitoring is performed within the first week after implantation to assess proper pacemaker function throughout the day, not just for a brief period during pacemaker interrogation. For those children old enough to undergo exercise testing, this is always accomplished within the first 2 weeks after implantation. Transtelephonic ECG monitoring is done monthly during this period.

Intermediate Follow-Up

The intermediate follow-up period, defined as 3 months to 5 years after implantation, tends to be a period during which there is a small incidence of electrode or generator malfunction. During this time, pacing systems tend to be more stable and do not require as frequent re-evaluation. Our current

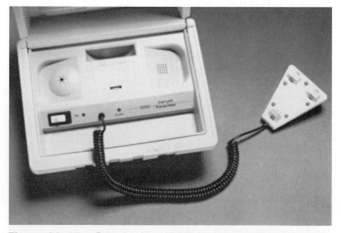

Figure 36–47. Example of a transtelephonic transmitter particularly well suited for use in children. It consists of a cradle in which the phone receiver is placed and a small unit that can easily be held against that child's chest with one hand while the other hand is free to steady and calm the child during transmission.

Strength-duration Curve Changes With Time

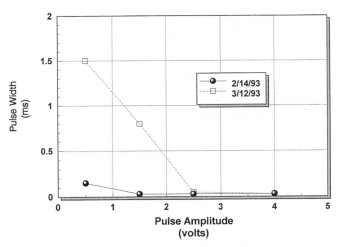

● 2/14/93
□ 3/12/93

Figure 36–48. Example of a change with time of the strength–duration curve of a patient showing changes not necessarily apparent if thresholds had been determined only at pulse amplitudes above 2.5 V.

protocol is to see patients semiannually for pacemaker interrogation and threshold testing and to obtain yearly 24-hour ambulatory ECG recordings. Transtelephonic ECG monitoring is done bimonthly in the absence of complicating features believed to require more frequent monitoring. In addition, patients and their parents are encouraged to send transmissions whenever there is a question about proper pacemaker function.

Late Follow-Up

Between 5 years after implantation and the time for pacemaker replacement is the period during which generator failure is more likely than electrode failure. Although electrode failure does occur, the thresholds, in general, tend to be stable, and most electrode failures during this period are a consequence of acute lead fracture and not exit block. There tends to be no warning preceding lead fracture, and no follow-up method currently used has been shown to be useful in predicting such events. However, a depletion of the generator's battery can be adequately detected early through the use of monthly transtelephonic ECG monitoring. Ambulatory ECG recordings are still obtained yearly.

■ IMPLANTABLE DEFIBRILLATOR USE IN CHILDREN

The use of ICDs in children has been limited by many factors, including uncertainty of the indications for its use, device size, and the difficulty initially of implanting the epicardial electrodes. With additional experience in the adult population and a decrease in size of the devices and the electrodes—both epicardial and endocardial—the pediatric use of ICDs is increasing. Silka and colleagues[75] reported on a large multicenter experience on initial use in children

ranging in age from 1.9 to 20 years. More recently, Hamilton and associates[76] reported on 11 children ages 4 to 16 years of age in a single-center experience. Kron and coauthors[77] reported on the use of nonthoracotomy electrode systems in 17 children ages 12 to 20 years of age. The issues surrounding use of ICDs in children involve (1) appropriate patient selection, (2) selection of epicardial versus endocardial implantation and the techniques involved, (3) appropriate tachyarrhythmia detection and therapy programming, and (4) appropriate follow-up.

Patient Selection

In all series, all patients had experienced a syncopal or sudden death episode documented to be a ventricular arrhythmia or had an inducible ventricular arrhythmia at electrophysiologic study following their syncopal or sudden death event. In the study of Silka and colleagues,[75] 76% of children were survivors of a sudden cardiac death episode, whereas 10% had experienced a syncopal episode with inducible sustained ventricular tachycardia. The remainder had drug refractory ventricular tachycardia. The underlying diagnoses were hypertrophic cardiomyopathy, long QT syndrome, dilated cardiomyopathy, or repaired congenital heart disease. Less than half had depressed ventricular function. In general, any child who has survived a sudden cardiac death episode or has a condition that can result in such an episode should be considered for ICD implantation. Medical therapy should always be employed, but one must decide if this alone will completely eliminate the likelihood of a repeat episode. For example, the patient with long QT syndrome who has experienced a sudden death episode should be treated medically and undergo ICD placement. Conversely, the child with congenital complete heart block and a documented episode of ventricular fibrillation may only require permanent pacing.

Although cardiomyopathies and primary electrical diseases constitute the most common diagnoses requiring ICD placement, children following repair of congenital heart disease are beginning to present with malignant ventricular arrhythmias. The most common lesions are tetralogy of Fallot and transposition of the great arteries after Mustard's repair.[75] In our experience, 15% of all patients receiving ICDs had undergone prior repair of tetralogy of Fallot. Children with this diagnosis accounted for 22% of patients in the report of Silka and colleagues.[75] Any child following surgery who requires a ventriculotomy or repair of a coronary artery abnormality is at potential risk for ventricular arrhythmias.

One unresolved issue is whether children who are potentially at risk for a sudden death episode but who have not experienced one should undergo ICD placement. In our practice, symptom-free children with long QT syndrome and a family history of sudden death are treated medically unless ventricular arrhythmias can be evoked at electrophysiologic study.

Implantation Approaches

Two decisions affect ICD implantation—the choice of epicardial versus endocardial electrode placement and subclavicular versus abdominal device placement. Each can be made independently of the other. Epicardial electrode placement was initially used exclusively in children, owing to the very large size of the transvenous electrode and the inappropriate shocking coil spacing or the need to place a second electrode. Even with transvenous electrode improvements, which are discussed later, it remains the preferred method for smaller children. The smallest child to receive an endocardial system in the study of Kron and associates[77] weighed 32 kg and in the study of Hamilton coauthors[76] weighed 27 kg. In our center, the smallest child weighed 20 kg. Therefore, we still use epicardial patches in children weighing less than 20 kg or in whom there is no venous access to the ventricle.

Patches are generally placed to maximize the distance between them and to maximize exposure of the myocardium to the defibrillation energy. They are sutured to the pericardium rather than the epicardial surface to minimize growth effects and patch distortion (Fig. 36–49). With time, however, distortion can develop, but it does not necessarily have an adverse effect on the defibrillatory thresholds. The leads are then tunneled to the abdomen, and the pocket is created as for implantation of an epicardial pacemaker system. In one case of a child with absent abdominal musculature, the device was placed intrathoracically.

With the development of smaller-diameter transvenous electrodes and with use of the device can as the second defibrillation electrode, a transvenous system can be used in most children. The currently available electrodes, both single- and dual-coil, can be introduced using a 10.5F introducer. The intercoil spacing in the dual-coil electrode, however, is in general too great to be employed in children. Positioning the second coil properly requires buckling of the electrode within the right atrium (Fig. 36–50), potentially

dislodging the electrode tip. Use of the single-coil electrode eliminates this problem. Even with such electrode buckling, the superior vena cava coil remains close to the clavicle, placing it at risk for fracture.

Use of a single coil electrode requires use of the device can as the second electrode or use of a second electrode—either a second intravascular coil or a subcutaneous array. Initially, use of the active can was restricted to implantation of the device under the left clavicle. In our institution, however, we have implanted the device in an upper left quadrant abdominal pocket with the single coil, bipolar pacing, steroid-eluting electrode introduced into the left subclavian vein and tunneled subcutaneously to the device pocket (Fig. 36–51); this technique is similar to the method proposed by Molina and colleagues[78] for transvenous pacemaker implantation in small patients. This approach has been used in children as small as 20 kg in weight in our center. Defibrillatory thresholds have been less than 10 J in all cases, even though the electrode area is reduced.[79] No patient has required an additional electrode—either subcutaneous array or second transvenous electrode.

Programming Considerations

The issues of appropriate programming are similar to those in the adult patient. The major concern is the higher sinus rates that can occur in the child. Initially, β-blockers were employed to reduce the maximal sinus rate. However, this approach often resulted in significant exercise intolerance. Although β-blockers may be indicated to treat the underlying disease (i.e., long QT syndrome), their use solely to reduce the maximal sinus rate is no longer necessary. Current de-

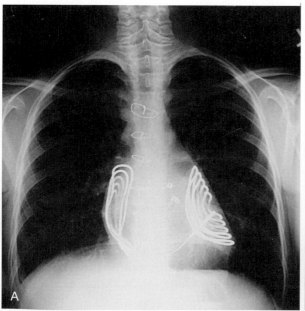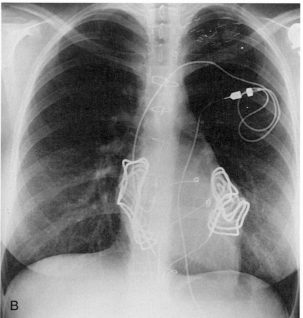

Figure 36–49. *A,* Chest radiograph taken after acute placement of epicardial defibrillation patches in a child. *B,* Chest radiograph in the same child 4 years after implantation, showing buckling of the patches; however, defibrillatory thresholds remain low. Note also the placement of a transvenous atrial electrode tunneled to the device in the abdomen using a lead extender because the device had been upgraded to a dual-chamber pacemaker-defibrillator. The epicardial ventricular pacing and sensing electrodes placed originally continue to be used.

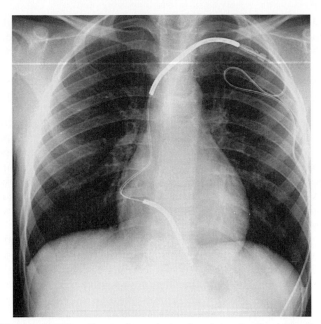

Figure 36–50. Chest radiograph showing placement of a dual-coil single-lead transvenous defibrillator system with the lead tunnel to the abdomen. Note the buckling of the lead within the atrium necessary to place the distal coil properly within the innominate vein. This can potentially dislodge the right ventricular coil and still leaves the distal coil near the clavicle–first rib space.

vices can now be programmed to very high rates as a criterion of ventricular tachycardia and can also employ other markers, such as increased QRS duration and sudden onset. Yet for most children, use of high rate alone is usually sufficient to detect fibrillation. Also, many children have wide QRS complexes as a consequence of prior cardiac surgery, making this criterion difficult to use. In practice, we program the device to a detection cycle interval that is 50 msec greater than the documented fibrillation cycle interval consistent with the approach of Hamilton and coauthors.[76] QRS duration is only used when cycle interval alone has been unable to prevent inappropriate therapy delivery.

Follow-Up Procedures

All children undergo induction of ventricular fibrillation 1 week after implantation to ensure that detection and therapy are appropriate. This is especially crucial for transvenous implants because small shifts in the electrode position can significantly alter the detection and therapy properties.

At each subsequent clinic visit, the device is interrogated, and each recorded event is inspected for cycle length and QRS morphology. Pacing thresholds are also determined as for pacemaker patients. After each therapy delivery, the child is seen and the device is interrogated to be sure that the therapy was appropriate. This is particularly crucial because inappropriate therapies are not rare. Also, the medical therapy is re-evaluated to ensure that it does not require alteration. Finally, the psychological aspects of the child's reaction to the therapy are evaluated, and support is offered as needed. Assessing the need for long-term support is extremely important and is discussed later.

■ PROPHYLACTIC MEDICATION

There has been significant controversy concerning the need for prophylactic anticoagulants or antibiotic agents for the prevention of subacute bacterial endocarditis in children with pacemakers. The current recommendations of the American Heart Association do *not* suggest the use of antibiotics for children with pacemakers.[80] However, most of these children have other underlying structural diseases that do require the use of antibiotics for prophylaxis. Our current practice is to prescribe antibiotics for prophylaxis of subacute bacterial endocarditis for all children who have endocardial electrodes if there is any AV valve regurgitation present by physical examination or echocardiography. Children with epicardial pacing systems without associated structural cardiac lesions do not require such prophylaxis.

Prophylactic anticoagulation has not been shown to be useful in children who have endocardial pacing systems. Only those children with chronic atrial flutter or fibrillation are routinely anticoagulated. We believe that the risk to the active child from chronic anticoagulation is significant and the benefit derived minimal.

■ PSYCHOSOCIAL ADJUSTMENTS IN CHILDREN WITH PACEMAKERS

Comprehensive care of the child with a pacemaker requires awareness of the psychosocial issues faced by children and families. Although there are issues specific to having a pacemaker, such as dependence on a mechanical device and the certainty of periodic surgeries throughout life, overall, the challenges are similar to those faced by children with other types of chronic illness. Treatment goals include facilitation of positive child and family adjustments with preven-

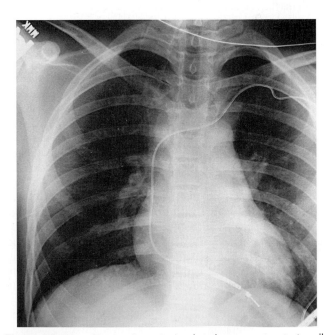

Figure 36–51. Chest radiograph showing placement of a single-coil transvenous defibrillator system with the lead tunneled down the lateral chest wall to the device, which also serves as the second defibrillation electrode, placed in a left upper quadrant abdominal pocket.

tion of avoidable negative psychosocial outcomes. Important illness-related tasks for parents of children with pacemakers include participating in the treatment plan, preserving emotional well-being for themselves and their children, and preparing for an uncertain future.[81] Children at high risk for emotional or behavioral adjustment problems may benefit from early identification and intervention.[82]

Currently, curative therapies are not available for the arrhythmias treated by pacemakers; hence these children, by definition, have a chronic illness.[83] Because of the underlying disease and the lifelong need for a pacemaker, the children and their families are chronically subjected to stressful experiences, including repeated surgeries, body image changes, and exposure to the possibility of death.[84] Prognoses and disease-imposed physical limitations vary considerably in this population, ranging from the adolescent athlete with congenital complete heart block to the child with severe cardiomyopathy. Although disease severity varies, most of the children can anticipate many fruitful adult years, and many are anticipated to have a normal or nearly normal life-span.

In one of the few studies examining the psychosocial outcomes for children with pacemakers, no significant differences were found between the children with pacemakers and comparison children on standardized measures of trait anxiety, self-competence, and self-esteem.[85] Children with pacemakers were more external in their locus of control orientation than healthy controls but were not significantly different on this measure from children with comparable heart disease but without a pacemaker.[85] Interview data from the same study suggest that comparison children were likely to report negative stereotypes about children with pacemakers. These findings are consistent with other studies indicating that most chronically ill children make positive adjustments, although there is an increased risk for psychosocial problems.[86] The incidence of problems is not insignificant; epidemiologic studies suggest that up to 30% of children with chronic illness may demonstrate secondary psychosocial impairment by 15 years of age.[87]

The risk for psychosocial problems in this population can be understood as a response to chronic stress that challenges the adaptive capacities of the children and their families.[88, 89] Consistent with this model, negative adjustments are likely to occur when stress exceeds the child's adaptive capacities. Certainly, there is wide variation in children's adaptations, and some children are able to make positive adaptations despite extremely stressful circumstances.[90, 91]

Considerable research has aimed to identify the biomedical, age-specific, and social-environmental factors linked with children's adjustments. Many of the factors identified reflect a continuum, with one end representing a protective factor and the other a risk factor. For example, family functioning that is cohesive and adaptable is associated with positive adaptations in children, whereas family functioning that is disengaged and rigid is associated with emotional and behavioral problems in the children.[92]

Disease-related biomedical factors anticipated to affect children's adjustments include diagnosis (disease severity, prognosis, treatment), functional impairment, cognitive abilities, and visibility (physical changes).[93, 94] For children with a chronic illness, diagnosis and disease severity are less important predictors of child adjustment than are other fac-

tors[93]; however, the diagnosis of heart disease during childhood may pose particular challenges for reasons not well understood.[95] Biomedical factors that may negatively influence psychosocial outcomes for children with heart disease include early mother–infant attachment problems,[96] neuropsychological changes,[97] learning disabilities,[98] and exclusion from competitive sports.[99]

Inherent child factors that may affect adjustment include temperament, developmental stage, and competency.[83, 93] For example, an academically gifted child may experience opportunities for self-esteem, socialization, and social recognition that ameliorate the negative effects of having a chronic illness, whereas a child with a learning disability who has a chronic illness is at increased risk for serious adjustment problems.[100]

Social-environmental factors linked with children's adjustments include family environment, mothers' psychological functioning, family economic resources, and children's peer relationships. Families that are adaptive, cohesive, and communicate effectively support positive adjustments for children.[101, 102] Maternal adjustment may play a particularly important role in children's adjustment,[103, 104] and persistent maternal distress (e.g., symptoms of anxiety or depression) warrants intervention.[93] Economic resources appear to be powerful moderators of children's adjustment to stressful life circumstances.[90, 91, 105] The quality of children's friendships is also important because positive peer relationships are linked with pro-social behavior, academic achievement, stress resistance, and later, adolescent competence.[106–108] Conversely, negative child peer relationships are associated with academic failure, aggressive behavior,[107, 109] and general psychopathology, which persists during adulthood.[110] Social isolation and feelings of loneliness are a potential source of emotional distress for chronically ill children and family members.[83]

Coping methods are the processes used by children and families to accomplish disease-related tasks, maintain normal function, and minimize family disruption. Adaptive parental coping strategies include maintaining family integrity through cooperation and maintenance of an optimistic outlook; maintaining social support, self-esteem, and psychological stability; and understanding the medical situation through communication with other parents and health care providers.[111] Coping is a dynamic process that may promote or hinder positive adjustments.[112] Coping methods can be categorized as problem focused or emotion focused, and generally, both methods are used by individuals responding to stress.[112] Problem-focused coping methods involve actions taken to address a stressful situation, whereas emotion-focused methods are those coping methods that change the emotional reaction to an event, such as altering the perception of the experience, blunting, or denial. There are differences in the coping strategies employed by fathers and mothers, which may be a source of distress within the marriage.[113] Children's coping strategies reflect developmental stage, and problem-focused strategies precede emotion-focused strategies during childhood.[114]

Implications for Health Care Providers

Knowledge of the factors associated with child and family adjustments, illness-related tasks, and coping methods guide comprehensive treatment for the child with a pacemaker and can be used by providers to clarify what can be realistically influenced within their practices. Comprehensive management of the child with a pacemaker is based on assessment of the child and family, with identification of areas of strength and vulnerability. As described previously, considerable data suggest that key areas to include in the assessment are child functional impairment, school achievement and peer relationships, maternal distress, family functioning, and socioeconomic status. If these factors are favorable, there is a high likelihood that the child will make a positive adjustment to having a pacemaker. Significant problems in any of these areas suggest the need for further assessment, intervention, and possible referral to a mental health professional.

Provider–Family Interactions: Opportunities for Education, Support, and Intervention

Provider–family interactions afford key opportunities for education, support, and intervention aimed at facilitating positive child adjustments. The time of initial implantation and the time of pacemaker replacement are stressful times for children and families when many questions and concerns arise. Families are generally more relaxed during routine follow-up visits, making this an optimal time to further the provider–family relationship, explore lifestyle issues, and affirm successes in the child's life. Because questions often arise between visits, ready phone access to experienced pacemaker professionals is important.

Communication with providers about the child's prognosis, appropriate activities, and restrictions is necessary for parents and children to adjust to life with a pacemaker. At the time of the initial implantation, many parents are unfamiliar with the use of pacemakers in children and may assume that needing a pacemaker means the child's "heart is getting worse" or that the child "won't live long because only old people get pacemakers." Conversations with providers about what the pacemaker means for the child's future are important because emotional well-being is predicated on a hopeful outlook—one that permits belief in a personal and meaningful future.[115]

As identified previously, feelings of loneliness and social isolation are potential sources of emotional distress for children with pacemakers and family members. Providers can furnish opportunities for social support, both informally by introducing families in the clinic or hospital and formally by sponsoring support groups. Providers can also link families with state and national family support networks and reputable on-line support groups. Children may benefit from meeting other children with pacemakers in the clinic or by having a "pacemaker pen pal." One child who attends our clinic was feeling isolated because he "never met other kids who have pacemakers." A one-time social gathering was arranged with the child, his parents, and three other families who agreed to participate. A pediatric psychologist facilitated the discussion, and the distressed child experienced a more positive mood after the meeting.

Education is necessary so that parents can adhere to monitoring protocols, use medical resources effectively, and provide appropriate activities for their children. Areas to be addressed include the symptoms of pacemaker malfunction, appropriate use of transtelephonic monitoring systems, precautions, activity recommendations, and the need for periodic pacemaker replacement. It is our practice to recommend cardiopulmonary resuscitation (CPR) training for all parents, and parents with pacemaker-dependent children receive CPR training in the hospital before discharge. Education of the children varies based on developmental stage, among other factors. Children who undergo initial pacemaker implantation in infancy or early childhood need ongoing education regarding their disease and treatment to fill in age-related gaps in their understanding. When developing a teaching plan, it is important to remember that children's social networks may include nontraditional family members, school personnel, and extended family.

Surgery, whether for the initial pacemaker or at the time of replacement, is a stressful time for children and families. Parents often have questions about when to talk to their child about the upcoming surgery and what content they should include. The aim of preoperative education is to facilitate the child's ability to cope with the stress of surgery. The timing, content, and methods used to educate children vary with developmental stage and must be individualized. In general, upcoming surgery should be discussed with young children close to the surgery, within 24 to 48 hours. Young children often respond enthusiastically to short play sessions during the preoperative visit, with hospital articles such as anesthesia masks, plastic syringes, and other masks.

An important functional outcome for children with pacemakers is successful integration into the school community. Although there is realistic concern about negative stereotyping by school personnel,[83] some data suggest that parents believe that school personnel should be informed about their child's illness and that health professionals are the most appropriate people to provide this education.[116] To facilitate school integration, we have used a variety of interventions, including participation in parent–teacher meetings at the child's school, visiting the child's classroom, and making pacemaker models and other materials available to the child for school presentations.

■ PSYCHOSOCIAL ADJUSTMENTS IN CHILDREN WITH IMPLANTABLE CARDIOVERTER-DEFIBRILLATORS

Minimal data are available regarding the adjustments of children and adolescents after ICD implantation. In study of nine patients, ranging in age from 13 to 49 years, Vitale and Funk[117] reported difficulty sleeping, low energy, and interruptions in planned activities. Problems reported for older patients after ICD implantation include increased anxiety levels, excessive anger, psychological disturbances, sexual abstinence, restricted physical activities, and restricted social activities.[118, 119] Some newer studies, however, emphasize that most older adults appear to make positive adjustments after ICD implantation.[120]

Although the data are lacking, this population would appear to be at risk for the development of psychosocial problems due to disease-related factors, including disease severity, functional impairment, and body image changes. Disease severity is significant because the children have survived, or are at high risk for, a lethal arrhythmia. **Many** of the children are survivors of out-of-hospital cardiac arrests with the fear, drama, and exposure to the possibility of death that this experience entails. The incidence of anoxic encephalopathy after cardiac arrest is not insignificant, and if present, is anticipated to affect later adjustment. Visibility is also an issue because the devices are still large in relationship to a child's body mass. The treatment delivered by the device is another source of distress for patients, with ramifications exceeding the pain and potential embarrassment at the time of therapy (an issue that is more fully discussed later). Finally, many of the children who require ICD implantation have inherited diseases, such as long QT syndrome, familial dilated cardiomyopathy, and hypertrophic cardiomyopathy. Therefore, health-related concern extends beyond that child to other family members who may be affected. Because of the hereditary nature and severity of these diagnoses, many families have experienced the death of one or more family members, which adds to feelings of grief, anxiety, and guilt.

It has been our experience that the potential for a life-threatening arrhythmia and receiving a shock are sources of considerable anxiety, particularly for adolescents. Conscious shocks, particularly repeated conscious shocks, have been very traumatic. Three adolescent patients in whom we have implanted ICDs have experienced conscious (appropriate) shocks, and two of these patients experienced repeated conscious shocks. After these events, all three patients experienced severe anxiety that persisted longer than a month. In two patients, school phobias developed. The other patient was home for summer vacation and, very uncharacteristically, would not participate in usual summer activities, preferring to stay at home. One young patient demonstrated classic symptoms of post-traumatic stress disorder, including intrusive thoughts re-experiencing the traumatic event, suicidal thoughts, feelings of detachment, and high levels of anxiety. All three young people required professional counseling, and one was treated with antidepressant medication and biofeedback. All have since returned to school; two are now in college and one in high school. It is important to note that none of the adolescents had a history of psychiatric problems before the ICD implantation.

The body of literature concerning conditioned learning can facilitate our understanding of the effect of unpredictable, conscious shocks on young people. It is known that repeated unpredictable aversive stimuli, in addition to producing fear and avoidance behavior, can have long-term debilitating effects.[121] Many of the experiments done on the effects of aversive conditioning actually used unpredictable electric shocks as the source of the stimuli. Maier and Seligman[122] have proposed that in such circumstances, people may develop the expectation that their behavior has little effect on their environment, and this expectation may generalize to a wide range of situations. This behavior mode, referred to as *learned helplessness,* has been linked with human depression.[122]

Complicating the situation for patients with tachyarrhythmias is the catecholamine release that occurs secondary to anxiety. The increased heart rate is often perceived as the possible onset of the arrhythmia, leading to increased anxiety and feelings of loss of control. Relaxation under these conditions can present a challenge for young people. Potential therapies, in addition to counseling, include relaxation methods and biofeedback.[123]

Support groups have shown to be helpful in promoting positive adjustments to chronic illness in a family member.[124] Factors associated with support group participation that may be therapeutic for patients and family members include sharing of information, instilling of hope, universality, altruism, and interpersonal learning.[124] Although an effective intervention, the use of support groups by this population so far appears to be limited. Professionals working with these patients report that many younger patients do not participate in ongoing ICD patient support groups because the groups do not address issues of personal concern, such as work, intimate relations, childbirth, school, friends, and dating. Also, the relatively small numbers of young defibrillator patients in any one geographic area have limited the ability to initiate support groups specifically for this population.

In an attempt to address the needs of this unique population, we have collaborated with the adult electrophysiology service at our hospital on two "Youth and Young Adult Support seminars" for ICD patients in their 30s and younger. In addition to educational workshops on topics of interest to young patients, there were professionally facilitated support groups divided by age, gender, and role (patient, spouse, parent). It is our belief that the children and adolescents benefit from interactions with young adult ICD patients because they can see firsthand that a meaningful future is possible for them. Evaluations revealed that many of the patients had never met another young person with a defibrillator before the conference.

School re-entry after ICD implantation has been a source of considerable concern for parents and school professionals. Education of school personnel by clinic staff regarding the child's arrhythmia, how the device works, what to do if therapy is given, and development of an emergency plan for school personnel is routine after implantation. Parental permission is always obtained before the school is contacted, and parents are included as important participants in all school-based meetings. During the meetings, it has been helpful to emphasize the protection afforded by the device and that the purpose of undergoing device implantation is to permit the child to live, as much as possible, a normal life.

The long-term outlook of children requiring either ICD or pacemaker implantation continues to improve. Thus, a positive attitude must be conveyed to the child, the parents, and the caregivers to allow the child to lead as normal a life as possible.

REFERENCES

1. Moquin PM, Vaysse J, Durand M, et al: Implantation d'un stimulateur interne pour correction d'un bloc auriculo-ventriculo-ventriculaire chirurgical chez une enfant de 7 ans. Arch Mal Coeur Vaiss 55:241, 1962.
2. Shearn RPN, Flemming WH: Fourteen years of implanted pacemakers in children. Ann Thorac Surg 25:144, 1978.
3. Simon AB, Dick M II, Stern AM, et al: Ventricular pacing in children. PACE 5:836, 1982.
4. Walkens JJS: Cardiac pacemakers in infants and children. Pediatr Cardiol 3:337, 1982.
5. Ector H, Dhooghe G, Daenen W, et al: Pacing in children. Br Heart J 53:541, 1985.
6. Serwer GA, Mericle JM: Evaluation of pacemaker pulse generator and patient longevity in patients aged 1 day to 20 years. Am J Cardiol 59:824, 1987.

7. Walsh CA, McAlister HF, Anders CA, et al: Pacemaker implantation in children: A 21-year experience. PACE 11:1940, 1988.

8. Brownlee JR, Serwer GA, Dick M II, et al: Failure of electrocardiographic monitoring to detect cardiac arrest in patients with pacemakers. Am J Dis Child 143:105, 1989.

9. McCue CM, Mantakas ME, Tingelstad JB, Ruddy S: Congenital heart block in newborns of mothers with connective tissue disease. Circulation 56:82, 1977.

10. Kangos JJ, Griffiths SP, Blumenthal S: Congenital complete heart block: A classification and experience with 18 patients. Am J Cardiol 20:632, 1967.

11. Dorostkar P, Serwer GA, LeRoy S, Dick M II: Long-term course of children and young adults with congenital complete heart block. J Am Coll Cardiol 21:295A, 1993.

12. Michaelsson M, Riesenfeld T, Jonzon A: Natural history of congenital complete atrioventricular block. PACE 20: 2098, 1997.

13. Kugler JD, Danford DA: Pacemakers in children: An update. Am Heart J 117:665, 1989.

14. Karpawich PP, Gillette PC, Garrison A, et al: Congenital complete atrioventricular block: Clinical and electrophysiologic predictors of need for pacemaker insertion. Am J Cardiol 48:1098, 1981.

15. Winkler RB, Freed MD, Nadas AS: Exercise-induced ventricular ectopy in children and young adults with complete heart block. Am Heart J 99:87, 1980.

16. Gillette PC, Wampler DG, Shannon C, Oth D: Use of cardiac pacing after the Mustard operation for transposition of the great arteries. J Am Coll Cardiol 7:138, 1986.

17. El-Said G, Rosenberg HS, Mullins LE, et al: Dysrhythmias after Mustard's operation for transposition of the great arteries. Am J Cardiol 30:526, 1972.

18. Eldor M, Griffin JC, Abbott VA, et al: Permanent cardiac pacing in patients with long QT syndrome. J Am Coll Cardiol 3:600, 1987.

19. Dreifus LS, Fisch C, Griffin VC, et al: Guidelines for implantation of cardiac pacemakers and antiarrhythmic devices. J Am Coll Cardiol 18:1, 1991.

20. Rishi F, Hulse LE, Auld DO, et al: Effects of dual-chamber pacing for pediatric patients with hypertrophic obstructive cardiomyopathy. J Am Coll Cardiol 29:734, 1997.

21. McGrath LB, Gonzalez-Lavin L, Morse DP, Levett JM: Pacemaker system failure and other events in children with surgically induced heart block. PACE II:1182, 1988.

22. Serwer GA, Mericle JM, Armstrong BE: Epicardial ventricular pacemaker electrode longevity in children. Am J Cardiol 61:104, 1988.

23. Serwer GA, Uzark K, Dick M II: Endocardial pacing electrode longevity in children. J Am Coll Cardiol 15:212A, 1990.

24. Serwer G, Dick M II, Eakin B: Cardiac output response to treadmill exercise in children with fixed-rate pacemakers. Circulation 84:II-514, 1991.

25. Karpawich PP, Perry BL, Farooki ZQ, et al: Pacing in children and young adults in nonsurgical atrioventricular block: Comparison of single-rate ventricular and dual-chamber modes. Am Heart J 113:316, 1987.

26. Karpawich PP, Justice CD, Cavitt DL, Chang CH: Developmental sequelae of fixed-rate ventricular pacing in the immature canine heart: An electrophysiologic, hemodynamic, and histopathologic evaluation. Am Heart J 119:1077, 1990.

27. Preston TA, Fletcher RD, Luechesi BR, et al: Changes in myocardial threshold: Physiologic and pharmacologic factors in patients with implanted pacemakers. Am Heart J 74:235, 1967.

28. Serwer GA, Uzark K, Beekman R, Dick M II: Optimal programming of rate altering parameters in children with rate-responsive pacemakers using graded treadmill exercise testing. PACE 13:541, 1990.

29. Yabek SM, Wernly J, Check TW, et al: Rate-adaptive cardiac pacing in children using a minute ventilation biosensor. PACE 13:2108, 1990.

30. Gillette PC, Shannon C, Blair H, et al: Transvenous pacing in pediatric patients. Am Heart J 105:843, 1983.

31. Ward DE, Jones S, Shinebourne EA: Long-term transvenous pacing in children weighing ten kilograms or less. Int J Cardiol 15:112, 1982.

32. Spotnitz HM: Transvenous pacing in infants and children with congenital heart disease. Ann Thorac Surg 49:495, 1990.

33. Gillette PC, Zeigler V, Bradhaus GB, Kinsella P: Pediatric transvenous pacing: A concern for venous thrombosis? PACE 11:1935, 1988.

34. Yakvevich V, Alogen D, Papo J, Vidne BA: Fibrotic stenosis of the SVC with widespread thrombotic occlusion of its major tributaries. J Thorac Cardiovasc Surg 85:632, 1983.

35. Sunder SK, Ekong EA, Sevalingram K, Kumar A: SVC thrombosis due to pacing electrodes. Am Heart J 123:790, 1992.

36. Wilkoff BL, Byrd CL, Love CJ, Hayes DL, Sellers TD, Schaerf R, Parsonnet V, Epstein LM, Sorrentino RA, Reiser C: Pacemaker lead extraction with the laser sheath: results of the pacing lead extraction with the excimer sheath (PLEXES) trial. J Am Coll Cardiol 33:1671, 1999.

37. Kantharia BK, Kutalek SP: Extraction of pacemaker and implantable cardioverter defibrillator leads. Curr Opin Cardiol 14:44, 1999.

38. Sharifi M, Sorkin R, Lakier JB: Left heart pacing and cardioembolic stroke. PACE 17:1691, 1994.

39. Levin AR, Spach MS, Boineau JP, et al: Atrial pressure-flow dynamics in atrial septal defects (secundum type). Circulation 37:476, 1968.

40. Serwer GA, Armstrong BE, Anderson PAW, et al: Use of contrast echocardiography for evaluation of right ventricular hemodynamics in the presence of ventricular septal defects. Circulation 58:327, 1978.

41. Westerman GR, Van Revanter SH: Surgical management of difficult pacing problems in patients with congenital heart disease. J Cardiovasc Surg 2:351, 1987.

42. Moak JP, Friedman RA, Moffat D, et al: Dual-chamber pacing in children: The optimal lead configuration—unipolar or bipolar? J Am Coll Cardiol 17:208A, 1991.

43. Breivik K, Danilovic D, Ohm OJ, et al: Clinical evaluation of a thin bipolar pacing lead. PACE 20:637, 1997.

44. DeLeon SY, Ilbawi MN, Koster N, Idriss FS: Comparison of the sutureless and suture-type epicardial electrodes in pediatric cardiac pacing. Ann Thorac Surg 33:273, 1982.

45. Michalik RE, Williams WH, Zorn-Chelten S, Hotches CR: Experience with a new epimyocardial pacing lead in children. PACE 7:83, 1984.

46. Kugler J, Minsour W, Blodgett C, et al: Comparison of two myoepicardial pacemaker leads: Follow-up in 80 children, adolescents, and young adults. PACE 11:2216, 1988.

47. DeLeon SY, Ilbawi MN, Becker CL, et al: Exit block in pediatric cardiac pacing. Thorac Cardiovasc Surg 99:905, 1990.

48. Hamilton R, Gow R, Bahoric B, et al: Steroid-eluting epicardial leads in pediatrics: Improved epicardial thresholds in the first year. PACE 14:2066, 1991.

49. Karpawich PP, Harkini M, Arciniegas E, Cavitt DL: Improved chronic epicardial pacing in children: Steroid contribution to porous platinized electrodes. PACE 15:1151, 1992.

50. Johns JA, Fuh FA, Burger JD, Hammon JW Jr: Steroid-eluting epicardial pacing leads in pediatric patients: Encouraging early results. J Am Coll Cardiol 20:395, 1992.

51. Serwer GA, Dorostkar PC, LeRoy S, Dick M II: Comparison of chronic thresholds between differing endocardial electrode types in children. Circulation 86:I-43, 1992.

52. Rosenthal E, Bostock J: VDD pacing in children with congenital complete heart block: Advantages of a single pass lead. PACE 20:2102, 1997.

53. Robertson JM, Hillel L: A new technique for permanent pacemaker implantation in infants and children. Ann Thorac Surg 44:209, 1987.

54. Ulicny KS Jr, Detterbeck FC, Starek PJK, Wilcox BR: Conjoined subrectus pocket for permanent pacemaker placement in the neonate. Soc Thorac Surg 53:1130, 1992.

55. Ott DA, Gillette PC, Cooley DA: Atrial pacing via the subxiphoid approach. Tex Heart Inst J 9:149, 1982.

56. Lawrie GM, Seale JP, Morris GC Jr, et al: Results of epicardial pacing by the left subcostal approach. Ann Thorac Surg 28:561, 1979.

57. Brenner JI, Gaines S, Cordier J, et al: Cardiac strangulation: Two-dimensional echo recognition of a rare complication of epicardial pacemaker therapy. Am J Cardiol 61:654, 1988.

58. Perry JC, Nihill MR, Ludomirsky A, et al: The pulmonary artery lasso: Epicardial pacing lead causing right ventricular outflow obstruction. PACE 14:1018, 1991.

59. Serwer GA, Dick M II, Uzark K, et al: The value of redundant ventricular epicardial electrode placement in children. PACE 9:531, 1988.

60. Gillette PC, Edgerton J, Kratz J, Zeigler V: The subpectoral pocket: The preferred implant site for pediatric pacemakers. PACE 14:1089, 1991.

61. Hayes DC, Holmes DR Jr, Maloney JD, et al: Permanent endocardial pacing in pediatric patients. J Thorac Cardiovasc Surg 85:618, 1983.

62. Hoyer MH, Beerman LB, Ettedgui JA, et al: Transatrial lead placement for endocardial pacing in children. Ann Thorac Surg 58:97, 1994.

63. Serwer GA, Dorostkar PC, LeRoy S, et al: Evaluation of rate variable pacemaker function at maximal exertion in children and young adults. PACE 16:899, 1993.

64. Serwer GA, Kodali R, Eakin B, et al: Changes in pacemaker threshold with exercise in children and young adults. J Am Coll Cardiol 17:207A, 1991.

65. Gillette PC, Zinner A, Kratz J, et al: Atrial tracking (synchronous) pacing in a pediatric and young adult population. J Am Coll Cardiol 9:811, 1987.

66. Frohlig G, Blank W, Schwerdt H, et al: Atrial sensing performance of AV universal pacemakers during exercise. PACE 11:47, 1988.

67. Ross BA, Zeigler V, Zinner A, et al: The effect of exercise on the atrial electrogram voltage in young patients. PACE 14:2092, 1991.

68. Bricker JT, Barison A, Traveek MS, et al: The use of exercise testing in children to evaluate abnormalities of pacemaker function not apparent at rest. PACE 8:656, 1985.

69. Jain P, Kaul U, Wasir HS: Myopotential inhibition of unipolar demand pacemakers: Utility of provocative manoeuvres in assessment and management. Int J Cardiol 34:33, 1992.

70. Strathmore NF, Mond HG: Noninvasive monitoring and testing of pacemaker function. PACE 10:1359, 1987.

71. Kerstjens-Frederikse MWS, Bink-Boelkens MTE, de Jongste MJL, Homan van der Heide JN: Permanent cardiac pacing in children: Morbidity and efficacy of follow-up. Int J Cardiol 33:207, 1991.

72. Jarosik DL, Redd RM, Buckingham TA, et al: Utility of ambulatory electrocardiography in detecting pacemaker dysfunction in the early postimplantation period. Am J Cardiol 60:1030, 1987.

73. Vincent JA, Cavitt DL, Karpawich PP: Diagnostic and cost effectiveness of telemonitoring the pediatric pacemaker patient. Pediatr Cardiol 18:86, 1997.

74. Shepard RB, Kam J, Colvin EC, et al: Pacing threshold spikes months and years after implant. PACE 14:1835, 1991.

75. Silka MJ, Kron J, Dunnigan A, Dick M, II: Sudden cardiac death and the use of cardioverter-defibrillators in pediatric patients. Circulation 87:800, 1993.

76. Hamilton RM, Dorian P, Gow RM, Williams WG: Five-year experience with implantable defibrillators in children. Am J Cardiol 77:524, 1996.

77. Kron J, Silka MJ, Ohm O-J, et al: Preliminary experience with nonthoracotomy implantable cardioverter defibrillators in young patients. PACE 17:26, 1994.

78. Molina LE, Dunnigan AC, Crosson JE: Implantation of transvenous pacemakers in infants and small children. Ann Thorac Surg 59:689, 1995.

79. Halperin BD, Reynolds B, Fain ES, et al: The effect of electrode size on transvenous defibrillation energy requirements: A prospective evaluation. PACE 20: 893, 1997.

80. Committee on Rheumatic Fever, Endocarditis, and Kawasaki Disease: Prevention of bacterial endocarditis: Recommendations by the American Heart Association. JAMA 264:2919, 1990.

81. Moos RH, Tsu UD: The crisis of physical illness: An overview. In RH Moos (ed): Coping With Physical Illness. New York, Plenum, 1977, p 3.

82. Satin W, LaGreca AM, Zigo MA, Skyler JS: Diabetes in adolescence: Effects of a multifamily group intervention and parent simulation of diabetes. J Pediatr Psychol 14:259, 1989.

83. Eiser C: Growing up with a chronic disease. London, Jessica Kingsley, 1993.

84. Gamble WJ, Owens JP: Pacemaker therapy for conduction defects in the pediatric population. In Roberts N, Gelband H (eds): Cardiac Arrhythmias in the Neonate, Infant, and Child. New York, Appleton-Century-Crofts, 1977, p 469.

85. Alpern D, Uzark K, Dick M II: Psychosocial responses of children to cardiac pacemakers. J Pediatr 114:494, 1989.

86. Wallander JL, Thompson RJ: Psychosocial adjustment of children with chronic physical conditions. In Roberts MC (ed): Handbook of Pediatric Psychology, 2nd ed. New York, Guilford Press, 1995, p 124.

87. Pless IB, Roghmann KJ: Chronic illness and its consequences: Observations based on three epidemiologic surveys. J Pediatr 79:351, 1971.

88. Rolland J: Chronic illness and the life cycle: A conceptual framework. Fam Proc 26:203, 1987.

89. Wallander JL, Varni JW: Adjustment in children with chronic physical disorders: Programmatic research on a disability-stress-coping model. In LaGreca AM, Siegal L, Wallander JL, Walker CE (eds): Stress and Coping With Pediatric Conditions. New York, Guilford Press, 1992, p 279.

90. Garmezy N, Tellegen A: Studies of stress-resistant children: Methods, variables, and preliminary findings. In Morrison F, Lord C, Keating D (eds): Advances in Applied Developmental Psychology, vol 1. New York, Academic Press, 1984, p 231.

91. Werner EE, Smith RS: Vulnerable but invincible: A longitudinal study of resilient children and youth. New York, McGraw-Hill, 1982.

92. Wallander JL, Varni JW, Babani L, et al: Family resources as resistance factors for psychological maladjustment in chronically ill and handicapped children. J Pediatr Psychol 14:157, 1989.

93. Thompson R, Gustafson K: Adaptations to chronic childhood illness. Washington, DC, American Psychological Association, 1996.

94. Stein RE, Jessop DJ: A noncategorical approach to chronic childhood illness. Pub Health Rep 97:354, 1982.

95. Lavigne JV, Faier-Routman J: Psychological adjustment to pediatric physical disorders: A meta-analytic review. J Pediatr Psychol 17:133, 1992.

96. Goldberg S, Simmons RJ, Newman J, et al: Congenital heart disease, parental stress, and infant-mother relationships. J Pediatr 119:661, 1991.

97. Miller G, Tesman JR, Ramer JC, et al: Outcome after open-heart surgery in infants and children. J Child Neurol 11:49, 1996.

98. Wright M, Nolan T: Impact of cyanotic heart disease on school performance. Arch Dis Child 71:64, 1994.

99. Gutgesell HP, Gessner IH, Better VL, et al: Recreational and occupational recommendations for young patients with heart disease. Circulation 74:1195A, 1986.

100. Werner ME, Smith R: Kauai's Children Come of Age. Hawaii, University of Hawaii Press, 1982.

101. Hamlett KW, Pellegrini DS, Katz KS: Childhood chronic illness as a family stressor. J Pediatr Psychol 17:33, 1992.

102. Blechman EA, Delamater AM: Family communication and type 1 diabetes: A window on the social environment of chronically ill children. In Cole RE, Reiss D (eds): How Do Families Cope With Chronic Illness? Hillsdale, NJ, Lawrence Erlbaum, 1993, p 1.

103. Demaso D, Campis L, Wypij D, et al: The impact of maternal perceptions and medical severity on the adjustment of children with congenital heart disease. J Pediatr Psychol 16:137, 1991.

104. Lyons-Ruth K, Zoll D, Conell D, Grunebaum HV: The depressed mother and her one year old infant: Environment, interaction, attachment and infant development. In Field T, Tronick E (eds): Maternal Depression and Infant Disturbance. San Francisco, Jossey-Bass, 1986, p 61.

105. Masten AS, Garmezy N, Tellegen A, et al: Competence and stress in school children: The moderating effects of individual and family qualities. J Child Psychol Psychiat 29:745, 1988.

106. Green KD, Forehand R, Beck SJ, Vosk B: An assessment of the relationship among measures of children's social competence and children's academic achievement. Child Dev 51:1149, 1980.

107. Masten AS, Morison P, Pellegrini DS: A revised class play method of peer assessment. Dev Psychol 21:523, 1985.

108. Morison P, Masten AS: Peer reputation in middle childhood as a predictor of adaptation in adolescence: A seven year follow-up. Child Dev 62:991,1991.

109. Pelham WE, Milich R: Peer relationships in children with hyperactivity/attention disorder. J Learn Disabil 17:560, 1984.

110. Cowen EL, Pederson A, Babigian H, et al: Long term follow-up of early detected vulnerable children. J Consult Clin Psychol 41:438, 1973.

111. McCubbin HI, McCubbin MA, Patterson JM, et al: CHIP: Coping-health inventory for parents: An assessment of parental coping patterns in the care of the chronically ill child. J Marr Fam 45:359, 1983.

112. Lazarus RS, Folkman S: Stress, appraisal, and coping. New York, Springer, 1984.

113. Affleck G, Tennen H, Rowe J: Mother, fathers, and the crisis of newborn intensive care. Infant Mental Health 11:12, 1990.

114. Compas BE, Worsham NL, Ey S: Conceptual and developmental issues in children's coping with stress. In LaGreca AM, Siegal LJ, Wallander JL, Walker CE (eds): Stress and Coping in Child Health. New York, Guilford Press, 1992, p 7.

115. Yarcheski A, Scoloveno MA, Mahon N: Social support and well-being in adolescents: The mediating role of hopefulness. Nurs Res 43:288, 1994.

116. Andrews SG: Informing schools about children's chronic illness. Pediatrics 88:306, 1991.

117. Vitale MB, Funk M: Quality of life in younger persons with an

implantable cardioverter defibrillator. Dimen Crit Care Nurs 14:100, 1995.

118. Cooper DK, Luceri RM, Thurer RJ, et al: The impact of the automatic implantable cardioverter defibrillator on quality of life. Clin Prog Electrophysiol Pacing 4:306, 1986.

119. Kuiper R, Nyamathi A: Stressors and coping strategies of patients with automatic implantable cardioverter defibrillators. J Cardiovasc Nurs 5:65, 1991.

120. Luderitz B, Jung W, Deister A, Manz M: Patient acceptance of implantable cardioverter defibrillator devices: Changing attitudes. Am Heart J 127:1179, 1994.

121. Mazur JE: Learning and Behavior. Upper Saddle River, NJ, Prentice Hall, 1998, p 187.

122. Maier SF, Seligman ME: Learned helplessness: Theory and evidence. J Exp Psychol Gen 105:3, 1976.

123. Stoyva JM, Carlson JG: A coping/rest model of relaxation and stress management. *In* Goldberger L, Breznitz S (eds): Handbook of Stress: Theoretical and Clinical Aspects: New York, Free Press, 1993, p 724.

124. Teplitz L, Egenes KJ, Brask L: Life after sudden death: The development of a support group for automatic implantable cardioverter-defibrillator patients. J Cardiovasc Nurs 4:20, 1990.

Index

Note: Page numbers in *italics* refer to illustrations; page numbers followed by t indicate tables.

Q

R